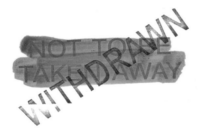

**Gregory's
Pediatric
Anesthesia**

This book is dedicated to all of the patients and house staff who have taught me most of what I know. GAG

This book is dedicated to the faculty of the Department of Anesthesiology at Texas Children's Hospital. Their continued clinical and academic excellence, and daily compassion for our patients and their families, are a constant source of inspiration. DBA

Gregory's Pediatric Anesthesia

EDITED BY

George A. Gregory

MD
Professor Emeritus
Department of Anesthesia and Perioperative Care
and Department of Pediatrics
University of California San Francisco (UCSF)
San Francisco, CA, USA

Dean B. Andropoulos

MD, MHCM
Chief of Anesthesiology
Texas Children's Hospital
Professor, Anesthesiology and Pediatrics
Baylor College of Medicine
Houston, TX, USA

FIFTH EDITION

WILEY-BLACKWELL

A John Wiley & Sons, Ltd., Publication

Library of Congress Cataloging-in-Publication Data

Gregory's pediatric anesthesia / edited by George A. Gregory, Dean B. Andropoulos. – 5th ed.
    p. ; cm.
  Pediatric anesthesia
  Rev. ed. of: Pediatric anesthesia / [edited by] George A. Gregory. 4th ed. c2002.
  Includes bibliographical references and index.
  ISBN-13: 978-1-4443-3346-6 (hard cover : alk. paper)
  ISBN-10: 1-4443-3346-1 (hard cover : alk. paper)
  ISBN-13: 978-1-4443-4515-5 (ePDF)
  ISBN-13: 978-1-4443-4518-6 (Wiley Online Library)
  [etc.]
  1. Pediatric anesthesia. I. Gregory, George A., 1934- II. Andropoulos, Dean B. III. Pediatric anesthesia.
  IV. Title: Pediatric anesthesia.
  [DNLM: 1. Anesthesia. 2. Child. 3. Infant. WO 440]
  RD139.P4 2012
  617.9'6083–dc23

                                    2011027299

A catalogue record for this book is available from the British Library.

Wiley also publishes its books in a variety of electronic formats. Some content that appears in print may not be available in electronic books.

Set in 9.5/12pt Palatino by Toppan Best-set Premedia Limited, Hong Kong
Printed and bound in Singapore by Markono Print Media Pte Ltd

1 2012

Contents

Part 4 Quality, Outcomes, and Complications in Pediatric Anesthesia

List of Contributors

Warwick Ames
MBBS, FRCA
Assistant Professor of Anesthesiology and
Pediatrics
Duke University Medical Center
Durham, NC, USA

Robert Bart III
MD
Assistant Professor
Department of Anesthesiology Critical Care
Medicine
Children's Hospital Los Angeles
University of Southern California
Keck School of Medicine
Los Angeles, CA, USA

Loren A. Bauman
MD
Associate Professor
Department of Anesthesiology
Wake Forest University School of Medicine;
Pediatric Anesthesiologist
Wake Forest University Baptist Medical
Center
Winston-Salem, NC, USA

James Bennett
MBBS, FRCA
Consultant Anaesthetist
Birmingham Children's Hospital and
Honorary Consultant Anaesthetist
Liver Unit
Queen Elizabeth Hospital
Birmingham, UK

Charles Berde
MD, PhD
Sara Page Mayo Chair in Pediatric Pain
Medicine
Chief, Division of Pain Medicine
Department of Anesthesiology, Perioperative
and Pain Medicine
Children's Hospital Boston;
Professor of Anaesthesia (Pediatrics)
Harvard Medical School
Boston, MA, USA

Robert A. Berg
MD
Professor of Anesthesiology and Critical Care
Medicine
The University of Pennsylvania School of
Medicine;
Russell Raphaely Endowed Chair
Division Chief, Critical Care Medicine
The Children's Hospital of Philadelphia
Philadelphia, PA, USA

Bruno Bissonnette
MD
Professor of Anesthesia
Department of Anesthesia
University of Toronto;
President and Founder
Children of the World Anesthesia
Foundation
Toronto, Ontario, Canada

Adrian T. Bosenberg
MB,ChB, FFA(SA)
Director of Anesthesia
Seattle Children's Hospital;
Professor, Department of Anesthesiology and
Pain Management
University of Washington
Seattle, WA, USA

Ken M. Brady
MD
Associate Professor
Department of Anesthesiology and Pediatric
Baylor College of Medicine;
Texas Children's Hospital
Houston, TX, USA

Claire Brett
MD
Professor of Anesthesia and Perioperative
Care
Department of Anesthesia and Perioperative
Care
University of California San Francisco
San Francisco, CA, USA

Peter N. Bromley
MBBS, FRCA
Consultant Anaesthetist
Birmingham Children's Hospital;
Honorary Consultant Anaesthetist
Liver Unit
Queen Elizabeth Hospital;
Honorary Senior Lecturer in Clinical
Medicine
University of Birmingham
Birmingham, UK

William Browne
MBBS, FANZCA
Department of Aneasthesia and Pain
Management
Royal Children's Hospital
Parkville, Australia

Stefan Budac
MD
Acting Assistant Professor
Department of Anesthesiology and Pain
Medicine
University of Washington School of
Medicine;
Attending Anesthesiologist
Seattle Children's Hospital
Seattle, WA, USA

James Edward Caldwell
MB ChB
Professor and Vice Chair
Department of Anesthesia and Perioperative
Care
University of California San Francisco
San Francisco, CA, USA

Danton Charr
MD
Instructor of Anesthesiology
Department of Anesthesia
Stanford Hospital and Clinics
Stanford University
Stanford, CA, USA

Michael Chen
MD
Department of Anesthesia
Stanford Hospital and Clinics;
Assistant Professor of Anesthesia
Stanford University
Stanford, CA, USA

Andrew Davidson
MD, MBBS, FANZCA
Associate Professor
Department of Anaesthesia and Pain
Management
Royal Children's Hospital
Parkville, Australia

Jayant K. Deshpande
MD, MPH
Professor of Pediatrics and Anesthesiology
University of Arkansas for Medical Sciences
Arkansas Children's Hospital
Little Rock, AR, USA

James A. DiNardo
MD
Senior Associate in Anesthesia
Cardiac Anesthesia Service
Children's Hospital Boston;
Associate Professor in Anaesthesia
Harvard Medical School
Boston, MA, USA

Burdett S. Dunbar
MD
Professor, Anesthesiology and Pediatrics
Baylor College of Medicine;
Former Chief, Pediatric Anesthesiology
Texas Children's Hospital
Houston, TX, USA

R. Blaine Easley
MD
Associate Professor
Department of Anesthesiology and Pediatrics
Baylor College of Medicine;
Texas Children's Hospital
Houston, TX, USA

Claude Ecoffey
MD
Chairman
Service d'Anesthésie-Réanimation
Chirurgicale
Hôpital Pontchaillou
University of Rennes
Rennes, France

Ross Fairgrieve
MBChB, FRCA
Consultant in Paediatric Anaesthesia and
Pain Management
Royal Hospital for Sick Children
Glasgow, Scotland, UK

John E. Fiadjoe
MD
Assistant Professor of Anesthesiology
University of Pennsylvania School of
Medicine;
Attending Anesthesiologist
The Children's Hospital of Philadelphia
Philadelphia, PA, USA

Randall Flick
MD
Consultant, Department of Anesthesiology
Mayo Clinic;
Assistant Professor of Anesthesiology
College of Medicine
Rochester, MN, USA

Maria Victoria Fraga
MD
Department of Anesthesiology and Critical
Care Medicine
The University of Pennsylvania School of
Medicine;
Neonatology Fellow
The Children's Hospital of Philadelphia
Philadelphia, PA, USA

Jeffrey Galinkin
MD, FAAP
Department of Anesthesiology and Pediatrics
The Children's Hospital;
Associate Professor, Anesthesiology and
Pediatrics
University of Colorado at Denver
Aurora, CO, USA

Priscilla J. Garcia
MD
Assistant Professor
Anesthesiology and Pediatrics
Baylor College of Medicine;
Staff Pediatric and Obstetric Anesthesiologist
Texas Children's Hospital
Houston, TX, USA

Christine Greco
MD
Director, Acute Pain Services
Department of Anesthesiology, Perioperative
and Pain Medicine
Children's Hospital Boston;
Assistant Professor (Anesthesia)
Harvard Medical School
Boston, MA, USA

Patrick J. Guffey
MD
Department of Anesthesiology
University of Colorado School of Medicine;
Children's Hospital Colorado
Aurora, CO, USA

Harshad Gurnaney
MBBS
Assistant Professor of Anesthesiology and
Critical Care
The University of Pennsylvania School of
Medicine;
Anesthesiologist
The Children's Hospital of Philadelphia
Philadelphia, PA, USA

Susan H. Guttentag
MD
Department of Anesthesiology and Critical
Care Medicine
The University of Pennsylvania School of
Medicine;
Associate Professor of Pediatrics
The Children's Hospital of Philadelphia
Philadelphia, PA, USA

Walid Habre
MD, PhD
Associate Professor
Department of Anaesthesiology,
Pharmacology and Intensive Care
University Hospitals
Geneva, Switzerland

Jeanne E. Hendrickson
MD
Aflac Cancer Center and Blood Disorders
Service
Associate Medical Director
Blood and Tissue Services
Children's Healthcare of Atlanta;
Assistant Professor of Pediatrics and
Pathology
Emory University School of Medicine
Atlanta, GA, USA

Robert S. Holzman
MD, FAAP
Senior Associate in Anesthesia
Department of Anesthesiology, Perioperative
and Pain Medicine
Children's Hospital Boston;
Associate Professor of Anaesthesia
Harvard Medical School
Boston, MA, USA

Anita Honkanen

MD
Service Chief, Anesthesia
Clinical Professor of Anesthesia
Department of Anesthesia
Stanford Hospital and Clinics;
Associate Professor of Anesthesia
Stanford University, Stanford, CA, USA

Philipp J. Houck

MD
Assistant Professor of Anesthesiology
Columbia University College of Physicians
and Surgeons
New York, NY, USA

Kelly Howard

BSc(Hons), MPsych (Clinical Child), PhD
Department of Anaesthesia and Pain
Management
Royal Children's Hospital
Parkville, Australia

Todd J. Kilbaugh

MD
Assistant Professor of Anesthesiology and
Critical Care Medicine
The University of Pennsylvania School of
Medicine;
The Children's Hospital of Philadelphia
Philadelphia, PA, USA

Cathy Lammers

MD
Director, Pediatric Anesthesiology
UC Davis Children's Hospital;
University of California
Davis, CA, USA

Ira S. Landsman

MD
Monroe Carell Jr Children's Hospital at
Vanderbilt
Department of Anesthesiology
Vanderbilt University Medical Center
Nashville, TN, USA

Peter C. Laussen

MBBS
Senior Associate in Anesthesia
Children's Hospital Boston;
Professor of Anaesthesia
Harvard Medical School
Boston, MA, USA

Jerrold Lerman

MD, FRCPC, FANZCA
Clinical Professor of Anesthesiology
Women and Children's Hospital of Buffalo
State University at Buffalo
Buffalo and Strong Memorial Hospital
University of Rochester
Rochester, NY, USA

Ronald S. Litman

DO
Professor of Anesthesiology and Pediatrics
University of Pennsylvania School of
Medicine;
Attending Anesthesiologist
The Children's Hospital of Philadelphia
Philadelphia, PA, USA

Andreas W. Loepke

MD, PhD
Departments of Anesthesia and Pediatrics
Cincinnati Children's Hospital Medical
Center;
Associate Professor of Clinical Anesthesia &
Pediatrics
University of Cincinnati College of Medicine
Cincinnati, OH, USA

Ursula Lopez

DIPPsych
Psychologist
Department of Anaesthesiology
Pharmacology and Intensive Care
University Hospitals
Geneva, Switzerland

Shobha Malviya

MD
Professor of Anesthesiology and Pediatrics
Division of Pediatric Anesthesiology
University of Michigan Health System
Ann Arbor, MI, USA

David Mann

MD
Assistant Professor
Anesthesiology and Pediatrics
Baylor College of Medicine;
Staff Pediatric and Obstetric Anesthesiologist
Texas Children's Hospital
Houston, TX, USA

Lynn D. Martin

MD, FAAP, FCCM
Director
Department of Anesthesiology & Pain
Medicine
Medical Director
Bellevue Clinics and Surgery Center
Seattle Children's Hospital;
University of Washington School of Medicine
Seattle, WA, USA

Markus Martini

Dr. med, Dr. med. dent
Department of Maxillo-Facial Surgery
Bonn University Hospital
Bonn, Germany

Keira P. Mason

MD
Senior Associate in Anesthesia
Department of Anesthesiology, Perioperative
and Pain Medicine
Children's Hospital Boston;
Associate Professor of Anaesthesia
(Radiology)
Harvard Medical School
Boston, MA, USA

Jean X. Mazoit

MD, PhD
Paediatric Anaesthetist
Université Paris-Sud
Paris, France

Grant McFadyen

MBChB, DA(SA), FRCA
Acting Assistant Professor
Department of Anesthesiology and Pain
Medicine
University of Washington School of
Medicine;
Attending Anesthesiologist
Seattle Children's Hospital
Seattle, WA, USA

Martina Messing-Jünger

MD, PhD
Department of Pediatric Neurosurgery
Asklepios Klinik Sankt Augustin
Sankt Augustin, Germany

Bruce E. Miller

MD
Director, Pediatric Cardiac Anesthesiology
Children's Healthcare of Atlanta;
Associate Professor of Anesthesiology
Emory University School of Medicine
Atlanta, GA, USA

Wanda C. Miller-Hance

MD
Professor of Pediatrics and Anesthesiology
Baylor College of Medicine;
Associate Director for Pediatric
Cardiovascular Anesthesia
Director of Intraoperative Echocardiography
Texas Children's Hospital
Houston, TX, USA

Anthony Moores
MBChB, FRCA
Consultant in Paediatric Anaesthesia
Royal Hospital for Sick Children
Glasgow, Scotland, UK

Neil S. Morton
MD, FRCA, FRCPCH, FFPMRCA
Reader in Paediatric Anaesthesia & Pain
Management
Royal Hospital for Sick Children
Glasgow, Scotland, UK

Vinay M. Nadkarni
MD, MS
Associate Professor of Anesthesiology and
Critical Care Medicine
The University of Pennsylvania School of
Medicine;
Endowed Chair, Pediatric Critical Care
Medicine
The Children's Hospital of Philadelphia
Philadelphia, PA, USA

Olubukola O. Nafiu
MD
Division of Pediatric Anesthesiology
University of Michigan Health System
Ann Arbor, MI, USA

Kirsten C. Odegard
MD
Senior Associate in Anesthesia
Cardiac Anesthesia Service, Children's
Hospital Boston;
Associate Professor in Anaesthesia
Harvard Medical School
Boston, MA, USA

Olutoyin A. Olutoye
MD
Associate Professor
Anesthesiology and Pediatrics
Baylor College of Medicine;
Staff Anesthesiologist
Texas Children's Hospital
Houston, TX, USA

Ellen Rawlinson
FRCA
Clinical Fellow in Paediatric Anaesthesia
Birmingham Children's Hospital,
Liver Unit
Queen Elizabeth Hospital
Birmingham, UK

Michael Richards
BM, MRCP, FRCA
Assistant Professor
Department of Anesthesiology and Pain
Medicine
University of Washington School of
Medicine;
Attending Anesthesiologist
Seattle Children's Hospital
Seattle, WA, USA

David Robinowitz
MD
Assistant Professor
Department of Anesthesia and Perioperative
Care
University of California San Francisco
San Francisco, CA, USA

Mark D. Rollins
MD, PhD
Assistant Professor of Anesthesia and
Perioperative Care
University of California San Francisco
San Francisco, CA, USA

Mark A. Rosen
MD
Professor of Anesthesia and Perioperative
Care
Professor of Obstetrics, Gynecology and
Reproductive Sciences
Director of Obstetric Anesthesia
University of California San Francisco
San Francisco, CA, USA

Allison Kinder Ross
MD
Associate Professor of Anesthesiology and
Pediatrics
Duke University Medical Center
Durham, NC, USA

Patrick A. Ross
MD
Assistant Professor of Clinical
Anesthesiology and Pediatrics
Department of Anesthesiology Critical Care
Medicine
Children's Hospital Los Angeles
University of Southern California
Keck School of Medicine
Los Angeles, CA, USA

Venkata Sampathi
MD
Clinical Instructor
Associate Program Director for Residency
Department of Anesthesiology
SUNY Upstate University Hospital
Syracuse, NY, USA

Neeta R. Saraiya
MD
Assistant Professor of Anesthesiology
Columbia University College of Physicians
and Surgeons
New York, NY, USA

Joseph A. Scattoloni
Clinical Lecturer
Division of Pediatric Anesthesiology
University of Michigan Health System
Ann Arbor, MI, USA

Ehrenfried Schindler
Dr. med
Professor and Head
Department of Pediatric Anesthesiology
Asklepios Klinik Sankt Augustin
Sankt Augustin, Germany

Laura Schleelein
MD
Assistant Professor of Clinical
Anesthesiology and Critical Care
The University of Pennsylvania School of
Medicine;
Anesthesiologist
The Children's Hospital of Philadelphia
Philadelphia, PA, USA

Mark S. Schreiner
MD
Associate Professor
Department of Anesthesiology and Critical
Care Medicine
The University of Pennsylvania School of
Medicine;
The Children's Hospital of Philadelphia
Philadelphia, PA, USA

Alan Jay Schwartz
MD, MSEd
Professor of Clinical Anesthesiology
and Critical Care
Perelman School of Medicine
University of Pennsylvania;
Senior Attending Anesthesiologist
The Children's Hospital of Philadelphia
Philadelphia, PA, USA

Thomas L. Shaw
MD
Assistant Professor
Anesthesiology and Pediatrics
Baylor College of Medicine;
Staff Anesthesiologist
Texas Children's Hospital
Houston, TX, USA

Sulpicio G. Soriano
MD
Department of Anesthesiology, Perioperative and Pain Medicine
Children's Hospital Boston;
Associate Professor of Anaesthesia
Harvard Medical School
Boston, MA, USA

Stephen A. Stayer
MD
Professor, Anesthesiology and Pediatrics
Baylor College of Medicine;
Associate Chief of Anesthesiology
Medical Director of Perioperative Services
Texas Children's Hospital
Houston, TX, USA

Paul A. Stricker
MD
Assistant Professor of Anesthesiology
University of Pennsylvania School of Medicine;
Attending Anesthesiologist
The Children's Hospital of Philadelphia
Philadelphia, PA, USA

Lena S. Sun
MD
Professor of Anesthesiology and Pediatrics
Columbia University College of Physicians and Surgeons
New York, NY, USA

Robert M. Sutton
MD, MSCE
Assistant Professor of Anesthesiology and Critical Care Medicine
The University of Pennsylvania School of Medicine;
The Children's Hospital of Philadelphia
Philadelphia, PA, USA

Joseph D. Tobias
MD
Chairman
Department of Anesthesiology and Pain Medicine
Nationwide Children's Hospital;
Professor of Anesthesiology and Pediatrics
The Ohio State University
Columbus, OH, USA

Joseph R. Tobin
MD
Professor and Chairman
Department of Anesthesiology
Wake Forest University School of Medicine;
Pediatric Anesthesiologist
Wake Forest University Baptist Medical Center
Winston-Salem, NC, USA

Alexis A. Topjian
MD
Assistant Professor of Anesthesiology and Critical Care Medicine
The University of Pennsylvania School of Medicine;
The Children's Hospital of Philadelphia
Philadelphia, PA, USA

Donald C. Tyler
MD, MBA
Associate Professor of Anesthesiology and Critical Care Medicine
The University of Pennsylvania School of Medicine;
Anesthesiologist
The Children's Hospital of Philadelphia
Philadelphia, PA, USA

David B. Waisel
MD
Senior Associate in Anaesthesia
Department of Anesthesiology, Perioperative and Pain Medicine
Children's Hospital Boston;
Associate Professor of Anaesthesia
Harvard Medical School
Boston, MA, USA

Ewan Wallace
MBChB, FRCA
Locum Consultant in Paediatric Anaesthesia
Royal Hospital for Sick Children
Glasgow, Scotland, UK

Mehernoor F. Watcha
MD
Associate Professor
Anesthesiology and Pediatrics
Baylor College of Medicine;
Staff Anesthesiologist
Texas Children's Hospital
Houston, TX, USA

Stacey Watt
MD
Associate Professor of Anesthesiology
Program Director Pediatric Anesthesiology Fellowship
Department of Anesthesia
Women and Children's Hospital of Buffalo
State University at Buffalo
Buffalo and Strong Memorial Hospital
University of Rochester
Rochester, NY, USA

Randall C. Wetzel
MB, MBA
Chairman Department of Anesthesiology and Critical Care Medicine
Director of the Lorna P and Leland K. Whittier Virtual PICU
Professor of Pediatrics, Anesthesiology and Critical Care Medicine
Department of Anesthesiology Critical Care Medicine
Children's Hospital Los Angeles
University of Southern California
Keck School of Medicine
Los Angeles, CA, USA

Glynn Williams
MD
Pediatric Cardiovascular Anesthesiology
Lucille Packard Children's Hospital at Stanford;
Associate Professor of Anesthesia
Stanford University School of Medicine
Palo Alto, CA, USA

Ivan Wilmot
MD
Attending Pediatric Cardiologist
All Children's Hospital Heart Institute
St Petersburg, FL, USA

Cecile Wyckaert
MD
Pediatric Anesthesiology
UC Davis Children's Hospital;
University of California
Davis, CA, USA

Myron Yaster
MD
Richard J Traystman Professor
Departments of Anesthesiology, Critical Care Medicine and Pediatrics
The Johns Hopkins University
Baltimore, MD, USA

Laura N. Zeigler
MD
Assistant Professor of Clinical Anesthesiology
Monroe Carell Jr Children's Hospital at Vanderbilt and Department of Anesthesiology
Vanderbilt University Medical Center
Nashville, TN, USA

Preface

Many changes have occurred in the practice in pediatric anesthesia during the past few years. This, the fifth edition of *Pediatric Anesthesia*, reflects these changes. The book is now the work of multiple new authors from several continents and many countries, which gives all of us the opportunity to broaden our view of pediatric anesthesia. It is also the work of Dean Andropoulos who is now the co-editor of this book. Both the authors and Dean have helped move the book to a new and higher level.

The book is divided into several parts that include: Principles of Pediatric Anesthesia; Pediatric Anesthesia Management; Practice of Pediatric Anesthesia; and Quality, Outcomes, and Complications in Pediatric Anesthesia. The latter part includes new chapters addressing important contemporary issues, including anesthetic neurotoxicity; simulation; databases and outcomes research; electronic anesthesia and medical records; and operating room safety, communication, and teamwork. Also included are appendices on drug dosing and normal laboratory values. This edition is published in full color, to better present the myriad images that illustrate the unique features of pediatric anesthesia. New with this edition are online videos of common anesthesia procedures that concisely and effectively show how to do the procedures. There are also cases presented at the end of each clinical chapter that highlight the main concepts presented in that chapter. One goal of the book has not changed, i.e., to provide pharmacological and physiologi-cal data pertinent to each chapter. Without this information, the clinician often must provide care by rote. Many children do not respond well to rote! If the clinician understands the pharmacology and physiology of the situation, he/she can effectively respond to problems. Knowledge of physiology and pharmacology also allow better planning for anesthesia and surgery.

We thank Rob Blundell and Helen Harvey of Wiley-Blackwell for their constant support and help in the production of this book. Their clear understanding of our vision has provided the guidance necessary to produce the book in the way we envisioned.

And last but not least, we thank the residents and fellows for teaching us as much, or more, than we taught them. Their insightful questions, thoughts, and prodding is what academic medicine is about. This probing forces everyone to get out of her/his comfort zone and think differently. We also thank the surgeons and nurses for their support. Most of all, we thank the patients for giving us the privilege of caring for them and for their continuing to teach us every single day. They are the best teachers!

George A. Gregory
Dean B. Andropoulos

List of Abbreviations

3-D	three-dimensional	AHG	antihuman globulin
5HT3	5-hydroxytryptamine-3 receptor	AHI	apnea-hypopnea index
6-MP	6-mercaptopurine	AHRQ	Agency for Healthcare Research and Quality
α1-ATD	α1-antitrypsin deficiency		
AA	artery-to-artery	AICD	automatic implantable cardiac defibrillator
AAA	asleep-awake-asleep		
AAG	α1-acid glycoprotein	AIMS	anesthesia information management system
AAP	American Academy of Pediatrics		
ABA	American Board of Anesthesiology	AKI	acute kidney injury
ABC	ATP-binding cassette	ALI	acute lung injury
ABG	arterial blood gases	ALL	acute lymphocytic leukemia
ABP	arterial blood pressure	ALT	alanine aminotransferase
ACA	anterior cerebral artery	AML	acute myeloid leukemia
ACD	active compression-decompression device	AMM	anterior mediastinal mass
		AMPA	alpha-amino-3-hydroxy-5-methyl-4-isoxazole-propionic acid
ACE	angiotensin-converting enzyme		
ACEi	angiotensin-converting enzyme inhibitor	ANA	antinuclear antibody
		ANH	acute normovolemic hemodilution
ACGME	Accreditation Council for Graduate Medical Education	ANP	atrial natriuretic peptide
		AoDP	aortic diastolic blood pressure
ACh	acethylcholine	AP	anterior–posterior
ACP	antegrade cerebral perfusion	APL	adjustable pressure limiting
ACRM	anesthesia crisis resource management	APS	acute pain services
ACS	acute chest syndrome/abdominal compartment syndrome/American College of Surgeons	APSF	Anesthesia Patient Safety Foundation
		APTT	activated partial thromboplastin time
		AQI	Anesthesia Quality Institute
		AR	adrenergic receptor
ACTH	adrenocorticotropic hormone	ARDS	adult/acute respiratory distress syndrome
ADH	antidiuretic hormone		
ADP	adenosine diphosphate	ARF	acute renal failure
ADPKD	autosomal dominant polycystic kidney disease	ARRA	American Recovery and Reinvestment Act
ADT	admission, discharge, and transfer		
AED	automated external defibrillator	ASA	American Society of Anesthesiologists
aEEG	amplitude-integrated EEG	ASC	ambulatory surgery center
AFP	α-fetoprotein	ASCA	anti-*Saccharomyces cerevisiae*
AGA	appropriate for gestational age	ASD	atrial septal defect/autism spectrum disorder
AGP	α1-acid glycoprotein		
AHA	American Heart Association	ASIS	anterior superior iliac spine
AHCPR	Agency for Health Care Policy and Research	ASO	arterial switch operation
		AST	aspartate aminotransferase

AT	antithrombin
ATG	antithymocyte globulin
ATP	adenosine triphosphate
AUC	area under the curve
AV	arterial-venous/atrioventricular
AVM	arteriovenous malformation
AVP	arginine vasopressin
BBB	blood–brain barrier
BC	bronchogenic cyst
BDNF	brain-derived neurotrophic factor
BHR	bronchial hyper-responsiveness
BiPAP	bi-level positive airway pressure
BIS	Bispectral Index
BMD	Becker muscular dystrophy
BMI	Body Mass Index
BOS	bronchiolitis obliterans syndrome
BP	blood pressure
BPCA	Best Pharmaceuticals for Children Act
BPD	bronchopulmonary dysplasia
bpm	beats/minute
BPS	bronchopulmonary sequestration
BSA	body surface area
BSEP	bile salt export pump
BSI	bloodstream infection
BT	bleeding time
BU	Bethesda units
BUN	blood urea nitrogen
CA	cardiac arrest
CA-BSI	catheter-associated bloodstream infection
cAMP	cyclic adenosine monophosphate
CAS	central anticholinergic syndrome
CAV	coronary artery vasculopathy
CAVH	continuous arteriovenous hemofiltration
CBC	complete blood count
CBCL	Child Behavior Checklist
CBF	cerebral blood flow
CBFV	cerebral blood flow velocity
CBV	cerebral blood volume
CCAM	congenital cystic adenomatoid malformation
CCL	cardiac cycle length
CDH	congenital diaphragmatic hernia
cEEG	continuous EEG
CF	cystic fibrosis/clubfoot
CFTR	cystic fibrosis transmembrane conductance regulator
cGMP	cyclic guanosine monophosphate
CGRP	calcitonin gene-related peptide
CHB	complete heart block
CHCT	caffeine-halothane contracture test
CHD	congenital heart disease
CHEOPS	Children's Hospital of Eastern Ontario Pain Scale
CHF	congestive heart failure
CIOMS	Council of International Organization and Medical Sciences
CK	creatine kinase
CKD	chronic kidney disease
CLD	chronic lung disease
CLE	congenital lobar emphysema
cLMA	classic laryngeal mask airway
CL/P	cleft lip and palate
CMA	chromosomal microarray
C_{max}	maximum plasma concentration
CME	continuing medical education
$CMRO_2$	cerebral metabolic rate of O_2
CMV	cytomegalovirus
CN	cranial nerve
CNI	calcineurin inhibitor
CNS	central nervous system
CO	cardiac output/carbon monoxide
COX	cyclo-oxygenase
CP	cerebral palsy
CPAP	continuous positive airway pressure
CPB	cardiopulmonary bypass
CPOE	computerized physician order entry
CPP	coronary/cerebral perfusion pressure
CPR	cardiopulmonary resuscitation
CrCL	creatinine clearance
CRF	chronic renal failure
CRI	chronic renal insufficiency
CRM	crew resource management
CRP	C-reactive protein
CRPS	complex regional pain syndrome
CRRT	continual renal replacement therapy
CSF	cerebrospinal fluid
CSI	Cerebral State Index
CT	closure time/computed tomography
CUF	conventional ultrafiltration
CVA	cerebrovascular accident
CVC	central venous catheter
CVP	central venous pressure
CVR	cerebral vascular resistance/coronary vascular resistance/CCAM volume ratio
CVVHF	continuous venovenous hemofiltration
CXR	chest x-ray
CYP	cytochrome P450
DA	dopaminergic
dBA	decibel
DBS	deep brain stimulator
DC	direct current
DDAVP	1-deamino-8-D-arginine vasopressin
DEB	dystrophic EB
DHCA	deep hypothermic circulatory arrest
DI	diabetes insipidus
DIC	disseminated intravascular coagulation
DKA	diabetic ketoacidosis

DLCO	diffusing capacity for carbon monoxide	FDAMA	FDA Modernization and Accountability Act
DLT	double-lumen tube	FETO	fetal endoscopic tracheal occlusion
DMD	Duchenne muscular dystrophy	FEV_1	forced expiratory volume in 1 second
DO	distraction osteogenesis	FFP	fresh frozen plasma
DPPC	dipalmitoyl phosphatidylcholine	FHF	fulminant hepatic failure
DRG	diagnosis-related group	FHR	fetal heart rate
DS	Down syndrome	FISH	fluorescence *in situ* hybridization
DSMB	data safety monitoring board	FLACC	Face, Leg, Activity, Cry, Consolability Scale
DUF	dilutional ultrafiltration	fMRI	functional MRI
EA	emergence agitation/esophageal atresia	FNHTR	febrile non-hemolytic transfusion reaction
EACA	ε-aminocaproic acid	FOB	fiber-optic bronchoscope
EAT	ectopic atrial tachycardia	FRC	functional residual capacity
EB	epidermolysis bullosa	FRF	filter replacement fluid
EBL	estimated blood loss	FVC	forced vital capacity
EBM	evidence-based medicine	FWA	Federal Wide Assurance
EBV	estimated blood volume/Epstein–Barr virus	GA	gestational age
ECC	emergency cardiovascular care	GABA	γ-aminobutyric acid
ECG	electrocardiogram	GABAA	γ-aminobutyric acid receptor, A subunit
ECLS	extracorporeal life support	GCP	Good Clinical Practice
ECMO	extracorporeal membrane oxygenation	GERD	gastroesophageal reflux disease
E-CPR	extracorporeal cardiopulmonary resuscitation	GFR	glomerular filtration rate
ECW	extracellular water	GI	gastrointestinal
ED	emergency department	HAS	Hospital Administrative Service
EDV	end-diastolic volume	HAV	hepatitis A virus
EEG	electroencephalography	HbF	fetal hemoglobin
EELV	end-expiratory lung volume	HBV	hepatitis B virus
EGD	esophagogastroduodenoscopy	HCFA	Health Care Financing Administration
EHR	electronic health record	HCG	human chorionic gonadotropin
ELBW	extremely low birthweight	Hct	hematocrit
ELISA	enzyme-linked immunosorbent assay	HCUP	Healthcare Cost and Utilization Project
EMA	European Medicines Agency	HCV	hepatitis C virus
EMG	electromyography	HD	hemodialysis
EMLA	eutectic mixture of local anesthetics	HFHNC	high-flow humidified nasal cannula
EMR	electronic medical record	HFOV	high-frequency oscillatory ventilation
EMS	emergency medical services	HFPS	high-fidelity patient simulation
EMT	emergency medical technician	HH	hand hygiene
ENS	enteric nervous system	HIE	hypoxic-ischemic encephalopathy
ENT	ear, nose and throat	HIPAA	Health Insurance Portability and Accountability Act
EP	evoked potential	HITECH	Health Information Technology for Economic and Clinical Health Act
EPO	erythropoietin	HIV	human immunodeficiency virus
ERCP	endoscopic retrograde cholangiopancreatography	HLA	human leukocyte antigen
ERF	established renal failure	HLHS	hypoplastic left heart syndrome
ESR	erythrocyte sedimentation rate	HME	heat and moisture exchanger
ESRD	end-stage renal disease	HMWK	high molecular weight kininogen
ESRT	evoked stapedius reflex threshold	HOCM	hypertrophic obstructive cardiomyopathy
ESS	endoscopic sinus surgery	HPS	hepatopulmonary syndrome
$ETCO_2$	end-tidal carbon dioxide	HPV	hypoxic pulmonary vasoconstriction/human papillomavirus
ETT	endotracheal tube		
EXIT	*ex utero* intrapartum treatment		
FAP	functional abdominal pain		
FCC	fetoscopic cord coagulation		
FDA	Food and Drug Administration		

HR	heart rate	LPS	lipopolysaccharide
HSA	human serum albumin	LR	lactated Ringer's (solution)
HTLV	human T-lymphotrophic virus	L-R	left-to-right
HTR	hemolytic transfusion reaction	LST	life-sustaining treatment
HUS	hemolytic uremic syndrome	LV	left ventricle
IBD	inflammatory bowel disease	LVEDP	left ventricular end-diastolic pressure
ICD	implantable cardioverter-defibrillator	MAC	minimum alveolar concentration
ICN	intensive care nursery	MAET	multidrug and toxin extrusion
ICP	intracranial pressure		transporter
ICU	intensive care unit	MAP	mean arterial pressure
ICW	intracellular water	MCA	middle cerebral artery
ID	internal diameter	MDCT	multidetector computed tomography
I:E	inspiratory:expiratory	MDR	multidrug-resistant
IHPS	idiopathic hypertrophic pyloric stenosis	MEG	magnetoencephalography
IJ	internal jugular	MELD	model for end-stage liver disease
IJV	internal jugular vein	MEP	motor evoked potential
IL	interleukin	MET	medical emergency teams
IM	intramuscular	MH	malignant hyperthermia
IND	Investigational New Drug	MI	myocardial infarction
iNO	inhaled nitric oxide	MIS	minimally invasive surgery
INR	international normalized ratio/	MMC	migrating motor complex/
	interventional neuroradiology		myelomeningocele
IO	intraosseous	MMF	mycophenolate mofetil
IOM	Institute of Medicine	MOCA	Maintenance of Certification in
IOP	intraocular pressure		Anesthesiology
IPPV	intermittent positive pressure	MODY	maturity-onset diabetes of the young
	ventilation	MODS	multiple organ dysfunction syndrome
IRB	investigational review board	MPA	mycophenolic acid
ISHLT	International Society of Heart and Lung	MPAP	mean pulmonary artery pressure
	Transplantation	MPD	maximum permissible dose
ISI	International Sensitivity Index	MPOG	Multicenter Perioperative Outcomes
ISPAD	International Society for Pediatric and		Group
	Adolescent Diabetes	MPP	myocardial perfusion pressure
IT	iliotibial	MRA	magnetic resonance angiography
ITD	impedence threshold device	MRI	magnetic resonance imaging
IU	international unit	MRP	magnetic resonance perfusion
IV	intravenous	MRT	magnetic resonance therapy
IVC	inferior vena cava	MRV	magnetic resonance venography
IVH	intraventricular hemorrhage	MTD	maximal tolerated dose
JET	junctional ectopic tachycardia	mTOR	mammalian target of rapamycin
JRA	juvenile rheumatoid arthritis	MUF	modified ultrafiltation
LA	local anesthetic/left atrium	MVA	motor vehicle accident
LAS	lung allocation score	MVO_2	mixed venous oxygen saturation
LCR	laryngeal chemoreflex	MW	molecular weight
LDH	lactate dehydrogenase	NAC	N-acetylcysteine
LDLT	living donor lobar transplant	NAD	nicotinamide adenine dinucleotide
LED	light-emitting diode	NADPH	nicotinamide adenine dinucleotide
LES	lower esophageal sphincter		phosphate
LGA	large for gestational age	NAT	nucleic acid testing
LHR	lung to head ratio	NCA	nurse-controlled analgesia
LiDCO	lithium dilution cardiac output	NCS	non-convulsive seizures
LMA	laryngeal mask airway	NDA	New Drug Application
LOH	loss of heterozygocity	NE	norepinephrine
LOR	loss of resistance	NEB	neuroendocrine bodies

NEC	necrotizing enterocolitis	PBS	prune belly syndrome
NEHI	neuroendocrine hyperplasia of infancy	PCA	patient-controlled anesthesia/ postconceptual age
NFκB	nuclear factor κ B		
NGT	nasogastric tube	PCRA	patient-controlled regional anesthesia
NIF	negative inspiratory force	PCS	patient-controlled sedation
NIPPV	nasal intermittent positive pressure ventilation	PCWP	pulmonary capillary wedge pressure
		PD	pharmacodynamic/peritoneal dialysis
NIRS	near infrared spectroscopy	PDA	patent ductus arteriosus
NIS	Nationwide Inpatient Sample	PDE	phosphodiesterase
NIV	non-invasive ventilation	PEA	pulseless electrical activity
NMB	neuromuscular blockade	PEEP	positive end-expiratory pressure
NMBA	neuromuscular blocking agent	PEFR	peak expiratory flow rate
NMDA	N-methyl-D-aspartate	PEG	percutaneous endoscopic gastrostomy
NNT	number needed to treat	PELD	pediatric end-stage liver disease
NO	nitric oxide	PELOD	pediatric logistic organ dysfunction
NPH	nephronophthisis/neutral protamine Hagedorn (insulin)	PET	positron emission tomography
		PEVPPS	Preverbal, Early Verbal Pediatric Pain Scale
NPO	nil per os		
NPPE	negative pressure pulmonary edema	PFC	persistent fetal circulation
NRBS	non-rebreathing systems	PFIC	progressive familial intrahepatic cholestasis
NRL	natural rubber latex		
NRP	Neonatal Resuscitation Program	PFO	patent foramen ovale
NSAID	non-steroidal anti-inflammatory drug	PFT	pulmonary function test
NSQIP	National Surgical Quality Improvement Program	PG	prostaglandin
		PGD	primary graft dysfunction
OAT	organic anion transporter	P-gp	P-glycoprotein
OATP	organic anion transporting polypeptide	PHBQ	Post Hospitalization Behavior Questionnaire
OAVS	oculo-auriculovertebral spectrum		
OBRA	Omnibus Budget Reconciliation Act	PHI	protected health information
OCT	organic cation transporter	PICC	percutaneously inserted central catheter
OELM	optimal external laryngeal manipulation	PICU	pediatric intensive care unit
		PIPP	Premature Infant Pain Profile
OI	osteogenesis imperfecta	PIV	peripheral intravenous catheter
OLT	orthotopic liver transplantation	PK	pharmacokinetic/prekallikrein
OLV	one-lung ventilation	PLE	protein-losing enteropathy
OMS	oral maxillofacial surgery	PLV	protective lung ventilation
OPTN	Organ Procurement and Transplant Network	PN	parenteral nutrition
		PNAM	presurgical nasal alveolar molding
OR	operating room	PNEC	pulmonary neuroendocrine cells
OSA	obstructive sleep apnea	PO	per os
OSAS	obstructive sleep apnea syndrome	POAH	preoptic anterior thalamus
P4P	pay-for-performance	POBD	postoperative behavior disorder
PA	pulmonary artery/pulmonary atresia	POCA	Pediatric Perioperative Cardiac Arrest Registry
PABD	preoperative autologous blood donation		
		PONV	postoperative nausea and vomiting
PAC	premature atrial contractions	POV	postoperative vomiting
PACU	postanesthesia care unit	POVL	postoperative visual loss
PAED	pediatric anesthesia emergence delirium	PPH	portopulmonary hypertension
		PPHN	primary pulmonary hypertension of the newborn
PAI	plasminogen activator inhibitor		
PALS	pediatric advanced life support	PPIA	parental presence at induction of anesthesia
PaO$_2$	partial pressure of oxygen in arterial blood		
		PPV	positive pressure ventilation
PAS	periodic acid-Schiff	PR	pulmonary regurgitation/per rectum

PRA	panel reactive antibody	RSV	respiratory syncytial virus
PRAN	Pediatric Regional Anesthesia Network	RV	right ventricle/residual volume
PRBC	packed red blood cells	RVOT	right ventricular outflow tract
PREA	Pediatric Research Equity Act	SAE	serious adverse event
PRIS	propofol infusion syndrome	SAH	subarachnoid hemorrhage
PRISM	Pediatric Risk of Mortality Score	SaO_2	percent arterial oxyhemoglobin saturation
PRS	Pierre Robin sequence		
psi	pounds per square inch	SAR	specific absorption rate
PSRC	Pediatric Sedation Research Consortium	SBE	subacute bacterial endocarditis
PT	prothrombin time	SCD	sickle cell disease
PTFE	polytetrafluoroethylene	SCFE	slipped capital femoral epiphysis
PTLD	post-transplant lymphoproliferative disorder	SCh	succinylcholine
		SCT	sickle cell trait/sacrococcygeal teratoma
PTP	post-transfusion purpura	SD	standard deviation
PTSD	post-traumatic stress disorder	SE	status epilepticus
PTT	partial thromboplastin time	SFLP	selective fetoscopic laser photocoagulation
PUBS	percutaneous umbilical blood sampling		
PUV	posterior urethral valves	SGA	small for gestational age
PV	postoperative vomiting	SIADH	syndrome of inappropriate secretion of antidiuretic hormone
PVB	paravertebral block		
PVC	premature ventricular contractions	SIDS	sudden infant death syndrome
PVOD	pulmonary vascular obstructive disease	SIRS	systemic inflammatory response syndrome
PVR	pulmonary vascular resistance		
RA	right atrium	$SjvO_2$	oxygen saturation in jugular venous bulb
RAP	right atrial pressure		
RAS	renin-angiotensin-aldosterone system	SLC	solute carrier
RBC	red blood cell	SMR	standardized mortality ratio
RCM	radiocontrast media	SNP	sodium nitroprusside
RCP	regional cerebral perfusion	SOS	Shikani optical stylet
RCT	randomized controlled trial	SPA	Society for Pediatric Anesthesia
RDI	respiratory disturbance index	SPECT	single photon emission computed tomography
RDS	respiratory distress syndrome		
REE	resting energy expenditure	SSEP	somatosensory-evoked potential
REM	rapid eye movement	SSI	surgical site infection
RF	rheumatoid factor	SSRI	selective serotonin reuptake inhibitor
RFA	radiofrequency ablation	SVC	superior vena cava
RFCA	radiofrequency catheter ablation	SVL	Storz video laryngoscope
RFID	radiofrequency identification	SVR	systemic vascular resistance
rFVIIa	recombinant activated factor VII	SVT	supraventricular tachyarrhythmia/supraventricular tachycardia
RHA	rhabdomyolysis		
RIPA	ristocetin-induced platelet aggregation assay	TA	tranexamic acid
		T&A	tonsillectomy and adenoidectomy
R-L	right-to-left	TACO	transfusion-associated circulatory overload
RLFP	regional low flow perfusion		
ROP	retinopathy of prematurity	TAFI	thrombin-activatable fibrinolysis inhibitor
ROSC	return of spontaneous circulation		
RPGN	rapidly progressive glomerulonephritis	TA-GVHD	transfusion-associated graft-versus-host disease
R-R	R to R interval		
RRT	renal replacement therapy	TAP	transversus abdominis plane
RSBI	Rapid Shallow Breathing Index	TB	tuberculosis
RSI	rapid-sequence induction	TBI	traumatic brain injury/total body irradiation
RSII	rapid-sequence induction and intubation		
		TBV	total blood volume
rSO_2	regional oxygen saturation	TCD	transcranial Doppler ultrasound

TCI	target-controlled infusion
TCOM	transcutaneous CO_2 monitoring
TCPC	total cavopulmonary connection
TCS	Treacher Collins syndrome
TeamSTEPPS®	Team Strategies and Tools to Enhance Performance and Patient Safety
TEE	transesophageal echocardiogram
TEF	tracheo-esophageal fistula
TEG	thromboelastography
TF	tissue factor
TFPI	tissue factor pathway inhibitor
TGF	transforming growth factor
THAM	tris-hydroxymethyl amino-methane
TIA	transient ischemic attacks
TIVA	total intravenous anesthesia
TLC	total lung capacity
TLR	Toll-like receptor
TLV	total lung volume
T_{max}	time to maximum concentration
TMJ	temporomandibular joint
TNF	tumor necrosis factor
TOF	tetralogy of Fallot/train-of-four
TOI	tissue oxygenation index
TOMS	team-oriented medical simulation
tPA	tissue plasminogen activator
TPN	total parenteral nutrition
TR	tricuspid regurgitation
TRALI	transfusion-related acute lung injury
TRAP	twin reversed arterial perfusion sequence/thrombin receptor agonist peptides
TRIM	transfusion-related immunomodulation
TSC	tuberous sclerosis complex
TT	thrombin time
TTP	thrombotic thrombocytopenic purpura
TTTS	twin–twin transfusion syndrome
TV	tricuspid valve
TXA	tranexamic acid
UAC	umbilical arterial catheter
UBF	uterine blood flow
UDP	uridine diphosphate
UDPGA	uridine diphosphate glucuronic acid
UDPGT	uridine diphosphate glucuronyltransferase
UDT	undescended testes
UGT	UDP-glucuronosyltransferase
UNOS	United Network for Organ Sharing
UPJ	ureteropelvic junction
URI	upper respiratory infection
URTI	upper respiratory tract infection
US	ultrasound
USCOM	ultrasonic cardiac output monitor
UTI	urinary tract infection
UVC	umbilical venous catheter
UVJ	ureterovesical junction
VA	veno-arterial/Veterans Administration
VACTERL	vertebral, anal, cardiac, tracheo-esophageal, renal and limb anomalies
VAD	ventricular assist devices
VAP	ventilator-associated pneumonia
VAS	visual analog scale
VATS	video-assisted thoracoscopic surgery
VCFS	velocardiofacial syndrome
VEGF	vascular endothelial growth factor
VF	ventricular fibrillation
VHL	von Hippel–Lindau
VIP	vasoactive intestinal polypeptide
VMI	visual motor integration
VP	ventriculoperitoneal
VSD	ventricular septal defect
VT	ventricular tachycardia
VUR	vesicoureteric reflux
VV	vein-to-vein/veno-venous
vWD	von Willibrand disease
vWF	von Willibrand factor
vWF:RCo	ristocetin co-factor assay
WB	whole blood
WBC	white blood cell
WEB	wire-guided endobronchial blocker
WHO	World Health Organization
WOB	work of breathing
WPW	Wolff–Parkinson–White
WS	Williams syndrome
ZBUF	zero-balance ultrafiltration

CHAPTER 1
Ethical Considerations

David B. Waisel

Department of Anesthesiology, Perioperative and Pain Medicine, Children's Hospital Boston, and Harvard Medical School, Boston, MA, USA

Introduction

Although physicians may think of medical ethics in dramatic terms – withdrawing life-sustaining therapy, allocating organs for transplant – medical ethics floods our daily practice. Consider an anesthesiologist who recommends postponing surgery in an infant because of a borderline upper respiratory infection (URI) [1]. How should the anesthesiologist respond to a parental request to proceed? These decisions are often framed as medical decisions based on the characteristics of the URI and the surgery. But within the decisions lie the ethical components of informed consent and obligations to the child and family. How do we decide how much weight to give the parents' strong desire to proceed? Does it matter why they want to proceed (convenience because grandma is in town to care for siblings? concern about being able to get time off from work again? scheduling because the child spends the summer with an out-of-town parent, effectively delaying the operation until fall? etc.). Should we even consider the effects on the family? What if there is concern that the parents will not reschedule surgery?

Ethical dilemmas occur when a physician is faced with "oughts" – that which a physician is bound by duty to do – that conflict. In the above example, anesthesiologists ought to base proceeding with surgery solely on the child's best interest. Anesthesiologists also ought to ensure that a child receives necessary healthcare within the realistic complexities of family life. Medical ethics provides the process by which to resolve these apparently conflicting "oughts."

Resolving ethical dilemmas is not solely a matter of being a moral person. Identifying, diagnosing and managing ethical conflicts requires the same extent of expertise that is required to identify, diagnose, and manage myocardial ischemia. Training and experience in resolving ethical dilemmas enable ethics consultants to identify critical facts, apply ethical principles and case-based analysis, articulate precise questions, and have the moral imagination to create more palatable solutions.

Ethics committees and their consultation services provide the resources to help resolve dilemmas. Anesthesiologists may find consultation services particularly helpful with concerns about disagreements among

Gregory's Pediatric Anesthesia, Fifth Edition. Edited by George A. Gregory, Dean B. Andropoulos.
© 2012 Blackwell Publishing Ltd. Published 2012 by Blackwell Publishing Ltd.

patients and clinicians, appropriate decision-making roles for adolescents, and decisions about end-of-life care. A typical free-standing children's hospital has between six and ten ethics consultations each year, but some perform as many as 50 consultations annually [2].

Members of ethics committees include representatives throughout the hospital such as chaplains, administrators, social workers, nurses, and physicians. Many committees also include a local community representative. Depending on local practice, consultations may be performed by an individual, a small group or the entire ethics committee. Most ethics consultation services permit patients, parents and anyone with standing to request a consultation. Standing is defined broadly as participating in the care of the patient. Most services enter a written report into the clinical record. The standard of care is that ethics consultation services advise only and have no formal authority [3]. A committee with a strong record, however, does have substantial informal authority. The case study at the end of the chapter provides an example of an ethics consultation.

The law is not a desirable substitute for resolving ethical dilemmas. Most importantly, the law represents a lower boundary for acceptable behavior, whereas ethics articulates a standard to which we should aspire. Pragmatically, the law does not provide clear guidance because most law surrounding ethical dilemmas is case law. In addition, the frequently adversarial legal process may pollute future relations. Crude statutes and regulations are unable to govern complex medical care. Consider the Baby Doe regulations regarding withdrawing therapy for neonates. The rigid regulations devastated the ability to apply thoughtful, tailored therapy to individual neonates [4–6].

Ethics committees also provide formal education sessions, ward ethics rounds, and institutional consultation. An example of an institutional consultation would be to determine and implement the necessary infrastructure to ensure compliance with an adolescent's refusal to receive transfusion therapy.

Informed consent process for pediatric patients

The doctrine of informed consent centers on the belief that patients have a right to self-determination [7]. The right to self-determination is actualized through the legal concept of competency. Except in specific situations, minors are not legally competent to consent for healthcare. But minors do have varying degrees of decision-making capacity, and should be included in medical decision making to the extent permitted by the child and situation (Box 1.1).

Box 1.1 Elements of consent and assent as defined by the American Academy of Pediatrics Committee on Bioethics [7]

Consent

1. Adequate provision of information including the nature of the ailment or condition, the nature of the proposed diagnostic steps or treatment and the probability of their success; the existence and nature of the risks involved; and the existence, potential benefits, and risks of recommended alternative treatments (including the choice of no treatment).
2. Assessment of the patient's understanding of the above information.
3. Assessment, if only tacit, of the capacity of the patient or surrogate to make the necessary decisions.
4. Assurance, insofar as it is possible, that the patient has the freedom to choose among the medical alternatives without coercion or manipulation.

Assent

1. Helping the patient achieve a developmentally appropriate awareness of the nature of his or her condition.
2. Telling the patient what he or she can expect with tests and treatment.
3. Making a clinical assessment of the patient's understanding of the situation and the factors influencing how he or she is responding (including whether there is inappropriate pressure to accept testing or therapy).
4. Soliciting an expression of the patient's willingness to accept the proposed care.

The process of pediatric informed consent depends on the age of the child (Table 1.1). The concepts of best interest, informed permission and assent are used when considering pediatric informed consent. For convenience, the term "parent" will be used to describe the child's surrogate decision maker. Parents are not always the legal surrogate decision maker and parental authority may be limited in adolescents. The term "decision maker" will refer to those involved in the specific decision and may include parents, children. and their advisors.

The primary lesson of this chapter should be to respect the experiences and opinions of children. The American Academy of Pediatrics emphasizes that "no one should solicit a patient's views without intending to weigh them seriously. In situations in which the patient will have to receive medical care despite his or her objection, the patient should be told that fact and should not be deceived" [7].

Informed permission and the best interest standard

To recognize the fact that ethical informed consent only can be given by the patient, the American Academy of

Table 1.1 Graduated involvement of minors in medical decision making [7,9]

Age	Decision-making capacity	Techniques
Under 6 years	None	Best interest standard
Age 6–12 years	Developing	Informed permission Informed assent
Age 12–18 years	Mostly developed	Informed assent Informed permission
Mature minor	Developed, as legally determined by a judge, for a specific decision	Informed consent
Emancipated minor	Developed, as determined by a situation (e.g. being married, in the military, economically independent)	Informed consent

This broad outline should be viewed as a guide. Specific circumstances always must be taken into consideration. When children are in the upper range of an age bracket, limited or full inclusion of a higher technique, such as the use of assent for a 6 year old, may be appropriate.

Pediatrics uses the term "informed permission" for when the parent provides legal consent and ethical decision making for the child [7]. This conceptual framework highlights the limits of parental decision making. It does not affect the legal obligation to obtain informed consent from the parents as defined by local statutes.

Children younger than the age of 7 years have insufficient decision-making capacities to effectively participate in the informed consent process. When children cannot participate, the best interest standard guides decision making. Best interest does not mean the best care as defined by the clinicians. There are often several acceptable options, and clinicians rely on parents to determine what is in the child's best interest. Parents are given considerable latitude in decision making because society values the role of family, parents want the best for their children, and families often have to live with the result of the choices. Parental values are also a reasonable approximation of the child's future values [4].

Parental decisions should be scrutinized if they appear to fall outside the boundaries of acceptable care. Boundaries are determined by the extent and likelihood of potential harms arising from the intervention or its absence, the likelihood of success, and the overall risk-to-benefit ratio. When parents appear to choose unacceptable treatments, anesthesiologists should seek other clinicians to assess the acceptability of the decision and, if necessary and appropriate, to participate in the discussion [8]. Anesthesiologists should seek to resolve disagreements without resorting to legal intervention. However, the state has an interest in protecting those who cannot protect themselves. If other options have failed, anesthesiologists should report parents they believe to be choosing unacceptable treatments to child welfare authorities for possible legal action.

Informed assent: the role of the patient

Children should participate in decision making to the extent their development permits [7]. For children between the ages of 7 and 13, anesthesiologists should seek both informed permission from the parent and assent and participatory decision making from the child. Common decisions in which children participate include whether a 6 year old wants sedation prior to an inhalation induction, whether a 10 year old wants inhalation or intravenous induction of anesthesia and whether a 12 year old wants an epidural for postoperative analgesia.

Anesthesiologists should assume that adolescents older than 13 years have sufficient decision-making capacity to fulfill the ethical obligations of informed consent. Adolescents have likely developed adult levels of abstract thought, complex reasoning and abilities to foresee and anticipate outcomes. However, adolescent decision-making abilities are limited by emotional impulsiveness and a tendency to undervalue long-term consequences. For these reasons, the influence an adolescent has on decision making is tempered by their maturity and the risks of the decision. Decisions are considered higher risk when they include an increased likelihood of permanently lost opportunities that have noteworthy consequences. For example, delayed scoliosis surgery may increase the extent of the curve, subsequently impairing cardiopulmonary function. These impairments can affect the quality of life, future morbidity, and lifespan. In determining the extent of risk in a decision, the quality and relevance of the data must be rigorously considered. This is particularly important when predicting future outcomes for infants.

Emancipated minors and the mature minor doctrine

Emancipated minors are minors who have a statutory right to legally consent for their own healthcare decisions. States often award this status to patients who are in the military, who are married, who have children and who are economically independent. To be declared a mature minor, the patient must be determined by a judge to be legally and ethically capable of giving legal consent in a specific situation. Judges consider mature minor status based on the extent of the risk in the decision and the developmental maturity and age of the child [9].

Disclosure

The reasonable person standard, the legal standard for most of the United States, requires that the information disclosed satisfies the hypothetical reasonable person. For the most part, however, the exact information to be disclosed to decision makers is not itemized. Further, preferences vary for the extent of disclosure and the desire to participate in decision making [10,11]. For example, in one typical survey, 74% of parents wanted to know all possible risks of anesthesia, while 24% wanted to know only those likely to occur, and 2% wanted to know only those that may result in a significant injury [12]. Rather than rely on a rote informed consent process, anesthesiologists should seek to satisfy the needs of the decision makers by meeting their information and decision-making needs. Because sociodemographic characteristics do not reliably predict preferences for disclosure and decision making, anesthesiologists should seek to meet the needs of the decision makers through patient-driven interactions. Anesthesiologists can do this by informing decision makers about that which the anesthesiologist feels must be communicated and about options that affect the perioperative experience (e.g. regional versus general anesthesia). The anesthesiologist can then ask if the decision makers wish to know more. Patient-driven interactions likely reduce malpractice lawsuits. The likelihood of being sued based on informed consent malpractice issues is very rare [13]. But the improved satisfaction that comes from patient-driven interactions (or, more simply, from listening to and responding to the decision makers' needs and requests) leads to decreased complaints and lawsuits in general [14,15].

Informed refusal

Informed refusal of a recommendation requires anesthesiologists to more fully inform decision makers about the risks, benefits and alternatives than if the decision makers were following the recommendation. This helps ensure that decision makers are as knowledgeable as possible about the risks of selecting a less desirable path. Anesthesiologists who believe parents are refusing necessary care for a child without decision-making capacity should use the best interest standard.

Children with significant decision-making capacity (perhaps around the age of 10 years but certainly by the age of 13 years) might refuse non-emergency procedures. Anesthesiologists should respect this refusal of assent and conscientiously avoid pressuring the child. Coercing or manipulating a child into having a procedure damages the child's trust of the medical profession and impairs future co-operation with their care. Maintenance of trust is particularly important in children with chronic medical conditions.

Strategies for resolving conflicts center on maintaining communication, clarifying misunderstandings about the anesthetic and surgical experience, and decreasing the anxiety of both the child and parents. The goal is to resolve the problem without impairing the relationships among clinicians, patient, and parents. Anesthesiologists may want to emphasize that nothing will happen without the child's approval, *but only if that is true*. Moving the discussion away from the preoperative area or letting the child dress in street clothes will often reduce stress and improve communication.

Anesthesiologists should recognize the distinction between using pharmacological agents to calm an anxious adolescent to enable proceeding and using pharmacological agents to manipulate the adolescent into proceeding. Consider the 15 year old who becomes overwhelmingly anxious and refuses surgery. It would be inappropriate to unilaterally administer midazolam for the purpose of getting the patient to co-operate. On the other hand, it is wholly appropriate to seek the patient's assent to receive sufficient anxiolysis so that upon return to the preoperative area, the patient is able to undergo the procedure. Time, respect, and simple strategies often resolve issues satisfactorily and efficiently.

Confidentiality for adolescents

Physicians are obligated to protect patient information from unauthorized and unnecessary disclosure. With adolescents, confidentially is crucial for even the banal. Adolescents concerned about confidentiality withhold pertinent information and defer necessary treatment [16]. Anesthesiologists may want to ask sensitive questions without the parents present. Squarely addressing confidentiality concerns often improves truthfulness.

Anesthesiologists in possession of sensitive information should encourage the adolescent to share the relevant information with the parents. It is useful to engage adolescent specialists or social workers to enable the adolescent to communicate successfully with the parents and to ensure future care. However, anesthesiologists should honor the adolescent's right to confidentiality. It is ethically justifiable to breach confidentiality only when complying with reporting statutes or when breaching confidentiality will prevent serious harm to the child or another. Anesthesiologists should confer with legal counsel to determine if a presumed legal obligation requires breaching confidentiality.

State statutes may limit the anesthesiologist to informing only the adolescent about a positive pregnancy test [17]. In addition to ethical principles and practical reasons, these statues are specifically present to address concerns about child abuse in pregnant adolescents.

The ethical complexity increases logarithmically when a pregnant adolescent does not want to inform her parents and it is appropriate to postpone the procedure. Even though anesthesiologists must postpone the case in a manner that does not breach confidentiality, the details of how the postponement is communicated affects the ability to maintain confidentiality. For example, anesthesiologists can issue a terse communiqué to the parents that the procedure will be postponed. While this approach avoids explicit lying, its oddness may confuse parents and trigger a cascade of questions, leading to a loss of confidentiality. On the other hand, anesthesiologists may choose to deceive more actively. These clinicians would argue that if parents have no right to that information, then their obligations to the adolescent demand their best effort to maintain confidentiality.

Although peculiar in a medical textbook, perhaps a short course in deception is useful. Anesthesiologists should deceive in ways that will be successful, not require diagnostic or therapeutic interventions and not unduly worry parents. For example, while intimating about unavailable operating room space and emergency surgeries may be useful, the excuse is rather weak if stated in the morning, when the family could offer to wait until something is available. Using a "new murmur" as an excuse may worry parents and cause unnecessary consultations. More simple deceits, such as postponement due to concerns about inadequate fasting or upper respiratory infections, tend to minimize unintended consequences.

The rules surrounding parental involvement in elective abortions are confusing [18]. Although many states require either parental consent or notification prior to an elective abortion, the exceptions to parental involvement make it prudent to consult with hospital counsel. In general, though, parental consent requires permission from parents while parental notification only requires informing parents. There are times when parental involvement in abortion may harm adolescents [18,19]. To ensure that adolescents can seek an abortion confidentially in states with parental involvement laws, states must have a judicial bypass procedure to preclude parental involvement. In a judicial bypass hearing, the judge interviews the adolescent to determine if she is sufficiently mature to consent for an abortion. Even if the judge determines

that the adolescent is insufficiently mature, the judge may grant permission for the abortion if the judge believes it is in the adolescent's best interest.

Emergency care

Emergency therapy is considered desirable and should be given to the minor who does not have a parent available to give legal consent or informed permission [20]. Anesthesiologists should err on the side of treating if they are unsure whether to wait for parental consent.

Emergency therapy becomes more complex when adolescents nearing the age of majority refuse to assent to care. Urgency may not permit the extended evaluation necessary to determine whether the minor has sufficient decision-making capacity. Anesthesiologists should use the best interest standard to guide therapy acutely. Consider a 15 year old with an acute cervical fracture who refuses emergency stabilization, which may cause irrevocable harm. The typical adolescent's decidedly short-term outlook and overvaluation of physical abilities make it unlikely that the adolescent possesses sufficient decision-making capacity in the acute situation. It is hard to imagine honoring an adolescent's refusal of emergency therapy in this case.

Children of Jehovah's Witnesses

Jehovah's Witnesses interpret biblical scripture to mean that anyone who takes blood will be "cut off from his people" and not receive eternal salvation [21,22]. Adults may refuse potentially life-sustaining transfusion therapy. The presumption is that they are making an informed and voluntary decision. But the courts routinely authorize transfusion of children of Jehovah's Witnesses. The courts base these decisions on the doctrine of *parens patriae*, the obligation of the state to protect the interests of incompetent patients.

Anesthesiologists should directly address transfusion therapy when caring for a child of Jehovah's Witnesses. The patient and family should be informed that, as with all patients, attempts will be made to follow the family's wishes within the standard of care. Because refusal of transfusion therapy is deemed a "matter of conscience," the anesthesiologist should clarify acceptable interventions. Deliberate hypotension, deliberate hypothermia, and hemodilution are often acceptable techniques. Synthetic colloid solutions, dextran, erythropoietin, desmopressin, and preoperative iron are usually acceptable. Some Jehovah's Witnesses will accept blood removed and returned in a continuous loop, such as cell saver blood. The family should be informed that in critical situations, the anesthesiologist will transfuse while concomitantly seeking legal authorization. Anesthesiologists should be familiar with the hospital's preferred mechanism for obtaining legal authorizing. In instances where the likelihood of requiring blood is high or the local judiciary is not that familiar with case law for Jehovah's Witnesses, anesthesiologists may choose to obtain the court order preoperatively if there is a likelihood of transfusion.

Elective procedures may be postponed until the child is of sufficient age and maturity to decide about transfusion therapy. But delays may increase the risk of morbidity or the quality of outcome. Factors affecting whether to proceed include the quantitative and qualitative changes in risks and benefits.

Consent for pediatric procedures without direct benefits

Pediatric anesthesiologists may encounter children undergoing bone marrow donation for siblings who would benefit from hematopoietic stem cell transplantation [23]. The stem cell donor receives no direct medical benefit from the donation. The major risks of donation are the anesthetic and the potential need for transfusion.

The benefit of donation is commonly considered to be the psychosocial benefit of helping a family member and pediatric donors report that the benefits of donations outweigh the physical harm [24]. As can be expected in such a complex dynamic, however, donation can result in moderate post-traumatic stress. Some donors felt they did not have a choice about being a donor and that they may be responsible for unsuccessful transplants.

Given the risks and benefits and the unique position of families in society, the American Academy of Pediatrics believes it is ethically permissible for minors to donate bone marrow when certain requirements are met, including a close relationship between donor and recipient, a likelihood of benefit to the recipient and an absence of a suitable medically equivalent adult relative.

The temporarily impaired parent

Chemically intoxicated parents may be disruptive, dangerous, and incapable of fulfilling surrogate responsibilities. Anesthesiologists should use the least restrictive means to protect patient and parent confidentiality while ensuring the safety of the child, the impaired parent, and others present [25].

Although it seems ethically and legally prudent to postpone routine treatment until informed permission and legal consent can be obtained from an unimpaired parent, anesthesiologists will have to weigh the benefits of postponement with the risk that impaired parents may not reliably return. It may be in the child's best interests to proceed with a routine procedure even thought the impaired parent is unable to give informed permission and legal consent. Anesthesiologists should consult with legal and risk management colleagues for guidance.

Molecular genetic testing

The combination of genetic testing and electronic medical records permits anesthesiologists to be aware of testing used to confirm a diagnosis, determine carrier status or for asymptomatic testing for disorders of late onset [26]. While genetic testing provides substantial benefits, it can also do harm by informing people about their genetic lineage without the patient's consent or adequate preparation.

Whether to test is particularly hazardous with minors. Genetic testing may affect personal psychosocial development and business opportunities and removes the opportunity to choose whether to obtain that genetic information. Testing should be performed only when there are immediate medical benefits to the child or when there are medical benefits to a family member and no expected harm to the child. Otherwise, testing should be deferred until the child can display an understanding of the consequences of genetic testing [26].

Forgoing potentially life-sustaining therapy

Do-not-resuscitate orders

Do-not-resuscitate orders enable patients to forgo potentially life-sustaining treatment (LST) because the likely burdens outweigh the potential benefits. Benefits of receiving LST may include prolongation of life (understanding that the continuation of biological existence without consciousness may not be a benefit); improved quality of life after the life-sustaining medical therapy has been applied (including reduction of pain or disability); and increased "physical pleasure, emotional enjoyment, and intellectual satisfaction" [27]. Burdens should be viewed from the patient's perspective and may include "intractable pain; irremediable disability or helplessness; emotional suffering; invasive and/or inhumane interventions designed to sustain life; or other activities that severely detract from the patient's quality of life" [27]. Benefits and burdens should be considered in terms of both short- and long-term goals.

Children with do-not-resuscitate orders seek benefits from procedures that decrease pain, provide vascular access, enable living at home or treat an urgent problems unrelated to the primary problem (e.g. fractures). Potential burdens from procedures may be due to either the resuscitation attempt or to function or cognitive decrements that may follow resuscitation.

The American Society of Anesthesiologists, the American Academy of Pediatrics and the American College of Surgeons recommend mandatory re-evaluation of the do-not-resuscitate order before going to the operating room [28–30].

Re-evaluating the order prior to surgery requires clarifying the goals for the procedure and end-of-life care through discussion with the patient, parents, and relevant clinicians such as surgeons and primary care physicians. Children should be involved in a developmentally appropriate manner. In practice, the re-evaluation of the do-not-resuscitate order for the perioperative period should result in either full resuscitation or a goal-directed approach toward perioperative resuscitation.

Discussions with the relevant decision makers should emphasize the differences between the operating room and the ward. Perioperative care permits a more personalized, real-time determination of whether resuscitation efforts would be consistent with the end-of-life goals. In the operating room, specific clinicians care for the patient for a defined period of time. Detailed knowledge of the goals for end-of-life care permits anesthesiologists and surgeons to tailor the extent of resuscitation to the likelihood of achieving those goals. In the dynamic surgical environment, the ability to respond flexibly, based on goals, is necessary to allow clinicians to thoughtfully enact limits on resuscitation. Additional information to give decision makers is listed in Box 1.2 [30].

Box 1.2 Components of the discussion to re-evaluate do-not-resuscitate orders for the perioperative period [29,30,32]

- Planned procedure and anticipated benefit to child
- Likelihood of requiring resuscitation
- Reversibility of likely causes that require resuscitation
- Description of potential interventions and their consequences
- Chances of successful resuscitation, including differences between outcomes to witnessed and unwitnessed arrests
- Ranges of outcomes with and without resuscitation
- Discussion of the response to iatrogenic events
- Intended and possible venues and types of postoperative care
- Postoperative timing and mechanisms for resuscitation and for re-evaluation of limitations on resuscitation
- Establishment of an agreement through a goal-directed approach or revocation of the DNR order for the perioperative period
- Documentation

Do-not-resuscitate directives that list acceptable interventions (e.g. tracheal intubation, chest compressions, etc.) are impractical in the operating room. Reaching an agreement can be difficult because of unclear distinctions between anesthetic practice and resuscitation [31]. Inflexible directives increase the chance that physicians will get "caught" in a technicality that is inconsistent with the patient's desires. For example, a restriction on tracheal intubation that is intended to limit a lengthy intensive care unit stay is not intended to refuse a presumably short-term tracheal intubation resulting from opioid-induced apnea during monitored anesthesia care. This "do what I mean, not what I say" dissonance leads to physicians using their reasonable beliefs to violate directives. But using a system that requires physicians to violate patient directives to fulfill patient wishes will eventually result in unnecessary and harmful violations. In addition, it inexorably weakens the perceived importance of following policies and directives.

Goal-directed approaches permit patients to guide therapy by prioritizing outcomes (e.g. "I don't want to suffer in the ICU for 2 weeks before I die"). After decision makers define goals, operating room physicians can use their clinical judgment to determine whether and to what extent resuscitation will help achieve these goals. The decision about whether to use a certain intervention, such as chest compressions, will likely be more consistent with the end-of-life goals if the decision is made when the etiology of the event is known. This model encourages the ethically redoubtable strategy of trialing therapies. A trial of chest compressions that do not achieve specific goals provides evidence that continuing the therapy would be inconsistent with the goals of end-of-life care. Witnessed arrests in the operating room often have a better outcome than unwitnessed arrests due to the more immediate intervention and the greater likelihood that the cause of the arrest is known [29,32]. For these reasons, decision makers may choose to modify their previous limits on resuscitation for the perioperative period.

From clinical experience, the vast majority of decision makers that choose to use a goal-directed approach authorize temporary therapeutic interventions to manage quickly and easily reversible events, but reject those interventions that will likely result in permanent sequelae, such as neurological impairment or dependence upon life-sustaining technology [29]. For example, a brief bradyarrhythmia that responds to intravenous epinephrine and chest compressions would be consistent with the authorization to treat events that are temporary, easily reversible and unlikely to have significant sequelae. On the other hand, if the bradyarrhythmia resulted in an extended resuscitation, continued therapy would require unacceptable burdens that in any case would be unlikely to achieve the patient's return to previous functional status. In that case, it would be appropriate to cease resuscitation efforts.

This common goal-directed preference can be documented as "The patient desires resuscitative efforts during surgery and in the PACU only if the adverse events are believed to be both temporary and reversible in the clinical judgment of the attending anesthesiologists and surgeons."

The goal-directed approach requires determining the appropriate extent of postoperative therapy. Patients may want a trial of therapy before concluding that the burden of continuing therapy outweighs the benefits. In pediatrics, precisely defining and documenting postoperative plans is often less essential, because parents are often available in the postoperative period to make decisions regarding therapy. Parents are often cognitively capable of participating in discussions of withdrawal of therapy because they have already grappled with analyzing the benefits and burdens of end-of-life care. The presence of parents permits greater trials of perioperative resuscitation while still respecting the decision to limit the burdens.

Barriers to honoring perioperative limitations on life-sustaining therapy

Barriers to honoring perioperative limitations on LST center on insufficient knowledge about policies, law, and ethics. Many anesthesiologists and surgeons still believe that do-not-resuscitate orders must be revoked when patients come to the operating room.

Others worry, wrongly, that honoring limitations on LST may result in being sued. Statutes that address requirements for do-not-resuscitate orders often include immunity provisions that protect physicians from liability [33]. Indeed, the risk of liability for honoring an appropriately documented do-not-resuscitate order is likely to be lower than the risk of not honoring it [33].

Perhaps a more subtle barrier to honoring these directives is the response of clinicians to iatrogenic events [34]. Some anesthesiologists will initiate resuscitation solely because the etiology was iatrogenic rather than the patient's disease [35-37]. But by instituting perioperative limitations on LST, decision makers have declared that their sole concern is the physical and mental status following the arrest [38]. Anesthesiologists should initiate and continue resuscitation based solely on achieving the patient's goals.

Attitudes affect end-of-life care [39-41]. Clinicians are more likely to honor a refusal of resuscitation for a palliative procedure than for an elective procedure [30]. Clinicians prioritize imminence of death when considering the appropriateness of a patient's desire to limit LST while patients, on the other hand, prioritize functional status when choosing to refuse LST [34]. This dissonance

affects the ability of clinicians to implement perioperative LST.

Concepts of inadvisable care and futility

Most of the confusion surrounding the concept of futility comes from imprecise terminology [42]. Futile therapy should be considered as treatments that cannot accomplish a specific, intended goal. In that sense, dilemmas about whether to use futile therapy rarely arise. Treatments with low likelihood of success, on the other hand, may be considered inadvisable because of the benefits and burdens of proceeding, but they cannot be considered futile. A treatment may be considered inadvisable because of burdens to the child, cost or uncertain benefit.

At the clinician level, discussions about inadvisable care center on the benefits and burdens to the child. Qualitative and quantitative considerations should be defined carefully and physicians should explain whether the information used to form the estimation is based upon intuition, clinical experience or rigorous and sufficiently relevant scientific studies. Complicating matters is the dubiety in predicting the likelihood and range of outcomes of therapeutic interventions in very young children. In the end, in the absence of national standards, *decision making for a child near the end of life should be based on the best interests of the child and not on cost.*

Hospitals should have established processes for resolving conflicts. However, the ethical underpinnings of conflict resolution prioritize parental preferences as determined by the President's Commission for the Study of Ethical Problems in Medicine and Biomedical and Behavioral Research (Table 1.2) [4]. Clinician preferences only supersede parental preferences if a therapy is clearly beneficial.

Table 1.2 Suggested grid for resolving disputes about appropriate care (modified) [4]

	Parents prefer to accept treatment	Parents prefer to forgo treatment
Physicians consider treatment clearly beneficial	Treat	Provide treatment during review process
Physicians consider treatment to be of ambiguous or uncertain benefit	Treat	Forgo
Physicians consider treatment to be inadvisable	Review	Forgo

Withdrawing mechanical ventilation therapy

The extent and type of sedation given when mechanical ventilation therapy is being withdrawn should be based on benefits and burdens. The benefits of administering sedation to minimize discomfort and suffering usually outweigh the burdens of an ever-diminishing likelihood of survival. Providing skillful withdrawal therapy is difficult and anesthesiologists should not assume that without training or experience they can provide high-quality end-of-life care [43–45]. Anesthesiologists should not use paralytic agents to hide patient movements during withdrawal of therapy [46]. Even though patient movements may upset parents, use of paralytic agents will hide the signs of distress that physicians use to titrate analgesia and sedations. Explaining this to family members may help them tolerate otherwise upsetting movements or event.

Other topics in pediatric anesthesiology

Research in pediatric patients

The anesthesiologist Henry K. Beecher was one of the first to recognize that research in pediatric patients requires greater oversight than research in adults [47]. Research subjects requiring surrogate consent are vulnerable to abuse. Pediatric research exposes children to unknown risks of long-term harm because research interventions occur during growth and development of the child.

The increased risk of harm and lack of direct benefit to the child increase the obligation to obtain the developmentally appropriate assent from the child. This obligation is not always met, particularly in diseases that have a strong emotional overlay, like cancer [48,49]. Assent may be waived if there is the prospect of direct benefit to the child that is available only through participation of research. Although undesirable, assent also may be waived if the study exposes the child to no more than minimal risks or if the study could not sensibly proceed without the waiver [50,51].

Federal guidelines define four categories of pediatric research (Box 1.3). The hallmark of these categories is that potential benefits must increase commensurate with potential risks. Most controversy about pediatric research relates to the interpretations of minimal risk and minor increase over minimal risk [52].

Minimal risk is defined as "the probability and magnitude of harm or discomfort anticipated in the research are not greater in and of themselves than those ordinarily encountered in daily life or during the performance of routine physical or psychological examinations or tests"

Box 1.3 Federal classifications for pediatric research [50]

Research not involving greater than minimal risk

(a) Institutional review board (IRB) determines minimal risk
(b) IRB finds and documents that adequate provisions are made for soliciting assent from children and permission from their parents or guardians

Research involving greater than minimal risk but presenting the prospect of direct benefit to the individual subject

(a) IRB justifies the risk by the anticipated benefit to the subjects
(b) The relation of the anticipated benefit to the risk is at least as favorable as that presented by available alternative approaches
(c) Adequate provisions for assent and permission

Research involving greater than minimal risk and no prospect of direct benefit to individual subjects, but likely to yield generalizable knowledge about the subject's disorder or condition

(a) IRB determines the risk represents a minor increase over minimal risk
(b) The intervention or procedure presents experiences to subjects that are reasonably commensurate with those inherent in their actual or expected medical, dental, psychological, social or educational situations
(c) The intervention or procedure is likely to yield generalizable knowledge, which is of vital importance for the understanding or amelioration of the subject's disorder or condition
(d) Adequate provisions for assent and permission

Research not otherwise approvable which presents an opportunity to understand, prevent or alleviate a serious problem affecting the health or welfare of children

---

[50,51]. The common interpretation is that minimal risk refers to risks encountered by healthy children, such a playing sports and riding in a car [53,54]. Some use a more relative interpretation, basing the standard of "daily life" on the events to which children enrolled in the research are routinely exposed. In other words, if a child enrolled in the study routinely receives lumbar punctures as part of therapy, then it may be acceptable to expose a child to the risk of a lumbar puncture for study purposes.

The category *"greater than minimal risk* and no prospect of direct benefit to individual subjects, but likely to yield generalizable knowledge about the subject's disorder or condition . . . which is of vital importance"* defines when it is acceptable to expose a child to a "minor increase over minimal risk" [50]. *"Minor increase over minimal risk"* has been interpreted as pain, discomfort or stress that is transient, reversible and not severe [53]. Risk assessment is based on the combined exposure to risks throughout the study and the relationship between the risks and the patient population. For example, although drawing blood in healthy 15 year olds may be considered acceptable, drawing blood from 15 year olds with severe autism spectrum disorder may be unacceptable because their inability to understand may cause intolerable stress [55].

"Condition" is used to mean characteristics "that an established body of scientific or clinical evidence has shown to negatively affect children's health and wellbeing or to increase the risk of developing a health problem in the future" [53,55]. For example, consider a protocol to assess insulin resistance in obese children who do not have type II diabetes. If the investigator presented sufficient scientific support to the institutional review board that obese children are at increased risk of developing diabetes because of their obesity, then those obese children would be acceptable research subjects for this study. Svelte children would not be acceptable, because they would not be considered at risk for developing diabetes [55].

Stringent regulations certainly hinder necessary and beneficial research [56,57]. But regulations are often responses to previous transgressions. At some point, relaxation of regulations will reanimate the abuses that beget the regulations. It is difficult to identify that line until it is crossed.

Improving the institutional review board process may minimize the inaccurate estimations of risk that hinders appropriate research and permits inappropriate research. An individual's intuition about the risk level of an activity is hampered by cognitive biases, such as familiarity, control of activity and reversibility of the potential harms [54]. Systematizing evaluation of research risks may reduce inaccurate estimations of risk. One approach is to use a standardized scale to categorize the extent and likelihood of each potential harm and then compare the potential harms with comparative activities [58].

Advocacy and good citizenship

Physicians owe their ability to train, practice and thrive to society's largesse. The implicit social contract therefore obligates physicians to manage matters within their sphere of influence, with a special obligation to address issues that "directly influence individuals' health" in the physician's community [59,60]. "Community" may refer to a physical location or a type of patient to whom the physician is particularly obligated. Pediatric anesthesiologists have a special obligation to further pediatric healthcare.

Pediatric anesthesiologists have actively taken up this obligation (Fig. 1.1). One of the more notable activities has been the development of specialty organizations, like the Society for Pediatric Anesthesia and the American Academy of Pediatrics Section on Anesthesiology and Pain Medicine. Organizing engages the wisdom and energy of like-minded individuals to identify concerns, define goals and implement solutions. For example, the pediatric anesthesiology fellowship programs advocated becoming an ACGME-accredited fellowship to ensure a standard for training programs for pediatric anesthesiologists [61].

Collaborative projects gather data about rare events to help determine ways to prevent them. The Pediatric Perioperative Cardiac Arrest Registry began in 1994 and has provided useful information in understanding the causes of pediatric cardiac arrest. Wake Up Safe is a similar registry designed to assess serious adverse events and recommend how they can be prevented. It is every anesthesiologist's obligation to participate in efforts like these.

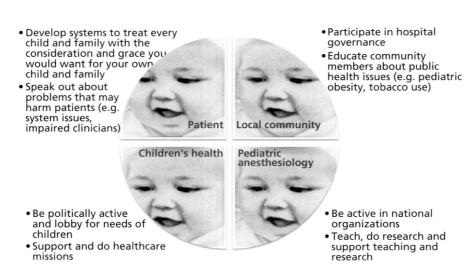

• Develop systems to treat every child and family with the consideration and grace you would want for your own child and family
• Speak out about problems that may harm patients (e.g. system issues, impaired clinicians)

Patient   Local community

•Participate in hospital governance
•Educate community members about public health issues (e.g. pediatric obesity, tobacco use)

Children's health   Pediatric anesthesiology

• Be politically active and lobby for needs of children
• Support and do healthcare missions

•Be active in national organizations
•Teach, do research and support teaching and research

Figure 1.1 Obligations of pediatric anesthesiologists. Pediatric anesthesiologists are obligated to these four communities. Individual anesthesiologists are not expected to fulfill every obligation. "Units" of anesthesiologists such as private practice groups, academic departments, and state societies should fulfill these obligations collectively. A few examples are given.

Physicians should fulfill obligations to society by participating in activities that are consistent with the individual's "expertise, interests and situations" [60]. For pediatric anesthesiologists, one appropriate approach would be to participate in the initiatives of relevant professional organizations. Anesthesiologists should consider addressing relevant public health issues such as pediatric obesity, pediatric tobacco use and second-hand smoke, and socio-economic disparities in healthcare and healthcare access [60,62–64].

Safety and quality care initiatives

Anesthesiologists have an obligation to foster patient safety. This obligation requires participation in surveillance data collection and compliance with policies intended to improve care, such as perioperative time-outs to ensure the right patient is receiving the right procedure [65,66]. Implementation of seemingly unnecessary policies often meets with resistance but it is difficult for individual physicians to appreciate the broad perspective from their individual perches. Anesthesiologists need to accept the limitations of their vantage point and willingly incorporate safety activities to further the common good. But they also should voice concerns through appropriate channels about poor or inadequate policies. Resorting to workarounds prevents policy remediation and encourages selective following of policies, which in turn causes more medical errors.

Apology and disclosure

Parents wish to be informed about medical errors that harm or may harm their children [67,68]. They also wish to receive appropriate apologies. Yet clinicians discount these clear desires. Barely half of pediatricians would disclose a serious error and fewer than a quarter would apologize for the same error [69]. Principles of respect of autonomy and truth-telling require physicians to be forthright about medical errors.

Most arguments against apology about and disclosure of errors center on increasing the risk of being successfully sued and on protecting the patient from unnecessary anxiety regarding the event or future care. Upon examination, these arguments are weak. An apology is an expression of regret or sorrow. A sincere apology followed by actions consistent with regret is invaluable; an insincere apology is costly. Even though more than half the states have laws prohibiting the admission of apology or sympathy as evidence of wrongdoing, it is conceivable that an apology may increase the risk of being sued or losing a suit [70]. But lore and literature indicate that the best protection against being sued is a good patient–doctor relationship [14]. Hiding, dissembling or being indifferent about an event will likely do more to galvanize a lawsuit and destroy trust than a sincere apology.

For example, some recommend apologizing for the effect on the patient but not to take responsibility for the actual event. This apology is appropriate for a rash caused by an appropriately administered antibiotic but it seems bizarre not to take responsibility when an anesthesiologist errantly injects a neuromuscular blocking agent instead of an anticholinesterase agent when attempting to antagonize muscle relaxation. Common sense suggests that not taking responsibility in that case (unless there was a good reason) would aggravate parents.

Thoughtful full disclosure should commence upon recognition of the problem [71,72]. Ethics aside, anesthesiologists should ignore the temptation to withhold disclosure. Parents will eventually learn what happened and will wonder, likely with animosity, why such information was withheld. Anesthesiologists should share what is known but should not make assumptions about what is not known, particularly about fault. Decision makers should be informed about the medical implications of the event and any necessary treatment. Because disclosure is a process over time, the patient and family should be given a contact person who will be available to answer questions, arrange meetings, explain the results of the investigation and describe the plan to prevent comparable events.

Parents are naturally sensitive about the perioperative experiences of their children. Anesthesiologists should consider apologizing or at least sympathizing about unpleasant experiences such as multiple, painful attempts to insert an intravenous catheter or an out-of-control inhalation induction of anesthesia. These discussions can include an acknowledgment that it was a bad experience and recommendations for the future. For example, an anesthesiologist could say, "I am sorry the intravenous catheter took so many sticks" and "Next time, we should probably give oral sedation prior to attempting the intravenous catheter." These comments simply acknowledge what happened, express regret and educate the family for the future.

Production pressure

Production pressure is the ubiquitous "internal or external pressure on the anesthetist to keep the operating room schedule moving along speedily" [73]. As a consequence, anesthesiologists may feel pressure to curtail preoperative discussions, inadvisably proceed with cases or prematurely extubate the trachea to speed turnover. Anesthesiologists should be aware of pressures to provide anesthesia inconsistent with their level of skill or to permit surgery in inappropriate settings. For example, the "routine" tonsillectomy for a child with achondroplastic dwarfism may be too complex for some anesthesiologists or some surgery centers. Anesthesiologists have an obligation to their patients and to themselves to only provide care for which they are competent and to recognize when economic and administrative pressures induce them to do otherwise.

Suspicion of child abuse

Physicians are legally obligated to report even the suspicion of child abuse [74,75]. It is natural to downplay concerns because of a hesitancy to inform authorities, particularly if the parents are from a socio-economic class similar to the physician's. But child abuse should never be minimized as a one-time event. Early intervention minimizes disastrous consequences.

Anesthesiologists may be the first to recognize child abuse because evidence of abuse frequently occurs on the arms, hands, head, face, neck, and mouth [76,77]. Signs of abuse include bruises or burns in shapes of objects, injuries that fit a biomechanical model (e.g. a handprint), fractures in infants and developmentally inappropriate injures that are not explained by the offered history. Anesthesiologists should be aware that child abuse might occur in the hospital during diagnostic or therapeutic care [78,79]. Munchausen by proxy is a type of abuse in which parents either cause or fictionalize clinical problems in their children [80]. The signs and symptoms of the resultant diseases are often difficult to explain coherently.

CASE STUDY

This case study is designed to emphasize that superficially defining cases such as "a 17 year old wants to refuse transfusion therapy" overlooks relevant complexities; to examine the process and relevant factors in determining maturity for medical decision making in an adolescent; to provide an example of how dilemmas may be evaluated; and to provide an example of the content in an ethics consultation. Characteristics of consultations include clarifying medical issues, identifying stakeholders and their relative extent of influence, defining the ethical questions and issues, and providing an assessment and recommendation.

Summary

Seventeen-year-old Candace has a rare type of rhabdomyosarcoma. She presents for resection of a tumor intertwined with major blood vessels. Candace is a Jehovah's Witness and wants to refuse transfusion therapy during and after the resection of the tumor.

Medical questions

This type of rhabdomyosarcoma is too rare to be able to reliably predict outcome. The best guess, though, is a 5-year survival of 5–10%. While there is a low likelihood of significant bleeding during the operation, the position of major blood vessels presents the possibility of sudden, rapid and substantial bleeding.

Family

Candace is the daughter of Linda and Larry. Through a friend, Larry began exploring the Jehovah's Witness community 9 years ago and became baptized as a Jehovah's Witness 6 years ago. Linda describes herself as spiritual but has no interest in organized religion. She very much supports the authority of Candace's decision making.

Candace "was very skeptical the first month of learning about [the Jehovah's Witness religion]. I had friends who had 'found' religion . . . but it never made sense to me." Jehovah's Witness "made sense to me, in an easy to understand manner. This is it, this is the right religion." Following thorough study, at age 14 she chose to become a baptized member to show her dedication to being a Jehovah's Witness.

Candace leads an active high school life. She is a starting wing on the field hockey team and she frequently participates in school theater productions. She leads bible study and weekly youth group meetings. She is an accomplished public speaker, speaking to groups "over 100 people" about being a Jehovah's Witness.

Linda and Larry like the person Candace has become. Candace, Linda and Larry share decision making about family matters. They have the normal disputes about things like curfew.

Candace is an active participant in her care. She asks appropriate and extensive questions about options and short- and long-term implications.

In private discussions with Candace, she emphasized that she did not want to die. However, because she believes that Bible and God forbid taking blood, receiving blood would fill her with incredible guilt and sadness because she had disappointed her God. While she was concerned that taking blood would separate her from God, her primary concern was the overwhelming sense of failing her God. When asked whether being transfused forcibly or while unconscious would ease her conscience, she answered that she would feel the same because she had actively put herself in a position in which she could involuntarily receive blood. She equated being transfused forcibly while unconscious as "rape." She stated in a factual and calm way that "if I woke up and found I was getting blood, I would rip it out of my arm."

Candace coherently articulates her religious and spiritual faith. Her beliefs are consistent with the teachings of her chosen faith community. She views herself as able to reason and be responsible for acting on personal moral judgments. She can imagine separating from the Jehovah's Witness community if so guided by her conscience.

Ethical questions

1. If individuals of majority age have the right to refuse potentially life-sustaining transfusion therapy, do minors have this right?
2. What characteristics and criteria can be used to determine whether a minor possesses sufficient decision-making capacity and maturity to make this decision?
3. What issues should be discussed to ensure that their desired blood therapy wishes be followed?

Maturing adolescents are granted increasing authority in decision making. Relevant characteristics that give evidence of adolescent maturity and decision-making capacity include an understanding of their options and associated consequences, an internally coherent rationale, an ability to articulate their positions, an intellectual and emotional freedom to entertain alternative perspectives, and an indication of mature relationships with older individuals. Not all characteristics need to be present for an adolescent to be considered mature. The threshold for the evidence necessary to have decision-making capacity for a specific decision increases as the consequences of the decision increase.

The case of Phillip Malcolm describes a child without decision-making capacity. Phillip and his parents were not permitted to refuse transfusion when the almost 18-year-old Phillip was acutely diagnosed with severe anemia and cancer [81]. Transfusions were recommended to stabilize his clinical status. The court learned that although the family had joined the religion 3 years earlier, Phillip did not become interested until 1 year ago. Phillip understood the "basic tenet of the religion's prohibition regarding blood transfusions" but had rudimentary knowledge about the Bible. He did not consider it a sin if the court ordered a transfusion. Phillip had not shown independent or shared decision making in his relationship with his parents.

Legitimate concerns about adolescents being overly influenced by short-term consequences should not be tainted by less relevant concerns that preferences may change as adolescents become older. Mature individuals are able to change their minds based on experience and

evidence. That adolescents may change their mind as they mature does not invalidate current choices inasmuch as sufficient decision-making capacity is present.

Pragmatism affects considerations about whether to force adolescents to receive undesired healthcare. Adolescents are most capable of physical protest, either by yanking intravenous catheters or by not presenting for therapy. For example, Billy Best, a 16 year old with Hodgkin lymphoma, ran away so that he would not have to complete his chemotherapy regimen [9]. On the other hand, following an accident, 16-year-old Greg Novak was thought to urgently require transfusion therapy [82]. Being Jehovah's Witnesses, Novak and his parents refused transfusion therapy. However, a court-appointed guardian requested transfusion therapy. Novak was physically restrained and transfused.

Assessment

The advisory committee believes that Candace meets the requirements of being a mature individual with substantial decision-making capacity who understands the gravity of her choice. Her active participation outside the Jehovah's Witness community indicates a wider view of the world rather than a more narrow view that may be present with exposure only to the Jehovah's Witness community. Given her beliefs and her extensive missionary and teaching activities, we believe that she has thoughtfully chosen to become a Jehovah's Witness. She has a loving and comprehensive relationship with her parents. Although her refusal of potentially life-sustaining therapy may lead to significant morbidity or death, we believe she exceeds the criteria to make these decisions.

Recommendations

1. The committee believes that Candace should be considered primary decision maker.
2. We are aware that the surgeon requests a court order permitting Candace to be able to consent for refusal of potentially life-sustaining transfusion therapy. We encourage Candace and her family to seek as much information about this process as possible, including the process of seeking this status, the possible drawback of pursuing and securing mature minor status, the role of the parents after achieving this status and the use of healthcare proxies. A court order may minimize chances that wayward individuals may transfuse Candace.
3. To ensure fidelity in regard to the hospital's implicit promise to honor her preferences, a cadre of clinicians committed to honoring Candace's wishes must be identified. Necessary clinicians include operating room nurses and technicians, anesthesiologists, trainee

Continued

anesthesiologists and surgeons, and postoperative nurses and physicians, particularly ICU physicians. Arrangements must be made to ensure willing clinicians in case of an emergency reoperation. The needs of these clinicians (e.g. to meet Candace) should be met.

4. This consultation is solely advisory. Our comments are restricted to the ethical interpretation of the issues facing Candace, her family and the care team. You may wish to contact the Office of Legal Counsel for their input on existing regulations as well.

Postscript. A court order granted Candace the authority to make decisions about transfusion therapy. In informal conversation later, the judge declared that one of his primary considerations aside from Candace's maturity was the very low likelihood of survival. If her possible survival had been higher, he would have been much less likely to grant her the legal authority to make decisions about transfusion therapy.

Annotated references

A full reference list for this chapter is available at:
http://www.wiley.com/go/gregory/andropoulos/pediatricanesthesia

7. Committee on Bioethics, American Academy of Pediatrics. Informed consent, parental permission, and assent in pediatric practice. Pediatrics 1995; 95: 314–17. This article is the fundamental explanation of informed consent for children. Pay particular attention to the introduction, in which Dr William Bartholome (in absentia) exhorts clinicians to respect "the experience, perspective and power of children."

9. Will JF. My God my choice: the mature minor doctrine and adolescent refusal of life-saving or sustaining medical treatment based upon religious beliefs. J Contemp Health Law Policy 2006; 22: 233–300. This article provides a thorough explanation of the ethical and legal subtleties of mature minors.

27. Committee on Bioethics, American Academy of Pediatrics. Guidelines on forgoing life-sustaining medical treatment. Pediatrics 1994; 93: 532–6. This article gives a clear explanation of what constitutes benefits and burdens in children.

30. Fallat ME, Deshpande JK. Do-not-resuscitate orders for pediatric patients who require anesthesia and surgery. Pediatrics 2004; 114: 1686–92. This article is a complete explanation of perioperative do-not-resuscitate orders for children.

42. Consensus Statement of the Society of Critical Care Medicine's Ethics Committee regarding futile and other possibly inadvisable treatments. Crit Care Med 1997; 25: 887–91. This article explicates the

importance of recognizing the ethical and clinical differences between futile treatment and other inadvisable treatments and expands on the classifications used in this chapter.

59. Waisel DB. Nonpatient care obligations of anesthesiologists. Anesthesiology 1999; 91: 1152–8. This article describes the obligations of anesthesiologists to the specialty of anesthesiology and to society. The origin of the obligations, how to fulfill them and the consequences of not fulfilling them are reviewed.

60. Gruen RL, Pearson SD, Brennan TA. Physician-citizens – public roles and professional obligations. JAMA 2004; 291: 94–8. This article provides a thoughtful perspective on the obligations of physicians.

61. Rockoff MA, Hall SC. Subspecialty training in pediatric anesthesiology: what does it mean? Anesth Analg 1997; 85: 1185–90. This article explains the reasoning underlying the formalizing of specialty training in pediatric anesthesiology. The reasoning exemplifies the touchstone that should be at the forefront of policy decisions about peditric medicine: to benefit children.

83. Greene NM. Familiarity as a basis for the practice of anesthesiology. Anesthesiology 1976; 44: 101–3. A précis of the patient care obligations of anesthesiologists. Greene disdains "do-what-you-are-familiar-with" anesthesia and declares that the complete anesthesiologist "orchestrates and selects anesthetic drugs and procedures to assure that each of his . . . patients recives the best that modern anesthesia has to offer."

84. Kon AA. Answering the question: "Doctor, if this were your child, what would you do?" Pediatrics 2006; 118: 393–7. This article helps anesthesiologists understand and answer this frequent and deceptively simple question.

CHAPTER 2
History of Pediatric Anesthesia

Burdett S. Dunbar & Dean B. Andropoulos

Department of Anesthesiology and Pediatrics, Baylor College of Medicine, and Texas Children's Hospital, Houston, TX, USA

Introduction

Any examination of the history of pediatric anesthesiology requires considering the general history of the specialty of anesthesiology as well as the contexts in which changes in the specialty have occurred over time. We shall review the relatively short time over which today's widely recognized subspecialty began, grew and matured, mostly within the past 60 years. Early pediatric anesthesiology practitioners, some still living today, will be noted. These can fairly be termed pioneers or foundation makers. It is also necessary to describe the close interplay between pediatric anesthesiology practitioners and their colleagues in general and cardiovascular surgery, neonatology, critical care medicine and pain medicine. Although short by most historical standards, the specialty's history is rich in achievement, whether one considers the beginnings from the 1840s to the 1940s, the acceleration of growth from about 1950 to 1990, or the maturation of our specialty into its current status. We continue to expect further accomplishments in children's healthcare in the 21st century.

The first 100 years

Inhalation of ether marked the initiation of modern anesthesia. The person who gave the first anesthetic is no longer in doubt; it was Dr Crawford Long (Fig. 2.1) in Jefferson, Georgia, in 1842. His report of his activities was delayed until 1849 [1]. Thus, the dentist William T.G. Morton (Fig. 2.2) is recognized as the first to publicly demonstrate ether anesthesia in Boston in October, 1846 [2]. The published report of this success, by the Boston physician Henry J. Bigelow, spread around the world both in knowledge and practice in less than 1 year [3].

Inhalation anesthesia in children began with Dr Long whose third patient in 1842 was an 8-year-old boy who underwent a toe amputation; this is reported in his 1849 publication. In London, John Snow (Fig. 2.3), now recognized as a founder of the specialty of anesthesiology, reported on inhalation anesthesia in both adults and children and marked the changes from ether inhalation to chloroform inhalation. He reported in 1857 a series of over 100 children less than 1 year of age. It is to Dr Snow that we owe the recorded observation that onset and

---

Gregory's Pediatric Anesthesia, Fifth Edition. Edited by George A. Gregory, Dean B. Andropoulos.
© 2012 Blackwell Publishing Ltd. Published 2012 by Blackwell Publishing Ltd.

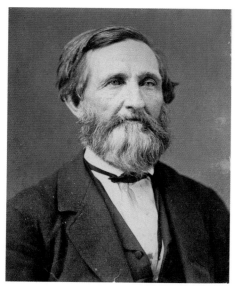

Figure 2.1 Crawford W. Long MD. Reproduced with permission from Crawford T. Long Museum, Jefferson, GA, USA.

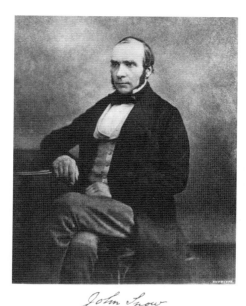

John Snow

Figure 2.3 John Snow. Reproduced with permission from US National Library of Medicine, Bethesda, MD, USA.

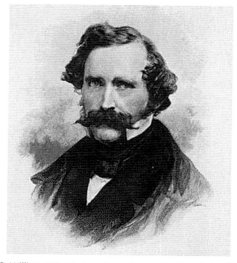

Figure 2.2 William T.G. Morton. Reproduced with permission from US National Library of Medicine, Bethesda, MD, USA.

effect of inhaled anesthetics, in this case chloroform, occurred "more quickly" in infants and children than adults [4].

For the next 100 years it appears that large numbers of children were anesthetized successfully by both inhalation and regional techniques [5]. Chloroform inhalation, especially in unskilled hands, proved dangerous, even deadly. Its use, especially in the United States, was largely replaced by diethyl ether, commonly "ether." It was usually given by the "open drop" method, where the liquid ether was poured (dripped) onto a mask device

covered in gauze mesh, which covered the patient's nose and mouth, so the patient's breathing vaporized the ether.

It required 75–80 years before sufficient technology developed to produce more accurate flow meters and more reliable vaporizers, making possible the shift from open drop to more sophisticated inhalation techniques.

Children in this era were treated like small adults. An evolutionary change in this attitude occurred only as the subspecialty of pediatric surgery began to develop in the late 1930s into the 1940s.

Surgery and anesthesiology for children

Major advances in surgery for children developed in the hands of only a few, but one surgeon, William E. Ladd MD, at Boston Children's, can fairly be said to have laid the foundation for the development of pediatric surgery [6]. His work as a teacher and clinician was carried on by Robert M. Gross MD who first ligated a patent ductus arteriosus in 1939 [7]. While a signal accomplishment, the legacy of Ladd and Gross is probably best defined by the many surgeons whom they trained. This next generation had skills and ambitions which coupled well with developing skills of pediatricians to advance the surgical care of infants and children. This progress compelled further refinement in the techniques and skill needed by anesthesiologists.

The 1940s and 1950s

In the decade before World War II, fundamental changes occurred which accelerated and matured in the decade after the end of the war. The most important major step was the establishment of the first academic anesthesia department at the University of Wisconsin under Ralph Waters. Waters-trained anesthesiologists became the leaders of the specialty in the 1950s, 1960s, and 1970s. The emphases in Waters' program were on clinical excellence, research, and education, a tradition carried on today among the "second and third generation" of Waters-influenced leaders. Waters himself published his early experiences with a forerunner of outpatient anesthesia in his downtown anesthesia clinic [8]. He also contributed a device which allowed exhaled CO_2 adsorption by soda lime so that cyclopropane, a common anesthetic gas used well into the 1960s and 1970s, could be administered by to-and-fro breathing [9]. Although a now archaic method, the Waters canister added portability, reliability and utility for surgery lasting more than an hour. Its size was easily scaled down for pediatric practice and it was widely used through the 1960s.

Few anesthesiologists devoted themselves solely to pediatric practice prior to the 1950s [10]. In North America, Charles Robson (Fig. 2.4) at Toronto Sick Children's Hospital, starting in 1919, and in London, Robert Cope (Fig. 2.5) at the Hospital for Sick Children, Great Ormond Street (appointed 1937), were recognized pediatric anesthesiologists prior to World War II. These practitioners and their few trainees added clinical experience to the emergence of new knowledge about children's physiology and pathology, providing the basis for finally defining that infants and children were not small adults.

Dr M. Digby Leigh (Fig. 2.6), who trained with Waters before World War II, became the anaesthetist-in-chief at Montreal Children's Hospital in 1940. In 1947, he published, with his associate Kay Belton, the English language text *Paediatric Anaesthesiology*, a first [11]. Dr Leigh moved to Vancouver in 1947 and organized the University Department of Anesthesia from the existing clinical departments at Vancouver General Hospital and the Infants' and Children's Hospitals. In 1954, he became

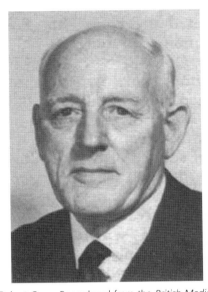

Figure 2.5 Robert Cope. Reproduced from the *British Medical Journal*, Obituaries: RW Cope, 15 May 1976, p.1223 with permission from BMJ Publishing Group Ltd.

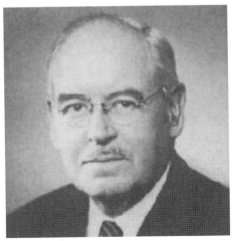

Figure 2.4 Charles Robson. Reproduced from Conn AW. History of Canadian anaesthesia: Dr. C.H. Robson (1884–1969). Can J Anaesth 1990; 37: 579 with permission from Springer.

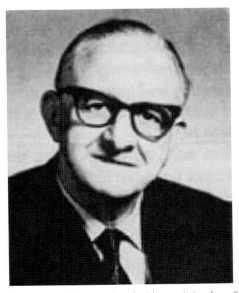

Figure 2.6 M. Digby Leigh. Reproduced with permission from Springer.

Director of Anesthesia at the Children's Hospital Los Angeles, and Professor of Anesthesiology at the University of Southern California. Dr Leigh continued for another two decades to be an outspoken teacher as well as an advocate for children, until his retirement in 1970. His contributions included descriptions of the use of spinal anesthesia in children, a low dead space, non-rebreathing valve and a scaled-down CO_2 absorber circle system, endotracheal anesthesia with avertin for cleft palate surgery, and bradycardia following succinylcholine in children. The annual teaching conference devoted to pediatric anesthesia at the Children's Hospital Los Angeles began under Dr Leigh's direction, and continues to this day.

The importance of Leigh's and colleagues' contributions, which established, maintained and taught high standards of anesthesia care for children, cannot be over-stated. They resulted in significant early advances in the US, United Kingdom and Canada in the care of children undergoing surgery in the late 1940s, especially in the areas of airway care and respiratory physiology.

Another important evolution occurred in pediatric surgery: the earlier and better recognition of the complementary role required between anesthesiologists and surgeons. This mutual co-operation was essential to overcome the many and often previously unrecognized technical problems arising as surgical skills advanced and anesthetic techniques and agents improved. As events moved into the 1950s, the stage was set for explosive growth and change.

World War II (1941–1945 for the US) provided young physicians – both surgeons and anesthesiologists – with experience under widely varying conditions, but nearly all practiced with the growing confidence that technical hurdles could be overcome with skill and even daring. As this cadre of physicians returned to civilian practice, many sought further specialty training. These men, and almost all were men at the time, became the staff members of departments of surgery and anesthesiology in the 1960s and 1970s. Surgeons led by Ladd, Gross, and C. Everett Koop tackled increasingly complex pediatric problems requiring surgery. Robert M. Smith at Boston Children's (Fig. 2.7), Robert McQuiston at Chicago Children's and Herbert Rackow at Columbia in New York City began work in postwar departments which advanced training and practice in pediatric anesthesiology [12–15]. G. Jackson-Rees in Liverpool, England, developed the techniques of endotracheal nitrous oxide-oxygen inhalation with muscle relaxants (Liverpool technique), which Rees felt was especially useful in sick children and neonates [16]. Jackson-Rees modified a T-tube non-breathing system originally devised by Ayre for use with an endotracheal tube in cleft palate repair [17] (Fig. 2.8). Versions of the Jackson-Rees system are in use today. The

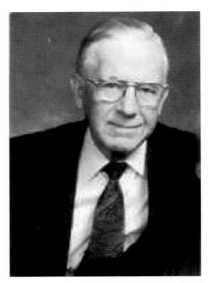

Figure 2.7 Robert M. Smith. Reproduced with permission from Children's Hospital, Boston, MA, USA.

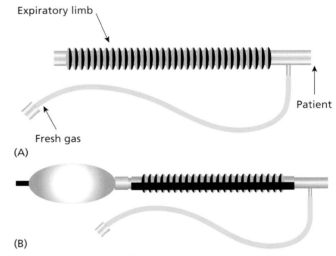

Figure 2.8 (A) Operation of the Ayre's T-piece. During inspiration, the patient inspires fresh gas from the reservoir tube. During expiration, the patient expires into the reservoir tube. Although fresh gas is still flowing into the system at this time, it is wasted because it is contaminated by expired gas. In the expiratory pause, fresh gas washes the expired gas out of the reservoir tube, filling it with fresh gas for the next inspiration. In the reservoir tube, the volume must be greater than the patient's tidal volume, otherwise the inspired gas will be contaminated by the surrounding air. (B) Jackson-Rees modification of the Ayre's T-piece. Reproduced with permission from Ayre's T-Piece: Anesthesia Service and Equipment. http://asevet.com/resources/circuits/ayres.htm.

Ayre's T-piece and Jackson-Rees systems are valveless non-rebreathing systems (NRBS). Another, valved NRBS, much less frequently used today, also arose during this period: the Mapleson systems, in A-D versions, well recalled and equally loathed by several generations of candidates attempting to pass their American Board of Anesthesiology certifying exams [18].

The results of these early successful attempts to better control airway management and ventilation improved surgical outcomes further, raising expectations and demands for more anesthesiologists to continue or expand this level of care. Related evolutions in blood banking, fluid administration, thermal homeostasis and circulatory control or support all advanced interdependently with advances in surgical and anesthesia care. Examples of congenital problems successfully approached in this era include congenital heart disease, congenital diaphragmatic hernia (CDH) and problems in patients' developing gut, such as omphalocele, malrotation, and pyloric stenosis. The separation of conjoined twins began in this era as advancing techniques in diagnostic imaging became more accurate. It is further testament to the improved care of these infants that they are no longer brought to the operating room *in extremis* for urgent surgical correction.

Mortality remained high for these patients into the 1990s but with the application of extracorporeal membrane oxygenation (ECMO) to patients with CDH, mortality overall has been reduced in the last decade. However, problems, often severe, remain related to underdeveloped lung tissue on the herniated side. Anesthesia care for the patient with congenital heart defects has become a specialty of its own, with ever more complex procedures carried out on sicker and younger infants, with the expectation that mortality will remain low. It is beyond the scope of this chapter to address the progress that continues to be made in solving complex problems in this group of patients. However, early attempts at cardiac surgery by surgeons such as Blalock in Baltimore required skilled anesthesia care. This new era required thinking about circumstances that had never occurred before. Despite this, reports like those of Harmel on the care of patients undergoing repair of congenital pulmonary stenosis noted generally favorable outcomes under primitive conditions [19].

Pediatric anesthesiology, firmly established in the 1960s, continued to lead the field of general anesthesiology in the areas of monitoring vital function, airway control, sedation, and pain management. Equipment modification by manufacturers increased as large numbers of children required anesthesia care. Hand-fashioning basic equipment such as blood pressure cuffs as described by Dr Smith and others before him became a thing of the past [20]. It is worth noting that in many instances, the equipment modifications were often done by nurse anesthetists in the eras before 1960. Tracheal intubation, the indications and need for which continued to be argued into the late 1960s, became commonplace and a standard of care in infants and children [21]. Care of the wounded during the Vietnam conflict along with the development of non-reactive plastic polymers for producing endotracheal tubes finally laid the arguments pro and con to rest, although problems with prolonged intubation were recognized in the mid-1960s [22]. Postintubation hoarseness ("croup"), a concern during the use of red rubber tubes, became less so with plastic tubes and is a rarity now. Pediatric precordial stethoscopy has been a hallmark of monitoring in anesthesia care since the 1950s, supplanted only in the last decade with the current monitoring applied to children, especially pulse oximetry.

Thermal homeostasis, with warm rooms, overheated surgeons, warm humidified respiratory gases and limb and head wraps, began in the 1950s; with the advent of forced warm air circulating blankets, temperature control is now much easier but remains a hallmark of quality patient care. The use of controlled hypothermia in cardiac surgery has a history of its own, beginning with McQuiston's report of its use in 1949 to reduce oxygen consumption [14].

Unique contributions to pediatric anesthesia, neonatal, and intensive care: 1950s to 1970

The introduction of halothane

As new agents were introduced to practice, especially halothane in 1958, a new era emerged which permitted better control of perioperative conditions by the anesthesiologist [23]. Flammable agents were abandoned by the 1970s. Electrocautery became a primary mode for hemostasis, driving down past dangers of exsanguination in such conditions as the excision of sacrococcygeal teratoma.

Premedication

Premedication of the anxious child prior to the 1980s involved diverse agents and combinations of drugs administered by a variety of routes, which had a mixed history of consistent success in smoothing the transition from parents' arms to the operating room. Bachman and colleagues in Philadelphia advocated the use of a parenteral combination of pentobarbital, morphine and scopolamine to circumvent preoperative anxiety and its consequence: the screaming, agitated child [24]. Work published with his colleague, Freeman, followed earlier work by Eckenhoff in documenting regression of behavior postoperatively in the unpremedicated child [25]. Those early experiences, even though with a markedly different inhalation agent from those used now, seem to continue to resonate with current experience about the preoperatively agitated child.

Neonatal and pediatric intensive care

The perioperative experience modified and supported by the practices of pediatric anesthesiologists built on experiences in these major areas: fluid requirements, antibiotic use, oxygen regulation and airway humidification. The era of polio epidemics in the 1950s showed the need for effective ventilation and respiratory care. The demonstrated effectiveness of continuing the airway control techniques from the operating room into the then new postanesthesia care unit illustrated the need to co-ordinate anesthesia practice methods, medications, and equipment beyond the operating room [26]. The growth of specialty practice pediatricians' ability to care for ill newborns, especially those with respiratory distress syndromes (RDS), produced neonatologists and the neonatal care unit, with early emphasis on respiratory support using intubation, oxygen supplementation and subsequently endotracheal ventilatory support. These efforts progressed into the late 1960s. Among the leaders were pediatric anesthesiologists Alan Conn in Toronto and Bachman and Downes in Philadelphia [27,28]. Gregory in San Francisco established early that continuous positive airway pressure (CPAP) was effective in improving survival in infants with RDS [29]. The stage was set for the rapid evolution of intensive care units.

First established in 1955 by Feychtung in Sweden, multidisciplinary pediatric intensive units were opened in Liverpool and Melbourne between 1960 and 1964. John Downes established the first North American unit in 1967 at the Children's Hospital of Philadelphia, and in the following 4 years, such units were established in Pittsburg, New Haven, Boston (Massachusetts General Hospital), and Toronto [30].

Diverse contributions from fields outside pediatrics greatly influenced and improved care of critically ill pediatric patients. In the 1950s and 1960s, the development of transistors and integrated circuits permitted large improvements in miniaturization of equipment, and the development of ventilators with complex cycles to better support ventilation. Primary pediatric ventilator computers allowed real-time monitoring and trend analysis with ever more compact equipment. The development of nonreactive extrudable plastic polymers produced better tracheal tubes and more effective and smaller means for vascular access equipment.

Virginia Apgar: the Apgar score

Virginia Apgar (Fig. 2.9) was a pediatric and obstetric anesthesiologist at Columbia University in New York City, trained under the auspices of Ralph Waters in Wisconsin and Emery Rovenstein at Bellevue Hospital. Using the skills of astute clinical observation so common in the pioneers of that era, she devised the famous Apgar score to assess the circulatory and respiratory status of

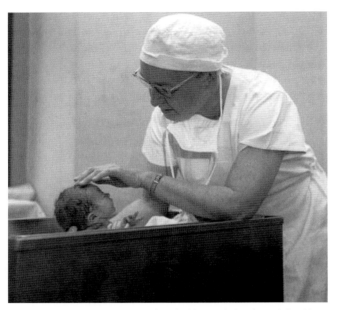

Figure 2.9 Virginia Apgar. Reproduced with permission from Columbia University Library. http://library.cpmc.columbia.edu/hsl/archives/HSTimeline.html, accessed August 8, 2010.

the newborn infant, which is universally utilized today throughout the world and has improved the assessment, research, and care of neonates ever since. It is appropriate that her first report of the Apgar score was published in the journal *Anesthesia & Analgesia* [31].

Box 2.1 summarizes some of the major developments in pediatric anesthesiology from 1842 until the late 1960s.

The modern history of pediatric anesthesia: major pediatric anesthesia research and clinical advances, late 1960s to 2010

Since the late 1960s there have been a number of seminal contributions by pediatric anesthesiologists that have greatly advanced our knowledge of the pathophysiology of conditions encountered in pediatric anesthesiology, surgery, and intensive care and significantly improved the outcomes and experiences for patients. These achievements further spurred the development of the subspecialty of pediatric anesthesia and define the modern history of the field. Several of the important advances are detailed in this section.

Malignant hyperthermia

The familiar story of the 21-year-old young man with the tibial and fibula fracture who underwent halothane anesthesia in 1960 in Melbourne, Australia, and had the first recognized case of malignant hyperthermia (MH) led

Box 2.1 Major developments in pediatric anesthesia, 1842–late 1960s

- First description of general anesthesia in a child by Long (1842)
- Snow's series of general anesthesia: over 100 infants less than 1 year (1857)
- Robson becomes Chief of Pediatric Anesthesia at Toronto Sick Children's Hospital (1919)
- Ayre's T-piece developed (1938)
- Harmel and Lamont's first description of anesthesia for congenital heart disease (1946)
- Smith appointed director of anesthesia at Children's Hospital Boston (1946)
- Leigh and Belton publish first textbook of pediatric anesthesia (1947)
- Apgar devises and publishes newborn resuscitation score (1953)
- Jackson-Rees produces his modification of the Ayre's T-piece, studies curare and develops the Liverpool technique of controlled endotracheal ventilation with muscle relaxation for surgical anesthesia (1950–55)
- Keats' descriptions of anesthesia for open heart surgery in infants (1955–60)
- Denborough's description of malignant hyperthermia (1960)
- Establishment of multidisciplinary pediatric intensive care units (1955–67)

to the recognition by 1970 of a number of additional cases, and a realization that children under the age of 18 comprised the majority of patients [32]. In the ensuing 40 years, the work of anesthesiologists, both pediatric and adult, as well as basic scientists and geneticists has made major advances in discovering the etiology, triggering agents, prevention, testing, and treatment of this disease.

The discovery that all potent halogenated inhalation agents and succinylcholine are triggering agents has allowed anesthesiologists to avoid these drugs. The widely published clinical descriptions, case series, and grading scales have increased early recognition of this disorder, and the discovery that dantrolene treatment can control the hypermetabolic state has greatly reduced the mortality of an MH episode. The advent of the halothane-caffeine contracture test to help determine susceptibility, and the genetic mutation of the ryanodine receptor on chromosome 19 present in some MH patients, has greatly improved identification of susceptible patients [33]. All these advances have decreased the rate of an MH episode with general anesthesia from approximately 1:5000 anesthetics in the 1970s to 1:100,000 today. In addition, when an MH episode does occur, the mortality rate has decreased from 70% to 5% or less. The MH success story is an excellent example of anesthesiologists recognizing a significant problem and, through basic, translational, and clinical research, transforming this disease into one that is manageable.

Postanesthetic apnea

With the advent of neonatal intensive care in the 1960s and 1970s, more premature infants required anesthesia and surgery. The special set of problems occurring in this fragile group of patients soon became evident. In 1981, Gregory reported that 25% of preterm infants had apnea after general anesthesia [34]. In 1982, Steward reported that six of 33 premature infants experienced apnea [35] and in 1983, Liu et al, in the first prospective study of 41 premature and 173 full-term infants, reported that six of the premature infants had postanesthetic apnea [36]. These reports resulted in widespread awareness of the problem, and in yet larger clinical studies that defined a risk profile, including anemia, pre-existing apnea, younger gestational age at birth and during anesthesia, and use of IV sedation during regional anesthesia. The resulting improvement in perioperative outcomes in premature infants has been significant, and the change in anesthetic practice to avoid elective anesthetics in vulnerable patients, and to institute postoperative cardiorespiratory monitoring in those who must undergo anesthesia, has prevented a large number of adverse events in these patients.

High-dose fentanyl for neonatal anesthesia

Another problem that became evident with the advent of neonatal intensive care was the patent ductus arteriosus (PDA) in the premature infant, which would lead to congestive heart failure, pulmonary edema, and respiratory insufficiency. Once again, pediatric anesthesiologists had a major role in the recognition of this condition and its treatment. The neonatal intensive care physicians at the University of California in San Francisco, including Gregory, were the first to publish a series of patients with this condition, including diagnosis and surgical treatment [37]. However, it was evident in those early days that even with successful surgical closure, these premature infants had a high mortality rate postoperatively, with nine of 21 dying of respiratory insufficiency or bowel ischemia. Of the 21 infants, 10 received halothane, nine fluroxene, and two ketamine. Other anesthetic regimens in use at that time for PDA ligation included N_2O, oxygen, and d-tubocurarine.

Responding to the concerns over hemodynamic instability from halothane or insufficient anesthesia when only N_2O was used, Robinson and Gregory published a series of 10 premature infant PDA ligations using 30–50 μg/kg of fentanyl as the anesthetic [38]. This anesthetic prevented an increase in systolic blood pressure and heart rate in response to incision and provided excellent hemodynamic stability. This publication ushered in the era of high-dose opioid anesthesia for unstable premature and full-term neonates, exemplified by the pioneering work of Anand and Aynsley-Green who demonstrated with a controlled study design that the addition of fentanyl to nitrous oxide anesthesia dramatically reduced the hormonal stress response in premature neonates undergoing PDA ligation [39]. This was followed by a controlled trial of halothane-morphine versus high-dose sufentanil in full-term neonates undergoing complex cardiac surgery with cardiopulmonary bypass, demonstrating a similar reduction in stress response, and a significantly lower mortality, with opioids [40]. These contributions permanently changed the practice of neonatal anesthesia.

Age and anesthetic requirement

Halothane became available in 1958 and as the advantages of this agent were evident, including minimal pungency and airway irritation, allowing for a smooth inhalation induction in children, there were reports that young children required higher inspired halothane concentrations for induction and maintenance of anesthesia. In 1969, Gregory, Eger, and Munson published their landmark paper entitled "The relationship between age and halothane requirement in man" and for the first time there were data substantiating the clinical impression that young children did require more anesthesia, and an objective measure, the minimum alveolar concentration (MAC), was used to demonstrate this [41]. (That the elderly required less anesthetic was also reported in this paper.) This model became the framework for the more detailed and precise study of later anesthetic gases including isoflurane, desflurane, and sevoflurane, including specific studies of the full-term neonate less than 30 days and also the premature infant [42]. The important knowledge that different agents behave differently, and that the premature infant requires dramatically reduced concentrations of the halogenated agents, arose out of these early data, generated by a pediatric anesthesiologist who was an expert clinician, precise observer, and clinical scientist who devised rigorous studies to answer this important clinical question.

Latex allergy

In the late 1980s case reports and case series began to appear describing severe anaphylactic reactions, some fatal, apparently in patients sensitized to natural latex proteins from surgical gloves and other medical devices and equipment [43]. Many of these were pediatric or young adult patients with a history of multiple surgical procedures during childhood, with procedures such as myelomeningocele repair or other surgeries where a mucosal surface had prolonged exposure to the surgeon's gloves. By the early to mid 1990s there was widespread recognition of this problem and through the efforts of

many pediatric anesthesiologists, allergist-immunologists, and others, the at-risk patient population was better defined, skin and serum testing was developed and validated, and protocols for pretreatment and for the provision of latex-free environments for at-risk patients were developed [44]. With advocacy by pediatric anesthesiologists, patient groups, and others, latex products were gradually replaced with latex-free substitutes and at the present time the operating room and anesthetic environment are virtually latex free, and the problem of anaphylaxis to latex has essentially disappeared. Overcoming the latex allergy problem is another example of the leadership of pediatric anesthesiology in identifying and solving problems to improve patient care and outcomes.

Out-of-operating room anesthesia

Since 1990, the rapid and sustained increase in diagnostic and therapeutic procedures in children done outside the operating room setting has necessitated that children undergo sedation and anesthesia with increasing frequency, especially for procedures such as magnetic resonance imaging (MRI) examination. Pediatric anesthesiologists worldwide have assumed a major role in both providing these services and in developing and supervising hospital programs for non-anesthesiologists to provide this sedation. Pediatric anesthesiologists have been leaders in establishing safe guidelines for monitoring, drugs and doses, recovery and discharge, and screening, evaluation, and triage of patients [45–47]. These efforts have greatly increased the safety of these procedures and improved outcomes. Indeed, up to 25% or more of anesthetics delivered by many pediatric anesthesia programs are now outside the operating room and have extended to such areas as endoscopy and bronchoscopy suites, interventional radiology, bone marrow aspiration/intrathecal chemotherapy, auditory brainstem-evoked responses, botulinum toxin injections, and many other locations and modalities. These developments in the recent history of pediatric anesthesia have permanently changed practice as the advantages of expertise in providing pain-free and minimally stressed experiences for children have been recognized.

Pediatric Perioperative Cardiac Arrest Registry

The Pediatric Perioperative Cardiac Arrest Registry (POCA) was formed in 1994 under the auspices of the American Academy of Pediatrics Section on Anesthesiology and the American Society of Anesthesiology [48]. Its purpose was to investigate the causes of cardiac arrest under or soon after anesthesia in children, with the eventual goal of preventing these devastating events. As such, the POCA was a pioneer of a multi-institutional outcomes registry and database, with voluntary anonymous reporting of major adverse events in great detail, with a panel of experts assigning a cause. In a series of landmark reports, the POCA has demonstrated that infants under 1 year of age account for the majority of anesthesia-related cardiac arrests [48], and that halothane was a major cause of medication-related cardiac arrests, which diminished greatly after the drug was replaced by sevoflurane [49].

Cardiovascular causes account for about 40% of cardiac arrests [49]. In addition, the dramatically higher number of reports of cardiac arrest in patients with underlying congenital heart disease, as well as the lower rate of successful resuscitation, has highlighted the vulnerability of this group of patients [50]. The early leadership of pediatric anesthesiology in pioneering this approach to improving quality and outcomes qualifies the POCA Registry for a place in the recent history of the specialty.

Pediatric cardiac anesthesia

Congenital heart disease is present in about eight per 1000 babies born worldwide, and is one of the most common birth defects, and is the most common defect requiring invasive treatment, including surgery. As such, the development of congenital heart surgery in the 1950s obligated the development of the field of pediatric cardiac anesthesia. The most prominent early pioneer in this field was Arthur S. Keats MD (Fig. 2.10), working at Texas Children's Hospital with the surgeon Denton A. Cooley. From 1955 to 1970, this team performed more surgeries for infants and children than any in the world, and Keats' numerous publications of anesthetic techniques and surgical outcomes from that era give us an important perspective of the daunting task facing these physicians. The descriptions of approaches to premedication, airway management, induction and maintenance of anesthesia, arrhythmias and their intraoperative treatment, perfusion, and the invention of a postoperative mechanical ventilator in 1958 set the standard for many of our modern practices [51–53]. Among other Keats landmark descriptions was anesthesia for cardiac catheterization in children in 1958 and the reversal of heparin with protamine in 1959 [54,55]. The importance of these early contributions by Keats and colleagues to the development of pediatric cardiac anesthesia as a subspecialty cannot be overstated.

In the 1970s and 1980s Hansen and Hickey at Children's Hospital, Boston, encouraged by the surgical leadership of Dr Aldo Castaneda, established the first anesthesia service dedicated solely to providing care to infants and children undergoing surgery, and other procedures in infants and children with cardiac disease. Among their many contributions was the description of anesthesia for

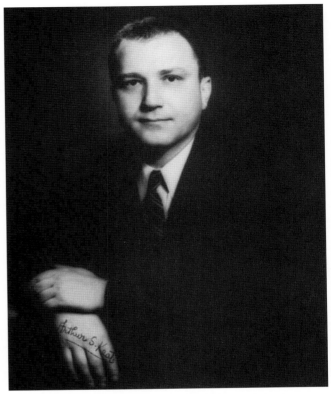

Figure 2.10 Arthur S. Keats MD. Reproduced with permission from Baylor College of Medicine, Houston, TX, USA.

the first Norwood Stage I palliation of hypoplastic left heart syndrome, high-dose fentanyl and sufentanil for complex neonatal cardiac surgery and its ablation of the stress response leading to improved survival, a description of anesthetic complications, and a recognition of, and treatment strategies for, severe perioperative pulmonary hypertension in infants undergoing congenital heart surgery [56–59].

In the late 1980s and early 1990s Greeley and co-workers at Duke were among those pediatric anesthesiologists making important contributions to the field of congenital cardiac anesthesia and surgery. The first was a landmark series of clinical studies using Xe^{133} technology to measure cerebral oxygen consumption during cardiopulmonary bypass and deep hypothermia, including circulatory arrest. These investigators conclusively demonstrated the vulnerability of the brain to prolonged periods without oxygen delivery and correctly extrapolated the "safe" duration of circulatory arrest [60]. In addition, this group was the first to demonstrate the efficacy of intraoperative echocardiography, and that the correction of residual defects during the initial repair in the operating room led to decreased mortality and morbidity, an approach that became a cornerstone of the surgical treatment of congenital heart disease [61].

Throughout the 1990s and early 2000s, many centers developed specialized pediatric cardiac anesthesia services, and efforts to provide ongoing education and forums for discussion began at the major anesthesia meetings in North America and Europe. The rapid advances in the field, including emphasis on primary complete repair of complex congenital heart lesions in the neonatal period, highlighted the difficulty and complexity of mastering the knowledge base in the pathophysiology of the cardiac condition, the neonate, and the technical aspects of invasive monitoring, echocardiography, and pharmacological management of the circulation during open heart procedures. In 2004 the Congenital Cardiac Anesthesia Society was formed under the auspices of the Society for Pediatric Anesthesia in the United States, which has grown to a membership of over 600, including representation from Europe, Australia, and Asia. This society holds a successful annual meeting with over 250 attendees, and has recently published recommendations for fellowship training in pediatric cardiac anesthesia [62].

Anesthetic neurotoxicity

In 1999 Olney et al published a paper in *Science* describing neuroapoptosis in the developing rat brain in response to ketamine, commonly used for sedation and analgesia in pediatric patients [63]. This paper was little noticed at the time by the pediatric anesthesia community, but the follow-up paper by this group in 2003, describing widespread apoptosis to commonly used anesthetic agents interacting with the GABA receptor, including isoflurane, midazolam, and nitrous oxide, certainly gained widespread attention in the pediatric anesthesia field, and anesthesiology in general. The longer term persistent learning deficits in these animals were particularly concerning [64]. This problem has led to an explosion of research, both in the animal and tissue culture laboratories as well as clinical research, to determine the extent of this issue in the clinical setting, as well as strategies to ameliorate this problem. These include the use of regional anesthesia alone, different anesthetic agents (opioids, dexmedetomidine), neuroprotective strategies, and the avoidance of elective sedation and anesthesia in the neonatal and early infancy periods altogether. This problem has led to the formation of a public–private partnership in the US to study this problem, involving the Food and Drug Administration, International Anesthesia Research Society, Society for Pediatric Anesthesia, and the National Institute of Child Health and Development [65]. This vitally important question potentially affecting the millions of children who undergo anesthesia and sedation annually around the world will likely be the prime driver of research and change in clinical practice for the next generation of pediatric anesthesiologists [66].

Teaching, research and professionalism through the 1980s and beyond

By the early 1980s the stages had been set and many of the players were in place to take the next steps in specialty development and maturation. Clinical practices continued to improve. Airway management became more consistent. Ability to monitor peripheral oxygen saturation and exhaled gases added precision to the administration of newer inhaled agents such as sevoflurane and desflurane, which had less cardiac depression, especially during induction [67,68]. Halothane is now largely abandoned in North American clinical practices. Fluid management and blood replacement guidelines became more standardized. Increasing numbers of individuals were attracted to advanced training for 6 months to 2 years in pediatric anesthesia and pediatric critical care, insuring a supply of practitioners devoted solely to the anesthetic care of children. These changes paralleled the continuing advances in surgery such as cardiac surgery in infants, transplantation of solid organs and increasingly complex and lengthy procedures to correct congenital anomalies of the face and skull. Attention turned more and more to the outpatients, the patient requiring anesthesia outside the operating room, sedation, pain management and regional techniques.

Teaching programs evolved, increased in size and became more rigorous. "Fellowship" training beyond the required training for certification by the American Board of Anesthesiology began in the 1970s and continues to grow. This prompted a lengthy, detailed examination of many variables which could better define the needs of children undergoing anesthesia and surgery as well as addressing the growing concerns about how better to recognize the practitioners who anesthetize children and institutions where that is done. Led by Hackel at Stanford and Gregory in San Francisco, this work produced the publication of guidelines for requirements that hospitals needed to meet in order to safely provide anesthesia to children [69,70]. Hackel and many others pursued a parallel effort which led to the recognition and accreditation of training programs in pediatric anesthesia [71].

Teaching and scholarly pursuits best characterize a maturing specialty area such as pediatric anesthesiology. From a single text in the nascent field in 1945, there are now dozens devoted to the specialty. Another hallmark of maturity is the quality and quantity of investigative work produced by pediatric anesthesiologists. Using only one criterion, there is remarkable activity. In the past 15 years the annual meeting data of the American Society of Anesthesiology (ASA) shows growth from about 20 pediatric anesthesia scientific abstracts in 1995, to 66 in 2000, to 106 in 2010 [72].

In addition, a vital, well-attended specialty meeting is held twice a year: once for a day in connection with the ASA annual meeting each fall and once in late winter/early spring with 3 days devoted entirely to pediatric anesthesiology. Two US specialty groups recognize pediatric anesthesia practitioners. The older of the two is a fellowship section of anesthesiology of the American Academy of Pediatrics (AAP) begun in the late 1960s [21]. This group requires that a major part of one's practice must be pediatric. In the 1980s the Society for Pediatric Anesthesia was established with a more encompassing goal: a member must have an interest in pediatric anesthesia, but need not practice it exclusively or even part time [21]. Obviously the two groups' members overlap and share similar goals. It is testimony to their willingness to share, not compete, that the annual spring meeting combines both groups and was attended in 2010 by over 700 practitioners.

In the US, fellowship training in pediatric anesthesiology was formally recognized in 1997 by the Accreditation Council on Graduate Medical Education, with the requirements that it be a 12-month fellowship with a specified didactic curriculum, supervision and clinical teaching by qualified faculty, and expertise and exposure to a wide variety of clinical components in pediatric anesthesia [71]. There are currently 46 programs accredited in the United States [73]. In 2009, the American Board of Anesthesiology Directors voted to support the development of an examination process that would lead to subspecialty certification in pediatric anesthesiology, further evidence of the recognition and support for organized anesthesiology in this field.

International development of pediatric anesthesiology

In parallel with and even preceding professional society development in the US, pediatric anesthesiology has developed as an organized subspecialty in Canada, Europe, Asia, and Australia/New Zealand, and is beginning in Africa. A partial listing of societies of pediatric anesthesiology includes the Asian Society of Paediatric Anesthesiologists (2000), Japanese Society of Pediatric Anesthesiology (1971), the Canadian Pediatric Anesthesia Society (2004), the Association of Paediatric Anaesthetists of Great Britain and Ireland (1973), the European Society of Paediatric Anaesthesia (2009), Association des Anesthetistes Reanimateurs Pediatriques d'Expression Francaise (1998), the Italian Society of Neonatal and Paediatric Anaesthesia and Reanimation (1995) , and the Society for Paediatric Anaesthesia in New Zealand and Australia (1998). The pervasiveness of the internet and the increasing ease of and opportunity for international travel have greatly increased international collaborations among these societies, and a number of joint meetings

Box 2.2 Major developments in pediatric anesthesia, late 1960s–2010

- Gregory and Eger's description of age and halothane requirement (1969)
- Gregory and colleagues' description of continuous positive airway pressure for neonatal respiratory distress syndrome (1971)
- Organization of the Association of Paediatric Anaesthetists of Great Britain and Ireland (1973)
- Reports of postanesthetic apnea in the premature infant (1981–83)
- Robinson's and Gregory's description of high-dose fentanyl anesthesia for PDA ligation in the premature infant (1981)
- Anand's report of fentanyl's dramatic reduction of stress response to PDA ligation in prematures (1987)
- Founding of the Society for Pediatric Anesthesia in the US (1988)
- First reports of latex allergy in pediatric patients undergoing anesthesia (1989)
- Greeley and colleagues study of cerebral physiology with cardiopulmonary bypass and deep hypothermic circulatory arrest (1991)
- Formation of the Pediatric Perioperative Cardiac Arrest Registry (1994)
- Accreditation Council for Graduate Medical Education accreditation of pediatric anesthesia fellowships in the US (1997)
- Hackel and colleagues' publication of the guidelines for the perioperative environment for pediatric anesthesia (1999)
- Olney and colleagues' first description of anesthetic neurotoxicity in the developing rodent brain (1999)
- Founding of the Congenital Cardiac Anesthesia Society (2004)
- American Board of Anesthesiology votes to support development of an examination for subspecialty certification in pediatric anesthesiology (2009)

have been held in the last decade. The international makeup of the editorial board of a major clinical journal, *Paediatric Anaesthesia*, and the wide geographic contribution of the scientific and clinical articles, editorials, and letters to the editor in this and other major international journals are evidence of the ongoing international development of pediatric anesthesiology.

Box 2.2 summarizes some of the major developments in pediatric anesthesiology from the late 1960s to 2010.

Conclusion

As stated at the beginning of this chapter, pediatric anesthesiology has a short history but is long in achievement and success. The accomplishments have a broad base now, although the foundation 60–70 years ago was narrow. It is important to recognize our indebtedness not only to the pioneers chronicled here but also to others, often unheralded, whose continuing efforts on behalf of children underpin the progress to date and our hopes for the future. Expectations are that the upward trajectory will continue as the 21st century progresses.

Annotated references

A full reference list for this chapter is available at:
http://www.wiley.com/go/gregory/andropoulos/pediatricanesthesia

1. Long C. An account of the first use of Sulphuric ether by inhalation as an anesthetic in surgical operations South Med J 1849; 5: 705–13. The description of the first use of ether for anesthesia.

10. Costarino AT, Downes JJ. Pediatric anesthesia historical perspective. Anesthesiol Clin North America 2005; 23: 573–95. A very thorough, well-researched and well-written account of the history of pediatric anesthesia.

14. McQuiston WO. Anesthetic problems in cardiac surgery in children. Anesthesiology 1949; 10: 590–600. One of the very first papers reporting anesthesia for pediatric cardiac surgery.

25. Eckenhoff JE. Relationship of anesthesia to post-operative personality changes in children. Am J Dis Child 1953; 86: 587–91. A remarkably prescient paper, written 30 years before the problem received widespread attention.

29. Gregory GA, Kitterman JA, Phibbs RH et al. Treatment of the idiopathic respiratory distress syndrome with continuous positive airway pressure. N Engl J Med 1971; 284: 1333–40. The description of the treatment that ushered in the era of modern neonatal intensive care.

30. Downes JJ. The historical evolution, current status, and prospective development of pediatric critical care. Crit Care Clin 1992; 8: 1–22. A thorough account by one of the founders of pediatric critical care.

31. Apgar V. Proposal for a new method of evaluation of the newborn infant. Anesth Analg 1953; 32: 260–7. The classic paper describing the Apgar score now used worldwide.

38. Robinson S, Gregory GA. Fentanyl-air-oxygen anesthesia for ligation of patent ductus arteriosus in preterm infants. Anesth Analg 1981; 60: 331–4. The classic description of high-dose fentanyl anesthesia that began this era in critically ill neonates.

41. Gregory GA, Eger EI 2nd, Munson ES. The relationship between age and halothane requirement in man. Anesthesiology 1969; 30: 488–91. The classic paper describing the marked differences in anesthetic requirement, using the now universal measure of potency, the minimum alveolar concentration.

52. Keats AS, Kurosu Y, Telford J, Cooley DA. Anesthetic problems in cardiopulmonary bypass for open heart surgery; experiences with 200 patients. Anesthesiology 1958; 19: 501–14. The first large series of open heart surgery anesthetics in infants and children by one of the pioneers of pediatric cardiac anesthesia.

CHAPTER 3

Educating Pediatric Anesthesiologists: What's Best for the Kids?

Alan Jay Schwartz
Department of Anesthesiology and Critical Care Medicine, Perelman School of Medicine, University of Pennsylvania, and The Children's Hospital of Philadelphia,

Philadelphia, PA, USA

If you want to learn something, read about it. If you want to understand something, write about it. If you want to master something, teach it. *Yogi Bhajan* [1]

Education (is) an essential leg for anesthesiology's four-legged stool! [2]

Introduction: why pediatric anesthesiology education? The needs assessment

Educating anesthesiologists about pediatric patients is essential if children are to receive the most effective and efficient anesthesia care. The importance of this concept was one of the major impetuses for the push to develop accredited subspecialty educational programs in pediatric anesthesiology [3]. What specifically justifies the existence of a special subspecialty of anesthesia patient care devoted to children and the need for education specially focused on this clinical care area?

Pediatric patient care data alone are a compelling justification. The Federal Census Bureau has projected that by July 2011, the US population will include >79,000,000 people from birth through 18 years of age [4]. This number represents 25% of the US population projected to total

>311,00,000 in the same time period [4]. In 2007, birth statistics documented newborns as a growing segment of the US population (Box 3.1) [5]. While more recent trends indicate a small decrease in the total number of births and the birth rate, it is obvious from the data that a large number of babies are born each year. An appreciable portion of these newborns present with clinically significant morbidity necessitating surgical and non-surgical diagnostic and therapeutic procedures which can only be accomplished with the assistance of pediatric anesthesia patient care.

Approximately 1 in 33 babies born in the US has a birth defect [6]. While these defects may be minor abnormalities, others may significantly affect the infant's physiology. One in every 100–200 babies has a congenital cardiac defect, which constitutes between 25–33% of all birth deformities [6]. Neural tube, orofacial and urinary tract abnormalities represent some of the other significant pathphysiological birth defects. Birth anomalies predispose newborns to a greater chance of acute illness and long-term disability than babies without birth defects and are the leading cause of more than 20% of all infant deaths (Box 3.2) [6,7].

On a yearly basis, up to 25% of children (>39,000/day) sustain an injury mandating medical attention [8], a clinically significant number of which will need diagnosis and

---

Box 3.1 Births in the United States: preliminary data for 2007 [5]

- Number of births: 4,317,119
- Birth rate: 14.3 per 1000 population
- Fertility rate: 69.5 births per 1000 women aged 15–44 years
- Percent born low birthweight (less than 2500 grams): 8.2%
- Percent preterm births (infants delivered at less than 37 weeks of gestation): 12.7%
- Percent unmarried: 39.7%

Box 3.2 The 10 leading causes of infant death (2007) [7]

1. Congenital malformations, deformations and chromosomal abnormalities (congenital malformations)
2. Disorders related to short gestation and low birthweight, not elsewhere classified (low birthweight)
3. Sudden infant death syndrome (SIDS)
4. Newborn affected by maternal complications of pregnancy (maternal complications)
5. Accidents (unintentional injuries)
6. Newborn affected by complications of placenta, cord and membranes (cord and placental complications)
7. Bacterial sepsis of newborn
8. Respiratory distress of newborn
9. Diseases of the circulatory system
10. Neonatal hemorrhage

---

therapy requiring pediatric anesthesia patient care. For older, healthy children, pediatric anesthesia patient care needs also exist. Contact sports are the primary cause of trauma in children [9]. Data on sports injuries include children 6 years and older and indicate, for example, that basketball is associated with an injury rate of 1 in 525 children engaging in this sport (1900 injuries/1,000,000 times children play this sport); approximately 180 of these children fracture bones and 160 will require surgery [9]. Football is even more risky, being associated with an injury rate of 1 in 250 children engaging in this sport; approximately 910 of these children fracture bones and 270 will require surgery [9].

The number of children needing anesthesia patient care is large yet the distribution of pediatric patients in hospitals is quite uneven. There are more than 5800 hospitals in the US [10]. There are 57 children's hospitals performing an estimated 640,000 operations each year [11]. The full range of resources specifically geared to pediatric patients (pharmaceuticals, equipment and knowledgeable, skilled and psychologically savvy physicians and paraprofessionals) is obviously more plentiful in hospitals that only care for children and their families.

In a 2005 report in the Newsletter of the American Society of Anesthesiologists (ASA) [12], Hackel and Gregory highlighted the clinical practice dilemma for everyone to ponder. It is recognized that pediatric patients and their anesthesia patient care needs are clearly different from those of the adult population; recognition and acceptance of this resulted in the development of special practice guidelines for pediatric anesthesia patient care, published in 1999–2004 by the ASA, American Academy of Pediatrics (AAP) and the Society of Pediatric Anesthesia (SPA) [13–15]. Yet most community hospitals, with less than the full complement of pediatric resources, are faced with a need to care for children, albeit a small number of such patients each year.

In all pediatric patient care settings, pediatricians, pediatric surgeons and pediatric subspecialists want anesthesiologists who are knowledgeable and skillful in pediatric anesthesia patient care. As the public has become more informed about pediatric healthcare, with understandable health information easily accessed on publicly available Internet websites (see Appendix 3.1), parents have also requested, and in some instances demanded, anesthesia patient care for their children provided by anesthesiologists knowledgeable and skillful in pediatric practice. "Data from other areas of medicine support this demand and show that fewer complications arise the more often practitioners perform a procedure" [12,16].

The intuitive assumption is that all of this is transferable to pediatric anesthesia patient care and this requires sufficient manpower (anesthesiologists with pediatric anesthesiology expertise) and sufficient sophistication (fully educated as pediatric anesthesiologists) to care for all of the children (all acuity, patient care scenarios).

What constitutes pediatric education for anesthesiologists (the curriculum) and how is the need for pediatric anesthesia patient care met? (accredited pediatric anesthesiology education)

In the US, the Accreditation Council for Graduate Medical Education (ACGME) is the organization that assures uniform education of physicians after completing their undergraduate education from an accredited medical school and embarking upon specialty practice education. Each specialty develops, implements, and evaluates its specialty educational process through an ACGME Residency Review Committee (RRC). Program requirements for the specialty education are developed through a peer review process based upon established standards and guidelines; program requirements grow through a consensus building process. What pediatric anesthesiology education does the Anesthesiology RRC sponsor via its program requirements? The answer to this question depends upon whether the pediatric anesthesiology education is for anesthesiology graduate trainees learning the basics of anesthesia practice (core residency 4-year continuum) or those who have successfully completed the basic anesthesiology education and are devoting additional time (1-year fellowship) to education exclusively devoted to the subspecialty aspects of pediatric anesthesia patient care [17].

The Anesthesiology RRC defines the program requirements in pediatric anesthesia patient care for the core education of residents in the following manner [18].

Int.B.2.b). (4)

> During the 36 months of clinical anesthesia training, there must be a minimum of two identifiable one month rotations in . . . pediatric anesthesia . . . If the program director judges that a resident has gained satisfactory skills and experience in clinical anesthesia in . . . [the subspecialty] . . . before completion of the second required month, the resident may pursue other experiences that augment learning of perioperative care in the subspecialty during the time remaining in the second month. For example, a resident who has gained sufficient experience in [pediatric] anesthesia (see IV.A.5.a) Patient Care) before completion of the second month of a [pediatric] anesthesia rotation may benefit from other perioperative experiences [in pediatric related clinical settings] . . .

Int.B.2.b). (5)

> Additional subspecialty rotations are encouraged, but the cumulative time in any one subspecialty may not exceed six months during the CA-1 through CA-3 years [36 months].

IV.A.5.a). (1). (c)

> Care should be provided for: 100 patients less than 12 years of age undergoing surgery or other procedures requiring anesthetics. Within this patient group, 20 children must be less than three years of age, including five less than three months of age.

The core resident therefore need only complete two of 36 months or 6% of their full clinical anesthesia educational program learning pediatric patient care and only care for 20 children less than 3 years of age, of which only five need be less than 3 months of age. Successful completion of the examination requirements of the American Board of Anesthesiology (ABA) therefore only guarantees that a certified anesthesiologist has been exposed to this relatively limited pediatric anesthesiology experience.

Subspecialty (fellowship) education in pediatric anesthesiology provides a 1-year immersion in the full depth and breadth of anesthesia care of children added to what has already been experienced during the prerequisite core residency pediatric anesthesiology education described above.

I.B.

> The clinical training in pediatric anesthesiology [fellowship] must be spent caring for pediatric patients in the operating rooms, other anesthetizing locations, and in intensive care units. The training will include experience in providing anesthesia both for inpatient and outpatient surgical procedures and for non-operative procedures outside the operating rooms, as well as pre-anesthesia preparation and post-anesthesia care, pain management, and advanced life support for neonates, infants, children, and adolescents. [19]

The Anesthesiology RRC has not specified minimum numbers of cases that a fellow must complete in specific pediatric anesthesia patient care settings as it has done for the core residency. The Anesthesiology RRC has been collecting case log data from all pediatric anesthesiology fellows on a yearly basis to document their experiences. The data document the average experience for a pediatric anesthesiology fellow in specified categories of clinical care, i.e. "index cases" (Table 3.1) [20]. The fellowship program requirements do elucidate an extensive array of clinical and didactic components for the curriculum in pediatric anesthesiology (see Appendix 3.2) [19].

The question that everyone (anesthesiologists, the patients they care for, the families of these patients, the pediatricians and pediatric surgeons caring for the patients, the hospital administrators in whose institutions this care takes place and the public) must answer is what type of pediatric anesthesiology education is appropriate and sufficient for the best care of children; pediatric anesthesiology education that is 6% of the total anesthesiology educational curriculum or pediatric anesthesiology education that is one full year of education focused exclusively on the care of pediatric patients? What makes this question difficult to answer is that there are varying degrees of acuity of pediatric patients; it seems very appropriate for anesthesiologists who are ABA certified, having completed the core residency education, to care for somewhat older, otherwise healthy pediatric patients, even if on a less frequent and inconsistent basis and for anesthesiologists who are graduates of the full year accredited pediatric anesthesiology subspecialty fellowship and have ongoing pediatric anesthesia experience to care for the youngest, very high-acuity pediatric patients, on a regular and consistent basis. There are extensive data supporting the view that better care is provided when a

Table 3.1 Pediatric Anesthesiology Graduating Residents (Fellows) Report (Abridged), 2008–2009 reporting year, Residency Review Committee, administered anesthetics

	Average	Maximum
Type of surgery		
Cardiac – with cardiopulmonary bypass	34	290
Cardiac – without cardiopulmonary bypass	18	69
Intrathoracic non-cardiac (intracavitary)	10	26
Intracranial neuro (excluding shunts)	14	42
Intra-abdominal (intracavitary)	35	262
Solid organ transplant – kidney	1	4
Solid organ transplant – heart	1	6
Solid organ transplant – liver	1	8
Solid organ transplant – lung	1	1
Major orthopedic surgery	13	57
Craniofacial surgery	7	35
Airway surgery	16	42
Neonatal emergencies – TEF	2	28
Neonatal emergencies – gastroschisis	3	31
Neonatal emergencies – diaphragmatic hernia	2	6
Neonatal emergencies – necrotizing enterocolitis	4	12
Neonatal emergencies – other	19	330
Other	145	541
Age of patient		
Neonates	36	87
1–11 months	66	183
1–2 years	62	176
3–11 years	126	399
12–17 years	70	265
Techniques for anesthesia		
General	348	994
Epidural/caudal	28	364
Intrathecal	4	200
Peripheral nerve block	12	200
Procedures		
Central venous cannulation	27	90
Arterial cannulation	56	127
Flexible fiberoptic intubation	10	117
Pain management outside OR		
Consultations	30	135
Patient-controlled analgesia	41	372
Peripheral nerve blocks	11	250
Central neuraxis blocks	12	200
Percentage of patients ASA 3 or greater	33	100

OR, operating room; TEF, tracheoesophageal fistula.
Number of residents (fellows), 118.

consistent and sufficient volume of similar patients (case types) are cared for by specialty and subspecialty educated physicians who, therefore, have more frequent opportunity to hone and apply their specialized knowledge, skills and attitudes [12,16]. The SPA supports subspecialty certification in advanced pediatric anesthesiology to "... provide a means to gauge the knowledge and problem-solving ability of those practicing in a distinct and very well-defined area of medicine. There can be no doubt that once subspecialty certification in pediatric anesthesiology exists, it will raise the bar for all practicing within the specialty. That, in turn, can only benefit [pediatric] patients" [21].

Pediatric anesthesiology education during residency and fellowship is very important yet insufficient. To remain current, lifelong education is essential. Reviewing and refreshing knowledge, skills and attitudes is the way to assure that anesthesiologists stay current; this is especially true for anesthesiologists who do not care for a large volume or a broadly diverse population of pediatric anesthesiology patients. Learning new knowledge, skills and attitudes that came into existence after an anesthesiologist's primary education will only take place through a continuing medical education (CME) process.

American Board of Anesthesiology certification prior to 2000 was without a time limit; since 1 January 2000, ABA certification has had a 10-year limit. To address the time-limited certification and provide for continuing education and lifelong learning, the ABA's Maintenance of Certification in Anesthesiology (MOCA) has been developed for anesthesiologists as similar maintenance of certification programs have been developed for all American Board of Medical Specialties disciplines [22]. The MOCA consists of four components: assessments of professional standing, cognitive expertise (knowledge test), and practice performance, and participation in and documentation of lifelong learning and self-assessment [21,23]. While not solely devoted to a single subspecialty within the discipline of anesthesiology, the MOCA is the vehicle that incentivizes all anesthesiologists, including pediatric anesthesiology subspecialists, to stay current and benefit from the many CME programs offered in their areas of practice expertise.

What are the fundamental principles of education for all aspects of anesthesia patient care? The educational design [24–28]

Education is change in behavior based upon experience

This definition speaks to the essential ingredients of education: individuals (students and teachers), behaviors (the student's baseline knowledge, skills and attitudes and the teacher's curriculum) and experiences (the activities that constitute the learning, i.e. student–teacher interaction and the environment in which this takes place). The ingredients, when mixed properly, result in effective and efficient education. The proper mixing of the ingredients is addressed with answers to the question: "How shall who teach what to whom for what purpose now and in the future?" (DE Greenhow, personal communication, 1982). This question asks for answers about what defines the teaching goals and describes the students, the teachers and the teaching methods.

The *teaching goals* for pediatric anesthesiology have been outlined above; the student learns specific information unique to the care of children to become a knowledgeable and skilled provider of anesthesia patient care to this special patient population, the ultimate goal being the provision of the best outcomes possible for the patients.

The *student of pediatric anesthesiology* is an adult learner [29]. When providing medical care, everyone agrees that children are not small adults. An analogous concept applies when it comes to education: *adult learners are not large children*. Adult learners are unique and very different from child learners [29]. Adult learners:

- are highly motivated to seek out goal-directed learning (want to learn pediatric anesthesiology for future medical practice opportunities)
- tend to pick and choose some, not necessarily all, of the educational activities available because their learning is goal oriented toward relevant life-centered needs (a future anesthesiology patient care practice)
- enter new learning possessing vast knowledge gained prior to the current learning (have successfully completed a minimum of 4 years of undergraduate medical education and the 4-year continuum of anesthesiology resident education)
- interact with teachers who are physician peers. [29]

Adult learners have life commitments and specific intentional attachments including, among others, marriage, child rearing, financial responsibility that often includes debt incurred for medical education up to the time of residency or fellowship and coping with aging parents, all of which affect how their decisions are made about whether and for how long additional education will be embarked upon. Education must provide for the inherent differences among adult learners that tend to increase with aging and include, among others, differences in style, time, place, and pace of learning. The time factor for adult learners is especially crucial. Adults perceive that time passes rapidly; to the adult learner there is less time available to learn, or do anything, for that matter. With time perceived to be in short supply, adult learners tend to be selective in their learning so they use what time

they have more efficiently. The pediatric anesthesiology learner may devote time to learning in the operating room and weekly departmental case conference but may choose to skip the journal club to spend time with their family [24].

Recognizing and acknowledging the unique characteristics of adult learners enable teachers to tailor their educational programs to these special students, resulting in a welcoming environment for a better educational outcome than would occur if the teacher imposed on the learner what the teacher alone thinks is right.

The most current data for graduate medical education in the US (2008–2009) document 108,176 residents in all specialty education programs, of which 5208 (5%) are core anesthesiology residents and 296 (0.003%) are subspecialty anesthesiology fellows; included in the fellow group are 129 (0.001%) pediatric anesthesiology fellows [30].

The *teachers of pediatric anesthesiology* comprise a small group within the total teaching faculty for the specialty. Pediatric anesthesiology is taught by physician anesthesiologists, many of whom have themselves completed fellowship education in this subspecialty. Full-time anesthesiology faculty positions in United States medical schools in 2007–2008 numbered 6117 [31]. Anesthesiologists represent 5.5% of the clinical teachers and 4.8% of all American medical school teaching faculty [31]. The 6117 anesthesia faculty in medical schools (as of 1 December 2007) assumed the major responsibility for teaching some or all of the 70,349 enrolled undergraduate medical students, the 5222 graduate trainees in anesthesiology residency and fellowship educational programs, as well as many of the approximately 106,012 physician house staff trainees [31]. The actual number of anesthesiologists who devoted the majority or all of their educational commitment to pediatric anesthesiology is unknown and contained within the 6117 total anesthesiology faculty positions in the US.

Teachers of pediatric anesthesiology, like almost all medical teachers, are ill equipped for this responsibility [32]. While these physicians are experts in their medical practice discipline, they, like almost all physicians, have never formally learned how to be a teacher; they have learned how to teach from their teachers who have role modeled teaching, although they too have never studied education in a formal manner. It is as though watching someone change an automobile transmission "qualifies" the observer to teach someone else how to accomplish this task and they in turn will be "qualified" to teach others what they have observed. It is doubtful that one would feel safe driving the vehicle in which a new transmission was installed under these conditions; it is very curious that we do feel safe to accept medical care from individuals who have been educated under these conditions. It is also very curious that a major portion of the teaching responsibility falls upon the shoulders of the relatively inexperienced junior faculty as opposed to more senior experienced faculty [33].

Physicians need not feel they are without resources that would help them learn to become effective teachers of medicine and pediatric anesthesiology in particular. Physicians can look to the medical literature for the latest "science" about education and teaching just as they would read the journal *Anesthesiology,* for example, to learn the latest science about anesthesia patient care.

Academic Medicine is the official, peer-reviewed journal of the Association of American Medical Colleges. The journal serves as an international forum for the exchange of ideas, information, and strategies to address the major challenges facing the academic medicine community as it strives to carry out its missions in the public interest. The journal's areas of focus include: education and training issues . . . [34]

Effective teaching has been studied and the principles identified (Box 3.3) are clearly applicable to teaching pediatric anesthesiology [35].

An example of how studying education may improve learning outcome for the student deals with the student–teacher relationship and philosophy of education. There are at least two student–teacher relationships with associated philosophies: teacher in total control (Tylerian approach [36]) or student in a peer position as partner with the teacher (Dewey's progressive education approach [37]). It becomes intuitively obvious that for students of pediatric anesthesiology, a philosophy of education that values a student–teacher partnership will be more effective.

An example of these two philosophies put into action clarifies their differences. Let us consider teaching/learning how to manage a patient who is being mechanically ventilated in the operating room. The Tylerian teacher might lecture to the [fellows] on how to use the ventilator. It is hoped that the [fellows] will remember what they heard and be able to put what they learned into action. In contrast, the teacher using Dewey's approach might create a patient simulation exercise in which [fellows] can "experiment" with differing ventilator setups to infer what might occur clinically. A much more meaningful learning environment might be provided by the simulation – coupled with the anesthesiologist faculty member's reactions to and guidance about how the [fellows] tinkered with the ventilator – than might be provided by the lecture format. In addition, the teacher using Dewey's philosophy might be more likely to encourage the student with prior experience, like [fellows] who used different types of ventilators during their internship [and residency], to share their know-how with other, less experienced, peers. [24]

Anesthesiologists who study pediatric anesthesiology are often students of pediatrics as well. Many have successfully completed a 3-year pediatric residency. They enter pediatric anesthesiology fellowship as very knowledgeable and skilled pediatricians with a wealth of prior pediatric understanding upon which to build their new anesthesiology subspecialty education. If they are lucky enough to have teachers who understand the concepts of adult learning and Dewey's philosophy, their prior knowledge will be accepted by their teachers and their learning will flourish.

The teaching methods available for effective pediatric anesthesiology education include, among others, the tried and true standards such as formal didactic lectures, interactive conferences, problem-based learning discussions (PBLD), journal club discussions to consider the classic and current literature, interactive patient care teaching in clinical settings such as the operating room, intensive care unit, and pre-anesthesia evaluation clinic, computer-based "surfing the Web" and simulation exercises.

To be the most effective teachers, physicians must learn the nuances of the standard teaching methods. How to ask a student a question so that the student will demonstrate the full extent of their understanding, as an example, depends upon teachers understanding the difference between closed and open questions [38]. There is a huge difference between the question "What is the dose of lidocaine for a caudal block of a 7 kg baby?" compared to

---

Box 3.3 Characteristics of an effective clinical teacher

- Allocates dedicated time for teaching
- Creates a trusting learning environment
- Demonstrates clinical credibility
- Provides an initial orientation and final evaluation for the teaching event
- Engages learners by expecting them to present cases, the pertinent details and educational benefit of which are managed by the teacher
- Enhances clinical case material with complementary didactic sessions
- Role models physician–patient relationships through bedside teaching
- Encourages student consideration of and interactive discussions about the psychosocial aspects of medical care
- Transfers the teaching responsibility to the students who are the future medical educators

Modified from Schwartz [24].

"Why would you perform a caudal block on a 7 kg baby undergoing inguinal hernia repair?". Teaching psychomotor skills is another example of a standard teaching method that requires an intricate understanding of the component steps and their proper sequencing [38]. The "See one, do one, teach one" method of teaching delicate skills, especially those to be performed upon the tiniest and highest acuity premature babies, is an unacceptable way to teach and learn pediatric anesthesiology skills [38].

There is a vast array of print materials (textbooks and journals) providing information about pediatric anesthesiology and its related subjects. Although there is a constant attempt to update textbooks, it is almost impossible to have current, complete and up-to-date print material. The internet solves the problem of potentially being out of date with one's print resources. Search engines, databases, and Internet links make an encyclopedic amount of up-to-date information available to the learner of pediatric anesthesiology (see Appendix 3.1). A caution reminds the viewer of internet resources to be discerning of materials that may not be accurate, peer reviewed or impartial, i.e. always consider the source of the material. It would be nice to state that the list of web-based resources in Appendix 3.1 is all-inclusive but by its very nature, the internet is constantly changing. The pediatric anesthesiology teacher, student, and practitioner are encouraged to use the listing in Appendix 3.1 as a springboard to continually explore this vast educational reservoir as a lifelong learning exercise.

Simulation is the most current, new teaching methodology (see Chapter 42), which has been embraced by most medical educators. Simulation permits imitation of a real-life clinical situation using a mannequin. This allows learning experiences, in repetitive fashion if desired, with zero risk [39]. A great number and variety of simulation devices for medical education have been developed over the past several decades, many of which are directly applicable to education of pediatric anesthesiologists.

> Evidence has been accumulated that simulation results in a better educational outcome for the learner. Schwid and colleagues [40] randomized anesthesiology residents and faculty into two learning groups (textbook reading versus computerized ACLS [Advanced Cardiac Life Support] simulation education) preparing for performance evaluation at an ACLS mock resuscitation. Computer simulation-prepared learners were judged to perform better than textbook-prepared learners during standardized mega codes that required treatment protocols for clinical simulation of cardiovascular life-threatening scenarios with supraventricular tachycardia, ventricular fibrillation, and second-degree type II atrioventricular block. [25]

Arrhythmia recognition and treatment is an example of a very pertinent simulation activity that can be geared to pediatric anesthesiology education.

Simulation augments clinical education by adding a more sophisticated aspect to the learning, i.e. teamwork and improved processes of care. By employing simulation exercises as the teaching vehicle, multidisciplinary teams can learn to work effectively together to develop the best care for patients. Crew resource management (CRM) concepts can be effectively learned using group simulation exercises [25,41]. Holman [42] and Grogan [41] have demonstrated that CRM (anesthesia crisis resource management) enhances interpersonal communication, situational awareness, and appropriate management of available patient care resources [42] and fatigue management, adverse event recognition, team decision making, and performance feedback [41]. CRM is so timely a topic that an entire supplement issue of *Quality and Safety in Health Care* entitled "Simulation and Team Training" [43], described the state of the art [25].

Simulation is ideal for addressing the concern that the teaching-learning situation presents in pediatric anesthesiology.

> Atul Gawande has made a critically important medical education dichotomy and dilemma transparent to the public in his book *Complications: A Surgeon's Notes on an Imperfect Science* in the chapter entitled "Education of a Knife," writing that there is an ". . . imperative to give patients the best possible care and [at the same time] to provide novices with experience" [44]. To accomplish these two conflicting imperatives in the past, learning clinical care (pediatric anesthesia, for example) was most often a process of application of knowledge and trial of techniques, both new to the student, on high acuity/low physiologic reserve patients in real-time patient care settings. This scenario was characterized by high anxiety for the student and significant risk of complications to the patient cared for by the novice. For the present and future, Gawande makes it clear that the traditional medical education paradigm is no longer acceptable:

> "By traditional ethics and public insistence (not to mention court rulings), a patient's right to the best care possible must trump the objective of training novices" [25,44].

> The aviation industry long ago recognized this dilemma when teaching pilots. Acknowledging the high-stakes nature of flying, simulation technology was instituted to teach and evaluate a pilot's competence rather than allow her/him to fly a jumbo-jet and risk loss of hundreds of lives. Learning to apply the knowledge and perform the techniques before entering the "cockpit"

reduces the risk of a "crash disaster." Medical care in general and anesthesia patient care in particular, especially of very high-risk [narrow margin pediatric anesthesiology] patients, is analogous to the jumbo-jet situation and logically calls for a similar approach to education, that is, use of simulation [45]. The public is no longer willing to accept teaching on patients [25,46].

How do we know that the educational activity is effective? Evaluation of the educational process

Undertaking an educational activity requires that several essential steps be accomplished:
- defining that education is necessary, i.e. completing a needs assessment
- characterizing the participants in the learning setting, i.e. understanding who the students and teachers are
- designing and implementing an educational experience, i.e. developing the curriculum and transmitting it via teaching methods.

Like the classic medical model (diagnosis = the need of a patient, prescription = therapy for the problem, monitoring = assessment of the effect of the treatment, and disposition = maintaining or adjusting therapy), the teaching/learning process is incomplete without an evaluation to maintain or modify the educational activity.

The ACGME requires that its educational programs, such as fellowship programs in pediatric anesthesiology, be evaluated on an ongoing basis and in multiple ways (faculty evaluate fellows, fellows evaluate faculty, and everyone evaluates the program) [19]. The primary assessment method is a program's voluntary request to be evaluated against ACGME program "standards" (program requirements). Accredited programs participate in this assessment every 5 years or sooner [47]. The component parts of the ACGME accreditation and reaccreditation process include the program's completion of a Program Information Form (PIF) describing and quantifying the program components and experiences, the ACGME's site visit to view the program and interview representatives of the program and others who interact with the program, and based on review of the PIF and report of the site visit, the ACGME Anesthesiology RRC assesses, evaluates, and makes decisions about and recommendations to the program [19,47].

Evaluation of the pediatric anesthesiology fellow's performance during the course of (formative evaluation) and at the conclusion of (summative evaluation) their education is the basis upon which judgments can be put forth on the quality of the fellow's mastery of knowledge, skills, and attitudes important for the subspecialist to acquire and upon which the quality of the educational program can be gauged. The ACGME program require-

ments for education in pediatric anesthesiology explicitly outline evaluation of fellows.

X.A.

> Faculty responsible for teaching subspecialty [fellows] in pediatric anesthesiology must provide critical evaluations of each [fellow's] progress and competence to the pediatric anesthesiology program director at the end of 6 months and 12 months of training. These evaluations should include attitude, interpersonal relationships, fund of knowledge, manual skills, patient management, decision-making skills, and critical analysis of clinical situations. [19]

At the present time, ABA certification of pediatric anesthesiologists does not exist. However, as of this writing, the American Board of Medical Specialties has approved the ABA's request for subspecialty examination and certification in Pediatric Anesthesiology, and certification is expected to be available within the next several years. Therefore, there is no standardized test that must be passed by each fellow to evaluate their knowledge base in the subspecialty. The data that are collected document the pediatric anesthesiology clinical case experience (see Table 3.1) which allows evaluative inferences to be made about the quantity and diversity of cases that each fellow completes compared to the average for their peer group. No data exist that specify the minimum number of cases that, when successfully completed, will define a competent pediatric anesthesiologist.

Evaluating the quality of the teaching is vital to the recognition of outstanding faculty. A recent study of teaching effectiveness demonstrates that systematic collection and analysis of data about education of anesthesiology residents will define who the best teachers are and these teachers can in turn become the teachers of others with a pronounced positive ripple effect on educational process and outcome [48,49].

Whether the evaluation is of the program, the learners or the teachers, it is only through some type of formalized and standardized assessment process that pediatric anesthesiology fellowships can be recognized as being on a par with or better than similar programs elsewhere. It is also true that the recognition of program deficiencies (of the learners, teachers and/or the curriculum and teaching methods) may never occur to guide corrective measures if an evaluation system is not in place.

Educating pediatric anesthesiologists: what's best for the kids? The conclusion = the starting message

Anesthesiology education is a vibrant activity. The enterprise is vast. In the USA in 2007 and 2008, (a) accredited Graduate Medical Education (GME) programs included 129 core anesthesiology residencies and 126 subspecialty fellowship programs educating 5208 residents and 296 subspecialty anesthesiology fellows; included in the fellow group are 129 pediatric anesthesiology fellows, (b) 70,349 medical students received some modicum of anesthesiology education, (c) 6117 full-time clinical anesthesiology faculty were responsible for providing anesthesiology education and (d) 100,690 GME trainees in non-anesthesiology specialties [including pediatrics and pediatric subspecialties] (an 8% increase from 2002) clamored for anesthesiology related education (e.g. airway management, vascular access, safe local anesthetic use). [2]

Education *is* an essential leg for anesthesiology's four-legged stool! Starting with this premise is essential for the most effective and efficient education of physicians wanting to learn anesthesia patient care; it is equally important for anesthesiologists wanting to learn sophisticated subspecialty anesthesia care for pediatric patients. While it is true children are resilient and that they do not "break" easily, the margin of safety when caring for them is narrow. Systematic, standardized, practice parameter-driven care based on evidence-based pediatric anesthesiology medical understanding provides the best opportunity for pediatric anesthesiologists to learn the best care possible for this patient population. Including education in the topics for pediatric anesthesiologists to learn will given our discipline the best possible opportunity to provide both the best care for children and the best education for their anesthesiologists.

Annotated references

A full reference list for this chapter is available at:
http://www.wiley.com/go/gregory/andropoulos/pediatricanesthesia

2. Schwartz AJ. Education. An essential leg for anesthesiology's four-legged stool! Anesthesiology 2010; 112: 3–5. An editorial emphasizing the importance of education to the specialty of anesthesiology.
3. Rockoff MA, Hall SC. Subspecialty training in pediatric anesthesiology: what does it mean? Anesth Analg 1997; 85: 1185–90. An explanation of subspecialty fellowship training in pediatric anesthesia.
14. Section on Anesthesiology, American Academy of Pediatrics. Guidelines for the pediatric perioperative anesthesia environment. Pediatrics 1999; 103: 512–15. An important document describing guidelines for the environment for anesthetic care of children.
42. Holzman RS, Cooper JB, Gaba DM et al. Anesthesia crisis resource management: real-life simulation training in operating room crises.

J Clin Anesth 1995; 7: 675–87. A description of the importance of simulation and crisis management training in anesthesiology.
48. Baker K. Clinical teaching improves with resident evaluation and feedback. Anesthesiology 2010; 113: 690–703. A study concluding that learner feedback to the teacher will improve operating room teaching in anesthesiology.

Further reading

Barrows HS. Simulated (Standardized) Patients and Other Human Simulations. Chapel Hill, NC: Health Sciences Consortium, 1987.

Bunker JP (ed). Education in Anesthesiology. New York: Columbia University Press, 1967.

Dick W, Reiser RA. Planning Effective Instruction. Englewood Cliffs, NJ: Prentice-Hall, 1989.

Epstein J (ed). Masters: Portraits of Great Teachers. New York: Basic Books, 1981.

Gagné RM, Briggs LJ. Principles of Instructional Design, 2nd edn. New York: Holt, Rinehart and Winston, 1979.

Greenberg LW, Jewett LS. Commitment to teaching: myth or reality? South Med J 1983; 76: 910.

Greene NM. Anesthesiology and the University. Philadelphia: JB Lippincott, 1975.

Joyce B, Weil M. Models of Teaching. Englewood Cliffs, NJ: Prentice-Hall, 1980.

Lear E (ed). Virtual reality in patient simulators. American Society of Anesthesiologists Newsletter 1997; October: 61.

Lyman RA. Disaster in pedagogy. N Engl J Med 1957; 257: 504.

McGaghie WC, Frey JJ (eds). Handbook for the Academic Physician. New York: Springer-Verlag, 1986.

McGuire CH, Foley RP, Gorr A et al. Handbook of Health Professions Education. San Francisco: Jossey-Bass, 1983.

McKeachie WJ. Teaching Tips: A Guidebook for the Beginning College Teacher, 7th edn. Lexington, MA: DC Heath, 1978.

Miller GE. Adventure in pedagogy. JAMA 1956; 162: 1448.

Miller GE (ed). Teaching and Learning in Medical School. Cambridge, MA: Harvard University Press, 1961.

Miller GE. Educating Medical Teachers. Cambridge, MA: Harvard University Press, 1980.

Popham WJ, Baker EL. Establishing Instructional Goals. Planning an Instructional Sequence. Englewood Cliffs, NJ: Prentice-Hall, 1970.

Schwenk TL, Whitman NA (1984) Residents as Teachers: A Guide to Educational Practice. Salt Lake City, University of Utah.

Schwenk TL, Whitman NA. The Physician as Teacher. Baltimore, MD: Williams and Wilkins, 1987.

Segall AJ, Vanderschmidt H, Burglass R et al. Systemic Course Design for the Health Fields. New York: John Wiley, 1975.

Whitman NA. There is No Gene for Good Teaching: A Handbook on Lecturing for Medical Teachers. Salt Lake City, UT: University of Utah, 1982.

Whitman NA, Schwenk TL. A Handbook for Group Discussion Leaders: Alternative to Lecturing Medical Students to Death. Salt Lake City, UT: University of Utah, 1983.

Whitman NA, Schwenk TL. Preceptors as Teachers: A Guide to Clinical Teaching. Salt Lake City, UT: University of Utah, 1984.

Appendix 3.1 Pediatric anesthesiology internet resources

Organizations

www.acgme.org: Accreditation Council for Graduate Medical Education (ACGME)
www.aap.org: American Academy of Pediatrics (AAP)
www.aabb.org: American Association of Blood Banks
www.abanes.org: American Board of Anesthesiology (ABA)
www.abim.org: American Board of Internal Medicine (ABIM)
www.abms.org: American Board of Medical Specialties (ABMS)
www.abp.org: American Board of Pediatrics (ABP)
www.absurgery.org: American Board of Surgery (ABS)
www.americanheart.org: American Heart Association (AHA)
www.ama-assn.org: American Medical Association (AMA)
www.apsf.org: Anesthesia Patient Safety Foundation (APSF)
www.auahq.org: Association of University Anesthesiologists
www.cdc.gov: Centers for Disease Control and Prevention (CDC)
www.fda.gov: Food and Drug Administration (FDA)
www.faer.org: Foundation for Anesthesia Education & Research (FAER)
www.jcaho.org: Joint Commission on Accreditation of Healthcare Organizations
www.nih.gov: National Institutes of Health (NIH)
www.prb.org/: Population Reference Bureau

Specialty societies

www.acc.org: American College of Cardiology
www.asahq.org: American Society of Anesthesiologists (ASA)
www.amsect.org: American Society of Extra-Corporeal Technology
www.acta.org.uk: Association of Cardiothoracic Anaesthetists
www.aagbi.org: Association of Anaesthetists of Great Britain and Ireland
www.apagbi.org.uk: Association of Paediatric Anaesthetists of Great Britain and Ireland
www.asa.org.au: Australian Society of Anaesthetists
www.cas.ca: Canadian Anesthesiologists' Society
www.eacta.org: European Association of Cardiothoracic Anaesthesiologists
www.iars.org: International Anesthesia Research Society (IARS)
www.rcoa.ac.uk: Royal College of Anaesthetists
www.sambahq.org: Society for Ambulatory Anesthesia (SAMBA)
www.scahq.org: Society of Cardiovascular Anesthesiologists (SCA)
www.sccm.org: Society of Critical Care Medicine (SCCM)
www.seahq.org: Society for Education in Anesthesia (SEA)
www.snacc.org: Society of Neurosurgical Anesthesia and Critical Care (SNACC)
www.soap.org: Society for Obstetric Anesthesia and Perinatology (SOAP)
www.pedsanesthesia.org: Society for Pediatric Anesthesia (SPA)
www.pedsanesthesia.org/ccas/: Congenital Cardiac Anesthesia Society (CCAS)
www.sts.org: Society of Thoracic Surgeons
www.nda.ox.ac.uk/wfsa: World Federation of Societies of Anaesthesiologists

Journals

www.anesthesia-analgesia.org: *Anesthesia and Analgesia*
www.anesthesiology.org: *Anesthesiology*
http://ats.ctsnetjournals.org/: *Annals of Thoracic Surgery*
www.asa-refresher.com: American Society of Anesthesiologists Refresher Courses in Anesthesiology
www.bja.oupjournals.org: *British Journal of Anaesthesia*
http://bmj.bmjjournals.com/: *British Medical Journal*
www.cja-jca.org: *Canadian Journal of Anesthesia*
http://circ.ahajournals.org/: *Circulation*
www.cardiosource.com/jacc.html: *Journal of the American College of Cardiology*

http://jama.ama-assn.org/: *Journal of the American Medical Association*
www.jcardioanesthesia.com: *Journal of Cardiothoracic and Vascular Anesthesia*
www.journals.elsevierhealth.com/periodicals/JCA: *Journal of Clinical Anesthesia*
http://jtcs.ctsnetjournals.org/: *Journal of Thoracic and Cardiovascular Surgery*
www.nejm.org: *New England Journal of Medicine*
www.blackwellpublishing.com/journal.asp?ref=1155-5645: *Paediatric Anaesthesia*
www.pediatrics.org: *Pediatrics*

Literature search sites

The Review Group
www.cochrane-anaesthesia.suite.dk: Cochrane Anaesthesia Review Group
www.ncbi.nlm.nih.gov: National Center for Biotechnology Information
www.nlm.nih.gov: National Library of Medicine
www.pubmed.gov: National Library of Medicine
http://medlineplus.gov/: Medline Plus

Educational resource sites

http://depts.washington.edu/asaccp/: American Society of Anesthesiologists Closed Claims Project
American Society of Anesthesiologists (ASA) Closed Claims Project – home page links to:
http://depts.washington.edu/asaccp/ASA/index.shtml: ASA Closed Claims Project
http://depts.washington.edu/asaccp/POCA/index.shtml: Pediatric Perioperative Cardiac Arrest (POCA) Registry
http://depts.washington.edu/asaccp/eye/index.shtml: Postoperative Visual Loss Registry
http://depts.washington.edu/asaccp/prof/index.shtml: ASA Committee on Professional Liability
   MD, University of California San Francisco
www.pediheart.org: Congenital heart disease information site
www.theanswerpage.com: family of educational websites for the medical professional – anesthesiology, pain management, hospital and CCM, newborn
   medicine and ob-gyn. Specialty sites feature Question of the Day with a peer-reviewed, referenced answer
www.healthfinder.gov: health information site
www.ucsf.edu/teeecho: intraoperative TEE: a web based video primer
www.medscape.com: medical information from WebMD
www.guideline.gov: National Guideline Clearinghouse – a public resource for evidence-based clinical practice guidelines. The NGC is sponsored by the
   Agency for Healthcare Research and Quality (formerly the Agency for Health Care Policy and Research) in partnership with the American Medical
   Association and the American Association of Health Plans
www.ncbi.nlm.nih.gov/omim/: Online Mendelian Inheritance in Man (database catalog of human genes and genetic disorders) (syndrome clinical
   synopsis)
www.sickkids.ca/Anaesthesia/pac_list.asp: Paediatric Anaesthesia Conference – Discussion Group: Hospital for Sick Children, Toronto, Canada
www.picucourse.org: pediatric critical care education site
http://pedsccm.wustl.edu: PedsCCM is a collaborative, independent, information resource and communication tool for professionals caring for critically
   ill and injured infants and children
http://pedsccm.wustl.edu/All-Net/english/mainpage/contents/cardanesth.html: pediatric cardiac anesthesia section of picuBOOK, an on-line resource for
   pediatric critical care
www.pacep.org: Pulmonary Artery Catheter Education Project
www.ssih.org: Society for Simulation in Healthcare

Practice guidelines and advisories

www.asahq.org/publicationsAndServices/practiceparam.htm: ASA practice parameters
www.asahq.org/publicationsAndServices/pulm_artery.pdf: practice guidelines for pulmonary artery catheterization
www.asahq.org/publicationsAndServices/tee.pdf: practice guidelines for perioperative TEE
www.asahq.org/publicationsAndServices/Difficult%20Airway.pdf: practice guidelines for management of the difficult airway

Research resource sites

www.scs.uiuc.edu/suslick/seminaronseminars.html: collection of points on how to (and how not to) give a good research seminar
www.niaid.nih.gov/ncn/grants: NIH tutorial on the do's and don'ts for grant writing
www.niaid.nih.gov/ncn: useful information on other sections of an application including human subjects, training grants, and budgets

(Continued)

Pharmacology resource sites

www.epocrates.com: medication information
www.pdr.net: Physician's Desk Reference

General search engines

www.altavista.com: internet search engine
www.google.com: internet search engine
www.lycos.com: internet search engine
www.msn.com: internet search engine
www.yahoo.com: internet search engine
www.searchengineguide.com/searchengines.html: search engine guide

Computer-palm resource sites

www.aether.com: AetherPalm
www.handheldmed.com: Handheld Med
www.palm.com/us: Palm
http://dir.yahoo.com/Health/medicine/anesthesiology/: Yahoo Anesthesiology

---

Appendix 3.2 Abridged Program Requirements for Graduate Medical Education in Pediatric Anesthesiology [19]

V.B. Clinical components

The subspecialty resident in pediatric anesthesiology should gain expertise in the following areas of clinical care of neonates, infants, children, and adolescents:

V.B.1.   Preoperative assessment of children scheduled for surgery
V.B.2.   Cardiopulmonary resuscitation and advanced life support
V.B.3.   Management of normal and abnormal airways
V.B.4.   Mechanical ventilation
V.B.5.   Temperature regulation
V.B.6.   Placement of venous and arterial catheters
V.B.7.   Pharmacologic support of the circulation
V.B.8.   Management of both normal perioperative fluid therapy and massive fluid and/or blood loss
V.B.9.   Interpretation of laboratory results
V.B.10. Management of children requiring general anesthesia for elective and emergent surgery for a wide variety of surgical conditions including neonatal surgical emergencies, cardiopulmonary bypass, and congenital disorders
V.B.11. Techniques for administering regional anesthesia for inpatient and ambulatory surgery in children
V.B.12. Sedation or anesthesia for children outside the operating rooms, including those undergoing radiologic studies
V.B.13. Recognition, prevention, and treatment of pain in medical and surgical patients
V.B.14. Consultation for medical and surgical patients
V.B.15. Recognition and treatment of perioperative vital organ dysfunction, including in the postanesthesia care unit
V.B.16. Diagnosis and perioperative management of congenital and acquired disorders
V.B.17. Participation in the care of critically ill infants and children in a neonatal and/or pediatric intensive care unit
V.B.18. Transport of critically ill patients between hospitals and/or within the hospital
V.B.19. Psychological support of patients and their families

In preparation for roles as consultants to other specialists, subspecialty residents in pediatric anesthesiology should have the opportunity to provide consultation under the direction of faculty responsible for teaching in the pediatric anesthesiology program. This should include assessment of the appropriateness of a patient's preparation for surgery and recognition of when an institution's personnel, equipment, and/or facilities are not appropriate for management of the patient.

V.C. Didactic components

The didactic curriculum, provided through lectures and reading, should include the following areas, with emphasis on developmental and maturational aspects as they pertain to anesthesia and life support for pediatric patients:

V.C.1.   Cardiopulmonary resuscitation
V.C.2.   Pharmacokinetics and pharmacodynamics and mechanisms of drug delivery

V.C.3.   Cardiovascular, respiratory, renal, hepatic, and central nervous system physiology, pathophysiology, and therapy

V.C.4.   Metabolic and endocrine effects of surgery and critical illness

V.C.5.   Infectious disease pathophysiology and therapy

V.C.6.   Coagulation abnormalities and therapy

V.C.7.   Normal and abnormal physical and psychological development

V.C.8.   Trauma, including burn, management

V.C.9.   Congenital anomalies and developmental delay

V.C.10. Medical and surgical problems common in children

V.C.11. Use and toxicity of local and general anesthetic agents

V.C.12. Airway problems common in children

V.C.13. Pain management in pediatric patients of all ages

V.C.14. Ethical and legal aspects of care

V.C.15. Transport of critically ill patients

V.C.16. Organ transplantation in children

V.C.17. All pediatric anesthesiology residents should be certified as providers of advanced life support for children.

Subspecialty conferences, including morbidity and mortality conferences, journal reviews, and research seminars, should be regularly attended. Active participation of the subspecialty resident in pediatric anesthesiology in the planning and production of these conferences is essential. However, the faculty should be the conference leaders in the majority of the sessions. Attendance by residents at multidisciplinary conferences, especially those relevant to pediatric anesthesiology, is encouraged.

CHAPTER 4

An Introduction to the Ethical Design, Conduct, and Analysis of Pediatric Clinical Trials

Myron Yaster[1], Jeffrey Galinkin[2] & Mark S. Schreiner[3]

[1]Departments of Anesthesiology, Critical Care Medicine and Pediatrics, The Johns Hopkins University, Baltimore, MD, USA
[2]Department of Anesthesiology and Pediatrics, The Children's Hospital, University of Colorado at Denver, Aurora, CO, USA
[3]Department of Anesthesiology and Critical Care Medicine, The University of Pennsylvania School of Medicine, and The Children's Hospital of Philadelphia, Philadelphia, PA, USA

Introduction

Pharmacology and physiology, drug behavior and organ function are the fundamental underpinnings of perioperative anesthetic practice. At our core, anesthesiologists are physiologists and pharmacologists; we titrate drugs against an individual patient's response to achieve a desired therapeutic goal. Understanding the pharmacokinetics (uptake, distribution, elimination, and sensitivity of a drug's effects in an individual patient) and pharmacodynamics (clinical effects of the drug on effector sites; hemodynamic, respiratory, renal, and central nervous system function) of the drugs we administer is essential for the safe provision of anesthesia. But more fundamentally, how do we know if a therapy will be effective in the first place? Or if we are given a choice of therapies, which one is best? Further, although we titrate drugs to an individual patient's response, how do we know the population kinetics on which to determine how much drug to administer to produce the average or typical response?

Or, over what period of time should a drug be administered and be expected to last? Equally important, how are outcomes determined or tested and over what period of time?

Historically, most studies involving anesthetic drugs and techniques look at the perioperative period as the time frame for outcome. However, what if the effects of these drugs or techniques only reveal themselves weeks or years later? At one time, this would have been considered preposterous. However, we now know from long-term studies where follow-up was years rather than days that the consequences of how an anesthetic was delivered can have profound effects years later [1]. Studies examining the effect of variations in perioperative anesthetic management of adults with coronary artery disease and newborn infants undergoing anesthesia have revealed significant effects years after the anesthetic was provided [1–3].

The randomized, double-blind, placebo-controlled trial (RCT) is the "gold standard" for determining the efficacy

Screen for eligibility

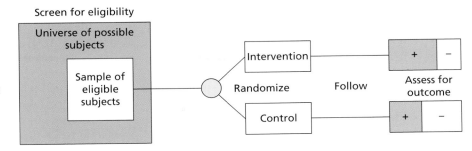

Figure 4.1 A clinical trial is a planned experiment that involves administration or implementation of an intervention to a sample group of subjects who are representative of the general population and is intended to determine the efficacy and safety of the intervention.

and safety of therapeutics. No other study design can provide better evidence for cause and effect between an intervention and an outcome. Unfortunately, ethically acceptable RCTs are very difficult to design when children are participants and there are numerous impediments to practical implementation. When a RCT is not feasible, clinicians must rely on weaker forms of evidence from other trial designs such as cohort studies, case–control studies, and even anecdote. While all of these are valuable, their results are less convincing due to confounding and bias.

No matter what the specifics of the study design, performing a clinical trial is challenging, often expensive and, when done to Good Clinical Practice (GCP) standards, excruciatingly difficult to perform [4]. Clinical trials strain resources and patience and are often viewed by investigators as an ordeal to overcome rather than as a welcomed ally.

New therapies approved for adults rapidly assume the mantle of the "standard of care" for pediatric patients, increasing the barrier to conducting an RCT and encouraging off-label prescribing which is rampant in pediatric practice [5–9]. Psychologically, this creates a very narrow window of time during which investigators are willing to conduct clinical trials of new therapies for children. When either clinicians or patients accept a therapy as effective, they do not want to participate in a study with the risk of enrolling into a placebo or control arm. However, using drugs off-label in children exposes them to ineffective care and untoward side-effects. Children who receive off-label drugs during an inpatient hospitalization have nearly double the likelihood of having an adverse drug reaction [10–12]. It is well established that children can have unique responses to drugs (e.g. weight gain, decreased growth), require different dosages and delivery methods, and often fail to show a therapeutic response even when the therapy provided is very effective for identical problems in adults (e.g. the use of triptans for migraine headaches or selective serotonin reuptake inhibitors (SSRIs) for depression) [13,14].

Given that it is not possible to predict whether children from neonates to adolescents will respond to drugs in the same way as adults, RCTs remain essential. The alterna-

tive to evidence is perpetual uncertainty with acceptance of unproven therapies as if they were effective. In this chapter, we will provide an introduction to clinical trials and discuss the special problems of performing them in infants, children, and adolescents.

What is a clinical trial?

A clinical trial is a planned experiment that involves administration or implementation of an intervention to a group of subjects and is intended to determine the efficacy and safety of the intervention (Fig. 4.1). Although vital, for the purposes of this chapter, we will not discuss clinical trials that involve a single group, such as pharmacokinetic studies. The intervention need not be limited to drugs, biological agents or devices, but could include diets (e.g. preoperative fasting interval), a method or processes of delivering care, or any other procedure that can be manipulated by the investigator. At a defined point in time, the outcomes between one or more groups of subjects who receive the test intervention are compared with those of one or more parallel comparable populations of subjects in a control group.

Common impediments

Nothing can be more frustrating for investigators than to realize that there is a clinical question that requires an RCT for a definitive answer but to be unable to address the question because of organizational, design or execution issues. This can be true not just for investigator-initiated single-center trials; obstacles can also impede industry- or government-sponsored multicenter trials as well. Common impediments in all trials include inadequate planning, protocol development issues, unavailability of subjects, and lack of funding. Furthermore, almost all clinical trial investigators, both in industry and in academia, have unrealistic or overly ambitious timelines for study completion. Indeed, data from the National Institutes of Health (NIH) indicate that 85% of clinical trials fail to complete on time.

Overly ambitious objectives or rushed timelines also result in the need for multiple revisions to protocols, an inability to get contracts between trial sponsors and centers finalized, and investigational review board (IRB, also referred to as research ethics committee) approval delays [15]. (A sponsor or sponsoring agency is the institution, organization or foundation that provides the fiscal and often the administrative and scientific support for a given clinical trial or project.) Inappropriate subject selection and incomplete data collection due to inadequate instructions or collection forms can result in unnecessary adverse events that can compromise the entire study. Unrealistic or overly ambitious timetables may also raise doubts in the minds of the investigators about their ability to participate, forcing them to opt out rather than taking part in the trial. These factors result in approximately 30% of sites in multicenter studies failing to enroll even a single subject. Alternatively, some investigators who are frustrated by the time required to perform a proper trial may begin an inadequately designed trial before all the necessary procedures and support systems have been adequately tested and developed. This not only endangers the trial but, worse, exposes subjects to unnecessary risks of a trial that produces unusable data.

Getting started

To avoid many of these pitfalls, an organized step-wise approach, involving teamwork and an understanding of clinical trials methodology, is necessary [16–18]. More than ever, clinical research is a collaborative venture between clinicians, research methodologists, statisticians, study co-ordinators, IRBs and study participants.

Defining the research question
Research begins with the research question that derives from a clinical problem. The research question is a general formulation and addresses the global question of interest such as "does this drug or medical procedure or device work?" This is insufficient by itself and needs to be refined and translated into specific study objectives. It can take considerable time and negotiation between investigators and sponsors to arrive at mutually agreed study objectives and endpoints and to create universally acceptable definitions for the study measurements. Nevertheless, the time it takes to do this is vital for the success of a trial. The efforts expended upfront will avoid disappointment and potential failure later on.

After collectively reading thousands of protocols, it is clear to the authors that there is confusion about the meaning of three related but distinctly different terms – objectives, endpoints, and hypotheses. The study *objectives* serve as a statement of the general purpose of the clinical trial. In general, they are written in the form "to determine the . . ." and this is followed by the thing to be

determined such as "the efficacy of the study drug for the treatment of . . . or "the pharmacokinetics of oral study drug . . ." An example may help. Assume that a clinical trial will test a new antihypertensive drug and the primary objective could be to determine the efficacy of the study drug for the treatment of moderate-to-severe hypertension in adults age 18–65 years of age. The primary objective serves as the basis for the sample size calculation (see below) while the secondary objectives are often exploratory (inadequate sample size to definitely address the objective).

The study *endpoints* convert each objective into an explicit operational definition that clearly defines how the objective will be measured and achieved. The endpoints specify the comparison groups, the time points at which the comparison will be made, and the exact measurements or evaluation that will be used for the comparison. In our antihypertensive example, the primary endpoint might be the difference in the change in non-invasively measured systolic (or diastolic) blood pressure in mmHg at 4 weeks compared to baseline in the study drug group compared to the placebo control group.

Lastly, there is frequent confusion about where to place the study *hypotheses*. They are often mistakenly included with the study objectives but in reality belong in the protocol statistical method section. The hypotheses are expressed in statistical terms as a null hypothesis and as an alternative hypothesis (see below).

After development of the objectives and endpoints, the next question in any clinical trial is simply: "Is it worth the effort to mount a trial in the first place?" The answer to this question is predicated on the following questions: What is already known about the research question? Is this question worth the time and effort to answer? If I had the results today how would it change my practice? Is it ethically permissible to conduct this study in humans? and finally, Is it feasible to answer this research question with a clinical trial or would an alternative approach be better?

Choice of control group
The choice of the test and control treatments is the obvious and most important next step in designing a clinical trial [19]. The groups must differ from one another and investigators and subjects must be willing to enroll into both. The principle of equipoise is one approach for determining whether or not it is ethically permissible to conduct a comparative trial [20]. When low-quality evidence accumulates suggesting that one treatment may be superior to another, investigators may be reluctant to participate in the trial because they are unwilling to randomize their patients. However, even when the investigator is convinced that the experimental intervention will be superior to the alternative, provided that there is genuine

uncertainty within the clinical community based on the available evidence, then the research question is in a state of equipoise and it is ethical to proceed. There is a long history of unexpected results in clinical trials, often with the placebo group having a survival advantage compared to what was perceived as the preferred treatment [21]. In 50% of the Children's Oncology Group clinical trials, the new study drug fails to outperform the standard treatment arm, emphasizing that frequently we are in a state of true equipoise [22].

By the time pediatric clinical trials begin, data from adults frequently suggest that the drug is active and effective, at least to some extent, for the proposed indication. In this situation, there may not be a state of equipoise. The requirement for true equipoise can be quite constraining and a number of alternative formulations have been proposed to substitute for it [23–25]. Many ethicists contend that in this situation, the decision about whether or not it is ethical to conduct the trial hinges on the risks associated with assignment to the control group (the less advantageous arm of the study). When the potential harms are minor and temporary then it may still be ethical to conduct the trial [26]. For example, a trial of a drug to replace acetaminophen for tension headache or a new treatment for allergic rhinitis could be ethically conducted because in neither situation would subjects suffer undue harm from assignment to a placebo.

The control group may be historical or concurrent and assignment to groups may be via a randomized or non-randomized process. While it is tempting to simply use an historical control to compare to a study intervention, the practice should be avoided. Considerable experience has shown that trials using historical controls are much more likely to conclude that a new therapy is more effective than those using concurrent controls [27].

Choices for concurrent controls include placebo, different doses of the same intervention (dose-ranging or dose–response studies), a different intervention (active control) or a combination of all of the above. The International Conference on Harmonization (ICH) "Choice of Control Group and Related Issues in Clinical Trials" document provides an extensive discussion of the advantages and disadvantages of each of these options [19].

The use of placebo controls remains a contentious and controversial topic [24,28–32]. The US Food and Drug Administration (FDA) has a clear mandate from Congress to only approve drugs, biologics, and devices that have proven to be safe and effective. In making their determinations, it is obvious that the FDA's clear preference is for placebo-controlled trials. Active controlled trials that seek to demonstrate equivalence suffer from the conundrum that if no difference is found between the two intervention arms, then it is possible that neither worked or both worked. As many as 40% of clinical trials for drugs for the treatment of depression, pain, and hypertension (amongst other conditions) fail to demonstrate superiority to placebo, contributing to the reluctance of the FDA to rely on active-controlled trials [32]. Placebo provides assay sensitivity, which means the ability to distinguish an active drug from an inactive one. Placebos also allow an accurate estimation of the magnitude of effect and help distinguish low-frequency adverse events caused by the intervention from background.

While a more complete discussion of this issue is beyond the scope of this chapter, in general, it is ethically permissible to use a placebo control in the following circumstances: whenever there is no proven treatment for the condition or disease, if the available treatments work poorly or have undue toxicities, if the participant has failed to respond to existing alternative therapies, or if there will be no undue discomfort or serious or permanent morbidity as a consequence.

Receipt of placebo is not usually equivalent to the absence of treatment. Frequently subjects receive standard care plus or minus the study intervention. In addition to standard care, there are two other methods that can be included to provide a margin of safety. First is an option for early escape – the study ends when the subject reaches an endpoint rather than after a fixed duration; the second is the use of immediate rescue treatment [19]. For example, in placebo-controlled pain studies, intravenous (IV) patient-controlled analgesia (PCA) morphine has been used as a rescue if the placebo (or study drug or procedure) is ineffective. The use of the rescue, the time to rescue, and the difference in the amount of rescue treatment have been used in some trials as the study endpoints rather than pain scores [33].

For many clinical trials involving anesthetic agents, it is not possible to use a placebo control but it often is for adjuvant therapies. As a result, trials of many anesthetic drugs focus on pharmacodynamics rather than efficacy. For example, trials of a muscle relaxant focus on dose–response, the time of onset and duration of effect rather than on comparisons in efficacy between agents.

Ensuring validity: randomization and allocation concealment

Clinical trials rely on two processes for their validity: masking (or blinding) of allocation assignment and randomization [34]. Masking has two components: concealment of the allocation assignment at the time of randomization and prevention of discovery of the assignment during the trial. We prefer the term masking to blinding because blinding has the potential for confusion, particularly when used in conjunction with a trial where loss of vision is the outcome measure or in a trial involving patients who have lost their vision. Indeed, a common phrase in many studies that we find comical is "the investigators were blinded . . ." It doesn't really mean that the investigators were actually "blinded," rather, it means that the allocation groups were masked. Randomization assures that all confounding variables, known and unknown, are distributed at random and hopefully equally between the two groups. A variety of techniques can be used to generate the treatment assignment including use of a table of random numbers or computer-generated sequences [35–37].

Simple random assignment can result in large imbalances in the number of subjects between the two groups in a trial. There are alternative techniques that ensure that the randomization sequence keeps the number of subjects in both groups relatively equal, both for the study as a whole and, for multicenter trials, within centers [38]. The most frequent approach is to randomize subjects in blocks such as groups of two, four or six subjects, to ensure that the number of subjects is equal within each block. For example, if the block size is two, then subjects are randomized to treatments A and B in the order AB or BA. However, if the treatment assignment is discoverable (e.g. the masking is incomplete), then knowledge of the first subject assignment in each block could permit prediction of what the next subject's assignment would be. Using a larger block size increases the number of possible treatment assignment combinations and makes it harder to predict the subject's assignment.

Another method used to ensure balance between the study groups is permuted block sizes. In this technique, two different size blocks are used at random, making it very difficult to predict treatment allocation. For example, some blocks would consist of four subjects and some would include six. Without knowledge of the block size, it becomes impossible to predict the next subject's treatment group assignment.

The treatment group allocation process must not only be random but the outcome must be concealed, which is the first part of masking. If the investigator knows the group assignment for the next subject, then this can affect their willingness to enroll the subject, can bias the consent process or could lead to measures to manipulate procedures to influence the assignment. There are reports of studies where investigators have held sealed envelopes up to bright lights or found other measures to defeat the randomization schedule to choose the subject's group assignment.

To prevent discovery of the treatment assignment, the statistician should not reveal either the randomization schedule or the block size to any member of the investigative team. In a single-center trial, someone other than the investigator should generate and maintain the randomization sequence. If the study is a drug trial, having a pharmacist not otherwise associated with the trial prepare the study drug for administration is a very effective way of concealing assignment.

When the outcome measure is subjective, the subject, the investigator, and the statistician should ideally all be masked to the subject's treatment assignment. Concealment of treatment assignment after start of the intervention limits expectation bias on the part of the subject and biased assessments by the investigator. If the outcome measure is unbiased, for example death, then it may be less important to maintain masking. Since concealment is key to a valid study, an assessment should be made and included in any publication of the extent to which the masking was preserved during the clinical trial [39].

In comparing two active treatments, it may not be possible to disguise the drugs because of method of administration, size or color of the drug. Using a double dummy approach where both active treatments have matching placebos can be an effective alternative. Each subject takes one of the two active treatments and a placebo to match the other treatment.

For many anesthesia and pain studies, it may be quite difficult to mask the treatment if it involves a volatile anesthetic whose concentration must be monitored or if the intervention is invasive (e.g. an epidural nerve block). When treatment assignment cannot be concealed from the investigator, it may still be possible to prevent the subject from discovering their treatment assignment and to have someone other than the investigator perform the assessments of outcome to minimize bias.

Outcomes measures

Meaningful clinical trial outcomes include clinical events that change an individual's health in some discrete and meaningful way, e.g. prevention of death, prolongation of life, prevention of morbidity, change in quality of life or an improved economic endpoint [40]. All other outcomes, such as change in a physiological variable or a biological measure, are surrogate endpoints [41]. Surrogate endpoints are frequently used in place of clinical events because the variable measured is believed to be correlated to the clinical outcome of interest and because of its perceived utility in detecting treatment differences. Surrogates may be easier to assess but unless proven to predict the outcome of interest, they are poor substitutes for pivotal trials. In the Cardiac Arrhythmia Suppression Trial (CAST), those patients receiving encainide or flecainide had less ventricular ectopy (surrogate outcome) but nearly three times the number of deaths as the placebo group [21].

In a hypothetical clinical trial designed to determine which of several different anesthetics had the best outcome for children with upper respiratory infection, hemoglobin-oxygen saturation <94% would be considered a surrogate measure of adverse respiratory outcome compared to pneumonia requiring hospitalization, brain injury or death. However, the relationship of hemoglobin-oxygen saturation <94% to death, morbidity, quality of life or cost is in fact very tenuous. Therefore, it is always better to select an outcome directly related to something that matters to the patient or the healthcare system (cost).

Sample size and power

Even an experienced investigator must consult with a biostatistician early in the protocol development process. As experienced an investigator as David Sackett has sagely advised that "If you don't start looking for a biostatistician co-principal investigator the same day that you start formulating your study question, you are a fool, and deserve neither funding nor a valid answer" [17].

A key decision in any clinical trial is to determine the number of patients needed to detect a clinically important difference in outcome with specified type I and II error protection [18,42]. A type I error is the probability of rejecting the null hypothesis when it is true and is usually designated in most formulas by the Greek letter alpha (α). The null hypothesis postulates no underlying difference in the population or groups being compared with the factor, trait, characteristic or condition of interest. In clinical trials this means that the true underlying effect of the test treatment, as expressed by a specified outcome measure, is no more or less than that for the control treatment. A type II error is the probability of accepting the null hypothesis as true when it is false and is usually designated in most formulas by the Greek letter beta (β) with power defined as 1-β. Power in this context is the probability of rejecting the null hypothesis when it is false. Thus, calculations based on type I and II error and power will determine the number of patients needed in a trial and will often determine a trial's feasibility, cost, and the number of study sites needed to perform the study.

Typically power is chosen as either 0.8 or 0.9, which means that if a real difference exists of the magnitude specified, the trial has an 80% or 90% chance of detecting that difference. The variables in the power calculation include the magnitude of the clinically important difference, the number of events observed, and the variability (standard deviation). The greater the difference or the number of events anticipated, the fewer the number of subjects required. The greater the variability in outcome of interest (i.e. the wider the standard deviation), the greater the number of subjects required in a trial. Unfortunately, few treatments have as dramatic an effect as most investigators presuppose. Indeed, a 25% effect is large [43]. Overestimating the efficacy of the new treatment will result in an underpowered trial and has enormous ethical impact. If a trial is underpowered, the study

cannot achieve its stated objectives and exposing/enrolling patients into it is considered ethically unacceptable because it exposes patients to unnecessary risk [44,45].

In our experience, the variables that enter into the power calculation are amongst the most manipulated and debated elements in a study design. Often, when the number of patients needed is large, event rates are adjusted or the magnitude of the anticipated effect is exaggerated. With or without these manipulations, in worse-case situations, if the number needed to study is so large, it may make the study impossible to perform and will force cancellation of the study in its entirety. On the other hand, if the study is manipulated to make it easy to perform by manipulating the pre-trial assumption regarding the number or outcome events, the results of the study may become inconsequential or invalid. Many have called for a re-evaluation of the methods used to estimate sample size, preferring the use of the width of confidence intervals or effect sizes rather than simply performing power calculations. This further underlines the importance of collaborating closely with a biostatistician during the initial planning phases of a trial [44,45].

Deciding on the number of subjects needed for a trial may take months of interactions between the investigators, biostatisticians and, when a new drug is being used, the pharmaceutical sponsor and the regulatory agencies supervising the study. Although it is beyond the scope of this chapter to discuss the details of how one calculates for type I and II errors or estimates the required sample size, we have referenced several good reviews and textbooks that will provide an overview [46–48]. Interestingly, the choice of type I and II error protection is somewhat arbitrary. At first blush, the study team may want a trial that prevents both types of error. In reality, this may not be possible and the final decision as to which factor should take precedence may depend on the medical and practical implications of the two kinds of errors. Thus, relatively high error rates ($\alpha = 0.10$ and $\beta = 0.2$) are usually used for preliminary trials that are likely to be replicated. On the other hand, smaller error rates ($\alpha = 0.01$ and $\beta = 0.05$) are used when replication is unlikely.

Single center versus multicenter

Anesthesiologists (the authors included) have most frequently resorted to single-center trials because they are relatively easy to mount and carry out. The research personnel are all located within the same institution, know each other, and can achieve a higher degree of uniformity in the execution of the study procedures and data collection. Perhaps most importantly, they are significantly less expensive and more efficient to perform because the bureaucratic structure required to design, execute, and supervise a multicenter trial is unnecessary.

The publication and academic promotion issues that are so critical for academic investigators are more clear-cut and without conflict.

Indeed, in our opinion, publication and the recognition investigators receive for publication are amongst the most important driving forces creating resistance to participation in multicenter pediatric clinical trials; it is also one of the least publically discussed issues. Promotion at most academic institutions is based on the number, quality, and originality of, and authorship position in published papers. In single-center trials, the investigator's name will be listed and may even be the first or senior author, the most prized position for academic promotion. On the other hand, in multicenter trials, pharmaceutical sponsors often base authorship on recruitment success and not on intellectual contribution. Indeed, most investigators are often only listed in the footnotes of the journal article within the membership of the study group. Furthermore, if the study is an industry-sponsored trial, authorship is often considered "tainted." Some have advocated abandoning authorship for contributorship, where each individual's role in the research is listed at the end of the publication rather than perpetuating the current inaccurate system [49]. Academic centers and promotion committees would need to agree to reward contributions listed rather than just authorship for this model to take hold.

While most academicians prefer the single-center model, there are serious limitations to this model. One center, with only a few investigators, may find it difficult, if not impossible, to recruit enough participants in a timely fashion. Further, when all the subjects come from within the same geographic area and are treated by a small group of clinicians, the results may have internal validity but may lack external validity, making them less generalizable to other practice settings [50]. Medical care has fortunately also reduced the number of poor outcomes, making differences in discrete clinical events that much harder to detect. For example, survival for childhood cancer has improved dramatically. Similarly, death related to anesthesia has dropped precipitously over the past 30 years. As a result of these successes, the size of the expected differences in outcome between two treatment groups has grown smaller. Since power is based on the number of events, not the number of subjects, better outcomes overall have translated into the need for larger and larger sample sizes.

The only realistic way to conduct many trials that address vital questions is to collaborate on large, simple trials, with multiple sites involved in enrolling, treating, and following up subjects using a common study protocol and data collection tool [51]. Obviously, the physical separation between sites requires a more systematic approach to documentation and data collection and an administrative and organizational structure to make it all happen, all of which are very expensive [52]. The NIH has been creating a mechanism to facilitate multicenter trials through networks such as the Clinical Translational Science Award centers (CTSA), and various subspecialty component groups focusing on rare diseases and at-risk populations have done so as well (e.g. cystic fibrosis, sickle cell disease, Marfan syndrome, etc.). Additionally, multicenter data management software has made computerization and standardization of data entry much easier. Before embarking on a clinical trial, it is important for the investigator to check for these institutional resources because they can be invaluable (and often free) in setting up a clinical trial.

Funding

All clinical trials cost money, lots of money. Where the money comes from and how much there is to spend are two of the key stumbling blocks in all clinical trials. Ideally, funding should come from a mix of private and public sources, including the government, the drug and device industry, and health insurance companies. Unfortunately, this ideal is rarely met and much of the funding comes from the government, private grants, and the pharmaceutical industry. The NIH, the primary healthcare research funding agency of the US government, rarely funds perioperative anesthetic research. Indeed, there is no specific institute within the NIH for anesthesiology. Further, the NIH cannot possibly bear the full burden of anesthesia-based research because of its priorities to primarily fund basic science research. Also, until very recently, industry was also unwilling to mount pediatric clinical trials because the pediatric market was viewed as too small to justify the return on investment, particularly because, as we will discuss shortly, most drugs used in pediatrics are used off-label anyway.

There is no easy answer to the lack of funding conundrum in pediatric perioperative anesthetic and analgesic trials. Despite the difficulties, it is essential to try. Giving up without a significant effort only assures failure. It has been our experience that if the project is worth doing, funding will be found either from traditional sources like the government and industry or from not so traditional sources like private and public foundations or local philanthropists. Often overlooked, there are anesthesia-specific foundations and societies that fund both novice and well-established investigators. These include the Foundation for Anesthesia Education Research (FAER), the Anesthesia Patient Safety Foundation (APSF), the International Anesthesia Research Society (IARS), and the subspecialty anesthesia societies, such as the Society for Pediatric Anesthesia (SPA). Additionally, many public foundations, such as the Mayday Fund and the Bill and

Melinda Gates Foundation, provide research funding for pediatric clinical trials, particularly pain trials.

Another funding source that is closer to home, and one that is often poorly mined by anesthesiologists, requires raising funds from within the community in which the trial will take place. Within every locality there are philanthropists, corporations, and community organizations that can be recruited to support anesthetic research, education, and patient care. Although hospitals in general and children's hospitals in particular are very good at this, anesthesia departments are notoriously poor at it.

Developing and raising money for research endowments or endowed chairs specifically designed to provide seed money for young and established investigators is essential for clinical trials and for our specialty.

Finally, regardless of how one obtains funding, the funding source(s) must always be disclosed to the IRB, the institutional conflict of interest office, and to the public when patients are being recruited to enter into the trial and when the data and conclusions generated by the trial are presented in public forums or published in the lay or scientific press.

Phases of testing a new drug

A considerable proportion of anesthesia research involves testing of drugs. All studies involving investigational new drugs require an Investigational New Drug (IND) application issued by the FDA before testing can move from animals to humans.

The first stage of testing a new drug is called phase I (Fig. 4.2). Phase I trials generate preliminary information on the absorption, distribution, metabolism, elimination and safety of a drug. Phase I studies typically involve 20–80 subjects and are usually conducted in healthy adult human volunteers. However, some phase I trials, for example chemotherapeutics targeted to pediatric cancer, may need to be conducted in children. In contrast to phase I studies in adults, pediatric participants must have the target disease or condition. Phase I studies are rarely if ever done with a comparison group; if one is included, it is typically the study drug at a different dose.

After phase I studies have established the basic pharmacology and safety profile for the new drug, testing proceeds to phase II. These trials explore the efficacy in individuals with the disease or condition of interest, usually using surrogate measures of efficacy (e.g. decrease in blood pressure or reduction in tumor size rather than mortality). These are well-controlled trials designed to provide preliminary evidence of efficacy, explore the useful dosage range of the drug, and supplement the data about the safety profile of the drug. They often include additional pharmacokinetic testing during repeat dosing and at the anticipated therapeutic dose. Phase II trials frequently involve a few hundred individuals.

Phase I and II studies frequently explore the relationship between the dose administered and the physiological response. Typically, five or six doses are needed to establish the complete range of responses – ranging from the highest no-response dose, the lowest dose with a meaningful response and up to the dose beyond which either no further effect or undue side-effects are seen. When only two or three doses are studied, then the trial is more appropriately termed a dose-ranging trial. Given the expected intraindividual variation, dose-ranging trials generally require dosages that are a factor of 3–4 to clearly distinguish one dose from the other. Failure to establish the correct dose prior to conducting efficacy studies can result in failed efficacy trials or unnecessary toxicity [53].

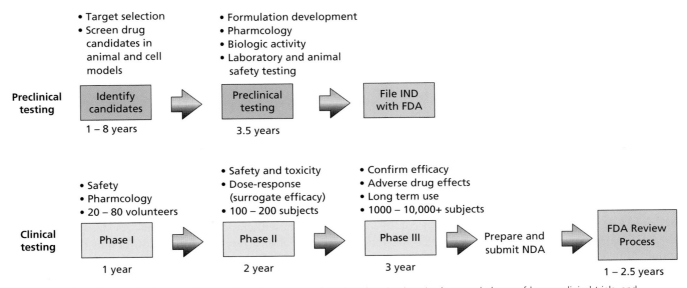

Figure 4.2 All studies investigating new drugs go through a process of preclinical testing in animals, several phases of human clinical trials, and culminate in a new drug application and approval by the FDA. The process takes years, with failure possible all along the way.

At the end of phase II testing, preliminary evidence of efficacy and safety has been established. For chemotherapeutic drugs, it is also necessary to identify the maximal tolerated dose (MTD). Based on dose–response studies, the dosage for confirmatory trials of efficacy is selected. At the end of phase II testing the sponsor and the FDA meet to establish the endpoints to be used for the phase III or pivotal trials.

Phase III trials are the final stage of new drug development and are designed to enable drug approval and labeling by the FDA. The drug label, distributed as a package insert, is the document approved by the FDA and furnished by the manufacturer of a drug for use when dispensing the drug. It lists a summary of the basic information about the pharmacology of the drug, its approved uses (conditions, populations, recommended dosage), contraindications, and potential side-effects.

Phase III trials are usually large, randomized, controlled clinical trials designed to confirm both the efficacy and safety of the drug. It is a given that all drugs provide a trade-off between their benefits and their side-effects. The results must be generalizable to the wider population. Surrogate measures of efficacy are no longer sufficient to support a labeling indication. For a cancer chemotherapy drug, improved survival would need to be established rather than simply reduction in tumor size. A new pain medication would need to not only demonstrate a statistically significant difference in pain score between groups, the difference would need to be large enough to be considered clinically important.

When the sponsor believes that they have established the efficacy and safety of the drug for a specific indication, they submit a New Drug Application (NDA) to the FDA to label and market the drug to the public. Of every 1000 drugs that enter preclinical testing, only 100 drugs enter phase I testing in humans, approximately 70 go on to phase II testing and 30–40 make it into phase III testing. Only about 12–15 result in an NDA submission and of those, only nine or 10 are approved (see Fig. 4.2).

Once a drug is approved, the sponsor must continue to conduct postmarket surveillance. Surprisingly, many serious adverse drug effects and interactions are only discovered after a drug has been approved for use and released into the marketplace. In reality, this shouldn't be surprising at all. At the time of initial approval, most newly approved drugs have actually been tested in only 1000–5000 people. Although to investigators and sponsors this is a huge number of people, in reality it is too small to detect rare but potentially very important side-effects. Most rare but serious side-effects occur in less than 1:10,000 individuals [54]. Obviously, this incidence would be below the radar and will not be reliably detected at the time of drug approval if less than 5000 people were studied. This underscores the importance of postmarket surveillance and explains the headline-making news accompanying the withdrawal of an approved drug from the marketplace, a process that occurs in approximately 1.5–5% of all newly approved drugs, depending on the epoch [55].

Some of the recently withdrawn drugs include rofecoxib, a COX-II inhibitor removed because of an increased risk of myocardial infarction, rapacuronium, a short-acting muscle relaxant, removed because of severe or fatal bronchospasm, hydromorphone extended-release because of the risk of accidental overdose, and ximelagatran, removed because of hepatotoxicity. Rare cases of idiosyncratic hepatotoxicity and increased risk of myocardial infarction may be difficult to detect in phase III trials. The safety of rosiglitazone has recently been the subject of considerable public debate, due to increased risk of cardiac events [56]. The absence of large, well-controlled trials focused on detecting increased cardiac risk contributed to the FDA's decision not to withdraw the drug from the market and only restrict marketing. However, the drug has been withdrawn in Europe.

None of the risks associated with these drugs was detected during initial testing and the risks came to light from postmarketing surveillance rather than as the result of phase IV trials. However, when common patterns emerge, the FDA and its European counterpart the European Medicines Agency (EMA) can impose additional requirements for the approval of all new drugs. For example, as the result of several drugs (e.g. astemazole, terfenadine and cisapride) being withdrawn due to cardiac arrhythmias in the 1990s, all new drugs are now tested for possible effects on prolonging the QTc interval.

To ensure and evaluate the long-term safety and efficacy of the newly approved drug following FDA approval and drug licensure, the FDA may require phase IV trials [57]. The pharmaceutical sponsor may also choose to explore additional indications for the drug or to study the drug in wider populations than studied in the phase III trials. Unfortunately, many phase IV studies do not have sound scientific designs and are funded by the pharmaceutical sponsor as seeding trials to increase interest in the drug and to generate sales.

Timing of pediatric clinical trials

Ideally, all new therapeutic interventions would be rigorously tested before introduction into clinical practice. The reality is far different, with clinical adoption of new therapies far outstripping a solid evidence base on which to make these therapeutic judgments. As stated previously, there is often a very narrow window of time during which it is feasible to test a new therapy, particularly for children. After introduction into practice, interventions approved for adults become "standard of care" for children, even without the benefit of adequate evidence of their efficacy or safety in children. Indeed, this is one of the ongoing conundrums of small case reports, case series, and other forms of uncontrolled trials that flood the medical literature. The recent mandate to conduct clinical trials in children has clearly demonstrated that trials are not only feasible but also essential. Children have been shown to experience unique adverse effects (e.g. growth impairment and suicidality), require different dosage levels or formulations, and may fail to respond to a drug in the same way that adults do, even when the disease is the same (e.g. triptans for migraine headache and SSRIs for depression) [13,14]. Clearly, the adage that "children are not small adults" has been proven true over and over again.

Therefore, the ideal time to start pediatric trials is before or just after a new treatment is first approved, before preconceived notions regarding its merit develop. Unfortunately, this is rarely the case because as we will describe, the planning, organization, and structure of a proper trial take a fair amount of time, patience, discipline, and money – qualities that many investigators unfortunately lack.

Anesthetic and pharmacological research in pediatrics

Although most children can't swallow pills, few drugs are available in liquid formulations. While pharmacies can make extemporaneous formulations, these must be used without information about bio-availability or palatability. Changes in formulation and route of administration affect uptake, distribution, and ultimately efficacy in unpredictable ways. "Inadequate information exposes children to age-specific adverse reactions, ineffective treatment due to inappropriate dosing, and lack of access to new drugs because physicians tend to prescribe less effective known medications" [58]. Additionally, insurance companies and other third-party payers may refuse payment for off-label use of medications. Indeed, in the past, so little pharmacokinetic and pharmacodynamic testing was performed in children that by 1968 they were termed "therapeutic orphans" [59].

To remedy the lack of appropriate labeling in children and in pediatric subpopulations (newborns, infants, school age, and adolescents), the US Congress enacted the FDA Modernization and Accountability Act (FDAMA) of 1997, its successor, the Best Pharmaceuticals for Children Act (BPCA, 2002) and the Pediatric Research Equity Act (PREA, 2003). Taken together, these laws were intended to promote standards and requirements for the use and labeling of drugs in children. The FDAMA and BPCA offered pharmaceutical companies incentives to study pediatric indications for approved drugs while the PREA required that all new drugs and biologics, all new formu-

lations and indications for approved drugs be tested and studied in children. The PREA and BPCA were reauthorized into a single law as part of the FDA Amendments Act (FDAAA, 2007). These programs have been tremendously successful, with labeling changes documented for well over 100 drugs and counting [12–14,60,61].

Despite the major advances in labeling drugs for children made since 1997, most of the drugs used in infants, children, and adolescents during the perioperative period are still administered off-label, that is, they have not been thoroughly tested for efficacy or safety in pediatric trials. One of the main reasons for this is that most anesthetic and pain management drugs are older and had no patent life or exclusivity remaining at the time the FDAMA was signed into law. However, some drugs, including desflurane, ondansetron, midazolam, milrinone, oxycodone, tramadol and sevoflurane, have been studied under the FDAMA or BPCA. Looking forward, all new drugs must be studied under the PREA.

Unfortunately, off-label administration of older medications to pediatric patients often goes beyond the indications on the approved label and by routes of administration neither tested nor approved even in adults. It is hard to extrapolate the data available from the relatively healthy adult participants in most phase III trials to chronically ill adults, the aged, pregnant women, infants, children, adolescents, and to both adult and pediatric critically ill patients without consideration of the maturation of drug-metabolizing enzymes or alterations in sites of action over the normal course of aging. To deal with the issue of older drugs, the BPCA included funding for off-patent drugs under a partnership between the NIH and the FDA. Studies are under way for nitroprusside and lorazepam but progress has been quite slow.

Ethical aspects of clinical trials

Overview

There is a long history of shame involving human research, from the Nazi war crimes in which lethal medical experiments were conducted on Jews and other subjugated people, to the Tuskegee syphilis study, which was conducted by the US Public Health Service from 1932 to 1972, in which minority men with syphilis were enrolled to study natural disease progression without being informed that they had the disease and were not treated after penicillin became available.

In the United States, the Belmont Report written by the National Commission for the Protection of Human Subjects of Biomedical and Behavioral Research identified beneficence, respect for persons, and justice as the essential ethical principles that should underpin research involving human subjects [62]. These principles are not merely ideals; they have been translated into the federal research regulations known as the Common Rule (45 CFR 46) and into the FDA research regulations (21 CFR 50 and 56). An excellent review has proposed that there are seven requirements for ensuring the ethical conduct of clinical research, referring back to the fundamental principles articulated in the Belmont Report [63]. Despite considerable progress, the death of Jesse Gelsinger in a gene transfer trial at the University of Pennsylvania in 1999 served to increase the attention on compliance with federal regulations, conflicts of interest in research, and clinical trials oversight by institutions [64]. For more information concerning federal regulations, we refer the reader to the federal websites [65–67].

Investigational review board review and approval

All institutions in the United States who receive federal funding for research must have a Federal Wide Assurance (FWA) issued by the Office for Human Research Protections (OHRP). The FWA is the institution's assurance to the government that it will follow the federal regulations guiding human research. Worldwide, the Declaration of Helsinki first adopted by the World Medical Association in 1964 and amended repeatedly (most recently in 2008) serves as an important expression of clinical research ethics worldwide. The Declaration is important for international trials but does not supersede American law and federal regulations. The FDA has recently adopted the International Conference on Harmonisation Guidelines on Good Clinical Practice to supplant the Declaration [68]. Other organizations with important clinical research ethics statements include the Council of International Organization and Medical Sciences (CIOMS) guidelines on the ethical conduct of clinical trials and the World Health Organization (WHO) operational guidelines for ethics committees that review biomedical research. Some organizations have produced more specific guidelines for pediatric clinical trials, including the EMA [69]. All these organizations share a common ethical perspective, namely, that the well-being of the individual research subject must take precedence over all other interests.

A fundamental principle of all clinical research mandated by US federal regulations (as well as by the CIOMS, WHO, EMA and the Declaration of Helsinki internationally) is the requirement for independent review and approval by a research ethics committee prior to initiation of any research protocol involving human subjects. In the United States these ethics committees are known as institutional review boards (IRBs) and consist of five or more individuals with diverse backgrounds in clinical research, medicine, law, research ethics, biostatistics, nursing, and, when children are involved, pediatrics [70]. To ensure independence and outside perspectives, at least one member of the IRB must be unaffiliated with the institution in which the research takes place and at least one member must be a non-scientific person, who preferentially is representative of the community surrounding the trial site's institution. Research that is no more than minimal risk can be reviewed using expedited procedures with review by just the chair of the IRB. Some types of minimal risk research are even eligible for waiver of informed consent (Box 4.1). In reality, most clinical trials are greater than minimal risk and require review by the convened board of the IRB. IRBs generally have a very formal application process that requires extensive documentation of the elements of the trial. Assembling and preparing this documentation is laborious, time consuming, and expensive, with many IRBs charging a fee for submission that can run into thousands of dollars. This cost and the cost of preparing the documentation for submission are often overlooked in trial design and implementation.

Typically, the documentation required by the IRB includes copies of the protocol, the informed consent form and assent documents (see below), copies of any advertisements and brochures that will be used to recruit

---

Box 4.1 Waiver or alteration of consent for minimal risk research

To approve such a waiver or alteration, the IRB must find and document that:

- the research involves no more than minimal risk to the subjects
- the waiver or alteration will not adversely affect the rights and welfare of the subjects
- the research could not practically be carried out without the waiver or alteration
- whenever appropriate, the subjects will be provided with additional pertinent information after participation.

Source: *US Department of Health and Human Services Regulations: 45 CFR 46.116(d)*

Examples of minimal risk research not requiring informed consent from patient, parent, or guardian:

- retrospective medical record review of anesthetic techniques for several hundred patients, where the process of finding patients and obtaining consent would prevent the study from being done
- retrospective medical record review of hundreds or thousands of anesthetics for complications, e.g. laryngospasm
- research from already existing large databases, i.e. state Medicaid databases, University Health Consortium, U.S. Agency for Healthcare Research and Quality Kids' Inpatient Database (KID), Child Health Corporation of America (CHCA) Database
- research involving only materials (data, documents, records, or specimens) that have been collected, or will be collected solely for non-research purposes (such as medical treatment or diagnosis). Examples: excess waste blood or urine for a novel biomarker assay technique; height and weight data from a large population of children to determine incidence of obesity in a given population presenting for anesthesia.

study participants, study data collection instruments, the investigational drug Investigators' Brochure, funding sources, and revelation of any conflicts of interest by the study investigators. Increasingly, many IRBs also require a detailed plan for data management, genetic specimen security and for how protection of subject privacy and confidentiality of data will be maintained. Finally, many institutions require documentation confirming that participating investigators have taken and passed institutionally mandated courses in research ethics, patient safety, billing, and confidentiality protection.

For multicenter research studies, a "central" IRB offers many potential time-saving, organizational efficiencies, and cost advantages [71]. A central IRB acts on behalf of a local IRB by reviewing and approving a trial proposal. Its organizational composition and process of review are identical to a local IRB. However, unlike a local IRB, the central IRB can simultaneously serve as the IRB of record for numerous sites. Central IRBs can be located either in an academic center or, as is most common, in one of many for-profit centers. Although the cost of submission and processing is often higher than a local institution's IRB, it is both much cheaper in the short and long term because of its center-by-center cost and is much more time efficient. Some have even advocated that the ethical oversight is superior when just one IRB takes responsibility for the trial [72]. Indeed, nothing is more expensive in a trial than not being able to start and enroll patients while awaiting IRB approval. Because of this, it is a favored method of the pharmaceutical industry.

Regardless of how a proposal is reviewed, the process often takes 3 months or more. For many investigators and sponsors, this delay becomes a source of friction and frustration. Although this is understandable, it can be made significantly more onerous if the IRB submission itself is inadequate or poorly conceived and written. It is our experience that many IRB reviews are prolonged by sponsor or investigator revisions, amendments, and by the rush to submission itself. Our mantra in protocol development and submission is to "measure twice and cut once." The trial planning process should ensure that there is sufficient time for both the initial IRB review as well the review of the IRB's requested modifications to the application, protocol, and consent documents. Finally, contracting issues also take time and are more frequently the rate-limiting step in getting a trial started. Again, it is our experience that it is far better and more efficient to do these in tandem than sequentially.

Special considerations when children are participants

The principle of respect for persons, which encompasses the right of the individual to self-determination, requires that investigators obtain the informed consent of participants prior to enrolling them in a clinical trial. Since children cannot legally give their consent and may be unable to comprehend the information about the trial, they are considered a vulnerable population in clinical research. Subpart D of both the Common Rule (45 CFR 46) and the FDA research regulations (21 CFR 50 and 56) contains additional protections for children. Extraordinary risk of harm is permissible when those risks are outweighed by the prospect for direct benefit, such as in an oncology trial. When the research offers no prospect of direct benefit, Subpart D limits the amount of risk to which the child can be exposed. It also delineates the requirements for parental permission and child assent. There are four ascending categories of risk/benefit that have corresponding increased levels of scrutiny (Box 4.2) (45 CFR 46 and 21 CFR 50: Subpart D).

Box 4.2 Federal classification for pediatric research

§46.404 and § 50.51: Research not involving greater than minimal risk

- IRB determines minimal risk
- Adequate provisions are made for soliciting assent from the child and consent from the parent or guardian
- In the State of Maryland, even this level of study must be of direct benefit to the patient

§46.405 and §50.52: Research involving greater than minimal risk but presenting the prospect of direct benefit to the child

- IRB justifies the risk by anticipated benefit to the child
- The anticipated benefit-to-risk ratio is at least as favorable as the current available alternative therapy
- Adequate provisions are made for soliciting assent from the child and consent from the parent or guardian

§46.406 and §50.53: Research involving greater than minimal risk and no prospect of direct benefit to the child but likely to yield generalizable knowledge about the disorder or condition

- IRB determines that the risk represents a minor increase over minimal risk
- The intervention or procedure presents experiences to subjects that are reasonably commensurate with those inherent in their actual or expected medical, dental, psychological, social or educational situations
- The intervention or procedure is likely to yield generalizable knowledge which is of vital importance for understanding or amelioration of the subject's disorder or condition
- Adequate provisions are made for soliciting assent from the child and consent from the parent or guardian

§46.407 and § 50.54: Research not otherwise approveable that presents an opportunity to understand, prevent or alleviate problems affecting the health and welfare of children

Informed consent is not simply a document that requires a signature; it is a process that involves detailed ongoing explanations regarding the purpose of the trial, the nature of the procedures, the risks and potential benefits, and the alternatives to the research intervention and procedures. Components of the informed consent process include an assessment by the physician of the competence and decision-making capacity of the subject, disclosure, and the assurance, as much as is possible, that the individual has the freedom to choose the medical alternatives without coercion or manipulation. Further, subjects must be told explicitly that they can withdraw their consent and discontinue trial participation at any time without affecting the quality of their care and by whom and where it is provided.

Since children cannot legally or developmentally provide consent, the child's parents or guardians serve as surrogate decision makers for them and provide permission to participate. Just as in clinical care, there is an expectation that parents will make their decision for research participation based on the best interests of their child. Studies that have greater than minimal risk (see Box 4.2) without prospect for direct benefit to the child must be approved under the provisions of §46.406 or 407 or §50.53 or 54. These regulations require an added protection: the need to get the permission of both parents (when it is practical to do so).

The assent of the child is required whenever the child is deemed capable of comprehending the required information [73,74]. Assent must be active and affirmative; failure to disagree does not constitute assent. In contradistinction to the requirements for consent, assent does not require the child to make a risk/benefit assessment. The assent process should disclose the purpose of the research, the nature of the procedures, and the right to withdraw assent at any time. Obtaining the assent of child participants requires an awareness of the child's cognitive abilities and the investigator's ability to describe the therapy, procedure, and trial objectives in terms that the child or adolescent can understand in age-appropriate language. In general, children less than 7 years of age are thought to be incapable of decision-making capacity and of providing assent. Children between 7 and 14 are in a gray zone and IRBs are quite variable in their requirements. In practice, we try to obtain assent for research trials in all mentally competent children older than 7 years of age. When assent is required, the requirement for documentation will be determined by the local IRB. Some require a separate written assent form and others just documentation of assent on the consent form [75,76].

Level of acceptable risk

Perhaps the unique aspect of pediatrics clinical research concerns the limits of acceptable risk. The definitions of minimal risk and a minor increase over minimal risk are key to understanding when research is approvable. When a clinical trial has risks that are no greater than minimal, any child can take part (§46.404 and §50.51). However, if the risks are more than a minor increase above minimal, than the trial is not possible unless there is a prospect for direct benefit to the child (§46.405 and §50.52). The definition of minimal risk is inherently confusing because embedded in it are two separate standards: the routine examination standard and the daily life standard. While the risks of routine examination are essentially trivial, the risks of daily life are considerable [77]. Almost all IRBs will consider a clinical trial involving administration of an investigational drug, no matter how innocuous, to be at least a minor increase above minimal risk.

It is ironic that the gravest risk for a considerable proportion of pediatric research is the risk of auto accident during the trip to the clinic. The risk of death from a car ride (adult driver) varies from 0.06 to 0.6 per million car trips. The daily cumulative likelihood of death, predominantly from car accidents and drowning, is 1.5 per million children per day. The likelihood of hospitalization and an emergency department visit varies between 1.0–2.1 and 6.4–64 per million children per day depending on the age of the child [77]. American Society of Anesthesiologists physical status I or II children undergoing general anesthesia currently have an estimated risk of death of approximately 4–5 per million (1:200,000). Thus, riding in a car, which is part of the risks of daily life, would be considered minimal risk, whereas receiving a general anesthetic, which is riskier, is at least a minor increase above minimal risk.

To avoid the possibility of exposing children to too high a level of risk, some within in the research ethics community believe that there should be just a single standard for risk and generally they favor risks closer to the routine examination standard [78]. Adoption of this unified standard would have a chilling effect on pediatric research. Part of the discrepancy between various IRBs in their decision making is due to the difference in their threshold for these two definitions.

Benefits

Benefits in clinical research can be direct, indirect or both. Research offers a prospect for direct benefit when there is a reasonable and plausible expectation, based on prior research, preclinical data or other basis, that participants will receive a meaningful clinical benefit [78]. Clinical trials that have greater than a minor increase above minimal risk are only permissible for studies that offer a prospect for direct benefit. As long as the prospects for benefit outweigh the risks and are at least as good as the alternatives available outside the research, the IRB can approve the research (§46.405 and §50.52).

If the research or a component of the research is purely for research purposes and is not for the participants' direct benefit, the IRB can only approve the research if the risks are limited to a minor increase above minimal risk (§46.406 or §50.53). Since the definition of minimal risk is controversial, it should be expected that the definition of minor increase is controversial too. Rid et al have recently proposed a rubric for assessing risk which requires that all the probabilities for all negligible, small, moderate, significant, major, severe, and catastrophic harms be defined for each intervention and then compared to the risks of daily life [79]. Investigators know much more about the procedures proposed than the IRB. It is their responsibility to provide the IRB with as much data as possible about the probability and magnitude of all possible harms from the procedure or intervention to assist the IRB in making its determination.

States also differ in what is permissible. In the extreme, Maryland does not allow non-therapeutic pediatric research unless there is a prospect for direct patient benefit, even for minimal-risk research. In an important case involving one of the author's (MY) medical institutions (Grimes v. Kennedy Krieger Institute 366 Md 29, 782, A2d, 807, 2001), the plaintiffs were children enrolled in a study to evaluate different methods of lead paint exposure and abatement in Baltimore city homes [80]. The plaintiffs alleged that they were encouraged to remain in the study houses so that their lead levels could be monitored, even if the houses still had lead paint. In the study, one child had elevated blood lead levels but his parents were never informed of this finding. The Maryland court of appeals ruled that "otherwise healthy children should not be subjects of non-therapeutic research that has the potential to be harmful to the child. It is first and foremost the responsibility of the researcher to see to the harmlessness of such non-therapeutic research. Consent of parents can never relieve the researchers of this duty." Litton and Miller express the more common view that there are differences and limits to the duties of an investigator compared to a clinician [81].

Coercion and undue inducements

Recruiting subjects can create or cross a very real line between persuasion and coercion. Coercion of subjects can include manipulating or misusing information, or instilling fear that non-participation will result in withdrawal of or inferior medical care. Many institutions consider it coercive to be both the principal investigator and also the individual's primary physician. Coercion is a threat and should be distinguished from undue inducement, a reward so generous that subjects ignore their better judgment and assume risks that they would not otherwise be willing to endure.

Undue inducement means payment so excessive that it makes it hard for subjects with limited means (economically vulnerable subjects) to decline participation. Examples of inducements can include indirect benefits of participation such as increased access to care or excessive financial remuneration. Indirect benefits of participation such as access to clinical experts, reduced waiting time for clinic visits, door-to-door transportation, and free care including study drugs during and after the trial can be quite persuasive incentives. The provision of free care and drugs and shortened wait times can be very powerful incentives to participate indeed.

There can be a fine line between fair subject payment and undue inducement. Reasonable compensation is ethical and gives all individuals the opportunity to take part in research without experiencing financial hardship. There is no evidence that moderate payment negatively affects subjects' judgment [82]. The object in designing a budget should be to try to make payment neutral.

Payments can be broken down into four components: reimbursement for expenses, compensation for time and effort, gifts of appreciation, and incentives [83]. Incentives are almost universally forbidden by IRBs. Appreciation gifts to subjects should be of nominal value. If participation imposes no travel or other burdens, then it may be inappropriate to include any payment. When subjects must return to the hospital or clinic for follow-up, payment of travel costs (reimbursement) and lost work time of the parents (compensation) is absolutely fair and expected [84]. When the child participant has to complete procedures, such as diaries, or must forego leisure activities, it is fair to compensate them for their time and effort as well as their parents [85,86]. Payments to children need to be age appropriate; children less than 9 years generally don't understand the relationship between the amount of effort and size of payment and should be paid with a fixed-size payment [73].

Operational planning and trial execution

As with any large-scale project, a clinical trial has several stages that must be managed for the trial to be run and completed successfully. Each has specific features and timelines for completion and each is associated with pitfalls that, if not dealt with, will lead to failure and frustration. For most clinical trials, the stages include initial design, feasibility assessment, protocol development, data management and document preparation, subject recruitment/screening and enrollment, study treatment and follow-up, close-out and study termination and an optional post-trial follow-up (Fig. 4.3). Once the enrollment and follow-up are complete, the data must be

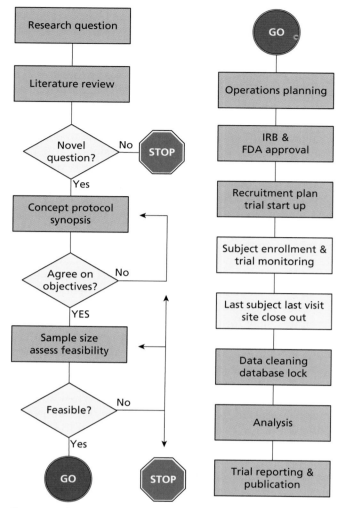

Figure 4.3 The primary stages of a clinical trial. Each major phase shown as a diamond has components shown as rectangles that are shared across the clinical trial.

the answer to the research question is known is also unethical [63].

In our experience, the best approach is to start by creating a synopsis or concept protocol. This is a 2–4-page document that outlines the primary and most important secondary objectives, the proposed study population (inclusion and exclusion criteria), the details of the proposed intervention(s) (study drug, device or other procedure), the choice of control group, the method of assignment to study treatment arms and the methods of concealing treatment allocation. The primary and secondary endpoints should be formalized, the required sample size estimated, and the statistical plan for the analysis of the primary endpoint specified. Only when all members of the protocol development team have agreed on the synopsis should the study planning proceed.

As the details of the concept protocol are being finalized, the details of the recruitment plan should also be considered to determine how many sites would be needed for the study. A preliminary timetable for the trial, the organizational structure, subject safety, and plans to ensure data integrity, quality, and security all need to be developed and implemented. Finally, it is at this point that funding proposals are sought, written, and submitted.

Feasibility and recruitment planning

With the protocol synopsis in hand, the principal investigators next need to assess whether the plans are operationally feasible. A realistic appraisal of the likely number of available subjects will determine whether or not the study can be conducted at a single site or whether other institutions will be needed to increase the pool of available subjects. Starting a clinical trial is a time-consuming process and unless the proposed study is feasible, it should not be started. Most ethicists consider underpowered or unfeasible studies unethical and many IRBs will not approve a study that has no hope of being completed [87].

If it has not already been done, it is at this moment of protocol planning that the principal and co-investigators must include and obtain the advice of their clinical co-ordinators. The study co-ordinator co-ordinates and administers research study-associated activities. The co-ordinator will either make or break a study. The co-ordinator assists in project planning and ensures that pre-established work scope, study protocol, and regulatory requirements are followed. The co-ordinator recruits and co-ordinates research subjects, as appropriate, and serves as principal administrative liaison between the study's administrative co-ordinating center and the local site. Finally, the co-ordinator oversees and co-ordinates the provision of administrative and staff services to the

checked to ensure that they are accurate (data cleaning) and only then can analysis commence. Obviously, there is overlap across each of these stages.

Initial design stage

The initial design stage specifies the rationale, purpose, and objectives of the clinical trial. A literature review is essential to identify pertinent background information about the target disease or condition and the proposed study intervention. Pharmaceutical trials compile this information in an Investigators' Brochure but it is up to the investigators to establish what is already known about the safety and efficacy of the intervention. Although confirmation of previous results has some value, it is usually a waste of time and resources to repeat work that has been done previously. Exposing subjects to risk when site investigators and maintains record-keeping systems, regulatory binders, and procedures.

Recruitment planning requires the input and planning of each study site and is often a collaborative effort between the study investigator and co-ordinator. The first step is to review the potential available population, keeping in mind the inclusion and exclusion criteria. If it appears that there will be insufficient numbers of potential participants, then the options are to loosen the inclusion/exclusion criteria to increase the available pool of subjects, increase the number of sites participating, or plan for an advertising campaign to widen the potential audience (see Fig. 4.3). In general, investigators greatly overestimate their ability to enroll subjects and the majority of trials fail to complete enrollment on time. In our experience of co-ordinating multicenter trials, a quarter to a third of sites fail to enroll even a single subject while the best 25% of the sites enroll 75–90% of the subjects. Since it is very difficult to predict which sites will successfully enroll subjects, it is usual to recruit more sites than would be expected to ensure study completion.

During the actual recruitment process, the study co-ordinator should track all subjects from screening to completion. The 2010 CONSORT guidelines provide an excellent resource on how and why patients should be tracked through the recruitment process and includes a recruitment table that should be provided in any randomized controlled trial for publication [88,89].

The nature of the study will determine how, when, and by whom prospective subjects will be approached. For anesthesia and pain trials, this could include review of the operating room schedule, solicitation in surgeons' offices or one or more publicity schemes, such as advertising in print, on the internet or radio.

Protocol development and operational planning

If the planned study appears feasible without modification, the next step is to flesh out the synopsis or concept into a complete protocol. It is at this stage that the nuts and bolts of the protocol are elaborated and put into writing ("cast in stone"). The objectives, endpoints, and inclusion and exclusion criteria will come from the study synopsis. However, many other items need to be specified, such as the time windows for screening and follow-up examinations, procedures for management of known or suspected complications related to the disease or therapy, and treatment algorithms for how the individual patient is to be monitored and treated if complications arise. Box 4.3 presents an example of a protocol table of contents for a clinical trial.

Most protocols provide very detailed scientific background sections but are left wanting when it comes to detailing the actual study procedures. The mark of a well-written protocol is that the study co-ordinator can read the protocol and know which procedures to perform and how to perform them for each study visit, the data manager can design the requisite case report forms, and the biostatistician can perform the study analyses.

The study procedures section should contain a visit schedule listing each and every measurement that is to be made during that encounter. Often, a simple bullet point list will do and usually a summary table is created as well. Having a complete list of visit-by-visit procedures is key to ensuring that all measurements are made as required at each time point. For clinical trials that take place in the operating room, the visits might be separated by minutes or hours rather than by days.

To assist with this, the study evaluations and measures section should specify how each evaluation will be performed. Continuing with our previous example of a clinical trial of an antihypertensive drug, it is not enough to state that systolic blood pressure will be measured. Rather, the protocol must describe exactly how it will be measured (which arm, which device, whether the subject is to be seated, lying or standing, after how many minutes of rest, and how many measurements will be averaged).

When completed, the protocol becomes the blueprint for the study execution and once put into place, its recipe must be followed to the letter, if the trial is to be successful. Indeed, it is this "cast in stone" rigidity that so befuddles many clinicians and represents the fundamental difference between a clinical trial and routine clinical care [81]. In routine clinical care, physicians use their best judgment to make treatment decisions. On the other hand, in a clinical trial, the investigator's responsibility is strict adherence to the protocol, not to his or her own judgment. This is absolutely essential to ensure the fidelity of the trial. For example, if a 6-year-old postoperative patient has an oxygen saturation of 92% in the post-anesthesia care unit (PACU), some clinicians might decide to watch and wait, whereas others may prescribe and administer supplemental oxygen. However, if a study protocol treatment algorithm requires a subject to receive oxygen if their oxygen saturation decreases below 94%, then oxygen must be administered even if this is not the investigator's individual clinical practice. Put another way, if a study protocol requires that subjects eat green Jell-O, the clinician/investigator must provide green Jell-O, even if they would prefer red.

Data management and document preparation

When the protocol is finalized, the informed consent and assent forms and the case report forms (CRF), paper or electronic, can be developed. Data should be recorded first in the source document, which is a medical chart,

Box 4.3 An example of a protocol table of contents for a clinical trial

anesthesia record or data collection form, and then transferred to the CRFs. If data collection forms will be used, they should be tested for usability. The data management team should be organized and must develop the data storage, back-up, and security plans. In multicenter trials, the data team will produce the randomization and treatment allocation schedules and develop protocols for data transfer from each site to the data center.

All clinical trials need a data quality control plan. If the study is conducted at a single site, the principal investiga-tor will be responsible. For a multicenter trial, the sponsor or contract research organization (CRO) will be responsible for site monitoring and for reviewing performance and outcomes during the course of the trial. These procedures establish the plan for collecting, processing, and verifying study data accuracy and for on-site monitoring to ensure that the protocol is being adhered to and that the data forms actually are being completed correctly.

Finally, the data monitoring group must develop guidelines for data security and access to study data by investigators within and outside the study and this access must be weighed by the rights of patients to privacy and confidentiality. The co-ordinating center may also be responsible for ancillary documents for the study staff to help ensure that the study procedures are followed precisely as well as to prepare any diaries or instructions for participants.

The Standards for Privacy of Individually Identifiable Health Information (the Privacy Rule) established, for the first time, a set of national standards for the protection of certain health information. The US Department of Health and Human Services (HHS) issued the Privacy Rule to implement the requirement of the Health Insurance Portability and Accountability Act of 1996 (HIPAA). The Privacy Rule standards addressed the use and disclosure of individuals' health information (called "protected health information") by organizations subject to the Privacy Rule (called "covered entities"), as well as standards for individuals' rights to understand and control how their health information is used. Within HHS, the Office for Civil Rights (OCR) has responsibility for implementing and enforcing the Privacy Rule with respect to voluntary compliance activities and civil money penalties. The effect of the Privacy Rule on the conduct of clinical trials has not been major and largely involves expansion of the mandated confidentiality language in the informed consent document.

Informed consent document

The principal investigator is usually responsible for the development of the informed consent template document. The consent forms must follow the federal regulatory required elements of informed consent (45 CFR 46.116(a) and 21 CFR 50.25). The document should be written in plain language, with a target reading level of 6–8th grade. Approximately 12% of Americans have a below Basic health literacy proficiency and 22% are at the Basic level. Thus, if the informed consent form is written at greater than 8th-grade level, over a third of the participants will be unable to comprehend what they are reading [90].

Safety monitoring plan

All clinical trials require monitoring of unanticipated problems involving risks to subjects or others, including serious adverse events (SAEs). In multicenter studies, SAEs are usually reported promptly to the study sponsor. The sponsor is responsible for reporting these events to the regulatory agency overseeing the study. However, not all SAEs have to be reported to the IRB. Both the FDA and the OHRP have published guidelines on reporting of adverse events to the IRB [67,91]. Regardless of the guidelines, investigators need to adhere to the policies in place at their local institution.

Safety monitoring should be tailored to the complexity of the study and the potential for harm to subjects. For a single-center study with a relatively low level of risk, the principal investigator's oversight should suffice. For a single-center trial with a moderate level of inherent risk, an internal data safety monitoring committee (DSMC) made up of the principal investigator and other knowledgeable individuals unassociated with the study would be advisable. For multicenter trials involving life-threatening conditions or risky therapies, an independent DSMC would be appropriate [92–95].

For all drug trials enrolling pediatric subjects, the American Academy of Pediatrics strongly recommends a DSMC for monitoring [96]. When the intervention has a track record of safety in adults and the condition of interest is not life-threatening, this level of oversight can be an unnecessary burden and adds substantially to the overhead costs of the study. Regardless of the oversight mechanism, meeting schedules and endpoints for interim analyses (if any) need to be defined and agreed upon. For trials involving life-threatening conditions, the protocol should contain stopping rules and procedures for early termination of the trial if serious unanticipated risks emerge. Only rarely should a trial be stopped for benefit and then only when one arm demonstrates a large margin of superiority [97,98].

Authorship and registration

Deciding exactly how the results of the study will be disseminated and by whom is a step often overlooked in the pretrial planning process. In our experience, failure to make this decision before embarking on a trial often leads to bad blood and ill will amongst the study investigators. As stated previously, for many investigators, authorship is essential for academic promotion. The order of authorship for study papers (and for ancillary studies) should be established and agreed upon by all investigators before starting a study. Ideally, a formal steering committee should be charged and entrusted with acting impartially on behalf of all the investigators early in a study design. The steering committee should establish procedures for review and approval of all publications and presentations made by members of the investigative group before professional and lay scientific committees. At this stage it is also important to clarify trial roles. Some journals now request the exact role of each investigator at the time of publication. Finally, it is also important to establish safeguards that protect against premature disclosure of study results or the publication of the study results by a "minority" within the study group.

The final step within the protocol development stage is establishing the budget and staffing requirements for the trial. Does each prospective participating center have the manpower and skills to safely, effectively, and efficiently conduct the trial? Do they have enough potential participants to enroll in a timely manner? How will oversight be performed and by whom? How will study drugs be packaged, labeled, distributed, and safeguarded? How will the study be funded and by whom? Who will do all the regulatory work required for the trial?

Funding and projected budgets are the keys to successful and unsuccessful trials. Inadequate funding, just like undercapitalization of a business, leads to failure. Indeed, it has been our experience that the real costs of conducting a study, including protocol development and site approval, are often underbudgeted which often results in contract delays and misadventures.

Because many if not all of the studies conducted by pediatric anesthesiologists involve drugs, and most if not all have invariably not been approved for use in children, approval by the FDA and its European counterpart the EMA may be required. It is beyond the scope of this chapter to discuss the process of obtaining an IND Application from the FDA but several useful sources are available at the FDA website (www.FDA.gov/CDER).

Finally, all phase II, III and IV trials require prospective registration in a national trial registry, such as www.clinicaltrials.gov in the United States. These registries are often funded by government entities and are designed to keep investigators from manipulating study endpoints by prespecifying the study objectives, intervention, subject population, sample size, and analysis plan of a trial before a trial is started. The databases are publically available and are searchable. Most journals use and require trial registration for any trial submitted for publication.

Trial execution: treatment and follow-up

It is only after all the preliminary development, feasibility assessments, protocol development, and regulatory approval have been organized that the investigators are ready for subject recruitment and actually conducting the trial. For all multicentered trials there is usually an investigators' meeting held before the first subject is enrolled at which required training, standard operating procedures, and data management are finalized.

For most perioperative pediatric anesthesia trials, the local investigator or his or her study co-ordinator recruits subjects from an in- and an outpatient operative list. Viewing and accessing these lists are subject to HIPAA rules and must be cleared with the IRB and the HIPAA compliance office within the institution. Advertising and liaisons with medical and lay societies that are so important in other adult and pediatric trials are often unnecessary. On the other hand, it is essential to inform the surgeons and the local referring pediatricians whose patients could be enrolled about the study and to get their tacit approval prior to recruiting subjects into the trial.

When it will be difficult to obtain consent and assent on the day of surgery, one approach is to screen the operative schedule and send letters to prospective study participants to inform them in general terms of the study objectives and procedures. Obviously, these letters are part of the regulatory binder and must be part of the IRB approval process. Without this prescreening and notification, there can be insufficient time to allow prospective participants to consider the risks, benefits, and alternatives to more complicated studies, making an informed decision difficult if not impossible. Thus, a successful recruitment plan often requires the investigator and coordinator to screen and recruit in the surgeon's or pediatrician's office.

Before agreeing to take part in a clinical trial, both the investigator and the prospective participant need to understand that care provided during research is different from usual clinical care. The investigator's obligation is to adhere to the protocol and not to individualize care to the participant's need. It is not known whether or not the participant will benefit directly from their participation; to promise benefit is to presuppose the outcome from the trial. Failure to understand the difference between clinical care and research is termed "therapeutic misconception" [99–101]. The investigator must ensure that the prospective participant understands the difference so that expectations are aligned with reality.

The data quality review, site monitoring visits, and meetings of the study steering committee, DSMC and other study committees take place at regularly scheduled intervals. At these meetings, recruitment progress and projected time lines for completion of the study are reviewed to ensure that the study is meeting its goals.

Close-out and termination stage

Once the last subject has had their last visit and the final data queries issued by the data management team are resolved, sites can be closed. In practice, low-enrolling sites are closed well before this point so that there are sufficient monitoring resources to rapidly lock the study database. The site monitoring team will direct the disposition of equipment, supplies, drugs and other stored materials. Once all data queries are resolved, the database can be locked, which means that no further changes will be made, even if small errors are discovered. As long as subject identifiers remain in the database used for analysis, the study must remain open and be approved by the IRB. For multicenter trials, most sites can submit a request for study closure once the sponsor has conducted the close-out visit.

The study's statisticians might or might not conduct the planned analyses blinded to treatment assignment. The statistician prepares results summarized in tables and figures. A formal study report is usually prepared and investigators and participants can be informed of the study's findings. The results of the study are submitted for publication and to regulatory agencies. Finally, if indicated, this is the time to plan for follow-up studies.

Conclusion

The randomized, blinded, placebo-controlled clinical trial is the indispensable "gold standard" in determining the efficacy of therapeutics. Trials are time consuming, maddeningly difficult and often very expensive to perform, and frustrating from inception to execution to completion. However, the failure to properly perform a trial results in perpetual uncertainty. Performing a proper trial takes time to develop a protocol, create and test the data collection forms, obtain support and funding and establish the structure for data intake and analysis. Once completed, the results of the trial must be published and made available to the public and regulatory agencies. Finally, above all else, all aspects of trial conduct must adhere to accepted ethical standards.

Annotated references

A full reference list for this chapter is available at:

http://www.wiley.com/go/gregory/andropoulos/pediatricanesthesia

26. Miller FG, Brody H. Clinical equipoise and the incoherence of research ethics. J Med Philos 2007; 32: 151–65. A discussion of the concept of clinical equipoise by investigators and clinicians with respect to enrolling patients in research trials.

32. Temple R, Ellenberg SS. Placebo-controlled trials and active-control trials in the evaluation of new treatments. Part 1: ethical and scientific issues. Ann Intern Med 2000; 133: 455–63. An important discussion of control groups, whether placebo or active controls, in clinical research.

50. Tunis SR, Stryer DB, Clancy CM. Practical clinical trials: increasing the value of clinical research for decision making in clinical and health policy. JAMA 2003; 290: 1624–32. A call for clinical trials with practical designs and outcomes that have the potential to effect actual clinical practice.

60. Klassen TP, Hartling L, Craig JC, Offringa M. Children are not just small adults: the urgent need for high-quality trial evidence in children. PLoS Med 2008; 5: e172. An important statement regarding the need for proper research in children, and not merely extrapolating adult data to pediatric practice.

70. Parvizi J, Tarity TD, Conner K, Smith JB. Institutional review board approval: why it matters. J Bone Joint Surg Am 2007; 89: 418–26. A discussion of the importance of proper institutional review board review for clinical research.

75. Kimberly MB, Hoehn KS, Feudtner C et al. Variation in standards of research compensation and child assent practices: a comparison of 69 institutional review board-approved informed permission and assent forms for 3 multicenter pediatric clinical trials. Pediatrics 2006; 117: 1706–11. An important study of child assent, and compensation for research in pediatric trials, with a discussion of this important issue in conducting ethical research.

77. Wendler D, Belsky L, Thompson KM, Emanuel EJ. Quantifying the federal minimal risk standard: implications for pediatric research without a prospect of direct benefit. JAMA 2005; 294: 826–32. A discussion of the problem of what constitutes minimal risk in pediatric research and how this concept relates to research without the possibility of a direct benefit.

87. Halpern SD, Karlawish JH, Berlin JA. The continuing unethical conduct of underpowered clinical trials. JAMA 2002; 288: 358–62. An important paper addressing the ethical problem of performing clinical research without doing a sample size and power analysis before the trial begins.

89. Schulz KF, Altman DG, Moher D, CONSORT Group. CONSORT 2010 statement: updated guidelines for reporting parallel group randomized trials. PLoS Med 2010; 7: e1000251. The updated guidelines for reporting clinical research enrollment, following protocols, subject dropout and crossover, and intention to treat analysis.

96. Shaddy RE, Denne SC, Committee on Drugs and Committee on Pediatric Research. Clinical report – guidelines for the ethical conduct of studies to evaluate drugs in pediatric populations. Pediatrics 2006; 125: 850–60. An important document laying out guidelines for ethical conduct of medication studies in pediatric patients.

97. Pocock SJ. Current controversies in data monitoring for clinical trials. Clin Trials 2006; 3: 513–21. An important discussion of the problems of data and safety monitoring for clinical trials.

CHAPTER 5

Developmental Physiology of the Cardiovascular System

Wanda C. Miller-Hance[1], Ivan Wilmot[2] & Dean B. Andropoulos[1]

[1]Department of Pediatrics and Anesthesiology, Baylor College of Medicine, and Texas Children's Hospital, Houston, TX, USA
[2]All Children's Hospital Heart Institute, St Petersburg, FL, USA

Introduction

The understanding of both normal and abnormal cardiac development and physiology is crucial in providing anesthetic care to infants and children. The explosion of knowledge over the past several decades regarding the extensive changes in the cardiovascular system during fetal, neonatal, and early childhood periods requires thorough review so the anesthesiologist can apply these complex principles to patient care. This chapter will first present normal cardiac embryology and development, and then review the abnormal cardiac development that results in the most common congenital cardiac defects recognized clinically. Then the normal physiological changes from the fetus to the neonate, and from infancy to childhood, will be reviewed. Finally, the pathophysiology of congenital heart disease, regulation of systemic and pulmonary vascular tone, and receptor signaling in disease states will be presented.

Cardiac embryology and normal development

The pathogenesis of congenital heart disease is not completely understood. Developmental mechanisms that include cell migration, hemodynamic function, cell death, and extracellular matrix proliferation have all been proposed in the etiology of cardiovascular malformations. Multiple genetic pathways have been identified that contribute to cardiac development and whose disruption

Gregory's Pediatric Anesthesia, Fifth Edition. Edited by George A. Gregory, Dean B. Andropoulos.
© 2012 Blackwell Publishing Ltd. Published 2012 by Blackwell Publishing Ltd.

may result in structural defects [1–6]. These genetic controls influence cardiac-specific mechanisms such as cardiogenesis, looping of the heart tube, chamber specification, cardiac septation, conotruncal and aortic arch development, valvular formation, and ventricular function [4,7].

A foundation in human embryology and, in particular, in the areas of cardiac morphogenesis and normal development provides a window into the complex series of events that may result in abnormalities of the cardiovascular system. As such, a basic understanding of embryology and critical events during the various stages of cardiac development should be of relevance to those who care for infants and children, in particular those affected by congenital heart disease.

This section provides an overview of the normal developmental program of the cardiovascular system, highlighting important events during cardiac morphogenesis and consequences of abnormal development, as relevant to the practice of pediatric anesthesiology. The data presented derive from a combination of descriptive or classic embryology, experimental work on other species, and current knowledge regarding human cardiac development.

The heart represents the first functional organ in the embryo. Cardiac development in most vertebrates is considered to follow a similar pattern from the formation of the cardiogenic plate to the complex fully developed organ, with minor variations across species.

The critical stages of cardiovascular development in the human encompass events between the second and eighth weeks of gestation (Fig. 5.1). The review that follows emphasizes main aspects of embryological development of the heart and great vessels during this period. To facilitate this discussion, a perspective that focuses on the origin and evolving changes of the major cardiovascular structures throughout embryonic development has been selected over a strict chronological approach. For a more exhaustive review of the subject, the reader is referred to several outstanding resources [8–14].

Early cardiogenesis

The earliest developmental stage of the heart and vascular system is seen following the second week of gestation. On the 15th day of gestation, mesoderm is derived from ectoderm. The "middle skin" or mesoderm will in turn give rise to the various cardiovascular structures. On the 18th day of gestation, the mesoderm-derived cardiogenic crescent forms the precursor to the heart (Fig. 5.2A). Cavitation of the mesoderm results in formation of the intraembryonic celom, from which all body cavities, including pericardial, pleural, and peritoneal, will eventually derived.

Straight heart tube

On the 15th day of gestation, the cardiogenic crescent has developed into the primitive heart tube [15]. Blood in this midline tube enters caudally via the inflow and exits cranially via the rudimentary outflow tract. The linear heart tube will eventually give rise to the atria, ventricles, bulbus cordis, and truncus arteriosus (Fig. 5.2B). The bulbus cordis and truncus arteriosus contribute to formation of the ventricles and great vessels respectively.

Cardiac looping

On the 21st day of gestation, cardiac loop formation takes place. The straight heart tube is fixed at both ends (the sinus venosus and truncus arteriosus segments) by pericardium. Differential growth of the straight heart tube results in the sinus venosus portion being positioned posteriorly, the common ventricle anteriorly, and the bulbus cordis anteriorly and superiorly. This accounts for cardiac looping and the ventricular relationship.

Looping of the heart tube to the right gives rise to the normal ventricular relationship (d-loop), where the right ventricle is ultimately positioned rightwards (Fig. 5.2C). In contrast, looping to the left results in an abnormal ventricular relationship (l-loop), where the right ventricle is positioned leftwards (l-looped ventricles) (Fig. 5.2D). Molecular cues determining cardiac looping remain poorly understood.

Atrial septation

Atrial septation begins in the fourth week of gestation and continues into the fifth week (Fig. 5.3). Ingrown tissue along the superior aspect of the atria initially results in a septum primum. In a curtain-like fashion, this septum primum extends inferiorly towards the embryonic endocardial cushions. Two foramina are associated with the septum primum: the superior foramen or ostium secundum and the inferior foramen primum. The foramen secundum arises from perforations in the septum primum and remains open until birth. The foramen primum is transient, as continued growth of the septum primum and endocardial cushions obliterates this communication.

The septum secundum forms during the fifth and sixth weeks of gestation, arising to the right of the septum primum. Similarly to the septum primum, the septum secundum extends inferiorly. The foramen secundum is closed by the inferiorly extending septum secundum. The superior septum secundum and inferior septum primum create the foramen ovale.

The foramen ovale acts as a one-way valve in fetal life, allowing oxygenated blood from the inferior vena cava to course from the right atrium to the left atrium. Functional closure of the foramen ovale occurs postnatally as a result of increased pulmonary blood flow and left atrial pressure exceeding that of the right atrium. This occurs as the

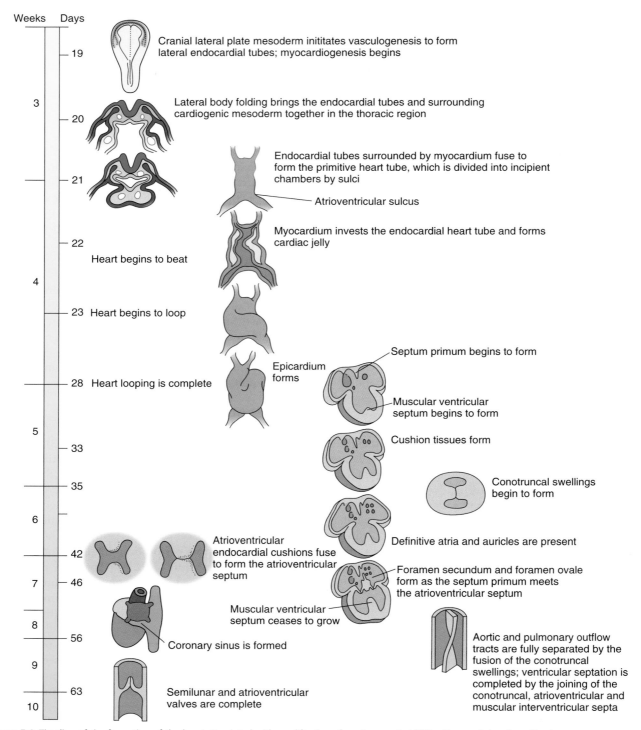

Figure 5.1 Timeline of the formation of the heart. Reprinted with modifications from Larsen et al [13] with permission from Elsevier.

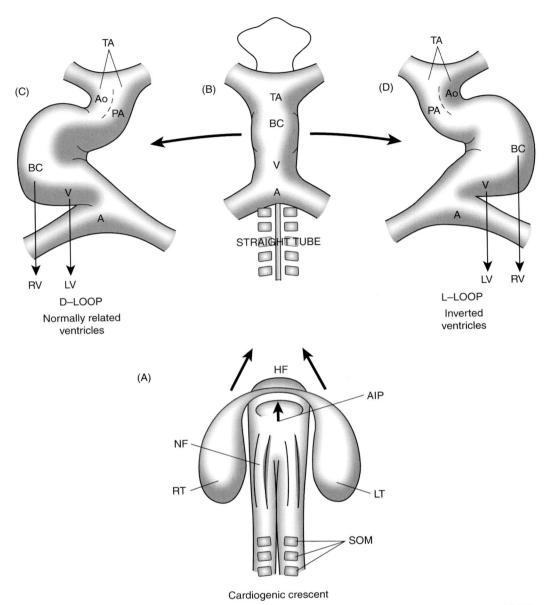

Figure 5.2 Cardiac loop formation. (A) Cardiogenic crescent of precardiac mesoderm. (B) Straight heart tube or preloop stage. (C) D-loop, with normally related ventricles. (D) L-loop, with inverted (mirror image) ventricles. A, atrium; AIP, anterior intestinal portal; Ao, aorta; BC, bulbus cordis; HF, head fold; LT, left; LV, morphological left ventricle; NF, neural fold; PA, main pulmonary artery; RT, right; RV, morphological right ventricle; SOM, somites; TA, truncus arteriosus. Reprinted from Van Praagh et al [156] with permission from Lippincott, Williams and Wilkins.

septum primum moves against the septum secundum. Fusion of the septum primum and septum secundum following birth results in anatomical closure of the foramen ovale and complete atrial septation.

Development and incorporation of the sinus venosus

Initially, the segment corresponding to the sinus venosus is positioned in the midline of the posteriorly positioned primordial atrium. On the 26th day of gestation, the right and left horns of the sinus venosus develop (Fig. 5.4A). The right horn is connected to the right umbilical, vitelline, anterior cardinal and common cardinal veins, and inferior vena cava. The left horn is connected to the left umbilical, vitelline, anterior and common cardinal veins. There is a progressive shift of drainage of venous blood from left- to right-sided structures. This result in an enlarging right horn and the sinoatrial orifice moving rightwards, towards the primordial atrium. This process culminates in the incorporation of the right horn of the sinus venosus into the future right atrium (Fig. 5.4B).

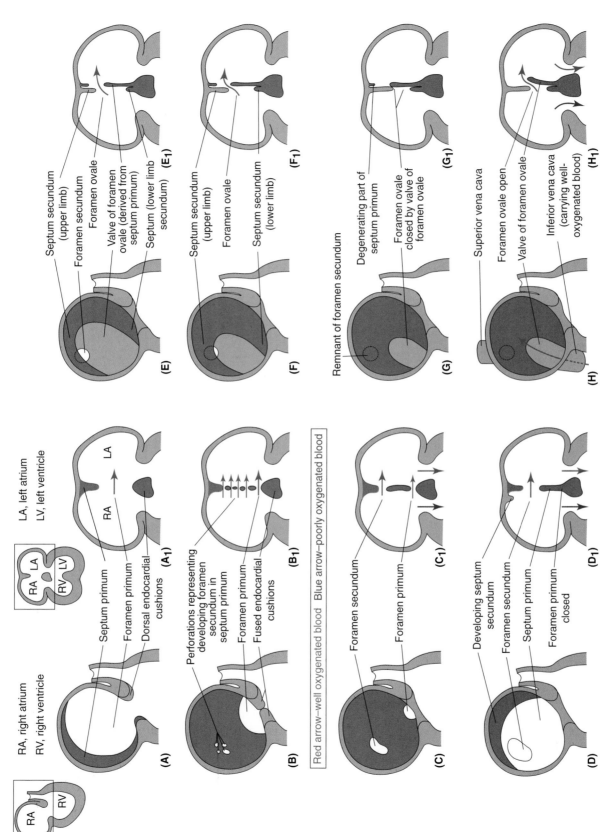

Figure 5.3 Atrial septation. Representation of the progressive stages involved in septation of the primordial atrium. (A–H) Sketches of the developing interatrial septum as viewed from the right side. (A₁–H₁) Coronal sections of the interatrial septum. As the septum secundum extends inferiorly, it overlaps the opening in the septum primum (foramen secundum). G₁ and H₁ depict the valve of the foramen ovale. When right atrial pressure exceeds that in the left atrium, blood moves from the right to the left side of the heart. When pressures are equal or higher in the left atrium, the flap closes (H₁). Reprinted from Moore and Persaud [12] with permission from Elsevier.

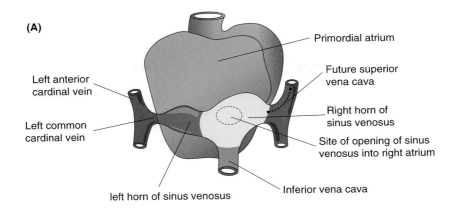

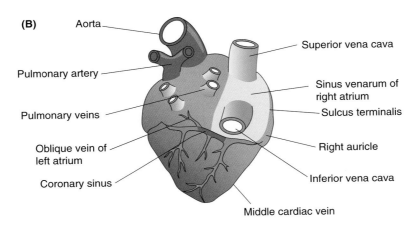

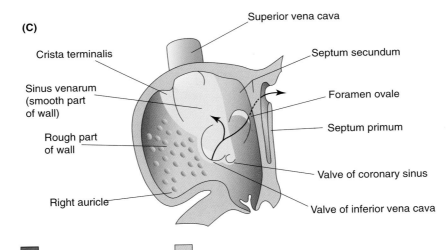

Figure 5.4 Fate of the sinus venosus. (A) Dorsal view of the heart (approximately 26 days) demonstrating the primordial atrium and sinus venosus. (B) Dorsal view at 8 weeks after incorporation of the right sinus horn into the right atrium. The left sinus horn has become the coronary sinus. (C) Internal view of the fetal right atrium showing: (i) the smooth part of the wall of the right atrium (sinus venarum) derived from the right sinus horn and (ii) the crista terminalis and the valves of the inferior vena cava and coronary sinus derived from the right sinoatrial valve. The primordial right atrium becomes the right auricle, a conical muscular pouch. Reprinted from Moore and Persaud [12] with permission from Elsevier.

The smooth portion of the mature right atrium, the sinus venarum, is derived from sinus venosus (Fig. 5.4C). The rough atrial appendage and conical muscular pouch of the right atrium are derived from the primordial atrium. Internally, the demarcation between the smooth sinus venarum posteriorly and the rough primordial atrium anteriorly is evidenced by a ridge of cardiac muscle tissue referred to as the crista terminalis. This is also marked externally by a groove, the sulcus terminalis. Both the right anterior cardinal and common cardinal veins contribute to the formation of the superior vena cava during the eighth week of gestation. The right horn receives all the blood from the head and neck via the superior vena cava, and from the caudal regions and placenta through the inferior vena cava. The smaller left horn eventually becomes the coronary sinus.

The sinus venosus contributes to the conduction system of the heart. The sinoatrial node develops from the sinus venosus during the fifth week of gestation. This is located along the high right atrium at the junction between the right atrium and superior vena cava. The atrioventricular node develops from the inferior portion of the sinus venosus in combination with cells from the atrioventricular region. The atrioventricular node arises slightly superior to the endocardial cushions (discussed below) with the atrioventricular bundle coursing into the ventricles.

Development of the systemic veins

The development of the venous structures associated with the heart occurs during the fourth week of gestation. Three paired veins drain blood into the tubular heart: the vitelline, umbilical, and common cardinal veins (Figs 5.5, 5.6A, 5.7).

The vitelline veins return poorly oxygenated blood from the yolk sac. The umbilical veins carry oxygenated blood from the placenta to the sinus venosus portion of the developing heart. As the liver develops, the umbilical veins lose their connection with the heart (Fig. 5.6B). The left umbilical vein courses through the liver. The inferior portion of the left umbilical vein becomes the ductus venosus, bypassing the liver parenchyma, and enters the inferior vena cava. The right umbilical vein degenerates at the end of the embryonic period.

The cardinal veins return deoxygenated blood from the body of the embryo to the sinus venosus. The superior and inferior cardinal veins join to form the common cardinal vein. The superior vena cava eventually develops from the right anterior cardinal vein and common cardinal vein as previously indicated (Fig. 5.6C). The subcardinal and supracardinal veins subsequently largely replace the posterior cardinal veins. The subcardinal veins give rise to several structures, including a segment of the inferior vena. During the seventh week of gestation, the supracardinal veins appear. The cranial portions of the supracardinal veins give rise to the azygous and hemiazygous veins. The caudal portion of the left supracardinal veins degenerates, with the right portion becoming the inferior portion of the inferior vena cava.

The inferior vena cava develops as a result of a shift of primordial venous drainage from the left to right side of the body (see Fig. 5.7). The inferior vena cava is composed of four main segments, each originating

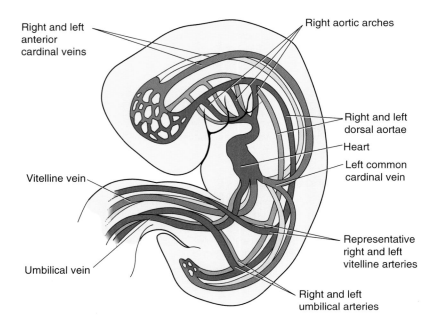

Right and left anterior cardinal veins

Right aortic arches

Right and left dorsal aortae

Heart

Left common cardinal vein

Vitelline vein

Umbilical vein

Representative right and left vitelline arteries

Right and left umbilical arteries

Figure 5.5 The embryonic vascular system in the middle of the fourth week. At this stage, the heart has begun to beat and circulate blood. The outflow tract is now connected to four pairs of aortic arches and the paired dorsal aortae that circulate blood to the head and trunk. Three pairs of veins, umbilical, vitelline, and cardinal, deliver blood to the inflow region of the heart. Reprinted from Larsen et al [13] with permission from Lippincott, Williams and Wilkins.

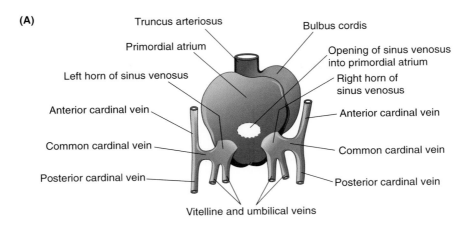

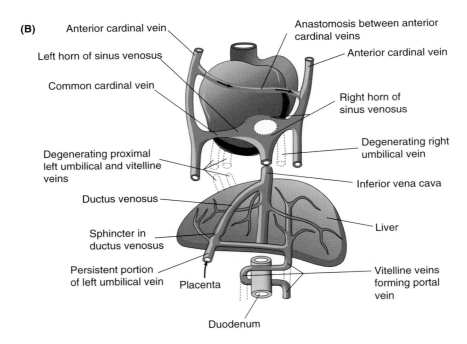

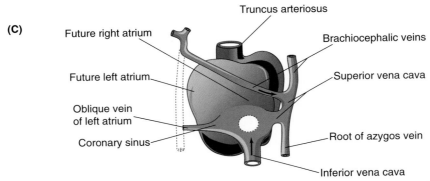

Figure 5.6 Dorsal views of the developing heart. (A) During the fourth week (approximately 24 days), showing the primordial atrium, sinus venosus and venous drainage. (B) At 7 weeks, illustrating the enlarged right sinus horn and venous circulation through the liver (organs are not drawn to scale). (C) At 8 weeks, indicating the adult derivatives of the cardinal veins. Reprinted from Moore and Persaud [12] with permission from Elsevier.

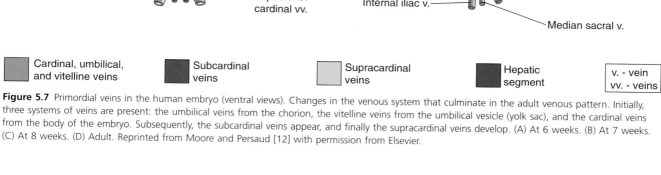

Figure 5.7 Primordial veins in the human embryo (ventral views). Changes in the venous system that culminate in the adult venous pattern. Initially, three systems of veins are present: the umbilical veins from the chorion, the vitelline veins from the umbilical vesicle (yolk sac), and the cardinal veins from the body of the embryo. Subsequently, the subcardinal veins appear, and finally the supracardinal veins develop. (A) At 6 weeks. (B) At 7 weeks. (C) At 8 weeks. (D) Adult. Reprinted from Moore and Persaud [12] with permission from Elsevier.

from primordial venous structures. This includes the hepatic segment (derived from the right vitelline vein), prerenal segment (derived from the right subcardinal vein), renal segment (derived from the subcardinal and supracardinal anastomosis), and postrenal segment (derived from the right supracardinal vein).

Development of the pulmonary veins

Pulmonary development begins as a ventral outgrowth from the foregut, termed the respiratory diverticulum. The respiratory diverticulum develops with its most caudal segments represented by lung buds. A capillary plexus called the splanchnic plexus surrounds the lung buds (Fig. 5.8).

The primitive pulmonary veins arise from the splanchnic plexus. The pulmonary venous plexus shares venous drainage with the splanchnic plexus, which is connected to the cardinal and umbilical venous systems in early embryonic development. Consequently, the initial pulmonary venous drainage is via the cardinal and umbilical venous systems [16,17]. A primordial endocardial outgrowth from the superior margin of the left atrium forms the primordial pulmonary vein. It is the connection of this primordial pulmonary vein with the pulmonary venous plexus that allows pulmonary venous blood to flow into the left atrium. Once this connection to the left atrium is established, the pulmonary venous plexus loses its connection with the cardinal and umbilical veins. The eventual lack of obliteration of these connections is considered to result in anomalies of pulmonary venous drainage [18].

The left atrium is largely derived from the incorporation of the pulmonary veins. As the primordial pulmonary vein and its branches are incorporated into primordial atrium, the four pulmonary veins incorporate into the left atrial wall. Areas of the left atrium derived from the pulmonary veins are smooth, whereas those derived from primordial atrium (left atrial appendage) have a rough surface.

Development of the atrioventricular valves

Development of mesenchymal tissue swellings, otherwise known as endocardial cushions, along the atrioventricular canal begins in the fourth week of gestation (Fig. 5.9). The superior and inferior endocardial cushions are located in continuity with the interatrial and interventricular septa [19]. The formation of separate right and left atrioventricular valves is the result of simultaneous ingrowth of the lateral endocardial cushions. In addition to the endocardial cushions, additional embryonic structures that contribute to the formation of the atrioventricular valves include the dextrodorsal conal crest and the ventricular walls.

The cushions perform a valve-like function, preventing blood flow from the ventricle into the atria during systole,

thus facilitating forward blood flow (Fig. 5.10) [20]. Initially these regions are muscular in nature, and through a process of cellular differentiation they become thin and membranous [21].

Ventricular development and septation

Ventricular septation begins in the fifth week and continues into the seventh week of gestation (Fig. 5.11). The primordial interventricular septum arises from a median muscular ridge between the right and left ventricular masses. Increased growth and dilation of the ventricles, combined with fusion of the medial ventricular wall, result in enlargement of the muscular ventricular septum. A crescentic interventricular foramen between the free edge of the septum and endocardial cushion exists up until the seventh week of gestation. Closure of the primary interventricular foramen (bulboventricular foramen) results from tissue ingrowth from the right and left bulbar ridges, and the endocardial cushion.

The membranous portion of the septum is derived from tissue ingrowth from the right side of the endocardial cushion to the muscular region of the interventricular septum. The atrioventricular septum, or region of the septum that separates the right atrium from the left ventricle, originates from the inferior cushion of the atrioventricular canal.

Cavitation of the ventricular walls begins during the fifth week of gestation. This leads to an increase in the ventricular sizes. Several of the remaining muscle bundles will form the trabeculae carneae (muscle bundles on the ventricular free wall), whereas others will eventually give rise to the future papillary muscles and their chordal attachments to the atrioventricular valves. With respect to the embryological origin of the ventricles, it has been suggested that the inlet region originates from the endocardial cushions, the trabecular area from the primordia of the trabecular portion of the ventricles, and the outlet region from conal tissue [22]. Other studies propose that the inlet and trabecular components are derived from the same primary ventricular septum [23].

Partitioning of the bulbus cordis and truncus arteriosus

Extensive experimental work in the chick embryo has provided insights into the development of the conus and truncus arteriosus [24–26]. These observations strongly suggest that these developmental sequences are similar in the chick and the human.

Neural crest cells originating in the posterior rhombencephalon are known to migrate into the pharyngeal arches. Continued migration of these cells contributes to the formation of the conus and great arteries (aorta, aortopulmonary septum), aortic arch branches, ductus arteriosus, and cardiac ganglia [27–30]. It is thus not surprising

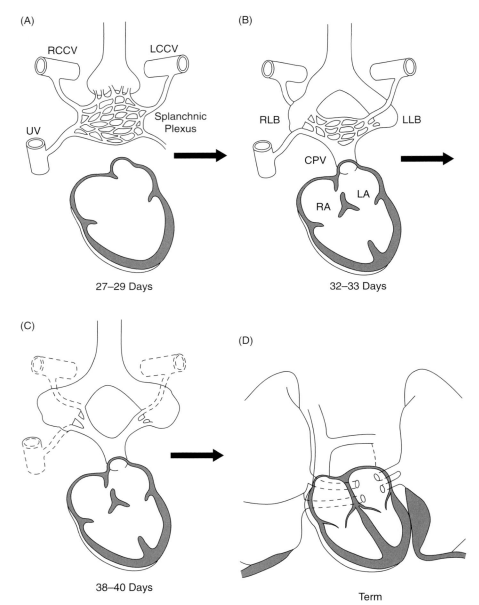

Figure 5.8 Development of the pulmonary veins. (A) At 27–29 days of gestation, the primordial lung buds are enmeshed by the vascular plexus of the foregut (splanchnic plexus). No direct connection to the heart is present at this stage. Instead, the multiple connections are present to the umbilicovitelline and cardinal venous systems. A small evagination can be seen in the posterior wall of the left atrium to the left of the developing septum secundum. (B) By the end of the first month of gestation, the common pulmonary vein establishes a connection between the pulmonary venous plexus and the sinoatrial portion of the heart. At this time, the connections between the pulmonary venous plexus and the splanchnic venous plexus are still patent. (C) Subsequently the connections between the pulmonary venous plexus and the splanchnic venous plexus involute. (D) The common pulmonary vein (CPV) incorporates into the left atrium so that the individual pulmonary veins connect separately and directly to the left atrium. LA, left atrium; LCCV, left common cardinal vein; LLB, left lung bud; RA, right atrium; RCCV, right common cardinal vein; RLB, right lung bud; UV, umbilical vein. Reprinted from Geva and van Praagh [56] with permission from Lippincott, Williams and Wilkins.

that the neural crest has been implicated in the pathogenesis of several cardiovascular anomalies [31].

Partitioning of the bulbus cordis and truncus arteriosus begins in the fifth week of gestation (see Fig. 5.11). Neural crest cells migrate into both the bulbus cordis and truncus arteriosus, forming bulbar and truncal ridges respectively. These ridges undergo 180° of rotation, causing the formation of a spiral aortopulmonary septum. Development of these ridges into the aortopulmonary septum divides the future aorta from the main pulmonary artery. The bulbus cordis contributes to the development of both ventricles. In the right ventricle, it forms the conus

(A)

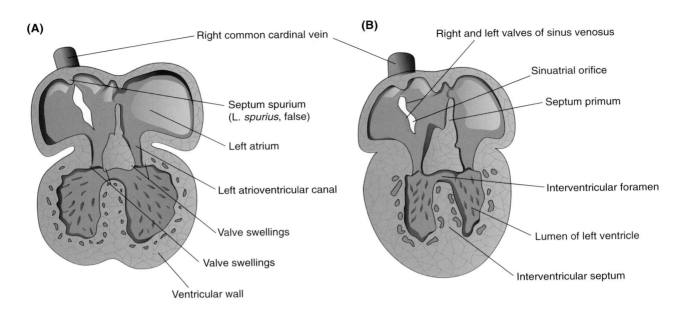

- Right common cardinal vein
- Septum spurium (L. *spurius*, false)
- Left atrium
- Left atrioventricular canal
- Valve swellings
- Valve swellings
- Ventricular wall

(B)

- Right and left valves of sinus venosus
- Sinuatrial orifice
- Septum primum
- Interventricular foramen
- Lumen of left ventricle
- Interventricular septum

(C)

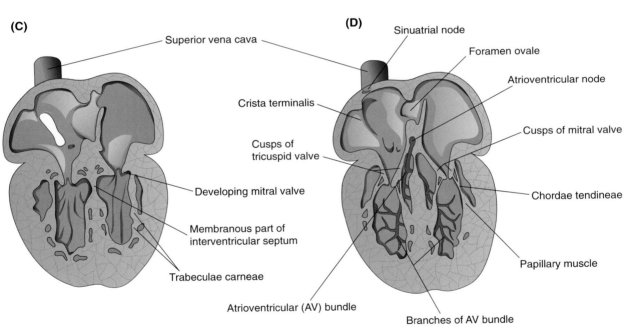

- Superior vena cava
- Crista terminalis
- Cusps of tricuspid valve
- Developing mitral valve
- Membranous part of interventricular septum
- Trabeculae carneae
- Atrioventricular (AV) bundle

(D)

- Sinuatrial node
- Foramen ovale
- Atrioventricular node
- Cusps of mitral valve
- Chordae tendineae
- Papillary muscle
- Branches of AV bundle

Figure 5.9 Sections of the heart illustrating successive stages in the development of the atrioventricular valves, tendinous cords, and papillary muscles. (A) At 5 weeks. (B) At 6 weeks. (C) At 7 weeks. (D) At 20 weeks. Reprinted from Moore and Persaud [12] with permission from Elsevier.

arteriosus or infundibulum that gives rise to the pulmonary trunk. In the left ventricle, it forms the aortic vestibule or aortic region inferior to the aortic valve. Partitioning of the bulbus cordis and truncus arteriosus nears completion in the sixth week of gestation.

At the end of the fifth week of gestation, the interventricular foramen is still patent (ventricular septal defect). The heart is largely septated into a double or parallel circulation at this stage. The third, fourth, and sixth aortic arches are present. The dorsal aorta and ductus arteriosus are formed. Continued neural crest cell migration aids in the formation of the infundibulum and great vessels. The ventricles continue to develop at this stage. The mitral valve, left ventricle, and aorta align with the interventricular foramen. On the 32nd day of gestation, the main pulmonary artery and ascending aorta septate, and

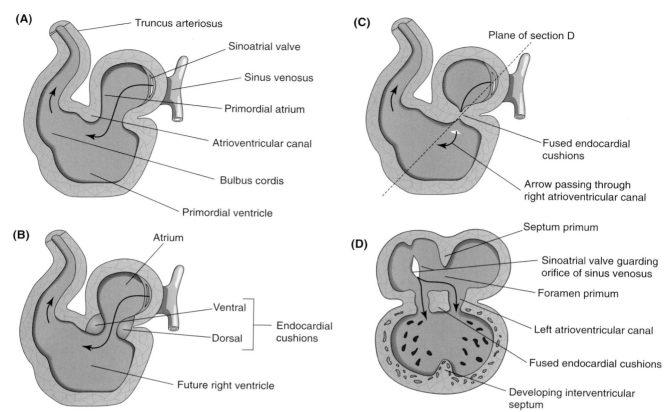

Figure 5.10 Sagittal sections of the primordial heart during the fourth and fifth weeks illustrating blood flow through the heart and division of the atrioventricular canal. (A–C) The arrows are passing through the sinoatrial orifice. (D) Coronal section of the heart at the plane shown in C. Note that the interatrial and interventricular septa have started to develop. Reprinted from Moore and Persaud [12] with permission from Elsevier.

shortly thereafter the atrioventricular valves septate. The right ventricle enlarges at this time with concurrent movement of the interventricular septum leftwards. The interventricular septum aligns underneath the atrioventricular canal as it moves leftwards. Failure of this interventricular alignment has been implicated in the etiology of double outlet right ventricle.

Semi-lunar valve development and great artery relationships

The semi-lunar valves originate from subendocardial tissue swellings in the aortic and pulmonary trunk. These swellings subsequently become hollow and form the valve cusps.

On the 30th day of gestation, the pulmonary valve begins its movement to its final position, anterior and leftwards of the aorta. This migration continues through the 36th day of gestation. During the course of this complex process, various observations have been made regarding the position of the great arteries with respect to each other that resemble known pathological relationships. On days 30–32 of gestation, the semi-lunar valve relationship is similar to that of *d*-transposition of the

great arteries. On the 33rd day of gestation, the semi-lunar valve relationship is side by side, similar to that seen in Taussig–Bing malformation. On the 34th day of gestation, the semi-lunar valve relationship resembles that seen in tetralogy of Fallot.

Fates of the vitelline and umbilical arteries

Development of the dorsal aortae, vitelline, and umbilical arteries is complete by the fourth week of gestation. The vitelline artery, supplying the yolk sac, will in turn supply the primordial gut. In the mature fetus, the vitelline artery will form the celiac, superior mesenteric, and inferior mesenteric arteries. The umbilical arteries transport poorly oxygenated blood from the body of the fetus to the placenta. These paired umbilical arteries will in turn form the internal iliac arteries (proximally), superior vesical arteries (proximally), and degenerate distally to form the medial umbilical ligament.

Development of the aortic arches

The mature aortic arch evolves from contributions of the aortic sac, aortic arches, and dorsal aortae (Fig. 5.12). Six pairs of aortic arches have been identified in the human

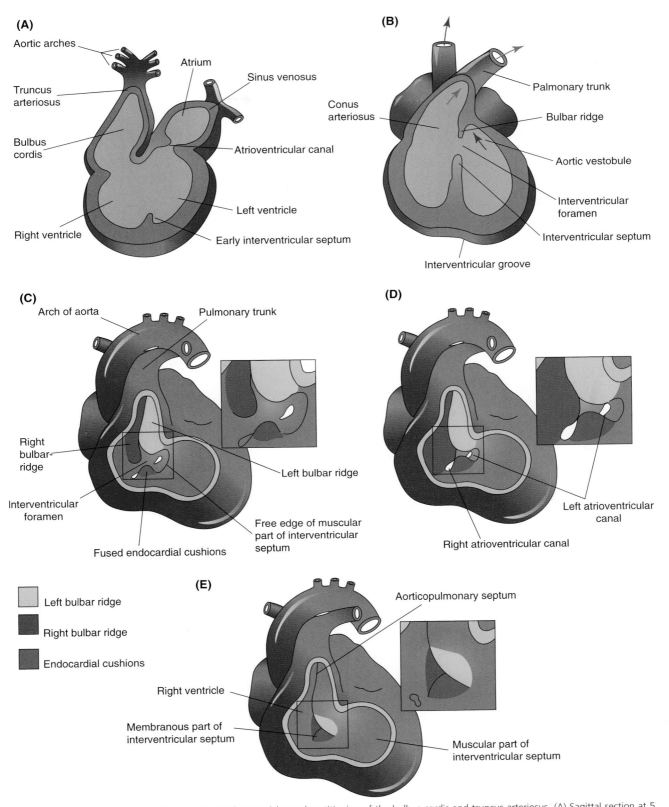

(A)

Aortic arches

Atrium

Sinus venosus

Truncus arteriosus

Bulbus cordis

Atrioventricular canal

Right ventricle

Left ventricle

Early interventricular septum

(B)

Palmonary trunk

Conus arteriosus

Bulbar ridge

Aortic vestobule

Interventricular foramen

Interventricular septum

Interventricular groove

(C)

Arch of aorta

Pulmonary trunk

Right bulbar ridge

Left bulbar ridge

Interventricular foramen

Free edge of muscular part of interventricular septum

Fused endocardial cushions

(D)

Left atrioventricular canal

Right atrioventricular canal

Left bulbar ridge

Right bulbar ridge

Endocardial cushions

(E)

Aorticopulmonary septum

Right ventricle

Membranous part of interventricular septum

Muscular part of interventricular septum

Figure 5.11 Incorporation of the bulbus cordis into the ventricles and partitioning of the bulbus cordis and truncus arteriosus. (A) Sagittal section at 5 weeks showing the bulbus cordis as one of the segments of the primordial heart. The primordial interventricular septum is noted. (B) Schematic coronal section at 6 weeks, after the bulbus cordis has been incorporated into the ventricles to become the conus arteriosus (infundibulum) of the right ventricle and the aortic vestibule of the left ventricle. The arrow indicates the direction of blood flow. The interventricular septum and interventricular foramen are depicted. (C-E) Closure of the interventricular foramen and formation of the membranous portion of the interventricular septum. The walls of the truncus arteriosus, bulbus cordis, and right ventricle have been removed. (C) At 5 weeks, showing the bulbar ridges and fused endocardial cushions. (D) At 6 weeks, showing how proliferation of subendocardial tissue diminishes the interventricular foramen. (E) At 7 weeks, showing the fused bulbar ridges, the membranous region of the interventricular septum formed by extensions of tissue from the right side of the endocardial cushions, and closure of the interventricular foramen. Reprinted from Moore and Persaud [12] with permission from Elsevier.

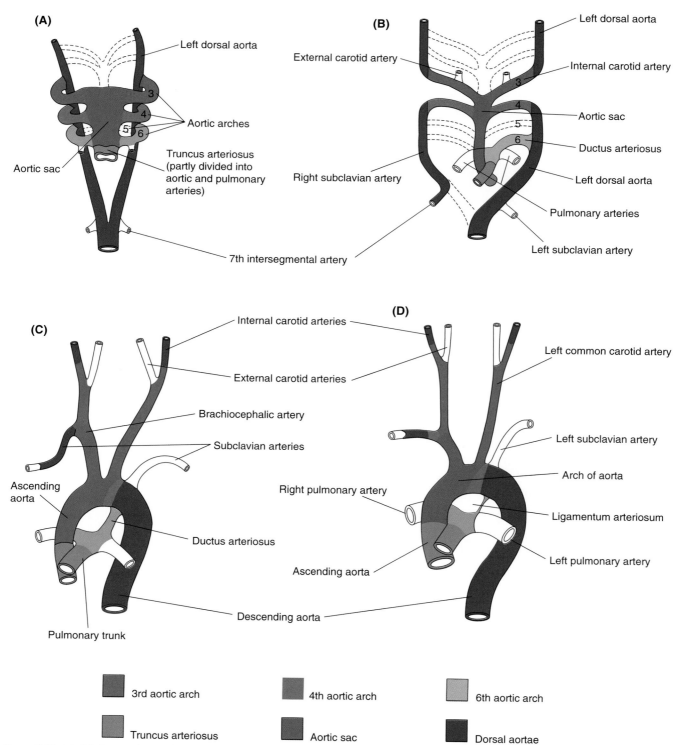

Figure 5.12 Arterial changes that result during transformation of the truncus arteriosus, aortic sac, pharyngeal arch arteries, and dorsal aortas into the adult arterial pattern. (Vessels not colored are not derived from these structures.) (A) Pharyngeal arch arteries at 6 weeks; by this stage, the first two pairs of the arteries have largely disappeared. (B) Pharyngeal arch arteries at 7 weeks; the parts of the dorsal aortae and pharyngeal arch arteries that normally disappear are indicated with broken lines. (C) Arterial arrangement at 8 weeks. (D) The arterial vessels of a 6-month-old infant. Note that the ascending aorta and pulmonary arteries are considerably smaller in C than in D. This represents the relative flow through these vessels at the different stages of development. The ductus arteriosus normally becomes functionally closed within the first few days after birth, eventually becoming the ligamentum arteriosum, as shown in D. Reprinted from Moore and Persaud [12] with permission from Elsevier.

embryo. Aortic arch development begins with the first pair of arches forming in the beginning of the fourth week of gestation. By the 26th day of gestation, the first aortic arches have involuted. A portion of these contributes to the development of the maxillary and external carotid arteries. At this time the second and third arches are formed, and the fourth and sixth arches are beginning to form. The second aortic arches eventually disappear; only a dorsal portion persists, giving rise to the stapedial artery. The third aortic arches contribute to the development of the carotid arteries.

During the sixth and seventh weeks of gestation, the arch and its branching pattern is established. If altered, these series of events can lead to vascular anomalies. The fourth aortic arch forms a portion of the aortic arch, innominate and proximal right subclavian arteries. The fifth aortic arch regresses during normal development. The first, third, fourth, and sixth aortic arches contribute to the formation of the mature arch. The sixth aortic arch forms the proximal left and right pulmonary arteries, and ductus arteriosus. The seventh intersegmental artery gives rise to the left subclavian artery. A summary of the aortic arches and their future vascular structures can be found in Table 5.1.

Normally various interruptions of the aortic arch system occur, resulting in a left aortic arch. These include involution of the right ductus arteriosus or sixth arch, the ductus caroticus (dorsal aorta segment between the third and fourth arches), and the right dorsal aorta distal to the seventh intersegmental artery (part of the embryonic right subclavian artery) [32].

Aortic arch sidedness is defined by the course of the arch over the mainstem bronchus. A left aortic arch courses over the left mainstem bronchus. Arch sidedness is determined by regression of the dorsal aortic arches. If the left dorsal aortic arch persists, the result is a left aortic arch; if the right dorsal arch persists the result is a right aortic arch. If both arches persist, the result is a double aortic arch.

Intersegmental arteries

The aortic arch arises from the aortic sac as a paired structure. The paired dorsal aortae soon fuse, caudal to the pharyngeal arches, to form a single dorsal aorta. Arising from the dorsal aorta are at least 30 intersegmental arteries, providing blood supply to anterior body structures. The anterior intersegmental arteries in the neck join to form the vertebral arteries. The majority of the connections between the intersegmental arteries and dorsal aorta eventually regress. In the thorax, however, the dorsal intersegmental arteries persist as intercostal arteries. In the abdomen, several of these persist as lumbar arteries, where the fifth pair of lumbar intersegmental arteries forms the common iliac arteries.

Development of the coronary arteries

The coronary arteries appear relatively late during cardiac development. During early cardiac morphogenesis, nutrients to the cardiac mass are derived directly from surrounding circulating blood, and subsequently from intramyocardial communications, also termed sinusoids. The appearance of subepicardial vascular networks during the fifth week of development is thought to give rise to the distal coronary vasculature.

Theories regarding the origin of the proximal coronary arteries are more controversial [33]. Several different mechanisms have been implicated [34–37]. These include penetration of the subepicardial vascular networks across the aortic wall to reach the aortic sinuses and the existence of coronary buds around the arterial trunks that eventually communicate with the subepicardial vascular network. The former concept is considered most likely to be the case.

Defects resulting from abnormal cardiac development

Defects of cardiac positioning

The position of the normal heart with the cardiac mass in the left thorax and apex pointing to the left is known as levocardia. Cardiac malpositions may result from extrinsic or intrinsic factors [38]. Dextrocardia, a positional abnormality, is considered to result from rightward rotation of the cardiac mass. This may or may not be associated with other defects. Dextrocardia with situs solitus (also known as isolated dextrocardia) is frequently seen in the context of severe cardiac anomalies that include atrioventricular discordance (*l*-looped ventricles), single

Table 5.1 Derivatives of the aortic arches

Aortic arch	Derivative
First aortic arch	Maxillary artery, external carotid arteries
Third aortic arch	Common carotid arteries Internal carotid arteries
Fourth aortic arch	Proximal right subclavian artery Transverse aortic arch (between left common carotid and left subclavian artery)
Sixth aortic arch	Proximal left and right pulmonary artery Ductus arteriosus
Seventh intersegmental artery	Distal right subclavian artery Left subclavian artery

ventricle, transposition of the great arteries, and heterotaxy syndrome. Dextrocardia with situs inversus is less likely to be accompanied by cardiac defects.

Defects of atrial septation

Defects resulting from the abnormal formation of the atrial septum represent a large proportion of congenital heart lesions [39]. Atrial septal defects can occur in isolation or may be seen in association with other cardiovascular malformations. Communications at the interatrial level include the following: patent foramen ovale, ostium secundum defect, ostium primum defect, sinus venosus defect, and common atrium.

A patent foramen ovale may be found in up to a fourth to a third of the population. This results from failure of fusion of the primum and secundum septae. Ostium secundum defects are the most common type of communications at the interatrial septum. They are typically located centrally in the interatrial septum. These defects result from a combination of excessive resorption of the septum primum and large foramen ovale defects. Ostium primum defects are seen in up to 20% of children with Down syndrome. These are communications in the lower portion of the atrial septum and are associated with a cleft in the mitral valve. These defects are considered a form of endocardial cushion defect. Primum defects result from lack of fusion of the primum septum with the absent endocardial cushion. Sinus venosus defects, located near the entrance of either the superior or inferior vena cava into the right atrium, result from defects in the sinus venosus portion of the atrial septum. They are associated with partial anomalous pulmonary venous connections. Complete absence of the atrial septum results in a common atrium. This may be part of the heterotaxy syndrome.

Defects of the atrioventricular canal and atrioventricular valves

Atrioventricular canal defects, also referred to as atrioventricular septal defects or endocardial cushion defects, result from failure of fusion of the superior and inferior endocardial cushions [21,40]. These defects can vary in severity and complexity [41]. The pathology involves a combination of the following: an atrial communication, a ventricular communication, and abnormal development of the atrioventricular valves. The complete form of the defect involves all three of these components and a common atrioventricular valve. The less severe forms involve only one or two of the above defects. Children with canal-type defects may have displacement of the conduction system, an important issue that has surgical implications. Atrioventricular septal defects are frequently associated with Down syndrome. In fact, nearly 80% of all infants with atrioventricular septal defects

have a chromosomal anomaly, syndrome, non-syndromic organ anomaly or deformation [42].

Tricuspid and mitral valve defects result from failure of normal formation of the two separate valves, chordae tendinae, and ventricular cavitation. Ebstein anomaly is characterized by an apically displaced tricuspid valve with an atrialized portion of the right ventricle. The tricuspid valve is often dysplastic and regurgitant [43]. Valve stenosis may be seen. Isolated mitral valve anomalies in children are relatively rare.

Defects of ventricular septation

Ventricular septal defects are one of the most common types of congenital heart lesions [44]. These defects encompass four major portions of the ventricular septum: membranous, muscular, inlet, and outlet. Defects in the membranous region (referred to as membranous or perimembranous) predominate. These result from failure of fusion of endocardial tissue ingrowth, aorticopulmonary septum, and muscular septum. Muscular defects are the second most common type of defects in the ventricular septum. These can be single or multiple and can be located anywhere along the muscular or trabecular portion of the septum. Multiple muscular defects in close proximity or that may coalesce together are colloquially referred to as "Swiss cheese" defects. Defects in the inlet septum are associated with endocardial cushion defects. These result from failure of fusion of the medial endocardial cushions and formation of the inlet ventricular septum. Outlet defects may also be referred to as conal, supracristal, subarterial or doubly committed defects. These are located in the right ventricular outflow tract immediately below the pulmonary valve. When examined from the left ventricular aspect, these defects lie just below the aortic valve. This anatomical relationship is a substrate for aortic valve prolapse or herniation of the valve cusps into the defect and may lead to aortic insufficiency.

Defects of conotruncal development and semi-lunar valve formation

Defects of conotruncal development and semi-lunar valve formation account for a large number of congenital heart defects [45,46]. These include truncus arteriosus, d-transposition of the great arteries, tetralogy of Fallot, and aortopulmonary window. Several of these conotruncal malformations have been linked to abnormal aortopulmonary septation under the influence of the neural crest [28,47,48].

Truncus arteriosus results from failed formation of the truncal ridges and aorticopulmonary septum. A single aorticopulmonary trunk with underlying ventricular septal defect (VSD) gives rise to the pulmonary, coronary, and systemic circulations [49]. Several subtypes of this anomaly exist with variants based on the anatomical origin of the pulmonary arteries.

Failure of spiral septation of the aorticopulmonary septum can result in several congenital cardiac defects. Both transposition of the great arteries and tetralogy of Fallot can be explained by this mechanism. Transposition of the great arteries is thought to be the result of failed spiral septation. This results in the pulmonary artery arising from the posterior left ventricle and the aorta originating from the anterior right ventricle [50]. Tetralogy of Fallot results from unequal partitioning of the aorta and pulmonary artery. Anterior deviation of the conal septum results in a diminutive right ventricular outflow tract, over-riding aorta, and secondary right ventricular hypertrophy [51]. Failure of fusion of the conal septum with the bulbus cordis results in the ventricular level communication in this malformation. Pulmonary atresia is considered within the spectrum of tetralogy of Fallot as a severe form. Extreme anterior deviation of the aorticopulmonary and conal septae in this case results in lack of a pulmonary outflow tract.

An aortopulmonary window results from failed aorticopulmonary septation. In this defect there is a communication between the aorta and pulmonary artery, but typically no ventricular septal defect is present [52].

Defects in aortic arch development

Normal aortic arch development relies on sequential development and regression of the aortic arches. Failure of these processes can lead to a number of aortic arch anomalies.

Two developmental events that can result in aortic arch obstruction include hypoplasia of the arch and the presence of ductal tissue in the aorta at its site of insertion. The aortic arch is derived proximally from the aortic sac, distally from the fourth aortic arch, and at the isthmus from the fourth and sixth aortic arches. Failure of development of each of these segments can lead to underdevelopment of the aortic arch or interruption. Although the specific level of arch obstruction is variable among these lesions, perfusion to the lower body is often dependent on patency of the ductus arteriosus.

Aortic arch anomalies can result in a vascular ring, double aortic arch or pulmonary artery sling [53]. These variations in the arrangement of the great arteries can be further explained by considering the embryological development of the aortic arch and pulmonary arteries.

The embryonic aortic arches encircle the embryonic foregut (trachea and esophagus). Normal development results in regression of the right sixth aortic arch and involution of the right dorsal aorta, thus avoiding formation of a vascular ring. Failure of this normal development or regression can lead to variations in pathological anatomy that result in vascular encirclement or compres-

Table 5.2 Aortic arch anomalies

Anomaly	Cause
Left aortic arch with retroesophageal right subclavian artery (aberrant right subclavian artery)	Absence of right fourth aortic arch
Left aortic arch with retroesophageal diverticulum of Kommerell	Absence of right fourth aortic arch, persistence of right sixth arch (right ligamentum arteriosum)
Right aortic arch with mirror image branching	Absence of left dorsal aorta
Right aortic arch with diverticulum of Kommerell	Absence of left fourth aortic arch, persistence of left sixth arch (left ligamentum arteriosum)
Right aortic arch with retroesophageal left subclavian artery (aberrant left subclavian artery)	Absence of left fourth and sixth aortic arches
Double aortic arch	Persistence of right and left fourth aortic arches

sion of the trachea and/or esophagus, in some cases associated with obstructive symptoms.

Selected defects in aortic arch development are listed in Table 5.2. We initiate this discussion reviewing variants associated with a left aortic arch. The formation of a left aortic arch with an aberrant or retroesophageal subclavian artery (branching pattern: right carotid, left carotid, left subclavian, and anomalous right subclavian artery) is the result of abnormal regression of the right fourth aortic arch. This is the most common arch variant occurring in 0.5% of the general population. The right sixth aortic arch regresses normally in this defect, and no vascular ring is formed. In contrast, a left aortic arch with retroesophageal diverticulum of Kommerell also has abnormal regression of the right fourth aortic arch, but persistence of the right sixth aortic arch as the right ligamentum arteriosum. This defect results in a vascular ring encircling the trachea and esophagus.

The formation of a right aortic arch with mirror image branching is the result of regression of the left dorsal aorta. The branching pattern in this case is as follows: first arch vessel, left innominate artery that branches into left subclavian and left carotid arteries; second vessel, right carotid artery; and third vessel, right subclavian artery. This substrate is almost invariably associated with intracardiac disease.

A right aortic arch with a retroesophageal diverticulum of Kommerell results from regression of the fourth aortic arch, persistence of the left sixth arch as the ligamentum arteriosus and of the left dorsal aorta. This results in a vascular ring. A right aortic arch with aberrant subclavian artery (branching sequence: left carotid, right carotid, right subclavian, and anomalous left subclavian artery) can be accounted for by regression of the left fourth and sixth aortic arches. The absence of the left sixth arch, or ductal arch, prevents formation of a vascular ring. Many of these children have conotruncal malformations. The formation of a double aortic arch is the result of persistence of both the right and fourth aortic arches. The presence of both arches results in a vascular ring and frequently the left arch is atretic. This anomaly is associated with symptomatology in infancy related to tracheal and esophageal compression.

A cervical aortic arch occurs when the arch extends into the soft tissues of the neck, above the level of the clavicle. This rare anomaly has also been referred to as "high aortic arch." Various arrangements including normal and anomalous arch branching patterns, in addition to pathology such as aortic arch obstruction, have been reported in affected patients. A number of embryological explanations (atresia of the fourth primitive aortic arch associated with persistence of the third arch, failure of normal caudal aortic arch migration) have been proposed to account for the various subtypes.

Defects in coronary artery development

The coronary arteries arise from epicardial blood islands in the sulci of the developing heart. These in turn connect to the sinuses of Valsalva and form capillary networks with veins connected to the coronary sinus. Buds from the pulmonary arteries also connect to the coronary arteries, but regress during normal development.

Persistence of this pulmonary connection can lead to anomalous origin of the left coronary artery from the pulmonary artery [54]. Affected children become symptomatic as the pulmonary vascular resistance declines following birth. The diminished perfusion pressure of the left coronary artery accounts for myocardial ischemia and ventricular dysfunction.

Defects of the venous system

Defects of the superior and inferior vena cava rarely occur [55]. Among systemic venous anomalies, persistence of the left superior vena cava draining into the coronary sinus is most common. This is due to persistence of the left anterior and common cardinal veins. Interruption of the inferior vena cava with azygous and hemiazygous continuation of flow into the right atrium may be seen, most frequently in the setting of complex congenital heart disease. In these patients the inferior vena cava is interrupted above the renal veins and blood eventually enters the heart via alternative venous pathways. Failure of for-

mation of the hepatic portion of the inferior vena cava is thought to account for these anomalies.

Defects in pulmonary venous drainage

During the early stages of human development, the vascular plexus of the foregut, also known as the splanchnic plexus, which forms the pulmonary vasculature, has no direct connection to the heart. Defective development or regression of the pulmonary venous plexus and its connection to the primordial or common pulmonary vein can lead to anomalous pulmonary venous connections and/or drainage.

Anomalous pulmonary venous drainage can occur in a total or partial manner, meaning that all veins or a selected number do not enter the left atrium [56]. In total anomalous pulmonary venous drainage, the pulmonary veins drain into the right atrium or other vascular structures either above or below the liver. In partial anomalous pulmonary venous drainage, at least one vein empties normally into the left atrium with one or more pulmonary veins draining elsewhere. In some instances, mixed anomalous drainage may be present, with pulmonary venous connection to various sites.

Developmental cardiac physiology and pathophysiology

The circulatory system in congenital heart disease continually changes and develops in response to both normal and pathological stimuli. Response to anesthetic and surgical interventions must be understood within this framework, and is often radically different from the usual, expected pediatric and adult situations with a "normal" cardiovascular system. This section will review developmental changes of the cardiovascular system from fetal life through adulthood, both in the normal and pathophysiological states associated with congenital heart disease. As little is known about the development of the normal and diseased human heart, much of the information discussed in this chapter is derived from animal models. Undoubtedly, new information will be discovered as more studies on human myocardiocal tissues are undertaken.

Development from fetus to neonate
Circulatory pathways

The fetus receives oxygenated and nutrient-rich blood from the placenta via the umbilical vein, and ejects desaturated blood through the umbilical arteries to the placenta, and thus the placenta, not the lung, serves as the organ of respiration. Blood flow thus largely bypasses the lungs *in utero*, accounting for only about 7% of the fetal combined ventricular output [57]. Pulmonary vascular

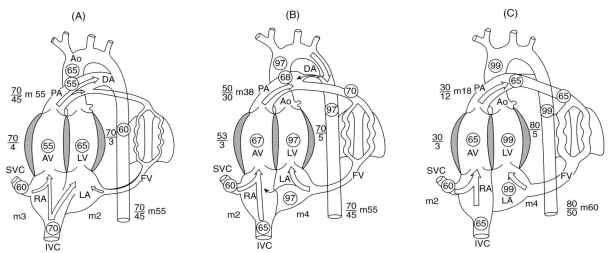

Figure 5.13 Transition from fetal to mature circulation. (A) Fetal circulation. (B) Transitional circulation. (C) Mature circulation. Circled numbers are oxygen saturations, uncircled numbers are pressures in mmHg. M, mean pressure; RV, right ventricle; LV, left ventricle; RA, right atrium; LA, left atrium; DA, ductus arteriosus; Ao, aorta; PA, pulmonary artery; SVC, superior vena cava; IVC, inferior vena cava; PV, pulmonary vein. Reproduced from Rudolph [149] with permission from Year Book Medical Publishers.

resistance is high, and the lungs are collapsed and filled with amniotic fluid. This is the basis for the fetal circulation, which is a parallel one, rather than the series circulation seen postnatally. Three fetal circulatory shunts exist to carry better oxygenated blood from the umbilical vein to the systemic circulation: the ductus venosus, ductus arteriosus, and foramen ovale (Fig. 5.13A). Approximately 50% of the umbilical venous blood, with an oxygen tension of about 30–35 mmHg, passes through the ductus venosus and enters the right atrium. There, it streams preferentially across the foramen ovale, guided by the valves of the sinus venosus and Chiari network into the left atrium. Thus the brain and upper body preferentially receive this relatively well-oxygenated blood, which accounts for 20–30% of the combined ventricular output. Blood returning to the inferior vena cava represents about 70% of the total venous return to the heart, and two-thirds of this deoxygenated blood passes into the right atrium and ventricle. About 90% of the blood flows through the ductus arteriosus to supply the lower fetal body.

With inflation of the lungs and increasing arterial oxygen tension at birth, there is a dramatic fall in pulmonary vascular resistance and increase in pulmonary blood flow. The placental circulation is removed and all these changes lead to closure of the ductus venosus, constriction of the ductus arteriosus, and reversal of pressure gradients in the left and right atria, leading to functional closure of the foramen ovale. This results in a state called the transitional circulation (Fig. 5.13B), characterized by high pulmonary artery pressures and resistance (much lower than *in utero*, however), and a small amount of left-to-right shunting through the ductus arteriosus. This is a

labile state, and failure to maintain lower pulmonary vascular resistance can rapidly lead to reversal to fetal circulatory pathways, and right-to-left shunting at the level of the ductus arteriosus and foramen ovale. This maintenance of fetal circulatory pathways is necessary for survival in many congenital heart lesions, particularly those dependent on patency of the ductus arteriosus for all or a significant portion of systemic or pulmonary blood flow, or in the settings of atresia of atrioventricular valves. Maintenance of ductal patency with prostaglandin E1 is essential in these lesions. In the two-ventricle heart with a large intracardiac communication, maintenance of the fetal circulation leads to right-to-left shunting at the foramen and ductal levels, and thus arterial desaturation.

Conversion to the mature circulation (Fig. 5.13C) in the normal heart occurs over a period of several weeks, as pulmonary vascular resistance falls further, and the ductus arteriosus permanently closes by thrombosis, intimal proliferation, and fibrosis. Factors favoring the transition from the fetal to a mature circulation include normal oxygen tension and physical expansion of the lungs, normal pH, nitric oxide, and prostacyclin. Factors favoring reversion to fetal circulation include low oxygen tension, acidosis, lung collapse, and inflammatory mediators (leukotrienes, thromboxane A2, platelet activating factor) as seen in sepsis and other related conditions, and endothelin A receptor activators [58].

Myocardial contractility
The fetal myocardium is characterized by a poorly organized cellular arrangement, and fewer myofibrils with a

random orientation, in contrast to the parallel, well-organized myofibrillar arrangement of the adult myocardium [59] (see below). Fetal hearts develop less tension per gram than adult hearts because of increased water content and fewer contractile elements. Calcium cycling and excitation-contraction coupling are also very different, with poorly organized T-tubules and immature sarcoplasmic reticulum, leading to more dependence on free cytosolic ionized calcium for normal contractility in the fetal heart. Despite this immature state, the fetal heart can increase its stroke volume in a limited fashion up to left atrial pressures of 10–12 mmHg according to the Frank–Starling relationship, as long as afterload (i.e. arterial pressure) is kept low [60]. These features continue throughout the neonatal and early infancy period.

Development from neonate to older infant and child

At birth, the neonatal heart must suddenly change from a parallel circulation to one in series, and the left ventricle in particular must adapt immediately to dramatically increased preload from blood returning from the lungs, and increased afterload as the placental circulation is removed. The very high oxygen consumption of the newborn necessitates a high cardiac output for the first few months of life. However, animal models have demonstrated that the fetal and newborn myocardium develops less tension in response to increasing preload (sarcomere length), and that cardiac output increases less to the same degree of volume loading [61,62]. Resting tension, however, is greater in the newborn compared to the mature heart. These data suggest that the newborn heart is operating near the maximum of its Frank–Starling curve, and that there is less reserve in response to both increased afterload and preload. This observation is borne out clinically in newborns after complex heart surgery, who are often intolerant of even small increases in left atrial pressure or mean arterial pressure. The newborn myocardium also has only a limited ability to increase its inotropic state in response to exogenous catecholamines, and is much more dependent on heart rate to maintain cardiac output than is the mature heart. One reason for this is the high levels of circulating endogenous catecholamines that appear after birth, necessary to make the transition to extrauterine life [63]. As these levels decrease in the weeks after birth, contractile reserve increases.

The neonatal myocardium is less compliant than the mature myocardium, with increased resting tension as noted above, and a significantly greater increase in ventricular pressure with volume loading [64]. This implies that diastolic function of the neonatal heart is also impaired compared to the mature heart [65]. The myofibrils of the newborn heart also appear to have a greater sensitivity to calcium, developing a greater tension than

adult myofibrils when exposed to the same free calcium concentration *in vitro* [66].

It must again be emphasized that nearly all of these data are derived from animal work, and although the information appears to agree with what is observed clinically, there is a need for non-invasive studies of normal human hearts from the neonatal period through adulthood to confirm these impressions of developmental cardiovascular physiology.

Innervation of the heart

Clinical observations in newborn infants have led to the hypothesis that the sympathetic innervation and control of the cardiovascular system are incomplete in this age group compared to older children and adults, and that the parasympathetic innervation is intact [59]. Examples of this include the frequency of bradycardia in the newborn in response to a number of stimuli, including vagal and vagotonic agents, and the relative lack of sensitivity in the newborn to sympathomimetic agents. Histological studies in animal models have demonstrated incomplete sympathetic innervation in the neonatal heart when compared to the adult, but no differences in the number or density of parasympathetic nerves [67,68].

Autonomic cardiovascular control of cardiac activity can be evaluated by measuring heart rate variability in response to both respiration and beat-to-beat variability in systolic blood pressure [69]. The sympathetic and parasympathetic input into sinoatrial node activity contribute to heart rate variability changes, with greater heart rate variability resulting from greater parasympathetic input into sinoatrial node activity [70]. Studies using these methodologies for normal infants during sleep suggest that the parasympathetic predominance gradually diminishes until approximately 6 months of age, coinciding with greater sympathetic innervation of the heart similar to adult levels [71].

Development from child to adult

Beyond the transition period from fetal to newborn life and into the first few months of postnatal life, there is limited human or animal information concerning the exact nature and extent of cardiac development at the cellular level. Most studies compare newborn or fetuses to adult animals [72]. Cardiac chamber development is assumed to be influenced by blood flow [73]. Large flow or volume load in a ventricle results in ventricular enlargement. Small competent atrioventricular valves, as in tricuspid stenosis, result in decreased blood flow and ventricular hypoplasia. Increases in myocardial mass with normal growth, as well as in ventricular outflow obstruction, are mainly due to hypertrophy of myocytes. Late gestational increases in blood cortisol are responsible for this growth pattern, and there is concern that antenatal glucocorticoids to induce lung maturity may inhibit cardiac myocyte proliferation. In the human infant, it is assumed that the cellular elements of the cardiac myocyte, i.e. adrenergic receptors, intracellular receptors and signaling, calcium cycling and regulation and interaction of the contractile proteins, are similar to the adult by approximately 6 months of age. Similarly, cardiac depression by volatile agents is greater in the newborn, changing to adult levels by approximately 6 months of age [74].

Normal values for physiological variables by age

It is useful for the anesthesiologist to be aware of normal ranges for physiological variables in premature and full-term newborns of all sizes, and in infants and children of all ages (Fig. 5.14). Obviously, acceptable ranges for these variables are highly dependent on the individual patient's pathophysiology, but the wide range of "normal" values may reassure the practitioner to accept "low" blood pressure, for example, if other indices of cardiac function and tissue oxygen delivery are acceptable.

Cardiomyocyte receptor function in normal and diseased hearts

The adrenergic receptor

The adrenergic receptors (AR) are part of a large super-family of receptors that mediate their biological responses

through the coupling of a specific guanine nucleotide regulatory protein or G protein [75]. This superfamily of receptors shares a common structural motif, character-ized by seven hydrophobic domains spanning the lipid bilayer. The seven domains are attached by three internal loops and three external loops between the amine termi-nus and the cytoplasmic carboxy terminus. The function of this receptor family is dependent on a specific agonist (or ligand) binding to the receptor, which causes a con-formational change in the receptor. This structural change permits the interaction between the intracellular portion of the receptor and guanine nucleotide regulatory protein (or G protein). This interaction, also referred to as cou-pling, inevitably links the activated receptor to a specific biological response. The regulation of the biological response is initiated by the specificity of the receptor for a particular extracellular agonist and the coupling of a specific G protein to that activated receptor.

Once an extracellular ligand (or agonist) is specifically recognized by a cell surface receptor, the receptor under-goes conformational changes that expose a specific region of the receptor complex to the intracellular side of the plasma membrane [76] (Fig. 5.15). This confirmation change triggers the interaction of the G protein with the amino acids of the third intracellular loop of the receptor, hence leading to G protein activation. There are three dif-ferent G proteins: stimulatory G protein (Gs), inhibitory G protein (Gi) and Gq (heterotrimeric G protein). Under

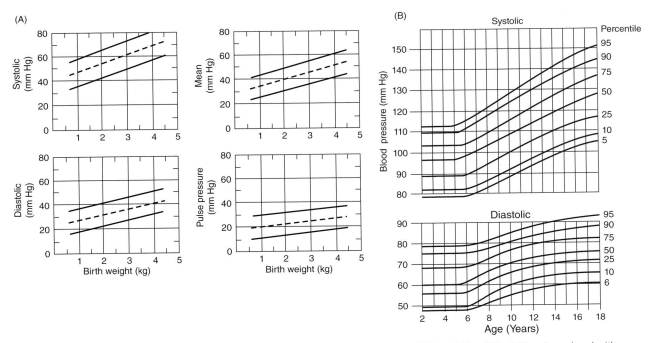

Figure 5.14 (A) Blood pressure measured in the umbilical artery of infants in the first 12 hours of life weighing 600–4200 g. Reproduced with permission from Versmold et al. [150]. (B) Blood pressure percentiles, age 2–18 years. Reproduced from Blumenthal [151] with permission from the American Academy of Pediatrics.

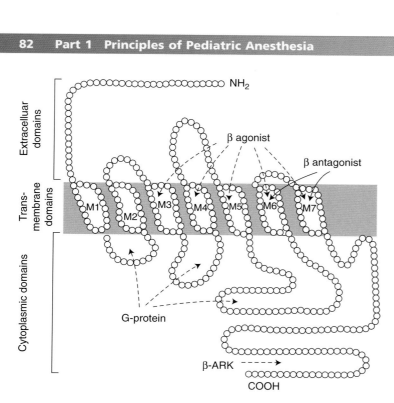

Figure 5.15 Molecular structure of the β-adrenergic receptor, demonstrating its three domains. The transmembrane domains serve as ligand-binding pockets for agonists (*dashed arrows*) and antagonists (*solid arrows*). The cytoplasmic domains interact with G proteins and β-adrenergic receptor kinases. Reproduced from Moss and Renz [75] with permission from Elsevier.

normal conditions, all the adrenergic β receptors interact with Gs, α1 interacts with Gq and α2 interacts with Gi. Each G protein is a heterotrimer made up of three subunits: α, β, and γ. The activation of the G protein-coupled receptor causes an exchange of bound guanosine diphosphate (GDP) for guanosine triphosphate (GTP) within the α subunit and initiates the dissociation of the β/γ subunit from the α subunit. The GTP-activated α subunit modulates the activity of a specific effector enzyme within a specific signaling pathway by catalyzing the hydrolysis of GTP to GDP and inorganic phosphate. This causes the transference of a high-energy phosphate group to an enzyme and in turn causes the deactivation of the α subunit. This process will eventually lead to the deactivation of the α subunit and the reassociation with the β/γ complex. This cycle is continuously repeated until the agonist becomes unbound from the receptor. Downstream of enzyme activation, the production of a second messenger regulates the biological response.

Adrenergic receptors have been subdivided into two principals, α and β, based on the results of binding studies using a series of selective agonists and antagonists [77]. This has been validated repeatedly with the development of drugs that function to selectively antagonize the α receptor with no effect on the β receptor. Soon after the distinction between the α and β receptor type was recognized, it became more evident that the separation of these receptors was not sufficient to explain pharmacological studies using rank order of potency for an antagonist, differing from an agonist because it blocks the biological response. With the advent of radioligand-labeled antago-

nists and new molecular cloning techniques examining receptor gene expression, it became clear that the two principal receptor groups could be further subdivided into additional subtypes.

To date, within the β adrenergic group, four different subtypes have been identified: β1, β2, β3, β4. Pharmacologically, β1 and β2 are differentiated by their affinities for different catecholamines: epinephrine, norephinephrine, and isoproterenol. β1 has similar affinity for epinephrine and norepinephrine, while β2 has a higher affinity for epinephrine than norepinephrine. Both β1 and β2 have the same affinity for isoproterenol. The β3 and β4 receptors have minor roles in cardiovascular function and will not be discussed further here.

The expression and distribution of each receptor subtype are highly dependent on the organ, which adds another level of specificity. Distribution of a particular receptor in two different tissue types may result in two different functions. When examining cardiovascular response to adrenergic stimulation, the β1 receptor is predominantly expressed in heart tissue. The stimulation of the receptor subtype leads to both inotropic and chronotropic effects on cardiac function, resulting in an increase in the myocardial contractile force and a shortening of contractile timing, respectively. While β2 can also be found in the heart, it is mostly expressed in vascular smooth muscle tissue. The distribution and function relevance of this receptor subtype in the heart are controversial and may change with alterations in cardiac function. The percentage of β2 receptors in the non-failing heart averages about 20% in the ventricle [78] and 30% in the atrium. The percentage of β1 to β2 receptors is approximately 75%:25% in the ventricles of younger hearts [79,80].

Each signaling pathway is specific to each adrenergic receptor. Once the agonist binds to the β1 receptor, causing the coupling of the G protein, the G protein α subunit becomes activated, followed by an increase in adenylate cyclase (AC) activity, which induces the conversion of ATP to cyclic adenosine monophosphate (cAMP). The second messenger, cAMP, phosphorylates protein kinase A (PKA). The function of a kinase is to phosphorylate other target proteins which initiate a biological response (see Fig. 5.15). PKA phosphorylates many effector proteins and the phosphorylation of each one functions to increase the concentration of intracellular calcium.

The β2 receptor has also been shown to function through the cAMP signaling pathway, causing the activation of PKA, but not nearly to the extent of β1 in cardiomyocytes [81]. The response of this stimulation appears to have a larger effect on smooth muscle, for example the vascular smooth muscle. In this tissue type, the stimulation of β2 and the subsequent increase in cAMP promotes the vasodilation of vascular smooth muscle and may lead to alterations in blood pressure. In these tissues, the effect of β1 stimulation appears to be minimal, due to lack of β1 receptors in the smooth muscle.

Similar to the β receptor, the α receptors can be pharmacologically subdivided into α1 and α2. The α1 receptor is distributed in most vascular smooth muscle and to a lesser extent the in the heart. The α2 receptor has been found in some vascular smooth muscle but its major functional importance is as a presynaptic receptor in the central and peripheral nervous systems. The use of molecular techniques has identified three additional subtypes of the α1 receptor (α1A, α1B, and α1D) and three additional subtypes of the α2 receptor [75]. Binding of an agonist to an α1 receptor in the heart or vascular smooth muscle results in activation of the Gq subunit of the G protein, which activates phospholipase C (see below), producing diacylglycerol and inositol-1,4,5-triphosphate, which releases calcium from the sarcoplasmic reticulum and increases vascular smooth muscle tone or cardiac contractility. A schematic classification of adrenergic receptors incorporating recent knowledge of molecular pharmacology and signal transduction is presented in Figure 5.16 [75].

The adrenergic receptor concentration in cardiac tissue is very small and measured as femtomoles per milligram of protein. However, the response to stimulation of the receptor is greatly amplified by the signal that occurs downstream of the receptor. In rat ventricular myocytes, the ratio between the β receptors and the next two downstream signaling components (β receptor: G protein: adenylate cyclase) is 1:200:3 [82]. This demonstrates how a large response can be initiated by the activation of a small number of receptors. In addition, it also demonstrates that the rate-limiting component that ultimately regulates intracellular production of cAMP is receptor density and the enzyme concentration of adenylate cyclase.

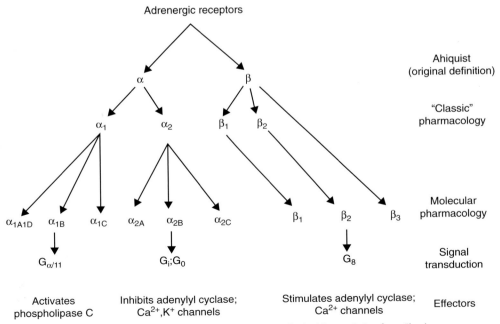

Figure 5.16 Classification of adrenergic receptors. Reproduced from Moss and Renz [75] with permission from Elsevier.

Developmental changes in adrenergic receptor signaling

Information concerning changes in adrenergic receptor function during the transition from neonatal to more mature myocardial development is limited to a few animal studies. As noted above, the neonatal heart has a limited inotropic response to catecholamine administration.

β-adrenergic receptor density is higher in the ventricular myocardium of neonatal versus adult rabbits, but the inotropic response to the same concentration of isoproterenol is significantly greater in adult tissue [83]. In the neonatal rat, the mechanism of β-adrenergic mediated increase in contractility is entirely due to β2 stimulation, whereas in the adult rat it is due solely to β1 receptor activation. Coupling of the β2 receptor to Gi protein action is apparently defective in the neonatal rat, because the ratio of Gi to Gs subunits is much higher in the neonate. The relative proportion of β1 and β2 receptors is the same in neonatal and adult hearts (17% β2), and approximates the ratio measured in children with simple acyanotic congenital heart disease, which is about 22% [84].

There is animal and human evidence to indicate that α-adrenergic receptor-mediated chronotropic and inotropic effects on the cardiac myocyte change with development. In the neonatal animal model, α stimulation produces positive inotropic and chronotropic effects, whereas in the adult it produces negative effects [85,86]. The chronotropic response to α1 stimulation diminished with increasing age in children being evaluated for autonomic dysfunction after vagal and sympathetic blockade [87].

Calcium cycling in the normal heart

Calcium assumes a central role in the process of myocardial contraction and relaxation, serving as the second messenger between depolarization of the cardiac myocyte and its contraction mediated by the actin-myosin system. The role of calcium in this excitation-contraction coupling in the normal mature heart will be reviewed briefly before discussion of developmental changes and changes with heart failure [88].

Cardiac muscle cell contraction depends on an increase in intracellular calcium above a certain threshold, and relaxation ensues when intracellular calcium falls below this threshold. Two major regions of calcium flux occur: across the sarcolemmal membrane (slow response), and release from internal stores: the sarcoplasmic reticulum (rapid release and reuptake) [89] (Fig. 5.17). The primary site of entry of calcium through the sarcolemmal membrane is through the L-type or low voltage-dependent calcium channels, which occurs in two types: a low-threshold, rapidly inactivating channel and a higher threshold, more slowly inactivating channel [90]. Depo-

larization of the sarcolemmal membrane triggers opening of these channels, resulting in the release of large amount of calcium from the sarcoplasmic reticulum (SR), the major internal calcium storage organelle. Calcium entry through the slowly inactivating channels serves to fill the SR with adequate calcium stores. Removal of calcium from the cytoplasm to the exterior of the cell occurs via two major mechanisms: the sodium–calcium ($NaO–Ca^{2+}$) exchanger and the calcium-ATPase pump. The $NaO–Ca^{2+}$ exchanger usually serves to exchange three sodium ions (moving into the cell) for one calcium ion (moving out of the cell), although the reverse action, as well as a 1:1 exchange, are possible [91]. The calcium-ATPase pump actively transports calcium (in a 1:1 Ca^{2+}/ATP ratio) out of the cell in an energy-dependent high-affinity but low-capacity manner [92]. The affinity of the sarcolemmal calcium-ATPase pump is enhanced by calmodulin, which binds free cytoplasmic calcium.

Although the calcium movement through the sarcolemma plays an important role in balancing internal and external calcium concentrations and in supplying calcium to replenish SR calcium stores, and in initiating the calcium-induced release of calcium from the SR, it is important to recognize that the amount of calcium flux is far less than across the SR, the far more important mechanism for excitation-contraction coupling in the mature heart [93]. The sarcolemmal calcium flux mechanisms play a much more important role in the excitation-contraction coupling of the neonatal (immature) heart.

The massive release and reuptake of calcium responsible for activation and deactivation of the actin-myosin complex and cardiocyte contraction and relaxation occur at the level of the SR. This is a closed, intracellular membranous network that is intimately related to the myofilaments responsible for contraction [94] (Fig. 5.18). The SR is connected to the sarcolemmal membrane via the transverse tubule (T-tubule) system. Depolarization of the sarcolemmal membrane leads to transfer of charge down the T-tubules to the SR, resulting in the opening of SR calcium channels and the release of large amounts of calcium into the cytoplasm, where it can then bind to troponin and initiate the actin-myosin interaction. The SR is divided into longitudinal SR and terminal cisternae; the latter connect to the T-tubules. The terminal cisternae are primarily involved in the release of calcium, and the longitudinal SR in its reuptake [95].

The primary calcium release mechanism of the SR is the ligand-gated calcium release channels that bind to the drug ryanodine (also known as the ryanodine receptors). The channels are activated by two primary mechanisms: depolarization via the T-tubules and binding of intracellular calcium itself; the predominance of one mechanism over the other differs in cardiac versus skeletal muscle. The close proximity of the L-type sarcolemmal calcium

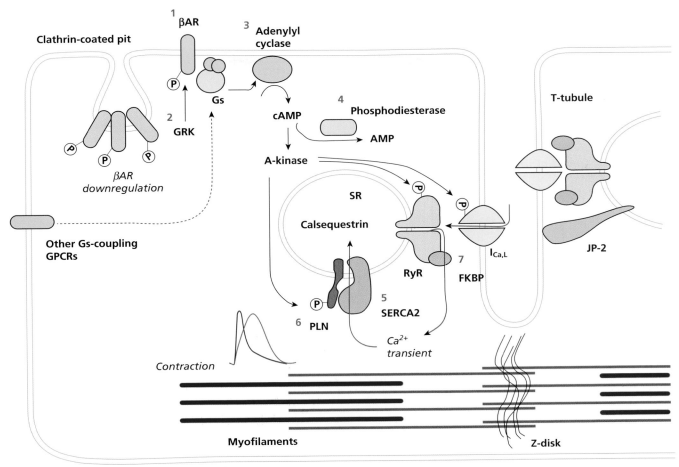

Figure 5.17 Calcium cycling and its relationship to the β-adrenergic receptor system and myocyte myofilaments. See text for discussion. β-AR, β-adrenergic receptor; Gs, stimulatory G protein; GRK, G-receptor kinase; cAMP, cyclic AMP; A-kinase, protein kinase A; SR, sarcoplasmic reticulum; RyR, ryanodine receptor; SERCA2, sarcoplasmic reticulum calcium-ATPase; PLN, phospholamban; $I_{Ca,L}$, L-type calcium channel; FKBP, FK-506 binding protein; JP-2, junctophilin-2; GPCR, G-protein coupling receptor. Encircled P represents sites of phosphorylation by the various kinases. Numbers 1 through 7 represent targets for pharmacological therapy in cardiac failure. Reproduced from Hoshijima and Chien [152] with permission from the American Society of Clinical Investigation.

channels in the T-tubules to the ligand-gated calcium release channels allows the depolarization to rapidly allow calcium into the cell and open the SR calcium channels. These ligand-gated calcium release channels close when the cytosolic calcium concentration increases; normally it opens at $0.6\,\mu M$ Ca^{2+} and closes at $3.0\,\mu M$ Ca^{2+}.

The reuptake and sequestration of calcium leads to relaxation of the cardiac myocyte, and is an active transport mechanism, primarily involving hydrolysis of ATP by the sarcoplasmic reticulum calcium-ATPase (SERCA), located in the longitudinal SR [96]. It binds two calcium ions with high affinity and rapidly transports them to the inside of the SR. This transport system differs from the sarcolemmal membrane: it has higher affinity, allows for more rapid transport, and is not sensitive to calmodulin. Calcium is stored in the SR by calsequestrin, a high-capacity, low-affinity protein that acts as a calcium sink.

There are two other proteins with essential roles in the regulation of calcium flux: phospholamban and calmodulin [97,98]. Phospholamban is associated with the SERCA, and can be phosphorylated by at least four different protein kinases (see above): cAMP dependent, calcium / calmodulin dependent, cyclic guanosine monophosphate (cGMP) dependent, or protein kinase C. When phosphorylated, phospholamban increases the affinity of the SERCA for calcium, facilitating calcium flux back into the SR, thus affecting the inotropic and lusitropic state of the heart. Phospholamban plays an important role in the β-adrenergic mediated increase in the inotropic state of the heart. Calmodulin is a calcium storage protein with four binding sites, found in the cytoplasm, which interacts with the sarcolemmal calcium ATPase (increasing its affinity for calcium), the SR ligand-gated calcium release channel (inhibits its activity at optimal cytoplasmic

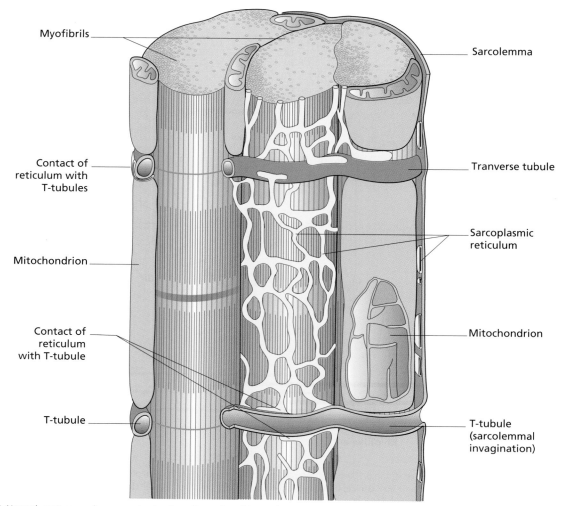

Myofibrils

Sarcolemma

Contact of
reticulum with
T-tubules

Tranverse tubule

Sarcoplasmic
reticulum

Mitochondrion

Contact of
reticulum
with T-tubule

Mitochondrion

T-tubule

T-tubule
(sarcolemmal
invagination)

Figure 5.18 Normal, mature cardiac myocyte structure. Reproduced from Bloom and Fawcett [153] with permission from Elsevier.

calcium), and binds to the calcium/calmodulin-dependent protein kinase [98].

The increase in intracellular cytoplasmic calcium initiates the contractile process. Myosin is the major component of the thick filaments, which make up the microscopic structure of the myofibril, and its interaction with actin (the major component of the thin filaments) provides the mechanical basis of cardiac muscle cell contraction [99]. Actin and myosin make up approximately 80% of the contractile apparatus, and are arranged in a parallel, longitudinal fashion, projecting from a Z-line or band (Fig. 5.19) to form the basic contractile unit called the sarcomere. A three-dimensional lattice is formed, consisting of interdigitated thick and thin filaments in a hexagonal array with three thin filaments in close proximity to each thick filament. The actin and myosin are linked by projections on the myosin protein called S1 cross-bridges,

which bind to actin and, via an energy-dependent hinge-like mechanism, produce the sliding filament cross-bridge action that is thought to produce sarcomere shortening and lengthening. The lattice is held together by connecting proteins such as titin, nebulin, and α-actinin [100].

The actin-myosin interaction is initiated when calcium binds to troponin, a protein closely connected to actin which consists of three subunits: a calcium binding subunit (TNC), a tropomyosin binding unit (TNT), and an inhibitory subunit (TNI). TNC can bind up to four calcium ions and this produces a conformational change on the thin filament, which allows the S1 myosin head cross-bridges to attach [101]. This also changes the TNI subunit's conformation and allows tropomyosin, another protein integral in filament interaction, to move aside and expose the binding sites on actin, allowing the strong binding to the S1 cross-bridges. With calcium

(A)

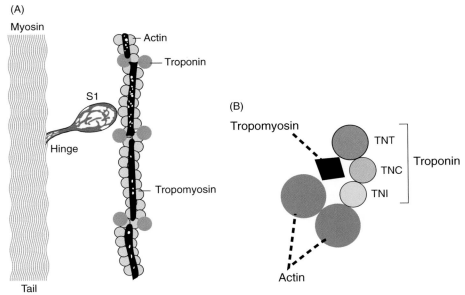

Figure 5.19 (A) Single thick and thin filament showing the S1 cross-bridge and hinge mechanism. (B) Relationship of actin to tropomyosin and the three troponin subunits. See text for explanation. Reproduced from Michael [154] with permission from Lippincott, Williams and Wilkins.

present, actin causes myosin ATPase to hydrolyze one ATP molecule, providing energy that causes the S1 myosin head to pull on the thin filament, resulting in sarcomere shortening. Troponin C is the most important aspect of the regulation of cardiocyte contraction, and has a steep response curve to local levels of calcium. The reuptake of calcium into the SR causes calcium levels to decline rapidly and the inhibitory form of the troponin-tropomyosin-actin complex returns, resulting in reversal of the cross-bridge binding and thus sarcomere relaxation.

Besides calcium, many other regulatory mechanisms exist to influence the interaction and sensitivity of calcium binding to troponin. These mechanisms include β-adrenergic stimulation, thyroid hormone, and phosphorylation by cAMP-dependent protein kinases.

Developmental changes in calcium cycling

Several aspects of the excitation-contraction system are unique in the immature heart. The T-tubule is not fully formed [102], the SR has less storage capacity and less structural organization [103], less mRNA expression [104,105], and less responsiveness to chemical blockade [106,107]. The inhibitory subunit of troponin (TNI) changes from a predominantly cAMP-insensitive form to a cAMP-responsive form by 9 months of age, an additional factor contributing to the increased responsiveness seen with β-adrenergic stimulation after the neonatal period [107]. All of this information has led to the theory that the neonatal cardiac myocyte is more dependent on

free cytosolic calcium fluxes than is the mature heart, and more susceptible to blockade of the L-type calcium sarcolemmal channels as a mechanism of myocardial depression. The latter is thought to be the mechanism producing greater myocardial depression observed with halothane in neonatal rat models compared with sevoflurane, and the same phenomenon seen clinically [108]. A summary of the major differences in cardiac development and function between the neonatal and mature heart is presented in Table 5.3.

Thyroid hormone

Tri-iodothyronine (T3) has a critical role in both the development of the cardiovascular system, and also in acute regulation and performance. Normal T3 levels are essential for normal maturation and development of the heart through expression of genes responsible for the production of the cardiac contractile proteins, elements of the calcium cycling apparatus, and development and density of β-adrenergic receptors [109]. There are cell nucleus-mediated effects from exogenous T3 that occur via an increase in protein synthesis and require at least 8 h to develop. These include an upregulation of β-adrenergic receptors, increase in cardiac contractile protein synthesis, mitochondrial density, volume, and respiration, and SR calcium-ATPase mRNA, and changes in myosin heavy chain isoforms. However, there are acute effects of T3 on cardiac myocytes that occur in minutes from interactions with specific sarcolemmal receptors, and include stimulation of L-type calcium pump activity, stimulation of SR

Table 5.3 Summary of major differences between neonatal and mature hearts

Feature	Neonatal	Mature
Physiology		
Contractility	Limited	Normal
Heart rate dependence	High	Low
Contractile reserve	Low	High
Afterload tolerance	Low	Higher
Preload tolerance	Limited	Better
Ventricular interdependence	Significant	Less
Calcium cycling		
Predominant site of Ca^{2+} flux	Sarcolemma	Sarcoplasmic reticulum
Dependence on normal iCa^{2+}	High	Lower
Circulating catecholamines	High	Lower
Adrenergic receptors	Downregulated, insensitive	Normal
	$\beta2$, $\alpha1$ predominant	$\beta1$ predominant
Innervation	Parasympathetic predominant	Complete
	Sympatheticpredominant	Incomplete
Cytoskeleton	High collagen/water content	Lower collagen/water content
Cellular elements	Incomplete SR	Mature SR
	Disorganized myofibrils	Organized myofibrils

SR, sarcoplasmic reticulum.

calcium-ATPase activity, increased protein kinase activity, and decrease in phospholamban [110]. Cardiac surgery and cardiopulmonary bypass interfere with the conversion of thyroxine (T4) to T3, and serum levels decrease significantly after cardiac surgery in infants and children [111]. T3 infusions improve myocardial function in children after cardiac surgery and reduce intensive care unit stay [112].

Regulation of vascular tone in systemic and pulmonary circulations

The regulation of vascular tone is an important consideration in the understanding and treatment of congenital heart disease. Both the systemic and pulmonary circulations have complex systems to maintain a delicate balance between vasodilating and vasoconstricting mediators in normal patients. Abnormal responses may develop which lead to pulmonary or systemic hypertension or, conversely, vasodilation. A schematic representation of some of these mediators is shown in Figure 5.20. To some extent, the control mechanisms reviewed are present in both the systemic and pulmonary circulations; however, certain mechanisms are more important in one circulation. For example, the endothelial-mediated systems (nitric oxide-cGMP pathways, etc.) predominate in the pulmonary circulation (low-resistance circulation), and

the phospholipase systems in the systemic circulation (high-resistance circulation).

Pulmonary circulation

Vasoactive metabolites of arachidonic acid, called eicosanoids, are produced in cell membranes. Eicosanoids metabolized via the lipoxygenase pathway will form leukotrienes, and those metabolized via the cyclo-oxygenase pathway form the prostaglandins (PG). Important vasodilating prostaglandins include PGE1, which also promotes and maintains patency of the ductus arteriosus. Prostacyclin, PGI2, is a potent pulmonary vasodilator [113]. Prostaglandins act in vascular smooth muscle of the systemic and pulmonary circulations by binding to receptors in the smooth muscle cell membrane, activating adenylate cyclase and increasing cAMP concentrations, which lead to lower calcium levels and a reduction of vascular tone. Thromboxane A2 is a potent leukotriene that has the opposite effect to the prostaglandins, producing vasoconstriction and platelet aggregation. Imbalance in this system caused by chronic hypoxia can lead to chronic pulmonary hypertension.

Nitric oxide (NO) is an endothelium-derived factor that causes relaxation of vascular smooth muscle cells after diffusing into the cell and activating guanylate cyclase, increasing the concentration of cGMP, leading

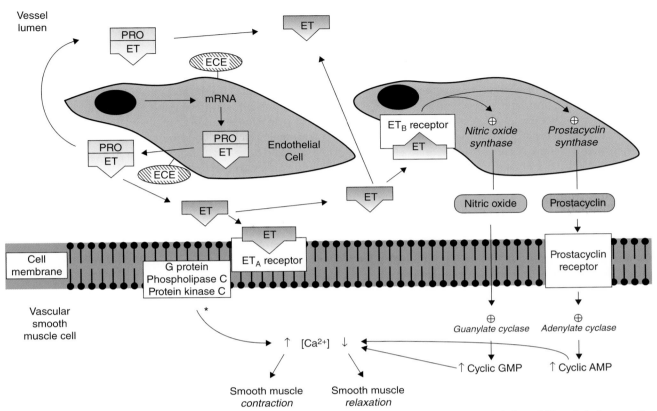

Figure 5.20 Some major mediators of vascular tone in the pulmonary circulation. ET, endothelin-1; PROET, proendothelin-1; ECE, endothelin converting enzyme. See text for explanation. Reproduced from Haynes and Webb [155] with permission from Portland Press.

to a reduction in the local concentration of calcium and thus reducing vascular tone [114]. Calcium-sensitive potassium channels contribute to the vasodilation caused by NO via a cGMP-dependent protein kinase [115]. NO is formed from L-arginine by NO synthase, and is almost immediately inactivated by binding to hemoglobin. Phosphodiesterase V breaks down cGMP, so the phosphodiesterase-inhibiting drugs, like sildenafil, potentiate NO-mediated vasodilation [116].

Endothelins are powerful endothelium-derived vasoactive peptides, and endothelin-1 (ET-1) is the best characterized. ET-1 is produced from proendothelin-1 by endothelin-converting enzymes in the endothelial cells of systemic and pulmonary vasculature. Increased pressure, shear stress, and hypoxia can lead to increased production of ET-1 in the pulmonary circulation. Two ET-1 receptors, ETA and ETB, mediate effects on smooth muscle vascular tone [117]. The ETA receptor is found on the smooth muscle cell membrane and mediates vasoconstriction, while the ETB receptor is located on the endothelial cell itself and results in increased NO synthase activity, producing vasodilation. The primary activity of ET-1 appears to be to stimulate the ETA receptor, and indeed

increased levels of ET-1 are found in many pulmonary hypertensive states such as Eisenmenger syndrome and primary pulmonary hypertension [118].

Systemic circulation

There are multiple levels of control over the peripheral circulation. Neural control by the sympathetic and parasympathetic nervous systems is produced by stimulation of receptors on the afferent limb such as stretch receptors within the walls of the heart, and baroreceptors in the walls of arteries, such as the aortic arch and carotid sinuses. Stretch in the arterial wall stimulates the baroreceptors, producing vasodilation and heart rate slowing mediated by the vasomotor centers of the medulla [119]. Atrial stretch receptors inhibit secretion of vasopressin from the hypothalamus.

The efferent limb of the autonomic nervous system consists of sympathetic and parasympathetic nerve fibers. The sympathetic nerves can be divided into vasoconstrictor and vasodilator fibers. When stimulated, the vasoconstrictor fibers release norepinephrine activating α-adrenergic receptors and producing vasoconstriction. The vasodilator fibers release acetylcholine or epinephrine, and are mainly present in skeletal muscle. Parasympathetic fibers are vital in control of heart rate and function, but have only a minor role in controlling the peripheral circulation [120].

Hormonal control and receptor-mediated intracellular signaling are other important mechanisms. Norepinephrine primarily stimulates peripheral α receptors and causes vasoconstriction. It is secreted by the adrenal medulla and by sympathetic nerves in proximity to the systemic blood vessels. Epinephrine is also secreted by the adrenal medulla, but its primary action is to stimulate the $\beta2$ receptors in the peripheral circulation, causing vasodilation through cAMP-mediated reductions in intracellular calcium concentrations.

Angiotensin II is produced by activation of the renin-angiotensin-aldosterone axis in response to reduced flow and pressure sensed by the juxtaglomerular apparatus in the kidney. Renin produces antiotensin I by cleaving angiotensinogen, and angiotensin II is produced by angiotensin-converting enzyme when angiotensin I passes through the lung. Angiotensin II is a potent vaso-

constrictor and also induces the hypothalamus to secrete vasopressin (antidiuretic hormone), which also has vasoconstrictor properties.

Atrial natriuretic factor (ANF) is released from atrial myocytes in response to stretch (elevation of right or left atrial pressure) on the atrium. ANF has vasodilatory and cardio-inhibitory effects, and leads to sodium retention from decreased tubular reabsorption of sodium in the kidney [121]. B-type natriuretic peptide (BNP) is released by ventricular myocardium, also in response to stretch, and causes an increase in cGMP, leading to vasodilation in both arterial and venous systems. In addition, it increases urinary sodium and water excretion [122].

Second messenger systems affect the activation of receptors on systemic vascular cell membranes, leading to changes in vascular tone. The phosphoinositide signaling system is the common pathway for many of these agonists[119] (Fig. 5.21). Membrane kinases phosphorylate phosphatidylinositol, which is an inositol lipid located mainly in the inner lamella of the plasma membrane, producing phosphatidylinositol 4,5 biphosphate.

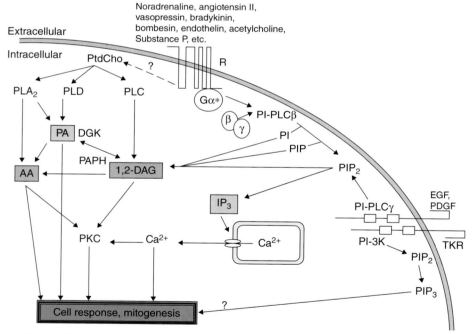

Figure 5.21 Phospholipase C system. The major receptor-activated pathways for production of inositol 1,4,5-triphosphate (IP3) and 1,2-diacyglycerol (1,2-DAG). The binding of an agonist to a receptor R with seven membrane-spanning domains results in the activation of the phosphatidylinositol-specific phospholipase Cβ (PI-PLCβ), whereas the stimulation of tyrosine kinase receptors (TKR) by polypeptide growth factors will activate phosphatidylinositol-specific phospholipase Cγ (PI-PLCγ). Both pathways will result in the hydrolysis of phosphatidylinositol 4,5-biphosphate (PIP2) and the formation of IP3 and 1,2-DAG. In addition, agonists that act on the heterotrimeric receptors may stimulate phosphatidylcholine (PtdCho) hydrolysis, and activation of tyrosine kinase receptors will stimulate the production of phosphatidylinositol 3,4,5-triphosphate (PIP3). DGK, diacylglyceral kinase; PAPH, phosphatidic acid phosphohydrolase; G*, activated G protein subunit; β subunits; PLD, phospholipase D; PKC, protein kinase C; PI-3K, phosphatidylinositol 3-kinase; PI, phosphatidylinositol; PIP, phosphatidylinositol 4-phosphate; EGF, epidermal growth factor; PDGF, platelet-derived growth factor; PLA2, phospholipase A2; AA, arachidonic acid. Reproduced from Izzard et al [119] with permission from Lippincott, Williams and Wilkins.

The second messenger, inositol 1,4,5-triphosphate, is produced from this compound by the action of the enzyme phospholipase C (PLC) [123]. The sequence begins with the binding of an agonist, such as angiotensin II, vasopressin, norepinephrine or endothelin, to a receptor with seven membrane-spanning domains. This receptor is linked to the activated Gq protein subunit, which in turn stimulates phosphatidylinositol-specific PLC (PI-PLC) to produce inositol 1,4,5,-triphosphate, which causes release of calcium from the SR, activating the actin-myosin system in the smooth muscle cells and thus producing vasoconstriction. Another second messenger, 1,2-diacylglycerol, is also produced, which goes on to activate protein kinase C, which in turn has a role in mitogenesis and thus proliferation of smooth muscle cells.

There are many isozymes of PLC; the form implicated in this series of events is the PLCβ form. The PLCγ isoform is activated when cell growth factors such as platelet-derived growth factor bind to their receptors on the cell surface and active tyrosine kinases. This results in the production of phosphatidylinositol 3,4,5-triphosphate, which is also implicated in mitogenesis.

Vasodilation of the systemic circulation results from the formation of NO by nitrovasodilators, or by activation of β2-adrenergic receptors in the peripheral vasculature, both of which result in the activation of guanylate cyclase and the production of cGMP, which reduces intracellular calcium concentrations, producing vasodilation [124].

The vascular beds in various peripheral tissues differ in the amount of local metabolic control of vascular tone. For example, pH has much more influence on the pulmonary circuit, with low pH leading to vasoconstriction and higher pH leading to vasodilation, than in the vascular tone of other tissues. Local CO_2 concentration is much more important to central nervous system vasculature, with high levels leading to vasodilation. Decrease in oxygen tension will often lead to vasodilation, as adenosine is released in response to the decreased oxygen delivery; however, decreased oxygen tension increases tone in the pulmonary circulation. Autoregulation, or maintaining relatively constant blood flow over a wide range of arterial pressures, predominates in the cerebral circulation but is not as critical in other tissue beds. Autoregulation and CO_2 responsiveness are both blunted in the fetal and immature brain [125].

Receptor signaling in myocardial dysfunction, congenital heart disease, and heart failure

A discussion of receptor signaling and calcium cycling in myocardial dysfunction is useful to serve as the basis for understanding many of the therapies discussed later in this text, and this section will focus on receptor physiology and calcium flux in three settings: acute myocardial

dysfunction as seen after cardiac surgery and cardiopulmonary bypass, changes seen as responses to chronic cyanotic heart disease, and those seen with chronic congestive heart failure and cardiomyopathy.

Receptor signaling in acute myocardial dysfunction

Acute myocardial dysfunction, such as that sometimes seen after cardiopulmonary bypass, is often treated with catecholamines. These drugs may not be effective, especially when used in escalating doses. In children, the number and subtype distribution of β-adrenergic receptors in atrial tissue are not affected by cardiac surgery with bypass; however, the activation of adenylate cyclase by isoproterenol is significantly reduced after bypass [126]. There is an uncoupling of β-receptors from the Gs protein-adenlyate cyclase complex. Densensitization to moderate or high doses of catecholamines may occur after only a few minutes of administration, because increased cAMP concentrations results in uncoupling from the Gs protein [127].

Only a few minutes of high-dose catecholamine administration may result in inactivation of the phosphorylated adrenergic receptors from sequestration. These receptors can be sequestered by endocytosis, in a process involving a protein called β-arrestin, which binds to the receptor, and a sarcolemmal protein called clathrin (Fig. 5.22). These sequestered receptors may be either recycled back to the cell membrane surface or destroyed by lysosomes [128]. This permanent destruction and degradation of receptors occurs after hours of exposure to catecholamines, and is accompanied by decreased mRNA and receptor protein synthesis, resulting in prolonged decrease in adrenergic receptor concentrations, which is reversed by decreasing exogenous catecholamines, but only as fast as new receptors can be synthesized.

Neonatal hearts may exhibit a different response to the acute or prolonged administration of catecholamines. Instead of desensitization, neonatal animal models demonstrate an enhanced β-adrenergic receptor response, accompanied by an increase in adenylate cyclase activity [129]. Desensitization as described above occurs later in development. The exact translation of these data to humans is not clear.

Treatment with catecholamines may also increase the concentration of Gi protein subunits, decreasing the sensitivity of the β-adrenergic receptor. This relative decrease in the ratio of Gs to Gi protein subunits has been demonstrated in rat and dog models [130,131]. Another possible mechanism of catecholamine-induced desensitization of the neonatal myocyte was demonstrated in a rat model, where prolonged exposure to norepinephrine caused an initial increase in functional L-type calcium channels on the sarcolemmal membrane. Continued exposure caused

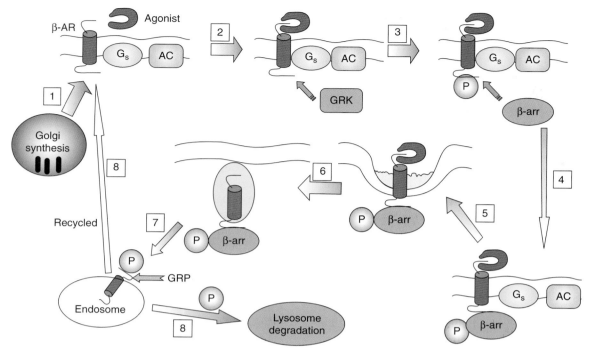

Figure 5.22 Desensitization and downregulation of the β adrenoreceptor (β-AR). (1) Agonist binding. (2) Phosphorylation of the β-AR by G protein-coupled receptor kinases (GRK). (3) β-arrestin binds to the GRK-phosphorylated β-AR, which is bound to the Gs protein. The receptor is then sequestrated to the endosomal compartment (4–7) to be dephosphorylated, and then either recycled back to the sarcolemma (8) or translocated to lysosomes for further degradation (8). AC, adenylate cyclase; GRP, G protein-coupled receptor phosphatase; P, inorganic phosphate groups; β-arr, β-arrestin. Reproduced from Booker [76] with permission from Wiley-Blackwell.

a decrease in L-type calcium channel mRNA to 50% of control values [132]. Sarcoplasmic reticulum calcium-ATPase concentrations are reduced with chronic norepinephrine administration in the dog [133]. Finally, exposing adult or neonatal rat myocytes to high concentrations of catecholamines for 24h leads to increased apoptosis of myocardial cells, a genetically programmed energy-dependent mechanism for cell death and removal [134,135]. This effect was mediated through β-adrenergic receptors in the adult model and α receptors in the neonatal model.

All these studies provide the theoretical basis for the argument that administration of catecholamines to patients with acute myocardial dysfunction should be limited in dose and duration. Obviously, this is difficult to accomplish in the setting of weaning a hemodynamically unstable patient from cardiopulmonary bypass. Strategies that may limit catecholamine dose include administering low doses of catecholamines together with phosphodiesterase inhibitors, as well as adding corticosteroids, tri-iodothyronine, and vasopressin [136].

Receptor signaling in congenital heart disease
In the past decade, new information has become available concerning adrenergic receptor signaling in patients with

congenital heart disease. A study of 71 infants and children undergoing cardiac surgery used tissue from the right atrial appendage to study β-adrenergic receptor density, distribution of β1 and β2 receptor subtypes, and coupling to adenylate cyclase [137]. This study found that patients with severe or poorly compensated acyanotic (e.g. congestive heart failure) or cyanotic (e.g. severe cyanosis) disease had significantly reduced β-adrenergic receptor densities. Outside the newborn period, this downregulation was β1 selective but in newborns with critical aortic stenosis or transposition of the great arteries, there was additional significant downregulation of the β2 subtype. In patients with tetralogy of Fallot, those treated with propranolol had a significant increase in the number and density of β-adrenergic receptors, when compared with untreated patients. β-adrenergic receptor downregulation correlated with increased circulating norepinephrine levels. Finally, in severely affected patients, adenylate cyclase activity was reduced, demonstrating a partial decoupling, as noted above.

Other studies have determined that symptomatic tetralogy of Fallot patients, i.e. those with cyanotic spells, have a significantly greater number of β-adrenergic receptors in their right ventricular outflow tract muscle, and their adenylate cyclase activity was greater when compared to patients without cyanotic spells [138]. α1-Adrenergic receptors are also affected by congenital heart disease. A study of atrial tissue excised at surgery in 17 children evaluated α- versus β-adrenergic receptor stimulation with pharmacological agents. The α component was responsible for 0–44% of the inotropic response, and β stimulation for 56–100% of the response, with the degree of right ventricular hypertrophy and pressure load correlating with the amount of α stimulation found [139].

Receptor signaling in congestive heart failure and cardiomyopathy

Like adults with heart failure, children with congestive heart failure due to chronic left-to-right shunting and volume overload have elevated levels of circulating norepinephrine. This leads to a downregulation in β-adrenergic receptor density [140]. The degree of elevation of pulmonary artery pressure and amount of left-to-right shunting correlate with the plasma catecholamine levels, and are inversely correlated with β-adrenergic receptor density. All these abnormalities return to normal levels after corrective surgery.

The degree of receptor downregulation in congestive heart failure correlates with postoperative morbidity in infants and children. Children with an intensive care unit stay of greater than 7 days or those who died during the early postoperative period (nine of the 26 in a published report) had significantly less β1 and β2 mRNA gene expression than those who had better outcomes [141]. In addition, children receiving propranolol for treatment of their congestive heart failure had higher β-adrenergic receptor mRNA levels and tended to have improved outcomes. Finally, children with dilated cardiomyopathy also have a reduced response to catecholamines, with one study showing no significant increase in ejection fraction during a dobutamine stress test, with infusion of dobutamine at 5 and then 10 μg/kg/min [142].

The preceding has been a brief discussion of receptor signaling in pediatric heart disease. This emerging field has many implications for treatment strategies, and the reader is referred to excellent reviews for more detailed information on this subject [143].

Myocardial preconditioning

Myocardial preconditioning refers to the finding that repeated, brief exposure of the myocardium to ischemia, volatile anesthetics or other stresses induces a protective effect against a later (i.e. 12–24 h), more prolonged, ischemic insult, resulting in decreased myocardial infarction size and improved myocardial function after the insult [144]. Chronic cyanosis also induces a similar protective effect in the myocardium, although the effect size is smaller and more long-lasting, i.e. beyond 24 h.

The mechanisms of myocardial preconditioning are complex but are thought to involve release of various neurohormonal agents and peptides such as adenosine, bradykinin, and nitric oxide via a cGMP-dependent mechanism, which then triggers a series of signal transduction events within the cardiomyocyte that confer a "memory" effect that protects the myocardium from future ischemic insults. The signal transduction effects include protein kinase C, tyrosine kinases, mitogen-activated protein kinases, glycogen synthase kinase 3β, and other enzymes [145]. This series of events allows activation of mitochondrial and sarcolemmal potassium-ATP channels, which leads to the preconditioning by elusive mechanisms.

One recently discovered candidate for this end effector is the mitochondrial permeability transition pore (MPTP) [145]. This is a non-specific channel that spans both mitochondrial membranes and when opened for a prolonged period, leads to dissipation of mitochondrial electrical potential, inhibition of ATP synthesis, and ultimately mitochondrial swelling, rupture, failure of cellular energy metabolism, and cell death. Agents and stimuli that confer myocardial preconditioning have been found to keep the MPTP closed, thus possibly elucidating further the subcellular mechanisms involved.

Several studies in pediatric cardiac surgical patients have been published elucidating the potential effects of myocardial preconditioning, which could have the beneficial effect of ameliorating the myocardial stunning observed in infants after surgical interventions that required long aortic cross-clamp times [146]. In a study of 90 infants randomized to sevoflurane, propofol or midazolam anesthesia for maintenance, plus a sufentanil infusion for analgesia, patients receiving sevoflurane had a very strong trend toward lower troponin T concentrations in the first 24 h after surgery, potentially signifying less myocardial injury due to the pre-bypass exposure to sevoflurane [147].

In a novel variation of myocardial preconditioning, remote ischemic preconditioning (RIPC) produced by inflating a blood pressure cuff on a lower extremity to produce a 5-min period of limb ischemia, for four cycles before cardiopulmonary bypass, was studied in 37 children undergoing cardiac surgery. Patients who underwent RIPC had lower peak troponin I levels (17 versus 22 μg/L, p = 0.04), and lower inotrope score in the RIPC group at both 3 and 6 h post bypass [148]. This interesting phenomenon of RIPC may work through modulation of the inflammatory response through some as yet unknown humoral mechanism. The entire area of myocardial preconditioning, whether ischemic, anesthetic induced, remote or other variation, is an important field of future study that may well have several translations into clinical care.

Acknowledgments

Portions of this chapter were previously published as (1) Wilmot I, Miller-Hance WC. (2010) Embrology, development, and nomenclature of congenital heart disease. In: Andropoulos DB, Stayer SA, Russell IA, Mossad EB (eds.) Anesthesia for Congenital Heart Disease, 2nd edn. Wiley-Blackwell, Oxford, pp. 37–54, and (2) Andropoulos DB. Physiology and molecular biology of the developing circulation. In: Andropoulos DB, Stayer SA, Russell IA, Mossad EB (eds.) Anesthesia for Congenital Heart Disease, 2nd edn. Wiley-Blackwell, Oxford, pp. 55–76.

Annotated references

A full reference list for this chapter is available at:
http://www.wiley.com/go/gregory/andropoulos/pediatricanesthesia

6. Sander TL, Klinkner DB, Tomita-Mitchell A et al. Molecular and cellular basis of congenital heart disease. Pediatr Clin North Am 2006; 53: 989–1009. An excellent review of the modern understanding of the genetic and molecular pathways resulting in altered cardiac development which result in congenital cardiac defects.

31. Van Mierop LH, Kutsche LM. Cardiovascular anomalies in DiGeorge syndrome and importance of neural crest as a possible pathogenetic factor. Am J Cardiol 1986; 58: 133–7. An important paper linking chromosome 22 anomalies associated with congenital heart disease with their neural crest abnormalities.

38. Stanger P, Rudolph AM, Edwards JE. Cardiac malpositions. An overview based on study of sixty-five necropsy specimens. Circulation 1977; 56: 159–72. A review of the cardiac malpositions based on a significant number of autopsy specimens.

57. Rudolph AM. Distribution and regulation of blood flow in the fetal and neonatal lamb. Circ Res 1985; 57: 811–21. A classic article resulting in the fundamental understanding of fetal, transitional, and neonatal circulations.

59. Baum VC, Palmisano BW. The immature heart and anesthesia. Anesthesiology 1997; 87: 1529–48. An excellent review of the physiological basis for anesthetic care of the patient with an immature heart; discusses the principles which are still current.

61. Friedman WF. The intrinsic physiologic properties of the developing heart. Prog Cardiovasc Dis 1972; 15: 87–111. A now classic review of the animal data that form the basis for our understanding of changes in physiology of the developing heart.

73. Rudolph AM. Myocardial growth before and after birth: clinical implications. Acta Pediatr 2000; 89: 129–33. An excellent review, by one of the founders of the specialty of pediatric cardiology, of the morphological changes in the myocardium in health and disease.

76. Booker PD. Pharmacological support for children with myocardial dysfunction. Paediatr Anaesth 2002; 12: 5–25. An outstanding review of the physiological basis for choosing particular agents for myocardiac dysfunction in children.

108. Prakash YS, Seckin I, Hunter IW et al. Mechanisms underlying greater sensitivity of neonatal cardiac muscle to volatile anesthetics. Anesthesiology 2002; 96: 893–906. An excellent article reviewing the understanding of why the neonate's myocardium is more sensitive to volatile anesthetic-induced myocardial depression.

148. Cheung MM, Kharbanda RK, Konstantinov IE et al. Randomized controlled trial of the effects of remote ischemic preconditioning on children undergoing cardiac surgery: first clinical application in humans. J Am Coll Cardiol 2006; 47: 2277–82. A fascinating proof of concept study describing that the simple technique of inflating a blood pressure cuff on an extremity for prescribed periods in the pre-cardiopulmonary bypass period improves inflammatory response, myocardial function, and some clinical parameters.

CHAPTER 6

Developmental Physiology of the Respiratory System

Susan H. Guttentag[1], Maria Victoria Fraga[1] & Dean B. Andropoulos[2]

[1]Department of Anesthesiology and Critical Care Medicine, The University of Pennsylvania School of Medicine, and The Children's Hospital of Philadelphia, Philadelphia, PA, USA
[2]Department of Anesthesiology and Pediatrics, Baylor College of Medicine, and Texas Children's Hospital, Houston, TX, USA

Introduction

Aerobic cellular respiration is critical for survival and requires the efficient exchange of oxygen for carbon dioxide at the alveolar surface. The alveolar surface area must be able to accommodate the tremendous range in oxygen consumption – from 250 mL/min at rest to 5500 mL/min at peak exercise [1]. As a result, the gas exchange surface area of the adult lung will attain 50–100 m^2 with a final total lung capacity of 2.5–3.0 L. Lung organogenesis expands the lung surface area to meet these needs. This chapter will discuss the development of lung, chest wall, and diaphragm structure, development of the pulmonary vasculature, lung fluid physiology, transition in pulmonary function and circulation at the time of birth, and the postnatal development of lung structure and pulmonary function. Then the developmental pathophysiology of three diseases commonly encountered by the anesthesiologist will be presented: asthma, bronchopulmonary dysplasia, and cystic fibrosis.

Embryology of the lungs, chest wall, and diaphragm

Prenatal lung development

Lung formation begins early in human gestation and growth extends well into childhood [2,3]. Although lung development is organized into stages (embryonic, pseudoglandular, canalicular, saccular, and alveolar), there is considerable temporal overlap of each stage that can be modified by prenatal and postnatal events (Fig. 6.1).

The embryonic phase of lung development is marked by the formation of the lung bud and initial branches of the airways. The primordial lung is a foregut derivative,

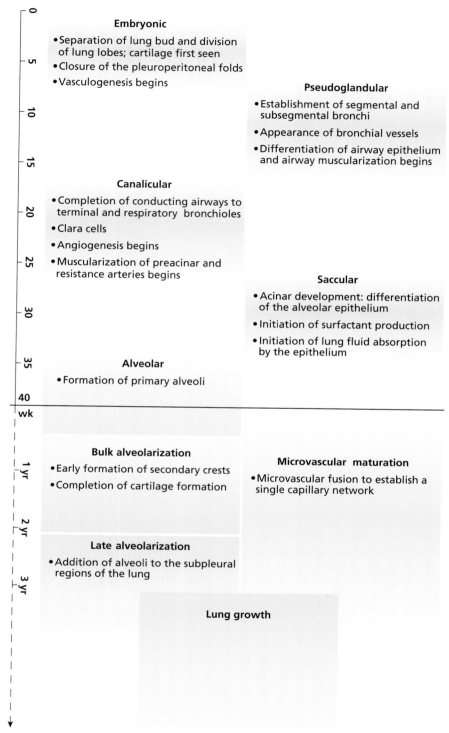

Embryonic
- Separation of lung bud and division of lung lobes; cartilage first seen
- Closure of the pleuroperitoneal folds
- Vasculogenesis begins

Pseudoglandular
- Establishment of segmental and subsegmental bronchi
- Appearance of bronchial vessels
- Differentiation of airway epithelium and airway muscularization begins

Canalicular
- Completion of conducting airways to terminal and respiratory bronchioles
- Clara cells
- Angiogenesis begins
- Muscularization of preacinar and resistance arteries begins

Saccular
- Acinar development: differentiation of the alveolar epithelium
- Initiation of surfactant production
- Initiation of lung fluid absorption by the epithelium

Alveolar
- Formation of primary alveoli

Bulk alveolarization
- Early formation of secondary crests
- Completion of cartilage formation

Microvascular maturation
- Microvascular fusion to establish a single capillary network

Late alveolarization
- Addition of alveoli to the subpleural regions of the lung

Lung growth

Figure 6.1 The fetal and postnatal stages of lung development.

first recognizable at 25 days in the human fetus as a laryngotracheal groove in the ventral foregut. The more distal aspect of the groove closes, resulting in the only remaining connection between foregut in the region of the developing hypopharynx and larynx. Failure of closure results in a spectrum of tracheo-esophageal fistulas, from the most common proximal esophageal pouch with a distal fistula between trachea and esophagus, typically at the level of the carina (87%), to the less common isolated esophageal atresia (8%), H-type fistula (4%), and esophageal atresia with either proximal (1%) or proximal plus distal (1%) fistula [4]. Upon closure of the laryngotracheal groove, the lung bud begins a series of dichotomous divisions that give rise to the conducting airways and five primordial lung lobes (two left and three right). Failure of the lung bud to divide can result in pulmonary agenesis, most typically of the right lung.

The pseudoglandular stage of lung development marks the establishment of the large conducting airways of the lung. Divisions that establish the trachea, segmental and subsegmental bronchi are completed by 7 weeks in the human fetus, and all bronchial divisions are completed by 16 weeks. It is important to remember that although the conducting airways will enlarge as the fetus and newborn grow (airway diameter and length increase 2–3-fold between birth and adulthood), large airway branching ceases after 16 weeks of gestation.

The canalicular phase of lung development is marked by completion of the small conducting airways through the level of the terminal bronchioles, the last airways with cartilaginous support. Respiratory bronchioles no longer invested with cartilage mark the beginning of the gas exchange region of the lung. A respiratory bronchiole and all its associated alveolar ducts and alveoli constitute an acinus, which is the basic gas exchange unit of the lung. A terminal bronchiole with all its associated acinar structures constitute a lobule. Branching of the terminal and respiratory bronchioles during the canalicular phase will ultimately result in a total of 23 airway subdivisions, and completes the branching of the airways.

The saccular phase of lung development begins at roughly 24 weeks of human gestation and continues until just prior to term gestation. During this phase there is evolution of the relationships between the airspaces, capillaries and mesenchyme, although the alveolocapillary membrane (the distance from the lumenal surface of the airspace/alveolus to the lumenal surface of the capillary) is sufficient to participate in gas exchange (0.6 μm) by approximately 24 weeks. Beyond this point, the efficiency of gas exchange is determined by the available surface area, not by the width of the alveolocapillary membrane. Lengthening and widening of the smooth-walled airspaces of terminal sacs expand the gas exchange surface area which remains invested with a double capillary network.

The alveolar phase of lung development is the final stage that is initiated during fetal lung development, but alveolarization will not be completed until much later (see Postnatal lung development). While branching morphogenesis establishes the conducting airways of the lung, alveolarization will establish the large surface area involved in gas exchange [5]. This process will result in a 20-fold increase in surface area between birth (with between 0 and 50 million alveoli) and adulthood (>300 million alveoli). Primitive saccules develop low ridges (primary septa) that subdivide the saccule into an alveolar duct containing primary alveoli, and outpouchings between the ridges (secondary septa) that establish secondary alveoli. Regions destined for secondary septation exhibit increased elastin deposition [6], and elastin localizes to the tips of the secondary crests as they form. Septae contain a connective tissue core separating two capillary membranes, suggesting that the septum is formed by the folding of a capillary on itself. Septation also leads to the development of the pores of Kohn, allowing gaseous continuity between acini. Formation of secondary crests and the maturation of the microvasculature are critical elements of this stage of lung development, which only begins at roughly 36 weeks gestation in the human. Thus, the human lung is not fully mature structurally, even at term delivery. The completion of alveolar development is discussed below.

Development of the chest wall and diaphragm

Formation of the ventral body wall is initiated in the fourth week post fertilization with the formation of the lateral body wall folds. The folds consist of lateral plate mesoderm and overlying ectoderm, and the folds will move ventrally to meet in the midline of the developing embryo [7]. Failure of closure may occur anywhere along the midline, resulting in congenital malformations of the thoracic body wall (ectopia cordis, sternal cleft) and abdominal body wall (omphalocele, bladder exstrophy). The sternum arises from parallel bands of condensed mesenchyme in the 6th week and will fuse in the 10th week [8]. Formation of cartilage appears in the sternum immediately but ossification will not begin until the 6th month. Ossification of the ribs begins in the 7th week of gestation and will be completed by early adulthood. Equally important are changes in the configuration of the chest wall. The orientation of the ribs is horizontal in infancy and will begin to slope downwards so that by age 10 years the ribs have reached the adult configuration. As a result, the contraction of the diaphragm and intercostal muscles, lifting the ribs like a bucket handle, is more effective in increasing intrathoracic volume, and thus negative pressure, in adulthood than it is in infancy.

The diaphragm is critical for separating the developing lung within the thorax from the abdominal cavity with the developing gut and solid organs of the abdomen. Closure of the pleuroperitoneal folds is initiated in the pseudoglandular phase, and is completed by 7 weeks in the human fetus. During this time, the midgut resides within the umbilical cord and returns to the peritoneal cavity at 10 weeks. Thus, failure of diaphragm formation results in continuity between thoracic and peritoneal cavities, allowing peritoneal contents (stomach, intestine, and/or liver) to migrate into the thoracic cavity. This restricts the space into which the lung grows, leading to pulmonary hypoplasia of the lung ipsilateral to the diaphragmatic defect. Pulmonary hypoplasia can also extend to the contralateral lung due to shifting of the mediastinum as abdominal viscera accumulate within the thorax.

Owing largely to ossification of the rib cage and increasing chest wall muscle mass, the chest wall stiffens with age. Compliance of the chest wall in infants is 2–6 times higher than the compliance of the lung tissue, even more so in preterm infants, but will decrease to nearly equal lung tissue compliance in childhood and adulthood. Unchecked, this leads to problems in maintaining adequate lung volume at end-expiration in infancy. As a result, term infants actively maintain resting lung volume by prolonging expiratory time constants via a braking maneuver. A given percentage of passively exhaled breath will require a constant time for exhalation regardless of the starting lung volume, given constant lung mechanics. This is the time constant of the lung (τ) and is the product of airway resistance (R_{aw}) and lung compliance (C). Braking consists of interrupting expiratory flow before full relaxation of respiratory muscles, thus prolonging τ, and is no longer necessary beyond 1–2 years of age due to stiffening of the chest wall [9].

Development of the pulmonary vasculature and its relationship to alveoli

The pulmonary vasculature consists of the vascular supply to the acini and the bronchial circulation [10]. During early fetal life, the airways act as a template for pulmonary blood vessel development. Early pulmonary blood vessels form by vasculogenesis, which is *de novo* differentiation of mesenchymal cells into endothelial cells and then capillaries. As each new airway buds into the mesenchyme, a new plexus forms and adds to the pulmonary circulation, By 5 weeks of human gestation, a capillary network surrounds each bronchus and circulation of blood between the right ventricle and the left atrium via this network is evident. By the canalicular stage of lung development, new blood vessels form from pre-existing vessels via angiogenesis in which endothelial cells proliferate and sprout from established vessels. Vasculogenesis is the primary mode of pulmonary vascular development until the 17th week of gestation when all preacinar airways are complete, whereas angiogenesis becomes the predominant mode in the later stages of lung development. Interconnections between vascular networks arising from both angiogenesis and vasculogenesis increase in the saccular phase of lung development.

In the human lung, a second circulatory system, the bronchial circulation, arises from the dorsal aorta supplying systemic blood. The bronchial vasculature develops after the pulmonary circulation, with bronchial vessels first apparent by 8 weeks. The network of bronchial vessels is extensive, with bronchial arteries demonstrated as distal as the alveolar ducts in the adult respiratory tree. The inappropriate branching of bronchial vessels from the dorsal aorta is implicated in the formation of bronchopulmonary sequestration, a space-occupying lung malformation that can result in hypoplasia of the ipsilateral lung.

Vasculogenesis and angiogenesis are the primary mechanisms of vascular development throughout intrauterine life. The human lung at term contains only a small portion of the adult number of alveoli, and the airspace walls are represented by a thick "primary septum" consisting of a central layer of connective tissue surrounded by two capillary beds, each of them facing one alveolar surface [3]. This double capillary network is not present in the adult lung. As alveolar architecture changes with the appearance of secondary septa, folding of one of the two capillary layers occurs within the secondary septa. Microvascular maturation involves fusion of the double capillary network into a single capillary system. The expansion of surface area and luminal volume compresses the interstitium, bringing the capillary networks in close proximity to potential airspaces and thereby promoting both alveolar surface area expansion and capillary bed fusion. By the third postnatal week, lung volume increases by 25% and there is a 27% decrease of the interstitial tissue volume that is believed to promote microvascular fusions. Subsequently, there is preferential growth of fused areas that continues until ~3 years of age. Lung volume increases about 23-fold between birth and young adulthood, while capillary volume expands 35-fold. It has been recently shown that this increase in capillary volume occurs by insertion of capillaries in the absence of capillary sprouting. This new concept in capillary network growth has been named *intussusceptive microvascular growth* and involves the formation of transluminal tissue pillars within existing vessels that then expand to increase capillary surface area [3].

Muscularization can be detected early in development of the pulmonary arteries [10]. Initially the muscular investment of the vasculature is derived from the migration of bronchial smooth muscle cells from adjacent airways. Muscularization of preacinar and resistance arteries of the pulmonary vasculature begins in the canalicular stage and continues through the remainder of gestation. This second phase of smooth muscle cells investing pulmonary vessels develops from the surrounding mesenchyme. A third phase of vascular muscularization has been described, largely in the very distal lung, in which capillary endothelial cells undergo a process of endothelial-mesenchymal transition that encompasses endothelial cell division, separation and migration from the endothelial layer, and expression of smooth muscle cell markers. Normal muscularization of pulmonary arteries extends down to the level of the terminal bronchiole, and is minimal to absent in vessels surrounding respiratory bronchioles. Abnormal extension of smooth muscle along arterioles supplying acinar structures occurs in infants dying from persistent pulmonary hypertension of the newborn and in severe bronchopulmonary dysplasia.

Recent evidence suggests that the pulmonary capillary bed actively promotes normal alveolar development and contributes to the maintenance of alveolar structures throughout life [11]. The observation that combined abnormalities in the airways and vasculature occur in bronchopulmonary dysplasia supports this hypothesis. Intra-acinar arteries and veins continue to develop after birth by angiogenesis as long as alveoli continue to increase in number and size. This may well be a reciprocal process because vascular growth around the distal airspaces suggests an inductive influence from the alveolar epithelial cells.

Lung fluid physiology

Fetal lung fluid is a product of the epithelial cells lining the developing lung [12], and averages 4–6 mL/kg/h. Laryngeal abduction creates resistance to the passage of lung fluid out into the amniotic fluid, providing end-expiratory pressure of approximately 2–4 cmH$_2$O. As a result, fetal lung fluid accumulates to a total volume of 20–30 mL/kg during gestation. The composition of fetal lung fluid is distinct from both amniotic fluid and plasma, as illustrated in Table 6.1. The increased chloride content of fetal lung fluid, as compared to serum, is the result of active chloride secretion by the tracheal and distal pulmonary epithelium. Fetal lung fluid secretion can be enhanced by prolactin, keratinocyte growth factor, and prostaglandins E2 and F2, while it is inhibited by a variety of mediators, including β-adrenergic agonists, vasopressin, serotonin, and glucagon.

While fetal lung fluid is an essential component of lung development, it presents a significant obstacle to the transition to air breathing upon delivery. Three important events must occur to decrease the amount of fetal lung fluid and its potential impact on alveolar surface tension: absorption, bulk removal, and maturation of pulmonary surfactant. Conversion of the epithelial surface from secretory to absorptive is largely due to enhanced sodium transport across the alveolar epithelium during the third trimester [12]. Much evidence suggests that induction of components of the epithelial sodium channels (ENaC) around the time of birth is a major factor in promoting sodium transport with water passively following the movement of sodium. Induction of ENaC components occurs at a transcriptional level in response to changes in extracellular matrix components, glucocorticoids, aldosterone and oxygen. By comparison, agents that increase intracellular cAMP levels (i.e. β-agonists, phosphodiesterase inhibitors and cAMP analogs), while not increasing the number of sodium channels, increase the probability of a channel being open to sodium transport. Glucocorticoids and thyroid hormones play an important role in priming the lung epithelium to the actions of β-adrenergic agonists on sodium transport across lung epithelia near term. Water channels consisting of aquaporins are also induced during the late fetal period to facilitate fluid movement, but their importance remains unclear.

Conversion to an absorptive surface is not sufficient to minimize the fetal lung fluid at the time of term delivery. The absence of uterine contractions is associated with an increased incidence of retained fetal lung fluid in infants delivered by cesarean section without the benefit of labor. Upon delivery of the head and neck, continued uterine contractions on the fetal thorax promote expulsion of bulk fluid from the fetal lung. However, animal studies have shown that the magnitude of the benefit of thoracic compression during labor is only modest [13]. The primary mechanism by which labor facilitates clearance of lung fluid is through hormonal effects on fluid clearance, especially through catecholamine-induced changes in the open probability of ENaC. The onset of air breathing with increased intrathoracic negative pressure assists in the clearance of residual fetal lung fluid into the loose interstitial tissues surrounding alveoli. Fluid is then reabsorbed via lymphatics and pulmonary blood vessels. The amount of residual liquid in the lung after transition is approximately 0.37 mL/kg bodyweight.

Table 6.1 Composition of human fetal lung fluid compared to other body fluids

Component	Lung fluid	Interstitial fluid	Plasma	Amniotic fluid
Sodium (mEq/L)	150	147	150	113
Potassium (mEq/L)	6.3	4.8	4.8	7.6
Chloride (mEq/L)	157	107	107	87
Bicarbonate (mEq/L)	3	25	24	19
pH	6.27	7.31	7.34	7.02
Protein (g/dL)	0.03	3.27	4.09	0.10

Pulmonary cell types, development and release of surfactant

Proximal airways

The proximal airway epithelium is tall and columnar, decreasing to a more cuboidal appearance distally [14,15]. The endodermal epithelial lining cells of the trachea and bronchi partition into four cell types: undifferentiated columnar, ciliated, secretory/goblet, and basal cells. Ciliated cells critical to the process of mucus clearance are first apparent between 11 and 16 weeks of human gestation and become less prevalent in more distal airways. Three types of secretory cells – those with largely mucous granules, those with serous granules, and some with both types of granules – can be seen as early as 13 weeks. The number of mucin-producing goblet cells in airways peaks at midgestation in the fetus, and declines into adulthood. Finally, immature basal cells expressing epidermal keratin have been noted as early as 12 weeks of gestation.

Cartilaginous support of the tracheobronchial tree proceeds in a centrifugal fashion, beginning in the primitive trachea at 4 weeks of human gestation, reaching the main bronchi by 10 weeks, and proceeding to the most distal terminal bronchioles by approximately 25 weeks. Cartilaginous investment of airways is complete by the second month postnatally. Submucosal glands are found in the interstitium between the cartilaginous tissue and surface epithelium, and play a major role in airway host defense. The airways of infants and children contain relatively more submucous glands than adults. The glands are lined by mucous cells proximally and serous cells more distally, the latter comprising 60% of the total epithelial cell content of the glands. Serous cells secrete water, electrolytes, and proteins with antimicrobial, anti-inflammatory, and antioxidant properties, while the mucous cells produce primarily mucins. In addition to this host defense role, submucosal glands also contain a population of basal cells that respond to injury of the airway by replenishing the airway epithelium.

Muscular investment of the airways begins as early as 6–8 weeks of gestation as smooth muscle cells are identifiable around the trachea and large airways. Fetal airway smooth muscle is innervated and able to contract during the first trimester. It is also responsive to methacholine challenge that is reversible with β-adrenergic agonists. Muscularization increases through fetal life and childhood such that there is an increase in the amount of smooth muscle relative to airway size compared to adults. Furthermore, there is a rapid increase in bronchial smooth muscle immediately after birth, whether born at term or prematurely.

Pulmonary neuroendocrine cells (PNEC) are found throughout the airways, often in innervated clusters known as pulmonary neuroendocrine bodies (NEB) located at branch points in the bronchial tree [16]. Solitary PNEC are sensitive to stretch- and hypoxia-mediated secretion, producing both amines (i.e. serotonin) and peptides (i.e. bombesin) that are important in regulating bronchial tone. Pathological conditions recently associated with PNEC/NEB, most often characterized by hyperplasia, include bronchopulmonary dysplasia, disorders of respiratory control (congenital central hypoventilation syndrome and sudden infant death syndrome (SIDS)), cystic fibrosis, and pulmonary hypertension. Neuroendocrine hyperplasia of infancy (NEHI) is a rare form of interstitial lung disease of infancy associated with expansion of the number of PNEC and NEB, but little is known about the mechanism of disease.

Distal airways

The bronchiolar epithelium differs from the more proximal airway epithelium and contains progressively fewer ciliated cells and goblet cells, which are ultimately absent from the terminal bronchioles. Clara cells are found in increasing numbers and density down the conducting airways, such that they are the most abundant cell of the terminal bronchiole [14]. Clara cells are first evident by 16–17 weeks of human gestation, initially exhibiting large glycogen stores that are replaced by secretory granules. Between 23 and 34 weeks there is a dramatic increase in Clara cell numbers in distal bronchioles. Clara cells play an important role in host defense and in the detoxification of gaseous components of the air we breathe. This specialized cell produces the highest levels of cytochrome P450 and flavin mono-oxygenases in the lung. While critically important in detoxification, these enzymes participate in the bio-activation of procarcinogens as well, placing the Clara cell at risk as a target of toxic metabolites. The Clara cell also plays an important role in immunoregulation in the distal airways. Important host defense products of the Clara cell include Clara cell secretory protein (CCSP or CC10), surfactant proteins A, and D, leukocyte protease inhibitor, and a trypsin-like protease. The secretion of antiproteases from Clara cells suggests that they modulate the protease–antiprotease balance in the distal lung.

Alveoli

During the 4th through 6th months of gestation the epithelial cells lining the acini begin to differentiate further [17]. The cuboidal epithelial cells accumulate large glycogen stores and develop small vesicles containing loose lamellae. The large glycogen pools provide a ready source of substrate required for the production of increasing amounts of surfactant phospholipids, and they decrease in size as surfactant production advances in the fetal lung. In cells destined to become type 2 cells, lamellar bodies become larger, more numerous and more densely packed with surfactant phospholipids and proteins, whereas those cells destined to become type 1 cells, upon losing their relationship to mesenchymal fibroblasts, lose the prelamellar vesicles and become progressively thinner, thereby adopting a phenotype more suitable for gas exchange. Alveolar type 1 and 2 cells are readily identified early in the saccular stage of fetal lung development. There remains considerable controversy regarding the origin of type 1 cells. In culture, these cells demonstrate very slow turnover, with a doubling time estimated to be between 40 and 120 days, suggesting that *in vivo* they are functionally terminally differentiated. In response to epithelial damage, type 2 cells proliferate to re-establish epithelial continuity, and then lose phenotypical features such as lamellar bodies while acquiring markers of type 1 cells, suggesting that rapid repopulation of type 1 cells requires a type 2 cell intermediary.

There is increasing appreciation that the alveolar type 1 cell is more than a passive membrane for gas exchange [18]. The large surface area and small cytoplasm/nucleus ratio provides for a thin alveolocapillary membrane to facilitate gas exchange. However, this large surface area also provides a large absorptive surface in the lung. The presence of water and ion channels, some distinct from those in type 2 cells, helps to ensure that the alveolus remains relatively dry. Type 1 cells may also regulate cell proliferation locally, signal macrophage accumulation, and modulate the functions of local peptides, proteases and growth factors.

While most notable for its role in surfactant production, the alveolar type 2 cell provides additional important functions in the alveolus [19]. Alveolar type 2 cells are local progenitor cells, as mentioned previously. Like type 1 cells, alveolar type 2 cells contain specialized ion and water channels as well as ion pumps in both the apical and basal membranes that contribute to the movement of water and ions across the epithelium. Type 2 cells also produce important antioxidants (SOD-1, -2, -3, glutathione) and molecules of innate host defense (SP-A, SP-D, lysozyme) to participate in detoxification and sterilization of the alveolar microenvironment.

More recently, it is becoming clear that alveolar type 2 cells may also play a part in exacerbating alveolar pathology. The type 2 cell participates in the coagulation–fibrinolysis cascade through the production of fibrinogen, urokinase-type plasminogen activator, and tissue factor, especially under pathological circumstances. Type 2 cells are increasingly recognized as a source of cytokine and chemokine production in the lung, as well as growth factors that can promote fibrosis. Finally, cross-talk between epithelial cells, cell matrix, interstitial cells, and local inflammatory cells can foster the resolution of injury and inflammation, or prolong lung remodeling after injury with detrimental effects such as lung destruction and fibrosis. Therefore, while previously heralded as the defender of the alveolus, the alveolar type 2 cell plays a much more complex role in alveolar health and disease.

Surfactant

Pulmonary surfactant is essential to alveolar health. A thin layer of liquid is constantly secreted into the alveolar lumen to protect the delicate alveolar epithelium. The surface tension generated by this aqueous layer opposes alveolar inflation and promotes alveolar collapse at the end of expiration owing to the Law of LaPlace, which states that the collapsing pressure on the alveolus is directly proportional to the surface tension while inversely proportional to the radius of curvature of the alveolus. The presence of pulmonary surfactant at the air–liquid interface lowers surface tension as alveolar surface area decreases, thereby preventing end-expiratory atelectasis, maintaining functional residual capacity, and lowering the force required for subsequent alveolar inflations.

Pulmonary surfactant is a complex mixture of phospholipids (80% by weight), neutral lipids (10%), and proteins (10%) that is synthesized, packaged, and secreted by alveolar type 2 cells [20]. Storage of surfactant occurs in the lamellar body, a lysosome-derived membrane-bound organelle that undergoes regulated secretion in response to a variety of stimuli, including stretch. In the alveolus, surfactant phospholipids transition through an extracellular storage form, tubular myelin. Phospholipid and protein components are recycled out of the surfactant monolayer at the air–liquid interface, and taken back into the alveolar type 2 cell where they can be repackaged into lamellar bodies. Alveolar macrophages engulf and degrade surfactant components as well.

Saturated phosphatidylcholine makes up 45% of surfactant by weight, with unsaturated phospholipids accounting for 25% of surfactant and other phospholipids (most notably phosphatidylglycerol at 5%) contributing 10%. The predominant saturated surfactant phospholipid is dipalmitoyl phosphatidylcholine, or DPPC. DPPC is the only surface-active component of lung surfactant capable of lowering surface tension to nearly zero. The presence of unsaturated phospholipids and other lipid components like cholesterol enables the monolayer to remain fluid at body temperature during the respiratory cycle. The phospholipid content of the developing fetal lung increases with advancing gestation due to increased activity of enzymes responsible for phospholipid synthesis within alveolar type 2 cells. The expression and activity of enzymes of the choline incorporation pathway, the predominant pathway for surfactant phospholipid synthesis, are not only developmentally regulated but are also induced by hormones. The inductive hormones that have direct clinical relevance are glucocorticoids and agents that increase intracellular cAMP, such as the β-adrenergic agonist (and tocolytic) terbutaline.

Surfactant contains a group of specific proteins important for surfactant function and host defense that contribute up to 5% of surfactant by weight; the remaining 5% of the protein content of surfactant comes largely from serum proteins. The four surfactant proteins, SP-A, -B, -C, and -D, are subdivided based upon their physical characteristics into either hydrophobic (SP-B and -C) or hydrophilic (SP-A and -D) proteins. The hydrophobic surfactant proteins play a major role in the surface-active properties of surfactant, whereas the primary roles of the hydrophilic surfactant proteins are in host defense, immunomodulation, and surfactant clearance and metabolism.

Together, the hydrophobic proteins facilitate the mobilization of surfactant phospholipid from tubular myelin to the surface monolayer, promote spreading of phospholipids in the surfactant film, and assist in film stability at end-expiration [20]. SP-B plays a central role in alveolar health due to its critical function in surfactant homeostasis. It is a secretory protein that exhibits strong association with membranes, unlike SP-C which contains a membrane-spanning domain and covalently attached fatty acids (palmitate) that render it integral to phospholipid membranes [21]. Both SP-B and SP-C are synthesized as large precursor proproteins that undergo extensive post-translational processing as they pass through the secretory pathway, ultimately reaching the lamellar body. SP-B is essential for the process of lamellar body formation, and the alveolar type 2 cells of infants with inherited deficiency of SP-B are devoid of lamellar bodies. Because the lamellar body is where SP-C processing is completed, infants with inherited deficiency of SP-B are also deficient in mature SP-C, instead accumulating a larger, non-functional precursor of SP-C. Thus, patients with inherited deficiency of SP-B, despite having relatively normal surfactant phospholipid profiles, make a pulmonary surfactant with very poor surface tension properties due to the absence of both SP-B and SP-C. Conversely, because SP-C does not play either a direct nor indirect role in SP-B protein processing, animals with SP-C deficiency have normal SP-B, normal lamellar bodies, and relatively normal surfactant function, and exhibit no perinatal lethality due to surfactant dysfunction.

Like the enzymes of surfactant phospholipid production, SP-B and SP-C exhibit developmental and hormonal regulation of expression [22]. In human fetuses, SP-C mRNA is detected as early as 12 weeks of gestation and SP-B mRNA by 14 weeks, yet the mature proteins are not detectable in fetal lung tissue until after 24 weeks. SP-B protein is not detectable in amniotic fluid until after 30 weeks' gestation, increasing towards term [23]. This is due to developmental regulation of post-translational events in the proteolytic processing of proSP-B and proSP-C [24]. Consequently, infants delivered prematurely have reduced levels of both surface-active components of surfactant, phospholipid and hydrophobic surfactant proteins, due to the developmental regulation of surfactant proteins and the enzymes of phospholipid production in alveolar type 2 cells. The rate of type 2 cell differentiation, and secondarily surfactant production by the fetal lung, is modulated by levels of endogenous corticosteroids and is accelerated by administration of antenatal glucocorticoid to women in preterm labor. The response of the surfactant system to glucocorticoid involves all the lipid and protein components, and occurs primarily through increased gene expression, thus representing precocious maturation mimicking the normal developmental pattern. Endogenous thyroid hormones, prostaglandins, and catecholamines also have stimulatory effects on type 2 cell maturation as well as on clearance of lung fluid at birth. Certain proinflammatory cytokines (e.g. tumor necrosis factor and transforming growth factor β) inhibit surfactant production in experimental systems and may downregulate surfactant in conditions such as sepsis and inflammation.

Physiological changes in lung and pulmonary blood flow at birth

Two critical events in fetal development play a major role in the adaptation to air breathing that occurs at birth: removal of fetal lung liquid and changes in fetal circulation. Each is considered separately below but they are interdependent in the process of neonatal transition.

While fetal lung fluid is critical for early lung development, it is essential that fluid is cleared in preparation for the onset of air breathing [25]. Because fluid reabsorption depends largely upon regulation of the sodium channel, management options during labor and delivery that impair the catecholamine-induced maturation of ENaC (i.e. cesarean section without the benefit of labor) can impair lung fluid clearance, resulting in retention of fetal lung fluid, known as transient tachypnea of the newborn. Transient tachypnea of the newborn is a relatively benign condition generally requiring supportive care in the form of supplemental oxygen to allow for drainage of the excess fluid via lymphatics, or continuous positive airway pressure (CPAP) to facilitate clearance of lung fluid from the alveoli. It is important to recognize that retained fetal lung fluid can complicate other neonatal respiratory conditions such as meconium aspiration syndrome and bacterial and viral pneumonias. Furthermore, retained fetal lung fluid may complicate the transition from fetal to adult circulatory physiology and thereby contribute to the development of persistant pulmonary hypertension of the newborn described below.

The other critical event during neonatal transition is the adaptation of the circulatory pattern. During fetal life, the organ of gas exchange is the placenta. Thus, the circulatory pattern of the fetus is adapted to optimize blood flow to/from the placenta and minimize blood flow to/from the lungs to 5–10% of cardiac output. This is achieved through the low resistance/high capacitance of the placenta, the high resistance of the pulmonary vasculature, and the ductus arteriosus. The large surface area and lacunar structure of the placenta contribute to the low resistance/high capacitance of this organ. The low partial pressure of oxygen in the fetal lung and circulating vasoconstrictors, such as endothelin-1, leukotrienes, and Rho kinase, in the face of low production of vasodilators, including nitric oxide and prostacyclin, contribute to high pulmonary vascular tone [26]. As a result, pulmonary and systemic pressures are roughly equivalent. The high pulmonary vascular resistance and equivalent pulmonary and systemic pressures together favor the flow of oxygenated blood returning from the placenta (via the umbilical vein and ductus venosus) to the right atrium across the foramen ovale to the left atrium and out to the systemic circulation. The ductus arteriosus, a blood vessel developing from the sixth aortic arches, bridges between the pulmonary artery and the aorta at the bifurcation of the left pulmonary artery, and approximately at the level of the left subclavian artery as it branches from the aortic arch. The high pulmonary vascular resistance and low systemic vascular resistance *in utero* favor flow of oxygenated blood passing from right atrium to right ventricle and pulmonary artery, through the ductus arteriosus, and into the aortic arch to supply the systemic circulation. In addition to optimizing flow of oxygenated blood systemically, the combination of atrial and ductal level shunts allows for sufficient blood flow to all the chambers of the heart, facilitating their development during fetal life, and this explains the greater muscularization of the right ventricle in the newborn period relative to the left ventricle.

In the transition to air breathing, the circulatory pattern must undergo change to establish the lung as the organ of gas exchange [27]. Clamping and transection of the umbilical cord at delivery removes the placenta from the systemic circulation, resulting in a precipitous increase in systemic vascular resistance. This has at best a modest effect on changing blood flow centrally, instead improving blood flow to the lower body. Initiation of air breathing inflates the lungs and increases oxygen tension across the alveolar capillary bed, facilitating a precipitous decrease in pulmonary vascular resistance. Pulmonary stretch receptors elicit reflex dilation of the pulmonary vasculature independently of the effects of enhanced oxygen tension. The net effect of these events is that left atrial pressure becomes higher than right atrial pressure, leading to functional closure of the foramen ovale. These changes also reduce flow through the ductus arteriosus by 24% soon after birth, but are not sufficient to eliminate ductal flow for 48 h after birth. Cessation of ductal blood flow and ultimately scarring of this structure, which becomes the ligamentum arteriosum, occur over the first 2–3 weeks of life. Increasing hypoxemia of the muscle media of the ductus due to reduced blood flow through the ductal lumen promotes vasoconstriction of the ductus. Ductal constriction enhances muscle media hypoxia by collapsing the vasa vasorum, the other source of oxygen to the ductus. Together, these adaptations lead to the adult circulatory pattern with the lung in series with the systemic circulation, enabling efficient oxygenation.

These physiological changes are dynamic and capable of reverting to a fetal pattern over the first days of life. While pulmonary vascular resistance decreases precipitously in the first minutes to hours of life, it does not achieve adult levels for weeks to months postnatally, and the pulmonary vasculature is prone to vasoconstriction in response to hypoxia and acidosis during that time. In addition, events associated with reduced systemic vascular resistance, such as septicemia, can lower systemic vascular resistance enough so that even the normal pulmonary vascular tone in the first days of life can lead to pulmonary pressures becoming suprasystemic, leading to enhanced right-to-left blood flow.

Persistent pulmonary hypertension of the newborn, also known as persistent fetal circulation, can occur in association with other neonatal diseases such as septicemia or meconium aspiration, or can be idiopathic in nature [26]. The disorder is characterized as suprasystemic right ventricular pressure, right-to-left flow of deoxygenated blood through the ductus arteriosus, and severe hypoxemia. Primary pulmonary hypertension of the newborn (PPHN) can result from lung parenchymal disease leading to pulmonary vasoconstriction, from pulmonary vascular remodeling in the absence of lung parenchymal disease, or from primary or secondary pulmonary hypoplasia. Animal studies have elucidated pathways for targeted therapies such as nitric oxide/cGMP, prostacyclin/cAMP, and endothelin to lower pulmonary vascular resistance. Optimization of oxygenation and ventilation while providing specific pulmonary vasodilatation with nitric oxide has lowered the morbidity and mortality of this disorder and reduced the need for more aggressive therapies such as extracorporeal membrane oxygenation (ECMO).

Ductal patency can also complicate the management of prematurely born infants [28,29]. The ductus arteriosus of premature infants is thin-walled and thus depends only on luminal blood flow for oxygenation. As a consequence, the ductal muscle media does not become as hypoxic with constriction of the premature ductus, thus contributing to a prolonged delay in anatomical closure. As pulmonary vascular resistance decreases in preterm infants in response to lung inflation and surfactant administration, the high systemic vascular resistance favors left-to-right flow across a patent ductus arteriosus resulting in pulmonary edema. Both are responsive acutely to elevated positive end-expiratory pressure. The pulmonary overcirculation can also be associated with vascular steal from the cerebral and mesenteric vasculatures, increasing the risk of intraventricular hemorrhage and intestinal ischemia. Closure of a patent ductus arteriosus can be achieved by treatment with agents that reduce prostaglandin synthesis, such as indometacin and ibuprofen, but success is inversely related to gestational age. When repeated indometacin therapy fails and the patent ductus arteriosus is felt to be a major factor in pulmonary symptoms, surgical ligation through a left thoracotomy approach is possible. There is some controversy regarding the long-term morbidity of surgical ligation of a patent ductus arteriosus.

Lung development after birth

As with fetal lung development, postnatal lung development can be subdivided into several stages, also illustrated in Figure 6.1 [3]. True alveoli containing secondary septae (described above) become evident as early as 36 weeks in the human fetus, initiating the alveolar phase of fetal lung development which extends through 1–2 years of age. Postnatal alveolarization begins with a phase of bulk alveolarization occurring within the first 6 months postnatally, with a more modest addition of secondary alveoli through the remainder of this period. The alveoli of the infant lung are different from adult alveoli. These immature secondary alveoli contain a double capillary bed, whereas adult alveoli are invested by a single capillary bed. Microvascular maturation, the next phase of postnatal lung development, occurs between the first few postnatal months of life through 3 years of age (discussed above).

There is considerable controversy regarding when the lung ceases to add alveoli. Estimates have ranged from as early as 2 years to as late as 20 years in humans. This is further complicated by the observation that alveolar expansion can occur in response to pneumonectomy in adult animals and humans. The acquisition of alveoli after the maturation of the microvasculature has been termed late alveolarization. This activity has been most often demonstrated in subpleural regions of the lung and likely invokes mechanisms similar to the formation of secondary alveoli.

The addition of alveoli is not the only means of expanding the surface area of the lung. While alveolarization wanes over the first 3 years of life in the human, growth of the lung continues to expand the gas exchange surface. Between 2 years of age and adulthood, lung tissue expands with lung volume roughly proportional to the increase in bodyweight of the child. Thus, owing to the combined processes of prenatal lung development, postnatal lung development, and lung growth, there is tremendous potential for expansion of the gas exchange surface area that is developmentally programmed into the fetal lung to account for the growing needs of the infant, child, and adult for aerobic cellular respiration. The extent to which these developmental mechanisms can be harnessed after premature birth, with or without superimposed lung injury, is a topic of active investigation.

Normal values for pulmonary function with age

In neonates and children, developmental changes discussed above lead to rapid transformations in the mechanical properties of the respiratory system and influence pulmonary function. Unlike many physiological parameters that do not vary with age (i.e. arterial pH), predicted values of pulmonary function depend upon age, height, gender, and race [30]. Consistent normalization of pulmonary function test results, based on weight or height, is important to the interpretation of results and for comparison to reference values. When tests rely on the subjective effort of an infant or young child, technique can have profound effects on measurements and efforts to standardize pulmonary function testing. For example, several studies have compared compliance measurements from preterm infants with and without bronchopulmonary dysplasia to term infants to determine their diagnostic or prognostic value. However, there was a large overlap between the groups, with the majority of infants with bronchopulmonary dysplasia (BPD) having compliance measurements within the 95% confidence interval of the control group [31]. This observation suggests that measurements in individual infants are of limited value as a diagnostic or prognostic tool. However, in a research setting, consistency can best be obtained in a pulmonary function laboratory, although infant and pediatric ventilators now provide opportunities to make measurements in the intensive care setting. The discussion below presents an outline of basic parameters and descriptions of how pulmonary function changes with age where applicable, including normal references only where they are considered consistent standards (Table 6.2).

Table 6.2 Standards for lung mechanics and pulmonary function in infants, children, and adults

	Infant	Child	Adult
Compliance (cc/cmH₂O/kg)	1.5–2.0	2.5–3.0	0.1 L/cmH₂O[a]
Resistance (cmH₂O/L/s)	20–40	20–40[b]	1–2
Functional residual capacity (cc/kg)	20–25	20–25[c]	1.9–2.4 L[a]
Tidal volume (cc/kg)	4–8[d]	4–8	6–8
Respiratory rate (breaths/min)	20–60	20–30	12–20
Minute ventilation (cc/kg/min)	240–480		5–8[a]

[a]note different units; [b]up to 2 years; [c]up to 18 months; [d]preterm 3–5 mL/kg.

Compliance

The elastic characteristics of the lung are described by the changes in volume (V) per unitary change in transpulmonary pressure (PL) under conditions of zero flow, or lung compliance ($CL = \Delta V/\Delta PL$). The systematic change in both pressure and volume during inflation and deflation allows a static pressure–volume curve of the lungs to be plotted. Lung compliance ranges from 1.5 to 2 mL/cmH₂O/kg in newborns to 2.5–3 mL/cmH₂O/kg in children and adults [32].

Resistance

Airway resistance (R_{aw}) reflects the non-elastic airway and tissue forces resisting gas flow. Lung resistance is determined predominantly by frictional resistance to inspiratory and expiratory air flow in the larger airways (80%), while tissue resistance (19%) and inertial forces (1%) also contribute [33]. By definition, resistance to airflow is equal to the resistive component of driving pressure (ΔP) divided by the air flow (Q), $R_{aw} = \Delta P/Q$ with units of cmH₂O/L/s. Poiseuille's Law states that resistance to flow increases by a power of 4 with any decrease in airway diameter ($R_{aw} = 8\eta L/\pi r^4$, where η is the gas viscosity, L is length and r the radius of the airway). Resistance is also dependent on the number of airways, lung volume, and respiratory rate. The diameter of airways in infants and children is much smaller than adults, resulting in increased R_{aw}. Airway resistance in normal healthy infants up to 2 years of age ranges from 20 to 40 cmH₂O/L/s, whereas R_{aw} in adults is 1–2 cmH₂O/L/s.

Total lung capacity

Measurement of total lung capacity (TLC) is effort dependent and thus cannot be obtained readily in infants. Postmortem studies have demonstrated that lung volume is linearly related to body length during childhood [34]. On average, girls reach their maximal height and lung volume earlier than boys [35,36]. However, for any given age and stature, boys have larger lung volumes than girls as a result of increased numbers of alveoli and respiratory bronchioles. These sex-dependent differences are absent below 2 years of age.

Functional residual capacity

Functional residual capacity (FRC) is defined as the static resting volume of the lung. Functionally, FRC is achieved when the opposing forces resulting from the outward elastic recoil of the chest wall and the inward elastic recoil of the lung, which determine the static resting volume of the lung, are balanced. The balance of the elastic recoil forces of the lung and chest wall in the infants predicts a supine FRC of only 10% of TLC, whereas in adults FRC accounts for approximately 50% of TLC in the upright position [32]. This intuitively seems incompatible with appropriate stability and patency of the peripheral airways to achieve gas exchange. As described above, infants incorporate laryngeal braking during expiration to maintain FRC, and will initiate inspiration before achieving balance between elastic recoil of chest wall and lung tissue. In infants, the postinspiratory activity of the inspiratory muscles and the laryngeal control of expiratory flow ("grunting") modify respiratory mechanics to maintain the patency of small airways and alveoli. The net result of these breathing strategies is that measured values of FRC (i.e. using gas dilution technique) in infants remain approximately 40% of TLC. Mean values for FRC range from 20 to 25 mL/kg in infants up to 18 months of age [32].

Tidal volume

Tidal volume is the volume of each breath and is measured during inhalation or exhalation, or averaged for the entire respiratory cycle. The value should be normalized to bodyweight or length. During spontaneous breathing, normal values in healthy neonates range from 5 to 10 mL/kg, although >8.5 mL/kg has been generally accepted as overdistension [37]. Very small preterm infants may have spontaneous breathing tidal volumes as low as 3–5 mL/kg.

Minute ventilation

Minute ventilation is the product of tidal volume and respiratory rate. The respiratory rate of most preterm and term infants is 20–60 breaths/min, and the normal range for minute ventilation is 240–480 mL/kg/min [37].

Pathophysiology of important respiratory diseases affecting infants and children

Asthma

Asthma is a chronic, recurrent disease characterized by reversible bronchoconstriction, accompanied by inflammation and increased mucus production in the small airways. Asthma exacerbations are manifest by expiratory wheezing and obstruction to expiratory and sometimes inspiratory airflow, cough, and varying degrees of respiratory distress. Because of the broad definition and heterogeneous nature of the disease prevalence estimates vary, but 6–9 million children in the United States have asthma, making it the most common chronic respiratory disease and a condition commonly encountered by the pediatric anesthesiologist [38,39]. Total asthma prevalence in the United States in 2009 was 8.2%, with 9.6% of children aged 0–17 years having the disease. Children 5–15 years of age have a particularly high prevalence, with 12–13% of males in this age group suffering from this condition. About half of these patients have an asthma attack annually, and in 2007 157,000 children were hospitalized for asthma, and there were 185 asthma deaths in children in the US [40].

For many children, the disease originates in infancy. Many infants wheeze with viral upper and lower respiratory tract infections, particularly with respiratory syncytial virus (RSV) and rhinovirus. Many of these children will only wheeze during their preschool years, and thus do not develop chronic asthma. In some children, RSV infection is felt to increase the risk of developing chronic asthma, through a combination of genetic, environmental, and immune response mechanisms that are not clearly elucidated. Those who have recurrent bronchospasm events after age 6 years are diagnosed with asthma; many of these patients will have their disease resolve completely or greatly diminish after adolescence. Those with asthma persisting into adolescence often have an atopic/allergic component to their disease. Up to 75% of young children who wheeze with viral respiratory tract infections will have complete resolution of symptoms by adulthood [39–42].

The inciting events for an episode of bronchospasm are legion. As noted above, viral respiratory infections, especially with RSV, are a frequent inciting event in children. Other viruses known to be associated with asthma exacerbations include rhinovirus, influenza, parainfluenza, and coronavirus. Allergic sensitization and innate immune response to the virus exposure play a role in these exacerbations [39]. Other infections, such as chlamydia, mycoplasma, and bacterial infections of the respiratory tract, can provoke asthma exacerbations. Allergic responses with antigen-specific IgE antibodies to aeroallergens is another important mechanism that usually does not occur until at least 2–3 years of age. This mechanism increases during later childhood and adolescence, and peaks in the second decade of life. Dust mites, animal dander, trees and grass pollens are among the most frequent inciting factors for allergic asthma. Another very important risk factor for childhood asthma is exposure to tobacco smoke, which is thought to be the single most important environmental factor for asthma exacerbation in infants and children [42]. Other factors for asthma exacerbation, particularly in older children, include exercise-induced asthma, allergy to non-steroidal anti-inflammatory agents, including aspirin (5–10% of adult asthmatics), gastroesophageal reflux, and psychosocial stressors.

The genetic components of asthma are complex and multifactorial, and although the atopic phenotype has a familial component, recent genome-wide association studies and other gene candidate studies have had limited success in elucidating the genetic origins of asthma. Several groups have reported markers on chromosome 17q21 that were reproducibly associated with childhood-onset asthma in families from the United Kingdom and Germany, and other populations. This association appears to be strongest in young children with tobacco smoke exposure. There are several candidates identified, but as yet no definitive asthma genes have been designated [43].

The pathophysiology of an asthma exacerbation is complex, keeping in mind that it is an acute episode superimposed upon an abnormal airway with chronic changes of inflammation, increased airway smooth muscle resulting in airway remodeling and chronic loss of lung function, and increased mucus production. In addition, the asthma phenotype has been divided into a number of subphenotypes. Airway inflammation is a fundamental abnormality in asthma pathogenesis, with mast cells, eosinophils, neutrophils, CD4$^+$ T-lymphocytes all playing a role. In allergic asthma, antigen exposure in the airway to IgE-specific antibodies incites a T-helper cell 2 (Th2) type lymphocyte response, which in turn generates a cytokine response. The cytokine response attracts mast cells, eosinophils, and basophils, which in turn are activated and release mediators of airway smooth muscle tone, including histamine, leukotrienes (including slow reacting substance of anaphylaxis), and prostaglandins, and resulting in acute

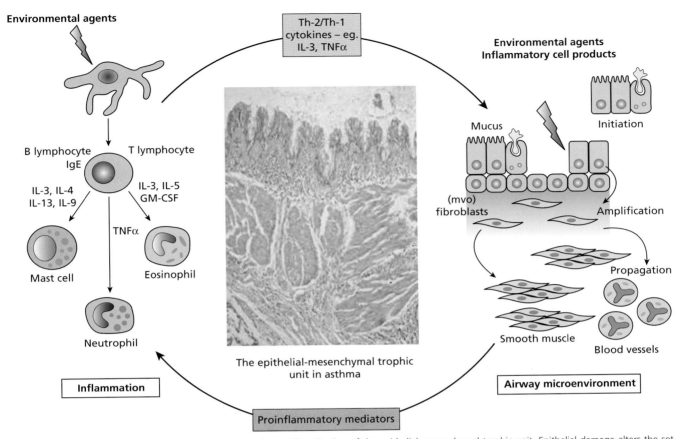

Figure 6.2 Inflammatory and remodeling responses in asthma with activation of the epithelial mesenchymal trophic unit. Epithelial damage alters the set point for communication between bronchial epithelium and underlying mesenchymal cells, leading to myofibroblast activation and increase in mesenchymal volume, and induction of structural changes throughout the airway wall. Reproduced from Holgate and Polosa [45] with permission from Elsevier.

bronchospasm [44]. The chronic inflammation effects on the airway epithelium are now known to be crucially important to asthma pathogenesis. Bronchial biopsies in moderate-to-severe asthma show areas of epithelial metaplasia, thickening of the subepithelial basal membranes, increased numbers of myofibroblasts, and evidence of airway remodeling including hypertrophy and hyperplasia of airway smooth muscle, mucus gland hyperplasia, angiogenesis and an altered deposition and composition of extracellular matrix proteins [44,45] (Fig. 6.2). This means a chronically abnormal airway characterized by increased smooth muscle, an immune system primed to respond to allergen exposure, and airways chronically narrowed by this inflammation and mucus production will constrict further with acute airway smooth muscle constriction. Particularly in small pediatric patients, the narrow small airways diameter means that a relatively small degree of airway smooth muscle

constriction can result in more severe bronchospasm symptoms, given that resistance to airflow is inversely proportional to the fourth power of the airway radius with laminar flow, and the fifth power of the radius with turbulent flow.

Evaluation of asthma in young children involves careful history of frequency and severity of episodes, response to treatment, and ascertaining environmental allergens and exposures. Clinical examination is important, and active wheezing in the preanesthetic period is cause for concern and should merit cancellation of elective surgery. Pulmonary function testing, particularly forced expiratory volume in 1 sec (FEV_1) and forced expiratory flow at 25–75% of the expiratory volume (FEF_{25-75}), is important in older children, to gauge both baseline status and response to treatment during an acute exacerbation. Obviously, young children will not co-operate for pulmonary function testing so clinical examination and history are the primary methods for evaluation. Chest radiography is important to assess degree of hyperinflation and rule out infectious causes.

Treatment of asthma depends on the age of the patient and the severity of the asthma. Acute exacerbations of asthma are usually treated with a short-acting β-agonist by inhalation route (nebulized or metered dose inhaler), such as levalbuterol, which will enhance the action of cyclic AMP and thus relax airway smooth muscles. Halogenated inhaled anesthetics are well known to relax airway smooth muscle via inhibition of Ca^{2+} influx. (See Chapter 9 for a complete discussion of the pharmacology of inhaled anesthetics.) In the rare case of acute severe bronchospasm with general anesthesia where gas exchange is so compromised that any inhaled agent does not reach the airways, intravenous β-agonists (epinephrine, isoproterenol), as well as intravenous magnesium sulfate, can acutely relax airway smooth muscle and allow inhaled agents to reach the airways. The US National Institutes of Health published evidence-based asthma evaluation and treatment guidelines in 2007 [46]. For intermittent asthma, episodic treatment with short-acting β-agonists as needed is recommended. As the severity and chronicity of asthma increase, additional chronic treatments such as inhaled corticosteroids, cromolyn (mast cell stabilizer), montelukast (leukotriene receptor inhibitor), longer acting β-agonists or oral corticosteroids are added (Fig. 6.3).

Bronchopulmonary dysplasia

Bronchopulmonary dysplasia (BPD) was described over 40 years ago by Northway et al, in a series of 32 preterm infants following mechanical ventilation for respiratory distress syndrome (RDS). The disease featured prominent interstitial fibrosis, alveolar overdistension alternating with regions of atelectasis, and airway abnormalities, including squamous metaplasia and excessive muscularization [47]. In those early days of survival of preterm infants, ventilator therapy often included high FIO_2 and high ventilating pressures and volumes, features now known to cause significant lung injury and which contributed to the severe chronic lung disease in many early BPD patients. In recent years, with survival of more and more premature infants, and recognition of pulmonary oxygen toxicity and the adverse effects of excessive pressures and volumes with mechanical ventilation, the BPD phenotype has changed to a histological pattern of arrest of airway and alveolar development: alveolar numbers are reduced and the alveoli are larger than normal in diameter; the more severe changes are absent [48,49] (Fig. 6.4). The most common current definition of the "new" BPD is a premature infant who had a diagnosis of RDS, and requires supplemental oxygen at 36 weeks postconceptional age, whether or not they required mechanical ventilation. A joint US National Institute of Childhood Health and Development/National Heart Lung and Blood Institute workshop further classified mild BPD as the need for supplemental oxygen at ≥28 days' but not at 36 weeks' postconceptional age; moderate BPD was defined as the need for supplemental oxygen at 28 days, in addition to supplemental oxygen at FIO_2 ≤0.30 at 36 weeks' postconceptional age; and criteria for severe BPD included the need for supplemental oxygen at 28 days' and at 36 weeks' postconceptional age, and the need for mechanical ventilation and/or FIO_2 >0.30 [48].

The incidence of BPD varies by center, but in recent studies of infants born at 24–31 weeks' gestation at 500–1500 g, BPD rates average 25–30% using the definition of oxygen requirement at 36 weeks, but intercenter variability means these rates vary from about 5% to 60% [48]. The overall incidence of BPD is stable or actually increasing slightly, presumably due to increasing survival of more premature infants. Risk factors for BPD include lower gestational age and birthweight, intrauterine growth retardation, male sex, family history of asthma, not receiving antenatal glucocorticoids, and likely a genetic component that is not yet fully elucidated.

Theories about pathogenesis of the new BPD include lung injury in very preterm infants at critical stages of lung development during the late canalicular and saccular phases (see above), resulting in arrested development of lung structures and disrupted repair at critical stages [50]. Proposed risk factors for this lung injury include chorio-amnionitis and fetal inflammatory response, ventilator-induced lung injury (volutrauma, pressure trauma, stretch trauma), oxygen toxicity (oxygen free radical production and lipid perioxidation), lack of surfactant, and disruption of vasculogenesis (inhibition of vascular endothelial growth factor (VEGF) pathways) [50].

Strategies to reduce the incidence and severity of BPD include non-invasive forms of ventilation, in lieu of endotracheal intubation in prematures with RDS. Both nasal CPAP and nasal intermittent positive pressure ventilation (NIPPV), delivered via specially designed nasal prongs, have been used for this purpose. As a primary treatment for respiratory failure secondary to RDS, non-invasive ventilation may avoid endotracheal intubation in some infants, but so far trials have not shown a consistent ability to reduce the incidence of BPD with these modalities. Non-invasive ventilation is well established as a postextubation therapy to reduce the duration of endotracheal intubation and mechanical ventilation. However, these modalities used after extubation have not been conclusively demonstrated to reduce the incidence of BPD [49]. Modern conventional

Assessing severity and initiating therapy in children who are not currently taking long-term control medication

Components of severity		Classification of asthma severity (0–4 years of age)			
			Persistent		
		Intermittent	**Mild**	**Moderate**	**Severe**
Impairment	Symptoms	≤2 days/week	>2 days/week but not daily	Daily	Throughout the day
	Nighttime awakenings	0	1–2x/month	3–4x/month	>1x/week
	Short-acting beta$_2$-agonist use for symptom control (not prevention of EIB)	≤2 days/week	>2 days/week but not daily	Daily	Several times per day
	Interference with normal activity	None	Minor limitation	Some limitation	Extremely limited
Risk	Exacerbations requiring oral systemic corticosteroids	0–1/year	≥2 Exacerbations in 6 months requiring oral systemic corticosteroids, or ≥4 wheezing episodes/1 year lasting >1 day AND risk factors for persistent asthma		
		← Consider severity and interval since last exacerbation. Frequency and severity may fluctuate over time. →			
		Exacerbations of any severity may occur in patients in any severity category.			
Recommended step for Initiating therapy **(See figure 6–3c for treatment steps.)**		Step 1	Step 2	Step 3 and consider short course of oral systemic corticosteroids	
		In 2–6 weeks, depending on severity, evaluate level of asthma control that is achieved. If no clear benefit is observed in 4–6 weeks, consider adjusting therapy or alternative diagnoses.			

Key: EIB, exercise-induced bronchospasm

Notes

■ The stepwise approach is meant to assist, not replace, the clinical decisionmaking required to meet individual patient needs.

■ Level of severity is determined by both impairment and risk. Assess impairment domain by patient's/caregiver's recall of previous 2–4 weeks. Symptom assessment for longer periods should reflect a global assessment such as inquiring whether the patient's asthma is better or worse since the last visit. Assign severity to the most severe category in which any feature occurs.

■ At present, there are inadequate data to correspond frequencies of exacerbations with different levels of asthma severity. For treatment purposes, patients who had ≥2 exacerbations requiring oral systemic corticosteroids in the past 6 months, or ≥4 wheezing episodes in the past year, and who have risk factors for persistent asthma may be considered the same as patients who have persistent asthma, even in the absence of impairment levels consistent with persistent asthma.

(A)

Figure 6.3 Classifying asthma severity and initiating treatment in (A) children 0–4 years of age, (B) children 5–11 years of age. Stepwise approach for managing asthma in (C) children 0–4 years of age, (D) children 5–11 years of age. Reproduced from National Institutes of Health, National Heart, Lung, and Blood Institute Asthma Treatment Guidelines [46] with permission from NHLBI.

Assessing severity and initiating therapy in children who are not currently taking long-term control medication

Components of severity		Classification of asthma severity (5–11 years of age)			
				Persistent	
		Intermittent	Mild	Moderate	Severe
Impairment	Symptoms	≤2 days/week	>2 days/week but not daily	Daily	Throughout the day
	Nighttime awakenings	≤2x/month	3–4x/month	>1x/week but not nightly	Often 7x/week
	Short-acting beta₂-agonist use for symptom control (not prevention of EIB)	≤2 days/week	>2 days/week but not daily	Daily	Several times per day
	Interference with normal activity	None	Minor limitation	Some limitation	Extremely limited
	Lung function	• Normal FEV$_1$ between exacerbations • FEV$_1$ >80% predicted • FEV$_1$/FVC >85%	• FEV$_1$ = >80% predicted • FEV$_1$/FVC >80%	• FEV$_1$ = 60–80% predicted • FEV$_1$/FVC = 75–80%	• FEV$_1$ <60% predicted • FEV$_1$/FVC <75%
Risk	Exacerbations requiring oral systemic corticosteroids	0–1/year (see note)	≥2/year (see note) ⟶		
		⟵ Consider severity and interval since last exacerbation. ⟶ Frequency and severity may fluctuate over time for patients in any severity category.			
		Relative annual risk of exacerbations may be related to FEV$_1$.			
Recommended step for initiating therapy (See figure 6–3d for treatment steps.)		Step 1	Step 2	Step 3, medium-dose ICS option	Step 3, medium-dose ICS option, or step 4 and consider short course of oral systemic corticosteroids
		In 2–6 weeks, evaluate level of asthma control that is achieved, and adjust therapy accordingly.			

Key: EIB, exercise-induced bronchospasm; FEV$_1$, forced expiratory volume in 1 second; FVC, forced vital capacity; ICS, inhaled corticosteroids

Notes

- The stepwise approach is meant to assist, not replace, the clinical decisionmaking required to meet individual patient needs.

- Level of severity is determined by both impairment and risk. Assess impairment domain by patient's/caregiver's recall of the previous 2–4 weeks and spirometry. Assign severity to the most severe category in which any feature occurs.

- At present, there are inadequate data to correspond frequencies of exacerbations with different levels of asthma severity. In general, more frequent and intense exacerbations (e.g., requiring urgent, unscheduled care, hospitalization, or ICU admission) indicate greater underlying disease severity. For treatment purposes, patients who had ≥2 exacerbations requiring oral systemic corticosteroids in the past year may be considered the same as patients who have persistent asthma, even in the absence of impairment levels consistent with persistent asthma.

(B)

Figure 6.3 (*Continued*)

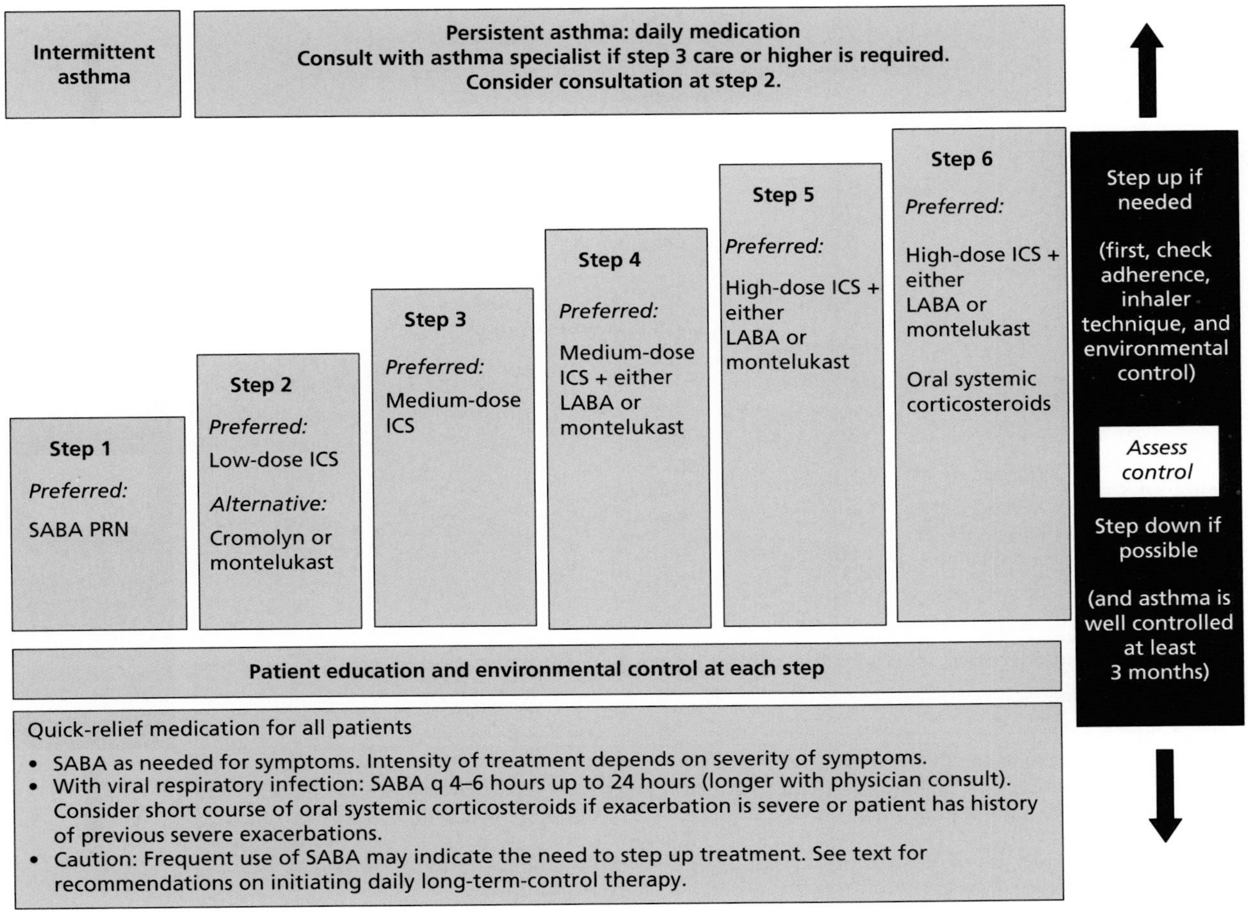

Intermittent asthma	Persistent asthma: daily medication Consult with asthma specialist if step 3 care or higher is required. Consider consultation at step 2.

Step 6
Preferred:
High-dose ICS + either LABA or montelukast
Oral systemic corticosteroids

Step 5
Preferred:
High-dose ICS + either LABA or montelukast

Step 4
Preferred:
Medium-dose ICS + either LABA or montelukast

Step 3
Preferred:
Medium-dose ICS

Step 2
Preferred:
Low-dose ICS
Alternative:
Cromolyn or montelukast

Step 1
Preferred:
SABA PRN

Step up if needed
(first, check adherence, inhaler technique, and environmental control)

Assess control

Step down if possible
(and asthma is well controlled at least 3 months)

Patient education and environmental control at each step

Quick-relief medication for all patients
- SABA as needed for symptoms. Intensity of treatment depends on severity of symptoms.
- With viral respiratory infection: SABA q 4–6 hours up to 24 hours (longer with physician consult). Consider short course of oral systemic corticosteroids if exacerbation is severe or patient has history of previous severe exacerbations.
- Caution: Frequent use of SABA may indicate the need to step up treatment. See text for recommendations on initiating daily long-term-control therapy.

Key: **Alphabetical order is used when more than one treatment option is listed within either preferred or alternative therapy.** ICS, inhaled corticosteroid; LABA, inhaled long-acting beta$_2$-agonist; SABA, inhaled short-acting beta$_2$-agonist

Notes:

- The stepwise approach is meant to assist, not replace, the clinical decisionmaking required to meet individual patient needs.

- If alternative treatment is used and response is inadequate, discontinue it and use the preferred treatment before stepping up.

- If clear benefit is not observed within 4–6 weeks and patient/family medication technique and adherence are satisfactory, consider adjusting therapy or alternative diagnosis.

- Studies on children 0–4 years of age are limited. Step 2 preferred therapy is based on Evidence A. All other recommendations are based on expert opinion and extrapolation from studies in older children.

(C)

Figure 6.3 (*Continued*)

Intermittent asthma	Persistent asthma: daily medication Consult with asthma specialist if step 4 care or higher is required. Consider consultation at step 3.

Step 1

Preferred:

SABA PRN

Step 2

Preferred:
Low-dose ICS

Alternative:
Cromolyn, LTRA, nedocromil, or theophylline

Step 3

Preferred:
EITHER:
Low-dose ICS + either LABA, LTRA, or theophylline
OR
Medium-dose ICS

Step 4

Preferred:
Medium-dose ICS + LABA

Alternative:
Medium-dose ICS + either LTRA or theophylline

Step 5

Preferred:
High-dose ICS + LABA

Alternative:
High-dose ICS + either LTRA or theophylline

Step 6

Preferred:
High-dose ICS + LABA + oral systemic corticosteroid

Alternative:
High-dose ICS + either LTRA or theophylline + oral systemic corticosteroid

Step up if needed

(first, check adherence, inhaler technique, environmental control, and comorbid conditions)

Assess control

Step down if possible

(and asthma is well controlled at least 3 months)

Each step: patient education, environmental control, and management of comorbidities.

Steps 2–4: Consider subcutaneous allergen immunotherapy for patients who have allergic asthma (see notes).

Quick-relief medication for all patients
- SABA as needed for symptoms. Intensity of treatment depends on severity of symptoms: up to 3 treatments at 20-minute intervals as needed. Short course of oral systemic corticosteroids may be needed.
- Caution: Increasing use of SABA or use >2 days a week for symptom relief (not prevention of EIB) generally indicates inadequate control and the need to step up treatment.

Key: **Alphabetical order is used when more than one treatment option is listed within either preferred or alternative therapy.**
ICS, inhaled corticosteroid; LABA, inhaled long-acting beta$_2$-agonist, LTRA, leukotriene receptor antagonist; SABA, inhaled short-acting beta$_2$-agonist

Notes:

■ The stepwise approach is meant to assist, not replace, the clinical decisionmaking required to meet individual patient needs.

■ If alternative treatment is used and response is inadequate, discontinue it and use the preferred treatment before stepping up.

■ Theophylline is a less desirable alternative due to the need to monitor serum concentration levels.

■ Step 1 and step 2 medications are based on Evidence A. Step 3 ICS + adjunctive therapy and ICS are based on Evidence B for efficacy of each treatment and extrapolation from comparator trials in older children and adults—comparator trials are not available for this age group; steps 4–6 are based on expert opinion and extrapolation from studies in older children and adults.

■ Immunotherapy for steps 2–4 is based on Evidence B for house-dust mites, animal danders, and pollens; evidence is weak or lacking for molds and cockroaches. Evidence is strongest for immunotherapy with single allergens. The role of allergy in asthma is greater in children than in adults. Clinicians who administer immunotherapy should be prepared and equipped to identify and treat anaphylaxis that may occur.

(D)

Figure 6.3 *(Continued)*

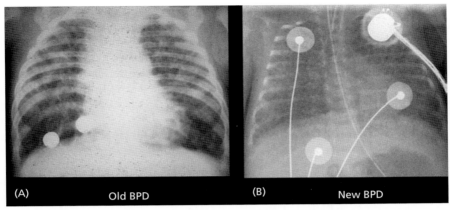

Figure 6.4 Radiographic picture of bronchopulmonary dysplasia (BPD). (A) Old BPD: areas of atelectasis and hyperinflation. (B) New BPD: diffuse opacification of lung fields. Reproduced from Gupta et al [49] with permission from Elsevier.

mechanical ventilation techniques employ microprocessor technology, allowing patient-triggered synchronized ventilation, volume-targeted ventilation, and flow-cycled ventilation, all of which are proving to have advantages in reducing the incidence of ventilator-induced lung injury. Permissive hypercapnia reduces the duration of mechanical ventilation but the incidence of BPD with this technique is unchanged. High-frequency oscillatory ventilation is often used in preterm infants with RDS; this strategy has also been found to reduce the incidence of BPD in some studies [49]. Oxygen toxicity has been postulated to have an important role in the pathogenesis of worsening RDS and BPD, and in recent studies, targeting an SpO_2 in the 85–89% range, rather than the 94–97% range, appears to have some effect in reducing the severity of lung injury and of BPD; meta-analysis of combined trials is underway to further elucidate the magnitude of this effect [51].

Drug therapies used to reduce the severity of RDS include a single course of antenatal glucocorticoids (dexamethasone or betametasone) to accelerate the maturation of the surfactant system in the fetal lung; there is no evidence that this intervention reduces the risk of BPD, probably because of an increase in survival. Surfactant therapy significantly reduces the incidence and severity of RDS, but again does not reduce the incidence of BPD likely because of the survival benefit. Caffeine therapy, originally used to reduce apnea of prematurity, also reduces the incidence of BPD. Inhaled nitric oxide (iNO), the potent pulmonary vasodilator, has been used in prematures with hypoxemic respiratory failure, but in randomized controlled trials has demonstrated an inconsistent effect on survival and incidence of BPD in premature infants, and is not recommended as routine therapy in RDS. Other drug therapies that have been used in infants with RDS and evaluated to reduce the incidence of BPD

include systemic or inhaled corticosteroids, furosemide, β-receptor agonist or anticholinergic inhaled drugs, indometacin and ibuprofen, vitamin E, and superoxide dismutase; these agents have not reduced the incidence of BPD. Therapies shown to be effective at reducing BPD incidence include vitamin A and inositol supplementation in the diet [51].

When caring for a patient with a diagnosis of BPD, the anesthesiologist must thoroughly review the history and current chest radiographs. The severity of BPD, according to the criteria noted above, should be assessed. Severe "old" BPD in a chronically ventilated infant with a tracheostomy is rare in the modern era. Examination often reveals an infant receiving supplemental oxygen by endotracheal tube, nasal CPAP or conventional nasal cannula, with varying degrees of tachypnea, intercostal and subcostal retractions, and signs of increased lung water or bronchial reactivity such as fine rales and expiratory wheezing. It is important to understand the patient's baseline oxygen saturation and $PaCO_2$, often available from capillary or venous blood gases. Ventilatory strategies in the operating room should be designed to minimize barotrauma, volutrauma, and oxygen toxicity, and allow permissive hypercapnia to the patient's normal $PaCO_2$. Decreases in lung compliance, increases in resistance, and the increased risk for postoperative mechanical ventilation must all be anticipated and planned for in the infant with BPD. Additional doses of diuretics or bronchodilators may be needed to optimize perioperative pulmonary outcomes.

Cystic fibrosis

Cystic fibrosis (CF) is an autosomal recessive disorder caused by a defect in the cystic fibrosis transmembrane conductance regulator (CFTR) gene. It is present in approximately 30,000 children and adults in the United

States, with about 1000 new cases diagnosed annually. With improvements in early diagnosis and care, life expectancy has increased markedly over the past several decades, with median life expectancy at more than 37 years [52]. CFTR is an adenosine triphosphate (ATP)-binding protein that regulates chloride and bicarbonate transport across epithelial cells via cyclic adenosine monophosphate (cAMP). CFTR also regulates the airway surface liquid depth through regulation of other proteins, most prominently the epithelial sodium channel. Absent or dysfunctional CFTR results in abnormal electrolyte and fluid content on the epithelia of the lung, pancreas, intestine, hepatobiliary tract, sweat gland, and vas deferens. Patients with CF have thick, dehydrated, hyperviscous mucus that severely deters effective mucus clearance (Fig. 6.5). Patients with CF are susceptible to chronic infection with pathogens such as *Staphylococcus aureus* and *Pseudomonas aeruginosa* that are nearly impossible to eradicate once established. Inflammation occurs

both secondary to chronic infection and independent of microbial disease. Chronic infection and inflammation precipitate a cycle of tissue destruction, bronchiectasis, and airway obstruction, a process that eventually leads to respiratory failure. Slowly progressive lung injury is often accompanied by episodic pulmonary exacerbations, followed by periods of relative disease stability [53] (Fig. 6.6).

Standard therapies for CF include daily airway clearance maneuvers with chest physiotherapy by vibropercussion, hand-administered therapy or specially designed vests which assist with mucus clearance. Inhaled nebulized recombinant human DNase thins excessive DNA debris in sputum that accumulates due to the bacterial burden and the large influx of neutrophils into the airway lumen. This therapy improves pulmonary function, decreases the frequency of CF exacerbations, and improves quality of life [52]. Nebulized hypertonic saline has also been shown to be effective in some

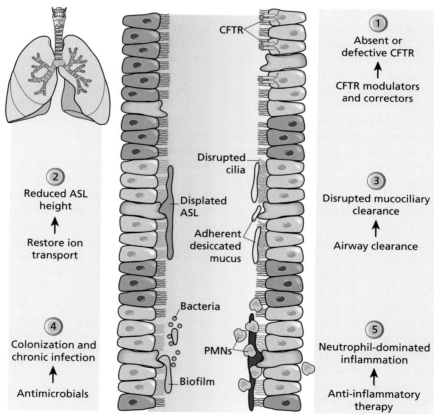

Figure 6.5 Pathogenesis of cystic fibrosis lung disease is characterized by absent or dysfunctional cystic fibrosis transmembrane conductance regulator (CFTR) at the epithelial surface (1), resulting in disordered ion transport and a depleted airway surface liquid layer (2). This contributes to delayed mucociliary clearance (3), setting the stage for colonization and chronic infection with bacterial pathogens (4) and a robust inflammatory response (5). Therapeutic approaches to each feature are indicated. ASL, airway surface liquid; PMN, polymorphonuclear cell. Reproduced from Rowe and Clancy [52] with permission from Lippincott Williams and Wilkins.

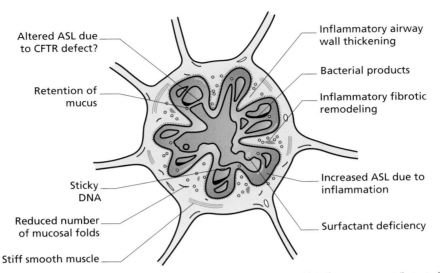

Figure 6.6 Factors that may contribute to small airways obstruction in early CF lung disease. Multiple factors can contribute to filling of the interstices between the folds. ASL, airway surface liquid; CFTR, cystic fibrosis transmembrane conductance regulator. Reproduced from Tiddens et al [53] with permission from Wiley-Blackwell.

trials. Early and aggressive antimicrobial therapy targeted at the patient's specific organisms and susceptibilities is believed to be responsible for a large component of the improvement in quality of life and reduction in exacerbations in patients with CF in recent years. Regular parenteral antibiotic therapy (i.e. every 3 months) is used in some centers, with agents including aminoglycosides, ceftazidime, and meropenem. Antibiotic resistance is a major problem, especially with resistant *Pseudomonas* species, and other resistant organisms such as *Burkholderia cepacia*. Inhaled nebulized tobramycin has been shown to be effective at preventing CF exacerbations. Anti-inflammatory therapy with low-dose corticosteroids or non-steroidal anti-inflammatory agents is also used in some patients [52]. CFTR-modulating drugs are under development and in some clinical trials; gene transfer therapy would be the ideal treatment but faces significant obstacles and clinical use is not imminent. Lung transplantation is reserved for patients with severe CF and a life expectancy of 2 years or less.

Cystic fibrosis patients present to the anesthesiologist for a variety of procedures, including vascular access procedures, lung biopsies, bronchoscopy, feeding gastrostomy, endoscopic sinus surgery, and lung transplantation. A very thorough review of history, medications, diagnostic testing, and physical examination is important.

Annotated references

A full reference list for this chapter is available at:
http://www.wiley.com/go/gregory/andropoulos/pediatricanesthesia

3. Burri PH. Structural aspects of postnatal lung development – alveolar formation and growth. Biol Neonate 2006; 89: 313–22. This review

article discusses the stages of fetal and postnatal lung development with emphasis on newer concepts of alveolarization, including microvascular maturation and late alveolarization.

5. Galambos C, Demello DE. Regulation of alveologenesis: clinical implications of impaired growth. Pathology 2008; 40: 124–40. This article provides a comprehensive view of the process of alveolarization with particular attention to the regulation of alveolarization by growth factors, transcription factors, cell–cell communication, and cell–matrix interactions.

10. Hislop A. Developmental biology of the pulmonary circulation. Paediatr Respir Rev 2005; 6: 35–43. This review article presents the major events and concepts in the development of the pulmonary vasculature in the context of the stages of fetal lung development.

14. Jeffrey PK. The development of large and small airways. Am J Respir Crit Care Med 1998; 157: S174–80. This review article discusses in detail the development of airways in the fetus and the differentiation of airway epithelial cells.

17. Mallampalli RK, Acarregui MJ, Snyder JM. Differentiation of the alveolar epithelium in the fetal lung. In: McDonald JA (ed) Lung Growth and Development. New York: Marcel Dekker, 1997, pp. 119–62. This chapter is a review of alveolar epithelial differentiation. In addition to a discussion of markers that readily distinguish alveolar type 1 from type 2 cells, there is a discussion of surfactant composition and function.

20. Zuo YY, Veldehuizen RA, Neuman AW et al. Current perspectives in pulmonary surfactant – inhibition, enhancement and evaluation. Biochim Biophys Acta 2008; 1778: 1947–77. This review article provides a historical perspective on surfactant and its biophysical properties.

25. Jain L, Eaton DC. Physiology of fetal lung fluid clearance and the effect of labor. Semin Perinatol 2006; 30: 34–43. This review article discusses the physiological mechanisms underlying fetal lung fluid absorption, illustrates how delivery management influences fetal lung fluid reabsorption, and explores potential strategies for facilitating neonatal transition to air breathing.

27. Aschner JL, Fike CD. New developments in the pathogenesis and management of neonatal pulmonary hypertension. In: Bancalari E (ed) The Newborn Lung. New York: Saunders Elsevier, 2008, pp.

241–99. This is a comprehensive, well-referenced review of circulatory adaptations that occur in the process of neonatal transition and how they are related to the development of pulmonary hypertension. In addition, there is a discussion of therapeutic strategies for the management of primary pulmonary hypertension of the newborn.

29. Noori S, Seri I. The Very low birth weight neonate with a hemodynamically significant ductus arteriosus during the first postnatal week. In: Kleinman CK, Seri I (ed) Hemodynamics and Cardiology. New York: Saunders Elsevier, 2008, pp. 178–94. This chapter discusses the physiology and pathophysiology of the ductus arteriosus during neonatal transition with particular focus on maladaptation of the ductus arteriosus in the premature infant.

32. Schramn C, Grunstein M. Pulmonary function tests in infants, In: Chernick V, Boat T, Wilmott R, Bush A (eds) Kendig's Disorders of the Respiratory Tract in Children. New York: Elsevier Saunders, 2006, pp. 129–67. This chapter presents a thorough discussion of pulmonary function testing in infants and young children, and includes reference data on pulmonary mechanics and lung function tests.

CHAPTER 7

Developmental Physiology of the Central Nervous System

Ken M. Brady[1], R. Blaine Easley[1] & Bruno Bissonnette[2]

[1]Department of Anesthesiology and Pediatrics, Baylor College of Medicine, and Texas Children's Hospital, Houston, TX, USA
[2]Department of Anesthesia, University of Toronto, and the Children of the World Anesthesia Foundation, Toronto, Ontario, Canada

Introduction

The child is not merely a small adult. At birth, central nervous system (CNS) development is incomplete and will not be mature until the end of the second year of life. Because of this delay in maturation, several specific pathophysiological and psychological differences ensue. Neurodevelopment follows a complex interplay between timed genetic events and activity-dependent structural modifications. The vigorous cellular plasticity of the brain is in contrast to its unforgiving metabolic vulnerability when exposed to conditions of substrate deprivation. Care of the critically ill child susceptible to neurological injury is best carried out with a comprehensive understanding of the physics of the intracranial compartment, vascular physiology of the brain and developmental peculiarities of the nervous system.

Embryology of the developing brain and spinal cord, changes from fetus to neonate to child

Embryogenesis of the brain

The CNS development begins from a relatively simple single layer of cells and progresses to a very complex, multilayered central structure that eventually connects with every part of the body. The processes of CNS embryogenesis follow three steps: (1) neurulation, (2) canalization, and (3) retrogressive differentiation (Table 7.1).

Within 2 weeks of conception, a groove is formed in a plate of embryonic ectoderm, which contains the cells that will become brain and spinal cord. By 1 month, *neurulation* is complete and the lateral edges of this groove are fused to form the neural tube (Fig. 7.1). At this time, neural crest cells are excluded from the tube closure and subsequently

Table 7.1 Central nervous system embryogenesis

Phase	Gestational age (days)	Outcome
Neurulation	16–28	Brain, spinal cord through L2–L4
Canalization	30–52	Sacrococcygeal segments of the spinal cord
Retrogressive differentiation	46–birth	Filum terminale

migrate and differentiate to populate diverse neuronal structures such as the sympathetic chain ganglia, the enteric neuronal plexi, the dorsal root ganglia and adrenal medulla, in addition to becoming melanocytes in the skin.

Rostrally, the neural tube undergoes differential growth, expansion and folding, to form the three primary brain vesicles: the prosencephalon, mesencephalon and rhombencephalon. Caudally, the neural tube and surrounding mesoderm retain segmental characteristics and form the portion of spinal cord from the medulla to the midlumbar segments. Secondary brain vesicles are

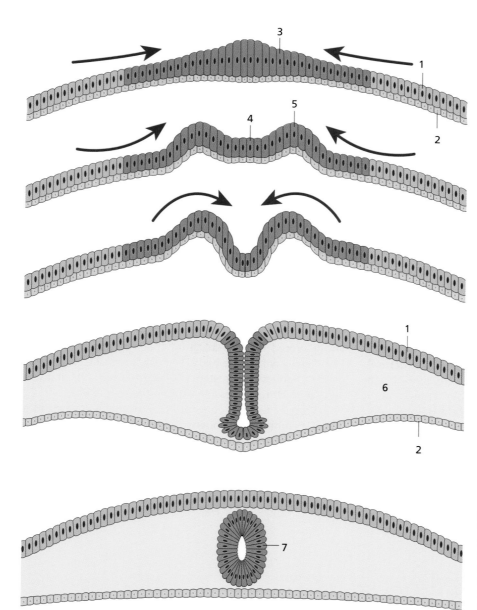

Figure 7.1 Neurulation (see text for details). The arrows indicate the direction of cell movement. (1) Embryonic ectoderm. (2) Embryonic endoderm. (3) Neural ectoderm. (4) Neural plate with neural groove. (5) Neural fold. (6) Mesoderm. (7) Neural tube. Modified from Karfunkel [156] with permission from Elsevier.

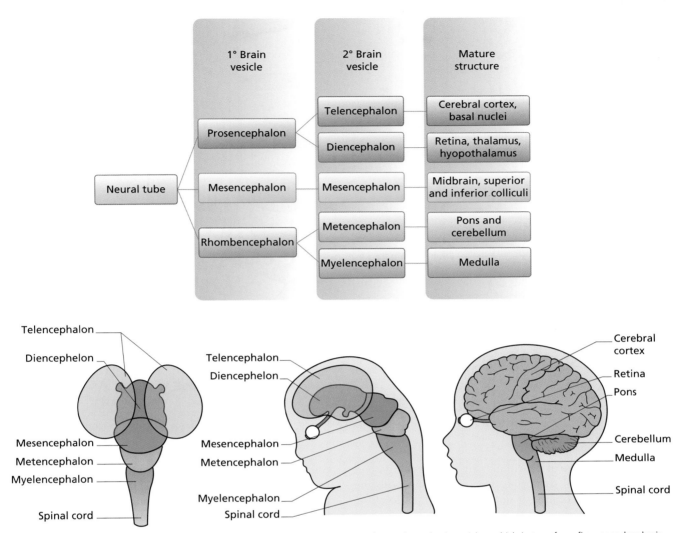

Figure 7.2 Brain development from the neural tube. The neural tube gives rise to three primary brain vesicles, which in turn form five secondary brain vesicles before completing development into the mature brain.

formed as the primary vesicles subdivide. The prosencephalon divides into the telencephalon (cerebral cortex and basal nuclei) and the diencephalon (thalamus, hypothalamus and retinae). The mesencephalon (midbrain) does not subdivide. The rhombencephalon divides into the metencephalon (pons and cerebellum) and the myelencephalon (medulla) (Fig. 7.2).

Embryogenesis of the spinal cord

The spinal cord from the medulla to the midlumbar segments is derived from the caudal portion of the neural tube. The posterior neuropore closes within a month of gestation, and subsequently elongates to form the distal spinal cord and conus medullaris. *Canalization* is the fusion of the notochord and neural epithelium into a caudal cell mass to form sacral and coccygeal segments

between 1 and 2 months of gestation. Microcysts develop and coalesce within this mass. *Retrogressive differentiation* is the necrosis of excess cells formed by canalization in the caudal neural tube, leaving the filum terminale and cauda equina, a process that continues into the early postnatal period. Vertebral column growth exceeds spinal column growth, resulting in ascension of the conus medullaris from the L3 vertebral segment at birth to the L1 vertebral segment at adulthood (Fig. 7.3).

Neural tube defects

A neural tube defect is any defect that may occur during the development of the CNS. Defects occurring during neurulation can be classified into (1) those involving the brain and spinal cord, (2) those involving the brain only and (3) those involving the spinal cord only. For example,

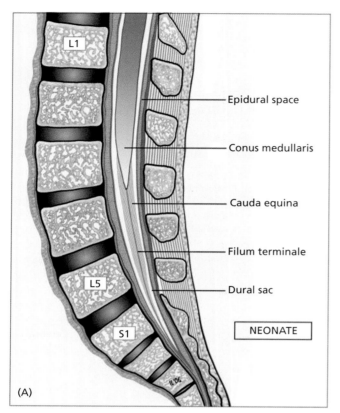

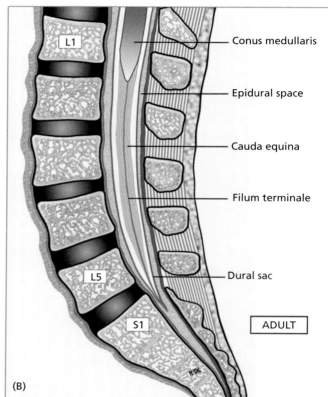

Figure 7.3 Asymmetric growth of the spine and its vertebral canal causes a change in the position of the conus medullaris with respect to the vertebral column with growth from neonate (A) to adult (B).

when there is failure of neurulation in early development, a condition of total dysraphism occurs within both the brain and spinal column. If only the brain fails to close, the condition is termed anencephaly.

Later in development, many malformations of the brain can occur which have clinical relevance for the pediatric anesthesiologist, including congenital hydrocephaly. Abnormal neuronal migration results in cortical malformations that may be appreciated on gross surface anatomy [1].

Schizencephaly (clefts in the cerebral wall), pachygyria (sparse, broad gyri), and polymicrogyria are examples of anomalies strongly associated with migrational abnormalities. Lissencephaly (smooth brain) is a severe anomaly that may be produced by either migrational anomalies or earlier disruptions in neurogenesis. Partial or complete agenesis of the corpus callosum may be associated with any of the above anomalies but it is believed to be a migrational abnormality in and of itself. Failure of canalization results in a myelocele if the lesion is flat or myelomeningocele if there is an additional dorsal outpouching of the meninges/neural tissue.

Proliferation and migration

The second month of brain development, following closure of the neural tube, is marked by an exponential cellular proliferation, and this continues into the second trimester. The second trimester is, therefore, a time when the central nervous system is prone to global insult from teratogen exposure. Radial migration is a robust element of cortical development and has been well characterized. Cells destined to populate the neocortex, as both glial and neuronal varieties, originate from the rapidly dividing periventricular cell layer and migrate along a glial network. They populate the six-layered cortex by migrating past the last formed layer, such that the youngest cells are found at the outermost layers. At term, cellular proliferation in the cortex is largely completed. However, when an infant is born prematurely, especially at the limits of viability near the beginning of the third trimester, residual germinal matrix is present in the caudothalamic groove adjacent to the lateral ventricles. This ongoing germinal activity is accompanied by a transient network of fragile vascular overgrowth, and is a site of hemorrhage in the premature neonate [2,3].

Synaptogenesis and myelination

The third trimester of neuronal development starts a period of neuronal growth, synaptic proliferation, axonal growth, and myelination. The myriad interneuronal connections forming an incomprehensible network of logical units in the human brain are the result of interplay between genetically determined anatomic directives and environmentally determined plasticity. The basic strategy of the network formation is to excessively populate and interconnect neuronal networks and then thin cell populations by apoptotic mechanisms, prune inactive synapse formations, and reinforce functional, active connections. The viability of neurons and synaptic connections is determined by their activity patterns. The resultant functionality of the network is, therefore, dependent on sensory and environmental input, and some of these inputs are known to be time sensitive.

Amblyopia is the most striking example of synaptogenesis gone awry for lack of appropriate sensory input during a critical stage of development. Spatially organized and synchronized neuronal activity along the visual pathway is required for normal development of the occipital cortex. Activity-dependent synapse reinforcement of the occipital cortex begins in darkness, *in utero*, as waves of electrical activity spontaneously pass across the retina, reinforcing spatially co-ordinated synaptic connections throughout the visual pathway [4]. After birth, further synaptic reinforcement is dependent on light-mediated excitation in the retinae. If the retinae receive inadequate or disconjugate light stimulus through the critical development period up to 2 years of age, the corresponding cortical network is irreversibly pruned and the result is permanent blindness of the affected eye [5–7].

Critical periods for other neurodevelopmental processes are less well defined, but the perinatal surge in synapse formation is known to continue through early childhood to the preteen years. The existence of a critical period distinguishes developmental, primary synaptogenesis from other forms of neural plasticity, which continue throughout life. The relative permanence of synaptogenic modulation during infancy and childhood is even postulated to create a critical period for development of intellect, behavior, and affect. Environments rich in stimulation, interaction and socialization promote increased synapse retention, whereas neglectful, stimulus-poor developmental environments yield synapse-depleted cortical networks, and may lead to permanent cognitive deficits [8–11]. The dendritic arborization of cortical pyramidal neurons has been shown to be environment dependent even in the mature mammalian brain (Fig. 7.4). Furthermore, the introduction of a consistently noxious environment during critical developmental stages may yield undesirable affective changes.

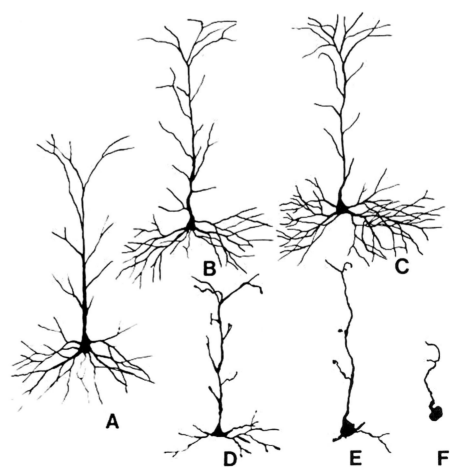

Figure 7.4 Age-related patterns of dendritic arborization of cortical pyramidal neurons. Mature pyramidal neurons (A) can undergo a stimulus-dependent process of stabilization and even increase in synaptic interconnection and dendritic branching (B,C). Alternatively, without stimulus input, the mature neuron can undergo synaptic pruning and regressive loss of dendritic arborization (D–F). Reproduced from Diamond [155] with permission from Academia Brasileira de Ciencias.

Myelination

Myelination and axonal maturation also start in the third trimester, with a peak density of immature oligodendrocytes in the cortical white matter between 23 and 32 weeks' gestation, a time of white matter vulnerability in the premature infant [12]. Myelination continues through childhood and into the teen years, mirroring brain growth. The brain is 450 grams at birth, 1000 grams at 1 year, and 1400 grams at 18 years, growth that is accounted for by myelination and increases in cell size and organization, not cellular proliferation. Developmental milestones are also observed to follow patterns of myelination. For instance, myelination of the corticospinal tract begins at 36 weeks' gestation and is completed at around 2 years of life. Myelination of this tract progresses from short to long fibers, giving an anatomic explanation for the head-to-toe disappearance of hyper-reflexia and increased tone seen in normal development. Axonal maturation of the speech-dominant frontotemporal pathway continues through late childhood and adolescence, along with the development of increasingly sophisticated language competency [13]. As with synaptogenic processes, myelination patterns are activity dependent [14].

Immature patterns of myelination are seen on magnetic resonance imaging (MRI) of term infants with congenital heart disease. An estimated 25% of infants with congenital heart disease have lesions on MRI before undergoing bypass, and brain immaturity is a risk factor for new MRI lesions after cardiopulmonary bypass. Many of these lesions are diffuse white matter injury, similar in nature to periventricular leukomalacia seen in preterm infants [15].

Development of pain pathways and responses

The relatively new specialty of pediatric anesthesia has arguably made its greatest contribution in the understanding of nociception and the effects of "pain" on the developing infant and child. The nociceptive systems develop during the second and third trimesters of gestation with further maturational changes occurring during the first 2 years of life. Historically, pediatric pain was undertreated during the neonatal period and infancy due to a belief that the pain system was underdeveloped during these times [16]. However, although a "verbal" response to pain may not be present, the "physiological" responses were recognized and prompted a careful exploration into the physiological basis of nociception.

Nociception begins with the sensation of the stimulus at the level of the peripheral nervous system [17]. Unlike the adult-specific sensations of touch, pressure, heat or cold, there are no specific pain sensors in the developing fetus. Rather, the "pain" stimulus is sensed by free non-specific nerve endings. Rapidly adapting pressure receptors are the first to appear during fetal life, followed by the development of slowly adapting pressure receptors, and then rapidly adapting mechanoceptors. The depolarization responses of these receptors to mechanical injury, chemical irritants, and inflammatory mediators are similar to those of adult receptors [18]. Cutaneous sensory receptors appear in the perioral area at 7 weeks' postconceptual age (PCA), spread to the hands and feet by 11 weeks' PCA, and are present at all cutaneous and mucous surfaces by 20 weeks PCA [19,20]. The development of these sensory reflexes is preceded by synaptogenesis between afferent fibers and sensory neurons in the dorsal horn of the spinal cord.

The sensation of pain is mediated via free nerve endings of A- and C-fibers. These fibers do not demonstrate fatigue, but rather repeated or continuous stimulation *increases* the ease of transmission of the impulse. Histological studies show that the density of nociceptive nerve endings in the newborn skin is similar to that of adult skin [21]. More importantly, the neurophysiological properties of the earliest nociceptors are also similar to those of adults. Myelinated fibers are the first to grow into the developing spinal cord and form connections with deeper layers of the dorsal horn, with collaterals to neurons in the substantia gelatinosa. With the ingrowth of C-fibers (unmyelinated fibers) and synaptogenesis with superficial dorsal horn neurons, these collaterals undergo developmental degeneration. Nociceptive stimuli in fetal life (and in the extremely premature neonate) are transmitted by myelinated A-fibers until the maturation of C-fiber connections [22].

The first-order neuron, whose cell body lies in the paravertebral ganglion, carries the nociceptive input into the dorsal horn of the spinal cord. The first-order neuron synapses with a second-order neuron in the dorsal horn of the spinal cord. The second-order neuron then crosses the midline and ascends in various pathways, including the spinothalamic tract, synapsing in the thalamus with a third-order neuron which projects to the sensory cortex [23]. In the dorsal horn of the spinal cord, nociceptive input is modified (amplified and inhibited) by descending fibers from the central nervous system and interneurons within the dorsal horn. This modulation is mediated via various chemical compounds (substance P, adrenergic agents, serotonin, and endogenous opioids), which bind to the first- or second-order neuron via specific receptor systems (Fig. 7.5).

In the first trimester of pregnancy, development of the spinal cord and central nervous system begins with the closure of the neural canal. At this time, the dorsal horn begins to appear. Electron microscopic and immunochemical studies demonstrate that the development of the various neuronal cell types in the dorsal horn, with their laminar arrangement, interneuronal connections, and

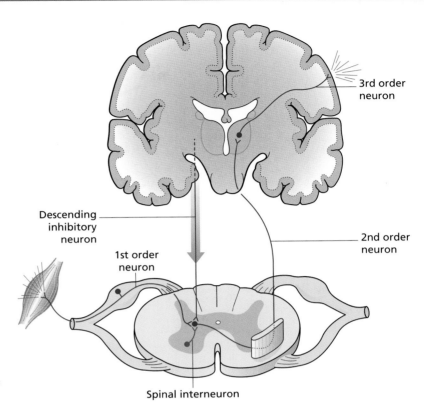

Figure 7.5 Pain transmission is modulated by descending inhibitory pathways and spinal interneurons at the level of the spinal cord.

expression of specific neurotransmitters and receptors, begins before 13 weeks of gestation and is completed by 30–32 weeks PCA. Initially, the receptive fields of dorsal horn neurons are very large with an extensive overlap between the receptive fields of adjacent neurons. As maturation occurs, the receptive fields of individual dorsal horn cells progressively decrease and can be more precisely defined [24]. On a cellular level, the transmission of nociceptive impulses through the dorsal horn of the spinal cord is mediated and modulated via the release of excitatory neurotransmitters (Fig. 7.6), such as substance P, glutamate, calcitonin gene-related peptide (CGRP), vasoactive intestinal polypeptide (VIP), neuropeptide Y, and somatostatin. Modulation of this nociceptive transmission occurs by the release of metenkephalin from local interneurons and norepinephrine, dopamine, and serotonin from descending inhibitory axons.

These descending inhibitory axons originate in supraspinal centers and terminate at all levels of the spinal cord and brainstem. During the first and second trimesters and up until the latter half of the third trimester, there is an imbalance between the mechanisms that favor the facilitation rather than the inhibition of nociceptive input. Of the nociceptive neurotransmitters, substance P, CGRP, and somatostatin are expressed in the dorsal horn by 8–10 weeks' PCA. Glutamate, VIP, and neuropeptide Y appear at 12–16 weeks' PCA. Modulation of incoming noxious

stimuli in extremely premature infants may occur through the local release of metenkephalin, which is first expressed at 12–16 weeks' PCA. However, this mechanism is unlikely to be effective in diminishing the transmission of intensive painful stimuli. In the latter half of the third trimester, with the maturation of the descending inhibitory pathways from supraspinal centers, inhibition of incoming sensory stimuli can occur with the release of dopamine and norepinephrine in the dorsal horn of the spinal cord. These neurotransmitters are first expressed at 34–38 weeks of human gestation followed by serotonin, which develops during the postneonatal period [25,26].

Conduction of nociceptive impulses to the supraspinal centers occurs via the spinothalamic, spinoreticular, and spinomesencephalic tracts located primarily in the anterolateral and lateral white matter tracts of the spinal cord. Lack of or decreased myelination in these tracts was previously proposed as an index of immaturity of the neonatal CNS and was used to support the argument that neonates cannot feel pain or do not react to it in the same manner as adults. This argument was widely supported despite the common knowledge that incomplete myelination does not imply lack of function, but merely imposes a slower conduction velocity in the central nerve tracts of neonates. Additionally, any slowing in the central conduction velocity would be completely offset by the shorter interneuronal distances that must be traveled by the

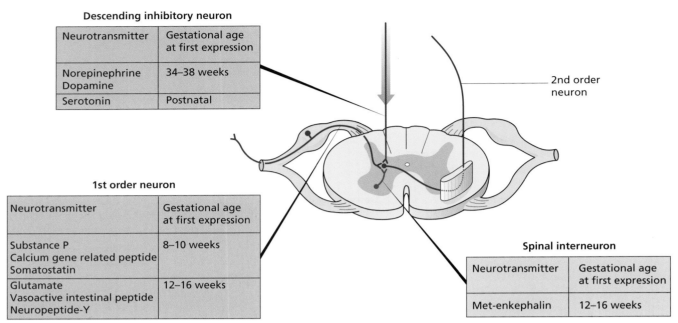

Figure 7.6 Neurotransmitters found in the spinal cord modulating activity of the pain pathway are shown with the gestational age at which they are first expressed.

impulse when comparing an infant to the much larger (and longer) adult [27]. The nociceptive tracts to the brainstem and thalamus are completely myelinated by 30 weeks of human gestation and the thalamocortical pain fibers are fully myelinated by 37 weeks. The timing of the thalamocortical connection is of crucial importance for cortical perception since the majority of sensory pathways to the neocortex have synapses in the thalamus. In the primate fetus, thalamic neurons produce axons that arrive in the cerebrum before midgestation. These fibers remain just below the neocortex until migration and dendritic arborization of cortical neurons are complete and finally establish synaptic connections at 20–24 weeks' PCA [27].

The functional maturity of the cerebral cortex is suggested by the presence of fetal and neonatal electroencephalographic (EEG) patterns and by the behavioral development of neonates. Intermittent EEG bursts in both cerebral hemispheres, first seen at 20 weeks' PCA, become sustained at 22 weeks and are bilaterally synchronous at 26–27 weeks' PCA. By 30 weeks, the distinction between wakefulness and sleep can be made on the basis of EEG patterns [28,29]. Cortical components of somatosensory, auditory, and visually evoked potentials have been recorded in preterm babies before 26 weeks' PCA [30]. Several forms of behavior imply cortical function during fetal life. Well-defined periods of quiet sleep, active sleep, and wakefulness occur even *in utero*, beginning at 28 weeks' PCA. In addition to specific behavioral responses to pain, neonates have various cognitive, co-ordinative,

and associative capabilities in response to visual and auditory stimuli, attesting to the presence of cortical function and intact processing of nociceptive input. Several lines of evidence suggest that the complete nervous system is active during prenatal development and that detrimental or developmental changes in any part can affect the entire system [23].

Development of the response to pain stimulation

The human fetus is capable of spontaneous movements and complex responses early in gestation. Reflex movement in response to direct stimulation begins at 7.5 weeks' PCA, initially localized to the head and neck region [31]. Sensitivity develops in a craniocaudal direction with the lower limbs responding by 14 weeks' PCA. Data from the immature rat and other animals show that responses to stimulation are initially inconsistent, non-specific, and poorly localized [32]. However, if a response is achieved, it can be extremely exaggerated and long-lasting [33]. These observations tie in well with neurophysiological data in animals and clinical work with preterm human infants.

Single cell studies from the dorsal root ganglion of the rat show that cutaneous receptive fields are present in the hindlimb as soon as innervation to the skin has taken place [34]. The firing rates and durations are lower than those in the adult but even at this stage, different classes of afferent responses to noxious stimuli can be demonstrated. Initially stimulation of cutaneous afferents fails to produce suprathreshold excitation in dorsal horn cells but by birth, depolarization can be produced from light touch alone [32]. However, while the synaptic linkage remains weak at birth, suprathreshold stimulation provokes a long-lasting hyperexcitable state in the dorsal horn cells [34].

Polymodal nociceptors which pass to the dorsal horn via C-fibers show fully mature responses to pinch, heat, and chemical stimulation by birth [35]. However, despite their observed anatomic connections, these C-fiber afferents fail to evoke activity in the dorsal horn cells until a week after birth. Thus, while the C-fiber connections remain immature at birth and fail to directly transmit their nociceptive input, they may greatly increase the response to other noxious (A-fibers) and non-noxious inputs. Together with the large receptive fields observed in dorsal root ganglion cells, this may increase the likelihood of a central response from the relatively immature nervous system. The lack of functional descending inhibitory pathways from higher centers also contributes to the potentially excitable and poorly damped responses to afferent inputs.

Central integration of afferent inputs

In the human, complex central integration of afferent sensory and nociceptive input is present at 30 weeks' gestation. Visual and auditory evoked potentials are present and complex EEG reactions to external influences are seen at this time [28,29]. Klimach and Cooke demonstrated the presence of somatosensory evoked potentials (SSEPs) in the preterm neonate [30]. In fact, SSEPs have been measured in infants as young as 28 weeks' gestation. These investigators also demonstrated that the velocity of both peripheral nerve conduction and central conduction increased with gestational age. However, there was considerable variability in peripheral velocity and central processing in the younger infants, suggesting that there are large individual differences in maturation rates. SSEPs continue to mature during infancy [36]. Subarachnoid injections of lidocaine in the ex-premature infant cause rapid loss of SSEPs corresponding to the onset of motor and sensory blockade. The offset of the block can be monitored with the return of SSEPs and shortening of the latency back to the baseline [37]. Positron emission tomography scans in the infant have shown that glucose utilization is maximal in the sensory areas of the cerebral cortex, implying a high level of activity [38].

There is also recent evidence to suggest that cortical activation occurs after painful stimuli in preterm neonates [39]. Bartocci et al, using near infrared spectroscopy in preterm infants 28–36 weeks' PCA, have demonstrated increased blood flow in the somatosensory cortex, but not the occipital cortex, after venepuncture [40]. In a similar study, Slater and colleagues recorded cortical activation after heelpricks in 18 infants between 25 and 45 weeks' PCA [41]. No cortical response was noted after tactile stimulation even when this stimulation was accompanied by reflex limb withdrawal. Taken together, these studies provide additional evidence that the conscious sensory perception of painful stimuli is present even in preterm newborns. Table 7.2 summarizes the behavioral and physiological nociceptive responses of the neonate.

Interneuronal connections

The impression that emerges from these and related human studies is that even the very preterm infant has complex interneuronal connections capable of integrated responses to tactile or nociceptive input. These infants also show inconsistent responses to external stimuli, which may reflect the late functional connections of sensory afferents (particularly C-fibers) within the spinal cord. However, the combination of larger receptive fields, recruitment of non-nociceptive afferents, and reduced inhibitory controls results in "underdampened" responses (long-lasting, exaggerated and poorly localized) once afferent stimuli have achieved central activation above a threshold level. Inconsistency of response to more complex noxious stimuli may also reflect the profound effects that conscious state and other external responses have on behavior [42,43].

Molecular basis of pain perception

Studies of developmental cytochemistry in the animal models have focused on substance P, opioid peptides and receptors, N-methyl-D-aspartate (NMDA) receptors, and the expression of the *C-fos* gene. While transmitters can be demonstrated to be present early in gestation, their concentrations are usually very low and they may not always be found at sites that suggest a functional role [44]. By contrast, receptors are often seen in higher

Table 7.2 Main physiological responses to pain

Assessment	Effect of pain stimulation
Middle cerebral artery pulsatility index	Decrease
Intracranial pressure	Increase
Systemic blood pressure	Increase
Heart rate	Increase (inconstant in neonates)
Transcutaneous oxygen tension	Decrease
Vagal tone (amplitude of sinus arrhythmia)	Decrease
Palmar sweating	Increase
Near infrared spectroscopy	Decrease

densities and have a more widespread distribution than in adult life, which may facilitate responses at a time when only low levels of transmitter are available [17]. The transient appearance of receptor populations that have ceased to be expressed by birth remains puzzling and demonstrates that a large gap still exists between the *in vitro* cytochemical findings and our understanding of *in vivo* nociception [45]. Opioid receptors change both in numbers and in receptor type during development. Zhang and Pasternak demonstrated that in newborn rats, high-affinity binding sites for a tritiated enkephalin ligand increased up to threefold in the first 2 weeks of life while during this period, a large rise in analgesic response to morphine occurred [46]. In contrast, the effects of morphine on ventilatory drive during this period (2–14 days after birth) were constant. Other studies have confirmed the increase in the number of opioid receptors and changes in their binding affinities during *in utero* and postnatal development [47].

The ability to evaluate and analyze gene and protein expression on a cellular and tissue level has led to a more systems-based approach to the adaptation to nociceptive triggers, resulting in new insights into the physiological responses to painful stimulus. The implication of such varied responses in rodent models allows us to assess the earliest alterations in gene expression within peripheral nerves, the spinal cord, and brain in both acute and chronic pain response models [48]. The results of proteomic and microarray techniques have demonstrated previously unrecognized alterations in actual transcribed and activated proteins from within a specific cell line and/or tissues [25,49]. One important example of these techniques is the identification of genetic variations and altered expression within the opioid receptor. Following the studies of Pasternak et al, these techniques have identified gene-splice variants as well as single nucleotide polymorphisms within animal and human populations that can better explain the clinical variability in analgesia seen between drugs based on altered opioid-binding kinetics and molecular responses [46,50]. Future directions in molecular pain research will develop molecular signatures of neuronal and receptor responses that correlate with our phenotypical definitions of acute and chronic nociception as well as leading to more personalized pain treatments based on these molecular characterizations (pharmacogenomics) [51].

The intracranial compartment

The mature brain is both protected and threatened by its bony encasement. The brain cannot tolerate acute mass effect because of the lack of elasticity of the skull and dura. The risks of herniation and stroke from elevated intracranial pressure (ICP) have been described for nearly two centuries as the Monro–Kellie doctrine [52,53]. Elastance in the skull is not linear, as in the normal brain there is a reserve mechanism of cerebrospinal fluid movement from the brain into the spinal canal. When this reserve compliance is exhausted, further increases in intracranial volume cause blood volume to be pushed out of the skull, and finally, terminal increases in intracranial volume cause herniation of brain matter.

Historically, intracranial elastance was estimated by injections of small volumes of artificial cerebrospinal fluid into patients while intracranial pressure was monitored. Now, most practitioners are content with simple intracranial pressure monitoring when indicated. Recently, an analysis of the pulse amplitude behavior of the intracranial pressure waveform has been developed to delineate three clinical states of intracranial elastance. The correlation coefficient (R) between the pulse frequency amplitude (A) and the mean pressure value (P) of the intracranial pressure wave across periods of slow change in mean intracranial pressure gives an index termed the RAP [54,55]. In the normal state, RAP is near zero because the pulse amplitude of intracranial pressure is low and unchanging within a compliant skull. As compliance reserve is exhausted and the elastic properties of the skull and dura begin to dominate, the pulse frequency amplitude of the intracranial pressure becomes passive to slow changes in mean intracranial pressure and RAP trends toward 1. Finally, when intracranial pressure is terminal and herniation is imminent, further increases in intracranial pressure push blood out of the skull and diminish the pulse amplitude of the intracranial pressure, so the RAP becomes negative (Fig. 7.7). Patients with critical ICP have improved elastance as estimated by the RAP when they undergo decompressive craniectomy [56].

Eight major bones separated by eight suture lines and six fontanelles form the intracranial compartment. Delayed ossification of these bones permits deforming *compression* of the skull by the birth canal during parturition. The corollary concept that fontanelles allow *expansion* of the cranial vault in the setting of acute mass effect is erroneous. Slow growth and expansion of the sutures and fontanelles can occur in the setting of subacute mass effect, but the fibrous interosseous connections are not compliant, nor do they accommodate mass added acutely to the intracranial compartment. Although it serves no protective role in the setting of acute intracranial mass effect, physical examination of the anterior fontanelle is an important monitor of intracranial pressure. Tonometry has been applied to the anterior fontanelle to measure ICP non-invasively when ICP monitoring is desirable but not invasively accessible [57]. By 2 years of age, the fontanelles are closed and suture lines are replaced with bone, but the fibrous sutures permit ongoing bone growth.

Figure 7.7 Intracranial pressure waves are schematized as a product of fixed cardiac stroke volume pulsations, occuring at different positions on the intracranial pressure–volume curve. Intracranial compliance reserve can be delineated with RAP: correlation (R) between intracranial pressure pulsation amplitude (A) and mean intracranial pressure (P). Three states of intracranial compliance reserve have been defined with this method. (1) RAP = 0, intracranial pressure pulse amplitude does not change with increases in mean intracranial pressure, volume changes are easily absorbed by intracranial compliance reserve. (2) RAP = 1, intracranial pressure pulse amplitude is correlated to changes in mean intracranial pressure. Patients on the ascending portion of the intracranial pressure–volume curve have diminished compliance reserve. (3) RAP < 0, intracranial pressure pulsations are inversely correlated to changes in mean intracranial pressure. When the RAP is negative, intracranial compliance reserve is exhausted and herniation is imminent.

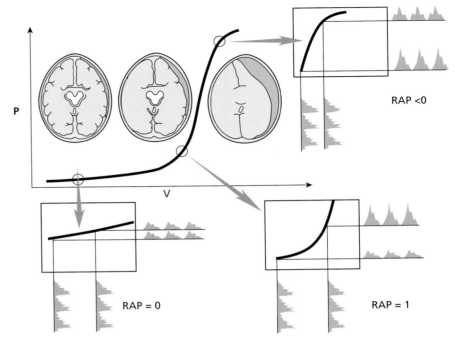

The intracranial compartment is subdivided by the tentorium, a dural separation between the brainstem and cerebellum posteriorly and cortex and diencephalic structures anteriorly. Because many children have posterior compartment neoplasms, and ICP is monitored in the anterior compartment, it is important to know that the pressures in the two compartments can be distinct. Posterior compartment mass effect causes deformation of the brainstem, with signs of coma, bradycardia, and hypertension that can exist without bulging fontanelles or elevated anterior compartment pressures.

Cerebrospinal fluid

Derangements of cerebral spinal fluid production, flow and reabsorption account for significant morbidity in the pediatric population. Normal cerebrospinal fluid physiology is well described in adults who have an average 150 mL of cerebrospinal fluid (CSF), 30–40 mL contained in the ventricles, and produce 20 mL/h CSF at the choroid plexus. This causes a replacement of the entire volume of CSF 3–4 times a day. The flow of CSF through the extracellular spaces of the brain and reabsorption through the arachnoid granulations are driven by a constant small pressure gradient between the spinal fluid space and the sagittal sinus. Age-dependent rates of cerebrospinal fluid production have been described in children with external ventricular drains. Given the pathologies associated with the clinical need for drain placement, it is not surprising that a wide range of cerebrospinal fluid production was documented. Nevertheless, spinal fluid

production was seen to increase logarithmically during the first year of life and reaches 60% of adult production levels at 2 years of age [58].

Vascular anatomy of the central nervous system

Brain vascular anatomy

A healthy 3 kg infant with a normal, 500 g brain has a cardiac output of 250 mL/kg/min, and a cerebral blood flow of 25 mL/100 g/min (= 42 mL/kg/min). The infant brain therefore consumes 17% of cardiac output, but also accounts for 17% of the body mass. For comparison, a healthy, 50 kg teenager with a 1400 g brain and a cardiac output of 100 mL/kg/min would have a normal cerebral blood flow of 22 mL/kg/min. The mature brain therefore comprises just over 2% of total body mass, but utilizes 25% of the cardiac output.

Blood flow is supplied to the brain by an extensive network of arteries originating from paired internal carotid and vertebrobasilar arteries. These arteries branch into the anterior cerebral arteries and the posterior cerebral arteries, respectively, which anastomose with each other on the ventral surface of the brainstem to create the anterior and posterior segments of the circulus arteriosus cerebri (circle of Willis), which is completed by the anterior and posterior communicating arteries. The circle of Willis provides collateral blood flow to the brain parenchyma; therefore, damage to any one vessel typically does not result in clinically significant ischemia. However, incomplete formation, damage or obstruction of any one of the major cerebral vessels may result in a cerebrovascular accident (CVA). The vessels comprising the circle of Willis are prone to the formation of berry aneurysms, which are congenital birth defects related to defective arterial wall formation. Although these berry aneurysms are present at birth, they rarely rupture until early to middle adulthood.

Another congenital vascular abnormality of significance is arteriovenous malformation (AVM), which is the most frequently occurring cerebrovascular malformation. AVM results in the shunting of blood from the arterial to the venous side secondary to anomalous dilated capillaries. Fifty percent of patients will present with seizures or neurological deficits as a result of compression or a steal phenomenon, while the other 50% will present with hemorrhage. The vast majority of AVMs occur in the supratentorial compartment (typically in a lobar region), while only 10% occur in the infratentorial region.

The cerebral veins run in the pial layer while the large collecting veins run in the subarachnoid layer. They eventually traverse the subdural space and open into the cranial venous sinuses. The venous drainage system of the brain is primarily made up of the venous sinuses located between the dura mater and the cranial periosteum. The walls of the venous sinuses lack both valves and muscle. Although the brain is insensitive to pain, the cerebral dura mater demonstrates nociceptive responsiveness, particularly around the venous sinuses.

There are other sinuses within the venous drainage system that may be of importance to the anesthesiologist, including the superior sagittal sinus which, because of its relatively superficial midline location, is particularly vulnerable to damage during surgical correction of craniosynostosis or during a morcellation craniectomy. The superior sagittal sinus ends by becoming continuous with the right transverse sinus 60% of the time, while in the remaining 40% it becomes continuous with the left. The transverse sinus courses laterally to the sigmoid sinus superior to the tentorium cerebelli. The S-shaped sigmoid sinus (hence its name) is located within the posterior cranial fossa and eventually enters the venous enlargements known as the internal jugular venous bulbs. Most of the venous drainage system empties into the sigmoid sinuses and subsequently into the internal jugular vein, excluding the inferior petrosal sinuses, which enter the internal jugular veins directly. The sigmoid sinus is separated anteriorly from the mastoid antrum and mastoid air cells by only a thin plate of bone. The occipital sinus, which lies along the foramen magnum, ends in the confluence of sinuses. The cavernous sinus, which surrounds the sella turcica, joins the superior petrosal sinuses draining into the transverse sinus.

Spinal cord vascular anatomy

The arterial supply of the spinal cord primarily arises from a single anterior spinal artery and two posterior spinal arteries, both originating from the vertebral artery. Supplemental blood flow is also received from radicular arteries originating from spinal branches of the ascending cervical, deep cervical, intercostal, lumbar and sacral arteries. The anterior spinal artery supplies the ventromedial aspect of the spinal cord that includes the corticospinal tracts and motor neurons. The two posterior spinal arteries, forming a plexus-like network on the cord surface, supply the dorsal and lateral aspects of the spinal cord, which includes the sensory tracts responsible for such sensations as proprioception and light touch [59].

The anterior spinal artery courses ventrally on the spinal cord to supply the white matter tracts and penetrates the cord parenchyma where it divides in the gray matter. However, the anterior spinal artery is not functionally continuous along the length of the spinal cord, so frequently one of the anterior radicular branches which arises from the aorta, called the arteria radicularis magna (great radicular artery of Adamkiewicz) which has a variable origin and is most commonly located between T9 and L5, on the left side, is responsible for supplying blood to as much as the lower two-thirds of the spinal cord. The ventral spinal cord is quite dependent on collateral flow through radicular arteries as there is essentially no collateral blood flow between the anterior and posterior circulations (Fig. 7.8). Only 6–8 of the 62 radicular vessels present during intrauterine development persist into adulthood and up to 45% of the general population have less than five. Generally, most individuals possess 1–2 cervical, 2–3 thoracic, and 1–2 lumbar radicular arteries. This results in a spinal cord that is particularly susceptible to ischemia at the upper thoracic and lumbar areas, especially during aortic or spinal surgery and following trauma.

The venous return of the spinal cord consists of two median longitudinal veins, two anterolateral longitudinal veins, and two posterolateral longitudinal veins, which drain into the vertebral venous plexus [60]. The venous drainage consists of an internal and external plexus, which communicate with each other as well as with the segmental systemic veins and the portal system. The internal plexus, consisting of thin-walled, valveless veins, connects to a vein from the spinal cord and basivertebral vein at each spinal segment and communicates through the foramen magnum with the occipital and basilar sinuses. The internal plexus empties into the intervertebral veins that pass through the intervertebral and sacral foramina to the vertebral, intercostal, lumbar and lateral sacral veins. The external plexus is formed by joined veins that exit from each vertebral body to form the anterior

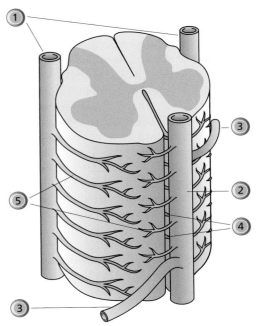

Figure 7.8 Spinal cord blood supply. (1) Posterior spinal arteries. (2) Anterior spinal artery. (3) Anterior radicular artery. (4) Sulcal branch arteries. (5) Pial arterial plexus.

vertebral plexus. The posterior vertebral plexus is formed by the veins that pass through the ligamentum flavum.

Cerebral vascular physiology

Normal adult cerebral blood flow is considered to be 50–75 mL/100 g/min, an average of diverse values that have been collected over decades following the ground-breaking work of Kety and Schmidt [61–64]. Wide variability between subjects in these reports is not due to imprecision of the methods, but because cerebral blood flow itself is variable and substrate delivery is tightly matched to the cerebral metabolic rate of oxygen consumption. The adaptation of the technique for children 3–10 years old showed that the preteen child has a cerebral blood flow nearly twice that of adults [65]. Subsequent measurements in the healthy infant and preterm infant without respiratory distress syndrome (RDS) showed that, at birth, cerebral blood flow is roughly one-third of adult values, and in many infants appeared to hover near the ischemic threshold of 20 mL/100 g/min [66–69]. The normal developmental changes in cerebral blood flow across age are depicted in Figure 7.9.

The cerebral blood flow developmental pattern recapitulates the trend of cellular growth, synaptogenesis, and myelination that occur in the first years of life. When global cerebral metabolism was quantified as a function of age, the same trends persist: infants have rates of cer-

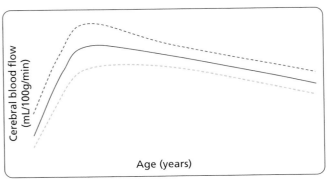

Figure 7.9 Developmental changes in cerebral blood flow. At birth, blood flow to the brain is low compared with adult levels of cerebral blood flow. During the first years of life, blood flow rates increase sharply to a peak at 4 years of age and then taper off during adolescence to adult values.

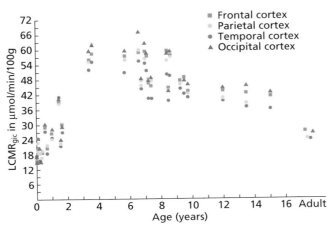

Figure 7.10 Cerebral metabolism, quantified by the local cerebral metabolic rate of glucose (LCMR$_{glc}$) utilization, is low at birth, increases in the first years of life and tapers during adolescence. This pattern recapitulates and explains the developmental pattern of cerebral blood flow changes.

ebral metabolism that are 30% lower than adults, and between birth and 4 years of age, cerebral metabolism increases to exceed adult rates by twofold [70,71] (Fig. 7.10).

The brain lacks appreciable glycogen stores and is intolerant to the pH changes associated with anaerobic metabolism. The brain is therefore unique among organs in its requirement of a constant supply of oxygen and glucose. Paradoxically, the brain is also injured by excessive cerebral blood flow due to the elastance of the intracranial compartment. Several layers of servo-mechanisms contribute to the homeostasis of cerebral metabolic demand and substrate delivery. These mechanisms operate at different frequencies, with distinct precision, and with varying regional specificity in the brain. This chapter presents four separate mechanisms of cerebral blood flow control. The first three are presented sequentially as increasingly precise mechanisms working in concert to fine-tune cerebral blood flow in a dynamic pressure flow system: the systemic vasoconstrictive response, pressure autoregulation and neurovascular coupling. Next, the cerebral vascular responses to homeostatic perturbations of arterial carbon dioxide, oxygen and glucose concentration are discussed. Developmental considerations of the mechanisms are considered independently.

Neurovascular regulation as a generic principle requires complete vascularization and development of muscular arterioles capable of reactivity. The term brain has a fully functional vascularity, but cerebral vasculature is both anatomically incomplete and underdeveloped in infants born at the current limits of viability. As mentioned above, persistence of the germinal matrix is accompanied by a fragile periventricular vascular overgrowth in the premature infant that is prone to hemorrhage. Penetrating arterial growth from the pial surface into deep white matter structures is also incomplete in the premature neonate. The adult brain has a redundant arterial network in the white matter circulation where the premature infant has poorly anastamosed white matter circulation that is vulnerable to ischemic injury [72,73]. According to studies in fetal sheep, vasoreactivity to arterial pressure changes occurs at 2/3 of gestation, which would correspond to the current limits of viability. However, the limits of reactivity are much closer to resting blood pressure than in the term animal [74]. Development of the muscularis layer of arteries and arterioles involved in vasoreactivity occurs during the third trimester first in larger, pial vessels, and then in progressively smaller arterioles. This anatomy would predict that vasoreactivity would be coarse in the extremely preterm infant and more fine-tuned with increasing gestational age. Apparently normal preterm infants have been shown to spend significant portions of time with pressure-passive circulation, a state seen in adults with shock or intracranial pathology [75].

Systemic vasoconstrictive response

The most blunt of the mechanisms that preserve cerebral blood flow is the systemic vasoconstrictive response, which renders cerebral blood flow independent of cardiac output. Decline in cardiac output results in increased sympathetic tone, activation of the renin-angiotensin-aldosterone axis, and increased vasopressin activity. All three of these axes exert a vasoconstrictive response that is differentially asserted between the systemic and cerebral circulations. The net effect is to preserve cerebral perfusion at the expense of systemic perfusion [76–79]. For example, normotensive shock can result in renal failure and necrotizing enterocolitis without neurological sequelae. When systemic vasoconstrictive responses are functional, the brain takes a variable percentage of total

cardiac output to maintain cerebral blood flow [80–82]. Even during cardiopulmonary bypass, cerebral blood flow is preserved as long as perfusion pressure is adequate, regardless of the flow rates [83].

Because of the systemic vasoconstrictive response, it is said that the brain is not dependent on cardiac output, and it is also said that what is good for the brain is not good for the splanchnic organs. The antagonistic relationship between cerebral and systemic perfusion is seen in profoundly septic patients who lose digits and renal function after pressor therapy titrated to maintain cerebral perfusion. This balance is also relevant in the care of children with cardiac disease, as afterload reduction is a mainstay of therapy and increases survival in the setting of congestive heart failure. In this setting, the clinician must balance reduction of systemic vascular resistance against the need for adequate cerebral perfusion pressure. Even adult patients (for whom the limits of cerebral perfusion pressure are more defined) suffer symptoms of cerebral hypoperfusion when aggressively treated for cardiomyopathy. The pediatric patient has the same risk, but is less likely to report presyncopal symptoms. Infants on cardiopulmonary bypass are frequently maintained at critically low perfusion pressures with vasodilator therapy. This strategy is associated with improved renal and splanchnic perfusion and survival, but also with predictably decreased cerebral perfusion [84–86]. The impact of this therapy on the high incidence of neurological injury in this population has not been elucidated (Fig. 7.11).

The sympathetic nervous system develops early in gestation, and the parasympathetic nervous system develops and increases parasympathetic tone near term [87]. Preterm vasculature has less reserve in the systemic vasoconstrictive response, and consequently has less ability to maintain perfusion pressure to the brain. The preterm heart also has limited ability to modulate output, operating near maximal contractility and at elevated heart rates. Hence, the preterm infant is vulnerable at birth due to lack of the first homeostatic cerebral blood flow mechanism: maintenance of perfusion pressure. This is manifest as hypotension, especially in the first hours and days of life, when transition from the low-resistance placental circulation places afterload on the underdeveloped myocardium [88].

Pressure autoregulation

The next layer of cerebrovascular control is commonly referred to as pressure autoregulation – the maintenance of constant cerebral blood flow across a range of cerebral perfusion pressure. Pressure autoregulation, like the systemic vasoconstrictive response, allows the brain to steal and shunt blood flow to and from the systemic vasculature. Pressure autoregulation is a function of reactivity of

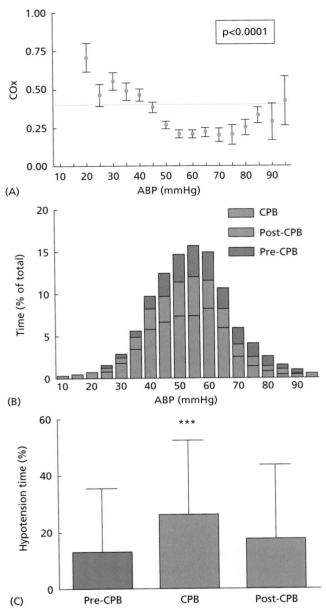

Figure 7.11 Cerebrovascular pressure autoregulation was quantified in children during cardiac surgery by correlation between arterial blood pressure and cerebral oximetry (COx), which indicates pathological pressure passivity with increasingly positive values. (A) When normotensive, subjects showed intact pressure autoregulation that was increasingly disturbed with progressive hypotension. (B) The majority of time during the recordings was from normotensive periods with intact autoregulation. (C) Hypotensive recordings with impaired autoregulation occurred most frequently during cardiopulmonary bypass.

the cerebral vasculature to changes in arterial pressure, in contrast to the systemic vasoconstrictive response, which is responsive to changes in both arterial pressure and cardiac output. Response times for pressure autoregulation are much faster than systemic vascular responses, occurring within 4–10 sec of a change in arterial blood

pressure in an adult study, and within 2 sec of a change in blood pressure in a study of neonates [89,90]. Pressure autoregulation allows changes in cerebral blood flow at the pulse and respiratory frequencies, but acts as a high-pass filter, preventing fluctuations of cerebral blood flow that persist longer than 10–20 sec.

Autoregulatory activity can be seen in physiological recordings of intracranial pressure, blood volume, blood flow, blood flow velocity, and oxygenation during slow changes of arterial blood pressure lasting between 20 and 300 sec. In the normal autoregulating brain, blood volume and intracranial pressure are inversely related to blood pressure at these low frequencies. This inverse relationship is caused by reactive dilation and constriction of the resistance arterioles mediating autoregulation. The result is constant cerebral blood flow, flow velocity, and oxygenation during slow blood pressure changes. At blood pressures below the lower limit of autoregulation, unresponsive cerebral vasculature dilates and constricts passively to changes in arterial blood pressure. In this setting, cerebral blood volume, intracranial pressure, cerebral blood flow, flow velocity and oxygenation are all positively correlated with slow changes in arterial blood pressure. These distinctions between intact and perturbed autoregulation form the basis of physiological monitoring of the state of autoregulation [91–94] (Fig. 7.12).

Pressure autoregulation response times and limits of operation are variable and influenced by CO_2 tension. The lower limit of autoregulation, originally described at 50 mmHg in adults by Lassen, is now understood to have a wide interpatient and situational variability [64,95] (Fig. 7.13).

The lower limit of autoregulation has not been well defined for pediatric populations, but infants on cardiopulmonary bypass have shown a lower limit between a mean arterial blood pressure of 30 and 40 mmHg [84,86]. Preterm infants have shown intact pressure autoregulation at surprisingly low pressures, and many have a lower limit somewhere between 25 and 30 mmHg mean arterial pressure [96,97]. Absolute safe arterial blood pressure recommendations cannot be made for specific ages because the data do not exist. Such recommendations would likely not be applicable to critically ill populations, as clinical factors related to critical illness may impair autoregulatory function and shift the limits of intact pressure autoregulation. For instance, newborn piglets without intracranial pathology have an average lower limit of autoregulation at a cerebral perfusion pressure of 30 mmHg, and piglets with hydrocephalus have an average lower limit of autoregulation at 50 mmHg [98]. Even monitoring intracranial pressure would not account for the shift in autoregulation function seen in that study. Without information about the state of autoregulation, blood pressure and cerebral perfusion pressure

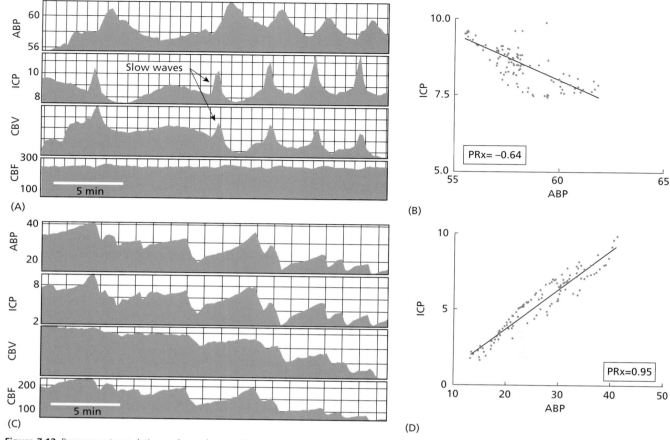

(A)   (B)

(C)   (D)

Figure 7.12 Pressure autoregulation and vascular reactivity can be quantified and monitored. Recordings from a normotensive piglet (A,B) of arterial blood pressure (ABP), intracranial pressure (ICP), cerebral blood volume (CBV) and cerebral blood flow (CBF) show intact autoregulation. Slow waves of ABP cause reactive dilation and constriction of resistance arterioles, which is reflected in both CBV and ICP as slow waves that are inverted when compared with the ABP tracing. CBF is constant in this state of intact autoregulation. The pressure reactivity index (PRx) quantifies the inverted ICP–ABP relationship with a negative Pearson's coefficient of correlation, indicating healthy vascular reactivity. In a hypotensive piglet (C,D), ABP, ICP, and CBV are all in phase at the slow-wave frequency, indicating pathological pressure passivity. CBF is fluctuant in this state of impaired autoregulation, and the PRx is positive.

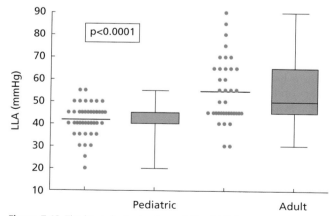

Figure 7.13 The lower limit of autoregulation (LLA) is not necessarily 50 mmHg. Individual determinations of the LLA were made for pediatric and adult populations during cardiac surgery. The blood pressure threshold associated with pressure-passive cerebral oximetry was determined for each subject in the study. Pediatric patients, in general, tolerated lower blood pressures than adult patients, and intersubject variability was high, suggesting that a single blood pressure threshold is not adequate for hemodynamic management guidelines [86].

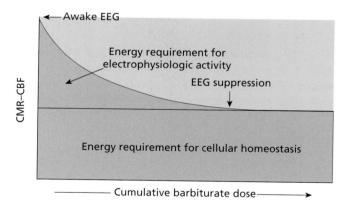

Figure 7.14 More than half of cerebral metabolism (CMR) is utilized for the maintenance of voltage gradients discharged during neuronal activity. EEG silence, induced with barbiturate administration, ablates this metabolic activity and results in a concomitant reduction of cerebral blood flow (CBF) as flow–metabolism coupling is maintained.

management is still crudely applied to the protection of the pediatric brain.

Impairment of pressure autoregulation is a state of vulnerability to secondary injury of the brain from hypoperfusion and hyperemia. Patients are more likely to survive traumatic brain injury with intact pressure reactivity [99]. This finding has been verified in pediatric patients, and pressure autoregulation has been shown to be a function of blood pressure management [100,101].

Neurovascular coupling

In 1890, 54 years before the Kety–Schmidt technique was first applied to measure cerebral blood flow, a relationship between neuronal activity and cerebral blood flow was observed.

> We conclude, then, that the chemical products of cerebral metabolism contained in the lymph which bathes the walls of the arterioles of the brain can cause variations of the calibre of the cerebral vessels: that in this re-action the brain possesses an intrinsic mechanism by which its vascular supply can be varied locally in correspondence with local variations of functional activity. Roy and Sherrington, 1890 [102]

The method employed by Roy and Sherrington to show activity flow coupling in the brain was a direct measurement of a regional brain volume change brought about by electrical stimulation of exposed sensory nerves in dogs. Since then, with the advent of sensitive regional blood flow measurement techniques, neurovascular interactions have been a major focus of research. The model currently used to explain activity-dependent flow is a neurovascular unit in which an astrocyte anatomically bridges a collection of synapses and penetrating arterioles [103]. From these studies, we have learned that neurovascular coupling is a fast response, affecting vascular diameter change within 1 second of neuronal activation, and it is spatially specific, affecting only flow in the immediate region of neuronal activation. Neurovascular coupling is a finer control of cerebral blood flow when compared to the relatively slow and global pressure autoregulation mechanism.

Metabolic regulation of cerebral blood flow can cause large changes in cerebral blood volume, as seen with the induction of barbiturate coma for treatment of elevated intracranial pressure. Cerebral oxygen consumption and cerebral blood flow decrease concomitantly with increasing doses of barbiturate. At doses sufficient to produce EEG silence, cerebral blood flow and volume are half of awake values. Further increase in barbiturate dosing does not further reduce cerebral blood flow (Fig. 7.14) [104].

Similar effects are seen with propofol administration to burst suppression [105]. This technique is helpful for reduction of brain volume to improve the surgical field, and to decrease intracranial pressure in patients with acute intracranial mass effect. When temperature reduction is used to suppress brain metabolism, the plateau at EEG silence is not observed, and reductions in temperature continue to reduce both cerebral blood flow and volume because of slowing of cellular metabolism not related to the discharge and maintenance of membrane voltage potentials. The moderately hypothermic brain has a cerebral blood flow that is half that of the normothermic brain, and deep hypothermia yields a cerebral blood flow that would be below the critical threshold for ischemia in a normothermic brain [106–108].

Both hypothermia and electrical suppression therapies maintain and utilize the coupling of metabolism and cerebral blood flow. When hypocarbia is used to reduce cerebral blood flow, however, cerebral blood flow is reduced below metabolic demand. Uncoupling metabolism and cerebral blood flow creates an ischemic vulnerability, and patients with head trauma have worse outcomes when prophylactic hypocarbia is applied [109].

Flow response to homeostatic derangements

The three mechanisms of cerebral blood flow control outlined above are flow and pressure control mechanisms, which are over-ridden during states of non-physiological chemical perturbation. Examples, which have been well characterized, are disturbances of arterial carbon dioxide, oxygen and glucose. It is logical that the brain would have fail-safe vascular compensations during states of inadequate substrate delivery, even when perfusion pressure is adequate.

Cerebrovascular response to carbon dioxide

Acute decreases in arterial carbon dioxide tension cause vasoconstriction of the cerebral vasculature while acute increases in arterial carbon dioxide tension cause cerebral vasodilation. The carbon dioxide response of the cerebral vasculature is most active across the physiological range of carbon dioxide and is correlated with changes in cerebrospinal fluid pH. Neuronal function is adversely affected by low pH in the cerebrospinal fluid, and the blood–brain barrier is impermeable to hydrogen ions. However, carbon dioxide diffuses freely into the cerebrospinal fluid.

Cerebrospinal fluid pH is tightly regulated by a combination of two mechanisms. First, there is robust metabolic buffering by rapid spinal fluid turnover with high carbonic anhydrase activity in the ependymal cells of the choroid plexus. Second, the coupling of cerebral blood flow to arterial carbon dioxide tension modulates the removal of carbon dioxide from the cerebral spinal fluid. The time course of cerebral blood flow responses to changes in carbon dioxide is partially explained by spinal fluid buffering. The initial vasoreactive response to a change in arterial carbon dioxide is mediated within seconds and reaches steady state within 10 min. This is followed by a gradual return toward baseline cerebrovascular resistance over 3–6 h, consistent with the time course of pH regulation [110,111]. Persistent hypercapnia results in late hyperemia, not explained by this model, that does not return to normal after normalization of serum carbon dioxide.

The use of arterial carbon dioxide as a drug to effect change in the cerebral blood flow is a common practice in pediatric anesthesia. Decreasing cerebral blood volume by hyperventilation facilitates craniotomy in the presence of elevated intracranial pressure. The use of hyperventilation to manage intracranial volume is done at the expense of cerebral blood flow, and disrupts normal metabolic coupling to cerebral blood flow. Ischemic injury occurs in pediatric patients with traumatic brain injury when hyperventilation is used prophylactically to manage intracranial pressure and that practice is contraindicated by the Brain Trauma Foundation except for transient use during surgery or to prevent impending herniation.

Conversely, hypercarbia is often employed in the management of the patient who has a single ventricle and a large left-to-right shunt. In this setting, serum hypercarbia and acidosis increase pulmonary vascular resistance, but hypercarbia and acidosis in the cerebrospinal fluid cause decreased cerebral vascular resistance. The combination effect is to mitigate pulmonary overcirculation and enhance cerebral oxygen delivery.

When arterial carbon dioxide modulation is used as a therapy to change cerebral blood flow, the effect is mediated by changes in spinal fluid pH. Because of the rapid CSF turnover and high range of responsiveness of carbonic anhydrase during CSF production, the duration of a pH change in the CSF is blunted after 3–6 h. Because serum and spinal fluid buffers are separated by the blood–brain barrier, the brain pH returns to normal even if the serum pH remains abnormal. Buffering of the spinal fluid limits the duration of effectiveness of carbon dioxide-modulating therapies. Furthermore, caution should be exerted when normalizing the serum pH of a patient after prolonged respiratory acidosis or alkalosis. For instance, low serum pH and high serum carbon dioxide tensions at the time of initiating rescue cardiopulmonary bypass are associated with stroke and hemorrhage [112–114].

Cerebrovascular response to oxygen delivery

Arterial oxygen tensions between 60 mmHg and 300 mmHg do not appreciably change cerebrovascular tone. However, when oxygen delivery is impaired by arterial hypoxia or anemia, cerebral vascular resistance is decreased and cerebral blood flow increases [115–117]. The response of the cerebral vasculature is in contrast to the carbon dioxide response, which is most active in the normal physiological range of arterial carbon dioxide tension. There is no vascular response to fluctuations of arterial oxygen delivery within the physiological range, and it is only when oxygen delivery reaches a critical threshold that the autoregulatory mechanisms are disrupted by global hypoxic vasodilation.

Cerebrovascular response to glucose delivery

Although adult brain metabolism is 7.5 times that of the average tissue metabolism, the brain has very little stored glycogen, only about 2 minutes' worth in neurons. The lack of a local glucose buffer makes the brain dependent on a constant capillary supply. Insulin is required for glucose transport from the serum to the intracellular space in most cells, but glucose diffuses readily into neurons even in the absence of insulin. Glucose deprivation in the adult brain leads to vasodilation only after unconsciousness and EEG changes have occurred, but in the newborn brain the vasodilatory response has a higher threshold, with vasodilatory changes occurring at serum glucose levels of 30 mg/dL, without loss of consciousness or EEG changes [118–120].

Electroencephalogram

Electroencephalogram (EEG) monitoring has been used perioperatively to identify abnormalities and potential periods of cerebral injury or malfunction. When appropriately applied, the EEG provides a continuous recording of electrical activity between reference electrodes placed at specific positions on the scalp. This electrical activity is thought to originate from the postsynaptic potentials of the dendrites of cortical neurons. The EEG waveforms are classically divided according to frequency as δ (1–3/sec), θ (4–7/sec), α (8–12/sec) and β (13–20/sec) (Fig. 7.15). These waveforms are altered by many factors including age, state of awareness/alertness, tasks (like eye opening), medications, and various disease states. In particular, sleep can manifest in unique alterations, like sharp waves (K complexes) and sleep spindles (regular 12–14/sec) confined to the central electrodes. Seizure or epileptiform activity is characterized by combinations and locations of spike and slow-wave activity and may interfere with processed EEG validity. Therefore, adequate interpretation of continuous EEG tests requires good lead contact and continuous analysis by a trained technician/clinician.

Because of these limitations, comprehensive and continuous EEG monitoring has only had limited usage in the intensive care unit (ICU) and operating room (OR) despite results demonstrating potential for clinical benefit

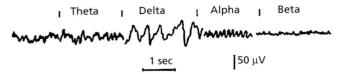

Figure 7.15 The electroencephalographic (EEG) waveforms are classically divided according to frequency as δ (1–3/sec), θ (4–7/sec), α (8–12/sec) and β (13–20/sec). Notice that δ waves are also characterized by a higher amplitude (>75 μV), while β waves have a very low amplitude (<10 μV). These waves are interpreted based on the clinical state of the patient (i.e. level of arousal or seizure activity). The propensity and distribution of these various waveforms change throughout life and during different mental activities. For example, sleeping adult subjects monitored with EEG have increased δ wave activity while adult subjects who are awake and thinking have more α and β wave activity.

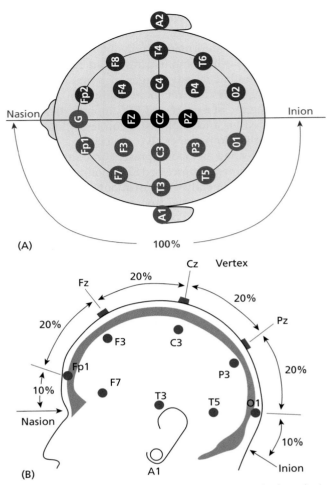

Figure 7.16 The standardized placement of scalp electrodes for a classic EEG recording has become common since the adoption of the 10/20 international system. (A) In the sagittal view, the "10/20" orientation of the electrodes can be related to the relative percentages of distance between the nasion-inion and other fixed points. These points are marked as the frontal pole (Fp), central (C), parietal (P), occipital (O), and temporal (T). The midline electrodes are marked with a subscript z, which stands for zero. (B) In the coronal view, subscripted odd numbers are used to indicate positions over the left hemisphere and even numbers over the right.

and management. For instance, EEG has been used during cardiopulmonary bypass to titrate cooling strategies, detect intraoperative events, and monitor for seizures postoperatively. The EEG is affected by maturation of the brain and by a host of environmental factors, such as anesthetic agents, pain, cerebral metabolism, and temperature. Preoperative EEG monitoring has been used in premature infants to detect seizure and ischemic events. These studies have utilized both comprehensive as well as processed EEG [121].

In most patients, EEG is isoelectric during cardiopulmonary bypass (CPB) [122]. With deep hypothermic cardiac arrest, waiting to achieve an isoelectric EEG during cooling before initiating circulatory arrest is potentially neuroprotective [123]. There is much interpatient variability in the degree of hypothermia required to induce electrocerebral silence. Temperatures at which electrocerebral silence on EEG occurs are lower than when evoked potentials disappear, making EEG a more reliable method of neuromonitoring during cooling [124].

Electroencephalogram activity resumes upon cerebral reperfusion and rewarming. The temperature at which continuous EEG activity returns is predictive of postoperative neurological dysfunction as this appears to be related to intraoperative brain injury. In adult studies, the risk of postoperative confusion or stroke significantly increases with every degree higher at which continuous EEG activity resumes [125].

In addition, perioperative EEG monitoring detects seizures that clinically would be missed due to pharmacological neuromuscular blockade and sedation, including subclinical seizure activity [126]. Seizures may occur secondary to cerebral injury and worsen pre-existing or ongoing neuronal damage. Clancy et al performed EEG monitoring on 183 infants after cardiac surgery and identified that 11% of the patients had EEG-detected seizure activity postoperatively, though there were no clinically apparent seizures [126]. Most recently, postoperative, diffuse EEG slowing has been reported in children during the first 48 h following cardiac surgery. However, EEG slowing was not associated with neurological deficits or MRI changes [127] (Fig. 7.16).

Processed EEG monitoring

Processed EEG monitoring was pioneered in clinical anesthesia practice by Maynard and Prior. Multiple studies described the use of comprehensive and processed EEG signals to help in the identification and management of patients at risk for adverse perioperative events. Prior and Maynard divided the clinical applications of such neurophysiological monitoring into three categories: (1) where it had been shown conclusively to reduce the risk of iatrogenic harm to an at-risk patient during elective procedures; (2) where it had provided additional useful information not obtainable by other means; and (3) where monitoring could have been of potential value but its advantages in terms of reduced morbidity or mortality remained unproven [128,129]. However, the use of a processed EEG monitor that eliminates the need for a technologist/neurologist interpretation is appealing to perioperative clinicians.

These studies and methods represent fundamentally the current development of processed EEG monitoring devices used today in perioperative care of infants and children. A recent publication by Davidson provides an excellent review of this monitoring principle in children [130]. For the purposes of this text, we will focus on the available techniques/technologies in current clinical practice.

Amplitude-integrated EEG (aEEG) uses the P3–P4 positions and ground Fz to monitor the vulnerable watershed region in neonates. The signal is amplified and passed through an asymmetrical band-pass filter that strongly attenuates activity below 2 Hz and above 15 Hz in order to minimize artifacts from such sources as sweating, muscle activity and electrical interference. Additional processing includes semi-logarithmic amplitude compression, rectification and time compression. aEEG recordings with a cerebral function monitor, such as the "BraiNZ" monitor (Natus Medical Incorporated, San Carlos, CA, USA), obtained continuously from two biparietal electrodes, have also been shown to be useful in the early prediction of the severity of brain injury. Of 35 infants with a moderately abnormal or suppressed tracing and/or seizures, 27 died or survived with neurological abnormalities on follow-up at 18–24 months. Of 21 babies with normal amplitude, 19 were normal on follow-up [131]. One of the challenges of the aEEG is training of the bedside clinician to recognize and interpret the background amplitudes and to correlate the pattern with the clinical status of the patient [128].

Continuous comprehensive EEG can be technically difficult to use and interpret in the operating room. However, limited channel EEG-based technologies with automated interpretation have correlated electrical brainwave activity with depth of anesthesia and awareness in adults. Commercially available devices are the Bispectral Index® (BIS) monitor (ASPECT Medical Technologies, Norwood, MA, USA) and most recently the SEDLine™ monitor (SEDLine Inc., Irvine, CA, USA). These monitors use algorithm-based analysis of multiple EEG characteristics and integrate these into a single dimensionless number. Unlike routine EEG, these monitors utilize placement of a single sensor containing multiple electrodes positioned easily on the forehead and temple in a specific pattern. The BIS utilizes a unilateral sensor array, while the SEDLine utilizes a bilateral sensor. Glass et al demon-

strated that BIS recorded from several different electrode arrangements (or montages) provided similar results [132]. They used a frontal (Fp1 and Fp2) to CZ electrode montages, as well as an alternative placement (FPz–At) that approximates the BIS sensor electrode positions. At this time, only the BIS has an approved pediatric probe.

The SEDLine uses a bilateral four-channel frontal array (FP1, FP2 and F7, F8) to generate the Patient State Index or PSI.

Although these monitors have US FDA approval to assess anesthetic depth, there have been multiple reports of additional applications of these monitors (i.e. burst suppression, sedation monitoring) throughout the perioperative period [130,133,134]. The PSI and BIS indices both range from 0 (isoelectric EEG or electrocerebral silence) to 100 (awake) although studies have demonstrated differences in the actual interpretation of these scales in relation to depth of anesthesia. For instance, there are multiple studies correlating increased BIS values (>80) with awareness and decreased BIS values with depth of anesthesia and hypothermia during bypass [135] while similar studies evaluating the range of PSI values from 25 to 50 have been demonstrated to provide protection from awareness while avoiding issues of delayed emergence (PSI <25) [136,137].

There are limited studies to date evaluating the SEDLine in children. However, recent studies have evaluated the utility of the BIS monitor in children younger than 2 years of age and demonstrated good correlation with prior adult studies in predicting depth of anesthesia, despite the BIS algorithm being based on adult subjects [138].

There are many other processed EEG monitors available with similar functionality but differing lead array placement and signal analysis. The Cerebral State Monitor™ (Danmeter A/S, Odense, Denmark) is a handheld wireless device that also uses a proprietary algorithm and a 0–100 scale, with 40–60 indicating an adequate depth of hypnosis. The Cerebral State Index (CSI) that is calculated by the device is derived from the time and frequency domain analysis, which inputs into a fuzzy logic inference system that calculates the index. In a comparative study, both the BIS and the CSI had a predictive probability statistic for depth of anesthesia of 0.87, which demonstrates good performance. The CSI performed better for deeper levels of anesthesia than the BIS, which was better at lighter levels [139].

The Narcotrend™ monitor (MonitorTechnik, Bad Bramstedt, Germany) is another monitor that processes raw EEG signals using one-channel or two-channel recordings from different electrode positions. Early models graded the depth of hypnosis into five stages from A (awake) to F (very deep level of anesthesia). The latest Narcotrend software (version 4.0) now calculates the Narcotrend Index, another dimensionless 0–100 scale that is similar to those calculated by the monitors described above. When compared with BIS, the performance of the Narcotrend Index in terms of prediction probability of depth of sedation was slightly better than BIS (predictive probability statistic 0.88, as compared with 0.85) [140].

Additional approaches to brain monitoring in the ICU and OR include response entropy and state entropy [141]. The irregularity of the EEG signal can be quantified and, by using an algorithm that is in the public domain, quantified to reflect depth of sedation. This Entropy™ Monitor (GE Healthcare, Fairfield, CT, USA) utilizes the electromyography (EMG) signal, which may provide information useful for assessing whether a patient is responding to an external stimulus, for instance a painful stimulus. The combination of EEG and EMG is presented as the response entropy, and the lower frequency EEG signals alone are presented as the state entropy. The prediction probability values of the entropy indices for differentiating between consciousness and unconsciousness are high and comparable with those for BIS [142]. Noxious stimulation does increase the difference between response entropy and state entropy, but an increase in the difference does not always indicate inadequate analgesia [143].

Evoked potential monitoring

Assessment of the integrity of the neural pathways, both ascending and descending, can be undertaken with a variety of evoked potential (EP) monitoring methods. An EP is an electrical response that follows stimulation of the CNS by a specific stimulus of the visual, auditory, sensory or motor system. The perioperative EP assessment tools and their application are summarized in Table 7.3.

Perioperative electrophysiological monitoring

Germane to this chapter, the complex and sometimes dynamic interaction between patient-related factors and clinical management necessitates an understanding of the basic neurophysiology of these tests [144–153]. Like the EEG, state of arousal, presence of various anesthetic agents, metabolic derangements, and temperature can dramatically affect these monitoring modalities. For ascending (dorsal/posterior) pathway monitoring, a stimulus is applied peripherally and supracortical monitors detect the change in cortical electrical activity. This allows for assessment of amplitude, latency and decay. The experience of the team and availability of resources to perform continuous evoked potential monitoring limit its consistent utilization. Certainly with spine surgery, SSEPs have become a widely accepted practice standard.

For assessment of the descending (anterior) pathways, the cerebral cortex is stimulated and the resulting peripheral motor response is assessed. Motor evoked potentials or MEPs can be done in conjunction with SSEP monitoring to provide dual assessment of anterior and posterior spinal cord integrity. The use of intraoperative MEP is a growing practice in pediatric anesthesiology, but like other EP monitoring modalities, it is susceptible to alterations based on the neurodevelopment of the patient, along with other operative and anesthetic factors. In a retrospective study of children aged 2–12 undergoing surgery for idiopathic scoliosis, a strong correlation between MEP thresholds and age was demonstrated [147]. Although the exact mechanisms responsible for this finding are subject to debate, it agrees with the prior observations of Parano et al [154] who hypothesized that delayed conduction and decreased EP amplitudes were significantly diminished in the youngest children secondary to delayed neuronal maturational changes with age, specifically multifactorial issues of ongoing synaptogenesis, incomplete nerve integration, and decreased myelination. This dynamic difference makes empiric numbers less useful, and often forces clinicians to use each patient as their own baseline. In addition, the impact that various anesthetic agents have on these monitoring modalities is also highly variable and changes with both the age of the patient and agent used. Because of these issues, many centers favor intravenous anesthetic techniques to minimize or eliminate the use of inhalational agents [147,148].

Table 7.3 Perioperative electrophysiological monitoring [144–153]

Monitor	Procedures	Current practice
EEG	AVM repair/clipping	Used in most centers
	Cardiopulmonary bypass	Used in some centers
	Level of consciousness	Used in some centers
BAEP	Acoustic neuroma	Monitoring recommended
	CN V decompression	Used in some centers
	CN VII decompression	Used in some centers
	Level of consciousness	Used in some centers
SSEP	Spine surgery	Monitoring recommended
	Aortic surgery	Used in some centers
MEP	Spine surgery	Used in some centers
	Aortic surgery	Used in some centers
VEP	ICU care of TBI	Used in some centers
	Optic surgery	Research

AVM, arteriovenous malformation; BAEP, brain stem auditory evoked potential; CN, cranial nerve; ICU, intensive care unit; MEP, motor evoked potential; SSEP, somatosensory evoked potentials; TBI, traumatic brain injury; VEP, visual evoked potentials.

Conclusion

For safe and effective perioperative care of infants and children at risk of neurological injury, the pediatric anesthesiologist must have a working knowledge of the unique neurodevelopmental events and neurophysiological principles relevant to the pediatric patient. Our specialty has contributed to the growing body of knowledge that will reduce the toxicity of critical illness to the developing human brain. We can expect further refinement of anesthetic practices designed to protect normal neurodevelopmental processes. Neuromonitoring modalities will continue to adapt, and provide an increasingly complex real-time data set to the anesthesiologist caring for a critically ill child. When this information is combined with an understanding of neurodevelopmental principles, the physics of the intracranial compartment, and neurovascular physiology, we will more effectively choose care practices that yield improved outcomes for our patients.

Annotated references

A full reference list for this chapter is available at:
http://www.wiley.com/go/gregory/andropoulos/pediatricanesthesia

12. Back SA, Luo NL, Borenstein NS et al. Late oligodendrocyte progenitors coincide with the developmental window of vulnerability for human perinatal white matter injury. J Neurosci 2001;21:1302–12. A developmental explanation of the vulnerability of white matter to injury in the premature neonate.

16. Lee SJ, Ralston HJ, Drey EA et al. Fetal pain: a systematic multidisciplinary review of the evidence. JAMA 2005;294:947–54. A review of the evidence for the development of fetal pain pathways from early in gestation.

20. Clancy B, Darlington RB, Finlay BL. Translating developmental time across mammalian species. Neuroscience 2001;105:7–17. A bioinformatics approach to equating developmental stages of brain development across different animal species.

30. Klimach VJ, Cooke RW. Maturation of the neonatal somatosensory evoked response in preterm infants. Dev Med Child Neurol 1988;30:208–14. Very interesting study demonstrating the maturation of evoked potentials in preterm infants.

50. Uhl GR, Sora I, Wang Z. The mu opiate receptor as a candidate gene for pain: polymorphisms, variations in expression, nociception, and opiate responses. Proc Natl Acad Sci USA 1999;96:7752–5. An early study of genetic polymorphisms as an explanation for differential responses to opioids, establishing the field of pharmacogenomics.

57. Taylor RH, Burrows FA, Bissonnette B. Cerebral pressure–flow velocity relationship during hypothermic cardiopulmonary bypass in neonates and infants. Anesthes Analg 1992;74:636–42.
    A careful study describing the loss of pressure–flow autoregulation with deep hypothermia in children undergoing cardiopulmonary bypass procedures.

63. Kety SS, Schmidt CF. The effects of active and passive hyperventilation on cerebral blood flow, cerebral oxygen consumption, cardiac output, and blood pressure of normal young men. J Clin Invest 1946;25:107–19. The classic paper describing the cornerstones of cerebral vascular physiology.

98. Brady KM, Lee JK, Kibler KK et al. The lower limit of cerebral blood flow autoregulation is increased with elevated intracranial pressure. Anesthes Analg 2009;108:1278–83. An important study demonstrating in patients that autoregulation is modified by increased intracranial pressure.

106. Greeley WJ, Kern FH, Ungerleider RM et al. The effect of hypothermic cardiopulmonary bypass and total circulatory arrest on cerebral metabolism in neonates, infants, and children. J Thorac Cardiovasc Surg 1991;101:783–94. The now landmark study describing cerebral physiology during hypothermic bypass and circulatory arrest in infants and children.

130. Davidson AJ. Measuring anesthesia in children using the eeg. Paediatr Anaesth 2006;16:374–87. A thorough review of EEG techniques for monitoring anesthetic depth in children.

CHAPTER 8

Developmental Physiology of the Liver, Gastrointestinal Tract, and Renal System

Peter N. Bromley, Ellen Rawlinson & James Bennett
Birmingham Children's Hospital and Liver Unit, Queen Elizabeth Hospital, Birmingham, UK

The liver

The embryological development of the liver, its subsequent transition at birth and maturation in infancy constitute a hugely complicated subject. Hypoglycemia, jaundice and impaired drug metabolism are common in the first weeks of life. Knowledge of the principles of hepatic development allows the anesthesiologist to understand the susceptibility of the liver to disease in infancy.

Embryology of the liver

The liver and gastrointestinal tracts arise from modifications of the primitive gut (see embryology of the gastrointestinal tract, later in this chapter) [1,2]. The liver develops from a thickening of the endoderm on the ventral surface of the foregut. These endodermal cells proliferate to form the hepatic diverticulum, which gives rise to cords of hepatoblasts within the mesenchyme of the transverse septum. The hepatoblasts are undifferentiated cells which can become hepatocytes, bile canaliculi or hepatic ducts under the influence of Notch signaling; abnormalities of this process are associated with Alagille syndrome, described towards the end of this section. The hepatocytes divide rapidly and arrange themselves around vitelline veins to form hepatic sinusoids.

The transverse septum is an important area and develops at a junctional site in the embryo – internally between foregut and midgut, and externally where the endoderm of the yolk sac meets the ectoderm of the amnion. The mesenchyme of the transverse septum also gives rise to the stromal cells which provide the serous and fibrous tissues of the liver, such as the liver capsule and the falciform ligament. The various connective tissues and smooth muscle of the biliary tracts also form from this mesenchymal tissue.

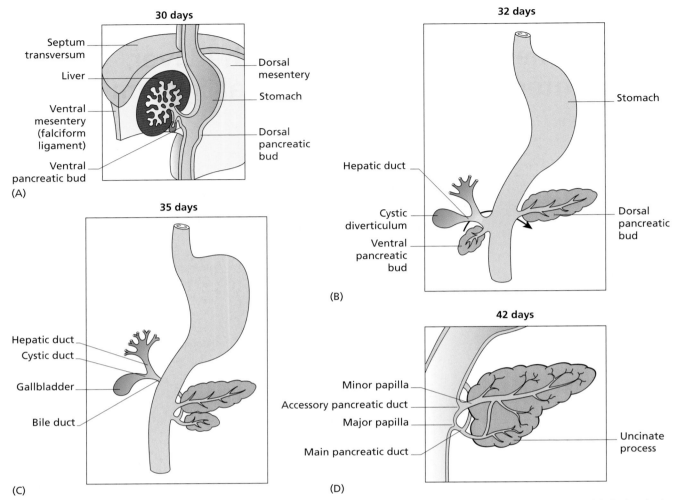

Figure 8.1 Development of the liver, gallbladder and pancreas and their duct systems from endodermal diverticula of the duodenum. (A) The liver bud sprouts during the 4th week and expands in the ventral (anterior) mesentery. (B) The cystic diverticulum and ventral pancreatic bud also grow into the ventral mesentery, whereas the dorsal pancreatic bud grows into the dorsal mesentery. (C) During the 5th week, the ventral pancreatic bud migrates around the posterior side (former right side) of the duodenum to fuse with the dorsal bud. (D) The main duct of the ventral bud ultimately becomes the major pancreatic duct, which drains the entire pancreas. Reproduced from Schoenwolf et al [1] with permission from Elsevier.

The gallbladder and cystic duct originate from a thickened portion of the ventral duodenum just below the hepatic diverticulum at around 4 weeks; this is known as the cystic diverticulum. As the connection between the hepatic diverticulum and foregut (duodenum) narrows, the hepatic ducts form. The cystic duct and hepatic ducts form the common bile duct which enters the duodenum, initially anteriorly, later from the left (see gut rotation). The growth of the liver and biliary tracts is rapid and by the 9th week the liver accounts for about 10% of the weight of the fetus (Fig. 8.1).

Fetal hematopoiesis

Hematopoietic stem cells capable of producing erythrocytes, megakaryocytes and macrophages migrate from the yolk sac to the liver, where hematopoiesis begins [3].

There is a second influx of hematopoietic stem cells originating from mesoderm surrounding the dorsal aorta. These cells are later programmed to migrate to the bone marrow and other lymphatic tissue. The immature fetal erythrocytes are bigger than mature red cells and, like white cells and platelets, they increase in number throughout gestation.

Development of the circulation in the fetal liver

The circulation in the fetal liver is complex and the reader is advised to refer to Chapter 5.

The arterial supply to the liver, like the rest of the foregut, originates from the vitelline arteries arising from the yolk sac [4]. A plexus of arteries between the vitelline vessels and the dorsal aorta coalesces to form three distinct arteries, supplying the whole of the gut from the aorta as the yolk sac shrinks. The celiac artery supplies the foregut, the superior mesenteric artery supplies the midgut and the inferior mesenteric artery supplies the hindgut. The arterial supply to the liver and gallbladder is the common hepatic artery, which originates from the celiac artery.

Venous blood is received into the two horns of the sinus venosus from three bilaterally symmetrical venous systems: the vitelline veins return blood from the developing gut, the umbilical veins return oxygenated blood from the placenta and the cardinal veins return blood from the embryo.

The vitelline veins originate as a network of vessels in the yolk sac, which in time form the venous drainage of the primitive gut. A plexus of vessels arises between the paired vitelline veins in the septum transversum, and as the hepatic diverticulum expands in the transverse septum, hepatic cords arrange themselves around this venous plexus to form primitive hepatic sinusoids. Caudal to the liver, the vitelline veins form numerous anastomoses; the left vitelline vein receives blood from the splenic and superior mesenteric veins, and the distal right vitelline vein regresses. The anastomosis between the left and right vitelline veins becomes the distal part of the portal vein. The proximal part of the portal vein is formed from the proximal right vitelline vein. The proximal left vitelline vein disappears at the time when the left sinus horn regresses to form the coronary sinus, and a series of transverse anastomoses carry blood to the right vitelline vein. Cephalad to the liver, an enlarged right vitelline vein returns all of the blood to the heart, which in time will become the inferior vena cava.

The two umbilical veins receive blood from the chorionic villi of the placenta and thus deliver oxygenated blood, rich in nutrients, to the developing fetus. In the second month of development the right umbilical vein regresses; possibly abnormalities in this process can cause abdominal wall defects (see Chapter 21 for clinical management of abdominal wall defects). The remaining left umbilical vein carries oxygenated blood to the fetus, entering the ductus venosus and then, via the inferior vena cava, the right atrium. Early in the neonatal period, the umbilical vein atrophies since blood is no longer flowing through it, forming the ligamentum teres. The atrophic ductus venosus forms the ligamentum venosum. In the presence of portal hypertension these ligamentous remnants can recanalize.

Functional development

The liver constitutes 10% of the weight of the fetus at 9 weeks' gestation, decreasing to 4% of the neonate and around 2% of adult bodyweight. The fetal hepatocytes are smaller than the mature cells, lack many enzyme systems and are deficient in glycogen.

Carbohydrate metabolism

Neonatal hypoglycemia is a common problem and highlights the crucial role that the liver plays in glucose metabolism. The fetus receives all its glucose from the mother, via the placenta; following birth, the newborn rapidly acquires the ability to maintain independent glucose homeostasis [5]. By the 9th week of gestation the fetal hepatocytes are able to synthesize glycogen. At term, stores of glycogen are high (40–60 mg/g of liver), providing some reserve for the neonate until milk production and digestion start. A healthy term baby can withstand a fast of 12 hours by the liver generating and releasing glucose by glycogenolysis [6]. Glycogenolysis is catalyzed by glycogen phosphorylase, the activity of which is promoted by glucagon and epinephrine. Following delivery, there is a rise in glucagon and a fall in insulin levels. Premature neonates lack the ability to effectively store and break down glycogen and so are at greater risk of hypoglycemia.

Following birth and before the establishment of effective feeding, glucose is in short supply and ketogenesis has yet to commence. The neonate depends on gluconeogenesis from lactate and pyruvate, which is thought to be stimulated by the high circulating levels of glucagon and catecholamines following delivery.

Gluconeogenesis is insignificant in the fetal liver [7], probably due to high insulin levels and low levels of the rate-limiting enzyme phosphoenolpyruvate carboxykinase, the activity of which rises rapidly following birth. Similarly, levels of hepatic galactokinase, the enzyme responsible for phosphorylation of galactose, increase near term. This allows the newborn to metabolize galactose in its diet. Interestingly, the utilization of glucose by the fetal liver is low, using amino acids and lactate for energy instead. Following birth, there is little glucose utilization by the liver of the neonate; instead, galactose is preferred for carbohydrate synthesis, and glucose is utilized preferentially by peripheral tissues. Glucose-6-phosphatase activity, needed to convert glucose-6-phosphate into glucose, is low in the fetal liver. Thus glucose production is low, promoting the storage of glycogen to the required high level. Levels of this enzyme also increase near term.

The transition of glucose metabolism from the fetus to the newborn is highly complex and the controls of the enzyme systems responsible for glucose metabolism are still a matter of research. Delivery and suckling also have a role in the initiation of glucocorticoid pathways and the decrease in insulin levels.

Amino acid metabolism

The majority of protein catabolism occurs in the liver, producing amino acids which may be used for protein synthesis. Amino acids may also be deaminated by aminotransferases and used to produce glucose, ketones or fatty acids. Ammonia is produced as a product of deamination and is converted into urea.

Animal studies suggest that amino acids provide about 40% of the energy requirements of the fetus, with even essential amino acids utilized as fuel. *In utero*, the fetal liver has a high uptake of amino acids, which declines following delivery. The urea cycle enzymes are well established in the second trimester, and the fetal liver accounts for the majority of ammonia clearance. Accumulation of ammonia is toxic and contributes to the raised intracranial pressure and encephalopathy seen in acute liver failure.

Nearly all amino acids cross the placenta from mother to fetus by active transport, the exceptions being glutamate, serine and aspartate which are produced by the fetal liver. The enzyme systems necessary for the regulation of amino acids are expressed at birth, but the appearance of p-hydroxyphenyl pyruvate oxidase may be delayed. This enzyme is responsible for the breakdown of tyrosine, and may account for a transient tyrosinemia following delivery.

Lipid metabolism

The oxidation of fatty acids provides a major source of energy for the developing fetus [8]. Fatty acids may be synthesized by the fetus, non-esterified fatty acids may diffuse from the placenta or, in the case of some long chain fatty acids, undergo active transport across the placenta to the fetus. Free fatty acids are stored in the liver and adipose tissue, but are not used by peripheral tissues.

Animal models suggest relatively low levels of acetyl coenzyme A carboxylase (responsible for fatty acid synthesis) in the fetal liver, as compared to adults. Ketones and glucose from the mother may act as precursors for fatty acid synthesis in the fetus.

Following birth, the accumulated fat in the fetal liver is mobilized for oxidation to produce energy as adenosine triphosphate (ATP), and for ketone body formation, which may be used peripherally in tissues. This ability to oxidize fatty acids matures rapidly in the first few days of life, in response to falling insulin and rising glucagon levels. The liver is the most important source of ketone bodies (acetoacetate, 3-hydroxybutyrate and acetone). Fat stores are particularly important for preterm infants, due to immature glucose metabolism.

Following birth, the newborn suckles and takes milk, which is relatively high in fat but low in carbohydrate compared to solid foods (see below). Long and medium chain fatty acids in the diet stimulate gluconeogenesis, by increasing the supply of gluconeogenic substrate for the liver. Weaning increases the amount of carbohydrate in the infant's diet, and the ability of the liver to produce fat is again increased.

Drug metabolism

The liver's central role in the metabolism of substances absorbed by the gut means that it has many of the enzyme systems necessary to alter alien substances (xenobiotics), such as drugs. Liver immaturity may alter the ability to clear drugs, as well as rendering it susceptible to damage from them and their breakdown products. Infant drug metabolism is complex as it depends on liver mass (usually relatively greater than in adults), protein binding and blood flow, as well as enzymatic metabolism and clearance processes.

The metabolism of most drugs involves chemical processes to modify their structure, followed by conjugation to make them more polar (water soluble), so allowing excretion. These are termed phase 1 and phase 2 reactions. Phase 1 reactions are the result of electron transfers carried out by the cytochrome P450 enzymes – nicotinamide adenine dinucleotide phosphate (NADPH) and NADPH-cytochrome c reductase. They cause oxidation by electron removal or sometimes reduction by electron addition. Phase 1 reactions also include hydrolysis of esters and amides, sulfation, dehalogenation, N-dealkylation and O-demethylation.

Cytochrome P450 (CYP) is a group of iron-containing membrane-bound enzymes found in endoplasmic reticulum and mitochondria. There are at least 57 human CYP genes producing enzymes which are classified according to the degree of amino acid homogeneity shown [9]. There are at least 18 families of CYP enzymes; they are named "CYP" plus the family number, followed by a letter, then a final number. Great variation is therefore possible between individuals, explaining some differences in drug handling.

Phase 2 reactions involve conjugation with a substrate to form a more polar and water-soluble conjugate, for example a glucuronide, sulfate or acetylated derivative. Glucuronidation involves the addition of an activated form of glucose (uridine diphosphate glucuronic acid, UDPGA) by the enzyme glucuronyl transferase. The glucuronide compounds so formed are readily excreted in urine or, in the case of larger compounds, in bile. Bilirubin is excreted in this way; however, glucuronyl transferase activity is low in the newborn, so a significant amount of hemolysis will overload the conjugating capacity of the enzyme and result in an unconjugated hyperbilirubinemia. Phenobarbital may be used to induce the enzyme.

The expression of CYP enzymes is an important factor in the development of drug metabolism in the fetus and newborn. CYP enzymes are active in the human liver early in intrauterine development; indeed, many systems are available for xenobiotic metabolism before 8 weeks' development. There is a gradual increase in activity throughout fetal development, and a major increase following birth.

To analyze the development of all the CYP enzymes is beyond the scope of this chapter, so we will attempt to highlight some examples of the CYP enzyme groups. The CYP 3A family serves as a good example of development; it is the most abundant of the CYP enzymes and is involved in the metabolism of many common drugs [10]. CYP 3A7 is the most abundant CYP enzyme in the fetus, is present during organogenesis and plays a role in steroid metabolism. Expression of this enzyme ceases at delivery. Conversely, CYP 3A4 is the most abundant member of the CYP 3A family following birth and is involved in the metabolism of over 70 drugs; its expression is low in the fetus but increases to 50% of adult levels by 1 year of life. CYP 2E1 is involved in the metabolism of alcohol and is responsible for the conversion of acetaminophen to the hepatotoxic metabolite N-acetyl-P-benzoquinone-imine. CYP 2E1 expression is low in the fetus, increasing to around 40% of adult levels at 1 year of age and is not fully expressed until 10 years.

The development of the phase 2 enzymes is less well understood; however, there are significant differences in gene expression between infancy and adulthood, as well as genetic polymorphism. The uridine glucuronyl transferase enzymes catalyze the glucuronidation of bilirubin, as well as agents such as morphine and acetaminophen. In the midterm fetus the glucuronidation of morphine is only 10–20% of adult levels. Following birth, morphine glucuronidation reaches mature levels at around 2–6 months, but this may be delayed until 2 years of age. Similar polymorphism has been identified for other glucuronyl transferase enzymes. Abnormalities of uridine glucuronyl transferase 1A (UGT1A) are responsible for Crigler–Najjar syndrome and Gilbert syndrome, which are described later in this chapter.

Development of bile formation and secretion

The liver is responsible for the excretion of bilirubin, bile acids and xenobiotics with bile into the small intestine, for ultimate elimination in the feces. It plays an important role in nutrition, as excretion of bile acids into the intestinal lumen is involved in the absorption of long chain fatty acids and fat-soluble vitamins as well as a number of drugs and hormones. This is of particular importance in the nutrition and thus growth of infants with cholestasis.

The immaturity of bile synthesis and secretion is clinically apparent in the susceptibility of the sick neonate to develop cholestasis in response to sepsis, administration of parenteral nutrition (PN), as well as the phenomena of physiological jaundice and breast milk jaundice in the healthy baby. However, understanding of the development of bile formation and secretion in the fetus is limited.

The composition of bile in the newborn is different to that in the adult, with higher concentrations of hyocholic acid as well as some unusual bile acids. Soon after birth, the concentrations of the bile acids cholate and chenodeoxycholate increase rapidly. Bile secretion starts at 4 months' gestation and thereafter the biliary system always contains bile, which secreted into the gut gives meconium its distinctive color [11]. Bile secretion appears to be low in the neonate and increases throughout infancy. Similarly, the ability of the gallbladder to empty in response to a test feed occurs soon after birth, but is reduced in preterm neonates of 27–32 weeks' gestation.

Bile flow is driven by the secretion and enterohepatic circulation of bile acids. Bile acids absorbed from the small intestine are taken up from portal blood by the Na-dependent bile salt importer proteins. They are rapidly transported across the hepatocyte cytoplasm, and then secreted into the bile canaliculi by the bile salt export pump (BSEP), against a steep concentration gradient. Mutation of the gene responsible for BSEP is responsible for progressive familial intrahepatic cholestasis 2 (PFIC 2); this and related conditions are described in the section concerned with metabolic causes of conjugated hyperbilirubinemia.

Conjugated bilirubin is secreted into bile by means of a separate transporter protein, MRP2, mutation of which leads to Dubin–Johnson syndrome. This autosomal recessive condition results in a mild conjugated hyperbilirubinemia with normal liver function tests. Dubin–Johnson syndrome is asymptomatic, and affected individuals have a normal lifespan (Fig. 8.2).

Cholestasis

Cholestasis is classically regarded as due to an anatomical blockage or obstruction of part of the biliary tree. However, the various constituents of bile are secreted by different transporter proteins and thus deficiencies, or abnormalities, of these may cause cholestasis. The hepatocyte is the main cell responsible for the manufacture and secretion of bile acids and bile; thus the liver is the organ most likely to be damaged by bile acid retention, when bile flow is reduced. The intracellular accumulation of bile acids appears to be the most significant pathological consequence of cholestasis.

Obstruction of the biliary tree, as in biliary atresia, or impaired secretion by the hepatocyte (e.g. PFIC2) can lead to a high concentration of bile acids in the hepatocyte cytoplasm. Bile acids exert their deleterious effects by a number of mechanisms; they may act as detergents which alter membrane structure and function, or by altering

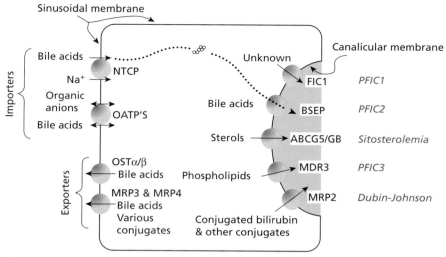

Figure 8.2 Roles for critical hepatic transporters in the formation of bile and adaptation to cholestasis. On the left is a representation of the sinusoidal surface and on the right, a canalicular surface. Diseases associated with defects in specific canalicular transporter genes are noted in italics. Note that bile acids have several means of transport across the sinusoidal membrane, both import and export, whereas there is one canalicular bile acid transporter, BSEP. These transporters allow for fine-tuning of intracellular bile acid concentrations as a way of adapting to a variety of cholestatic conditions. The principal means for bile acid flux across the hepatocyte is shown by the dotted line. NTCP, Na+ /taurocholate co-transporting polypeptide; OATP, organic acid transporting polypeptide; OST, organic solute transporter; MRP, multidrug resistance-related protein; FIC1, familial intrahepatic cholestasis 1; BSEP, bile salt export pump; MDR, multidrug resistance protein; PFIC, progressive familial intrahepatic cholestasis. Official gene designations: *FIC1 (ATP8B1), BSEP (ABCB11), MDR3 (ABCB4), and MRP2 (ABCC2)*. Reproduced from Karpen [12] with permission from Cambridge University Press.

cellular signaling pathways and gene expression. CYP 450 pathways are activated to detoxify the liver; Kupffer cells, stellate cells and myofibroblasts are also activated, potentially leading to fibrosis [12].

Neonatal jaundice
The following section deals with jaundice in infancy; it is not intended to be an exhaustive list of differential diagnoses but rather an illustration of the pathophysiological mechanisms described previously. Some of the conditions are rare, and a few only become manifest later in childhood; however, the jaundiced baby is a problem commonly encountered by the pediatric anesthesiologist. Neonatal jaundice has a variety of causes which may require investigation, and of crucial importance is the diagnosis of treatable conditions, such as biliary atresia. The causes of neonatal jaundice described below are divided into unconjugated and conjugated hyperbilirubinemia.

Unconjugated hyperbilirubinemia
The excretion of bilirubin, a breakdown product of heme, is one of the principal roles of the liver. Bilirubin is a toxic molecule, and diffusion of its free form into neural tissue, particularly the basal ganglia, can cause kernicterus in the premature neonate. As bilirubin is bound tightly to albumin, the usually low free levels may be increased by hypoalbuminemia or by drugs which dis-place bilirubin from its binding sites, e.g. sulfonamides and furosemide.

Physiological jaundice
Transient neonatal jaundice occurs in around 50% of babies in the first week of life [13,14]. It is due to immaturity of glucuronyltransferase, leading to an unconjugated hyperbilirubinemia. Occasionally the jaundice may be significant, with a serum bilirubin over 12mg/dL, which may be associated with prematurity, bruising and breast feeding. Physiological jaundice peaks at day 3 of life and declines thereafter, but the hyperbilirubinemia may persist for as long as 14 days. Treatment is usually unnecessary as the jaundice is self-limiting; however, if it is slow to clear, phototherapy can be used, which is an effective treatment.

Breast milk jaundice
Unconjugated hyperbilirubinemia associated with breast feeding is common. Jaundice tends to occur after day 4 of life, may overlap with physiological jaundice, and can sometimes be protracted. The etiology is still to be elucidated but hypotheses include enhanced enterohepatic recirculation of bilirubin due to free fatty acids in breast milk, and the action of β-glucuronidase causing deconjugation of bilirubin. The diagnosis is clinical and no treatment is usually required, other than reassurance and exclusion of more sinister causes of liver disease.

Crigler–Najjar syndrome

Crigler–Najjar syndrome is an autosomal recessive condition resulting from deficiency of the enzyme bilirubin uridine diphosphate glucuronyltransferase (UDPGT). The syndrome is divided into two types: type 1 has no UDPGT present, and in type 2 levels of the enzyme are reduced. Consequently, type 1 is the more severe condition and presents in the newborn with rising unconjugated bilirubin levels, with the risk of kernicterus.

Management of type 1 Crigler–Najjar syndrome often involves phototherapy. Acute exacerbations may be precipitated by sepsis and require plasmapheresis or exchange transfusion. Liver transplantation is a long-term option to avoid neurological deterioration. Type 2 Crigler–Najjar syndrome follows a more benign course.

Gilbert syndrome

Gilbert syndrome is a condition leading to mild unconjugated hyperbilirubinemia and results from a defect of the UDPGT gene. The affected individual, usually male, has mild jaundice worsened by intercurrent illness. Presentation is typically in teenage years, but heterozygotes for the genetic defect may present in the neonatal period. Treatment is unnecessary.

Conjugated hyperbilirubinemia

The identification of conjugated hyperbilirubinemia essentially allows the clinician to distinguish jaundice which is due to liver disease from the more common but generally more benign causes, which present with unconjugated hyperbilirubinemia.

The liver synthesizes all of the clotting factors except for the von Willebrand fraction of factor VIII, which is derived from vascular endothelium. Factors II, VII, IX and X require vitamin K for their synthesis, so their levels are liable to fall if there is any biliary obstruction, because the fat-soluble vitamin K is poorly absorbed from the gut, unless dietary fat is emulsified by bile salts. Vitamin K deficiency bleeding (VKDB) occurs in 1:10,000 babies. It may occur on the first day or in the first week of life (classic). In around half of cases it may occur after the first week, and is usually associated with breast feeding or liver disease. The risk of intracranial hemorrhage is high in this group. Vitamin K supplementation at birth is routine in Europe and North America.

Acquired cholestasis
Cholestasis associated with sepsis

Sepsis originating outside the liver is the most common cause of cholestasis in infants. It appears not to involve damage to hepatocytes but is rather an impairment of hepatocyte function, perhaps explaining the particular susceptibility of the immature liver to various insults. In animal models the administration of endotoxin lipopolysaccharide invariably leads to a sustained reduction in bile flow. The mechanism appears to be due to endotoxin-mediated cytokine release from Kupffer cells, inducing signaling changes in the sinusoidal membranes of neighboring hepatocytes to reduce bile formation [15]. There are also endotoxin receptors on the membranes of hepatocytes, implying a direct action of endotoxin.

The liver also plays a central role in the acute-phase response to infection and injury. This is mediated by endotoxin, and results in expression of genes coding for a host of proteins and enzymes necessary to fight infection and repair tissue, whilst suppressing expression of hepatocyte transport proteins. Within an hour of endotoxin exposure, both BSEP and MRP2 proteins are reduced significantly, thus reducing bile secretion.

Cholestasis secondary to parenteral nutrition

Cholestasis associated with PN administration is particularly common in the neonatal population. The clinical scenario is familiar to the pediatric anesthesiologist – a premature neonate, who has undergone extensive bowel resection, is in trouble with sepsis and requires PN administration.

The mechanisms of PN cholestasis are unclear but prematurity, infection, short gut and toxic or missing components in the PN regimen all probably play a role. The inherently immature ability of the neonatal liver to produce bile and handle drugs suggests that neonatal livers are particularly susceptible to cholestatic insults. It is interesting that PN-associated cholestasis is rare in older children and adults. Recurrent central venous catheter infections will often provoke acute rises in serum conjugated bilirubin. A lack of oral intake interrupts the enterohepatic circulation of bile acids and may contribute to cholestasis, possibly secondary to abnormal gut hormone secretion. Bacterial overgrowth in the small intestine may lead to bacterial translocation and endotoxin production. The absence or presence of certain constituents within PN remains an attractive explanation but to date, there is little strong evidence to implicate any particular compound. However, PN regimens low in lipid and supplemented with taurine and carnitine may be associated with less cholestasis.

The striking feature of PN-associated cholestasis is the association with prematurity, intestinal failure and sepsis [16]. This provides the clinician with a therapeutic rationale to support the infant nutritionally, allowing growth and development while avoiding the progression of cholestasis to liver cirrhosis. Attention to strict aseptic technique is crucial to avoid central venous catheter infections. Innovative intestinal surgical techniques may lessen the chance of bacterial translocation and reduce the risk of sepsis. If possible, an increase in enteral feeding is

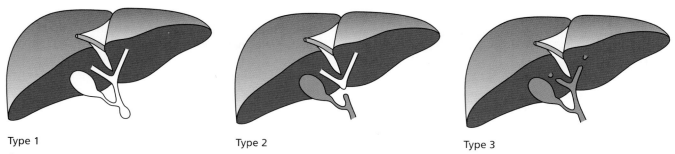

Type 1   Type 2   Type 3

Figure 8.3 Classification of biliary atresia. Type 1: atresia affecting the common bile duct, often associated with proximal biliary cyst. Type 2: atresia affecting the common hepatic duct. Type 3: obliteration and atresia affecting the whole of the extrahepatic biliary tree. Reproduced from Millar [17] with permission from Wiley-Blackwell.

encouraged, to reduce PN administration, stimulate gut hormone secretion and support the enterohepatic circulation. The PN formulation should contain sufficient trace elements, amino acids and essential fatty acids.

Structural abnormalities
Biliary atresia
Biliary atresia accounts for about a third of cases of neonatal cholestasis. It is an important condition, as delay in diagnosis and treatment can result in irreversible liver damage. It remains the most common indication for liver transplantation in children [17].

Biliary atresia is characterized by a progressive inflammation and destruction of the extrahepatic bile ducts, as well as damage to intrahepatic bile ducts; if left untreated, hepatic fibrosis and biliary cirrhosis develop. The most accepted classification system is based on the anatomical location of the damage (Fig. 8.3).

The condition has an incidence of around 1:10,000–15,000 in the United Kingdom and the United States. The etiology of biliary atresia remains obscure but the association with other anomalies makes an embryological hypothesis attractive (syndromic biliary atresia). Approximately 10% of infants with biliary atresia have associated anomalies including polysplenia, abnormal portal vein, interrupted inferior vena cava and cardiac defects.

Infants with biliary atresia are typically healthy term babies who initially appear normal, but soon develop persistent jaundice and pale stools. Lethargy, pruritus and poor weight gain soon become apparent. Hepatomegaly is often noted and as the condition progresses, signs of portal hypertension such as splenomegaly and ascites appear.

On confirmation of the diagnosis, the surgical treatment is the Kasai portoenterostomy, which involves excision of the atretic portion of the biliary tree, formation of a Roux-en-Y loop of jejunum and its anastomosis to the transected tissue at the porta hepatis, to allow bile drain-

age. As biliary atresia is a progressive inflammatory condition, many children proceed to liver cirrhosis despite achieving apparently adequate bile drainage. The success rate is much worse in those older than 8 weeks or with advanced hepatic fibrosis or established cirrhosis. The Kasai procedure achieves some biliary drainage in 70% of infants which may be adequate to ensure survival to 5 years in around 60% of cases; however, in around 30% of infants, the symptoms and signs of hepatic dysfunction occur despite successful surgery [18,19].

Many children progress to cirrhosis and suffer symptoms of portal hypertension, which include splenomegaly, variceal hemorrhage and ascites. Liver transplantation offers excellent results in this group of children. See Chapter 27 for a discussion of the anesthetic management of liver transplantation.

Choledochal cyst
Choledochal cysts are congenital localized swellings of the bile ducts with an incidence of 1:100,000; they are more common in girls (female:male ratio 5:1). Interestingly, the condition is more prevalent in Japan. The position of the cysts is variable, leading to a number of classification systems; they are most frequently found on the common bile duct, but may occur anywhere along the biliary tree (Fig. 8.4). The etiology of the cysts remains obscure.

Presentation may occur at any age and antenatal diagnosis on antenatal scanning sometimes occurs. Symptoms are classically of pain and jaundice with a palpable abdominal mass. Diagnosis is confirmed by ultrasound scanning or magnetic resonance cholangiopancreatography. Secondary stone formation, cholangitis, pancreatitis and spontaneous rupture may occur; the cysts also have a potential for malignant change in the long term. Portal hypertension may occur due to portal vein compression or as a result of cirrhosis. Treatment is by surgical excision of the cyst with biliary drainage via a Roux-en-Y anastomosis. The prognosis is generally very good and reversal of portal hypertension has been reported.

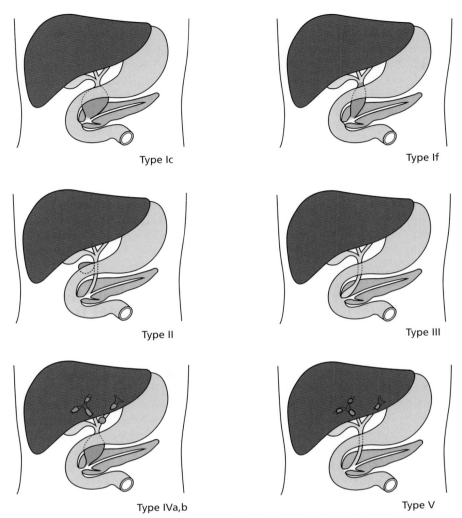

Figure 8.4 Classification of choledochal cysts. Type I dilations may be cystic (Ic) or fusiform (If) and typically associated with pancreaticobiliary malunion. Other types are II (diverticulum), III (choledochocele), IVa (multiple cystic dilations of the extrahepatic and intrahepatic ducts), IVb (multiple extrahepatic cysts), and V (single or multiple intrahepatic duct cysts). Reproduced from Millar [17] with permission from Wiley-Blackwell.

Alagille syndrome

Alagille syndrome is a rare autosomal dominant disorder affecting 1:100,000 deliveries and is characterized by the paucity of interlobular bile ducts. It is caused by a mutation of the *Jagged1* gene [20], which encodes for proteins involved in the Notch signaling pathway. The syndrome is characterized by triangular facies, butterfly hemivertebrae and peripheral pulmonary stenosis often leading to pulmonary hypertension. The cardiac abnormalities are variable and may include hypoplastic pulmonary arteries, pulmonary valve stenosis and ventricular septal defect. The affected infants are often developmentally delayed and short in stature. The severity of the liver disease is variable, with many children having mild disease, but pruritus is often severe.

Treatment is supportive with management of pruritus, nutritional support and in some cases corrective cardiac procedures. Liver transplantation is an option for those with decompensated liver disease or in whom pruritus is intolerable; however, the outcome following transplantation may be affected by the associated cardiac disease, and careful planning and assessment are necessary.

Metabolic conditions
α1-Antitrypsin deficiency

α1-Antitrypsin deficiency (α1-ATD) is the most common inherited disorder causing neonatal jaundice, with an incidence of 1 in 1600 livebirths. Only a few patients with the deficiency develop liver disease, but it is a common cause of emphysematous lung disease in adults

[21]. α-1-antitrypsin is a protease inhibitor produced by the liver, which is an acute-phase reactant and responsible for inactivation of leukocyte elastase. Deficiency is due to mutation of its gene which is found on chromosome 14. Over 70 phenotypes are described but the PiZZ phenotype (Pi stands for protease inhibitor, ZZ is the isoelectric focusing banding pattern of the abnormal α-1-antitrypsin protein) is the most significant, with homozygous PiZZ individuals at risk of progressive liver disease. The pathogenesis of the condition remains obscure and is associated with a build-up of an abnormal α1-antitrypsin molecule in the hepatocyte. However, as not all individuals with the genetic defect develop liver disease, other pathophysiological processes are likely to be important.

The clinical presentation is similar to biliary atresia: a jaundiced baby with pale stools and hepatomegaly. Infants who are homozygotes have a low serum α1-antitrypsin level. Liver biopsy reveals histological findings of neonatal hepatitis and periodic acid–Schiff (PAS)-positive granules within the hepatocytes. Management consists of nutritional support, fat-soluble vitamin supplementation and treatment of pruritus. The prognosis is variable; many individuals do well, but a proportion progress to cirrhosis and may deteriorate precipitately, requiring liver transplantation. The outcome following liver transplantation in α1-antitrypsin deficiency is good.

Progressive familial intrahepatic cholestasis

Progressive familial intrahepatic cholestasis (PFIC) is a group of autosomal recessive disorders associated with abnormalities of bile canalicular transport proteins [22]. PFIC-1 is caused by mutation of the *FIC* gene, which is expressed in the bile canaliculi; it is characterized by cholestasis, diarrhea and pancreatitis presenting in the first months of life. Bile duct paucity is seen on liver biopsy. Treatment is generally supportive but external biliary diversion has been used in some cases. Liver cirrhosis occurs in early childhood and may progress to require liver transplantation. PFIC-2 is due to deficiency of the bile salt export pump and is similar to PFIC-1, except pancreatitis is not seen. It has a worse prognosis and children often require liver transplantation in the first decade of life. PFIC-3 is due to a defect in the canalicular phospholipids transporter MDR3, presents with intrahepatic cholestasis but with an elevated γ-GT, unlike PFIC-1 and PFIC-2. The condition is similar to PFIC-1, but presentation is often delayed into adult life and the prognosis is variable.

Cystic fibrosis

Cystic fibrosis affects around 1:3000 livebirths and is the most common life-threatening autosomal recessive condition. It affects the lungs, pancreas, sweat glands and liver.

There is great variation in the severity of liver disease; it affects one-third of individuals with cystic fibrosis but is the most important non-pulmonary cause of death. Liver disease usually presents in the teenage years but may rarely present in infancy with neonatal cholestasis, inspissated bile ducts or meconium ileus [23]. The latter presentation is particularly important, as it may be associated with sepsis and PN administration. The neonatal cholestasis usually resolves spontaneously, and appears not to predict future liver disease.

The reader should understand that although the causes of liver disease are varied, the pattern of progression to advanced liver disease may be similar. Therapeutic advances in hepatology and transplantation offer much hope to children with liver disease, but present an array of challenges to the pediatric anesthesiologist.

Developmental physiology of the gastrointestinal tract

Overview

Anesthesiologists tend not to take much notice of the gastrointestinal tract, except perhaps to wonder if the preoperative *nil per os* (NPO) period has been long enough. It probably merits more attention than this. The proper functioning of the gastrointestinal tract is fundamental to the well-being of the organism, in some ways as much as the cardiovascular, respiratory and renal tracts, on which we concentrate so much, quite rightly. It is true that problems in the gastrointestinal tract may take longer to show their full impact, but we all know from experience of our own physiology how little we notice our gastrointestinal tract when it functions well and how ill we feel when it does not. Some of the sickest patients the anesthesiologist will ever encounter are in this desperate condition as a result of problems which have arisen in the gastrointestinal tract.

The great majority of animals, and all of those regarded as the more complex, conform to the same basic body plan: they are modified tubes and the inner surface is, or originates from, the gastrointestinal tract. The importance of this collection of structures and organs is indicated by the degree to which the developmental plan is conserved across classes of organisms which otherwise vary enormously. The genetic scientist can learn a great deal about the gastrointestinal tract of the human by studying that of the fruit fly or the nematode.

We are not so much interested in the details of the genetics of development, although the understanding of this topic has grown amazingly in the recent past, and our realization of its complexity similarly. This section will describe the embryology of the gastrointestinal tract in outline, and show how the anomalies which the anesthesiologist will encounter may have arisen. Relatively more attention will be given to those points which have a relevance to the diseases and conditions which may be seen by the practical pediatric anesthesiologist, but the management of these conditions will be covered in other chapters.

The development of the gastrointestinal tract is dictated by an unavoidable deadline. By the time a baby is born, the gastrointestinal tract must be ready to supply fully the baby's needs for fluid and electrolyte intake, to digest its food, initially completely milk, to provide sufficient energy and biochemical raw materials for extremely rapid growth and development, and to do so efficiently enough not to upset the immature homeostatic control mechanisms. At the same time, a sudden onslaught of pathogenic organisms and potential poisons has to be resisted. Within a few months of birth, the gastrointestinal tract has to be ready for weaning from its comforting milk diet to whatever the environment can be made to provide – one of the first crucial steps to independent existence. Thereafter, the demands made on the gastrointestinal tract do not alter so radically, and although there is a lot of growing to be done and full functional maturity will not be attained for some years, the processes remain more or less unchanged for the rest of the individual's life. This timescale means that the pace of development *in utero* is hectic, and after birth many of the remaining functional changes normally happen soon.

It will be obvious that physiological experiments on the developing gut are difficult to carry out, even in animal models, so there are gaps in scientific knowledge, sometimes glaring enough to be obvious to the non-specialist. Some (maybe even much) of what is known is extrapolated from data from other species, and although the homogeneity of gastrointestinal tract design means that this may often be accurate, some of it may not.

Basic gastrointestinal tract physiology

An abbreviated account of the physiology of the gastrointestinal tract follows. It is merely intended as an *aide-mémoire*. The interested reader is referred to standard physiology texts for a more complete account.

The gastrointestinal tract epithelium comprises four basic types of cell: enterocytes, goblet cells (secreting mucus), endocrine cells, and Paneth cells. The 'basic' gastrointestinal tract cell is the enterocyte, which has a brush border of microvilli facing in to the gut lumen and tight junctions with its neighboring enterocytes. It sits on a basement membrane, beneath which capillaries and lacteals provide access to the circulation and lymphatic systems. Above the basement membrane, between adjacent cells, the basolateral surfaces border the fluid-filled paracellular space, which is crucial to the handling and transport of fluid and electrolytes. The enterocytes are

arranged on villi, tiny finger-like mucosal projections into the gut lumen (Fig. 8.5).

The mass of crowded villi give the healthy gut luminal surface a velvety macroscopic appearance. Between villi, pits project down into the gut submucosa – these are known as crypts (of Lieberkühn). Enterocytes originate from stem cells in the crypts and there is a continuous procession of maturing cells from the crypts out and up on to the villi, gradually working their way to the tips of the villi, from where they are shed into the lumen.

The enterocyte has numerous digestive and absorptive functions. Substances can be taken into the cell by pinocytosis, passive diffusion, facilitated diffusion, and active transport. Enormously complex neural networks coordinate activity. This is explored in more detail in the section on the development of motility.

Basic gastrointestinal tract embryology

An understanding of basic embryology is necessary to make sense of the common structural anomalies.

By day 5 after fertilization, the late blastocyst consists of a hollow ball of cells. The outer cells will go on to form the trophoblast, and later the structures that will make the fetal component of the placenta. An inner cell mass forms a small mass lying against the side of the blastocyst. The inner cell mass soon develops into a bilayered structure: on one side, ectodermal cells border the amniotic cavity and on the other, the endoderm borders the yolk sac. The plate-like embryo starts to curl round and over, side to side and head to tail, so that the endoderm becomes more and more the lining of the inner side, and cells migrating inwards from the primitive streak on the ectodermal side become mesodermal cells, which surround the endoderm. The endoderm still communicates with the yolk sac which lies outside the middle part of the embryo. By day 25, the caudal and cephalic ends of the endoderm have invaginated at the anterior and posterior intestinal portals to form the blind-ending tubes of the primitive gut. The gut has buds which grow out to form, in order from head to tail, the thyroid, the tracheobronchial bud, the liver, the pancreas, and the allantois, a hollow endodermal projection which still lies outside the embryo.

It is customary to describe the gut in four parts: the pharynx, which extends as far as the tracheobronchial bud; the foregut, from there as far as the liver bud; then the midgut, as far as the posterior intestinal portal, which is where the caudal blind-ending tube starts in the early embryo – in the adult, this point will be two-thirds of the way along the transverse colon. From here onwards is the hindgut.

The gut becomes an open tube at both ends; cephalad, a pit develops, which is closed by the buccopharyngeal membrane. This meets the pharynx and perforates to

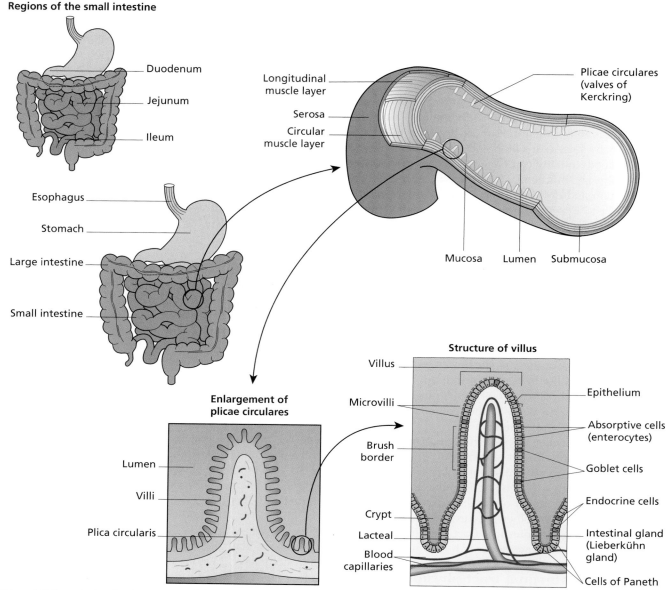

Figure 8.5 The gut, showing the structure of the small intestine from macroscopic to microscopic. Reproduced from reference [134] with permission from Encyclopaedia Britannica.

form the proximal opening. At the end of the hindgut a similar pit grows inwards to meet the hindgut and form the common opening of the gut and urogenital system, the cloaca. In the foregut, the tracheobronchial bud develops ventrally; normally the only communication between the two is where the larynx opens into the oropharynx. The esophagus elongates as the tracheobronchial bud grows downwards and the heart descends [24].

The most common congenital defect in this area is esophageal atresia and tracheo-esophageal fistula which occurs about 1:4000 births [25]. The cause is unclear. In the most common form (over 80% of cases), the upper esophagus ends as a blind tube and the distal esophagus

opens into the trachea posteriorly near the level of the carina. Other combinations are seen but esophageal atresia or stenosis without any fistula into the respiratory tract is unusual. Chromosomal abnormality (e.g. trisomy 21) is sometimes associated, but in most cases there is no other anomaly (Fig. 8.6).

The stomach starts as a dilation in the foregut. It rotates round clockwise so that the left side becomes anterior and the right side becomes posterior; as this process occurs, its mesentery is dragged behind and forms a pocket of peritoneum behind the stomach – the lesser sac. The stomach is therefore surrounded by peritoneum, preventing its fixation and allowing for the necessary movement

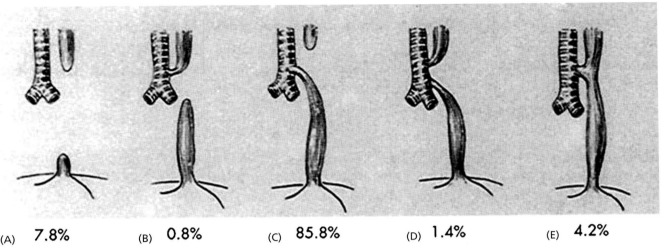

(A) **7.8%**   (B) **0.8%**   (C) **85.8%**   (D) **1.4%**   (E) **4.2%**

Figure 8.6 Anatomical classification of anomalies of the esophagus and trachea, with approximate incidences. Type A: esophageal atresia without tracheoesophageal fistula (TEF); Type B: esophageal atresia with proximal TEF; Type C: esophageal atresia with distal TEF; Type D: esophageal atresia with proximal and distal TEF; Type E: H-type TEF without esophageal atresia. Reproduced from Gross [135] with permission from Elsevier.

and expansion. The posterior wall (now left side) grows faster than the right, causing the distal part to be pushed out to the right. The liver bud develops from the ventral part of the duodenum; it grows up and forwards, so its upper surface lies in contact with the septum transversum and this structure, part of which gives rise to the diaphragm, is all that separates it from the base of the right lung and the heart. The duodenum also participates in this left-to-anterior rotation, so that the connection with the liver, which is drawn out into the thin common bile duct, is pulled behind the duodenum and ends up opening into the duodenum on the left side, at the papilla (see Figure 8.1).

There are two pancreatic buds, ventral and dorsal. The ventral bud is also pulled round behind the duodenum and ends up touching and partially fusing with its dorsal counterpart. It is still recognizable in the adult as the uncinate process of the pancreas, which normally lies a little below the main body. The pancreatic ducts generally fuse to form a common pancreatic duct, which opens, with the common bile duct, into the duodenum at the papilla.

From here on, the midgut grows enormously, forming a long loop. Its blood supply, the superior mesenteric artery, is pulled out in the mesentery. The midgut undergoes rotation so the distal part is pulled upwards and to the right counterclockwise, so that the dilation which will form the cecum ends up in the right upper quadrant in front of the rest of the gut and the liver. As this part later elongates to form the ascending colon, it drops down towards the right lower quadrant, so the final rotation ends up approximating 270° (Fig. 8.7).

The small bowel loops repeatedly as it lengthens, whereas the colon does not. The growth of the midgut is so rapid that it cannot be accommodated in the abdominal cavity, so it herniates out. As the abdominal cavity

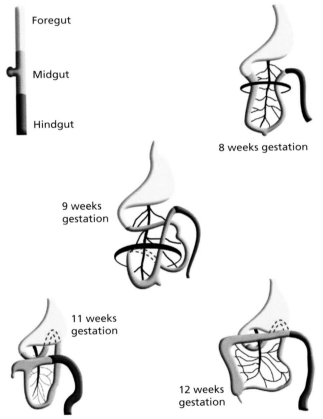

Figure 8.7 Rotation of embryonic gut. Reproduced from reference [136] with permission from Health Education Assets Library.

becomes more spacious because of the growth of the whole fetus and the lifting up of the heart and liver, the midgut is gradually retracted back into the abdominal cavity by 11 weeks' gestation, the yolk sac obliterates and the abdominal wall closes over it, leaving only the umbilical cord and its vessels passing out of the body cavity. At the point where the involuted yolk sac meets the midgut, a remnant may persist (Meckel's diverticulum) which may contain ectopic stomach epithelium, or there may be a fibrous cord, sometimes containing a vitelline cyst, tethering it to the anterior abdominal wall.

The hindgut is separated from the urogenital opening by the downward growth of the urogenital septum, which meets the cloacal membrane, dividing it into two: the anterior part, derived from the allantois, which will form the urinary bladder and genital tract, and the posterior part which forms the rectum. By 9 weeks' gestation, the ectodermal anal pit perforates into the rectum, opening the distal end of the gut.

Imperforate anus occurs in around 1:5000 births and ranges from a thin membrane across the anus to complete failure of the formation of the anal canal and associated sphincters. There may be other defects in urogenital structures, and the anomaly may be associated with spinal defects, omphalocele, and aganglionosis [26].

Congenital abdominal wall defects: gastroschisis and omphalocele (exomphalos)

In gastroschisis, there is a defect in the abdominal wall, generally to the right of the umbilicus, and usually less than 5 cm across. The etiology is uncertain; there may be more than one causative factor [27]. It could be that a failure of mesenchymal cell migration means that the abdominal wall never completely closes over the defect left by the physiological herniation of the gut, which is normally retracted into the abdominal cavity around the 10th week of gestation, and so as growth of the gut progresses, the gut reherniates. Possibly in some cases a weakness or ischemia of the abdominal wall causes it to rupture, having initially closed. The position to the right of the umbilicus may indicate defective involution of the right umbilical vein. Sometimes the liver is also herniated. The herniated gut is not covered and is exposed to amniotic fluid, and is necessarily exposed after birth. The blood supply to the herniated part can be compromised, and the ischemic gut can be reduced to fibrous bands or may contain segments of atresia. Even if this is not the case, the gut may not develop normally and its function may be impaired. Sometimes the gut is covered with a fibrinous "peel" which may form as a response to gut contents which have leaked into the amniotic fluid bathing the exposed gut; the presence of a peel predicts a worse outcome [28].

In omphalocele (also known as exomphalos), the gut herniates through the umbilical ring itself, which is wide open. The gut is covered by amnion, the membrane which surrounds the umbilical cord, which forms a sac, although this may rupture, especially if it is large. The size is variable; there may be anything from only a small amount of bowel in the sac to most of the small bowel, liver and spleen.

The incidence of the two abdominal wall defects together is around 1:2000 births but the proportion of each varies by region and in many places is changing over time, the general trend in the developed world being that gastroschisis is becoming more common while omphalocele remains the same or is declining slightly, so that in many areas, gastroschisis is seen slightly more frequently than omphalocele. Gastroschisis is related to young maternal age but is often the only abnormality, just 17% or so having other congenital abnormalities, whereas in omphalocele over 60% have anomalies elsewhere [29].

Congenital umbilical hernia resembles omphalocele but in this case, the abdominal wall originally closed normally, so when the hernia occurs, it is covered by peritoneum as well as amnion.

Prune belly syndrome is an uncommon condition, occurring in less than 1:30,000 births, almost always in boys [30]. The muscles of the anterior abdominal wall are replaced by thickened collagenous bands, perhaps due to defective migration of mesenchymal elements which normally give rise to striated muscle. The abdomen therefore looks lax, the shapes of loops of bowel can be made out beneath the wrinkled skin, which gives the condition its name, and there may be visible peristalsis. The musculature of the bladder and renal tract is also affected and there may be a large thick-walled bladder, hydroureter and renal dysplasia. The very rare megacystis-microcolon intestinal hypoperistalsis syndrome presents a similar appearance.

Malrotation

When the embryo's midgut is outside the abdominal cavity before the 10th week of gestation, the gut rotates through 270° so that the cecal bud, which would lie at 6 o'clock if there were no rotation, comes first to lie at 12 o'clock with the first 180° of rotation, and then finally round at 9 o'clock with a further 90°, which brings the cecal bud to lie in the right upper quadrant, next to the liver, and means that the colon lies over (anterior to) the duodenum. The gut loops on the left return first, so that as the cecal bud descends with the growth of the ascending colon, these structures lie on the right. Where the gut mesentery comes to lie on the peritoneum, it may fuse and so fix the gut at that point; normally the C-loop of the duodenum, ascending and descending colon become fixed, and the small bowel loops and transverse colon retain a mesentery.

In malrotation, the gut rotation sometimes amounts to just 90°; if the left-sided structures return to the abdomen first, this will mean the distal parts will return first and the colon (all of it) will lie on the left and the small bowel loops will lie on the right.

If the malrotation is 90° clockwise instead of counterclockwise, then the duodenum will overlie the colon rather than the other way around.

The problems with malrotations are that the gut can be obstructed by the abnormal positioning or, lacking the normal fixation of parts of the gut to the retroperitoneum, the mesenteries can twist (volvulus), causing ischemic damage, or the abnormal peritoneal bands can themselves cause obstruction. This can commonly occur when the cecum lies to the left of the duodenum, so that the fibrous bands to the cecum lie over the duodenum (Ladd's bands) [31]. Sometimes the malrotated gut can function perfectly normally, and volvulus or obstruction occurs later in life, or it may cause no trouble and never be discovered, or only incidentally as a result of imaging or surgical exploration carried out for unrelated reasons. However, over 70% of cases present before the age of 1 year, and a similar proportion will have congenital abnormalities elsewhere. Malrotations are quite common, occurring in 1:500 births.

Intestinal atresias, stenoses and webs

The duodenum is thought to pass through a solid phase in development, the lumen being re-established by the coalescing of vacuoles in week 8–10 of gestation (there is some doubt about this account [32]). If recanalization is incomplete then a stenosis, web or atresia occurs, or if there is no connection to the lumen at all, a duplication cyst may result. Duodenal atresia is frequently (50%) associated with intrauterine growth retardation, polyhydramnios, prematurity and congenital anomalies elsewhere which may be part of the VACTERL association (vertebral, anal, cardiac, tracheo-esophageal, renal and limb anomalies [33]). Sometimes a duodenal stenosis can be surrounded by a ring of pancreatic tissue (annular pancreas), but it is not clear whether this is the cause of the stenosis or a result of it [34].

Jejunoileal atresias may be due to *in utero* interruptions in blood supply to a portion of the gut at a much later stage of development than duodenal atresias. They vary from stenosis, through cases where a small length of bowel is replaced by a fibrous band, to multiple atresias with long sections of missing gut and defects in the mesentery. Sometimes the interrupted gut may be supplied by a marginal blood vessel, and therefore a length of progressively tapering hypoplastic gut winds around it in a spiral shape, giving rise to the "apple peel" or "Christmas tree" malformation (type IIIb) [35] (Fig. 8.8). They are not particularly associated with other abnormalities. Often the gut may be dilated proximal to the obstruction and collapsed or hypoplastic distal to it,

although some stenoses may show distal dilation (windsock deformity).

Colonic atresias may occur by similar mechanisms but are more unusual – less than 15% of all intestinal atresias.

Functional development of the gastrointestinal tract – vesicles, carbohydratase enzymes, transmembrane transporters

The epithelium of the gut changes from stratified to simple columnar between the 9th and 10th weeks of gestation [36]. Some absorptive processes are possible at the stratified stage, but significant functional capability does not become evident until the columnar stage. Maturation is not uniform, either between types of cell or between regions of the gut. In general, absorptive cells mature first, then goblet and endocrine cells, and Paneth cells last. Development also proceeds from proximal to distal. Villi appear first, proliferating to such a degree that the lumen may be obliterated. Crypts develop later. Epithelial cells differentiate from stem cells in the proliferative zone, which comes to lie in the crypts; Paneth cells migrate down into the crypts, all the others up towards the tips of the villi. There are therefore two axes of development: vertically on the crypt–villus axis and along the gut on the proximo-distal axis. The interaction between the endoderm-derived epithelium and the mesodermal elements which migrate into position beneath is crucial to the organized development of the gut [37]. The villi tend to be tallest in the jejunum and get shorter more distally. The mature colon does not have villi, only crypts, but there are villi in the immature colon.

A fundamental property of absorptive cells is that they can take up substances from the lumen in vesicles. Specialized proteins associated with vesicles (e.g. clathrins and caveolin) allow for selective absorption and onward intracellular distribution of substances from the gut lumen [38,39].

Developing enterocytes are structurally different from mature ones –at around 17 weeks' gestation, giant lysosomes can be seen in the ileum. There are more lysosomes in the adult gut than in the neonate, but no giant ones [40]. The developing gut needs to absorb more macromolecules undigested (growth factors, hormones, immunoglobulins) from amniotic fluid and milk, and is therefore more permeable to these, which may account for a greater susceptibility to pathogens and allergies at this stage.

Apical carbohydratase enzyme development has been studied in some depth, particularly lactase and the double complex sucrase/isomaltase [41]. Neither enzyme appears until the epithelium becomes columnar. Thereafter levels gradually increase. From 32 weeks' gestation there is a sudden large increase in lactase and

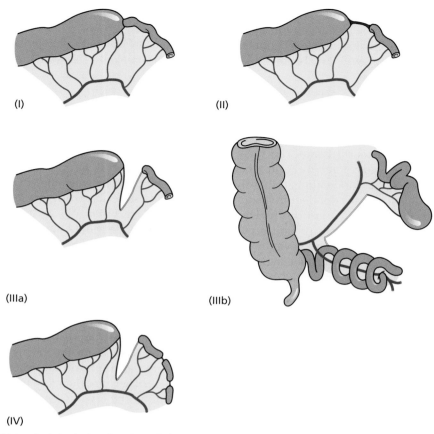

(I)   (II)

(IIIa)   (IIIb)

(IV)

Figure 8.8 Classification of jejunoileal atresia describes the pathology as type I (mucosal web), type II (fibrous cord), type IIIa (mesenteric gap defect), type IIIb ("apple peel") or type IV (multiple atresias). Reproduced from Welch et al [137] with permission from Elsevier.

sucrase activity. In most mammals (and most humans), lactase activity declines sharply after weaning (later childhood in humans), typically to 10% or so of its peak, leaving most adult humans lactose intolerant [42]. Lactase is the only enzyme capable of cleaving the disaccharide lactose into its component glucose and galactose moieties. Lactose intolerance is by far the most common disaccharide intolerance. Other disaccharide intolerances are much rarer and are the result of transporter defects, not enzyme deficiency. In those of northern European ancestry, lactase activity usually persists into adulthood. These populations often have a tradition of consuming domesticated animal milk and milk products, and may at one time have been dependent on it or at least, its availability conferred a survival advantage. Mutations reducing or eliminating the decline in lactase activity with age may have originated separately in several different human populations. The distribution of the enzymes also varies along both crypt–villus and proximo-distal axes; lactase is concentrated to more proximal regions of the small bowel, and towards the tips of the villi, where it is vulnerable to being sloughed off if there is any inflammatory

process. Sucrase is evenly distributed up the villus and further along the small bowel, but neither enzyme is found in the adult colon [43].

Development of transporters

The principal carbohydrate transporters are SGLT-1 which is a brush border (apical) sodium co-transporter for glucose and galactose, GLUT-5, which is a brush border facilitative transporter for fructose, and GLUT-2, which is a basolateral facilitator for all hexoses. Carbohydrate transporters start to be expressed during gestation, the number and density increasing and accelerating as term approaches. At birth, SGLT-1 is found along the whole length of the villus whereas in adults, it is found only on the third nearest the tip. Therefore the absorptive capacity per unit area of intestine tends to decrease with age but the total intestinal area of course increases, approximately proportional to the bodyweight after the neonatal period or slightly less [44]. The transporters are much more numerous proximally, where high carbohydrate concentrations would be expected. At the time of weaning, the transport capacity for sugars declines further and is at least in part genetically programmed, as it occurs even if a totally milk diet persists.

Amino acid transporters are more complicated; there are more types, absorbing different groups of amino acids, although their affinities may overlap with each other somewhat. Small peptides (mostly 2 and 3 amino acids) also have their own transporters.

There are specific transporters for bile salts which, unlike the other transporters, are much more numerous in the ileum. Curiously, they do not appear until weaning; presumably before that bile salts are absorbed passively all along the small bowel, as an enterohepatic circulation certainly exists during the suckling stage [45]. It may be that it is important for the development of colonic bacterial flora that bile salts enter the colon during suckling.

Carbohydrate malabsorption can be a dangerous problem. The consequences are that sugars reach the colon, where they cause an osmotic diarrhea. The sugars are fermented by colonic bacteria and hydrogen, methane and carbon dioxide are produced. By far the most common cause is a loss of the brush border carbohydratase enzymes, the most common being lactase deficiency. Congenital lactase deficiency in infants was usually fatal before the advent of lactose-free milk substitutes. Genetic defects in the other carbohydratase enzymes are very rare, but acquired deficiency can be caused by a range of factors which may cause mucosal damage, including inflammatory, ischemic or allergic processes.

Defects in nutrient transporters are rare. Glucose-galactose malabsorption is due to defective synthesis of SGLT-1.

The enteric nervous system

The enteric nervous system (ENS) is essential for the functioning of the gastrointestinal tract. All the nerves of the ENS are derived from neural crest cells and are broadly arranged into two plexuses: the inner submucosal plexus, situated as its name suggests, and the myenteric plexus, which lies between the inner circular smooth muscle layer and the outer longitudinal one. The ENS is much more than an extension of the parasympathetic branch of the autonomic nervous system. It contains a vast number of neurons (as many as the spinal cord) and many different cell types, and it is capable of functioning without any input at all from outside. Its neurons, which may be sensory, motor (both muscular and secretory) or interneurons, include types which resemble those found in the central nervous system: glial cells, astrocytes, and so on. One could go as far as to say that the complexity of the ENS, and its independence, allow it to be considered a "second brain." The largest share of the relatively tiny number of nerve connections to other systems comes from the vagus nerve, and 90% of those fibers are sensory

– so perhaps in some respects the ENS controls the CNS more than the other way around.

Among the properties of the neural crest cells which find their way into the ENS are that they are highly migratory, highly pluripotent, and they originate from restricted areas – the vagal neural crest of the hindbrain supplies cells which populate the whole of the gut, starting proximally and eventually reaching the whole hindgut. Some neurons which derive from other parts (neural tube and sacral somites) also contribute to the ENS, and functioning ganglia cannot be generated anywhere without all the normal components in a favorable matrix. The factors which control this migration and differentiation are extremely complex.

Hirschsprung disease is a congenital defect in the development of the ENS where ganglia are absent from a variable length of the gastrointestinal tract starting from the distal end (although occasionally, and disastrously, it may be complete). The presentation is of obstruction usually associated with megacolon. The fundamental defect is a failure of neuronal migration, and several different factors may be involved. The gene coding for a tyrosine kinase (c-RET) is clearly implicated, as are glial-derived growth factor and an endothelin receptor, ENDRB. Other genes which have a role in regulating development in neurons, SOX-10 and MASH-1, can have mutations which mimic Hirschsprung in animals [46]. Clearly, the process of getting the right neuron in the right place is extraordinarily complex, and far from completely understood.

Motor function in the developing gut

The functionality of the immature gut is perhaps more limited by deficiencies in the motor function of the gut than by the lack of structural elements, cell types, or digestive enzymes and secretions. The development of motor function rather lags behind these other factors. It is at least 2 years before the system can be considered mature. The main movements which are required are swallowing, sucking, mixing and propulsion of gut contents, and evacuation. The esophagus, and those parts proximal to it, are striated muscle and under voluntary control. The muscle of the rest of the gastrointestinal tract, until the external anal sphincter, is smooth muscle and although neural projections and humoral influences from higher centers can modify its function, it is essentially autonomous and regulated by its own enteric nervous system and humoral factors.

Swallowing

Swallowing movements are evident in the fetus at 16 or 17 weeks' gestation, and there is a steady increase in the volume of amniotic fluid swallowed, from less than 20 mL daily at 20 weeks to around 450 mL daily at term [47]. There is much more to this than just "practice"; amniotic fluid contains nutrition and growth factors, and the development of the gut is promoted by it. An interruption of fetal swallowing can lead to polyhydramnios. In the premature infant, propulsive pressures in the esophagus are lower than at term, and the movement may not be completely or properly co-ordinated, and complications due to reflux and aspiration are more likely. The function of the lower esophageal sphincter (LES) is particularly important in this. Although the lower LES pressure found in premature neonates would seem to make reflux more likely, reflux episodes appear to be more related to transient relaxations in the LES [48], the causes of which are not fully clear, than to inadequate resting LES pressure.

Sucking movements can be seen from 28 to 30 weeks' gestation but effective co-ordination with swallowing and breathing is generally not achieved until 37 weeks or so. Babies more premature than this may still be able to suckle by stopping breathing for short periods and then resting.

In both stomach and small bowel, the smooth muscle shows a typical pattern of slow-wave electrical activity, the periodicity of which is controlled by the pacemaker activity of the interstitial cells of Cajal. A muscle contraction is caused by a spike potential causing an additional depolarization on top of the slow wave and over the threshold for muscle contraction.

In the mature stomach and small bowel, in the fasting state the characteristic feature is the migrating motor complex (MMC), which is a wave of contraction passing from the stomach to the rectum. In the adult, these are seen every 90 min or so. Feeding abolishes them and for 3 or 4 h only segmentations and short peristaltic waves are seen, before the MMC re-establishes. A fully developed MMC is not seen until nearly full term [49,50] but this mature electromyographic pattern is not essential for successful enteral feeding. Gastric emptying can be seen up to 6 weeks before the appearance of the MMC, and contractile activity long before that, but in more premature infants nasojejunal feeding may be needed to overcome inadequate gastric emptying. It is clear that enteral feeding promotes the development of effective motor activity and so in conditions where full enteral feeding is impossible, at least some enteral feed is beneficial. Certainly in some animals, bacterial colonization is also required for normal gut development.

The rate of gastric emptying is of course of great interest to the anesthesiologist wishing to provide safe anesthesia for his or her patient. Unfortunately, it is highly variable. Very dogmatic adherence to a protocol NPO period before anesthesia rather implies a lack of understanding of gastrointestinal physiology. The half-time for gastric emptying in premature infants is usually 20–40 minutes, rather slower than it is for term babies, and it will be slower for formula feed than for breast milk.

The colon also shows propagated waves of contraction when mature, and the passage of fecal material into the rectum may lead to reflex relaxation of the internal anal sphincter and defecation. The frequency of these contraction waves decreases with age from several times per hour in the term infant, especially just following a feed, to once or twice per day in the adult. Most babies pass their first stool within 2 days of birth, but it may be longer than that in the case of prematurity. There is normally no passage of meconium into the amniotic fluid *in utero*, and evidence of it is often considered a sign of fetal distress.

Many factors can interrupt the normal process of gastrointestinal tract motor maturation, including some which appear to be outside the gut; babies with hypoxic brain injury are much more likely to have problems with reflux and experience delays in establishing enteral feeding.

Meconium ileus is most commonly seen in infants with cystic fibrosis. Cystic fibrosis (CF) is caused by a defect in the gene coding for a protein which forms a cAMP-dependent chloride channel (cystic fibrosis transmembrane conductance regulator, CFTR). The disease is characterized by abnormally thick, viscid mucus, which typically causes blockage and infection in the respiratory tract or causes pancreatic insufficiency. There are other changes in CF goblet cell secretions and intestinal mucus apart from lack of chloride – for example, it contains more protein, specifically more albumin. The result is that the sticky meconium causes an intestinal obstruction. Rare cases which occur without CF may be due to motility disorders, for instance defective interstitial cells of Cajal.

Immunity in the gastrointestinal tract

The very purpose of the gastrointestinal tract is to take substances in from the environment and transport them into the organism; it follows that this process is a major liability when that environment teems with potential pathogens. To protect the organism effectively from these myriad threats requires an extremely sophisticated multimodal defense system.

Innate immunity

The goblet cells secrete a mucus which forms a physical barrier, which also contains antimicrobial compounds, protecting the mucosa from pathogens. The number of goblet cells increases in inflammatory conditions and in response to some parasites. The enterocytes may contribute to immunity by an unusual mechanism [51]. The lifespan of enterocytes after birth is short, around 3–5 days. As these cells die and are shed into the lumen, they release histones, which are components of the cell nucleosome but which also seem to have significant antimicrobial activity (similar compounds are present in macrophages). So many enterocytes are shed into the lumen that this could be an effective protection, and it is not otherwise apparent why their lifespan needs to be so short; Paneth cells (originating from the same precursors) live much longer, as do fetal enterocytes in their sterile environment. Enterocytes therefore seem to have an immune function which is secondary to their main function but for Paneth cells, their primary function is immunological. Paneth cells secrete a range of bactericidal compounds. They contain numerous granules (like neutrophils), and the granules seem remarkably similar, containing lysozyme, phospholipase A_2, and peptides known as α-defensins. All these components show antimicrobial activity. Most, and possibly all, of the Paneth cell granules are released into the lumen and so their antimicrobial activity occurs outside the cell, unlike neutrophils and macrophages, and also unlike those cells of myeloid lineage, Paneth cells are fixed, in the epithelium of the crypts. Paneth cells can be detected in humans at about 13–14 weeks of gestation and produce low levels of defensins straight away. The levels increase markedly around the time of birth but still, defensin levels are several times lower in neonates than in adults.

Acquired immunity

A detailed account of the mechanism of cellular and humoral immunity is outside the scope of this chapter, so we will assume some knowledge of these systems. The fundamental problem that the gastrointestinal tract poses to the immune system is that while the organism must be capable of defending itself against a vast array of pathogens which may attack by this route, it is unavoidable that the ingestion of food will also present an enormous range of foreign antigens and to respond to every one would be unfeasible, wasteful, detrimental and potentially disastrous. Therefore there must be an accurate and subtle method for inducing tolerance to antigens which are harmless (and may be required), whilst maintaining immune vigilance against genuine threats. Perhaps needless to say, the precise and complete details of how this is achieved are not known and anyway, the complexities of what is known need not trouble us too much for the purposes of this account.

Lymphocytes appear in the gastrointestinal tract in three broad areas – as intraepithelial lymphocytes, in Peyer's patches, and in the lamina propria.

Intraepithelial lymphocytes appear at around 11 weeks' gestation and increase continuously, so by 27 weeks about 70% of the infant level is reached [52]. In the lamina propria, B- and T-cells are present from 12 to 14 weeks' gestation, and similarly increase their number towards birth. The cell subsets present are distinctly different in these two areas and cell proliferation is seen throughout, whereas in the adult, proliferation is confined to the

Peyer's patches: these can be seen from around 18 weeks' gestation, mostly in the ileum, as in adults. There are typically around 100 at birth, increasing to 250 or so in teenagers, thereafter gradually declining. As soon as they appear, the epithelium overlying the patches changes from columnar to cuboidal, and the enterocyte-derived M-cells appear – their function is to transport antigens from the lumen and present them to lymphocytes [53]. Mature M-cells are surrounded by clusters of lymphocytes.

In utero, the sterile conditions do not test the immune system but at birth there is a sudden influx of antigens. Premature infants are capable of mounting both humoral and delayed hypersensitivity-type reactions, but the response is less reliable than in term babies. After birth, the immune system continues to develop quickly, at least in part stimulated by luminal antigen (the process is less effective in parenterally fed infants), and normally after 1 year of age there are three times as many intraepithelial lymphocytes as in the neonate.

B-cells and the immunoglobulins they produce are crucial to the protection of the huge mucosal surface of the gastrointestinal tract. Peyer's patches are fundamental to the production of activated plasma cells. The clonal expansion of specific cell lines is carried out there, and the maturing cells disperse out into the circulation and so are distributed to the whole of the lamina propria. Immunoglobulin-secreting plasma cells produce predominantly IgA which is packaged with a secretory component and exported into the lumen by the enterocytes. In the neonate, significant amounts of IgA are supplied by the mother's breast milk, compensating to some extent for the immature humoral immune system.

Breast milk, the suckling period, and bacterial colonization

Breast milk is considered to provide many advantages over artificial alternatives [54]. The composition of human breast milk alters as the baby ages, is not uniform during a single feed, and varies quite a bit between individuals. For the first few days postpartum, colostrum is produced; the volume is rather lower and its composition different from more mature milk.

Milk proteins

There are a very large number of milk proteins, which are classified into two groups according to whether they clot, forming a curd on exposure to acid (caseins), or not (whey). Caseins form micelles in the watery milk environment, containing ions, especially calcium and phosphorus. The principal caseins in human milk are β- and κ-casein. Of the whey proteins, those with the highest concentrations are α-lactalbumin, lactoferrin, secretory IgA (sIgA), and serum albumin.

Secretory IgA (90% of milk immunoglobulin) has an obvious immunological utility; the clonal varieties will be directed against antigens that the mother has encountered and are therefore tailored to the probable local environment. Immunoglobulins are resistant to degradation in the infant gut.

In addition, there are small amounts of important enzymes in milk, such as bile salt-activated lipase, which assists in the digestion of milk fat content. This enzyme, and the plasma membrane which encloses milk lipid droplets as they are secreted in the mammary gland, ensures that milk fat is particularly easily digestible.

Some growth factors, for example insulin-like growth factor, transforming growth factor and epidermal growth factor, promote gastrointestinal tract cell proliferation, which can be extremely rapid after the first feed, intestinal mass as much as doubling within 3 days in piglets [55].

Hormones present in milk include insulin, thyroxine, and glucocorticoids and these, and other factors such as nucleotides, may have important roles in gut maturation.

Cytoprotective substances such as prostaglandins and phospholipids are also present.

Non-protein components of milk

Mature human milk (produced at least 3 weeks postpartum) contains typically [56] 4% fat, almost all triglycerides of medium- or long-chain fatty acids, 7% carbohydrate, almost all lactose, and 1–1.5% protein (about 40% caseins, 60% whey).

Colostrum contains less fat and carbohydrate (about 75% of that in mature milk) and much more whey protein (about double) which includes up to 5–12 times as much sIgA, as well as high concentrations of trophic factors, especially in the first day or two [57,58]. By comparison, cow's milk is very different – it contains about half as much lactose, a little less fat, about three times as much caseins, and has a higher electrolyte concentration.

The infant stomach does not produce much acid – the pH in the neonate's stomach is 4–5, so pepsin activity and hence protein digestion are very limited. The stomach is much more important in the digestion of milk fat. Gastric lipase activity is very high in the neonate (even if premature) and it seems that this enzyme is required to start the breakdown of the membrane-coated milk fat globule, which otherwise resists the activity of bile-salt activated lipase (a milk constituent).

Initially there is significant transport of macromolecules unaltered across the gut mucosa. This certainly occurs *in utero*, and factors present in amniotic fluid appear in the fetal circulation. Later, the gut becomes much less permeable, a process known as closure. The precise timing of closure is difficult to determine; it happens rather earlier in humans than in some other mammals – in the rat, closure occurs long after birth. Certainly the human gut is more permeable in the neonatal period, and factors in breast milk may promote closure; this may be protective against infection.

Bacterial colonization is clearly an important event in the neonate, and is inevitable within a few days of birth. The neonatal gut is relatively more aerobic and this suppresses colonization by obligate anaerobes. The first organisms found are usually bifidobacteria, *Escherichia coli*, Enterobacter, and staphylococci. It might seem intuitive that these organisms are derived from the mother's gut flora but in fact, this is not always the case, even in unhygienic conditions. The infant gut is often colonized by organisms which are rarely found in the adult gut, such as Klebsiella and Citrobacter. Clostridia are found more often in babies than in adults, and are not necessarily pathogenic – up to 30% of healthy babies carry them. Bacteroides and lactobacilli generally appear later [59]. Usually the flora in formula-fed babies resembles that of adults more than breast-fed babies, and breast feeding confers some protection against urinary tract infection, septicemia, diarrhea and necrotizing enterocolitis. Weaning promotes the transition to an adult-type gut flora. Infants are, however, much more susceptible to infection by Salmonella, Campylobacter and pathogenic *E. coli* strains than adults. The use of antibiotics, and just being in a hospital environment, tends to disturb the establishment of a normal gut flora, and makes diarrheal illness more likely.

Recently, interest has been aroused in the proposition that inadequate exposure to bacteria increases the risk of food allergy and atopic illnesses. It is true that components of *E. coli* can improve the induction of immune tolerance to food protein, and that rates of allergy and atopy are much higher in hygienic Western countries.

Necrotizing enterocolitis

Necrotizing enterocolitis (NEC) is the most common gastrointestinal disorder found in the neonate. Despite its frequency, and a large volume of research, the causes remain obscure [60]. It is much more prevalent in premature babies, affecting about 10% of babies born less than 1500 g, and the more prematurely the baby is born, the more likely it is to develop NEC. The condition is unusual in babies born later than 35 weeks' gestation. When it does occur in a term neonate, the onset is typically within a few days, but may be several weeks after birth in very premature babies.

It is attractive to ascribe an infective cause and it is true that in advanced severe cases, the clinical picture is of sepsis. Cases also sometimes cluster, suggesting an epidemic etiology. However, it is clear that no one particular organism is responsible. Many cases of NEC show heavy gut colonization with Clostridia, but these are commonly found in healthy babies and this finding is not universal. In a breast-fed infant, bifidobacteria tend to predominate, and counts of these species are lower in NEC cases; possibly giving probiotics to enhance their growth may be protective [61]. Breast milk has a protective effect against NEC and contains anti-inflammatory substances, sometimes in higher concentrations in the milk of mothers of premature babies [62]. It seems likely that NEC is a result of a combination of gut ischemia, bacterial translocation, an inflammatory response and defective immune modulation of that response.

The clinical picture is often of a premature baby who may initially progress well on enteral feeds but then becomes feed intolerant, and may have abdominal distension and vomiting. Apneas are common, and the baby may seem lethargic or appear to be uncomfortable. Radiographs may show dilated bowel loops and gas in the gut wall or, if the condition progresses to full-thickness ischemia and intestinal perforation, free gas in the peritoneum. Systemic signs may be hypothermia, acidosis and other electrolyte disturbances, and eventually cardiovascular collapse and multiorgan failure.

Treatment is to rest the gut (parenteral nutrition may be required), general supportive measures and antibiotic therapy, and celiotomy if the condition worsens. Sections of ischemic gut may have to be resected, and stoma formation may be necessary. Mortality remains high, up to 50% in babies weighing less than 1500 g at birth. Survivors may run into trouble later as a result of short gut or malabsorption disorders.

Developmental physiology of the renal system

Developmental abnormalities of the kidney and urinary tract are the most common cause of childhood renal failure in the United States [63]. Defects occur in as many as 1:100 livebirths and range from benign, asymptomatic duplications to lethal conditions such as bilateral renal agenesis [64].

Embryology and development
Kidney and urinary tract
The definitive kidney has two embryonic precursors: the pronephroi and mesonephroi. Although ultimately both degenerate, they are essential for normal renal development. The pronephroi arise from intermediate mesoderm early in the 4th week and are rudimentary, non-functional kidneys, composed of simple tubules in the neck region [63]. The pronephroi drain into bilateral ducts, precursors of the Wolffian (nephrogenic) ducts, which elongate caudally to fuse with the cloaca. The mesonephroi develop caudally to the pronephroi at the end of the 4th week. They comprise well-developed nephrons and vascular glomeruli that drain into the Wolffian duct and function as interim kidneys for about 4 weeks. They regress at the end of the first trimester although they have several adult derivatives in the male [65].

Development of the permanent kidneys begins early in the 5th week. A diverticulum known as the ureteric bud arises from the caudal end of the mesonephric duct and is the precursor of the ureter and renal collecting system (Fig. 8.9). It penetrates a specialized area of intermediate

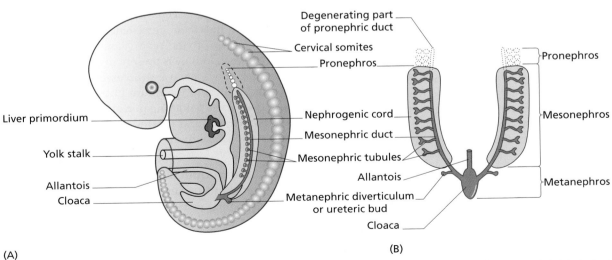

Figure 8.9 The three sets of excretory systems in an embryo during the 5th week. (A) Lateral view. (B) Ventral view. The mesonephric tubules have been pulled laterally; their normal position is shown in (A). Reproduced from Moore and Persaud [65] with permission from Elsevier.

(a)

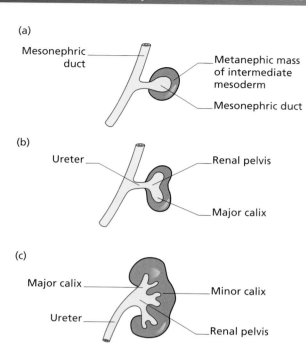

(b)

(c)

(d)

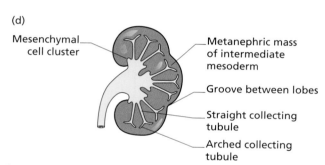

Figure 8.10 Development of the permanent kidney. (A–D) Successive stages in the development of the metanephric diverticulum or ureteric bud (weeks 5–8). Observe the development of the ureter, renal pelvis, calices, and collecting tubules. Reproduced from Moore and Persaud [65] with permission from Elsevier.

mesoderm at the level of the hindlimb termed the metane-phric mass, which is the precursor of the renal paren-chyma. The ureteric bud elongates to form the ureter and branches to form calices and collecting tubules. The end of each collecting tubule induces cells of the metanephric mass to form vesicles that elongate to become definitive tubules (Fig. 8.10).

Nephron development commences around the 8th week. It occurs in a centrifugal pattern with cortical nephrons formed after juxtamedullary ones. The rate of development increases rapidly after 18 weeks' gestation and is complete by 34–36 weeks, with each kidney pos-sessing between 800,000 and 1,000,000 nephrons [66]. Renal growth after this is mainly due to elongation of the proximal convoluted tubule and an increase in interstitial

tissue. Premature and low-birthweight infants have fewer nephrons, leading to high nephron filtration rates and glomerular hypertrophy [67]. These changes are associated with the development of hypertension, cardiovascular disease and increased susceptibility to renal disease in later life [68,69]. Abnormalities in ure-teric bud induction of nephrogenesis underlie many congenital defects; details of common ones are given in Table 8.1.

Urinary bladder

The cloaca is partitioned by the urorectal septum into a ventral urogenital sinus and dorsal rectum. The bladder arises mainly from the vesical part of the urogenital sinus, with the trigone derived from the caudal ends of the mesonephric ducts. As the ducts are incorporated, so the ureters come to open into the bladder, their orifices moving superolaterally as a result of "traction" from the ascent of the kidneys. The bladder is initially contiguous superiorly with the allantois (a vestigial structure) which constricts to become the urachus, represented in adults by the median umbilical ligament. If fetal bladder empty-ing is obstructed, the urachus may remain patent, allow-ing urine to leak out around the umbilicus.

Renal migration and blood supply

The kidneys initially lie close to each other in the pelvis and attain their abdominal, retroperitoneal adult position by the 9th week. This apparent migration is due to embry-onic growth caudal to the kidneys rather than movement of the kidneys themselves, and abnormalities in this process are common (see Table 8.1).

Renal arteries and veins start as branches of the common iliac vessels; as the kidneys ascend, they receive new branches from successively more superior points of the aorta and inferior vena cava. Inferior vessels usually degenerate but their persistence explains much of the variation seen in the renal vasculature. A single renal artery to each kidney is present in only 75% of adults, and 25% of kidneys have 2–4 accessory arteries [70]. These usually drain into the hilum but accessory arteries may be end-arteries, rendering portions of a kidney vulnerable to ischemia, and those to the lower pole may obstruct the ureter and cause hydronephrosis [71].

Fetal urine production and the oligohydramnios sequence

Urine production by the fetal kidney begins by week 10 and is responsible for 90% of amniotic fluid volume by week 20. Production increases from 0.1 mL/min at 20 weeks to 1 mL/min at 40 weeks' gestation, which is far in excess of urine production rates in the term neonate [72]. The absence of adequate amniotic fluid gives rise

Table 8.1 Common abnormalities of the urinary tract and their embryological origins

Condition	Embryological etiology	Clinical effects
Renal agenesis	Failure of ureteric bud to contact metanephric mesoderm	Unilateral – 1:1000 livebirths. Usually detected incidentally, may be associated with higher risk of chronic kidney disease in later life
	Complete involution of a severely dysplastic kidney	Bilateral – 1:10–30,000 livebirths. Absence of fetal urine leads to oligohydramnios sequence (see text). Usually fatal
Urinary tract duplication	Ureteric bud division	Bifid ureter with either a divided kidney or a supernumerary kidney
	Duplication of ureteric bud	Two ureters each with their own kidney on the affected side
Renal ectopia	Arrested or aberrant migration +/- fusion while kidneys lie in fetal pelvis	Pelvic kidney – unilateral failure to ascend. No symptoms but may be confused with tumors or damaged during surgery
		Crossed renal ectopia – one kidney migrates to contralateral side. May occur with fused kidneys
		Discoid or "pancake" kidney – complete fusion in pelvis. Kidney mass lies above bladder with short ureters
		Horseshoe kidney – 1:500 livebirths (7% of those with Turner syndrome). Fusion of kidney poles (usually inferior). U-shaped kidney lies in hypogastrium as normal ascent is prevented by root of inferior mesenteric artery. Usually no symptoms
Dysplastic or hypoplastic kidneys	Failure of induction of nephrogenesis by the ureteric bud	From small kidneys with low numbers of normal nephrons to normal-sized kidneys with a wide variety of tubular defects. Dysplastic kidneys may also be multicystic – these often involute spontaneously *in utero* or the first few years of life. Together, the most common cause of established renal failure worldwide. Molecular mechanisms are being elucidated [75]
Wilms tumor	Nephrogenic rests: abnormal structures arising from failure of mesenchyme differentiation	Kidney malignancy affecting 1:10,000 children. Nephrogenic rests are found much more frequently in children with Wilms tumors [76]

to the oligohydramnios sequence. Characteristic facial features, known as Potter's facies, include micrognathia, wide-set eyes, flattened nasal bridge, and large, low-set ears which lack cartilage [73]. Skeletal anomalies associated with oligohydramnios include club feet, hip dysplasia, scoliosis, torticollis, and contractures. Amniotic fluid is also essential for normal lung development; pulmonary hypoplasia is the main reason for the high mortality associated with significant oligohydramnios [74]. The fetus swallows significant volumes of amniotic fluid daily which is absorbed by the intestine. However, fetal waste products are transferred across the placenta for excretion by maternal kidneys. The kidneys do not assume their excretory role until after birth [75,76] (see Table 8.1).

Developmental physiology
Glomerular filtration
Glomerular filtration is the process whereby water and solutes cross the glomerular membrane. Ultrafiltrate is virtually identical to plasma apart from containing very little protein. The rate of ultrafiltration is governed by four factors: the balance of Starling forces across the capillary wall; plasma flow rate; glomerular capillary wall permeability; and total surface area of the capillaries.

Quantifying glomerular filtration rate (GFR) is important for the rational prescribing of drugs and in monitoring chronic kidney disease. Comparing direct measurements from small infants to adults requires scaling to a standard of reference. Although kidney weight cannot be directly measured, both kidney weight and absolute GFR correlate well with body surface area (BSA). Adjusting GFR for BSA removes the variability caused by the variation in pediatric body size [77]. BSA in children and adolescents may be calculated from the formula [78]:

$$\text{BSA (m}^2\text{)} = 0.024265 \times \text{Weight}^{0.5378} \times \text{Height}^{0.3964}$$

The most common method of measuring GFR is based on the concept of clearance. The renal clearance of a substance x (C_x) is expressed by the formula:

$$C_x = U_x V / P_x$$

where U_x is the urine concentration, P_x the plasma concentration and V the urine flow rate. If a substance is freely filtered and not metabolized, synthesized or transported by the kidney then its clearance is equal to GFR.

Despite the importance of GFR, accurate measurement remains problematic. Renal clearance of inulin is still the gold standard in all age groups. However, its utility is compromised by availability, difficult assays and the practical problems of collecting urine samples in children. Urine volumes are inaccurate in the presence of vesicoureteric reflux and conditions which preclude complete voiding [79]. Creatinine is routinely measured and hence used frequently to estimate GFR in pediatric populations. It is freely filtered and secreted by tubular cells but the technique is inaccurate in children with reduced muscle mass, and tends to overestimate GFR in the presence of renal dysfunction when extrarenal clearance of creatinine is markedly increased [80]. The common and easily used Schwartz formula, which incorporated serum creatinine, height and an age- and sex-dependent constant, now appears inaccurate with newer and more precise assays for creatinine [81]. Radiolabeled isotopes are accurate but not ideal agents in children, particularly for repeated assessments.

There are two newer agents that are showing promise for measurement of GFR. Iohexol is a non-ionic contrast agent already used at higher doses for radiological procedures even in the presence of renal dysfunction. Equations utilizing iohexol plasma clearance provide good estimates of GFR [82]. Further, results from blood spots collected on filter paper correlate well with venous samples which may facilitate late sampling by patients at home and the use of iohexol as an epidemiological tool [83]. The endogenous cysteine protease inhibitor cystatin C is produced constantly, independent of inflammatory conditions, sex, muscle mass and age above 1 year, and is freely filtered [84]. Estimations of GFR using serum cystatin C appear very accurate although assays are currently not widely available [82].

Glomerular filtration begins in the fetus during the 9th week. GFR reaches $12\,mL/min/1.73\,m^2$ in the premature infant at 30 weeks and $20\,mL/min/1.73\,m^2$ by term. Maturation continues rapidly in the postnatal period with a doubling of GFR by 2 weeks, a proportional rise that is seen in both premature and low-birthweight babies [85,86]. Adult values of GFR (corrected for BSA) are reached by 18–24 months of age [87]. Low GFR is primarily mediated by vasoconstriction through the renin–angiotensin system (see below) and may represent a necessary adaptation to prevent excessive fluid and electrolyte loss secondary to tubular immaturity [88].

Tubular function
Sodium

Fractional excretion of sodium (FE_{Na}) falls from 12.8% at 30 weeks to 3.4% at 38 weeks and 1% in the normal adult [89]. Prematurity is associated with significant salt wasting and a risk of hyponatremia. Term neonates have a limited capacity both to conserve sodium necessary for growth and to excrete a sodium load. Excessive administration of sodium to term neonates may cause extracellular volume expansion, edema and significant hypernatremia [90]. Sodium excretion usually exceeds oral intake (breast or formula milk) in the first few days of life, leading to negative sodium balance with associated weight loss. As FE_{Na} falls further and oral intake increases, birthweight is regained in 5–7 days. The ability to excrete a sodium load matures by around 1 year [91].

Sodium is reabsorbed along the entire nephron length via different mechanisms. A key component is the Na-K-ATPase enzyme, located on the basolateral membrane of tubular cells, which actively transports sodium out of the cell into interstitial fluid and the peritubular capillaries, creating an electrochemical gradient for the movement of sodium out of the tubular lumen (Fig. 8.11). This movement often occurs via specific transporter proteins to which the transfer of many other electrolytes and

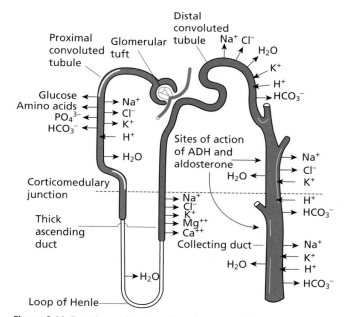

Figure 8.11 Excretion and reabsorption of water and electrolytes. Water is reabsorbed in the proximal tubule together with glucose, amino acids, phosphate, sodium and bicarbonate, and from the distal nephron under the influence of antidiuretic hormone and the hypertonic medulla. In the distal tubule sodium is reabsorbed under the influence of aldosterone with associated excretion of potassium and hydrogen ions. Reproduced from Cumming and Swainson [138] with permission from Elsevier.

compounds are coupled. In the neonate, reabsorptive mechanisms in both the proximal and distal convoluted tubule are immature. The postnatal enhancement of sodium conservation is brought about mainly by increased numbers of Na-K-ATPase and other transporter proteins in both locations [88].

Water

Infant nutrition is entirely liquid, so a high urine flow rate is necessary to maintain fluid balance. This is achieved with a high fractional excretion of water (FE_{H2O}). Water reabsorption in the proximal convoluted tubule is isotonic. Neonates have reduced plasma protein, so the hydrostatic and osmotic forces acting from lumen to capillary are reduced, resulting in decreased proximal water reabsorption. Distally, water reabsorption is under the influence of antidiuretic hormone (ADH), to which even preterm babies are sensitive. Neonates are able to adjust water excretion appropriately from day 2 of life and can achieve FE_{H2O} of up to 13% (a similar value in adults would produce 20 L of urine per day) [92].

While minimum urine concentration equals adults levels of 50 mmol/kg at birth, maximum urine concentration is 600–800 mmol/kg, which is about half that of older children. This reflects both shorter loops of Henle and reduced tonicity of the medullary interstitium (urea levels are low, reflecting the anabolic state of the growing infant). Assuming a solute load of 10–15 mosmol/kg, the minimum urine flow rate required to prevent solute retention is 25 mL/kg/day [93]. This approximates to 1 mL/kg/h and is the basis for the use of this figure as an indication of renal failure.

Potassium

The immature kidney has a reduced capacity to excrete potassium; neonates excrete 9% of the filtered potassium load whereas children and adults excrete around 15% [94]. The main site of potassium excretion is the distal convoluted tubule and cortical collecting ducts. Aldosterone acts on the principal cells of these regions to enhance the activity of the Na-K-ATPase pump on the basolateral membrane, which elevates intracellular potassium. It also increases the permeability of the luminal membrane to potassium, thus promoting its excretion. Aldosterone levels are high in infants but the cellular response is attenuated [95]. In addition, lower tubular flow rates lead to higher potassium concentrations, reducing the gradient for diffusion. Normal values are achieved by around 3 months of age. The reduced ability of infants to excrete potassium is only likely to be of significance in cases of excess administration or pathological cellular release, where hyperkalemia may ensue more rapidly.

Glucose

Glucose is completely reabsorbed in the early portion of the proximal convoluted tubule by a stereo-specific transported protein. The process involves secondary active transport and is saturable (see Fig. 8.11). Term infants have a threshold for glucose that is equal to older children and adults when corrected for GFR. However, premature infants demonstrate significant glucose wasting, which may be due to reduced nephron numbers, reduced basolateral Na-K-ATPase pump activity or changes in the expression and density of the transporter proteins [96].

Phosphate

Rapid growth requires the normal infant to be in positive phosphate balance; plasma phosphate is high *in utero* and in infancy and decreases with age. Neonates demonstrate a reduced fractional excretion of phosphate that is not attributable to reduced load from a lower GFR. Rather, the immature kidney has an increased ability to reabsorb phosphate in both the proximal and distal convoluted tubules that is independent of parathyroid hormone activity and dietary phosphate. Growth hormone may have a regulatory effect, suggesting that this represents an appropriate physiological response to the need for phosphate, rather than an immature system [97].

Acid–base balance

Neonates have a reduced capacity to maintain acid–base status for a number of reasons, including a reduced ability to reabsorb bicarbonate, secrete organic acid and produce ammonia and a low level of titratable acid, specifically phosphate. Bicarbonate is usually 85–90% reabsorbed in the proximal convoluted tubule, an energy-dependent process requiring the secretion of hydrogen ions in exchange for sodium. The renal threshold for bicarbonate (the level at which it appears in the urine) is 18 mEq/L in the premature infant, approximately 21 mEq/L in the term neonate, rising to adult levels of 24–26 mEq/L by around 1 year [95]. Decreased bicarbonate reabsorption may be due to immature luminal Na-H antiporters or a reduced activity of the Na-K-ATPase pump which lowers the driving force for sodium.

The main site of hydrogen ion secretion is the distal convoluted tubule which in maturity can excrete hydrogen against a gradient of as much as 1000:1 (compared to gradients of 4–10:1 by secondary active transport in the proximal convoluted tubule) [98]. The ability to acidify urine is acquired by 1 month, even in premature infants, suggesting that distal tubular hydrogen ion secretion is inducible independent of the gestational age of the kidney. By 2 months, the response to an ammonium chloride load is the same as for older children and adults (once corrected for GFR) [99].

Amino acids

Infants demonstrate a transient physiological aminoaciduria in the first few weeks of life. This is unlikely to represent a generalized disorder as not all are wasted to a similar degree [100]. Amino acids are freely filtered at the glomerulus; adults reabsorb 98–99% in the proximal convoluted tubule, against a concentration gradient, using secondary active transport across the luminal membrane and facilitated diffusion across the basolateral membrane (see Fig. 8.11). These specific transport systems exist from birth but do not function at full capacity for reasons which remain unclear [101]. Neonates and infants are more susceptible to dietary protein inadequacies. For example, taurine, which is important for retinal development, has been shown to be low in plasma of low-birthweight infants receiving parenteral nutrition without supplementation [102].

Control systems

Plasma renin is high in the fetus and is approximately twice adult levels at term. Levels increase for the first few weeks of life and then start a gradual decline until adult levels are reached at around 6–9 years of age. As renin is the rate-limiting step in angiotensin II (AII) production, levels of the latter follow a similar pattern. AII has important trophic effects on the developing renal system. Maternal administration of angiotensin-converting enzyme inhibitors (ACEi) during the second and third trimesters results in renal dysplasia, renal failure, oligohydramnios and pulmonary hypoplasia [103]. AII is a potent systemic vasoconstrictor in adults; it reduces renal blood flow but preserves GFR by constriction of efferent arterioles. This pressor response is present but reduced in neonates, possibly due to high occupancy of AII receptors by existing high levels of AII.

Renal blood flow

The proportion of cardiac output distributed to the kidneys is 2–3% in the fetus, 4–6% in the first 12 hours of life and 8–10% by 1 week. Effective renal plasma flow reaches adult levels (corrected for BSA) by 12–24 months [104]. The neonatal kidney can autoregulate its blood flow at appropriately lower systemic perfusion pressures although the response appears to be less efficient. Intrarenal blood flow is distributed differently, with a higher proportion of neonatal blood flow going to juxtamedullary nephrons, leaving cortical nephrons at higher risk of ischemia. The rise in renal blood flow with maturation is probably due to alterations in cardiac output, perfusion pressure and renovascular resistance. While AII seems important in maintaining a basal tone, other vasoactive agents may also play a role, including ADH, atrial natriuretic peptide, adenosine and endothelin [105].

Pediatric renal disease
Acute kidney injury

Acute kidney injury (AKI) is characterized by the inability of the kidney to fulfill its excretory functions and manage fluid and electrolyte balance appropriately. Causes of AKI may be divided into prerenal injury, intrinsic renal disease and obstructive uropathies (Table 8.2). Etiology is age dependent; cortical necrosis and renal vein thrombosis are more common in neonates, whereas hemolytic uremic syndrome (HUS) is more

Table 8.2 Etiology of acute kidney injury in neonates and children

Type	Etiology

Pre-renal	Decreased intravascular volume
	  – dehydration
	  – salt wasting renal or adrenal disease
	  – hemorrhage
	  – third space losses – sepsis, trauma
	Renal hypoperfusion (with normal intravascular volume)
	  – cardiac failure/ tamponade
	  – hepatorenal syndrome

Intrinsic renal disease	Acute tubular necrosis
	  – ischemic/ hypoxic injury
	  – drug induced, e.g. aminoglycosides, contrast agents
	  – toxins
	    – endogenous, e.g. hemoglobin, myoglobin
	    – exogenous, e.g. methanol, ethylene glycol
	Interstitial nephritis
	  – drug induced, e.g. penicillins, NSAIDs, sulphonamides
	  – idiopathic
	Rapidly progressive glomerulonephritis
	Vascular lesions
	  – renal artery or vein thrombosis
	  – cortical necrosis
	  – hemolytic-uremic syndrome
	Uric acid nephropathy and tumor lysis syndrome
	Congenital abnormalities
	  – hypoplasia/ dysplasia with or without obstruction
	    – idiopathic
	    – maternal drugs, e.g. ACEi, NSAIDs
	  – polycystic kidney disease

Obstructive uropathy	Congenital malformations
	  – posterior urethral valves
	  – ureteroceles
	  – vesicoureteric reflux
	  – prune belly syndrome
	Acquired obstruction
	  – kidney stones
	  – tumors, e.g. sacrococcygeal

ACEi, angiotensin converting enzyme inhibitor, NSAIDs, non-steroidal anti-inflammatory drugs.

common in young children, and rapidly progressive glomerulonephritis (RPGN) is generally found in older children and adolescents.

Acute kidney injury in hospitalized children is likely to be multifactorial, with prerenal as well as hypoxic/ischemic and nephrotoxic insults being important; children receiving stem cell transplants and undergoing cardiopulmonary bypass are at particular risk.

The incidence of AKI has been estimated at 0.8 per 100,000 population [106] and rates appear to be increasing [107]. However, the precise incidence and causes of AKI are difficult to establish in children because no epidemiological studies have been conducted using an established definition of AKI [108]. The majority of definitions in use include a change in serum creatinine levels, although it is accepted that this is an insensitive and delayed marker. More sensitive biomarkers are required to allow development and implementation of early preventive measures. Most promising are panels of investigations including plasma cystatin-C and neutrophil gelatinase-associated lipocalin, and urinary interleukin-18 and kidney injury molecule-1 [109].

Prerenal injury

Prerenal injury occurs when blood flow to the kidneys is reduced. If prolonged, this may result in a hypoxic/ischemic acute tubular necrosis. However, this process is not sudden and the insult is reversible provided the kidney is intrinsically normal [110]. Compensatory mechanisms include the relaxation of afferent arterioles under the influence of intrarenal prostaglandins, a response which may be impaired by administration of cyclo-oxygenase inhibitors. The use of indomethacin for ductus arteriosus closure in premature newborns is associated with a significant risk of renal insufficiency [111].

Urinary parameters may assist in distinguishing prerenal from intrinsic renal injury. In response to decreased perfusion, functioning tubules will appropriately conserve sodium and water, producing concentrated urine with osmolality 400–500 mosmol/L, urinary sodium 10–20 mEq/L and fractional sodium excretion of less than 1%. The renal tubules of neonates are relatively immature so corresponding values for renal hypoperfusion are osmolality >350 mosmol/L, sodium <20–30 mEq/L and fractional excretion <2.5%.

Tubules which have sustained injury are unable to conserve sodium in this manner, producing dilute urine with osmolality <350 mosmol/L, sodium 30–40 mEq/L and fractional sodium excretion of >2%. However, these values require that initial tubular function was normal and urinary indices are difficult to interpret in those with pre-existing renal disease or who have received diuretics [112].

Intrinsic renal disease

Hypoxic/ischemic AKI is characterized by early vasoconstriction followed by patchy tubular necrosis, although the mechanism of cellular injury is not yet clear. ATP depletion occurs early and leads to disruption of the cytoskeleton and loss of cellular polarity, with Na-K-ATPase found on the luminal as well as the basolateral membrane. The same mechanism has been shown to contribute to kidney dysfunction in transplanted kidneys [113]. Alteration of vascular tone regulation by nitric oxide and endothelin, as well as the generation of reactive oxygen and nitrogen molecules, may also play a role [114].

Nephrotoxic injury may be caused by a wide variety of agents. Aminoglycoside toxicity is common and thought to be related to lysosomal dysfunction of proximal tubules. The incidence is dose and duration dependent, but is reversible once therapy is discontinued. Hemoglobin or myoglobin in urine produces tubular injury via several mechanisms, including vasoconstriction, precipitation in the tubular lumen and/or heme protein-induced oxidant stress [115].

Uric acid nephropathy and tumor lysis syndrome are most commonly seen in children with acute lymphocytic leukemia and B-cell lymphoma. The pathogenesis is complex, but an important mechanism relates to the precipitation of uric acid crystals in either tubules or the renal vasculature. The rapid breakdown of tumor cells can also cause severe hyperphosphatemia, and the precipitation of calcium phosphate crystals may also contribute to AKI.

Prognosis

Outcome in AKI is dependent upon the underlying cause. Mortality is higher when AKI is a component of multisystem failure, compared with prerenal or intrinsic renal disease. Renal function recovers in the majority of cases, although one study revealed that 34% of 176 children had reduced renal function or were dialysis dependent on discharge from a tertiary center after an episode of AKI [116]. However, even when renal function recovers initially, children with AKI are at risk of subsequent renal impairment. This is true for all ages and not only for conditions associated with significant nephron loss, such as HUS and cortical necrosis, but also for hypoxic/ischemic and nephrotoxic insults [117,118].

Chronic kidney disease

Chronic kidney disease (CKD) is defined as either kidney damage or GFR <60 mL/min/1.73 m² for >3 months [119]. It is characterized by progressive decline in renal function associated with significant morbidity and mortality. CKD may present at any age from the antenatal period onwards; because of the renal role played by the placenta, even

Table 8.3 Etiology and prevalence of established renal failure in children in the UK

Etiology	Percentage
Renal dysplasia with or without reflux	33
Glomerular diseases	19
Obstructive uropathy	15
Congenital nephrosis	8
Tubulo-interstitial disease	8
Renovascular disease	4
Metabolic diseases	4
Unknown	4
Polycystic kidney disease	3
Malignancy	1
Drug nephrotoxicity	1

Source: Ansell et al [120].

lethal malformations may not result in biochemical disturbance for several days. Causes of established renal failure (ERF) are given in Table 8.3 [120].

Cardiovascular disease is much more common in children with ERF than age-matched controls, and accounts for around 20% of deaths in children undergoing dialysis [121]. Growth retardation is proportional to the decrement in GFR, and is more common in children undergoing dialysis than those being treated conservatively or with a transplant. Factors contributing to poor growth include metabolic acidosis; renal osteodystrophy; malnutrition; glucocorticoid therapy; and reduced responsiveness to growth hormone [122]. A variety of neurocognitive deficits have been identified, from severe developmental delay to more subtle verbal and attention deficits; improvements in dialysis, correction of malnutrition and decreased aluminum exposure have improved outcomes.

Treatment of CKD in children is not easy; dialysis and the access it requires pose particular problems (see Chapter 29). Renal abnormalities often occur with other congenital defects or as part of a syndrome and these may have a bearing on the appropriateness of treatment.

Polycystic kidney disease

Autosomal dominant polycystic kidney disease (ADPKD) is the most common hereditary renal disease and affects 1:400–1000 livebirths. It causes 5–10% of cases of ERF worldwide and affects all races equally [123]. Two genes are responsible for the majority of cases: *PKD1* on chromosome 16 and *PKD2* on chromosome 4 account for 85% and 15% respectively. The genes encode transmembrane proteins polycystin 1 and 2 which interact with each other, and possibly the cytoskeleton, although their precise roles remain obscure [124].

Autosomal dominant polycystic kidney disease usually presents in adult life, but 2% of cases present with severe manifestations in childhood, and prenatal diagnosis has been reported [125]. Epithelial-lined cysts arise from about 5% of tubules and detach from the parent tubule (usually at >2 cm). There is massive enlargement of the kidneys secondary to cyst growth, and progressive renal impairment. Associated features include hepatic cysts and intracerebral aneurysms. Presentation is usually with hematuria, hypertension or renal impairment. The decline in renal function is variable but survival on dialysis and post transplant is better with ADPKD than with other forms of ERF [126].

Autosomal recessive polycystic kidney disease affects 1:10–40,000 livebirths and is caused by mutations of the *PKHD1* gene on chromosome 6 which encodes a protein polyductin. Renal cysts arise from the distal collecting duct and cause progressive renal impairment without renal enlargement. Congenital hepatic fibrosis is a universal feature. Presentation is variable, with renal symptoms more common in early life and hepatic complications later. Renal failure *in utero* may lead to presentation with the oligohydramnios sequence, and those who present with severe renal disease in infancy have a high mortality. In older children, features of hepatic fibrosis and portal hypertension tend to dominate the clinical picture. Combined renal and hepatic transplantation is used successfully.

Renal cysts also occur in other disease states. Nephronophthisis (NPH) is a chronic tubulointerstitial nephritis. The infantile form is characterized by cortical microcysts and progression to ERF by 5 years of age, whereas cysts occur much later in the juvenile form [127]. Up to 20% of patients with tuberous sclerosis complex (TSC) will have multiple, bilateral renal cysts. The gene *TSC2*, which accounts for around 75% of sporadic cases of TSC, is found within 48 base pairs of *PKD1* on chromosome 16.

Prune belly syndrome

Prune belly syndrome (PBS) occurs in 1:29,000 to 1:40,000 livebirths [128]. It is 20 times more common in males, four times more common in twins [129], and infants of younger mothers appear to be at greater risk [130]. The syndrome comprises a triad of abnormal abdominal muscles, bilateral cryptorchidism and dilated ureters [131]. It takes its name from the characteristic wrinkled and prune-like appearance of the abdominal wall in which normal musculature fails to develop. Urinary tract abnormalities include a dilated, thick-walled bladder, tortuous, dilated and thick-walled ureters, and kidneys which may be hydronephrotic or dysplastic.

The mechanism by which PBS occurs remains unclear. Some theories emphasize early urethral obstruction which leads to bladder distension, degeneration of the abdominal wall musculature and prevention of testicular descent. However, a more convincing theory proposes abnormal mesenchymal development, termed mesodermal arrest, between weeks 6 and 10 as the underlying abnormality. This is supported by findings of abundant collagen, smooth muscle, fibrous and connective tissue throughout the renal tract, features which are difficult to explain with a purely obstructive lesion [132].

Mortality has traditionally been high, but the use of *in utero* vesicoamniotic shunts appears to be improving matters. Renal failure occurs in around 30% of survivors due to renal dysplasia and from scarring secondary to infections. The abdominal wall abnormalities do not appear to increase the complication rate associated with peritoneal dialysis if it is required [133].

Annotated references

A full reference list for this chapter is available at:
http://www.wiley.com/go/gregory/andropoulos/pediatricanesthesia

1. Schoenwolf G, Bleyl S, Brauer P, Francis-West P (eds). Larsens's Human Embryology, 4th edn. Edinburgh: Churchill Livingstone, 2008. An excellent standard text of human embryology, beautifully illustrated and well referenced.

12. Suchy FJ, Sokol RJ, Balistreri WF (eds). Liver Disease in Children, 3rd edn. Cambridge: Cambridge University Press, 2007. This textbook provides a detailed description of the development of the liver as well as excellent guidance on the diagnosis of liver disease.

13. Kelly D (ed). Diseases of the Liver and Biliary System in Children, 3rd edn. Oxford: Blackwell Publishing, 2008. An excellent textbook which provides practical guidance on the diagnosis and management of pediatric liver disease.

43. Sanderson IR, Walker WA (eds). Development of the Gastrointestinal Tract. Hamilton, Ontario: BC Decker, 1999. A very detailed account of the topic, including a lot of genetics and molecular biology – not so much on anatomical embryology. Now becoming a little dated in a very fast-moving field.

65. Moore KL, Persaud TVN. The Developing Human: Clinically Orientated Embryology. Philadelphia: Saunders, 2007. An established textbook, covering all aspects of embryology with excellent pictures. The clinical implications of developmental abnormalities are well described.

77. Schwartz GJ, Work DF. Measurement and estimation of GFR in children and adolescents. Clin J Am Soc Nephrol 2009;4:1832–43. A comprehensive review of factors affecting the measurement of GFR in children and potential new approaches from a leading researcher in the field.

101. Jones DP, Chesney RW. Development of tubular function. Clin Perinatol 1992;19:33–57. A detailed summary of tubular function and its maturation throughout childhood.

107. Goldstein AL, Devarajan P. Progression from acute kidney injury to chronic kidney disease: a pediatric perspective. Adv Chronic Kidney Dis 2008;15:278–83. An overview of the etiology and changing demographics of kidney disease in children, the link between acute and chronic kidney disease and an assessment of future challenges.

Further reading

Johnson LR (ed). Gastrointestinal Physiology 7th edn. Philadelphia: Mosby Elsevier, 2007. Excellent, fairly concise account of gastrointestinal physiology. No pediatric or developmental emphasis, nothing on embryology or immunology.

Commare CE, Tappenden KA. Development of the Infant Intestine: Implications for Nutrition Support. Nutrition Clin Pract 2007; 22: 159–173. Good review article of most aspects of the physiology of intestinal development, with a clinical angle on the principles of enteral nutrition for premature neonates.

CHAPTER 9

Pharmacology

Jean X. Mazoit

Université Paris-Sud, Paris, France

Introduction

Children are not small adults. Their body hydric volumes, content, and its partition between central and peripheral blood, their metabolic rates, their pulmonary volumes and cardiac and hemodynamic variables markedly differ from those of adults. However, *children are also small adults* in that they have the potential of their future in their genes. Some phenotypic expression may be absent in early life, but most genetic traits are fully expressed at birth.

Development of uptake, distribution, protein binding, metabolism and excretion systems for drugs in the fetus, newborn, infant and child [1]

Uptake, disposition and elimination
Volumes, flows, rates

Body composition differs markedly among neonates, infants and adults (see Chapter 10). This is particularly important for total body water, which decreases from 80–85% of bodyweight in 26 and 31 week' gestation infants to 75% at full term and to 60% in adolescents. The extracellular compartment, which is mainly regulated by the sodium intake after birth, decreases from 65% of bodyweight at 26 weeks' gestation to 40% at full term and 20% by 10 years [2,3]. Therefore, the volume of distribution of hydrophilic drugs, e.g. succinylcholine, is higher in newborn and infants than in older children. Membranes are also immature at birth. For example, drug efflux systems are not fully mature at birth, making cerebral bio-availability of numerous hydrophobic (the term "hydrophobic" will be used instead of "lipophilic" throughout the text) drugs higher in newborns than in children or adults [4,5]. Cardiac output is also different and is closely related to body surface area. The volume of the central compartment of volatile anesthetics is higher in neonates than in adults on a weight basis.

Scaling [6]

Until recently, the only way of correcting for these differences was to use the rule of three, i.e. to divide by 70 kg or 1.73 m² and multiply by the weight or surface area of

Gregory's Pediatric Anesthesia, Fifth Edition. Edited by George A. Gregory, Dean B. Andropoulos.
© 2012 Blackwell Publishing Ltd. Published 2012 by Blackwell Publishing Ltd.

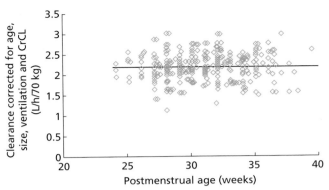

Figure 9.1 Predicted vancomycin clearances in individual premature babies. The data are standardized to a 70 kg person, using allometric scaling, and corrected for age and creatinine clearance (CrCL) (NONMEM). Simple co-variates included in the model markedly decreased interindividual variability. Reproduced from Anderson et al [10] with permission from Blackwell Publishing Ltd.

the subject. Different approaches are used today [7–9]. Allometric scaling considers that extensive parameters, such as metabolic rates or clearances, are related to the corresponding adult parameters raised to an empirical power:

$$CL_{Ped} = CL_{Adult}\left(\frac{BW_{Ped}}{BW_{Adult}}\right)^{x}$$

where CL_{Ped} and CL_{Adult} are the pediatric and adult parameters respectively (clearance in this example) and BW_{Ped} and BW_{Adult} are the pediatric and adult bodyweight respectively; x is the empirical scaling factor. This approach has excellent predictive powers, when incorporated into pharmacokinetic (PK) or pharmacodynamic (PD) models (Fig. 9.1) [10]. Allometric scaling cannot account for all the changes observed during development. Therefore, other approaches, such as physiological models, may provide more accurate results [9,11].

Uptake and absorption

The gastric pH rapidly increases from 1–3 to 5–7 immediately after birth and remains basic during the first month of life [12]. Gastric emptying and intestinal transit time are also slower in newborns than in infants and adults. The rate and extent of gastric and intestinal absorption are variable, due to immature membrane transport, pancreatic enzyme activity, and bile salt secretion. Oral medications may have erratic bio-availability and absorption rates in this age group. Also, the first-pass effect is often reduced in neonates due to immature liver metabolism. Consequently, drug potency may increase in some cases.

Absorption by other routes is often rapid in infants and children. For example, after topical anesthesia of the pharynx and larynx, peak concentrations of lidocaine may appear 2–4 min later [13]. Lidocaine toxicity has occurred following infiltration of the drug for laceration repair in young patients. Because the rate and extent of absorption depend on the drug and site of injection, this topic will be discussed in the PK section for each drug.

Transport of molecules across membranes: the effect of transporters

Drugs are small molecules that are susceptible to passive or active transport through biological membranes. Uptake and elimination transporters are found in all cell membranes. Two superfamilies of transporters, the solute carrier (SLC) and ATP-binding cassette (ABC), control molecular traffic across membranes [4,14]. While SLC transporters are usually for uptake, some are involved in bidirectional transport. ABC transporters are efflux pumps that remove chemicals from the cell.

The organic anion transporting polypeptides (OATPs), the organic cation transporters (OCTs), and the organic anion transporters (OATs) are the principal solute carrier transporters. These membrane proteins are localized to the sinusoidal boundary in heart, liver, brain, kidney, and placenta. One SLC family, the multidrug and toxin extrusion transporters (MAETs), excretes oxaliplatin, cimetidine, metformin, and procainamide from cells.

ATP-binding cassette transporters comprise the P-glycoprotein (P-gp), which is encoded by a variety of multidrug-resistant (MDR) genes, and the MDR-associated proteins. These are excretion pumps that transport endo- and xenobiotics such as unconjugated bilirubin and anticonvulsants. Like SLC transporters, these transporters are ubiquitous in the blood–brain barrier (BBB), blood–cerebrospinal fluid (CSF) barrier, gut and intestinal wall, hepatocytes, and renal tubular cells. P-gp is located at the luminal membrane of endothelial and epithelial cells. It appears in human brain as early as 22 weeks' gestational age (GA) and is almost totally mature at birth [15]. All these transporters are highly polymorphic. In conjunction with polymorphism of the 3A4 and 2C9/19 isoforms of the cytochrome P450 or of UDP-glucuronosyltransferase (UGT) 1A and 2B, polymorphism of P-gp increases resistance to most antiepileptic drugs (phenytoin, carbamazepine, phenobarbital, gabapentin, felbamate, topiramate, lamotrigine, valproic acid, diazepam, lorazepam).

To date, little is known about the ontogeny of these transporters. The human fetal liver has only a small number of transporters. mRNA expression of SLC and ABC transporters increases from birth to 4 years of age and full expression is attained by 7 years [16]. Similar findings have been reported in the kidneys and gut.

P-glycoprotein has been detected as early as 22–26 weeks of human gestation in some parts of the brainstem.

By term, P-gp seems to be fully functional. Multiple drug resistance protein 1 (MRP1) is detected in the fetus at 22–26 weeks' gestation and has almost the same intensity as in adults. This is consistent with observations that the choroid plexus and tight junctions are mature before birth, which makes the blood–CSF barrier functional [5,17]. Lipids and possibly small hydrophobic molecules can cross the barrier with less selectivity until 6 months of age.

Disposition of drugs: transport in the blood and distribution

After administration, drugs disperse within the body. Because cardiac output and the central compartment volume are larger than those of adults, distribution of drugs to target organs occurs more rapidly in young patients. Sophisticated models that tentatively explain the relationship between age, volumes, clearance, and the dose required to produce anesthesia have been described. However, population PK-PD models using age as a covariate and parameters such as the exit rate constant from the effect compartment (ke0) and the pseudo-steady state concentration leading to half maximum effect (Cpss50 or Ce50) are now used to characterize the disposition of drugs from the central to the effect compartment and the resulting effect [18,19]. The ke0 is equivalent to the rate constant for transfer from the central compartment to the effect compartment at steady state. This parameter (or T½ke0, the corresponding half-life) is the best indicator of a drug's rate of accessing its target. It is directly related to time to peak action. Ce50 is the concentration of the drug in the (virtual) effect compartment and is approximated by Cpss50, the drug concentration in the effect compartment at steady state. Drugs also distribute in deeper compartments, depending on plasma and tissue protein binding, hydrophobicity, pKa, steric bulk, and clearance when steady state is not attained. This distribution process is important because it is the main factor that causes differences in delay of awakening after short or prolonged administration of drugs (volatile anesthetics, propofol). This has led to the concept of context-sensitive half-time [20]. In addition, distribution of drug into deep compartments (including gastric and bowel contents) may cause recirculation of drugs like fentanyl when cardiac output and body temperature increase after surgery.

Protein binding

Many drugs are bound to serum proteins, mostly albumin (human serum albumin – HSA) and α1-acid glycoprotein (AGP). Acidic drugs like thiopental and propofol bind preferentially to HSA and basic drugs to AGP. Protein-bound molecules may or may not cross barriers, depending on factors such as the nature of binding (rate of association-dissociation to the receptor) and the organ transit time [21,22]. In the liver, the presence of the Disse space slows transit times. Clearance of drugs metabolized by the liver is frequently independent of protein binding [23]. In organs with rapid transit times, such as the brain and heart, protein binding often controls the amount of drug absorbed by the organ.

Serum albumin is the most abundant protein in plasma (approximately 0.6 mM). It contains three homologous helical domains (I–III) with binding pockets. HSA has two major high-affinity binding sites with association constants in the range 10^4 to 10^6 M^{-1} [24,25]. Site 1 binds warfarin, thiopental, propofol, and many other drugs. Site 2 binds endogenous carboxylic acids (eicosanoids, fatty acids), propofol, volatile anesthetics and most non-steroidal anti-inflammatory drugs (NSAIDs), often in a stereospecific and allosteric manner. Some metabolites of NSAIDs bind covalently, leading to permanent occupation of the site. Bilirubin also binds to multiple sites on HSA [26]. Drugs such as propofol can displace bilirubin, increase the amount of free bilirubin, and possibly produce kernicterus in newborns [24].

α1-Acid glycoprotein, also called orosomucoid (ORM), is an acute-phase protein. At birth, AGP concentrations are about one-third to one-fourth of adult concentrations and increase slightly over the next 9–12 months [27,28]. The first consequence of reduced AGP is increased free drug that can cross barriers (blood–brain, blood–heart), causing increased drug effects. The second consequence of the increased amount of free drug is a greater apparent total hepatic clearance than is expected for drugs with low hepatic clearance, e.g. bupivacaine. AGP has 2–3 high-affinity sites that mostly bind basic drugs [29,30]. However, some acidic drugs (e.g. phenylbutazone) and neutral drugs also bind to AGP. Three genetic variants (A, F1 and S) cause two main forms (F1S and A) that differently bind xenobiotics. During inflammatory processes, the AGP concentration and its affinity for drugs markedly increase. During the postoperative period, the AGP concentration almost doubles (Fig. 9.2). For drugs with low to moderate hepatic extraction ratios, such as bupivacaine, this may produce time-dependent changes in total clearance (but not in the intrinsic clearance of the free drug) after surgery (Fig. 9.3) [31]. Like most basic drugs, local anesthetics and phenylpyperidine opioids (fentanyl, sufentanil, alfentanil) are primarily bound to AGP.

Protein–drug adducts [32,33]

Binding of drugs to proteins may be entropy driven (passive phenomenon, as with xenon) or enthalpy driven (usually exothermic). This causes strong binding of the drug (covalent, van der Waals forces). Covalent binding of drugs or their metabolites to tissue or plasma proteins produces mostly toxic protein–drug adducts. These adducts often induce immunological reactions that cause

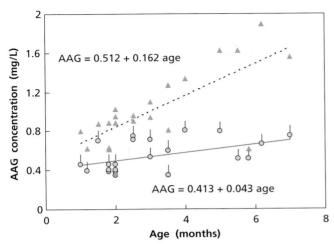

Figure 9.2 α1-Acid glycoprotein (AAG) concentrations in infants according to their age. AAG concentrations are very low at birth and progressively increase with age. The concentration of AAG increases rapidly after an inflammatory insult. Circles are individual values measured before surgery and triangles are the values measured 2 days later. AAG concentrations increased in all patients after surgery. Reproduced from Meunier et al [27] with permission from Lippincott Williams and Wilkins.

hypersensitivity. The toxicity of halothane, paracetamol (acetaminophen), diclofenac, sulfonamides, and valproic acid is the result of adducts.

During cardiopulmonary bypass, the concentration of unbound propofol increases significantly due to decreased protein binding [34]. This is probably true for most drugs with strong protein binding.

Metabolism and clearances including genetic polymorphism [35]

Renal function (glomerular filtration rate and tubular function) is immature at birth. Therefore, elimination of most renally excreted drugs and their active metabolites is impaired until 2–3 years of age. For example, theophiline and caffeine have very low clearances at birth. In the same way, morphine-6-glucuronide, which is an active metabolite of morphine, accumulates in premature and full-term infants, increasing the risk of respiratory depression [36–38]. Drugs such as aminoside antibiotics may also be toxic. Prostaglandin concentrations are elevated in newborns to maintain an effective glomerular filtration rate. By blocking the effects of prostaglandins, NSAIDs may induce renal hypoperfusion and renal failure [3].

Hepatic metabolism

Most drugs used for anesthesia, preoperative care, and pain control are metabolized by the liver. Hepatic metabolism of xenobiotics is by phase 1 and phase 2 reactions [39]. Phase 1 reactions are characterized by microsomal oxidative metabolism that inactivates or sometimes acti-

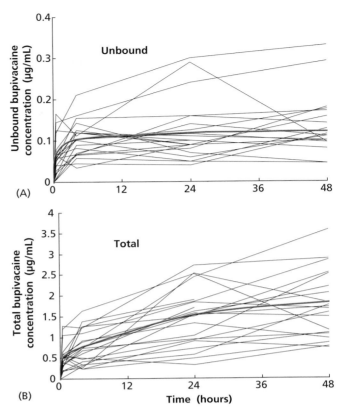

Figure 9.3 Unbound (A) and total (B) bupivacaine concentration in plasma after epidural administration (bolus at T0 followed by a continuous infusion of 0.375 mg/kg/h for 2 days). Black lines are individual data and blue lines are population value fitted using NONMEM. The unbound concentration reaches steady state in less than 12 hours whereas the total concentration has not reached steady state 48 hours after initiating the infusion. The continuous increase in α1-acid glycoprotein concentration caused by the inflammatory process increases protein binding. However, the unbound concentration, which is the toxic moiety, is at steady state because intrinsic hepatic clearance remains constant. Reproduced from Meunier et al [27] with permission from Lippincott Williams and Wilkins.

vates the drug (Table 9.1). Phase 2 reactions involve conjugation and take advantage of the electrophilic properties of either the original drug or of the product of phase 1 metabolism (Table 9.2) [40,41]. Phase 2 reactions occur mainly in the liver but can occur in the gut wall, the kidney parenchyma, and the lung. Enzymes involved in phase 1 reactions are located primarily in endoplasmic reticulum, while phase 2 conjugation enzyme systems are primarily cytosolic.

Cytochrome P450 is a family of enzymes located primarily in the centrilobular portion of hepatic lobules. CYP3A4 is the most abundant isoform (Fig. 9.4) [42–46]. Two factors characterize the importance of an isoform for metabolizing a given molecule: the capacity, i.e. the abundance of the enzyme, and the affinity and rate of metabolism (Km and vm in the Michaelis–Menten equation). Xenobiotics may be substrates for, inhibitors of or

Table 9.1 Hepatic metabolism of the agents used in anesthesia and perioperative care. Phase I metabolism

	Cytochrome P450 isoform					
	1A2	2A6	2B6	2D6	2E1	3A4/5[(1)] (3A7)
Early expression in liver	1 mo	1 mo	1 yr	1 w	Birth	
50% of adult activity	1 yr	1 yr		6 mo	1 yr	
90% of adult activity	4–6 yrs				4–6 yrs	
Variability between subjects due to polymorphism	Up to 60-fold			Up to 60-fold	Up to 50-fold	Up to 60-fold
Halogenated agents						
Halothane		++			++ [(2)]	++
Isoflurane		+/−	?		+	
Sevoflurane			+/−		+ [(3)]	
Desflurane			?		+/− [(3)]	
Propofol[(4)]			+++	I	II	I
Ketamine			+++			++ I
Midazolam			+			+++
Opioids						
Fentanyl						+++
Alfentanil						+++
Sufentanil						+++
Tramadol[x]				+++		+
Codeine				+++		
Amide local anesthetics						
Lidocaine	++		+/−			++
Bupivacaine	+					+++
Ropivacaine	+++		+/−			++
Acetaminophen	+				++	+
Caffeine	+++				+	+

Other isoforms involved: 2C8/9: most NSAIDs, phenytoin, barbiturates, ketamine and to a small extent caffeine; 2C19: diazepam, barbiturates and proton pump inhibitors. CYP2C19 is subject to important polymorphism. The isoform(s) involved in the metabolism of thiopental and etomidate remain(s) to be characterized.

Abbreviations: +, substrate for the CYP isoform; I, inhibitor of the CYP isoform; mo, month after birth; yr, year after birth; w (GA), week (gestational age).

(1) CYP3A7 is active in the fetus as early as 50–60 days after gestation, with a progressive switch to CYP3A4 after birth.

(2) The 2E1 isoform is responsible of the formation of toxic metabolites involved in hepatic toxicity.

(3) Desflurane is the least metabolized agent; sevoflurane metabolism is very low before the age of 4 yrs because of immaturity of CYP2E1.

(4) Propofol is also metabolized by CYP2C to a lesser extent.

inducers of the reaction and cause drug–drug interactions that have clinical consequences. Maturation of these enzymes is variable and occurs from early in intrauterine life to several years of age. For example, morphine elimination via UGT is impaired until 9 months of age [36,37,47] whereas fentanyl, which is metabolized by the CYP3A4/3A7 isoform of cytochrome P450, is adequately metabolized by very young preterm infants [48]. Ropivacaine metabolism by CYP1A2 is not fully mature before the age of 4–6 years [49].

Children are small adults [50]

Individuals have the potential of their future in their genes. Some phenotypic expression may be absent early in life, but most genetic traits are fully expressed at birth. The most common factors influencing drug dosing are related to genetic polymorphism of metabolizing enzymes [51–57].

Polymorphism of CYP2D6 may increase rates of biotransformation of tramadol to the opioid receptor agonist O-desmethyl tramadol (M1) [57,58]. Codeine is also metabolized to morphine by the CYP2D6 [59,60]. One death is suggested to have occurred when a breast-feeding mother extensively metabolized codeine to morphine postoperatively [61]. The increased amounts of morphine in breast milk caused severe apnea and death of the infant. Toxic events have also been reported in infants and young children treated with codeine for more

Relative CYP content   Contribution to drug metabolism

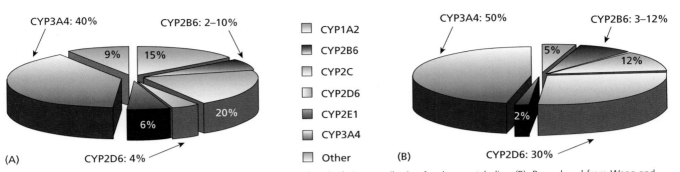

Figure 9.4 Cytochrome P450 isoforms in the liver. Relative content (A) and relative contribution for drug metabolism (B). Reproduced from Wang and Tompkins [286] with permission from Bentham Science Publishers Ltd.

Table 9.2 Hepatic metabolism of the agents used in anesthesia and perioperative care. Phase II metabolism

	NAT2	SulfoT	Uridine 5'-diphosphate (UDP)-glucuronosyltransferases (UGT)					
			1A1	1A3	1A6	1A8	1A9	2B7
Early expression in liver	1 T	Early in the fetus	Birth	2 T	Birth			10–20% <1 T
50% of adult activity				2 yr	6 mo			1 mo
90% of adult activity			3–6 mo		Puberty			6 mo
Bilirubin			+++ (1)					
Morphine				+ in the neonate		+		+++
Codeine								+++
Buprenorphine			+	+++				+
Propofol						++	+++	
Acetaminophen		++ in the fetus			+++		++	
Isoniazid	+++							
Sulfonamides	+++							
NSAIDs			+	++			++	+++

NAT2, N-acetyltransferase type 2; SulfoT, sulfotransferase.

Diazepam strongly inhibits the metabolism of morphine and codeine; ketamine inhibits the metabolism of morphine; ranitidine inhibits the metabolism of morphine and acetaminophen. Rifampin is an inducer of metabolism of codeine, morphine, acetaminophen, lamotrigine, and propafenone. Phenobarbital (and possibly thiopental) and phenytoin are inducers of acetaminophen metabolism, which may enhance its toxicity.

(1) Lack of the 1A1 isoform induces the autosomal recessive Crigler–Najjar and Gilbert syndromes.

Abbreviations: T, trimester of intrauterine life; +, substrate for the isoform; I, inhibitor of the isoform; mo, month after birth; yr, year after birth.

than one day or children with renal failure [62]. On the other hand, about 5–8% of Caucasians and 20–25% of Japanese metabolize codeine poorly and do not receive analgesic effects from the drug [63].

Pharmacokinetics and pharmacodynamics of inhaled drugs

Gases and vapors were the first agents used for general anesthesia (ether in 1842, nitrous oxide in 1844 and chlo-

roform in 1847). Their mechanism of action is far from fully elucidated, even today [64,65]. A thermodynamic effect on biological membranes has long been thought to be their mode of action. Now specific effects of these drugs on ion channels and receptor are favored. However, a body of facts leads one to think that there is a complex combination of these actions. The Meyer–Overton theory (and other related theories) is based on the observation that anesthetics non-specifically disturb the physical organization of membranes by solubilizing into lipids. There is still debate on the validity of the Meyer–Overton rule [66,67]. Interestingly, xenon, which is a rare gas, binds non-specifically to proteins, mainly by weak van der Waals forces [68,69].

A unified theory combining non-specific thermodynamic effects on the lipid bilayer and direct inhibition on excitatory neuronal channels is emerging, tentatively explaining the specific effect of anesthetics on the spinal cord [70,71]. Indeed, all anesthetic agents provoke immobility, even when noxious stimuli induce sympathetic responses. In addition, isobolographic analysis and response-surface curves of a combination of agents (both IV and volatile) show only additivity, which is a strong argument for a common mechanism of action [72–74].

In the usual conditions of pressure and temperature, nitrous oxide and xenon are gases whereas halogenated anesthetic agents are in liquid form (desflurane boils at 22.8°C, thus necessitating special vaporizers) (Table 9.3). N_2O is now the single most important ozone-depleting substance emitted [75]. In addition, halogenated volatile anesthetics (and N_2O) are greenhouse gases. Twenty-year global warming potential (GWP (20)) values and the carbon dioxide equivalent calculated at 1 minimum alveolar concentration (MAC) show a ratio of 2.2, 1 and 26.8 for isoflurane, sevoflurane and desflurane respectively [76].

Nitrous oxide

Nitrous oxide (N_2O) is a gas with a molecular weight of 44 Da and a blood/gas distribution ratio of 0.47. At an inhaled concentration of 70%, rapid equilibrium takes place between the inspired and expired fractions of N_2O [77–80]. The kinetics of N_2O is rapid; the deep peripheral compartment is no greater than 8–10 L. Severinghaus first recognized this when he demonstrated that N_2O does not follow the Kety principle, thus leading to the first description of context-sensitive times. When administration is discontinued, elimination is rapid. Even after several hours of administration, elimination is only slightly delayed. In addition, because N_2O is rapidly diffusible, the phenomenon of diffusion hypoxia or "Fink effect" may occur when room air is administered to patients previously breathing a mixture of N_2O and O_2 [81,82]. Because of its ability to diffuse into cavities, N_2O should be used with caution when middle ear or bowel pressures are critical. N_2O has a MAC of at least 104% [83] and an additive effect with volatile and IV anesthetics. In addition, it has euphoric, neuroprotective, analgesic and anti-hyperalgesic properties, probably because of its effect on the N-methyl-D-aspartate (NMDA) receptor [84,85]. This is why a 50% mixture of N_2O and O_2 is often used outside the operating room for sedation and analgesia. Like all anesthetics, N_2O has vasodilating properties. It moderately increases CBF (cerebral blood flow) and decreases vascular resistances. The net effect on intracranial pressure (ICP) varies, but it usually increases [86].

Xenon

Xenon (Xe) is the heaviest non-radio-active natural noble gas (molecular weight (MW) 131.3) [87]. It is colorless, odorless, and non-flammable. It is a dense monoatomic gas with a density of 5.76 and a high viscosity of 2.3 Pa/s (both under normal conditions). The high viscosity may theoretically render its use difficult in patients with increased airway resistance and in premature infants [88]. Its blood/gas distribution ratio is 0.14; its MAC is 70%. Xenon crosses biological barriers easily and reaches 90% equilibrium between inspired and alveolar gas concentration after 5 min of administration.

Despite its classifications as a noble gas, xenon binds to proteins but does not undergo biotransformation [89]. Because of its large atomic polarizability, xenon binds within cavities in all proteins [69,90]. This is why xenon has been considered to act by physical properties, such as the Meyer–Overton rule or the London dispersion forces (or weak van der Waals forces). Like N_2O, xenon acts as a low-affinity use-dependent NMDA receptor antagonist, but while xenon inhibits ketamine-induced c-fos expression in the rat cortex, nitrous oxide enhances it [91,92]. In addition, xenon is a potent antinociceptive agent. This effect is thought to be independent of the opioid or adrenergic pathways. The mechanisms involved seem different from those implicated in neuroapoptosis caused by ketamine or halogenated agents.

Altogether, these data have led to the suggestion that xenon, uniquely among compounds with known NMDA receptor antagonist properties, may exhibit neuroprotective action without co-existing neurotoxicity. In preliminary studies, xenon successfully protected the brain following neonatal asphyxia [93]. Another interesting property of xenon is cardiovascular stability and cardioprotection. Xenon does not alter myocardial contractility nor does it markedly change vascular tone. Xenon preconditioning before an ischemic insult has been observed at both the neuronal and myocardial levels. Like local anesthetics, xenon modulates the inflammatory response of the immune system by decreasing the production of tumor necrosis factor (TNF)-α and interleukin (IL)-6 by monocytes in response to stimulation by lipopolysaccharide (LPS) [91]. However, further studies are needed to assess these beneficial effects. The problem of industrial production and cost will certainly limit the use of xenon in the foreseeable future.

Halogenated agents

Halogenated agents are small molecules with MW from 168 to 200 Da (see Table 9.3) [79,94–96]. They are mildly hydrophobic and dissolve rapidly in blood and tissue. Halothane is an alkane substituted with bromide, chloride and fluoride. Isoflurane, sevoflurane and desflurane are ethers, substituted with chloride and

Table 9.3 Gases and volatile anesthetics. Physicochemical properties and pharmacokinetics

	Halothane	Isoflurane	Desflurane	Sevoflurane	N₂O	Xe
Molecular weight (Da)	197	184	168	200	44	133
Partition coefficient (*)	200	126	398	631	3	
Density (air = 1.29, helium = 0.18) (g/L, 0°C, 760 mmHg)		1.50	1.46	1.5	1.94	5.89
Viscosity (air = 1.83, helium = 1.97) (Pa/s, 25°C, 760 mmHg)					1.46	2.3
Boiling point (°C at 760 mmHg)	50	48	23	57	−88	−108
Vapor pressure (mmHg at 20°C)	244	238	669	170	57.9	−
Pressure at critical point					71.7 at 36.4°C	58 at 16.5°C
Blood/gas partition coefficient	2.40	1.40	0.45	0.65	0.47	0.12
Brain/blood partition coefficient	1.9	1.6	1.3	1.7	1.1	
Percent metabolized	15–20	0.2	0.02	3.0	0.004	<0.001
Vss (L)#	148	69	19	38		
MAC in adult (vol %)	0.76	1.15	6.0	2.0	104	63
Ce50 (%)	−	0.60–1.3	4.0–6.0	1.12–1.5	170	
T½ke0 (min)	−	3.2–4.3	0.9–1.3	2.0–3.5		

* from the LogP.
# Vss, the total volume of distribution is for an average adult weighing 70 kg, with a cardiac output of 5 L.
T½ke0 from BIS, Shannon or approximate entropy or from the Narcotrend give similar results.

fluoride (isoflurane) or only fluoride (desflurane and sevoflurane). Halothane, enflurane and isoflurane are chiral drugs, i.e. they have an asymmetric carbon, and they are marketed as racemic mixtures. Sevoflurane is non-chiral. Degradation of sevoflurane with CO_2 absorbents induces the formation of compound A, which is toxic for the kidney of rats [97]. However, the risk in humans seems almost non-existent [98].

Mode of action

The principal effect of anesthetic agents is to provoke immobility through effects that occur at the spinal cord level. Apart from the Meyer–Overton theory (see general considerations above), the mechanism of action of halogenated agents is thought to be related to interactions with ion channels and receptors in spinal cord and brain [64,65,99]. They simultaneously enhance the activity of gamma-aminobutyric acid (GABA) and glycine receptors and inhibit glutamate receptors ((2-amino-3-(5-methyl-3-oxo-1, 2-oxazol-4-yl)propanoic acid) (AMPA), kainate and NMDA receptors). They also inhibit the neuronal

nicotinic receptors, a mechanism that is common with N_2O and xenon. NMDA inhibitors are known to protect against ischemia reperfusion and to suppress the hyperalgesia induced by surgery. However, they also promote apoptosis through the mitochondrial pathway, particularly in the developing brain [100–102].

Pharmacokinetics

All halogenated agents bind to HSA in the following order: desflurane>isoflurane>halothane>sevoflurane [99,103–105]. HSA binds approximately 3 moles of anesthetic/mole of HSA.

Halogenated agents are absorbed and eliminated by the blood–alveolar interface. These agents, which are hydrophobic, distribute in deep compartments, and trace amounts can be measured in expired gases several weeks after anesthesia. Their hydrophobicity allows rapid transfer to the effect compartment and absorption by the fat. The agents with low solubility (see Table 9.3) rapidly reach saturation, i.e. pseudo-steady state [95,106]. The consequence is a more rapid induction of anesthesia and less context-sensitive increase in decrement time. Because an important amount of data is available on the solubility of these molecules in organs, as well as regional blood flows and volumes, physiological kinetic models have often been used to describe the time-course of halogenated agents in the body. Classic compartmental models are now preferred, mainly because they allow simple interpretation of basic parameters such as volumes, clearance and half-times, and easy application to clinical situations [107–112].

The pharmacokinetics of halogenated agents is best described by first-order kinetics, using linear mammillary models. After inhalation of a gas containing the vapor, transfer from alveolar gas to blood is rapid, and distribution to peripheral compartments, including brain (effect compartment), occurs. Elimination occurs via the same route, except for the variable amount of drug that is metabolized by the liver. The alveolar fraction of vapor (FA) is considered to reflect the arterial concentration and the inspired fraction (FI) the concentration in the invasion compartment. During induction of anesthesia, the FA/FI ratio (alveolar to inspired fraction) versus time reflects the rate of invasion (wash-in). After drug administration is discontinued, the ratio of alveolar fraction to alveolar fraction at the time of discontinuation (FA/FAo) reflects elimination (wash-out). The end tidal fraction (FET) (%) or end tidal partial pressure (mmHg) usually approximates FA.

The uptake and elimination of volatile anesthetics depend on cardiac output and the extent of ventilation. As always in pharmacokinetics, there is no direct correspondence between physiological and kinetic compartments. The volume of the central compartment depends on cardiac output and clearance; clearance depends on both minute ventilation and cardiac output. In an analogy with hepatic clearance of drugs eliminated by liver metabolism, ventilation is equivalent to intrinsic (metabolic) clearance and cardiac output (CO) to hepatic blood flow. Because CO is a major scaling factor, it would be interesting to have data relating CO to uptake and elimination in pediatrics [113]. It is also important to remember that 40% of halothane entering the body is eliminated by hepatic metabolism [107,108,114,115].

Context-sensitive decrement times [116]

Because the kinetics is multicompartmental (steady state is not attained before several days of administration, mainly because intercompartmental clearances are very slow), the observed decline is highly context sensitive [72,110]. After a short period of administration (less than 30 min), the decline of FA/FAo of sevoflurane or desflurane is faster than that for N$_2$O. This is due to the fact that N$_2$O reaches near steady state by 20–30 min whereas sevoflurane or desflurane are at about 60–80% of steady state by this time. After 90 min, the difference between agents becomes clinically significant (Fig. 9.5). As for the

effects of minute ventilation and cardiac output on kinetics, pediatric data describing decrement times as a function of age are lacking. Moreover, most articles are now based on data files generated with the aid of software (GasMan®) and do not verify their adequacy with data from patients.

Pharmacodynamics

The measure of anesthetic action has been the subject of research for more than 40 years. The initial criterion was the MAC, leading to a specific effect in 50% of the patients studied [117]. The MAC is the equivalent of Ce50 for IV agents. The concept of the MAC is based on the strong assumption that alveolar concentration is almost immediately in equilibrium with the cerebral concentration and adequately reflects the concentration at the neuronal effect site. MAC is defined as the alveolar concentration of volatile anesthetic agent (in oxygen or in a mixture of oxygen and N$_2$O) that abolishes 50% of the response to skin incision. One may also consider other effects, such as the cardiovascular depression induced by these agents, depression which is particularly important in neonates and in infants. The MAC has a great number of variations that have appeared over time: MACINT, which is the MAC for tracheal intubation, MACBAR, which is the MAC for abolition of sympathetic response to incision (tachycardia and increase in blood pressure), MACEXT, which is the MAC for deep tracheal extubation, etc. [118–122].

The MAC of isoflurane was found to be lower in preterm babies than in term neonates. This relatively low MAC in immature babies is thought to be a general phenomenon of all volatile anesthetics, although we lack data in this age group. At birth and during the first months of life, MAC is at its peak value for all drugs (except for halothane, which attains its peak value several months after birth). After the first year of life, there is a reversal in the relationship between age and MAC; MAC decreases with age (Fig. 9.6). In summary, infants aged 6 months have a MAC 1.5–1.8 times that observed for a mean adult aged 40 years [123–126]. Also, preterm infants are supposed to be more sensitive to cardiac depression than neonates, who are also more susceptible than older children and young adults [127].

The MAC gives the probability of inappropriate anesthesia in an average patient. The possibility of modulation of anesthesia depth in line with the patient's status now exists using several indexes obtained by EEG monitoring, such as the BISpectral Index (BIS) and the spectral entropy or Narcotrend Index [128–131]. In adults, numerous studies have shown that the population value of T½ke0 given by these indices was similar and close to the values expected from clinical experience (see Table 9.3) [132–136]. However, great interindividual variability has been observed, which is similar to that observed with

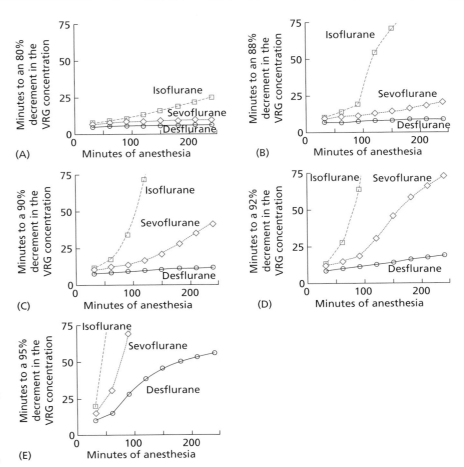

Figure 9.5 Context-sensitive decrement times in the rich vascularized compartment (VRG), i.e. brain, heart, kidney, liver, according to the duration of volatile anesthetic administration. Reproduced from Eger and Shafer [72] with permission from Lippincott Williams and Wilkins.

propofol, for example. In addition, the correlation between different MAC methods is difficult because, as with IV agents, all these EEG-derived algorithms are perturbed because hypnosis and analgesia are measured simultaneously. In children older than 2 years, it appears that the correlation between BIS IC50 and the different MAC measures is similar to that of adults [133,137]. To date, none of these monitors can correctly predict hypnosis in infants, perhaps with the exception of using regional and general anesthesia together (Fig. 9.7) [138–141].

Effects of volatile anesthetics on the different functions

Isoflurane and desflurane are pungent and can cause airway irritation during induction of anesthesia [142]. Only halothane – which is less and less used because of its lower margin of safety compared to other agents (see below) – and sevoflurane are used for anesthesia induction. This pungency does not increase the risk of laryngospasm after induction.

Specific action on the central nervous system

Volatile anesthetics depress neuronal activity in a concentration-dependent manner. High concentrations depress the electroencephalogram (EEG) and burst suppression occurs at concentrations greater than 2 MAC [143]. Sevoflurane induces epileptic activity with epileptiform discharges at concentrations usually greater than 1. 5 MAC, but this also occurs at lower concentrations in some patients [144]. Convulsion-like movements may accompany these EEG signs. The morbidity of these manifestations is unknown, and no sequelae have yet been reported. However, it is recommended not to use sevoflurane concentrations in excess of 6% for induction of anesthesia and to maintain anesthesia with concentrations not higher than 1.5 MAC.

Volatile anesthetics are often associated with agitation during emergence from anesthesia and for many minutes afterwards [145,146]. Emergence agitation is more frequent with newer agents such as sevoflurane. Concomitant administration of opioids, propofol, regional anesthesia or ketamine may prevent emergence agitation [147]. Awareness is more frequent in children than in adults, but implicit memory seems to be less of a concern in pediatric patients [148,149]. Both midazolam and propofol inhibit conscious memory, but midazolam does not prevent implicit memory if present [150].

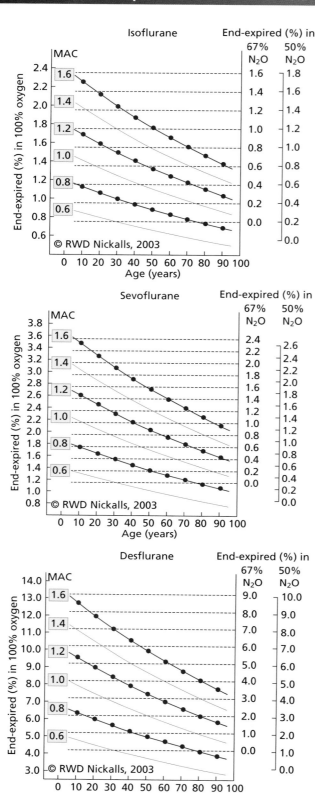

Figure 9.6 Minimum alveolar concentration of isoflurane, sevoflurane, and desflurane according to age. Premature infants have a lower MAC than neonates. Reproduced from Nickalls and Mapleson [126] with permission from Oxford University Press.

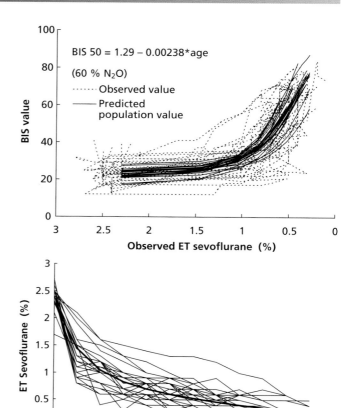

Figure 9.7 BIS values in 6 (mean) ± 3 (SD) year old children as a function of end-tidal (ET) sevoflurane. All patients had a regional block. Dotted lines are individual values and solid lines are Bayesian values calculated using NONMEM. Interestingly, in the absence of a nociceptive signal, the relationship between BIS value and ET sevoflurane is excellent and exhibits a negative correlation with age. Data from Kern et al. [141].

Apart from the possible neuroapoptosis induced by volatile anesthetics in infants and young children (see above), volatile anesthetics exert a protective effect on the nervous system that is similar to that observed for the heart [148–151]. This effect seems to be independent of the inhibition of the NMDA receptor. In addition to a direct neuroprotective effect, preconditioning with isoflurane, sevoflurane, and desflurane appears efficacious in protecting against focal ischemia and apoptosis induced by ischemia or hypoxia reperfusion. This effect seems related to the activation of various two-pore potassium channels and to the activation of inducible NO syntheses. Preconditioning seems to be particularly promising for neonatal cardiac surgery.

All volatile anesthetics increase CBF [152,153]. This increased blood flow is accompanied by a marked increase in intracerebral blood volume, which explains why increases in ICP are greater in children receiving volatile anesthesia than with IV anesthesia. Desflurane increases

ICP more than isoflurane or sevoflurane. However, autoregulation is depressed in a dose-dependent manner, and the administration of less than 1–1.5 MAC seems to preserve enough autoregulation for clinical purposes, inasmuch as the main factor causing a decrease in cerebral perfusion pressure is the arterial pressure, which should be preserved [154–158].

Effect on the respiratory system [159–161]

All volatile anesthetics depress ventilation by reducing tidal volume, which is not compensated for by a parallel increase in respiratory rate. Interestingly, halothane depresses the ventilatory response to CO_2 less than the other agents. However, the important clinical issue is the response to acute hypoxia, which is more depressed by halothane than by isoflurane. Sevoflurane and desflurane are the least depressive agents. In case of a sudden decrease in PaO_2, desflurane and sevoflurane are safer agents. During one-lung anesthesia, no difference between isoflurane, desflurane and sevoflurane has been noticed. Also, no difference is reported between propofol and volatile anesthetics. At 0.5 MAC, all agents are bronchodilators. At higher concentrations, bronchoconstriction appears with desflurane at concentrations >0.5 MAC and with sevoflurane at concentrations higher than 1–1.5 MAC. Only isoflurane maintains its bronchodilating properties at 2 MAC. However, in children with airway susceptibility, for instance those with recent upper respiratory tract infection, desflurane markedly increases bronchial resistances, whereas sevoflurane exerts a bronchodilating effect [162,163].

Effect on the cardiovascular system [164–170]

All anesthetics depress contractility and inhibit sympathetic tone. Halothane significantly does so at 1 MAC, whereas isoflurane, desflurane and sevoflurane only do so at concentrations above 1.5 MAC. In addition, halothane causes marked bradycardia, whereas sevoflurane has almost no effect on cardiac rhythm below 1.5 MAC. Isoflurane and desflurane have been shown to increase heart rate in adults, but an increase in heart rate is not as critical in pediatric patients. Interestingly, depression caused by halothane is poorly corrected by atropine, whereas it increases contractility in infants and children who are anesthetized with the other three agents. This difference between halothane and other agents (mainly sevoflurane has been studied) has been observed in patients without cardiopathy or with various congenital heart diseases. This is true also in patients breathing spontaneously. In addition, only halothane significantly potentiates epinephrine-induced cardiac arrhythmias. Halothane, isoflurane and sevoflurane depress the autonomic control of arterial pressure in a similar manner. However, the bradycardia caused by halothane should be

considered. Premature infants, who have an immature baroreflex, are particularly sensitive to the depression induced by anesthetics. In conclusion, halothane should be avoided when possible in infants and children, as halothane overdose has been associated with deaths in this age group.

Isoflurane, desflurane and sevoflurane possess cardioprotective effects, and both desflurane and sevoflurane have been shown to decrease postoperative mortality in adults suffering from coronary artery diseases. Indeed, the cardiac depressive effect reduces oxygen demand and may protect during ischemia. However, there is evidence of a specific effect related to pre- and post-conditioning. This may be beneficial for cardiac procedures in infants and children [165,171,172].

Effect on muscle relaxation

Volatile anesthetics have an intrinsic effect on muscle relaxation [173–175]. Their prejunctional effect decreases the firing rate of motor fibers. In addition, they my also affect the sensitivity of the motor endplate. Volatile anesthetics interact with muscle relaxants. They do not interact with the kinetics of non-depolarizing muscle relaxants, but decrease Ce50 [176]. The dose of rocuronium or atracurium needed to achieve similar effect is decreased by about 25–30% in patients anesthetized with sevoflurane compared to those anesthetized with propofol [177]. At similar MACs, all volatile anesthetics enhance the action of pancuronium, vecuronium, rocuronium, atracurium, and cisatracurium to a similar degree [178].

Malignant hyperthermia (see Chapter 40)

All volatile anesthetics may induce malignant hyperthermia (MH) [179–181]. Succinylcholine increases its severity. This genetic disorder of the ryanodine receptor of the skeletal muscle has a prevalence estimated at between 1:3000 and 1:8500. Indeed, the prevalence largely varies between populations. The incidence of MH associated with general anesthesia is estimated at between 1:30,000 and 1:100,000. Patients with various myopathies may be susceptible to MH [182]. Central core disease and hypokalemic periodic paralysis are particular risks [183,184].

The usual clinical presentation is an uneventful induction of anesthesia, progressive development of tachycardia and hyperthermia, and a rise in end-tidal CO_2 tension. The associated muscle rigidity is a direct sign of impaired intracellular calcium regulation. In patients spontaneously breathing, a progressive rise in minute ventilation is also observed. Acidosis and hyperkalemia, a serum creatinine kinase >10,000 IU/L, are the main biological manifestations. If untreated, MH may be rapidly lethal. These manifestations are not always typical, and there is a risk that the diagnosis will be missed because MH may progressively develop after discharge of the patient from the operating room or because a lethal episode may occur during a future anesthetic.

Dantrolene is the specific treatment (2–3 mg/kg up to 10 mg/kg as a bolus). Clinical signs determine the dose of dantrolene needed. Following treatment, the signs and symptoms of MH may recur, making it necessary to reinject dantrolene. This is why dantrolene must always be readily available. Dantrolene must be dissolved in sterile water (possibly warmed to 40°C), because dissolution is very difficult. It is important to change the anesthesia machine and the entire circuit, to cool the patient if necessary, and to correct acidosis if necessary. The diagnosis is ascertained by a muscle biopsy, which should always be performed. Prevention of MH in susceptible subjects consists of preparing the anesthesia machine by removing the vaporizers and changing the circuit. Total intravenous anesthesia is used and succinylcholine is avoided.

Pharmacokinetics and pharmacodynamics of intravenous drugs

Benzodiazepines

Benzodiazepines interact with a specific site on the GABA$_A$ receptor, increasing the affinity of the receptor for GABA [185,186]. GABA$_A$ is the principal inhibitory neurotransmitter which increases the frequency of opening of the chloride channel. In normal conditions, chloride concentration is lower inside the cell than outside. Opening of the channel increases the concentration of chloride inside the cell and hyperpolarizes the membrane. Benzodiazepines have hypnotic and sedative properties. They are potent anticonvulsants. They are also anxiolytic and provoke antegrade amnesia. Although they are weak muscle relaxants (a central effect), they do not notably interact with peripherally acting muscle relaxants.

Pharmacokinetics

Benzodiazepines are weak bases bound to serum proteins, mainly AGP (Table 9.4) [187,188]. Only midazolam is water soluble. Benzodiazepines rapidly cross the BBB and quickly access the receptor: their $T\frac{1}{2}ke0$ is less than 3 min, except for lorazepam [189–192]. Conversely, the duration of action mainly depends on affinity to the receptor. Midazolam, clonazepam and lorazepam have an affinity constant to the receptor 20 times higher than diazepam and the duration of action is as follows: diazepam 2 hours, midazolam 2–4 hours, clonazepam 24 hours, lorazepam 24–72 hours.

Benzodiazepine metabolism takes place in the liver via the CYP3A4 isoform of the cytochrome P450, with the exception of lorazepam, which is metabolized by the UGT [193–195]. There is no phase 1 metabolism. Diazepam has active metabolites, mainly N-desmethyldiazepam which may accumulate in intensive care unit (ICU) patients with kidney failure. Midazolam has an active metabolite, α1-OH-midazolam, but the ratio between metabolite and parent drug remains constant, even in ICU patients. Because all these molecules have low hepatic extraction ratios, their elimination mainly depends on the hepatic function; in case of liver failure, the clearance of benzodiazepines is markedly decreased.

After oral administration, absorption of midazolam is rapid; its bio-availability is 50% and its T_{max}, the time to peak concentration, occurs 40–50 min after administration. Absorption is very rapid after rectal administration. In children, T_{max} is 10 and 15 min for diazepam and midazolam respectively. After rectal administration, bio-availability is 50–80% for diazepam and 20–50% for midazolam. The IM route has been abandoned because of unpredictable absorption. The volume of distribution is large (1–2 L/kg) and the terminal half-life long (see Table 9.4) [196–199].

Apart from some inhibitors of HIV replication, such as ritonavir, few interactions between benzodiazepines and other drugs metabolized by the CYP3A4 have been described. Because of immaturity of CYP3A4, midazolam clearance is very low in preterm infants and during the first 2–3 months of life [200,201].

Pharmacodynamics
Action on the central nervous system

Benzodiazepines cause sedation through their effect on GABA$_A$ receptors. Their indications include premedication and sedation in the ICU [202]. When used as a premedicant, a paradoxical agitation reaction to benzodiazepine sometimes occurs. However, their sedative, anxiolytic and amnesic effects make midazolam one of the preferred drugs for premedication, particularly for unco-operative children or patients who have undergone multiple procedures. However, the effect on anterograde amnesia and implicit memory remains controversial [150]. Benzodiazepines have almost no effect on the CBF, ICP or cardiovascular system, which makes these drugs suitable for sedation in the ICU, particularly in neonates and in patients with head trauma, when long-term propofol administration is a risk [203].

Action on the respiratory and cardiovascular systems

Midazolam depresses ventilation by decreasing sensitivity to CO$_2$ [204]. Narcotics potentiate this effect. Diazepam and midazolam produce only mild cardiovascular depression and a minimal reduction in blood pressure, due to a decrease in vascular resistance [205]. This effect is increased when the drug is administered concomitantly

Table 9.4 Benzodiazepines and IV anesthetics. Physicochemical properties and pharmacokinetics

Drug	Molecular weight (Da)	pKa	Distribution ratio (octanol/buffer)	Protein binding %		T½ (h)	CL (mL/kg/min)	Vc (L/kg)	Vss (L/kg)	T½ke0 (min)	Ce50 (µg/mL)
Midazolam	326	6.1	475	96	Adult:	3–8	1.3–4	–	1.1	3.2	–
Diazepam	284	3.3	580	98	Adult:	40	0.4–0.6	–	–	1.6	–
Thiopental	242	7.4	209	80	Adult:	12–15	3.1	0.28	2.1	1.2	–
					5 mo–4 yrs:	6	6.6	0.4	2.1	–	–
Propofol	178	11	6900	99%	Adult:	6–8	20	0.15	5	2.6 (LOC)–4.2(BIS$_{50}$)	1.8(LOC)–5.2(BIS$_{50}$)
–	–	–	–	–	1 yr:		50	1.0	10	0.8(BIS$_{50}$)	5.2(BIS$_{50}$)
–	–	–	–	–	5 yr:	12–15	30	0.4	8	–	–
–	–	–	–	–	Premature:		15	1.3	6	–	–
Etomidate	244	4.5	1000	75	Adult:	3.5–4.6	10	0.3	2.5–4	1.55(BIS$_{50}$)	0.53(BIS$_{50}$)
–	–	–	–	–	7–13 yr:	4	17	0.66	5.6	–	–
Ketamine	238	7.5	750	60	Adult S(+):	2.5–5.3	21–36	0.2–0.4	3.4	–	–
–	–	–	–	–	Adult R(-):	2.6	19	0.4	3.0–8.0	–	–
–	–	–	–	–	8 yr:	6–8	30	0.4	8.0	0.2	0.52 (arousal)

Ce50 is for loss of consciousness (LOC) or for a 50% decrease in the BIS value (BIS$_{50}$). BIS, entropy, and various measures based on EEG give similar results.

with narcotics or other sedatives. When given to ICU patients for several days, midazolam has no significant effect on liver or adrenal function. Tolerance and tachyphylaxis may occur, particularly with longer term infusions (≥3 days). Benzodiazepine withdrawal syndrome occurs with high-dose/long-term midazolam infusions [206].

Dosing

For premedication in infants and children after the age of 3–6 months, midazolam 0.3–0.5 mg/kg orally (or rectally if the oral route is not possible) 30–40 min before induction of anesthesia, diazepam (if midazolam is not available) 0.1 mg/kg 60 min before surgery. As an adjunct for the induction of anesthesia, use 0.15 mg/kg. As the sole agent for anesthesia induction, use 0.3–0.6 mg/kg IV. The infusion dose of midazolam in critically ill patients is 0.03–0.3 mg/kg/h (30–300 µg/kg/h). The dose of midazolam is adjusted in ICU patients according to the patient's clinical condition (use of a sedation score by the attending nurse is highly recommended).

Flumazenil, a specific benzodiazepine antagonist, reverses all the effects of benzodiazepines. However, its

rapid elimination kinetics makes continuous infusion of the drug necessary to maintain therapeutic efficacy [207]. The dose by IV bolus is 5–10 µg/kg/min up to 40–50 µg/kg. It may be necessary to follow this titrated dose with a continuous infusion of the drug at a rate corresponding to the titrated dose given over an hour.

Thiopental

Thiopental is still an important drug for induction of anesthesia in the younger patients. Like propofol, thiopental modulates the GABAA and glycine receptors, but thiopental mainly acts at the spinal cord level and preferentially on the glycine receptor [186,208–210].

Pharmacokinetics

Thiopental is a weak acid (with a pKa of 7.6) and an octanol/buffer distribution ratio of 490 (LogP = 2.69) (see Table 9.4) [96,211]. It is a racemic mixture of two stereoisomers (S-(+) and R-(–)), the S-(+) isomer being twice as potent as the R-(–) isomer. Thiopental binds to HSA with an average free fraction of 15% in adults and 28% in neonates [212,213]. Binding is enantioselective with the R-(–) slightly less bound than the S-(+) enantiomer.

Thiopental is metabolized by the cytochrome P450 system, but the precise pathway(s) remain(s) to be characterized [214]. Its terminal half-life is very prolonged [215–220]. After a bolus injection, the drug distributes rapidly, making its effect transient. Following a single injection, thiopental's pharmacokinetics is best described by a two-compartment linear model, with a terminal half-life of ≈12 hours in adult patients. Intrinsic unbound clearance and volumes of distribution of the unbound fraction are similar for both enantiomers. The rate of administration markedly influences the total dose needed to achieve a predetermined effect: because of rapid redistribution of the drug, the higher rate of administration leads to high but transient peak concentration, which is unable to correctly cross the BBB; a minimum duration of plateau concentration is needed to achieve clinical efficacy. This is consistent with an equilibration half-time (T½ke0) of 2.4 min between the central and effect compartments (see Table 9.4). Disposition of the drug is similar in infants, children, and adolescents. In pediatric patients older than 6 months, clearance is higher than in adults, and the average T½ is 6.1 hours (see Table 9.4) [221]. With prolonged administration (for example, in patients with critically increased ICP), thiopental exhibits non-linear (Michaelis–Menten) kinetics, with an apparent terminal half-life of 15 hours [215,217]. In neonates and young infants, kinetics are not profoundly altered but the pharmacodynamics are likely different, with an ED50 (the dose leading to loss of lid reflex in 50% of children) of 3.4, 6–7, 5.5 and 4.2 mg/kg in patients aged 0–14 days, 1–6 months, 6–12 months and older than 1 year respectively [222]. Interestingly, the curve representing ED50 versus age is very similar to that of MAC versus age for halogenated agents. Studies considering allometric scaling are lacking.

Pharmacodynamics
Effect on the central nervous system
Thiopental is still the drug of choice for sedation of patients with increased ICP because it does not increase CBF and may decrease ICP (although the cerebral perfusion pressure may not significantly change). The very prolonged elimination that is the result of Michaelis–Menten kinetics must be taken into account in these patients.

Effect on the respiratory and cardiovascular systems
Thiopental depresses ventilation, likely because of decreased sensitivity to CO_2. In adults, more critical respiratory events occur in the immediate postoperative period with thiopental use than with propofol, although both cause similar changes in functional residual capacity (FRC) [223]. This increase in the number of events is likely related to the higher residual sedation associated with thiopental.

Thiopental decreases arterial blood pressure. Contrary to propofol, this decrease is related not only to decreased vascular tone but also to decreased myocardial contractile force [224]. Consequently, thiopental must be used with care in patients with cardiac failure.

Other effects
Thiopental, like other barbiturates, may induce porphyria. Its use is absolutely contraindicated in patients susceptible to such pathology. The acidity of thiopental solutions may cause necrosis at the injection site if extravascular diffusion occurs. Inadvertent arterial injection has caused severe necrosis.

Dosing
Because the risk of necrosis is high following inadvertent extravascular injection, the use of dilute solutions is recommended (2.5% in children and adults, 1% in infants). When adjuncts (opioids) are used for induction of anesthesia, the usual dose of thiopental is 2.5–3 mg/kg in neonates <10 days of age, 6–7 mg/kg in infants, and 5 mg/kg in children.

When ICU patients have thiopental infused for prolonged periods of time, thiopental kinetics becomes non-linear, in both adults and children. It may then be important to monitor thiopental plasma concentrations if the rate of thiopental administration exceeds 4–5 mg/ kg/h.

Propofol
Propofol is progressively replacing thiopental for induction and maintenance of anesthesia. This latter indication is likely related to the emergence of computer-driven systems for drug administration, since propofol kinetics and dynamics have been extensively studied [225]. Propofol enhances gating of the GABAa receptor by GABA and slows desensitization of the receptor [208,209]. In addition, propofol presynaptically depresses excitatory synaptic transmission and decreases glutamate release. It also enhances activation of the glycine receptor by glycine.

Pharmacokinetics
Propofol is a weak acid with a pKa of 11.5 and an octanol/ buffer distribution ratio around 6500 [96]. Because of its high hydrophobicity, propofol is "solubilized" in lipid emulsions, initially in Intralipid®. Propofol binds to red blood cells and serum albumin, and the free fraction is <1% [226–228]. Binding is markedly decreased in patients on cardiopulmonary bypass [229] and those in ICUs who have decreased serum concentrations of HSA.

The pharmacokinetics largely varies with age, explaining the differences in dosing between infants, children, and adults (see Table 9.4) [230–233]. When one compares a typical 20 kg, 5-year-old child and a typical 70 kg, 30-year-old adult, the main findings are: (1) an elimination clearance moderately higher in children than in adults, and (2) more importantly, volumes (both the central (Vc) and peripheral (Vss) compartments) are between 2 and 2.5 times greater in children than in adults, and the associated intercompartmental clearances are 1.5 greater in children than adults. When allometric scaling is performed, clearance is constant across species and age in humans: CL = 71 * (BW/70) ^ 0.78 L/min, where BW is bodyweight and 70 the standard bodyweight for adult humans [234].

Propofol exhibits marked multicompartmental kinetics and context-sensitive decrement times (Fig. 9.8) [235]. Altered kinetics (decrease in elimination clearance) has been reported in ICU patients and in neonates [233]. In premature infants less than 38 weeks' postmenstrual age, clearance is very low since maturation of metabolism occurs at birth. Interestingly, there are almost no differences in pharmacodynamic parameters across age [236–241]. The differences are mainly kinetic, i.e. Ce50, the concentration in the effect compartment needed to achieve a desired effect, is nearly similar among infants, children, and adults. Conversely, T½ke0 and the time to peak effect are shorter in younger patients than in adults, and the difference is identical to the difference measured for volumes and intercompartmental clearances (see Table 9.4). Interestingly, the effects on ventilation and arterial blood pressure do not have the same kinetics [242,243]. In adult patients, T½ke0 for respiratory depression is 2.6 min, similar to that for hypnosis, whereas T½ke0 for a half decrease in systolic blood pressure from baseline to

80 mmHg is 6 and 11 min in 20- and 75-year-old patients respectively.

Pharmacodynamics
Specific action on the central nervous system
Propofol has little effect on CBF or ICP when normocarbia is present [244]. This is why propofol is so popular in ICUs for sedation of patients with increased ICP [245]. Propofol is also used to treat seizures, mainly in cases of status epilepticus [246].

Effect on the respiratory and cardiovascular systems
Like all hypnotic agents, propofol depress ventilation by decreasing sensitivity to CO_2. This effect is central since the T½ke0 of respiratory depression is similar to the T½ke0 of hypnosis [243]. Propofol and thiopental decrease the functional residual capacity by similar amounts [247].

Propofol has a direct negative inotropic effect at very high (supratherapeutic) concentrations [224]. At therapeutic concentrations, its effect on contractility is insignificant [248]. The main cardiovascular effect of propofol is on vascular tone, probably because it inhibits the sympathetic nervous system. The prolonged T½ke0 on vascular tone strongly suggests that the effect is at least partly peripheral [242]. Propofol protects the myocardium against ischemia reperfusion injury through its ability to inhibit the mitochondrial permeability transition pore and its antioxidant and free radical scavenging properties [249,250].

Propofol infusion syndrome
After more than 2 days of propofol infusion in ICU patients, severe toxic effects have occurred [251,252]. This "propofol infusion syndrome" is likely caused by the uncoupling effect of propofol on the respiratory chain in the mitochondria. The clinical presentation includes lactic acidosis, rhabdomyolysis, and cardiovascular collapse (bradycardia, sometimes Brugada-like ECG, asystole). Green or red urine has been described in some patients [253]. This syndrome was initially described in children and adults with head trauma who received high-dose propofol for sedation. If sedation with propofol seems to benefit the patient, it is recommended to give <4 mg/kg/h for less than 48 hours. Close monitoring of acid–base status, serum lactate and creatine kinase concentrations should be performed. The use of propofol for total intravenous anesthesia (TIVA) for several hours has not been reported to cause adverse effects in children.

Presentation and dosing
Propofol is available as a 1% or 2% emulsion. The carrier emulsion was originally Intralipid® but other

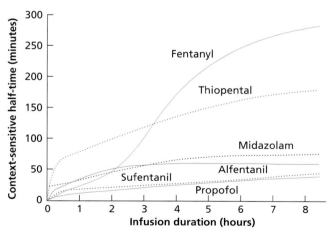

Figure 9.8 Context-sensitive decrement times of the principal agents used intravenously. Remifentanil is not depicted in this figure since its decrement times are constant. Reproduced from Hughes et al [20] with permission from Lippincott Williams and Wilkins.

lipid emulsions are used in generic preparations. Propofol contains EDTA, sodium metabisulfite or benzyl alcohol as antimicrobial agent. Pain at the site of injection is common and may be attenuated by lidocaine (0.5–1 mg/kg), either injected before the propofol or in the same syringe with the drug. Propofol should not be prepared in advance, since bacteria grow rapidly in the emulsion. Postoperative nausea and vomiting occur less frequently with propofol than with other agents (e.g. volatile anesthetics). To achieve similar plasma concentrations in children and in adults, the initial dose must be 2–3 times greater in children [254]. Because the volume at steady state is also markedly different, the initial 15–60 min of an infusion must be higher in children than in adults [255]. However, the significant hemodynamic effect of propofol must be taken into account, and balanced anesthesia with adjuncts seems preferable for induction of anesthesia. The usual doses for anesthesia induction are <1 month 4 mg/kg, 1 month to 3 years 5–6 mg/kg, 3–8 years 3–5 mg/kg, >8 years 3 mg/kg. Loss of consciousness lasts for 5–10 min after a single injection. The dosing scheme for continuous infusion of the drug is provided in Table 9.5.

Table 9.5 Propofol and ketamine infusion scheme

Propofol infusion dosing in infants and children. After induction of anesthesia with propofol (3–5 mg/kg), anesthesia is maintained with the following scheme. Anesthesia needs to be complemented with fentanyl/alfentanil/sufentanil or regional anesthesia. Adapted from RJ Steur et al. Ped Anesth 2004; 14: 462–7.

	Time (min)					
Age	First 10	10–20	20–30	30–40	40–100	>100
<3 months	25	20	15	10	5	2.5
3–6 months	20	15	10	5	5	2.5
6–12 months	15	10	5	5	5	2.5
1–3 years	12	9	6	6	6	6
Adult	10	8	6	6	6	4

Ketamine infusion scheme for children weighing 12–40 kg. Depending on the procedure, adjuncts may be given. Adapted from D Dallimore et al. Paediatr Anaesth 2008; 18: 708–14.

	Infusion rate (mg/kg/h)				
Loading dose	0–20	20–40	40–60	60–120	>120
2 mg/kg	11	7	5	4	3.5

Etomidate

Etomidate is a carboxylated imidazole that is highly hydrophobic, has hypnotic properties, and has little effect on the cardiovascular system. It is often used for induction of anesthesia in patients with critical hemodynamic conditions, despite its suppressive effect on adrenal steroid synthesis [256,257]. Etomidate has a high degree of enantioselectivity. The R-(+) enantiomer is 10 times more potent than the S-(–) enantiomer [258,259]. The commercial preparation is the pure R-(+) enantiomer. Like propofol, etomidate interacts with the GABAA receptor, but the actions of these two drugs on the different subunits of the receptor differ [260–262]. Etomidate causes marked *in vitro* endothelium-dependent vasodilation. However, this effect is less than that observed with propofol and is reversed by adrenergic stimulation [258].

Pharmacokinetics

Etomidate is a weak base, hydrophobic (the active molecule is "solubilized" in propylene glycol or in a lipid emulsion), and is bound to AGP. Protein binding is decreased in patients with kidney and liver failure, which may increase the sensitivity of these patients to the drug [259,263].

Etomidate is metabolized in the liver by the cytochrome P450 system, but the specific isoform(s) involved remain(s) to be characterized. CYP3A2 may be involved because etomidate decreases antipyrine clearance [264]. Clearance of etomidate is decreased in cirrhotic patients [265–267]. Metabolites are inactive. In children, the volume of the central compartment is more than twice that of adults (0.66 versus 0.27 L/kg) [268]. Clearance is also higher. However, the volume of the central compartment depends on the cardiac output. If, indeed, children with normal cardiovascular function need a greater dose of drug for induction of anesthesia, those with impaired hemodynamics may require less [269,270].

Pharmacodynamics
Specific action on the central nervous system
Etomidate has no intrinsic action on CBF. It decreases ICP. Cerebral perfusion pressure is likely unchanged because of the etomidate-induced slight decrease in arterial blood pressure, which may explain the decrease in CBF and subsequent decrease in ICP.

Effect on the respiratory and cardiovascular systems
Etomidate induces moderate respiratory depression by reducing sensitivity to CO_2.

Etomidate is mainly used for induction of anesthesia (particularly in emergency cases) because of the hemodynamic stability observed [224,258,271–273]. Etomidate has no effect on heart rate, and contractility is only moderately impaired. *In vitro* and *in vivo* studies in animals and humans have shown that etomidate has an intrinsic negative inotropic effect that is similar to the effects observed with ketamine and midazolam. This effect is totally reversed by β-adrenergic stimulation. More importantly, etomidate only moderately impairs vascular tone. Baroreflex control is preserved, in contrast to propofol and thiopental.

Effect on adrenal function

Etomidate blocks 11-β-hydroxylase, thus inhibiting conversion of cholesterol to cortisol [274]. After an induction dose of etomidate, adrenal suppression lasts for about 24 h. This effect may be clinically relevant, particularly in patients with septic shock who have compromised adrenal function.

Formulation and dosing

Two formulations are distributed, depending on the solvent used. The initial formulation uses propylene glycol (35% vol/vol), and the second uses a lipid emulsion (propofol) as the carrier. Both preparations are painful on injection, but the propylene glycol preparation is particularly irritating because of its osmolality (4640 mOsm/L).

For induction of anesthesia in the emergency department, 0.2–0.3 mg/kg is used in children with compromised cardiovascular function and 0.3–0.6 mg/kg in patients in a stable condition. Myoclonus may occur with injection of the drug. In pediatric patients, rectal induction of anesthesia is possible with a dose of 6–8 mg/kg. Continuous administration of the drug is not recommended because it suppresses cortisol synthesis.

Ketamine

Ketamine has hypnotic, analgesic, and antihyperalgesic properties and produces "dissociative anesthesia," profound analgesia, and marked sympathomimetic reactions [275]. However, ketamine has unwanted side-effects, such as hallucinations, confusion, delirium, hypersalivation and bronchial hypersecretion. Ketamine anesthesia is characterized by rapid immobility and cataleptic appearance, mydriasis, nystagmus, and increased muscular tone. Emergence from anesthesia is characterized by a state of confusion, often with hallucinations. This state, which is amplified by light and noise, is less frequent in younger children than in adults and may be prevented by administering adjunct drugs such as benzodiazepines. Ketamine has moderate effects on the cardiovascular system. It has an asymmetric carbon, with two enantiomers: R-(−)- and S-(+)-ketamine. The S-(+) enantiomer is about four times more potent than the R-(−) enantiomer [276].

Ketamine acts mainly as a non-competitive NMDA receptor antagonist. It inhibits presynaptic release of glutamate and potentiates GABAᴀ. Ketamine also has opioid and muscarinic properties. The effects on the NMDA receptor include both the neuroprotective and proapoptotic effects of ketamine [277–281].

Pharmacokinetics

Ketamine is 50% ionized and 50% non-ionized at pH 7.4. Both the parent drug and its metabolite norketamine are bound to serum proteins, with a free fraction of 40% and 50% respectively [282]. Ketamine is metabolized by CYP2B6 and 3A4 [283–286]. N-demethylation produces norketamine, which has about 30% of the activity of ketamine. Norketamine undergoes almost the same metabolism as ketamine (hydroxylation by CYP2B6 and glucuroconjugation) and has a terminal half-life of similar duration (≈4–6 hours) [287–296]. Norketamine is then considered to be responsible for some of the effects of ketamine. Access to the receptor is very rapid, with a T½ke0 of <1 min (see Table 9.4). Drug redistribution occurs rapidly (the initial distribution half-life is <15 min), and after a single 1 mg/kg IV injection, anesthesia lasts 6–10 min. Because of the multicompartmental nature of ketamine's pharmacokinetics, decrement times are markedly context sensitive.

Pharmacodynamics

Specific action on the central nervous system

Ketamine has specific effects on the CNS [294,295]. It enhances EEG activity and increases CBF and cerebral metabolic rate of O_2 ($CMRO_2$). Because the arterial pressure increases, there is an increase in ICP that is proportional to the increase in CBF. However, when adjuncts are used with ketamine and, more importantly, when normocarbia is maintained, ICP does not increase. Thus ketamine is often used in neurologically impaired patients. Ketamine has neuroprotective effects through its action on the mitochondria. However, the effects of ketamine on the ATP-sensitive mitochondrial K+ channel remain a subject of debate. On the other hand, ketamine also induces apoptosis via the mitochondrial pathway. This is considered a major issue in neonates and infants. The neurotoxicity of ketamine on the brains of developing animals seems clear. Consequently, this agent should probably be used with care in younger patients.

Effect on the respiratory and cardiovascular systems

Ketamine does not depress ventilation, and the CO_2 response remains intact [296]. Tidal volume and respiratory rate are unchanged. Ketamine does not alter FRC, even at high doses, but it does induce moderate bronchodilation. The pharyngo-laryngo-tracheal reflexes are partly conserved, leading to a relative airway protection.

Ketamine has minimal effects on myocardial contractility [297–300]. It preserves sympathetic activity and baroreflex activity. In healthy subjects, ketamine raises arterial blood pressure slightly, increases the myocardial contractile force, and increases cardiac output. However, in patients with decreased cardiac reserve, negative inotropic effects of the drug can be unmasked when myocardial contractility fails to increase with β-adrenergic stimulation. In addition, the increase in mixed venous oxygen saturation (MVO_2) may be deleterious in patients who have insufficient coronary reserve. It has been reported that ketamine inhibits ischemic preconditioning via its inhibition of ATP-sensitive K+ channels, but this is still in debate. The S-(+) enantiomer is undoubtedly less deleterious on both contractility and loss of ischemic preconditioning of the myocardium than the R-(−) enantiomer.

Antihyperalgesic effect of ketamine

By its anti-NMDA action, subanesthetic doses of ketamine are potently antihyperalgesic [301]. Ketamine limits opioid-induced hyperalgesia and has potent morphine-sparing effects. These effects are observed when ketamine is used early in the time-course of nociceptive stimulation, i.e. in the perioperative period. When ketamine is used only in the postoperative period, even when used with patient-controlled anesthesia (PCA), the results are not so clear. In pediatric patients, these effects need to be confirmed. The use of ketamine before the age of 2–4 years is still controversial because of possible neurotoxicity.

Effects on immune function and inflammation

Like local anesthetics, ketamine has potent immunomodulatory and anti-inflammatory properties. Ketamine decreases nuclear factor κ B (NFκB) activation and Toll-like receptor (TLR)4 expression and is more frequently used in septic and trauma patients [302]. These anti-inflammatory properties have not been shown in pediatric patients. Further studies are needed to assess the beneficial effect of ketamine in septic or cancer patients.

Formulations and dosing

Ketamine has various formulations. The initial preparation of the racemic mixture contains benzethonium chloride as a preservative. Both the R-(−) enantiomer and the preservative are neurotoxic. In numerous countries, the S-(+) enantiomer without preservative is available because it is less toxic. However, even the pure S enantiomer may be neurotoxic at high concentrations, and its use is

not being recommended as an adjuvant for epidural injection.

Numerous routes for ketamine delivery are used. For IV induction of anesthesia, 1–2 mg/kg are used. For maintenance anesthesia, 2–4 mg/kg/h of ketamine is infused. However, because of the context-sensitive half-time of the drug, it may be better to use an adapted regimen (see Table 9.5). Ketamine may also be injected intramuscularly at a dose of 5–8 mg/kg. The onset of anesthesia is slower (5–10 min) and its duration is prolonged (20–30 min). Ketamine may also be given rectally at the same dose.

The low-dose regimen used to prevent postoperative hyperalgesia consists of an IV loading dose of 0.15–0.30 mg/kg before surgery and a continuous infusion of 0.1–0.3 mg/kg/h for 24 hours. As an adjunct to PCA, the dose is 1 mg ketamine per mg of morphine. However, most pediatric studies do not show a benefit to low-dose ketamine.

Opioids

Opioids interact with specific opiate receptors (μ, δ, κ). Their major sites of action include the spinal cord, the medulla, and the periaqueductal gray matter [303,304].

Two main families of opioids are currently available. Long-lasting hydrophilic drugs, mainly used for postoperative or chronic pain relief, and short-acting drugs of the phenylpiperidine chemical family, used preferentially for perioperative analgesia. However, short-acting drugs are being used more and more commonly outside the operating room. These are almost pure μ receptor agonists. Except for remifentanil, the liver metabolizes phenylpiperidines.

Phenylpiperidines
Pharmacokinetics

Phenylpiperidines are weak bases that bind to AGP [28,305,306]. They are exclusively metabolized in the liver by the CYP3A4 isoform, with the exception of remifentanil, which is degraded in plasma by non-specific cholinesterases [307–310]. These cholinesterases are ubiquitous; their deficiency is lethal. Thus, all patients are able to metabolize remifentanil. Clearance of remifentanil is very rapid in neonates. The drug's clearance decreases slightly thereafter (Table 9.6). These molecules have no active metabolites. Fentanyl, alfentanil, and sufentanil undergo hepatic metabolism, which rapidly matures (Fig. 9.9) [48]. Sufentanil is a suitable choice for opioid administration by target-controlled infusion (TCI) because it has shorter, predictable context-sensitive half-times than fentanyl or even alfentanil (see Fig. 9.8) [311]. The decrement times of remifentanil are very short and almost constant,

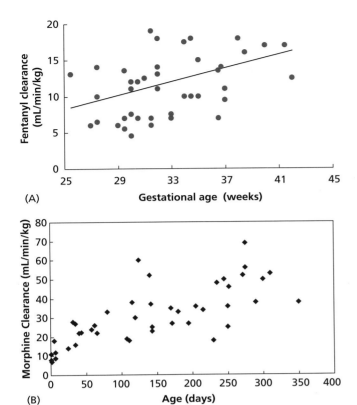

(A)

(B)

Figure 9.9 (A) Fentanyl and (B) morphine clearance as a function of age. In the younger premature infants, fentanyl clearance is relatively high (about half the liver blood flow). Maturation occurs rapidly and is almost complete at 42 weeks. Morphine clearance, on the other hand, is low at birth and maturation is complete only at the end of the first year of life. Reproduced from Saarenmaa et al [48] (part A) and Lynn et al [47] (part B) with permission from Elsevier.

whereas the decrement times of fentanyl markedly increase with duration of administration [20].

Effect on the central nervous system

None of these agents have a deleterious effect on cerebral hemodynamics, provided the CO_2 tension is normal. With normal CO_2, neither cerebral blood flow nor ICP is increased [312–314].

Effect on the respiratory and cardiovascular systems

All narcotics depress ventilation. Muscle rigidity may be a problem in younger patients, especially when the drug is rapidly injected [315]. At equipotent doses, all phenyl-piperidines reduce FRC to the same extent [316,317]. When injected slowly, these agents do not significantly decrease chest wall compliance, which allows them to be used in ICUs. Interestingly, muscle rigidity has been described following remifentanil injection in the mother [318].

All phenylpiperidines have depressant effects on myocardial contractility and vascular tone [169,319–322]. They provoke marked bradycardia. Atropine does not totally restore myocardial contractility. Remifentanil causes more bradycardia than the other drugs but at equi-analgesic doses, all four drugs probably have similar effects. The incidences of respiratory depression, nausea and vomiting, pruritus, and rarely urinary retention are similar for all opioids [303] (see below).

Fentanyl

Fentanyl is the oldest of these agents [48,323–328]. Its half-life is very long, particularly when it is used to sedate patients in ICUs. Fentanyl's hepatic extraction ratio is greater than 70–80% in children. Soon after birth, fentanyl's clearance from the body exceeds 50% of hepatic blood flow (see Fig. 9.9). Unfortunately, its important volume of distribution and slow intercompartmental clearance lead to rapid increases in context-sensitive decrement times with increased duration of administration. Moreover, fentanyl is secreted into gastric fluid, and recirculation of the drug from gastric contents and deep compartments can occur long after recovery from anesthesia. The usual dosing is 2–4 μg/kg as a bolus injection and 1–2 μg/kg for reinjections. The same dose, 1–2 μg/kg/h, is used for continuous IV infusion. Continuous infusion of fentanyl is not recommended during surgery if the plan is to extubate the trachea shortly after surgery. The time to peak effect is 5–6 min.

Alfentanil

Alfentanil has a short half-life, limited distribution into deep compartments, and high clearance (see Table 9.6) [326,328,329]. After an IV bolus dose of drug, alfentanil's peak effect occurs in 1–2 min. Following a prolonged infusion, decrement times increase moderately. The usual bolus dose of 10–20 μg/kg is followed by reinjections of 5–10 μg/kg for procedures of short duration.

Sufentanil

Sufentanil's half-life is of intermediate duration [326,328,330–334]. Its effect is prolonged the least by prolonged administration of the drug, which is why its use has become very popular. Sufentanil's time to peak effect is 2–4 min. The usual bolus dose is 0.2–0.4 μg/kg at the time of anesthesia induction, followed by either reinjections (0.1–0.25 μg/kg) or an infusion of 0.1–0.5 μg/kg/h.

Remifentanil

Remifentanil is a very potent opioid that has a rapid onset (<1 min) and a very short half-life [328,335–340]. Its decrement times are constant. The context-sensitive half-time, i.e. 50% decrement time, is close to 4 min no matter how long the drug is administered. When given with propofol

(3–4 mg/kg) or sevoflurane (0.5–1 MAC), excellent intubating conditions are produced in children in 20–30 sec after a bolus of 2–3 µg/kg. However, bolus doses of remifentanil are not recommended in neonates and infants because they may develop significant bradycardia and hypotension [319,320]. When given with 0.5–1 MAC of volatile anesthetic, a continuous infusion of 0.15–0.25 µg/kg/min (in neonates and infants) or 0.50 µg/kg/min (in children) gives excellent analgesia and stability, even for neonates who are more susceptible to the heart rate and blood pressure effects. However, care should be taken to (1) provide quality analgesia upon awakening and in the postoperative period because the analgesic effects of remifentanil are very short once the drug infusion is discontinued, and (2) look for occurrence of the postoperative hyperalgesia syndrome, which follows the administration of large doses of opioids. Remifentanil and sufentanil are the drugs of choice for TIVA. The usual dose of remifentenil is 0.10 µg/kg/min in infants and 0.25 µg/kg/min in children.

Morphine

Morphine is a natural alkaloid derived from *Papaver somniferum*. It is an ampholyte, with a MW of 285 (free base), pKas of 9.85 and 7.87, an octanol:water distribution ratio of 1.42 at physiological pH, and is 35% protein bound to HSA. Morphine has four isomers, with little difference between them (codeine has the same isomeric distribution and morphine-6-glucuronide (M-6-G), the active metabolite of morphine, has two isomers).

Pharmacokinetics

Morphine (like hydromorphone) does not undergo phase 1 metabolism by cytochrome P450, but undergoes direct phase 2 metabolism by the 2B7 and to a lesser extent the 1A3 isoforms of the UGT [38,40,341,342]. About 40% of morphine metabolism is extrahepatic, explaining why clearance is markedly greater than hepatic blood flow [343]. However, in patients with either a prothrombin time <40% or a liver mass that decreases functional liver by 50%, dosing must be halved (titration is unchanged) [344–346]. Although less than 10% of morphine is transformed to M-6-G, it has major importance because M-6-G has 2–8 times the potency of morphine and because its clearance is critically low [347,348]. In cases of renal failure, M-6-G elimination is impaired, and the risk of respiratory depression increases when the creatinine clearance (CrCL) is below 30 mL/min/1.73 m² [349]. Because the production of M-6-G is delayed, its concentration rises long after morphine administration is discontinued (Fig. 9.10). In patients with a CrCL of 15–30 mL/min/1.73 m², the dose of morphine should be halved. Drugs other than morphine should be given if the CrCL is <15 mL/min/1.73 m². Naloxone is efficacious for the treatment of narcotic-induced respiratory depression, but at times it must be

infused for hours or even days. Peritoneal dialysis is poorly efficacious for removal of morphine, but hemodialysis (and usually hemofiltration) removes M-6-G. However, M-6-G may accumulate between dialysis sessions. Fentanyl and sufentanil are eliminated by hemofiltration, and require the use of alternative agents in ICU patients undergoing hemofiltration.

Phase 2 metabolism is immature at birth and slowly increases during the first 6–9 months of life (see Fig. 9.9) [37,47]. This fact, together with the opioid receptor immaturity during the same period of time, explains why morphine dosing is different in young infants than in older infants and children (see Table 9.6) [36,37,350–353].

Morphine is hydrophilic and does not easily cross biological membranes. Its effect concentration peaks 20 min after an IV injection (see Fig. 9.10). However, morphine concentration in the effect compartment reaches 80% of peak concentration 6 min after an IV bolus. It remains above this concentration for 80 min. Morphine's duration of action is much longer than that of fentanyl or sufentanil.

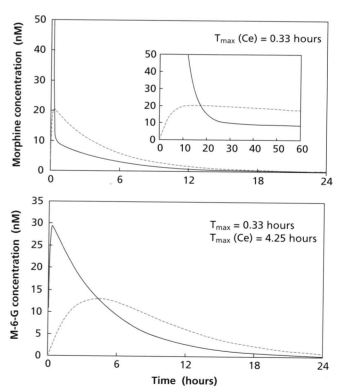

Figure 9.10 Morphine (*top*) and M-6-G (*bottom*) concentrations in the central compartment (*solid lines*) and in the effect compartment (*dotted lines*) after a single IV injection of morphine. After an IV bolus injection, morphine concentration peaks at 20 min because this hydrophilic drug slowly crosses the blood–brain barrier. M-6-G, which is more hydrophilic, peaks more than 4 hours after the morphine injection. This phenomenon explains why the effect of oral morphine is delayed (part of the effect is due to M-6-G because of the first-pass effect). Data from Mazoit et al [347].

Table 9.6 Opioids. Physicochemical properties and pharmacokinetics

Drug	Molecular weight (Da)	pKa	Distribution ratio (octanol/ buffer)	Protein binding %		T½ (h)	CL (mL/kg/ min)	Vc (L/kg)	Vss (L/kg)	T½ke0 (min)
Fentanyl	336	8.4	860	70–85		6–8	10–20	–	4–5	5
Alfentanil	–	6.5	130	65–90		1–2	10–15	–	0.4–1	1.5
Sufentanil	387	8.0	1750	80–90		2–3	4–9	–	2–3	2–4
Remifentanil	–	7.1	18	–		0.1	90–46	–	0.45–0.24	<1
Morphine	285	8.0#	6	30–35		1.5–2	30–40	–	2–4	100
Tramadol	263	9.4	250	20	Adult:	5.5	6.3	–	2.7–4.1	–
					2–8 yrs:	2.8–3	10.3	–	2.2	100–200
					Neonate	–	5.7	–	–	–
Codeine[1]	299	8.2	12	–		1.7	8.5	–	–	–
Acetaminophen	151	9.5	3	–	Adult:	2	3.8	0.5	0.9	–
					2–15 yrs:	2	3.3	0.34	0.82	–
					Prem babies and neonates (IV) CL = 0.5–1.5 mL/kg/min (27–46 week PMA)					

\# Morphine is a zwitterionic ampholyte with a principal pKa of 7.9.

1 Codeine is metabolized to morphine, which is the active molecule.

CL = Total Body Clearance, PMA = Postmenstrual Age.

Pharmacodynamics

Respiratory depression is a frequent side-effect of narcotics in neonates and infants. Respiratory rates decrease progressively, and respiratory depression increases. Depression is more associated with episodes of desaturation than with hypercarbia because of the associated sedation. However, sedation is difficult to appreciate in infants, because they normally sleep much of the time. Monitoring by transcutaneous pulse oximetry is recommended for infants, but clinical observation is also necessary, probably in the PACU (Post Anesthesia Care Unit) or an ICU (Intensive Care Unit). Apart from respiratory depression, the other side-effects of morphine include nausea and vomiting, urinary retention, pruritus, and constipation after 2–3 days of drug administration. Dexamethasone, droperidol or a 5-HT3 receptor inhibitor like ondansetron best prevent postoperative nausea and vomiting (PONV).

Dosing

Morphine should be titrated in infants and young children. In neonates and infants younger than 3 months of age, a continuous IV infusion of the drug is usually sufficient. The doses are between 10 and 30 μg/kg/h and are adjusted according to desired effect and the respiratory rate. Infants <3 months of age are very sensitive to the respiratory depressive effect of morphine. In infants older than 3–6 months and children <10 kg BW, IV titration of the drug is begun by injecting a loading dose of 50 μg/kg before the age of 12 months or 100 μg/kg thereafter. The loading dose is followed by 25 μg/kg every 5 min until the desired effect is reached. Children <40 kg usually receive 75 μg/kg every 5 min until the effective dose is reached. Children weighing more than 40 kg may receive the adult regimen, i.e. 3 mg as a bolus every 5 min.

Before the age of 6–7 years, it is not appropriate to use a PCA device with the parents injecting the boluses, because of safety issues. Even after this age, this method has its limits and only a few teams continue to practice parent-controlled analgesia. Continuous infusions of narcotics have shown similar benefits and limits as PCA, i.e. the lack of efficacy on pain with movement. The infusion regimen is between 20 and 40µg/kg/h. After the age of 6 or 7 years, children are able to understand the principle of PCA. The dosing and rules of administration for children are similar to those for adults, i.e. boluses of 15–20µg/kg every 5–10min. Continuous infusion of morphine along with the PCA has long been used, but this practice may induce respiratory depression. In patients receiving a continuous infusion of drug, nurse-controlled analgesia allows the injection of small boluses of drug and/or the modification of the infusion rate of morphine by increments or decrements of 5µg/kg and is used in numerous centers. This is a good practice, provided all team members (including doctors and nurse) are well trained and follow rigorous protocols.

When pumps for continuous drug infusion or for PCA are not available, the intramuscular or (better) subcutaneous route can be used but when this is done, the blood concentration exhibits peaks and troughs. The oral route is also possible but when this route is used, the hepatic first-pass effect needs to be taken into account because part of the morphine dose is metabolized before reaching the general circulation. Only 10% of the metabolites are active (M-6-G). The concentration of M-6-G in the effect compartment is not significant before 6–9h after initial administration of the drug (see Fig. 9.10). The oral dose of morphine is 0.2–0.4mg/kg, with a maximum dose of 20mg every 6 hours.

Other opioids
Tramadol
Tramadol, a centrally acting analgesic, is a racemic mixture of cis and trans isomers that have few differences in activity, binding or metabolism. It is a weak µ opioid receptor agonist that inhibits norepinephrine and serotine reuptake [354–356]. The (+) enantiomer has greater affinity for the µ receptor and preferentially inhibits serotonin uptake while enhancing serotonin release. The (-) enantiomer preferentially inhibits norepinephrine reuptake by stimulating α2-adrenergic receptors. The O-desmethyl metabolite (M1) is active and (+)M1 is the principal active molecule.

Pharmacokinetics
Tramadol is metabolized primarily by the CYP2D6, which is immature at birth [58,357,358]. Formation of M1 is impaired *in utero* and has important polymorphisms. The affinity of M1 for the µ receptor is 300–400 times greater than that of tramadol [358]. Both forms have similar half-lives [359–361]. Because M1 is at least as efficacious as the

parent drug, there is a lag-time between its administration and effect. This is why the tramadol dose–effect relationship is flat and why it provides inadequate analgesia when injected immediately after surgery [362]. Hepatic failure markedly decreases the clearance of tramadol. Renal failure slightly decreases its clearance, but markedly decreases M1 clearance. CYP2D6 polymorphism may lead to inadequate analgesia in 5–6% of Caucasians because tramadol metabolism and M1 formation are reduced. In contrast, ultra-fast metabolizers of tramadol are at risk of respiratory depression. After oral administration, bio-availability of the drug is 70–90% after an oral dose. The T_{max} is 1–2 hours, depending on the formulation (drops are more rapidly absorbed).

Pharmacodynamics
Respiratory depression with tramadol is less common than with morphine. Other side-effects include nausea, vomiting, dizziness, sweating, dry mouth, and drowsiness.

Dosing
Tramadol is mainly used to treat mild to moderately severe postoperative pain and for intraoperative analgesia, although its analgesic properties are weaker than those of phenylpiperidines or morphine. Giving 2–3mg/kg IV at the beginning of surgery can provide effective postoperative analgesia for many patients. Continuous infusions of tramadol are not recommended because the lag-time for M1 formation is long. Oral tramadol 1–3mg/kg is given every 6–8 hours.

Codeine
Codeine is a natural alkaloid from opium. It mainly acts by producing morphine, which is a minor metabolite (≈5–6% of codeine is transformed into morphine in most Caucasian subjects) [59,63]. The main metabolite, codeine-6-glucuronide, does not appear to be active. Because of CYP2D6 polymorphism, there are large variations in morphine production. For example, about 20–25% of East Asians do not metabolize codeine to morphine; 5–6% of Caucasians fail to do so. In those adults who metabolize codeine extensively, the absorption of 50mg codeine leads to morphine and M-6-G production with C_{max}(maximum observed concentration) = 27 ± 23 and 41 ± 33nM at T_{max}(time to Cmax) = 0.7 and 1.8 hours respectively. The corresponding areas under the curve (AUC) compare with those obtained after 3–6mg of oral morphine. However, some ultra-fast metabolizers have CYP2D6 gene duplication and may produce exaggerated amounts of morphine [60]. Fatalities have been reported in babies breast fed by their ultra-fast metabolizing mothers, in infants and young children treated with codeine for more than one day, or children with renal

failure in whom M-6-G production was dramatically increased [61,62,363].

Dosing

Codeine is sometimes used in combination with acetaminophen. In children older than 6 months of age, dosing is 1 mg/kg/6–8 h. For day case surgery, parents should be warned about the possible lack of effect or the very rare possibility of overdosage with drowsiness or even coma and bradypnea [364].

Acetaminophen (paracetamol)

Acetaminophen has anti-inflammatory, antipyretic, and analgesic properties. Its mechanism of action is central and partly unknown [365,366]. Acetaminophen inhibits the COX-3 variant of cyclo-oxygenase. In addition, an active metabolite (p-aminophenol) may exert an effect through cannabinoid receptors.

Acetaminophen is poorly soluble in water. Mixing acetaminophen with mannitol and cysteine improves its solubility and stability. The time to peak plasma concentration is 30–60 min and 1–2 hours after oral and rectal administration respectively (see Table 9.6) [367–373]. Bioavailability after oral administration is 85–95% and is usually <80% after rectal administration. Metabolism of the drug is by CYP2E1, CYP1A2, and CYP3A4 in the liver (see Table 9.1). N-acetyl p-benzoquinone imine (NAPQI) is a toxic metabolite that causes hepatotoxicity by binding to cellular proteins and forming drug adducts [33,373]. Exposure to acetaminophen in infancy and early childhood may be a cause of the increasing incidence of asthma [374]. However, the role of confounding factors cannot be excluded. Neonatal icterus reduces clearance by 40%.

Dosing

Acetaminophen is available as tablets, an oral solution, suppositories, and as a solution for IV infusion [371,372]. The latter formulation is not available in all countries. For IV and oral administration, dosing is 10 mg/kg/6 h in premature infants and neonates. However, because of the considerable variability in clearance caused by CYP polymorphism, measurement of aminotransferase is required in premature infants and neonates. Oral dosing is 15 mg/kg/6 h from 1 month to 2 years and 20 mg/kg/6 h from 2 to 15 years. By the rectal route, the first dose is 40 mg/kg.

Muscle relaxants

The main two classes of muscle relaxants are depolarizing and non-depolarizing. Succinylcholine is the only depolarizing muscle relaxant still in use. Non-depolarizing agents include non-steroidal and steroidal agents. Both classes are non-competitive antagonists of acetylcholine (ACh).

Neuromuscular transmission

Muscle contraction is elicited by release of ACh in the synaptic cleft of the neuromuscular junction [375,376]. Calcium-dependent mechanisms are responsible for release of ACh from stores in presynaptic vesicles. In the synaptic cleft, ACh is rapidly degraded by acetylcholinesterases. There is also reuptake of some of the ACh by motor nerve endings. ACh works by stimulating opening of muscle nicotinic acetylcholine receptors (nAChR), which allows sodium and calcium to enter the cells. The signal is further transmitted by sodium channels ($NA_V1.4$) [377], which are particularly abundant around endplates. $NA_V1.4$ density is lower in neonatal muscle. Seventeen subunits assemble numerous nAChR subtypes. Two variants of muscle type receptors, the adult $\alpha1\beta1\varepsilon\delta$ and the fetal $\alpha1\beta1\gamma\delta$, are present in humans (Fig. 9.11). During the first 2–4 years of life, the adult subtype progressively replaces the fetal subtype. Fetal receptors respond more slowly to ACh. Interestingly, fetal subtypes are re-expressed in ICU patients during prolonged periods of immobilization and inflammation. Neonates, infants, and young children also release less ACh into synaptic clefts than adults. However, the response of infants and children to muscle relaxants depends on numerous factors, such as the pharmacokinetics of the muscle relaxant and the binding capacity of the receptor. For example, the volume of distribution of succinylcholine and most non-depolarizing agents is increased in infants.

Monitoring neuromuscular blockade [378]

The only way to directly and reliably determine and prevent residual muscular blockade is by neuromuscular

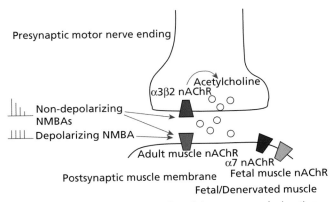

Figure 9.11 A schematic representation of the neuromuscular junction. The effect of neuromuscular blocking agents (NMBA) on the postsynaptic and presynaptic nicotinic acetylcholine receptor (nAChR) is depicted. The fetal muscle type nAChR has lower affinity and rate of response than the usual adult receptor. Reproduced from Fagerlund and Eriksson [376] with permission from Oxford University Press.

stimulation by acceleromyography. Acceleromyography measures the contraction of muscles in response to stimulation of their motor nerve. Single twitch measures the response height elicited by a single impulse. The train of four (TOF) measures the response to four successive supramaximal stimuli at 0.5 sec intervals, and the height of the fourth to the first response is determined (T4/T1 ratio, that measures the amount of fade after repetitive stimulations). This ratio measures the decrease in response (fade) to repeated stimuli and is a measure of the amount of fade. Tetanic stimulation, the result of high-frequency stimulation, causes tetanic muscle contraction. Double-burst stimulation (DBS) consist of two short tetani (three impulses at 50 Hz) separated by an interval long enough to allow relaxation (usually 750 msec). Post-tetanic stimulation is the response to a single twitch or a TOF after a tetanic facilitation. Presynaptic neuronal nAChR is not inhibited by succinylcholine. Fade observed with non-depolarizing agents is related to the effect on presynaptic receptors; succinylcholine has no effect on these receptors so no fade is observed with this agent. This may explain why there is a lack of effect with TOF and tetanic fade

[379]. All non-depolarizing drugs, on the other hand, inhibit neuronal nAChR and exhibit fade.

The most common monitoring sites are the adductor pollicis (thumb), orbicularis oculi (eyelid), and corrugator supercilii (superciliar arch). The latter is used to test for blockade of the laryngeal adductor muscles. The time course of blockade of the different muscles varies (Fig. 9.12) [380–383]. The abdominal wall and laryngeal muscles exhibit rapid onset and offset of neuromuscular blockade compared to the adductor pollicis. In addition, laryngeal adductors require higher doses of non-depolarizing drugs to achieve complete blockade than the adductor pollicis. The diaphragm is the muscle most resistant to blockade; its onset and recovery from blockade are similar to those of the adductor pollicis. The differences in T½ke0 at different sites reflect differences in muscle physiology (Table 9.7; see Fig. 9.12) [384]. Low degrees of neuromuscular blockade cause sufficient pharyngeal dysfunction to allow easy tracheal intubation [385]. Consequently, the corrugator supercilii is the best indicator of ease of tracheal intubation, and the adductor pollicis is the best indicator of early recovery from the block. One response out of four

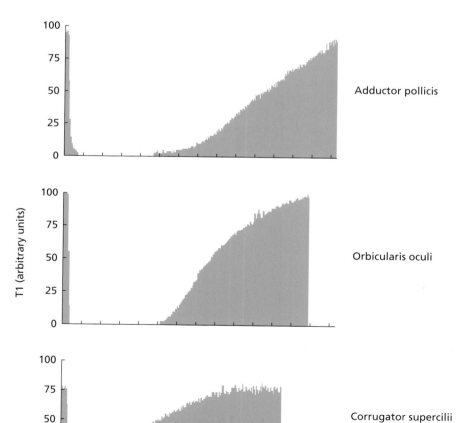

Adductor pollicis

Orbicularis oculi

Corrugator supercilii

Figure 9.12 Difference in pharmacodynamics of muscles after injecting rocuronium into a patient. Train-of-four stimulations were repeated every 15 sec and the T1 response is depicted in the figure. Clearly, the corrugator supercilii has a shorter delay of response, but is more resistant. Its kinetics is close to that of the laryngeal muscles. This is in perfect accordance with the 2–4-fold difference in T½ke0 reported for the adductor pollicis and laryngeal muscles after vecuronium or rocuronium injection. Reproduced from Plaud et al [380] with permission from Lippincott Williams and Wilkins.

Table 9.7 Muscle relaxants. Physicochemical properties and pharmacokinetics

Drug	Molecular weight (Da)	Distribution ratio (octanol/buffer)	Protein binding %	T½ (min)	CL (mL/kg/min)	Vc (mL/kg)	Vss (mL/kg)	T½ke0 Adductor Pollicis (min)	Larynx (min)	Ce50 (ng/mL)
Succinylcholine	290	7×10^{-5}	20	1.01	37	9	40	12	–	746
Pancuronium	–	–	–	107	1.81	–	275	5.1	–	–
Vecuronium	558	0.15	70	–	4.9	40	200	5.8	1.2	166
Rocuronium	546	0.02	45	71	3.2	47	210	4.4	2.7	820–1420
Infant (1–10 mo):				–	–	35	230	2.8	–	650
Child (2–6 yrs):				46	7.1	35	165	3.6	–	–
Atracurium	929	1×10^{-4}	37	–	–	–	–	6.8	–	–
Cisatracurium	929	1.9×10^{-4}	20	26	4.1	35	94	3.9–9.8	–	98–153
Child (1.5–6 yrs)					6.8	87	207	6.0	–	129
Mivacurium	1029	3×10^{-3}	30							
Cis–cis				68	3.8	–	227	–	–	–
Cis–trans				2.0	106	–	278	–	–	–
Trans–trans				2.3	57	–	211	–	–	–
Neostigmine	223	32	–	110	9.2–10	80	1700–1860	–	–	–
Edrophonium	166	63	–	126	8.3–12.1	50	810–900	–	–	–
Infant (3–7 mo):				73	17.8	150	1180	–	–	–
Child (1–4 yrs):				99	14.2	170	1220	–	–	–
Sugammadex	2178	–	–	136	75–138	50	160–200	1.0 (rocuronium)	–	720
								1.7 (vecuronium)	–	62

(TOF) means that the muscular force is <10% of control. When the fourth response reappears, the force of the tested muscle has reached at least 25% of control. In clinical practice, the recovery of T4/T1 to >90% indicates that non-significant residual block remains. Reversal of muscle blockade is usually only possible if two of four responses of the TOF are present.

Succinylcholine

Despite succinylcholine (SCh) being the only depolarizing muscle relaxant available, its precise mechanism of action remains unclear. Its injection induces massive exocytosis of ACh and muscle fasciculation. The ensuing paralysis involves complex mechanisms that include desensitization of the receptor and inactivation of the sodium channels. SCh has a rapid onset and short duration of action, which makes it the agent of choice for rapid sequence induction.

Succinylcholine has low affinity for the presynaptic nAChR and causes a phase I block (decreased twitch amplitude, absence of fade, absence of post-tetanic potentiation). Large doses of SCh cause tachyphylaxis and a phase 2 block that resembles a non-depolarizing block.

Pharmacokinetics

Succinylcholine has two molecules of ACh linked by an ester bond. It is highly hydrophilic (see Table 9.7) [386].

Like cocaine, heroin, and ester local anesthetics, SCh is hydrolyzed in serum, red blood cells, and liver by nonspecific esterases (butyrylesterases or pseudocholinesterases) [387,388]. There are many plasma cholinesterase genotypes that are responsible for wide variations in plasma cholinesterase activity. Some patients have reduced blood pseudocholinesterase activity. More than 20% of Caucasians are heterozygous for the main atypical variant. Patients with this variant have elimination halflives that are nearly double those of patients without the variant. Patients who are homozygous for this abnormal variant may remain paralyzed for hours to days following a single injection of SCh. Determining the dibucaine number is the test for lack of pseudocholinesterase. However, lack of sensitivity, specificity, and cost make its routine use unlikely. Eskimos or Australian aborigines share the same genotype and have greater risk for prolonged paralysis with SCh.

Succinylcholine rapidly accesses the neuromuscular junction. It is rapidly degraded due to its small volume of distribution and to elimination from both the central and peripheral compartments (see Table 9.7) [389]. The elimination half-life of SCh is 1 min. However, the $T\frac{1}{2}ke0$ for blockade of the adductor pollicis is 12 min and is similar to that for non-depolarizing agents. The short onset of the drug's effect is aided by the high dose injected. Unfortunately, no recent data for infants and children are available [390–392]. Infants require 3 mg/kg and children 2 mg/kg to produce the same intubating conditions. It is highly probable that these differences in drug dosage are the result of different volumes of distribution in the two groups. SCh is very hydrophilic. PK-PD data are needed in newborns, infants and children, and should be correlated using allometric scaling.

Pharmacodynamics

Succinylcholine has numerous side-effects that have caused some anesthesiologists to abandon its use.

Effects on the central nervous system

Succinylcholine is said to increase ICP. However, recent studies have shown that this is not the case if normocapnea is maintained. It has also been thought to increase intraocular pressure by causing contraction of the extraocular muscles. Recent evidence has shown that intraocular pressures do not increase when the trachea is rapidly intubated and the lungs are ventilated [393].

Effects on the cardiovascular system

Succinylcholine can cause either tachycardia or bradycardia, but bradycardia seldom occurs with the first dose of SCh. It occurs much more commonly after a second or third dose of the drug. Bradycardia is easily prevented by atropine [394]. Although not well documented, SCh-induced fasciculations are said to increase cardiac output and $CRMO_2$. This effect does not appear to have clinical relevance.

Potassium release, effects on muscles, and malignant hyperthermia

Succinylcholine causes potassium release that usually is minimal and has no clinical consequence, unless the patient is hyperkalemic. Patients with Duchenne muscular dystrophy and other myopathies, paralysis (usually of spinal origin), rhabdomyolysis, and burns have a significant risk for developing arrhythmias with SCh due to receptor upregulation and phenotype changes in denervated muscle [395,396].

Succinylcholine may cause masseter spasm and incomplete relaxation of the jaw, particularly when it is given during halothane anesthesia. Some authors argue that this occurs because the dose of SCh was inadequate. SCh can trigger malignant hyperthermia (see the section on volatile anesthetics and Chapter 40). This is more likely when it is used with halothane or sevoflurane.

Non-depolarizing muscle relaxants

Non-depolarizing muscle relaxants compete with ACh at both muscle and nAChR. Non-depolarizing relaxants are either aminosteroids (pancuronium, vecuronium and rocuronium) or benzylisoquinoliniums (atracurium, cisatracurium and mivacurium) [397]. All these drugs produce a block of <40 min duration. Mivacurium's duration of action is the shortest.

Pharmacokinetics

All neuromuscular relaxants are highly water soluble and have small volumes of distribution [386]. They are best described by two- or three-compartment linear kinetics (see Table 9.7) [397–407]. The volume of the central compartment is no larger than the plasma volume, and the volume of distribution at steady state (Vss) is equal to one-quarter of the bodyweight. Clearance of nondepolarizing muscle relaxants is usually relatively low, except for mivacurium, which is hydrolyzed by the same cholinesterases as SCh.

Metabolism

Aminosteroids are principally eliminated unchanged in urine and bile by carrier-mediated processes [408,409]. Transport is by the OCT and, to a lesser extent, by the P-gp.

Pancuronium has major renal transport and limited hepatobiliary transport [398,410]. As much as 25% of a dose of pancuronium can be recovered as 3-hydroxy metabolite, which has blocking properties half as potent as those of pancuronium. Patients with renal and/or liver failure have delayed elimination of pancuronium.

Vecuronium is excreted unchanged in urine and in bile (>50% is transported in bile) [411]. Patients who have cholestasis have reduced clearance of vecuronium. Renal failure has less effect. However, patients with end-stage renal failure also exhibit decreased clearance of vecuronium and a slightly higher sensitivity to the drug than normal subjects. Small amounts of 3-desacetyl vecuronium, a moderately active metabolite, were found in plasma after prolonged administration of vecuronium.

Rocuronium, a derivative of vecuronium, has a rapid onset and duration of action that are similar to those of vecuronium. Rocuronium is excreted unchanged in urine and feces; its metabolism is minimal. Rocuronium's elimination is only slightly impaired by renal failure. Excretion by transporters is less impaired than that by metabolism. For example, patients with cirrhosis have greater volumes; patients with cholestasis and jaundice have decreased clearance. The order of clearance is pancuronium < vecuronium ≈ rocuronium, which explains their durations of action.

Atracurium has ten stereo-isomers [412]. The 1R-cis, 1'R-cis isomer is called cisatracurium. Both atracurium and cisatracurium are spontaneously degraded in plasma by Hofmann elimination and to a small degree by carboxylesterase activity. The Hofmann reaction is rate limited and temperature and pH dependent. The main end-product of atracurium and cisatracurium is laudanosine, which is toxic and may cause seizures. However, serum concentrations of laudanosine are always below the toxic threshold. Because cisatracurium is 3–5-fold more potent than atracurium, cisatracurium causes less histamine release and has less potential for causing convulsions.

Mivacurium is hydrolyzed in plasma by the same pseudocholinesterases that hydrolyze SCh [413,414]. It is a mixture of stereo-isomers; the cis-trans and the trans-trans both have similar potency. A third isomer, the cis-cis, accounts for <6% of the total amount of metabolites and is about one-thirteenth as potent as the other two isomers. Unfortunately, the cis-cis isomer is poorly cleared; its T½ is about 20–30 times longer than that of the other two isomers. Patients who are heterozygous for plasma cholinesterase (those with the atypical AA variant, i.e. 20% of the Caucasian population) clear the major isomers 50% less well and have a prolonged T½ [388]. Patients who are homozygous for AA or other variants can have prolonged neuomuscular blockade. Clearance of mivacurium is moderately decreased by renal failure [414].

Pharmacodynamics

For neuromuscular blocking agents, ke0 is strongly correlated with logD, the distribution coefficient. Highly hydrosoluble molecules rapidly access their receptors, producing a rapid onset of action. Ce50 is inversely correlated to logD and to MW. Highly hydrosoluble molecules and those with low MW are more potent [386]. The duration of action depends on the rate of receptor access (T½ke0) and on affinity for the receptor. Interestingly, there is a great difference between the different sites of action. T½ke0 is much slower for adductor pollicis muscles than for the laryngeal muscles [380,383]. Drug access to the laryngeal muscles is 4–6 times more rapid than to the adductor pollicis and the diaphragm. The onset of action is dose dependent. Drugs with relatively short durations of action, like rocuronium, may require relatively large doses for onsets of action to be rapid. Rocuronium has the shortest T½ke0 and a rapid onset of action. Because of its intermediate duration of action, it is possible to use high doses of rocuronium to provide excellent intubating conditions 1 min after its injection.

Specific effect on organs

Non-depolarizing agents have little effect on cerebral blood flow or intracranial pressure. Atracurium, cisatracurium, and mivacurium release histamine which, when injected rapidly, can induce bronchoconstriction, hypotension, and tachycardia [415]. Pancuronium (and occasionally rocuronium) blocks muscarinic receptors and induces moderate tachycardia.

Interactions

Volatile anesthetics and neuromuscular blocking drugs interact [416–418]. The mechanism for this potentiation remains unclear, but is likely an additive effect on the nAChR [416]. For example, sevoflurane shortens the onset and prolongs the duration of a rocuronium-induced block in children. T½ke0 and Ce50 are decreased by 60%, and the recovery time to T1 = 5% is prolonged by 25%. Acid–base disturbances, hypokalemia, and hypothermia may prolong the duration of action of muscle relaxants. Numerous drugs (volatile anesthetics, antimicrobials like gentamicin, lithium, and calcium channel blockers) interact with neuromuscular blocking agents and enhance the block. Magnesium sulfate potentiates the action of non-depolarizing agents by decreasing ACh release. Resistance to neuromuscular blocking drugs can be caused by phenytoin, carbamazepine, and other anticonvulsants. Giving SCh after a non-depolarizing agent prolongs the block.

Allergy to muscle relaxants

Neuromuscular blocking agents can cause severe anaphylaxis, which is different from the release of histamine commonly observed when atracurium, cisatracurium or mivacurium is injected rapidly [419–421]. Anaphylaxis is rare in neonates and infants. The incidence of anaphylaxis increases with age and reaches its maximum in 30–60-year-old patients. Based on skin tests, rocuronium is said to cause more allergic reactions than the other drugs, but skin testing may not be the best way to determine this. Grade III (bronchospasm ± urticaria) reactions occur in about 75% of cases.

Dosing

Pancuronium 0.08–0.1 mg/kg has an onset time of 3–5 min and duration of action of more than 60 min. The reinjection dose 0.02 mg/kg is given when T2 of the TOF returns. *Vecuronium* 0.1–0.2 mg/kg has an onset time of 1–3 min and duration of action of 30–40 min. The reinjection dose is 0.1 mg/kg. A continuous infusion at 1–1.2 µg/kg/min is used for maintenance. *Rocuronium* 0.4–0.6 mg/kg has an onset of 1–2 min and duration of action of 40–60 min. The reinjection dose is 0.1–0.15 mg/kg. A continuous infusion of 5–15 µg/kg is often used for maintenance. *Atracurium* 0.4–0.8 mg/kg has an onset of 2–3 min and duration of action of 40–60 min. The reinjection dose is 0.1–0.2 mg/kg. A continuous infusion of 5–15 µg/kg/min is used for maintenance. *Cisatracurium* 0.1–0.2 mg/kg has an onset of 2–3 min and duration of action of 40–60 min. The reinjection dose is 0.03–0.5 mg/kg. A continuous infusion of 1–3 µg/kg/min is used for maintenance. *Mivacurium* 0.2 mg/kg has an onset of 1–3 min and duration of action of <30 min.

Tracheal intubation

The intubating dose of SCh is 1 mg/kg in adults, 3 mg/kg in infants, and 2 mg/kg in children. The intramuscular dose of SCh for emergency tracheal intubation is 5 mg/kg [422].

The intubating dose for rocuronium is 0.6 mg/kg in both infants and children. This dose produces excellent intubating conditions in <1 min. Older children often require the adult dose 1.2 mg/kg for rapid-sequence induction of anesthesia. This dose of drug provides excellent intubating conditions, but its duration of action is prolonged.

Reversal agents

Two different classes of antagonists are used to reverse neuromuscular blockade: the quaternary ammonium-reversible acetylcholinesterase inhibitors and sugammadex.

Acetylcholinesterase inhibitors

Acetylcholinesterase inhibitors (neostigmine and edrophonium) are quaternary ammoniums and are hydrophilic, ionized compounds.

Pharmacokinetics

Neostigmine and pyridostigmine are tertiary ammonium compounds that bind covalently to acetylcholinesterase and form inactive carbamylated complexes that degrade slowly (T½ ~30 min) [423]. Edrophonium forms a weak complex that degrades more rapidly, which explains why its effects are shorter than those of neostigmine. Its half-life is shorter than that of either neostigmine or edrophonium. Neostigmine is rapidly metabolized at the neuromuscular junction by acetylcholinesterases and by erythrocytes. The nearly inactive metabolites are conjugated and eliminated by the kidney [424]. Edrophonium is metabolized to an inactive glucuronide conjugate. Interestingly, although the pharmacokinetics of both drugs is poorly understood, their terminal half-lives are longer than those of all neuromuscular blockers, including pancuronium (see Table 9.7) [425,426]. In anephric patients, elimination of neostigmine is impaired (T½ = 181 versus 80 min). The time to reach T1, T4/T1 and T2 is always faster in children than in adults. Moreover, recovery occurs more quickly with edrophonium in children than with neostigmine [427–434]. This is true for all blocking agents studied. Neostigmine is about 12–18 times more potent than edrophonium. In pediatric patients, the doses of edrophonium required for either 50% or 80% recovery of twitch height are comparatively greater (on a weight basis) than in adults. It is unclear if this is true for neostigmine.

Pharmacodynamics

Acetylcholinesterase inhibitors have numerous side-effects that are mostly related to their muscarinic effects [415]. These include bradycardia, salivary and intestinal secretions, miosis, and bronchoconstriction. Atropine or glycopyrrolate administration can prevent or reverse these effects. In pediatric patients, atropine-induced tachycardia is rarely a problem, but bradycardia may be a problem, particularly in neonates and infants. Edrophonium causes less bradycardia than neostigmine and is preferred in pediatric patients. The bronchoconstriction induced by these drugs may be a problem, particularly in patients with asthma.

Dosing

In infants and children, the dose of neostigmine required to reverse the block varies between 0.03 and 0.07 mg/kg, depending on the neuromuscular blocking agent used. The author recommends a bolus of 0.05 mg/kg. The drug's peak effect occurs 10 min after injection. Edrophonium 0.75–1 mg/kg is given as a bolus. Its peak effect occurs 2–3 minutes after injection. Atropine 0.10–0.15 µg/kg should be given *before* either drug to prevent bradycardia. Glycopyrrolate 4 µg/kg in children and up to 8 µg/kg in neonates and infants effectively prevents bradycardia.

Sugammadex

Sugammadex is a cyclodextrine that can encapsulate aminosteroid neuromuscular blockers. It has both an outer hydrophilic structure and an inner hydrophobic core. The drug was designed to specifically encapsulate rocuronium and vecuronium and, to a lesser extent, pancuronium. Sugammadex has no effect on benzylisoquinoliniums (atracurium, cisatracurium, and mivacurium). No serious side-effects have been reported, but anaphylaxis is possible.

Pharmacokinetics

Sugammadex is eliminated unchanged by the kidney [435]. Its half-life exceeds that of all neuromuscular blockers [436,437]. Its clearance is 75–138 mL/min, which approximates the glomerular filtration rate (GFR). In patients with renal failure, the decreased sugammadex clearance is similar to the decrease in renal clearance [438,439]. The affinity of sugammadex for vecuronium and rocuronium differs. T½ke0 for vecuronium is twice that of rocuronium (see Table 9.7). This difference in the rate of access is consistent with the difference in Kd, the equilibration dissociation rate constant (0.1 µM for rocuronium versus 0.175 µM for vecuronium). However, the binding capacity is similar for both drugs (the ratio of Ce50 for the sugammadex effect site is similar to the ratio of Ce50 for the neuromuscular junction effect site). After a dose of rocuronium, 2 mg/kg of sugammadex is injected at reappearance of T2. The time to 90% recovery of TOF occurs after 0.6 min in infants, 1.2 min in children, and 1.2 min in adults. Doses >2 mg/kg do not hasten recovery.

Dosing

For routine reversal of a block after reappearance of T2, 2 mg/kg of sugammadex is adequate. However, in an emergency (e.g. failure to intubate the trachea after a large dose of rocuronium), sugammadex doses as high as 12 mg/kg may be required.

Anticholinergic agents

Two anticholinergic agents are clinically available: atropine and glycopyrrolate [440–446]. These are non-selective competitors for ACh at the muscarinic receptors and have little or no action on nicotinic receptors.

Atropine is a natural alkaloid of *Atropa belladonna*. It is a tertiary amine with a pKa of 9.9. It is highly ionized at physiological pHs and rapidly diffuses in water compartments (Vd 4.9 L/kg). Atropine has a chiral carbon (the R form is almost inactive).

Glycopyrrolate is a synthetic quaternary ammonium salt that is totally ionized at physiological pHs. Its volume of distribution is small: 0.60 L/kg. In adults, the terminal half-life of atropine is 3–4 times longer than that of glycopyrrolate (2.3–3.7 versus 0.8 h). In infants and children, glycopyrrolate's T½ is very short (20 min) due to its greater clearance (22 mL/kg/min (infants and children) versus 9 mL/kg/min (adults)). Atropine's clearance is 15.4 mL/kg/min in adults. The larger volume of distribution in neonates and infants makes the T½ slower than in adults. Atropine is metabolized in the liver; one of its metabolites, 1-hyoscyamine, is active. Glycopyrrolate is not extensively metabolized and is rapidly excreted unchanged in urine. Elimination of glycopyrrolate is impaired by renal failure. Unlike atropine, glycopyrrolate does not cross the blood–brain barrier.

Anticholinergic agents increase heart rate, inhibit secretions, and induce bronchodilation. Atropine induces mydriasis while glycopyrrolate does not. At very low doses, both drugs can cause bradycardia. Glycopyrrolate's heart rate effects are delayed compared to those of atropine (2–3 min versus 1 min). Toxicity (tachycardia, restlessness and excitement, hallucinations, delirium, and coma with paralysis) occurs at supratherapeutic doses of atropine. Hypotension and circulatory collapse may also occur.

Dosing

The IV dose of atropine is 10–15 µg/kg. That of glycopyrrolate is 4 µg/kg for children and up to 9 µg/kg for infants 1 month to 2 years old. Some preparations of glycopyrrolate contain benzyl alcohol, which is toxic to neonates and infants and should not be repeated.

Following intramuscular injection, T_{max} occurs in 15–30 min. However, drug absorption by this route varies widely. IM doses are similar or slightly higher than IV doses.

Local anesthetics

Local anesthetics (LA) block propagation of impulses along nerve fibers by inactivation of voltage-gated sodium channels, which initiate action potentials [447]. Some toxins (tetrodotoxin (TTX)) act on the outside of cells to block action potentials; local anesthetics have their effects on the cytosolic side of phospholipid membranes. Two main chemical compounds have been synthesized and used clinically as LAs: amino esters (2-chloroprocaine, procaine, tetracaine) and amino amides (lidocaine, bupivacaine, ropivacaine). Amino esters are degraded by pseudocholinesterases in plasma; they undergo minimal hepatic metabolism. Amino amides are more stable and are metabolized exclusively by the liver.

Table 9.8 Physicochemical properties of local anesthetics

Drug	Molecular weight (Da)	pKa*	Distribution coefficient†	Protein binding	Onset of action	Duration of action	Potency‡
Esters							
Procaine	236	8.9	1.7	6%	Long	1 h	0.5
Chloroprocaine	271	9.1	9.0	?	Short	½ h–1 h	0.5–1
Amides							
Lidocaine	234	7.8	43	65%	Short	1 h 30–2 h	1
Prilocaine	220	8.0	25	55%	Short	1 h 30–2 h	1
Mepivacaine	246	7.7	21	75%	Short	1 h 30–2 h	1
Bupivacaine **	288	8.1	346	95%	Intermediate	3 h–3 h 30	4
Ropivacaine	274	8.1	115	94%	Intermediate	3 h	3.5–4

*pKa at 37°C.

**Bupivacaine = levobupivacaine.

†Octanol:buffer partition.

‡Potency is relative to lidocaine.

Pharmacokinetics [448]

Local anesthetics are weak bases with molecular weights of 236–288 Da (Table 9.8). The pKa of all LAs is between 7.6 (mepivacaine) and 9.1 (chloroprocaine). At a pH of 7.40, 60–85% of the molecules are ionized and diffuse in the body's water compartments. LAs are also soluble in lipids and cell membranes. Bupivacaine is 10 times more soluble in membranes than lidocaine; ropivacaine is twice as soluble as lidocaine. With the exception of lidocaine, all amide LAs possess an asymmetric carbon. Although the physicochemical properties (pKa, distribution ratio) of the isomers are identical, the enantiomers have different affinities for the biological effectors (channels, receptors, proteins). Ropivacaine and levobupivacaine are pure S-(–) enantiomers. LAs are marketed as hydrochloride salts in water at pHs of 4–5 to prevent them from coming out of solution. The salts precipitate when bicarbonate is added to the solution to increase its pH.

Like most weak bases, amide LAs bind to serum proteins and red cells, which may be clinically important, especially in neonates and young infants. Neonates who have hematocrits >45% may have less unbound drug. In serum, LAs bind to both α1-acid glycoprotein and to albumin. Despite its low concentration in serum (less than 1 g/L in adults), AGP is the major protein that binds LAs. During the first 6–9 months of life, AGP concentrations progressively increase and reach adult levels by 1 year of age (see Fig. 9.2) [27]. When this occurs, the free fraction of LAs decreases [449], which may protect from LA toxicity. However, the concomitant decrease in hepatic clearance of free drug may leave clearance unchanged (see Fig. 9.3). LAs also bind to HSA, but with a very low affinity. It is only because HSA is the most abundant protein in serum that its binding capacity is significant.

Absorption

After applying topical anesthesia to the upper airway, LAs are rapidly absorbed and can cause toxicity, particularly in children less than 4 years old. This is why it is important to use nozzles that deliver no more than 10 mg with each squeeze [450]. EMLA® (Eutectic Mixture of Local Anesthetics) cream contains equal amounts of lidocaine and prilocaine and is not absorbed in significant amounts, except in premature babies [451]. Prilocaine produces methemoglobinemia in neonates and infants, especially if they are also treated with trimethoprim-sulfamethoxazole [452]. The cream may not work in premature babies because of their very high skin blood flow.

Amide LAs have a bio-availability of 1 (metabolism is exclusively hepatic). Since these drugs are hydrophobic, they bind to tissues, which delays their absorption. This delay varies depending on the local conditions. For example, absorption occurs more rapidly after an ilio-inguino-iliohypogastric block than after a caudal block. In adults, 3 hours after an epidural injection, only 70% of a dose of lidocaine and 50% of a dose of bupivacaine or of ropivacaine is absorbed, which is a safety factor [453]. From adult studies, it is clear that the speed of drug absorption decreases from head to foot and from the thoracic to the caudal portion of the epidural space. Lidocaine and bupivacaine concentrations peak about 30 min after caudal or lumbar injection in infants and adults. The T_{max} for ropivacaine is much longer in infants than in children and in children than in adults, probably because CYP1A2, which metabolizes lidocaine and ropivacaine, is immature before 4–7 years of age [454]. This phenomenon is less important with levobupivacaine because it is metabolized by CYP3A4/7 [455].

Epinephrine reduces the peak concentrations of LAs. The usual concentration used in clinical practice is 5 mg/L (1/200,000), which is optimal in adults. It is possible that this concentration of epinephrine may decrease spinal cord blood flow in some infants and produce neurological deficits. Therefore, some authors suggest using no more than a 1/400,000 concentration of epinephrine in infants <1 year of age, since this concentration is also efficacious [456].

Distribution

The volume of distribution of local anesthetics at steady state (Vss) is slightly less than 1 L/kg (Table 9.9) [453–455,457–467]. Because drug absorption is delayed, volumes calculated after administration by non-IV routes are markedly overestimated. Terminal half-lives are also increased compared to values obtained after an IV injection. Total body clearance of the drug is only measured accurately following extravascular administration, but sampling must take place over a prolonged period of time. It is highly probable that LAs distribute into large volumes in neonates, infants, and adults, thus preventing high serum drug concentrations from occurring after a single injection. However, this is not the case following several injections. Ropivacaine's volume of distribution is smaller than that of bupivacaine in adults and probably in pediatric patients. At similar doses, the C_{max} of ropivacaine is higher than that of bupivacaine, despite ropivacaine's delayed T_{max}.

Elimination

Liver cytochrome P450 enzymes metabolize all amide local anesthetics. Bupivacaine is predominantly metabolized into pipecoloxylidide (PPX) by CYP3A4/7 [468]. Ropivacaine is predominantly metabolized to 3'- and 4'-OH-ropivacaine by CYP1A2 and to a minor extent to PPX by CYP3A4 [49]. These enzymes are not fully mature at birth and have important differences in their developmental expression (see above). The extraction ratios for lidocaine (0.65–0.75) are relatively high. Lidocaine is flow limited rather than rate limited for its elimination. Therefore, any decrease in cardiac output decreases

Table 9.9 Bupivacaine, levobupivacaine and ropivacaine pharmacokinetics after different routes in infants and children compared to adults

		fu	Vss#	CLT /f	CLU /f	T½#
			(L/kg)	(mL/min/kg)	(mL/min/kg)	(h)
Bupivacaine						
IV adults		0.05	0.85–1.3	4.5–8.1	≈100	1.8
Epidural adults		–	–	4–5.6	–	5.1–10.6
Infants caudal single shot		0.16 (0.05–0.35)	3.9	7.1	–	–
Children (5–10 yrs)		–	2.7	10	–	–
Infants epidural prolonged		(0.06–0.24) *	–	5.5–7.5 *	36–73	–
Levobupivacaine						
IV adults		0.045	0.72	4.2	116	2.6
Caudal, infants 0.6–2.9 months		0.13	2.87	6.28	51.7	–
Ropivacaine						
IV adults		0.05	0.5–0.6	4.2–5.3	≈100	1.7
Epidural adults		–	–	4.0–5.7	≈70	2.9–5.4
Caudal single shot	Neonates	0.07	–	–	50–58	–
	Infants	0.05–0.10	2.1	5.2	–	–
	Children	5.2 (1.3–7.3)	2.4	7.4	151	–
Epidural prolonged	Neonates	–	2.4	4.26	–	–
	Infants	–	2.4	6.15	–	–
	Children	0.04	–	8.5	220	–

fu, free fraction; Vss, volume of distribution at steady state; CL/f, total body clearance over bio-availability (T, total fraction, U, unbound fraction); T½, terminal half-life.
For adults, a mean bodyweight of 75 kg has been assumed.
#apparent value.
T½ and volumes measured after non-IV injections are overestimated because of a flip-flop effect (i.e. because absorption lasts longer than elimination).
* After 3 h infusion.
‡ After 48 h infusion, CLT decreases with time because protein binding increases.

hepatic clearance of lidocaine. The resultant increase in plasma concentration of LA may be toxic. Bupivacaine and ropivacaine, on the other hand, have a relatively low hepatic extraction ratio (0.30–0.35) and are rate limited for their elimination. Thus, hepatic clearance and free fraction are major determinants of total clearance. After surgery, serum AGP concentrations increase, which increases protein binding. This decreases total clearance but not intrinsic clearance. This resets the total serum concentration, without changing the unbound concentration (see Fig. 9.3). Bupivacaine clearance is low at birth and increases slightly during the first 6–9 months of life. Ropivacaine clearance, which is also low in neonates and infants, increases during the first 2–6 years of life [454,463,465,466]. Despite the low clearance, ropivacaine concentrations remain below toxic levels, even in younger patients.

Pharmacodynamics

Local anesthetics cross membranes as free bases (unionized). Inside the cells, they become ionized and bind to specific amino acids within sodium channel pores and mechanically block the pores [447]. LAs also block potassium and calcium channels, but this requires slightly higher drug concentrations than those needed to block sodium channels. Voltage-gated potassium channels initiate repolarization. Some of these channels (including the human ether-à-go-go (hERG) related gene channel) are responsible for genetically induced arrhythmias, such as the long-QT, short-QT or Brugada syndromes. These channels are blocked by LA concentrations just slightly higher than those needed to block sodium channels [469,470]. Unlike the CNS and heart, peripheral nerves only express a small number of potassium channels. Both sodium and potassium channel blockade are stereospecific. The S enantiomers induce a lesser block than R enantiomers. LAs bind to L-type calcium channels, but it is unclear if blockade of these channels affects the cardiotoxicity of long-lasting LAs.

Nerve fibers are either myelinated or unmyelinated. The action potential of unmyelinated fibers propagates continuously. After initial depolarization, the sodium channels become unreceptive to stimulation (refractory period), which prevents backward propagation of impulses. Sodium and potassium channels are evenly distributed along the fibers. Conduction velocity of small fibers is low. Myelin insulates myelinated nerves, and this layer is interrupted regularly by the nodes of Ranvier. Sodium channels are situated at the node of Ranvier in concentrations of ≈200,000 channels/cm² [471,472]. Potassium channels are distributed along the myelin sheet with a higher concentration present in the juxtaparanodal region. The sudden depolarization of the node induces an electrical field, which extends to 2–3 nodes.

Action potentials "jump" rapidly from one node to the next. Because the distance between nodes is greater in heavily myelinated fibers (there are 3–4 nodes/cm in Aα fibers and 20–30 nodes/cm in Aδ fibers), the conduction velocity is faster in motor and small sensory fibers than in fibers that conduct pain signals. Because the electrical field extends over a relatively long distance, nerve fibers must be "bathed" over a relatively long distance by LAs. This progressive extinction of the signal is called decremental conduction. Fortunately, the phasic block that is induced by the high firing rate of nerves reinforces the block. Small Aδ lightly myelinated fibers are blocked by less drug than is needed to block heavily myelinated fibers. This phenomenon, called differential nerve block, is explained by differences in internode distance between fibers [473]. It is unknown to what extent concentration gradients across the myelin sheet also participate in this phenomenon.

Myelinization begins during the third trimester of pregnancy and is incomplete at birth. After birth, myelinization increases rapidly and is almost complete by 3–4 years of age [471,472]. In rats, the nodes of Ranvier are fully mature at 2–3 weeks of age. Interestingly, the internode distance is similar between 2-week-old and adult rats. This may explain why infants and young children require larger volumes of LAs per kilogram than older children or adults (Fig. 9.13) [474]. Fortunately, lower concentrations of LA are needed to cause the block. Infants and children need larger volumes of solution with lower

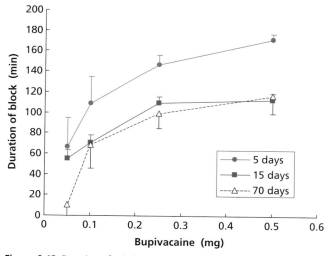

Figure 9.13 Duration of sciatic nerve blocks in rats after an injection of bupivacaine. The block is more protracted in newborn than in older rats. Duration of the block in 2- and 10-week-old rats was similar despite a marked difference in size and weight. It appears that the distance between nodes of Ranvier, which is fixed at its adult value by the age of 1–2 weeks, is the main determinant of the motor blockade. Data from Kohane et al [474].

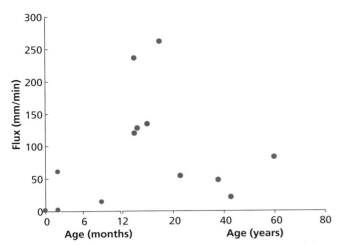

Figure 9.14 Cerebrospinal fluid flux according to age. Flux is initially low in infants, and then rapidly increases and becomes maximal in older children. Thereafter, it decreases regularly. Data from Greits and Hangers, Am J Neuroradiol 1996; 17: 431–8.

concentration of LAs to achieve blocks of similar intensity and duration as adults. Surprisingly, infants require larger doses of LAs for spinal anesthesia. Despite this, the duration of the spinal block is shorter. Some authors have attributed this difference to a larger volume and a more rapid turnover of CSF in neonates and infants than in older children and adults. Unfortunately, the pharmacokinetics of LAs in the CSF is particularly unknown in pediatric patients. The brain CSF volume and CSF turnover are lower in neonates and infants than in children and adults (Fig. 9.14) [475,476]. The major factor responsible for this rapid effect seems to be pharmacodynamic. The intensity and duration of the block depend on the number of nodes of Ranvier blocked (differential block). The distance between nodes is fixed soon after birth [471,472]. When this occurs, the short duration of spinal anesthesia in infants is not surprising.

Effects on the central nervous system and cardiovascular systems

Like all inhibitors of sodium channels, low doses of LAs are anticonvulsive, which is why lidocaine is still used to treat intractable epilepsy in children [477]. However, the therapeutic ratio is low and the margin of safety does not favor lidocaine. At higher doses, LAs may produce convulsions and coma. At similar concentrations to those that cause convulsions, long-lasting LAs can induce cardiac arrhythmias. With the exception of nodal conduction, which depends on calcium channels, impulse conduction in the heart depends on sodium channels. This is why lidocaine is a chief class Ib antiarrhythmic agent. LAs prolong the refractory period, but the balance between the increase in effective refractory period and the decrease

in the ventricular conduction velocity does not favor LAs. Long-lasting LAs, like bupivacaine, profoundly decrease ventricular conduction velocity [478]. This phenomenon is markedly amplified by tachycardia [479]. In neonatal and adult animals, the intensity of the block is similar at similar heart rates [480]. However, because neonates and infants normally have higher heart rates than adults, they are more sensitive to local anesthetic-induced blocks than adults. LAs also impair myocardial contractility. However, to obtain the same decrease in contractile force, it is necessary to infuse 10 times more bupivacaine than is required to impair ventricular conduction.

Apart from the effect of the central block-induced sympathetic blockade, LAs have direct vasoactive properties. The S enantiomers (ropivacaine and levobupivacaine) have mild vasoconstrictive properties. These properties have been suggested as the cause of ischemia after penile block, but a direct relationship between ropivacaine and ischemia in this report seems doubtful [481].

Stereo-specificity

Mepivacaine, prilocaine, bupivacaine, and ropivacaine have an asymmetrical carbon. Because binding to serum proteins, hepatic enzymes, or ion channels may be asymmetrical, different stereo-specific properties are expected. Protein binding, pharmacokinetics, and nerve blocks have little stereoselectivity, which is why levobupivacaine has almost the same blocking properties as its racemic counterpart. In the heart, conduction is markedly stereo-specific, whereas contractility is unaffected by steroselectivity.

Local anesthetics have anti-inflammatory properties and inhibit platelet aggregation [482]. They decrease leukocyte priming and the production of free radicals [483–485]. Systemically administered lidocaine has antinociceptive effects, particularly on neuropathic pain [486]. Consequently, LAs are now used peroperatively to prevent postoperative hyperalgesia in adults [487]. Interestingly, LAs can prevent and even treat complex regional pain syndrome in adults and children by limiting the neuropathic inflammatory processes [488,489].

Toxicity of local anesthetics

At the site of injection, the minimum concentration required to produce a nerve blockade is 300–1500 μM for lidocaine and 100–500 μM for bupivacaine. In adults these concentrations of lidocaine occasionally cause cauda equina syndrome but are more likely to cause transient neurological symptoms following spinal anesthesia. LAs can also be toxic to muscles, bupivacaine being the most toxic [490,491]. Muscle toxicity is not enantioselective. Care should be taken when regional anesthesia is provided for eye surgery in adults, for children with myopathies (bupivacaine is an *in vitro* model of Duchenne myopathy), and perhaps for children with mitochondrial cytopathy. Peripheral blocks are more dangerous than central blocks because it is easier to inject drug directly into muscle with peripheral blocks.

After both local and regional anesthesia, the blood concentration of LAs rises rapidly and can cause neurological or cardiac toxicity. Neurological toxicity occurs in about one case per 1000 patients [492]. Because of their low protein binding and intrinsic clearance, infants are more prone to LA toxicity than adults. General anesthesia may conceal the early signs of LA toxicity in children. In addition to pharmacokinetic factors, the rapid heart rate of children increases LA toxicity. Ropivacaine and levobupivacaine (S-(–) enantiomers) are appropriate choices for younger patients because both drugs should produce less tonic block. Even if toxic events occur with ropivacaine, small doses of epinephrine should cause rapid recovery. Impaired ventricular conduction is the primary manifestation of LA toxicity. QRS widening, bradycardia, and torsades de pointe are followed by either ventricular fibrillation and/or asystole [493]. The slight decrease in myocardial contractility caused by LAs is usually not a major problem. Treatment includes oxygenation, cardiac massage, correction of acidosis, and epinephrine (which is given in small incremental boluses beginning with 2–4 µg/kg) [494]. If ventricular fibrillation persists, defibrillation (2–4 joule/kg) is performed.

Although resuscitation measures must be initiated immediately, the specific treatment of LA toxicity is rapid administration of Intralipid®. Numerous case reports have shown that rapid bolus injections of a lipid emulsion reverse the toxic effects of LAs [495–497]. Because one mole of Intralipid® binds >3000 times more molecules of bupivacaine than a mole of buffer, the volume of distribution suddenly increases [498,499]. The recommended dose of 20% Intralipid® for pediatric patients is 5 mL/kg by IV bolus. If cardiac function does not return, this dose (up to 10–12 mg/kg) is repeated. Rather than institute a maintenance infusion of Intralipid®, patients are closely monitored and given more Intralipid® as needed. The lipid emulsion decreases LA elimination, so the cardiac effects may recur later.

Prevention of toxicity includes slow injection of small amounts of drug and frequent catheter aspiration. Some authors recommend injecting a solution that contains epinephrine. Continuous administration of LAs for postoperative pain is better than bolus injections because the latter may cause peaks and troughs of drug concentration and pain relief. If the catheter migrates into a blood vessel, continuous administration is safer. In older children, patient-controlled regional anesthesia (PCRA – see Chapter 33) works well. Also, the size of the boluses is small enough to avoid toxicity.

Adjuvants

Adjuvants are often used to prolong the duration of analgesia. Epinephrine (5 µg/mL = 1/200,000) decreases C_{max}, without affecting the time to peak concentration. In infants <6 months old, 2.5 µg/mL 1/400,000 epinephrine has been recommended [456]. However, the drug is less efficacious with long-acting S-(–)- enantiomers and has limited use with these solutions. Plain solutions of LAs *must* be used for penile, interdigital, and eye blocks.

Clonidine 1–2 µg/kg, either IV or in the epidural space, prolongs the duration of caudal blocks [500]. More than 2 µg/kg may lead to hypotension. Clonidine is not recommended for infants <3 months of age because it can cause apnea in this age group.

Some clinicians use ketamine as an adjuvant for epidural block [501]. Both the R-(–) enantiomer and the preservative are highly neurotoxic. Even the S(+) enantiomer can be toxic. Thus it may be wise to avoid the use of ketamine as an adjuvant for epidural blocks [502,503].

Opioids are often used as adjuvants for epidural block. After 6–9 months of age, adding opioids to LAs prolongs epidural analgesia for up to 24 hours. Hydrophobic agents (fentanyl, sufentanil) must be placed at the metameric level where the pain will occur [504,505]. Preservative-free morphine easily spreads rostrally and can be placed at a lower metameric level, but the risk of respiratory depression is theoretically higher. The bolus dose of morphine is 25–30 µg/kg in the epidural space, which is followed by a continuous infusion of 1 µg/kg/h. When continuous epidural administration of fentanyl or sufentanil is combined with local anesthetics, the doses are 0.2 µg/kg/h and 0.1 µg/kg/h respectively. Morphine 5–10 µg/kg can be used as the sole agent for spinal analgesia during general anesthesia.

Formulation and dosing

Plain solutions of amide LAs are preservative free; only solutions containing epinephrine include metabisulfite [506]. The S enantiomers (ropivacaine and levobupivacaine) are safer and cause similar quality and duration of analgesia and less motor blockade than a racemic mixture of bupivacaine. When regional analgesia is used during general anesthesia, low concentrations of LAs (2–2.5 mg/mL, i.e. 0.2–0.25%) are used. The maximum dose is 2–2.5 mg/kg for the initial caudal injection, 1.2–1.7 mg/kg for lumbar or thoracic epidural injections, and 0.5 mg/kg for peripheral blocks. Continuous infusion of LAs for postoperative analgesia uses low concentrations of drug (0.625–1 mg/mL) at a maximum rate of 0.20 mg/kg/h in neonates, 0.30 mg/kg for 1–6 months old, and 0.40 mg/kg beyond 6 months of age.

CASE STUDY

A full-term newborn weighing 3520 g was scheduled for esophageal atresia (type 3) repair 16 h after birth. Cardiac, abdominal, and renal echography was normal. A small amount of stridor was noticed. An ENT surgeon was asked to evaluate the child and perform laryngoscopy prior to surgery. All blood tests were normal for the age, except the activated coagulation test, which was slightly prolonged (45 sec versus 35 sec for control). Factors VIII and IX were subsequently found to be normal, as was a preoperative thromboelastogram. The physical examination showed an apparently healthy boy who was spontaneously breathing and had mild stridor. A peripheral venous catheter was in place. A suction catheter was present in the upper esophagus to aspirate saliva. Anesthesia was induced with sevoflurane (6% inspired) with spontaneous ventilation. The ENT surgeon sprayed the larynx with 10 mg of 2% lidocaine without epinephrine. No airway abnormality was found, and the trachea was intubated.

Following tracheal intubation, the patient was given sufentanil (0.5 μg) and atracurium (1 mg) over 1 min. The lungs were mechanically ventilated. An epidural was performed using levobupivacaine. Because lidocaine had been administered 30 min earlier for examination of the larynx, the initial bolus of LA was reduced (5 mg or 2 mL of a 2.5 mg/mL solution). The bolus was immediately followed with a continuous infusion of 0.85 mg/h, i.e. 1.4 mL/h of a 0.0625% solution. Anesthesia was maintained with sevoflurane 1.5–2% (0.5–0.6 MAC without N₂O). Surgery was uneventful and the trachea was extubated after reversal of the muscle relaxant (neostigmine 350 μg, atropine 75 μg). In addition to the epidural, IV acetaminophen (50 mg bolus plus 25 mg every 6 h) was given (IV acetaminophen is approved in approximately 80 countries, including Europe, and has recently been launched in the US as Ofirmev). Unfortunately, the epidural catheter was dislodged 5 hours after surgery. The anesthesiologist prescribed a continuous IV infusion of morphine 40 μg/h but because drugs already given through the epidural catheter would provide pain relief for 1–2 more hours, no loading dose of morphine was given. Six hours later, the patient's respiratory rate progressively decreased to 16 bpm. The infusion of morphine was decreased to 30 μg/h and the respiratory rate returned to normal. The remainder of his postoperative course was uneventful.

Key points

1. Because lidocaine was used for the laryngeal examination, a smaller dose of LA was given into the epidural space. Lidocaine is rapidly absorbed following topical application to mucous membranes and may interact with levobupivacaine given for blocks.

2. Sevoflurane was used to induce anesthesia because it, plus the topical anesthesia, provided excellent condition for the laryngopharyngeal examination. Following tracheal intubation, a phenylpiperidine opioid and a muscle relaxant were slowly injected to prevent a "stiff" chest from developing. The drugs were also injected slowly to prevent the profound hypotension that sometimes occurs when sufentanil and atracurium are injected rapidly.

3. The epidural was performed (1) to provide postoperative analgesia, allow rapid tracheal extubation, and avoid postoperative mechanical ventilation, and (2) to reduce the amount of halogenated agents used and prevent their possible deleterious CNS effects. At this age, MAC is higher than that of adults. However, MAC may differ for different variables (e.g. hemodynamic variables). Balanced anesthesia with opioids and regional anesthesia is a good choice. Levobupivacaine was chosen over ropivacaine because it is metabolized by CYP3A4/3A7, which is more mature at birth. Ropivacaine is metabolized by CYP1A2, which is immature until 4 years of age. Pure S enantiomers (ropivacaine and levobupivacaine) are less toxic and induce less motor blockade, a significant problem in infants. Because the volume of distribution of hydrophilic local anesthetics is large in newborns and infants, the initial bolus dose/kg is usually the same as in older children. Since LA toxicity is additive, and because a topical spray of lidocaine was used less than a hour before the epidural block, limited amounts of levobupivacaine (1.4 mg/kg) were injected into the epidural space. This initial bolus was followed by a continuous infusion of the drug. The infusion dose was reduced because the volume of distribution would be filled after 4–5 half-lives; at that point, clearance rapidly becomes the only factor governing drug concentration. Because clearance of the unbound fraction, which is responsible for LA toxicity, is low at birth and progressively increases with age, the dose varies with age. Fortunately, <4–6 month olds have excellent pain relief with smaller doses of LAs.

4. Postoperative pain control is critical, not only to relieve the pain but also to reduce respiratory complications (hypoventilation). In addition to regional anesthesia, this patient received paracetamol (acetaminophen). Because metabolism of this drug is reduced during the first month of life, the child was given about half the dose of paracetamol given to older patients. No loading dose was given.

Annotated references

A full reference list for this chapter is available at:
http://www.wiley.com/go/gregory/andropoulos/pediatricanesthesia

1. Kearns GL, Abdel-Rahman SM, Alander SW et al. Developmental pharmacology – drug disposition, action, and therapy in infants and children. N Engl J Med 2003; 349: 1157–67. This excellent review outlines the major factors leading to differences in drug action between neonates, children, and adults. In the era of genomics, it is important to remember that simple factors, such as body composition or relative blood flows of organs, are the primary determinants of absorption, distribution, and elimination.

6. Anderson BJ, Allegaert K, van den Anker JN et al. Vancomycin pharmacokinetics in preterm neonates and the prediction of adult clearance. Br J Clin Pharmacol 2007; 63: 75–84. Population pharmacokinetics allows accurate individualized prediction of PK parameters. Using sparse sampling (604 routine clinical assays in 214 subjects), mixed-effect modeling allows the incorporation of co-variates such as weight, postmenstrual age, creatinine clearance, and the need for artificial ventilation and inotropic drugs to accurately predict drug clearance (see Fig. 9.1). The use of a personal digital assistant or a computer to determine drug dosage and effect in a given patient seems necessary in the near future to customize dosing and avoid drug interactions.

35. Hines RN. The ontogeny of drug metabolism enzymes and implications for adverse drug events. Pharmacol Ther 2008; 118: 250–67. This is a comprehensive review of a complex subject. The author usually updates or produces a variant of this paper every 2–4 years to make new developments on this rapidly changing subject available to the reader. It is impossible to memorize all the information, and in the future computer-aided prescribing that incorporates this information will be the rule.

50. Wilkinson GR. Drug metabolism and variability among patients in drug response. N Engl J Med 2005; 352: 2211–21.This review gives some examples of environmental and genetic factors leading to interindividual variability in drug absorption, disposition, and elimination. The importance of the environment, such as the diet, is highlighted.

102. Mellon RD, Simone AF, Rappaport BA. Use of anesthetic agents in neonates and young children. Anesth Analg 2007; 104: 509–20. This is a good summary of questions raised by the use of anesthetic agents in neonates and infants. Clearly, agents with NMDA antagonist properties have potential neurodegenerative actions, but it is not known if this is clinically relevant. Other factors, such as blood pressure, may also contribute to ischemia-reperfusion in younger subjects.

116. Bailey JM. Context-sensitive half times and other decrement times of inhaled anesthetics. Anesth Analg 1997; 85: 681–6. This paper explores the pharmacokinetics of inhaled agents through a semi-physiological, semi-compartmental model and clearly shows the importance of the duration of administration in the speed of recovery. Compartmental models derived from the principles of chemical kinetics are now used. Their empirical aspect allows calculation of simple parameters, such as clearance, volumes or times, without the need to know the precise characteristic of each of the physiological compartments. More relevant co-variates, such as cardiac output or age, may be incorporated in the same way as in the study of Anderson et al. [6].

162. Von Ungern-Sternberg BS, Saudan S, Petak F et al. Desflurane but not sevoflurane impairs airway and respiratory tissue mechanics in children with susceptible airways. Anesthesiology 2008; 108: 216–24. What to do with the child with airway problems is a daily dilemma. Should we anesthetize this child with upper respiratory tract infection for this particular surgery or not? Interestingly, this paper shows that sevoflurane has beneficial effects on airway resistances as compared to desflurane.

235. Hughes MA, Glass PS, Jacobs JR. Context-sensitive half time in multicompartment pharmacokinetic models for intravenous anesthetic drugs. Anesthesiology 1992; 76: 334–41. Context-sensitive decrement times for volatile anesthetics have been long recognized. However, the concept and the use of context-sensitive half-times are fully explained in this paper. This concept is at the basis of all computer-driven, pharmacokinetic-based administration of drugs.

384. Plaud B, Debaene B, Donati F. The corrugator supercilii, not the orbicularis oculi, reflects rocuronium neuromuscular blockade at the laryngeal adductor muscles. Anesthesiology 2001; 95: 96–101. This paper explains why T½ke0 for muscle relaxants may be so long when compared to our clinical impressions. The onset of effect and recovery times are different from one muscle to another. For example, T½ke0 of vecuronium is four times longer for the adductor pollicis than for the laryngeal muscles. Whether one wants to monitor the onset of action for tracheal intubation or the recovery for adequate ventilation, the muscle of interest should be different. Because it is not possible in daily practice, it is important to understand this concept to adapt our understanding of the observed phenomenon.

498. Mazoit JX, Le Guen R, Beloeil H, Benhamou D. Binding of long-lasting local anesthetics to lipid emulsions. Anesthesiology 2009; 110: 380–6. Lipid rescue. This *in vitro* study shows that long-acting local anesthetics are rapidly (less than 30 sec) adsorbed in lipid particles by a passive (entropy-driven) phenomenon. At 37°C and pH 7.40, the mole fraction of bupivacaine between Intralipid® and buffer was 3100, i.e. 3100 molecules of bupivacaine distribute in a mole of emulsion for every one molecule found in a mole of buffer. The consequence is an immediate increase in the volume of distribution of the local anesthetics and a lower elimination rate. Recurrences of toxicity may then occur, inasmuch as the half-life of the chylomicrons is very short (6–7 min). Close patient monitoring for several hours after lipid rescue appears mandatory.

CHAPTER 10
Fluids, Electrolytes, and Nutrition

Claire Brett[1] & Danton Charr[2]

[1]Department of Anesthesia and Perioperative Care, University of California San Francisco, San Francisco, CA, USA

[2]Department of Anesthesia, Stanford Hospital and Clinics, Stanford University, Stanford, CA, USA

Introduction

Mammals maintain electrolyte balance over a wide range of physiological states. In his review of early investigations of fluid and electrolyte physiology and its translation into clinical practice [1], Holliday quoted from Walter Cannon's book *The Wisdom of the Body* [2]. Cannon introduced the term "homeostasis" into fluid and electrolyte physiology and discussed the mechanisms for maintaining stability in spite of "dangerous conditions in the outer world, and equally dangerous possibilities within the body . . . and yet they continue to live and carry on their functions with relatively little disturbance . . . somehow the unstable stuff of which we are composed had learned the trick of maintaining stability." By his awareness of the history of our current principles of fluid and electrolyte management, Holliday encourages continued, critical, open-minded investigation and re-evaluation of clinical practice.

The ability to manage fluids and electrolytes requires an in-depth understanding of a wide range of topics encompassing renal, hepatic, cardiorespiratory, endocrine, and central nervous system physiology. Electrolyte derangements both evolve from and cause multiorgan dysfunction. For example, electrolyte and acid–base abnormalities are associated with primary renal, neurological, hematological, and/or hepatic injury and often accompany myocardial or pulmonary failure. On the other hand, fluid and electrolyte imbalance of any etiology can produce electrophysiological abnormalities that have profound simultaneous effects on multiple organ systems. Age-related differences in organ function and pharmacodynamic responses in infants and children, coupled with congenital anomalies and genetic abnormalities, add to the complexity of fluid and electrolyte management of these patients.

In this chapter, the newborn is discussed separately from the infant and child because managing perioperative fluids and electrolytes in infants requires understanding of the unique developmental aspects of distribution of total body water and of age-related renal, hepatic, cardiorespiratory, and central nervous system physiology. Following discussion of the newborn, principles of perioperative fluid and electrolytes for the older infant and child are considered. For both the newborn and the older infant/child, background information will be translated into specific recommendations and guidelines for preoperative evaluation, intraoperative monitoring, and

Gregory's Pediatric Anesthesia, Fifth Edition. Edited by George A. Gregory, Dean B. Andropoulos.
© 2012 Blackwell Publishing Ltd. Published 2012 by Blackwell Publishing Ltd.

delivery of glucose, crystalloid, and colloid. In all age groups, meticulously anticipating and responding to the preoperative and intraoperative events sets the stage for a smooth transition to stable postoperative fluid and electrolyte status.

General considerations

Intravenous (IV) fluids replete water and electrolyte losses when oral intake is inadequate or absent. Intravenous fluid administration has at least four components: (1) replacing deficits caused by being nil per os (NPO) or from excessive losses (e.g. treating dehydration/hypovolemia), (2) calculating requirements associated with "maintenance" water and electrolytes (e.g. insensible and urinary losses), (3) estimating ongoing fluid losses (e.g. diarrhea/vomiting, bleeding, intraoperative events), and (4) identifying additional derangements (e.g. hypo- or hyperglycemia, acid–base abnormalities, pathophysiological states, such as birth asphyxia, excessive secretion of arginine vasopressin (AVP)). Although this framework for analyzing fluid delivery applies to the entire spectrum of ages from newborn to the elderly, the unique developmental physiology of the newborn and young infant alters aspects of each component. For example, estimating "maintenance" fluid depends on gestational and postnatal age and the changes in normal glucose requirements that are age dependent. Finally, derangements in fluids and electrolytes accompany many disease-induced problems, but responses to a given insult vary depending on developmental stage.

At all ages, sodium is the primary cation in the plasma and chloride is the major anion. Potassium, calcium, and magnesium comprise the remainder of the cations in the extracellular space; bicarbonate, chloride, and proteins are notable anions. The intracellular fluid primarily consists of potassium and magnesium (cations) and proteins and organic/inorganic phosphate (anions) (Table 10.1).

The regulation of the extracellular compartment is closely inter-related with cardiovascular function. Blood pressure and intravascular volume, as well as serum sodium concentration, are sensed by baro- and osmoreceptors. The responses of the heart, peripheral vasculature, kidneys, and brain to changes in pressure and osmolarity are tightly regulated by complex interactions between hormones and mediators (e.g. renin-angiotensin-aldosterone system (RAS), arginine vasopressin (AVP) (also known as antidiuretic hormone (ADH), atrial natriuretic peptide, catecholamines). Other mediators fine-tune these regulatory hormones. Thus, a variety of hormones regulates the volume and composition of the extracellular compartment, primarily by effects on renal sodium and water balance and on cardiac and peripheral

Table 10.1 Composition of the extracellular and intracellular fluid compartments

	Extracellular fluid	Intracellular fluid
Osmolality (mOsm)	290–310	190–310
Cations (meq/L)	155	155
Sodium (Na⁺)	138–142	10
Potassium (K⁺)	4.0–4.5	110
Calcium (Ca⁺⁺)	4.5–5.0	–
Magnesium (Mg⁺⁺)	3	40
Anions (meq/L)	155	155
Chloride (Cl⁻)	103	2
Bicarbonate (HCO₃⁻)	27	8
Hydrogen phosphate (HPO₄⁻²)	–	10
Phosphate (PO₄⁻²)	3	149
Organic acids	6	Variable
Protein	16	40

vasculature. For example, if the extracellular volume expands in patients with normal physiology, urine output increases in response to increased renal blood flow and glomerular filtration; as a result, extracellular volume and osmolarity are relatively normal. However, in the presence of pathology (e.g. sepsis), the blood volume and/or arterial blood pressure may not increase in response to an expanded extracellular volume due to increased capillary permeability and widespread edema and organ dysfunction (e.g. pulmonary edema).

Tight regulation of the extracellular fluid compartment ultimately determines the intracellular volume space. That is, if the osmolality of the extracellular compartment changes, water moves into or out of cells; water readily equilibrates across cell membranes in response to changes in solute concentrations. In contrast, movement of a solute depends on the permeability of the solute in a specific membrane and on hydrostatic and osmotic gradients. The mathematical relationship (Starling equation) [3] describing net water movement across a membrane includes factors for oncotic and hydrostatic pressures on either side of the membrane (e.g. interstitium and the intravascular space):

$$J_v = KF ([P_C - P_I] - \delta[\pi_c - \pi_I])$$

where J_v = the net flow across the membrane, K_F = fluid filtration coefficient of the membrane, P_C = hydrostatic pressure (e.g. capillary), P_I = hydrostatic pressure (e.g. interstitial), δ = solute reflection coefficient (permeability of solute across a specific membrane), π_c = oncotic pressure (e.g. capillary), and π_I = oncotic pressure (e.g. interstitial). Fluid moves as a function of the product of the permeability of the membrane and net driving pressure (hydrostatic pressure minus oncotic pressure). If this relationship is disturbed (e.g. when membrane trauma decreases the reflection coefficient for proteins), the interstitial compartment may expand (i.e. edema develops). In the normal patient, oncotic and hydrostatic pressures are balanced but with various disease states, the interstitial space expands at the expense of the intravascular space. For example, increased capillary permeability during sepsis (trapping protein in the interstitial space, increasing π_I) or increased venous pressure with positive pressure ventilation (increasing P_C) may produce edema and/ or decrease intravascular volume.

The newborn: developmental aspects of fluids and electrolytes

Developmental changes in fluid compartments and distribution of water

In the newborn, total body water accounts for $78 \pm 5\%$ of total bodyweight. It decreases to 60% (mostly due to loss from the extracellular fraction) by 6 months and to 57% later in childhood. Total body water is distributed into both the intracellular (ICW) and extracellular (ECW) fluid compartments (Fig. 10.1). In the fetus, the extracellular compartment predominates, contributing ~62% of bodyweight during the first trimester but only ~43% at term. At the same time, ICW increases from 25% to 32% of bodyweight [4,5]. Because the ratio of surface area to

volume decreases with maturation, the total body water actually increases after the first month of extrauterine life. However, ECW and plasma volume remain constant as a function of surface area.

With their larger surface area, premature infants have a greater percentage of their bodyweight as total body water and a larger ECW compartment than infants born at term. The change in total body water distribution, as a function of weight, continues postnatally so that by 3 months of life, the intracellular compartment is larger than the extracellular compartment. The adult ratio of ECW to ICW is achieved by about 1 year of age. ECW is divided into plasma and interstitial compartments. The plasma compartment remains constant throughout life, comprising ~5% of bodyweight. Although two additional body compartments (slowly exchangeable areas (e.g. bone and cartilage) and transcellular) are actually extracellular, neither is a clinically important site for water exchange under normal circumstances.

The values for blood volume of normal infants and children [6] and low-birthweight infants [7] measured 4–5 decades ago remain the accepted norms for estimating a wide variety of clinically important therapy, such as blood loss and transfusion of blood products, distribution of drugs, etc. The blood volume gradually decreases (as a function of weight) with growth and development. Thus, the blood volume for premature infants is ~100 mL/ kg, for full-term infants is 85–90 mL/kg, for 2 year olds is 80 mL/kg, and for older infant and adolescents is 75–80 mL/kg.

Insensible water loss

Insensible water loss occurs primarily through evaporation from the skin (~70%) and from the respiratory tract (~30%). The total volume and source of this loss vary with ambient temperature and relative humidity [8] and are directly proportional to the exposed surface area. Because the ratio of skin surface area to bodyweight increases as gestational age decreases, most premature infants lose large amounts of water transcutaneously. Other factors, including increased permeability of and blood flow to the skin and lesser amounts of subcutaneous fat, augment transcutaneous water loss. The cornified layer of extremely low-birthweight (ELBW) infants (<1000 g) consists of only 2–3 cell layers, which provides a less effective barrier to diffusion of water, especially during the first days after birth [9]. The newborn's higher minute ventilation increases insensible water loss from the lungs. Tachypnea further exaggerates transpulmonary water loss.

Neutral thermal environment

In a neutral thermal environment (skin temperature 36–36.5°C with an environmental temperature of 32–34°C) [10], newborns expend the least amount of energy to

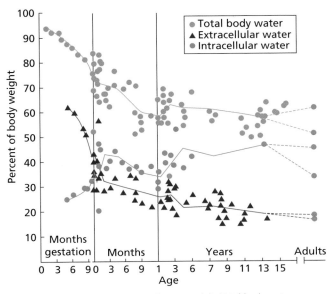

Figure 10.1 Body compartments: fetus to adult. Total body water, extracellular water, intracellular water as a percentage of bodyweight. Reproduced from Friis-Hansen [5] with permission from the American Academy of Pediatrics.

maintain a normal body temperature, which improves growth [11]. For decades, eliminating "cold stress" has been correlated with improved survival of premature infants [12,13]. Overhead radiant warmers provide stable environmental temperatures and allow easy access to critically ill infants, but they also increase transcutaneous insensible water loss, at least during the first 2–4 days of life [14]. Despite having higher fluid requirements than infants cared for in incubators, infants cared for under overhead warmers have similar long-term weight gain, length of hospital stay, and incidence of adverse outcomes (e.g. chronic lung disease, necrotizing enterocolitis, intraventricular hemorrhage). Phototherapy for treatment of hyperbilirubinemia of the newborn also increases transcutaneous water loss. Recently, investigators suggested that providing a humidified environment improves fluid and electrolyte balance and growth, especially in ELBW infants [15].

Surgery performed in either the intensive care nursery (ICN) or the operating room often necessitates moving the patient from a protected and/or humidified environment to an open bed. Overhead warming and enclosed humidifying devices cannot be used during surgery because they limit access to the patient. These warmers also cannot be used during transport of infants to an operating room for lack of electricity. To minimize heat and fluid loss during transport and surgery, newborns should be covered with plastic shields, polyethylene blankets or semi-occlusive skin barriers (e.g. Seran Wrap™), and a hat. In addition, portable warmers placed under the infant help maintain body temperature during transport, and a variety of electrical warming devices are utilized intraoperatively.

Developmental physiology
Various aspects of age-related characteristics of renal, cardiac, hepatic, hematological, and neurological function directly affect fluid and electrolyte balance in the newborn. Each will be discussed briefly.

Renal physiology: glomerular filtration rate, tubular function (see Chapter 8)
Maintenance of normal extracellular fluid volume, electrolyte concentrations, and water balance is inter-related and undergoes significant postnatal changes that are highly dependent on renal function. By 35–36 weeks' gestation, neonates have approximately the adult number of nephrons. Thereafter, both the glomeruli and tubules increase in size. The renal vasculature matures in parallel with the nephrons. In general, fetal and neonatal renal function is characterized by low renal blood flow (high vascular resistance), low glomerular filtration rate (GFR), low excretion of solids, and limited ability to concentrate the urine.

Filtration of solutes and electrolytes across the renal capillaries is the first step in urine formation. Glomerular filtration is present as early as the 10th week of gestation and increases steadily throughout fetal life (10–13 mL/min/$1.73\,m^2$ at 25–28 weeks' gestation and 20–25 mL/min/$1.73\,m^2$ after 34 weeks' gestation [16]) and after birth. It reaches adult levels at 1–2 years of life (~125 mL/min/$1.73\,m^2$, although values vary between men and women). Urine production also increases steadily throughout gestation (2–5 mL/h at 20 weeks' gestation, 10–12 mL/h at 35 weeks' gestation, and 35–50 mL/h at 40 weeks' gestation) [17].

In spite of differences in normal vascular resistance, arterial blood pressure, blood flow, and the responses to a variety of physiological stimuli (e.g. blood loss, sepsis, hypoxia) at various stages of development, GFR always depends on the difference between hydrostatic and oncotic pressures across the renal capillaries (see General considerations, above). At any filtration pressure, GFR is a function of plasma flow and of surface area and permeability of the capillaries. As the number and size of nephrons increase during fetal life, GFR steadily increases until ~35 weeks' gestation. After birth, GFR increases dramatically, approximately doubling in the first 2 weeks of life and tripling 3 months after full-term gestation. GFR increases at a slower rate in preterm infants, especially in the ELBW infant [18]. The change in GFR reflects increasing capillary surface area and filtration pressure (arterial blood pressure) and decreasing afferent and efferent vascular resistance.

Serum creatinine is commonly used as a surrogate marker for GFR. However, at birth the infant's creatinine concentration reflects that of the mother and is higher than stable, normal values of 1–2-week-old normal term neonates (0.4 mg/dL). In fact, plasma creatinine is higher in preterm than in term infants during the first 4 weeks of life [19]. Serum creatinine concentrations did not differ at birth among 27–32-week gestation neonates and increased in all groups over the first 3 days of life, after which it gradually decreased to <0.5 mg/dL [20]. Creatinine clearance increases in all groups but increases more slowly in <27-week gestation infants.

In addition to dramatic increases in GFR and renal blood flow during fetal and postnatal life, unique and critical developmental changes occur in the renal tubules. The plasma ultrafiltrate formed from glomerular filtration is presented to the proximal tubules, which play a major role in regulating the serum concentrations of a wide variety of molecules (e.g. sodium, chloride, potassium, phosphate, acid, glucose, amino acids) and water excretion. Depending on the nutrition and metabolic state of the patient, this tightly controlled activity results in salvage or excretion of the solutes. Neonates, especially prematures, neither excrete nor reabsorb sodium as well as more mature infants. For example, 5% of the filtered sodium load is excreted by a <30-week gestation infant, but only 0.2% of filtered sodium appears in the urine of term infants [21]. Premature newborns maximally concentrate their urine to 245–450 mOsm/L, while term infants can achieve 600–800 mOsm/L; adults concentrate their urine to 1200–1400 mOsm/L. Response to 1-desamino-8-D-arginine vasopressin (DDAVP) follows a similar pattern: 30–35-week gestation infants achieve an osmolality of 520 mOsm/L, a 1-month-old term infant, 570 mOsm/L, and a 1–2-year-old child, 1300–1400 mOsm/L. After 35 weeks' gestation, infants can dilute their urine to adult levels (50 mOsm/L); <35-week gestation newborns can only dilute their urine to 70 mOsm/L [16].

Tubular immaturity accounts for other acid–base and electrolyte features of the newborn. The Na^+-K^+-ATPase pump exists in all mammalian cells and is critical for maintaining the normal intracellular/extracellular distribution of sodium and potassium. Located on the basolateral membrane, activity of this enzyme accounts for approximately 70% of renal oxygen consumption. The enzyme exchanges three sodium ions for two potassium ions by an active transport process (utilizes ATP). Moving sodium extracellularly maintains the inwardly directed sodium gradient, which is the driving force for several secondarily active membrane transport proteins. These transporters mediate reabsorption of glucose, amino acids, and other nutrients across the brush border membranes of the renal proximal tubules. Thus, sodium-dependent transporters salvage amino acids, glucose, phosphate, and other molecules from the glomerular filtrate that enters the proximal tubules. Sodium is co-transported down its concentration gradient, which provides the energy to move the substrate from the filtrate into the cell against a concentration gradient. At birth, the activity of the Na^+-K^+-ATPase transporter increases 5–10-fold [22]; the increase is often blunted in preterm infants. Similar developmental changes in other transporters (e.g. Na^+/H^+ antiporter [23]) may account in part for differences in acid–base balance in newborns and older infants, children, and adults.

Due to immaturity of the renal tubules, reabsorption of glucose is impaired, and glucosuria occurs in preterm infants at serum glucose concentrations as low as 100 mg/dL. Similarly, bicarbonate loss due to incomplete tubular reabsorption leads to decreased serum bicarbonate concentrations (12–16 mEq/L, <26–28 weeks' gestation; 18–20 mEq/L, 30–35 weeks' gestation; 20–22 mEq/L, term infant; 25–28 mEq/L, adult) [24]. As usual, mild hyperkalemia co-exists with metabolic acidosis (i.e. intracellular potassium moves extracellularly in exchange for protons that move intracellularly).

The newborn's renal function changes with both gestational and postnatal age. Due to rapid maturation after birth, the 3-week old, ex-27 week gestation infant usually demonstrates more mature renal function than a 1-day-old term infant. It appears that exposure to solute improves filtration and tubular function.

Arginine vasopressin

Arginine vasopressin (AVP) modulates maintenance of normal osmolality by increasing free water reabsorption by insertion of water channels (vasopressin-sensitive water channel (aquaporin 2)) into the distal tubule and collecting ducts [25,26]. In addition, AVP induces peripheral vasoconstriction that is often associated with a rise in arterial blood pressure. The concentration of AVP is elevated in the newborn, and this has been correlated with the neonate's low urine output during the first 24–48 h of life. Hypoxia, lung injury (bronchopulmonary dysplasia), and central nervous system injury (intraventricular hemorrhage) increase AVP secretion in both term and preterm infants [27] which, through its effects on free water reabsorption, can cause hyponatremia. In some cases, the etiology of hyponatremia is due to abnormal release of and response to AVP (ADH). This leads to the syndrome of inappropriate secretion of antidiuretic hormone (SIADH), the diagnosis of which should be reserved for cases where circulating AVP concentrations are elevated despite the absence of both osmotic and baroreceptor-mediated stimuli [26].

Because of their limited ability to concentrate urine, newborns are also at increased risk for hyponatremia from the non-osmotic secretion of AVP (e.g. pain, nausea and vomiting, positive pressure ventilation) (see sections on Physiology of hyponatremia, Clinically relevant concepts, and Intravenous fluids and hyponatremia: current controversy). Renally produced prostaglandins (PG) counterbalance the effects of AVP. Specifically, PGE2, PGD2, and PGI2 increase renal blood flow, free water clearance, urine flow, and natriuresis [28].

Renin-angiotensin-aldosterone system

The juxtaglomerular apparatus (which consists of smooth muscle cells in the wall of the afferent arteriole) responds to various inputs (e.g. decreased sodium or chloride in the distal nephron (macula densa), decreased renal blood flow, sympathetic nervous system input) by secreting renin. Renin stimulates production of angiotensin I from angiotensinogen, and angiotensin-converting enzyme mediates formation of angiotensin II from angiotensin I. The direct effects of angiotensin II include vasoconstriction, release of catecholamines from the adrenal glands, sodium and water reabsorption, and the release of aldosterone [29]. Aldosterone induces potassium secretion and sodium reabsorption in the distal tubule. Thus, AVP's role is primarily to preserve normal osmolality whereas that of the RAS system is to maintain extracellular fluid volume. However, the newborn kidney has decreased capacity to respond to either and this accounts, in part, for the high levels of these hormones over the first few weeks of postnatal life [30].

Renin is present as early as 5 weeks' gestation. While plasma renin concentration and activity are high *in utero*, they increase further postnatally and then slowly decrease during infancy. Similarly, the concentrations of aldosterone and angiotensin II are high in both fetuses and neonates, and plasma renin activity and aldosterone are markedly elevated in the early postnatal period in preterm infants. The increased activity of the RAS in both newborns and infants, along with the low GFR, are responsible for much of the physiology of sodium balance in the preterm, neonatal, and infant kidney. Similar to the responses to AVP, prostaglandins partly counterbalance the vasoconstricting effects of aldosterone, angiotensin, and renin. Of note, the renal dysfunction that sometimes follows the administration of indometacin (a prostaglandin inhibitor) to close a patent ductus arteriosus has been attributed to the unopposed vasoconstrictive effects of angiotensin and AVP and the absence of the vasodilatory effects of prostaglandin [28].

In addition to their vasoactive roles, angiotensin II and angiotensin-converting enzyme also mediate renal growth and development. Inhibition of angiotensin has teratogenic effects, as occurs when angiotensin-converting enzyme inhibitors are given to mothers during the second and third trimesters of pregnancy. The effects of these drugs include fetal hypotension, renal tubular dysplasia, anuria/oligohydramnios, growth restriction, hypocalvaria, and death [31].

Atrial natriuretic peptide

This hormone counterbalances the effects of the RAS through its direct vasodilatory and naturiuretic effects and by inhibiting the release of renin and aldosterone [32]. The concentration of atrial natriuretic peptide (ANP) in newborn humans has been correlated with atrial size, status of the ductus arteriosus, and extracellular volume [33].

Thus, interactions of the renal and cardiovascular systems regulate the child's fluid and electrolyte status. Clearly, the highly variable blood pressures and intravascular volumes of critically ill newborns may elicit dramatic and even pathological responses via AVP, aldosterone, and the RAS.

Cardiovascular physiology: cardiac output, heart rate, calcium flux

At birth, elimination of the placental circulation and initiation of ventilation decreases pulmonary vascular resistance and increases pulmonary blood flow. At the same time, systemic vascular resistance increases. Left atrial pressure rises, which functionally closes the foramen ovale. These events, and the closure of the ductus arteriosus and ductus venosus, are the most critical aspects of the cardiovascular transition from intra- to extrauterine life.

Cardiac output per kilogram bodyweight is higher in newborns than at any other age. Nonetheless, at any developmental stage, ventricular function is determined by the same factors: preload, afterload, contractility, and heart rate. However, the ability to compensate for abnormalities is narrow in the newborn, especially in the ELBW infant. That is, in preterm infants (some of whom are born at midgestation), the immature myocardium and the peripheral circulation are at significant disadvantage when the low-resistance placenta is abruptly replaced with the higher resistance pulmonary and systemic vascular beds and interventions such as positive pressure ventilation and inotropic support are introduced at birth. While volume loading the immature ventricle increases cardiac output, it does so to a far lesser extent than at older ages [34]. Finally, since the resting heart rate of the newborn is high, increasing the heart rate above normal has less effect on cardiac output. Decreasing heart rate drastically reduces cardiac output.

Differences in myocardial ultrastructure (e.g. receptors, channels, transporters, pumps, contractile proteins) and the immaturity of various intracellular structures (e.g. myofibrils, sarcoplasmic reticulum, microtubules) influence clinical management of fluids and electrolytes, especially in the often unstable perioperative period. For example, the volume of the sarcoplasmic reticulum and its ability to pump calcium increases *in utero* and postnatally. In addition, the various subtypes of sarcoplasmic reticulum are less differentiated functionally in the immature heart [35]. Probably because of these differences, immature hearts are more sensitive to calcium channel antagonists [36], and maximal contractility is more dependent on extracellular calcium [37] than in adults.

The relationship between arterial blood pressure (BP), cardiac output (CO), and systemic vascular resistance (SVR) remains the same throughout life: $BP = CO \times SVR$. That is, pressure and flow are not equal but are related via resistance. Thus, flow to an organ may increase, decrease or remain constant over a wide range of blood pressure, depending on changes in vascular resistance. Because of the unique physiology of the ELBW infant, measuring cardiac output and defining "normal" for parameters such as arterial blood pressure and heart rate are difficult. Marked variability in the quantity of blood flowing across the foramen ovale and ductus arteriosus adds to the complexity of monitoring the cardiovascular function of the premature infant. For example, defining hypotension is not simple [38,39]. Although the normal

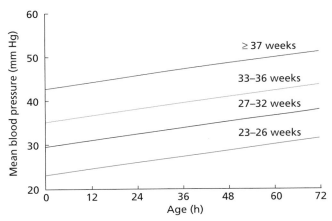

Figure 10.2 Predicted lower limit of mean blood pressure in newborns (initial 72 h of life). Reproduced from Engle [126] with permission from Elsevier.

ranges for blood pressure correlate with gestational age [40,41], the definition of hypotension remains elusive. One study noted that mean blood pressures that were below the gestational age in weeks were correlated with the 10th percentile for arterial blood pressure [42]. They recommended this criterion as a definition of hypotension (Fig. 10.2).

Nonetheless, the variability in "normal" arterial blood pressures and heart rates among infants of the same gestational and/or postnatal ages creates a dilemma in the clinical care setting, especially during the commonly unstable perioperative period. Recognizing that neither arterial blood pressure [43,44] nor capillary refill time [45] reliably correlates with left ventricular output in preterm infants, flow in the superior vena cava has been suggested to estimate systemic blood flow to the brain (and upper body). This eliminates the need for considering the influence of shunting through the ductus arteriosus or the foramen ovale on the accuracy of the measurement [46]. Of interest, neither dopamine nor dobutamine increased contractility when the drug was given to treat low superior vena cava blood flow [47]. Unfortunately, "functional echocardiography" requires sophisticated equipment and experience so that its use as a routine bedside monitor remains impractical.

Thus, until bedside monitoring allows direct measurement of flow, assessing acid–base status and intravascular volume of infants to define appropriate fluid administration requires integrating readily available cardiovascular parameters (e.g. arterial blood pressure, heart rate) with renal, hepatic, central nervous system, and respiratory function. For example, electrolyte concentrations, pH, pCO_2, and urine output must be interpreted in the context of an infant's overall clinical condition (e.g. sepsis, bleeding, neurological status) as well as specific trends in arterial blood pressure, heart rate, and peripheral perfusion

over multiple hours. Changes over time provide more useful information than isolated measurements.

Central nervous system physiology: autoregulation of cerebral blood flow

Although cerebral vascular autoregulation is present in both preterm and term neonates after birth, the range of arterial blood pressures over which flow is regulated is narrower for preterm infants and seems to be easily disrupted [48,49]. In addition, the blood pressure of preterm infants is normally close to the lower autoregulatory limit, especially in the ELBW infant [49–52]. The upper range of autoregulation has not been clearly established in the newborn [49]. Of importance, autoregulation seems to be disturbed or disrupted by hypoxia, acidosis, seizures, and by the low diastolic blood pressures of patients with a patent ductus arteriosus [50,51]. Rapid increases in arterial blood pressure (e.g. from overly aggressive fluid administration) can rupture the fragile immature brain vessels, while hypotension and low cerebral perfusion pressures may produce cerebral ischemia. More than at any other developmental stage, the intravascular volume status of the neonate, especially preterm neonates, may have rapid and significant effects on the brain.

Hepatic physiology: glucose and coagulation

To discuss hepatic function from the perspective of neonatal fluids and electrolytes, two topics are most relevant: glucose homeostasis and coagulation of blood.

Glucose homeostasis

The transplacental supply of glucose to the fetus is abruptly interrupted at birth, which requires neonates to convert their liver glycogen stores to glucose by glycogenolysis or to produce glucose by gluconeogenesis. Compared to adults, the liver of term infants is larger and has a greater store of glycogen [53]. Thus, after the first day of life, most term infants can maintain a normal serum glucose concentration during a 10–12-h fast. Since glycogen storage and the capacity for its degradation mostly occur during the last trimester of pregnancy, infants born in the second or early third trimester often develop hypoglycemia, especially in the first 24–48 h of life. The fetal liver apparently does not produce glucose by gluconeogenesis [54], but a variety of hepatic enzymes required for this process (e.g. glucose-6-phosphatase) develop rapidly after birth.

Glucose concentrations in the fetus remain constant (~50–55 mg/dL) during the third trimester of pregnancy if maternal carbohydrate metabolism is normal. In experimental animals, glucose utilization at midgestation is ~9.5 mg/kg/min and decreases to ~5 mg/kg/min at term [55]. These data provide estimates of normal serum glucose requirements for premature infants of similar gestation. Of note, the rates of glucose production

Table 10.2 Normal values of coagulation function in newborns compared with adults

	Prothrombin time (sec) (range)	Partial thromboplastin time (sec) (range)	Thrombin time (sec) (range)
Adults	13.0 (11.2–14.5)	44.0 (36.8–50.0)	10 (9.0–11.1)
Term infants	13.6 (12.8–14.4)	65.2 (50.0–84.0)	12.5 (10.0–15.0)
ELBW infants	15.4 (14.6–16.9)	108 (80.0–168)	14.9 (11.0–17.8)

ELBW, extremely low birthweight.
From Barnard DR, Simmons MA, Hathaway WE. Coagulation studies in extremely premature infants. Pediat Res 1979; 13: 1330–5.

(7–10 mg/kg/min) by stable preterm infants who are receiving intravenous alimentation [56] are similar to those of fetal animals. The brain consumes ~4–5 mg/kg/min, protein synthesis ~2–3 mg/kg/min, and other organs (e.g. liver, heart, muscle) utilize the remaining glucose. A surge in the concentration of catecholamines, glucagon, and cortisol (e.g. during birth or stress) increases glycogenolysis and gluconeogenesis, often resulting in hyperglycemia. In high-risk newborns (e.g. large or small for gestational age, premature infants, asphyxiated infants), glucose concentrations must be monitored and infusion rates adjusted to maintain normoglycemia.

Initially, glucose should be infused at rates of ~5–6 mg/kg/min in NPO newborns (e.g. 10% dextrose, 4 mL/kg/h = 6.6 mg/kg/min of glucose) and the rates adjusted to maintain serum glucose concentrations of 60–90 mg/dL. For infants who are stable on a well-established regimen, the glucose infusion rates in the operating room should mimic those used in the ICN and should be altered if hypo- or hypergylcemia develops. In many cases, especially in small infants, obtaining a blood sample may be difficult without an arterial or central venous catheter in place. Currently available devices allow glucose measurements on a single drop of blood, which can be obtained from a finger, toe or ear lobe.

Monitoring glucose intraoperatively is particularly relevant in critically ill newborns, because their symptoms of hypoglycemia are sometimes absent and often vague. The non-specific symptoms of hypoglycemia include irritability, jitteriness, and apnea in this age group, which are masked by general anesthesia. Hypoglycemia can have devastating effects on the central nervous system through effects on cerebral blood flow. Magnetic resonance imaging (MRI) of the brain of hypoglycemic newborns demonstrates white matter abnormalities, and clinical evaluation at 18 months of age revealed persistent central nervous system injury [57]. Older pediatric patients with abnormal glucose metabolism also have increased morbidity and mortality [58].

Coagulation

Coagulation factors do not efficiently cross the placenta. Although these factors are produced by the fetus, their plasma concentrations and the laboratory tests used to monitor their function (prothrombin time (PT), activated partial thromboplastin time (APTT)) differ markedly in both normal term and preterm infants and adults (Table 10.2). Concentrations of vitamin K-dependent proteins (factors II, VII, IX, X), factors XI and XII, prekallikrein, and kininogen are about 50% those of adults. On the other hand, the levels of fibrinogen, factors V and VIII are similar to those of adults [59,60]. Coagulation disturbances associated with liver dysfunction are linked to decreased synthesis of clotting and fibrinolytic factors and with abnormal platelet function. PT correlates with availability of factor VII. APTT primarily reflects the amount of thrombin generated. The concentration of thrombin in newborns is about 50% that of adults.

In spite of the differences in liver function between newborns and adults, clinically significant bleeding is uncommon in normal neonates with adequate vitamin K levels. On the other hand, sepsis and/or asphyxia-induced disseminated intravascular coagulation (DIC) increase the risk for bleeding. Both asphyxia and sepsis deplete coagulation factors (e.g. fibrinogen, factors V and VIII, and platelets) and produce fibrin degradation products. To compensate for abnormal levels of coagulation factors, especially if accompanied by cardiovascular instability and ongoing blood loss, administering specific blood components not only improves clotting function but may also replete intravascular volume.

Hematological physiology

In otherwise normal appropriate for gestational age (AGA) fetuses, hemoglobin concentration varies with gestational age (14 g/dL at 25 weeks' gestation, 16 g/dL at 30 weeks, 17 g/dL at 35 weeks, 18 g/dL at term) [61] but not with gender. The higher concentration of hemoglobin of small for gestational age (SGA) infants at birth may compensate for intrauterine hypoxia and may represent a response to elevated concentrations of erythropoietin [62]. In contrast, compared to both SGA and AGA infants, preterm infants have lower concentrations of hemoglobin at birth. In addition, the normal postnatal decrease in hemoglobin occurs more rapidly in premature infants [63].

Indications for transfusion of red blood cells or other blood components pre-, intra- or postoperatively must be defined in the context of the patient's cardiorespiratory status, ongoing blood and fluid losses, and response to delivery of crystalloid and colloid.

Neonatal perioperative fluids: general concepts

For the first 2–3 h of life, the neonate's electrolyte concentrations reflect those of the mother and of perinatal events (e.g. asphyxia, placental or umbilical cord hemorrhage). Afterwards, the electrolyte concentrations reflect a balance between normal metabolism, cardiovascular, renal and hepatic function, and ongoing metabolic derangements (e.g. sepsis, congenital metabolic diseases, complex cyanotic congenital heart disease, etc.). Until adequate tissue perfusion is established and wash-out of accumulated acid and other metabolic byproducts of anaerobic metabolism occurs, metabolic acidosis may persist in depressed newborns, especially those who were severely asphyxiated and required resuscitation.

Sodium is seldom added to intravenous maintenance fluids of term and late preterm infants during the first 24 h of life. During this time, urine output is usually low (see section on Renal physiology, above), despite the fact that 30 mL/kg of fluid must be mobilized from the lungs during and after birth [64]. On day 2 of life, sodium (2–6 meq/kg/day) is added to the intravenous fluids. In the ELBW infant, sodium-containing fluid is often required as early as 12–24 h of life to maintain adequate intravascular volume, especially when there is evidence for excessive transcutaneous fluid losses (see section on Insensible water loss, above). After the first few days of life, adequate sodium intake is essential for infants of all gestational ages to sustain normal growth and weight gain. Poor skeletal and tissue growth, as well as adverse neurodevelopment, are associated with chronic sodium deficiency [26].

Ensuring normal fluid and electrolyte balance in the newborn in the presence of the high metabolic rate associated with growth, marked insensible water losses, and the limited ability to salvage and excrete water and solutes requires accurate monitoring of fluid loss (i.e. urine, gastrointestinal, cerebrospinal fluid, blood sampling) and electrolyte concentrations to guide the quantity and quality of replacement fluid. Frequent measurements of bodyweight will document excessive gain or loss and these data should be correlated with simultaneous trends in serum electrolyte concentrations (e.g. decrease or increase in sodium). Especially in the premature infant, surgery and anesthesia have dramatic effects on distribution of water and electrolytes and on organ function (e.g. cardiovascular, hepatic, renal).

Based on the complex interactions between illness and immaturity, the anesthesiologist must consider the following when determining appropriate fluid and electrolyte management in the newborn (see Table 10.3).

- The normal postnatal diuresis contracts the extracellular space in all newborns, and to a greater degree in preterm infants. During the first few days after birth, negative fluid and electrolyte balance occurs normally in healthy term infants, but prematurity and/or hemodynamic instability may require aggressive intravascular fluid administration.
- Transepidermal fluid loss is inversely related to gestational age and can be as much as 60–100 mL/kg/day in ELBW infants. During the first few postnatal days, naked preterm infants lose 15 times more water by evaporation than naked term infants [65].
- Providing a warm, humidified environment and/or the use of plastic shields reduces transepidermal fluid loss, especially in the ELBW infant. Shielding devices are difficult or impossible to use during surgery but should be used during transport of the patient to and from the operating room and in the operating room before and after surgery.
- The hypothesis that overhydration or hyper- or hyponatremia increases the incidence of patent ductus arteriosus, necrotizing enterocolitis, and chronic lung disease should be considered, but data documenting a strong correlation with these variables are inconsistent.
- An intravenous infusion of calcium is usually required in preterm, asphyxiated or large for gestational age (LGA) or small for gestational age (SGA) infants until they establish adequate enteral nutrition. Ideally, calcium is infused into a central venous catheter. Infiltration of calcium into subcutaneous tissue usually causes extensive tissue necrosis.

Preoperative evaluation of the neonate

The focus of any preoperative assessment includes identifying aspects of the patient's history and physical examination that are relevant to the surgery/procedure and anesthetic management. For example, in the case of newborns, this includes consulting with the staff in the intensive care nursery to identify the normal variability in the heart rate and blood pressure and the cardiovascular responses to interventions such as change in positioning, fluid administration or positive pressure ventilation. Details of labor and delivery are critical to analyze in the first 2–3 days of life, but they become less relevant as the baby gets older and recovers from her/his adaptation to the effects of *in utero* events. For example, the effects of a placental hemorrhage or severe asphyxia may have a dramatic impact on fluid management during the first day of life but will have less impact at 2 weeks of age. The 2

Table 10.3 Intraoperative fluids: newborn

Thirty-week gestation infant, 5 days old, 1.2 kg at birth, now 1.0 kg, with bowel perforation associated with necrotizing enterocolitis, is scheduled for open laparotomy. Her abdomen is distended, nasogastric tube in place. She requires ventilatory support (18/4, rate of 50, FIO₂ = 0.40). Urine output has decreased from 2 mL/kg/h to 0.5 mL/kg/h. Two peripheral IVs and an umbilical artery catheter are in place. BP 50/24, heart rate 160 bpm, stable after multiple boluses of normal saline, platelets, fresh frozen plasma, fibrinogen. Dopamine infusing, 8 μg/kg/min. D10 with protein and electrolytes infusing at 5 mL/h.

- Arterial blood gas: pH 7.35; pO_2 62; pCO_2 37.
- Electrolytes: Na^+ 135; K^+ 4.6; Cl^- 106; HCO_3^- 18; Ca^{++} 1.0; glucose 100 mg/dL.
- Renal function: BUN 32/creatinine 0.9.
- Hemoglobin 15; platelets 75,000; PT 18 sec; PTT 85 sec; fibrinogen 90.

Deficit	Maintenance	Ongoing losses
0 mL	• 5 mL/h D10 infusing	• Blood products available in operating room: RBCs, fresh frozen plasma; platelets available • Infuse crystalloid, 10–50 mL/kg/h or more; boluses to maintain hemodynamic instability • RBCs for blood loss (1 mL for each 2–3 mL of blood loss). Fresh frozen plasma infusion/boluses in response to bleeding/laboratory values • Monitor Hg, PT/PTT, platelets

The same patient, now 2 months old, now dependent on total parenteral nutrition (TPN) secondary to "short gut" after surgery for necrotizing enterocolitis scheduled for hernia repair. No ventilatory support, no meds. No enteral intake; D15 with protein and electrolytes infusing at 25 mL/h; weight 4.2 kg; hemoglobin 10 g/dL; glucose 90 mg/dL; open herniorrhaphy.

Deficit	Maintenance	Ongoing losses
0 mL	• According to "formula", 17 mL/h • Tolerating 25 mL/h in ICN; continue 25 mL/h intraoperatively	• Insignificant • Bolus of crystalloid only in response to hemodynamic instability • Transfusion unnecessary unless unexpected blood loss; postoperative apnea may prompt transfusion

BUN, blood urea nitrogen; ICN, intensive care nursery; PT, prothrombin time; PTT, partial thromboplastin time; RBC, red blood cell.

week old may have residual but stable renal failure and neurological and hepatic insults, but it is likely he or she will have recovered from asphyxia-induced cardiac depression. Understanding how fluids and electrolytes were managed before surgery will help avoid dangerous and unnecessary alterations in therapy (e.g. rate of glucose delivery). Of course, intraoperative events, such as general anesthesia, blood loss, and increased insensible losses (e.g. open abdomen with exposed intestine), often require changes in the volume and type of fluid delivered. Developing an effective relationship with the intensive care nursery staff facilitates intraoperative consultation with the primary medical team, if necessary.

The following summarizes the most significant aspects of preoperative evaluation of the newborn.

1. Review of labor and delivery; documentation of appropriate fetal growth (AGA, LGA or SGA).
2. Review of systems.
   - Trend in weight (daily or more frequent)
   - Trend in intravenous and oral intake and urine output and specific gravity
   - Trend in other output (gastrointestinal, cerebrospinal fluid, etc.)
   - Composition of intravenous fluid (glucose, sodium, calcium) correlated with corresponding trends in plasma concentrations of these electrolytes
   - Hemodynamic instability: trends in heart rate, arterial blood pressure, peripheral perfusion; presence and effect of patent ductus arteriosus or other cardiovascular dysfunction (e.g. tricuspid regurgitation after asphyxia)
   - Current hemoglobin concentration and recent trend correlated with hemodynamic function; determine if this patient "requires" a minimum level of hemoglobin (e.g. increased heart rate or acidosis if the hemoglobin is <10 g)
   - Central nervous system insult (presence of intraventricular hemorrhage)

- Current coagulation status, history of bleeding, and trends and requirements for blood components; availability of blood products.
3. Adequacy of intravenous access and monitors (functioning arterial, venous or central venous catheters).
4. Estimate "allowable blood loss" as part of the preoperative evaluation. For example, blood volume in a 3-day-old, 1 kg infant is 100 mL/kg, or 100 mL. A loss of 20 mL of blood is 20% of the blood volume. Anticipating the need for transfusion depends on the current hemoglobin concentration and history of tolerance for decreasing blood volume and/or hemoglobin.

Intraoperative fluid management

During transport from the ICN to the operating room, intravenous infusions, ventilatory support, body temperature, and monitoring of hemodynamic status/oxygenation must be maintained. At a minimum, heart rate and oxygen saturation should be continuously monitored, and more invasive hemodynamic monitoring (e.g. arterial blood pressure) may be required depending on the clinical condition of the patient. The infant's head and body should be covered with semi-occlusive material and/or blankets to reduce evaporation and heat loss. Portable warming devices are often placed under the infant. Intravenous infusions that will be used in the operating room should be available and functioning before leaving the ICN. For example, the extensions on the intravenous and intra-arterial tubing should be long enough to allow their easy access with the surgical drapes in place.

Initially in the operating room, glucose infusion should continue at the same rate used in the intensive care nursery to maintain normoglycemia. Often, simply continuing the infusion of "maintenance" fluid or total parenteral nutrition is appropriate. In surgical procedures lasting longer than 1 h, monitoring glucose concentrations is needed to ensure normoglycemia. In most cases, additional non-glucose containing fluid must be delivered to compensate for intraoperative events and losses of blood and fluid. To avoid hyperglycemia and its side-effects (e.g. osmotic diuresis, central nervous system injury), glucose-containing solutions should never be used to replace volume losses. A variety of techniques allows the anesthesiologist to separate delivery of glucose (e.g. maintenance fluid) from intravenous crystalloid and/or colloid needed to replace intraoperative losses (e.g. multiple peripheral intravenous catheters or several access ports inserted into one peripheral or central line).

As always, anesthesia agents should be titrated to maintain appropriate hemodynamic status during induction of anesthesia. Newborns, especially premature newborns, vary enormously in their responses to anesthetic agents and are prone to hypotension. For example, an older infant or child may tolerate high concentrations of sevoflurane briefly for induction of anesthesia, but the same concentration of drug in a newborn often results in marked hemodynamic instability. Rapid delivery of intravenous agents to neonates may also cause significant cardiovascular instability. Often, dramatic hemodynamic responses to anesthetics (e.g. hypotension, tachycardia) require prompt rapid delivery of a bolus of normal saline or lactated Ringer's solution (5–10 mL/kg or more).

As surgery proceeds, blood loss and coagulation abnormalities often require the administration of various blood components to maintain intravascular volume and hemodynamic stability, and to restore the levels of coagulation factors to normal. Ideally, monitoring of the levels of coagulation factors (e.g. fibrinogen, platelets, prothrombin time, partial thromboplastin time), acid–base status (e.g. pH, pCO_2), hemoglobin, and/or electrolytes will guide intravenous therapy. Monitoring blood loss requires meticulous observation of the surgical field, since small volumes of blood loss are difficult to track and are easily hidden in drapes and body cavities. Since the blood volume of a 1 kg infant is only 100 mL, a 10–20 mL blood loss can induce significant hemodynamic instability. Theoretically, urine output should be monitored but in the smallest of infants, measuring small urine volumes accurately often proves difficult or impossible. That is, placing a tube into the bladder and attaching the tube to a drainage system often requires the infant to produce more than 5 mL of urine before the anesthesiologist can see any urine. In addition, the small catheter and drainage system are often soft and are easily compressed, kinked or occluded during positioning of the patient.

Inspired gases should be warmed and humidified to near body temperature. Overhead, servo-controlled warmers should be used during preoperative preparation (e.g. adjusting intravenous lines and ventilatory devices, preparation of the surgical site). The surgical bed should include a warming device (varies among institutions), and the room temperature should be adjusted to minimize the occurrence of hypothermia. Once the child is draped for surgery, the room temperature can be adjusted, depending on the response of the infant's body temperature to the surgery and to decreases in the environmental temperature. Intravenous fluids and blood products should be warmed, especially if large volumes of either are required.

The following summarizes the most significant aspects of intraoperative fluid management in the newborn (see case study, Table 10.3).
1. Ensure that the intravascular volume is adequate before induction of anesthesia.

2. Determine the intraoperative need for blood products before the start of anesthesia/surgery. This process should begin in the intensive care nursery.

3. In spite of normovolemia, the newborn may respond to judicious doses of either inhaled or intravenous anesthetic agents with dramatic changes in heart rate, arterial blood pressure, and peripheral perfusion. Fluid and/or colloid boluses or infusions may be required to maintain hemodynamic stability.

4. Glucose infusion should continue at the same rate used in the intensive care nursery to maintain normoglycemia. This can be considered the "maintenance" component of fluid administration. The infusion should be adjusted, based on intraoperative measurements of glucose.

5. In most cases, delivering crystalloid compensates adequately for insensible losses, but the required rate of delivery depends on the type of surgery. For example, during a laparotomy to treat necrotizing enterocolitis, 10–50 mL/kg/h (or more) of non-glucose containing crystalloid may be required to compensate for insensible losses from inflamed, exposed bowel and peritoneum. During less invasive procedures (e.g. inguinal hernia repair), less crystalloid is required (0–5 mL/kg/h). At some point after delivering large volumes of crystalloid (30–40 mL/kg/h) for several hours (sometimes longer, sometimes shorter, depending on cardiovascular and clotting status), colloid may be a more appropriate intravenous therapy (see points 6 and 7).

6. Most critically ill newborns, especially those who are premature, seem to be more hemodynamically stable (e.g. less apnea and bradycardia) when their hematocrit is >40%. In those cases, frequent packed red blood cell transfusions (and/or erythropoietin) are required in the ICN. Infants who have been in the ICN for days to weeks and who are stable and undergoing elective surgery (e.g. inguinal hernia repair) often tolerate lower concentrations of hemoglobin. For example, an ex-26 week gestation infant undergoing an inguinal hernia repair at 10 weeks of age may have no cardiorespiratory problems (i.e. no apnea/bradycardia, tachycardia or hypotension) associated with a hematocrit of 30%. In contrast, a 5 day old who has a patent ductus arteriosus and necrotizing enterocolitis, and requires mechanical ventilatory support usually has improved perfusion and metabolic status with a hematocrit >40%. The hematocrit required by infants in the ICN provides the initial guideline for the appropriate perioperative level.

7. Many newborns, especially critically ill newborns, respond more promptly to colloid delivery than to crystalloid after losing 10–20% of their blood volume. Colloid may include packed red blood cells, fresh frozen plasma or fibrinogen, depending on the coagulation status and hemoglobin concentration.

8. Monitoring urine output, arterial blood pressure and/or central venous pressure guides intravenous fluid therapy.

9. Heat and insensible fluid loss should be minimized during transport of the infant to and from the operating room.

The older infant and child

Introduction
Unlike the newborn, older infants and children often present for elective surgery with a clearly defined medical and/or surgical history. That is, congenital anomalies and metabolic/genetic abnormalities have been identified and a specific, stable treatment plan has been established. Outside of trauma, accidents or development of an acute new illness (e.g. malignancy, gastrointestinal event, systemic or localized infection, etc.), emergent or urgent surgery is usually required to treat complications of a recognized anomaly or because diagnostic evaluations are needed to assess an underlying illness.

As in all age groups, preoperative evaluation of the fluid and electrolyte status of older infants and children requires assessing intravascular volume, reviewing cardiorespiratory/renal/hepatic/central nervous system status, and noting relevant laboratory studies. Fine-tuning fluid and electrolyte abnormalities must be balanced against the urgency of the surgery. When devising a rational plan for intraoperative fluid management, one must determine maintenance fluid requirements, replacement for ongoing losses, and the need to correct specific abnormalities (e.g. glucose, potassium, calcium, coagulation). In some cases, plans must be made for monitoring laboratory values (e.g. ensuring easy access to central venous, arterial or a large-bore peripheral intravenous catheter during surgery).

Maintenance fluid: classic concepts
Maintenance fluids are defined as those containing appropriate amounts of water and electrolytes to replace urine, gastrointestinal, sweat, breathing, and skin evaporation losses. Oral, intravenous, and other routes can be used to supply maintenance fluid.

The contributions of Gamble [66] and Darrow [67] are often the starting point for understanding evidence-based fluid and electrolyte therapy. Gamble introduced the critical concept of the extracellular space and defined the role of the kidney in fluid maintenance by measuring loss of electrolytes during fasting and other stresses [66]. He emphasized the importance of maintaining the extracellular fluid space, especially in cases of excessive fluid

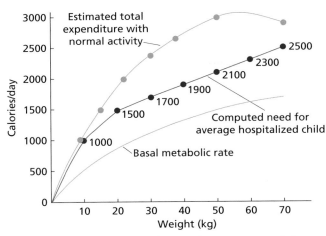

Figure 10.3 Based on Holliday and Segar's data, energy expended (calories) is the approximately the same as requirement for fluid (mL). Although caloric expenditure varies (basal rate versus normal activity), three linear sections are easily identified (0–10 kg, 10–20 kg, >20 kg). Energy expended by hospitalized patients was estimated to be approximately between that for basal and normal activity. From the curve for the hospitalized patient, a 10 kg infant expends 1000 calories (requires 1000 mL/day, 100 mL/kg) and a 20 kg child, 1500 calories (requires 1500 mL/day, 100 mL/kg for 10 kg + 50 mL/kg for 10 kg). Reproduced from Holliday and Segar [68] with permission from American Academy of Pediatrics.

Table 10.4 Calculating maintenance fluid: the "4–2–1 rule"

Weight (kg)	Hourly rate	Daily volume
<10	4 mL/kg	100 mL/kg
10–20	40 mL + 2 mL/kg (for each kg between 10–20)	1000 mL + 50 mL/kg (for each kg between 10–20)
≥20	60 mL + 1 mL/kg (for each kg >20)	1500 mL + 20 mL/kg (for each kg >20)

losses, such as with diarrhea. Darrow recognized the effects of potassium loss and developed regimens for replacing deficits of sodium, chloride and potassium in children with diarrhea [67]. He also estimated deficits in extra- and intracellular volume.

Finally, any discussion of "maintenance" fluids and electrolytes inevitably notices the report of Holliday and Segar: "The maintenance need for water in parenteral fluid therapy" [68]. These authors simplified the calculation of fluid requirements by correlating insensible loses to the metabolic rate of healthy children at rest and during activity (Fig. 10.3). They noted that the requirements for water paralleled those for energy, and that the metabolic rate correlated with weight: <10 kg, 100 kcal/kg; 10–20 kg, 1000 + 5 kcal/kg; >20 kg, 1500 + 2 kcal/kg. For a 10 kg child, they calculated a net loss of ~34 mL/kg/day of insensible loss (i.e. evaporative loss of water from the skin and respiratory tract) and ~66 mL/kg/day of urine, for a total of 100 mL/100 kcal/day (~4 mL/kg/h) of maintenance fluid for the ≤10 kg patient. In the normal, non-premature infant, ~30% of insensible loss is via the lungs and 70% via skin. Based on curves generated from plots of weight versus estimated calories expended/day, the authors estimated that required maintenance fluid is100 mL/kg/day up to 10 kg, an additional 50 mL/kg/day (~2 mL/kg/h) for each kilogram between 10 and 20 kg, and 20 mL/kg/day (1 mL/kg/h) for each kilogram beyond 20 kg. This is the basis for the "4–2–1" formula

widely used to calculate the rates of hourly maintenance intravenous fluid requirement (Table 10.4).

Assuming that electrolytes in intravenous fluid should mimic those in breast milk, Holliday and Segar estimated the amount of sodium and potassium in 100 mL of human milk and used those concentrations of electrolytes to determine daily requirements based on the volume of maintenance fluid (i.e. ~3–4 meq/kg/day for sodium and ~2 meq/kg/day for potassium). This led to the practice of adding 0.2% saline to 5% dextrose for routine intravenous fluid. However, clinicians should be mindful that Holliday and Segar's recommendations are estimates and intravenous fluid should be considered an "invasive therapy" or a "medication" rather than an exact replacement for breast milk, formula or other oral fluids. That is, patients who require intravenous fluid often have a significant illness, hormonal imbalance or physiological derangement (e.g. renal or hepatic disease, chronic lung disease) that complicates the maintenance of adequate intravascular volume and electrolyte balance. Therefore, a single "protocol" for delivering intravenous fluids/electrolytes is not appropriate for all patients or all clinical scenarios. Holliday reminds us, "When fluid therapy extends beyond the first day, monitoring is needed to adapt orders to special cases, avoiding the consequences of "one plan fits all" [69].

Although the principles proposed by Holliday and Segar for calculating routine intravenous fluid have been in place for over 60 years and are widely accepted, adhering to these formulas has been challenged recently (see section on Intravenous fluids and hyponatremia: current controversy, below). Clearly, variability of fluid and electrolyte needs from patient to patient requires the clinician to view the principles of Holliday and Segar as a starting point for "maintenance" [69]. The information gained by clinical assessment and monitoring of serum electrolytes often necessitates significant departures from the "4–2–1" formula. Furthermore, some authors have suggested that predicting fluid requirements (i.e. fluid losses) based on energy expenditure in hospitalized patients overestimates the need for maintenance fluid [70].

Physiology of hyponatremia: clinically relevant concepts

Hyponatremia signifies an excess of water, with or without a deficit of sodium, in the presence of AVP. In most cases, hyponatremia is caused by water rather than sodium imbalance. Despite the fact that many clinical settings are associated with oversecretion of AVP (e.g. surgery, diuretic therapy, central nervous system abnormalities), hyponatremia is rare without an excess of water. Large volumes of hypotonic intravenous fluid are one obvious source of excess water. Moritz, on the other hand, claims that a neurological complication related to the use of 0.9% normal saline in a patient without underlying central nervous system disease has not been reported [71].

Sodium, more than any other molecule, establishes osmolality (normal, 280–290 mOsm/L) in the extracellular space (plasma osmolality $= 2 \times [Na^+] + [glucose]/18 + [BUN]/2.8$). Consequently, sodium contributes significantly to maintaining extracellular fluid volume, blood volume, and perfusion pressure. Through activation of mechanoreceptors in the left ventricle, carotid sinus, aortic arch, and renal afferent arterioles (see section on Renal physiology, above), hypovolemia stimulates the renin-angiotensin system (i.e. synthesis of renin and release of angiotensin II), non-osmotic (or osmotic) release of AVP, and thirst. Aldosterone increases sodium salvage and AVP decreases water excretion; both effects are primarily exerted in the renal tubules.

Sodium cannot freely move across cell membranes. Stable concentrations of sodium in the extracellular space depend on the energy-dependent activity of Na^+-K^+-ATPase (see section on Renal physiology, above). On the other hand, water freely passes through cell membranes in response to osmolar gradients (see section on General considerations, above). Thus, isotonic solutions do not change cell volume but intravenous hypotonic solutions can increase movement of water intracellularly and hypertonic solutions can increase movement of water extracellularly and alter cell volume, if compensatory physiological responses (e.g. changes in renal sodium and water excretion/reabsorption) are not prompt or are incomplete.

The etiology of hyponatremia (plasma Na^+ <135 meq/L) may be multifactorial and complex. Hyponatremia may be isotonic (e.g. with bladder irrigation during laparoscopic surgery) or hypertonic (e.g. with hyperglycemia) but in most cases it is hypotonic. That is, hyponatremia decreases extracellular osmolality, permitting water to freely move from the extracellular to the intracellular space to maintain osmotic equilibrium. Although hypotonic hyponatremia is caused by myriad disorders (congestive heart failure, adrenal insufficiency, diuretics, cerebral salt wasting, etc.), the most relevant etiologies in the perioperative setting include excessive losses (e.g. vomiting, gastrointestinal (GI) suction) and "third-spacing" of fluids (e.g. peritonitis, burns).

Clinical symptoms of hyponatremia develop in proportion to the rapidity of its development. Mild hyponatremia is usually asymptomatic but severe, rapidly developing hyponatremia (Na^+ <120 meq/L) may produce life-threatening cerebral edema and encephalopathy [72]. In some cases the morbid consequences are due to pontine and extrapontine myelinolysis [73]. Compared to acute hyponatremia (developing in less than 48h), chronic hyponatremia is often associated with fewer clinical symptoms because the brain has gradually accommodated to the changes in osmolality.

Complex regulatory systems in the brain, including glial cells, astrocytes/astrocyte foot processes, and aquaporin water channels interact to maintain normal water balance. Astrocytes protect neurons from a hyposmolar insult, in part because of their high number. Glia play a key role in the response to hyposmolality by actively transporting sodium from the intracellular to the extracellular space via Na^+-K^+-ATPase, allowing water to exit the cell. Swelling of cells induces a variety of other protective mechanisms, including potassium and anion channels, the Na^+/Ca^{2+} transporter, and Ca^{2+}-ATPase.

Menstruant women seem to be predisposed to severe consequences of hyponatremia secondary to high concentrations of estrogen. Because the structure of estrogen resembles that of ouabain, an inhibitor of Na^+-K^+-ATPase, women have decreased capacity to adapt to hyponatremia. In addition, AVP vasoconstricts cerebral vessels of women more than it does in men. The resulting decreased availability of cerebral oxygen delivery impairs the energy-dependent mechanisms required to maintain intracellular volume [74]. AVP also directly promotes water entry into cells, especially in the brain, beyond its effects on hyponatremia alone [75].

Although no gender differences are apparent in children, prepubescent children also seem to be at high risk for hyponatremia-induced neurological complications for several reasons, including their high ratio of brain (fully grown by age 6) to cranium (not fully grown until adulthood), the higher intracellular concentration of sodium [76], and the lower activity of Na^+-K^+-ATPase [77]. During the first year of life, the open fontanelle may in part explain why infants have better neurological outcomes following hyponatremia [78].

Intravenous fluids and hyponatremia: current controversy

Over the last two decades, reports of hyponatremia-induced morbidity and mortality have provoked heated debate about whether hypotonic or isotonic crystalloid should be used routinely as maintenance fluid, especially in the perioperative period. Non-osmotic stimuli for AVP secretion are commonly encountered perioperatively (e.g. pain, nausea and vomiting, narcotic administration, inhalation anesthetic agents, positive pressure ventilation), which increases the risk for hyponatremia. Some suggest that all surgical patients are at risk for hyponatremia, especially postoperatively [71,79], if there is central nervous system injury [80] or if the patient underwent scoliosis repair [81,82].

Burrows [81] noted that serum sodium concentration decreased postoperatively in patients who were given either hypotonic or isotonic fluids, but more so after hypotonic solutions. Arief and others described that hyponatremia for elective surgery resulted in respiratory arrest, seizures, and death or permanent brain injury in healthy women [83–85]. The same phenomenon has been noted in children, many of whom were postsurgical. Administering hypotonic intravenous fluid in the presence of AVP was hypothesized to precipitate hyponatremia and death or permanent brain injury in some children [86,87]. Because the incidence of hyponatremia in both adults (~1–2.5%) and children is high [88–91], awareness of this disorder is critical, especially in high-risk groups. Infants and children who are at high risk for hyponatremia include those with meningitis, encephalitis, head injury, bronchiolitis, chronic lung disease, and those who are postsurgery [92]. In addition, malignancies (lung, brain, leukemia, lymphoma, thymoma), various chemotherapeutic agents (vincristine, cyclophosphamide), and diuretics are also associated with hyponatremia. Finally, infants and children who require surgery are more likely to have significant medical illnesses that predispose them to AVP secretion (e.g. leukemia/chemotherapy, congenital heart disease/diuretic therapy, chronic lung disease/ex-premature infant).

Holliday continues to suggest that rapidly restoring intravascular volume with a bolus of 20–40 mL/kg of normal saline, followed by oral rehydration therapy or maintenance fluid containing 0.25% normal saline, represents the most "physiological" approach to fluid and electrolyte therapy, including for patients who are dehydrated preoperatively [93,94]. However, several prospective randomized studies [95–97], as well as smaller observational reports [98] and a recent review [99], have noted that administering 0.9% sodium chloride postoperatively prevents significant hyponatremia, whereas administering hypotonic solutions may not. The rate of fluid delivery is apparently less important than the concentration of sodium delivered [96,97]. Hyponatremia developed even when hypotonic solutions were administered at one-half to two-thirds of the traditional maintenance rates; others report that administering excessive volumes of hypotonic intravenous fluid causes hyponatremia [98,100]. Hypernatremia did not develop even when 0.9% sodium chloride was delivered at rates as low as one-half standard maintenance [97]. Death or neurological injury was reported in 30% of severely hyponatremic children [100].

Based on these data, many suggest that isotonic solutions are appropriate for postoperative maintenance fluids with the proviso that serum electrolytes are monitored frequently and the rate and electrolyte composition of the intravenous fluid are adjusted as needed. As Bailey notes, "No single IV fluid can be used safely in all situations" [99]. Excessive delivery of any solution to patients with cardiovascular or renal failure could be disastrous. Finally, hypotonic intravenous solutions may be required to compensate for excessive free water loss (e.g. diabetes insipidus).

Preoperative assessment and intraoperative fluid management in older infants and children

Whether to vigorously replace a preoperative fluid deficit induced by fasting, bleeding, excessive gastrointestinal losses, etc. depends on several factors, including the nature of the surgical procedure and its indications (e.g. acute trauma secondary to a gunshot wound versus elective craniotomy), current clinical status (e.g. hemodynamically stable), and co-existent medical problems (e.g. renal failure, chronic lung disease). In many cases, preoperative hypovolemia can be corrected by giving boluses of normal saline or lactated Ringer's (10–20 mL/kg). In other cases (e.g. traumatic hemorrhage), fluid resuscitation initiated before surgery must be continued intraoperatively. Once hemodynamic stability has been achieved, intravenous fluid delivery should revert to maintenance fluids plus sufficient crystalloid/colloid to replace the ongoing fluid losses and to maintain hemodynamic stability. Intraoperatively, either normal saline or lactated Ringer's solution is routinely used for both maintenance fluids and replacement of volume deficits and ongoing fluid losses. Glucose, if needed, is given separately.

When prolonged preoperative fasting was in vogue, some experts recommended simply calculating the maintenance fluid for the number of hours the patient had been without oral intake [101] and delivering half that volume during the first hour of surgery and the other half over the subsequent 2 h. Since clear liquids are now given orally up to 2 h before the induction of anesthesia, children are seldom fasted preoperatively for more than 3–4 h [102]. Thus, significant intravascular volume deficits due to prolonged fasting are uncommon, and any preoperative dehydration is more likely due to an underlying disease state. One must assess the current physical status of the patient rather than simply calculate the time of fasting before induction of anesthesia.

Table 10.5 Intraoperative fluids: beyond infancy

Three-year-old, previously healthy child is scheduled for excision of a Wilms' tumor. NPO × 3 h; weight 15 kg; hemoglobin 13 g/dL; open laparotomy.

Deficit	Maintenance	Ongoing losses
150 mL	50 mL/h	• 10–20 mL/kg/h (or more) to compensate for insensible losses via exposed bowel • Until transfusion, replace EBL with crystalloid (volume 2–3 times the EBL) • Consider RBCs if Hgb <8 g/dL and/or hemodynamic instability/or massive ongoing losses

Six-year-old healthy boy hit by car while riding his bicycle. He is alert, oriented with an isolated fracture right femur. Past medical/surgical history is unremarkable. A 22 g angiocath is infusing 0.9 normal saline. Weight 25 kg; hemoglobin 12 g/dL; no urine; scheduled for pinning of the fracture in the operating room under general anesthesia.

Deficit	Maintenance	Ongoing losses
• Full stomach • Blood pressure 70/40, heart rate 150 • Deliver boluses of 0.9 normal saline, 10 mL/kg before induction • Monitor hemoglobin, urine output	70 mL/h	• Monitor Hgb, PT/PTT if bleeding persists • Consider transfusion of packed RBCs if Hgb <7 g/dL after crystalloid infusion to establish adequate intravascular volume or to replete ongoing blood loss and/or treat hemodynamic instability

EBL, estimated blood loss; Hgb, hemoglobin; NPO, nil per os; RBC, red blood cell, PT, prothrombin time; PTT, partial thromboplastin time.

If preoperative assessment suggests hypovolemia or if hypotension develops during the induction of anesthesia, an intravenous bolus of lactated Ringer's solution or normal saline is appropriate initial treatment for patients of any age. After a 4–6 h (or longer) fast, older infants or children without significant cardiorespiratory or renal disease usually have no evidence of intravascular compromise. If the preoperative fast was appropriate and/or there is no evidence for intravascular fluid deficit or hemodynamic response to induction of general anesthesia, administration of IV fluids beyond maintenance rates may be unnecessary or may be deliberately avoided (e.g. stable patient undergoing neurosurgery).

Rapidly administering intravenous fluids before, during or after the induction of anesthesia should be based on need and need alone. Both before and during surgery, the anesthesiologist must differentiate between fluids administered to treat hypovolemia and those administered for "maintenance" (e.g. to compensate for NPO status). Boluses of either lactated Ringer's solution or normal saline are appropriate for correction of hypovolemia (i.e. hemodynamic instability, poor perfusion).

In the perioperative period, one indication for giving hypotonic fluids is excessive loss of free water, which must be diagnosed and monitored by simultaneously determining serum and urine electrolyte concentrations. Meticulous monitoring of the patient's clinical status and serum electrolytes is essential to avoid perpetuating or inducing electrolyte abnormalities.

Intraoperative glucose delivery in the older infant/child (see Table 10.5)

In the era of prolonged preoperative fasting, hypoglycemia was common [103,104]. Today, with more liberal NPO regimens, the incidence of hypoglycemia is 0–2.5% and occurs almost exclusively in patients who have been fasted for inappropriately long periods (8–19 h) [105]. Nonetheless, in spite of its rare occurrence, the consequences of both hypo- (see section on Glucose homeostasis) and hyperglycemia can be catastrophic. For example, administering glucose-containing fluid at high rates during surgery often leads to hyperglycemia, glucosuria, and an osmotic diuresis. Of greater significance, hyperglycemia has been associated with increased mortality and infection in both adults and children in ICUs [106,107]. In the absence of an underlying metabolic derangement (e.g. diabetes, methylmalonic acidemia), intraoperative glucose administration is usually not necessary.

The patient with diabetes: perioperative management

Although there are no controlled studies of perioperative management of pediatric patients with diabetes, the recommendations of an excellent recent review [108] were reaffirmed by the International Society for Pediatric and Adolescent Diabetes (ISPAD) in both its 2007 and 2009 consensus guidelines for both pediatric and adolescent patients [109]. The following discussion and recommendations are consistent with these reports.

The incidence of both type 1 and type 2 diabetes mellitus has increased in the pediatric population, both in the United States and worldwide [110,111]. Because of its common occurrence and the devastating multisystem complications of this disease, aggressive efforts have been undertaken to minimize morbidity. This includes maintaining tight glycemic control by continuous insulin infusion and administering long and rapidly acting insulin analogs. Tight glycemic control benefits both short-term surgical outcomes (wound healing, fluid and metabolic derangements) and long-term health [112–114]. On the other hand, tight glycemic control increases the risk for developing hypoglycemia. Anesthesiologists encounter diabetic patients frequently and must have knowledge of their increasingly complex treatment regimens.

Most pediatric patients with diabetes fall into one of two categories. Type 1 is usually caused by immune-mediated pancreatic β-cell destruction that causes insulin deficiency. Type 2 is caused by a combination of insulin resistance and relative insulin deficiency [115]. Rarer forms of diabetes include genetic defects of β-cell function, genetic syndromes and systemic endocrine disorders, and those that develop secondary to other diseases or their treatment (e.g. cystic fibrosis, steroid administration, chemotherapy) [116].

The stress response caused by trauma and surgery elicits cortisol and catecholamine production and release, which increases blood glucose concentrations by catabolizing protein and fat. Patients with insulin deficiency are unable to increase insulin production sufficiently to counter the rise in glucose concentration; this causes profound hyperglycemia and ketoacidosis. Hyperglycemia impairs wound healing by hindering collagen production, decreasing the tensile strength of the wound, and adversely affecting neutrophil phagocytosis and bactericidal killing. Reducing sympathetic nervous stimulation is critical for preventing the release of catecholamines and their negative effects on glycemic control. A comprehensive flexible intra- and postoperative plan for pain control should be developed and understood by the nurses, anesthesiologists, and surgeons in order to reduce sympathetic activation.

In a study of perioperative infections that included ~23,000 adult patients, the rate of postoperative clean wound infections was 1.8% in patients without diabetes and 10.7% in those with diabetes [117]. However, this report failed to provide data on perioperative glucose control. A more recent study in adult vascular patients reported no difference in the risk for postoperative wound infection in diabetic and non-diabetic patients when the blood glucose was maintained between 122 and 168 mg/dL [118]. In cardiac surgery patients, when the blood glucose levels were maintained below 200 mg/dL for 48 h postoperatively, the risk of sternal wound infection decreased [119]. In adult patients requiring intensive care, tight postoperative glycemic control (80–110 mg/dL) with an insulin infusion significantly decreased mortality and morbidity. However, 5.2% of the "tight control" group had hypoglycemic episodes (though none were severe) compared to 0.8% of controls [120].

For major surgery, the data in adults support tight perioperative control of glucose. A reasonable similar target in pediatric patients is a blood glucose concentration of <200 mg/dL. Because insulin therapy is often needed to achieve tight control, glucose concentrations must be monitored at least once an hour during surgery if patients are receiving insulin to ensure prompt detection and correction of hypoglycemia. General anesthesia masks the symptoms of hyperglycemia. Similarly, if the glucose concentration is maintained between 100 and 200 mg/dL, the risks associated with hyperglycemia (e.g. osmotic diuresis, dehydration, electrolyte imbalance, metabolic acidosis, and infection) are minimized. The data for brief and minor surgical procedures are less clear, but the goal of maintaining perioperative blood glucose levels below 200 mg/dL [109] seems appropriate.

Given the complexity and variability in treatment options, the need for tight glycemic control, and the variable effects of different surgeries and postoperative courses, a perioperative plan for every patient with diabetes should be devised in advance, ideally in consultation with an expert in diabetes management [108]. The perioperative approach should be based on two primary factors: the regimen followed by the patient chronically and the type of surgical procedure.

If a patient with diabetes must fast for any surgery or procedure, the following points should be borne in mind.

- Maintain the blood glucose concentration between 100–200 mg/dL. Preoperative monitoring should ensure stable glucose control for at least several weeks before surgery. Then a specific preoperative regimen can be developed for each patient that reflects her/his recent history of glycemic control. For example, patients who have stable insulin schedules and predictable glucose concentrations may only require a single preoperative determination of glucose concentration. Brittle diabetics with widely fluctuating glucose levels require more intense preoperative evaluation. It is important to remember that even a long-standing stable preoperative course may be disrupted by surgery and anesthesia. Establishing an approach to various intraoperative scenarios and having access to a diabetologist during surgery are essential components of preoperative planning.
- Children with diabetes should be admitted to hospital early on the morning of the procedure to measure their

blood glucose concentrations and to repeat them as needed. If necessary, an intravenous infusion is started. If the surgery is delayed for several hours, monitoring of blood glucose concentrations will help prevent both hypo- and hyperglycemia [108].

- If the blood glucose is >250 mg/dL, a conservative dose of regular (short-acting) insulin should be given to restore relative normoglycemia. This is best achieved by using the child's usual sliding insulin scale or a "correction factor." The insulin correction factor is the decrease in the blood glucose concentration expected after administering 1 U of short- or rapid-acting insulin. It is calculated by using the "1500 rule" (1500/child's usual total daily dose of insulin). For example, a child who typically takes 30 U of insulin daily would have a correction factor of 50 (1500 ÷ 30). Thus, giving 1 U of rapid-acting or short-acting insulin would be expected to decrease the blood glucose concentration by approximately 50 mg/dL [108].
- The treatment regimen of pediatric patients with type 2 diabetes may include insulin and/or one of several oral antihyperglycemic drugs. Metformin is commonly used and should be discontinued 24 h before a procedure because its half-life is long and there is a remote risk of lactic acidosis in patients with renal or cardiac failure [121]. In fact, renal failure is a contraindication for the use of metformin.
- Other oral drugs, such as sulfonylureas and thiazolidinediones, may be discontinued on the morning of the procedure [122].

For minor/short procedures

- Most pediatric patients with diabetes who are stable on a subcutaneous regimen of insulin can continue this mode of therapy.
- Since intermittent intravenous boluses of regular insulin seem to offer comparable effectiveness to continuous infusions in adults with type 2 diabetes, a similar approach is justified in pediatric patients. Patients with Type 2 diabetes can often be managed without continuously infusing insulin [123,124].
- During minor procedures that last <2 h, patients typically continue to receive their usual basal rate of insulin for that time of day via their pump. However, when using this approach, the anesthesiologist must measure intraoperative glucose concentrations and be comfortable with using an insulin pump. Otherwise he/she must seek consultation with and have intraoperative access to a pediatric endocrinologist or other skilled personnel prior to inducing anesthesia.
- If the child can drink soon after a brief procedure, he/she may not need an intravenous glucose infusion. If the fast is likely to be prolonged, an intravenous infusion should deliver glucose at a maintenance rate

(see section on Maintenance fluid: classic concepts, above).

- Patients with stable glucose and normal serum potassium concentrations have minimal risk for electrolyte imbalance (e.g. acidosis, hypokalemia).

For longer/more complex procedures

- For procedures lasting more than 2 h, patients with insulin pumps should receive intravenous insulin, either by the pump or by a separate infusion.
- Children with diabetes undergoing major surgical procedures should receive their usual insulin dose on the day prior to the procedure. On the morning of the procedure, an intravenous infusion of 5% or 10% dextrose (depending on a patient's relative risk for hyper- or hypoglycemia) in half-normal saline should be started at a maintenance rate (see section on Maintenance fluid: classic concepts, above). The rate of insulin infusion should be adequate to maintain blood glucose concentration between 100–200 mg/dL.
- Because prepubescent children are relatively more sensitive to insulin than pubertal adolescents [108], the insulin dose necessary for children varies with age. In prepubescent children with type 1 diabetes, the insulin requirement is typically 0.6–0.8 U/kg/d, compared to 1.0–1.5 U/kg/d for adolescents. Patients with type 2 diabetes often have higher insulin requirements because they have resistance to insulin. A suitable ratio of intravenous regular insulin to glucose for prepubescent children is 1 U per 5 g of intravenous glucose and 1 U per 3 g of intravenous glucose for adolescents (>12 years old) [108].
- Intraoperative maintenance fluids for children with diabetes should contain glucose if the case is long and/or complex. However, intraoperative volume losses (e.g. blood, excessive insensible losses) should be replaced with non-glucose containing lactated Ringer's solution or normal saline. *To avoid hyperglycemia and its potentially disastrous consequences, glucose-containing solutions should not be used to replace intraoperative fluid losses!*
- Patients undergoing longer or emergency surgeries are at greater risk for metabolic decompensation. Their electrolytes should be assessed intraoperatively and corrected as needed. In all cases, blood glucose concentration should be measured hourly and, if abnormal, the amounts of insulin and glucose adjusted to maintain the blood glucose concentrations between 100–200 mg/dL [108].

As soon as the patient can resume normal oral intake after surgery, her/his usual diabetes regimen (insulin and/or oral drugs) should be reinstituted, and any glucose infusions discontinued. Normal renal function should be documented before restarting metformin. Patients who are unable to tolerate adequate oral intake require infusions of intravenous glucose, electrolytes, and regular insulin to maintain normal electrolytes and glucose concentrations of 100–200 mg/dL. Frequent monitoring of blood glucose and blood or urine ketone bodies is essential because the interplay of postsurgical events, including surgical trauma, inactivity, pain, nausea or vomiting, poor oral intake, and medications is complex. *Before* discharge, patients require appropriate teaching about how to contact experts if glucose and insulin therapy must be altered.

Conclusion

Holliday's perspective on the contributions of Gamble, Darrow, Howland and others provides an exciting historical document [1]. He notes, "The development of body fluid physiology and fluid therapy in pediatrics has special importance in the history of medicine because this development introduced physiology into clinical practice" (and eventually enabled the explosion in surgical innovation). James Gamble and Dan Darrow were leaders in this enterprise. Holliday emphasizes, "Pediatrics, medicine, and surgery are all indebted to the research of each, which emphasized the value of basic physiology in clinical practice." Clearly, the foundation of current principles of fluid and electrolyte therapy is easily traced to these pioneers. However, these principles continue to evolve and should be revised when new evidence appears. Darrow advised in his address to the American Pediatric Society in 1957 that "research is the process by which teachers and students are forced to deal with the lively facts of medical science rather than rules of the trade" [1,125]. As we move forward in the era of clinical trials and evidence-based medicine, our practices for delivery of maintenance fluid, crystalloid for replacement of intraoperative fluid losses, and various synthetic colloids, as well as other practices, should be responsibly reviewed and revised based on rigorous investigation and data.

Annotated references

A full reference list for this chapter is available at:
http://www.wiley.com/go/gregory/andropoulos/pediatricanesthesia

1. Holliday MA. Gamble and Darrow: pathfinders in body fluid physiology and fluid therapy for children, 1914–1964. Pediatr Nephrol 2000; 15: 317–24. As a respected pediatric nephrologist who has contributed enormously to our understanding of pediatric fluids and electrolytes, Malcolm Holliday aptly chronicles the contributions of Gamble and Darrow to the development of the physiological basis of clinical management of electrolyte derangements.

5. Friis-Hansen B. Body water compartments in children: changes during growth and related changes in body composition. Pediatrics 1961; 28: 169–81. This lecture delivered in 1960 summarizes the changes in total body water and its distribution between the extracellular and intracellular compartments. This reference invariably is included in reviews, chapters, and other scholarly publications related to pediatric fluids and electrolytes.

44. Groves AM, Kuschel CA, Knight DB et al. Relationship between blood pressure and blood flow in newborn preterm infants. Arch Dis Child Fetal Neonatal Ed 2008; 93: F29–F32. These investigators had earlier documented that SVC flow correlated with left ventricular output (see ref. 46). SVC flow reflects systemic perfusion. Such flow rather than blood pressure may be a more reliable clinical variable in the newborn. However, blood flow in four different vessels did not correlate with blood pressure.

49. Greisen G. To autoregulate or not to autoregulate – that is no longer the question. Semin Pediatr Neurol 2009; 16: 207–15. This review of history of studies of autoregulation of cerebral blood flow in the newborn written by an internationally recognized expert eventually leads to a discussion of the concept of autoregulation as a "quantity rather than a quality."

68. Holliday MA, Segar WE. The maintenance need for water in parenteral fluid therapy. Pediatrics 1957; 19: 823–32. The origin of the "4–2–1 rule" resides in this manuscript after Holliday and Segar correlated energy expenditure with fluid requirements, noting that the needs of the "average hospitalized patient" reside between those associated with "basal metabolic rate" and those of the normal individual during normal activity. The authors also describe maintenance electrolyte requirements.

71. Moritz ML, Ayus JC. Water water everywhere: standardizing postoperative fluid therapy with 0.9% normal saline. Anesth Anal 2010; 110: 293–5. This brief but comprehensive overview of risks for perioperative hyponatremia presents cogent evidence that "there can be no justification for administering hypotonic fluids in the perioperative setting." The report accompanies Bailey's (ref. 99) review of perioperative fluid management.

76. Arieff AI, Ayus J, Fraser C. Hyponatremia and death or permanent brain damage in healthy children. BMJ 1992; 304: 1218–22. The authors retrospectively reviewed 24,412 <16-year-old pediatric admissions. Sixteen patients with symptomatic hyponatremia are described who developed hyponatremia after receiving hypotonic intravenous therapy. Authors discuss pediatric CNS adaptation to hyponatremia, document the significant mortality, and emphasize the critical role of early recognition and treatment.

97. Neville KA, Sandeman DJ, Rubinstein A et al. Prevention of hyponatremia during maintenance intravenous fluid administration: a prospective randomized study of fluid type versus fluid rate. J Pediatr 2010; 156: 313–19. This prospective study documents that the risk for hyponatremia is associated with the type of fluid (hypo- vs isotonic) rather than the rate of administration in the surgical pediatric patient.

99. Bailey AG, McNaull PP, Jooste E et al. Perioperative crystalloid and colloid fluid management in children: where are we and how did we get here? Anesth Anal 2010; 110: 375–90. While providing a historical review of perioperative fluid management, the authors also analyze current controversies, and present the limited evidence-based data that exist to guide clinical practice. They also discuss currently available colloids.

108. Rhodes ET, Ferrari LR, Wolfsdorf JI. Perioperative management of pediatric surgical patients with diabetes mellitus. Anesth Analg 2005; 101: 986–99. This document provides the basis for a recommended algorithm for the perioperative management of both type 1 and type 2 diabetics. The review focuses on the pediatric age group but borrows extensively from the literature/evidence in adults.

CHAPTER 11

Coagulation, Bleeding, and Blood Transfusion

Bruce E. Miller[1] & Jeanne E. Hendrickson[2]

[1]Pediatric Cardiac Anesthesiology, Children's Healthcare of Atlanta and Department of Anesthesiology, Emory University School of Medicine, Atlanta, GA, USA
[2]Aflac Cancer Center and Blood Disorders Service, Children's Healthcare of Atlanta and Department of Pediatrics and Pathology, Emory University School of Medicine, Atlanta, GA, USA

Introduction

The hematological system is unique among all the systems in the body. It is composed of multiple components, each of which engages in a very specific and unique function that is critical for life. This chapter will focus on one of those functions: coagulation. New concepts describing the coagulation pathway, maturational factors affecting coagulation in neonates and infants, tests of and defects in the coagulation system, and principles of transfusion therapy and blood conservation will be discussed.

The coagulation pathway

The coagulation system is a complex interplay of cellular elements and plasma proteins that functions to stop bleeding from an injured blood vessel and then to re-establish patency of that vessel. The process which stops bleeding is understood to occur in two phases. Primary hemostasis arrests bleeding by inducing vasoconstriction in the injured vessel and by causing the formation of a platelet plug. Secondary hemostasis then involves the circulating plasma coagulation factors and results in the formation of a fibrin clot at the site of blood vessel damage. While it is easy to think of these two phases as separate, distinct, and sequential, they are in fact highly co-ordinated, interdependent, and concurrent. In the end, the fibrinolytic system removes clot to re-establish blood flow and to allow wound healing [1].

Primary hemostasis is triggered by damage to a blood vessel wall. This disruption exposes subendothelial collagen to the bloodstream. Platelets become immediately involved and respond by adhesion to the wall of the damaged blood vessel, by activation, and by aggregation to each other. Platelet adhesion is mediated by von Willebrand factor (vWF). Circulating vWF binds to the exposed subendothelial collagen of the damaged blood vessel wall and then to the glycoprotein Ib receptor on platelet surfaces. This results in platelet adhesion to the blood vessel at the point of damage. Platelet activation then occurs, resulting in release of platelet agonists (adenosine diphosphate (ADP) and serotonin) and coagulation factors (vWF and factor V) from platelet storage granules and in changes in the shape and surface function of the platelets. Arachidonic acid from activated platelet membranes is converted into substances that cause vasoconstriction of the injured vessel by a series of enzymatic reactions involving cyclo-oxygenase. Changes in the shape of platelets allow the expression of glycoprotein

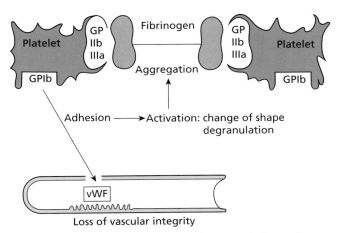

Figure 11.1 Primary hemostasis: platelet adhesion, activation, and aggregation. Reproduced from Hardy [180] with permission from Springer.

Table 11.1 Coagulation factor numbers and synonyms

Roman numeral	Synonyms
I	Fibrinogen
II	Prothrombin
III	Thromboplastin Tissue factor
IV	Calcium
V	Proaccelerin Labile factor
VII	Proconvertin Stable factor
VIII	Antihemophilic factor (AHF) Antihemophilic globulin (AHG) Antihemophilic factor A Factor VIII : C
IX	Plasma thromboplastin component Antihemophilic factor B Christmas factor
X	Stuart factor Prower factor Stuart–Prower factor
XI	Plasma thromboplastin antecedent Antihemophilic factor C
XII	Hageman factor Contact factor Surface factor Glass factor
XIII	Fibrin stabilizing factor Laki–Lorand factor

IIb/IIIa surface receptors. Platelet aggregation then occurs as fibrinogen binds these exposed receptors on adjacent platelets (Fig. 11.1). Finally, the phospholipid membrane of activated platelets provides the surface on which the process of secondary hemostasis occurs [2].

Secondary hemostasis involves the interaction of coagulation factors to form a fibrin clot. Roman numerals are used to designate most of these factors in order to provide an international code for clear communication [3] (Table 11.1). The clotting factors exist in inactive precursor forms before being converted to active enzymes upon initiation of secondary hemostasis [4]. Most coagulation factors (I (fibrinogen), II (prothrombin), V, VII, VIII, IX, X, and XI) and some anticoagulants (antithrombin and proteins C and S) are predominantly produced by the liver. Endothelial cells participate in the production of many anticoagulants (thrombomodulin, tissue factor pathway inhibitor, tissue plasminogen activator, heparan, nitric oxide, and cyclo-oxygenase) as well as some procoagulants (vWF, plasminogen activator inhibitor type 1, thromboxane, and possibly tissue factor) [1].

Our attempts at understanding secondary hemostasis began in the 1960s with a waterfall or cascade model of what came to be known as the "intrinsic" pathway of coagulation [4,5]. This pathway was described *in vitro* in cell-poor plasma and was termed "intrinsic" because all required factors existed in the plasma. An "extrinsic" pathway was subsequently described that involved tissue factor (TF), a protein in the blood vessel wall that is extrinsic to blood. Both of these pathways were determined to converge on a "common" pathway leading to thrombin generation and subsequent fibrin formation (Fig. 11.2). However, questions from several clinical and laboratory scenarios led to the recognition that the intrinsic and extrinsic coagulation pathways do not operate independently *in vivo*. Additionally, even the early descriptions of coagulation recognized the significant role of phospholipid acting as a surface catalyst for coagulation and postulated that the phospholipid might be derived from platelets during the clotting process [5].

Subsequently, a cell-based model has been proposed to explain secondary hemostasis. This model emphasizes the importance of cell surfaces as the platform upon which the previously described extrinsic pathway initiates and then amplifies the beginning of secondary coagulation with subsequent fibrin formation by factors of the classic intrinsic pathway [6].

The cell-based model describes three overlapping phases of secondary coagulation: initiation of coagulation on TF-bearing cells, amplification of the procoagulant signal by thrombin generated on the TF-bearing cells, and propagation of thrombin generation on platelet surfaces.

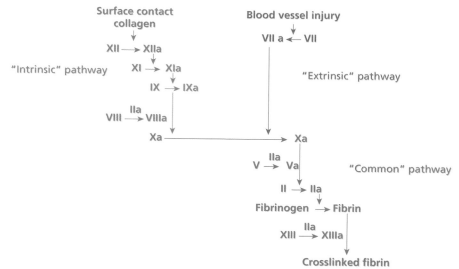

Figure 11.2 Secondary hemostasis: the coagulation cascade.

Initiation of coagulation occurs when TF, a transmembrane protein that acts as a receptor and co-factor for activated factor (F) VII, is exposed on cells at the site of a blood vessel injury. FVIIa normally circulates in the blood in low concentrations, "patrolling" the circulation for damaged blood vessels with exposed TF. Once FVIIa and TF meet, the resulting FVIIa/TF complex catalyzes the activation of FX and FIX on the surface of the TF-bearing cells. FXa then interacts with FVa on the cell surface. This cell-bound FVa may come from the degranulation of nearby activated platelets or may originate from non-coagulation proteases. The Xa/Va interaction generates small amounts of thrombin (Fig. 11.3A). This thrombin is insufficient in quantity to lyse fibrinogen but it is sufficient to stimulate the second phase of the cell-based coagulation model. The FIXa formed by the FVIIa/TF complex diffuses from the TF-bearing cells to nearby activated platelets to play a later role in thrombin formation. However, the activity of FXa is restricted to the TF-bearing cell on which it was formed because tissue factor pathway inhibitor (TFPI) or antithrombin (AT) will inhibit any FXa that dissociates from the cell surface. This initiation phase of the cell-based coagulation model has been compared to the classically described extrinsic coagulation pathway (Fig. 11.4A).

In the subsequent amplification step, the initial thrombin produced on the TF-bearing cell surfaces activates more nearby platelets and FV, FVIII, and FXI. The activated platelets provide the phospholipid surfaces on which large amounts of thrombin are subsequently generated in phase three. The newly activated coagulation factors will become vital co-factors in this subsequent phase (Fig. 11.3B).

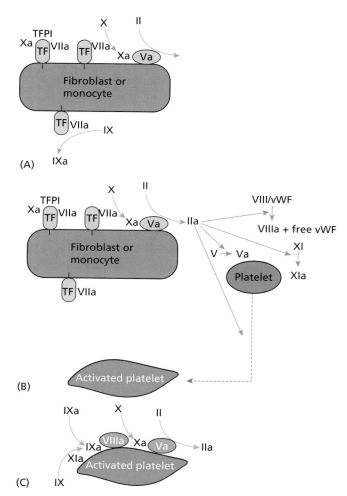

Figure 11.3 Secondary hemostasis: the cell-based model. Reproduced from Hoffman and Monroe [6] with permission from Elsevier.

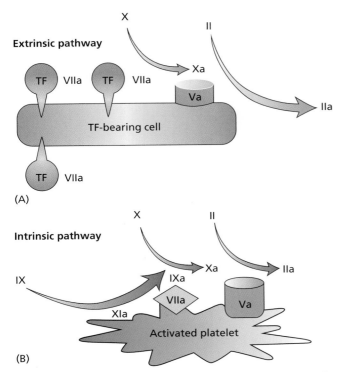

Extrinsic pathway

(A)

Intrinsic pathway

(B)

Figure 11.4 Comparison of the coagulation cascade and the cell-based model of secondary hemostasis. Reproduced from Hoffman and Monroe [6] with permission from Elsevier.

The third phase is propagation of thrombin generation on the surfaces of activated platelets. In this phase, FVIIIa from the amplification phase forms a complex with FIXa from the initiation phase on the surfaces of nearby activated platelets. FXIa from the second phase also binds to nearby platelets and can activate more circulating FIX to join surface-bound FVIIIa. The FVIIIa/IXa "tenase" complex then activates FX. The FXa joins with FVa from the second phase on activated platelet surfaces. This FXa/Va "prothrombinase" complex finally catalyzes the large-scale conversion of prothrombin into thrombin (Fig. 11.3C). These actions have been compared to those outlined in descriptions of the intrinsic coagulation pathway (Fig. 11.4B). Unlike the small quantity of thrombin produced by TF-bearing cells, the quantity of this platelet-produced thrombin is sufficient to cleave fibrinogen to fibrin. It also functions to stabilize the fibrin clot by activating FXIII to cross-link the fibrin monomers and to link thrombin-activatable fibrinolysis inhibitor (TAFI) and α2-antiplasmin to the fibrin in order to inhibit the fibrinolytic process and thus prevent clot dissolution [6,7].

After clotting has occurred and bleeding has been stopped, activation of the fibrinolytic system allows patency of the involved blood vessel eventually to be restored so that wound healing can proceed. Tissue plas-

minogen activator (tPA) is released from endothelial cells in response to the presence of thrombin and venous occlusion. Both tPA and its substrate, plasminogen, bind to lysine residues on fibrin surfaces. Fibrin-bound tPA then converts this localized plasminogen to its active form, plasmin. Plasmin dissolves a fibrin clot by cleaving fibrin at specific lysine and arginine residues to eventually re-establish blood flow through the vessels [6,7].

The hematological system constantly balances the ability to keep blood flowing through undamaged vessels with the ability to stop bleeding from damaged blood vessels. Under normal circumstances, the luminal surface of undamaged blood vessels is non-thrombogenic because of the constitutive presence of thrombomodulin, AT, and heparan sulfate [8]. Thrombomodulin binds circulating thrombin, resulting in activation of protein C. Activated protein C, with its co-factor protein S, then attenuates thrombin production by inactivating FVa and FVIIIa. AT, catalyzed by endothelial cell-produced heparan sulfate, neutralizes circulating FIXa, FXa, FXIa, and thrombin to prevent fibrin formation [9]. Intact vessel walls also release nitric oxide and prostacyclin to inhibit platelet activity and release tPA to promote fibrinolysis [8]. Thus, undamaged blood vessels have protective mechanisms to prevent clot formation. Vascular damage not only exposes TF but also downregulates thrombomodulin and AT, thus creating an environment conducive to clot formation [8].

The hematological system is also constantly challenged to localize its coagulation process only to areas of blood vessel damage. Exposure of TF only on cells in areas of blood vessel damage and subsequent activation only of nearby platelets allows the coagulation process to stay localized to areas of blood vessel injury. Additionally, each activated coagulation factor that participates in the secondary hemostasis process is balanced by a naturally occurring anticoagulant in order to maintain control and to balance hemostasis: TFPI neutralizes the FVIIa/TF/Xa complex on TF-bearing cells; AT inhibits thrombin and circulating FIXa, FXa, and FXIa; and protein C, with its co-factor protein S, inhibits FVa and FVIIIa [1,7]. The fibrinolytic system is also balanced by inhibitors in order to control the extent of fibrinolysis. The activity of any circulating tPA is inhibited by plasminogen activator inhibitor (PAI) type 1. Ongoing formation of plasmin is prevented when TAFI cleaves the lysine residues from degrading fibrin to which tPA and plasminogen must bind in order to interact and form plasmin. Finally, circulating plasmin itself is inhibited by α2-antiplasmin [6–8]. In the end, under normal conditions, coagulation and fibrinolysis occur only where they are needed and are prevented from becoming pathological generalized problems by procoagulant and anticoagulant factors that delicately balance the system.

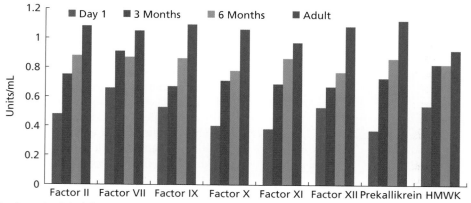

Figure 11.5 Coagulation factor levels in full-term infants and with age. HMWK, high molecular weight kininogen. Modified from Andrew et al [13].

Maturation of the coagulation system

Coagulation proteins, platelets, and fibrinolytic proteins do not cross the placental barrier but their synthesis by the fetus begins at approximately 11 weeks of gestational age. During the remainder of fetal development, maturation of the coagulation and fibrinolytic systems parallel each other so that a delicate hemostatic balance is maintained [10,11]. However, despite this ongoing maturation, both quantitative and qualitative deficiencies exist in these systems at birth.

Plasma levels of coagulation factors and coagulation inhibitors have been documented in detail in both healthy premature infants (30–36 weeks' gestational age) and full-term infants (>37 weeks' gestational age) from birth through 6 months of age [12,13]. Plasma levels of the vitamin K-dependent coagulation factors (II, VII, IX, and X) and the contact factors (XII, XI, high molecular weight kininogen (HMWK), and prekallikrein (PK)) at 1 day of age in the premature and full-term infants studied were all less than 70% of adult values. Additionally, levels of several of these factors (IX, XI, and XII) were significantly lower in the premature infants compared to the full-term infants. By 6 months of age, levels of all these coagulation factors in both premature and full-term infants had risen to within adult ranges (Fig. 11.5).

On the other hand, levels of fibrinogen, FV, FVIII, and FXIII, and vWF were all greater than 70% of adult values on the first day of life in both premature and full-term infants. Fibrinogen levels were lower in premature infants than in full-term infants while levels of FV were higher in premature infants than in full-term infants at 1 day of age. Levels of vWF on day 1 of life were higher than adult values in both groups of infants, dropping to adult range between 3 and 6 months of life [12,13] (Fig. 11.6). Finally, platelet counts in the neonatal period have been shown to be similar to those found in adults and not to differ between premature and full-term neonates [14].

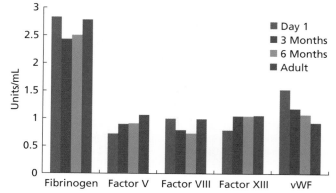

Figure 11.6 Coagulation factor levels in full-term infants. vWF, von Willebrand factor. Modified from Andrew et al [13].

The inhibitors of coagulation showed similar developmental patterns. At 1 day of age, plasma levels of AT, protein C, and protein S were lower in both groups of infants than levels in adults and levels of all three of these coagulation inhibitors were lower in premature infants than in full-term infants. In both groups at 6 months of age, levels of AT and protein S had risen to within adult ranges while protein C levels remained low [12,13] (Fig. 11.7).

In the fibrinolytic system, plasminogen levels were significantly lower on the first day of life in both premature and full-term infants than those seen in adults and were significantly lower in premature infants compared to full-term infants. These values remained low during the first 6 months of life [12,13]. tPA levels in term newborns have also been found to be significantly lower than adult levels while PAI levels were similar to those measured in adults [15]. As these findings would predict, plasmin generation and fibrinolysis are suppressed in infancy. Thus, if thrombolytic therapy is needed in infants, higher doses of activator will need to be administered [15].

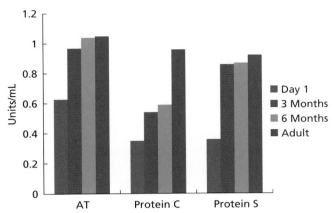

Figure 11.7 Coagulation inhibitor levels in full-term infants. AT, antithrombin. Modified from Andrew et al [13].

In addition to these quantitative issues in development of the hemostatic system, qualitative issues exist as well. The concept of a "fetal fibrinogen" has been proposed [16,17] and evidence of impaired fibrinogen function in infants has been postulated based on thromboelastography data [18] and on differences between measured activity and antigen levels of fibrinogen [19]. Comparison of the biological activity and the plasma levels of FXII, PK, protein C, and plasminogen has suggested that these factors may also exhibit qualitative deficiencies [10,20–22] but the data are not absolute [15,19]. Finally, impairment of platelet aggregation has been documented in neonates in the first 48 h of life [23].

Coagulation tests have also been studied in infants. Activated partial thromboplastin time (aPTT) has been shown to be the most prolonged coagulation test in both premature and full-term infants on day 1 of life compared to adults, being 1.2–1.5 times longer in term infants and 1.4–2.4 times longer in preterm infants [12,13,24]. This prolongation has been attributed to the quantitative and qualitative deficiencies of contact factors described above. In full-term infants, aPTT values were similar to adult values by 3 months of age. In premature infants, this equalization occurred by 6 months of age. Values of pro-thrombin time (PT) are less prolonged, with reported values ranging from being not significantly different from adult values to being 1.15–1.3 times longer in term infants and 1.3 times longer in preterm infants [12,13,24]. Although FVII levels are low at birth, their levels are more preserved than those of other coagulation factors and may prevent excessive prolongation of the PT in early infancy. Thrombin times (TT) are approximately 1.16–1.4 times longer than adult values in term infants and 1.31–1.5 times longer in preterm infants [12,13,24]. The existence of dysfunctional fibrinogen may explain this prolongation. If prolonged at birth, PT and TT values reach adult ranges within several days of age [11–13].

Interpretation of these maturational issues of the hemostatic system is complex. There is no evidence that neonates, infants or children have an increased risk of bleeding spontaneously, after trauma or during surgery, compared to adults. In fact, thromboelastograms have shown intact coagulation systems even in neonates [25]. However, the alterations in coagulation factors and coagulation inhibitors in young infants result in a reduced ability to generate thrombin as well as a significant delay in thrombin generation once the coagulation system is triggered. On the other hand, deficiencies in the fibrinolytic system result in decreased plasmin generation and impairment of fibrinolysis [22,26]. Fortunately, maturation of coagulation and fibrinolysis proceeds in tandem and in accordance with gestational age, and the net effect apparently strikes the necessary balance to maintain a competent hemostatic picture. Nevertheless, while quantitative and qualitative immaturities resolve during the first year of life, normal values for plasma levels of most coagulation factors, coagulation inhibitors, and fibrinolytic proteins in young infants must be recognized to be different from those values considered normal for adults.

Evaluation of the coagulation system

Anesthesiologists and surgeons usually employ laboratory tests of the coagulation system to screen patients preoperatively for inherited or acquired hemorrhagic disorders or to diagnose the cause(s) and monitor the treatment of intraoperative or postoperative bleeding [27]. None of the available tests is perfect because each either reports a quantitative count with no consideration of qualitative function or is performed *in vitro* in environments that are not equivalent to what actually occurs *in vivo*. This section will describe available laboratory tests and their indications and limitations.

Evaluation of primary hemostasis

Evaluation of primary hemostasis includes quantitative and functional analysis of platelets and vWF. Platelet counts are measured by automated systems on whole-blood samples. The range of normal for platelet counts is typically 150,000–400,000/μL. Platelet counts, however, do not assess the functional capacity of the available platelets. The bleeding time (BT) and the closure time (CT) of the platelet function analyzer (PFA-100, Siemens Diagnostics, Marburg, Germany) have been developed for this purpose. The BT was described in 1910 as "a method for studying hemorrhage" [28] and attempted to assess primary hemostasis *in vivo*. The BT is performed by making a skin cut on the volar surface of the patient's forearm [29] and standardization is attempted by using commercially available spring-loaded devices to make the skin incision and by maintaining a constant forearm venous pressure of 40 mmHg using a sphygmomanometer cuff [30]. Typical reference ranges for BT are 6–11 min [30]. The BT is operator dependent [27], is not a useful predictor of hemorrhage risk with surgery in the absence of a bleeding history, and a normal value cannot exclude the possibility of excessive hemorrhage with invasive procedures [29]. Furthermore, the BT is a poor diagnostic and prognostic test for vWD [31] and does not reliably identify platelet dysfunction produced by aspirin or nonsteroidal anti-inflammatory drug (NSAID) use [29]. For these reasons, the BT has largely been replaced with *in vitro* tests such as the PFA.

In the PFA, whole blood is aspirated at high shear rates across an aperture cut in a membrane coated with collagen and either ADP or epinephrine. The collagen, along with the high shear rates employed and the patient's level of vWF, causes platelet adhesion to the membrane while the ADP or epinephrine stimulates platelet aggregation. Closure time, the amount of time required for a platelet plug to form and occlude the aperture in the membrane, is measured and is dependent on platelet number and function as well as on functional vWF. Thus, the PFA is a better screening test than the BT for vWD [32]. Normal CTs in children are 91 ± 13 sec for ADP cartridges and 117 ± 23 sec for epinephrine cartridges and these values are similar to those found in adults. Neonates have shorter CTs (56 ± 6 sec for ADP cartridges and 81 ± 17 sec for epinephrine cartridges), probably because of their elevated levels of vWF or presence of the larger, more hemostatically active multimers of vWF [32,33]. The CT is prolonged in patients with platelet counts below 50,000/µL or hematocrits below 25% and in patients with severe platelet dysfunction (Bernard–Soulier syndrome (Gp Ib receptor defect) and Glanzmann thrombasthenia (Gp IIb/IIIa receptor defect)), and severe vWD (types 2 and 3). CT is also prolonged by aspirin, NSAID or Gp IIb/IIIa inhibitor use [27,30,34]. The most reliable use of the PFA is in patients with severe bleeding where a normal CT excludes quantitative deficiencies of platelets or vWF, severe platelet function disorders, and severe vWD [30,35]. However, the PFA has a low sensitivity as a screening test for platelet function defects so its usefulness as a preoperative screening tool is questionable [35].

While abnormal results of BT or PFA-100 CT indicate a problem in primary hemostasis, definitive investigation and identification of the specific problem are accomplished by sophisticated tests such as platelet aggregometry, platelet secretion assays, and platelet flow cytometry. Platelet aggregometry is considered the gold standard for global platelet function testing. Platelet secretion assays use highly technical methodology to measure the release of substances from platelet granules. Platelet flow cytometry uses monoclonal antibodies to diagnose defects in platelet surface glycoproteins (Bernard–Soulier syndrome and Glanzmann thrombasthenia) [34]. Appropriate use of these tests requires extensive expertise in diagnosing hemostatic disorders and thus should be under the guidance of a hematologist.

Quantification of vWF levels (vWF:Ag) is obtained from plasma samples using an enzyme-linked immunosorbent assay (ELISA), a latex immunoassay or the Laurell immunoelectrophoretic assay [36,37]. The accepted standard for measuring functional vWF activity is the ristocetin co-factor assay (vWF:RCo). The antibiotic ristocetin induces the binding of vWF to the adhesive Gp Ib receptor on platelets. Therefore, addition of ristocetin to a mixture of patient plasma and formalin-fixed normal platelets should induce platelet agglutination that can be detected by aggregometry. The extent of platelet agglutination is proportional to the functional activity of vWF in the patient's plasma [37].

Evaluation of secondary hemostasis

Evaluation of secondary hemostasis involves examining the steps in thrombin generation and fibrin formation. Available tests include quantitative measurements of coagulation factor levels and analyses of the interactions of these factors in the coagulation process.

Measurement of fibrinogen level is the most common quantitative test performed. In the most commonly used measurement method, the sample plasma is diluted 10-fold and excess thrombin is added. Time to clot formation is then measured. The 10-fold plasma dilution ensures that the amount of fibrinogen remaining in the sample is the rate-limiting step in clotting. Time to clot formation is thus inversely related to fibrinogen concentration and, therefore, a fibrinogen level can be derived. Fibrin degradation products or other inhibitors of fibrin formation can cause artificially low results but, since excess thrombin is added to the test plasma, small amounts of heparin do not interfere with the results [38]. Normal values for fibrinogen level range between 150 and 400 mg/dL.

The interactions of coagulation factors are commonly measured with the PT, aPTT, and TT. The PT is classically used to examine the factors involved in the "extrinsic" and common pathways of coagulation and thus is sensitive to factors VII, X, V, II (thrombin), and I (fibrinogen) (Fig. 11.8). Thromboplastin, a mixture of TF, phospholipids, and calcium, is used to initiate coagulation. Changes in optical density of the plasma are then used to detect and time the formation of clot. The PT is expressed in seconds (usual range 10–14 sec) but the result will vary depending on the potency of the thromboplastin preparation used to initiate coagulation. Each batch of thromboplastin is assigned an International Sensitivity Index (ISI) value by its manufacturer which ranges from 1.0 to 2.0 based on comparison to an International Reference

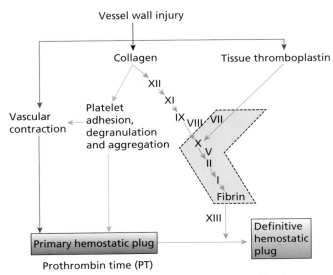

Figure 11.8 Portion of the coagulation cascade examined by the prothrombin time (PT). Reproduced from Bleyer et al [11] with permission from Elsevier.

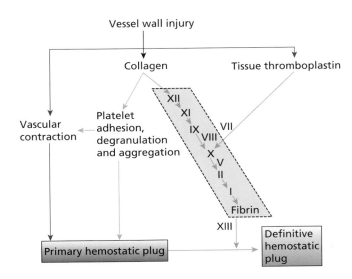

Figure 11.9 Portion of the coagulation cascade examined by the activated partial thromboplastin time (aPTT). Reproduced from Bleyer et al [11] with permission from Elsevier.

Preparation. An international normalized ratio (INR) is then obtained by the following formula: INR = (PT$_{test}$/PT$_{normal}$)^{ISI}. The INR thus allows a more accurate comparison of PT values [38]. Falsely prolonged PT values can be seen when too little sample is drawn or when too little plasma is available in a given sample (such as in polycythemic patients). The PT is useful in the detection of coagulation defects due to vitamin K deficiency, intestinal malabsorption, hepatic failure, dilutional or consumptive coagulopathies, and isolated deficiencies of the factors noted above, especially factor VII. Anticoagulation with oral vitamin K antagonists (warfarin) is monitored using the PT and INR [27].

The aPTT is described as a test to evaluate the "intrinsic" and common coagulation pathways (Fig. 11.9). Only the phospholipid part of thromboplastin is used to activate factor XII, hence the term "partial thromboplastin" time, and coagulation is accelerated for this test using an activator (celite, kaolin, silica or ellagic acid), hence the term "activated" PTT. The normal range for the aPTT is 21–35 sec but this range varies from laboratory to laboratory. The aPTT is prolonged by deficiencies of the contact coagulation factors (XII, XI, HMWK, and PK), factors VIII and IX, and factors of the common pathway (X, V, II (thrombin), and I (fibrinogen)). It is also prolonged in the presence of heparin, inadequate sample (or inadequate plasma), and lupus anticoagulants.

Lupus anticoagulants belong to the broad family of antiphospholipid antibodies and were initially thought to occur exclusively in patients with autoimmune disorders. However, they are now known to occur in up to 1% of the normal population. They inhibit the proper assembly of lipid-dependent coagulation complexes such as the factor VIIIa/IXa tenase complex and the factor Xa/Va prothrombinase complex. While their presence is probably the most common cause of a prolonged aPTT [39], they do not increase the risk of bleeding. In fact, their predominant clinical manifestation is the development of thrombosis secondary to their effect on platelet–endothelial interactions and their interference with protein C and protein S activity. Initial differentiation of a prolonged aPTT may be made by using a 50:50 mixture of the plasma being tested and normal plasma. Subsequent correction of the aPTT indicates a factor deficiency whereas ongoing prolongation suggests the presence of an inhibitor such as heparin, lupus anticoagulants or a coagulation factor-specific inhibitor [27,38]. Immediate correction followed by prolongation at 1 h may indicate a FVIII inhibitor. If heparin contamination is responsible for prolongation of the aPTT, treatment of the sample with hepzyme (an enzyme that neutralizes heparin) should correct the value.

Activity levels of most individual coagulation factors can be obtained by using the PT or aPTT to measure clotting in mixtures of patient plasma and commercially available plasma known to be deficient in the specific coagulation factor being assayed. The observed clotting times are proportional to the amount of the specific factor in the patient plasma and are then converted into units of factor activity using a reference curve constructed from the control plasma. PT-based assays are used to measure activity levels of factors II, V, VII, and X while aPTT-based assays are used for measurement of activity levels of factors VIII, IX, XI, and XII and of HMWK

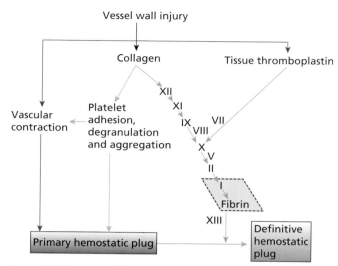

Figure 11.10 Portion of the coagulation cascade examined by the thrombin time (TT). Reproduced from Bleyer et al [11] with permission from Elsevier.

and PK. Factor antigen levels may be detected with immunological methods, including monoclonal antibodies. However, factor activity assays are typically most clinically relevant. FXIII function cannot be tested by the PT or aPTT but may be screened using 5M urea clot stability testing.

The TT is the time required for the conversion of fibrinogen to fibrin after a patient's plasma is exposed to exogenous thrombin (Fig. 11.10). The reference range for the TT is typically 10–15 sec. The TT is prolonged in the presence of heparin, antibodies to thrombin, hypofibrinogenemia, dysfibrinogenemia, fibrin degradation products, lupus anticoagulants, and amyloidosis [38]. In the presence of heparin, the TT can be modified to assess fibrin formation by using reptilase, a substance derived from snake venom. Reptilase, like thrombin, will stimulate the conversion of fibrinogen to fibrin but, unlike thrombin, it is not inhibited by heparin. The TT can also be prolonged by thrombolytic therapy since the action of these drugs decreases circulating levels of fibrinogen and fibrin.

Evaluation of fibrinolysis

The occurrence of fibrinolysis can be determined either by measuring the endproducts of fibrin degradation or by directly measuring clot lysis by viscoelastic tests [38]. When fibrinolysis occurs in response to the activation of the coagulation system, plasmin degrades the resulting fibrin clots into fibrin degradation products including D-dimers, a breakdown product composed of two of the "D" fragments of fibrin cross-linked together [40]. When plasmin is activated in the absence of coagulation activation, as may occur during liver transplantation or exog-

enous administration of tPA, fibrinogen is broken down into various fibrinogen degradation products (X, Y, D, and E fragments but mostly non-clotted X fragments) [38,41]. The presence of D-dimers thus specifically indicates the breakdown of FXIII cross-linked fibrin, as may be seen with disseminated intravascular coagulation (DIC), so the presence of D-dimers may indicate a pathological condition that can cause organ damage [42]. Assays for fibrin and fibrinogen degradation products and for D-dimers can be performed by automated methods, by ELISA or by mixing serial dilutions of the patient's plasma with antibody-coated latex beads and observing for the subsequent agglutination [39]. Assays for fibrin and fibrinogen degradation products are usually performed in reference laboratories while D-dimer assays can be performed in many hospital laboratories.

Viscoelastic tests assess hemostasis from clot formation to clot retraction and lysis [43]. These tests can identify both hypercoagulable and hypocoagulable scenarios as well as the occurrence of fibrinolysis. Thromboelastography (TEG®), rotational thromboelastography (ROTEM®), and Sonoclot® are the available viscoelastic tests. Some advantages of these tests are that they are performed on small samples of whole blood, not only making testing technically simpler but also allowing interactions between platelets, red blood cells, and coagulation factors to be taken into account. These tests can be performed in the operating room at the patient's bedside and, with the use of specific coagulation activators, can provide very rapid results that can be used to immediately influence patient care [44]. With the use of certain modifiers, the contributions of platelets and fibrinogen to the clotting process also can be assessed [45,46]. Additionally, the effects of coagulation product transfusions [25], recombinant factor VIIa [47,48], antifibrinolytics, antiplatelet therapies [49] and direct thrombin inhibitors [50] can all be monitored with modifications of these tests. These tests have proven very useful in managing the coagulation problems associated with liver transplantation and cardiac surgery [25,51,52] and have been used to develop algorithms to guide post-cardiopulmonary bypass (CBP) transfusion therapy [53,54]. Drawbacks to these tests include difficulty in standardization and the need for special training for clinicians to perform these tests and interpret their results. An additional concern is that the contribution of blood vessel endothelium is not considered by these tests because they are performed in an *in vitro* cuvette at low shear stresses [55].

Use of laboratory tests

Coagulation tests typically have been used to screen patients preoperatively in an attempt to predict perioperative bleeding problems. The rationale for obtaining preoperative coagulation tests in patients with significant systemic illnesses and in those undergoing procedures such as liver transplantation or cardiac surgery is straightforward and understandable. However, obtaining preoperative coagulation tests routinely on healthy patients who are undergoing routine procedures and have no history or physical signs to suggest an underlying bleeding diathesis is controversial. The main reason for obtaining screening tests in this population is to detect previously undiagnosed inherited bleeding disorders such as vWD or hemophilia [56]. However, because of the infrequent occurrence of these disorders [56,57], the routine use of coagulation tests for preoperative screening in the absence of a significant bleeding history seems unjustified from an economic standpoint [56]. Furthermore, the tests used for preoperative screening of patients (platelet count, BT, PFA, PT, aPTT) do not provide data that reliably predict perioperative bleeding [58]. Limitations of the platelet count, BT, and PFA in screening for defects of primary hemostasis have already been described. The PT screens only the "extrinsic" coagulation pathway and thus will not detect either type of hemophilia. Finally, the aPTT has not been found to predict postoperative bleeding in patients with no clinical indicators of bleeding problems [59].

The use of preoperative screening coagulation tests has been intensely scrutinized in children undergoing tonsillectomy and adenoidectomy (T&A). Approximately 2–4% of patients undergoing this surgery experience postoperative hemorrhagic complications [60,61]. These children are usually otherwise healthy and this surgery is often a child's first significant hemostatic challenge. Results from many studies have shown no ability of the PT or aPTT to predict which children will bleed postoperatively [56,60–62]. Additionally, there are a large number of initially abnormal routine tests that return to normal on retesting, thus causing unnecessary concern for parents, unnecessary delays in surgery, and increased costs [63,64]. Findings such as these have led some authors to state that in the absence of suspicions raised from a patient's history or physical exam, preoperative laboratory screening contributes little to patient care and should not be done [56,63,65–68]. Indeed, the practice advisory published by the American Society of Anesthesiologists on preanesthesia evaluation discourages the use of preoperative laboratory testing in asymptomatic patients unless indicated by findings on history or physical exam [69]. Additionally, the American Academy of Otolaryngology, Head and Neck Surgery recommends performing coagulation studies only in those patients undergoing T&A whose medical histories or physical exams may indicate coagulation problems [70].

Preoperative evaluation of the coagulation system should, therefore, start with a pertinent history and physical examination. A sample of questions to ask parents

---

Box 11.1 Questions regarding bleeding history

- Does your child have trouble with any of the following:
  - Easy bruising (larger than 2 inches)?
  - Gum bleeding with tooth brushing?
  - Frequent nose bleeds?
  - Oozing a long time from cuts or scrapes?
  - Abnormally heavy menstrual periods?
  - Bleeding into joints or muscles?
- Has your child had trouble with bleeding after:
  - Loss of teeth or dental extractions?
  - Previous surgery (including circumcision)?
  - Previous injuries?
  - When his/her umbilical cord came off?
- Is your child taking:
  - Antihistamines?
  - Aspirin?
  - Ibuprofen or other non-steroidal anti-inflammatory drugs?
  - Other over-the-counter medicines for headaches, colds or menstrual cramps?
- Does your child take any prescribed medicines or have any chronic medical problems requiring a doctor's ongoing care?
- Has your child ever received a blood transfusion?
- Is there a family history of easy bruising or unusual bleeding after surgeries, injuries or childbirth?
- Does anyone in your family have hemophilia, von Willebrand disease, low platelets or any other blood disorder?

---

and older children is outlined in Box 11.1 [56,71,72]. Pertinent findings on physical exam include petechiae, purpura, and ecchymoses with no antecedent injury [71,73]. Clinicians must always be aware, though, that the accuracy of histories and physical exams depends on the clinician performing them and the parent and/or child answering the questions. The ability of parents and children to understand and answer medically related questions appropriately may be lacking, memories and interpretations of previous events may not be perfect or accurate, family histories may be overinterpreted, knowledge of a child's personal or family history by foster or adoptive parents may be deficient, ingestion of medications may be forgotten, and exams may be incomplete [71,72]. Additionally, negative family histories may occur in up to 40% of cases of inheritable bleeding disorders because of spontaneous mutations or variable expression of the disorders in relatives. Also, young children may not have experienced an injury, undergone previous surgery or have had other experiences that would allow a bleeding problem to be revealed [64,71].

Currently, the opinion of most authorities remains that preoperative laboratory tests should only be obtained in the face of indicative histories and/or physical exams. However, one's clinical experience and judgment must be applied to the content and quality of the information obtained from the history and physical exam to make final decisions about obtaining preoperative laboratory tests.

In cases of active bleeding, quantitative assessments of platelet counts and fibrinogen levels and qualitative assessments of clotting with PT and aPTT have limitations. First, there are few agreed-upon absolute values at which transfusion of blood components is indicated. Second, these tests are usually done in a central lab with a relatively long turnaround time. Therefore, by the time results are obtained, the clinical picture may have changed. With advances in technology, point-of-care tests have been developed and allow results to be available to the bedside clinician significantly faster. Platelet counts, fibrinogen levels, PT, aPTT, and TT can all be obtained with this methodology but the accuracy and validation of these against conventional laboratory tests await confirmation [27]. The viscoelastic tests (TEG®, ROTEM®, and Sonoclot®) can also provide immediate data to clinicians and have been extensively studied as aids to manage post-CPB bleeding in children [25,74].

While the use of point-of-care tests ameliorates the timeliness problem, absolute trigger values that dictate intervention are still lacking. Therefore, transfusion decisions still are heavily influenced by the clinical situation and the appearance of the operative field (and the opinions of those observing it!) while coagulation tests are used to monitor trends in the coagulation status as therapy is administered.

Congenital hematological disorders

Congenital disorders of hemostasis can present major perioperative management challenges to anesthesiologists that extend well beyond the time when the patient is anesthetized in the operating room. Knowledge of the more common of these disorders will allow intelligent conversations with hematologists and surgeons in preparing to provide appropriate care to affected children.

Von Willebrand disease

Von Willebrand disease (vWD) is an inherited hemorrhagic disorder caused by quantitative or qualitative abnormalities in von Willebrand factor (vWF) [37,75,76]. It is the most common inherited bleeding problem, occurring in up to 2% of the population. However, its true incidence is difficult to establish because its highly heterogeneous nature and variable expression leave many cases undetected or undiagnosed. vWF serves two roles. It promotes the formation of a platelet plug during primary hemostasis by binding to components of exposed subendothelium and to platelet Gp Ib receptors, thus causing platelet adhesion to an injured blood vessel wall.

It also acts as a carrier protein for coagulation factor VIII, thus preventing the rapid clearance of FVIII from the circulation. vWF is synthesized in endothelial cells and megakaryocytes in a precursor form that is cleaved into monomers which are then assembled into multimers through disulfide-linked bonds. The larger multimers are necessary to promote platelet adhesion to injured vessels. vWF is stored in the Weibel–Palade bodies of endothelial cells and in the α-granules of platelets.

The inheritance of vWD follows an autosomal pattern, with the vWF gene located on chromosome 12. Three major types of vWD are generally identified. Type 1 is characterized by decreased amounts of vWF that otherwise is normal in structure and function. This type accounts for 70–80% of the cases of vWD and is inherited as an autosomal dominant trait. When interpreting vWF levels, however, it must be remembered that people with type O blood have mean vWF levels that are only approximately 75% of that seen in people with other blood types. Type 2 is caused by various qualitative defects in vWF, especially in the larger multimers, where there is failure of multimer assembly or increased proteolysis of mutant multimers (2A), increased binding of abnormal large multimers to the Gp Ib receptors of circulating platelets not actively involved in primary hemostasis (2B), decreased binding of vWF to platelets because of an abnormal vWF binding site for platelet Gp Ib receptors (2M), or an abnormal vWF binding site for FVIII leading to increased clearance of free FVIII with subsequent decreased plasma levels (2N). Type 3 is the most severe form of vWD and is characterized by a complete absence of vWF and an autosomal recessive or compound heterozygous inheritance. Finally, a "platelet-type" or "pseudo" vWD has been described where abnormal platelets demonstrate an enhanced affinity for normal vWF. This type of vWD, as well as type 2B, results in varying degrees of thrombocytopenia and the absence of large multimers of vWF in plasma due to spontaneous *in vivo* binding of vWF and platelets with subsequent consumption of the large multimers and platelets.

Clinical manifestations of types 1 and 2 vWD are typically relatively mild and are mostly those of mucous membrane bleeding: epistaxis, gingival bleeding, gastrointestinal bleeding, menorrhagia, excessive postpartum bleeding, cutaneous bleeding, easy bruising, and excessive bleeding after dental extractions, tonsillectomy and adenoidectomy, or minor surgeries or traumas. Type 3 vWD, however, can lead to the hemarthroses and muscular hematomas commonly seen with hemophilia and even to intracranial bleeding.

Screening tests for vWD, including aPTT, BT, and PFA, lack sensitivity and specificity so assays of vWF quantity, function, and structure are required for definitive diagnosis. Measurement of vWF:Ag determines vWF levels and measurement of vWF:RCo assesses vWF function. The "ristocetin-induced platelet aggregation assay" (RIPA) uses lower doses of ristocetin than are used in the vWF:RCo assay to detect the hyper-responsive binding of vWF to platelets that is seen in type 2B and platelet-type vWD. Electrophoresis is used to determine the structure of the vWF multimers present in a patient's plasma in order to help differentiate the subtypes of type 2 vWD. Finally, it may be useful to measure FVIII activity levels since significantly decreased levels are seen in types 2N and 3 vWD. Repeated testing may be required to establish the diagnosis of vWD because the results of these tests can vary considerably from time to time in individuals with vWD [77] and are influenced by factors such as stress (as may be induced while obtaining these tests in children!) and inflammation.

The goals of treatment of vWD are to restore the normal platelet adhesion of primary hemostasis and to increase abnormally low levels of FVIII. vWF:RCo and FVIII:C levels of 40–50% are considered sufficient for minor surgery or bleeding or for tooth extractions. Levels of 80–100% are desired for major surgery or life-threatening hemorrhage with maintenance of levels greater than 50% for at least 3 days for vWF:RCo and for 5–7 days for FVIII:C. DDAVP (desmopressin), a synthetic vasopressin analog, releases vWF from endothelial cells and platelets and increases plasma levels of vWF and FVIII. It is effective in treating patients with type 1 vWD. It will also restore plasma levels of FVIII and vWF in many patients with type 2 vWD but the vWF will still be qualitatively deficient so primary hemostasis may continue to be abnormal. However, DDAVP is contraindicated in type 2B and platelet-type vWD since the release of vWF will exacerbate the thrombocytopenia common to these conditions. DDAVP can be given intravenously at a dose of $0.3\,\mu g/kg$ bodyweight or intranasally at a dose of $150\,\mu g$ (one puff) for children weighing less than $50\,kg$ and $300\,\mu g$ (two puffs) for those weighing more than $50\,kg$. Problems with water retention may be encountered so fluid restriction is recommended for $24\,h$ following DDAVP dosing. Tachyphylaxis may also develop with repeat dosing. A trial dose of DDAVP with measurement of the subsequent vWF:RCo response is recommended before a child with vWD encounters a hemostatic challenge in order to guide its use. Replacement of vWF and FVIII may be required perioperatively in patients with type 3 vWD and in those with type 2 vWD who do not respond to DDAVP.

Several plasma-derived FVIII concentrates are commercially available and carry minimal risk of viral transmission. However, only one, Humate-P® (CSL Behring, Marburg, Germany), is licensed by the FDA for use in treating vWD since it is the only product that contains adequate amounts of the larger vWF multimers. Cryoprecipitate contains both vWF and FVIII so may be useful in instances where Humate-P is not available. Finally, antifibrinolytics can be used as an adjunct therapy, especially with bleeding from oral and nasal mucous membranes, to prevent clot lysis after hemostasis has been achieved by DDAVP, replacement therapy or local measures [37,75,76]. Antifibrinolytics are typically given for 3–7 days following surgical procedures in patients with vWD. It is obvious that the management of a child with vWD who is undergoing a surgical procedure must involve consultation with a hematologist, ideally at least a month prior to scheduled surgery, to allow time for appropriate testing and treatment planning.

Hemophilia

Two types of hemophilia are typically discussed: hemophilia A (classic hemophilia) results from a deficiency of FVIII while hemophilia B (Christmas disease) results from a deficiency of FIX. Bleeding occurs in patients with either type of hemophilia because adequate amounts of thrombin cannot be generated since the factor VIIIa/IXa "tenase" complex cannot be formed on activated platelets. Both types of hemophilia usually are transmitted as X-linked recessive traits; therefore, most affected patients are males. However, approximately 30% of patients with hemophilia have negative family histories and appear to be affected by spontaneous mutations. Multiple gene mutations have been described as causing each of these diseases. Hemophilia A occurs more frequently than hemophilia B (1 in 10,000 versus 1 in 60,000 people). Classification of both types of hemophilia is based on levels of FVIII or FIX activity and is described as severe (levels < 1%), moderate (levels 1–5%) or mild (levels >5–40%) [78,79].

The clinical manifestations of hemophilia are those of delayed bleeding that particularly involves joints and muscles or occurs with surgery or other injuries. This is in contrast to the immediate bleeding most commonly involving mucocutaneous surfaces seen in vWD. This difference is due to interference with primary hemostasis in vWD versus interference with secondary hemostasis in hemophilia. The severity of bleeding in hemophilia is determined by the severity of clotting factor deficiency and manifests as bleeding after surgery or trauma in mild and moderate disease and as spontaneous bleeding in severe disease. In neonates, bleeding occurs after heel-sticks, injections, and circumcision. Therefore, boys born to mothers known to be carriers of hemophilia should not be circumcised until it has been determined that they do not have the disease.

As children grow older, excessive bruising, mouth bleeding after tooth loss, muscle hematomas, joint hemorrhages, and even intracranial bleeding may become evident. One of the more debilitating problems encountered by affected children is the development of a progressive arthropathy in a "target joint." A target joint is one in which recurrent bleeding has occurred at least four times in 6 months or 20 total times. Iron from the blood extravasated into the joint accumulates in synovial cells, triggers inflammation, and results in the proliferation of friable synovial villi. This predisposes to further intra-articular bleeding and joint damage. In severe cases, these synovial villi may require arthroscopic removal or radio-active sclerosis.

The diagnosis of hemophilia is made by demonstrating low plasma activity levels of FVIII or FIX. Screening tests such as the aPTT are not consistent, sensitive or specific enough to be useful as diagnostic tools. Results of factor assays are expressed as "% activity" with one unit of factor per mL of plasma being equivalent to 1% activity. In families with a history of hemophilia, newborns can be diagnosed by testing plasma from cord blood, and fetal diagnosis can even be made as early as 20 weeks gestation.

Treatment of hemophilia focuses on factor replacement, typically with recombinant or plasma-derived FVIII or FIX. These products currently undergo multiple viral and pathogen inactivation steps, thus virtually eliminating infectious complications of HIV, hepatitis B or hepatitis C. Historically, cryoprecipitate was used to treat hemophilia A, with fresh frozen plasma used at times as well. However, large infusion volumes and infectious disease risks have made these therapies essentially obsolete in the United States.

Factor replacement therapy can be administered prophylactically or "on demand." Prophylactic therapy may be given 1–4 times per week to prevent bleeding. "On-demand" therapy is used to treat acute bleeding episodes, with the desired plasma factor level depending on the location and severity of the bleeding. A minimum level of 40% should be targeted for minor oral, nasal or urinary tract bleeding and should be maintained for several days. For bleeding in more critical anatomical areas such as the brain, retropharynx or target joints and for severe bleeding in the gastrointestinal tract or muscle, levels of 80–100% should be achieved and then maintained for 3–14 days (depending on the severity of bleeding). When replacing FVIII, 1 unit/kg of replacement product will increase plasma levels of FVIII by 2%. The average half-life of the products is 12h. For FIX, 1 unit/kg of replacement product will increase plasma levels of FIX by 1% with an average half-life of 20–24h.

A complication of treatment with factor replacement is the development of inhibitory antibodies to FVIII (or, more rarely, to FIX). Inhibitors develop in up to 20–30% of patients with hemophilia A and can make treatment quite complicated [79,80]. The titer of inhibitory antibodies is expressed in Bethesda units (BU), with one BU denoting the level of antibody that decreases the plasma factor level by 50%, and in logarithmic fashion. Elimination of these antibodies by immune tolerance induction therapy, where large and frequent (usually daily) doses of FVIII or FIX are administered with or without immunosuppressants, is successful in approximately 70% of these patients. Bleeding in the setting of high-titer inhibitors typically requires treatment with either high doses of recombinant FVIIa or with activated prothrombin complex concentrates [78,79,81].

Desmopressin may be useful in minor bleeding in patients with mild hemophilia A since it releases FVIII from endothelial cells and platelets. It will not be effective as a sole treatment with severe bleeding. As with vWD, the usefulness of DDAVP should be explored by documenting its effect on FVIII levels before depending on it to help treat bleeding. Antifibrinolytics may be helpful in preventing clot lysis after factor replacement has helped clotting to occur, especially after oral, intraocular or gastrointestinal bleeding. As is the case with managing a child with vWD, the expert help of a hematologist is crucial in providing the best perioperative care to children with hemophilia.

Thrombophilias

The thrombophilias are coagulation abnormalities which predispose to the development of thromboembolic events [82]. Many thrombophilic abnormalities are inherited, including deficiencies of natural anticoagulants (AT, protein C, and protein S), factor V Leiden mutation, prothrombin G20210A mutation, and hyperhomocysteinemia. While inherited deficiencies of AT, protein C, and protein S are the least common of these abnormalities, they result in the highest potential for thrombosis since their absence leaves the stimulated coagulation system unregulated and unchecked. Factor V Leiden results from a mutation in the FV gene that makes the mutant FV resistant to inactivation by activated protein C, thus allowing its persistent activity and an increased risk for thrombosis. The prothrombin G20210A mutation results from a glutamine-to-arginine transition at position 20,210 of the 3′ untranslated region of the prothrombin gene and leads to the production of increased levels of prothrombin with a subsequent increase in thrombin generation. Hyperhomocysteinemia results from a mutation in the gene coding for methylenetetrahydrofolate reductase which leads to an increased production of homocysteine with resultant endothelial cell damage [82–86].

Other thrombophilic abnormalities can be acquired, the most common of these being the presence of antiphospholipid antibodies such as anticardiolipin antibodies or the lupus anticoagulant. The lupus anticoagulant may be found in patients with autoimmune disorders such as systemic lupus erythematosus or in patients with malignancies or viral infections. The name is not accurate given that it is not exclusively associated with systemic lupus erythematosus nor is it truly an anticoagulant. Antiphospholipid antibodies may react with multiple components of the coagulation system and lead to alteration of platelet–endothelial interactions and inhibition of the protein C/protein S system that predispose patients to recurrent thrombotic events as well as recurrent fetal loss due to placental vascular insufficiency [82,86–88].

Although the presence of intrinsic prothrombotic abnormalities may set the stage for thrombosis, the imposition of additional clinical risk factors is usually necessary to cause thrombosis in children. The use of central venous lines is the most common thrombosis trigger in children with thrombophilia. Catheter-associated risk factors include the use of large-bore catheters, the use of percutaneously placed versus embedded catheters, location of the catheter tip in the right atrium, insertion in femoral or subclavian versus jugular veins, and the expertise of the physician placing the catheter. The use of heparin-coated catheters decreases thrombotic problems and the use of antibiotic-impregnated catheters decreases infective complications of thromboses. Other triggers include underlying medical conditions, most commonly systemic infection and cancer. Surgery, trauma, immobilization, autoimmune inflammatory diseases, congenital heart disease, vascular malformations, use of estrogen-containing oral contraceptives, and pregnancy may also play a similar role [83–86].

The frequent use of central venous catheters in neonates and infants, advances in medical care that allow the survival of children with chronic medical conditions, and improved diagnostic modalities for thrombosis are increasing the occurrence and recognition of thrombosis as well as the awareness of thrombophilia in children [84]. Peak incidences of thrombosis occur in neonates because of the use of central lines and the frequent existence of clinical risk factors and in adolescents with the onset of autoimmune inflammatory diseases and the use of oral contraceptives. Even in these two age groups, though, thrombosis still occurs significantly less frequently in thrombophilic children than in adults [82,84].

Non-invasive techniques used to diagnose thromboses include Doppler ultrasonography, echocardiography, computed tomography (CT) venography, and magnetic resonance (MR) venography. However, these techniques lack sensitivity and angiography of involved veins may be required for diagnosis. Treatment options for identified thrombi include observation without intervention, anticoagulation, thrombolytic therapy, and surgical thrombectomy, with ultimate decisions based on thrombus location, potential for future complications, and current clinical signs. Unfractionated heparin, low molecular weight heparin, warfarin, aspirin, and tPA are all available for use. While the optimal drug, dosage of that

drug, and duration of therapy for children with thrombosis have not been definitively established, recommendations have been outlined by several authors [84,89]. Regardless of the therapy employed, close monitoring of the thrombus for extension or regression and the input of a knowledgeable hematologist to help diagnose and manage thrombophilic children after a thrombotic complication are important.

Sickle cell disease

Hemoglobin molecules are composed of two pairs of globin chains, each possessing an Fe^{+2}-containing heme group. Hemoglobin A, composed of two α and two β chains, accounts for 95% of normal adult hemoglobin. Hemoglobin S contains abnormal β chains resulting from the substitution of the amino acid valine for glutamic acid in the sixth position of the 146-amino acid β chain. The alleles coding for the β chain are co-dominant so a person who is heterozygous for the normal and the sickle β chains produces both hemoglobins A and S. This predominantly benign carrier state, termed sickle cell trait (SCT), is found in more than 8% of African-Americans [90] and is felt to have persisted in this population because it offers protection from the fatal complications of *Plasmodium falciparum* malaria [91].

Homozygotes for the sickle β chain produce only hemoglobin S. This condition, termed hemoglobin SS disease, may be associated with significant clinical manifestations [92,93]. Hemoglobin S can also combine with hemoglobin C (Hb SC disease), abnormal β globin chains (HbSβ^0 or HbSβ^+ thalassemia) or other hemoglobin variants. The term sickle cell disease (SCD) encompasses all of these related abnormalities. HbSβ^0 thalassemia is a disease similar to HbSS disease, while HbSC and HbSβ^+ thalassemia typically are associated with milder disease. Hemoglobinopathies can be diagnosed by hemoglobin electrophoresis or high performance liquid chromatography. Patients with SCT as well as those with SCD will have a positive sickle dex screen. Currently, newborns in the United States are screened for SCD shortly after birth.

The pathophysiological consequences of hemoglobin S relate to it being less stable and less soluble than hemoglobin A as a result of altered electrical charge of the hemoglobin molecule. The decreased stability of hemoglobin S results in its accelerated denaturation and breakdown, leading to red blood cell (RBC) membrane damage and RBC rigidity. These rigid RBCs adhere to and damage endothelial cells, causing a chronic vascular inflammation. The decreased solubility of hemoglobin S leads to its rapid precipitation out of solution into long polymer strands when it is deoxygenated. This results in the characteristic deformation of RBCs into a sickled shape. Both vascular endothelial dysfunction and sickled RBCs play roles in the pathophysiology of SCD [93].

Intermittent painful vaso-occlusive crises are the clinical hallmark of SCD. Infection and surgical stress are frequent initiators although a triggering event is not found in over half of these crises. Activation of vascular endothelium and of inflammatory and coagulation systems leads to vaso-occlusion, trapping of RBCs, which subsequently deoxygenate and sickle, and ultimately ischemia, bone and organ infarctions, and pain. This often initially manifests in young children as dactylitis or painful swelling of the hands and feet. Management includes aggressive pain control with acetaminophen, NSAIDs, opioids, and possibly regional anesthetic techniques. Guidelines for pain management in children with SCD are available from the American Pain Society [94].

Acute chest syndrome (ACS) is another complication of SCD and is a leading cause of death. ACS is defined as a new pulmonary infiltrate in combination with fever, chest pain or respiratory symptoms. Etiologies include infections and fat emboli from necrotic bone marrow. Treatment includes the administration of a broad-spectrum antibiotic, the use of incentive spirometry, supplemental oxygen if hypoxia is present, and bronchodilators, adequate hydration and pain management, and transfusion if improvement is not achieved by initial interventions. Repeated episodes of ACS often lead to chronic lung injury.

Neurological complications, including transient ischemic attacks and stroke, are common with Hb SS disease. In instances of cerebral ischemic infarctions, emergency exchange transfusion to reduce the level of circulating hemoglobin S to less than 30% may be undertaken upon presentation. Chronic transfusion regimens are then useful to prevent recurrences.

Renal and genitourinary problems such as papillary necrosis, hyposthenuria, and enuresis can also occur in SCD. Priapism is a medical emergency and is treated with aggressive hydration, pain control, and possibly direct injection of α agonists into the corpora cavernosa. Avascular necrosis of the femoral and humeral heads, retinopathy, and cholelithiasis/cholecystitis are other complications of SCD. Finally, while some degree of baseline anemia is present in all patients with SCD, acute decreases in hemoglobin levels can be caused by splenic sequestration or aplastic crises. Splenic sequestration may occur in association with a viral illness and may result in hypovolemia and even shock. Treatment involves fluid resuscitation, potentially including RBC transfusion. A splenectomy may be indicated for recurrent episodes. Aplastic crises are usually the result of a parvovirus infection and may also result in the need for RBC transfusion [92,93,95].

The complications of SCD may necessitate a variety of surgical interventions. Cholecystectomy is the most frequently performed procedure. Splenectomy and orthopedic, neurosurgical, cardiac, and obstetric procedures are also commonly undertaken. Preoperatively, identification of the current activity and level of severity of the patient's SCD is important. Manifestations of chronic organ system dysfunction and evidence of active infection should be sought. Useful preoperative laboratory tests include hemoglobin and hematocrit, blood urea nitrogen (BUN) and creatinine, and a chest x-ray (CXR) [93]. Prophylactic preoperative RBC transfusions have been shown to decrease the incidence of perioperative complications by diluting the abnormal RBCs with normal ones. Aggressive transfusion regimens aim to decrease the hemoglobin S concentration to less than 30% while conservative regimens aim to increase the hemoglobin level to 10 g/dL without concern for hemoglobin S concentrations. The conservative regimen has been found to be as effective as the aggressive approach in preventing perioperative SCD-associated complications while significantly decreasing the number of RBC units transfused and the number of transfusion-associated complications [96]. This approach is currently recommended by the US National Institutes of Health [97]. Preoperative transfusion may be foregone in children undergoing minor superficial elective surgical procedures but is important prior to major surgical procedures (including thoracotomies, laparotomies, orthopedic procedures, and T&As) [98].

Red blood cells chosen for transfusion should be sickle negative and negative for all antigens against which the patient has pre-existing antibodies. Phenotypic matching of RBCs for C, E, and Kell antigens has been shown to decrease rates of RBC alloimmunization and ultimately to decrease rates of hemolytic transfusion reactions in patients with SCD [99]. Thus, RBCs chosen for transfusion should also ideally be phenotypically matched for these antigens. However, transfusing non-phenotypically matched RBCs (or RBCs from donors whose sickle status is not known) is acceptable in urgent situations.

Intraoperative anesthetic management includes exercising usual caution about adequate oxygenation, hydration, thermoregulation, and acid–base balance. No evidence exists to support the prolonged postoperative administration of supplemental oxygen in the absence of hypoxemia. However, pulse oximetry should be monitored and oxygen therapy should be used to maintain normal oxygen saturations.

Aggressive pulmonary toilet and early ambulation postoperatively may limit pulmonary complications. Adequate postoperative pain management is critical. Regional anesthetic techniques may be useful both intraoperatively as part of the anesthetic plan and postoperatively for pain control. Surgery on an outpatient basis is appropriate for superficial procedure on patients with stable disease [93]. The use of tourniquets for orthopedic procedures is controversial [100,101] but their uncomplicated use has been documented in patients after preoperative exchange transfusions [102]. Similarly, cardiac surgery involving CPB has been safely conducted after performing preoperative and intraoperative exchange transfusions [103,104]. No consensus exists on the appropriate body temperature to be maintained during CPB or on the use of cold cardioplegia, but the maintenance of normothermia seems intuitive.

Transfusion therapy

Transfusion medicine has played a major role in allowing the medical and surgical advances that benefit children in the 21st century, and the administration of blood components is an integral part of the practice of anesthesiology. This section will describe the basic principles of transfusion therapy, the blood products available for transfusion, the logistics of transfusion, the indications and triggers for administering blood products, and the potential adverse effects that can accompany transfusion of these products.

Principles of transfusion therapy
ABO blood group system

Blood is classified into groups or types based on the presence or absence of specific inherited RBC surface antigens. The International Society of Blood Transfusion recognizes 30 major blood group systems, the most important of which is the ABO system. Dr Karl Landsteiner is credited with the discovery of the ABO system in 1900 and was subsequently awarded the Nobel Prize in 1930 for his work.

The ABO system defines an individual's "blood type" by the presence or absence of A and/or B antigens on RBC surfaces. These antigens are produced by the modification of a precursor called the H antigen through the enzymatic actions of co-dominant A and B alleles at the ABO locus on chromosome 9. A third allele, termed the O allele, exists but lacks enzymatic activity and, therefore, does not modify the H antigen or produce a RBC surface antigen. The homozygous presence of the A allele or the heterozygous presence of the A and O alleles thus results in only the A antigen being expressed on RBCs and an individual having "type A" blood. Similarly, the homozygous presence of the B allele or the heterozygous presence of the B and O alleles results in the production of only the B antigen, with subsequent "type B" blood. The homozygous presence of the O allele results in no RBC surface antigen production for this blood system and thus in "type O" blood. Finally, the heterozygous presence of A and B alleles results in production

Table 11.2 ABO blood group system

	ABO type			
	A	**B**	**O**	**AB**
Allele combinations	AA AO	BB BO	OO	AB
ABO antigen present	A	B	None	A and B
ABO antibody present	Anti-B	Anti-A	Anti-A Anti-B	None

of both A and B antigens and "type AB" blood (Table 11.2). Ethnic and racial differences exist in the distribution of ABO blood groups across the world. In the United States, approximately 44% of the population has type O, 42% has type A, 10% has type B, and 4% has type AB blood [105].

Individuals develop antibodies against the ABO antigen(s) not present on their own RBCs. This occurs in the first years of life, even without exposure to blood transfusions, probably in response to exposure to antigens from bacteria, viruses or plants that are structurally very similar to the ABO antigens. Thus, those with type A blood develop anti-B antibodies (IgM type), those with type B blood develop anti-A (IgM type), those with type O blood develop both anti-A and anti-B (IgM and IgG types), and those with type AB blood develop no anti-ABO antibodies (see Table 11.2). IgG type anti-A and anti-B antibodies in type O mothers can cross the placenta and cause hemolysis in children with A or B antigens on their RBCs.

Rh blood group system

The Rh blood group system is second in importance after the ABO group. A RBC antigen in the Rhesus macaque monkey, designated as "Rh factor," was reported by Drs Karl Landsteiner and Alexander Wiener in 1940 after finding that the serum of rabbits immunized with RBCs from this monkey agglutinated about 85% of human RBCs. A serologically similar antigen was also found in humans and retained the name "Rh factor." Two sets of nomenclatures have been used to describe the human Rh blood group system but the CDE nomenclature of the Fisher–Race system is most commonly used today. Although 50 antigens have been discovered in this group, the five most important ones are C, c, D, E, and e. There is no d antigen. These antigens are encoded by two adjacent gene loci, one for D and the other for C, c, E, and e, on chromosome 1. Of these five antigens, D is the most immunogenic and the Rh status of an individual is based solely on its presence or absence. Inheritance of one D allele results in the production of the D antigen. The term "Rh positive" refers to the presence of the D antigen on the surface of RBCs whereas "Rh negative" indicates its absence. Approximately 85% of the United States population is Rh positive.

In contrast to the ABO blood group system, anti-Rh antibodies only develop in Rh-negative individuals after exposure to Rh-positive blood by a blood transfusion or by placental exposure during pregnancy. Once anti-Rh antibodies have developed, repeat exposure to Rh-positive RBCs can result in hemolysis. Since anti-Rh antibodies are of the IgG class, they can cross the placenta. This can be of grave importance to sensitized Rh-negative mothers carrying a Rh-positive child. These mothers may have been sensitized by the feto-maternal transfer of Rh-positive RBCs during a previous pregnancy with a Rh-positive child. Transplacental transfer of the sensitized mother's IgG anti-Rh antibodies to her second Rh-positive child can lead to hemolytic disease of the newborn (erythroblastosis fetalis) as the unborn child's Rh-positive RBCs are hemolyzed.

Transfusion compatibility between recipients and donors

The presence of RBC surface antigens and circulating plasma antibodies to these antigens mandates immunological compatibility between recipients and donors of blood products. Since whole blood (WB) contains both ABO antigens and antibodies, it can be transfused only to ABO-identical recipients. Packed RBCs (PRBCs) contain RBC surface antigens but minimal amounts of antibody-containing plasma so donors and recipients do not have to be ABO identical. However, patients can only receive PRBCs whose ABO surface antigens will not react with the patient's circulating anti-ABO antibodies. Type A patients with their anti-B antibodies can receive type A or type O PRBCs. Type B patients with their anti-A antibodies can receive type B or type O PRBCs. Type O patients with their anti-A and anti-B antibodies can receive only type O PRBCs. Finally, type AB patients with no anti-ABO antibodies can receive type AB, A, B or O PRBCs (Table 11.3). Therefore, when transfusing PRBCs, type O individuals are universal donors whereas type AB patients are universal recipients.

Conversely, plasma-containing products (including fresh frozen plasma and platelets) contain anti-ABO antibodies so patients can only receive plasma-containing products whose anti-ABO antibodies will not react with the patient's ABO surface antigens. Type A patients can receive type A or type AB plasma-containing products. Type B patients can receive type B or type AB plasma-containing products. Type O patients can receive type O, A, B or AB plasma-containing products. Finally, type AB

Table 11.3 ABO compatibility

	Recipient ABO type			
	A	**B**	**O**	**AB**
Compatible donor RBCs (contain antigens)	A O	B O	O	A B O AB
Compatible donor plasma-containing products (contain antibodies)	A AB	B AB	O A B AB	AB

patients can receive only type AB plasma-containing products (see Table 11.3). Therefore, when transfusing plasma-containing products, type AB individuals are universal donors whereas type O patients are universal recipients.

Rh factor status must also be considered when transfusing blood products. Rh-positive individuals may receive PRBCs from either Rh-positive or Rh-negative donors and plasma-containing products from donors without anti-Rh antibodies (either Rh-positive or previously untransfused Rh-negative donors).

Rh-negative individuals preferentially should receive Rh-negative PRBCs since exposure to Rh-positive RBCs invokes the production of anti-Rh antibodies in 30–80% of transfusion recipients. This is especially true if these recipients can be expected to receive further transfusions at future dates or if they are females who may bear children in the future. Although platelets contain ABO antigens, they do not contain Rh antigens. However, RBCs contaminate all platelet preparations to some extent. Thus, Rh-negative patients should preferentially receive Rh-negative platelets. If transfusion of Rh-positive platelets to Rh-negative recipients is necessary, Rho(D) immune globulin can be given within 72h to prevent the development of anti-Rh antibodies that may be induced by contaminating RBCs. Since fresh frozen plasma is devoid of Rh antigens, Rh-negative individuals can receive plasma from either Rh-positive or Rh-negative donors.

Available blood products
Collection techniques

A variety of blood products are available for transfusion and can be collected via two processes [106–108]. Whole blood can be collected from a single donor as a 450–500 mL aliquot. While being collected, the blood is mixed with 70 mL of an anticoagulant/preservative solution.

Basic "CPD" solutions contain citrate for anticoagulation, phosphate to buffer the acidosis that develops during storage, and dextrose to serve as a source of energy for the RBCs. These CPD anticoagulant/preservative solutions allow RBC-containing products to be stored for 21 days when kept at 1–6°C. The addition of adenine to the solution (CPDA-1) supports the synthesis of ATP by the RBCs and prolongs the shelf-life to 35 days. Newer adenine-saline additive solutions, such AS-1 (Adsol), AS-3 (Nutricel), and AS-5 (Optisol), add various additional amounts of phosphate, dextrose, adenine, mannitol, and saline and further extend the shelf-life to 42 days [107–109].

Most units of WB are subsequently separated into various components. This practice allows several patients to benefit from one blood donation, optimal storage of the different components, and focused administration of specifically indicated components [106]. Centrifugation of one unit of WB ultimately can provide one unit each of PRBCs, plasma, and platelets. In the majority of centers in North America, a unit of WB is separated initially into PRBCs and platelet-rich plasma. The platelet-rich plasma is then further separated into plasma and platelets. Cryoprecipitate can subsequently be obtained from plasma. Alternatively, individual components can be specifically collected from a donor by apheresis. In this process, blood from a donor is drawn into an external circuit, a specific component is separated by filtration or by centrifugation based on its specific gravity, and the remaining components are returned to the donor [106,107]. This process can be used to collect RBCs, platelets, plasma or granulocytes. Its use can minimize donor exposures for blood product recipients by providing larger quantities of a desired component from one donor than WB separation techniques can provide [107].

Whole blood

Products containing red blood cells include WB and PRBCs. Whole blood is obtained from donors with a hematocrit of at least 38% [108] and is used not only to support hemoglobin levels but also to provide coagulation factors [110]. The ability of WB to raise hemoglobin levels, however, is limited by the hemoglobin level of the donor. Its use may be advantageous in neonatal exchange transfusions and in controlling bleeding after complex cardiac surgeries requiring cardiopulmonary bypass in children less than 2 years old and after massive blood loss and transfusion [107,111]. However, only relatively "fresh" WB (i.e. less than 24–48h old) is useful in correcting coagulopathic bleeding. During storage at 1–6°C, the activities of the temperature-sensitive labile coagulation factors, V and VIII, progressively diminish in WB [107]. Additionally, storage at this temperature rapidly and dramatically alters platelet survival. After 3h of storage at

4°C, platelet viability drops to 62% then to 12% after 24h and to 2% after 48h [112]. However, the logistics of timely acquiring, testing, and transporting WB so that it is available for use at many facilities within 24–48h of its collection pose major barriers to its regular availability. Because of these practical considerations as well as the previously mentioned benefits of separating WB into components, WB is rarely used today [106].

Packed red blood cells

Packed red blood cells are the most common component used to raise hemoglobin levels and thus increase the oxygen-carrying capacity of blood [106,108,110]. They can be prepared by separation from WB or by apheresis. Like WB, PRBCs are stored at 1–6°C in an anticoagulant/preservative solution. If CPDA-1 is the solution used, the hematocrit of the unit of PRBCs is 65–80%, the volume is approximately 250mL, and the shelf-life is 35 days. If one of the additive solutions (AS-1, AS-3 or AS-5) is used, the volume of the unit is increased to approximately 350mL, the hematocrit is decreased to 55–65%, and the shelf-life is extended to 42 days [106–108]. PRBCs can be further processed by freezing, washing, irradiation or leukocyte reduction.

Packed red blood cells with unique phenotypes or RBCs collected for autologous use that need to be stored for more than 42 days can be frozen for up to 10 years at −65°C or lower after adding glycerol as a cryoprotective agent. After thawing these frozen PRBCs for transfusion, the glycerol must be removed by washing the RBCs with progressively lower concentrations of sodium chloride-containing solutions [106–108]. Washing RBC units also removes plasma proteins, inflammatory mediators such as cytokines, and other plasma contaminants. Washed RBCs are indicated to prevent severe recurrent allergic reactions caused by foreign plasma proteins, to remove excess potassium from older units of PRBCs or from those that have been irradiated, and to remove plasma IgA prior to transfusion to IgA-deficient patients who have developed anti-IgA antibodies. After washing, PRBC units must be used within 24h if stored at 1–6°C or within 4h if stored at 20–24°C since the hermetic seal of the unit will have been broken [106–108].

Irradiation of PRBCs (or WB) with γ-irradiation using a cesium (^{137}Cs) source or with x-rays using a linear accelerator is performed to inactivate viable lymphocytes, thus preventing transfusion-associated graft-versus-host disease. Irradiation is indicated when PRBC (or WB) recipients are immunocompromised, are first- or second-degree blood relatives of the donor or are neonates. The shelf-life of PRBCs after irradiation is reduced to 28 days if the anticoagulant/preservative-dictated shelf-life still exceeds 28 days at the time of irradiation. Potassium and free hemoglobin leak from the RBCs into plasma after irradiation so washing of irradiated PRBCs may be considered when there is an extended length of time between irradiation and transfusion [106–108,113].

Leukocyte reduction of PRBCs is performed to decrease the incidence of febrile non-hemolytic transfusion reactions, to decrease the incidence of alloimmunization of recipients to HLA antigens, to reduce the risk of transmission of cytomegalovirus (CMV) and other infectious diseases transmitted by white blood cells (WBCs), and possibly to reduce the effects of transfusion-related immunomodulation [106–108,114]. Leukocyte reduction can be performed before storage at the time of collection of the blood or after storage in the laboratory or at the bedside. Post-storage leukocyte reduction has been reported to cause unexpected severe hypotension in some recipients (especially those taking angiotensin-converting enzyme (ACE) inhibitors) due to bradykinin activation [108]. Additionally, inflammatory mediators released by leukocytes during storage are not removed by post-storage leukoreduction. Given these considerations, more than 80% of RBCs transfused in the United States are leukoreduced before storage, with leukoreduction filters removing more than 99% of leukocytes [106,107].

Plasma

Plasma is prepared by separation from the platelet-rich plasma component of WB or by apheresis. The volume of a unit of plasma derived from WB is 170–250 mL whereas a unit obtained by apheresis measures up to 500 mL. To be labeled as "fresh frozen plasma" (FFP), the plasma has to be stored at −18°C or colder within 8h of collection. This prevents the inactivation of the temperature-sensitive "labile" coagulation factors, V and VIII, and allows a shelf-life of 1 year [106,108]. If not frozen within 8h of collection, the activity of factors V and VIII will diminish but the plasma can still be frozen at or below −18°C within 24h, labeled "plasma frozen within 24 hours", and stored for up to 1 year [107,108]. By definition, each mL of FFP contains one international unit (IU) of each coagulation factor [108]. FFP also contains 2–4 mg of fibrinogen per mL [115]. No cryoprotectant is included in the unit and, therefore, the majority of leukocytes are killed or rendered non-functional. As a consequence, irradiation to prevent transfusion-associated graft-versus-host reaction and leukocyte reduction to prevent CMV infection are not necessary for FFP [107]. Prior to administration, FFP is thawed in a waterbath at 30–37°C for approximately 20–30 min. The unit should then be infused immediately or it may be stored at 1–6°C and transfused within 24h [107,108]. If it is not used within this 24-h window, it can be stored for an additional 4 days at 1–6°C but it must be relabeled as "thawed plasma" and it will have diminished, although still hemostatic, levels of factors V and VIII [106,108].

Cryoprecipitate

Cryoprecipitated antihemophilic factor, or "cryoprecipitate," is the cold-insoluble white precipitate that forms when a unit of FFP is thawed only to 1–6°C. Once prepared from FFP, cryoprecipitate must be refrozen at −18°C or colder within 1h and then has a shelf-life of 1 year. Each unit of cryoprecipitate contains concentrated amounts of fibrinogen (150–250 mg), factor VIII (80–150 IU), vWF (40–70% of original plasma concentration), factor XIII (30% of original plasma concentration), and fibronectin (30–60 mg) in approximately 5–15 mL of plasma. The plasma remaining after extraction of cryoprecipitate is relabeled as "cryoprecipitate-reduced plasma." Since this plasma is deficient in the above-mentioned coagulation factors, it should not be used as a substitute for FFP.

Once thawed in preparation for transfusion, cryoprecipitate must be administered within 6h to prevent loss of factor VIII activity. If several cryoprecipitate units are pooled, transfusion must take place within 4h to minimize risks from potential contamination. Since cryoprecipitate is stored, like FFP, at temperatures below −18°C, irradiation and/or leukocyte reduction are not necessary before cryoprecipitate transfusions. Additionally, since cryoprecipitate contains no RBCs and only small amounts of plasma (thus, minimal amounts of anti-ABO antibodies), ABO and Rh compatibility are not required before its use in adults [106–108,115,116]. However, the small amount of plasma in cryoprecipitate units may be significant relative to the blood volume of infants and young children, so pediatric centers often administer cryoprecipitate whose plasma is ABO compatible with the recipient.

Platelets

Platelets are prepared by separation from the platelet-rich plasma component or the buffy coat layer of WB or by apheresis. Platelet units prepared from WB are termed "random donor platelets" and contain a minimum of 5×10^{10} platelets in 50–70 mL of plasma. Platelet units obtained by apheresis are designated as "single donor platelets" and contain at least 3.5×10^{11} platelets in 200–400 mL of plasma. One single donor apheresis platelet unit is equivalent to 6–8 units of random donor platelets. Apheresis platelet units have become the primary source of platelets for transfusion in the United States since their use minimizes donor exposures to recipients. Platelet units are stored at 20–24°C with continuous gentle agitation to prevent aggregation. Because of the risk of bacterial contamination at this temperature, platelet units in the United States currently have a shelf-life of only 5 days [106,107]. Since platelet units are not subjected to the extremely cold temperatures at which plasma and cryoprecipitate are stored, they (like WB and PRBCs) must be irradiated to kill viable lymphocytes in clinical situations where transfusion-associated graft-versus-host disease is a concern and must be leukocyte reduced when transmission of CMV is a risk [106,108].

In adult centers, type compatibility may not be required between recipients and donors of platelet units for small-volume transfusions. However, platelets express multiple surface antigens, including ABO and platelet-specific antigens, so ABO-identical platelets may be needed if survival of ABO-incompatible platelets is decreased. With the significant amount of plasma contained in platelet units, though, compatibility between donor plasma and recipient ABO type is generally recommended in infants and children. Additionally, since a small amount of RBCs remain in both random and single donor platelets, Rh-negative patients preferentially should be transfused with platelets from Rh-negative donors to prevent Rh alloimmunization, especially in females or in patients who may receive future transfusions [106,107,117].

Logistics of transfusion
Typing, screening, and cross-matching

Preparation for transfusion begins with determining the blood type and Rh status of the intended recipient and the prospective donor unit. ABO group is defined using forward and reverse typing. Forward typing tests patient RBCs against reagents containing anti-A and anti-B antibodies while reverse typing tests patient plasma against reagent cells that carry A or B surface antigens. Therefore, blood group is defined by identifying the ABO antigen(s) and anti-ABO antibody(ies) present. Neonates typically do not develop anti-ABO antibodies until 4–6 months of age; therefore, forward tying is primarily utilized to determine their blood type. Rh status is defined by testing RBCs for the presence of the D antigen using anti-D containing reagent [106].

The plasma of the intended recipient is then screened for the presence of unexpected antibodies to antigens of any of the other blood group systems that can be present on RBC surfaces. This is accomplished by incubating the recipient's plasma with screening RBC panels composed of three or four group O RBCs selected in such a way that most common non-ABO antigens capable of inducing the production of significant antibodies that could cause hemolysis are represented on at least one screening cell. Antihuman globulin is then added to agglutinate any RBCs to which an antibody has attached (indirect Coombs test). If an antibody is detected, the screen is considered positive and further investigation must be undertaken to identify the specific antibody present [106]. Antibody screening must be repeated if RBCs are ordered and 3 days have elapsed since the last antibody screen. An exception is in neonates where, due to the immaturity of their immune systems, an initial negative screen does not

have to be repeated during the same hospitalization until after 4 months of age [107].

Cross-matching of recipient plasma and donor RBCs is the next step prior to PRBC transfusions. If the recipient has a negative antibody screen, only ABO compatibility between the recipient and the donor RBCs must be verified. This can be done with an immediate spin cross-match to provide serological verification or with an electronic cross-match that uses a series of computer algorithms to select a suitable PRBC unit that is in stock in the blood bank. Either of these cross-matching techniques can be used to have PRBCs ready for transfusion in 5–10 min for recipients with negative antibody screens. However, if the recipient has a positive antibody screen, a more detailed serological cross-match, called an antihuman globulin (AHG) or "full Coombs" cross-match, must be performed to verify compatibility of the recipient's plasma against clinically significant non-ABO antigens that may be present on donor RBC surfaces. This process requires up to 45 min to perform, although identifying the recipient antibody and finding compatible donor RBCs may take considerably longer [106].

In contrast to PRBCs, cross-matching is not necessary prior to plasma, cryoprecipitate or platelet transfusions. For each of these products, units whose plasma is ABO compatible with the recipient's RBCs are administered. FFP and cryoprecipitate can be thawed and available for transfusion in approximately 20–30 min. Since platelets are stored at room temperature, they can be immediately available for transfusion when required.

Administration of blood products

The process of transfusing blood products begins with the proper identification of the recipient, verification that the product to be transfused has been assigned to that recipient, and confirmation that the ABO type and Rh status of the blood product are appropriate for that recipient.

Red blood cell products transfused intraoperatively may need to be warmed since they will have been kept at 1–6°C in the blood bank or stored on ice in the operating room. This may be accomplished by warming the WB or PRBC unit in a temperature-controlled water bath or by warming the RBCs as they flow through the IV tubing by using circulating water, forced air or a heat exchanger. Warming these products prior to their administration attenuates not only the development of hypothermia but also any vasoconstriction and/or coagulopathy that may accompany hypothermia [118]. Care must be taken, however, to prevent excessive warming as this can lead to hemolysis [108]. FFP and cryoprecipitate will be warmed in the blood bank prior to their release and platelets are stored at room temperature so further warming is not usually necessary prior to their administration.

If PRBCs need to be diluted to expedite their flow through IV tubing, 0.9% NaCl (normal saline) should be used. Calcium-containing solutions such as Ringer's lactate must be avoided for this purpose because calcium in excess of the chelating ability of the citrate anticoagulant in the PRBC unit will cause the formation of small clots. Hypotonic solutions must also be avoided because they may cause hemolysis of the RBCs. No medicines or other IV solutions may be infused through the same IV tubing being used for any blood products [106,108].

Screening filters with pore sizes of 170–200 μm should be used in the transfusion of WB, PRBCs, FFP, cryoprecipitate, and platelets to remove clots and aggregates. These filters are incorporated into all standard blood administration sets. There are no firm indications for using microaggregate filters (pore size 20–40 μm) although these are commonly used when reinfusing blood processed through a cell saver device. Microaggregate filters will trap platelets so should definitely not be used when transfusing platelet units. Finally, once any blood product is accessed for transfusion, its administration should be completed within 4h to minimize the risk of bacterial contamination [106,108].

Indications/triggers for blood product transfusion

Blood products are used for the correction of anemia to improve oxygen-carrying capacity and for the treatment of coagulopathies to attenuate bleeding. The administration of blood products, however, is accompanied by infectious, immunological, and non-immunological risks that must be weighed against the anticipated benefits of their use. Therefore, insightful thought processes should guide any decision to transfuse these products [110].

Packed red blood cells

There is no single minimum hemoglobin level that serves as a transfusion trigger for all patients in all clinical scenarios [106,110,115,119]. To complicate this problem for pediatric caretakers, there is a dearth of randomized controlled trials on RBC transfusion thresholds for neonates, infants, and children [107]. Surveys of pediatric intensive care units (PICUs) have shown significant variations in hemoglobin levels that trigger RBC transfusion [120] as well as a variety of clinical factors other than hemoglobin level than are used to help make this decision [121]. The "10/30" rule for transfusion that was introduced in the 1940s has fallen into disfavor based on risk:benefit analyses [110], and hemoglobin levels are currently allowed to fall to levels much lower than 10 g/dL before PRBCs are administered in many clinical situations. Physiological signs such as tachycardia, hypotension and, if available, low mixed venous oxygen saturations or increased oxygen extractions ratios are useful in providing objective evidence of the need to correct a given level of anemia [106,110].

In addressing specific hemoglobin levels, data from adults have shown that at a hemoglobin level less than 6 g/dL, coronary artery blood flow reserve may be exceeded and oxygen extraction may be compromised [110]. Studies in both adults and children in intensive care units using a restrictive transfusion strategy of only administering PRBCs when hemoglobin levels drop below 7 g/dL have shown reductions in number of patients transfused and units given with unchanged or improved morbidity and mortality rates when compared to more liberal strategies of transfusing at hemoglobin levels of 9.5 or 10 g/dL [122,123]. With these data in mind, recommendations to transfuse PRBCs for hemoglobin levels less than 7 g/dL seem appropriate. Transfusion for levels greater than 10 g/dL are probably unnecessary in the absence of ongoing blood loss or complicated clinical scenarios. Transfusions for hemoglobin levels between 7 and 10 g/dL should be triggered by objective physiological signs of inadequate oxygen delivery to tissues [124]. These guidelines require modification for premature infants and for children with cyanotic congenital heart disease, congestive heart failure or significant co-morbidities. Indeed, although not without controversy [125], the use of a restrictive transfusion threshold in premature infants may be associated with an increase in neurological morbidities that have been postulated to result from decreased oxygen delivery to the brain [126]. Practice parameters for these infants and children are even less evidence based than those previously described.

It typically has been taught that transfusing 10–15 mL of PRBCs per kg of bodyweight will raise the hemoglobin level by approximately 3 g/dL or the hematocrit by 10% [106,107]. Formulas have been developed to add more precision to determinations of volume of PRBCs to be transfused. One such formula is:

Volume of PRBCs to be transfused = total blood volume × (desired hemoglobin − actual hemoglobin)/ hemoglobin of PRBC unit

Assumptions of total blood volume (TBV) are based on the age of the recipient: 90–100 mL/kg for preterm neonates, 80–90 mL/kg for full-term neonates, 80 mL/kg from 6 months to 2 years of age, and 70 mL/kg for children older than 2 years [127]. The hemoglobin of the PRBC unit depends on the anticoagulant/preservative solution used to store the unit [107]. The actual/predicted hemoglobin rise using this formula is 0.61–0.85 and is influenced by the TBV and PRBC hemoglobin values used. A new formula developed from a regression analysis of volume of PRBCs transfused versus bodyweight results in an actual/predicted hemoglobin rise of 0.95 that is valid across different age groups [128]:

Volume of PRBCs to be transfused
$$= 4.8 \times weight\ (kg) \times desired\ rise\ in\ hemoglobin\ (g/dL)$$
$$or = 1.6 \times weight\ (kg) \times desired\ rise\ in\ hematocrit\ (\%)$$

Use of this formula may minimize the need for repeat transfusions.

Plasma

Generally agreed upon indications for transfusing FFP include the treatment of active microvascular bleeding associated with an acquired coagulopathy (DIC, liver disease, massive transfusion, cardiac surgery or liver transplantation) in the presence of an INR >2.0 or an aPTT >1.5 times normal or when an INR and an aPTT cannot be obtained in a timely manner; replacement of rare congenital coagulation factor deficiencies (II, V, X, XI, XIII, protein C) when specific concentrates are not available; emergency reversal of the anticoagulant effects of warfarin; replacement of AT deficiency in patients with heparin resistance when AT concentrate is not available; and replacement of C1 esterase inhibitor in patients with hereditary angioedema [106,107,115,124,129]. FFP is not indicated for volume expansion, to augment albumin concentration or when specific factor concentrates are available to correct documented deficiencies [106,107,115,129]. "Cryoprecipitate-reduced plasma" is sometimes used in the management of thrombotic thrombocytopenic purpura (TTP), a condition where the breakdown of large multimers of vWF is inhibited, thus leading to microvascular thromboses and tissue infarctions. Transfusion of this plasma product, which is devoid of vWF, replenishes the deficient enzyme (ADAMTS13) responsible for cleaving vWF and ameliorates the complications of TTP [107,108,130].

Ten to 15 mL of FFP per kg of bodyweight is the conventional volume transfused for the above indications. This amount is reported to increase plasma levels of coagulation factors by 25–30% [106,115] and thus to exceed the factor level thresholds required for hemostasis (15% for factor V and 30% for all other factors) [131].

Cryoprecipitate

Transfusion of cryoprecipitate is indicated in the presence of microvascular bleeding when the fibrinogen level is <80–100 mg/dL or when the fibrinogen level cannot be measured in a timely fashion and in actively bleeding patients with congenital fibrinogen deficiencies. Cryoprecipitate is rarely indicated when the fibrinogen level exceeds 150 mg/dL but its use may be prudent with fibrinogen levels between 100 and 150 mg/dL when there

is a risk of bleeding into a confined space such as the brain or the eye. Cryoprecipitate is not indicated as a first-line treatment for hemophilia A or B, factor XIII deficiency or vWD but may be used when purified or recombinant factor concentrates are not available or when vWD is unresponsive to the administration of DDAVP [106,107,115,124]. In small children, 1 unit of cryoprecipitate per 5 kg of bodyweight is estimated to raise the fibrinogen level by 100 mg/dL [107]. In older patients, one unit per 10 kg should increase the fibrinogen level by approximately 50–70 mg/dL [106].

Platelets

Platelet transfusions may be required because of low platelet counts or because of abnormal platelet function regardless of the number of platelets present. Controlled trials are lacking, and only general guidelines are available to help guide platelet replacement therapy. In the face of active bleeding in the perioperative period, it is prudent to maintain platelet counts above 50,000/µL. When microvascular bleeding is present, this level should probably be raised to 100,000/µL. When active bleeding occurs in the setting of platelet dysfunction (uremia, thrombasthenias or ingestion of antiplatelet drugs), platelet transfusion will be required regardless of platelet counts. Even in the absence of bleeding, platelets are often transfused prophylactically when counts fall below 50,000/µL in the setting of sepsis, antibiotic use or other coagulopathies or when counts fall below 10,000/µL in patients who do not have these additional risk factors. Platelet counts greater than 30,000/µL are felt to be a safe level for most neonatal ICU patients if they have no other risk factors or previous intraventricular hemorrhage.

Prior to invasive procedures such as surgery, central line placement, thoracentesis, endoscopy or lumbar puncture, platelet counts should be raised to greater than 50,000/µL. For neurosurgical or ophthalmological procedures or if bleeding in the central nervous system has occurred, platelet counts above 100,000/µL are preferred. Platelet transfusions are not typically indicated prior to bone marrow biopsies or in scenarios of increased platelet destruction (idiopathic thrombocytopenic purpura). Platelet administration will increase the risk of thrombosis in patients with TTP and heparin-induced thrombocytopenia [106,107,115,124,129].

When transfusing random donor platelets, 5–10 mL of platelets per kg of bodyweight in neonates and 0.1–0.2 units/kg in older infants and children should result in a platelet increment of 50,000–100,000/µL. When single donor apheresis platelet units are being transfused, a general rule is to administer 10 mL/kg to neonates, ¼ unit to children <15 kg, ½ unit to children between 15 and 30 kg, and a whole unit to children >30 kg. Response to these transfused volumes varies among patients and according to the platelet content of the unit transfused. Failure to achieve expected platelet increments after transfusion should prompt a search for causes of platelet refractoriness and may require the use of phenotypically matched platelets for future transfusions [107].

Massive transfusion

Trauma-induced injuries are the most common scenarios that result in massive hemorrhage. Indeed, hemorrhage accounts for 30–40% of all trauma-related deaths. One to three percent of civilian trauma patients will require massive transfusion [132]. Massive transfusion is defined in children as the transfusion of one blood volume of PRBCs in a 24-h period [133]. However, more dynamic definitions such as the transfusion of 50% of blood volume in a 3h period may be more relevant [134]. Since the use of PRBCs with minimum plasma replaced the use of WB in the late 1980s and early 1990s, dilution of coagulation factors with massive transfusion using PRBCs has become a significant problem [134,135]. The "lethal triad" of coagulopathy, hypothermia, and acidosis may accompany massive transfusion, with each component of this triad then exacerbating the other two components and exsanguination and death often resulting [132,136]. The aim of transfusion therapy in this situation is to restore blood volume, maintain tissue oxygenation, and achieve hemostasis to prevent or interrupt the development of this lethal triad [118].

Military and civilian adult studies have shown improved survival after transfusing FFP, platelets, and cryoprecipitate along with PRBCs during massive transfusion [132,137]. Some argue that blood component therapy during massive transfusion should be guided by laboratory tests; however, this is practically difficult because of slow turnaround times for these tests [138]. Therefore, massive transfusion protocols have been developed as part of "damage control resuscitation" using predetermined ratios of blood products to rapidly treat coagulopathies, decrease crystalloid infusions, and minimize delays in having blood products ready for use [133]. The goals of massive transfusion protocols are to provide plasma support to keep coagulation factor levels at least 40% of normal while not compromising delivery of RBCs and to transfuse enough platelets to maintain platelet counts well above 50,000/μL [139]. Several massive transfusion protocols advocate using a 1:1:1 ratio of PRBCs, FFP, and random donor platelets after identifying massive hemorrhage [139,140]. If using apheresis platelets, one unit is given after every 10–12 units each of PRBCs and FFP, as is 10 units of cryoprecipitate. Laboratory tests can later be used to refine therapy after bleeding has been controlled. Use of such a massive transfusion protocol has been shown to reduce coagulopathy development and mortality in adult civilian trauma patients [141].

Box 11.2 Potential adverse effects of transfusion

- Transmission of infectious diseases
- Immune-mediated risks
  - Hemolytic transfusion reactions
  - Febrile non-hemolytic transfusion reactions
  - Allergic reactions
  - Transfusion-related acute lung injury
  - Transfusion-associated graft-versus-host disease
  - Post-transfusion purpura
  - Transfusion-related immunomodulation
  - Alloimmunization
- Non-immune-mediated risks
  - Septic transfusion reactions
  - Non-immune hemolysis
  - Transfusion-associated circulatory overload
  - Metabolic derangements
  - Red blood cell storage lesions
  - Mistransfusion

Potential adverse effects of transfusion

The transfusion of blood products is not without risks. Transmission of infectious diseases as well as non-infectious immune and non-immune mediated hazards of transfusion are sources of ongoing concern and investigation (Box 11.2). Advances in blood donor selection, infectious disease testing of donated blood products, use of leukoreduction filters, and irradiation of blood components in defined situations have made today's blood supply safer than ever [107,142,143]. Nevertheless, vigilance must be maintained to identify known risks and to anticipate emerging risks in today's blood supply.

Transmission of infectious diseases

While the public may be unaware of many of the risks of transfusion, the risk of contracting an infectious disease from a blood product transfusion has not escaped its attention. Potentially transmissible agents include viruses, bacteria, parasites, and prions (Box 11.3). Currently, donated blood products are regularly tested for human immunodeficiency virus (HIV), human T-lymphotrophic virus (HTLV), hepatitis B virus (HBV), hepatitis C virus (HCV), and *Treponema pallidum* [144] (Table 11.4).

Contraction of HIV or hepatitis is the major concern of patients (or parents of patients) when receiving blood component transfusions. Disease transmission by transfusions occurs primarily in the window period of a disease, i.e. the time after a blood donor has become infectious but before any donor screening tests are positive [114]. The advent of nucleic acid testing (NAT) in the last decade has shortened window periods and

Box 11.3 Infectious agents/diseases potentially transmissible by blood product transfusion

Viral

- HIV 1/2
- HTLV I/II
- Hepatitis A virus
- Hepatitis B virus
- Hepatitis C virus
- Hepatitis G virus
- Cytomegalovirus
- Epstein–Barr virus
- Parvovirus B-19
- Human herpesvirus-8
- West Nile virus
- Enterovirus

Bacterial

- Syphilis (*Treponema pallidum*)
- Rocky Mountain spotted fever (*Rickettsia rickettsii*)
- Contaminants

Parasitic

- Malaria (*Plasmodium* sp)
- Babesiosis (*Babesia* sp)
- Chagas disease (*Trypanosoma cruzi*)
- Toxoplasmosis (*Toxoplasma gondii*)
- Leishmaniasis (*Leishmania* sp)

Prions

- Variant Creutzfeldt–Jakob disease

Table 11.4 Infectious disease tests performed on donated blood components

Infectious agent	Tests
HIV	HIV nucleic acid amplification test Anti-HIV-1 Anti-HIV-2
HTLV	Anti HTLV-I/II
Hepatitis B virus	HBsAg Anti-HBc
Hepatitis C virus	HCV nucleic acid amplification test Anti-HCV
Treponema pallidum	Treponemal antibody test

Source: American Society of Anesthesiologists, Committee on Transfusion Medicine [106].

Table 11.5 Estimated residual risks of transfusion-associated infections

Infection	Risk
HIV	1 in 2.3 million
HTLV	1 in 2 million
Hepatitis B	1 in 350,000
Hepatitis C	1 in 1.8 million

Source: Hendrickson J, Hillyer C. Noninfectious serious hazards of transfusion. Anesth Analg 2009; 108: 759–69.

allowed earlier detection of several viruses than could be accomplished with serological tests [145]. As a result, transmission risks of these viruses have been decreased approximately 10,000-fold [146] and are so low that mathematical models are currently needed to estimate risks [114,147] (Table 11.5).

The first descriptions of transfusion-transmitted HIV infections occurred in late 1982 and early 1983. HIV antibody testing was begun in March 1985 with a resultant window period for HIV-1 of 22 days. HIV-2 testing of donor blood was implemented in 1992. Testing for the HIV p24 antigen was initiated in late 1995 and decreased the window period to 16 days. Currently, NAT for HIV RNA is performed on minipools of 16–24 donated units and has further reduced the window period to 11 days [114,148]. The current estimated residual risk for transfusion-associated transmission of HIV is 1 in 2.3 million [146].

The use of NAT has had an even more dramatic effect on decreasing transfusion-associated transmission of HCV. A serological test for HCV antibody was developed in 1990 and thus identified the cause of most cases of non-A, non-B hepatitis [147]. This significantly reduced the incidence of post-transfusion HCV infection but left a window period of approximately 70 days. Institution of NAT for HCV RNA in 1999 decreased this window period to 8–10 days and reduced the residual risk of HCV infection to 1 in 1.8 million [114,146,148].

The risk for post-transfusion HBV infection is approximately 1 in 350,000 [142,146]. HBsAg and anti-HBc testing are currently performed on all donated blood in the United States. NAT testing for HBV DNA is not currently routinely performed in the United States since its use would reduce the window period by just 2–7 days compared to the most sensitive HBsAg screening tests [114,142].

West Nile virus first appeared in the US in 1999 with the peak number of cases reported in 2003. It was subsequently recognized that this virus could be transmitted through transfusion of leukoreduced and non-leukoreduced PRBCs or platelets and through transfusion of FFP [149]. NAT methodology was quickly modified to test for this agent. NAT has been used in at-risk geographical regions since 2003 with subsequent dramatic reduction of transfusion-associated infection rates [147,150].

Hepatitis A virus is rarely transmitted by blood products since individuals are usually symptomatic when infected and thus excluded from donation, no chronic carrier state exists, and many people have developed antibodies either naturally from previous infection or by vaccination [106,114].

Cytomegalovirus is harbored in white blood cells and can be transmitted by transfusion of cellular products (WB, PRBCs, and platelets) that may contain functional white blood cells. Clinical disease after transmission is usually seen only in immunocompromised patients. The two approaches used in the United States to reduce the risk of CMV transmission in at-risk patients are the use of leukoreduced cellular blood products (termed "CMV safe") and the use of CMV-seronegative cellular blood products [106,114].

Donated blood products are routinely screened by serological tests for infection with *Treponema pallidum*, the causative agent of syphilis. In addition, this spirochete poorly survives storage in citrated blood at 4°C for longer than 72h so its transmission by transfusion is very infrequent [106,147].

A major concern is the transfusion-associated transmission of other infectious agents for which no screening tests are currently available. This includes human herpesvirus-8 (a causative agent of Kaposi sarcoma) and most of the parasitic diseases (malaria, babesiosis, Chagas disease, toxoplasmosis, and leishmaniasis) [115,142,143,151]. Fortunately, transmission of parasitic diseases is rare in developed countries. However, potential transmission of hepatitis G virus, other as yet unknown viruses, and the agent causing variant Creutzfeldt–Jakob disease is a significant concern [119,137].

Variant Creutzfeldt–Jakob disease is the human equivalent of bovine spongiform encephalopathy ("mad cow disease"). It is caused by a prion, an infectious agent composed mainly of protein that causes native proteins to refold and produce the clinical disease. The confirmed cases of transfusion-associated transmission have become evident 6–8 years after transfusion, with the donors not developing clinically apparent disease until 17–42 months after donation [142]. This long asymptomatic carrier state is of great concern since screening tests are not available [143]. Currently, potential blood donors who visited European countries affected by bovine spongiform encephalopathy between 1980 and 1996 are barred from donating [147]. New filtration processes to remove prions from donated blood products are being developed and offer hope for the future.

The risks of transfusion-associated transmission of infectious agents are not static because new agents continue to emerge and old agents change their properties and epidemiological patterns. New pathogen reduction technologies effective against most viruses, bacteria, and parasites are being developed to improve future safety, as are prion retention filters [147,151]. Nevertheless, currently used screening methods are effective enough that non-infectious hazards of transfusion have now emerged as the leading complication of transfusion therapy [114,146].

Immune-mediated hazards of transfusion

Immune-mediated transfusion risks include hemolytic transfusion reactions, febrile non-hemolytic transfusion reactions, allergic reactions, transfusion-related acute lung injury, transfusion-associated graft-versus-host disease, post-transfusion purpura, transfusion-related immunomodulation, and alloimmunization [146].

Hemolytic transfusion reactions

Immune-mediated hemolytic transfusion reactions (HTRs) are caused by the transfusion of RBCs to patients with pre-existing antibodies to antigens on those RBCs. The most serious HTRs are caused by the transfusion of ABO-incompatible RBCs and result in acute intravascular hemolysis. Clerical error is the most common cause of this mishap and, therefore, most are preventable. Awake patients may manifest chills, fever, nausea, anxiety, and chest and flank pain but these may be masked in anesthetized patients. Tachycardia, hypotension, microvascular bleeding, and hemoglobinuria may be seen but need to be recognized as resulting from a HTR as opposed to myriad other potential causes in anesthetized patients.

Once an acute immune-mediated HTR is suspected, the transfusion should be immediately stopped, the unit of blood should be returned to the blood bank for investigation, and steps should be taken to prevent or ameliorate acute renal failure and coagulopathy.

Delayed immune-mediated HTRs result from the transfusion of RBCs containing a non-ABO antigen to which the recipient has developed an antibody because of a previous transfusion or pregnancy. The antibody is usually present in such low levels that it is undetected during the screening procedure. However, a rapid anamnestic response follows the transfusion. A delayed HTR presents 3–10 days after transfusion as a falling hemoglobin level. No treatment is usually indicated but recognition of the problem, identification of the recipient's antibody, and future transfusion of blood negative for the corresponding antigen are necessary [106,107,115,146,147].

Febrile non-hemolytic transfusion reactions

A febrile non-hemolytic transfusion reaction (FNHTR) is defined as a 1°C increase in body temperature into the febrile range during or soon after a transfusion. These reactions are typically caused by leukocyte-derived cytokines that have been released into the blood product during storage or by the reaction of recipient antileukocyte antibodies (developed after previous transfusions or pregnancies) against donor leukocytes. They are most commonly seen in association with platelet transfusions but can also accompany RBC or plasma administration. FNHTR is a diagnosis of exclusion after other transfusion-associated causes of fever, such as acute HTRs, septic transfusion reactions or transfusion-related acute lung injury, have been ruled out. The use of prestorage leukocyte reduction has significantly reduced the occurrence of these reactions [106,107,146,147].

Allergic reactions

Allergic reactions are the most common of all acute transfusion reactions and result from the reaction of an antibody in the recipient to a soluble plasma antigen in the donor. Leukocyte reduction of cellular blood products, therefore, does not decrease the occurrence of these reactions. However, pretransfusion washing of PRBCs or platelets removes plasma and associated antigens and thus does decrease the occurrence of allergic reactions. Treatment of allergic reactions involves stopping the transfusion and administering antihistamines. Some of these reactions are anaphylactic in nature and will require aggressive treatment, including steroids, and epinephrine. IgA deficiency of the recipient should be considered after a severe allergic transfusion reaction has occurred. IgA-deficient individuals can develop anti-IgA antibodies that react with donor IgA, resulting in an anaphylactic reaction. Use of IgA-deficient plasma or washed cellular products will be necessary for any future transfusions to recipients known to have IgA deficiency and anti-IgA antibodies [106,107,146].

Transfusion-related acute lung injury

Transfusion-related acute lung injury (TRALI) has historically been a leading cause of transfusion-related deaths [146]. TRALI is defined as new acute lung injury occurring during or within 6 h after a transfusion with a clear temporal relationship to the transfusion in patients with or without alternative risk factors for acute lung injury [152]. TRALI can occur after the administration of all types of blood components but is more likely after the transfusion of plasma-rich components such as FFP and apheresed platelets [153].

Two pathophysiological mechanisms have been proposed. In the "classic antibody-mediated" mechanism (approximately 85% of cases), donor antileukocyte antibodies react with recipient leukocytes, resulting in the release of inflammatory mediators that damage pulmonary alveolar epithelium and vascular endothelium leading to non-cardiogenic pulmonary edema. In approximately 15% of cases, no antibody can be detected. Systemic inflammatory conditions secondary to clinical scenarios such as major surgery, sepsis, trauma, aspiration or massive transfusion lead to activation of leukocytes and pulmonary endothelium with subsequent leukocyte sequestration in the lungs. "Bio-active factors" such as cytokines, interleukins or lipids in transfused products may then activate these sequestered leukocytes, leading to lung injury and non-cardiogenic pulmonary edema [106,153].

The clinical presentation of TRALI mirrors that of acute respiratory distress syndrome (ARDS). Treatment is primarily supportive with recovery usually occurring within 96 h although the mortality rate is 5–10%. Diuresis does not improve symptoms and the role of steroids is unproven [106,115,153,154]. Plasma products from multiparous women have been implicated in the majority of cases of antibody-mediated TRALI because these donors may develop antileukocyte antibodies during pregnancy. Eliminating or minimizing the use of plasma products from these donors dramatically decreases the incidence of TRALI [107,153].

Transfusion-associated graft-versus-host disease

Transfusion-associated graft-versus-host disease (TA-GVHD) occurs when immunocompetent CD8$^+$ lymphocytes in transfused cellular blood products (RBCs, platelets or granulocytes) engraft in a recipient, proliferate, and attack host tissues. This occurs when the recipient is immunocompromised and cannot eliminate the donor lymphocytes or when the recipient does not recognize the donor lymphocytes as foreign (biologically related donors or HLA-matched products) and thus does not eliminate them. Clinical manifestations include fever, rash, diarrhea, liver dysfunction, and pancytopenia and occur 1–6 weeks after transfusion. The diagnosis can be made by detecting donor DNA in a skin biopsy or in circulating lymphocytes taken from the recipient. Irradiating RBCs and platelets before their administration renders donor lymphocytes incapable of proliferating and thus eliminates the risk of the development of TA-GVHD. TA-GVHD is nearly uniformly fatal, with mortality rates approaching 90% [106,146,147].

Post-transfusion purpura

Post-transfusion purpura (PTP) is the development of severe thrombocytopenia after a transfusion in recipients who have developed antibodies against platelet-specific antigens as a result of previous transfusions or pregnancies. While PTP is a rare event, it can occur 5–10 days after the administration of RBCs, FFP or platelets. Both transfused and autologous platelets are destroyed in this process, thus severely decreasing the recipient's platelet count, even to below 10,000/μL. Recovery is usually spontaneous although treatment with steroids and IV immune globulin is indicated, with plasmapheresis being a second-line intervention. Platelet transfusions are usually ineffective in raising the platelet count but, if felt necessary in the face of severe bleeding, may need to be administered in large doses since many of the transfused platelets also will be destroyed [106,146,155].

Transfusion-related immunomodulation

While the exact mechanism of transfusion-related immunomodulation (TRIM) has yet to be elucidated, modulation of the recipient's immune responses after transfusion may have both beneficial and harmful effects. Improved survival of transplanted kidneys has been documented in patients transfused before transplantation, as has survival of cardiac and liver transplant patients after pretransplant transfusion of donor-specific or HLA-DR shared RBCs. TRIM may also decrease the recurrence rate of Crohn disease and of miscarriages in women who share HLA antigens with their mates. Evidence linking increased incidences of postoperative infections and cancer recurrence with transfusions, however, is controversial and not definitely proven. Theories of the etiology of TRIM indict leukocytes as major participants so harmful effects of transfusion that are blamed on TRIM may be ameliorated by prestorage leukocyte reduction of blood products [119,146,156].

Alloimmunization

Alloimmunization is the development of antibodies to minor RBC antigens or to platelet or leukocyte antigens after exposure by transfusion or pregnancy. Subsequent transfusion of blood products containing these antigens results in delayed HTRs or platelet refractoriness. Approximately two-thirds of clinically significant alloantibodies are directed toward Rh and Kell antigens on RBC surfaces. Up to 40% of children with sickle cell disease who are managed with chronic transfusion protocols develop alloantibodies. These children, therefore, should undergo extended RBC antigen phenotyping prior to the initiation of chronic transfusion therapy. Provision of PRBCs phenotypically matched for Rh and Kell antigens has been shown to decrease rates of alloimmunization from 3% per unit transfused to 0.5% per unit transfused [99]. Similarly, HLA-matched platelet units may be necessary for patients with platelet refractoriness and anti-HLA alloantibodies. These matched platelets, however, must be irradiated prior to transfusion to eliminate the risk of TA-GVHD due to the HLA similarity between donor and recipient [107,146,147].

Non-immune mediated hazards of transfusion

Non-immune mediated hazards of transfusion include septic transfusion reactions, non-immune hemolysis, transfusion-associated circulatory overload, metabolic derangements, complications from red blood cell storage lesions, and mistransfusion [146].

Septic transfusion reactions

Transfusion-associated bacterial sepsis is another potential cause of transfusion-related deaths. Platelet units are by far the most frequently contaminated blood product since they are stored at room temperature. *Staphylococcus* species are the most common contaminants of platelet units whereas gram-negative bacteria such as *Yersinia enterocolitica* that can replicate at cold temperatures are more commonly found as contaminants in PRBC units. The major sources of contamination are the donor's skin at the venipuncture collection site, donor bacteremia that is asymptomatic or undetected, unsterile collection packs, and violations of sterility during processing procedures. The institution in 2004 of mandatory testing of platelet units for bacterial contamination has resulted in a significant decrease in the incidence of post-transfusion sepsis. Ongoing improvements in blood component collection techniques as well as detection and treatment of bacterial contamination of blood components provide hope for further reduction of this transfusion-related risk [106,114,115,144,146].

Non-immune hemolysis

Non-immune hemolysis of RBCs can result from incorrect storage of the blood unit, inadequate deglycerolization of frozen RBCs, thermal injury to RBCs by malfunctioning blood warmers, exposure of RBCs to hypotonic or hypertonic IV solutions, rapid transfusion through small-bore IV catheters or processing techniques used during RBC salvage. This problem is usually preventable by strictly following established guidelines for storing, preparing, and transfusing RBCs [106,146].

Transfusion-associated circulatory overload

Transfusion-associated circulatory overload (TACO) is the development of cardiogenic pulmonary edema from volume overload during transfusion. Infants and patients with cardiopulmonary compromise and renal failure are particularly susceptible to this risk. Diuretic administration, as well as slowing the blood administration rate, may minimize TACO symptoms [146].

Metabolic derangements

Hyperkalemia, hypocalcemia, and hypothermia can accompany the transfusion of blood products. Hyperkalemia is a potential problem with PRBC administration because RBCs leak potassium into their storage solution over time. Potassium concentrations reach an average of 12 mEq/L after 7 days of storage and 32 mEq/L after 21 days of storage. Hyperkalemia can be a particular problem when transfusing neonates, when using unwashed previously irradiated PRBCs, or in instances of massive transfusion because of the relative volume of PRBCs administered. Hyperkalemia causes tall peaked T waves on an electrocardiogram and can lead to ventricular dysrhythmias and cardiac arrest. The use of fresher PRBCs (<14 days old), transfusion into IV lines further away from the right atrium, correction of acidosis, administration of calcium to stabilize the myocardium, and administration of glucose and insulin to lower potassium levels are helpful with prevention and treatment. After transfusion is completed, excess potassium is gradually taken back into RBCs and normal metabolic activity is restored [132,146,157].

Hypocalcemia from "citrate toxicity" may be a problem with administration of large volumes of plasma and platelets. These components have high citrate concentrations in their anticoagulant solutions. Citrate exerts its anticoagulant effect by binding ionized calcium. Neonates and infants are particularly prone to the development of hypocalcemia since their intracellular calcium reserves are limited. Hypocalcemia can produce tetany, prolonged QT interval on an electrocardiogram, and decreased myocardial function. Treatment consists of the administration of calcium and slowing the infusion rate of the blood products. Citrate undergoes rapid hepatic metabolism so hypocalcemia associated with transfusion is a transient problem [132,146,157].

Hypothermia is a complication of the rapid infusion of large amounts of inadequately warmed blood products. Hypothermia not only potentiates the cardiac toxicity of hyperkalemia and hypocalcemia but also is a component of the "lethal triad" of coagulopathy, hypothermia, and acidosis that can occur during massive hemorrhage and transfusion. Therefore, its occurrence should be aggressively prevented and/or treated [146].

Red blood cell storage lesions
The ability to store RBCs for up to 42 days gives blood distribution centers significant flexibility in managing the blood supply [143]. However, during this storage period, detrimental changes occur in RBCs themselves and in the RBC product as a unit. RBCs lose their deformability and increase their adhesiveness so that their passage through capillaries is impaired. Levels of 2,3-DPG fall so that the oxygen affinity of hemoglobin increases, while some hemoglobin molecules are converted to methemoglobin which is incapable of binding oxygen. Finally, concentrations of nitric oxide fall, possibly impairing vasodilation of blood vessels. Therefore, even though raising the hemoglobin level by transfusing RBCs allows more

oxygen to be transported by blood, the sum of these effects may actually reduce the availability of this oxygen to tissues. These effects may be minimized by using PRBCs that are less than 14 days old [118,132,133,146,158].

Mistransfusion
Mistransfusion is the transfusion of the incorrect blood product to the incorrect recipient. It is the most common non-infectious complication of blood product transfusion. Approximately 30% of the errors leading to mistransfusion occur in the blood bank while 50% occur in clinical areas. Meticulous attention to detail when labeling blood samples and identifying blood products and recipients is critical to avoid the occurrence of this preventable hazard of blood transfusion [114,146].

Blood conservation

In light of the potential hazards posed by transfusing allogeneic blood products, efforts to minimize the necessity for transfusions should always be considered. These efforts may be especially important in patients who, for religious reasons (Jehovah's Witnesses), refuse blood product transfusion. Proactive blood conservation plans tailored to individual patients and their anticipated surgical procedures are essential for success but require significant forethought. Combining preoperative, intraoperative, and postoperative modalities will offer the best chance for a positive impact.

Preoperative modalities
Personal and family histories of bleeding disorders should be sought and investigated prior to surgery. Indicated laboratory tests should be performed well enough in advance to allow preoperative action based on the results. Causes of anemia should be investigated. Anticoagulant and antiplatelet drugs should be discontinued, if feasible, for an appropriate interval before surgery.

Preoperative anemia is a major risk factor in determining the need for perioperative allogeneic blood transfusion [119,159]. This risk may be reduced by the preoperative administration of erythropoietin, a hormone produced by the kidneys that acts on erythroblast precursor cells in the bone marrow to accelerate the production of mature erythrocytes and thus increase hemoglobin levels [160]. Recombinant human erythropoietin has been shown to increase preoperative hemoglobin levels in infants and children prior to a variety of surgical procedures [160–162]. However, it is expensive, it must be repeatedly injected intravenously or subcutaneously over a several week period preoperatively, and its use must be accompanied by iron supplementation. The most significant preoperative use of erythropoietin may be to increase hemoglobin levels in anticipation of preoperative autologous blood donation or intraoperative acute normovolemic hemodilution [162–165].

Preoperative autologous blood donation (PABD) is the preoperative collection of blood for transfusion back to the same donor in the perioperative period. PABD may be useful in children undergoing elective surgical procedures in which the likelihood of transfusion is substantial and in children who have rare blood groups or alloantibodies to high-incidence antigens. PABD decreases exposure to allogeneic blood products and has been used in a wide variety of surgical procedures in children [163,166–168]. As with erythropoietin, the use of PABD requires time and forethought. Depending on the size of the child and the anticipated surgical blood loss, several donations may be collected but the donations should be completed far enough in advance of surgery to allow the patient's hemoglobin level to recover prior to surgery. Estimations of the volume of blood to be collected at each donation have been based on a percentage (15%) of estimated blood volume (EBV), a defined amount (10 mL) per kg bodyweight, a weight-corrected proportion of an adult unit of blood ([weight/50 kg] × 450 mL), and on formulas to keep the child's postdonation hematocrit above 30% (EBV × [initial hematocrit – 30]/average hematocrit with average hematocrit = (initial hematocrit – 30)/2) [166]. PABD should not be used in children with active infections, anemia or limited cardiopulmonary reserves. Vascular access issues may limit the use of PABD in young infants [162,163]. This problem has been circumvented in some children prior to cardiac surgery by obtaining autologous blood from the large-bore vascular sheaths used during preoperative diagnostic cardiac catheterization [168]. The use of blood collected from PABD still carries risks from clerical errors and bacterial contamination, so appropriate indications should dictate its retransfusion while its automatic administration back to the donor without indications should be avoided [166].

Intraoperative modalities

Surgical technique obviously plays a role in limiting intraoperative blood loss and exposure to allogeneic blood transfusions. Direct control of bleeding vessels is essential and infiltration of local vasoconstrictors into surgical wound edges, use of tourniquets, patient positioning to elevate the surgical site, and use of topical clotting agents may all be important [159].

Anesthesiologists can also play helpful roles in minimizing perioperative exposure to allogeneic blood products. Maintenance of normothermia is important to prevent hypothermia-induced dysfunction of platelets and coagulation factors. Controlled hypotension techniques may help reduce intraoperative blood loss. Reinfusion of RBCs salvaged from the operative field may minimize effective

blood loss but should not be used during cancer surgery, in patients with active infections or after application of topical clotting agents. Tolerating lower hemoglobin levels and basing decisions to initiate transfusion on indicators such as the development of lactic acidosis or hemodynamic lability may avoid transfusion in some cases. Administration of increased inspired oxygen concentrations will increase dissolved oxygen in blood and help maintain adequate oxygen delivery to tissues when lower hemoglobin levels are being allowed. The use of acute normovolemic hemodilution (ANH) or pharmacological interventions may also be considered [119].

Acute normovolemic hemodilution involves the intraoperative collection of blood for reinfusion at the end of surgery. Blood is withdrawn from a patient after anesthetic induction while isovolemia is maintained by infusing crystalloid (3:1 volume replacement) and/or colloid (1:1 volume replacement). Subsequently, blood with a lower hemoglobin level is lost intraoperatively and safe, fresh autologous blood with a higher hemoglobin level and functioning coagulation factors and platelets is available for reinfusion once blood loss is controlled. The amount of blood to be withdrawn can be calculated using the formula EBV × (initial hematocrit – target hematocrit)/average hematocrit where average hematocrit = (initial hematocrit – target hematocrit)/2 [169]. ANH may be considered when surgical blood loss is anticipated to exceed 15% of a child's EBV and the child has a baseline hematocrit exceeding 35% and adequate cardiopulmonary reserve to tolerate lowering of the hematocrit [166]. ANH has been used in children in surgeries ranging from posterior spinal fusions to abdominal surgery, cancer surgery, and bone marrow harvesting [166]. It offers advantages over PABD in that it may be performed on the day of surgery for both elective and emergency procedures after adequate vascular access has been obtained in an anesthetized child, and it is associated with lower administrative costs [170]. Blood withdrawn during ANH may be stored for up to 8h at room temperature and, if more than one bag of blood was withdrawn, should be reinfused in the reverse order of collection [169]. Therefore, blood with the highest hematocrit (the first unit collected) will be reinfused after bleeding has been controlled.

Pharmacological interventions include antifibrinolytic agents and recombinant factor VIIa. Antifibrinolytic agents include aprotinin and the lysine analogs, ε-aminocaproic acid (EACA) and tranexamic acid (TA). Although aprotinin is remarkably effective in reducing perioperative blood loss and transfusion exposure, its marketing was suspended in 2007 after concerns about adverse renal, cardiovascular, and cerebrovascular effects and increased postoperative mortality were raised in adults in whom it was administered during cardiac surgery [171–174]. While studies in neonates and children undergoing cardiac surgery have not documented similar concerns [175–178], aprotinin currently remains unavailable for clinical use.

Thus, EACA and TA are the two clinically available antifibrinolytic agents. Both of these agents exert their antifibrinolytic effect most importantly by binding with the lysine-binding sites of plasminogen and plasmin. This reversible binding alters plasminogen's conformation, precludes its association with fibrin, and prevents its conversion to its active form, plasmin, while also inhibiting the activity of plasmin on fibrin [179,180]. These drugs have been shown to decrease blood loss and allogeneic blood transfusion in cyanotic children undergoing cardiac surgery [181–183], in children undergoing repeat sternotomies for cardiac surgery [184], and in children undergoing posterior spinal fusion for idiopathic or secondary scoliosis [185–187]. They have also been shown to have beneficial effects in adults undergoing liver transplantation [188,189] and total knee replacement [190,191] and thus would probably be beneficial for similar types of surgeries in children. These drugs may also be helpful in preventing clot lysis in patients with vWD or hemophilia after hemostasis has been achieved with appropriate factor replacement therapy, especially with bleeding from mucous membranes [37,78]. Evidence points to TA being more effective than EACA in its hemostatic effects [192]. Appropriate dosing regimens remain an unresolved issue for both of these drugs. While no thrombotic complications have been reported with their use, an increased incidence of postoperative seizures has been reported with TA use in adults undergoing cardiac surgery [193,194].

Recombinant activated factor VII (rFVIIa) promotes clot formation by enhancing thrombin generation. A TF-dependent mechanism involving saturation of exposed TF on injured blood vessels as well as a TF-independent mechanism involving direct interaction with activated platelets adherent to injured vessels may both be involved and confine the effects of rFVIIa to the injury site [195]. Resulting clot consists of a dense fibrin structure which is resistant to lysis because of concomitant increases in activation of the fibrin cross-linker, FXIII, and of TAFI [196]. rFVIIa is currently approved for use in patients with hemophilia A or B who have developed inhibitors to FVIII or FIX and in patients with acquired hemophilia to prevent or treat bleeding. It is also approved for the treatment of bleeding in patients with congenital FVII deficiency [197]. However, "off-label" applications are becoming increasingly frequent and include administration for reversal of warfarin-induced anticoagulation, management of inherited or acquired platelet function abnormalities, attenuation of hepatic dysfunction-induced coagulopathies, and control of intracerebral and gastrointestinal hemorrhage [198,199]. rFVIIa has been found to be beneficial during liver transplantation [200], cardiac surgery [201,202], and trauma surgery [203,204]. Its role is mainly that of a "rescue" therapy but the optimal dosing regimen is unclear and randomized, blinded, controlled studies are needed to define the appropriate clinical scenarios for its use. The potential for systemic thrombotic complications ("black box warning" issued for increased risk of arterial thrombosis), the lack of a validated laboratory monitor, and the significant cost of rFVIIa all remain concerns [199,202].

Postoperative modalities

Efforts to minimize exposure to allogeneic blood products should continue into the postoperative period. Useful strategies include limiting blood sampling to necessary tests and continued use of restrictive transfusion thresholds to trigger RBC transfusions. Reinstitution of postoperative anticoagulant or antiplatelet therapies should begin only after correction of coagulopathies acquired intraoperatively. Future considerations include development of appropriate coagulation test-based transfusion algorithms to guide blood component use and the development of safe artificial oxygen carriers to limit RBC transfusions.

Annotated references

A full reference list for this chapter is available at:
http://www.wiley.com/go/gregory/andropoulos/pediatricanesthesia

6. Hoffman M, Monroe DM. Coagulation 2006: a modern view of hemostasis. Hematol Oncol Clin North Am 2007; 21: 1–11. A comprehensive discussion of coagulation and fibrinolysis that describes the cell-based model of coagulation and contrasts it to the classic coagulation cascade explanation of the coagulation process.

10. Andrew M, Paes B, Johnston M. Development of the hemostatic system in the neonate and young infant. Am J Pediatr Hematol Oncol 1990; 12: 95–104. A compendium of Dr Andrew's classic work in defining quantitative maturational development of procoagulants, anticoagulants, and fibrinolytic components during the neonatal period and infancy.

75. Zimmerman TS, Ruggeri ZM. Von Willebrand disease. Hum Pathol 1987; 18– 140–52. A comprehensive review of the von Willebrand factor and the classification, diagnosis, and treatment of von Willebrand disease.

78. Dunn AL, Abshire TC. Recent advances in the management of the child who has hemophilia. Hematol Oncol Clin North Am 2004; 18: 1249–76. An interesting review of the history, pathophysiology, diagnosis, clinical presentation, management, and complications associated with hemophilia A and B.

84. Journeycake JM, Manco-Johnson MJ. Thrombosis during infancy and childhood: what we know and what we do not know. Hematol Oncol Clin North Am 2004; 18: 1315–38. A discussion of the risk factors for thrombosis in children, referencing both inherited thrombophilias and acquired clinical factors. Tables outline guidelines for treatment of thrombotic events in children and antithrombotic drugs doses.

93. Firth PG, Head CA. Sickle cell disease and anesthesia. Anesthesiology 2004; 101: 766–85. A detailed review of the genetics, pathophysiology, clinical features, and perioperative management of patients with sickle cell disease.

106. American Society of Anesthesiologists Committee on Transfusion Medicine. Questions and answers about blood management, 4th ed. 2008. www.ASAhq.org (accessed 26 February 2010). Answers to many questions an anesthesiologist might ask about the blood donation process, preparation of and indications for the administration of blood product components, adverse effects of transfusions, massive transfusion, coagulopathies associated with cardiac surgery and liver transplantation, and perioperative blood conservation techniques.

146. Hendrickson JE, Hillyer CD. Noninfectious serious hazards of transfusion. Anesth Analg 2009; 108: 759–69. A comprehensive summary of the non-infectious immune and non-immune mediated hazards of transfusion.

159. Goodnough LT, Shander A. Blood management. Arch Pathol Lab Med 2007; 131: 695–701. Discussion of useful preoperative, intraoperative, and postoperative blood conservation strategies including the use of pharmacological agents such as erythropoietin, recombinant FVIIa, antifibrinolytics, and desmopressin.

166. Murto KTT, Splinter WM. Perioperative autologous blood donation in children. Transfusion Sci 1999; 21: 41–62. Discussion of the application of preoperative autologous blood donation, normovolemic hemodilution, and intraoperative blood recovery in the pediatric arena. Includes discussion of the advantages, disadvantages, controversies, indications, contraindications, and techniques associated with each of these techniques.

CHAPTER 12
Cardiopulmonary Resuscitation

Todd J. Kilbaugh, Alexis A. Topjian, Robert M. Sutton, Vinay M. Nadkarni & Robert A. Berg
Department of Anesthesiology and Critical Care Medicine, The University of Pennsylvania School of Medicine, and The Children's Hospital of Philadelphia, Philadelphia, PA, USA

Introduction

Pediatric cardiac arrest is not a rare event. At least 16,000 American children (8–20/100,000 children/year) suffer a cardiopulmonary arrest each year [1–5]. More than half of these cardiac arrests probably occur in hospital [1,6]. With advances in resuscitation science and implementation techniques, survival from pediatric cardiac arrest has improved substantially over the past 25 years [7]. This chapter focuses on pediatric cardiac arrest, cardiopulmonary resuscitation, and other therapeutic interventions that have been specifically designed to improve outcomes from pediatric cardiac arrest.

Epidemiology of pediatric cardiac arrest

Cardiovascular disease remains the most common cause of disease-related death in the United States, resulting in approximately 1 million deaths per year [8]. It is estimated that more than 400,000 Americans will suffer a cardiac arrest each year, nearly 90% in prehospital settings. While data regarding the incidence of childhood cardiopulmonary arrest are less robust, the best data suggest that ~16,000 American children suffer a cardiac arrest each year (annual incidence: 8–20/100,000 children per year) [1–5,9]. For in-hospital arrests specifically, it is estimated that approximately 2–6% of all children admitted to pediatric intensive care units [5,10,11] and approximately 4–6% of children admitted to cardiac units will suffer a cardiac arrest [12,13]. In short, pediatric cardiac arrest is a critical public health problem.

Outcomes from pediatric cardiac arrest have improved significantly over the past 20 years. For example, survival to discharge from pediatric in-hospital cardiac arrest has increased from <10% in the 1980s [14,15] to >25% in the 21st century. Of the pediatric patients who survive to hospital discharge, nearly three-quarters will have favorable neurological function defined by specific pediatric cerebral outcome measures and quality of life indicators (Table 12.1) [7,12,16,17]. Factors that influence outcome from pediatric cardiac arrest include:
- the pre-existing condition of the child
- the environment in which the arrest occurs

Table 12.1 Summary of representative studies of outcome following in-hospital pediatric cardiac arrest

Author, year, reference	Setting*	Number of patients	ROSC	Survival to discharge	Good neurological survival
Raymond 2010 [178]	In hospital, E-CPR	199	N/A	87 (43.7%)	56 of 59 reported survivors (94.9%)
Meert 2009 [107]	In hospital	353		147 (48.7%)	132 (76% of survivors)
Tibballs 2009 [32]	In hospital, METS	23	Not reported	14 (73%)	Not reported
Prodhan 2009 [197]	In hospital, E-CPR	32	N/A	24 (73%)	75% no change PCPC from baseline
Thiagarajan 2007 [196]	In hospital, E-CPR	682	N/A	261 (38%)	Not reported
Tibballs 2006 [198]	In hospital	147	81 (73%)	40 (36%)	Not reported
Meaney 2006 [17]	All ICU patients <21	464	232 (50%)	102 (22%)	64 (14%)
Samson 2006 [179]	In-hospital CA (initial VF/VT rhythm)	272 (104)	125 (70%)	52 (35%)	46 (33%)
Nadkarni 2006 [7]	In-hospital CA	880	459 (52%)	236 (27%)	154 (18%)
Lopez-Herce 2005 [199]	Mixed in-hospital & OOH CA	213	110 (52%)	45 (21%)	34 (16%)
Reis 2002 [16]	In-hospital CA	129	83 (64%)	21 (16%)	19 (15%)
Parra 2000 [12]	Ped CICU CA	32	24 (63%)	14 (44%)	8 (25%)
Chamnanvanakij 2000 [200]	In-hospital intubated NICU pts with chest compressions for bradycardia	39	33 (85%)	CPR 20 (51%) CA 10%	CPR 5 (13%) (6 lost to follow-up)
Suominen 2000 [4]	In-hospital CA	118	74 (63%)	1-year survival 21 (18%)	Not reported
Young 1999 [3]	Meta-analysis in-hospital CA	544	Not reported	129 (24%)	Not reported
Torres 1997 [201]	In-hospital CA	92	Not reported	1-year survival 9 (10%)	7 (8%)
Slonim 1997 [5]	In-hospital PICU CA	205	Not reported	28 (14%)	Not reported
Tunstall-Pedoe 1992 [24]	Mixed in-hospital & OOH CA	3765	1411 (38%)	706 (19%)	Not reported
Zaritsky A 1987 [14]	In-hospital CA	CA 53	Not reported	CA 5 (9%)	Not reported

CA, cardiac arrest; E-CPR, extracorporeal membrane oxygenation-assisted cardiopulmonary resuscitation; METS, medical emergency teams (rapid response teams); OOH, out-of-hospital; NICU, neonatal intensive care unit; PCPC, pediatric cerebral performance category; PICU, pediatric intensive care unit; ROSC, return of spontaneous circulation; VF, ventricular fibrillation; VT, ventricular tachycardia.

- the initial electrocardiographic (ECG) rhythm detected
- the duration of no-flow time (the time during an arrest without spontaneous circulation or cardiopulmonary resuscitation; CPR)
- the quality of the life-supporting therapies provided during the resuscitation
- the quality of life-supporting therapies administered after resuscitation.

Not surprisingly, outcomes after pediatric out-of-hospital arrests are much worse than those after in-hospital arrests (Table 12.2) [2–3,10,18–25]. This may be due to the fact that there is a prolonged period of no flow in out-of-hospital arrests, where many of the pediatric cardiac arrests are not witnessed and only 30% of children are provided with bystander CPR. As a result of these factors, less than 10% of pediatric out-of-hospital cardiac arrests survive to hospital discharge, and among those who survive, severe neurological injury is common. These findings are especially troublesome given that bystander CPR more than doubles patient survival rates in adults [26].

An exciting prospective, nationwide, population-based cohort study from Japan similarly demonstrates more

Table 12.2 Summary of representative studies of outcome following out-of-hospital pediatric cardiac arrest

Author, year, reference	Setting*	Number of patients	ROSC	Survival to discharge	Favorable neurological survival
Kitamura 2010 [27]	OHCA Japan (age 1–17)	*Non-cardiac* No CPR (1293) Compression only (380) Conventional CPR (624) *Cardiac* No CPR (339) Compression only (158) Conventional CPR (282)	*Non-cardiac* No CPR (4.6%) Compression only (5.3%) Conventional CPR (9.9%) *Cardiac* No CPR (7.1%) Compression only (11.4%) Conventional CPR (12.1%)	*Non-cardiac* No CPR (6.9%) Compression only (8.9%) Conventional CPR (15.9%) *Cardiac* No CPR (10.6%) Compression only (16.5%) Conventional CPR (16.0%)	*Non-cardiac* No CPR (1.5%) Compression only (1.6%) Conventional CPR (7.2%) *Cardiac* No CPR (4.1%) Compression only (8.9%) Conventional CPR (9.9%)
Osmond 2006 [23]	OHCA Canada	503	Not reported	10 (2%)	Not reported
Donoghue 2005 [2]	OHCA Systematic review	5693	Not reported	689 (12%)	228 (4%)
Berg 2005 [202]	OHCA Shockable rhythm	13	13 (100%)	0 (0%)	0 (0%)
Young 1999 [3]	Meta-analysis OHCA	1568	Not reported	132 (8%)	Not reported
Sirbaugh 1999 [19]	OHCA	300	33 (11%)	6 (2%)	1 (<1%)
Suominen 1998 [203]	OHCA After trauma	41	10 (24%)	3 (7%)	2 (5%)
Suominen 1997 [18]	OHCA	50	13 (26%)	8 (16%)	6 (12%)
Schindler 1996 [20]	OHCA	80	43 (54%)	6 (8%)	0 (0%)
Kuisma 1995 [10]	OHCA	34	10 (29%)	5 (15%)	4 (12%)
Dieckmann 1995 [21]	OHCA	65	3 (5%)	2 (3%)	1 (1.5%)
Lopez-Herce 2005 [199]	Mixed in-hospital & OHCA	213	110 (52%)	45 (21%)	34 (16%)
Tunstall-Pedoe 1992 [24]	Mixed in-hospital & OHCA	3765	1411 (38%)	706 (19%)	Not reported

OHCA, out-of-hospital cardiac arrest; ROSC, return of spontaneous circulation.

than doubling of survival rates for children who have out-of-hospital cardiac arrests and receive bystander CPR either with conventional CPR (with rescue breathing) or chest compression-only CPR compared to no bystander CPR [27]. The same study then further stratifies outcomes for out-of-hospital cardiac arrest into "cardiac" and "non-cardiac" causes for arrest, and defines the relative value of rescue breathing during CPR by bystanders. Pediatric patients who have out-of-hospital cardiac arrests with non-cardiac causes and receive bystander conventional

CPR (including rescue breathing) had an association with higher frequency of favorable neurological outcomes at 1 month after arrest compared to compression-only bystander CPR or no bystander CPR. For pediatric arrests defined as "cardiac" in nature, bystander CPR (conventional or compression only) was associated with a higher rate of favorable neurological outcomes 1 month after arrest compared to no bystander CPR. Interestingly, the two types of bystander CPR (conventional or compression only) seemed to be similarly effective for pediatric cardiac arrests with cardiac causes, consistent with animal and adult studies [27].

Survival outcomes after in-hospital cardiac arrest are higher in the pediatric population compared with adults; 27% of children survive to hospital discharge compared with only 17% of adults [7]. For both children and adults, outcomes are better after arrhythmogenic arrests, from ventricular fibrillation/ventricular tachycardia (VF/VT). Importantly, pediatric in-hospital arrests are less commonly caused by arrhythmias (10% of pediatric arrests versus 25% of adult arrests), and approximately one-third of children and adults with these arrhythmogenic arrests survive to hospital discharge. Interestingly, the superior pediatric survival rate following in-hospital cardiac arrest

reflects a substantially higher survival rate among children with asystole or pulseless electrical activity (PEA) compared with adults (24% versus 11%). Further investigations have shown that the superior survival rate seen in children is mostly attributable to a much better survival rate among infants and preschool age children compared with older children [17]. Although speculative, the higher survival rates in children may be due to improved coronary and cerebral blood flow during CPR because of increased chest compliance in these younger arrest victims, with improved aortic diastolic pressure and venous return [28,29]. In addition, survival of pediatric patients from an in-hospital cardiac arrest is more likely in hospitals staffed with dedicated pediatric physicians [9].

Phases of resuscitation

The four distinct phases of cardiac arrest and CPR interventions are: (1) prearrest, (2) no flow (untreated cardiac arrest), (3) low flow (CPR), and (4) postresuscitation/arrest. Interventions to improve outcome of pediatric cardiac arrest should optimize therapies targeted to the time and phase of CPR, as suggested in Table 12.3.

Table 12.3 Phases of cardiac arrest and resuscitation

Phase	Interventions
Pre-arrest (Protect)	• Optimize community education regarding child safety • Optimize patient monitoring and rapid emergency response • Train in-hospital METs and rapid response teams • Recognize and treat respiratory failure and/or shock to prevent cardiac arrest • Transfer patients to skilled pediatric centers
Arrest (no-flow) (Preserve)	• Minimize interval to BLS and ACLS (organized response) • Minimize interval to defibrillation, when indicated
Low-flow (CPR) (Resuscitate)	• Push hard, push fast • Allow full chest recoil • Minimize interruptions in compressions (15:2) • Avoid overventilation • Titrate CPR to optimize myocardial blood flow (coronary perfusion pressures and exhaled CO_2) • Consider E-CPR if standard CPR/ACLS not promptly successful (within 5 min), if available
Post-resuscitation, short-term (Metabolic Delivery)	• Optimize cardiac output and cerebral perfusion • Treat arrhythmias, if indicated • Avoid hyperglycemia, hyperthermia, hyperventilation, hypoxemia, and hyperoxia • Consider mild postresuscitation systemic hypothermia (34–36°C in centers with dedicated protocols and pediatric critical care medicine) • Continual quality improvement for future responses to emergencies
Postresuscitation phase, longer-term rehabilitation (Regenerate)	• Early intervention with physical medicine and rehabilitation • Bio-engineering and technology interface • Possible future role for stem cell transplantation

ACLS, advanced cardiac life support; BLS, basic life support; E-CPR, extracorporeal membrane oxygenation-assisted cardiopulmonary resuscitation; METs, medical emergency teams.

Prearrest

The prearrest phase refers to any relevant pre-existing conditions of the child (e.g. neurological, cardiac, respiratory or metabolic problems) and precipitating events (e.g. respiratory failure or shock) uncoupling metabolic delivery and metabolic demand. Pediatric patients who suffer an in-hospital cardiac arrest often have changes in their physiological status in the hours leading up to their arrest event [30,31]. Therefore, interventions during the prearrest phase focus on preventing the cardiac arrest, with special attention to early recognition and targeted treatment of respiratory failure and shock.

Early recognition plays a key role in identifying a pre arrest state in children, who, unlike adults, may be able to mount a prolonged physiological response to a worsening clinical picture. Medical emergency teams (METs) (also known as rapid response teams) are in-hospital emergency teams designed specifically for this purpose. Front-line providers, and even parents, are encouraged to initiate evaluation by METs based on physiological protocol-driven parameters or even intuition. Patients are assessed by the METs and those at high risk of clinical decompensation are transferred to a pediatric intensive care unit if necessary, with the goal of preventing progression to full cardiac arrest or decreasing the response time to initiation of advanced life support, thereby limiting the no-flow state. Implementation of METs decreases the frequency of cardiac arrests compared with retrospective control periods before MET initiation [32–34].

While early recognition protocols cannot identify all children at risk for cardiac arrest, it seems reasonable to assume that transferring critically ill children to an ICU early in their disease process for better monitoring and more aggressive interventions can improve resuscitative care and clinical outcomes. The caveat is that prearrest states must be identified to initiate monitoring and interventions that may inhibit the progression to an arrest. While a significant amount of research dollars and resources are spent on the other phases of cardiac arrest, particular focus on the prearrest state may yield the greatest improvement in survival and neurological outcomes.

No flow/low flow

In order to improve outcomes from pediatric cardiac arrest, it is imperative to shorten the no-flow phase of untreated cardiac arrest. To that end, it is important to monitor high-risk patients to allow early recognition of the cardiac arrest and prompt initiation of basic and advanced life support. Effective CPR optimizes coronary perfusion pressure (by elevating aortic diastolic pressure relative to right atrial pressure) and cardiac output to critical organs to support vital organ viability (by elevating mean aortic pressure) during the low flow phase. Important tenets of basic life support are:

Push hard, push fast, allow full chest recoil between compressions, and minimize interruptions of chest compression.

The myocardium receives blood flow from the aortic root, mainly during diastole, via the coronary arteries. When the heart arrests and no blood flows through the aorta, coronary blood flow ceases. However, during chest compressions, aortic pressure rises at the same time as right atrial pressure and with the subsequent decompression phase of chest compressions, the right atrial pressure falls faster and lower than the aortic pressure, which generates a pressure gradient that perfuses the heart with oxygenated blood. Therefore, full elastic recoil (release) is critical to create a pressure difference between the aortic root and the right atrium. A coronary perfusion pressure (CPP) below 15 mmHg during CPR is a poor prognostic factor for return of spontaneous circulation (ROSC). Achieving optimal coronary perfusion pressure, exhaled carbon dioxide concentration, and cardiac output during the low-flow phase of CPR is consistently associated with an improved chance for ROSC and improved short- and long-term outcome in mature animal and human studies [35–42]. There is a critical need for research evaluating goal-directed CPR, in both immature animal models and pediatric patients.

Other measures essential for truncating the no-flow phase during ventricular fibrillation and pulseless ventricular tachycardia are rapid detection and prompt defibrillation. Clearly, CPR alone is inadequate for successful resuscitation from these arrhythmias. For cardiac arrests resulting from asphyxia and/or ischemia, adequate myocardial perfusion and myocardial oxygen delivery are the critical elements for return of spontaneous circulation.

Postarrest/resuscitation

The postarrest/resuscitation phase includes co-ordinated, skilled management of the immediate postresuscitation stage, the next few hours to days, and long-term rehabilitation. The immediate postresuscitation stage is a high-risk period for ventricular arrhythmias and other reperfusion injuries. Goals of interventions implemented during the immediate postresuscitation stage and the next few days include adequate tissue oxygen delivery, treatment of postresuscitation myocardial dysfunction, and minimizing postresuscitation tissue injury (e.g. preventing postresuscitation hyperthermia and hypoglycemia and, perhaps, initiating postresuscitation therapeutic hypothermia, preventing hyperglycemia and avoiding hyperoxia). This postarrest/resuscitation phase may have the greatest potential for innovative advances in the understanding of cell injury (excitotoxicity, oxidative stress, metabolic stress) and cell death (apoptosis and necrosis), ultimately leading to novel molecular-targeted interventions. The rehabilitation stage concentrates on salvage of injured cells, and support for re-engineering of reflex and voluntary communications of these cell and organ systems to improve long-term functional outcome.

The specific phase of resuscitation dictates the focus of care. Interventions that improve outcome during one phase may be deleterious during another. For instance, intense vasoconstriction during the low-flow phase of cardiac arrest improves CPP and the probability of ROSC. The same intense vasoconstriction during the postresuscitation phase increases left ventricular afterload and may worsen myocardial strain and dysfunction. Current understanding of the physiology of cardiac arrest and recovery allows us to only crudely manipulate blood pressure, oxygen delivery and consumption, body temperature, and other physiological parameters in our attempts to optimize outcome. Future strategies will likely take advantage of increasing knowledge of cellular injury, thrombosis, reperfusion, mediator cascades, cellular markers of injury and recovery, and transplantation technology, including stem cells.

Interventions during the cardiac arrest (no-flow) and cardiopulmonary resuscitation (low-flow) phases

Airway and breathing

Establishing an airway with effective gas exchange as soon as possible is critical for the success of resuscitation. Details of airway management are presented in Chapter 14. Establishing a patent airway with bag-valve-mask ventilation and 100% oxygen is an initial step in resuscitation, followed by endotracheal intubation as soon as possible, with minimal interruption in chest compressions. Colorimetric CO_2 detectors for exhaled gas are standard of care for pediatric CPR [43]. Absence of CO_2 in exhaled gas may mean the endotracheal tube is in the esophagus or that CPR is ineffective and there is no, or very low, pulmonary blood flow for gas exchange to occur. If CO_2 is absent, a direct laryngoscopy by an experienced clinician is performed immediately. If the tube is properly positioned in the trachea, attention is turned to effectiveness of chest compresions (see below). Persistence of adequate levels of end-tidal CO_2 during CPR is a favorable prognostic factor for ROSC [44,45].

During CPR, cardiac output and pulmonary blood flow are approximately 10–25% of those during normal sinus rhythm; therefore, a lower minute ventilation is necessary for adequate gas exchange from the blood traversing the pulmonary circulation. Animal and adult data indicate that hyperventilation ("overventilation" from exuberant rescue breathing) during CPR is common and can sub-stantially compromise venous return and subsequently cardiac output [46–48]. These detrimental hemodynamic effects are compounded when one considers the effect of interruptions in CPR to provide airway management and rescue breathing and may contribute to worse survival outcomes [49–52].

While overventilation is problematic, in light of the fact that most pediatric arrests are asphyxial in nature (90% of arrests begin with respiratory insufficiency), immediate initiation of *adequate* ventilation is still important. The difference between arrhythmogenic and asphyxial arrests lies in the physiology. In animal models of sudden VF cardiac arrest, acceptable PaO_2 and $PaCO_2$ persist for 4–8 min during chest compressions without rescue breathing [53,54]. This is in part because aortic oxygen and carbon dioxide concentrations at the onset of the arrest do not vary much from the prearrest state with no blood flow and minimal aortic oxygen consumption. The lungs act as a reservoir of oxygen during the low-flow state of CPR; therefore, adequate oxygenation and ventilation can continue without rescue breathing.

Several retrospective studies of witnessed VF cardiac arrest in adults have also shown that outcomes are similar after bystander-initiated CPR with either chest compressions alone or chest compressions plus rescue breathing [5]. However, during asphyxial arrest peripheral and pulmonary blood flow continues during the prearrest state, resulting in significant arterial and venous oxygen desaturation, elevated lactate levels, and depletion of the pulmonary oxygen reserve. Therefore, at the onset of cardiopulmonary resuscitation, there is substantial arterial hypoxemia and resulting acidemia. In this circumstance, rescue breathing with controlled ventilation can be a life-saving maneuver. In contrast, the adverse hemodynamic effects from overventilation during CPR combined with possible interruptions in chest compressions to open the airway and deliver rescue breathing are a lethal combination in certain circumstances such as VT/VF arrests. In short, the resuscitation technique should be titrated to the physiology of the patient to optimize patient outcome, with rapid, efficient, skilled airway management with minimal interruption of chest compressions a cornerstone of success in pediatric resuscitation.

Circulation
Optimizing blood flow during low flow cardiopulmonary resuscitation

When the heart arrests, no blood flows to the aorta and coronary blood flow ceases immediately [55]. At that point, provision of high-quality CPR (*push hard, push fast*) is vital to re-establish coronary flow. The goal during CPR is to maximize the myocardial perfusion pressure (MPP). Related by the following equation: MPP = aortic diastolic blood pressure (AoDP) – right atrial pressure (RAP), myocardial blood flow improves as the gradient between AoDP and RAP increases. During downward compression phase, aortic pressure rises at the same time as right atrial pressure with little change in the MPP. However, during the decompression phase of chest compressions, the right atrial pressure falls faster and lower than the aortic pressure, which generates a pressure gradient, perfusing the heart with oxygenated blood during this artificial period of "diastole." Several animal and human studies have demonstrated, in both VT/VF and asphyxial models, the importance of establishing MPP as a predictor for short-term survival outcome (ROSC) [41,56–59]. Because there is no flow without chest compressions, it is important to minimize interruptions in chest compressions. To allow good venous return in the decompression phase of external cardiac massage, it is also important to allow full chest recoil and to avoid overventilation (preventing adequate venous return because of increased intrathoracic pressure).

Based on the equation above, MPP can be improved by strategies that increase the pressure gradient between the aorta and the right atrium. As an example, the inspiratory impedance threshold device (ITD) is a small, disposable valve that can be connected directly to the tracheal tube or facemask to augment negative intrathoracic pressure during the inspiratory phase of spontaneous breathing and the decompression phase of CPR by impeding air flow into the lungs. Application in animal and adult human trials of CPR has established the ability of the ITD to improve vital organ perfusion pressures and myocardial blood flow [52,60–64]; however, in the only randomized trial during adult CPR, mortality benefit was limited to the subgroup of patients with PEA [62]. Additional evidence that augmentation of negative intrathoracic pressure can improve perfusion pressures during CPR comes from the active compression-decompression device (ACD). The ACD is a hand-held device that is fixed to the anterior chest of the victim by means of suction similar to a household plunger that can be used to apply active decompression forces during the release phase, thereby creating a vacuum within the thorax. By actively pulling during the decompression phase, blood is drawn back into the heart by the negative pressure [65]. Animal and adult studies have demonstrated that the combination of ACD with ITD acts in concert to further improve perfusion pressures during CPR compared to ACD alone [62].

In the end, while novel interventions such as the ITD and ACD are promising adjuncts to improve blood flow during CPR, the basic tenets of *push hard, push fast, allow full chest wall release, minimize interruptions, and don't overventilate* are still the dominant factors to improve blood flow during CPR and chance of survival.

Chest compression depth

The pediatric chest compression depth recommendation of at least one-third anterior–posterior (AP) chest depth (approximately 4cm in infants and 5cm in children) is based largely upon expert clinical consensus, using data extrapolated from animal, adult, and limited pediatric data. In a small study of six infants, chest compressions targeted to one-half AP chest depth resulted in improved systolic blood pressures compared to those targeted at one-third AP chest depth [66]. While only a small series with qualitatively estimated chest compression depths, this is the first study to collect actual data from children supporting the existing chest compression depth guidelines. In contrast, two recent studies using computed axial automated tomography (CT)[67,68] suggest that depth recommendations based on a relative percentage of AP chest compression depth are deeper than that recommended for adults, and that a depth of one-half AP chest depth will result in direct compression, to the point of fully emptying the heart and requisite shifting of heart because of inadequate AP diameter reserve in most children. Future studies that collect data from actual children and that associate quantitatively measured chest compression depths with short- and long-term clinical outcomes (arterial blood pressure, end-tidal carbon dioxide, return of spontaneous circulation, survival) are needed.

Compression/ventilation ratios

The amount of ventilation provided during CPR should match, but not exceed, perfusion and should be titrated to the amount of circulation during the specific phase of resuscitation as well as the metabolic demand of the tissues. Therefore, during the low flow state of CPR when the amount of cardiac output is roughly 10–25% of normal, less ventilation is needed [69]. However, the best ratio of compressions to ventilations in pediatric patients is largely unknown and depends on many factors, including the compression rate, the tidal volume, the blood flow generated by compressions, and the time that compressions are interrupted to perform ventilation. Recent evidence demonstrates that a compression/ventilation ratio of 15:2 delivers the same minute ventilation and increases the number of delivered chest compressions by 48% compared to CPR at a compression/ventilation ratio of 5:1 in a simulated pediatric arrest model [70,71]. This is important because when chest compressions cease, the aortic pressure rapidly decreases and coronary perfusion pressure falls precipitously, thereby decreasing myocardial oxygen delivery [55]. Increasing the ratio of compressions to ventilations minimizes these interruptions, thus increasing coronary blood flow. The benefits of positive pressure ventilation (increased arterial content of oxygen and carbon dioxide elimination) must be balanced against the adverse consequence of decreased circulation. These findings are in part the reason why the American Heart Association (AHA) now recommends a pediatric compression/ventilation ratio of 15:2 for two rescuers and 30:2 for a single rescuer.

Duty cycle

In a model of human adult cardiac arrest, cardiac output and coronary blood flow are optimized when chest compressions last for 30% of the total cycle time (approximately 1:2 ratio of time in compression to time in relaxation) [72]. As the duration of CPR increases, the optimal duty cycle may increase to 50%. In a juvenile swine model, a relaxation period of 250–300 msec (duty cycle of 40–50% at a compression rate of 120 per min) correlates with improved cerebral perfusion pressures compared with shorter duty cycles of 30% [73].

Circumferential versus focal sternal compressions

In adult and animal models of cardiac arrest, circumferential (vest) CPR has been demonstrated to dramatically improve CPR hemodynamics [74]. In smaller infants, it is often possible to encircle the chest with both hands and depress the sternum with the thumbs, while compressing the thorax circumferentially (thoracic squeeze). In an infant animal model of CPR, this "two-thumb" method of compression with thoracic squeeze resulted in higher systolic and diastolic blood pressures and a higher pulse pressure than traditional two-finger compression of the sternum [75]. Although not rigorously studied, our clinical experience indicates that it is very difficult to attain adequate chest compression force and adequate aortic pressures with the two-finger technique, so we fully support the AHA guidelines for healthcare providers to perform CPR on infants with the two thumbs plus encircling hands technique [76].

Open-chest cardiopulmonary resuscitation

In animal models, high-quality standard, closed-chest CPR generates myocardial blood flow that is >50% of normal, cerebral blood flow that is approximately 50% of normal, and cardiac output ~10–25% of normal [55,57,77,78]. By contrast, open-chest CPR can generate myocardial and cerebral blood flow that approaches normal. Although open-chest massage improves CPP and increases the chance of successful defibrillation in animals and humans [79–81], performing a thoracotomy to allow open-chest CPR is impractical in many situations. A retrospective review of 27 cases of CPR following pediatric blunt trauma (15 with open-chest CPR and 12 with closed-chest CPR) demonstrated that open-chest CPR increased hospital cost without altering rates of ROSC or survival to discharge. However, survival in both groups was 0%, indicating that the population may have been too severely injured or too late in the process to benefit from this aggressive therapy [82]. Open-chest CPR is often provided to children after open-heart cardiac surgery and sternotomy. Earlier institution of open-chest CPR may warrant reconsideration in selected special resuscitation circumstances.

Vascular access

Obtaining vascular access is obviously crucial to the success of resuscitation. Standard peripheral venous access is the first technique to consider. Details and techniques of peripheral venous access are presented in Chapter 17. Infants and children, especially hospitalized children and those with multiple previous medical interventions, often have poor peripheral venous access and it is not uncommon, even with in-hospital arrest, to encounter a patient without venous access. In this situation intraosseous (IO) infusion has become the recommended practice, supported by decades of animal study and clinical use [43,83]. Fourteen, 16, and 18 gauge specially made styletted intraosseous needles should be kept on all CPR carts, and the flat surface of the proximal tibia is utilized. The needle is placed perpendicular to the bone and inserted with a twisting, "boring" motion until loss of resistance heralding perforation of the bony cortex into cancellous bone. In infants and young children, active bone marrow hematopoiesis is occurring, and removal of the IO needle stylet and aspiration of bone marrow signifies successful placement. After rapid flush of 5–10 mL normal saline, resuscitation drugs and fluids can be administered IO, all followed by rapid flush with saline. These drugs include epinephrine, atropine, antiarrhythmic agents, naloxone, and dextrose. Fluids and blood can also be administered and blood samples can be obtained for laboratory studies. Caution must be exercised to detect extravasation of fluid into surrounding tissues. Standard venous access must be obtained as soon as possible. Central venous access is often difficult to obtain during resuscitation, and IO access is preferred. Venous access attempts should not interfere with chest compressions.

Medications used to treat cardiac arrest

While animal studies have indicated that epinephrine can improve initial resuscitation success after both asphyxial and VF cardiac arrests, there are no prospective studies to support the use of epinephrine or any other medication to improve survival outcome from pediatric cardiac arrest. A variety of medications are used during pediatric resuscitation attempts, including vasopressors (epinephrine and vasopressin), antiarrhythmics (amiodarone and lidocaine), and other drugs such as calcium chloride and sodium bicarbonate. Each will be discussed separately below.

Vasopressors

Epinephrine (adrenaline) is an endogenous catecholamine with potent α- and β-adrenergic stimulating properties. The α-adrenergic action (vasoconstriction) increases systemic and pulmonary vascular resistance. The resultant higher aortic diastolic blood pressure improves coronary perfusion pressure and myocardial blood flow even though it reduces global cardiac output during CPR, and as noted above, adequacy of myocardial blood flow is a critical determinant of ROSC. Epinephrine also increases cerebral blood flow during good-quality CPR because peripheral vasoconstriction directs a greater proportion of flow to the cerebral circulation [84–86]. However, recent evidence suggests that epinephrine can decrease local cerebral microcirculatory blood flow at a time when global cerebral flow is increased [87]. The β-adrenergic effect increases myocardial contractility and heart rate, and relaxes smooth muscle in the skeletal muscle vascular bed and bronchi; however, the β-adrenergic effects are not observed in the peripheral vascular beds secondary to the high dose used in cardiac arrest.

Epinephrine also increases the vigor and intensity of VF, increasing the likelihood of successful defibrillation. High-dose epinephrine (0.05–0.2 mg/kg) improves myocardial and cerebral blood flow during CPR more than standard-dose epinephrine (0.01–0.02 mg/kg) in animal models of cardiac arrest and may increase the incidence of initial ROSC [88,89]. However, prospective and retrospective studies have indicated that the use of high-dose epinephrine in adults or children does not improve survival and may be associated with worse neurological outcome [90,91]. A randomized, blinded, controlled trial of rescue high-dose epinephrine versus standard-dose epinephrine after failed initial standard-dose epinephrine in pediatric in-hospital cardiac arrest demonstrated a worse 24-h survival in the high-dose epinephrine group (one of 34 survived with high dose, versus 7 of 34 with standard dose, p = 0.05) [92]. Based on these clinical studies, high-dose epinephrine cannot be recommended routinely for either initial or rescue therapy. Importantly, these studies indicate that high-dose epinephrine can worsen a patient's postresuscitation hemodynamic condition and likelihood of survival.

Vasopressin is a long-acting endogenous hormone that acts at specific receptors to mediate systemic vasoconstriction (V$_1$ receptor) and reabsorption of water in the renal tubule (V$_2$ receptor). Vasoconstrictive properties are most intense in the skeletal muscle and skin vascular beds. Unlike epinephrine, vasopressin is not a pulmonary vasoconstrictor. In experimental models of cardiac arrest, vasopressin increases blood flow to the heart and brain and improves long-term survival compared with epinephrine. However, it can decrease splanchnic blood flow during and following CPR and can increase afterload in

the postresuscitation period, placing further strain on the left ventricle [77,93–96]. Adult randomized, controlled trials suggest that outcomes are similar after use of vasopressin or epinephrine during CPR [97,98]. A case series of four children who received vasopressin during six prolonged cardiac arrest events suggested that the use of bolus vasopressin may result in ROSC when standard medications have failed [99]. However, a more recent retrospective study of 1293 consecutive pediatric arrests from the National Registry of CPR (NPCRP) found that vasopressin use, while infrequent (administered in only 5% of events), was associated with a lower likelihood of ROSC.

Therefore, it is unlikely that vasopressin will replace epinephrine as a first-line agent in pediatric cardiac arrest. However, the available data suggest that its use in conjunction with epinephrine may deserve further investigation, especially in prolonged arrest unresponsive to initial epinephrine resuscitation.

Antiarrhythmic medications

See the section on ventricular fibrillation in children.

Calcium

Calcium is used frequently in cases of pediatric cardiac arrest, despite the lack of evidence for efficacy. In the absence of a documented clinical indication (i.e. hypocalcemia, calcium channel blocker overdose, hypermagnesemia or hyperkalemia), administration of calcium does not improve outcomes from cardiac arrest [100–108]. On the contrary, three pediatric studies have suggested a potential for harm, as routine calcium administration was associated with decreased survival rates and/or worse neurological outcomes [100–108]. Despite limited clinical data to support the use of calcium during CPR, it is reasonable to consider calcium administration during CPR for cardiac arrest patients at high risk of hypocalcemia (e.g. renal failure, shock associated with massive transfusion).

Buffer solutions

There are no randomized controlled studies in children examining the use of sodium bicarbonate for management of pediatric cardiac arrest. Two randomized controlled studies have examined the value of sodium bicarbonate in the management of adult cardiac arrest [109] and in neonates with respiratory arrest in the delivery room [110]. Neither study was associated with improved survival. In fact, one multicenter retrospective in-hospital pediatric study found that sodium bicarbonate administered during cardiac arrest was associated with decreased survival, even after controlling for age, gender and first documented cardiac rhythm [107]. Therefore, during pediatric cardiac arrest resuscitation, the routine use of sodium bicarbonate is not recommended. Clinical trials involving critically ill adults with severe metabolic acidosis do not demonstrate a beneficial effect of sodium bicarbonate on hemodynamics despite correction of acidosis [111,112]. This is somewhat surprising in light of data that severe acidosis may depress the action of catecholamines and worsen myocardial function [113,114]. Nevertheless, the common use of sodium bicarbonate during CPR is not supported by clinical data. Pediatric patients with implanted cardiac pacemakers may have an increased threshold for myocardial electrical stimulation when acidotic [115]; therefore, administration of bicarbonate or another buffer is appropriate for management of severe documented acidosis in these children. Administration of sodium bicarbonate also is indicated in the patient with a tricyclic antidepressant overdose, hyperkalemia, hypermagnesemia or sodium channel blocker poisoning.

The buffering action of bicarbonate occurs when a hydrogen cation and a bicarbonate anion combine to form carbon dioxide and water. Carbon dioxide must be cleared through adequate minute ventilation; thus, if ventilation is impaired during sodium bicarbonate administration, carbon dioxide build-up may negate the buffering effect of bicarbonate. Because carbon dioxide readily penetrates cell membranes, intracellular acidosis may paradoxically increase after sodium bicarbonate administration without adequate ventilation. Therefore, bicarbonate should not be used for management of respiratory acidosis.

Unlike sodium bicarbonate, tris-hydroxymethyl aminomethane (THAM) buffers excess protons without generating carbon dioxide; in fact, carbon dioxide is consumed following THAM administration. In a patient with impaired minute ventilation, THAM may be preferable when buffering is necessary to mitigate severe acidosis. THAM undergoes renal elimination, and renal insufficiency may be a relative contraindication to its use. Carbicarb, an equimolar combination of sodium bicarbonate and sodium carbonate, is another buffering solution that generates less carbon dioxide than sodium bicarbonate. In a canine model of cardiac arrest comparing animals given normal saline, sodium bicarbonate, THAM or Carbicarb, the animals given any buffer solution had a higher rate of ROSC than the animals given normal saline. In the animals given sodium bicarbonate or Carbicarb, the interval to ROSC was significantly shorter than in animals given normal saline. However, at the end of the 6-h study period, all resuscitated animals were in a deep coma, so no inferences regarding meaningful survival can be drawn [116]. It is premature to recommend either THAM or Carbicarb during CPR at this time.

Table 12.4 summarizes the recommendations for medication administration during pediatric CPR [43].

Postresuscitation interventions

Temperature management

Mild induced hypothermia is the most clinically promising recent goal-directed postresuscitation therapy for adults. Two seminal articles [117,118] have established that induced hypothermia (32–34°C) could improve outcome for comatose adults after resuscitation from VF cardiac arrest. In both randomized, controlled trials, the inclusion criteria were patients older than 18 years who were persistently comatose after successful resuscitation from non-traumatic VF [119,120]. Interpretation and extrapolation of these studies to children are difficult; however, fever within the first 48h following cardiac arrest, brain trauma, stroke, and ischemia is associated with poor neurological outcome. Emerging neonatal trials of selective brain cooling and systemic cooling show promise in neonatal hypoxic-ischemic encephalopathy (HIE), suggesting that induced hypothermia may improve outcomes [121,122].

The efficacy of therapeutic hypothermia following pediatric cardiac arrest is being evaluated in a randomized controlled trial (clinicaltrials.gov identifier NCT00880087); THAPCA: Therapeutic Hypothermia After Pediatric Cardiac Arrest (www.thapca.org). At a minimum, it is advisable to avoid hyperthermia in children following CPR. Using an approach of "therapeutic normothermia" with scheduled administration of antipyretic medications and the use of external cooling devices, while monitoring core temperature, may be necessary to prevent hyperthermia in this population. Notably, preventing hyperthermia is not easy. Many children become hyperthermic post arrest despite the intention to prevent hyperthermia [118].

Glucose control

Both hyperglycemia and hypoglycemia following cardiac arrest are associated with worse neurological outcome [123–126]. While it seems intuitive that hypoglycemia would be associated with worse neurological outcome, whether hyperglycemia *per se* is harmful or is simply a marker of the severity of the stress hormone response from prolonged ischemia is not clear. In critically ill adult patients, tight glucose control using an insulin infusion was associated with improved survival [127,128]. However, subsequent studies of non-surgical adult populations and neonatal/pediatric trials have demonstrated no survival benefit and the potential for harm from attempts at tight glucose control because of high rates of inadvertent hypoglycemia [123,129–135].

In summary, there is insufficient evidence to formulate a strong recommendation on the management of hyperglycemia in children with ROSC following cardiac arrest. If hyperglycemia is treated following ROSC in pediatric

Table 12.4 Medications for pediatric resuscitation and arrhythmias

Medication	Dose	Remarks
Adenosine	0.1 mg/kg (maximum 6 mg) Repeat: 0.2 mg/kg (maximum 12 mg)	Monitor ECG Rapid IV/IO bolus
Amiodarone	5 mg/kg IV/IO; repeat up to 15 mg/kg (maximum: 300 mg)	Monitor ECG and blood pressure Adjust administration rate to urgency (give more slowly when perfusing rhythm present) Use caution when administering with other drugs that prolong QT (consider expert consultation)

Atropine	0.02 mg/kg IV/IO
	0.03 mg/kg ET[a]
	Repeat once if needed
	Minimum dose: 0.1 mg
	Maximum single dose:
	   Child 0.5 mg
	   Adolescent 1 mg
		Higher does may be used with organophosphate poisoning

Calcium chloride (10%)	20 mg/kg IV/IO (0.2 mL/kg)	Slowly Adult dose: 5–10 mL
Epinephrine	0.01 mg/kg (0.1 mL/kg 1:10 000) IV/IO 0.1 mg/kg (0.1 mL/kg 1:1000) ET[a] Maximum dose: 1 mg/IV/IO; 10 mg ET	May repeat every 3–5 min
Glucose	0.5–1 mg/kg IV/IO	$D_{10}W$: 5–10 mL/kg $D_{25}W$: 2–4 mL/kg $D_{50}W$: 1–2 mL/kg
Lidocaine	Bolus: 1 mg/kg IV/IO Maximum dose: 100 mg Infusion: 20–50 µg/kg per min ET[a]: 2–3 mg/kg	
Magnesium sulfate	25–50 mg/kg IV/IO over 10–20 min; faster in torsades Maximum dose: 2 g	
Naloxone	<5 y or ≤20 kg: 0.1 mg/kg IV/IO/ET[a] ≥5 y or >20 kg: 2 mg IV/IO/ET	Use lower doses to reverse respiratory depression associated with therapeutic opioid use (1–15 µg/kg)
Procainamide	15 mg/kg IV/IO over 30–60 min Adult dose: 20 mg/min IV infusion up to total maximum dose 17 mg/kg	Monitor ECG and blood pressure Use caution when administering with other drugs that prolong QT (consider expert consultation)
Sodium bicarbonate	1 mEq/kg per dose IV/IO slowly	After adequate ventilation

[a]Flush with 5 mL of normal saline and follow with 5 ventilations. ET indicates via endotracheal tube.

ET, endotracheal; IO, intraosseous. Reproduced from Atkins et al [43] with permission from American Heart Association.

patients, blood glucose concentrations should be carefully monitored to avoid hypoglycemia.

Blood pressure management

A patient with ROSC may have substantial variability in blood pressure following cardiac arrest. Postarrest/resuscitation myocardial dysfunction is very common and is often associated with hypotension (see below) [119,120,136–145]. In addition, hypertension may occur, especially if the patient receives vasoactive infusions for postarrest myocardial dysfunction. Optimization of blood pressure post arrest is critical to maintain adequate perfusion pressure to vital organs that may have already been injured from the "no-flow" and "low-flow" states during initial cardiac arrest and CPR.

Cerebral blood flow in healthy patients is tightly controlled over a wide range of mean arterial blood pressure via the cerebral neurovascular bundle (autoregulation);

however, adults resuscitated from cardiac arrest have demonstrated impaired autoregulation of cerebral blood flow and this may also be the case in children [146]. Dysautoregulation of the cerebral neurovascular bundle following cardiac arrest may limit the brain's ability to regulate excessive blood flow and microvascular perfusion pressure, thereby leading to reperfusion injury during systemic hypertension. However, in animal models, brief induced hypertension following resuscitation results in improved neurological outcome compared with normotensive reperfusion [147,148]. Conversely, systemic hypotension may perpetuate neurological metabolic crisis following ischemic injury by uncoupling bio-energetic demand and delivery. Therefore, a practical approach to blood pressure management following cardiac arrest is to attempt to minimize blood pressure variability in this high-risk period following resuscitation.

Postresuscitation myocardial dysfunction

Postarrest myocardial stunning and arterial hypotension occur commonly after successful resuscitation in both animals and humans [119,120,136–145]. Animal studies demonstrate that postarrest myocardial stunning is a global phenomenon with biventricular systolic and diastolic dysfunction. Postarrest myocardial stunning is pathophysiologically and physiologically similar to sepsis-related myocardial dysfunction and postcardiopulmonary bypass myocardial dysfunction, including increases in inflammatory mediators and nitric oxide production [139,142,143,145].

Because cardiac function is essential to reperfusion following cardiac arrest, management of postarrest myocardial dysfunction may be important to improving survival. The classes of agents used to maintain circulatory function (i.e. inotropes, vasopressors, and vasodilators) must be carefully titrated during the postresuscitation phase to the patient's cardiovascular physiology. Although the optimal management of postcardiac arrest hypotension and myocardial dysfunction has not been established, data suggest that aggressive hemodynamic support may improve outcomes. Controlled trials in animal models have shown that dobutamine, milrinone and levosimendan can effectively ameliorate postcardiac arrest myocardial dysfunction [136,137,149,150]. In clinical observational studies, fluid resuscitation has been provided for patients with hypotension and concomitant low central venous pressure, and various vasoactive infusions, including epinephrine, dobutamine, and dopamine, have been used to treat the myocardial dysfunction syndrome [110–120,140–144]. In the end, optimal use of these agents involves close goal-directed titration, and the use of invasive hemodynamic monitoring may be appropriate.

General critical care principles suggest that appropriate therapeutic goals are adequate blood pressures and adequate oxygen delivery. However, the definition of "adequate" is elusive. Reasonable interventions for vasodilatory shock with low central venous pressure include fluid resuscitation and vasoactive drug infusions. Appropriate considerations for left ventricular myocardial dysfunction include euvolemia, inotropic infusions, and afterload reduction.

Neuromonitoring

Continuous neuromonitoring and goal-directed intervention following cardiac arrest is an exciting frontier with great promise for improving neurological outcomes post cardiac arrest [151]. Continuous EEG (cEEG) monitoring is an increasingly instituted modality for neuromonitoring of critically ill patients, especially to diagnose nonconvulsive seizures (NCS) and seizures in patients receiving muscle relaxants. cEEG monitoring is noninvasive, performed at the bedside, and permits continuous assessment of cortical function. Interpretation of cEEG is usually performed by a neurologist from a remote location, and not bedside critical care physicians. However, advances in quantitative EEG tools may allow bedside caregivers to identify important electrographic events, such as seizures or abrupt background changes, to potentially permit real-time analysis and intervention [152]. In a prospective study of cEEG in children, nonconvulsive seizures were detected in 39% (12 of 31) of children following cardiac arrest [153]. In a partially overlapping cohort of 19 children, NCS were common in children undergoing therapeutic hypothermia after cardiac arrest [153]. NCS seem to be a common occurrence following cardiac arrests in children.

Although the relationship of NCS to worse outcomes has not been established in pediatric patients following cardiac arrest, it has been associated with worse outcomes among critically ill adults and neonates [154–160]. We believe that cEEG should be considered for children post cardiac arrest and that patients with NCS (especially status epilepticus with NCS) should be treated with anticonvulsant medication. Further study is warranted to better establish frequency of NCS and potential benefit in outcomes with anticonvulsant therapy.

Oxidative injury may be greatest in the early phases of postresuscitation therapy following cardiac arrest [161]. Interestingly, the use of 100% oxygen (compared to room air) during and immediately following resuscitation in animal models may potentiate oxidative injury to key mitochondrial enzymes (pyruvate dehydrogenase or manganese superoxide) or mitochondrial lipids (cardiolipin) and is associated with worse neurological outcomes [162–165]. Experimental protocols in large animals using peripheral pulse oximetry to titrate oxygenation in the postresuscitation phase can reduce postresuscitation hyperoxia and significantly improve neuropathology and neurobehavioral outcomes [166]. Consistent with these experimental findings, arterial hyperoxia (PaO$_2$ ≥ 300 mmHg) was independently associated with in-hospital mortality compared with either hypoxia or normoxia in an observational study among critically ill adult patients admitted to the ICU within 24 h of a cardiac arrest [167]. We believe it is prudent to titrate oxygenation during and following pediatric cardiac arrest. Although the optimal SpO$_2$ is not known, we recommend titration of FiO$_2$ to the lowest amount necessary to assure SpO$_2$ > 94%.

Perhaps the future of postarrest care will include more aggressive neurocritical care monitoring, such as near infrared spectroscopy, cerebral microdialysis, brain tissue oxygen saturation (PbtO$_2$), cerebral blood flow, and even bedside analysis of mitochondrial dysfunction.

Other considerations

Quality of cardiopulmonary resuscitation

Despite evidence-based guidelines, extensive provider training, and provider credentialing in resuscitation medicine, the quality of CPR is typically poor. CPR guidelines recommend target values for selected CPR parameters related to rate and depth of chest compressions and ventilations, avoidance of CPR-free intervals, and complete release of sternal pressure between compressions [168]. Slow compression rates, inadequate depth of compression, and substantial pauses are the norm. An approach to *"push hard, push fast, minimize interruptions, allow full chest recoil and don't overventilate"* can markedly improve myocardial, cerebral, and systemic perfusion, and will likely improve outcomes [51]. Quality of postresuscitative management has also been demonstrated to be critically important to improving resuscitation survival outcomes [140]. Measuring the quality of CPR and avoiding overventilation during cardiac arrest resuscitation have recently been re-emphasized by consensus of the International Liaison Committee on Resuscitation and the American Heart Association [169]. Although the correct amount, timing, intensity, and duration of ventilation required during CPR are controversial, there is no controversy that measurement and titration of the amount of ventilation to the amount of blood perfusion are desirable. Thus, additional technology that is safe, accurate, and practical would improve detection and feedback of the "quality of CPR."

Recent technology has been developed that monitors quality of CPR by force sensors and accelerometers and can provide verbal feedback to the CPR administrator regarding the frequency and depth of chest compressions and the volume of ventilations. Recent pediatric data illustrate that intensive training and real-time corrective feedback can help chest compression quality approach age-specific AHA CPR guideline targets [170–172]. Moreover, improvements in postresuscitation care can improve resuscitation survival outcomes [140].

Extracorporeal membrane oxygenation-cardiopulmonary resuscitation

Extracorporeal cardiopulmonary resuscitation (E-CPR) has been reported to improve short-term and long-term survival outcomes following in-hospital and out-of-hospital cardiac arrest refractory to conventional therapy in observational studies [173–177]. Such studies are provocative and hypothesis generating, but can be criticized for small numbers, selection bias, and the lack of randomization to control for confounding by indication [178]. It is unlikely that there will ever be a randomized controlled trial (RCT) investigating the treatment effect of E-CPR for in-hospital cardiac arrest, because of the need for a large sample size, complexity of methodology, lack of blinding, and lack of equipoise among providers. Devoid of a RCT, E-CPR observational studies in children clearly suggest favorable early survival outcomes in children with primary cardiac disease when E-CPR protocols were in place at the time of the arrest [30,161–171]. For pediatric patients without primary cardiac disease, the data are less clear. Impressively, these studies consistently show that >1/3 of children provided with E-CPR survive to hospital discharge despite median durations of CPR of approximately 50 min prior to extracorporeal membrane oxygenation (ECMO) implementation. Importantly, 64% of patients who survived to discharge after E-CPR had favorable neurological outcomes [178].

Current guidelines recommend that extracorporeal CPR (E-CPR or rescue ECMO) should be considered in pediatric patients with in-hospital cardiac arrest that is refractory to initial resuscitation efforts when the cause of the arrest is believed to be reversible or amenable to heart transplantation [43]. Timely, quality E-CPR may be an exciting adjuvant to conventional CPR for pediatric patients. Future frontiers will define patient populations and optimize the clinical approach to extracorporeal support; however, clinicians providing CPR should consider E-CPR early in the course of a resuscitation not responding to conventional CPR. Perhaps after failure to attain ROSC within 5 min, clinicians should ask themselves: (1) Does the patient have a potentially reversible process? (2) Would ECMO be a "bridge" to a potentially good outcome? (3) Do we have the personnel and resources to provide EMCO promptly? If the answer to all three is "yes," prompt implementation of E-CPR should be considered.

Ventricular fibrillation and ventricular tachycardia in children

Pediatric VF or VT has been an underappreciated pediatric problem. Recent studies indicate that VF and VT (i.e. shockable rhythms) occur in 27% of in-hospital cardiac arrests at some time during the resuscitation [179]. In a population of pediatric cardiac intensive care unit patients, as many as 41% of arrests were associated with VF or VT [13]. According to the National Registry of Cardiopulmonary Resuscitation (NRCPR) database (www.nrcpr.org), 10% of children with in-hospital cardiac arrest had an initial rhythm of VF/VT. In all, 27% of the children had VF/VT at some time during the resuscitation [179]. The incidence of VF varies by setting and age [180]. In special circumstances, such as tricyclic antidepressant overdose, cardiomyopathy, post cardiac surgery, and prolonged QT syndromes, VF and pulseless VT are more likely.

The treatment of choice for short-duration VF is prompt defibrillation. In general, the mortality rate increases by 7–10% per minute of delay to defibrillation. Because VF must be considered before defibrillation can be provided, early determination of the rhythm by electrocardiography is critical. An attitude that VF is rare in children can be a self-fulfilling prophecy with a uniformly fatal outcome. The recommended defibrillation dose is 2 J/kg, but the data supporting this recommendation are not optimal and are based on old monophasic defibrillators. In the mid-1970s, authoritative sources recommended starting doses of 60–200 J for all children. Because of concerns about myocardial damage and animal data suggesting that shock doses ranging from 0.5 to 1 J/kg were adequate for defibrillation in a variety of species, Gutgesell et al evaluated the efficacy of their strategy to defibrillate with 2 J/kg monophasic shocks. Seventy-one transthoracic defibrillations in 27 children were evaluated. Shocks within 10 min of 2 J/kg resulted in successful defibrillation (i.e. termination of fibrillation) in 91% of defibrillation attempts [181]. More recent data demonstrate that an initial shock dose of 2 J/kg terminates fibrillation in <60% of children, suggesting that a higher dose may be needed [22,182,183]. Despite five decades of clinical experience with pediatric defibrillation, the optimal dose remains unknown.

Antiarrhythmic medications: lidocaine and amiodarone

Administration of antiarrhythmic medications should never delay administration of shocks to a patient with VF. However, after an unsuccessful attempt at electrical defibrillation, medications to increase the effectiveness of defibrillation should be considered. Epinephrine is the current first-line medication for both pediatric and adult patients in VF. If epinephrine and a subsequent repeat attempt to defibrillate are unsuccessful, lidocaine or amiodarone should be considered.

Lidocaine traditionally has been recommended for shock-resistant VF in adults and children. However, only amiodarone improved survival to hospital admission in the setting of shock-resistant VF compared with placebo [184]. In another study of shock-resistant out-of-hospital VF, patients receiving amiodarone had a higher rate of survival to hospital admission than patients receiving lidocaine [185]. Neither study included children. Because there is moderate experience with amiodarone use as an antiarrhythmic agent in children and because of the adult studies, it is rational to use amiodarone similarly in children with shock-resistant VF/VT. The recommended dosage is 5 mg/kg by rapid intravenous bolus. There are no published comparisons of antiarrhythmic medications for pediatric refractory VF. Although extrapolation of adult data and electrophysiological mechanistic information suggest that amiodarone may be preferable for pediatric shock-resistant VF, the optimal choice is not clear.

Pediatric automated external defibrillators

Automated external defibrillators (AEDs) have improved adult survival from VF [186,187]. AEDs are recommended for use in children 8 years or older with cardiac arrest [76,188]. The available data suggest that some AEDs can accurately diagnose VF in children of all ages, but many AEDs are limited because the defibrillation pads and energy dosage are geared for adults. Adapters with smaller defibrillation pads that dampen the amount of energy delivered have been developed as attachments to adult AEDs, allowing their use in children. However, it is important that the AED diagnostic algorithm is sensitive and specific for pediatric VF and VT. The diagnostic algorithms from several AED manufacturers have been tested for such sensitivity and specificity and therefore can be reasonably used in younger children.

Simulation and pediatric cardiopulmonary resuscitation

Simulation has achieved an increasingly important place in medical education and training in pediatric anesthesiology and critical care, with resuscitation scenarios among the most frequent programs provided by pediatric simulation centers [189]. Simulation scenarios can reveal gaps in knowledge and technique for physicians. In a study of 20 anesthesia residents in a scenario of hyperkalemic cardiac arrest during anesthesia for a craniotomy for tumor incision in a 1-year-old patient weighing 10 kg resulting in pulseless electrical activity, only one-third of the residents performed chest compressions properly, and administered the correct dose of epinephrine. Only one-fourth of the residents considered hyperkalemia as a cause of the arrest, and none asked for dosing aids [190]. In a study of *in situ* simulation training for effective chest compressions in a pediatric ICU, healthcare providers with more frequent exposure to these sessions correctly demonstrated proper chest compressions in significantly less time than those with less frequent exposure to these sessions [172]. See Chapter 42 for a thorough discussion of simulation in pediatric anesthesia.

Intraoperative cardiac arrest

See Chapter 40 for a detailed discussion of the causes of intraoperative cardiac arrest.

When should cardiopulmonary resuscitation be discontinued?

Several factors determine the likelihood of survival after cardiac arrest, including the mechanism of the arrest (e.g. traumatic, asphyxial, progression from circulatory shock), location (e.g. in-hospital or out-of-hospital), response (i.e. witnessed or unwitnessed, with or without bystander CPR), underlying pathophysiology (i.e. cardiomyopathy, congenital defect, drug toxicity or metabolic derangement), and the potential reversibility of underlying diseases. These factors should all be considered before deciding to terminate resuscitative efforts. Continuation of CPR has been traditionally considered futile beyond 15 min of CPR or when more than two doses of epinephrine are needed [191]. Presumably in part because of improvements in CPR quality and postresuscitation care, improved outcomes from in-hospital CPR efforts beyond 15 min or two doses of epinephrine are increasingly the norm [7,16]. The potential for excellent outcomes despite prolonged CPR has been highlighted by the E-CPR data noted above [192–197]. Conversely, the decision to discontinue CPR prematurely is final and cannot be rescinded. In the first decade of the 21st century, there is no simple answer to the important clinical question: when should CPR be discontinued?

Updated recommendations for pediatric CPR

In late 2010 the latest recommendations from the American Heart Association, European Resuscitation Council, and International Liaison Committee on Resuscitation were published [204]. The major changes from the previous recommendations published in 2005 are:

1. Additional evidence shows that healthcare providers do not reliably determine the presence or absence of a pulse in infants or children.

2. New evidence documents the important role of ventilations in CPR for infants and children. However, rescuers who are unable or unwilling to provide ventilations should be encouraged to perform compression-only CPR.

3. To achieve effective chest compressions, rescuers should compress at least one third the anterior-posterior dimension of the chest. This corresponds to approximately 1.5 inches (4 cm) in most infants and 2 inches (5 cm) in most children.

4. When shocks are indicated for ventricular fibrillation (VF) or pulseless ventricular tachycardia (VT) in infants and children, an initial energy dose of 2 to 4 J/kg is reasonable; doses higher than 4 J/kg, especially if delivered with a biphasic defibrillator, may be safe and effective.

5. More data support the safety and effectiveness of cuffed tracheal tubes in infants and young children, and the formula for selecting the appropriately sized cuffed tube was updated.

6. The safety and value of using cricoid pressure during emergency intubation are not clear. Therefore, the application of cricoid pressure should be modified or discontinued if it impedes ventilation or the speed or ease of intubation.

7. Monitoring capnography/capnometry is recommended to confirm proper endotracheal tube position.

8. Monitoring capnography/capnometry may be helpful during CPR to help assess and optimize quality of chest compressions.

9. On the basis of increasing evidence of potential harm from exposure to high-concentration oxygen after cardiac arrest, once spontaneous circulation is restored, inspired oxygen concentration should be titrated to limit the risk of hyperoxemia.

10. Use of a rapid response system in a pediatric inpatient setting may be beneficial to reduce rates of cardiac and respiratory arrest and in-hospital mortality.

11. Use of a bundled approach to management of pediatric septic shock is recommended.

12. The young victim of a sudden, unexpected cardiac arrest should have an unrestricted, complete autopsy, if possible, with special attention to the possibility of an underlying condition that predisposes to a fatal arrhythmia. Appropriate preservation and genetic analysis of tissue should be considered; detailed testing may reveal an inherited "channelopathy" that may also be present in surviving family members

The reader is advised that new guidelines are published every few years, and the most recent guidelines should be sought out and followed.

Summary

Outcomes from pediatric cardiac arrest and CPR appear to be improving. Perhaps the evolving understanding of pathophysiological events during and after pediatric cardiac arrest and the developing fields of pediatric critical care and pediatric emergency medicine have contributed to these apparent improvements. In addition, exciting breakthroughs in basic and applied science laboratories are on the immediate horizon for study in specific subpopulations of cardiac arrest victims. By strategically focusing therapies to specific phases of cardiac arrest, there is great promise that critical care interventions will lead the way to more successful cardiopulmonary and cerebral resuscitation in children.

CASE STUDY

A 5-year-old girl was found floating at the bottom of a swimming pool after not being seen by her parents for approximately 10 min. She was pulled from the water by a lifeguard. He noted that she was apneic and had no signs of life. Rescue breaths were given and chest compressions were initiated. The lifeguard gave rescue breaths co-ordinated with chest compressions at a cycle of 15:2 while the emergency medical services (EMS) were called. Upon arrival of the EMS, an endotracheal tube was placed while in-line neck stabilization was provided. Following intubation, the girl was hand ventilated at a rate of 10–12 breaths per min and received compressions at a rate of 100 per min simultaneously. An AED was placed and did not advise shocking. The EMS providers placed a cervical collar, and inserted an intraosseous needle in her proximal right tibia. They infused an intraosseous bolus of 2 mL epinephrine 1:10,000 (0.1 mL/kg based on a presumed weight of 20 kg) every 3 min × 3. She was transported to an outside hospital emergency department (ED), and return of spontaneous circulation was noted on arrival.

In the ED she had a rectal temperature of 36°C, a heart rate of 170 beats per min, a blood pressure of 120/60 and SpO_2 of 100% with $FiO2$ 1.0. Her end-tidal CO_2 was 65 mmHg. Her pupils were 4 mm bilaterally and reactive and she had intermittent extensor posturing with stimulation, but no purposeful movement. Two peripheral intravenous lines were placed. Her initial venous blood gas revealed a pH 6.9, PCO_2 65 mmHg, PaO_2 25 mmHg, bicarbonate 12 meq/L, a base deficit of −22 meq/L and an ionized calcium of 1.02 mmol/L. A complete blood count had a white blood cell count of 15,000/mm³, hemoglobin of 12 g/dL, and a platelet count of 242,000/mm³. A chemistry panel showed a sodium of 138 meq/L, potassium 7 meq/L, chloride of 103 meq/L, BUN of 15 mg/dL and a creatinine of 0.3 mg/dL. The glucose was 345 mg/dL. The initial chest x-ray showed an endotracheal tube in the mid trachea with bilateral hazy infiltrates. Secondary to hyperkalemia in the face of a severe metabolic and mild respiratory acidosis, the patient was hyperventilated at a rate of 22 breaths per min. She received 2 meq/kg of sodium bicarbonate as well as 50 mg/kg of calcium gluconate intravenously. She also received 20 mL/kg of normal saline, 20 μg of fentanyl, and 1 mg of midazolam for posturing and twitching, with resolution of her twitching. The head computed tomography scan showed no intracranial injury. She was then transferred to the ICU for further management.

On arrival in the ICU, her vital signs were rectal temperature of 35.5°C, a heart rate of 150 beats per min, a blood pressure of 90/40 and a SpO_2 of 100% on FiO_2 1.0 with hand ventilation. She had an end-tidal CO_2 of 50 mmHg. She was placed on initial ventilator settings of tidal volume 160 mL, a positive end expiratory pressure of 10 cmH$_2$O and a rate of 22 breaths per min with FiO_2 1.0. To avoid hyperoxia, her supplemental oxygen was weaned to maintain her SpO_2 >94%. Her ventilation rate was titrated to maintain normocarbia.

Simultaneously she had an esophageal and bladder temperature probe placed for core temperature monitoring. The esophageal probe was placed through the mouth and measured to terminate at the distal end of the esophagus. The temperature-sensing Foley catheter was placed for both urinary output monitoring as well as continuous core temperature monitoring. A 5 French, 12 cm triple-lumen right subclavian catheter was placed under sterile conditions. This was placed both for continuous medication administration as well as co-oximetry and central venous pressure monitoring. A repeat chest x-ray was obtained which showed the catheter terminating at the right atrial–superior vena caval junction. There was no evidence of pneumothorax and the esophageal probe terminated at the distal esophagus. She also had a right radial arterial line placed under sterile conditions for continuous arterial blood pressure monitoring and frequent lab sampling.

Following these procedures, the patient remained tachycardic with a heart rate of 140 bpm, and became hypotensive with a blood pressure of 70/40. Her central venous pressure was 2 cmH$_2$O, and her repeat venous blood gas was pH 7.13/PCO$_2$ 45/PO$_2$ 38/base deficit –12/lactate 6. She received another 20 mL/kg of normal saline × 2 with improvement in her central venous pressure to 6, but despite fluid boluses she remained persistently hypotensive at 80/40. At that time, the intensivist decided to initiate vasopressor therapy to improve her cerebral perfusion pressure. Dopamine was infused at 5 μg/kg/min, resulting in a blood pressure of 102/55 mmHg and a urine output of approximately 5 mL/kg/h.

Labs were sent to further evaluate end-organ perfusion. Her troponin was 1.5 μg/L, creatine kinase (CK) was 2023 units/L and her CK-myocardial band percentage was 7%. Her amylase, lipase, aspartate aminotransferase (AST) and alanine aminotransferase (ALT) were within normal limits. Her glucose was 327 mg/dL. She remained comatose with a Glasgow Coma Score of 6 Total (Eye opening 1, Verbal response 0 (intubated), Motor response 5).

At that time the clinical team placed her on a cooling blanket with the goal of maintaining her temperature between 36 and 37°C to avoid hyperthermia. She was initiated on maintenance fluids without dextrose due to hyperglycemia. An insulin infusion was ordered to start at 0.01 units/kg/h to maintain her glucose <180 and prevent excessive urine output from osmotic diuresis. Because of hypotension and the known risk of postcardiac arrest myocardial depression, an echocardiogram was obtained at the bedside, which showed a shortening fraction of 40% and a hyperdynamic myocardium. Because of intermittent posturing and tachycardia, which resolved after IV midazolam treatment, a continuous electroencephalogram was performed to monitor for postcardiac arrest seizure activity. The neurologist noted non-convulsive seizure activity on the electroencephalogram, and the patient was loaded with 20 mg/kg of intravenous fosphenytoin. She was sedated with fentanyl and midazolam infusions to decrease metabolic demand immediately post arrest.

During the 3 days following her cardiac arrest, her temperature was maintained between 36 and 37°C, her blood pressure was maintained within normal limits or age and she was weaned off dopamine, her PaCO$_2$ was maintained

in the 40s and her SpO$_2$ was maintained at >95%. Within 36 h post arrest, trophic feeds were initiated and slowly titrated to goal caloric needs via a nasoduodenal feeding tube. On postcardiac arrest day 3, her neurological exam revealed bilateral reactive pupils, a cough and gag, spontaneous respiratory effort, and she was localizing to noxious stimuli. Her seizures were controlled with phenytoin and EEG monitoring was discontinued at 72 h with no new seizures evident. On day 4 post arrest, her temperature-sensing Foley and esophageal probes were removed so that she could go to MRI for evaluation of her brain and cervical spine. Her cervical spine showed no evidence of bony or ligamentous injury and her cervical collar was removed by trauma surgery. Her brain MRI showed evidence of subtle acute hypoxic ischemic injury in the cerebral cortex bilaterally. On day 5 her sedation infusions were discontinued and she was extubated. On day 6 her central line and arterial line were discontinued and she was transferred to inpatient rehab for intensive therapies.

Three months following her cardiac arrest, she was verbal and interactive. She was able to ambulate with assistance. She had had no seizures and was maintained on phenytoin with plans to wean it off at 6 months post arrest if there was no new seizure activity.

Key points

1. The chain of survival includes early, good-quality CPR, early defibrillation if appropriate, aggressive postresuscitative care and rehabilitation services.
2. Prompt bystander CPR was provided with chest compressions and rescue breathing.
3. Postresuscitative care requires a multidisciplinary approach and focus on details of avoiding secondary injuries from hyperoxia, hyperthermia, hypotension and acidosis.
4. Post cardiac arrest, patients often exhibit intravascular volume depletion, and have a systemic inflammatory response syndrome (SIRS) and myocardial depression. Therefore, close hemodynamic monitoring and cardiovascular supportive care are necessary for optimal postresuscitative care.

Annotated references

A full reference list for this chapter is available at:
http://www.wiley.com/go/gregory/andropoulos/pediatricanesthesia

27. Kitamura T, Iwami T, Kawamura T et al. Conventional and chest-compression-only cardiopulmonary resuscitation by bystanders for children who have out-of-hospital cardiac arrests: a prospective, nationwide, population-based cohort study. Lancet 2010; 375: 1347–54. A very important study demonstrating that chest compressions alone are as effective as standard CPR in children with cardiac arrest from cardiac causes, concurring with the principle that has been demonstrated in adults and further underscoring the importance of effective chest compressions.

34. Sharek PJ, Parast LM, Leong K et al. Effect of a rapid response team on hospital-wide mortality and code rates outside the ICU in a children's hospital. JAMA 2007; 298: 2267–74. Demonstration that medical emergency teams, otherwise known as rapid response teams, decrease the frequency of cardiac arrest in a study at a large children's hospital.

43. Atkins DL, Berg MD, Berg RA et al. 2005 American Heart Association (AHA) guidelines for cardiopulmonary resuscitation (CPR) and emergency cardiovascular care (ECC) of pediatric and neonatal patients: pediatric advanced life support. Pediatrics 2006; 117: e1005–28. The latest guidelines for CPR and acute arrhythmia treatment in pediatric patients.

47. Aufderheide TP, Lurie KG. Death by hyperventilation: a common and life-threatening problem during cardiopulmonary resuscitation. Crit Care Med 2004; 32(9 Suppl): S345–51. An important explanation of the physiology of adverse effects of hyperventilation during CPR.

92. Perondi MB, Reis AG, Paiva EF et al. A comparison of high-dose and standard-dose epinephrine in children with cardiac arrest. N Engl J Med 2004; 350: 1722–30. An important prospective, randomized, blinded, controlled study demonstrating that high-dose epinephrine results in worse survival than standard-dose epinephrine in pediatric in-hospital cardiac arrest.

99. Mann K, Berg RA, Nadkarni V. Beneficial effects of vasopressin in prolonged pediatric cardiac arrest: a case series. Resuscitation 2002; 52: 149–56. A small series demonstrating that vasopressin may be effective in restoring circulation after prolonged pediatric cardiac arrest.

118. Hickey RW, Kochanek PM, Ferimer H et al. Hypothermia and hyperthermia in children after resuscitation from cardiac arrest. Pediatrics 2000; 106: 118–22. A seminal article demonstrating that hypothermia after pediatric cardiac arrest may be associated with better outcomes, that became the basis for current multicentered trials of therapeutic hypothermia after cardiac arrest.

179. Samson RA, Nadkarni VM, Meaney PA et al. Outcomes of in-hospital ventricular fibrillation in children. N Engl J Med 2006; 354: 2328–39. An important study demonstrating that 27% of children with in-hospital cardiac arrest had ventricular fibrillation at some point during the arrest and resuscitation.

188. Topjian AA, Berg RA, Nadkarni VM. Pediatric cardiopulmonary resuscitation: advances in science, techniques, and outcomes. Pediatrics 2008; 122: 1086–98. A comprehensive review article of the state of the art in pediatric CPR.

196. Thiagarajan RR, Laussen PC, Rycus PT et al. Extracorporeal membrane oxygenation to aid cardiopulmonary resuscitation in infants and children. Circulation 2007; 116: 1693–700. A large series of ECMO-CPR in pediatric patients with short- and medium-term outcome data.

CHAPTER 13

Preoperative Evaluation and Preparation, Anxiety, Awareness, and Behavior Change

Andrew Davidson¹, Kelly Howard¹, William Browne¹, Walid Habre² & Ursula Lopez²

¹Department of Anaesthesia and Pain Management, Royal Children's Hospital, Parkville, Australia
²Department of Anaesthesiology, Pharmacology and Intensive Care, University Hospitals, Geneva, Switzerland

Preoperative evaluation

Quality perioperative care begins with a comprehensive preanesthetic evaluation and preparation of the child and family. Healthcare providers should aspire to deliver healthcare that is safe, effective, patient centered, efficient, and equitable [1]. These principles should guide not just the preoperative evaluation but the entire perioperative process.

While the majority of children presenting for surgery are in excellent general health, many will have complex medical and/or psychological issues requiring careful assessment and planning. Pediatric co-morbid diseases are predominantly genetic, congenital or developmental. This contrasts to the largely acquired and degenerative diseases more common in adulthood. Accordingly, while the guiding principles are the same, the focus and approach of the preoperative evaluation for children and adults are often different.

This section outlines the rationale for and organizational aspects of the preoperative evaluation, key issues in history taking, physical examination and ordering investigations, and a review of current fasting guidelines and medical conditions commonly encountered in pediatric patients.

Goals of preoperative evaluation
Achieve optimal medical outcomes and minimize risk

The primary role of the preoperative evaluation is to identify the presence and severity of both known and previously undiagnosed conditions [2]. Untreated or poorly managed diseases can frequently be optimized prior to surgery. Of particular interest are conditions that complicate the provision of anesthesia and/or increase perioperative risk. Understanding perioperative risk is essential for developing an appropriate management plan aimed at achieving optimal outcomes and for providing

---

Gregory's Pediatric Anesthesia, Fifth Edition. Edited by George A. Gregory, Dean B. Andropoulos.
© 2012 Blackwell Publishing Ltd. Published 2012 by Blackwell Publishing Ltd.

appropriate preoperative counseling to the patient and family.

Neonates, infants, and young children are at increased risk of anesthesia-related morbidity and mortality compared to older children and adults [3–7]. Young age is associated with an increased incidence of both respiratory [8–10] and cardiac complications [11]. Age-independent risk factors for adverse outcomes include the presence of multiple co-morbidities and American Society of Anesthesiologists (ASA) physical status classification of III or more [5,11,12]. However, the ASA classification should be used with caution as a predictive tool, as it was not designed for use in children or as a predictor of their perioperative outcome and there is poor inter-rater reliability in the pediatric setting [13].

Respiratory complications predominate in children and include events such as laryngospasm, bronchospasm, hypoxia and postextubation stridor. Specific risk factors for respiratory complications include current or recent upper respiratory tract infection [8,10,14,15], asthma [16], obstructive sleep apnea [17], bronchopulmonary dysplasia, obesity [18–20], passive smoking [15,21], positive family history of asthma or atopy (in at least two members) [22] and specific conditions (e.g. Down syndrome) [23]. The preoperative evaluation should aim to identify these risk factors.

Identification of psychological issues

The perioperative period can be a stressful time for the child and family. Anxiety and behavioral stress are very common in children, and have been associated with adverse postoperative outcomes such as emergence delirium, increased pain, increased analgesia use, anxiety, and sleep problems [24,25].

The preoperative consultation provides an excellent opportunity to establish rapport with the child, identify high-risk patients, and develop a plan aimed at minimizing anxiety and distress. Effective preparation of the child for surgery is guided by the child's age and developmental level, and may include elements such as education, hospital tours, play therapy, hypnosis, relaxation techniques, and sedative/anxiolytic premedication. These will be discussed at greater length later in the chapter.

Education

It has been shown that children and parents want detailed information regarding the perioperative period [26–28]. While younger children may be more interested in the physical appearance of the operating room, older children may be concerned about the anesthetic technique, procedures, pain and potential complications [26].

Comprehensive information is also required for ethical and legal purposes in order for parents to make informed decisions about their child's care. The information should cover key topics such as the rationale for fasting, details of the anesthetic plan and the role of the anesthesiologist. Unfortunately, parental knowledge in these areas has frequently been shown to be lacking [29]. There may be a perception by some anesthesiologists that the provision of detailed information may increase parental anxiety but this has been shown not to be the case and may have the opposite effect of reducing anxiety levels [27,30,31].

Information can be communicated in a number of ways. Verbal information given during the preoperative evaluation can be effectively supplemented with written and audiovisual matter [30,31]. While formal parental education programs are known to improve knowledge and reduce anxiety in parents [32], educational programs for children may not provide a similar benefit [33]. Translation services must be available as appropriate for parents whose primary language is not English, and are not able to fully understand the perioperative information.

Perioperative planning

A comprehensive perioperative plan is essential for quality patient care. The complexity of planning is proportional to the patient and family's particular needs. Key considerations in the perioperative planning process include:

1. identifying an appropriate surgical setting
   - hospital type: tertiary pediatric versus peripheral hospital
   - operating theater location: "main" operating theater versus day unit
   - admission type: inpatient versus out
2. arranging appropriately skilled practitioners
   - a specialist pediatric anesthesiologist should ideally care for all children, particularly those at greater risk of adverse outcomes. The absence of a specialist pediatric anesthesiologist is an established risk factor for adverse perioperative outcomes [9,22]
   - some diseases warrant care from a subspecialized pediatric anesthesiologist, such as a cardiac anesthesiologist for children with complex cardiac issues
3. formulation of specific anesthesia plan
   - preparation and premedication
   - fasting prescription
   - induction: mode of induction, parental presence
   - intraoperative management: monitoring, analgesia
   - postoperative management: destination and special monitoring/observation requirements
4. identify special needs or equipment.

Hospital efficiency and economics

Thorough and timely preoperative evaluation and planning can reduce the incidence of day-of-surgery cancellations and delayed start times [34]. Reduced cancellations mean less wasted operating theater time and greater utilization of healthcare resources.

Organizational aspects of the preoperative evaluation

Organizational frameworks for preoperative assessment differ between institutions. High day-of-surgery admission rates necessitate the implementation of effective systems to process and evaluate patients in the preoperative period [35]. All children scheduled for surgery should be screened for significant issues, using either a written questionnaire or telephone interview [36]. This process identifies children who will benefit from further outpatient evaluation. Additionally, a phone call on the day prior to surgery confirms planned patient attendance and understanding of fasting policies, and identifies any new issues (e.g. upper respiratory tract infection).

Outpatient assessment clinics play an important role in the preoperative process and have been shown in adults to improve patient satisfaction and reduce the rate of cancellations, length of stay, patient anxiety, inappropriate referrals, and unnecessary investigations [34,37–41]. Most healthy pediatric patients do not, however, require outpatient evaluation and can be safely assessed on the day of surgery [42,43].

Outpatient preassessment clinics frequently adopt a multidisciplinary approach, with team members consisting of anesthesiologists, nurse practitioners, nurses, physiotherapists and child life specialists. Nurse practitioner-assisted models of preoperative evaluation have been successfully introduced in some institutions, allowing anesthesiologists more time in the operating theater [42,44]. Regardless of which professional evaluates the child, the ultimate responsibility for declaring "fitness for surgery" rests firmly with the anesthesiologist performing the case.

History

The preoperative evaluation should incorporate a thorough exploration of the patient's medical history. Information can be obtained from a variety of sources, including an interview with the patient and his/her parents; a review of medical records with an emphasis on previous anesthetic charts; and a discussion with the child's regular physician(s) and the proceduralist performing the scheduled surgery.

During interactions with patients and their parents, medical professionals often spend the majority of time interacting with parents and focus predominantly on medical talk [45]. It is important to involve the child in the discussion and to utilize the opportunity to build rapport and establish the confidence of the child.

The nature of the presenting condition and the details of the planned procedure should be established first. Knowledge of the presenting problem immediately identifies potential anesthetic issues, e.g. the child with obstructive sleep apnea presenting for adenotonsillectomy is at risk of airway complications and increased apnea incidence postoperatively. Understanding the surgeon's specific plans and potential concerns is crucial to planning safe anesthesia.

Background history should begin with a review of relevant obstetric and perinatal issues. Points of interest include the gestational age at birth and problems of prematurity, in particular the requirement for and duration of respiratory support and incidence of apnea. Growth and developmental history should then be assessed. Failure to reach or loss of developmental milestones should initiate diagnostic work to investigate the possibility of unrecognized neuromuscular conditions, many of which have profound anesthetic implications (e.g. Duchenne muscular dystrophy). Congenital and acquired medical conditions should also be reviewed with a focus on disease duration; severity; course and stability; current disease activity; past and current treatment (medical and surgical); complications of therapy; and long-term prognosis.

Family history is important in identifying the presence of genetic conditions of anesthetic interest. Important inherited conditions include malignant hyperthermia; pseudocholinesterase deficiency; muscular dystrophies; disorders of coagulation (e.g. hemophilia, von Willebrand disease); primary electrical diseases of the heart (e.g. Wolff–Parkinson–White syndrome, prolonged QT syndrome, Brugada syndrome and catecholaminergic polymorphic ventricular tachycardia) [46]; and metabolic conditions (e.g. porphyria).

Past surgical procedures should be investigated, with a particular focus on the anesthetic experience. Useful information includes the mode and success of previous anesthetic induction, the need for sedative premedication, anesthesia drugs and techniques employed, and complications. Anesthetic plans should be modified accordingly when adverse episodes in past experience have been identified, such as induction distress, emergence agitation or delirium, airway difficulties, awareness, adverse drug reactions (e.g. malignant hyperthermia, anaphylaxis), requirement for postoperative ventilation and severe postoperative nausea and vomiting (PONV). Risk factors for postoperative vomiting (PV) in children include age greater than 3 years, surgical duration of greater than 30 min, strabismus surgery and positive history of PV for the child or PV/PONV in first-degree relatives [47,48].

An appraisal of past pain experiences is critical, particularly in the setting of a complex medical history or multiple past procedures. Important aspects of the pain history include previous difficulties with pain management (e.g. uncontrolled pain or unacceptable adverse effects from analgesic medications), past or current chronic pain, and current analgesic requirements.

A systematic review searching for organ-specific conditions should be conducted, with a particular emphasis on the known associations of identified syndromes (e.g. congenital heart disease with Down syndrome) (Table 13.1). Chapter 38 outlines commonly encountered syndromes.

All current and recent medications should be identified, including prescription, "over-the-counter," herbal, and natural medications. Drug and environmental sensitivities and the nature of the adverse reaction are important in developing an appropriate treatment plan. Latex allergy is discussed in Chapter 40. Enquiry about recent immunizations is recommended. Although the interaction between anesthesia, surgery and vaccination is unclear, a delay between immunization and surgery of at least 2–3 days following an inactivated vaccine or 14–21 days following a live attenuated vaccine is recommended [49,50]. This practice avoids coinciding the time of peak incidence for systemic vaccine reactions with the perioperative period, minimizing confusion with postoperative complications [49].

Physical examination

The approach to clinical examination is tailored to the individual needs of the patient. Physical examination should be thorough, while minimizing patient exposure (for both modesty and thermoregulation) and distress. The primary focus is the airway, heart, and lungs.

Much valuable information can be obtained by direct observation of the child's physical appearance and behavior during the interview process. The quality of the child's interactions and level of co-operation with the examiner will shape the anesthesiologist's plans for anesthesia induction, including an assessment of the likely benefit of parental presence. Physical characteristics or signs that may be readily apparent during general observation include cyanosis, pallor, jaundice, nutritional state, work of breathing, oxygen requirement, conscious state, dysmorphic features (including specific syndromes), deformity (e.g. scoliosis), abnormal posture, movement disorders, and gross developmental level.

Baseline clinical observations should be recorded, including height, weight, heart rate, blood pressure, respiratory rate, oxygen saturation and temperature. Current bodyweight is essential for calculating appropriate drug doses. Weight-based dosing is simple and commonly used, despite the recognized non-linear relationship between weight and dose [51]. Calculation based on body surface area (BSA) is an alternative approach that may result in more accurate drug prescription [52]. Body Mass Index (BMI, weight [kg]/[height [m]^2]) is used to define overweight and obesity [53]. Childhood obesity is increasingly common and can lead to important pharmacokinetic changes, which further complicates accurate drug dose determination [54].

Co-operation during formal airway examination (as is conducted in adults) is unlikely to be forthcoming in small children. Furthermore, the parameters and scoring systems (e.g. Mallampati score) used in adult practice have not been validated in the pediatric setting. Assessment should seek to identify potential predictors of difficult intubation and/or ventilation such as limited mouth opening, stridor, obligate mouth breathing (suggesting adenoidal hypertrophy), loose teeth (risk of displacing into airway), mandibular hypoplasia/retrognathia, macroglossia, cleft or high-arched palate, tonsillar hypertrophy, restricted cervical spine movement and scars from previous neck surgery, radiotherapy or tracheotomy.

Cardiovascular signs of interest include presence of peripheral pulses (bilateral brachial and femoral), cardiac murmurs and evidence of cardiac failure (cyanosis, tachypnea, gallop rhythm, pulmonary rales and hepatomegaly). Respiratory examination should include an assessment of respiratory effort; presence of coryza (volume, purulence); the upper airway (see above); tracheal position; chest wall deformities (e.g. scoliosis, pectus excavatum) that can be associated with restrictive lung defects; and auscultation of the lungs to detect wheeze or crackles.

Preoperative evaluation should include an evaluation of peripheral veins and nomination of sites for application of topical local anesthetic cream. Indwelling vascular access devices (e.g. Portacath, Permacath) and surgically created arteriovenous fistulas (for hemodialysis or repeat infusions, e.g. hemophilia) are located and examined for patency and signs of infection. Caution is needed to prevent compression of fistulas with either blood pressure or pneumatic tourniquet cuffs. Other implanted devices that should be identified preoperatively include feeding tubes (e.g. percutaneous gastrostomy tubes) and electronic devices such as pacemakers, automatic implantable cardiac defibrillators (AICD), deep brain and vagus nerve stimulators. Electronic devices can malfunction in the setting of surgical electrocautery or strong magnetic fields (e.g. magnetic resonance imaging (MRI)), and may require reprogramming or modification of surgical plans.

Spinal anatomy should be examined if neuraxial techniques are planned. Evidence of spinal malformation, deformity, prior surgery or local skin infection may preclude such techniques. Any pre-existing neurological deficit should be documented prior to neuraxial or regional techniques. Where relevant, the operative site is examined in order to understand the nature of the surgical pathology and extent of the planned procedure.

Preoperative investigations

Routine preoperative blood screening of healthy children has long been abandoned from practice

Table 13.1 Review of common conditions by organ system

System	Preoperative considerations, associated disease and/or anesthetic implications
Cardiovascular	
Murmur	Clinical assessment, ECG, echocardiography, cardiology consultation
Congenital heart disease	Circulatory physiology (repaired, unrepaired, palliated), functional status, risk of endocarditis, anticoagulation, consultation with cardiologist
Pacemaker/AICD	Indication, mode, underlying rhythm/pacemaker dependence, date of last device check, risk of electrocautery interference, consider reprogramming to asynchronous mode and inactivate AICD for surgery
Respiratory	
Obstructive sleep apnea	Severity (polysomnography), cardiovascular complications, risk factors (young age, syndromal, airway surgery, opioid use), arrange postoperative monitoring
Prematurity	Respiratory (apnea, BPD, subglottic stenosis), cardiovascular (PDA, heart failure related to BPD), retinopathy of prematurity (caution with high inspired oxygen), see Chapters 20 and 21
Asthma	Severity and current control, recent URTI, consider short preoperative course of oral corticosteroids
Cystic fibrosis	Respiratory assessment (sputum, reactive airways, hospitalizations, exercise tolerance, pulmonary hypertension, right heart failure), nasal polyps, diabetes mellitus, malabsorption (pancreatic insufficiency), liver disease
Central nervous system	
Epilepsy	Seizure pattern and control, give regular medications, ketogenic diet (avoid glucose, potential metabolic acidosis), drug interactions, altered seizure threshold (surgery, stress, drugs, e.g. tramadol, meperidine)
Cerebral palsy	Seizures, communication difficulty, muscle spasm/contractures, poor swallowing, gastro-esophageal reflux, respiratory issues (recurrent pneumonia, poor cough, scoliosis with restrictive lung deficit)
Tumor	Raised intracranial pressure (altered conscious level, vomiting/aspiration risk), localized neurological signs (e.g. bulbar dysfunction secondary to posterior fossa mass)
Neuromuscular disease	
Muscular dystrophy	Respiratory function, cardiomyopathy, hyperkalemia with succinylcholine, volatile anesthetic-associated rhabdomyolysis
Gastrointestinal tract	
Chronic liver disease	Portal hypertension (splenomegaly, ascites, varices), coagulopathy, anemia, thrombocytopenia, hepatopulmonary syndrome, renal failure, encephalopathy, altered pharmacokinetics of anesthetic drugs
Endocrine & metabolic	
Chronic corticosteroids	Immunosuppression, hypertension, diabetes mellitus, obesity, adrenocortical suppression and potential for perioperative adrenal crisis
Diabetes mellitus	Define type of diabetes, control, complications, and treatment regime Potential problems: hypoglycemia, hyperglycemia (wound infection, osmotic diuresis, electrolyte imbalance), ketoacidosis
Obesity	Asthma, URTI, diabetes mellitus (type II), OSA, drug dosing
Renal	
Chronic renal failure	Define etiology, mode/frequency of dialysis and systemic complications (anemia, platelet dysfunction, fluid and electrolyte imbalance, metabolic acidosis, cardiovascular disease)
Hematological	
Anemia	Consider and investigate cause, severity dictates management (i.e. transfusion)
Coagulopathy	Increased bleeding risk. Replace platelets/factors in consultation with hematologist
Sickle cell disease	Anemia, vaso-occlusive disease (hyposplenism, pulmonary infarcts, stroke), cardiomegaly, renal and hepatic dysfunction. Role of perioperative transfusion unclear
Reproductive	
Possible pregnancy	Unknown risk of anesthesia in early pregnancy, consider pregnancy testing when pregnancy a possibility (follow local hospital protocol)

AICD, automatic implantable cardiac defibrillators; BPD, bronchopulmonary dysplasia; GER, gastro-esophageal reflux; OSA, obstructive sleep apnea; PDA, persistent ductus arteriosus; URTI, upper respiratory tract infection.

recommendations on the grounds that it provides little benefit to patients, has several potential disadvantages and rarely leads to alterations in patient management [55–61]. Thorough clinical assessment should instead lead to selective and targeted investigations that answer specific clinical questions. Indications for ordering investigations include diagnosing previously unrecognized conditions that may be suspected from the clinical assessment; assessing severity of known conditions; and establishing a "baseline" for parameters that may change during the treatment.

Every preoperative investigation should be carefully considered, and potential benefits balanced against inherent risk. Inappropriate testing causes unnecessary patient discomfort, wastes time and money, potentially delays surgery, can lead to additional invasive investigations in the event of false-positive results, and can have adverse medico-legal outcomes (routine tests are frequently not followed up appropriately) [62].

Hemoglobin

Asymptomatic anemia in the pediatric population is common yet difficult to detect clinically [57,63]. Mild-to-moderate anemia is of minimal consequence to healthy children having minor surgery and does not alter anesthetic management [64–66]. Routine testing is therefore not recommended. Severe anemia reduces oxygen-carrying capacity and can impair tissue oxygen supply. A safe lower limit for hemoglobin concentration in children undergoing surgery is unclear. Preoperative management of severe anemia is dictated by the urgency of the planned surgery.

Measuring preoperative hemoglobin should be considered in certain settings, including:
- severe anemia suspected from clinical assessment
- increased baseline risk of anemia (age <1 year, chronic disease, ethnicity)
- former preterm infants, whereby anemia increases the incidence of postoperative apnea [67,68]
- to establish a baseline before surgery with potential for major blood loss.

Sickle cell disease

Sickle cell disease is a relatively common hematological condition, particularly in children originating from central Africa, southern Italy, northern Greece, Turkey, Saudi Arabia, and central India [69]. Sickle cell disease has significant implications for the perioperative period and unless previously tested, children at high risk should be considered for preoperative screening (hemoglobin electrophoresis) [70–72]. It is noted that detection rates for sickle cell disease during preoperative screening are very low. A Canadian study that screened 1906 children diagnosed 4.1% (79 children) with the sickle cell trait and 0.16% (three children) with sickle cell disease [73]. Two of the three patients who tested positive had a known family history, emphasizing the importance of thorough clinical assessment.

Patients with known sickle cell disease require preoperative hemoglobin assessment to guide perioperative management. Preoperative transfusion is recommended prior to major surgery, aiming for Hb 8–10 g/dL and HbS <30% [74,75].

Blood group

Blood group and antibody screening are performed when the potential for perioperative blood transfusion is significant. To minimize patient distress, specimen collection and subsequent testing can be completed following anesthetic induction. In the patient with non-ABO red cell antibodies or a history of multiple transfusions, testing is performed in advance of surgery allowing time for antibody assessment and sourcing of blood products. In sickle cell disease, extended cross-matching should include Rhesus and Kell subgroups [76].

Coagulation studies

Concern commonly exists regarding the potential for undiagnosed bleeding disorders in patients presenting for major surgery or neuraxial blockade, particularly in younger children in whom significant haemostatic challenges may not have occurred previously [77,78]. There is no evidence, however, to support routine preoperative coagulation studies (activated partial thromboplastin time (APTT), prothrombin time (PT)) in low risk patients [59,77–81]. Coagulation tests have low sensitivity and positive predictive value, and neither exclude an underlying haemostatic disorder nor predict increased bleeding risk [77–79]. A study of children with prolonged APTT attending a hematology outpatient clinic found that in 65% of cases, the initial abnormality was attributable to a sampling or processing error and that only 2.4% of initially abnormal results were due to an underlying coagulopathy [79].

Recommendations regarding preoperative coagulation testing support a targeted approach aimed at those patients deemed to be at increased risk for an underlying bleeding disorder [82]. Despite the lack of evidence to support routine testing, isolated case reports of serious coagulation disorders detected by routine testing have prompted authors to advise caution in abandoning the practice [83]. Triggers for preoperative coagulation testing include:
- family history of bleeding disorders
- a personal history of easy bruising, bleeding after minor trauma and/or recurrent epistaxis

- an underlying condition associated with coagulopathy (e.g. liver disease, malabsorption, malnutrition)
- potentially as a "baseline" prior to major surgery with a large expected transfusion requirement likely to result in acquired coagulopathy.

Standard testing with APTT, PT and a platelet count will not reliably diagnose all underlying haemostatic disorders. Conditions such as factor XIII deficiency, some forms of von Willebrand disease, and disorders of platelet function may be missed [77]. Where there is concern regarding an undiagnosed bleeding disorder, consultation with a hematologist is useful and should result in a more comprehensive battery of tests, including platelet function, specific factor assays and assessment for von Willebrand disease [79].

Urea, electrolytes, and creatinine

Assessment of electrolytes and renal function will be dictated by the clinical history (e.g. pre-existing renal impairment, diabetes insipidus). A recent study examining electrolyte levels in children with cardiac disease and taking cardiac medications found a low overall incidence of abnormalities requiring treatment and recommended against routine screening in this group [84].

Chest radiography

Routine screening chest x-ray has no role in pediatric practice [85–87]. Chest x-ray should be considered for children with cardiac, respiratory and malignant diseases. In particular, children with suspected lymphoma require a chest x-ray to exclude a mediastinal mass. The presence of a mediastinal mass is associated with significant anesthetic morbidity, including complete airway obstruction and cardiovascular collapse, and warrants careful preoperative planning. Additional imaging such as computed tomography and echocardiography is recommended to assess for compression of the trachea, bronchi, heart or great vessels, all of which are associated with increased anesthetic morbidity [88]. Furthermore, respiratory function testing with flow-volume loops may be predictive of airway obstruction during anesthesia [89].

Fasting guidelines

Preoperative fasting aims to reduce the risk of gastric regurgitation and pulmonary aspiration by minimizing the volume of fluid and particulate matter in the stomach. While pulmonary aspiration is uncommon, when it does occur it can result in serious morbidity and rarely mortality [90]. Modern fasting guidelines (Table 13.2) are more liberal than previous recommendations,

Table 13.2 American Society of Anesthesiologists fasting recommendations

Ingested material	Minimum fasting period (hours)
Clear fluids	2
Breast milk	4
Infant formula	6
Non-human milk	6
Light meal	6

reflecting an increased understanding of both the potential adverse effects of prolonged fasting (e.g. dehydration, hypoglycemia, patient discomfort) and the differential rate of gastric emptying of various substrates (where clear liquids are emptied at a quicker rate than solids). With fasting, neonates and young infants may be more at risk of hypoglycemia compared to older children.

Clear fluids can be safely given until 2 h preoperatively with no increase in the gastric volume or reduction in pH [91]. Children allowed clear fluids are less likely to be dehydrated, less thirsty and hungry, more comfortable, and better behaved than children fasted for 6 h [91,92].

Breast milk clearance from the stomach is slower than clear fluids but faster than various formula preparations [93,94]. Mean gastric emptying time for breast milk in one study was 2.43 h (range 2–2.75) [95]. Despite the ASA recommendation of a 4-h fast for breast milk, some institutions have adopted a 3-h limit with no adverse clinical outcome [96].

Infants can safely consume formula until 4 h preoperatively with no increase in gastric fluid volume [97]. Fasting times for formula feeds in infants varies between institutions, ranging from 4 to 6 h [96,98,99]. The ASA recommends a 6-h fasting interval for formula [100]. The specific composition of the formula is also important, with factors such as osmolality, protein content, energy density, and pH all altering the rate of gastric emptying [101]. For example, whey-predominant formula empties more rapidly than casein-predominant formula [94].

Cow's milk separates into a liquid phase and a solid curd phase after mixing with acidic gastric fluid [97]. The high lipid content results in slow gastric emptying. Cow's milk is therefore treated in the same way as solid food, and a 6-h fast is recommended [100].

Fasting guidelines apply to healthy children undergoing elective surgery. The presence of factors known to delay gastric emptying should be considered when assessing aspiration risk. Gastric emptying may be reduced by trauma, pain, bowel obstruction, ileus and opioids [96,102]. Fasting recommendations vary between institutions and anesthesiologists need to be aware of local policies.

Specific conditions requiring careful preoperative evaluation

There are a number of common scenarios or conditions that merit particular attention in the preoperative evaluation. Cerebral palsy, congenital heart disease and the ex-premature infant are covered elsewhere.

Asthma

Asthma is a chronic inflammatory disorder of the airways characterized by recurrent episodes of bronchospasm and airflow obstruction, with symptoms of wheeze, breathlessness, and cough. The incidence of serious respiratory morbidity in asthmatic patients is reportedly low [103] but when bronchospasm does occur, it can be life-threatening [104]. Laryngoscopy and endotracheal intubation are potent airway irritants that can precipitate bronchospasm. Intraoperative complications are associated with recent asthma symptoms, recent need for bronchodilator use and recent hospitalization for asthma symptoms [103]. Acute or poorly controlled asthma should delay elective surgery. Bronchial hyper-responsiveness persists following an acute exacerbation and the risk of intraoperative airway events remains increased several weeks following resolution of symptoms [105,106].

History taking should focus on current and recent symptom control, nocturnal symptoms, bronchodilator requirements (including increasing use), recent hospitalizations, recent respiratory tract infection and prior mechanical ventilation for acute asthma (indicating severity of disease). Auscultation should ideally reveal no evidence of wheeze. If the child routinely monitors peak expiratory flow, then repeating this measurement is useful to assess current status.

A short course of corticosteroids reduces the incidence of perioperative bronchospasm [107] with no increased risk of wound infection or breakdown [108,109]. A suggested regime is oral methylprednisolone 1 mg/kg daily, commencing at least 48 h prior to surgery [110]. Administration of inhaled β2-agonists prior to induction also reduces the incidence of bronchospasm in both adults and children [111–113]. Regular bronchodilators are continued on the day of surgery and an additional dose of β2-agonist immediately before induction is prudent.

Diabetes mellitus

Diabetes mellitus is a metabolic disorder of multiple etiologies characterized by chronic hyperglycemia with disturbances of carbohydrate, fat and protein metabolism. Diabetes is classified into type 1 (insulin dependent, prone to ketosis); type 2 (non-insulin dependent, variable insulin resistance); gestational diabetes: and "other specific types" [114]. "Other specific types" include mono-genic diabetes (formerly maturity-onset diabetes of the young (MODY)); genetic defects of insulin action; disease of exocrine pancreas (e.g. cystic fibrosis); endocrinopathies (e.g. acromegaly); drug induced (e.g. corticosteroids); and associated with genetic syndromes (e.g. Prader–Willi, Down syndromes) [114].

The neuroendocrine response to surgery releases counter-regulatory hormones (e.g. cortisol, catecholamines) that result in hyperglycemia, and potentially ketoacidosis in type 1 diabetics. Fasting and the requisite reduction or omission of regular medications further compounds the situation. Perioperative hyperglycemia increases the risk of wound infection [115].

Evaluation and planning are best conducted in advance of surgery with endocrinology consultation. Assessment defines the type of diabetes, current treatment regime, quality of current control (including HbA_{1c}), presence of complications, planned surgery, and anticipated postoperative course.

Regular medications are administered on the day before surgery with the exception of metformin, which is withheld for 24 h. Where possible, surgery is scheduled for the first case of the day, minimizing fasting time (usual fasting guidelines) and facilitating planning. The aims of management are to avoid hypoglycemia, hyperglycemia (target blood glucose 90–180 mg/dL), fluid and electrolyte imbalance, and ketosis. Management of antidiabetes medication on the day of surgery is determined by the duration of surgery, usual treatment regime and local hospital protocols. A review by Rhodes et al outlines the algorithms used at the Children's Hospital Boston [116]. Regardless of the regimen (subcutaneous injection or insulin infusion), patients with type 1 diabetes must not have insulin withheld on the day of surgery. Intravenous dextrose infusion will reduce the risk of hypoglycemia. Regular glucose monitoring is mandatory in all patients throughout the perioperative period. An anesthetic that facilitates early oral intake postoperatively (e.g. regional analgesia) aids in re-establishing the usual treatment regime.

Epilepsy

Seizure disorders are common in children, particularly in those with abnormal brain structure and/or developmental delay (e.g. cerebral palsy). The incidence of perioperative seizures can be increased by surgical stress, fasting, interruption of usual medication regime and the administration of drugs that may alter the seizure threshold (e.g. tramadol, pethidine).

During the preoperative evaluation, it is important to establish the type and frequency of seizures, specific triggers and the quality of seizure control. Associated disease states may have particular anesthetic significance; for example, up to 50% of children with tuberous sclerosis have intracardiac rhabdomyomas, which can cause outflow obstruction or arrhythmias [117]. The patient's current treatment regime should be reviewed and may include pharmacological therapies, a ketogenic diet, vagal nerve stimulation and past surgical interventions. Chronic administration of anti-seizure medications, such as carbamazepine and phenytoin, has been associated with resistance to opioids and muscle relaxants [118–120]. Solutions containing glucose (e.g. sugary premedications) should not be administered to children who are treated with a ketogenic diet, as this may lower ketone levels and reduce the seizure threshold [121]. Vagal nerve stimulation is sometimes used to treat intractable epilepsy. Vagal nerve stimulators do not need to be reprogrammed or turned off preoperatively, but standard precautions with electrocautery should be adopted (as for permanent pacemakers) and the device's function should be checked postoperatively [122]. All regular medications should be administered on the day of surgery.

Heart murmur

The discovery of an undiagnosed cardiac murmur during the preoperative evaluation presents a common dilemma for anesthesiologists. Innocent cardiac murmurs are audible at some period of their life in up to 70% of children [123]. Innocent murmurs are those not associated with underlying structural or physiological abnormalities, and are therefore asymptomatic. On auscultation, they are predominantly systolic (Still's vibratory and pulmonary flow murmurs), but occasionally continuous (venous hum) [124]. While the overall incidence of structural heart defects is low, a murmur could still indicate underlying pathology with significant perioperative implications.

A pathological murmur is more likely in the presence of a positive family history (hypertrophic obstructive cardiomyopathy (HOCM), congenital heart disease); maternal diabetes, infection or drug ingestion; prematurity; chromosomal abnormality; and in the presence of symptoms such as poor feeding, failure to thrive, breathlessness, recurrent respiratory tract infections and reduced exercise tolerance [125]. General examination findings suggesting a pathological cause include low oxygen saturation/cyanosis, increased work of breathing, absent pulses and hepatomegaly. Innocent murmurs occur during early or mid systole, are usually soft (<grade III) and are associated with normal splitting of the second heart sound. They are not associated with an ejection click or palpable thrill. Typically innocent murmurs disappear or diminish with standing and increase with squatting [123]. Pansystolic or diastolic murmurs raise suspicion of underlying pathology. A normal 12-lead ECG is reassuring, while evidence of left axis deviation or left ventricular hypertrophy is cause for suspicion [126].

Differentiating innocent from pathological murmurs can be difficult, particularly when faced with an uncooperative, moving and/or crying child. Where doubt exists, surgery should be delayed and the child referred to a pediatric cardiologist [126]. If the decision is made to proceed with surgery, appropriate cardiology follow-up should occur postoperatively. Antibiotic prophylaxis is recommended only for children with unrepaired cyanotic congenital heart disease and various repaired defects [127]. Therefore very few children with a previously undiagnosed murmur who proceed with planned surgery will require antibiotic prophylaxis (i.e. cyanosis mandates further assessment).

Obstructive sleep apnea

Patients with obstructive sleep apnea (OSA) have episodes of partial and/or complete upper airway obstruction during sleep that can result in hypoxemia, hypercapnia, abnormal sleep patterns, and, if left untreated, pulmonary hypertension. OSA is common, especially in the setting of obesity, certain syndromes (e.g. Down syndrome) and in children with adenotonsillar hypertrophy.

The risk of perioperative respiratory complications is increased in OSA [17]. Preoperative assessment aims to detect OSA (although clinical diagnosis is unreliable), define disease severity and identify complications [128]. History taking should focus on identifying symptoms such as snoring, apnea, restless sleeping and behavioral problems. Physical examination of the upper airway and cardiorespiratory system should be performed. Overnight polysomnography is best practice for the diagnosis and classification of severity of OSA [129]. Echocardiography is recommended preoperatively for children with severe (SpO$_2$ <70%) or frequent desaturation events, systemic hypertension and/or evidence of right ventricular failure [129]. Children with severe OSA may benefit from preoperative continuous positive airway pressure (CPAP) [129].

During the preoperative phase, a plan should be made regarding postoperative destination (general ward versus intensive care unit) and monitoring requirements.

Oncology patient

Children with cancer require anesthesia for a variety of interventions, including the initial diagnostic evaluation (imaging, biopsies), long-term central venous access device insertion, tumor resection, radiotherapy, and intrathecal chemotherapy. Preanesthesia evaluation should identify pathophysiological manifestations of the malignancy, adverse effects of medical treatment and behavioral or psychological issues. Potential organ-specific effects to consider include airway compromise (tumor, post radiotherapy); respiratory involvement (mediastinal mass, pulmonary toxicity and radiotherapy changes); cardiac toxicity (e.g. anthracycline-related cardiomyopathy); bone marrow suppression (anemia, thrombocytopenia and neutropenia); immunosuppression; and gastrointestinal disease (mucositis, vomiting and aspiration risk). Children (and their parents) requiring repeated anesthesia often develop preferences regarding elements of the anesthetic technique such as the use of sedative premedication, the mode of induction (intravenous versus inhalational), use of antiemetics and techniques for avoiding emergence agitation. Preoperative evaluation should therefore focus on exploring prior anesthetic experience and seek to identify patient preferences.

A recent series of review articles by Latham et al is recommended for a comprehensive oncology overview [130–132].

Upper respiratory tract infection

The incidence of upper respiratory tract infection (URTI) in children presenting for surgery is high [133]. Anesthesiologists commonly face the difficult dilemma of deciding whether the proposed surgery should proceed or not. Active or recent URTI is a well-defined risk factor for perioperative respiratory complications [7,8,22,134], including laryngospasm [7,10,14,135], bronchospasm [136,137], desaturation [136,138,139], severe coughing and airway obstruction [22]. However, most of these events are manageable, and the likelihood of long-term sequelae is minimal [15,136,140].

Every patient with URTI symptoms should be assessed on their individual merits before a decision is made to proceed with surgery. Important principles for the clinician to consider in the decision-making process are outlined below.

- Severity of symptoms. Evidence of severe URTI or potential lower respiratory tract infection typically warrants postponing surgery [133]. Standard criteria for cancellation are:
  - fever >38 or 38.5°C
  - purulent nasal discharge
  - productive cough
  - systemically unwell (e.g. poor appetite, myalgia, lethargy, "not usual self" or "too unwell to go to school")
  - lower respiratory tract signs (wheeze, crepitations).
- Duration and course of URTI symptoms. Recent onset (24–48h) of URTI symptoms may herald the onset of a serious illness that has not yet revealed its full extent. A significant condition evolving in the perioperative period increases patient discomfort and risk. Conversely, an established URTI that is improving suggests a benign course.

- Differential diagnoses. While the majority of URTI-like symptoms are due to viral URTIs (i.e. the common cold), potential differential diagnoses to consider are:
  - non-infectious rhinitis (allergic or vasomotor)
  - viral infections such as influenza, laryngotracheobronchitis (croup), bronchiolitis, measles and varicella
  - bacterial infections such as epiglottitis, tonsillitis, pneumonia and meningitis [133,141].
- Presence of the specific risk factors for adverse outcomes in the setting of URTI. These include:
  - age <1 year old [141]
  - history of prematurity (<37 weeks old) [15]
  - asthma [15]
  - parental smoking [15,22,134]
  - children with congenital heart disease presenting for cardiac surgery (URTI increases respiratory complications, bacterial infections and length of ICU admission) [142].
- Clinical urgency of the planned surgical procedure. Emergency surgery proceeds regardless of an URTI because the benefits outweigh risk. For elective surgery (i.e. not time critical), the risk–benefit equation may favor cancellation.
- Type of surgery. Ear, nose and throat (ENT) and airway procedures (e.g. bronchoscopy) carry a higher risk of respiratory complications in children with and without a URTI [9,15,143]. Duration of anesthesia does not seem to be important [15].
- Anticipated plan for airway management. Facemask anesthesia is associated with the lowest risk of respiratory complications but its use is limited to certain cases [134]. Endotracheal intubation increases the risk of respiratory complications by up to 11 times [7,15]. Studies comparing endotracheal (ETT) intubation with laryngeal mask use have demonstrated an increase in the total number of respiratory complications in the ETT group [22,144]. If airway manipulation is unavoidable, some anesthesiologists may elect to defer surgery.
- Social and logistic considerations. Frequently families have made major commitments (e.g. time off work/school, interstate travel) to attend hospital for the scheduled surgery. While the child should not be put at risk to avoid inconvenience, in borderline cases this may be an important consideration. Cancellation has a significant social, emotional and economic impact on patients and their families [145].

An informed discussion involving the anesthesiologist, parent(s) and surgeon is essential. The potential risks and benefits of proceeding versus cancellation need to be well communicated, and all parties involved in reaching a decision. Cancellation is prudent if either the surgeon or family expresses significant concern. Details of any discussion should be clearly documented in the medical record.

In the case of procedure deferment, the optimal time to reschedule must be determined. It is established that bronchial hyper-responsiveness (BHR) persists beyond the duration of URTI symptoms, returning to baseline by 6 weeks [146,147]. A prospective study of 1078 children found an increased risk for 4 weeks following URTI [15], while a recent prospective cohort study of 9297 children found risk was increased for the first 2 weeks but lowered between 2 and 4 weeks post URTI [22]. No consensus exists regarding optimal timing for surgery after simple URTI but a delay of 2–4 weeks following resolution of symptoms seems reasonable.

Preoperative bronchodilators may be effective in reducing respiratory complications, although the evidence is unclear. A study by Elwood found no benefit in the administration of preoperative bronchodilators (albuterol or ipratropium) in a select population of children having non-airway, non-cavity surgery [148]. Importantly, the rate of respiratory complications in control and URTI groups was identical. A recent study demonstrated a 50% reduction in the rate of perioperative bronchospasm and severe cough in children with recent URTI who were given salbutamol 10–30 min before surgery [149].

Intraoperative management of the child with a URTI is discussed in Chapter 15.

Preoperative anxiety and psychological preparation of the child

Surgery and anesthesia can be frightening and stressful experiences for a child. Many children cry, scream, verbally express fear or sadness, protest, attempt to escape the procedure and/or physically or verbally resist mask placement for anesthesia [150]. Up to 40–50% of children experience high levels of anxiety in the preoperative period [150,151], which peaks during mask placement and may delay the induction process [150]. In cases of extreme distress and anxiety, it is not uncommon for children to be physically restrained during induction [152], which can be emotionally traumatic for children, parents, and medical staff and lead to dissatisfaction with the anesthetic experience [153]. Preoperative anxiety has implications for postoperative recovery, with research suggesting that high levels of preoperative anxiety are associated with increased pain, longer times to discharge, higher rates of emergence delirium and increased behavioral problems in the days and weeks following surgery [154–156]. Of particular concern, the nature of children's early experiences with anesthesia and surgery (whether positive or negative) may predispose them to better or

worse reactions to future surgical experiences [156,157]. Therefore it is critically important that we aim to minimize children's anxiety and distress during this vulnerable period in order to lessen adverse psychological reactions and increase children's and their parents' overall satisfaction with the experience.

Risk factors

The experience of having general anesthesia and surgery alone does not determine the amount of anxiety and distress children experience. Factors which influence distress include the child's age and developmental stage, individual temperament traits, coping style, parental anxiety, and previous medical experiences [151].

Research has shown that younger children (7 years or less) are particularly vulnerable to anxiety and distress during the preoperative period [150,151]. Young children find it hard to understand why they must have surgery. Some young children may believe that surgery, illness and hospitalization are punishments for being naughty or the result of a deliberate desire of the clinician to hurt them [158]. Further, young children tend to worry about separation from their parents and fear strangers. With advancing age, children are able to invoke some type of coping strategy and seek more information about their procedure. However, although high levels of anxiety are more common among younger children, up to 30% of school-aged children also show extreme levels of anxiety and distress during the preoperative period [150]. Older children may regress to a more basic level of reasoning when faced with the prospect of surgery and may be more upset with dealing with the medical practitioners themselves. Adolescents may fear health and body integrity.

Individual temperament traits and coping styles have also been suggested as placing a child at risk of anxiety during the preoperative period [154]. Specifically, research suggests that children with a "shy-inhibited" temperament are more likely to be highly anxious during this period [154,159]. Children with these temperament traits are predisposed to be more fearful of others and highly aroused and emotional in unfamiliar situations [160]. In addition, children who use avoidance behaviors as a way of coping with stress have also been found to be more likely to show higher levels of preoperative anxiety [161]. These children attempt to ignore the situation, withdraw, avoid information and use wishful thinking ("I wish I wasn't sick") as their primary means to cope with their stress. In contrast, children who engage in approach behaviors, such as information seeking, non-procedural talk, coping statements and humor, have been found to show less distress upon induction to anesthesia[150].

Multiple previous hospital admissions and surgeries have also been linked with high preoperative anxiety

[154]. Research suggests that children do not necessarily habituate to repeated procedures and past aversive experiences may increase the negative emotions associated with surgery and may thereby interfere with coping [154,162]. In comparison, for children with good-quality past surgery experiences, repeated experience may facilitate the development of adaptive skills and may lessen levels of preoperative anxiety. Therefore, what appears to be important is the quality of children's past medical experiences rather than just having a previous experience *per se*. Other factors, such as parental anxiety, have been shown to influence the relationship between multiple surgeries and anxiety. For example, Kain et al [163] found that on average, children's anxiety did not differ at their second surgery compared with their first, but at the second surgery parental anxiety was significantly lower.

Parental behavior and level of anxiety during the preoperative period have been found to have a strong influence on children's anxiety levels [154]. Anxious parents tend to elicit agitation and anxiety by their presence and this is especially the case when a parent is so distressed that they cannot assist their child to cope. In addition, parents who use emotion-focused behaviors (reassurance, apologies, empathy, and empathetic touch) are also more likely to elicit distress from their child [164]. This type of response or conversation tends to draw children's attention to the surgery and conveys the message that the surgery is something to worry about and be frightened of. In comparison, parents who use distracting behaviors (non-procedure related conversation and humor) or encourage the use of coping skills (e.g. "You're helping your whole body feel better by doing your breathing") are more likely to promote their child's ability to cope with the stress of surgery. This is because these behaviors convey the message that surgery and anesthesia are manageable.

Assessment of anxiety

Methods for assessing preoperative anxiety and distress have primarily relied on observational ratings of children's overt behaviors, such as facial expressions, crying, torso movements, kicking, verbal protest, and need for restraint. The most frequently used measures are the Yale Preoperative Anxiety Scale [165] (designed for use during induction of anesthesia) and the modified Yale Preoperative Anxiety Scale (Box 13.1) [166] (designed for use during the induction phase and in the preoperative holding area). On both versions of this scale, items fall into one of five categories of behavior (activity, emotional expressivity, use of parents, state of arousal and vocalization) and clinicians rate the behaviors they observe. The benefits of Yale scales are that they can be used with children as young as 2 years of age and are quick and easy to administer.

Box 13.1 Modified Yale Preoperative Anxiety Scale (m-YPAS). The child is scored for each domain and scores are then added giving a total score from 5 to 22 with a higher score representing more distress [166]

Activity

1. The child is looking around curiously, playing with toys, reading (or other age-appropriate behavior); moves around the holding area/treatment room to get toys or to go to parent; may move toward operating room.
2. Not exploring or playing, may look down, fidget with hands or suck thumb (blanket); may sit close to parent while waiting, or play has a definite manic quality.
3. Moving from toy to parent in unfocused manner, non-activity derived movements; frenetic/frenzied movement or play; squirming, moving on table; may push mask away or cling to parent.
4. Actively trying to get away, pushes with feet and arms, may move whole body; in waiting room, running around unfocused, not looking at toys, will not separate from parent, desperate clinging.

Vocalizations

1. Reading (non-vocalizing appropriate to activity), asking questions, making comments, babbling, laughing, readily answers questions but may be generally quiet; child too young to talk in social situations or too engrossed in play to respond.
2. Responding to adults but whispers, "baby talk," only head nodding.
3. Quiet, no sounds or responses to adults.
4. Whimpering, moaning, groaning, silently crying.
5. Crying or may be screaming "no."
6. Crying, screaming loudly, sustained (audible through mask).

Emotional expressivity

1. Manifestly happy, smiling or concentrating on play.
2. Neutral, no visible expression on face.
3. Worried (sad) to frightened, sad, worried or tearful eyes.
4. Distressed, crying, extreme upset may have wide eyes.

State of apparent arousal

1. Alert, looks around occasionally, notices or watches what anesthesiologist does (could be relaxed).
2. Withdrawn, sitting still and quiet, may be sucking on thumb or have face turned into adult.
3. Vigilant, looking quickly all around, may startle to sounds, eyes wide, body tense.
4. Panicked whimpering, may be crying or pushing others away, turns away.

Use of parents

1. Busy playing, sitting idle or engaged in age-appropriate behavior and doesn't need parent; may interact with parent if parent initiates the interaction.
2. Reaches out to parent (approaches parent and speaks to otherwise silent parent), seeks and accepts comfort, may lean against parent.
3. Looks to parent quietly, apparently watches actions, doesn't seek contact or comfort, accepts it if offered or clings to parent.
4. Keeps parent at distance or may actively withdraw from parent, may push parent away or desperately clinging to parent and not let parent go.

Table 13.3 Induction Compliance Checklist [167]

Checklist	Score
Perfect induction (does not exhibit negative behaviors, fear or anxiety)	
Crying, tears in eyes	
Turns head away from mask	
Verbal refusal, says "no"	
Verbalization indicating fear or worry, "where's Mommy?" or "will it hurt?"	
Pushes mask away with hands, pushes nurse/anesthetist with hands/feet	
Covers mouth/nose with hands/arms or buries face	
Hysterical crying, may scream	
Kicks/flails legs/arms, arches back, and/or general struggling	
Requires physical restraint	
Complete passivity, either rigid or limp	
Total score (number of categories checked, perfect score = 0)	

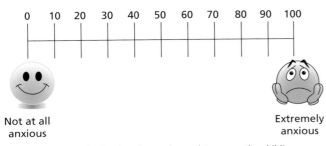

Figure 13.1 Generic visual analog scale used to assess the child's perception of their anxiety levels.

Observational methods of children's co-operation during induction have also been frequently used as a proxy measure of children's distress levels. The most commonly used is the Induction Compliance Checklist (Table 13.3) [167], which contains 10 possible negative or uncooperative behavioral responses to induction (such as crying, turning head away from mask, verbal refusal, verbalization of fear, physically resists mask, kicking and thrashing about, requires restraint, passive). The higher the number of negative behavior responses, the lower the rate of compliance, with a score of 0 representing a perfect induction.

Other less frequently used measures include self-report measures, such as a visual analog scale (VAS) [168], whereby children rate their anxiety on a scale from 0–100 (Fig. 13.1). As anxiety and distress are subjective experiences, self-reported measures are perhaps the most valid way to assess anxiety. However, for children undergoing induction of anesthesia, it is often not practical to obtain these ratings and self-report measures are also not suitable for very young children.

Physiological measures of anxiety and stress, such as levels of serum cortisol (a steroid hormone released in response to stress), have also been used in a small number of studies [169]. Serum cortisol levels are obtained immediately after induction of anesthesia via a blood sample. Ideally a baseline level of cortisol is needed to make sense of these findings, but it is not practical to sample children's blood prior to surgery. Other physiological indicators of anxiety such as heart rate and blood pressure are not suitable for this setting as they may be influenced by a range of other factors. These physiological indices are neither sensitive nor specific indictors of anxiety.

Non-pharmacological preparation programs

Knowledge of the growing literature for assisting children and their families facing surgical experiences is important for any anesthesiologist embarking on doing work with children. A number of different non-pharmacological interventions designed to reduce preoperative anxiety and increase compliance during induction have been described in the literature. Interventions have been targeted at the child, parent or both and include:

- cognitive or behavioral interventions, such as teaching coping skills, distraction, hypnosis, modeling and rehearsal, and shaping and exposure
- parenting interventions, such as acupuncture, psychoeducation and instruction on reinforcing children's coping behaviors during the procedure
- contextual interventions: parental presence, low sensory environment, use of induction room, patient retains own clothing, disguised anesthesia delivery systems.

With the exception of parental presence, the majority of evidence for specific non-pharmacological interventions is based on one or two single studies. Furthermore, published intervention trials often differ in terms of sample selection, blinding procedures and outcomes measures and often use a combination of interventions (e.g. parental presence and premedication). Such methodological differences have made it difficult to compare results across studies. Another limitation of current research is that few trials have stratified for age or examined adolescents. This is problematic given that past research has indicated that younger children are most at risk of preoperative anxiety [151], although even older children report high levels of anxiety during this stressful period [150]. Children with chronic illness, developmental delay, behavioral problems and previous surgical or hospitalization experiences have also been excluded from the majority of intervention trials. Given that these children may benefit most from interventions to reduce anxiety and increase co-operation and that these are the groups of children who present most often for surgery, exclusion of these children from studies represents a significant gap in the literature. With these limitations in mind, Yip et al [170] recently conducted a Cochrane Database review examining non-pharmacological interventions for assisting the induction of anesthesia in children. Their review included 17 trials involving 1796 children, their parents or both. Eight trials assessed parental presence and the remaining trials examined a range of different non-pharmacological interventions, directed at either children or parents. No evidence was found to support parental presence during induction or education of parents (i.e. in the form of pamphlets or videos) in reducing anxiety or improving co-operation of children. In comparison, based on single studies, promising evidence was found for acupuncture for parents, clown doctors, a quiet environment, video games and computer packages. The authors concluded that large randomized controlled trials are needed to determine the efficacy of these promising interventions.

Despite promising evidence to support a range of non-pharmacological interventions to reduce anxiety and increase co-operation in children, the translation of this research into practice has been limited. For example, in a study by O'Byrne et al [171] which surveyed a large sample of psychological experts, the majority rated coping skills, relaxation, and film as the most effective preparation procedures. Hospital tours, printed materials and narrative preparation were rated as the least effective. However, in a subsequent study surveying hospital staff, it was found that the least effective methods are actually the most frequently used in the "real world." They concluded that this is likely due to their ease of administration and cost-effectiveness whereas large-scale psychological interventions are often time consuming, expensive and not universally effective. Thus, the challenge is to find low-cost, easy-to-administer interventions and to target children who will most benefit from these types of non-pharmacological methods (rather than provide interventions to all children universally).

The finding that non-pharmacological interventions are not necessarily helpful for all children experiencing preoperative anxiety means that it is important that interventions are tailored to the individual child. Factors such as age, developmental level and past medical experiences have all been shown to affect the effectiveness of interventions aimed at reducing anxiety in children [162]. For example, Kain et al [162] found that the optimal timing of preparation depends on the age of the child. In their study, children aged 6 years or older were less anxious if prepared 5–7 days prior to surgery, and most anxious if presented with information within 24h of surgery. In comparison, children aged 3–6 years may benefit from preparatory information closer to the time of surgery. Children with past surgical experiences may not need the same level of preparation as those without past surgical experiences, as these children are likely to know what to expect. Research suggests that these children may benefit less from information-based preparatory programs and more from programs that focus on facilitating coping skills [162]. Further, the quality of children's past surgical experiences (whether positive or negative) needs to be taken into account when designing these programs [172].

Below we have briefly reviewed a number of non-pharmacological interventions.

Distraction

Distraction is a simple cognitive behavioral strategy that helps reduce children's distress. The goal is to focus the child's attention away from the upsetting aspects of the procedure and towards relatively more pleasant alternative stimuli. While a variety of distraction techniques exists, to be effective, the distraction technique must be age appropriate, and it must be appealing to the recipient.

Given their broad appeal, video games have been used in a variety of healthcare settings to distract children [173,174]. The benefit of video games is that they require active participation (as opposed to a passive activity such as watching television) and therefore are thought to engage sufficient attention resources of the child in order to distract them. To date, one study has utilized video games as a means of distraction during induction of anesthesia [175]. These authors found that children aged 4–12 years who played with a hand-held video game had less anxiety at induction compared with children who only had their parent present. No difference was seen in anxiety levels between children who played a video game and children who received premedication with midazolam.

Music therapy has been shown to achieve a significant reduction in preoperative anxiety at separation of parents and entry into the operating theater but not during induction of anesthesia [176]. Anxiety has been found to be at its highest during mask placement and it is possible that passive activities are not sufficient to engage children's attention during periods of extreme stress. Similarly, other more passive methods of distraction, such as use of novel toys, books and blowing bubbles, have not been found to reduce anxiety during induction compared with parental presence alone [177].

The presence of clown doctors during the induction of anesthesia has been shown to be an effective intervention for reducing anxiety for children in the preoperative waiting area in two studies [178,179]. However, the presence of clowns does not necessarily reduce anxiety during induction of anesthesia, with one study showing that anxiety in children accompanied by clowns actually peaks during this period and is greater than the anxiety found in children receiving midazolam or no intervention [179]. While further studies investigating the efficacy of this intervention are needed, it is interesting to note that Vagnoli et al found much resistance from staff regarding the use of clown doctors [178]. They found that while the majority of staff acknowledged the effectiveness of this technique, many were not in favor of utilizing clown doctors as it was believed that they would interfere with the operating room routine. This finding highlights the importance of considering the practicality of certain interventions.

Parental presence

Having a parent present during induction is thought to reduce the child's anxiety by providing comfort and eliminating separation anxiety [180]. As noted previously, parental presence during the induction of anesthesia has been the most extensively studied non-pharmacological intervention aimed at reducing anxiety and increasing co-operation in children. Most children prefer a parent to be with them and most parents prefer to be present during induction [181,182]. Further, an overwhelming proportion of parents believe that they were of some help to their child and the anesthesiologist during induction [169,181,183]. However, well-controlled randomized control trials have not shown this intervention to be effective for the reduction of children's preoperative anxiety or increase in children's compliance [170]. The reasons for this are not well understood, but some recent research has suggested that it may be what parents actually do and say during induction that is more critical to the reduction of children's anxiety than their mere presence. For example, parental behaviors such as criticism, excessive reassurance and commands have been associated with increased anxiety levels in children, whereas parenting behaviors aimed at distracting children or prompting coping skills have been associated with reduction in children's anxiety and distress [164]. Some research suggests that parents take their cues from anesthesiologists and nurses about how to behave during induction. When anesthesiologists use more non-procedural talk and humor, so do parents [164]. Thus, training medical staff may directly affect parents' behavior by engaging in higher rates of desirable behaviors themselves [150].

Hypnosis

Hypnosis uses relaxation, focused guided imagery, suggestions and therapeutic metaphors to build self-control over physical and emotional symptoms. Use of hypnosis is not recommended without appropriate training. Professionals using hypnosis as part of their treatment should have appropriate credentials from a recognized hypnotherapy association. In Australia, this association is known as the Australian Society of Hypnosis. To date, one study has evaluated the efficacy of hypnosis on anxiety versus midazolam [184]. It found that compared with midazolam, fewer children were anxious during induction in the hypnosis group compared to the midazolam group.

Acupuncture

Acupuncture is part of traditional Chinese medicine and involves inserting fine needles into specific points on the skin or applying various other techniques to the acupuncture points to bring about healing or relief from pain. One study has evaluated the efficacy of acupuncture in alleviating anxiety in parents of children undergoing surgery [185]. They found that children of parents who had anxiety reduction acupuncture prior to induction were less anxious and more co-operative during induction than children whose parents who received sham acupuncture. Parents' subjective ratings of anxiety were also less in the group who had anxiety reduction acupuncture rather than sham acupuncture.

Environmental modifications

The equipment, bright lights, the number of medical staff interacting with the child and high noise levels of the induction room are all believed to contribute to children's increased anxiety during induction of anesthesia. Few studies, however, have investigated the impact simple modifications to the environment may have on children's levels of anxiety and co-operation during induction. In one study, a low sensory input group (dimmed OR lights, only one person (the anesthesiologist) interacting with the child and soft classical music played in the background) was compared to a control group (usual practice) [186]. The authors found that children in the low sensory input group were less anxious and more co-operative during induction. However, it is unclear which aspect was most effective.

Educational programs

Preoperative education programs take various forms, including information leaflets and tours of the theater environment, videos depicting children going to theater, role play or psychological preparation. Educational programs may target parents or children or both. In studies investigating the effect of educational programs on parental anxiety, there has been some evidence to suggest that parents who participate in a preparation program or who view a preoperative video regarding anesthesia demonstrate reduced anxiety on the day of surgery [30,162]. Others, however, have found that this reduction in anxiety does not extend to the important and most stressful time of anesthetic induction [187].

Evidence for the efficacy of information-based programs designed for children to reduce their levels of preoperative anxiety has been mixed. Some studies have shown that information-based preparations (including tour of OR, watching a video showing a child from surgery to discharge and medical play with dolls for 30min) are successful at reducing anxiety in the preoperative holding area. However, this reduction in anxiety is temporary and does not extend to after separation from parents or induction of anesthesia. Others, however, have failed to find evidence for the efficacy of information-based programs for either the preoperative holding area or anesthesia induction. In a more recent study, an interactive computer program was used to prepare children for dental surgery and compared to a cartoon strip or no preparations [188]. Preparation with interactive computer packages (in addition to parental presence) was more effective in making children more co-operative during induction compared to parental presence alone.

Pharmacological interventions for reducing anxiety

Goals of premedication

There is no doubt that pharmacological premedication is an important, and often the best strategy to reduce anxiety in children. As stated in an early editorial, "if anxiolysis is the objective, premedication is the treatment" [189]. Other non-pharmacological strategies do not always provide a reliable and constant effect on preoperative level of anxiety. The aim of sedative premedication is to decrease the preoperative level of anxiety in children, facilitate parental separation, enhance the child's collaboration at induction of anesthesia, and improve recovery and postoperative outcome.

The decision to premedicate a child should not be based on set recipes or routine prescriptions for all children, but should be integrated within a global assessment of the child's needs and be part of the overall preoperative preparation for anesthesia. Medication should not be the rescue solution to a lack of proper preoperative assessment and interaction with the child and family. Premedication should be a supplemental strategy to reduce the child's anxiety and facilitate parental separation.

Pros and cons of premedication

There is controversy over the use of premedication, particularly over its routine use, for every child [190]. The arguments in favor of administering premedication stem from concern that preoperative anxiety and stress lead to negative postoperative outcomes such as emergence delirium, negative postoperative behavior changes, and increased postoperative pain [25,154,190]. Moreover, preoperative anxiety enhances neurohumoral response to stress, which further contributes to adverse postoperative outcomes [191]. Those who support systematic premedication highlight the impact of preoperative anxiety on these adverse outcomes and thus the potential benefit of an anxiolytic and sedative agent such as midazolam [192]. There is no doubt that many randomized controlled trials have highlighted the beneficial effect of midazolam in reducing preoperative anxiety and improving coping capabilities during induction of anesthesia [167,193]. Furthermore, the use of premedication is associated with reduced anxiety and improved satisfaction with the anesthesia management in the parents[167].

A reduction in postoperative behavior disorders (POBD) is one aim of premedication but there are conflicting data in the literature regarding the real benefit of this premedication in preventing the occurrence of negative postoperative behavior. While some authors have shown a higher incidence of arousal distress [194] and POBD after midazolam premedication [184,195], others have demonstrated no effects [155] or a slight decrease and limited in time [196]. More strikingly, preparing children with a non-pharmacological hypnotic strategy led to a significantly lower incidence of POBD than those who received midazolam [184]. The reason for this discrepancy may be due to a negative effect of the anterograde amnesia induced by midazolam in children [197,198]. Midazolam exerts a dissociative effect on memory by inhibiting explicit memory while implicit memory is preserved [199]. As implicit memory is involved in behavior, midazolam may potentiate POBD by not protecting the child from unconscious memory of preoperative events with a negative and emotional content. The child may be unable to report these memories consciously in the postoperative phase but rather express them postoperatively with negative behavior. The potentially negative effect of midazolam on memory and the recent development of successful cognitive behavioral therapies to reduce preoperative anxiety reinforced the arguments against the use of systematic premedication in children.

The development of a specific child-friendly environment [190], specific preoperative programs based on a multimodal information strategy [33,190,200], and extending the indications for parental presence at induction [169,190,201] have contributed to a reduction in preoperative anxiety and hence reduced the need to rely solely on pharmacological approaches. However, one should keep in mind that there will still be some children (especially preschool children) who may need a sedative premedication despite the application of all other strategies described. Sedative premedication should be given selectively and at the discretion of the anesthesiologist.

Most commonly used drugs

The sedative premedications used vary from one country to another but midazolam and clonidine are the most popular and most studied drugs with midazolam being the most widely and frequently administered sedative agent in children. The intravenous solution of midazolam allows administration by different routes (intranasally at 0.3 mg/kg, orally 0.25–0.5 mg/kg, rectally 0.5 mg/kg, and sublingually 0.3 mg/kg) and, being highly lipophilic in physiological pH, midazolam provides beneficial pharmacokinetic properties with rapid onset of action. In recent studies, the level of sedation and anxiolysis was considered as satisfactory in more than 75% of children after 7.7 ± 2.4 min, 12.5 ± 4.9 min and 16.3 ± 4.2 min respectively following intranasal, oral or rectal administration [202,203].

The oral route is the most popular and recommended administration mode. The nasal route is uncomfortable and seems to be associated with a potentially higher risk for paradoxical reactions [204,205]. The rectal route has also been largely abandoned since the absorption and concentration levels are unpredictable.

The half-life of midazolam can be very variable since the drug is essentially metabolized by the liver by the CYP450 enzyme system, particularly the subtypes 3A3 and 3A4 which have been found to be very variable between patients [206,207]. Moreover, many drugs can affect the CYP450 activity and contribute to the prolongation of the half-life.

Despite a relatively high safety profile, there are clinical situations where midazolam should be administered with caution because of the risk for airway obstruction, such as in children with large tonsils [208] and/or with obstructive sleep apnea. In addition, it has been recently demonstrated in children that midazolam induces a decrease in functional residual capacity, which may affect gas exchange in those with cardiopulmonary disease [209].

Clonidine, an $\alpha2$-adrenoceptor agonist, is nowadays the best alternative agent to midazolam [210]. It provides anxiolysis and sedation [211] without affecting cognitive function or memory [212]. In addition, its analgesic properties can be beneficial in children [213]. Furthermore, studies have demonstrated the beneficial effect of clonidine premedication in preventing agitation at induction of anesthesia with sevoflurane [214], and a decrease in the incidence of emergence delirium [215]. Clonidine can be administered by the intravenous, intramuscular, transdermal, oral and rectal routes [216]. It is mostly administered via the oral route at a dose of 4 μg/kg. Pharmacokinetic studies in children confirm that following oral administration, the bio-availability is relatively low (55%) and the maximum concentration level is obtained after 1 h [217]. Clonidine should be administered at least 60 min prior to induction to be effective. The elimination half-life of clonidine in children is similar to that observed in adults, at around 9 h [216]. This explains the longer sedative effect seen in children premedicated with clonidine. This prolonged sedation may be seen as a benefit or a problem postoperatively, with children better sedated and calmer but slower to leave the postanesthesia care unit (PACU). The sedative-anxiolytic effect of clonidine is mediated by the hyperpolarization of the ascending noradrenergic neurons in the locus ceruleus consequent on the inhibition of calcium entry into calcium channels in nerve terminals and change in membrane ion conductance [218].

Clonidine has a good therapeutic profile with very few contraindications to its administration. While the best indication could be children with obstructive sleep apnea syndrome, clonidine should be used with caution in children treated on a long-term basis with methylphenidate (Ritalin®) since this latter may also blunt sympathetic response and an association with clonidine may lead to a bradycardia and cardiovascular collapse at induction of anesthesia [219].

Ketamine is also used occasionally for premedication. It needs to be administered at a high dosage (5–10 mg/kg intrarectally or orally) to be effective and thus may induce a greater incidence of adverse events [220] and prolong postoperative sedation [221]. Intramuscular administration of ketamine (4 mg/kg) provides a dissociative sedation within 5–20 min but may have a higher incidence of respiratory adverse events and laryngospasm and should be performed under close monitoring [222]. Some authors have suggested adding midazolam 0.5 mg/kg to ketamine at 3 mg/kg orally to decrease the incidence of adverse events, shorten the onset time and decrease the recovery time [223]. In spite of the above concerns, there is still a place for ketamine, particularly intramuscular ketamine, in extremely anxious and unco-operative children who refuse to take premedication orally and in those who are unwilling to have any contact with health providers who are not part of their usual environment, such as autistic [223] or hyperactive children treated by meth-ylphenidate (Ritalin®).

Recently, new interest has been focused on melatonin but there are conflicting data in the literature regarding the anxiolytic effect of this agent [224,225]. Studies have demonstrated that oral melatonin at a dose of 0.2–0.4 mg/kg reduces the incidence of emergence delirium [225] and may prevent the occurrence of sleep disturbance at week 2 postoperatively [224].

Finally, one should not forget premedication with non-sedative drugs such as paracetamol to initiate pain treat-ment [226], salbutamol in children with bronchial hyper-responsiveness [149], and antibiotics as recom-mended by the American Heart Association [127].

In summary, it is important to reduce preoperative anxiety in children. Pharmacological premedication is one aspect of the multimodal approach that includes non-pharmacological interventions such as behavioral prepa-ration programs, parental presence at induction, and distraction techniques. There is no single medication that fits all children of all ages and pharmacological premedi-cation should be administered according to the interac-tion between the child, the parents and the anesthesiologist during the preoperative assessment.

Awareness and recall in pediatric anestheisa

Recently awareness has become a topic of major interest to the pediatric anesthesiologist. This is largely because of several studies which have shown a relatively high rate of awareness in children compared to adults [227–231]. Although the data are scarce, these studies may also suggest that the causes and consequences of awareness may be different in children.

What is awareness?

The usual definition of awareness is the explicit recall of an event that occurred during anesthesia. However, it is also possible to be awake during anesthesia without recall, and it is also possible to form implicit memory during anesthesia. Explicit recall is memory which is con-sciously recalled. Implicit memory is memory which leads to alterations in behavior with no conscious recollection.

The maturation of memory processes

Before discussing awareness in children, it is useful to have a brief understanding of what memory and con-sciousness are, and how they develop.

Consciousness

The study of consciousness is a controversial topic. From a philosophical perspective, being conscious involves having your own private world of sensations which are linked in a single being and which connect with other past experiences beyond the immediate physical sensa-tion [232,233]. Anesthesiologists tend to take a more prac-tical view of consciousness. Being conscious is being aware of the environment, and is often measured by seeking evidence of cognition or a coherent response to command. Being awake during an anesthetic is being conscious during the anesthetic.

Memory

Memory is divided into short-term (working) memory and long-term memory. Long-term memory is further classified as implicit or explicit. Explicit memory may contain semantic knowledge (facts) or episodic knowl-edge (what you remember doing). There are four basic steps to memory: encoding, consolidation, storage and retrieval. Encoding is the process of attending to informa-tion and associating it meaningfully and systematically with established memory. Memory is more easily encoded if it "fits in" easily and if there is a stronger motivation for encoding. Consolidation is the process of shaping the new information to enable long-term storage. Retrieval is the process of bringing memory back into working or short-term memory. Retrieval is most effective when the cues or context for retrieval closely resemble those present at encoding.

Implicit memory

Implicit memory is memory that unconsciously alters behavior. It does not require conscious processing for encoding or retrieval. Types of implicit memory include non-associative habituation or sensitization, and associa-tive learning such as classic or operative conditioning.

Development of memory and consciousness

The point at which a human becomes conscious is con-troversial but certainly relevant to pediatric anesthesiolo-gists. Evidence for consciousness can be assumed if there is evidence of thought or of a sense of self. Infants do show signs of thinking. If you show an infant an attractive object and suddenly plunge them into darkness, they will still search for the object [234]. Similarly, an infant will show greater attention to situations inconsistent with pre-vious knowledge, such as objects that when released seem to defy gravity. Evidence for self is harder to determine but in the toddler clear evidence of self can be seen in the use of the pronouns such as "I" and "we."

While all agree that infants are indeed conscious, it is hard to find good measures for precisely when an infant or toddler is conscious or unconscious from an anesthesiologist's perspective. Loss of response to command is used as a standard measure of consciousness in adult anesthesia. This requires language, understanding and motivation – all of which may not be possible in small children.

If we look back from adulthood, we cannot remember much about what happened before we were 3 years of age. This is known as "infantile amnesia." This, along with poorly developed language, makes the assessment of memory difficult in young children. There is, however, good evidence of memory from an early age. Implicit memory develops before explicit memory. Non-associative memory has been demonstrated in the fetus. A newborn will respond to their mother's voice, which they have heard during the last weeks of pregnancy, but not their father's [235,236]. Associative memory can be demonstrated in a neonate's response to painful stimuli such as heelprick [237].

The development of explicit memory is probably linked to the development of language. Good evidence for explicit memory can be found from around 3 years of age [238] and continues to develop throughout childhood. With increasing age, children can store increasing numbers of items in their working memory, and encoding, consolidation and retrieval are faster and more accurate as the child has a better understanding of events and increasing depth of experience. These factors must be borne in mind when considering how we assess explicit recall and awareness under anesthesia in children.

Measuring awareness in children

The measurement of awareness is inherently imprecise and subjective; it is even more so in children. If we simply ask a child if they remembered anything during the anesthesia, then they may not be able to differentiate between memories formed during anesthesia and those formed in the PACU. Similarly, they may report dreams or other forms of inaccurate or false memories. In adult awareness studies, researchers have sought to standardize studies by using an interview similar to that originally described by Brice [239]. However, its structure is unsuitable for children [228]. Children have poorer memory encoding, consolidation and retrieval strategies. Without carefully building context during questioning, children may not retrieve an awareness memory. Open-ended or temporally inconsistent questions such as used in the Brice interview could lead to an underestimate of awareness in children. Awareness may also be underestimated as confirmation of awareness relies on the richness of the memory. Children's memory may contain errors which make such confirmation more fraught with difficulties.

Children also have poorer source monitoring; they are more likely to confuse the origin or place of a memory. This is particularly likely if leading or repeated questions are used, which may implant memory. This may overestimate the incidence of awareness in children. Thus poor interview techniques can result in awareness being either under- or over-reported in children [240].

Children being awake during anesthesia

The isolated forearm technique involves inflating a tourniquet around the arm of a patient, before any neuromuscular blocking agents are given, and then repeatedly asking the patient to squeeze the researcher's hand. Isolated forearm technique studies in the adult population have demonstrated that patients may be awake and paralyzed during routine anesthesia with few clinical signs of being awake [241]. Typically, few of these patients have any explicit recall of being awake. Byers and Muir also used an isolated forearm technique during induction of anesthesia in children and found that many children responded to commands, though none had subsequent explicit recall [242]. Andrade et al performed a similar study during anesthesia but found that very few children responded to command [243].

Awareness in adults

Before looking more closely at awareness in children, it is useful to quickly recap what we know about awareness in adults. In adults, most studies find an incidence of awareness during routine anesthesia of roughly 1:2000 cases [244–247]. Lower or higher incidences may be due to different populations or ways in which awareness is assessed [248,249]. Risk factors include presence of paralysis or significant cardiovascular compromise, anesthesia for trauma, bronchoscopy, obstetrics and cardiac surgery, and a family history of awareness [246,248,250–257]. It is unclear if total intravenous anesthesia is also a risk factor [258–260]. Awareness is often not volunteered unprompted and there may be some delay in reporting [246]. In adults, awareness is usually auditory but may also include pain or feelings of paralysis. Awareness may be associated with tachycardia or hypertension but these signs are often present without awareness [261]. In adults, awareness is most commonly due to inadvertent light anesthesia after mishap or misjudgment [248,262]. Awareness under light anesthesia may also occur where the patient cannot tolerate larger doses of anesthesia (such as trauma or caesarean section).

Most adults who are aware do not enjoy the experience [263]. Many show anxiety postoperatively, some may avoid future anesthesia and some may develop post-traumatic stress disorder (PTSD) and other significant and persistent psychological disturbances [264–269]. In adults, principles of prevention are paying attention to good technique and reducing risk of error. Bispectral Index (BIS) monitoring has been shown to be superior to standard practice in reducing awareness in high-risk adults [250].

Frequency of awareness in children

A survey of the pediatric anesthesia community found that 27% of respondents had at least one case of pediatric awareness in their practice [270]. There are three old [271–273] and five newer cohort studies [227–231] designed to determine the incidence of awareness in children. Some other studies primarily designed to test for wakefulness or implicit memory formation also made some measure of explicit recall [242,243,274–277]. There are also three case series describing consequences of awareness which include some adults who would have been children when the awareness occurred [267–269]. A recent case report also describes two clear cases of awareness in children [278].

In 1973, McKie and Thorp interviewed 202 children aged 7–14 years and found 10 cases of definite awareness (5%) [272]. In 1988, O'Sullivan et al reported the effect of pretreatment with tubocurarine on the incidence of dreaming in 144 children aged 5–14 years who received succinylcholine [273]. There were no cases of awareness. The same investigators later published a prospective study of dreaming and awareness in 120 day-case children aged 5–17 years [271]. Again there were no cases of awareness. These studies used a very limited assessment for awareness.

More recently, a cohort study in 864 children aged 5–12 years found seven cases of awareness (0.8%) [227]. In this study the anesthesiologists were unaware which children were being studied. Postoperatively, the children were interviewed three times (for two of these, the interview was a proxy interview by the parents) and where awareness was suspected, the child's verbatim responses were then sent to four independent pediatric anesthesiologists who judged each report as "no awareness," "possible" or "awareness". Awareness was judged to have occurred if all agreed it was "awareness." More recently, the same group published another cohort study in 500 children [230]. This used Brice's idea of increasing the specificity of assessment by playing particular noises to the subjects during anesthesia [239]. In this cohort, using the same system of adjudication as used above, only one child was classified as being aware (0.2%). Importantly, some children reported hearing sounds during the anesthetic that had been played to them before anesthesia, thus clearly demonstrating errors of source monitoring.

In 2007, Lopez et al reported a cohort study assessing awareness in 410 children aged 6–16 years and found five children (1.2%) to be aware [228]. The children were interviewed by trained psychologists within 36 h and 1 month after the procedure. In this study, the interview was carefully tailored to the cognitive ability of children. The reports were tape recorded and then reviewed by three independent adjudicators who classified the transcript as "awareness," "possible awareness" or "not awareness." Children were classified as aware if at least two adjudicators judged the case as 'awareness."

A cohort study from The Netherlands with 928 children aged 5–18 years found six awareness cases (0.6%) [229]. Similarly, a multicenter cohort study in the United States reported an awareness incidence of 0.8% in children aged 5–15 (14 of 1784 interviewed children) [231].

Lastly, there are three small studies assessing implicit memory formation in children which incidentally found no evidence for explicit memory [274–276]. Similarly, in two studies designed to detect wakefulness using the isolated forearm technique, evidence for wakefulness was found in both cases but there was no explicit recall [242,243].

The earlier studies reported wide ranges in incidence. The high rates may be due to outdated anesthesia practice and the low incidences may be due to poor interview techniques. The recent large cohort studies all report incidences just below 1% – an incidence appreciably higher than in adults. The reason for the higher incidence remains unclear.

Characteristics of awareness in children

While many of the characteristics of awareness in children are similar to those in adults, there are some differences. Any comparison, however, must be tempered by the fact that there are very few studies and reports on which to base these comparisons. As in adults, in children awareness is often not volunteered to hospital staff (though some reports found that children told their siblings) and may only be detected at the second or third interview. In adults, awareness is often auditory and may be accompanied by pain and intense fear. Although some children do describe experiences like this, children report more tactile experiences, less pain and the experience may be less distressing. The memories are often fragmentary and less detailed. This is consistent with the developmental aspects of memory described previously.

Causes of awareness in children

In the pediatric studies reported so far, repeated airway manipulation was the only factor found to be associated with awareness [228]. There are no other obvious causes for awareness and awareness occurred in what would be considered as low-risk groups. It remains unclear why awareness is more common in children compared to adults.

There are three possible explanations for the high incidence of awareness. First, the finding may be due to measurement error and implanted memory or false recall due to errors in source monitoring. This is indeed a possibility though there are equally strong arguments to suggest that measurement error could underestimate the incidence of awareness. It is, however, pertinent to note that in one study, children reported hearing a stimulus that was given in the preoperative holding area – clear evidence that error in source monitoring does occur [230].

The second possibility is that pediatric anesthesiologists use techniques that increase the risk of awareness. The use of induction rooms has been suggested to increase the risk of awareness [279]. Induction rooms are used widely in Europe and Australia to enable induction to occur in a quieter, friendlier environment where parents can accompany their child without having to enter the main operating room itself. If induction rooms are used, the child is disconnected from the circuit for transfer to the operating room. In theory, this may allow breathing room air, lightening of anesthesia and hence increase risk of awareness – particularly if the circuit in the operating room is not primed. While pediatric anesthesiologists who use induction rooms should always be aware of this risk, it is unlikely to be the main cause of awareness in children as induction rooms were not used in two of the studies [228,231]. Another possibility is that pediatric anesthesiologists just accept periods of lighter anesthesia in children. There is no evidence to support this suggestion, but it is interesting to note that when comparing the two studies done by Davidson et al [227,230] the incidence was lower in the study where the anesthesiologists knew an awareness study was being performed; thus it is possible that awareness is reduced simply by anesthesiologists being more careful to avoid it.

The third possible cause could be simple and fundamental differences in the pharmacology of anesthetics in children. Children do have a higher minimum alveolar concentration (MAC). MAC peaks in infancy then declines with increasing age [280,281]. The MAC-awake is the concentration at which 50% return to consciousness [282]. When considering awareness, MAC-awake may be the more relevant measure of potency of anesthesia. Like MAC, MAC-awake is higher in children and declines with age [283–286]. Thus children do need more anesthetic to ensure unconsciousness. It is possible that awareness is more common in children simply because anesthesiologists do not give enough anesthetic or allow enough time for effect site concentrations to become adequate. Interestingly, the degree to which the EEG is suppressed at 1 MAC does vary with age

[287–290]. The significance of this for awareness risk is unclear.

Lastly, some children might be at risk for awareness for exactly the same reasons as adults. Errors in drug delivery due to miscalculation or equipment failure or syringe swap are just as likely to occur in children. Similarly, some children who are extremely unwell may not be able to tolerate large doses of anesthetic and children having cardiac surgery will have cardiovascular signs of inadequate anesthesia ablated – just as in adults. These may be the causes of awareness seen in some children but in the recent cohort studies, aware children were not in these high-risk groups and as far as can be determined, errors were not the cause.

Consequences of awareness in children

In adults, the consequences of awareness vary. In prospective cohort studies in adults, the incidence of severe psychological disturbance has been described as 0%, 2%, 9% and 44% [264–269]. Severe disturbance may only be apparent some time after the event. Awareness in the setting of paralysis is associated with greater anxiety and risk of significant persistent psychological disturbance. In children, data are scarcer.

Three studies interviewed adults about their experiences of awareness. Some of these studies included adults who would have experienced the awareness when they were children. Samuelsson et al found 46 cases of awareness and of these, five were children at the time of the previous surgery (aged 7–12 years) [267]. Of the 46 cases, 15 had psychological symptoms but only one of the children. Schwender et al interviewed 45 people and eight would have been under the age of 18 years at the time of awareness [268]. Twelve of the 37 adults developed psychological symptoms while only one of the eight children did. Osterman et al interviewed 16 adults all of who had diagnostic criteria for post-traumatic stress disorder (PTSD) [269]. Three would have been children at the time of awareness. These studies confirm that there are still some children who can have significantly disturbing awareness.

Although some children do develop substantial anxiety and significant delayed psychological disturbance, the children described in the recent large cohort studies do not appear as distressed as adults. In one, there was no evidence for behavioral disturbance 1 month after the event and at later follow-up none had signs of PTSD [227,291]. Another study found no evidence for PTSD 1 year after the event [292].

Prevention and management

Without understanding the causes of awareness in children, it is difficult to know how to prevent it.

Obviously it would be prudent to apply many of the recommendations made in adult anesthesia to reduce risk of error. This includes labeling syringes carefully, checking anesthesia machines and in particular that vaporizers are well fitted and full. As mentioned before, care should be taken to ensure that anesthetic levels in children are not light during transfer and most importantly, it must always be remembered that children have fundamentally higher anesthesia requirements – give more and wait longer for adequate effect site concentration to be achieved. In particular, remember that there is a substantial delay between end-tidal concentration of a volatile anesthetic and brain concentration.

The role of depth of anesthesia monitors and awareness in children is unclear. Most EEG-derived depth monitors have been validated to some extent in children. The numbers tend to go up and down with loss and regaining consciousness and there is some rough correlation with anesthetic concentration. There are theoretical reasons why they may have poorer performance due to EEG maturation but apart from infants, their performance seems similar to that in adults. However, the proof of their utility lies in properly conducted trials. There are no trials assessing the use of EEG-derived depth monitors in preventing awareness in children and because of differences in awareness characteristics and possibly causes, adult studies cannot be extrapolated to children.

The management of awareness is supportive. Children who report being aware should be listened to and the anesthesiologist should be sympathetic. The child and family should be provided with a clear explanation of anything that may have contributed to awareness and while persistent psychological disturbance may be rare, further psychological counseling should be offered. Particular care should be taken to follow up children who report painful experiences while being paralyzed. It should also be remembered that PTSD may develop some months after the event.

Implicit memory in children during anesthesia

In adults, implicit memory can be detected for events that occur during anesthesia [293]. Unlike explicit memory, there is some weak evidence that implicit memory can be formed without periods of consciousness or wakefulness [294]. The relevance of implicit memory formation during anesthesia is uncertain. In awake subjects, implicit memory can result in reinforcement of an existing desire [293]. For example, subliminal priming with pictures of food will increase an existing hunger. It is thus often considered that negative conversation about a patient during anesthesia or negative experiences during anesthesia may increase a patient's existing perioperative anxiety

which can be manifest as increased stress or maladaptive behavior postoperatively. While fine in theory, this is hard to prove or detect in practice. Similarly, therapeutic suggestions may also improve postoperative state but once again this is hard to prove clinically.

It has been suggested that children have a high incidence of postoperative maladaptive behavior and that this may be partly due to implicit memory formation. It is known that implicit memory matures earlier than explicit memory but as in adults, the actual relevance of implicit memory for events during anesthesia is uncertain in children. Several studies have found no evidence for implicit memory for events during anesthesia in children [240,243,274–276,295].

Awareness in the very young

Awareness requires explicit memory and children begin to develop some form of explicit memory at around the age of 3 years. However, younger children could still form implicit memory or have periods of consciousness during anesthesia. There is very little research or discussion examining the effect of periods of consciousness or implicit memory formation during anesthesia in this age group.

There is, however, increasing evidence that untreated pain is detrimental to infants, resulting in morphological change in the spinal cord, persisting changes in behavior and worse clinical outcomes. Similarly, several landmark studies have suggested that providing adequate analgesia and anesthesia in neonates undergoing surgery reduces stress markers and improves clinical outcomes [296–298]. Thus at the very least, the very young should not be left to suffer pain, regardless of any discussion about implicit memory or consciousness.

It would also seem reasonable and humane to reduce any obvious signs of distress caused by surgery. This could involve regional anesthetic, sedation or rendering the child unresponsive (general anesthesia). Unfortunately, assessing whether or not an infant is unconscious can be difficult (especially if the infant is paralyzed). Similarly, we have no easy direct way to determine if they are forming implicit memory. This makes the titration of anesthesia particularly difficult in this age group.

Conclusion

Awareness can certainly occur in children and there is substantial evidence to suggest that it may be more common than in adults. The reasons for this are unclear. While awareness is often not distressing in children, there are well-documented cases where it has resulted in significant psychological disturbance. It is difficult to know how to prevent awareness in children until we know more about why it occurs in children.

Postoperative behavior disorders

There is increasing awareness of the potential lasting negative psychological impact of hospitalization, anesthesia and surgery in children. These are events that may be stressful for both children and parents. Three clinical phenomena have been associated with this psychological stress: preoperative anxiety, emergence delirium in the very early postoperative period, and negative postoperative behavior changes after discharge from hospital [299,300]. While postoperative behavior disturbance was first described as early as 1945 [301], there is still no clear definition of the concept of negative postoperative behavior change. Further, knowledge about this has been limited as its detection has tended to rely on just one questionnaire that presents several limitations [302]. It is probable that various postoperative psychological disturbances occur after a distressing hospitalization. Thus, rather than speaking of just negative behavior change as defined by the questionnaire most widely used, it may be more useful to consider a wider concept of postoperative behavior disorders.

Negative postoperative behavior changes
Measuring postoperative behavior changes

In the past decade, concerns have been expressed about the high incidence of negative postoperative behavior changes in the pediatric population [154,156,196,303]. In spite of such concern, only one tool is used in nearly all the medical literature for the measurement of these negative changes: the Post Hospitalization Behavior Questionnaire (PHBQ) [302]. This questionnaire was developed in 1966 by Vernon et al [302] and was designed to measure children's behavior after discharge from hospital. It is composed of 27 items that evaluate six categories of anxiety: general anxiety, separation anxiety, eating disturbances, sleeping disturbances, aggression toward authority, and apathy/withdrawal. For each item, parents have to compare the actual (posthospitalization) behavior of their child with the child's typical behavior before hospital admission on a 1–5 scale (much less than before – scored 1; less than before – scored 2; same as before – scored 3; more than before – scored 4 and much more than before – scored 5). High scores indicate negative behavior change and low scores suggest positive behavior change. In the original PHBQ study [302], the questionnaire was sent to parents 6 days after discharge and a total score was obtained by adding the scores of each item.

Psychometric properties of the PHBQ
As this tool is the one used in most studies, it is important to understand its limitations before reviewing the litera-

ture. The value of a psychometric tool can be considered in terms of validity and reliability.

Validity. The validity of the construct was evaluated by comparing the total score achieved from the PHBQ with psychiatric interviews of 20 children aged between 2 and 10.5 years who underwent tonsillectomy. There was a moderate correlation (r = 0.47) [302]. It should be noted, however, that the sample used to evaluate the validity of construct was very small and not representative of all age groups [302]. Moreover, most of the questions of the PHBQ were more suited to the behavior of the young child and could not be applied to older children. This issue is of great importance since postoperative behavior in children may differ considerably with age. Consistent with this, recently researchers found moderate correlations between the PHBQ and the Child Behavior Checklist (a well-validated tool that is used extensively in children for the assessment of behavioral and emotional problems [304,305]) in the 2–4 and 4–7-year age groups [306], but no correlation at all in children above 7 years of age.

Reliability. Two classes of reliability of the PHBQ were tested: the test–retest reliability and the internal consistency. The first one was tested by Cassell et al in 37 children undergoing cardiac catheterization, ranging in age from 3 to 11 years [307]. The second class of reliability, the internal consistency, was evaluated in the original PHBQ study of Vernon et al [302]. In this study, 387 children aged from 1 month to 16 years (mean age 5.68 ± 4.33 years of age) and having various type of surgery were recruited. The internal consistency (Cronbach's alpha) for the six factors varied between 0.46 (Eating disturbances) and 0.73 (General anxiety), and was 0.82 for the total score [302]. However, the internal consistency for the six categories of anxiety (Cronbach's alpha) was lower than the value recommended in the literature [308].

Thus, in summary, the validity and reliability of the PHBQ have only been partly established, especially in older children.

Despite all the limitations highlighted in the last paragraph, the PHBQ is still considered as the "gold standard" tool for assessing postoperative behavior changes [302,309]. Another issue is that, this questionnaire has been often modified and various versions have been used in the literature with alterations in the number of items, mode of collection (the absolute versus the relative form) and the timing of application in the postoperative period. None of these modified questionnaires has been validated.

The mode of collection of the PHBQ is the most obvious variant. Two different versions can be identified:
- the *original, relative form* developed by Vernon et al [302] in which the parent is asked to compare the

postoperative behavior with the preoperative behavior of their child

- the *absolute form*, in which the parent is asked to complete the questionnaire twice, before and after the operation. In this form, each item is rated on a four-point Likert scale from "never" to "always" and changes in behavior are determined for each item by comparing the postoperative score with the preoperative score. Thus, each item can indicate a positive or a negative change, or no modification.

While the relative form has been reported to be more sensitive than the absolute form, it is also possible that the absolute form is less subject to response bias and thus could be more appropriate [309].

Finally, in the original formulation, no cut-off score was determined to identify clinically significant negative postoperative behavior changes [302]. There is great variability in the literature with regard to the scoring system and the presence or not of a cut-off score for the confirmation of the presence of negative postoperative behavior changes. While the total PHBQ score and subscales (obtained respectively by summing the scores of all the items and by summing the items belonging to the subscale) were reported in the original publication by Vernon et al [302], recent studies used only the total score [309] or reported only the percentage of any negative behavior change [154]. Thus, the definition of "negative postoperative behavior changes" may differ between studies and is arbitrary given the fact that no investigations were conducted to specify this aspect [155,299]. For instance, Stargatt et al used a cut-off score of 7 to consider deterioration in behavior as significant [155], whereas other authors used no cut-off score and reported percentage of any negative change [154].

Also there usually is no reporting of how behaviors improve. In most studies, only negative behavior is considered, with no description of how this might be balanced by behaviors actually improving. A child may have a net improvement in behavior while the analysis only highlights the negative changes. This tends to overemphasize negative behavior change.

A final criticism of the PHBQ is that it is a crude score which gives little indication of the type of symptoms presented by the children, their severity and their consequences for the children's life and development. Thus, it is probable that this concept as determined by the PHBQ regroups symptoms of different severity, integrating benign symptoms, which reflect "a normal reaction" to a stressful event, and more severe symptoms, which could be more incapacitating for children and their families. Lastly, the PHBQ can only reveal the symptoms related to some aspects of behavior, namely anxiety.

In summary, the absence of standardization of the PHBQ makes comparisons between studies hazardous. If

we also consider the lack of validation and reliability of this questionnaire, and the limited scope of the tool, then the concept of "negative postoperative behavior changes" as detected by the mean of the PHBQ might be questionable. Given all these remarks, the results in the literature should be considered with caution.

Incidence and duration of negative postoperative behavior changes

The incidence of POBD varies considerably between studies, from no change [310] to almost 80% of children presenting some negative behavior changes [311,312]. As discussed above, this variability can be attributed to the various methodologies applied in the different studies, and also to the small samples selected and to their characteristics, such as the medical condition and the cultural differences of the children. Nevertheless, the most frequently reported incidence of significant negative behavior changes is between 15% and 40% of children [153,155,156,313,314].

Despite the high incidence of negative behavior changes, it is important to note that most negative behavior changes are generally limited in duration. A meta-analysis including 26 studies using the PHBQ revealed that negative behavioral changes diminished with time and largely disappeared 2 weeks postoperatively [309].

There is little evidence for the persistence of negative postoperative behavior changes beyond 2 weeks. Most studies that addressed this issue were either retrospective [315] or were performed more than 30 years ago and have potentially significant limitations [316,317]. For instance, it is striking to note that Douglas (1975) showed in a follow-up that children with repeated admissions to hospital before the age of 5 years were "more likely to be delinquent and more likely to show unstable job patterns" than those who had not been admitted to the hospital during this period of age [316]. This early finding has been challenged by a more recent longitudinal study performed on 1048 children, which did not show any significant correlation between hospitalization during the preschool years and the evaluation of the child's behavior at the age of 6 years old if social factors and life events were taken into account [318].

Risk factors for negative postoperative behavior changes

Younger children, and in particular preschool children, are at increased risk for experiencing negative behavioral changes following anesthesia [300]. Other risk factors such as the child's preoperative anxiety, temperament and history as well as parental anxiety were also found to correlate highly with the occurrence of emergence delirium and/or negative behavioral changes [300,303,319]. It has also been demonstrated that emergence delirium and negative behavioral changes may be linked with children being agitated on recovery being more prone to develop negative behavior postoperatively [300].

Pain is also a risk factor for negative postoperative behavioral changes. Children with pain have almost a 10 times higher risk for having negative behavioral changes following tonsillectomy [156,300,320]; and if an aggressive pain treatment is established, more positive than negative behavioral changes are observed in children undergoing adenoidectomy [321]. Typically, behavioral changes associated with acute postoperative pain peak within 24h and wane progressively thereafter.

In addition to these factors, there are still unanswered questions regarding the role of intraoperative awareness as a trigger for negative postoperative behavioral changes. Changes in behavior could also be due to episodes of intraoperative implicit memory of events. While recent studies failed to demonstrate any evidence for the persistence of implicit memory during general anesthesia, it is important to point out that such assessment can be difficult to achieve and is based on complex psychological tests that may not be adapted to the child's cognitive development [240,243]. The role of midazolam as a risk factor for negative postoperative behavioral changes is unclear [198]. While some authors demonstrated the usefulness of midazolam in reducing negative postoperative behavior changes consequent upon a reduction in preoperative anxiety [167,322], others failed to show any benefit [155] or even demonstrated a higher incidence of negative changes following midazolam premedication [195].

Finally, a recent study using the Child Behavior Check List to assess negative postoperative behavior changes demonstrated a higher incidence of negative behavioral changes when urological surgery is performed at an age less than 24 months [323].

These findings confirm the complexity of the negative postoperative behavioral changes, which are of multifactorial origin with a potential interaction between preoperative (child's and parental anxiety, temperament, culture, preparation for surgery, etc.), intraoperative and postoperative (agitation on recovery, pain, family environment, etc.) factors.

Summary and suggestions

Despite all the limitations highlighted above (the lack of consensus on the terminology, the evaluation, the incidence and the severity of negative postoperative behavior changes) one should still bear in mind that important psychological manifestations may occur postoperatively in children. Therefore, preoperative assessment and preparation for anesthesia should focus on the parental and child's anxiety in order to prevent possible psychological symptoms that could be generated by hospitalization, anesthesia and surgery. Parents should be warned

that some children may have behavior change and told that it is usually self-limiting. Parents should be encouraged to contact the anesthesia team in the presence of persistent negative changes after approximately 2 weeks postoperatively. In this case, it would be worth organizing a psychological assessment in order to better specify the symptoms and to offer the child psychological support.

Post-traumatic stress disorder

Post-traumatic stress disorder is a psychiatric disorder generally diagnosed by means of DSM-IV. To meet the DSM-IV criteria, a person must have been exposed to an "extreme" stressor, usually involving a threat to life or physical integrity. The response to that stressful event must include a specific number of symptoms from each of three broad categories:

- at least one re-experiencing symptom (the traumatic event can be re-experienced in various ways such as recurrent and intrusive memories, flashbacks and nightmares)
- three avoidance behaviors toward trauma-related stimuli (for example, hospital and doctors)
- two hyperarousal symptoms (such as irritability and hypervigilance).

Symptoms must be present for more than 1 month and must cause clinically significant distress or impairment in social and/or academic functioning or other important areas of functioning [324].

Since hospitalization can be a stressful experience, the potential development of PTSD is of great concern in the pediatric population. Two specific experiences, namely intraoperative awareness and a stay in the intensive care unit, have been associated with the development of PTSD. While this disorder has been largely investigated in adults, there is still a lack of knowledge on the incidence of PTSD following hospitalization in children.

Post-traumatic stress disorder following admission to a pediatric intensive care unit

The criteria for admission to the PICU are various and include respiratory distress, deterioration in neurological condition, traumatic injuries, acute illness, and postoperative care. These experiences can be very stressful due to the medical condition itself as well as the requisite ICU treatment, which may include invasive and/or painful procedures (intubation, catheterization, etc.). For these reasons, the potential development of PTSD is of great concern in this specific population.

In adults, various studies have been performed in order to investigate the long-term psychological outcomes of ICU-treated patients. Results showed that the prevalence of PTSD is high (approximately 20%) [325] and the symptoms seem to persist over time and may negatively affect quality of life. Various risk factors for the development of post-ICU PTSD have been identified. Studies have highlighted potential factors such as an excessive administration in ICU of benzodiazepines, post-ICU memories of terrifying and/or psychotic experiences occurring during their stay in ICU and the presence of a prior psychopathology. However, the severity of illness does not seem to be a significant predictor for the occurrence of PTSD.

Although many studies in the last two decades have focused on the experience of pediatric illness, these studies were mainly looking at the impact on the parents. Thus, there is still a lack of knowledge about the long-term psychological impact of the PICU stay on the children themselves and the nature of their recall. The literature looking at the incidence of PTSD in children is scarce [326–330], but authors report a similarly high proportion of post-traumatic stress symptoms to that reported in adults, even several months following discharge from an ICU [327,330]. However, little is known about the mechanisms underlying the development and maintenance of PTSD in the pediatric population. Accordingly, there is no clear information about the involvement of factors related to the children's stay in the ICU (such as length of admission, severity of illness, degree of pain, number of invasive procedures and various medications) in the development of PTSD. In addition, it is unknown whether factors related to the hospital stay are better predictors than other variables, such as cognitive factors (i.e. subjective appraisals of the trauma and nature of memories of the PICU stay). In fact, only one study tried to examine the relationship between the nature of the PICU memory and the symptoms of PTSD. The results showed a significant relationship between memory for delusional events (such as hallucinations) and PTSD symptoms, and in particular intrusive thoughts [327].

The studies with an interest in this subject have several methodological limitations, such as small sample size (≤60 children) [328–330], the use of screening questionnaires to evaluate PTSD rather than applying semi-structured interviews [327,329,330], and the lack of reference to the influential cognitive theories of PTSD, which would help to identify the risk factors [327–330].

Post-traumatic stress disorder has significant consequences for children's lives as it can interfere with normal childhood development, including learning capacity and the acquisition of socially appropriate behavior. Furthermore, if PTSD is left untreated, it may last for at least 5 years in more than one-third of the children [331]. Given the possibly high incidence of PTSD, any child admitted to the PICU should be followed, ideally with a 1-month follow-up becoming a standard of practice in order to detect any symptoms and to offer psychological support to both the child and parents if necessary. In contrast to the uncertainty about the concept of negative postoperative behavioral changes, PTSD is clearly defined in the literature with well-validated tools for the detection of its occurrence.

Post-traumatic stress disorder following hospitalization in children is still underinvestigated and underappreciated, and deserves both attention and further research.

CASE STUDY

A 5-year-old child arrives at the preoperative assessment clinic 2 days prior to a scheduled outpatient adenotonsillectomy. The family and child are nervous. The parents report that 1 year ago, the child had had ear tubes inserted and on that occasion had needed to be held down for an inhalational induction, and had been very unsettled in the PACU. On discharge, the child had shown some regressive behavior for a week.

Today the child appears reluctant to be examined and very shy, hiding behind his mother. He also has a cough and purulent runny nose.

Reviewing the record, it is noted that the child has "mild obstructive sleep apnea." The parents say a sleep study has been performed but the results are not in the child's notes.

On examination, the child has a fever of 38.5°C. The lungs are clear on auscultation but a soft systolic murmur is heard. No other abnormalities are found. The child has normal oxygen saturation and pulses. You think the child probably has a normal second heart sound.

Lastly, the mother reports that she is terrified of anesthesia as she clearly recalls being wide awake and paralyzed during a laparoscopic cholecystectomy performed 10 years earlier.

Notes

After discussion with the family, it is decided to delay the case for 3 weeks to allow the upper respiratory tract infection to clear and to give time for more evaluation and preparation. In the meantime, you organize a cardiac review and request the missing sleep study report. You also suggest the family comes back a week prior to the planned surgery to discuss anesthesia options and in particular to introduce the family to coping strategies to reduce anxiety at induction. Before they leave, you discuss the risk of awareness in children.

Annotated references

A full reference list for this chapter is available at:
http://www.wiley.com/go/gregory/andropoulos/pediatricanesthesia

22. Von Ungern-Sternberg BS. Risk assessment for respiratory complications in paediatric anaesthesia: a prospective cohort study. Lancet 2010; 376: 10. This large prospective observational study identifies multiple risk factors for perioperative respiratory adverse events in pediatric patients.

116. Rhodes ET, Ferrari LR, Wolfsdorf JI. Perioperative management of pediatric surgical patients with diabetes mellitus. Anesth Analg 2005; 101: 986–99. Authors describe the standardized algorithms used to manage diabetic patients during the perioperative period at the Boston Children's Hospital.

129. Schwengel DA, Sterni M, Tunkel D et al. Perioperative management of children with obstructive sleep apnea. Anesth Analg 2009; 109: 60–75. A comprehensive review of the evidence surrounding how best to manage the common pediatric problem of obstructive sleep apnea during the perioperative period.

130. Latham GJ, Greenberg RS. Anesthetic considerations for the pediatric oncology patient – part 1: a review of antitumor therapy. Paediatr Anaesth 2010; 20: 295–304.

131. Latham GJ, Greenberg RS. Anesthetic considerations for the pediatric oncology patient – part 3: pain, cognitive dysfunction, and preoperative evaluation. Paediatr Anaesth 2010; 20: 479–89.

132. Latham GJ, Greenberg RS. Anesthetic considerations for the pediatric oncology patient – part 2: systems-based approach to anesthesia. Paediatr Anaesth 2010; 20: 396–420. Three-part series exploring the numerous issues surrounding anesthesia for pediatric oncology patients – a thorough and up-to-date review of the topic.

150. Chorney J, Torrey C, Blount R et al. Healthcare provider and parent behavior and children's coping and distress at anesthesia induction. Anesthesiology 2009; 111(6): 1290–6. This large prospective observational study examines adults' and clinicians' behavior during induction of anesthesia in children when parents are present. Results from this study provide evidence that clinicians' and parents' behavior during induction influences children's level of distress, suggesting a new avenue for intervention research.

163. Chorney J, Kain Z. Behavioral analysis of children's response to induction of anesthesia. Anesth Analg 2009; 109(5): 1434–40. This study examined a wide range of observable behaviors in children undergoing anesthesia induction and highlights the importance of considering both distress and coping behaviors in the design of future trials.

170. Yip P, Middleton P, Cyna A, Carlyle A. Non-pharmacological interventions for assisting the induction of anaesthesia in children. Cochrane Database of Systematic Reviews 2009; 8(3): CD006447. This systematic review of the literature on non-pharmacological interventions identifies all the key intervention studies in the area to date.

227. Davidson AJ, Huang G, Czarnecki C et al. Awareness during anesthesia in children: a prospective cohort study. Anesth Analg 2005; 100: 653–61. The first recent study to show a high incidence of awareness in children.

228. Lopez U, Habre W, Laurencon M et al. Intra-operative awareness in children: the value of an interview adapted to their cognitive abilities. Anaesthesia 2007; 62: 778–89. An awareness study in children which highlights the need for careful interview.

231. Malviya S, Galinkin J, Bannister C et al. The incidence of intraoperative awareness in children: childhood awareness and recall evaluation. Anesth Analg 2009; 109: 1421–7. The largest US study looking at awareness in children which confirmed earlier reports of high incidence.

302. Vernon DT, Schulman JL, Foley JM. Changes in children's behavior after hospitalisation. Some dimensions of response and their correlates. Am J Dis Child 1966; 111: 581–93. The original description of a measure of behavior change after hospitalization.

CHAPTER 14
Pediatric Airway Management

John E. Fiadjoe, Paul A. Stricker & Ronald S. Litman
Department of Anesthesiology and Critical Care Medicine, University of Pennsylvania School of Medicine, and The Children's Hospital of Philadelphia, Philadelphia, PA, USA

Introduction

Expertise in airway management in infants and young children is the cornerstone upon which every subspecialist in pediatric anesthesia is based. This expertise consists of two major facets: a comprehensive knowledge and understanding of the developmental anatomy and physiology of the human upper airway from birth through adolescence, and the physical skills of airway management which occur only by experience over time. This chapter will provide the basis upon which knowledge of pediatric airway management is gained. The chapter is divided into three major sections: (1) Developmental

anatomy and physiology of the upper airway; (2) Procedures and techniques for management of the normal pediatric airway; and (3) Specialized techniques with which to manage the child with an abnormal upper airway that presents challenges in ventilation or tracheal intubation.

The human upper airway is loosely defined as the air-conducting passages from the nose to the carina [1]. Anatomically, the upper airway of the developing fetus, infant, and child is a moving target. Its developmental course during fetal life is relatively less known compared with other organ systems, since much of this understanding is gained from descriptive animal and human postmortem studies. The structures of the upper airway continue to change shape and properties until the latter part of the first decade of life. Furthermore, up to 3% of children may have congenital or acquired upper airway abnormalities [1].

From an evolutionary perspective, the human upper airway is relatively smaller than other related species, and is oriented in a more vertical position in the body. In humans, the facial bones and accompanying oral airway structures assume a more vertical position beneath the cranium (this mirrors the changes seen during human growth; see below). These changes were likely due to the acquisition of language for survival [2,3]. Diamond called this adaptation "the great leap forward" and postulated that it occurred approximately 40,000 years ago [4].

Many other species are able to produce sounds that are analogous to vowels, but only humans are able to produce consonants, the basis of the spoken language. The ability to form consonants, according to Shprintzen, is the result of the relatively smaller supralaryngeal tract that evolved in humans. This adaptation included the ability of humans to close off and separate the communication between the nasal and oral pharynx to facilitate speech of consonants. The unique human property of having large adenoid tissue facilitates this separation. It is notable that the peak age of adenoidal growth (3–5 years) is the same approximate age of the refinement of consonant sounds [3].

This anatomical adaptation necessarily confers a disadvantageous human property: the predisposition to upper airway collapse during sleep (i.e. obstructive sleep apnea syndrome; OSAS) or during artificially induced unconsciousness (i.e. sedation or general anesthesia). Other than brachycephalic dogs, such as the English bulldog [5], OSAS appears to only occur in humans.

Developmental anatomy

In embryological life, the upper airway develops within the structural framework of the cranium and the most cephalad ends of the digestive and respiratory systems. The following description of the embryological development of the human is based on writings and descriptions from a number of references [6–10]. On the lateral surface of the 5 week-old, 4.0 mm embryo, one can observe five or six pairs of narrow masses called *branchial arches* (Fig. 14.1). Each branchial arch contains characteristic types of ectoderm and mesoderm, the primordial precursors of epithelial (e.g. skin) and mesothelial structures (e.g. muscle, bone), respectively. The areas between the arches are called *branchial clefts*. The tissue underlying the branchial clefts contains outpouchings of the foregut region, the *pharyngeal pouches*. These consist of endoderm and will develop into corresponding endothelial structures of the upper digestive and respiratory systems. The developing structures of each branchial arch receive motor or sensory innervation from an adjacent cranial nerve. Regardless of where the primordial muscle cell migrates to, it will retain its original embryonic innervation.

Branchial arches
The first branchial arch will ultimately develop into the ramus of the mandible and the muscles of mastication. It

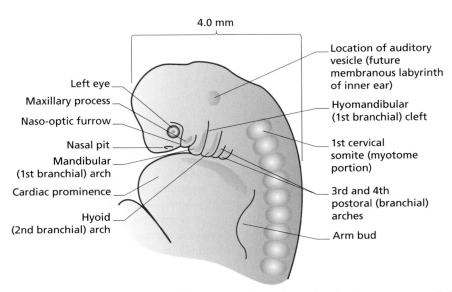

Figure 14.1 On the lateral surface of the 5-week-old, 4.0 mm embryo, one can observe five or six pairs of narrow masses called branchial arches.

also contributes to development of the middle ear bones and muscles between the ear and mandible, such as the tensor tympani, tensor veli palatini, and anterior belly of the digastric muscle. Motor and sensory innervation to the structures derived from the first arch is supplied by the trigeminal nerve.

The second branchial arch forms bony and muscular structures from the ear (proximally) to the hyoid bone (distally), including the muscles of facial expression that are innervated by the facial nerve (cranial nerve (CN) VII). In the developed human, the path of second branchial arch development can be traced from the styloid process, to the stylohyoid ligament, to the lesser cornu of the hyoid bone. Embryological abnormalities in the growth of the first and second branchial arches result in any one of a number of congenital airway syndromes involving the ear and jaw, such as Goldenhar syndrome.

The third branchial arch develops into the body and greater cornu of the hyoid bone and the stylopharyngeus muscle, which aids in elevating the pharynx during swallowing, and is innervated by the glossopharyngeal nerve (CN IX).

The fourth through sixth branchial arches contribute to the formation of the thyroid, cricoid, arytenoid, corniculate, and cuneiform laryngeal cartilages, as well as the muscles that form the pharynx, larynx, and upper half of the esophagus. These structures are innervated by the vagus (CN X) and accessory (CN XI) nerves. The earliest appearance of the future larynx is seen as a bud growing out from the ventral part of the foregut at approximately 4 weeks' gestation. The laryngeal and esophageal tracts are initially seen as one common tube that eventually separates into two adjacent, functionally different conduits. By 16 weeks' gestation, the larynx contains all its definitive elements in their proper proportions. During fetal and postnatal [11] growth, the development of the size of the larynx closely parallels the size of the surrounding bony and cartilaginous structures.

Pharyngeal pouches

The pharyngeal pouches are outpouchings of the lateral wall of the foregut that develop into the pharyngeal structures. Each pouch, at its lateral-most aspect, contacts the ectodermal epithelium of a branchial cleft. The first branchial cleft becomes part of the external auditory canal, but the remaining branchial clefts are remodeled and do not correspond to recognizable structures in the mature human. Nevertheless, abnormal formation of this area can lead to cysts or more significant malformations.

The first pharyngeal pouch becomes incorporated into the future temporal bone and forms the epithelial lining of the middle ear and the tympanic membrane. Adjacent to the first pharyngeal pouch, the first branchial cleft develops into the external auditory canal. The second

pharyngeal pouch develops into the tonsil. The superior portion of the third pharyngeal pouch differentiates into the inferior parathyroid and the inferior portion migrates caudad to become the thymus. The fourth pharyngeal pouch forms the superior parathyroid gland. The area roughly corresponding to the fifth and sixth pharyngeal pouches is incorporated into the thyroid gland.

Anatomical structures of the upper airway and their relation to the practice of pediatric anesthesia

The approach to airway management of infants and young children is influenced by developmental differences in head and neck anatomy. These differences are modified by two major growth spurts during childhood, the first at the time of the acquisition of permanent dentition (age 7–10 years), and the second during puberty in the teenage years, both of which contribute to the vertical growth of the facial structures. Thus, it is no coincidence that these two general age ranges are the approximate points in life in which certain persons without obvious anatomical deformities will become difficult to intubate.

Skull

When compared to the older child, the infant's skull (especially the occipital region) is relatively larger, such that neck flexion may not be required to attain the classic "sniffing" position that optimizes visualization of the glottic structures during laryngoscopy. At birth, the neurocranium to face size ratio is 8:1, and declines to 6:1 at 2 years of age, 4:1 at 5 years, and approximately 2:1 by adulthood [12,13]. The growth of the lower facial bones is proportionately linear from ages 1 to 11 years [11].

The mandibular arch of the infant is U-shaped and becomes more V-shaped during childhood until adolescence, when it is completely developed. The angle between the ramus and the body of the mandible is more obtuse in infants than in adults. This largely accounts for the relatively low incidence of difficult intubations in infants and young children compared with adults.

Nose

Overall, the most important difference in nasal anatomy between young children and adults is merely the smaller size. Small nasal passages are more likely to become obstructed with blood or secretions as a result of manipulations during general anesthesia. Young children are less likely to have occult nasal polyps or septal deviations when compared with adults [14]. The anatomical dimensions of the nasopharynx increase linearly between 1 and 11 years of age [11].

In the past, small infants were considered to be obligate nasal breathers and therefore predisposed to breathing difficulties during periods of nasal obstruction. However, this has largely been disproven [15] although infants with choanal atresia will often develop upper airway obstruction that results in varying degrees of hypoxemia [16].

Oral cavity

The infant tongue is relatively larger in proportion to the oral cavity when compared with the adult. Tongue volume increases linearly between 1 and 11 years [11]. Magnetic resonance imaging (MRI) studies of the upper airway during general anesthesia have demonstrated that, as in adults [17], upper airway obstruction occurs primarily at the levels of the soft palate and epiglottis, and not at the level of the tongue [18].

The 20 primary teeth are identified by a lettering system (Fig. 14.2A). They begin to erupt during the first year of life, and are shed at between 6 and 12 years of age. The 32 permanent teeth begin to appear at the same time as the primary teeth are shed and are identified by a numbering system (Fig. 14.2B).

Oropharynx

In newborns, the uvula and epiglottis are in close proximity, which makes possible the simultaneous acts of nasal breathing and oral ingestion of liquids. This anatomical relationship is maintained throughout most of the first year of life but during the second year, the larynx begins to descend as it adapts to its greater role in phonation.

Although mechanisms have not been elucidated, the pharynx of premature newborns is susceptible to passive collapse, especially during apnea, but may also collapse as a result of cervical flexion or nasal obstruction [19]. These effects are exacerbated by the administration of general anesthesia or sedatives, which decrease pharyngeal muscle tone. Furthermore, pharyngeal collapse often occurs in premature infants during application of cricoid pressure.

Of interest, the upper airway of a normal infant is smaller in both inspiration and expiration at 6 weeks of age compared to the neonatal period. This relative narrowing may be caused by postnatal growth of adenoid tissue or thickening of the mucous membrane lining in response to infection or second-hand smoke exposure. The linear dimensions of the soft palate and oropharynx increase linearly between 1 and 11 years of age [11,20].

Adenoidal and tonsillar tissue is minimal at birth, and then grows rapidly between 4 and 7 years of age. The growth of airway lymphoid tissue parallels the growth of the facial and cervical bony structures [11]. Hypertrophied tonsil and adenoid tissue is likely the most common cause of upper airway obstruction after administration of general anesthesia in children in this age group.

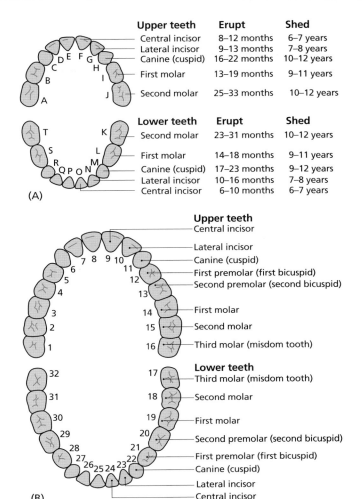

Upper teeth	Erupt	Shed
Central incisor	8–12 months	6–7 years
Lateral incisor	9–13 months	7–8 years
Canine (cuspid)	16–22 months	10–12 years
First molar	13–19 months	9–11 years
Second molar	25–33 months	10–12 years

Lower teeth	Erupt	Shed
Second molar	23–31 months	10–12 years
First molar	14–18 months	9–11 years
Canine (cuspid)	17–23 months	9–12 years
Lateral incisor	10–16 months	7–8 years
Central incisor	6–10 months	6–7 years

Figure 14.2 (A) Primary teeth (baby teeth). The picture is viewed as if the patient is facing the examiner with their mouth open. The 20 primary teeth are lettered A through T, beginning with the right upper molar and ending at the right lower molar. (B) Secondary teeth. The 32 permanent adult teeth are identified by a numbering system that begins at the right upper third molar and ends at the right lower third molar. Reproduced from [365] with permission from the American Dental Association.

The epiglottis of infants is relatively narrow and short, and angled into the lumen of the airway. The lower portion of the oropharynx at the level of the epiglottis is particularly compliant and prone to collapse during anesthetic or sedative-induced upper airway obstruction [21]. Therefore, obstruction at the epiglottic level can be significantly lessened by placing the patient in the lateral position [21].

The effect of gender on oropharyngeal length has been studied, with particular reference to an association between relatively longer airway length and the predisposition to obstructive sleep apnea [22]. Prior to the onset of puberty, boys and girls have relatively similar oropharyngeal length but after the onset of puberty, the oropharyngeal lengths in boys are greater than those of girls, even after correcting for height and weight (Fig. 14.3). The relatively longer upper airway length in males has been

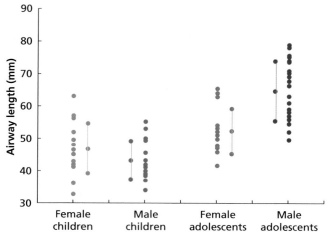

Figure 14.3 Prior to the onset of puberty, boys and girls have relatively similar oropharyngeal lengths but after the onset of puberty, the oropharyngeal lengths in boys are greater than those of girls, even after correcting for height and weight. Reproduced from Ronen et al [22] with permission from the American Academy of Pediatrics.

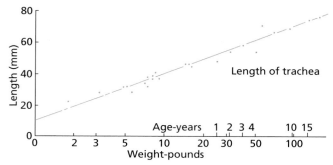

Figure 14.4 Distance between vocal cords and carina as a function of weight in pounds and age in years. Reproduced from Butz [30] with permission from the American Academy of Pediatrics.

implicated as a possible etiological factor in the greater disposition in males toward OSAS [23]. Thus, postpubertal boys may have a greater disposition toward upper airway collapse in response to administration of pharmacological agents that depress consciousness.

Larynx

During infancy, the relative position of the larynx is slightly higher in the neck than in older children and adults. Although its position relative to the cervical spine is complete by the age of 3 years (it descends from C2–C3 to C4–C5), it continues to descend relative to other facial structures such as the mandible [24]. The tip of the epiglottis proceeds in a gradual and linear descent from C2 to C3 from birth to 18 years of age [25]. This relative movement is unique to humans because of the shifting functionality from sucking and swallowing while breathing to the development of speech later in life. Early in life, a relatively high larynx facilitates simultaneous sucking and respiration due to the apposition of the epiglottis (as high as C1) and the soft palate. Additional differences in early life that protect against aspiration during feeding include relatively thicker aryepiglottic folds and larger arytenoids.

The chest wall of neonates and small infants is highly compliant and tends to collapse inward, thus reducing functional residual capacity (FRC) and promotion of atelectasis. To preserve FRC, the adductor muscles of the larynx act as an expiratory "valve" and restrict exhalation in order to maintain positive end-expiratory pressure. This is referred to as "laryngeal braking" [26,27].

The higher position of the larynx during infancy influences airway management to the extent that the glottic opening is more easily visualized using a straight, rather than a curved laryngoscope, and in infants less than 1 year of age, elevation of the base of the skull is usually not necessary [28].

In children with pharmacologically induced neuromuscular blockade, the cricoid cartilage is the narrowest portion of the upper airway because of its inability to distend in a similar manner to the vocal cords [29–31]. A tracheal tube that easily passes through the relatively compliant vocal cords may compress surface mucosa at the level of the cricoid cartilage and predispose to inflammation, edema, and subsequent scarring and stenosis [32–34]. Tracheal edema is more likely to increase airway resistance in smaller diameter airways since the resistance to flow through a tube is related to the fifth power of the radius of the tube (since this flow is largely turbulent). In non-intubated, sedated children without neuromuscular blockade, the adductor muscles of the vocal cords are active, and are the basis for the narrowest portion of the upper airway to occur at this level [35–37].

The relationship between the sizes of the structures along the upper airway remains relatively stable throughout growth and development [37]. Therefore, there appears to be no specific age during childhood at which the form or structure of the most appropriate tracheal tube (i.e. cuffed versus uncuffed) would require a change for the benefit of the child.

Some congenital conditions, notably trisomy 21, are associated with smaller than normal subglottic and tracheal diameters [38–42]. Therefore, appropriate tracheal tube sizes may be smaller than usual for age in these patients. Ultrasound examination of the subglottic region may be used to guide tracheal tube size selection [43].

Tracheal lengths (distance between glottis and carina) increase linearly during childhood [30,44]. A familiarity with these distances in infants will facilitate proper placement of the tracheal tube midway between the glottis and carina (Fig. 14.4). A shortened tracheal length (i.e. higher bifurcation) caused by a reduced number of tracheal cartilage rings is noted in certain conditions such as trisomy 21 [40] and myelomeningocele [39,45]. Therefore, in these patients, special attention is warranted to ensure proper tracheal tube position and avoidance of right bronchial intubation.

Developmental physiology of the upper airway

The human upper airway serves a concomitant function as a conduit for breathing and for the passage of food. This property, which is only found in higher evolved species, presents a unique problem, the basis of which is that the upper airway is integrally involved in the processes of breathing, speech, and eating, without the benefit of rigid cartilaginous support. In the conscious state, this requires rigorous neurological co-ordination between competing structures. Although relatively little is known about the development of neural control in the upper airway [1], it is this characteristic that renders the upper airway vulnerable to collapse during administration of sedatives or anesthetics.

The pharyngeal and laryngeal muscles that normally contract to maintain upper airway patency are activated in parallel with the diaphragm. Activation of pharyngeal abductor muscles prevents upper airway collapse in response to the brief challenge of negative pressure created by diaphragmatic contraction. Contraction of pharyngeal adductor muscles maintains lung volume during the exhalation portion of a breath [46].

Development of airway protective mechanisms

The term "airway protective mechanisms" encompasses two separate but inter-related functions of the upper airway: protection against aspiration of foreign material into the respiratory tree, and protection against airway collapse during sleep or states of pharmacologically impaired consciousness.

The mechanisms that protect against pulmonary aspiration of liquid or solid contents into the respiratory tree include a series of unconsciously controlled reflexes that include swallowing and cough (to transport substances away from the laryngeal inlet), and apnea and airway obstruction, which are attempts to prevent substances entering the respiratory tree [47]. Additional reflexes consist of laryngospasm and arousal [48]. Collectively, these have been termed the laryngeal chemoreflexes (LCR), and they mature throughout development [49]. The perinatal period represents a time of relatively high vulnerability to aspiration, as is clinically seen in the meconium aspiration syndrome, which occurs in 4% of all livebirths [50].

In the newborn, introduction of water into the larynx results in a characteristic set of responses that include swallowing, apnea, bradycardia, and peripheral vasoconstriction with shunting to the central vascular bed. These adaptive responses are prominent in preterm infants and lessen with advanced gestational age [47,51–56]. The apneic reflexes have been implicated in the etiology of sudden infant death syndrome (SIDS) [57]. Administration of sedatives and anesthetic agents is associated with prolongation of the apneic reflex [58–60]. The apneic reflex is also prolonged (and bradycardia worsened) during baseline hypoxemia [61,62], anemia [63] and respiratory syncytial virus (RSV) infection [64,65]. Conversely, the apneic reflex is shortened by administration of central stimulants such as theophylline [59]. Soon after the newborn period, the apneic portion of the LCR response disappears [66]. Cough is more prominent, and continues for the remainder of life when foreign substances enter the laryngeal area.

The effect of anesthetics and sedatives on the efficacy and potency of airway protective reflexes is clinically important to establish the safety of pharmacological agents administered to non-tracheally intubated children. The body of knowledge concerning these effects is beginning to develop. At predefined depths of general anesthesia, propofol appears to be a more potent inhibitor of the laryngospasm reflex than sevoflurane [67] and fentanyl does not appear to reduce the propensity toward laryngospasm in sevoflurane-anesthetized children [68]. Data are also emerging on the effects of anesthetics on upper airway patency. In adults, at similar depths of sedation or general anesthesia, propofol appears equal to isoflurane in promoting upper airway collapse [69,70] and both are more potent than equivalent levels of deep sedation attained with midazolam [71]. In children, the addition of 50% nitrous oxide promotes upper airway closure in those with enlarged tonsils who received oral midazolam [72] and halothane appears to preserve upper airway patency better than equipotent levels of sevoflurane [73].

Management of the normal pediatric airway

Preoperative airway assessment

Preoperative airway assessment will identify nearly all children who, when anesthetized, are likely to develop difficult mask ventilation or difficult tracheal intubation. Information gained from the preoperative history and physical examination will determine the method of anesthetic induction and the approach for maintaining a patent upper airway following loss of consciousness. Similarly, risk factors for postoperative respiratory complications are identified at this time, allowing for appropriate preparation or delay of anesthesia and surgery when appropriate. Common airway assessment techniques used in adults have not been validated for use in infants and children; however, modifications of these methods may yield valuable information.

History

In almost all cases, a review of the child's previous anesthetic records as well as discussion with parents will reveal potential airway management problems. A history of previous uneventful anesthetics is encouraging, but changes in growth and development may affect airway anatomy. A reliable history of unobstructed breathing during sleep, especially while supine, often predicts the ability to mask ventilate without difficulty. Conversely, loud snoring and/or obstructive apnea are excellent predictors of upper airway obstruction following anesthetic- or sedative-induced unconsciousness.

During the preoperative interview, children and parents should be asked about the presence of loose deciduous teeth. Chipped or missing teeth should be documented. Very loose teeth should be electively removed after induction of general anesthesia to avoid accidental dislodgment (and pulmonary aspiration) during airway manipulations. A loose tooth is removed by grasping it with a dry piece of gauze and pulling while rocking the tooth gently back and forth. Some bleeding is expected. This is performed immediately following induction of anesthesia or after tracheal intubation, depending on the location of the tooth and risk of dislodgment during direct laryngoscopy. If elective tooth removal is contemplated, it should be discussed with parents and caregivers during the preoperative visit to avoid an unpleasant surprise when they are reunited with their child in the recovery room.

Children with non-permanent orthodontic hardware that may be dislodged during airway management should have such devices removed whenever possible. Occasionally, preoperative orthodontic consultation may be required.

Co-existing diseases and airway management

A number of co-existing diseases may influence airway management. For example, children with tumors of the head or neck may have distorted airway anatomy. Previous radiation therapy which results in scarring of the tongue and submandibular tissues is often associated with difficult tracheal intubation secondary to poor mandibular soft tissue compliance. Radiation therapy may also cause mucosal tissues to be friable and prone to bleeding.

If a child presents with an unfamiliar syndrome or diagnosis, the anesthesiologist should obtain a comprehensive understanding of the condition as it relates to airway management. The anesthetic implications of a

number of common congenital syndromes and conditions are presented in Chapter 38.

The presence, type, and severity of pulmonary disease affect the advantages and disadvantages of different airway management techniques. For example, the child with limited pulmonary reserve may not tolerate anesthetic-induced hypoventilation and may require tracheal intubation and controlled ventilation for a procedure that would be performed with spontaneous ventilation and a natural airway in an otherwise healthy child. On the other hand, the child with highly reactive lower airways may benefit from a technique that is less stimulating to the airway.

In children with asthma, the severity, triggers, and current medication status should be assessed. Medical management should be optimized prior to surgery. This may include inhaled β-agonist therapy, inhaled corticosteroids or a course of systemic corticosteroids, depending on the severity of disease and the procedure being performed. Adequate preoperative preparation of asthmatic children results in decreased intraoperative bronchospasm [74]. Uncontrolled asthma may warrant postponement of elective surgery. Some children may have persistent lower airway obstruction despite maximal medical management. In such cases, the anesthetic plan should include provisions for limiting triggers that exacerbate bronchoconstriction.

Bronchopulmonary dysplasia is a chronic lung disease associated with prematurity. Currently, most cases occur in infants born at less than 30 weeks' gestational age and weighing less than 1200 g at birth [75]. Various factors contribute to the genesis of bronchopulmonary dysplasia, including mechanical ventilation-induced barotrauma and volutrauma, hyperoxia, infection, and genetic factors [75,76]. Although one study did not demonstrate an increased risk of postoperative respiratory complications [77], former preterm infants with pulmonary sequelae of prematurity may have a reduced tolerance of apnea and heightened airway reactivity, which can manifest as bronchospasm, oxyhemoglobin desaturation or laryngospasm.

Children with significant pulmonary disease may benefit from preoperative consultation with a pulmonologist. Conditions meriting such consultation include cystic fibrosis, severe asthma or pulmonary hypoplasia associated with congenital conditions such as congenital diaphragmatic hernia. Preoperative optimization of medical management and development of a postoperative care plan may decrease the incidence of postoperative complications.

Preoperative fasting and risk of aspiration

The adequacy of preoperative fasting and the risk of pulmonary aspiration of gastric contents should be assessed in every child. Current guidelines and recommendations for preoperative fasting in children are presented in Chapter 15. Children with high intestinal obstruction ideally should have gastric decompression prior to a rapid-sequence induction of general anesthesia. A history of gastroesophageal reflux disease warrants an assessment of its severity and response to therapy. Children with mild reflux disease or disease that has been effectively treated are candidates for inhaled induction of anesthesia. Children with esophageal motility disorders such as achalasia should be regarded as being at risk for pulmonary aspiration and managed accordingly.

Physical examination

Preoperative airway examination focuses on identification of physical features that suggest a difficult facemask ventilation or tracheal intubation. In adults, there are validated assessments that identify predictors of airway management difficulty [78–82]. Although seemingly useful (Fig. 14.5), similar validated assessments have not been published for infants and young children. Nonetheless, there are certain anatomical features that are consistently associated with airway difficulty in the pediatric population. These include limited mouth opening, limited neck mobility, maxillary hypoplasia, mandibular hypoplasia, and diseases associated with decreased compliance of the submandibular space. School-aged children and adolescents will co-operate with physical examination maneuvers to assess the airway but in toddlers and infants, the airway exam is limited to an assessment of external physical features. In infants, neck mobility can be assessed by watching the infant track a colorful object, and mouth opening is assessed during crying.

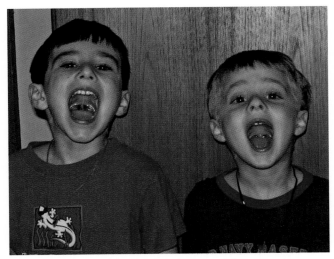

Figure 14.5 Although visualization of pharyngeal structures correlates with ease of intubation in adults, similar validation studies in pediatric patients have not been performed.

Routine airway management
Preoperative preparation of airway equipment

Airway-related equipment that should be prepared in the operating room prior to the arrival of the patient includes the appropriate sized facemask, laryngoscope handle and blade, tracheal tube, oral airway, laryngeal mask airway, and working suction catheter. If use of a laryngeal mask is planned, it should be prepared with lubricant and ready for insertion (see below).

A syringe of succinylcholine, 4–5 mg/kg, for intramuscular injection should be within reach in case laryngospasm or other type of upper airway obstruction occurs and immediate paralysis is required when intravenous access is absent. This dose should be calculated prior to the induction of general anesthesia.

Facemask ventilation

Proper positioning of the child during induction of general anesthesia is important in promoting upper airway patency and facilitating facemask ventilation and direct laryngoscopy. Because of the wide range of patient sizes encountered in pediatric practice, the adequacy of mask size and fit should be assessed prior to anesthetic induction. A properly fitting mask will cover the nose and mouth without covering the eyes or extending beyond the chin. A common mistake among trainees is to press the cephalad end of the mask onto the middle of the nose and unknowingly obstruct the airway. The cephalad end of the mask should be properly positioned on the bridge of the nose without pressing into the orbits. Introducing the mask to the child before it is connected to the anesthesia circuit provides a non-threatening opportunity for the child to acclimatize to it while giving the anesthesiologist an opportunity to assess fit.

Various types of pediatric facemasks are commercially available. While some have been designed to minimize dead space (attractive in the smallest patients), there are no data supporting the superiority of one mask type over another. Reusable black facemasks have largely been supplanted by transparent disposable facemasks. These disposable masks are advantageous in that the anesthesiologist can look through them during ventilation and assess the position of an oral or nasopharyngeal airway or identify regurgitated fluid or vomitus. Application of a fruit- or candy-scented lip balm to the interior of the unscented mask may improve the child's acceptance.

During inhaled induction of general anesthesia, the facemask is initially applied gently to the face. The hand holding the mask should be held in such a way that the child's field of view is not obstructed. The other hand may be placed on the child's head and kept ready to hold the head still during the excitement stage of anesthetic induction. As consciousness is lost, the position of the hand holding the mask is adjusted so that the third and possibly the fourth and fifth fingers are over the bony mandible. Special care must be taken in smaller children not to exert pressure on the submandibular tissues, which can create upper airway obstruction by posterior displacement of the tongue. Following loss of consciousness, 5–10 cmH$_2$O of continuous positive airway pressure (CPAP) is applied by partial closure of the adjustable pressure limiting (APL) valve, and a head tilt or chin lift maneuver is performed with the left hand holding the mask while the right hand holds the breathing bag to assess breath-to-breath adequacy of air movement. Adequacy of ventilation is also continuously assessed by visual inspection of chest rise and breathing bag movement, auscultation with a precordial stethoscope, and the presence of a capnographic waveform.

Chin lift, jaw thrust, and continuous positive airway pressure

Simple maneuvers such as performing a chin lift or mandibular protrusion (jaw thrust) can restore upper airway patency and relieve obstruction by increasing pharyngeal diameter at several levels [83–87]. The combination of either of these two techniques with the application of approximately 10 cmH$_2$O of CPAP is the initial treatment of airway obstruction in the spontaneously breathing child [88]. These combined maneuvers (jaw thrust with CPAP or chin lift with CPAP) increase the diameter and patency of the upper airway as well as that of the glottic opening [84]. While chin lift and jaw thrust have effects on tongue and epiglottis position, CPAP acts as a pneumatic splint to increase airway dimensions. Because jaw thrust combined with CPAP has not been shown to be superior to chin lift combined with CPAP, it has been suggested that chin lift with CPAP is preferable to a forceful jaw thrust, since this can result in postoperative discomfort [86]. In children with suspected cervical spine injuries, neck extension should be avoided; jaw thrust may be preferable in these cases.

Oral airway

After optimization of positioning, facemask application, and application of CPAP, the oral airway is usually the next intervention to restore patency of an obstructed upper airway in the anesthetized child. A variety of oral airways for pediatric patients with subtle differences in design are commercially available, with no literature supporting the superiority of one type or brand over another. However, those with hollow channels offer the advantage of being able to insert a suction catheter into the oropharynx with the oral airway inserted.

When inserting an oral airway, care must be taken to select the appropriate size. A properly sized airway should have its pharyngeal tip projecting just beyond the angle of the mandible when held next to the child's head

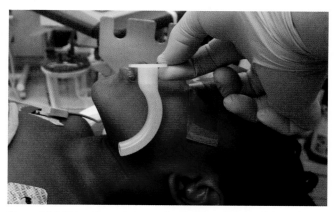

Figure 14.6 Sizing the oral airway, showing the pharyngeal tip projecting just beyond the angle of the mandible.

with the opposite end at the mouth (Fig. 14.6). Insertion of an undersized airway can push the tongue posteriorly and worsen obstruction, while an oversized airway can impinge on the epiglottis or glottis and worsen obstruction or trigger coughing and laryngospasm.

Oral airways are generally reserved for use in anesthetized children and are poorly tolerated by awake or lightly anesthetized children as they can stimulate gagging, coughing or laryngospasm. However, as a child emerges from anesthesia, it is best to leave an oral airway in place to prevent the child from biting on the tracheal tube and to maintain airway patency following extubation. Children will typically expel the device as they regain full consciousness.

Nasopharyngeal airway

A nasopharyngeal airway may be inserted to restore patency of the obstructed upper airway when the obstruction is suspected to be at the level of the upper pharynx or higher. Unlike an oral airway, a nasopharyngeal airway can be tolerated in the sedated or lightly anesthetized child and can be left in place postoperatively to maintain airway patency in selected circumstances such as following tonsillectomy for obstructive sleep apnea.

A disadvantage of nasopharyngeal airway insertion is occurrence of epistaxis, especially if the adenoid has been removed. This can be minimized by using a soft airway and adequate lubrication. If time allows, topical administration of a vasoconstrictor to the nasal mucosa is helpful. Hypertrophic adenoid tissue can impede passage and may result in bleeding. The proper size nasopharyngeal airway can be selected by holding it next to the face before insertion. With the flared external end at the position of the nasal opening, a properly sized airway will have the pharyngeal tip extending a finger breadth beyond the space between the angle of the mandible and the tragus (Fig. 14.7). A nasopharyngeal airway that is too

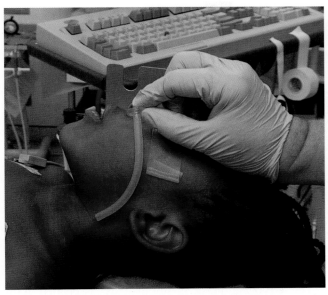

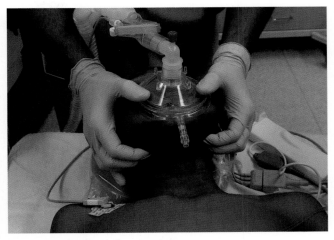

Figure 14.8 Two-handed mask technique.

Figure 14.7 Sizing the nasopharyngeal airway, showing the pharyngeal tip projecting just beyond the space between the angle of the mandible and the tragus.

short may not bypass upper airway obstruction, while one that is too long can impinge on the epiglottis and trigger coughing or laryngospasm.

Two-person, two-handed mask ventilation
When it is difficult to maintain a patent airway with the above techniques, having one provider apply the face-mask using two hands and simultaneously perform a chin lift and jaw thrust while another provider delivers breaths with the breathing bag is more effective than a single-handed mask ventilation technique (Fig. 14.8). Patients requiring a two-person technique should be considered difficult to ventilate by facemask [89,90].

Modified oral or nasal airway
The functionality of a standard oral or nasopharyngeal airway can be increased by inserting a 15 mm tracheal tube adaptor into the opening of the oral airway or the flared end of a nasopharyngeal airway (Fig. 14.9). The resulting modified airway can then be connected to the anesthesia circuit, and positive pressure can be delivered if the leaks around the airway are manually sealed. Positive pressure ventilation can be delivered by holding the mouth and opposite nasal passage closed [91]. This assembly with a nasopharyngeal airway is particularly useful in patients with limited mouth opening in whom oral airway or laryngeal mask insertion is not possible. The modified nasal airway is also a valuable adjunct to pediatric difficult airway management as a means of providing oxygen and inhaled anesthetic during oral

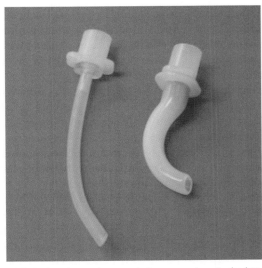

Figure 14.9 Oral and nasopharyngeal airways can be attached to a 15 mm tracheal tube adaptor to provide easy connection with an anesthesia machine circuit.

intubation while maintaining spontaneous respiration [92]. Similarly, a cut tracheal tube can also be used for the same purposes [93] but since it is made of stiffer material, it is more likely to cause trauma and bleeding during insertion.

Airway management with a facemask or natural airway
Maintenance of general anesthesia with a facemask is possible if a patent airway is easily achieved with or

without an oral or nasal airway. Generally, use of a face-mask is preferred for cases of shorter duration, and when the head of the operating room table is not turned away from the anesthesia machine. A natural airway that does not require the assistance of the anesthesiologist for patency is often used in conjunction with nasal cannula for supplemental oxygen administration, and the use of intravenous general anesthesia, such as propofol. Special cannulas designed to monitor exhaled carbon dioxide are commercially available or a standard cannula can be modified for this purpose. This technique is commonly used during total intravenous anesthesia for radiological or gastrointestinal endoscopy procedures.

Laryngeal masks and supraglottic devices

The introduction of the laryngeal mask airway (laryngeal mask) into clinical practice marked the beginning of a new era of anesthesia care for adults [94] and children [95]. Since that time, the laryngeal mask has functioned as an alternative to the facemask or the tracheal tube, depending on the clinical situation. Of equal importance is its use as an airway rescue device in patients with life-threatening upper airway obstruction, or as an aid to difficult tracheal intubation.

The laryngeal mask consists of an airway tube with an elliptically shaped cuff at the distal end that is inflated after insertion. When properly positioned, its distal aperture lies opposite the laryngeal inlet while the tip of the cuff rests in the proximal esophagus. The inflated cuff creates a seal with the lateral walls of the hypopharynx, the esophageal inlet, and the tongue base.

The classic sniffing position is used for routine laryngeal mask insertion. The deflated or partially inflated laryngeal mask is held in the dominant hand like a pencil, with the tip of the index finger at the junction of the cuff and the airway tube on the side of the laryngeal aperture. The mouth is opened and the tip of the device is pressed cephalad along the hard palate and into the oropharynx until a resistance is felt as the tip engages the esophageal opening. Because of anatomical differences in children (e.g. large tongue, cephalad larynx, tonsillar hypertrophy), this technique may result in a lower success rate than in adults. Therefore, alternative approaches have been devised (i.e. lateral and rotational insertion techniques) which may be more successful in children [96–101]. These studies were performed using the classic laryngeal mask; therefore it is unknown whether these results can be extended to other commercially available laryngeal masks and supraglottic airways that have alternate designs.

Airway management with the laryngeal mask is advantageous in a number of ways. Insertion of the device is simple and easily learned, and there is a high success rate with insertion even by inexperienced operators. Laryngeal mask insertion does not require muscle relaxation, can be performed at a lighter level of anesthesia compared to tracheal intubation, and is associated with fewer hemodynamic changes when compared to tracheal intubation [102,103]. However, when compared to adults, optimal positioning of the laryngeal mask becomes progressively more difficult in direct relation to the decreasing size of the child. Incorrect positioning of the laryngeal mask may lead to inadequate ventilation, airway trauma, mask dislodgment, and gastric insufflation. Fiberoptic assessment of laryngeal mask position is often useful to ascertain that the mask is properly positioned. A jaw thrust maneuver while inserting the smaller sized laryngeal masks may facilitate optimal positioning by lifting the epiglottis off the posterior pharyngeal wall and allowing the mask tip to slide into the upper esophageal sphincter without causing downfolding of the epiglottis.

The laryngeal mask is not usually associated with mechanical trauma to the tracheal mucosa and vocal cords. This is particularly relevant in children undergoing multiple anesthetics over a relatively short time interval (e.g. daily radiation treatment). Interestingly, the incidence of postoperative sore throat is equally as common compared with a tracheal tube [104]. The occurrence of postoperative sore throat in children appears to be correlated with laryngeal mask intracuff pressures above 40 cmH$_2$O [105]. The incidence of other less commonly reported complications from laryngeal mask use, such as lingual, hypoglossal or recurrent laryngeal nerve injury [106–109], may also be decreased by routine monitoring of laryngeal mask cuff pressures.

In the years following the introduction of the laryngeal mask, a variety of supraglottic airway devices have become available for use in children. The Cobra perilaryngeal airway (CobraPLA, Engineered Medical Systems, Indianapolis, IN) has a pharyngeal cuff rather than a laryngeal bowl and a leaf-shaped head with a slotted grill through which ventilation occurs. The CobraPLA has been demonstrated to perform as well as the Unique disposable laryngeal mask (Laryngeal Mask North America, San Diego, CA) in infants and children in terms of ease of insertion, airway sealing pressure, amount of gastric insufflation, and complications following removal. There is some evidence that its laryngeal positioning may not be optimal in infants less than 10 kg [110]. The i-Gel (Intersurgical Ltd, Berkshire, UK) has a non-inflatable bowl made of a heat-sensitive elastomeric gel whose shape conforms to fit the supraglottic airway. Although there exists a body of evidence supporting the efficacy and safety of the classic laryngeal mask and the ProSeal laryngeal mask in pediatrics, there are fewer data showing similar efficacy and safety of the similar supraglottic devices that are now available.

Like an oral airway, laryngeal masks and other supraglottic airways are poorly tolerated in awake or lightly anesthetized patients. Insertion at an inadequate plane of anesthesia can result in coughing, laryngospasm, gagging, and emesis. A number of studies have been conducted to determine optimal drug dosages to achieve adequate conditions for laryngeal mask insertion. Sevoflurane alone can be used to facilitate laryngeal mask insertion in children [111]; an effective concentration of 2.2 vol% provides satisfactory conditions in 95% of patients when 10 min are allowed to elapse for equilibration of brain and alveolar sevoflurane concentrations prior to insertion [102].

At approximately equipotent dose levels, propofol is a more potent suppressor of upper airway reflexes compared to thiopental [112] and is a superior induction agent for laryngeal mask insertion in terms of adverse respiratory events such as coughing or laryngospasm [113]. Propofol alone can be administered to facilitate laryngeal mask insertion. Doses exceeding 5 mg/kg are required to achieve satisfactory conditions in 90% of unpremedicated children [114]; however, such doses may result in undesirable hemodynamic effects and apnea. The combination of propofol with other drugs to facilitate laryngeal mask insertion is advantageous. For example, co-administration of lidocaine will result in less pain on injection of propofol [115–117] and may contribute to decreasing airway reflexes [118]. Opioids, such as fentanyl [119], alfentanil [115], and remifentanil [120] may also aid laryngeal mask insertion when co-administered with propofol.

In adults, the laryngeal mask was originally designed for removal as the patient awakens [94]. In children, there has been controversy over whether it is better to remove the laryngeal mask under deep general anesthesia or after awakening. Some studies show a higher incidence of respiratory complications (coughing, laryngospasm or oxyhemoglobin desaturation) when the laryngeal mask is removed when the child has largely regained consciousness [121,122] but others found a decreased incidence of such complications with awake removal [123,124] and some report no difference in complications based on removal technique [125,126]. One of the principal advantages of laryngeal mask removal under deep anesthesia is time efficiency – following laryngeal mask removal and assurance of a patent airway, the child can be transferred to the recovery room and allowed to emerge from anesthesia. If laryngeal mask removal under deep anesthesia is planned, the end-tidal sevoflurane concentration at which this can be safely performed in 95% of children without coughing, movement, laryngospasm or other airway complication is 2.2 vol% [127,128].

Laryngeal mask insertion may be tolerated in conscious newborns with severe upper airway obstruction, as occurs with the Pierre Robin sequence, Treacher Collins syndrome or Goldenhar syndrome [129–132].

The ProSeal laryngeal mask (Laryngeal Mask North America) is similar to a classic laryngeal mask with the addition of a channel through which a gastric drainage tube can be passed. The ProSeal mask is available in sizes appropriate for use in infants and children. Some practitioners avoid positive pressure ventilation with laryngeal mask use because of the possibility of gastric insufflation. Thus, the ProSeal mask may be preferred in patients who require positive pressure ventilation [133,134].

Pressure support ventilation decreases the work of breathing in spontaneously breathing children [135]. The advent of anesthesia machines with more sophisticated ventilators that can deliver pressure support ventilation has also made use of laryngeal masks more feasible as an alternative to tracheal intubation [136]. While work of breathing is improved with the application of CPAP [137], work of breathing is less and respiratory rate and end-tidal carbon dioxide are lower with pressure support ventilation compared to CPAP in children breathing with a laryngeal mask [138].

Laryngeal Tube

The Laryngeal Tube (VBM Medizintechnik, Sulz, Germany) is an extraglottic device that is inserted blindly in a manner similar to the laryngeal mask. When inserted, the distal end is positioned in the proximal esophageal opening. The device has an interconnected distal esophageal cuff and a proximal pharyngeal cuff, which results in equilibration of pressures between the two cuffs. Ventilation is delivered through numerous holes in the section of the tube between the esophageal and pharyngeal cuffs. This device is available in single-lumen and dual-lumen versions. The dual-lumen Laryngeal Tube has a channel that terminates in the esophageal end of the device. A catheter can be passed blindly through this lumen for gastric decompression. Indications for use of the laryngeal tube are similar to those for the laryngeal mask. However, unlike the laryngeal mask, this device cannot be readily used as a conduit for tracheal intubation.

Tracheal intubation

Indications for tracheal intubation are determined by the surgical procedure and the potential risk of aspiration of gastric contents. As a general rule, tracheal intubation is indicated for open cavity procedures of the abdomen or chest, intracranial procedures, and in cases where control of arterial PCO_2 is required. It is also indicated in cases where the anesthesiologist has limited access to the airway, such as procedures involving the head and neck or patients in the prone or lateral position.

Positioning for mask ventilation and tracheal intubation

In adults, the "sniffing position" (neck flexion and head extension) is classically described as the optimal head and neck position to facilitate direct laryngoscopy and tracheal intubation. The recommendation of this position is based on texts published between 1852 and 1944 [139]. Recently, a number of publications have suggested that the sniffing position in adults may offer no advantage over simple extension of the head for successful direct laryngoscopy [140–142]. Vialet et al compared the alignment of the oral, pharyngeal, and tracheal axes in children anesthetized for MRI scans of the head and neck, and found that there was better alignment achieved with simple extension of the head as compared to the sniffing position [143]. However, comparative trials examining the optimal position for laryngoscopy and intubation in children have not been done. The large occiput of an infant, when placed on a pillow, can flex the head and result in airway obstruction. Eliminating the pillow or placing a soft roll beneath the shoulders may improve upper airway patency.

Direct laryngoscopy

Direct laryngoscopy remains the most common method of tracheal intubation in children. Direct laryngoscopy using a straight Miller blade has traditionally been emphasized in infants and young children. This practice is largely based on anatomical studies [28] but comparative studies have not been performed [139,144,145]. The straight Miller blade may allow for greater control and displacement of the base of the tongue. The smaller size and lower profile of the straight blade may give the operator more room to pass the tracheal tube through the mouth and pharynx. When laryngoscopy is performed using a straight blade, the blade is advanced and used to directly lift the epiglottis to expose the larynx. The straight blade can also be directed into the vallecula and used to indirectly lift the epiglottis as is done with the standard curved blade. Miller's 1946 original description of the infant version of the blade states ". . . the epiglottis is visualized and raised slightly to expose the cords or, if the operator desires, the tip of the blade may be placed in front of the epiglottis and raised sufficiently to visualize the cords after the method of Macintosh" [146]. While direct laryngoscopy with the Miller blade may be more difficult to learn [147], there is evidence in adults that a superior view of the larynx can be achieved compared to the Macintosh blade [147,148].

If, during direct laryngoscopy, the visualization of the glottis is suboptimal, the laryngoscopist can optimize the glottic position by external manipulation of the thyroid cartilage. This practice was described by Benumof as optimal external laryngeal manipulation (OELM) [149].

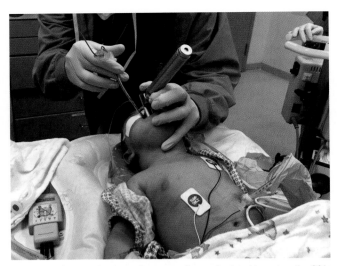

Figure 14.10 The glottis can be externally manipulated by using the fifth finger of the left hand that holds the laryngoscope.

The application of backward, upward, and rightward pressure on the thyroid cartilage (known as the BURP maneuver) [150] is an example of a specific type of OELM that many laryngoscopists employ as a first-line attempt at achieving optimal glottic exposure. In newborns and small infants, OELM can be performed using the fifth finger of the left hand (Fig. 14.10).

Hemodynamic response to laryngoscopy and tracheal intubation

Tracheal intubation in infants and children is an intensely stimulating procedure and can provoke tachycardia, hypertension, increased intracranial pressure, and bradycardia [151–155]. Tracheal intubation with flexible bronchoscopy does not result in a decreased pressor response compared to direct laryngoscopy [151]. Performance of intubation under deep anesthesia attenuates the pressor response to intubation; however, many of the agents used to achieve this can cause cardiovascular depression. The opiates fentanyl, remifentanil, and sufentanil have all been used for this purpose with success [156–158] while lidocaine does not appear to be effective [159].

Movement of the tracheal tube tip with neck movement

Flexion or extension of the neck results in predictable changes in location of the tracheal tube tip. In children, with both orotracheal and nasotracheal tubes, neck flexion results in caudad migration of the tube tip, while extension causes cephalad migration of the tube tip [160–162]. Therefore, bronchial intubation or extubation may result with neck movement after securing the tracheal tube.

Tracheal intubation without neuromuscular blockade

With the introduction into clinical practice of sevoflurane, propofol, and remifentanil, there has been increased interest in achieving tracheal intubation without neuromuscular blockade. Successful intubation can be accomplished with sevoflurane alone [163] although other drugs are commonly co-administered. Intubating conditions can be improved when sevoflurane is combined with propofol [164,165], lidocaine [118] and remifentanil [166,167].

"Awake" tracheal intubation

In select circumstances outside the obstetric delivery room, tracheal intubation may be performed in unpremedicated newborn infants who might not tolerate the cardiovascular depressant effects of anesthetic or sedative drugs. However, infants and neonates do experience the pain and discomfort from laryngoscopy; its performance without sedative premedication or general anesthesia has untoward cardiovascular (and behavioral) effects and should be avoided whenever possible. Furthermore, the administration of anesthetic, sedative, and neuromuscular blocking drugs improves conditions for intubation and decreases the likelihood of airway trauma [168–171]. A consensus statement published by the International Evidence Based Group for Neonatal Pain states "tracheal intubation without the use of analgesia or sedation should be performed only for urgent resuscitations in the delivery room or for life-threatening situations associated with the unavailability of intravenous access" [172].

Nasotracheal intubation

Before the advent of muscle relaxants, nasotracheal intubation was the preferred route for tracheal intubation; the technique was perfected by pioneering anesthesiologists such as Dr Ivan Magill (now memorialized for the forceps used for this purpose that bear his name) [173]. Following the introduction of muscle relaxants into anesthesia practice, orotracheal intubation became the favored technique. In current anesthesia practice, nasotracheal intubation is required for certain procedures (e.g. Lefort I osteotomy), while it is preferable for other procedures but not essential (e.g. oral rehabilitation). In other situations, such as in infants in the prone position, many anesthesiologists prefer a nasotracheal tube because of the possibility that it is more stable and secure than an oral tube. For children undergoing cardiac surgery, a nasotracheal tube may leave more room in the mouth for transesophageal echocardiography probe insertion. Nasotracheal intubation may be more comfortable than orotracheal intubation if postoperative tracheal intubation is expected.

Nasotracheal intubation is more challenging to perform than orotracheal intubation. The most common complication is epistaxis, especially in children with adenoidal hypertrophy. Other less common complications include retropharyngeal perforation [174,175], sinusitis [176], bacteremia [177–179] and turbinate avulsion [180,181]. Nasotracheal intubation is contraindicated in the setting of facial or skull fractures; intracranial tube placement has been reported following attempted nasotracheal intubation in this setting [182]. Oxymetazoline 0.05% can be applied to the nasal mucosa for vasoconstriction and to decrease the risk and severity of epistaxis. Cocaine (4–10%) and lidocaine with epinephrine have also been used for this purpose. Oxymetazoline is as effective as 10% cocaine and more effective than lidocaine with epinephrine for the prevention of epistaxis from nasotracheal intubation [183]. In a related study assessing vasoconstriction for endoscopic sinus surgery, oxymetazoline was preferable over both 0.25% phenylephrine and 4% cocaine [184]. To avoid triggering laryngospasm, topical vasoconstrictors should be sprayed after a deep plane of anesthesia has been reached or following administration of a neuromuscular blocking drug.

Topical vasoconstrictors used for nasal mucosal vasoconstriction are potent α-agonists that can be absorbed and exert systemic effects; these agents should be used judiciously. Life-threatening hypertension and pulmonary edema following the use of topical 0.5% phenylephrine have been described [184–186]. Severe hypertension and reflex bradycardia progressing to sinus arrest have also been reported following oxymetazoline administration [187,188].

The occurrence of nasal bleeding may also be reduced by softening the tracheal tube, which is achieved by soaking the tip in warm water or saline [189]. However, the use of a red rubber catheter to guide the tracheal tube through the nose into the pharynx is a more effective method of decreasing epistaxis compared to softening the tube tip in warm water [190–192].

Once inserted through the nose, the tube should be advanced so that its tip lies in the pharynx. Direct laryngoscopy is then performed, and the tip of the tracheal tube located in the pharynx. Once laryngeal exposure is optimized, the tube is gently grasped and guided into the trachea using Magill forceps as the tube is advanced. Care must be taken not to damage the cuff of a cuffed tube with the forceps.

Occasionally, it is difficult to advance the nasotracheal tube into the trachea despite an excellent view of the glottic inlet. This may occur because the natural curvature of the nasotracheal tube directs the tip anteriorly as it is advanced rather than in a direction parallel to the long axis of the trachea. Techniques to overcome this problem include neck flexion, directing the tube posteriorly with

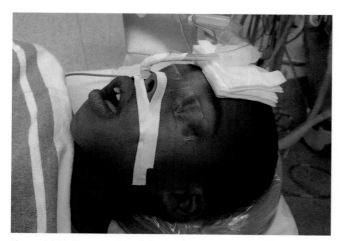

Figure 14.11 Proper taping of the nasal RAE tracheal tube to avoid pressure on the skin of the nasal alae.

the Magill forceps, rotating the tube so the narrowest part of the beveled tip is aligned parallel with the glottic opening, turning the head to the side, and rotation of the tube 180° as it is advanced to direct the natural curvature of the tube more posteriorly.

When securing a nasotracheal tube, it is important to tape the tube in a way that avoids excess pressure between the tube and the ala, as this can result in ischemia and subsequent ulceration (Fig. 14.11).

Tracheal tube selection

A variety of methods exist for determining the expected tracheal tube size in children, including formulas based on age, height–length ratio, ultrasound measurement [43] and qualitative methods such as comparison of tube size with the size of the fifth finger nail [193]. Although height is often used in the emergency department setting [194,195], age-based formulas are more commonly used by anesthesiologists. Uncuffed tube size is often determined by a modified Cole's formula: internal tube diameter (mm) = 4 + age/4 [193,196,197]. If a cuffed tube is to be used, a one-size smaller diameter tube should be selected to account for the small increase in external diameter created by the deflated cuff: internal tube diameter (mm) = 3 + age/4 [196].

RAE tubes

Oral and nasal tracheal tubes with a preformed bend (RAE tubes, named from the initials of the inventors Ring, Adair, and Elwyn) may be desirable in surgical procedures involving the eyes, oral cavity or face [198]. These tubes allow the anesthesia circuit to be directed away from the surgical field without kinking. The length of the preformed bend is fixed and varies with tube size. Sometimes the RAE tube that is the proper size for the child's tracheal diameter is too short or too long due to the fixed location of the bend. In cases where it is too long, a smaller size cuffed RAE can be used. In cases where it is too short, a standard straight tube may need to be substituted. For oral and nasal RAE tubes, a useful way of choosing the proper size based on length is to hold the tube next to the child's face and assess the location of the cuff or tube tip. In cuffed tubes, the cuff should lie at the level of the suprasternal notch; the tip of an uncuffed tube should lie at the level of the sternoclavicular junction.

Cuffed versus uncuffed tracheal tubes

Historically, uncuffed tracheal tubes were preferred in children up to the approximate age of 8–10 years. The lack of a cuff allowed for a greater internal diameter, which translated into lower resistance and decreased work of breathing during spontaneous ventilation, and greater ease of suctioning secretions. There was also concern that the use of cuffed tubes may be associated with a higher risk of subglottic injury. However, the use of modern tracheal tubes with high-volume, low-pressure cuffs has not been associated with an increased incidence of subglottic airway injury or of postextubation croup following their use in anesthetized children [199].

In 1951, Eckenhoff published a seminal article describing the anatomy of the infant and pediatric larynx [29]. The widespread teaching based on this article was that the infant larynx is funnel shaped with the widest portion at the glottic inlet and the narrowest portion at the cricoid ring. This has been disproven in a purely static anatomical measurement model using magnetic resonance imaging [35,37]; however, the cricoid ring remains *functionally* the narrowest portion of the airway because it is a complete ring and is non-distensible. These latter studies found the pediatric larynx to be slightly elliptical in cross-section, with a smaller transverse diameter and a larger anteroposterior diameter. Given this elliptical shape, an uncuffed tube of a size that effectively ablates an air leak would be expected to exert more pressure on the lateral walls of the larynx and trachea [200]. The cuff of a properly sized cuffed tracheal tube would conform to the shape of the trachea as it is inflated and pressure would be evenly distributed. The use of cuffed tubes in children is associated with a decreased incidence of post intubation stridor [201]. In addition to the anatomical factors described above, this may also be related to decreased need for repeat laryngoscopy and tube changes in cases where an uncuffed tube that is too small or too large is initially inserted.

Cuffed tracheal tubes provide a better seal to protect the trachea from macroaspiration, while simultaneously allowing for lower fresh gas flows (with associated economic advantages) and decreased operating room pollution. In cases such as tonsillectomy, use of a cuffed tube can limit escape of oxygen-enriched inspired gases and decrease the risk of intraoperative fires, although this does not obviate the importance of limiting inspired oxygen concentration in these cases. However, there is some evidence that the presence of a cuff may contribute to bronchoscopically proven airway injury [202].

In our clinical practice, uncuffed tracheal tubes are rarely used. However, they remain useful in certain situations where maximizing the internal diameter of the tube is important. Because resistance to airflow is inversely proportional to the fourth power of the radius of the tube (or fifth power with turbulent flow), the ability to ventilate can be impaired by selecting a cuffed tube that is a size smaller than the appropriate uncuffed tube. This effect is most clinically significant with smaller tube sizes used in preterm and very low-birthweight infants. Moreover, suctioning and pulmonary toilet are more difficult with the smallest tubes. An uncuffed tube is advantageous to achieve single lung ventilation by advancing and lodging it into the ventilated main bronchus. A separate bronchial blocker may be placed alongside the tube or within it, and because the bronchial blocker occupies a portion of the lumen, a larger lumen will help limit resultant increased resistance to airflow through the tube.

Determining proper endotracheal tube length

Like tracheal tube diameter selection, a variety of formulas have been created to predict the proper depth of orotracheal tube insertion. In infants and neonates, a commonly used rule of thumb is the "1234–78910 rule," where a 1 kg infant will have the tube taped at 7 cm at the maxillary alveolar ridge, a 2 kg infant taped at 8 cm, a 3 kg infant taped at 9 cm, and a 4 kg infant taped at 10 cm. In infants, when an uncuffed tracheal tube is used, it is common practice to advance the tube to achieve a deliberate right main bronchial intubation while auscultating the left chest. The centimeter depth at which breath sounds disappear (or become greatly decreased) is identified as the carina. The tube is then withdrawn midway between the carina and the vocal cords. Prior to performing this maneuver, it is useful to identify the centimeter marking relative to the gum or incisors following intubation and advancement of the cuff just beyond the vocal cords (or with an uncuffed tube, 1–2 cm beyond the vocal cords). Knowing the centimeter marking with this depth of insertion as well as the depth of the carina gives the anesthesiologist an idea of how much cephalad or caudad tube displacement can safely occur.

In older children, a good rule of thumb that is used to estimate the proper orotracheal tube depth in centimeters is to multiply the appropriate tube internal diameter (in millimeters) by 3. For nasotracheal intubation, multiplying the appropriate tube internal diameter by 4 is an effective method. When a cuffed tube is used, the ballotte technique can be used to place the cuff in its proper position at the level of the suprasternal notch. Identification of the depth of the tube relative to the maxillary alveolar ridge or maxillary incisors gives a more precise depth marking than identification relative to the lip.

Assessing tube size following endotracheal intubation

The appropriateness of the tracheal tube size selected must be verified in every child. A tube that is too large may exert excessive pressure on the tracheal mucosa, resulting in mucosal ischemia. In the short term, this can lead to mucosal edema and stridor following extubation, while in the long term it may contribute to the development of subglottic stenosis.

In some children, an oversized tube is identified by an inability to advance the tube into the trachea during the intubation attempt. The most common method to assess tube size after placement of the tube is the air leak test. After midtracheal positioning of the tube tip, the APL valve is closed and the circuit pressure is allowed to increase while a stethoscope is placed over the thyroid cartilage. The leak pressure occurs when air is heard escaping around the tube. The ideal leak pressure is between 20 and 30 cmH$_2$O. It is important to avoid a slow and prolonged leak test as this will have the hemodynamic consequences of a prolonged Valsalva maneuver. When a cuffed tube is used, the cuff inflation volume can be adjusted to achieve the desired leak pressure. For short cases, if the initial leak test is above 40 cmH$_2$O, some anesthesiologists will not exchange the tube for a smaller one in the interest of avoiding the trauma of repeated laryngoscopy. For longer cases, if the leak pressure is greater than 30–35 cmH$_2$O, exchange with a smaller tracheal tube may be preferred.

Rapid-sequence induction and intubation in pediatric patients

Rapid-sequence induction and intubation (RSII) is used to minimize the time from anesthetic-induced loss of consciousness and endotracheal intubation, to decrease the risk of pulmonary aspiration of gastric contents. RSII is often more challenging in pediatric patients when compared to adults because infants and small children have relatively higher oxygen consumption rates, reduced functional residual capacity (FRC), and elevated closing volumes and thus will develop oxyhemoglobin desaturation more quickly during periods of apnea.

Because of this propensity toward hypoxemia during RSII in children, and the lack of any feasible period of preoxygenation, many pediatric anesthesiologists perform a "modified" rapid-sequence induction [203]. In this modified technique, gentle facemask ventilation is performed using low inflation pressures (<10–$15\,cmH_2O$) while cricoid pressure is applied until enough time has elapsed for complete neuromuscular blockade to be established. In support of this practice, appropriately applied cricoid pressure has been shown to be effective in preventing gastric inflation during gentle bag-mask ventilation in anesthetized infants and children [204,205]. In older children and adolescents who can co-operate with adequate preoxygenation, a classic RSII may be preferred. If the initial attempt at intubation fails, gentle facemask ventilation through cricoid pressure should be performed. If ventilation is difficult with cricoid pressure despite the use of adjunctive devices (e.g. oral or nasopharyngeal airway, laryngeal mask), cricoid pressure should be lessened or released [206,207].

Cricoid pressure is contraindicated in the presence of active vomiting, suspected laryngeal or tracheal injury, and unstable cervical spine injuries [206,208]. In children, cricoid pressure applied below the cricoid ring can result in significant distortion of the larynx and trachea and increase the difficulty of ventilation or intubation [209]. A recent report of the complications of RSII in a large children's hospital population revealed an incidence of difficult intubation of 1.7%; however, it is unclear if these difficulties were related to presence of cricoid pressure [210].

Postoperative airway management

The first priority in the postoperative care of the child is ensuring a patent airway. Assessment should focus on residual effects of anesthetic agents, opioids, and sedatives in the context of the preoperative condition of the child, the course of intraoperative airway management, the surgical procedure, anticipated fluid shifts, and the expected postoperative course. During recovery, proper head and neck positioning promotes airway patency. In the supine position, a soft roll placed under the shoulders will extend the head and neck and help open the upper airway. Placing the child in the "recovery (lateral) position" increases upper airway size [21] and allows secretions to drain out of the mouth rather than backward into the pharynx. If airway obstruction fails to improve with positioning, and the child is semi-conscious, a soft nasopharyngeal airway can be inserted; if the child is still anesthetized, an oral airway may be preferred. If airway obstruction is incompletely relieved with a nasopharyngeal airway, a 15 mm tracheal tube adaptor

can be placed into the external flared end of a nasopharyngeal airway for the delivery of CPAP [91]. If one suspects that postoperative upper airway obstruction is caused by the residual effect of opioids, naloxone can be cautiously administered to test and treat this possibility. Incremental doses of 0.5–1 μg/kg can be carefully titrated to reverse respiratory depressant effects without reversal of analgesic effects. Children who fail these measures to restore airway patency may require tracheal reintubation.

Non-invasive respiratory support

In selected cases, non-invasive ventilatory support, such as CPAP or bi-level positive airway pressure (BiPAP), may be a useful option and can allow some patients to avoid tracheal intubation and mechanical ventilation in the postoperative period. Non-invasive support in older children is most often delivered by facemask or nasal mask, while nasal prongs are used in neonates and infants. Children and adolescents who use such devices preoperatively should receive respiratory support from these devices in the postoperative period. CPAP delivered by nasal prongs to neonates and infants is an effective way to improve respiratory function and prevent reintubation following extubation in the neonatal intensive care unit [211], as well as for treatment of apnea of prematurity [212,213].

Postoperative mechanical ventilation

If postoperative mechanical ventilation is required, a plan must be developed for transfer of the child's care from the operating room to the intensive care unit. Clear communication regarding the course of airway management should include discussion of the ease of facemask ventilation and direct laryngoscopy, tracheal tube size and insertion depth, current ventilator settings, and the reason why postoperative mechanical ventilation is necessary. The child will need to be transitioned from general anesthesia to an appropriate sedation regimen. If airway management was difficult, a plan should be in place in the event of accidental extubation. Keeping an appropriately sized laryngeal mask at the bedside is essential in such cases. If an oral RAE tube was used, this should be changed to a standard tracheal tube as protrusion of the tongue can easily result in extubation, and pulmonary toilet is more difficult with RAE tubes.

Upper airway complications and management

Laryngospasm
Laryngospasm is a prolonged glottic closure maintained beyond the initiating stimulus and is a protective reflex

that causes complete closure of the vocal cords to protect the trachea from aspiration of foreign material [214]. Prolonged laryngospasm can result in hypoxemia, bradycardia, postobstructive negative pressure pulmonary edema, regurgitation and aspiration of gastric contents, and cardiac arrest. Laryngospasm is more common in children than adults; it has been estimated to occur at a frequency from 1 per 1000 anesthetics to 17 per 1000 anesthetics [215–217]. While one belief has been that hypoxemia itself will result in abolition of this reflex, data from the Pediatric Perioperative Cardiac Arrest Registry reveal that laryngospasm continues to be a cause of cardiac arrest in children [218]. The incidence of laryngospasm appears to be increased in children with a history of active or recent upper respiratory tract infection [217,219–221].

Initial treatment of laryngospasm consists of CPAP delivered by facemask with 100% oxygen. Deepening the anesthetic may relieve the obstruction and can be achieved with intravenous propofol. If hypoxemia is occurring, the treatment of choice is immediate neuromuscular blockade with succinylcholine. In adults, low-dose succinylcholine (e.g. 0.1 mg/kg) is effective in treating laryngospasm [222]. However, larger doses may be preferred if reintubation is planned. When administering succinylcholine in children, some pediatric anesthesiologists prefer to co-administer an anticholinergic agent (i.e. atropine or glycopyrrolate) to prevent succinylcholine-induced bradycardia.

If laryngospasm develops prior to establishment of intravenous access, succinylcholine (4–5 mg/kg) may be administered via the intramuscular route [223]. Maximal twitch depression at the abductor pollicis following intramuscular injection of succinylcholine will develop in 3–4 min; however, clinical relief of airway obstruction occurs much sooner [224,225]. Succinylcholine-induced bradycardia is less likely with intramuscular administration [223,226]. Intralingual or submental administration of succinylcholine has been recommended because of its rapid onset of action [227,228]; however, many avoid this route because of concerns about intraoral bleeding. Intramuscular administration of 4–5 mg/kg of succinylcholine may result in a phase II block, and more than 20 min may elapse before neuromuscular blockade resolves [223].

Additional treatments for laryngospasm, such as pressure in the "laryngospasm notch" [229], digital elevation of the tongue [230], nitroglycerine [231] and doxapram [232] have been proposed but their efficacy in children has not been evaluated.

Laryngospasm accompanied by a strong inspiratory effort and hypoxemia may lead to negative pressure pulmonary edema with or without pulmonary hemorrhage [233–236]. The treatment depends on the severity of symptoms, and includes supplemental oxygen, furosemide, and positive pressure respiratory support.

Pulmonary aspiration of gastric contents

Pulmonary aspiration of gastric contents is a relatively uncommon event, although its incidence in children appears equal to or higher than that in adults [237–239]. The incidence in the pediatric population ranges from 1 in 2632 anesthetics [238] to 1 in 1000 anesthetics [239]. Death from anesthetic-related pulmonary aspiration is exceedingly rare. Children with clinically apparent pulmonary aspiration who did not develop symptoms within 2 h are unlikely to develop subsequent respiratory complications [238].

Factors associated with increased risk of pulmonary aspiration include emergency surgery, presence of bowel obstruction or ileus, younger age, and ASA physical status 3 or 4 [238,239]. Obesity is not associated with an increased gastric fluid volume or increased risk of pulmonary aspiration [240].

Postintubation croup

Postintubation croup presents as inspiratory stridor, hoarseness, a "barky" cough and, in severe cases, intercostal retractions and respiratory distress. Postintubation croup is thought to result from airflow restriction due to tracheal edema from mechanical trauma or mucosal ischemia related to endotracheal intubation. The site of greatest restriction is at the level of the cricoid ring. The incidence in children was reported to be 1% in 1977 [241]; however, more recent data suggest a lower incidence [242]. Postintubation stridor may develop shortly following tracheal extubation or several hours later. Upper airway obstruction from other causes must be investigated before the diagnosis is made. Treatment is initially supportive and is not unlike the treatment of infectious croup, which also results from subglottic edema. Delivery of humidified mist is first-line therapy. Physical exam findings determine the need for additional treatment. Nasal flaring, subcostal or intercostal retractions, or other features indicative of increased work of breathing are indications for pharmacological therapy. Dexamethasone, 0.5 mg/kg up to 10 mg, is an effective second-line treatment. Nebulized racemic epinephrine can also be administered but should be reserved for severe cases. Because of the potential for rebound edema after the racemic epinephrine has worn off, children should be observed to ensure that symptoms do not recur.

Airway management for tracheostomy insertion

Infants and children who require chronic ventilatory therapy will likely benefit from insertion of a tracheostomy tube. Diagnoses associated with the need for tracheostomy include neuromuscular impairment, chronic lung disease, trauma, upper airway anomalies, congenital heart disease, and prematurity [243]. Infants who have had long-term tracheal intubation and mechanical ventilation may develop subglottic stenosis and require tracheostomy to provide long-term ventilatory support. The in-hospital mortality in pediatric patients who undergo tracheostomy during their hospitalization is as high as 8.5% [243]. Most of these children present to the operating room with a secured airway (tracheal tube). In these cases the ease of previous mask ventilation and tracheal intubation must be determined preoperatively. Those children in whom direct laryngoscopy was difficult should have a plan developed in case accidental extubation occurs before tracheostomy completion. Such a plan might include leaving an airway exchange catheter in the trachea during completion of the tracheostomy or withdrawal of the tracheal tube to a position just above the tracheostomy incision, with the tip still between the vocal cords so that it can be easily advanced for reintubation should this be required. These cases require close vigilance and communication with the surgeon throughout the procedure. The risk of a surgical fire can be reduced by minimizing the inspired oxygen concentration and avoiding the use of nitrous oxide. The surgical team should avoid the use of cautery to enter the airway.

The choice of tracheostomy tube size and length depends on the indications for tracheostomy. Patients requiring chronic mechanical ventilation often benefit from low-pressure, high-volume cuffed tubes, often made with silicone or other soft material to minimize airway trauma. Patients with upper airway obstruction without significant lung disease often benefit from small uncuffed tracheostomy tubes, which are large enough to provide a patent airway, yet allow sufficient air leak to support vocalization. Consultation with the surgeon and pulmonologist is important to understand all the goals of the procedure and select the correct tracheostomy tube.

Certain children with upper airway congenital anomalies may not have an existing tracheal tube immediately prior to surgical tracheostomy. Airway management for tracheostomy may entail tracheal intubation with subsequent management as described above. Alternatively, a laryngeal mask may be used as an anesthetic airway conduit during tracheostomy insertion.

A newly placed tracheostomy requires 7–10 days for the stoma to be well formed; prior to this period, if a tube change is needed, it should be performed by an otolaryngologist. After healing, tracheostomy tubes should be changed every 1–2 weeks to reduce the formation of granulation tissue or mucus plugging of the tube. A tracheostomy bypasses the humidification and warming function of the nose and upper airway so an artificial humidification device is necessary. Heat and moisture exchangers (HMEs) are generally used to facilitate this function. They should be selected to minimize resistance to airflow, and minimize work of breathing [244].

Management of the child with a pre-existing tracheostomy

Tracheostomized children presenting for general anesthesia and surgery require a different approach to airway management. During the preoperative visit, the anesthesiologist should determine the type, size, and presence of a cuff on the tracheostomy tube. Parents and caregivers should be asked about the frequency of suctioning, as well as the suction catheter size and the depth it is inserted. The presence or absence of a leak around the tracheostomy tube as well as the amount of ventilator support the child requires should also be determined during the preoperative assessment. These children should come with emergency replacement supplies for their tracheostomy, which should be kept with them throughout their perioperative course.

Inhaled anesthetic induction is the most common induction technique in these children. It is often necessary to connect a flexible "accordion" extension from the end of the anesthetic circuit to the tracheostomy tube to increase the limited clearance between the clavicles and mandible, especially in infants. In those with a significant leak around the tracheostomy tube, inhaled induction may be prolonged due to mixing of air inspired from the upper airway with gases inspired through the tracheostomy tube. Following the loss of consciousness, holding the mouth and nose closed or applying a sealed facemask will help decrease mixing and facilitate ventilation through the tracheostomy.

For short procedures, it is often unnecessary to change the tracheostomy tube. For intracavitary or long procedures, if there is a significant leak around the tracheostomy tube, a standard cuffed tracheal tube will enable effective positive pressure ventilation. This can be achieved by exchange of the existing tracheostomy tube with the same-sized cuffed tracheal tube. With an established tracheal stoma, this is easily accomplished; however, consultation with an otolaryngologist may be useful in selecting the most appropriate tube and for performing the exchange, if necessary. Another option is replacement of the tracheostomy tube with a wire-reinforced tube. This lower profile alternative can be useful in cases where a standard tracheostomy tube would encroach on the surgical field. This tube can be secured to the chest with tape or sutured in place in selected circumstances. In cases where the tracheostomy site encroaches on the surgical field, the child's airway can be secured with an oral or nasal tracheal tube, and the tracheostomy site can be sealed with gauze and non-occlusive tape and dressing.

Tracheostomy tubes are available in a variety of sizes and lengths for pediatric use. They can be constructed from metal or plastic. Plastic tubes are most frequently used and are made from silicone or polyvinyl chloride. Some tracheostomy tubes are supplied with a tracheostomy disconnection wedge, which facilitates separation of connections to the tracheostomy. The internal and external diameters are usually marked on the flange of the tracheostomy tube. Several manufactured tubes have wire-reinforced designs, allowing flexibility without kinking, and some have long flexible proximal ends (e.g. FlexTend™), which place connections to the tube away from the child's neck, thus reducing the chance of tube obstruction in small patients.

Tracheostomy tubes are available in cuffed and uncuffed versions [245]. The cuff helps to protect the airway from secretions and facilitates positive pressure ventilation in children with poor lung compliance. Cuffed tracheostomy tubes have a high-volume, low-pressure cuff, a low-volume, high-pressure cuff, or a foam cuff, which is useful in patients with chronic aspiration. The Tight-To-Shaft tube (TTS™) has a low-volume, high-pressure cuff used for patients who need intermittent inflation such as during meals and at night. When deflated, the cuff assumes the profile of the tube and enables phonation and use of the upper airway. The cuff should be inflated with sterile water because it is gas permeable and will slowly deflate over time.

The Montgomery tube is a T-shaped silicone tube that has a short lumen projecting from its side at a 75° or 90° angle. It is typically used after tracheal reconstruction to stent the airway and can be left in place for months. The upper limb extends above the glottis and the short limb is brought out through the tracheostomy stoma.

The difficult pediatric airway

There are two broad categories of pediatric patients with a "difficult" airway: those who are difficult to mask ventilate, and those who are difficult to tracheally intubate by an experienced practitioner using standard direct laryngoscopy. Definitions for each of these categories have been proposed but are inconsistent throughout the literature. Therefore, in this chapter we focus on airway management techniques once a practitioner is faced with the expected or unexpected situation of inability to adequately perform mask ventilation or tracheal intubation despite the use of standard equipment, as described above in the section on management of normal pediatric airways.

There have been no systematic and validated studies that define predictors of difficult mask ventilation or tracheal intubation in the pediatric population. In adults, limited head extension, reduced mandibular space, and large tongue are predictive of difficult intubation [246]. These are also features in children with difficult intubations [247]. The mandibular space represents the area

available to displace the tongue and soft tissue. Adequate mandibular size is necessary for an easy direct laryngoscopic view of the glottis. Reduction of this space by anatomical anomalies (e.g. micrognathia) often makes laryngoscopy difficult. The mentum–hyoid distance provides an estimate of the mandibular space. In infants, the minimum mentum–hyoid distance for a "normal" airway should be 1.5 cm [247].

The diversity and complexity of craniofacial anomalies in children are vast; thus, an exhaustive review is not possible here. Nevertheless, children with craniofacial anomalies can be defined according to the anatomical compartment that relates to the airway difficulty. Craniofacial dysmorphisms may be defined as primary abnormalities of the maxilla, abnormalities of mandibular size, abnormalities of mandibular hinge and sliding function, and anatomical anomalies of the tongue and cervical spine. Classifying patients in this manner allows selection of the most appropriate equipment for addressing the airway anomaly (Table 14.1).

There is no device that represents a panacea for airway management and each device has unique strengths and weaknesses that need to be matched with the patient's condition and anatomical details. For example, a patient with limited mouth opening would be best managed with a flexible bronchoscope or optical/lighted stylet rather than a rigid video laryngoscope, whereas a patient with Robin sequence who presents with a potentially difficult mask ventilation may be best managed with a laryngeal mask followed by tracheal intubation through the mask, thus permitting ventilation during intubation. We use a simple acronym (AVAD: Anesthesia, Ventilation, Adjuncts, Devices) to guide the approach to airway management in known difficult airway patients (Fig. 14.12). Thinking about the patient in terms of these components facilitates the formulation of a primary and secondary plan, and dictates the necessary equipment for the chosen approach. The care provider should select an approach and device for each of the four components of the acronym.

As an example, let us consider a neonate with Pierre Robin sequence. The **A**nesthesia plan may include deep sedation with a secondary plan for general anesthesia. The **V**entilation plan may be spontaneous ventilation and the **A**djunct a modified nasal airway, with a secondary plan of controlled ventilation using a laryngeal mask. The **D**evice may be a video laryngoscope with the fiberoptic bronchoscope as a back-up device. The chart helps to ensure that all the critical aspects of the care plan are addressed, and horizontally represents increasing anesthetic and technical complexity. Nevertheless, practitioners should adopt a standard and consistent set of airway-related equipment and drugs for all anticipated difficult airway patients (Fig. 14.13).

When approaching the child with a known cause for a difficult airway, one of the first *a priori* decisions

Table 14.1 Congenital disorders and recommended devices based on anatomical abnormality

Primary anatomical area of abnormality	Maxilla	Mandible size	Tongue & soft tissue	Cervical spine	Larynx	Mandible sliding and hinge function
Associated disorders	Achondroplasia	Robin sequence	Down syndrome	Klippel–Feil syndrome	Laryngeal atresia	Fibrodysplasia ossificans progressiva
	Cleft palate	Goldenhar syndrome	Beckwith–Wiedemann syndrome	Goldenhar syndrome	Laryngeal web	Rheumatoid disease
	Nager syndrome	Treacher Collins syndrome	Lingual tonsillar hypertrophy	C-spine traumatic injury	Cri-du-chat syndrome	Gangrenous stomatitis
	Treacher Collins syndrome	Freeman Sheldon syndrome	Mucopolysaccharidosis	Oculodento-osseous dysplasia	Epiglottitis	
		Cri-du-chat syndrome	Arthrogryposis multiplex congenita			
		Cockayne syndrome				
Recommended devices	VL FFB	VL FFB LM + FFB	LM + FFB	OS VL FFB	OS FFB	OS FFB LW

FFB, flexible fiberoptic bronchoscope; LM, laryngeal mask; LW, lightwand; OS, optical stylet; VL, video laryngoscope.

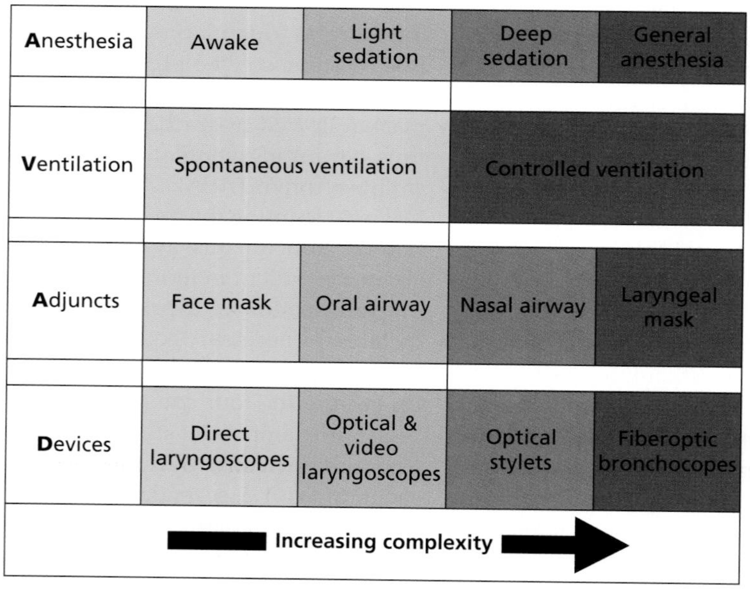

Anesthesia	Awake	Light sedation	Deep sedation	General anesthesia
Ventilation	Spontaneous ventilation		Controlled ventilation	
Adjuncts	Face mask	Oral airway	Nasal airway	Laryngeal mask
Devices	Direct laryngoscopes	Optical & video laryngoscopes	Optical stylets	Fiberoptic bronchocopes

Increasing complexity ➡

Figure 14.12 A simple acronym (AVAD: Anesthesia, Ventilation, Adjuncts, Devices) guides the approach to airway management in known difficult airway patients.

to be made is the anticipated level of consciousness during the airway management process. This largely depends on the anesthesiologist's confidence in their ability to avoid life-threatening hypoxemia in an anesthetized or sedated child using a facemask or a laryngeal mask.

"Awake" intubation

Tracheal intubation of an unco-operative child at a nearly conscious level is difficult and associated with complications [155,248]. Since the advent of the laryngeal mask, this approach has been largely abandoned for sedated or anesthetized techniques, with rare exceptions. For

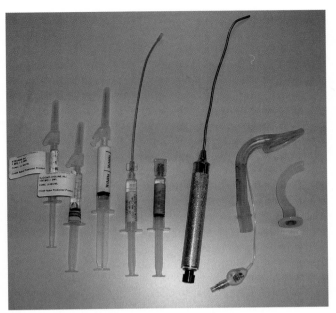

Figure 14.13 One example of a standard equipment and medication set-up for anticipated pediatric difficult airway. *From left to right*: atropine, succinylcholine, propofol, 2% lidocaine with mucosal atomizer attachment, vecuronium, lighted stylet, laryngeal mask, and oral airway.

example, neonates with Robin sequence (see below) are expected to have difficulty with mask ventilation; therefore, awake insertion of a laryngeal mask and confirmation of adequate ventilation can precede induction of general anesthesia [129,131].

Sedated intubation

Many children with anticipated difficult airways can be sedated to provide comfort and amnesia, yet retain spontaneous ventilation and upper airway patency during tracheal intubation attempts. A sedated technique is useful when life-threatening upper airway obstruction during induction of general anesthesia is anticipated, such as may be seen in children with a large cystic hygroma [249]. Although light sedation has been described for tracheal intubation in infants using opioids, amnestic agents, and incremental doses of induction agents, most children will require deeper levels of sedation to ensure optimal intubating conditions. This may also be accomplished using dexmedetomidine, as a sole agent or in combination with other agents [250]. Dexmedetomidine allows arousal with strong stimulation and maintenance of spontaneous ventilation, using a bolus dose of up to $2-4\,\mu g/kg$ over 10 min followed by a continuous infusion of $0.7\,\mu g/kg/h$. Dexmedetomidine can be combined with incremental doses of ketamine ($0.25\,mg/kg$) or midazolam (up to $0.1\,mg/kg$) to facilitate intubation without clinically significant respiratory depression [251,252]. There is little evidence for which to base the selection of drugs for sedated approaches to

intubation. Further studies are necessary to determine the optimal methods for preserving airway patency while minimizing reactivity during tracheal intubation.

Intubation under general anesthesia

The majority of children with a known or expected difficult intubation can receive general anesthesia during the intubation process. Many pediatric anesthesiologists will require an indwelling intravenous catheter prior to administration of general anesthesia but this is practitioner dependent. Upper airway patency may be facilitated by insertion of an oral or nasal airway. A nasal airway may be attached to a 15 mm tracheal tube adaptor, which allows connection to the anesthesia circuit for provision of anesthesia and oxygen, during intubation attempts (see Fig. 14.9) [92].

Ventilation of the patient with a difficult airway

The ultimate goal of any airway management strategy is to maintain adequate oxygenation and avoid life-threatening hypoxemia. It is critical that this overarching principle is not lost during attempts to secure the airway.

Facemask ventilation represents the first step in maintaining oxygenation between intubation attempts. The optimal ventilation strategy for the management of the difficult pediatric airway remains unknown. Traditional teaching advocates the maintenance of spontaneous ventilation during airway management because of the fear of loss of the ability to ventilate with multiple traumatic attempts and to preserve the ability to quickly awaken the patient if necessary. In children this concern is weighed against the possibility of coughing, and other movements if the level of anesthetic is too light. There is no plausible research that can examine this issue directly; much of the rationale for this strategy comes from case reports and clinical observations. Maintenance of spontaneous ventilation is it facilitates oxygenation during airway manipulation [253], it provides clues to the glottic location by way of the bubbling of secretions that can be observed breathing, and provides the anesthesiologist with increased uninterrupted time to accomplish the intubation. In addition, there may be greater upper airway patency and better visualization resulting from less soft tissue collapse when airway tone is preserved [254]. Although maintenance of spontaneous ventilation is preferred, some practitioners will attempt positive pressure ventilation and, if successful, will administer neuromuscular blockade to facilitate the intubation process. Although neuromuscular blockade often facilitates ventilation and intubation, there are reports in adults where the addition of neuromuscular blockade in itself has been reported to change the anatomical characteristics of the upper airway, and worsen ventilation or intubation conditions [255,256].

Topical anesthesia should be applied to the glottic structures to minimize airway reactivity and should be performed when an adequate depth of anesthesia is confirmed. An increase in heart rate, respiratory rate or physical movement when a 5 second jaw thrust is applied is usually a good indicator of adequate anesthetic depth for airway manipulation.

A total intravenous technique during intubation attempts will minimize operating room pollution from anesthetic gases. Various combinations of easily titratable intravenous agents (e.g. propofol, remifentanil) can be used for this purpose [257,258].

Impossible mask ventilation is unusual in the pediatric population. It is difficult to determine the true incidence because children suspected of impossible mask ventilation due to altered anatomy will undergo tracheal intubation using deep sedation and spontaneous ventilation. In an observational review of 22,000 adult anesthetics, the reported incidence of impossible mask ventilation was one in every 690 cases [259]. One-quarter of these patients were also difficult to intubate. Neck radiation was found to be the most significant predictor of impossible ventilation.

Indirect methods of tracheal intubation

There are many approaches to tracheal intubation in the child with a known or suspected difficult airway. In certain circumstances it may be appropriate to attempt direct laryngoscopy, if a reasonably long amount of time has passed since the previous intubation attempt and the anesthesiologist feels that the growth of the child has altered their airway anatomy in a favorable direction. If a direct method is deemed impossible, a variety of options exist for indirect tracheal intubation.

 ### Fiberoptic bronchoscopy (see Video clips 14.1–14.4)

The first article describing the use of flexible fiberoptic bronchoscopy in children appeared in 1978 [260] and despite many modifications in design, it remains the "gold standard" for accomplishing tracheal intubation in the difficult pediatric airway [92,248,252,253,261–291]. Limitations of fiberoptic intubation in children include the significant time necessary for skill acquisition, the processing and preparation time of the equipment, the fragility of the bronchoscope, and the high purchase and repair costs. Despite these limitations, the skill necessary to consistently perform a smooth fiberoptic intubation can be acquired during routine cases in children with normal airways. The introduction of the 2.2 mm and 2.7 mm ultrathin bronchoscopes allowed fiberoptic intubation of neonates and small children with tracheal tubes as small as 2.5 mm [292,293]. These ultrathin bronchoscopes did

not have a working channel and so functionality was limited in the presence of copious secretions; however, modern versions are available with functional working channels. Many larger bronchoscopes now incorporate a charge coupled device camera (CCD), which transmits the image from the tip of the scope to a screen, and replaces the fiberoptic bundles present in traditional scopes. This provides a high-clarity image without the honeycombing typically seen with standard fiberoptic bronchoscopes.

Fiberoptic intubation in children is performed in a similar fashion to adults but may be more challenging because of the small size of the scopes used, the short apnea time and the small size of the airway. The child is placed in a neutral position and the tongue elevated from the posterior pharyngeal wall by an assistant using a suction tubing or a gauze. The endoscopist places the scope in the midline in the pharynx and advances the scope in a deliberate manner following the tongue base and successively visualizing the uvula, palate, epiglottis and the vocal cords. A jaw thrust helps to elevate the epiglottis and allow for smooth passage of the scope. The thumb lever on the scope should be manipulated very slowly to allow for control of the scope position and adequate visualization of the airway structures. The scope should not be advanced if embedded in soft tissue as evidenced by a characteristic pink hue of the airway mucosa on the screen. After the scope is placed into the trachea, the tube is advanced along the scope into the trachea with the Murphy eye positioned anteriorly, this minimizes the incidence of hang up of the tracheal tube at the glottic opening by positioning the leading edge of the tube away from the right arytenoid, the most common location for hanging up of the tube.

Adult bronchoscopes can facilitate fiberoptic intubation in children. One method requires two providers. One places the bronchoscope at the glottic opening, while the other manipulates the tracheal tube independently into the trachea. This technique has the advantage over standard fiberoptic intubation of visualizing the passage of the tracheal tube through the vocal cords. A stylet in the tracheal tube will assist in directing the tube into the trachea [277]. A second technique involves the placement of a guidewire (e.g. 0.0035 in cardiac catheter guidewire, Mallinckrodt, St Louis, MO, USA) or tracheal tube exchanger into the trachea via the working channel of the bronchoscope. The bronchoscope is then removed and the tracheal tube advanced over the guidewire into the trachea [262,294–296].

In small children, the nasal route provides the most direct approach to the glottic opening with the flexible bronchoscope. This advantage has to be weighed against surgical considerations and the risk of nasal bleeding. Application of a vasoconstrictor such as oxymetazoline decreases this risk and visualizing the nasal passage prior to placing the tube may provide information as to the presence of polyps, adenoid tissue or narrowing that may impede advancement of the tracheal tube. The tracheal tube size should be matched closely to the fiberoptic bronchoscope size to reduce the incidence of impingement of the tracheal tube on glottic structures. Rotation of the tracheal tube 90° counterclockwise will orient the Murphy eye anteriorly, and may enhance placement through the glottic opening [297].

During fiberoptic intubation, ventilation can be enhanced using the Frei endoscopy mask, which incorporates a perforated silicone membrane that allows passage of the bronchoscope [298]. Alternatively, one may use the "mask mouth technique" in which the facemask is applied only to the mouth and one nare is occluded while the bronchoscope is advanced through the opposite nasal passage [299].

The laryngeal mask can serve as a conduit for intubation and an adjunct for ventilation in children with difficult airways. There are several manufactured designs and shapes but ideally the mask should provide full glottic exposure without encroachment of the epiglottis into the mask bowl. Prior to using a laryngeal mask as a conduit for intubation, it is critical to confirm that all components of the selected tracheal tube easily pass through the selected mask. Some masks will not accommodate the pilot balloon, particularly in smaller sizes [300,301].

To facilitate bronchoscopy through the laryngeal mask, a bronchoscope adaptor is placed on the 15 mm connector of the tracheal tube; the tracheal tube is then placed in the airway tube of the laryngeal mask and the cuff inflated. The anesthesia circuit is then attached to the tracheal tube and ventilation is established. An occlusive adhesive (e.g. Tegaderm™) can be applied to the bronchoscope adaptor to maintain a seal around the bronchoscope. Fiberoptic bronchoscopy is then carried out through the tracheal tube. When the trachea is entered, the tracheal tube cuff is deflated and the entire tube-bronchoscope adaptor unit is advanced into the trachea (Fig. 14.14) [302]. Removal of the laryngeal mask is challenging in children because the length of the tracheal tube is often similar to the length of the laryngeal mask tube. Techniques that may assist in laryngeal mask removal include using two tubes joined together to extend the working length, using a long pair of laryngeal forceps or using a tube stabilizer or exchanger.

Modified optical laryngoscopes

A variety of modified optical laryngoscopes have been developed to aid with direct visualization of the glottis in difficult airway pediatric patients. At the time of writing, there is not a sufficient body of knowledge with which to judge the comparative efficacy and complications of each of the devices. However, a number of case reports and case series have been published to date.

The Bullard laryngoscope (Circon ACMI, Stamford, CT) represents one of the earliest designs of optical laryngoscope. It consists of a curved metal blade with an integrated fiberoptic light source attached to an eyepiece. It provides an indirect view of the glottic opening and requires minimal mouth opening (0.64 cm) for insertion. Like many optical laryngoscopes, visualization may be limited by secretions. In a series of 93 children aged 1 day to 10 years, intubation was successful in 90 patients (97%). Two failures were attributed to excess secretions [303].

The Airtraq® (King Systems, Noblesville, IN) is an intubating device that consists of a curved blade with two adjacent channels. It is designed to provide glottic exposure without alignment of the oral, pharyngeal or laryngeal axes. One channel houses the optical system containing a series of prisms and lenses which end in a viewfinder (Fig. 14.15), while the second channel acts as a holder for the tracheal tube and a guide for advancing the tube into the trachea [304]. The infant Airtraq accepts tracheal tubes of internal diameter 2.5–3.5 mm, while the pediatric version accepts tubes of internal diameter 3.5–5.5 mm. The device is also available with the posterior surface removed to facilitate nasal

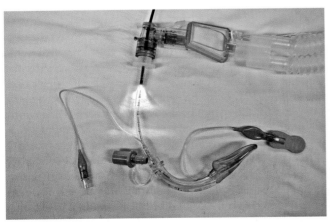

Figure 14.14 A bronchoscope adaptor is placed on the 15 mm connector of the tracheal tube, which is then placed in the airway tube of the laryngeal mask. This facilitates air exchange during bronchoscopic intubation.

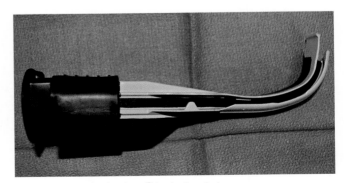

Figure 14.15 Pediatric Airtraq® intubating device.

intubation. After lubrication of the Airtraq channel and blade surface, the Airtraq is inserted in the midline of the pharynx and the tip placed in the vallecula. The device is adjusted so that the glottis is located in the center of the viewfinder, after which the tracheal tube is advanced into the trachea. After confirmation of successful tracheal intubation, the tracheal tube is moved laterally away from the Airtraq and the device slowly withdrawn. The Airtraq has been used successfully in patients with difficult direct laryngoscopy due to craniofacial anomalies such as Treacher Collins syndrome and Robin sequence [305]. In a series of 20 children managed with the Airtraq for elective surgery, one patient required the use of a malleable stylet to facilitate intubation because of difficulty aligning the glottis in the center of the view, and a second patient required two attempts to achieve successful intubation [306]. Other methods have been described to facilitate tracheal intubation with an Airtraq. These include the use of a gum elastic bougie, a flexible or malleable tracheal tube, and utilizing a fiberoptic bronchoscope [307,308]. Like many indirect devices for tracheal intubation, difficulty with tube passage is more common in infants and small children. This problem is also common with the non-channeled video and optical devices, and underscores the fact that the infant and neonatal airways are different from those of toddlers and older children [309].

The Truview EVO2 (Truphatek International, Netanya, Israel) is an indirect rigid laryngoscope with an angulated blade tip. The laryngoscope incorporates an optical lens that ends in an eyepiece that allows the operator to "see around the corner" and obtain an improved glottic view. It has an integrated oxygen port that allows oxygen administration during intubation. Tracheal intubation is achieved by placing the blade in the midline in the pharynx and following the curve of the tongue to the glottic opening. Once the glottis is visualized, the tracheal tube is advanced into the trachea. In a prospective comparison of intubation conditions between the Truview and the Miller laryngoscope in 60 neonates and infants, the Truview provided a statistically significant improvement in view with comparable intubation times [310]. In addition, since the Truview does not require neck extension for visualization and tracheal intubation, it can be used in patients with immobile cervical spines [311].

Video laryngoscopes

The miniaturization of video technology has fueled a revolution in laryngoscope design. There is a rapidly growing selection of video laryngoscopes available for pediatric use, such as the Glidescope®, the Storz Video Laryngoscope, the McGrath Scope, and the Pentax Airway Scope. This section will focus on devices with specific pediatric designs.

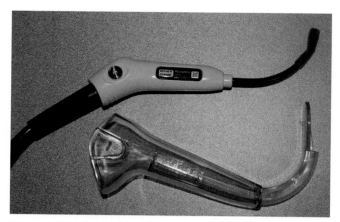

Figure 14.16 Glidescope® Cobalt and disposable plastic blade.

Glidescope® (see Video clip 14.5)

The Glidescope® (Verathon Medical, Bothell, WA) is a curved laryngoscope with an integrated miniature camera and a heated lens to minimize fogging during laryngoscopy. The device has evolved over the years from a bulky unit to a slim design (Glidescope® Cobalt, Fig. 14.16). The Cobalt consists of a camera stick that is inserted into a disposable plastic sheath. A high-resolution image is displayed on a small portable video screen. The blade of the device is placed in the midline of the pharynx and the tip placed in the vallecula. A styletted tracheal tube is usually necessary, and although the manufacturer recommends a 50–60° angulation of the tube, others report higher success in placing the tube with a 90° hockey-stick configuration [312]. Passage of the tracheal tube should be directly visualized during placement prior to its appearance on the video monitor to avoid injury to pharyngeal structures [313–319]. The Cobalt is available with a variety of blade sizes. When compared with direct laryngoscopy in difficult airway patients, it has been shown to improve the glottic view [319–321].

There remains a population of patients in whom significant difficulty is encountered with tracheal tube placement despite an adequate glottic view with the Glidescope. These difficulties can arise from a number of factors including the limited ability to manipulate the tube within the smaller pediatric pharynx, the acute angulation of the tracheal tube causing impingement on the anterior commissure or anterior trachea, and difficulty locating the tube in the pharynx after inserting the blade [322]. Some practitioners advocate placing the tracheal tube and Glidescope simultaneously as a single unit or placing the tracheal tube in the pharynx under direct vision prior to placing the Glidescope. If the tracheal tube impinges on the anterior trachea or anterior commissure, the Glidescope should be withdrawn slightly to decrease

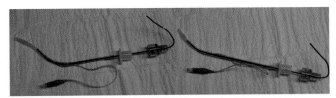

Figure 14.17 The tracheal tube on the left is "reverse loaded" by rotating the Murphy eye anteriorly on the stylet.

the anterior displacement of the glottis, allowing the axis of the tube and the trachea to become better aligned, and rotating the tube so that its concavity is oriented more posteriorly ("reverse loading", Fig. 14.17). The gum elastic bougie has also been utilized as a guide for tracheal intubation in children using the Glidescope [323].

There will always be certain patients in whom the Glidescope and other video laryngoscopes will fail so alternatives need to be readily available for difficult airway patients.

Storz video laryngoscope

The Storz video laryngoscope (SVL; Karl Storz Company, Tuttingen, Germany) incorporates a camera into various standard blades. The Storz DCI video laryngoscope is a rigid blade that integrates fiberoptics and a lens into the light source of Miller- and Macintosh-type blades [324]. The blades connect to a device-specific camera that transmits the image to a video monitor. The use of the SVL is similar to other video laryngoscopes in that the blade is placed in the midline followed by insertion of the tracheal tube. Advancing the tracheal tube along the shaft of the blade rather than from the right side of the pharynx as in traditional laryngoscopy facilitates quick visualization on the video monitor and avoids injury to the palatoglossal structures. The SVL has been successfully employed in intubating the trachea of patients with normal airways and has been reported to be more efficacious in pediatric difficult airway patients when compared to direct laryngoscopy. A one grade improvement in view (Cormack and Lehane) can be expected compared to Miller blade laryngoscopy [324–330]. Use of the SVL requires adequate mouth opening and practiced hand–eye co-ordination. The view through the SVL may be limited by fogging, which can be decreased by use of an anti-fog solution or prewarming the device.

Optical stylets

Optical stylets were first introduced into clinical practice in the 1970s and remain useful adjuncts in the management of the pediatric difficult airway. The optical stylet consists of a fiberoptic bundle within a rigid or malleable J-shaped stylet that ends in an eyepiece. They can displace pharyngeal soft tissue because of their rigid form and are more easily maneuvered than flexible scopes.

They often incorporate a port for insufflating oxygen to minimize secretions and fogging. However, we do not recommend oxygen insufflation even at low flow rates as pneumothorax and subcutaneous emphysema remain ever-present risks in infants [331–333]. Optical stylets are simple to assemble and their use involves a short learning curve. Furthermore, they are inexpensive when compared to fiberoptic bronchoscopes and video or optical laryngoscopes. The optical stylet allows visualization of the tracheal tube as it passes through the vocal cords because the stylet is recessed within the tracheal tube during intubation. However, their may be compromised by secretions or fogging.

Bonfils fiberscope

The Bonfils fiberscope (Karl Storz Company,Tuttingen, Germany) is a rigid fiberoptic stylet with a J-shaped 45° anterior-angulated tip. It provides a 90° angle of view and is available in all pediatric sizes. It is designed to be used via the retromolar approach, which brings the glottis into view rapidly and avoids negotiating the stylet around the bulk of the tongue. Once at the glottic opening, the preloaded tracheal tube is advanced through the vocal cords under direct vision. Some practitioners recommend the use of a rigid laryngoscope to create space for placement of the scope; however, some authors recommend against the use of this device in neonates [308,334–337]. The small optic aperture and significant 40-fold magnification render the visualization vulnerable to secretions [335]. In a simulated difficult pediatric airway, the Bonfils was easier to use and associated with better views of the larynx than direct laryngoscopy; however, intubation success rate and intubation times were similar [338].

Shikani Optical Stylet

The Shikani Optical Stylet (SOS; Clarus Medical, Minneapolis, MN) is a malleable, stainless steel J-shaped stylet with an enclosed fiberoptic bundle [339]. The pediatric SOS is 27cm long and can accommodate tracheal tubes as small as 2.5mm internal diameter. The SOS has been successfully used to intubate neonates and older children with a difficult airway. Extension of the head and application of jaw thrust facilitates elevation of the epiglottis off the posterior pharyngeal wall, which facilitates passage of the stylet [250,340–344]. The SOS is useful in patients who require maintenance of a neutral cervical spine during tracheal intubation [345]. Like the Bonfils, tracheal intubation can be accomplished efficiently and effectively with the assistance of the direct laryngoscope [346]. Use of the SOS is associated with minimal airway stimulation, permitting intubation in sedated children [131]. The SOS is lightweight, easily prepared and cleaned, and useful in managing the difficult airway in size ranges.

Lighted stylet

The lighted stylet allows tracheal intubation by observation of a transilluminated light in the neck. This often requires a darkened operating room to allow optimal visualization of the light. After loading the tracheal tube onto the lighted stylet, it is inserted orally in the midline of the pharynx while performing jaw thrust and the transilluminated light is located as a cone of light in the neck just above the suprasternal notch. It is critical that the light is located in the midline of the neck, as any deviation from the midline will direct the tube towards the esophagus. The centrally located light is then observed as the stylet is advanced caudally. Once the glottis is entered, the operator feels the stylet moving past the cords and observes an intensification of the light in the neck. Sometimes light is conducted down the trachea, creating a characteristic "cone of light" effect. The tracheal tube is then advanced off the stylet and tracheal placement confirmed by the usual means. Resistance during advancement of the stylet towards the glottis may suggest that the device is off midline or the tip may be entrapped in the vallecula or on the aryepiglottic fold. This requires retraction of the device and reinsertion while improving jaw thrust to elevate the epiglottis off the posterior pharyngeal wall [347].

Lighted stylet-guided intubation utilizes tactile and visual cues to successfully place the tracheal tube, it is a low-cost technique that is easily learned and remains useful in cases where visualization of the glottis is difficult or impossible. It can be employed in awake patients with difficult airways and can be successfully utilized via the nasal route [348–355]. In a cohort of patients with normal airways, the lighted stylet was as efficacious for tracheal intubation as the Airtraq® [356].

In 1957, Sir Robert Macintosh was the first to describe the use of a lighted stylet to facilitate intubation [357]. Since the advent of his 18-inch illuminated tracheal tube introducer, there have been many stylet designs. The fiberoptic lighted intubation stylet (Anesthesia Medical Specialties, Santa Fe, CA) is available in pediatric sizes, accommodating tracheal tubes as small as 3.5 mm internal diameter. Lighted stylets for use with tube diameters less than 3.5 mm can be fashioned by inserting a single fiberoptic light pipe adjacent to an appropriately sized stylet for the selected tracheal tube. The light pipe is illuminated by a fiberoptic light source and in this manner a lightwand can be created for any sized patient (Fig. 14.18).

Digital intubation

Digital intubation is a rarely taught technique that should be learned by pediatric anesthesiologists [358]. It predates direct laryngoscopy and may have been performed as early as the 1500s. It can be performed rapidly in patients

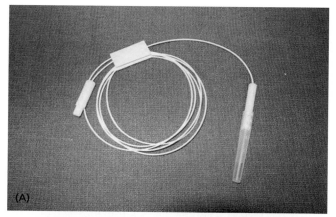

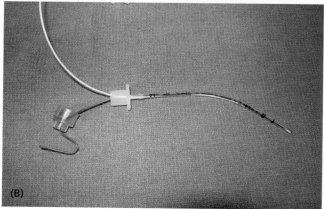

Figure 14.18 Lighted stylets for use with tube diameters less than 3.5 mm can be fashioned by inserting a single fiberoptic light pipe adjacent to an appropriately sized stylet for the selected tracheal tube. (A) Narrow gauge single fiberoptic light pipe. (B) Final assembly of fiberoptic light pipe, stylet, and endotracheal tube. See text for further explanation.

who may be difficult to intubate by direct laryngoscopy or who may be in a position that does not allow easy access to the airway (e.g. extubation in the prone position). To perform a digital intubation, the anesthesiologist stands at the side of the patient facing the head of the operating room table. The gloved non-dominant index finger is placed along the surface of the tongue in the midline and is advanced to feel the epiglottis, and then the finger is advanced further until the aryepiglottic folds are located. The dominant hand holds a styletted tracheal tube in a C-shaped configuration like a pencil and slides the tube alongside the non-dominant finger. The tip of the tracheal tube is directed through the glottis by the non-dominant finger and tracheal intubation is confirmed by the usual means. In a report of 39 digital intubations in 37 neonates, the mean time to intubation was 7 sec. All the patients were successfully intubated; one patient required two attempts [359].

Extubation of the difficult airway

Extubation of the difficult airway can occasionally be more challenging than the intubation and requires careful planning and preparation to avoid complications. The operating room should be prepared in a similar fashion to the set-up for intubation and the device successfully utilized in securing the airway should be available in the operating room. In selected cases, the use of an airway exchange catheter (Cook, Bloomington, IN) may be beneficial in the extubation of children with difficult airways. The Cook catheter is placed through the lumen of the tracheal tube into the trachea and is left in place after extubation. The catheter allows the administration of supplemental oxygen through a central hollow core. In a series of 20 pediatric difficult airway patients with an exchange catheter in place, five underwent successful reintubation over the catheter. No sedatives were required with the exchange catheter in place [360].

Surgical airway

On extremely rare occasions, the anesthesiologist may encounter a dire "can't ventilate/can't intubate" situation associated with prolonged hypoxemia which, if left untreated, would likely result in patient mortality. Therefore, every pediatric anesthesiologist should have a reasonable approach to obtaining a surgical airway should this rare event occur. Cricothyroidotomy was first described in 1969 [361]. There are three methods of achieving oxygenation via the cricothyroid membrane: the small cannula (often an intravenous angiocatheter) approach, the commercially available large cannula approach using the Seldinger technique, and the open surgical technique in which a tracheostomy tube is inserted. The techniques of choice for anesthesiologists and others not trained in open surgical tracheostomy are the needle cricothyroidotomy and Seldinger guided placement techniques.

Angiocatheter technique

The angiocatheter technique is probably the most plausible in pediatric patients requiring emergency surgical airway access. A needle cricothyroidotomy can be achieved using a 14, 16 or 18 gauge angiocatheter that is placed through the cricothyroid membrane. While extending the cervical spine, the angiocatheter connected to a syringe of saline is introduced in the midline in the lower half of the cricothyroid membrane at a 45° angle in an inferior and posterior direction [362]. The syringe attached to the angiocatheter is gently aspirated during insertion, and return of air confirms tracheal entry. The catheter is then advanced off the needle into the trachea. A high-pressure oxygen source (such as a wall oxygen supply or jet ventilator) is needed to overcome the resistance of the catheter in order to deliver effective oxygenation (ventilation is not readily achieved). The oxygen source can be connected to the catheter by a 3 mL syringe with the plunger removed and attached to a 15 mm tracheal tube adaptor. Barotrauma is a risk of ventilation through the angiocatheter, particularly in situations where exhalation is not possible because of upper airway obstruction. Structures at risk during the puncture are the superior thyroid artery along the lateral border of the membrane, the cricothyroid arteries, and the pyramidal lobe of the thyroid. The posterior tracheal wall could also be injured during the puncture attempt; thus, confirmation of correct placement is critically important as insufflation of high-pressure gas outside the trachea can cause life-threatening tension pneumomediastinum and tension pneumothorax. Even after correct placement, reassessment of positioning should occur frequently as children have little margin for error and a correctly placed catheter can become dislodged with minimal movement [363].

Large catheter Seldinger approach kits

Cricothyroidotomy kits based on the use of the Seldinger technique are now available for pediatric use. There are several manufactured kits that share common steps. A limited skin incision is made after identifying anatomical landmarks, a needle is inserted through the incision and cricothyroid membrane into the trachea, a guidewire is placed through the catheter and the catheter is removed leaving the guidewire in place. A dilator airway catheter assembly is advanced over the wire into the trachea and the guidewire and dilator are removed [364]. Ideally, pediatric anesthesiologists should develop expertise with this approach using an animal model or a specially designed patient simulator.

CASE STUDY

A 2-month-old, male former 31-week premature infant with Robin sequence presented for repair of bilateral large inguinal hernias, and open gastrostomy tube. Birthweight was 1600 g and it was evident after birth that the patient had significant micrognathia, with cleft palate. The patient had no other congenital anomalies, including no cardiac disease. He had moderate upper airway obstruction in the supine position without airway support. His airway had

Continued

been maintained with nasal CPAP of 5–7 cm H_2O, with FiO_2 0.21–0.30 and flows of 1–2 L/min. In addition, he was nursed in the lateral or prone positions. He had no major apnea/desaturation events, had grown slowly with nasogastric tube feeds and now weighed 1950 g. The multidisciplinary team of neonatologists, otolaryngologists, pulmonologists, and craniofacial anomaly specialists was considering tracheostomy to maintain airway patency. However, they were undecided at this point and wanted to address the hernias and a long-term feeding solution before attempting to wean the patient from CPAP and commiting him to a tracheostomy. The patient's trachea had never been intubated, and he had not had previous surgery or imaging procedures. Medications were multivitamins and iron, and he had no drug allergies. On physical examination, the patient had obvious significant micrognathia, normal cervical range of motion, and very mild retractions with no obvious upper airway obstruction on nasal CPAP of 5 cm H_2O, FiO_2 0.21. There was a small 6 Fr nasogastric tube in the right nare. The lungs were clear to auscultation bilaterally, there was no cardiac murmur, and a 2 Fr percutaneously inserted central catheter (PICC) was present in the right arm. SpO_2 was 96%, chest radiograph revealed clear lung fields, normal heart size and configuration, and the PICC was present in the midsuperior vena cava. Preoperative laboratory studies included hemoglobin concentration of 10.1 g/dL, a capillary blood gas of pH 7.36, $PaCO_2$ 44 mmHg, PaO_2 44 mmHg, and calculated base excess of +3 meq/L. After a discussion with the parents about the risks of difficult airway management and possible postoperative mechanical ventilation had occurred the day before, consent for anesthesia was obtained and the patient transported to the operating room.

The following equipment had been assembled in the OR: standard Miller 0 and 1 laryngoscope blades; styletted uncuffed endotracheal tubes of 2.5 and 3.0 mm sizes; oral airways size 000, 00, and 0; disposable straight laryngeal mask airways (LMA) size 1 and 1.5; Glidescope Cobalt® video laryngoscope with the small video baton and size 1 plastic laryngeal blade, and neonatal Magill forceps. Succinylcholine, 4 mg, and propofol, 6 mg were drawn up in syringes. After discussion with the pediatric anesthesia fellow, it was decided to use the LMA as a conduit for fiberoptic intubation. A second attending anesthesiologist was present for induction of anesthesia and tracheal intubation, and the patient's otolaryngologist, who was operating with a series of short cases in the adjacent OR, was alerted that the case was to start and was available for emergency back-up.

Standard monitors were placed, glycopyrrolate 0.02 mg was administered IV, the patient was preoxygenated with a facemask and FiO_2 1.0 for 3 min, and a #1 LMA, lubricated with 2% lidocaine gel, was inserted gently with the cuff

deflated and the patient awake. He tolerated this well, the cuff was inflated with 3 cc air, and the airway was patent with audible crying. After gentle awake assisted ventilation demonstrated good chest excursion, inhalation induction with sevoflurane, 2% inspired, and 5 L/min oxygen flow, was begun. Inspired sevoflurane was increased slowly to 4%, the patient had a patent airway throughout, and passed through stage II of general anesthesia without incident, and with manually assisted ventilation and end-tidal sevoflurane of 3% had SpO_2 99%, heart rate (HR) 135, and blood pressure (BP) 60/35. End-tidal carbon dioxide ($ETCO_2$) was 24 mmHg.

An extended 3.0 mm uncuffed ETT had been fashioned beforehand, made up of a standard 3.0 ETT with connector removed and the upper half of a second ETT taped with a single layer of clear plastic tape with the connector removed. The extended ETT was loaded onto a 2.2 mm pediatric fiberoptic bronchoscope (FOB), pushed up to the proximal end of the scope. The video image was displayed on three large screens in the OR. The FOB was lubricated, had antifog solution applied to the tip, and was inserted into the end of the LMA with a standard FOB elbow adaptor, and advanced easily down the shaft of the LMA, with the second anesthesiologist gently assisting ventilation and stabilizing the LMA. When the aperture of the bowl of the LMA was reached, the glottis was in clear view, with the epiglottis stented up by the LMA. Slight vocal cord abduction was observed with inspiration. Propofol 2 mg was administered to deepen anesthesia and produce apnea, and the FOB was advanced carefully, always with the airway lumen in view, until the vocal cords had been passed, and the cartilaginous tracheal rings and pars membranosa were clearly in view. The scope was advanced further to just above the carina, to avoid carinal stimulation. Then, the ETT was advanced down the scope, through the LMA, and very gently through the glottic opening, rotating the ETT so the beveled tip would be parallel to the vocal cord alignment. After passage of the ETT below the vocal cords, FOB position was checked and was still just above carina. The FOB was withdrawn slowly, and the ETT tip could be seen in mid trachea. The ETT connector was placed on the end of the extended ETT, and manual ventilation produced excellent chest rise, equal bilateral breath sounds, and persistent $ETCO_2$ of 45–50 mmHg. SpO_2 had decreased to 91% but quickly recovered to 99% after 30 sec of manual ventilation. HR was 120, BP slightly lower at 52/30, but with reduction in sevoflurane concentration to 2% and 10 mL lactated Ringer's solution bolus, returned within 2 min to 65/35. There was a leak around the ETT at 20 cm H_2O.

While grasping the ETT in the back of the oropharynx with the Magill forceps, the LMA cuff was deflated and the LMA removed gently over the extended ETT after the connector had been removed. The tape was removed from the extended ETT, producing a standard 3.0 ETT, the connector replaced, correct ETT placement and ventilation again verified, and the ETT secured in standard fashion. After the ETT was secured, a direct laryngoscopy was performed and a Grade IV Cormack and Lehane view was evident, even with external laryngeal manipulation. All airway procedures were detailed in the electronic anesthesia record, and a patient alert for difficult airway clearly noted. A caudal anesthetic and rectal acetaminophen were used for intra- and postoperative analgesia.

The case proceeded uneventfully and it was decided to transport the patient back to the neonatal intensive care unit (NICU) with the endotracheal tube in place. Analgesia was provided with morphine and the patient received 48h of mechanical ventilation, with good pain control. Extubation occurred in the NICU, with the patient awake, the anesthesiologist present at the bedside with LMA and fiberscope, and nasal CPAP ready to apply immediately after extubation. The patient was successfully extubated to nasal CPAP, spent another month in the NICU and was weaned from CPAP, with improved upper airway obstruction and good somatic growth, and was discharged home with pulse oximetry and apnea monitoring, without tracheostomy, at age 3 months. The parents were well aware of the difficulty with tracheal intubation.

Conclusions

This case illustrates the principles outlined in this chapter, including thorough discussion and preparation for the difficult airway, assembling all airway equipment and drugs beforehand, choosing one primary method of intubation with at least one back-up method available, having expert assistance immediately available, and planning for the difficult extubation. In addition, communication with other providers and parents, and documentation of airway procedures, are very important in the care of the patient with a difficult airway.

Annotated references

A full reference list for this chapter is available at:
http://www.wiley.com/go/gregory/andropoulos/pediatricanesthesia

1. Marcus CL, Smith RJ, Mankarious LA et al. Developmental aspects of the upper airway: report from an NHLBI Workshop, March 5–6, 2009. Proc Am Thorac Soc 2009; 6: 513–20. A contemporary evidence-based review of the development of the upper airway.
18. Litman RS, Weissend EE, Shrier DA et al. Morphologic changes in the upper airway of children during awakening from propofol administration. Anesthesiology 2002; 96: 607–11. A novel, important, and very interesting imaging study of airway morphology in children with emergence from anesthesia.
35. Dalal PG, Murray D, Messner AH et al. Pediatric laryngeal dimensions: an age-based analysis. Anesth Analg 2009; 108: 1475–9. A modern imaging study that challenges the classic notions of the anatomy and dimensions of the pediatric airway.
129. Markakis DA, Sayson SC, Schreiner MS. Insertion of the laryngeal mask airway in awake infants with the Robin sequence. Anesth Analg 1992; 75: 822–4. An early description of one of the most useful techniques for difficult intubation in small infants: awake LMA insertion followed by fiberoptic intubation.
143. Vialet R, Nau A, Chaumoitre K et al. Effects of head posture on the oral, pharyngeal and laryngeal axis alignment in infants and young children by magnetic resonance imaging. Paediatr Anaesth 2008; 18: 525–31. A contemporary imaging study challenging the classic teaching on the sniffing position, and delineating optimal head posture for alignment of oral, pharyngeal, and laryngeal axes in infants and young children.
144. Doherty JS, Froom SR, Gildersleve CD. Pediatric laryngoscopes and intubation aids old and new. Paediatr Anaesth 2009; 19(Suppl 1): 30–7. A comprehensive modern review of all of the intubation aids for pediatric patients.
164. Lerman J, Houle TT, Matthews BT et al. Propofol for tracheal intubation in children anesthetized with sevoflurane: a dose–response study. Paediatr Anaesth 2009; 19: 218–24. A modern controlled dose–response study of propofol for endotracheal intubation without muscle relaxation.
201. Weiss M, Dullenkopf A, Fischer JE et al. Prospective randomized controlled multi-centre trial of cuffed or uncuffed endotracheal tubes in small children. Br J Anaesth 2009; 103: 867–73. A modern well-designed trial of cuffed versus uncuffed endotracheal tubes in children.
221. Al Alami AA, Zestos MM, Baraka AS. Pediatric laryngospasm: prevention and treatment. Curr Opin Anaesth 2009; 22: 388–95. A contemporary review of laryngospasm and steps for prevention, recognition, and treatment.
321. Armstrong J, John J, Karsli C. A comparison between the GlideScope Video Laryngoscope and direct laryngoscope in paediatric patients with difficult airways – a pilot study. Anaesthesia 2010; 65: 353–7. A contemporary comparative study with one of the most widely used videolaryngoscopes, and conventional laryngoscopy in the difficult pediatric airway.

Video clips

This chapter contains the following video clips:

Video clip 14.1 Fundamentals of fiberoptic intubation.
Video clip 14.2 Oral fiberoptic intubation.
Video clip 14.3 Nasal fiberoptic intubation.
Video clip 14.4 Fiberoptic intubation via laryngeal mask airway.
Video clip 14.5 Videolaryngoscope intubation.
They can be accessed at:
http://www.wiley.com/go/gregory/andropoulos/pediatricanesthesia

CHAPTER 15

Induction, Maintenance, and Emergence from Anesthesia

Jerrold Lerman[1,2], Venkata Sampathi[3] & Stacey Watt[1,2]

[1]Department of Anesthesia, Women and Children's Hospital of Buffalo, [2]State University at Buffalo, Buffalo and Strong Memorial Hospital, University of Rochester, NY, USA

[3]Department of Anesthesiology, SUNY Upstate University Hospital, Syracuse, NY, USA

Evaluation of preoperative data

The preoperative assessment of a child for general anesthesia requires a focused and systematic review of the history and organ systems. The assessment should include details of the past medical history, current and recent medications, allergies, family history, nil per os (NPO) status, physical examination, and necessary ancillary testing.

Before beginning a detailed medical history, it is important to document a review of the child's vital signs, fasting status, and weight. A discussion of the fasting guidelines before surgery is found below. The child's weight should be assessed to determine whether he/she is normal weight, overweight or obese. An estimation of the child's ideal bodyweight may be calculated using the formulas:

For children ≤ 8 years of age: weight (kg)
$= 2 \times$ age (years) $+ 9$
For children > 8 years of age: weight (kg)
$= 3 \times$ age (years).

An estimate of the obese child's bodyweight for drug and fluid management should be based on the child's ideal bodyweight for age plus one-third the difference between the actual weight and the ideal weight.

The identity and legal status of the parent, guardian or person accompanying the child must be established preoperatively to ensure the consent for anesthesia and surgery is legal and appropriate medical information is available and accurate. If the patient is >18 years of age, he/she may consent for surgery. However, if the patient is cognitively challenged, a health proxy (i.e. legal guardian) is required to consent for surgery irrespective of the patient's age.

Family history of inheritable disorders or serious reactions that were potentially fatal under anesthesia should be solicited. Specific mention should be made of malignant hyperthermia and muscle wasting diseases, which are discussed below.

In reviewing the past medical history, the child's gestational age at birth is important, as infants who were born prematurely (i.e. <37 weeks' gestational age) may require overnight observation for perioperative apnea (see Premature Infant below) if their postconceptual age is currently <60 weeks. Furthermore, full-term neonates up to 4 weeks' postnatal age should not undergo general anesthesia on an ambulatory basis; they too should be admitted and monitored overnight.

A complete review of systems should be done during the assessment, including the cardiac, respiratory, gastrointestinal, genitourinary and renal organs, central nervous system, endocrine, and musculoskeletal systems.

Children with congenital heart disease, or their parents or guardians, should be questioned regarding the nature and status of the heart defect; whether the defect resolved spontaneously or required surgery; if surgery was performed; the nature and date of the surgery; recent admissions or physician visits related to following up the cardiac defect; and cardiac medications prescribed. In most instances, a recent cardiology evaluation should be available, including an updated echocardiogram to provide evidence of the heart's function and the need for antibiotic prophylaxis for subacute bacterial endocarditis. If the child's feeding, activity, color or vital signs have changed substantially since the last cardiac evaluation, consideration should be given to delaying the surgery for further cardiac evaluation.

If a murmur is detected during preoperative assessment, it is important to establish whether the murmur is new or old and whether its nature has changed. If there are no signs or symptoms of growth or activity delays, shortness of breath, blue spells, syncope or feeding problems, then a consultation with a cardiologist may be required based on the quality and duration of the murmur, whether and where it radiates, the presence of a diastolic murmur, and whether there is evidence of heart failure. If there is any uncertainty about the pathological nature of the murmur, a cardiologist should be consulted.

Illnesses affecting the respiratory system range from minor to life threatening. Discussions of the child with an upper respiratory tract infection (URTI) and respiratory compromise follow. Apart from congenital anomalies that may present in the perinatal period (such as congenital diaphragmatic hernia or congenital lobar emphysema), it should be determined whether the child has recently had serious croup or respiratory syncytial virus and whether the child was admitted to hospital for other respiratory ailments.

Children who present for tonsillectomy and adenoidectomy have either chronic infectious tonsillitis or obstructive sleep apnea (OSA). For the latter, most children have a clinical diagnosis based on the otolaryngologist's assessment of the severity of the symptoms. There are no clinical criteria that are diagnostic for OSA in children; thus the diagnosis of OSA can only be made by polysomnography [1]. Children with OSA are usually normal in

weight but snore loudly at night. They may stop breathing during their sleep and may arouse without actual awakening. They are often fatigued in the morning, despite having slept a full night. Many of them experience nocturnal enuresis and have attention deficit disorder and/or exhibit behavioral and learning difficulties at school. It is important to determine whether a polysomnogram was performed and if so, the oxygen saturation nadir during sleep. Children whose nadir is <85% show greater sensitivity to respiratory depression (apnea) with standard doses of opioids. If a polysomnogram was not done, opioid sensitivity can be evaluated during anesthesia by observing the child's respiratory responses to small doses of opioids while he/she breathes spontaneously. If apnea occurs in response to opioids, reduced doses must be administered cautiously during anesthesia and postoperatively to minimize the risk of perioperative adverse airway events.

Gastroesophageal reflux disease (GERD) is a national pandemic in children. Many children are diagnosed with reflux and treated with antireflux medication, even though they have no symptoms. Although most children undergo inhalational induction of anesthesia, including those with documented gastroesophageal reflux who undergo upper endoscopy, GERD does not appear to increase the risk for regurgitation and aspiration during anesthesia. Accordingly, we proceed with our usual anesthetic technique in children with gastroesophageal reflux.

Children with renal insufficiency or failure require a complete blood count and electrolyte panel preoperatively. If the child has renal failure, the type of dialysis and the timing of the last dialysis treatment, as well as how much fluid was removed, should be documented.

Children with Down syndrome present interesting challenges from a variety of perspectives. They range in cognitive function from very difficult behavioral problems to high-functioning, very pleasant children. It is important to obtain a complete cardiac history in these children because congenital heart disease (e.g. ventricular septal defect and endocardial cushion defect) is common. These children frequently have asymptomatic subglottic narrowing and require a tracheal tube sizes 0.5 to 1 mm ID smaller than expected for age. Much has been written about the instability of the cervical spine in these children despite the fact that there are only isolated reports of neurological sequelae associated with general anesthesia and surgery [2]. Evidence of a pre-existing neurological complaint, that the child suddenly favors one hand or foot over the other or has had a change in gait, complains of pain in the neck, is unable to turn the head to one side or the other, or complains of dizziness or fainting should be noted and are reason for concern regarding the integrity of the cervical spine. In such cases, a neurological investigation should be sought before proceeding with anesthesia. Although the American Academy of Pediatrics recommends cervical spine imaging in all 3–5-year-old children with Down syndrome, there is no evidence that these investigations are predictive of adverse neurological outcomes in the perioperative period. During anesthesia and tracheal intubation, the necks of these children should be maintained in a neutral position at all times.

Children with diabetes mellitus present a number of challenges in the perioperative period [3]. Those whose diabetes is controlled with diet or oral medications should have their morning blood sugar checked. These children do not usually require additional care and can resume their diet and medications postoperatively. Insulin-dependent diabetes presents a more complex management problem. A thorough history should detail their diabetes control, whether they experience hypo- or hyperglycemia, their typical HbA_{1c} concentration (typically <9%), the type and frequency of insulin, and whether they use an insulin pump. In many instances, the endocrinologist responsible for managing their diabetes provides a protocol to the patient and staff that recommends management of the diabetes in the perioperative period. Children who are prone to hypoglycemia should have a glucose infusion and measurement of periodic blood sugar concentrations (or finger pricks) during surgery and anesthesia. If the preoperative blood sugar is >250 mg%, a sliding scale of insulin should be started to reduce the blood sugar. Children who have insulin pumps should also have a fasting glucose measured and their pump set to basal rate during surgery; if the pump alarms with high or low blood sugars during surgery, a blood glucose should be determined to validate the alarm and appropriate action should be taken based on the result.

Children with muscle disorders, specifically malignant hyperthermia and the dystrophies and myopathies, are discussed below.

In adolescents, it is important to establish their use of tobacco and illicit drugs, which may not be possible until the child is separated from the parents. If there is any suspicion that illicit drugs, such as cocaine, crack or other cardiac and neurotoxins have been consumed recently, a toxicology screen should be obtained.

A list of medications, the frequency of their use, and when they were last taken should be compiled. Liquid medications may be taken on the morning of surgery. Children who take medication in pill form will often only take it when it is mixed with food. These medications, often antiepileptic drugs, should not be taken before surgery. β-Blockers and α2-agonists should be continued in the perioperative period, as suddenly stopping them may cause rebound effects. Since angiotensin-converting enzyme (ACE) inhibitors have been reported to cause severe hypotension in adults when taken on the day of surgery [4], their ingestion should be suspended for that day. Herbal medications, particularly St John's wort and most medications that begin with the letter "g" (e.g. garlic, gingko biloba), should be stopped at least 1 week before anesthesia [5,6].

Allergies present a very serious conundrum for anesthesiologists. Any drug reaction that a parent or child reports as abnormal is listed as an allergy in the chart. The reactions may be recognized effects of the drug (i.e. a flat skin rash after amoxicillin). Once a medication is listed as an allergy on a patient's chart, it is often difficult, if not impossible, to expunge it from the list. Examples of "allergic reactions" that are not allergic reactions that were reported to the authors while preparing this chapter include allergy to epinephrine because it causes headaches, a diaper rash from oral sulfonamide antibiotic, and a penicillin rash that occurred in the parent but was listed on the child's chart. Most allergies listed in the patients' charts have no immunological basis. Flat skin rashes produced by oral liquid antibiotics are almost certainly non-immunological in origin and warrant re-exposing the child to the antibiotic (if needed) if there was no re-exposure for 5 years. Egg allergy is not a contraindication to propofol [7]; soy and peanut allergies are contraindications only to propofol manufactured in Europe. Latex is commonly cited as an allergy. Skin (and hand) latex reactions are generally cited but are generally are non-immunological and do not proceed to systemic anaphylactic reactions. With the removal of latex from most medical products, children with spina bifida and congenital urological abnormalities are no longer exposed to latex products repeatedly and do not develop latex allergy [8]. These children are not born with a latex allergy, although one parent indicated that she was informed of such a predisposition in a spina bifida clinic. The most important question to ask regarding latex susceptibility is whether the child develops any reaction when he/she touches a toy balloon to her/his lips or the dentist inserts a rubber dam in the mouth. If the lips or tongue swell, then it is highly probable the child is immunologically allergic to latex. A latex-free environment in the operating room ensures safe care of children who are latex allergic.

Before any child is anesthetized, physical examination of the head and neck, chest, and heart must be performed. Physical examination of the head and neck includes the extent of mouth opening, ability to extend the tongue and neck and the state of the dentition, including loose teeth and any detachable plates or oral appliances. The latter must be removed before surgery. All metal piercings and objects must be removed to prevent aspiration (if they are within the oropharynx) or a skin burn if electrocautery is used [9].

Auscultation of the heart and lungs should be performed and recorded on the preoperative record. Any abnormal findings should be recorded and if necessary evaluated preoperatively.

Routine laboratory testing, such as complete blood counts, chemistry profiles, and urinalysis examination, is not indicated for most elective pediatric surgical procedures. However, if large blood loss is expected, a preoperative complete blood count and blood for type and screen or cross-match should be performed. In some children, it may be necessary to wait until they are anesthetized and intravenous access is established before sufficient blood can be obtained for the required tests.

The most recent recommendations by the ASA Task Force on Preanesthesia Evaluation state that "the literature is insufficient to inform patients or physicians on whether anesthesia causes harmful effects on early pregnancy. Pregnancy testing may be offered to female patients of childbearing age and for whom the result would alter the patient's management" [10]. We require a preoperative pregnancy test for all menarchal females who require anesthesia at our institution. If the test is positive, we inform the patient of the result and work towards a decision on whether to proceed with surgery and anesthesia. If we proceed with anesthesia, the optimal anesthetic technique for the mother and fetus must be reached by consensus with the pregnant mother.

The clinical value of a chest radiograph in a child about to undergo surgery is typically less than that of an oxygen saturation determination. An oxygen saturation reading of <95% is abnormal and may suggest deterioration of the child's pulmonary or cardiac status. This warrants further investigation.

Specialized tests such as electrocardiography and echocardiography can be invaluable clinical tools in a child with known congenital heart disease or myocardial dysfunction. These tests help to evaluate the cardiac anatomy, intracardiac shunting, ventricular function, right-sided heart pressures, valvular function, and the presence of pleural or pericardial effusions.

Radiological investigations, such as computed tomography (CT) or magnetic resonance imaging (MRI), may be useful not only to the surgical team but also to an anesthetist when evaluating the scope of the disease process, especially those involving airway anatomy.

Once all of the relevant preoperative data have been compiled, an assessment of the "ASA physical status" of the child should be performed. This metric is an assessment of the child's pre-existing diseases, but it is not intended as a measure of perioperative risk (Box 15.1).

Medical conditions
Malignant hyperthermia
Preparation of the anesthetic machine for an elective case of malignant hyperthermia (MH) begins with scheduling the child as the first case of the day as the concentra-

---

Box 15.1 ASA physical status classification system

P1. A normal healthy patient
P2. A patient with mild systemic disease
P3. A patient with severe systemic disease
P4. A patient with severe systemic disease that is a constant threat to life
P5. A moribund patient who is not expected to survive the operation
P6. A declared brain-dead patient whose organs are being removed for donor purposes

---

tion of inhaled anesthetics in the operating room is at its nadir if the room was unused overnight [11]. The vaporizers should be removed from the machine, the anesthetic circuit flushed, and the carbon dioxide canisters replaced with new ones to reduce the concentration of anesthetics in the machine to ≤10 ppm. Removing the vaporizers from the machine ensures that they cannot be inadvertently turned on during the anesthetic and that anesthetic cannot leak into the circuit. The anesthetic circuit should be purged of all residual inhalational anesthetic by flushing the machine with a fresh gas flow of 10 L/min (air/oxygen mixture) while the ventilator is operating.

Although the threshold concentration of vapor above which MH occurs is unknown, most studies suggest that the inhaled agent concentration in the machine should be reduced to ≤10 ppm. For Ohmeda Excel machines, a 10–15-min flush at 10 Lpm air/oxygen achieves this. For the newer anesthetic workstations from Siemens (Kion) and Drager (Primus and Fabius), a 75-min flush may be required to achieve ≤10 ppm of anesthetic. To reduce the flush times of the latter three machines to <10 min, one may replace the integrated breathing circuit with autoclaved circuit components or insert charcoal absorbent in the inspiratory and expiratory limbs of the breathing circuit [12]. Data for the wash-out of anesthetics from the new Ohmeda-GE machines are pending.

Once the breathing circuit has been flushed, a trigger-free anesthetic that includes propofol, opioids, non-depolarizing muscle relaxants, nitrous oxide, benzodiazepines, and regional anesthesia (all local anesthetics) may be used [11]. Monitoring must include end-tidal CO_2 (the earliest sign of a MH reaction) and temperature. IV dantrolene should be available in sufficient quantity to treat a reaction should it occur (2.4 mg/kg IV to stop most reactions, but 10 mg/kg may be necessary). The elimination half-life of intravenous dantrolene is 10 h; recrudescence may occur after 6 h when the blood concentration of dantrolene falls below the 3 μg/mL threshold [13]. Redosing half the original dose of dantrolene at this time will prevent recrudescence. New, rapidly soluble formulations of dantrolene are currently under investigation [13]. There is no longer any role for prophylactic preoperative dantrolene in children with MH.

Myopathies

The anesthetic management of children with the common myopathies, including Duchenne muscular dystrophy (DMD), Becker muscular dystrophy, and Emery–Dreifuss syndrome, should be tailored to avoid medications that are known to induce rhabdomyolysis, hyperkalemia, and myoglobinuria. In children <8 years of age, DMD is associated with unstable muscular membranes because they lack dystrophin. The administration of an inhalational anesthetic (halothane >> sevoflurane) with or without succinylcholine destabilizes the muscle membrane and releases the cellular contents, including myoglobin and potassium [14]. As the children reach adolescence, the muscle wasting in DMD abates and the predominant anesthetic concern is a progressive cardiomyopathy. In the case of Emery–Dreifuss, heart block may be the complicating presentation. Hence, preoperative echocardiogram and electrocardiogram are warranted before anesthetizing adolescents with DMD or Emery–Dreifuss syndrome.

The interaction between anesthetics and mitochondrial myopathies is far less clear [15]. Some children with myocardial myopathy develop lactic acidosis during infancy. Children with myopathies should receive normal saline for their intravenous solution as lactated Ringer's solution will increase lactate concentrations. Although MH is only associated with King–Denborough and central core diseases, rhabdomyolysis may theoretically occur in children with mitochondrial myopathies who receive an inhalational anesthetic. Hence, it is reasonable to flush the anesthetic machine before the child is anesthetized as if preparing for an MH patient. Even though many such children have been anesthetized with inhalational anesthetics without complications, it seems reasonable to recommend alternative anesthetics whenever possible, i.e. total intravenous anesthesia (TIVA).

Nil per os

All children scheduled for elective surgery should be fasted according to the ASA guidelines (Box 15.2) [16]. Note the fasting intervals are not age adjusted. Children who chew gum must expectorate the gum before induction of anesthesia. Although gum increases gastric fluid volume, the risk of regurgitation and aspiration pneumo-nia is not increased by chewing gum, therefore surgery need not be delayed [17].

The bowels of patients requiring emergency surgery cease peristaltic action as soon as the injury occurs. Peristalsis may further be impaired by the administration of opioids. Hence, all foods present in the stomach at the time of injury likely remain there until peristalsis resumes. The time until peristalsis resumes after an injury and after opioid administration is unpredictable. The only time interval that correlates inversely with the risk of aspiration pneumonitis (i.e. gastric fluid pH <2.5 and gastric volume >0.4 mL/kg) is the last oral intake-to-injury interval [18]. Bowel sounds alone do not confirm the resumption of intestinal peristalsis and gastric emptying, although passing of gas almost certainly indicates that peristalsis has resumed. We consider all children who undergo emergency surgery to be at risk for regurgitation and aspiration of gastric contents and take appropriate airway precautions.

Upper respiratory tract infection

Children who have had a recent upper respiratory tract infection (URTI) should not undergo non-emergency anesthesia for 4–6 weeks after the infection to ensure resolution of the pathological effects in the small airways. Because young children have 6–7 URTIs per year, most clinicians proceed with anesthesia 2–4 weeks after the original infection. When children present for elective surgery with a URTI, we recommend canceling the anesthetic if any one of the criteria in Box 15.3 is present[19] as each increases the risk of perioperative airway events.

Children with clear rhinorrhea, whether due to a mild URTI or allergic rhinitis, should receive 1–2 drops of oxymetazoline or neosynephrine (0.25%) per nostril to reduce nasopharyngeal secretions during anesthesia. We prefer to manage these children with a facemask to reduce the risk of airway reflex responses but if the airway must be manipulated, a supraglottic airway may trigger fewer airway reflex responses than a tracheal tube.

Asthma

Up to 20% of children have asthma or an asthmatic history, but many fewer present with severe asthma that may complicate anesthesia [20]. Children with a history of asthma must be in optimal pulmonary condition and

---

Box 15.2 Fasting intervals before elective surgery

• Clear fluids	2 h
• Breast milk	4 h
• Infant formula	6 h
• Solids	8 h

Box 15.3 Criteria for canceling elective surgery in a child with a URTI

1. Fever >38.5°C
2. Behavioral and eating changes
3. Mucopurulent secretions
4. Lower respiratory tract wheezing or rhonchi that do not clear with deep coughing

without a recent exacerbation or recent hospitalization with asthma to proceed with elective anesthesia and surgery [21]. The preoperative assessment should determine the age at onset of asthma, number of and date of the most recent hospital admissions for asthma, treatment (β2-agonists or steroids by inhalation), and current state of the asthma. Most children with asthma have never stayed overnight in hospital. If they have, the asthma is severe and should be carefully assessed. If oral steroids have been prescribed recently for an acute exacerbation of asthma, careful preoperative examination of the chest must be performed to ensure that there is no lingering reactive airway component.

On the morning of surgery, the child's lungs should be examined to check for wheezing. Preoperative bronchodilator therapy should be administered to non-wheezing children with mild-to-moderate asthma, as this reduces airway resistance during sevoflurane anesthesia and tracheal intubation by about 25% [22]. If wheezing is present, the child should be instructed to cough deeply to clear any airway secretions present, and bronchodilator therapy should then be administered. If the wheezing persists, the child should be referred to their pulmonologist for reassessment and the anesthetic deferred.

Preoperative bronchodilator therapy should be administered to children who are wheezing and present for emergency or urgent non-airway surgery. If tracheal intubation can be avoided, a facemask or laryngeal mask airway (LMA) should be used. An inadequate depth of anesthesia can cause laryngospasm when an LMA is in place. Equipment should be prepared to administer intraoperative bronchodilator therapy should the need arise (see Bronchospasm below).

Ex-premature infants

Infants who were born prematurely (<37 weeks' gestational age) and are <60 weeks' postconceptual age (defined as the sum of the gestational and postnatal ages) require 12–24 h of postanesthesia monitoring for apnea, irrespective of the surgery [23]. Factors that increase the risk of perioperative apnea in ex-premature infants include age (<60 weeks' postconceptual age), anemia (<12 g% Hb) and secondary diagnoses (e.g. intraventricular hemorrhage) [23,24]. Caffeine 10 mg/kg IV may be administered intraoperatively to reduce the frequency of perioperative apneas, but this may not completely eliminate apnea. Once the infant has been 12 h apnea free, he/she may be discharged home.

In contrast to general anesthesia, regional anesthesia does not appear to increase the risk of perioperative apnea and does not require perioperative monitoring, unless the infant was also sedated, has multisystem disease or a history of perioperative apneas [25]. Spinal or caudal anesthesia should provide sufficient anesthesia

to perform hernia surgery, the most common procedure in ex-premature infants [26]. If the infant is >44 weeks' postconceptual age, he/she may be discharged home from the postanesthesia care unit (PACU). If the parents have an apnea monitor at home and have been trained to manage apnea, the child may be discharged home in the parent's care.

Sickle cell disease

Sickle cell disease (SCD) or sickle cell anemia occurs primarily in children of sub-Saharan descent, with a frequency in North America of 1:5000. A point genetic mutation results in the replacement of the Hb AA with Hb SS in every red blood cell. Thus, 100% of the cells in children with SCD are at risk for sickling; these children have chronic low hemoglobin concentrations (6–8 g%), may have had acute vaso-occlusive crises, and may have received multiple red cell transfusions in the past. Vaso-occlusive crises involve a number of organs including bone, chest, and brain. They occur in some children and never in others, are unrelated to the presence of hypoxia, hypovolemia or hypothermia, and may be fatal [27]. Evidence now suggests that those with sickle cell disease and vaso-occlusive crises have markers of a systemic inflammatory response to the disease that upregulates endogenous factors, including an adhesive factor that traps sickle red cells in arterioles and precipitates occlusive crises [28]. Whether the traditional factors of hypoxia, hypovolemia, and hypothermia exacerbate the initial process or compound the inflammatory process has not been clearly established.

Sickle cell may also present in a heterozygote form, Hb AS, known as sickle trait. This disorder presents few problems during anesthesia and surgery provided extreme conditions, such as hypothermia, are not employed. Children with Hb AS have normal hemoglobin concentrations. Two additional hemoglobinopathies, Hb SC and Hb SD, occur less frequently than Hb SS but are equally likely to sickle. The hemoglobin concentrations are normal in children with Hb SC and SD.

The sickledex test determines whether the red cells can sickle. This test can be performed rapidly, inexpensively, and reliably in infants >6 months of age. In infants <6 months of age, the presence of Hb F interferes with sickling and renders the sickledex test non-confirmatory. In fact, infants <6 months of age rarely sickle because Hb F is present.

The definitive diagnostic test for SCD is the hemoglobin electrophoresis or high-performance liquid chromatography. These tests identify the specific normal and abnormal hemoglobins present in blood of infants and children of any age.

To attenuate the risk of a perioperative sickle crisis during elective surgery in children with SCD, some hematologists recommend transfusing packed red cells to increase the total hemoglobin to $10\,g\%$ [29]. This practice reduces the frequency of acute vaso-occlusive crises in children with SCD. Others disagree with both the practice of prophylactic blood transfusions and the need for transfusions in children undergoing *minor* surgery. The disadvantages of frequent transfusions in children who are at risk for sickle crises include sensitizing the recipient to minor antibodies (i.e. Kell and Duffy), iron overload, and transfusion reactions. It is important to consult local hematologists regarding the institutional management of children with SCD before the day of surgery to avoid surgical delays.

Anterior mediastinal mass

Children with anterior mediastinal mass (AMM) have a life-threatening risk for anesthesia when they present for a tissue (lymph node) biopsy, CT scan for diagnosis or indwelling central line for chemotherapy [30]. These tumors grow (on occasion very rapidly) in the small and confined space of the anterior mediastinum. Growing anterior mediastinal tumors can press on the tracheobronchial tree and/or right side of the heart (superior vena cava, right atrium or pulmonary artery). Four tissues can be found in AMMs in children: lymphomas, teratomas, thymomas, and thyroid. The most rapidly growing tumor in the anterior mediastinum is the lymphoblastic lymphoma, a non-Hodgkin lymphoma which has a doubling time of only 12–24h. These children may present with minor findings (e.g. night sweats) that rapidly progress over 1–2 days to life-threatening problems (e.g. orthopnea, superior vena cava syndrome). In children, investigating the effects of the tumor on the mediastinal structures, as well as acquiring tissue for the cell type, often requires anesthesia. The decision to proceed with local or general anesthesia depends on the age and level of co-operation of the child, the extent of mediastinal organ compromise, and the accessibility of the node or tumor being biopsied. A multidisciplinary team that includes the surgeon, anesthesiologist, and oncologist should review all radiological and preoperative data before embarking on the surgery.

In children who can tolerate local anesthesia and sedation, proceeding with the surgery is moot. However, for children who cannot tolerate local anesthesia with sedation and who have tumors that severely compromise the airway and/or pulmonary artery, a 12–24-h course of steroids should be considered to shrink the tumor (usually a lymphoblastic lymphoma). The risks associated with administering steroids include tissue necrosis, that may render diagnosis of the tumor cell type difficult, and cause tumor lysis syndrome. Some oncologists are reluctant to treat these children with steroids because of the potential difficulty of establishing the tissue diagnosis

should tumor necrosis occur. Establishing the tumor type is critical for determining which lymphoma regimen the child is to receive; the goal is to provide the most effective treatment with minimal treatment complications.

For most children who require radiological investigation, tumor biopsy or chemotherapy access, general anesthesia with spontaneous respiration is ideal. If the child cannot lie flat, anesthesia can be induced and the trachea intubated while the child is in the left lateral decubitus or sitting position. We intubate the trachea at induction of anesthesia to ensure a viable airway should it become necessary to turn the child prone because cardiovascular collapse occurs. Tracheal intubation is performed without muscle relaxation so spontaneous respiration can be maintained. It is important to recognize that the capnogram may be very helpful when establishing whether pulmonary circulation (and cardiac output) is present; sudden compression of the pulmonary artery will eliminate or markedly reduce the capnogram before systemic cardiovascular manifestations are present.

Endocarditis prophylaxis

The American Heart Association significantly revised the indications for bacterial endocarditis prophylaxis in 2007 [31]. The new recommendations were crafted for dental procedures and adopted by the dental societies. The American Heart Association no longer recommends endocarditis prophylaxis for children undergoing gastrointestinal, urological and genitourinary surgeries. However, many specialists in these areas continue to request endocarditis prophylaxis. Accordingly, it is incumbent upon the anesthesiologist to inquire of the specific specialist whether endocarditis prophylaxis should be administered.

For dental procedures, the only indications for subacute bacterial endocarditis (SBE) prophylaxis are those in Box 15.4. The antibiotic regimen for endocarditis prophylaxis has not changed since previously published [31].

Full stomach and rapid-sequence induction

The term "full stomach" refers to the presence of residual solid or liquid foods in the stomach at induction of

---

Box 15.4 Endocarditis prophylaxis

1. Prosthetic cardiac valve
2. Previous infective endocarditis
3. Cardiac transplantation children who develop a valvulopathy
4. Congenital heart disease (CHD)
   (i) Unrepaired cyanotic heart disease (incl. palliative procedures)
   (ii) Repaired CHD with prosthetic material or device during the first 6 months after procedure
   (iii) Repaired CHD with residual lead at or adjacent to prosthetic patch or device

anesthesia and is usually associated with hypokinetic or akinetic intestinal peristalsis. In such cases, the child is at risk for regurgitation and possibly aspiration of residual gastric contents into the lungs during anesthesia, a potentially fatal perioperative complication. A full stomach occurs most often in patients requiring emergency surgery, but also in children with gastric dysmotility syndromes and diabetes. In most cases of emergency surgery, the time interval between ingestion of food and induction of general anesthesia is too brief to ensure complete evacuation of the gastric contents. A full stomach due to the "trauma," pain, and stress of the injury is exacerbated by the administration of opioids, which increase gastric and intestinal paresis and further delay emptying of food from the stomach.

There are three important principles to remember in such cases.

- There is no safe time interval after an injury that guarantees that the stomach is empty of food.
- There is no safe time interval after an injury that guarantees that there is no risk of regurgitation of gastric contents.
- All children (even those treated with prokinetic motility medications) are at risk for regurgitation and aspiration during induction of, maintenance of, and emergence from anesthesia.

The interval between food ingestion and injury is the only variable that has been associated with an increased gastric fluid volume and decreased pH; the shorter the interval, the greater the risk that a larger gastric volume and lower pH is present. For example, if >8 h have passed between the last food ingested and the injury, the gastric fluid volume should be less and pH greater than if only 2 h had passed [18]. However, the risk in either case is not zero.

To protect the airways of children who are at risk for regurgitation and aspiration during induction of anesthesia, a rapid-sequence induction (RSI) of anesthesia secures the airway quickly and safely. Although there is no evidence that a RSI is the best strategy to use, it seems reasonable to induce anesthesia quickly and insert a tracheal tube into the larynx as quickly as possible. To perform a RSI, the appropriate equipment must be prepared (see Box 15.5).

In most institutions, a RSI is performed using intravenous anesthesia. Propofol is the most common induction agent (2–4 mg/kg), although ketamine (1–2 mg/kg) and etomidate (0.2–0.3 mg/kg) may be used for hemodynamically unstable children. We recommend succinylcholine 2 mg/kg for paralysis, although rocuronium 0.8–1 mg/kg has also been used. (NB: Recent concern regarding unexpected hyperkalemia and ventricular tachycardia in male children with undiagnosed muscle (wasting) diseases who received succinylcholine led the FDA to issue a black

---

Box 15.5 Rapid sequence induction for children

Preinduction

- Laryngoscope handle/blades sized for age
- Tracheal tubes appropriate for the age of the child, with a stylet
- Active Yankauer suction
- Preparation of induction agents and muscle relaxants in weight-appropriate doses
- Preoxygenation through a tight-fitting mask and breathing circuit (as tolerated)
- Position the head and neck optimally
- Suction and remove existing nasogastric tube

Induction

- Rapid intravenous induction of anesthesia using predetermined doses of drugs
- Maintain facemask with 100% oxygen; ventilation is usually avoided
- Once fasciculations are seen after succinylcholine or depression of the twitch response after a non-depolarizing relaxant, laryngoscopy and tracheal intubation are performed rapidly
- Insert a predetermined size tracheal tube
- If a cuffed tracheal tube is used, the cuff is inflated before the lungs are auscultated. Adjust cuff pressure once auscultation is performed

---

box warning of this complication. If succinylcholine is used, intravenous calcium chloride (10 mg/kg IV, repeat as necessary) must be immediately available to restore normal sinus rhythm. If the child has a muscle wasting disorder, rocuronium should be used if paralysis is required to secure the airway.) However, if the airway appears to be difficult or precarious, then alternative strategies to secure the airway should be considered, including an inhalational anesthetic or topical local anesthetic and TIVA sedation. If an inhalational induction is performed, the child may require emergency turning to the left lateral decubitus position if regurgitation occurs. It may be necessary to topicalize the airway during TIVA while maintaining spontaneous respiration to prevent coughing.

There is much debate regarding the importance and relevance of cricoid pressure in a RSI [32]. Currently, there is no evidence to support or refute the use of cricoid pressure for this purpose. However, there are some concerns regarding the application of cricoid pressure in infants. In both infants and children, the cricoid ring and trachea are mobile and deformable, and only 10 N of force are required to compress the airway by 50%. This is one-third the force recommended for cricoid pressure [33]. Cricoid pressure may also increase the level of difficulty of tracheal intubation by distorting tracheal anatomy or compressing the cricoid ring. Very few assistants are trained properly in the location of the cricoid ring and in the magnitude of the force required to occlude the esophagus. It remains our view that there is insufficient evidence for or against the use of cricoid pressure during RSI in children; the clinician should use their own best judgment in planning the optimal strategy to secure the airway rapidly and safely [32].

Preparation of operating room, equipment, monitors

Anesthetic machine

A complete machine check must be concluded before anesthesia commences. Modern anesthetic machines provide complete start-up checks that, for the most part, are completely automated. These will be machine specific, must be performed unless there is insufficient time to do so due to a pending emergency, and are not discussed further. Refer to the operations manual for the specific machine to conduct the machine check.

Before embarking on an anesthetic, the pressures in the emergency gas cylinders on the machine must be checked. An emergency oxygen cylinder is required on all machines to provide administration of oxygen if the line oxygen supply fails. Because oxygen is completely gaseous in these pressurized cylinders, the pressure in the tank decreases linearly as the tank is emptied. The volume (in liters) of oxygen present in the emergency E cylinder is the product of the ratio of the pressure within the tank to 2200 pounds per square inch (psi) (the pressure of a full cylinder of oxygen), and the number of liters of oxygen in a full cylinder (618 L). Thus, it is easy to calculate how many minutes of oxygen are available in the E cylinder for a given flow rate should the wall oxygen source fail. A source of air should also be available so that less than 30% oxygen can be delivered to infants at risk for oxygen toxicity and for those with congenital heart disease in whom excess oxygen may cause excess pulmonary blood flow. This is usually provided from a wall source, although an emergency air cylinder should be available. Supplementary nitrous oxide cylinders are not essential to maintain anesthesia if the wall source of N_2O fails. These tanks can be a source of operating room pollution and are costly to replace. Nitrous oxide in E cylinders contains both liquid and gaseous nitrous oxide at 750 mmHg pressure. The pressure within the cylinder remains constant until all the liquid nitrous oxide has evaporated. Up to that point, the content of nitrous oxide tanks can only be determined by weight. When the pressure gauge on the cylinder indicates that the pressure is decreasing, the cylinder is nearing empty and must be replaced quickly.

Box 15.6 SALTED mnemonic

S   Suction, stylet and solution (IV fluids RL or normal saline)
A   Airways oral and nasal – different sizes
L   Laryngoscope – Miller blades from sizes 0–3; MAC 2 or 3
T   Tubes – tracheal tubes of appropriate sizes, tape
E   Equipment – anesthesia machine with breathing circuit, McGill forceps, facemasks, back-up self-inflating AMBU bag, fluid warmer, venous cannulation kit, and standard monitors
D   Drugs (anesthesia and resuscitation drugs)

Anesthetic equipment

To ensure that the anesthetizing location is properly and completely prepared, it is useful to refer to a checklist such as the one shown in Box 15.6.

Appropriately sized equipment should be available for each child. A range of facemask sizes, oral airways, laryngoscope blades, tracheal tubes, and laryngeal mask airways should be present. We prefer cushioned clear facemasks that fit the contour of the child's face and permit rapid identification of either fluid or solid material within the mask. The importance of oral airways in establishing a patent upper airway in children has been supplanted in our practice with the jaw thrust maneuver (see below). We advocate the use of Miller and Wisconsin straight blades for tracheal intubation in infants and children because they align the axes of the mouth, pharynx, and larynx. A range of sizes of laryngoscope blades should be available in every anesthetizing location (Table 15.1). We advise against placing a roll under the shoulder of neonates and infants during laryngoscopy unless the laryngoscopist is seated; the shoulder roll raises the larynx, which is already anterior and cephalad in the neonate compared with older children, making it more difficult to align the axes while the laryngoscopist is standing. In neonates with limited oxygen reserve or when performing an awake tracheal intubation, the Oxyscope™, a straight blade fitted with a source of oxygen at the tip of the blade, may prevent oxygen desaturation during laryngoscopy. Macintosh blades are best suited for use in adolescents.

The classic laryngeal mask airway (cLMA) was introduced to replace facemasks in adults and has subsequently proven to be a versatile and useful airway device in children as well [34]. To fit pediatric airways, the dimensions of the adult cLMA were scaled down in size, although the mask was otherwise unmodified and made no compensation for the difference in laryngeal anatomy. The cLMA has proven to be effective in circumstances other than elective anesthesia, including neonatal resuscitation and fiberoptic intubation. A range of sizes of the cLMA should be available (see Table 15.1). Although effective, the cLMA does not "protect" the airway from

Table 15.1 Airway equipment

Laryngoscope blade size	
Age (years)	**Miller blade size**
0–0.5 years	Miller 0
0.5–2 or 3 years	Miller 1
2–4 years	Miller 1.5
3–8 years	Miller 2

Classic LMA size		
Weight (kg)	**LMA size**	**Max. ETT size**
0–5 kg	#1	3.5 mm ID
5–10 kg	1½	4.0
10–20 kg	2	4.5
20–30 kg	2½	5.0
30–50 kg	3	6.0

ETT, endotracheal tube; ID, internal diameter; LMA, laryngeal mask airway.

regurgitation and laryngospasm. Since the tone of the gastroesophageal sphincter is reduced in children compared with adults, children may be at greater risk for regurgitation in the presence of a full stomach or positive pressure ventilation. Hence, it is best to avoid LMAs in these clinical situations. Modifications of the cLMA to include a vent for regurgitant gas or liquid from the esophagus, as in the ProSeal supraglottic airway, may better protect the airway against aspiration.

Complications of the cLMA in children include gastric inflation, aspiration, airway obstruction, and laryngospasm. The frequency of complications with the cLMA in infants <1 year of age is greater than that in older children. Fiberoptic studies have demonstrated that the epiglottis folds down into the bowl of the cLMA in about 50% of children when the LMA is otherwise properly functioning; the relevance of this finding remains unclear.

A range of diameters of tracheal tubes appropriate for the child's age, as well as tubes 0.5 mm internal diameter smaller and larger, should always be available. The appropriate size uncuffed tracheal tube is based on the internal diameter (ID) of the tube. Guidelines for tracheal tube sizes in infants and children are: infant's weight (<1500 g, 2.5 mm ID; 1500 g–full-term gestation, 3.0 mm ID), neonate to 6 months postnatal age, 3.5 mm ID and 0.5–1.5 year, 4.0 mm ID. For children >2 years of age, the size of uncuffed tubes may be estimated using the formula: age (in years)/4 + 4 (or 4.5) mm ID. The size of cuffed tubes (mm ID) may be estimated using the formula: age (in years)/4 + 3 (for children <2 years) or +3.5 (for those >2 years).

The length of a tube from the lips to midtrachea in infants <1000 g in weight is 6 cm, 1000–2500 gm is 7–9 cm,

in term neonates 10 cm, and for infants and children, 10 + age (years) mm.

In the past, uncuffed tracheal tubes were used to secure the airway of children <8 years of age. The circular shape of the tracheal tube was similar to the shape of the lumen within the cricoid ring, which allowed for a good seal to form without the need for a cuff on the tube. Cuffs were avoided in children out of the concern that the loosely adherent pseudostratified columnar epithelium within the cricoid ring, the only solid cartilaginous ring in the upper airway, would swell and further encroach on this narrowest portion of the upper airway and cause stridor. Because airflow within the upper airway is turbulent, a 50% reduction in the radius of the airway would increase the resistance to airflow by the fifth power of the radius or 32-fold. This increase in resistance would rapidly lead to respiratory distress, fatigue, and ultimately respiratory failure in young infants and children, particularly if they were also septic. To preclude this potentially serious airway problem in the perioperative period, in addition to avoiding cuffed tubes, we carefully selected the tracheal tube in children so that it either passed through the cricoid ring without resistance or it did so with an audible leak at a peak inspiratory pressure of about 20 cmH$_2$O. If an audible leak were present at a peak airway pressure ≤10 cmH$_2$O, then the tracheal tube was changed to a half-size larger, otherwise ventilation may prove to be inadequate during the surgery. Before proceeding, the peak inspiratory pressure at which there was an audible leak would be retested. This process would be repeated until a satisfactory sized tube was present.

Recently, there has been a shift from uncuffed to cuffed tracheal tubes in children. This shift in practice has in no small part been facilitated by the introduction of the soft, high-compliance cuffed Microcuff® tube (Microcuff GMBH, Weinheim, Germany) [35]. These tubes have no Murphy eye, the cuff is positioned very close to the tip of the tube, the cuff material is polyurethane, and the shape is cylindrical (rather than spherical as in low-compliance cuffed tubes), mimicking the shape of the larynx. Several relatively small size studies have reported similar incidence of complications in children with high-compliance cuffed and uncuffed tubes. Microcuff™ tubes confer several additional advantages over traditional uncuffed tubes, including less contamination of the OR with anesthetic gases, fewer laryngoscopies and reintubations, and more consistent tidal volumes (as chest wall and abdominal compliance change during surgery) [36]. Overall, these factors substantially reduce the number of manipulations of the airway in children, OR costs, and OR pollution.

A functioning wall suction with suction tubing (that is long enough to reach the OR table) and a plastic Yankauer suction tip are mandatory. Yankauer suctions can cause trauma to oropharyngeal tissues that must be avoided. This is achieved in young children whose molar teeth have not come in by inserting the Yankauer between the cheek and the teeth and passing it behind the premolars to reach the hypopharynx. With this approach, the child cannot damage their central incisors by biting down on the suction while it is in the mouth. In addition, the suction should not remain in one position within the hypopharynx to avoid applying prolonged negative pressure to tissues (such as the uvula) and causing edema and bleeding. We prefer to use a Yankauer suction rather than a suction catheter in the OR because the former is capable of suctioning large volumes of blood, secretions, and/or vomitus expeditiously should the need arise; the latter is often difficult to pass into the hypopharynx.

The optimal ventilation strategy for infants and children during surgery has been the subject of much interest [37]. For many years, volume-controlled pressure-limited ventilators were used to ventilate the lungs of infants and children during surgery. However, these ventilators could not account for either the circuit compliance or the variable leak around the tracheal tube. There was additional concern regarding the shape of the inspiratory pressure tracing and the risk of delivering high pressures. Pressure-controlled ventilation has been used successfully in neonatal intensive care units (NICU) for many years, in part because it limits the peak pressure and decreases barotrauma with its constant inspiratory pressure pattern. It also provides a more even distribution of inspiratory gas in the lungs, reducing ventilation/perfusion (V/Q) mismatch.

Despite the advantages of pressure-controlled ventilators, many anesthesia ventilators were simply unable to compensate for decreases in abdominal and chest wall compliance caused by the surgeons or their instruments or by peritoneal insufflation of the abdomen or chest during laparoscopy. When this occurs, it is difficult to ensure reliable tidal volume ventilation. A new generation of anesthetic machines offers markedly improved ventilators and ventilation strategies that are hybrids of the best aspects of both volume- and pressure-regulated ventilation. These new ventilators may prove to be ideal for both preterm and term neonates. The hybrid pressure-regulated volume-controlled mode, which maintains a fixed tidal volume by taking into account the compressible volume of the breathing circuit, is used during controlled ventilation, and a pressure support mode is used once spontaneous respiration commences. It is essential to avoid causing barotrauma in small neonates by presetting weight-appropriate respiratory parameters on the ventilator before commencing ventilation.

Box 15.7 Basic mandatory monitoring for anesthesia and other monitors

- Electrocardiogram
- Arterial blood pressure
- Pulse oximetry
- End-tidal CO_2
- Temperature
- Secondary optional monitors
  - anesthetic depth monitoring
  - cerebral oxygenation monitoring
  - invasive monitors

Emergency drugs

Emergency drugs should always be available before inducing anesthesia. Syringes with a small-gauge (23 or 25 G) needle that contain weight-appropriate doses of atropine and succinylcholine should be immediately available to facilitate intramuscular or sublingual drug injection in an emergency. A syringe of propofol (1–2 mg/kg) should always be available to facilitate tracheal intubation or LMA insertion, as well as to break laryngospasm and increase the depth of anesthesia quickly [38]. Inotropic drugs are not routinely prepared for healthy children undergoing elective surgery.

Monitors

The ASA mandates basic patient monitoring during all anesthetics (Box 15.7). Monitoring children during anesthesia must include the standard five monitors: electrocardiogram, arterial blood pressure, oxygen saturation, capnogram, and temperature, as well as any additional monitors specific for the child's medical or anesthetic condition, e.g. depth of anesthesia monitor. Many infants and preschool age children fight the application of monitors while awake. Although induction of anesthesia is usually well tolerated and safe in expert hands, every effort should be made to apply at least a pulse oximeter before inducing anesthesia. The remaining monitors should be applied as soon as the child loses consciousness.

Electrocardiogram

A standard three- or five-lead electrocardiogram should be used in every anesthetic to detect arrhythmias (bradycardia) and peaked T waves or ST segment changes. The most common rhythm disturbance in healthy children is bradycardia that is usually caused by hypoxemia or vagal reflex stimulation (Box 15.8). Ventricular arrhythmias are exceedingly uncommon during sevoflurane anesthesia. The most common causes of ventricular arrhythmias in children are hyperkalemia and intravascular injection of amide local anesthetic.

Box 15.8 Causes of bradycardia

1. Hypoxia
2. Vagal reflex response (e.g. prolonged laryngoscopy, traction on the extraocular muscles)
3. Medication (e.g. succinylcholine)
4. Congenital heart defect, cardiac conduction defect, heart failure and cardiomyopathy
5. Raised intracranial pressure
6. Electrolyte imbalance (hyperkalemia, hypocalcemia)
7. Massive air embolism
8. Tension pneumothorax

Arterial blood pressure

Arterial blood pressure is usually measured non-invasively every 5 min with an automated Doppler technique during elective surgery. The cuff should cover approximately two-thirds the length of the humerus. In children, systolic pressure is used primarily as a measure of volume status and secondly as a measure of cardiac function. Diastolic pressure is not as closely regarded because peripheral vascular resistance is low in infants and children. Invasive pressures are usually reserved for prolonged surgeries, especially those associated with large blood loss, congenital heart disease or when sick children require inotropic support or repeated blood gas measurements.

Pulse oximetry

Pulse oximetry is used to determine the hemoglobin oxygen saturation (SaO_2) by measuring transmittance of two wavelengths of red light, 660 and 940 nM, through the blood in arterioles. The probe is commonly affixed to a digit but may also be applied to the earlobe, the hypothenar eminence or lateral aspect of the foot in infants. In addition to a visual display of SaO_2, current pulse oximeters have an audible tone whose pitch decreases when saturation decreases. Most oximeters use motion-artifact compensation software that enables them to measure the oxygen saturation even when the child is moving, e.g. during induction or emergence from anesthesia. Pulse oximetry accurately measures oxygen saturations between values of 70% and 100%. Most nail polishes do not interfere with the accuracy of oximeter readings, although we prefer to apply the oximeter to an unpainted surface. Pulse oximeters may fail to detect a pulse in the presence of a low cardiac output, low arterial blood pressure, hypothermia or vasculopathy. It should be noted that carbon monoxide is neither sensed nor measured by pulse oximeters in current use.

Capnography

Infrared analysis of the end-tidal carbon dioxide tension in the breathing circuit has been used to estimate the partial pressure of carbon dioxide in blood. Two distinct techniques are available to display end-tidal carbon dioxide tension. One continuously aspirates gas from the breathing circuit and determines the carbon dioxide tension in a remote sensor, known as side-stream capnography. The other analyzes the carbon dioxide tension directly in the breathing circuit and is known as mainstream capnography. The accuracy of side-stream capnometry improved dramatically when circle system breathing circuits replaced t-piece circuits because there is less dilution of expiratory gas. Side-stream capnometry using gas obtained from the elbow of the circle breathing circuit provides accurate data, even in neonates without cyanotic heart disease who have small tidal volumes. Mainstream capnography, on the other hand, is unpopular, particularly for infants and neonates, because it increases the dead space of the circuit and the sensors are bulky and heavy and may kink small tracheal tubes.

Recently, small dead-space, light mainstream capnography sensors have been developed for use with an oxygen facemask in children (personal communication, K. Miyasaka, Japan) although additional studies are required before they are available for clinical use. Capnography using gases obtained from the elbow of a circle circuit may also be accurately monitored while sedated children breathe through a facemask or through baffled nasal prongs.

Temperature

With induction of anesthesia, children undergo peripheral vasodilation and redistribute heat from their core to their periphery. In children, heat is lost from the body by four routes: 39% by radiation, 34% by convection, 24% by evaporation, and 3% by conduction [39]. The following strategies reduce/prevent substantial heat loss.

The temperature of the operating room should be increased to about 28°C (80°F) before non-febrile infants and young children enter the room. It is important to increase the room temperature as soon as the case is booked or the previous patient vacates the operating room because it may take more than an hour to sufficiently increase the room temperature. Increasing the temperature in the operating room raises the temperature of both the walls and ceiling and the air within the room, thereby reducing radiation and convection heat loss [39]. Forced air warmers are the single most effective strategy available to minimize heat loss by patients who undergo surgery lasting 1 h or more [40]. Although it is comforting to prewarm the air mattress before the child enters the operating room, doing so before the child is anesthetized does not alter the child's temperature at the end of surgery. Furthermore, it may predispose to airborne contamination and possible surgical infection [41]. Until further evidence is forthcoming, forced air warmers should not be used until the skin is prepped and draped for surgery.

Supplemental warming devices, such as warming blankets, overhead heat lamps, and fluid warmers, should also be used to maintain normothermia in neonates if the need arises.

The temperature of all children who receive anesthesia or sedation should be monitored continuously during the procedure and in the PACU. Core temperature is ideally measured in the midesophagus, immediately retrocardiac. The optimal location of the probe can be confirmed when using a combination esophageal stethoscope and thermistor, by inserting the stethoscope until the heart sounds are maximal. Alternative sites to measure core temperature include the rectum, nasopharynx, bladder and axilla, although each site has its limitations. Rectal temperature probes may yield inaccurate temperatures if the probe exits the rectum or is immersed in stool. Nasopharyngeal temperature may underestimate the core temperature if the probe is cooled by gas passing through the ventilation circuit. Axillary temperature may under- or overestimate core temperature because of IV fluid infused through the ipsilateral arm, because the probe is not positioned against the axillary blood vessels or because it is adjacent to the forced air warmer.

Anesthetic depth monitoring

Recently attention has been focused on reports of awareness, which occurs in about 1% in children who undergo elective surgery [42,43]. Most consider that this incidence of awareness is much greater than their experience, although postanesthesia interviews to determine the incidence of recall are not routine. Because children rarely self-declare their awareness, it is equally likely that our experience underestimates the true incidence of awareness.

Analysis of the reports of awareness in children suggests that many awareness episodes are attributable to local practices that expose children to low concentrations of anesthesia during periods of stimulation. In some cases, awareness occurred during the transport of children from the anesthesia induction room to the operating room [42], whereas in others the anesthesiologists deliberately decreased the anesthetic concentrations immediately after loss of eyelash reflex to reduce the risk of seizures [43]. These practices contrast with most of our practices where the anesthetic concentrations of sevoflurane are neither interrupted nor dramatically decreased until an adequate depth of anesthesia is achieved. We believe that the incidence of awareness during pediatric anesthesia is far less frequent than reported, that most instances are explicable by local practices, and do not justify routine depth of anesthesia monitoring in children.

The Bispectral Index (BIS) is the most widely studied anesthetic depth monitor in children in North America, although other monitors such as the Cerebral State Index and Spectral Entropy monitor are approved for clinical use. The BIS is purported to measure anesthetic depth continuously using a scale from 0 to 100; readings between 40 and 60 are considered adequate for general anesthesia. Thirty to 60 sec are required to display an index value. The probability that recall will occur is significantly increased if the BIS is >60 for more than 30 sec. A number of factors may influence BIS readings. First, BIS measurements vary with the anesthetic administered [44], For example, at comparable surgical depth, the BIS measurements during halothane anesthesia are 50% greater than those using sevoflurane. The difference may be explained in part by the very different EEG patterns of the two anesthetics. The EEG pattern associated with sevoflurane anesthesia consists of more slow waves and less fast-rhythm activity than halothane. Although the BIS measurements correlate generally with the sevoflurane concentration, the accuracy of the measurement is poor. BIS readings with nitrous oxide and ketamine do not reliably estimate the depth of anesthesia. Second, age affects the BIS readings [45,46] which in children <5 years of age are less reliable than those in children >5 years of age. The most likely explanation for this effect is related to maturation of the EEG from birth to school age. Third, the depth of anesthesia measurement is substantially affected by the extent of muscle relaxation. Recovery of the twitch response increases BIS readings, while paralysis decreases them. This effect complicates interpretation of the BIS reading. In non-paralyzed patients, the EMG component from spontaneous respiration may erroneously increase the BIS reading. Fourth, position may affect the BIS reading. Placing the patient in the Trendelenburg position (30° head down) increases the BIS by 20% [47].

There are few indications for the routine use of the BIS monitor in children, except for those who cannot tolerate general anesthesia because of hemodynamic instability, those in whom nitrous oxide is not used, and those anesthetized with total intravenous anesthesia (TIVA).

Methods for inducing anesthesia

Anxiolysis

A number of strategies may be used to allay anxiety in children before induction of anesthesia. These are summarized below.

Parental presence at induction of anesthesia

Two systematic reviews have summarized the published evidence on parental presence at induction of anesthesia (PPIA) and determined that PPIA reduced the anxiety of parents but not of children [48,49]. The popularity of PPIA has been facilitated in part by the use of induction rooms; parents accompany their children for induction of anesthesia in a non-sterile environment. Use of these rooms improves the efficiency of room changeover. Parents who are most insistent on being with their children during induction of anesthesia are often the most disruptive, least likely to calm their child, and actually provoke further non-compliant behavior in their child. Children 1–6 years of age are those for whom PPIA may be most beneficial. Separation anxiety rarely occurs before 8 months of age. Above all, parents should never be invited by healthcare personnel to accompany their child for a procedure lest both the hospital and the medical personnel be held responsible for any untoward outcomes to the parent. Rather, the parent should be told that they might be accommodated if they choose to accompany their child for the induction of anesthesia. Before a parent does this, everyone on the OR team must agree and understand that a parent will be present at induction, understand their role while the parent is present, and ensure that the parent understands that he or she must leave when asked to do so. Parents must be educated regarding the normal behavior of children during induction of anesthesia. They should be told that their child might cry, resist application of the mask (inhalation induction), experience noisy (and at times irregular) breathing, and demonstrate involuntary movements of the arms and/or legs, body twisting or frank lifelessness as anesthesia is induced. If the parent appears to be too emotional to cope with this situation, he/she should not be allowed to accompany the child to the induction. We believe that a blanket policy that all parents may accompany their child for induction of anesthesia should not be the standard for any anesthetic department. Rather, selection of parents to accompany their child for induction of anesthesia should be made carefully and on a case-by-case basis by the anesthesiologist only after determining that it is in the child's best interest for the parent/guardian to be present.

In cases of cognitively challenged adolescents and children, it may be difficult, if not impossible, to transfer the child to the operating room voluntarily without a parent. In such cases, it is imperative to ask the parents whether the child will come to the operating room unaccompanied. If not, then a parent must accompany the child. In children who are physically abusive and resistant to transfer to the operating room, intramuscular premedication can be used (see below).

Distraction techniques

There are a number of distraction and educational techniques that may be effective in reducing a child's anxiety. Preoperative coloring books, stories, videos, and websites have been developed to educate children of all ages about the appearance of the operating room, the equipment that will be used, and how they will be anesthetized. Operating room tours, usually on weekends, are popular in many children's hospitals. A staff representative dresses the family members and children in OR attire, they visit an operating room, and the child plays with anesthesia breathing circuits and facemasks. On the morning of surgery, child life providers may orient children who may be at risk for emotional instability and anxiety at the time of separation from parents and induction of anesthesia to the anesthesia mask. They may mark the inside of the mask with flavored lip balm before applying the mask to the child's face. Distraction techniques including video games, earphones, and portable internet devices all reduce preoperative anxiety [50]. To complement the above strategies, the circulating nurses and/or anesthesiologist should be skilled and trained to facilitate smooth and rapid separation of the child from the parents and then distract the child by pointing out wall designs, pictures, and other features as they travel to the operating room. Once the child enters the operating room, the anesthesiologist should establish rapport by telling a story, engaging them in conversation about a recent birthday, holiday or vacation, or by singing as they prepare for induction of anesthesia.

Pharmacological sedation

For some children, premedication is required to facilitate smooth separation from their parents. For some parents this is the first time the child and they have been separated, which can be extremely traumatic if the children and parents have been inadequately prepared.

Midazolam is the most widely used premedication for children in North America because it can be given orally, nasally, rectally, intramuscularly or intravenously to calm the child before induction of anesthesia. Whichever route of administration is used, midazolam premedication may depress respiration enough to cause apnea during induction of anesthesia with 8% sevoflurane.

The dose of oral midazolam increases with decreasing age [51]. We routinely give a maximum dose of 1.0 mg/kg (maximum dose 15–20 mg) to children 2–3 years of age to ensure a >95% success rate of sedating children in 10–15 min and administer a decreasing dose with increasing age and give 0.3–0.4 mg/kg for children ≥6 years of age [52,53]. This medication is an excellent anxiolytic and produces a smooth parent–child separation within 10–15 min of oral administration. However, even the commercial strawberry-flavored midazolam leaves a bitter aftertaste that adolescents complain about. To minimize the impact of the aftertaste, oral midazolam is best administered as a single swallow. We wash away the aftertaste by offering them a swallow or two of water. For younger children, midazolam should be instilled into the lateral gutters of the mouth via a needleless syringe. For older children, midazolam may be administered in a small medicine cup and followed by a sip of water. Obstructive sleep apnea is one of the few cautions regarding oral midazolam. About 3% of children with sleep apnea experience transient hemoglobin desaturation [54].

Alternative oral premedications include oral ketamine (5–6 mg/kg), although it offers few advantages over midazolam and may cause more postoperative vomiting [55]. Postoperative hallucinations and nightmares are extremely rare after oral ketamine. Some have combined oral midazolam and ketamine in a 50:50 mixture with good success. Other oral premedications include clonidine (2 µg/kg) [56] and dexmedetomidine (2 µg/kg) [57]. Although these α2-agonists provide effective premedication, they require 60–90 min for the onset of effect and may produce bradycardia and sedation that persist beyond the duration of the anesthetic. This onset time for sedation often exceeds the time the child is in the ambulatory unit. As a result, there is little role for these premedications in most ambulatory pediatric surgical practices.

Intranasal premedication is of limited interest in children because they dislike nasal administration of medications. Intranasal midazolam 0.1–0.2 mg/kg causes effective premedication, but the bitter burning aftertaste persists in the nasopharynx long after recovering from the anesthetic [58]. Intranasal sufentanil 2–4 µg/kg is also effective, although sufentanil is infrequently used in children. Its use may precipitate chest wall rigidity and necessitate succinylcholine administration. Most recently, intranasal dexmedetomidine (0.5–1 µg/kg) has been used for premedication [59] despite the fact that its onset of action is delayed and the sedation it causes may extend into the recovery period.

Intramuscular ketamine

For children who are cognitively challenged and have behavior problems, transfer to the operating room may be the greatest obstacle to completing the surgery. Even the parents may be unable to coax the child to participate and to facilitate the transfer. The typical child who presents in this manner is a muscular 75 kg or larger, autistic or Down syndrome child. He or she refuses to ingest or accept any premedication. If the child refuses transfer to the operating room under any conditions, the choice is either to cancel the surgery or premedicate the child with an intramuscular injection. In anticipation of the latter, the parent/caregiver and the child should be seated on a stretcher. Intramuscular ketamine 3–5 mg/kg (concentration 100 mg/mL) should be administered via a small-gauge needle into either the bare deltoid region of an arm or through the clothing in the same region [60,61]. The latter is not ideal, but in some instances it is our only

choice for achieving sedation. Once the ketamine is administered, it may take up to 5 min for the child to relax and stop resisting our efforts. This premedication is usually metabolized before the anesthesia and surgery are completed.

Induction techniques

Induction of anesthesia is defined as the transition from awake to anesthetized states. Anesthesia may be induced by one of several techniques, including inhalation, intravenous, intramuscular or rectal routes. The choice of technique depends on several factors, including the age of the child, the child's level of co-operation, clinical condition, and preoperative status. For some techniques, such as intravenous induction or single-breath induction, a qualified assistant is required.

Inhalational induction

The most common method of inducing anesthesia in children for elective surgery in North America is by inhalation. All infants and children, including those who are crying and upset, can undergo a smooth inhalational anesthesia induction if the atmosphere and attitude of the staff are appropriate. On many occasions we have engaged upset children in the operating room in a warm and reassuring manner and successfully induced anesthesia by mask. It is our belief that using "brutane" to hold children down and force a mask on their face has no place in pediatric anesthesia and may psychologically scar the child for life. We comfort children and achieve a successful induction of anesthesia by using this approach, even in children who have many emotional concerns and fears.

The greatest challenges at induction of anesthesia often occur in preschool-age children. In this age group, distraction techniques and premedication are key strategies for minimizing anxiety and distress during separation from parents and induction of anesthesia. Our induction strategy is designed to empower children during the induction and maximize their participation. Upon arrival in the operating room, we apply as many monitors as the child tolerates. The child chooses their favorite flavor from two or three choices of lip balm and then colors the inside of the mask with it, or if the child is too young (<3 years of age), we flavor the facemask for the child. With the child seated on the operating table with their back to our chest (or in our lap if a diaper is worn), we gradually and gently bring the facemask to the nose and mouth while flowing 5–7 L/min of 70% nitrous oxide in oxygen in the breathing circuit. We employ a 1 L reservoir bag in the pediatric breathing circuit to reduce the time required to wash in anesthetic into the circuit. It is critically important to ensure the adjustable pressure limiting (APL) valve is wide open so the child does not feel that they are unable to exhale as a tight-fitting facemask is applied.

During this time, we distract the child by singing a song or by telling a joke or a story until the end-tidal and inspired N_2O concentrations equilibrate or the child ceases to respond to verbal stimulation. At this time, the child has sufficient anesthesia that they cannot recall any malodorous gas, which allows us to increase the sevoflurane concentration to 8% in one stepwise move and reduce the total fresh gas flow to 3–4 L/min.

Once the child begins to lose consciousness (and their neck becomes too supple to hold up their head), we place them supine on the operating table while they continue to breathe 8% sevoflurane in 70% nitrous oxide. The remaining monitors are then applied. During this early period of the induction, we maintain silence in the operating room and the surgeons are not allowed to stimulate or manipulate the child. If the child becomes apneic during this period (as is often the case after premedication), ventilation should be assisted manually and gently. To reduce the risk of awareness, the concentrations of sevoflurane and nitrous oxide are maintained until intravenous access is established. Once IV access is established, an IV dose of propofol (1–2 mg/kg) is administered, the nitrous oxide is discontinued, and the laryngeal mask airway or tracheal tube is inserted [62]. Anesthesia is continued with 8% sevoflurane in 100% oxygen until we verify bilateral air entry in the chest. If apnea occurs after the airway is secured, the inspired concentration of sevoflurane is reduced by 25–35% or more until spontaneous ventilation resumes. If nitrous oxide is not contraindicated, it may be reintroduced at this time, along with an appropriate concentration of inhalational anesthetic. Only after the airway is secured should the surgeon examine the child.

Several alternative strategies may be used to achieve a deep level of anesthesia with sevoflurane, including increasing the inspired concentration of sevoflurane in a stepwise manner (2% per minute). Although this approach provides the same final outcome, its disadvantages are that it results in a longer induction time and excitement period.

Another distraction strategy that may be used is known as troposmia. Troposmia is a distorted perception of an odor that, in this case, can be attributed to the presence of inhalational anesthetics. The anesthesiologist asks the child their favorite flavor after applying a standard (e.g. strawberry) lip balm to the facemask. The child is then told that as they are anesthetized, the anesthetic will magically change the strawberry flavor to the child's favorite flavor. In one study, 80% of the children confirmed that they smelled their favorite flavor when they breathed the anesthetic gas [63].

The child with mask phobia poses a real challenge for those attempting to induce anesthesia by inhalation [64]. Besides refusing a mask, these frightened children often steadfastly refuse needles (and therefore an intravenous induction), leaving clinicians few options for inducing anesthesia. Several different solutions have been devised to address this problem, ranging from removing the mask from the breathing circuit to forcing the mask on the child's face (also known as "brutane") with 8% sevoflurane in the breathing circuit. We believe that induction of anesthesia with the former strategy is the preferred approach whereas induction with the latter approach is potentially traumatic and psychologically harmful, and it is not recommended.

There are many reasons why children may be fearful of facemasks, including the unappealing odor of 8% sevoflurane administered to an unpremedicated child, end-expiratory pressure that prevents the child from completely exhaling, and claustrophobia. Irrespective of the reason for the mask phobia, we hold to the philosophy that if the mask is the focal point of the fear, it should be eliminated from the induction. To induce anesthesia without a facemask, we interlace our fingers, with the breathing circuit elbow positioned between our fingers and deliver 70% nitrous oxide in oxygen. We cup our hands under the child's chin and gradually bring them closer and closer until they cover the child's mouth. Since nitrous oxide is heavier than air, our hands act as a reservoir for the nitrous oxide. Although this approach can be criticized for increasing operating room pollution, we believe this is the optimal approach for management of children with mask and needle phobias. Once the hands are tight over the mouth, we add 8% sevoflurane into the fresh gas flow. When the child is adequately anesthetized, we insert the elbow of the breathing circuit into the facemask and continue the anesthetic. When interviewing these children during the recovery period, they are thrilled that they avoided the "feared" mask.

Another way to deliver anesthesia by mask if the anesthesiologist insists on administering sevoflurane from the outset (i.e. without first using premedication or nitrous oxide) is to rotate the facemask 90° and use the balloon of the cuff to occlude the nares as anesthesia is induced. This eliminates/decreases the smell of sevoflurane and allows anesthesia to be induced smoothly.

Children who are older (usually >6 years of age) and understand how to hold their breath can perform a single-breath induction of anesthesia [65,66]. This is done by first priming the circuit with 8% sevoflurane (with or without 70% nitrous oxide) by flushing the circuit and reservoir bag 3–4 times. A 2 L reservoir bag is preferred because it limits the circuit volume and provides a sufficient reservoir in the event the child takes an additional breath. Before taking a single breath through the breathing circuit, the child practices vital capacity breathing, i.e. inhaling through their mouth and exhaling to residual volume through the mouth (by instructing the child to exhale until there is no air left in their lungs). Once the child has mastered the breathing maneuvers, they exhale to residual volume, at which point the facemask is applied tightly to the face. The child is instructed to take a single vital capacity breath through the mouth and hold it for as long as they can. While the child is holding their breath, the anesthesiologist counts aloud slowly. In general, the child loses consciousness before the count reaches 20 (sec), the head and neck are supported and the child placed in the supine position.

Intravenous induction

Most children eschew intravenous inductions because they fear the pain associated with establishing intravenous access. For children without intravenous access, anesthetic cream can be applied topically to the skin to obviate pain caused by the needle puncture. Several such creams are available, including the eutectic mixture of local anesthetics (EMLA®) cream (AstraZeneca, Wilmington, Delaware), which requires a 45–60-min application time to produce topical anesthesia, and Ametop® (Smith and New, Canada) and Synera® (Zars Pharma Inc, Salt Lake City, Utah) which require a 30-min application time and do not cause blanching of the skin or venoconstriction.

Once intravenous access has been established, intravenous anesthesia can be induced. Currently, the only induction agents routinely available in the US are propofol, ketamine, and etomidate; sodium thiopental is no longer available.

Propofol is the most widely available induction agent. It is available as Diprivan in a 1% solution that includes Intralipid (long-chain triglycerides from soy oil), EDTA, egg lecithin, and pH adjustment. Since propofol is a phenol derivative, it causes pain when injected into the small peripheral veins of children. Numerous strategies have been devised to attenuate or prevent this pain but two techniques appear to be the most effective: pretreatment with 70% nitrous oxide in oxygen by inhalation or a modified Bier block using 0.5–1 mg/kg of 1% lidocaine injected into a vein and occluding the vein for 30–45 sec [67].

Propofol is a very safe induction agent for children. When it was originally released, propofol was contraindicated in children with egg allergy. Egg lecithin is a phospholipid derived from egg yolk, a product to which children are not known to be allergic [7]. A second concern relates to children with soy allergy who may develop anaphylaxis to propofol. This theoretical concern has not been reported to occur in the literature, in part because all soy proteins are removed in the manufacturing of propofol, according to Astra Zeneca, North America. However, non-North American manufacturers caution against the use of propofol in children with soy and

peanut allergy, as children with soy allergy share epitopes with peanuts and develop peanut allergy [68]. Fortunately, >80% of children who claim to have peanut allergy are actually hypersensitive to peanuts, not immunologically allergic [69]. If children with "peanut allergy" have not been tested immunologically, then the clinician may either avoid propofol or administer a small aliquot of propofol to assess their allergic sensitivity to the drug.

Ketamine may be used for induction of anesthesia, although the concern of postoperative nightmares has relegated it to a second-tier anesthetic that is given for specific indications such as sepsis or cyanotic heart disease.

Etomidate has been neither studied in children nor approved for use in this age group. Its primary indication is for patients in septic shock. In adults, etomidate (0.3 mg/kg) suppresses adrenal function when administered as a continuous infusion, but comparable studies with etomidate have not been conducted in children to determine if they also develop adrenal suppression. Moreover, no dose–response relationship has been determined for etomidate and anesthesia in children. Etomidate may cause myoclonic jerking and pain upon intravenous injection. The latter may be prevented by pretreatment with intravenous lidocaine.

Sodium thiopental has been used for almost half a century as an intravenous induction agent, but in the past two decades it has been supplanted by propofol. Thiopental induces anesthesia very rapidly, and its effects are terminated equally rapidly, primarily by redistribution of the drug. Only 10% of thiopental is metabolized per hour, which delays emergence from anesthesia, particularly if supplemental doses are administered. Hence, this anesthetic is not suitable for continuous intravenous infusion. Most recently, thiopental has been in short supply and unavailable for clinical use.

Intramuscular induction

Intramuscular inductions of anesthesia are uncommon in children because they are painful and because the induction of anesthesia is delayed. The only anesthetic currently used for intramuscular injections is 3–5 mg/kg of ketamine (see above), and this is usually reserved for adolescent children who are cognitively impaired and unco-operative. The preferable location for an IM injection is the deltoid or triceps muscle, in part because there is little fat in the subcutaneous tissue, which causes a greater likelihood that the drug will be deposited into muscle rather than fat. The onset of sedation is approximately 3–5min and the duration of action is approximately 30–45min.

Rarely do children who require emergency securing of their airways present without intravenous access. When this does occur, any one of several approaches may be undertaken. Intravenous access may be established before induction of anesthesia, after anesthesia is induced with an inhalational agent or after IM injection of ketamine (3–5 mg/kg), atropine (0.02 mg/kg) and succinylcholine (4 mg/kg).

Rectal induction

Rectal induction of anesthesia was popular in young children (<5 years of age) in the past, particularly for those who were unwilling to take oral premedication or who were very frightened. Several regimens have been used for rectal induction: methohexital 15–25 mg/kg, midazolam 1.0 mg/kg, ketamine 5 mg/kg, or thiopental 30–40 mg/kg [70–72]. A number of problems were identified with rectal anesthesia inductions, including poor bioavailability of the induction agent (due to unpredictable rectal venous absorption or evacuation of the drug from the rectum), risk of laryngospasm (with methohexital), and possible delayed recovery from anesthesia. In immunocompromised patients, rectal administration of drugs may lead to sepsis. Today, rectal inductions are rarely employed. Most anesthetists prefer to involve the parents in managing the child's behavior at induction of anesthesia rather than administer a rectal medication.

Problems during induction of anesthesia

Oxygen desaturation

Healthy children breathing room air should have a SaO_2 >95% before induction of anesthesia, and this level of saturation should be maintained after induction of anesthesia and airway instrumentation, particularly with a FiO_2 ≥0.33. However some children decrease their SaO_2 to <94% in the early anesthesia period and do not increase it substantially, despite an increase in the FiO_2. In the presence of a normal capnogram, the foremost diagnosis is an endobronchial intubation, followed by asthma, mucus plug, and atelectasis. Once bilateral air entry is confirmed, no wheezing is detected, and suctioning the tracheal tube fails to produce purulent secretions, the next most probable diagnosis is segmental atelectasis. The mechanism for the atelectasis is the decrease in lung volumes and chest compliance that occur with induction of anesthesia plus reduced tidal volumes and respiratory effort. In this situation most of the pulmonary blood perfuses the basal segments of the lungs, whereas the upper lung segments receive most of the ventilation. This $\dot{V}/\dot{Q}$ mismatching is relatively unaffected by increasing the FiO_2 from 0.30 to 1.00 because of the sigmoidal shape of the oxyhemoglobin dissociation curve.

To restore the SaO_2 to >94%, the atelectatic alveoli must be reopened (or recruited) [73]. This is accomplished by manually inflating the lungs to 20–30 cmH_2O pressure for 20–30 sec (known as an alveolar recruitment maneuver). This maneuver should be applied cautiously if the child's circulation is unstable. The maneuver shifts ventilation up the pressure–volume curve where right-to-left shunting is minimal. The fresh gas used during this inspiratory pause may include any concentration of oxygen (including up to 70% nitrous oxide) as well as inhaled anesthetic to maintain general anesthesia. Once the inspiratory pause is completed, a physiological positive end-expiratory pressure (up to 10 cmH_2O) is applied and spontaneous respiration is allowed to resume.

Bronchospasm

Bronchospasm occurs infrequently in children during induction of anesthesia with sevoflurane and halothane [74] but is more common during induction with isoflurane and desflurane [75] and following tracheal intubation. Bronchospasm is defined as a sudden constriction of the airways. Wheezing, on the other hand, which literally means "hissing," is whistling (high- or low-pitched) noises in the airways. To keep these two terms distinct, remember the expression: "all that wheezes is not bronchospasm." Bronchospasm occurs more commonly in children with asthma, pulmonary infections, and anaphylaxis. Wheezing can occur at multiple airway levels, including the larynx (e.g. stridor), and can be intrinsic to the airway (e.g. asthma) or extrinsic to the airway (e.g. pneumothorax).

The factors that predispose to bronchospasm during anesthesia include a recent upper respiratory tract infection, asthma, foreign body in the airway (e.g. peanut or tracheal tube), first- and second-hand smoking, and GERD. Preoperatively, the chest is auscultated to detect wheezing. If new-onset wheezing is detected, elective surgery should be canceled and the child should be referred to the pediatrician or pulmonologist for further evaluation and treatment. Elective surgery should be canceled because wheezing is a sign of unstable pulmonary disease and increases the perioperative risks of general anesthesia. If the surgery is urgent/emergency, bronchodilator therapy should be instituted preoperatively, airway management should be directed towards avoiding a tracheal tube, and equipment should be prepared to provide intraoperative bronchodilator therapy (see below). If the child wheezes chronically despite maximum pulmonary therapy and there is no acute exacerbation of the disease, a dose of bronchodilator should be administered preoperatively and if possible, avoid using a tracheal tube.

If bronchospasm occurs after tracheal intubation, the cause should be determined and treated immediately. For the new onset of bronchospasm following induction of anesthesia and tracheal intubation, one should first rule out an endobronchial intubation by auscultating both lungs and verifying the depth of the tracheal tube tip in the airway. The tracheal tube should be suctioned to remove mucus plugs from the airways. Although passing a suction catheter down the tracheal tube does not rule out the presence of mucus or a defective ET tube cuff, it reduces the probability that either is present. If the bronchospasm is not resolved with either of these maneuvers, then albuterol should be administered via the tracheal tube. To deliver an aerosol of albuterol, the albuterol canister should be inserted into the barrel of a 30 mL syringe in the inverted position (after removing the syringe plunger) and the plunger should be reinserted on top of the canister and the syringe attached to the elbow of the breathing circuit. Pushing on the syringe plunger delivers albuterol into the circuit. Three to 12% of the aerosolized drug reaches the tip of the tracheal tube, depending on the internal diameter of the tracheal tube (from 3 to 6 mm ID) [76]. Hence, 5–10 activations may be required to deliver enough albuterol to alter bronchial tone. If these maneuvers fail and bronchospasm continues, 1–2 µg/kg epinephrine may be administered IV. If bronchospasm persists despite these treatments, then an extrinsic cause for the bronchospasm (e.g. pneumothorax) should be sought, investigated, and treated.

Laryngospasm

Laryngospasm is an infrequent but potentially life-threatening emergency in unintubated patients that most commonly occurs during induction or emergence from anesthesia. The frequency of laryngospasm in children varies dramatically from 0.4% to 10% among studies, the study populations, and predisposing factors [77–79]. Factors that increase the risk of laryngospasm in children are shown in Box 15.9 [79,80].

Laryngospasm is defined as reflex closure of the false and true vocal cords, although the precise pathogenesis of this reflex remains unclear. Complete laryngospasm is defined as closure of the false vocal cords and apposition of the laryngeal surface of the epiglottis and interarytenoids. This results in complete cessation of air movement or noisy breathing, lack of movement of the reservoir bag, and an absent capnogram. In contrast, incomplete (or partial) laryngospasm is defined as incomplete apposition of the vocal cords that leaves a small gap posteriorly that is sufficient to permit a persistent inspiratory stridor, limited movement of the reservoir bag, and progressively increasing respiratory effort. Some assert that incomplete laryngospasm is not laryngospasm at all, but for treatment purposes this is a moot point.

Laryngospasm begins as faint inspiratory stridor during induction of or emergence from anesthesia and is associated with suprasternal and supraclavicular indrawing due to increased inspiratory effort, increased diaphragmatic excursions, and flailing of the lower ribs. As greater inspiratory effort is expended, the intensity and volume of the stridor increase and the chest wall movement resembles that of a "rocking horse." As laryngospasm progresses, air movement through the almost closed glottis ceases and the inspiratory effort becomes completely silent. This is an ominous sign. If progression of the laryngospasm is not stopped, the limited reserve of oxygen in the lungs will be exhausted and oxygen desaturation will ensue. This will be followed immediately by a decrease in heart rate. This downward spiral must be interrupted as described below.

Management of laryngospasm requires a multifaceted and immediate response (Fig. 15.1) [78]. As soon as the diagnosis is suspected, a tight-fitting facemask should be applied to the child's face and 100% oxygen delivered with positive end-expiratory pressure (maximum 15–20 cmH₂O to limit gastric inflation). If the triggering event is blood, secretions or foreign material in the airway, these should be removed to take away the source of glottic stimulation.

As soon as the offending agent (if one is present) has been removed, a jaw thrust maneuver should be applied. The jaw thrust maneuver requires familiarity with the anatomy of the retromandibular notch, an area subtended by the condylar process of the ascending ramus of the mandible anteriorly, the mastoid process posteriorly, and the external auditory canal superiorly [81]. Bilateral digital pressure is applied to the most cephalad point on the posterior edge of the condylar process of the ascending ramus of the mandible, and the pressure is directed towards the frontal hairline. Pressure on the edge of the condylar process should be applied for 3–5 sec at a time and then released, all the while sealing the facemask tightly against the child's face. By applying and releasing pressure on the condylar processes, the repeated painful stimuli may cause sufficient pain to induce the child to

---

Box 15.9 Factors that increase the frequency of laryngospasm

- Young age (infants and young children)
- History of reactive airways disease
- Recent URTI (<2 wk)
- Exposure to second-hand smoke
- Airway anomalies
- Airway surgery
- Airway devices (tracheal tubes, possibly LMA)
- Stimulating the glottis during a light plane of anesthesia
- Secretions in the oropharynx (e.g. blood, excess saliva, gastric juice)
- Inhaled anesthesia (vs intravenous anesthesia)
- Inexperienced anesthesiologist

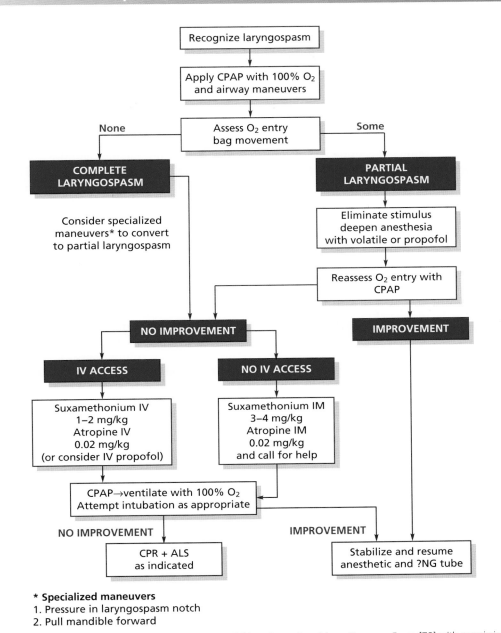

Figure 15.1 Algorithm for diagnosing and managing laryngospasm in children. Reproduced from Hampson-Evans [78] with permission from Elsevier.

cry. If the child cries, the vocal cords must open, which terminates the laryngospasm. In addition to delivering 100% oxygen and positive end-expiratory pressure to the upper airway, this maneuver confers the additional benefit of pain and the "flight and fright" response, which stimulates the respiratory effort and vocalization, possibly breaking the laryngospasm. Remember, laryngospasm cannot develop or persist if the vocal cords are moving and the child is vocalizing or crying.

If positive end-expiratory pressure, 100% oxygen, and the jaw thrust maneuver fail to quickly break the laryngospasm, further intervention should be undertaken

before desaturation and bradycardia develop. Appropriate treatment at this stage includes IV atropine (0.02 mg/kg) and IV propofol (<1 mg/kg) [38,82,83]. If the laryngospasm breaks, then ventilation should be assisted with 100% oxygen and an inhalational anesthetic. However, if the laryngospasm does not abate and the heart rate and oxygen saturation continue their downward courses, succinylcholine (1–2 mg/kg IV or 4–5 mg/kg IM) should be administered and the trachea intubated.

An interesting report suggests that gentle chest compressions effectively break laryngospasm in children [84]. Adding chest compressions to the management of laryngospasm requires a pair of free hands to perform the compressions. If no free hands are available, do not abandon the maneuvers described above. A free pair of hands may not be readily available but if they are, chest compression is worthy of consideration. The risks associated with performing chest compressions include sternal or rib fractures, which must be explained to the parents if they occur. Currently, it is our opinion that there is insufficient evidence to recommend routine use of chest compressions to relieve laryngospasm in children.

Bradycardia

Bradycardia is a slowing of the heart rate below age-defined limits. For infants (<1 year of age) this is 100 beats/minute (bpm), for young children 1–5 years of age, 80 bpm, and for children >5 years of age, 60 bpm. Since cardiac output of infants and children is heart rate dependent, a slow heart rate means a reduced cardiac output. If the heart rate decreases below these limits, corrective action should be taken to restore the heart rate, and if necessary cardiopulmonary resuscitation should be initiated.

Although hypoxia is the foremost cause of bradycardia in children, drug-associated causes include halothane and succinylcholine. Since sevoflurane has replaced halothane in developed countries, this cause of bradycardia has all but disappeared [74]. This is not the case in many developing countries. A single dose of succinylcholine remains a common cause of bradycardia in children but occurs much less commonly today because succinylcholine is not routinely used in children for tracheal intubation. Recently, it was reported that the incidence of bradycardia during the first 6 min of sevoflurane anesthesia in children with Down syndrome was fivefold greater than in matched controls [85]. Children who are rate dependent for cardiac output and develop bradycardia may require treatment with atropine or isoproterenol.

The causes of bradycardia in healthy children are listed in Box 15.8. To stop progressive slowing of the heart rate, the underlying cause of the bradycardia should be corrected (e.g. correct hypoxia when present and administer atropine 0.02 mg/kg). Atropine is only effective when myocardial electrical activity is present and the bradycardia is of vagal origin. If asystole occurs, however, atropine does not restore the heart rhythm, and the only definitive treatment is epinephrine (10 μg/kg). Secondary treatment should include isoproterenol.

Hypotension

The incidence of hypotension during induction of anesthesia in children is small. During minimum alveolar concentration (MAC) studies, we defined hypotension as a >30% decrease in systolic blood pressure from baseline

and at 1 MAC, the decrease in systolic blood pressure was <30% in both neonates and infants 1–6 months of age anesthetized with halothane [86] and in all children through adolescents who were anesthetized with sevoflurane or desflurane [87,88]. The decrease in systolic and mean arterial blood pressures in healthy children at >1 MAC sevoflurane and halothane was neither remarkable nor required intervention [65,66,89]. Induction of anesthesia with sevoflurane plus an intravenous bolus of propofol is a popular method of securing the airway of children. Recently, we determined that an intravenous bolus of 0–3 mg/kg of propofol given to 120 children anesthetized with 8% sevoflurane was associated with systolic blood pressures that were within the normal range [62].

In children, in addition to the effects of induction agents on blood pressure (BP), direct and indirect factors may cause hypotension during induction of anesthesia. Direct causes include a prolonged preoperative fast, bleeding, chronic vomiting or diarrhea, and anaphylaxis. Indirect causes of hypovolemia include coning of the brainstem, septic shock, cardiac tamponade, tension pneumothorax, major vascular compression (pulmonary arterial compression from an anterior mediastinal mass) and, rarely, hypothyroidism.

If hypovolemia is suspected, the initial treatment of hypotension is to restore euvolemia, rather than administer vasopressors. Balanced salt solutions, such as lactated Ringer's solution, should be administered in repeated 10–20 mL/kg boluses while reducing the inspired concentration of inhalational anesthetic.

Maintenance of anesthesia

Methods

The anesthetic management of infants and children during maintenance of anesthesia is most commonly accomplished with inhalational anesthetics. Over the past 150 years, the molecular structure of inhalational anesthetics has been refined to the point that today these anesthetics are effective, reliable, easy to deliver, offer favorable pharmacokinetics, and are safe. The vast majority of anesthetics in children are based on an inhalational anesthetic with intravenous supplementation of analgesics and antiemetics. One key advantage that distinguishes inhalational anesthetics from intravenous drugs is the ability to continuously measure end-tidal anesthetic concentrations of inhaled agents. This measurement provides invaluable knowledge regarding the accuracy of our delivery system and the patient's responses to the anesthetic.

Currently, three inhalational anesthetics are used to maintain anesthesia: isoflurane, sevoflurane, and desflurane. Although a discussion of the pharmacology of inhaled anesthetics is beyond the scope of this chapter (see Chapter 9), several key principles are summarized. All three anesthetics preserve cardiorespiratory homeostasis in healthy children. However, the use of desflurane in severe asthmatics and children exposed to second-hand smoke may be associated with more adverse respiratory events that are due to changes in pulmonary resistance during and after desflurane [90]. In addition, if desflurane is used for maintenance of anesthesia through an LMA, we remove the LMA when the child is awake to reduce the risk of adverse respiratory events [91].

The speed of emergence from isoflurane and sevoflurane anesthesia is similar when the anesthetic concentration is tapered during the maintenance phase. The speed of emergence after desflurane is more rapid than both isoflurane and sevoflurane, particularly if desflurane was the sole anesthetic used during the maintenance period, it was supplemented with short-acting opioids or non-opioid analgesics, and if the surgery was prolonged [92]. Alternatively, if large doses of opioids were used for analgesia, the sedative effects of the opioids may result in similar emergence times for all anesthetics.

Nitrous oxide is the oldest anesthetic still in use in developed countries and is commonly used during maintenance of anesthesia in children. Although it has several disadvantages, we believe none of them warrants its withdrawal from practice. However, there are several clinical scenarios (bowel obstruction, middle ear surgery, spine surgery with motor evoked potential and cardiopulmonary bypass) in which nitrous oxide is contraindicated. In other situations it has provided a background of anesthesia, sedation, and analgesia during painful procedures for decades. A meta-analysis of postoperative nausea and vomiting after anesthesia revealed that omission of nitrous oxide surprisingly yielded a 2% incidence of awareness [93]. Side-effects from nitrous oxide are common and include perioperative nausea and vomiting, expansion of air-filled cavities in the body, depression of methionine synthetase, and atmospheric pollution.

The environmental concern regarding nitrous oxide relates to its effects on depletion of the ozone layer and global warming. With an estimated life in the troposphere of 110 years [94], nitrous oxide is not environmentally green; however, <5% of the nitrous oxide released into the atmosphere originates from medicinal use. Fertilizers, fossil fuel combustion, and synthetic material manufacturing (nylon) are the top three anthropogenic sources of N_2O [94]. Anesthesia is not listed as a source of nitrous oxide in global environmental textbooks [94]. Methods to reduce the medical fingerprint on the troposphere include combining desflurane with nitrous oxide, reducing the use of desflurane, using sevoflurane or isoflurane with an oxygen/air fresh gas flow, and improved carbon dioxide absorbents [95].

Total intravenous anesthesia is used as a primary means of providing anesthesia for children with malignant hyperthermia, for those undergoing spine surgery requiring motor evoked potential monitoring, and for those with a history of severe perioperative nausea and vomiting. Propofol and ketamine are the primary general anesthetics used for TIVA. Propofol has few side-effects beyond pain on injection and a lack of analgesic properties. Pain on injection can be obviated by pretreatment with 70% nitrous oxide or by applying a modified Bier block for 30–45 sec with IV lidocaine (0.5–0.75 mg/kg) [67,96]. Propofol has anti-nausea effects that have been exploited in children with histories of nausea and vomiting. However, its major liability remains propofol infusion syndrome (PRIS), which in some jurisdictions has resulted in the anesthetic being proscribed for use as a sedative [97]. Propofol has caused PRIS in children sedated with >5 mg/kg/h of propofol for ≥48 h [97]. Between 1989 and 2004, more than 33 cases of PRIS were described in children during propofol sedation/anesthesia, as evidenced by an evolving lactic acidosis (for no apparent clinical reason) that reverted to a normal pH once the propofol infusion was discontinued or sudden death occurred [97–100]. Currently, continuous propofol infusions are used in North America to sedate children for medical and surgical procedures, but not in intensive care units when multiple days of sedation are required. Frequent blood gas determinations are prudent in all children who are sedated with propofol for prolonged periods. If an inexplicable lactic acidosis develops, propofol should be discontinued and appropriate resuscitation measures instituted.

Propofol infusion rates to prevent movement during MRI or surgery range from 200 to 400 µg/kg/min (12–24 mg/kg/h) in infants and children [101,102]. For surgery, supplemental medications, including opioids, muscle relaxants, and sedatives, are usually required. We have also noted that younger infants and those who are cognitively challenged require much greater propofol infusion rates to prevent movement during MRI than older children without cognitive impairment. A word of caution when using propofol infusions for infants <1 year of age: clearance of propofol is least in neonates and increases from neonates to infants 1 year of age. Thereafter, clearance remains unchanged into adulthood [103]. Thus, after the initial loading dose of propofol, the reduced drug clearance in young infants may necessitate lower infusion rates or recovery will be delayed.

To account for the differing pharmacokinetics of propofol (and other medications) over time and in children with differing physiology, target-controlled infusions were developed [104]. These infusion pumps incorporate software that automatically adjusts the infusion rate to the child's characteristics and to the desired blood concentration of propofol in that age group. To date, these infusion pumps have been modestly successful but are not widely available and are not expected to be available for use in humans in North America in the near future.

Supplemental analgesics are also used during both inhalational and intravenous anesthesia to prevent physiological responses and movement to pain. Remifentanil (with a zero context-sensitive half-life) 0.05–0.1 µg/kg/min can be administered as an infusion, whereas other opioids (fentanyl and morphine) are more often administered by intravenous boluses. Fentanyl (1–2 µg/kg) or morphine (0.05–0.1 mg/kg) can be administered intravenously; the dose is adjusted up or down depending on the child's exposure to opioids, the severity of the pain, and concomitantly administered analgesics.

Age versus minimal alveolar concentration

Minimal alveolar concentration (MAC) is defined as the minimum alveolar or end-tidal concentration of inhalational anesthetic at which 50% of subjects move in response to a noxious stimulus, usually a skin incision in humans. In children, the MAC values for most inhalational anesthetics increase with decreasing age, reaching a peak value during infancy. For example, the MAC of halothane and isoflurane increases with increasing gestational age and through early infancy, reaching its zenith in infants 1–6 months old. It then decreases with increasing age (Fig. 15.2) [105]. The MAC for desflurane, on the other hand, also increases during infancy but reaches its zenith later (6–12 months of age), and then decreases with increasing age [88]. In the case of sevoflurane, the rela-

tionship between MAC and age differs substantially from the aforementioned inhaled anesthetics [87]. The MAC of sevoflurane, interestingly, is constant at 3.2% in neonates and infants 1–6 months of age. It then decreases abruptly to 2.5% in late infancy to adolescence. The neurobiological reason(s) why MAC changes with age in childhood and why the relationships differ among the different anesthetics have not been explained, although several theories have been proposed, including differences in central nervous system development and neurohumoral factors.

The MAC concept includes the notion that all concurrently administered inhaled anesthetics contribute to the total MAC. Thus, 60% nitrous oxide with 1% isoflurane is equivalent to 0.6 + 1.0 or 1.6 MAC of inhalational anesthesia. This notion applies to isoflurane and halothane in children, as well as to all the inhalational anesthetics in adults. However, when the MAC of sevoflurane and desflurane was determined in children in combination with nitrous oxide, the MAC contribution of 60% nitrous oxide was only 20%, two-thirds less than the effect of nitrous oxide in the presence of isoflurane and halothane [87,106]. The reason for this substantially diminished effect of nitrous oxide with these two relatively insoluble anesthetics has not been explained.

A number of factors have been shown to influence the MAC of inhalational anesthetics. Approximately 90% of adults who are homozygous or heterozygous for the melanocortin-1 receptor gene (i.e. red heads) require 20% more anesthesia than those without this mutation [107]. Children with cerebral palsy and severe mental retardation require 25% less halothane than healthy children [108]. Chronic anticonvulsant therapy also reduces MAC.

In addition to the traditional nociceptive stimulus of skin incision, the MAC responses to other stimuli, including tracheal intubation and extubation, LMA insertion and removal, tracheal intubation/skin incision ratio, and wakefulness have been reported in children [109]. The tracheal intubation to skin incision ratio in children is about 1.33 for halothane and sevoflurane. MAC awake for sevoflurane in children 2–5 years of age is approximately 0.66% and is almost 50% greater than that in 5–12-year-old children, 0.44% [110].

Fluid management
General principles

Intravenous fluid administration sets should be prepared before the child arrives in the operating room. For young children, a 500 mL bag of lactated Ringer's solution with a buretrol is appropriate; for infants (<1 year) a 250 mL bag with a buretrol is preferable. All pediatric IV sets should include a manual controller, a one-way valve (to prevent medications from passing retrograde up the IV

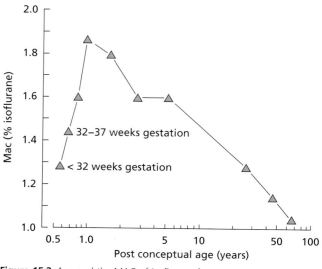

Figure 15.2 Age and the MAC of isoflurane from premature infants to adults. Reproduced from LeDez and Lerman [105] with permission from Lippincott Williams & Wilkins.

tubing), and needleless ports and/or three-way stopcocks for medication administration. For children >8 years of age, the IV infusion set may be prepared with a macro- or micro-drip without a buretrol and a 1000 mL bag of balanced salt solution.

For neonates and preterm infants from the NICU, we continue the clear maintenance infusion fluids from the NICU, i.e. 10% glucose and supplemental calcium. The infusion rate used in the NICU should be continued during surgery, since suddenly reducing this hyperglycemic infusion may cause hypoglycemia. If sequential blood glucose concentrations can be measured during surgery, the glucose infusion should be adjusted to maintain normoglycemia. Intralipid infusions from total parenteral nutrition are best discontinued before transfer to the OR to reduce the risk of contaminating the Intralipid and central venous access line by repeated line accessing.

Most IV fluids administered to healthy children during elective surgery now consist of a non-glucose containing isotonic salt solution, commonly lactated Ringer's solution in North America. These solutions replaced glucose-containing hypotonic solutions after reports of seizures, aspiration, and brain damage. Worldwide, the shift to isotonic solutions for intraoperative fluid maintenance in children has occurred more slowly [111]. Lactated Ringer's solution is slightly hypotonic (280 mOsm/L) and contains small concentrations of potassium and lactate. Normal saline (0.9% NaCl) is isotonic (308 mOsm/L) and contains no additional ionic moieties but has a pH of 5.0. It is not routinely used as the primary maintenance solution, since large volumes may lead to a hyperchloremic metabolic acidosis (non-anion gap type). We advocate glucose-containing solutions, such as 1% or 2.5% glucose in lactated Ringer's (LR) solution as a maintenance solution for full-term neonates and infants <6 months of age, and for young children who are cachectic, chronically malnourished, tolerate fasting poorly (maple sugar disease), and suffer from debilitating disease who may be at risk for hypoglycemia [112,113]. These solutions should not lead to intraoperative hyperglycemia or hyponatremia. Although the incidence of hyponatremia has been dramatically reduced with the shift to isotonic salt solutions, some specific surgeries may require intraoperative monitoring of serum electrolytes [114].

Children with specific medical conditions should have tailored intravenous solutions. For children in renal failure or renal insufficiency, normal saline is the preferred balanced salt solution because it contains no potassium. Children with a mitochondrial myopathy and who had lactic acidosis during infancy should be fasted for only brief periods (to avoid acidosis and hypoglycemia) and should receive only normal saline with glucose supplementation as needed.

Infants and children <2 years of age who may be hypovolemic should be assessed preoperatively to determine the magnitude of their fluid deficit: mild, moderate or severe [115]. The signs of mild dehydration (5% body-weight loss – approximately 50 mL/kg deficit) include poor skin turgor and dry mouth. The signs of moderate fluid dehydration (10% of bodyweight loss – 100 mL/kg deficit) include sunken fontanelle, tachycardia and oliguria in addition to the signs of mild dehydration. The signs of severe fluid dehydration (15% of bodyweight loss – 150 mL/kg deficit) include sunken eyeballs, hypotension, and anuria plus the signs of moderate dehydration.

Correction of hypovolemia requires a staged infusion of fluids. Approximately 50% of the deficit should be replaced in the first hour, 25% in the second, and 25% in the third hour. A balanced salt solution should be used to restore euvolemia.

Elective surgery

For minor elective surgery, the traditional calculation for the hourly fluid infusion rate has been based on replacing the triad of fluid deficit during fasting, ongoing maintenance, and blood and third space losses. In children, the calculation was predicated on the 4–2–1 mL/kg/h where 4 mL/kg is for the first 10 kg, 2 mL/kg is for the second 10 kg and 1 mL/kg is for the third 10 kg and any additional bodyweight thereafter hourly [116]. Initial blood loss may be replaced with balanced salt solution at a rate of 3 mL of solution for every 1 mL of blood loss. For third space losses, the replacement volume is based on the severity of the losses: 1–2 mL/kg/h for minor surgery, 2–5 mL/kg/h for moderate surgery, and 6–10 mL/kg/h for major surgery and large third space losses.

In a reappraisal of their 1957 4–2–1 fluid recommendations for children in the perioperative period, Holliday and Segar reviewed a series of reports of hyponatremia in children who had received hypotonic glucose-containing solution and evaluated the risks of using a balanced salt solution for maintenance fluids [117]. They determined that their original formula could lead not only to hyponatremia if excessive volumes were rapidly infused in young children, but to fluid and sodium overload in some children if the formula was used with a balanced salt solution. This was of particular concern in the postoperative period because pain and medications may lead to the syndrome of inappropriate antidiuretic hormone where an excess infusion of balanced salt solution might place some children at risk for congestive heart failure. They concluded that their previous 4–2–1 fluid formula used with hypotonic glucose-containing solutions should be replaced with a 2–1–0.5 formula for fluid management in children with balanced salt solutions. In this case, they recommended intraoperative rehydration with 20–30 mL/kg balanced salt solution in all children and postoperative maintenance using half their original formula or 2–1–0.5 mL/kg [117].

Although most pediatric surgeons are careful to minimize bleeding during surgery, it is important to remain vigilant to blood loss throughout the procedure. For procedures that are likely to result in significant tissue trauma or blood loss, appropriate size IV access must be provided for transfusion of the blood and blood products needed for volume replacement. Packed red cells cannot be rapidly infused through either #24 gauge intravenous catheters or peripherally inserted central catheters (PICC). A #22 gauge catheter is the smallest intravenous cannula through which blood can be infused rapidly. Every effort should be made to insert the largest intravenous catheter that the child's veins will accommodate. Initial blood loss is replaced with a balanced salt solution in a ratio of 3 mL of salt solution for every mL of blood loss. This replacement, together with the maintenance requirement, should be logged on the anesthetic record. As the combined volume of balanced salt solution approaches 75–100 mL/kg, it is important to consider the possibility of dilutional thrombocytopenia and dilution of coagulation factors; coagulation indices should be measured at this time.

The threshold for initiating packed red blood cell (RBC) transfusions in children has undergone a renaissance in the past decade as evidence is mounting that the outcome and complications associated with transfusion at 7 g% hemoglobin are similar to that with transfusion at 9 g% [118,119]. The estimated blood volume in children decreases with increasing age from 95–100 mL/kg in premature infants to 70 mL/kg in adults [120]. Note that the estimated blood volume of obese children is reduced 10% from that of non-obese children of similar age [120]. To estimate the allowable blood loss during surgery, the following equation based on hematocrit (Hct), may be used [120]:

Maximum allowable blood loss

= (starting Hct − target Hct)/(starting Hct)

× Estimated blood volume   (Equation 1)

Some use a modified version of equation 1 and replace the "starting Hct" in the denominator with the "average Hct." This increases the allowable blood loss before transfusion. Irrespective of which equation is used, the actual Hct should be determined before initiating blood transfusion to ensure that the Hct has actually decreased to the desired level. When initiating a blood transfusion in a child, two formulas provide rough estimates of the amount of blood required to increase the hemoglobin concentration 1 g%: 4 mL/kg packed cells and 6 mL/kg whole blood.

Postoperative vomiting

The incidence of postoperative vomiting (POV) in children depends on a number of factors that relate to the child (motion sickness history, age), the anesthetic (inhaled anesthetics, nitrous oxide, opioids, preoperative fluid administration, postoperative fluid ingestion), and the surgery (inguinal/orchidopexy, tonsillectomy and adenoidectomy, strabismus, and middle ear surgery). To predict the probability of POV in children, a validated score has been developed [121]. The risk of POV increases with the number of the risk factors present: age ≥3 years, duration of surgery ≥30 min, strabismus surgery, and a history of POV in the proband or immediate family [121,122].

Children should be fasted preoperatively for brief periods and not forced to drink oral fluids postoperatively until they request them [123]. Intraoperatively, the child should be hydrated with IV fluids and provided with regional anesthesia and non-steroidal anti-inflammatory agents instead of opioids when possible. If the child is scheduled for emetogenic surgery and has a history of POV, the optimal anesthetic regimen may include propofol oxygen/air and two antiemetics, although conflicting evidence exists regarding the role of substituting propofol and nitrous oxide in POV [124,125].

The optimal prophylactic antiemetic strategy to administer to children during anesthesia is dexamethasone and a serotonin receptor antagonist, such as ondansetron [126,127]. A dose of dexamethasone between 0.0625 and 1 mg/kg (maximum 24 mg) has been shown to be equally effective, although we limit our maximum dose to 10 mg [128]. One report suggested that dexamethasone is associated with an increased incidence of postoperative tonsil bleeding [129] but we question the validity of those data and continue to use dexamethasone routinely in tonsil surgery without complications. The dose of ondansetron we use for prophylaxis in children is 0.05–0.15 mg/kg.

Emergence and recovery from anesthesia

As surgery concludes, the inspired concentration of inhalational anesthetics or infusion rates of intravenous drugs should be reduced. Neuromuscular blockade should be antagonized and function of the neuromuscular junction assessed before extubation. Equipment should be available to manage the airway (facemask, 100% oxygen) as well as complications from the extubation (suction).

The primary focus of the entire anesthesia team at this time is to assess the child's airway, their ability to breathe, and their ability to protect their airway should bleeding or vomiting occur following extubation. It is our practice to remove the tracheal tube or LMA when the child has fully recovered airway reflexes and is awake. There are very few surgical or medical indications to remove the airway during deep levels of anesthesia and little evidence that this practice results in a better outcome. The greatest concern regarding deep extubations is that a child who is deeply anesthetized and transported with an unsecured airway relies totally on extremely high-quality nursing in the recovery room to manage the airway until emergence. In most instances, the anesthesiologist returns to the operating room and does not remain at the child's side during recovery in the PACU.

The evidence is mixed regarding the frequency of adverse airway events following deep tracheal extubation or awake extubation [130,131]. We transfer children to the PACU awake, with an intact airway rather than anesthetized with a potentially compromised airway. This approach ensures that the child's airway is protected, independent of the skill level of the PACU nurses. However, transferring children deeply anesthetized may be safe if the skill set of the nurses in PACU includes managing anesthetized children.

In our experience, children who have an LMA in their airway are at increased risk for developing progressive airway obstruction several minutes after emergence from anesthesia and removal of the device. Accordingly, we remove all LMAs in the operating room before transferring the child to PACU. In the case of desflurane, we found a substantially greater frequency of adverse airway reflex responses compared to isoflurane when the LMA was removed during a deep level of anesthesia than when it was removed awake [91]. We remove all LMAs when the child is awake, especially if desflurane has been administered.

The timing of tracheal extubation is critical for minimizing the risk of adverse airway events during emergence from anesthesia. The optimal time for extubation requires that children have sufficiently emerged from anesthesia and can support their own airway and that adverse airway events are unlikely to occur after extubation. Recognizing the optimal time for extubation requires that we appreciate the three phases of emergence from inhalational anesthesia in children: early, middle and late. Each of these phases may last for several minutes, depending on the anesthetic administered and the age of the child. During the early phase of emergence, the child first coughs intermittently, gags, struggles, and moves nonpurposefully. This phase passes relatively quickly as the child enters the middle or quiescent phase. During this phase, the child may adopt one or more of several appearances, including deeply anesthetized, apneic or "agitated" and may breath-hold, strain, and/or have oxygen desaturation, the latter necessitating manual ventilation of the lungs to restore the SaO_2 to >95%. As the child

resumes quiet, spontaneous respiration, they enter the third phase of emergence, which is characterized by purposeful movement, flexing the hips and coughing and gagging on the tracheal tube, all of which increase in intensity until the child grimaces and opens the eyes spontaneously. Removing the tracheal tube during either the early or middle phase markedly increases the risk of triggering an adverse airway event. It is only during this third phase of emergence that we are least likely to trigger adverse airway reflex responses when the tracheal tube is removed. Our residents are taught that if you think it is the correct time to remove the tube, don't! Leave the tube *in situ* for another minute (or two) until the child is definitely in the late or third phase of emergence, when the tracheal tube may be removed safely.

While children emerge from anesthesia, the practitioner can follow one of two strategies: either no-touch or stimulation. With the former technique, the child breathes 100% oxygen undisturbed and unstimulated while we await the third phase of emergence (as described above). When the end-tidal anesthetic concentration decreases to a level consistent with wakefulness (sevoflurane concentration <0.6%) [110], the eyes will open spontaneously, the child will reach for the airway, gag, and grimace, all of which indicate that it is time to remove the airway. With the latter technique, the initial recovery is the same as that with the no-touch technique; however, we speed the transition through the second and third phases by applying digital pressure to the posterior ramus of the condylar process, the most cephalad portion of the ascending ramus of the mandible, for 3–5 sec while directing the force toward the hairline [81]. This is done when the end-tidal anesthetic concentration of isoflurane is <0.25% or sevoflurane <0.6%. The child becomes highly aroused, gags on the tracheal tube, reaches for and removes the tube, and opens their eyes. Both strategies provide similar outcomes with safe and protected airways.

In the vast majority of children, emergence from anesthesia progresses smoothly as described above; there is increasing arousal, gagging, and rejection of the presence of the tracheal tube. However, in rare instances, this sequence of events fails to progress at all, or if it progresses, it is not smooth. Children who fail to emerge from anesthesia must be assessed for a variety of potential problems (Box 15.10). The most common causes of delayed emergence are drug overdose or failure to taper or reduce the dose of inhalational or intravenous anesthetic or the presence of hypothermia. However, rare but potentially catastrophic events such as unexpected hypoglycemia or intracranial bleeding may complicate the anesthesia and surgery and lead to prolonged coma. Laboratory tests may be required to diagnose the cause of the coma. Definitive treatment should be administered once the diagnosis is confirmed.

Box 15.10 Causes of delayed emergence from anesthesia

- Residual drug effects: inhalational anesthetics, opioids, propofol
- Non-anesthesia medications: recreational drug use (cocaine, crack), herbal medicines (valerian, St John's wort)
- Depressed neuromuscular junction: residual neuromuscular blockade or pseudocholinesterase deficiency
- Hypothermia
- Hypo- or hyperglycemia
- Electrolyte imbalance: hyper- or hyponatremia
- Acid–base disturbance
- Hypercapnia
- Cerebrovascular accident/hypoxia: check pupil size and responsiveness to light bilaterally, presence of a gag reflex, symmetrical limb reflexes

---

Complications during recovery

Approximately 5% of patients have complications in the PACU [132]. Of these, 77% are from vomiting and 22% from respiratory causes. The remaining 1% or less are due to cardiac problems. The age distribution of the complications is important: vomiting occurred more than twice as frequently in children >8 years of age, whereas respiratory complications occurred twice as frequently in infants <1 year of age.

Vomiting

The frequency of vomiting in the PACU has decreased dramatically following the introduction of prophylactic antiemetics for children at risk for postoperative nausea and vomiting (PONV). Routine use of dexamethasone and ondansetron reduces the perioperative incidence of vomiting by up to 80% or more [126]. Our experience is that few children vomit in the PACU; most children who vomit do so after ingesting their first fluids, in the car on the way home or at home. Hence, we encourage oral ingestion of liquids after surgery only when the child asks to drink [123]. If the child continues to vomit, there are few effective interventions that have been shown stop the vomiting. Oral fluids should be withheld. If the child is an ultra-rapid metabolizer of ondansetron, the antiemetic effect of this drug may be short-lived. CYP450 2D6 and CYP450 3A4 are responsible for degradation of 5-HT3 receptor antagonists such as ondansetron [133]. Single nucleotide polymorphisms of CYP450 2D6 have been reported to cause rapid metabolism of these drugs. A second dose of ondansetron may be given if at least 2 h have passed since the first dose.

Emergence agitation

The introduction of sevoflurane into pediatric anesthesia caused a recrudescence of emergence agitation (also known as emergence delirium, ED). Emergence delirium has been recognized as a sequela after anesthesia for several decades; the frequency increased every time a new, less soluble inhalational anesthetic was introduced. ED has a peak incidence in children (of both sexes) at 2–6 years of age, is more common after some anesthetics (sevoflurane > desflurane > isoflurane >> TIVA), lasts 10–15 min, and is terminated either spontaneously or following a single IV dose of propofol, midazolam, clonidine, dexmedetomidine, ketamine or opioids [134–137].

The challenge is to differentiate ED from pain in children in the PACU after surgery. To that end, ED was assessed in children undergoing MRI with either sevoflurane or halothane [138]. Since none of the children experienced pain after the MRI, any delirium must have resulted from the anesthetic. The authors found a fivefold greater incidence of ED after sevoflurane than after halothane.

A host of studies continued to report ED after a variety of surgeries using non-validated delirium scales, with and without adequate analgesia. This led to much confusion regarding the nature, cause, and treatment of ED. To clarify much of the confusion, the Pediatric Anesthesia Emergence Delirium (PAED) score was developed and validated as an objective measure of ED; a score >10 is indicative of the presence of ED but some have suggested that a score >12 may be more specific [139,140].

Laryngospasm, postoperative stridor, and negative pressure pulmonary edema

Laryngospasm, postoperative stridor, and negative pressure pulmonary edema occur both during induction of anesthesia and during or after emergence from anesthesia. Pulmonary edema, on the other hand, is more common after tracheal extubation than during induction of anesthesia. Factors that increase the risk of laryngospasm include removing the tracheal tube from the larynx prematurely, the presence of blood, secretions or foreign material within the pharynx, second-hand smoke, and a recent history of upper respiratory tract infection (see Box 15.9). For a full discussion of laryngospasm, please refer to the section on induction of anesthesia above.

Postextubation stridor may also occur upon tracheal extubation. Stridor occurs because the epithelium within the cricoid ring swells after the tracheal tube is removed, thus reducing the cross-sectional diameter of the airway. Because airflow in the upper airway is turbulent, the resistance to airflow increases as the fifth power of the radius decreases. That is, if the radius of the airway within the cricoid ring decreases by 50%, the resistance to airflow increases 32-fold. In infants with increased oxygen requirements and metabolic rates, residual opioids, muscle weakness, and anesthesia may further compromise their ability to maintain an increased work of breathing during stridor, which could hasten fatigue and respiratory failure. Children with Down syndrome have a greater risk of postextubation stridor [141]. Treatment of stridor includes humidified oxygen, dexamethasone (1 mg/kg IV) and nebulized racemic epinephrine (0.5 mL epinephrine in 2 mL saline). Rarely is it necessary to reintubate the trachea for persistent and severe stridor in the PACU. If hypoxemia or respiratory failure occurs, the trachea should be reintubated with a smaller size tube than the one originally used. To avoid further irritating the epithelium, an audible leak should be present after intubation. If a racemic epinephrine treatment is repeated more than twice, the child should be observed for rebound edema in either the PACU or a monitored unit.

Negative pressure pulmonary edema or postextubation pulmonary edema is an infrequent complication that usually occurs immediately or within several minutes after tracheal extubation in healthy, muscular adolescents and young adults, although it has been reported in infants [142–145]. Once the trachea is extubated, as the airway appears increasingly obstructed, the child appears somnolent and unresponsive. A cascade of events then rapidly occurs. Laryngospasm is present and may range in severity from very mild (i.e. hiccups) to severe. Contemporaneously, the oxygen saturation decreases, almost out of proportion to the severity of the airway obstruction. Ventilation by mask with 100% oxygen is usually insufficient and tracheal reintubation is required to restore the SaO_2 to normal values. Reintubation of the trachea is accomplished by using a muscle relaxant, propofol or both. Upon reintubation, pink frothy pulmonary edema fluid is suctioned from the tracheal tube. Positive pressure ventilation with a positive end-expiratory pressure and sufficient oxygen to restore the oxygen saturation to >94% should be maintained until oxygen and ventilation are no longer needed. Tracheal intubation is usually the only measure needed to treat the pulmonary edema. Sedation should be provided until the pulmonary edema resolves (usually 12–24h or more), after which time the trachea can be extubated.

The mechanism of the pulmonary edema postextubation is believed to be the result of extremely negative intrathoracic pressures generated against an obstructed airway (i.e. laryngospasm) and a marked increase in venous return. This excess fluid overloads the left ventricle and causes pulmonary edema.

Oxygen desaturation

Failure to maintain adequate oxygen saturation in the recovery room is a common problem. Evidence suggests that a single alveolar recruitment maneuver reduces the risk of post-extubation desaturation [146]. Unrecognized hypoxia may lead to deterioration in the child's clinical status and to sudden bradycardia and cardiac arrest. Continuous monitoring of the child's oxygen saturation is essential in the PACU to provide an early indication of this complication. The minimum acceptable oxygen saturation in the PACU is 94%. Administration of oxygen by facemask may be required to maintain the oxygen saturation, particularly if residual anesthesia or opioids are present, a craniofacial or muscular abnormality is present, or the child is obese or fluid overloaded. In healthy children, oxygen desaturation is generally indicative of hypoventilation and/or airway obstruction. Because there is no means of assessing ventilation in children in the PACU who do not have artificial airways, we rely on clinical signs to expeditiously diagnose and treat airway obstruction and hypoventilation.

Children should be weaned from oxygen dependency (assuming they did not require supplemental oxygen preoperatively) before they are discharged to the floor or the step-down unit. Some children remove their facemasks themselves when they awaken from anesthesia; if their oxygen saturation is >94% while breathing room air, then no additional oxygen is required. If the child requires supplemental oxygen by facemask, oxygen administration should be changed to nasal prongs. The prongs should subsequently be removed and the adequacy of SaO_2 in room air determined. If the child cannot maintain oxygen saturation after attempts to wean them from the oxygen, further investigation may be required (such as a chest x-ray) to rule out aspiration, pneumonia or pneumothorax.

Transport to the postanesthesia care unit and intensive care unit

Transferring children from the operating room to either the postanesthesia care unit (PACU) or the intensive care unit (ICU) has inherent risks that must be anticipated and assessed continuously.

Before commencing transport to the PACU, the child must have a stable airway, be able to maintain adequate oxygenation and ventilation, have stable heart rate and blood pressure measurements, and have adequate pain control. A vigilant expert who is trained to manage potential postoperative problems should accompany the child.

During transport to the PACU, most children breathe spontaneously without an oral airway in place. The optimal position for transfer of a child, particularly after airway surgery, is the lateral decubitus position, known as the "recovery position" [146]. In this position, the upper leg is flexed at the hip and the upper knee is resting on the bed in front of the lower leg. The child's upper hand should be placed under their lower cheek. This position facilitates drainage of secretions, blood or vomitus out of the mouth rather than onto the larynx, and the tongue falls to the lower cheek or out of the mouth rather than posteriorly onto the larynx. This position permits direct airway intervention should the need arise.

Supplemental oxygen may be administered during transport by nasal prongs or facemask; if the child is monitored with pulse oximetry, oxygen desaturation may not occur if the child hypoventilates. Some advocate pulling up the chin to feel air movement on their palms during transport. We do not encourage maneuvers that close the child's mouth because doing so often obstructs the airway. Instead, we recommend extending the child's neck with the base of the hand (thenar and hypothenar eminences) and holding the fingertips over the mouth/nose to sense expiration.

Others transport the child to the PACU in the supine position. This position undermines all of the advantages outlined for the decubitus position and facilitates posterior displacement of the tongue, which may obstruct the airway [147]. Opioids have been shown to depress hypoglossal motor nuclei centrally, which relaxes the genioglossus muscle [148]. If the child is positioned supine, relaxation of the genioglossus muscle may cause the tongue to obstruct the laryngeal inlet. When opioids are co-administered with inhalational anesthetics, the motor tone of the genioglossus muscle decreases, allowing the tongue to fall back and obstruct the airway. Thus, children who receive opioids and inhalational anesthetics should be transported in the lateral decubitus position to reduce the risk of airway obstruction during recovery.

Children who have recovered from anesthesia and who have normal heart and lungs generally do not have oxygen desaturation when breathing room air, unless their airway becomes obstructed. Administering oxygen en route to the PACU came into vogue about two decades ago at the same time as portable pulse oximetry became available for transport. Studies at that time demonstrated that children desaturate en route to the PACU. However, in most instances, the desaturation resulted from airway obstruction, not from desaturation during tidal respiration. Rather than administering oxygen during transport, the child should be positioned in the recovery position with the neck extended with the anesthesiologist's thenar and hypothenar eminences and should be carefully observed for evidence of upper airway obstruction. In this position, the anesthesiologist's fingertips are positioned over the child's mouth and nose to sense the warm air of expiration. If a facemask is used to deliver oxygen, observing moisture on the mask is the usual means of detecting respiration.

If the patient is scheduled for transport to the intensive care unit, additional planning is required before transfer. The medical and nursing staff in the intensive care unit must be given a verbal summary of the child's condition as it relates to anesthetic/drug infusions, cardiorespiratory status, and ventilation requirements before transport so they can prepare the appropriate equipment. The decision to transport the child with or without a tracheal tube should be made in conjunction with the intensive care team with a view to the child's longer-term management. Depending on the reason for admission to the ICU, the child should be transferred with appropriate monitoring, emergency drugs, and equipment to maintain cardiorespiratory stability, including equipment to re-establish the airway should it be lost during transport. Specifically, propofol, succinylcholine and atropine (and inotropes, depending on the child's needs) should be immediately available as well as a bag, facemask, second tracheal tube and a functioning laryngoscope.

In the case of neonates, particularly preterm infants, the distance between the operating room and the neonatal ICU is usually substantial and over several floors. Given the precarious nature of the neonate's airway and the need for adequate analgesia, it seems prudent to transfer these small infants with their airways secured with a tracheal tube and once in the NICU, a dialog should take place between the anesthesiologist and the neonatologist regarding the timing of tracheal extubation.

CASE STUDY

A 3-year-old child with loud snoring, brief periods of apnea during sleep, fatigue upon arousal in the morning, and attention deficit disorder presented to the otolaryngology service for possible ambulatory tonsillectomy. The child was small for his age, weighed 13 kg, and was otherwise healthy. The review of systems was unremarkable. He had an uneventful bilateral tympanostomy as an infant under general anesthesia. The child had no history of allergies to medications and was taking no medications. There was no family history of anesthesia-related complications or muscle diseases, although both parents had type II diabetes.

The child was appropriately fasted for surgery. To smooth separation from his parents, 10 mg oral midazolam was administered in a medicine cup and followed with a swallow of water. The nurse accompanied the child to the operating room where monitors were applied.

He chose a flavor of lip balm that we applied to color the inside of the clear facemask. The mask was then gently applied to his face while administering 70% nitrous oxide in oxygen. When he stopped responding to our conversation, 8% sevoflurane was added to the fresh gas. After intravenous access was established, a dose of propofol (1.5 mg/kg) was administered, and the trachea was intubated with an uncuffed RAE tube. After the mouth gag was inserted, the child spontaneously breathed a gas mixture of 70% nitrous oxide and 1% isoflurane. Dexamethasone (2 mg) and ondansetron (1 mg) were administered intravenously. Without a polysomnogram, it was unclear whether this child had oxygen desaturation at night and would be hypersensitive to opioids. To determine his sensitivity to opioids, we administered 20 μg/kg morphine. After a single intravenous dose, the child stopped breathing, his respiratory rate slowed from 35 to 18/min and his heart rate decreased from 125 to 96 beats per minute. A second dose of morphine was administered for a total of 40 μg/kg. At the conclusion of the anesthetic, the child breathed spontaneously but made no effort to reject the tracheal tube.

When the end-tidal isoflurane concentration had decreased to 0.2% and the child had not aroused, we became concerned. The doses of the propofol and opioids were rechecked to verify that an accidental overdose had not occurred. The ampoules for the dexamethasone and ondansetron were similarly rechecked. A venous blood sample was sent for blood gases, pH, electrolytes, and glucose concentration. All of the laboratory results were within normal limits. His vital signs were within normal limits. Help was summoned and a differential diagnosis of possible causes was explored. The parents were asked again about recent prescription or non-prescription (including herbal) medications that the child may have taken, but there were none.

No obvious cause for the comatose state was forthcoming until one of the anesthesiologists removed the tape from the child's eyes. Lifting the eyelid revealed a shocking finding. The child's left pupil was fixed and dilated and unresponsive to light.

The trachea remained intubated, and he was taken for an emergency computed axial tomography (CAT) scan that showed an intraventricular bleed, hydrocephalus, and a midline shift. Neurosurgery was consulted and they scheduled the child for insertion of a ventriculo-peritoneal shunt. Cerebral angiogram later demonstrated an arteriovenous malformation that was coiled by the interventional radiologist. The child made a slow but steady recovery after this completely unexpected and unpredictable neurological catastrophe.

Conclusions

This case shows how unexpected changes can occur during anesthesia without the usual changes in heart rate, arterial blood pressure, blood gases, and pH. It also demonstrates that anesthesiologists must look beyond the expected causes of a problem, here possible drug effects in a child who possibly had sleep apnea.

Annotated references

A full reference list for this chapter is available at:
http://www.wiley.com/go/gregory/andropoulos/pediatricanesthesia

1. Lerman J. A disquisition on sleep-disordered breathing in children. Pediatric Anesthesia 2009; 19(Suppl 1): 100–8. This review provides an in-depth description of the spectrum of sleep-disordered breathing in children, including clinical manifestations of obstructive sleep apnea that directly affect the perioperative conduct of anesthesia and patient management.

12. Kim TW, Nemergut ME. Preparation of modern anesthesia workstations for malignant hyperthermia-susceptible patients; a review of past and present practice. Anesthesiology 2011; 114: 205–12. An analysis of the studies published with recommendations on how to prepare anesthetic machines for children at risk for malignant hyperthermia. Addresses the salient issues in terms of old and new anesthetic machines.

37. Habre W. Neonatal ventilation. Best Practice Res Clin Anaesthesiol 2010; 24: 353–64. This update on past, present, and future ventilation strategies for neonates and infants is a very worthwhile read. Packed full of interesting aspects of ventilation strategies, it explains in uncanny detail everything the clinician needs to know about which ventilation strategy to use and why. A must-read.

97. Kam PCA, Cardone D. Propofol infusion syndrome. Anaesthesia 2007; 62: 690–701. Unraveling the pathogenesis of propofol infusion syndrome has been a challenge. This review provides a framework for understanding propofol infusion syndrome from a clinical and scientific perspective.

117. Holliday MA, Friedman AL, Segar WE, Chesney R, Finberg L. Acute hospital-induced hyponatremia in children: a physiologic approach. J Pediatr 2004; 145: 584–7. In this abstruse commentary on fluid administration in children, Holliday et al warn of the consequences of applying their 4–2–1 rule that was predicated on using glucose-containing hyponatremic solutions to balanced salt solutions. Their advice, albeit well concealed within the text, calls for us to revise our fluid management in children undergoing elective surgery to 20–30 mL/kg IV balanced salt solution during surgery followed by 2–1–0.5 mL/kg of a balanced salt solution postoperatively.

120. Barcelona SL, Thompson AA, Coté CJ. Intraoperative pediatric blood transfusion therapy: a review of common issues. Part II: transfusion therapy, special considerations, and reduction of allogenic

blood transfusions. Pediatr Anesth 2005; 15: 814–30. This is a classic paper that provides a comprehensive review of fluid and blood transfusions.

126. Engelman E, Salengros JC, Barvais L. How much does pharmacologic prophylaxis reduce postoperative vomiting in children? Calculation of prophylaxis, effectiveness, and expected incidence of vomiting under treatment using Bayesian meta-analysis. Anesthesiology 2008; 109: 1023–35. This study examines the contributions of single and multiple drug regimens for prophylaxis against PONV in children. Ondansetron and dexamethasone provided the greatest decrement in PONV, 80%.

CHAPTER 16

Postanesthesia Care Unit Management

Warwick Ames & Allison Kinder Ross

Department of Anesthesiology and Pediatrics, Duke University Medical Center, Durham, NC, USA

Introduction

The importance of the postoperative care unit in the safe, successful management of a child who has undergone anesthesia cannot be overstated. This phase immediately following surgery is beset with potential pitfalls and complications that require rapid assessment and treatment. Not only are there the basic needs that exist of a patient wakening from anesthesia, but in children there are additional unique aspects of postanesthesia care. Particularly in infants, perioperative anesthetic morbidity is higher than other age groups, which further underscores the importance of the dedicated pediatric postanesthesia care unit (PACU) [1]. The Pediatric Perioperative Cardiac Arrest (POCA) registry supports the importance of proper management in the postoperative period [2]. The increased incidence of adverse events mandates care and consideration of the design and staffing of a pediatric PACU in addition to the essential appropriate postoperative management of potential issues and complications.

Essentials of the postanesthesia care unit

Design

When determining the design of a recovery area, the ideal location of any PACU is adjacent to the operating rooms to minimize transfer time and distance for safety reasons. The floor plan or design of a pediatric PACU need not differ from any other PACU environment. Typically, a PACU will have an open plan to permit optimum visibility, although this may not be ideal for all recovering children. Not only can the audible distress of another patient be disruptive, but chatter and discourse of the medical staff have been noted as an unwanted feature of postoperative recovery [3]. The importance of lowering environmental stresses such as excessive noise is now being recognized in modern designs [3]. The presence of curtains between each bed space allows some visible privacy, but does nothing to change the noise pollution. Separate rooms would allow for a better sound barrier but they may be undesirable, as they do not allow for vigilant

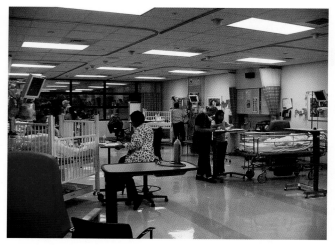

Figure 16.1 A modern pediatric postanesthesia care unit with open design, immediate adjacency to operating rooms, parents present, and ample staffing with experienced pediatric PACU nurses, and prompt availability of anesthesia providers to respond to emergencies.

monitoring by a nurse who is covering several patients and may also be more difficult to navigate in an emergency situation. A possible compromise occurs with rooms that have sliding glass dividers and curtains between them that allow flexibility between rooms but the ability to separate the rooms as needed. With any plan, separate isolation rooms are needed either for barrier purposes or reverse isolation. The number of beds in the PACU should reflect the surgical volume with a ratio of 2.5 beds to each operating room according to current perioperative environment design models (Fig. 16.1).

Equipment

The equipment in the pediatric PACU needs to have the ability to cover patients of all sizes. The American Academy of Pediatrics proposed guidelines for the pediatric perioperative anesthesia environment [4]. The essential components were identified to promote the safety and well-being of infants and children by reducing the risk of adverse events. In particular, all pediatric anesthesia equipment and drugs that are required in the operating room should be available for patients in the PACU. Every child admitted to the PACU must have their vital signs monitored which mandates monitoring equipment that is appropriate for all ages and sizes. Suction apparatus and oxygen delivery, via a flow meter to allow titration of inspired oxygen as required, must be available at each bedside. Equipment for intravenous fluid administration must allow for microadjustments of volume delivery. Particularly in the smallest children, placing the intravenous fluids on a pump to deliver set volumes on arrival to the PACU is advisable. Due to the increased risk of heat loss in children in the operating room, devices for the

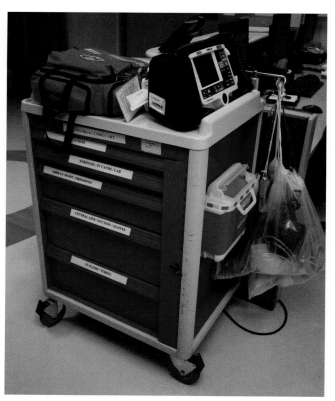

Figure 16.2 A standard emergency cart centrally located within the PACU with age-specific airway supplies and defibrillator on top.

maintenance of normothermia must be available and utilized.

The pediatric PACU should also have a focal, easily accessed location for the placement of portable emergency equipment. To prepare for the unexpected, a resuscitation cart with equipment appropriate for pediatric patients of all ages, including pediatric defibrillator paddles, must be immediately available. Specialized equipment for management of the difficult pediatric airway by a variety of techniques for airway control, intubation and ventilation, including emergency cricothyrotomy, is desirable. A dedicated airway bag that contains packets of age/weight-specific airway supplies should be a part of the resuscitation cart apparatus (Fig. 16.2). To simplify procedure in the event of an emergency, written pediatric doses for resuscitation drugs, and potentially pediatric advanced life support (PALS) algorithms, should be visible or immediately available. All emergency equipment must be frequently checked and regularly maintained with a checklist system.

Staffing

Staffing of the pediatric PACU is an important component for the success of the environment. For most patients, recovery from anesthesia is uneventful, but it is also a time when catastrophic events can occur. Pediatric-trained medical and nursing staff are required to be vigilant, caring and knowledgeable. In 1999 the American Society of Anesthesiologists assembled a task force to provide recommendations specifically for a pediatric PACU [4]. This task force recommended that in order to apply specific expertise in the provision of pediatric anesthesia services, an anesthesiologist or other physician trained and experienced in pediatric perioperative care, including the management of postoperative complications and pediatric cardiopulmonary resuscitation, must be immediately available to evaluate and treat any child in distress.

The intensity of nursing care is typically greater in a pediatric PACU than on the floor with assignments based on acuity. The requirements of PACU nursing will be institution dependent. Prior pediatric experience and PALS training would clearly be advantageous and is recommended. Mock codes, possibly to include scenarios using simulation, should be routinely performed with anesthesia and nursing staff so that the care is seamless in a true emergency. Although not stated by the task force, nursing staff should be pediatric trained, and ideally, with a background in pediatric intensive care. This would suggest confidence in the care of the unconscious child, ability to recognize a child in distress, ability to recognize a lost airway and having expertise in the safe administration of potent analgesics. To recognize the subspecialty expertise, pediatric PACU nurses are to be engaged as part of the perioperative team and be members of pediatric perioperative team meetings that include surgeons, anesthesiologists and nursing staff. This builds a cohesive group for the good of the pediatric perioperative environment.

Transport

Any hospital patient transport presents a period of significant risk of morbidity and mortality [5,6]. The transport of a child from the operating room (OR) to the PACU should not be considered routine. Apnea, loss of a patent airway, vomiting and emergence agitation are just a few of the potential problems encountered during transfer. To be prepared for these events, it is advisable for the anesthesia provider to have resuscitation drugs and airway equipment that are individualized for the patient or surgery that was performed. Children should be transferred on a bed or crib with guardrails. The lateral recovery position is often used because it facilitates a patent airway with gravity opening the airway and draining oral secretions and blood (Fig. 16.3). Oxygen must always be available along with a suitable delivery device such as nasal cannula, facemask or anesthesia circuit with mask. The use of a monitoring device depends on the status of the patient and distance to the recovery area.

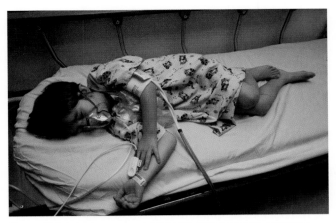

Figure 16.3 Lateral recovery position with airway open to encourage forward drainage of secretions. (Bed rail left down only for purpose of photo.)

Handover and assessment

The universal criteria by which patients are deemed suitable for the pediatric PACU are variable and dependent on many factors, including staffing and acuity. Some patients are easily considered candidates for PACU, including healthy outpatients for minor procedures, and others are clearly not suitable, such as the potentially hemodynamically unstable patient with cardiac disease. Other cases fall into a gray area that requires thought about the ultimate location for recovery. Skills and comfort level of the individual PACU and relationship with the floor or intensive care units may affect the decision of disposition post surgery. For example, following a repair of cleft palate, some centers will recover a patient in the PACU while other centers will prefer direct admission to the step-down or intensive care unit. Similarly, some PACUs may be comfortable with an intubated patient and the subsequent extubation procedure, while others may not [7,8]. Therefore, when determining admission parameters, it is important that there is a clear understanding by the surgical and anesthesia personnel about what location is suitable for the recovery of the individual child.

After the decision is made to admit to the PACU, it is important that there be good communication to the PACU from the operating room. Advance communication from the OR at the very least should include a phone call as the case nears completion. The call alerts the PACU to the new admission and should include details regarding the age, weight, stability of the patient, any intraoperative complications that would affect postoperative care, and any special needs. This initial call allows the nurses to target care, prepare medication and reorganize staff assignments as necessary. Once the patient arrives, the admitting staff should perform an 'initial assessment' prior to the handover from the anesthesia staff. This assessment must quickly determine airway patency, oxygen saturation, heart rate and rhythm, temperature and blood pressure. If all is well, it is then possible to proceed to the medical handover.

With regard to the communication between the anesthesia provider and PACU nurse, and in every aspect of medicine, the handover of patient care is critical. Patient safety is especially vulnerable when crossing professional boundaries. Misunderstanding can occur simply due to differences in culture, training, norms, attitudes, perspectives, goals, expectations, status, gender and socioeconomic status. Indeed, communication breakdowns are a leading cause of medical errors. In 2005, a US Joint Commission on Accreditation of Healthcare Organizations (JCAHO) analysis found that 70% of sentinel events were caused by communication breakdowns, half of those occurring during handovers [9]. To address the problem, the Joint Commission instituted a National Patient Safety Goal in 2006, calling on hospitals to implement a standardized approach to patient handovers. See Chapter 45 for more detail.

In order to improve the handover, it is important to recognize the process, a novel example of which was described at Great Ormond Street Hospital for Children in London [10]. The handover of patient and information from the operating room to the cardiac intensive care unit was actually reviewed by motor racing teams that likened the handover to a racing pit stop. Their recommendations and involvement resulted in standardized handovers, thereby eliminating variation and resulting in clear and concise instructions to ensure that even if team personnel changes, all members are absolutely clear about their responsibilities. Communication was noted as a critical factor in success. The same principles must be applied the handover of a patient from the OR to the PACU.

It has been advocated that training be instituted using interactive simulation-based sessions of standardized patients, clinicians, and manikin simulators with facilitated video debriefing to stimulate thought and reinforce positive behavior. Also, the introduction of mnemonics is useful to ensure timely, accurate and complete information about a patient's care plan, treatment, current condition and any recent or anticipated changes. Examples of these techniques include the "Five Ps" (patient name, problem list, plan of care, purpose of plan, precautions), as well as "I-SBAR" and the "I PASS the BATON" which are shown in Boxes 16.1 and 16.2. The hope is that the use of any of these measures will facilitate a consistent process, thereby improving patient safety.

Monitoring and patient safety

The American Society of Anesthesiologists has published standards for postanesthesia care, most recently updated in 2009 [11]. These standards are minimum requirements, and specify only that "The patient shall be observed and

Box 16.1 Examples of communication tools that use mnemonics for ease and consistency: I-SBAR communication tool

I	Introduction	Identify yourself and the patient
S	Situation	Patient age
		Gender
		Preop diagnosis
		Procedure
		Mental status preprocedure
		Patient stable/unstable
B	Background	Pertinent medical history
		Allergies
		Sensory impairment
		Family location
		Religion/culture
		Interpreter required
		Valuables deposition
		Meds given
		Blood given – units available
		Skin integrity
		Musculoskeletal restrictions
		Tubes/drains/catheters
		Dressings/cast/splints
		Counts correct
		Other – lab/path pending
A	Assessment	Vitals
		Isolation required
		Skin
		Risk factors
		Issues I am concerned about
R	Recommendation/ request	Specific care required immediately or soon
		Priority areas
		Pain control
		IV pump
		Family communication

monitored by methods appropriate to the patient's medical condition. Particular attention should be given to monitoring oxygenation, ventilation, circulation, level of consciousness, and temperature. During recovery from all anesthetics, a quantitative method of assessing oxygenation, such as pulse oximetry, shall be employed in the initial phase of recovery." Pulse oximetry is certainly used universally in pediatric anesthesia during the early phases of recovery but electrocardiographic (ECG) monitoring is not always used, with heart rate source being taken from the pulse oximeter or manual counting. An advantage of ECG monitoring is the ability to have a monitor of circulation when the pulse oximeter does not function due to patient movement or poor perfusion.

Additional benefits are the ability to diagnose non-sinus rhythms and to measure respiratory rate using impedence plethysmography. In addition, although the utility of capnography via a nasal cannula in non-intubated patients undergoing procedural sedation is well established, newer data suggest it may also be useful in some patient populations in the PACU, and this type of monitoring could become more frequent in the future [12].

Detailed nursing standards for postanesthesia care have also been published and are regularly updated [13]. Although the exact details of monitoring and assessment will be governed by regulatory agencies and local institutional policies and procedures, in general, a pediatric patient recovering from general anesthesia should have 1:1 nursing care for the initial recovery period, along with frequent monitoring of vital signs, i.e. every 5–15 min during the early recovery phases.

Regardless of the policies and guidelines in place, there is no substitute for well-trained PACU nurses with expertise and experience in pediatric anesthesia, who can recognize problems, institute treatment and call for help from their anesthesia and nursing colleagues. The anesthesiologist also must be mindful of the setting, i.e. busy children's hospital PACU with multiple available anesthesiologists and nurses available to address patient problems, versus a free-standing surgicenter with one or two operating rooms, PACU nurses with limited pediatric experience, and no readily available anesthesia providers for PACU problems because all are caring for patients in the operating rooms. The setting often determines the preferred treatment strategy, i.e. deep versus awake tracheal extubation, or the type or age of patient treated.

Parental presence

As previously stated, the primary goal of the pediatric PACU is to provide a safe environment for patients to return to their preanesthetic state. However, there is evidence that children may suffer negative behavioral changes following hospitalization for surgical procedures [14]. Although it is difficult to predict which child will do poorly, a 2006 cohort study revealed that particular individual, familial and procedural variables were able to identify the children at greatest risk of significant negative behavior change [15]. In particular, a factor that predicted negative behavior was increased parental anxiety. Other factors included younger age, overnight admission, lower birth order, and, surprisingly, having a discussion with the anesthetist preoperatively [15].

As part of the child's stress due to hospitalization and procedures, it would seem intuitive that separation from a parent may compound the problem. For this reason, many parents request to be present as their child recovers from anesthesia [16,17]. The policy of allowing parents into the PACU, however, is uniquely institutional and varies both culturally and nationally. It is not universally adopted, in part because there is little evidence that having a parent present during recovery from anesthesia results in a positive outcome, and as previously mentioned, parental anxiety may be counterproductive. However, in a recent randomized prospective study from Canada, a benefit of parental presence in the PACU for healthy children undergoing outpatient surgery was a decrease in negative behavior change at 2 weeks postoperatively [18]. There was no difference in acute distress (measured by "crying episodes") in the PACU between the group with a parent present and the group where no parent was present.

Despite these findings, parents may be successful with the non-pharmacological measures to relieve pain and distress. The non-pharmacological methods, that involve imagery, relaxation, breathing techniques and massage, may make pain more tolerable and give children a sense of control without the administration of drugs [19]. A qualitative interview study of children and parents following tonsillectomy noted that children have their own coping strategies. These included distraction, such as watching TV, thinking of something else, talking and reading, relaxing, eating ice cream, and simply having someone present [20].

The debate as to the value and appropriateness of parents in the PACU will continue. Most anesthesiologists have an anecdotal experience that colors their perspective on the matter. However, the emergence from anesthesia is obviously a potentially stressful time for the child. The sensation of pain, nausea and vomiting and waking in a strange and foreign environment are all contributors to this stress. The idealized benefit of a familiar and recognized caregiver is compelling although the actual evidence for such an advantage is poor. There are a significant number of studies on the effects of parental presence in the preoperative period and during induction of anesthesia, but the practice that includes presence of parents in the postoperative period and the PACU environment remains in need of additional study.

Discharge criteria

Discharge criteria have been created to permit an objective evaluation of children leaving the recovery unit. The criteria will depend upon the patient age, surgery performed and the subsequent destination (home versus floor versus intensive care). The two commonly used and cited scores in the literature are the Modified Aldrete score for inpatient care [21] and the postanesthetic discharge scoring systems (PADSS) for patients being discharged home [22]. Both scores use a selection of physiological variables to form an objective measure for discharge eligibility (Tables 16.1, 16.2). Whether the anesthesiologist must personally reassess the patient before discharge, or rely on a protocol with a physician order to discharge the patient when criteria are met, is governed by both regulatory agencies and local institutional policy and procedures.

The key components of scores like these include the following parameters: hemodynamic stability, respiratory sufficiency, neurological baseline, ability to maintain and protect the airway, absence of excessive bleeding, normothermia, minimal pain (patients should be observed for at least 30 min after the last dose of opioid), ability to ambulate if appropriate, and absence of excessive vomiting. The ability to drink clear liquids prior to discharge is not a discharge criterion, and forced ingestion of liquids is actually associated with a higher incidence of postoperative nausea and vomiting (PONV) [23].

Patient age is also a critical factor. Although actively debated, it is suggested that preterm infants should reach a minimum number of weeks postconceptual age (PCA) to be considered for outpatient surgery due to risks of postoperative apnea. Most institutions use conservative

Table 16.1 Discharge criteria using scoring systems. Modified Aldrete Score. Nine or more points are required for recovery to be confirmed

Category	Score = 2	Score = 1	Score = 0
Respiration	Breathes, coughs freely	Dyspnea, shallow or limited breathing	Apnea
O₂ saturation	SpO₂ > 92% in room air	Supplemental O₂ to maintain SpO₂ > 92%	SpO₂ < 92% with oxygen
Circulation	BP within 20 mmHg of preop	BP within 20–50 mmHg of preop	BP within 50 mmHg of preop
Consciousness	Awake and orientated	Wakes with stimulation	Non-responsive
Movement: voluntarily or on command	Four extremities	Two extremities	No extremities

Table 16.2 Post Anesthetic Discharge Scoring System (PADSS). At least nine points are required to be eligible for discharge

Category	Description of status	PADSS score
Vital signs	Within 20% range of preop	2
	Within 20–40% range of preop	1
	>40% range of preop	0
Ambulation	Steady gait/no dizziness	2
	Ambulates with assistance	1
	Not ambulating/dizziness	0
Nausea and vomiting	Minimal, treated with oral meds	2
	Moderate, treated with parenteral meds	1
	Continues after repeated treatments	0
Pain	Acceptable to patient	2
	Pain somewhat acceptable	1
	Pain not acceptable to patient	0
Surgical bleeding	Minimal: no dressing changes required	2
	Moderate bleeding: dressing change	1
	Severe bleeding: intervention required	0

criteria close to 50 weeks' PCA or a very conservative 60 weeks. However, 44 weeks can generally be considered the absolute minimum PCA for outpatient surgery based on when the true risk of apnea is considerable. Even in those infants who reach the minimum age criteria for discharge, an extended recovery time with observation during feeding and sleeping may be warranted [24]. Risk factors associated with apnea of prematurity are anemia, PCA and gestational age [24]. A separate entity known as apnea of infancy can occur in term infants but because of its rarity, term infants are not subject to the same postoperative monitored care unless other factors warrant it [25]. It is recommended that term infants, on the other hand, should be a minimum of 4 weeks of age to be eligible for same-day discharge. Although the risk of apnea in a full-term infant is extremely low, case reports suggest that it is not zero [26–28].

In addition to overall discharge criteria from anesthesia, there are also procedure-specific issues that may affect the time to discharge. For example, a child who receives a spinal anesthetic should show signs of resolution of both sensory and motor blockade prior to discharge. Children undergoing adenotonsillectomy typically would stay in PACU for 2 h and show an ability to take fluids. In a recent study to determine the factors that may delay discharge in children undergoing tonsillectomies, it was found that PONV and oxygen desaturation were the two major factors contributing to prolonged length of stay (LOS) [29]. The authors noted that the overall risk of prolonged LOS decreased with increasing age. Interestingly, LOS was not affected by the presence of an upper respiratory tract infection (URTI), leading the authors to suggest that patients with a URTI could be eligible for day case surgery.

Finally, handover of care for inpatients being discharged from the PACU to the floor or ICU needs to be as rigorous as with arrival. Full handover should include not only the intraoperative report but also the medications given and any PACU issues or special instructions. Prior to the final handover of the child to the accepting team, it should be confirmed that the intravenous infusions are placed on mechanized infusion pumps rather than free-flowing drips, a final examination of wound sites should be done, and an appropriate escort (nurse or doctor) who can give an accurate report to the accepting team needs to accompany the child for transport.

Potential postanesthesia problems and complications

Respiratory

Children are more likely to have airway-related problems rather than cardiovascular problems in the immediate postoperative period. Next to episodes of nausea and vomiting, the most frequent complications in the PACU are those that require airway support [30]. Maintenance of the airway following general anesthesia and sedation presents challenges due to the negative factors that occur during the perioperative period. Not only are the children still under the sedative influences of the anesthesia, but there are also risks of inadequate reversal of neuromuscular blockade, as well as diffusion hypoxia and the consequences of additional analgesic medications being administered in the PACU that can result in additional altered respiratory drive. The normal anatomy of a neonate or infant can render the airway vulnerable, and when side-effects of surgery are added, particularly surgery involving the airway, it is clear that a specialist's care and attention to detail may be required.

Although tracheal extubation occurs in the operating room in the vast majority of pediatric anesthesia programs and cases, the benefits and risks of extubation while deeply anesthetized versus "awake" continue to be debated [31]. The patient whose trachea has been extubated while deeply anesthetized will often be at increased risk of airway obstruction from airway muscle laxity, or emerging from anesthesia with increased risk for laryngospasm, during the early period after admission to the PACU, and so extra vigilance is required in this situation. In a minority of pediatric anesthesia programs, the patient is taken to the PACU with the endotracheal tube in place, in order to increase operating room efficiency. The trachea is extubated on the physician's order by protocol so that the PACU nurse can perform the extubation when criteria are met [7].

Hypoxemia is not uncommon in the pediatric patient who is recovering from anesthesia and surgery. In addition to mechanical issues that involve the airway, there are other intrinsic pulmonary events that lead to hypoxemia. The combination of higher oxygen consumption in the presence of a relatively reduced functional residual capacity and higher closing capacity puts the younger child at greater risk of oxygen desaturation. For all these reasons, postoperative patients should receive supplemental oxygen either by mask or by blow-by devices, and children are no exception. Children can be reluctant to accept any device to provide oxygen, but *purposeful* removal of the mask or blow-by device is often a good sign that it is no longer required. As oxygen is being delivered, the basics of airway support must still continue to be employed, including ensuring the airway is patent, there are clear breath sounds on auscultation with good chest excursion, no signs of respiratory distress (stridor, nasal flaring), no wheezing and a normal respiratory pattern devoid of apneic episodes.

A child may be best managed by placing them in the lateral recovery position and employing jaw thrust and mouth opening when airway obstruction is evident. Compared to the supine position, the lateral position will increase total airway volume by 45% in children who have been sedated for MRI, with the greatest change seen in the region between the epiglottis and vocal cords [32]. One must remember that neonates are obligate nasal breathers and the occlusion of the nares with assorted tubing or incorrect mask placement can lead to a compromised airway.

Residual neuromuscular blockade

Residual neuromuscular blockade has significant clinical implications for the patient in the PACU. These implications are due to changes in pharyngeal function with increased risk of aspiration, airway muscle weakness that can lead to airway obstruction, and attenuation of the hypoxic ventilatory response. In adults, there is evidence that up to 40% of patients exhibit a train of four ratio of <0.9 in the recovery area [33,34]. Although evidence would suggest that children have a more complete response to neuromuscular reversal and respond to lower doses of neostigmine significantly better than adults, the complications that can result from incomplete reversal can be devastating in a very young child [35,36]. When a child is admitted to the recovery area and exhibits the typical signs of incomplete reversal such as weakness or floppiness with the "fish out of water" appearance, this must be considered a cause and treated promptly before respiratory decompensation ensues. Administering additional neuromuscular blocking reversal is not necessarily the treatment of choice and should only be used if the maximum dose of neostigmine (0.07 mg/kg) has not already been administered as that dose should not be exceeded. Larger doses of neostigmine will lead to further muscular weakness and possible cholinergic crisis. Instead, care should be supportive, including reintubation if respiratory compromise is significant. The patient may then be sedated and ventilated until the neuromuscular blockade has subsided and extubation criteria are met.

Postextubation stridor or croup

One complication that is typically not seen until the PACU course is postextubation stridor (also known as postintubation croup). In 1977, the incidence of postextubation croup after anesthesia was reported at 1.6–6% [37]. Although these data are old, there is little evidence that the incidence has changed despite trends towards the use of cuffed endotracheal tubes. An editorial on the subject outlined the changes that have occurred over the last several decades based on recent literature, and how these changes have supported the use of cuffed endotracheal tubes in children [38]. It remains unclear what the overall outcome will be with changes in practice, and whether

eventually there will be a significant difference in the incidence of stridor in the PACU based on preference of endotracheal tube.

Postextubation stridor often may not need immediate treatment beyond humidified oxygen. However, if there are any sign of respiratory distress, nebulized racemic epinephrine (0.5 mL of 2.25% solution in 3 mL normal saline, for children over 6 months of age, 0.25 mL if less than 6 months) provides a rapid response. The mechanism of action of racemic epinephrine is through its stimulation of α-receptors resulting in vasoconstriction and secondary reduction in mucosal and submucosal edema. Due to the rebound effect of racemic epinephrine that may occur up until 2 h after administration, a child must remain in the PACU or in a monitored setting until this risk is no longer present as readministration may be necessary. Although it may take at least an hour to see results, a single dose of dexamethasone (0.15–0.6 mg/kg) can be administered for reduction of airway edema and the duration significantly outlasts racemic epinephrine with a half-life of over 30 h [39–41]. Despite the long half-life, dexamethasone dosing should be repeated every 6–12 h until resolution. In cases of significant respiratory distress, the child should be admitted to a monitored setting where heliox (60–80% helium:20–40% oxygen mixture) can be delivered [42]. Although heliox has no anti-inflammatory or bronchodilatory properties, its low density allows improved oxygen delivery and carbon dioxide elimination. In extreme cases, reintubation with an endotracheal tube at least 0.5–1 mm smaller than the original tube may be needed.

Laryngospasm

Laryngospasm, an event typically associated with intraoperative care, remains a potential complication in the PACU. Laryngospasm may occur due to irritation of the vocal cords, commonly from either saliva or blood, or simply from the child still being at risk while emerging from anesthesia with stage II being exhibited. Laryngospasm is the forceful closure of the vocal cords, resulting in total obstruction of the airway, and if untreated can be catastrophic. The first step must be the administration of oxygen by positive pressure mask with jaw thrust. In addition to simple jaw thrust, pressure applied to the "laryngospasm notch," located behind the lobule of the pinna of each ear, is anecdotally effective [43]. If the patient exhibits full airway obstruction without evidence of air movement, or if significant desaturations or bradycardia occur, succinylcholine is to be administered (or another rapid-acting muscle relaxant if succinylcholine is contraindicated). When laryngospasm occurs in the PACU, intubation is typically not necessary, and all that is needed for relaxation of the vocal cords is a small dose of intravenous succinylcholine (0.1–0.5 mg/kg). Small doses of propofol have also been reported for the treatment of laryngospasm in children [44]. The child will require bag/mask ventilation until good spontaneous respirations are restored. Atropine should be available in case either the succinylcholine or episode of hypoxia during the laryngospasm causes bradycardia.

Apnea

Although apnea may occur for many reasons in the PACU, apnea in the ex-premature infant requires careful consideration preoperatively during the work-up to guarantee that the appropriate postoperative destination is secured. With better survival of prematurely born infants, an increasing number of these patients appear on the operating schedule and so require care in the PACU. Typically, if the child is still in the intensive care nursery, then postoperative care will continue on the neonatal intensive care unit. However, if the child is on the ward or is an outpatient, individual consideration for the unique pathophysiology of a premature infant must be made to determine the postoperative disposition and level of monitoring.

Apnea is defined as a cessation of airflow for more than 20 sec, or the cessation of breathing for less than 20 sec if it is accompanied by bradycardia or oxygen (O_2) desaturation [45]. The frequency is inversely related to gestational age and the actual cause of apnea of prematurity is unknown, although it is likely to be multifactorial [46]. Depression or immaturity of the respiratory central generator located in the brainstem is most likely in addition to vulnerability to inhibitory influences such as hypoxia and temperature changes [47].

Beyond considerations that exist for infants with apnea of prematurity, the presence of obstructive sleep apnea (OSA) in any child presents significant risk in the postoperative period and is responsible for considerable morbidity, with a complication rate of up to 27% [48]. In fact, in 60% of children with severe OSA, nursing intervention in the postoperative period was required to treat complications that included desaturation to SpO_2 <90% [49]. The children also demonstrated signs of increased work of breathing and/or new radiographic findings of pulmonary edema, effusion, infiltrate, pneumothorax or pneumomediastinum.

Because of the potential complications that exist in this population, the American Society of Anesthesiologists in 2006 published practice guidelines for perioperative management that suggested that children with a history of OSA having adenotonsillectomy should be admitted for overnight stay if they are less than 3 years of age or if they have contributing medical conditions such as obesity [50]. If an otherwise well child greater than 3 years of age has mild-to-moderate OSA with an apnea-hypopnea index <10, same-day discharge may be considered. If the decision is made to discharge the child the same day as the procedure, it is best if the case is performed earlier in the day after a minimum PACU stay of 2 h [51].

Due to the chronic hypoxemia exhibited by children with OSA and its effects on respiratory drive, it is important to be cautious when ordering pain medication postoperatively. Children with a history of OSA have a higher incidence of apnea after administration of a typical 0.5 μg/kg dose of fentanyl when compared to children without OSA [52]. As a reference, children with sleep apnea who demonstrated an oxygen saturation <85% on polysomnography require only half the morphine dose to have the same analgesic effect as a child who did not have the same degree of desaturation [53].

When an infant or child is showing signs of OSA in the PACU, immediate maneuvers to stimulate the patient and open the airway are to be performed. These maneuvers include repositioning with a shoulder roll or to lateral position, performance of jaw thrust or insertion of a nasal or oral airway, and occasionally the administration of positive pressure by mask. If these measures are unsuccessful, the child may require tracheal intubation until they are fully recovered and able to maintain their own airway. In addition, the child who requires nasal continuous positive airway pressure (CPAP) or bi-level positive airway pressure (BiPAP) by mask at home during sleep may benefit from its application in the PACU.

Pulmonary edema

Pulmonary edema is rarely seen in children, but must be considered as a cause in the postoperative differential diagnosis of hypoxemia with desaturations in the PACU. Causes of pulmonary edema may be related simply to the delivery of a large volume of fluid or blood products in the operating room with or without significant fluid shifts, or to negative pressure pulmonary edema (NPPE). Clinical presentation is the same between these, but history will help delineate the cause. A history of forceful respirations against a closed airway such as laryngospasm, biting on the endotracheal tube or even long-standing history of upper airway obstruction from enlarged tonsils or epiglottis that has now been relieved with surgery, can lead to NPPE. The pathogenesis of NPPE from negative intrathoracic pressure causes decreased pulmonary capillary perivascular pressure, favoring hydrostatic transudation of fluid into the interstitial tissue. Although normal pleural inspiratory pressures are -2 to -5 cmH_2O, negative pressures from -50 to -100 cmH_2O are possible, particularly with young muscular males [54]. After the obstruction is relieved, there is a sudden increase in venous return and a redistribution of blood volume from peripheral to central circulation with a resulting increase in pulmonary hydrostatic pressure that is compounded by capillary leak.

In any of these scenarios, if significant pulmonary edema is present, the child will exhibit lower pulse oximetry readings, tachycardia, and tachypnea. Rales will be heard on chest auscultation and occasionally the child may exhibit pink frothy sputum. If otherwise stable and saturations are kept within normal range with supplemental oxygen, this may be all that is required. However, depending on the degree of pulmonary edema and respiratory distress, intubation with delivery of positive end-expiratory pressure (PEEP) may be necessary along with diuresis (furosemide 0.1 mg/kg with a maximum of 5 mg) to assist with the shift of fluid out of the lungs. In the case of NPPE, the use of PEEP is supported, but whether the delivery of diuretics is of benefit remains unclear [55].

Pulmonary aspiration

The risk of pulmonary aspiration in the perioperative period in children is low at approximately 0.1%, but it is not negligible and is at least two times higher than the risk in adults [56]. Particularly after airway surgery, the increased amount of secretions and blood puts the child at risk for aspirating these fluids during recovery from the sedative effects of anesthesia or pain medications. If aspiration is suspected, examination of the lungs may help to determine the diagnosis if significant rhonchi or coarse breath sounds are heard unilaterally, particularly on the right side. Treatment is supportive as sequelae are typically mild, although incidence and severity may correlate with the underlying medical condition of the child [56]. Pharmacological intervention with steroids or antibiotics for presumed aspiration is unwarranted.

Pneumothorax

Another cause of hypoxemia in the PACU is pneumothorax. Many surgical procedures, such as central line placement, ventriculoperitoneal shunts and any thoracic procedure, put the child at risk for intraoperative pneumothorax that may not manifest until the postoperative period. A thorough exam and chest radiograph will help determine the diagnosis. If the pneumothorax is significant and causing respiratory compromise, a chest tube will need to be inserted and the child sent to the appropriate postoperative setting. Lesser degrees of pneumothorax may be treated with 100% oxygen by non-rebreathing facemask, to hasten resolution by displacing nitrogen and allowing for faster resorption of the pneumothorax.

Cardiovascular factors

Although respiratory complications far outweigh hemodynamic issues in the typical recovering pediatric patient, children can decompensate rapidly and cardiovascular depression is a late and ominous sign.

Hypotension

Hypotension in the PACU, particularly in the presence of tachycardia, narrow pulse pressure, poor capillary refill (>3 sec) and low urine output (<0.5 mL/kg/h), is typically the result of hypovolemia. Depending on the nature of the procedure, the cause of the hypovolemia needs to be quickly determined in order to know whether to administer fluid or blood products. Attention to any blood accumulation in surgical drains allows for a rapid assessment. Isotoninc crystalloid fluid boluses (normal saline, lactated Ringer's solution or Plasmalyte®) should be administered in 5–10 mL/kg increments, depending on the degree of hypotension and ongoing losses with critical assessment in changes in blood pressure and heart rate in response to the fluid challenge. If there is any question as to the nature of the hypotension, blood should be drawn to check the acid–base status and base deficit as well as hemoglobin and/or hematocrit. If replacing blood loss, 10–15 mL/kg of packed red blood cells will raise the hemoglobin by 2–3 g/dL if no ongoing blood loss is occurring.

Other causes of hypotension that would be extremely uncommon in the PACU would be anaphylaxis from either latex exposure or delivery of postoperative drug, early signs of perioperative sepsis, or mechanical reasons such as pneumothorax or pericardial tamponade. Sympathetic block from central neuraxial anesthesia typically does not exist in a child below the age of 5 years due to lack of a significant peripheral vasodilation or venous pooling, and rarely would cause hypotension in a child older than 5 years with the typical low concentrations of local anesthetic that are used for postoperative infusions.

Hypertension

The presentation of hypertension in the postoperative period is typically the consequence of pain and is therefore usually associated with tachycardia and other outward signs of discomfort. If pain is suspected, appropriate treatment is necessary to alleviate the physiological responses in a rapid, safe manner. If not due to pain, the most common cause of hypertension may actually be the result of inaccurate readings due to a small blood pressure cuff, so this cause must be ruled out early on. Hypertension is rarely due to volume overload but some children are more susceptible than others to excessive intraoperative volume resuscitation, so the possibility does exist. Hypertension may also be the result of emergence agitation or bladder distension or, in patients with renal failure, rebound hypertension can occur because they are not taking their regular antihypertensive agent due to NPO status. In a child with moderate-to-severe hypertension in the PACU that is not attributable to pain, treatment may consist of intravenous agents such as hydralazine (0.25–0.5 mg/kg), labetalol (0.2 mg/kg), nitroprusside infusion (1–10 μg/kg/min) or nicardipine infusion (0.5–5 μg/kg/min). Close hemodynamic monitoring needs to occur if delivering any of these agents.

Tachycardia

Tachycardia is very non-specific in the PACU. As previously mentioned, when accompanied by hypotension, the combination suggests hypovolemia that needs to be promptly managed. Tachycardia and hypertension together suggest pain, anxiety or both. Tachycardia can also be secondary to drugs administered in the operating room such as atropine or glycopyrrolate and when no other factors are present, these causes should be considered and no further treatment is necessary. Rarely, tachycardia may be due to an underlying conduction abnormality, particularly in a child with a cardiac history, and these children will require a cardiology consult and/or admission to the ward to determine the significance. If an arrhythmia, i.e. supraventricular tachycardia, is suspected, it is crucial to record the abnormal rhythm, either by printout or electronically with as many leads as possible, and to record a standard 12-lead ECG, so that the consultant physicians will have adequate information.

Bradycardia

Bradycardia is often a more ominous sign than tachycardia and is often consequent to hypoxia. Indeed, the heart rate of a preterm infant will begin to fall within 30 sec of onset of apnea [57]. Therefore attention should be directed toward airway management and ensuring adequate oxygenation in the face of sudden, unexpected bradycardia. Having corrected hypoxia as a cause of bradycardia, other causes such as increased intracranial pressure or simple vagal response to airway maneuvers can be entertained. If bradycardia persists and is accompanied by low cardiac output or hypotension, atropine (0.02 mg/kg) should be administered. If unsuccessful and the patient remains in a low-output state, resuscitation efforts should then proceed with intravenous epinephrine and standard cardiopulmonary resuscitation (CPR) per pediatric advanced life support (PALS) protocol.

Other than tachy- or bradyarrhythmias, other arrhythmias are extremely rare in the PACU. With the reduction in the use of arrhythmogenic inhalational agents such as halothane, nodal or junctional arrhythmias are less frequent. However, a greater number of patients with congenital heart disease are surviving and requiring surgeries unrelated to the heart. These patients may have underlying defects in their conduction pathways that may become obvious in the PACU. A rhythm strip should be run in any child who has an unexpected change in heart rate to help determine any cardiac etiologies, and a cardiologist should be consulted prior to discharge from the PACU, if concern remains about significant cardiac pathology as a cause of the arrhythmia. Additionally, any hemodynamically significant arrhythmia requires basic resuscitation protocol.

Hypothermia and hyperthermia

Hypothermia

Hypothermia is defined as a core temperature of less than 36°C [58]. It is well documented that children lose heat more readily than their adult counterparts and anesthesia can further disrupt the patient's ability to thermoregulate [59]. Neonates and infants are at particular risk of developing hypothermia even during transport from the OR to the PACU. A working group established by the American Society of Anesthesiologists (ASA)/Physician Consortium for Performance Improvement noted that anesthetic-induced impairment of thermoregulatory control is the primary cause of perioperative hypothermia [60]. Even mild hypothermia (1–2°C below normal) has been associated in randomized trials with a number of adverse consequences, including increased susceptibility to infection, impaired coagulation and increased transfusion requirements, cardiovascular stress and cardiac complications, and postanesthetic shivering and thermal discomfort [61]. In addition, neonates are at risk of apnea and bradycardia when hypothermic.

Beyond the physiological issues, hypothermia also has an impact on efficiency of a PACU and is associated with an increased length of stay which has logistical and financial implications for a successful surgical unit [61].

It is therefore not surprising that perioperative temperature management is one of the five quality incentives established by the ASA as the Pay-for-Performance and Anesthesiology Quality Incentive [60]. The goal is to have measured at least one body temperature that is equal to or greater than 36°C (or 96.8°F) within the 30 min immediately before or the 30 min immediately after anesthesia end time, with some exceptions.

Temperature is to be measured as part of the initial assessment upon a child's arrival in the PACU. Measurements from different sites may not correlate particularly well because of compensatory mechanisms such as vasoconstriction that can change the relationship between the central and peripheral temperature. Core temperature must be estimated from peripheral sites and taken rectally, axillary, orally or via tympanic membrane. All of these sites have issues related to reliability, accuracy and flaws in measurement technique. Axillary temperatures in neonates and infants do correlate well with rectal temperature and thus remain the preferred method in many PACUs [62,63].

Acknowledging the importance of avoiding hypothermia has lead to the practice of prewarming of patients in the operating room [64,65]. When this has not occurred and the patient arrives hypothermic to the PACU, a number of measures are often employed. Simple and standard measures such as fluid warmers, warm blankets and infrared heat lamps are first line but may not be completely effective in treating hypothermia [66]. Only active warming devices such as convection or forced air warming devices have consistently been proven effective at treating hypothermia and are therefore recommended by the ASA for these circumstances [67].

Hyperthermia

Hyperthermia in the PACU is a very different entity. The typical cause of hyperthermia would be aggressive warming in the operating room. Although extremely rare, one must still have a high index of suspicion for a late presentation of malignant hyperthermia (MH) in a hyperthermic child, particularly if any other associated signs are present such as muscle rigidity, hyperventilation, and tachycardia. Aggressive diagnosis and treatment (see Chapter 40) should then ensue if a true case is suspected.

A more common concern would be how to recover the patient who may be MH susceptible but who has received a non-triggering anesthetic. Despite the seriousness of an episode of MH, it is reasonable for a patient who is at risk for MH to be admitted to the PACU and still be able to be discharged the same day as the procedure when they have not been exposed to potent inhaled anesthetics or succinylcholine [68]. In fact, there is no advantage to keeping a patient who is MH susceptible in the PACU for a prolonged period of time if there are no other complicating factors [69]. Based on a review of over 250 MH-susceptible patients, and per the Malignant Hyperthermia Association of the United States (MHAUS) website, a 1 h stay in the primary PACU with an additional 1–1.5 h in a step-down PACU, if indicated, is recommended [70].

Emergence agitation or delirium

It is not uncommon for children to emerge from anesthesia disoriented and frightened, resulting in negative behavior of restlessness, anxiety and inconsolability. As part of the assessment of this behavior, careful consideration must be given to an organic cause must be made. For example, hypoxemia, hypercarbia, hypotension, hypoglycemia, raised intracranial pressure or untreated pain should all be ruled out. Only after this has occurred can the phenomenon of emergence delirium (ED), also referred to as emergence agitation (EA), be considered.

In the modern era of the pediatric PACU, the issue of emergence delirium has become a popular topic of discussion. For example, a well-referenced analysis of perioperative morbidity published in 2004 failed to include ED as an adverse event as it seemingly was not considered a major issue at that time [1]. Defined as "a disturbance in a child's awareness of and attention to his/her environment with disorientation and perceptual alterations including hypersensitivity to stimuli and hyperactive motor behavior in the immediate postanesthesia period," ED can be stressful for the child, parents and caretakers [71].

There is a range of behavioral responses following anesthesia, from crying uncontrollably after emergence for more than 3 min (mild) to uncontrollable behavior requiring physical restraint for more than 3 min (major) [71]. With such a range of presentation, it is difficult to describe a precise incidence of ED as it may be as high as 80%, depending on how it is defined. The spectrum of clinical presentation has therefore lead to the creation of behavioral scales such as the Pediatric Anesthesia Emergence Delirium (PAED) scale (Table 16.3). When tested in 50 children for validity, the PAED scale revealed consistency and reliability [71].

The issue of emergence agitation/delirium was not truly evident until the practice of using sevoflurane started replacing the use of halothane. This suspicion that sevoflurane resulted in more frequent episodes of emergence delirium was reviewed in a meta-analysis which confirmed that sevoflurane was associated with a consistently higher incidence of agitation when compared to halothane [72]. In fact, ED is associated with both of the newer inhalational agents, desflurane and sevoflurane [73,74]. Because desflurane and sevoflurane have a greater incidence of emergence delirium compared to isoflurane

Table 16.3 Pediatric Anesthesia Emergence Delirium Scale (PAED)

Category	Score 4	Score 3	Score 2	Score 1	Score 0
Child makes eye contact	Not at all	Just a little	Quite a bit	Very much	Extremely
Child's actions are purposeful	Not at all	Just a little	Quite a bit	Very much	Extremely
Child is aware of surroundings	Not at all	Just a little	Quite a bit	Very much	Extremely
Child is restless	Extremely	Very much	Quite a bit	Just a little	Not at all
Child is inconsolable	Extremely	Very much	Quite a bit	Just a little	Not at all

or halothane, this results in the possible conundrum of the supposed benefit of shorter acting agents in promoting a quicker recovery and shorter discharge times possibly being negated by the increased incidence of ED from a rapid emergence. This concern was demonstrated to be valid in a study comparing recovery and discharge criteria between halothane and sevoflurane in children undergoing myringotomy tube placement. Emergence agitation was significantly higher in the sevoflurane group versus halothane group (57% versus 27%, respectively), and discharge times were similarly prolonged with the sevoflurane group [75].

However, it is simply not the fact that rapid emergence is responsible for ED. Delayed emergence by gradually decreasing the inhaled agent has no effect on the incidence of ED [76] and comparative anesthetics that offer quick emergence, such as propofol, still demonstrate that inhaled agents are associated with a greater incidence of ED [77]. This was shown in a randomized cross-over study where propofol was noted to have a zero prevalence of ED compared to sevoflurane as a maintenance agent [78]. The propofol group did have a longer recovery stay, but the parental satisfaction was higher with the propofol group than with the sevoflurane group.

In order to prevent emergence agitation or delirium, it is important to know the factors that predict its occurrence. First, ED may be associated with the type of surgery. An increased incidence is found after otorhinolaryngological and ophthalmological surgeries, at 26% and 28% respectively, when compared to other types of procedures [79]. In addition, there are patient factors that predict postoperative ED such as age less than 5 years, increased preoperative anxiety, and a temperament that is more emotional, more impulsive, less social, and less adaptable [80]. Clearly, these factors cannot necessarily be controlled preoperatively. There are also anesthesia factors, over and above what agent is used to induce and maintain anesthesia. For example, the smoothness of the induction is a predictor of emergence. Weldon et al studied 80 children less than 6 years of age receiving either sevoflurane or halothane [81]. All the children were premedicated with midazolam and received caudal regional anesthesia after their inhaled induction so that postoperative pain would not be a factor in their EA. Although the study was designed to compare the inhaled agents, and showed that children who received sevoflurane had a significantly higher incidence of EA than halothane at arrival to PACU (26% vs 6%), it also showed that the incidence of emergence agitation was higher in the children who had increased anxiety preoperatively per the Yale Preoperative Anxiety Scale [82,83]. In addition to an increased incidence of agitation on admission and more episodes of severe agitation, these same children also had a greater incidence of difficult mask inductions.

Early thoughts as to the cause of emergence delirium/agitation included the presence of pain. Although pain may be a contributing factor to an unsatisfactory emergence period, it has not been shown to be the cause of ED. In fact, ED has been shown to have a similar incidence after non-painful procedures such as MRI [75]. In children who have undergone sevoflurane anesthesia without surgical intervention, a small dose of fentanyl at 1μg/kg 10 min prior to emergence reduced emergence agitation from 56% to 12% with no increase in time to discharge [83]. Studies using caudal block in order to take the pain issue out of the equation of postoperative ED have shown inconsistent results as to the effectiveness of regional anesthesia in addition to sevoflurane for avoidance of agitation [81,84].

In addition to avoiding the agents that are commonly associated with emergence delirium such as sevoflurane and desflurane, other agents have been studied to determine if using them prophylactically will reduce the incidence of ED. In a recent meta-analysis, midazolam and 5-hydroxytryptamine-3 receptor (5HT3) inhibitors such as ondansetron were not found to have a protective effect against ED, whereas propofol, ketamine, fentanyl and α2-adrenoceptor agonists were all found to have a preventive effect [85].

The α2-adrenoceptor agonists are an emerging group of drugs used in the management of postoperative agitation. Clonidine causes sedation, analgesia and reduction in sympathetic tone and can be administered through many routes. An intravenous dose of 2μg/kg after anesthetic induction has been demonstrated to significantly reduce the incidence and severity of emergence agitation in boys undergoing circumcision with penile blocks under sevoflurane anesthesia [86]. This efficacy in the management of ED with clonidine has not been consistent at a dose of 1.5μg/kg when compared to the more efficacious tropisetron [87]. Dexmedetomidine, another α2-agonist, has both prophylactic and treatment potential for ED. When using dexmedetomidine as a single bolus dose immediately after inhalation induction, the incidence of emergence agitation in children who received sevoflurane with caudal block was significantly lower in a dose-dependent manner. The incidence of agitation in the group who did not receive dexmedetomidine was 37% whereas the group receiving 0.15μg/kg had an incidence of EA at 17% and a group who received 0.3μg/kg was 10% with no differences in time to discharge. Alternatively, infusion of dexmedetomidine at a rate of 0.2μg/kg/h infusion after induction and continuing 15 min into PACU is effective in reducing the incidence of ED [88,89]. The incidence of emergence agitation in the children who received dexmedetomidine infusion was 26% compared to 60.8% in the sevoflurane group with no differences in time to extubation or discharge from PACU.

In addition to the expected preventive measures and agents, melatonin, a hormone secreted by the pineal gland, when administered preoperatively has been demonstrated to be efficacious in the management of ED in a dose-dependent manner of up to 0.4 mg/kg (maximum 20 mg) when compared to midazolam [90]. Although doses of melatonin at 0.05 mg/kg and 0.2 mg/kg decreased ED, a dose of 0.4 mg/kg was the most efficacious and reduced the incidence of emergence delirium to 5.4%.

Beyond pharmacological intervention, parental presence has been evaluated in terms of its effect on emergence delirium. Although there was no measurable improvement on the incidence or duration of ED, the parents themselves had greater satisfaction with being present during the recovery phase [91].

Emergence agitation continues to be addressed, and additional work needs to be done to determine not only how to prevent its occurrence, but to improve the process by which it is diagnosed and treated when it occurs. These goals are necessary in order to make an otherwise uneventful perioperative course more pleasant for the child, family, and providers.

Seizures and myoclonus

Postoperative seizures are an uncommon event in the PACU but can be indicative of a more serious underlying problem. Regardless of the etiology of the seizure, supportive measures should be immediate and include the delivery of oxygen with airway maintenance and special efforts to avoid self-harm in the child. Depending on the severity and duration of the seizure, oxygen may be delivered by facemask or positive pressure ventilation, or require endotracheal intubation. A physician should be in attendance and determine the need for immediate pharmacological intervention, also depending on the severity or duration of the epileptic activity.

Causes of postoperative seizures are numerous, with significant consequences. Hypoxemia may be rapidly ruled in or out and treated as necessary with appropriate oxygenation and ventilation. If this is clearly not the cause, state laboratory tests should be obtained to rule out hypoglycemia and electrolyte disturbances such as hyponatremia and hypocalcemia must be sent, then rapidly interpreted and treated. A rare but potentially fatal cause of postoperative seizures is local anesthetic toxicity and the seizures may actually be a prelude to cardiovascular collapse. A thorough history of local anesthetic delivery should be assessed that includes last dose and total dosing if there is any suspicion of local anesthetic toxicity. If this is determined to be the cause, in addition to supportive measures, intravenous lipid emul-

sion should be delivered if cardiovascular arrest ensues [92]. PACU providers should be made aware of this possibility and be informed as to the location and delivery of lipid emulsion. See Chapter 40 for further discussion of this problem.

Beyond seizure activity, myoclonus may be observed in the PACU. Myoclonus is defined as the involuntary contraction of a muscle or muscle groups and has a variety of causes, including some anesthetic agents such as etomidate or as a prodrome to seizure activity. After other causes of myoclonus are ruled out, the possibility of central anticholinergic syndrome (CAS) should be entertained. CAS is secondary to the central antagonism of muscarinic cholingeric receptors and may be caused by medications that cross the blood–brain barrier, such as atropine or scopolamine [93]. The symptoms vary from agitation to actual coma, with myoclonus as a presenting sign. Slow delivery of physostigmine (10–30 µg/kg with maximum of 3 mg) is the treatment of choice.

Pain

Pain management does not begin in the PACU, but needs to be managed for the entire perioperative period and is the responsibility of every anesthesiologist. In the PACU, the recognition of postoperative pain becomes the duty of a recovery nurse as intraoperative analgesic medications wear off and the pain becomes more intense as the patient recovers. Although a complete discussion of pain is beyond the scope of this chapter and is presented elsewhere in this book (see Chapter 33), in the PACU environment it is important to consider how to assess the pain, what analgesics are appropriate, and what potential pitfalls and complications exist.

The assessment of pain in children remains a challenge in part because of the diversity of age range. No single assessment tool or score can possibly be applied equally to the newborn and the adolescent. Although of little benefit to children who are pre- and non-verbal, developmentally delayed or cognitively impaired, self-reporting is probably the most important single reliable indicator of pain. Children as young as 3 years of age can reliably score their own pain [94] provided that they are trained to use the chosen score prior to surgery. There are many validated pain intensity scales including visual analogs, faces scales, and numeric ratings, which are presented elsewhere. The OUCHER score utilizes photographs of a child's face exhibiting varying expressions of pain intensity alongside a numerical rating scale and allows the young child to self-report. Different ethnic versions are available and it has been validated in the 3–12-year-old age group, specifically in the PACU setting [95] (Fig. 16.4).

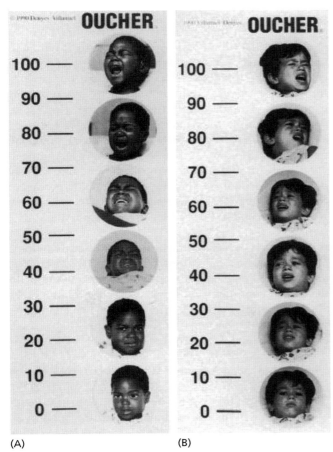

Figure 16.4 OUCHER pediatric pain scale for children age 3–12 years. (A) African-American version. (B) Hispanic version. Reproduced from Beyer and Knott [95] with permission from Elsevier.

Table 16.4 Faces, Legs, Activity, Cry, Consolability (FLACC) Scale [97]

Categories	Scoring		
	0	**1**	**2**
Face	No particular expression or smile	Occasional grimace of frown, withdrawn, disinterested	Frequent to constant quivering chin, clenched jaw
Legs	Normal position or relaxed	Uneasy, restless, tense	Kicking, or legs drawn up
Activity	Lying quietly, normal position, moves easily	Squirming, shifting back and forth, tense	Arched, rigid or jerking
Cry	No cry (awake or asleep)	Moans or whimpers; occasional complaint	Crying steadily, screams or sobs, frequent complaints
Consolability	Content, relaxed	Reassured by occasional touching, hugging or being talked to, distractable	Difficult to console or comfort

Each of the five categories (F) Face: (L) Legs; (A) Activity; (C) Cry; (C) Consolability is scored from 0–2, which results in a total score between zero and ten. Reproduced from Willis [97] with permission from Jannetti Publications.

In those children unable to provide a self report (age 3 years or less, or developmentally delayed), behavioral observational scales assist the caregiver in determining a level or degree of pain. The Children's Hospital of Eastern Ontario Pain Scale (CHEOPS) [96], the Face, Leg, Activity, Cry, Consolability Scale (FLACC) [97] (Table 16.4) and Preverbal, Early Verbal Pediatric Pain Scale (PEVPPS)[98] are all valuable tools but limited in that behavior varies significantly between individuals. These scales are not perfect as a paucity of abnormal behavior does not mean an absence of pain, and negative behavior does not necessarily indicate pain.

Finally, physiological signs, such as tachycardia, tachypnea, and hypertension, can be used as an indicator of pain but are the least sensitive and least specific markers [99]. Particularly in a child, these physiological signs can be present due to other stresses including anxiety or fearfulness, and need to be combined with other evidence that suggests pain as a cause. With all the different types of scales available, each institution needs to determine the ones that work best for their environment for the different age groups and keep it consistent for reliability across providers.

In the clinical setting, proving the existence of pain through a validated pain score is less important than actually understanding the potential degree of pain with knowledge of the surgery and actively managing symptoms and signs of distress. The PACU nursing staff have many pain management strategies available to them, both pharmacological and non-pharmacological, to ease pain and distress postoperatively [100]. Multimodal approaches are often the most effective and take advantage of non-opioid and opioid agents as well as other measures for comprehensive pain management.

Non-opioid pharmacological agents offer pain relief without some of the unfavorable side-effects such as nausea and vomiting and respiratory depression, and are therefore useful adjuncts to the postoperative pain management plan. Simple analgesics that require oral administration such as *acetaminophen* require patient co-operation and the absence of nausea and vomiting. Its mode of action is predominantly central by modulating dynorphin release through inhibition of cyclo-oxygenase (COX) [101] and recent findings suggest that it is highly selective for COX-2 [102]. Oral dosing is 10–15 mg/kg. Rectal administration of acetaminophen at 30–40 mg/kg is associated with a delayed (between 1 and 3 h) and varied uptake but offers an alternative route of administration in a child who must remain NPO or an unco-operative or nauseated child [103]. Daily cumulative dosing should be carefully monitored with previously administered doses and prescribed dosing clearly stated during handovers. Although oral dosing may be prescribed every 4 h, rectal dosing requires an every 6 h dosing scheme due to the delayed and unpredictable absorption. Maximum oral daily dosing limits are 100 mg/kg per day for children, 75 mg/kg for infants, 60 mg/kg for term and preterm neonates beyond 32 weeks of postconceptual age, and 40 mg/kg for preterm neonates from 28 to 32 weeks postconceptual age [104]. Injectable or intravenous acetaminophen (paracetamol) is now available in many countries and is undergoing clinical trials in children for perioperative use. In a prospective, placebo-controlled, double-blind study versus its older prodrug, proparacetamol, in 183 patients aged 1–12 years undergoing inguinal hernia repair, IV paracetamol was as effective as the older drug at relieving pain, with less injection site pain [105].

Other non-opioid agents such as the non-steroidal anti-inflammatory drugs (NSAIDs) can be delivered orally or intravenously. *Ibuprofen* at 10 mg/kg is given orally every 6 h and can be alternated with acetaminophen throughout the postoperative period. Another NSAID option is intravenous *ketorolac* at 0.2–0.5 mg/kg every 6 h with a single maximum dose of 15 mg and a maximum daily dosage of 90 mg [106]. Little difference in efficacy has been noted between the NSAIDs, and the mode of action is again by COX inhibition, similar to acetaminophen but predominantly peripherally in this case [107]. NSAIDs are invaluable in the successful management of pain and have been demonstrated to have a significant opioid-sparing effect of up to 46% [108,109]. Although widely used, caution should be exercised in children due to potential side-effects. Use in neonates and infants is not currently indicated due to the risk to the developing kidneys. There also remains controversial use in children due to the risk of bleeding from platelet dysfunction as well as the question of bone healing for certain orthopedic procedures [110,111]. *Aspirin* and other salicyclates can cause Reye syndrome in children and are therefore rarely recommended in this population of patients except for specific indications that do not include postoperative pain management [112].

Opioids continue to represent the mainstay of analgesia in the PACU. The popularity of these drugs stems from their efficacy, speed of onset and titratability. When non-opioid agents are ineffective by themselves for pain management, the addition of an opioid analgesic is required. Often fentanyl is the opioid intravenous analgesic of choice for the initial PACU period and for outpatients. Intravenous *fentanyl* 0.5–1.0 μg/kg every 3–5 min or *morphine* 0.05–0.1 mg/kg every 10–15 min have been extensively used and studied, but caution needs to be exercised as these medications have significant adverse potential, especially in children. In particular, neonates are prone to ventilatory depression, having immature and poorly developed responses to airway obstruction, hypercapnia and hypoxemia [113]. *Hydromorphone* at 10 μg/kg every 10–15 min may also be used for severe pain in the PACU setting.

Although typically administered intravenously, opioids have good bio-availability by other routes. For example, fentanyl can be given intranasally at 2 μg/kg without an increase in vomiting, hypoxemia or discharge times [114]. Short procedures such as myringotomy, when an intravenous line is not inserted, are ideally suited to this route of administration.

Opioids can also be administered through infusion devices, and patient-controlled analgesia (PCA) can be used for children typically 6 years and older [115]. Background or basal infusions should be used with caution and will require ongoing monitoring not only in the PACU but on the ward [116]. If a child is to receive PCA, it is advantageous to have this mode of analgesia started in the PACU with instructions so that it is fine-tuned and the child's pain is well under control prior to discharge to the ward.

For children who are going home from the recovery room, providing them with an oral dose of their prescribed medication prior to discharge will help the transition process from hospital to home. This allows the family additional time to get prescriptions filled and provides for a more comfortable ride home for the child. Before giving an oral medication, however, it needs to be clear that the child is alert enough to take the medication, able to maintain their own airway easily, and be free of nausea or vomiting prior to discharge. In addition, any oral medication that is made of a combination of the opioid with either acetaminophen or ibuprofen must be started only after the appropriate time interval has passed to keep those agents on an every 4 or every 6 h schedule.

Non-pharmacological analgesic remedies may include physical contact through cuddling, stroking, massage, holding and rocking. In addition, newborn infants can often be comforted with concentrated sugar water (24% dextrose 0.1–0.2 mL instilled intraorally or applied to a pacifier), perhaps due to the sucrose's release of endogenous opioids [117]. Older children may require more sophisticated methods using cognitive interventions along the lines of distraction, guided imagery and simple delivery of information. In addition, behavioral interventions such as biofeedback, positive reinforcement and relaxation exercises with controlled breathing can help alleviate pain in the postoperative period.

Postoperative nausea and vomiting

Postoperative nausea and vomiting (PONV) is a major cause of patient dissatisfaction in adults following anesthesia and surgery. Children have an even higher incidence of postoperative vomiting than adults [118] and nausea, which is difficult to diagnose in younger patients, is most likely under-reported. Effective management is important not simply for the humanitarian aspect but because length of stay (LOS) in the PACU is largely determined by PONV. Each episode of vomiting can result in a 28-min delay in children after adenotonsillectomy [23] and can be a major cause of unanticipated admission after outpatient surgery [119].

In 2003, the consensus guidelines for the management of PONV were developed as an evidence-based tool for clinicians [120]. In 2006, a multidisciplinary panel made further modifications, with attention to children due to their nearly doubled risk of postoperative vomiting (POV). The consensus guidelines focused on risk factors for PONV/POV, recommendations for prophylaxis, and the most effective treatment regimes.

Prophylactic management of pediatric POV typically requires drug intervention that may be costly or associated with unwanted side-effects [121]. It is therefore ideal to target those children at particular risk of POV. Risk factors for children are similar to those for adults, with a few differences. POV is rare under the age of 2 years but it increases with age until puberty, after which it decreases. A study in children under 14 years of age noted a sharp increase in PONV at age 3 years with a 0.2–0.8% increase per year [122]. There appears to be no gender difference in preadolescent patients, and a history of PONV or motion sickness in a child's parent or sibling may be a risk factor. Certain surgical procedures are associated with a higher incidence of POV in children such as adenotonsillectomy, orchidopexy, penile surgery, hernia repair, and especially strabismus repair [123].

The revised PONV consensus guidelines included a simplified risk score to determine the degree of POV risk in children. The degree of risk is based on the number of risk factors that are present from the following: duration of surgery ≥30 min; age ≥3 years; strabismus surgery; and history of POV or PONV among relatives. Risk of POV is elevated as the number of risk factors increase, with one risk factor representing a 10% risk and four risk factors representing a 70% risk for POV [122]. Of interest, this risk assessment analysis does not include tonsillectomy (with or without adenoidectomy) as a dominant risk factor for POV, when it is described by many as a significant cause of morbidity [124].

Having determined the children who represent a risk of POV, the next step is to address factors for reducing baseline risks such as promoting the use of propofol for total IV anesthesia (TIVA). Although not yet validated in pediatrics, in adults the avoidance of inhalation agents and use of straight regional techniques is recommended in those patients with a high risk for PONV. This is rarely applicable to children, but the use of regional anesthesia in addition to general anesthesia to minimize opiate requirement may reduce the incidence of pediatric POV [125]. In addition, although considerable hydration has been shown to reduce the frequency of PONV [126], insisting that children drink prior to discharge may actually increase the incidence.

Prophylactic drug therapies can either be monotherapy or a combination of medications. The prophylactic antiemetics recommended for pediatric patients include the 5HT3 antagonists ondansetron, dolasetron, granisetron, and tropisetron. Since the publication of the first guidelines, ondansetron (0.05–0.1 mg/kg up to 4 mg) was approved for use in children as young as 1 month of age and granisetron (40 μg/kg) and tropisetron (0.1 mg/kg) were added as therapeutic options [127]. Because the 5HT3 antagonists as a group have greater efficacy in the prevention of vomiting than nausea, these drugs are the first-line choice for prophylaxis in children.

Other therapies to prevent POV include dexamethasone (0.15 mg/kg), droperidol (0.05–0.075 mg/kg up to 1.25 mg), dimenhydrinate (0.5 mg/kg), and perphenazine (0.07 mg/kg). The revised guidelines specify a revised upper limit for the dose range of dexamethasone, reduced from 8 mg to 5 mg to address concerns over unwanted side-effects such as hypoglycemia, delayed wound healing and wound infection [128]. The timing of drug administration may also be a key factor in successful prophylaxis. For example, dexamethasone should be administered early in the anesthetic [128], while ondansetron has been shown to be more effective when given preoperatively [127].

The 2006 consensus guidelines recommend that children who are at moderate or high risk for POV should receive combination therapy with two or three prophylactic drugs from different classes. This differs from the recommendations for adults, where combination therapy should be reserved for "high risk" only. The combinations recommended in the revised consensus guidelines for children are ondansetron (0.05 mg/kg) with dexamethasone (0.15 mg/kg), ondansetron (0.1 mg/kg) with droperidol (0.015 mg/kg), or tropisetron (0.1 mg/kg) with dexamethasone (0.5 mg/kg). All of these combinations require intraoperative administration, and the particular drugs, doses and timing need to be conveyed during handover so that any breakthrough PONV/POV may be managed with that knowledge available.

The recommendations for treatment of PONV/POV when it occurs in the PACU, or when prophylaxis fails, include the use of an antiemetic chosen from a different therapeutic class than the agents used for prophylaxis. Droperidol can be used for pediatric patients who have failed all other therapies and are being admitted to hospital, although the potential for extrapyramidal side-effects exists. The United States Food and Drug Administration issued a "black box" warning on droperidol in 2001 for its association with QT prolongation. However, in the doses prescribed in the United States, the risk of cardiac effects from droperidol is no higher than other available antiemetics, but this possibility may still significantly reduce the willingness of physicians to prescribe it [129].

Non-pharmacological therapies have undergone some investigation in pediatrics. Acupuncture has been successfully used for POV prophylaxis in children undergoing strabismus repair, dental surgery and tonsillectomy [130]. Success using this technique in children has not been consistent [124].

With the options available and the fact that the incidence of POV is undoubtedly higher in children than in adults, a greater need for a better understanding and age-appropriate management of POV in children is necessary to reduce this unwanted side-effect in the perioperative period.

Medication errors

Medication errors in the PACU are a frequent occurrence, maybe possibly as high as 5% of all orders, and have significant potential to cause harm [131]. Medication errors may occur at any point from prescription to administration, and are the result of breakdowns in communication, calculation errors, decimal point errors, the use of a leading/trailing zero and/or knowledge deficit on the part of the health professional.

Children are at increased risk because almost all medications are prescribed on a weight basis and therefore require a calculation step. In fact, error rates for children have been found to be inversely related to the weight of the patient, with the greatest errors occurring in the smallest children [132]. Analgesic medications in particular are commonly involved in medication errors because of widespread use, split dosing and weight-based dosing regimen.

Although medication errors may occur at any time and for any of the previously stated reasons, most errors occur at the ordering stage in children often simply due to a result of poor handwriting [132–134]. For this reason, electronic prescribing systems are becoming increasingly frequent in the PACU and offer the clinician and patient the promise of safer prescribing. The American Academy of Pediatrics has recognized that within the hospital, computerized physician order entry (CPOE) can prevent medication errors, and this success is gaining increasing support in the literature [135,136]. Particularly in children, this additional safeguard may be an extra layer that will prevent potentially catastrophic events in the postoperative period.

Urinary retention

Urinary retention is often difficult to assess in the pediatric patient due to a child's inability to communicate the issue clearly, and it therefore may be underdiagnosed. In the adult population, urinary retention occurs at approximately 16% incidence and is associated with the amount of intraoperative intravenous fluid delivery and bladder volume on admission to the PACU as well as advancing age [137]. This would suggest that straight catheterization or bladder emptying prior to emergence in the operating room should occur in patients who have received a considerable amount of IV fluid in the operating room without a urinary catheter present. There is no association of urinary retention in the PACU with such factors as gender, urinary symptoms, type of surgery or anesthesia, intraoperative administration of anticholinergics or morphine. Postoperative urinary retention is not a significant factor after caudal anesthesia when compared to ilioinguinal/iliohypogastric block and does not delay recovery [138]. However, Metzelder et al demonstrated that children who undergo distal hypospadias repair and receive penile block are significantly less likely to exhibit postoperative urinary retention when compared to patients who receive caudal anesthesia (5/33 versus 15/27, respectively) [139].

Urinary retention, often forgotten as a possibility in children in the PACU, should be considered in any child who has otherwise unexplained tachycardia or signs of discomfort that cannot be attributed to the procedure.

Conclusion

The pediatric PACU requires careful planning and ongoing maintenance in order to provide a safe, efficient environment for the recovering pediatric patient. Despite widespread knowledge of the basic principles of postanesthetic recovery and the publication of general national standards, as this chapter indicates, specific practices are dictated by institutional experience and preference. Basic tasks such as recognizing and managing potential peri-operative complications are compounded by the nuances of taking care of pediatric patients of all ages and understanding the differences across these ages while also incorporating the parents into the experience.

CASE STUDY

The nursing staff in the pediatric PACU are notified by telephone from the operating room that a 4-year-old boy has just undergone a tonsillectomy and adenoidectomy and is ready for transfer to the PACU. The operating room nurse, using a checklist to ensure that all the important information is conveyed, gives the patient name, age and weight, identifies the surgeon responsible and gives a brief description of the operation. She also confirms with the anesthesia provider that there are no additional concerns or issues to be conveyed at the time of initial report. A pediatric-trained PACU nurse then prepares for the admission by establishing that the allocated bed space directly adjacent to her other patient is clean, that the monitoring is complete and working, and that there is an Ambu® bag and functioning suction.

The patient arrives in the PACU escorted by the anesthesia team and surgical resident. The patient is in the left lateral recovery position and has an oxygen mask applied that is connected to a full tank. On arrival, a rapid assessment is made by the PACU nurse which reveals a sleeping child with pink lips and patent airway. Monitors are placed and show an oxygen saturation of 100%, pulse (P) of 100 and blood pressure of 100/60. Temperature is 37°C.

Using the I-SBAR method, the nurse anesthetist introduces herself and the patient's identity is confirmed by name band with the PACU nurse. The remainder of the handover is as follows: the patient is a 4-year-old male weighing 20 kg with a history only significant for obstructive sleep apnea who underwent adenotonsillectomy and is currently stable. He has no known drug allergies and receives no current medications. The family are in the surgical waiting room and have spoken to the surgeon. The patient has undergone general anesthesia, with an inhalational induction of anesthesia, intravenous line placement and the insertion of a 4.5 cuffed RAE endotracheal tube. He received fentanyl 20 μg and no muscle relaxants. For antiemetic prophylaxis, he was given dexamethasone 2 mg and ondansetron 2 mg, as well as rectal acetaminophen 650 mg suppository. Fluid given was 400 mL of lactated Ringer's solution. The surgery took longer than anticipated due to excessive intraoperative bleeding. A deep extubation of the trachea was performed at the end of the case to avoid coughing and rebleeding. There were no drains and no labs were pending. Vital signs remained stable throughout the case with the exception of tachycardia that per-sisted throughout at a rate of 100–130 beats per minute. The patient's risk factors are his sleep apnea and risk of postoperative obstruction, and the nurse anesthetist states that she is also concerned about the risk of bleeding in the PACU in addition to the sleep apnea.

The nurse anesthetist has no additional specific care requirements to report, but the anesthesiologist has written postoperative orders including pain medication at a reduced dose, due to the apnea history. The IV is to be put on a pump and the family informed of the patient's arrival to the PACU.

Within 10 min after arrival in the PACU, the child wakes up crying and coughing. His parents are invited into the PACU to help pacify him and aid in the assessment of anxiety versus pain. The parents are immediately concerned over the amount of blood in the saliva and ask the PACU nurse if this is normal. The PACU nurse reassesses the patient and notes that there are indeed copious blood-filled secretions from the airway which require suctioning. The vital signs are measured and noted to be as follows: SpO_2 98%, P 140, and BP 90/60. The anesthesiologist is called with a brief report of the concerns and he comes immediately to the bedside to assess.

At this time the patient vomits what appears to be a large volume of blood. The anesthesiologist immediately determines the possibility of an ongoing tonsillar bleed and so instructs the PACU nurse to administer 10 mL/kg bolus fluid and to arrange for blood products to be delivered. The child is kept in head-down position to the side and frequent vital signs are measured. The anesthesiologist communicates his concerns to the surgeon in the operating room with an updated assessment of the current situation and a rapid plan of action is established.

During this time, other members of the PACU team bring the centrally located emergency cart with airway equipment to the bedside, along with emergency drugs for the induction of anesthesia. A second fluid bolus of 10 mL/kg is administered and a stat hemoglobin level sent for analysis, prompting the procurement of blood from the blood bank. The child is no longer vomiting and vital signs improve after the second delivery of volume, as noted by an increased blood pressure and reduced heart rate.

Resuscitation is deemed adequate and the patient is electively transported back to the operating room for re-exploration of the tonsillar bleed. The parents remain in the

Continued

PACU during this time and are informed of the events as they occur. The child undergoes a successful cauterization of the tonsillar bleed and makes an uneventful recovery.

Key points

This case illustrates several basic points.

1. Proper handover and communication in the PACU environment are essential. The Joint Commission has recently made the process of handover a key element of its assessment of a medical center or unit and evidence shows that good communication reduces the incidence of adverse events.

2. The PACU is an environment of constant vigilance and attention to detail. Regular patient assessment and attention to changes in condition require rapid management. Fully functioning monitoring with frequent measurements is imperative.

3. There must be a central core of emergency equipment supply and drugs and all team members should be familiar with what is present and available in the PACU. The ability of the PACU team to recognize the potential need for emergency airway care or volume resuscitation requires appropriate equipment and supplies that are readily available.

4. Even without issues such as pain, severe nausea and vomiting or emergence agitation, the PACU is an environment where a seemingly stable patient can become unstable and all team members need to act swiftly and appropriately.

Annotated references

A full reference list for this chapter is available at:
http://www.wiley.com/go/gregory/andropoulos/pediatricanesthesia

4. Hackel A, Badgwell JM, Binding RR et al. Guidelines for the pediatric perioperative anesthesia environment. American Academy of Pediatrics, Section on Anesthesiology. Pediatrics 1999; 103: 512–15. An important article articulating the standards for the pediatric perioperative environment, including the postanesthesia care unit.

21. Aldrete JA. The post-anesthesia recovery score revisited. J Clin Anesth 1995; 7: 89–91. Update of the classic paper describing the universally used PACU discharge scoring system, that now includes pulse oximetry.

22. Chung F, Chan VW, Ong D. A post-anesthetic discharge scoring system for home readiness after ambulatory surgery. J Clin Anesth 1995; 7: 500–6. An important addition to the discharge readiness literature, tailored for discharge home from ambulatory surgery.

24. Cote CJ, Zaslavsky A, Downes JJ et al. Postoperative apnea in former preterm infants after inguinal herniorrhaphy. A combined analysis. Anesthesiology 1995; 82: 809–22. A combined analysis stratifying the risk of postanesthetic apnea in former preterm infants, offering guidance as to gestational ages for admission and monitoring after anesthesia.

48. Schwengel DA, Sterni LM, Tunkel DE, Heitmiller ES. Perioperative management of children with obstructive sleep apnea. Anesth Analg 2009; 109: 60–75. A comprehensive review of the management of pediatric patients with this important problem being seen with increasing frequency.

85. Dahmani S, Stany I, Brasher C et al. Pharmacological prevention of sevoflurane- and desflurane-related emergence agitation in children: a meta-analysis of published studies. Br J Anaesth 2010; 104: 216–23. An important meta-analysis of available data on preventing emergence agitation with the newer inhaled agents.

91. Burke CN, Voepel-Lewis T, Hadden S et al. Parental presence on emergence: effect on postanesthesia agitation and parent satisfaction. J Perianesth Nurs 2009; 24: 216–21. An important study on the effect of parents' presence in the PACU.

97. Willis MH, Merkel SI, Voepel-Lewis T, Malviya S. FLACC Behavioral Pain Assessment Scale: a comparison with the child's self-report. Pediatr Nurs 2003; 29: 195–8. The description and validation of an important pediatric pain assessment scale for children.

104. Berde CB, Sethna NF. Analgesics for the treatment of pain in children. N Engl J Med 2002; 347: 1094–103. A classic review article on the pharmacological treatment of pain in children, including postoperative pain.

122. Eberhart LH, Geldner G, Kranke P et al. The development and validation of a risk score to predict the probability of postoperative vomiting in pediatric patients. Anesth Analg 2004; 99: 1630–7. An important study quantitating the risk score for postoperative vomiting in pediatric patients.

CHAPTER 17

Monitoring and Vascular Access

Dean B. Andropoulos

Department of Anesthesiology and Pediatrics, Baylor College of Medicine, and Texas Children's Hospital, Houston, TX, USA

Introduction

Vascular access and monitoring of circulation, respiration, the central nervous system, and other end organs is a central task for the pediatric anesthesiologist. The vast majority of cases will require simple peripheral venous access and standard non-invasive monitors. Extensive surgery or significant underlying disease may necessitate invasive cardiovascular monitoring, and procedures where the brain is at risk may require central nervous system monitoring. This chapter will address peripheral venous access and then invasive vascular access and monitoring, followed by monitoring of respiration, temperature, neuromuscular blockade and renal monitoring. Finally, central nervous system monitoring will be reviewed.

Venous access

Peripheral veins

Any visible peripheral vein, and many that are not visible, may be utilized for peripheral venous access. One strategy in pediatric patients is to cannulate a small superficial vein on the hand or foot with a small catheter (24 or 22 gauge) before induction or during inhalation induction of anesthesia to facilitate the early administration of intravenous agents and provide expeditious airway management. Later, with the airway secure and with an immobile patient, larger bore peripheral venous access can be achieved. Simple surgeries without blood loss require smaller catheters, but if significant fluid or blood administration is anticipated, larger catheter sizes should be utilized. Recommended sizes for major surgery are 22 or

Gregory's Pediatric Anesthesia, Fifth Edition. Edited by George A. Gregory, Dean B. Andropoulos.
© 2012 Blackwell Publishing Ltd. Published 2012 by Blackwell Publishing Ltd.

24 ga 1″ catheters for infants newborn through 6 months, 22 ga 1″ or 20 ga 1.25″ catheters for 6 months to 3 years, 20–22 ga or 18 ga 1.5″ for 3–12 years, and 16 or 14 ga 2″catheters for teenage or adult patients. Resistance to fluid flow predicted by Poiseuille's Law is proportional to the length of the catheter and the viscosity of the fluid, and inversely proportional to the fourth power of the catheter radius. When rapidly infusing the more viscous colloids or packed red blood cells, it is important to use a large-bore, short catheter in a large peripheral vein.

The saphenous vein at the ankle is large and in a constant anatomical position in patients of all ages. It can usually be cannulated even if it cannot be seen or palpated. A recommended technique is to apply a tourniquet below the knee, prepare the site antiseptically, and extend the ankle at the medial malleolus with one hand while puncturing the skin at a shallow angle of 10–30° with an angiocatheter 0.5–1 cm anterior and 1 cm inferior to the medial malleolus. Advance the catheter slowly in the groove between the malleolus and the tibialis tendon until blood return through the needle is established. Advance the needle and catheter together several millimeters, then advance the catheter over the needle into the vein with the index finger of the same hand that made the skin puncture, while maintaining extension of the ankle so that the saphenous vein is tethered straight in its course, to minimize the possibility of puncturing the posterior wall due to kinking of the vein. If the vein can be entered but the catheter will not advance its full length into the vein, a small flexible guidewire of 0.015″ or 0.018″ may be used to assist in cannulation of the saphenous or any other peripheral vein [1]. Other large peripheral veins may be found in infants and children on the dorsum of the hand, at the wrist superficial to the radial head, as branches of the cephalic or brachial venous system in the antecubital fossa or on the dorsolateral aspect of the foot. The latter site is especially prominent in many newborns.

The external jugular vein is often visible in infants and children undergoing anesthesia and surgery. This site can be used in cases of difficult access. A recommended technique is to choose the larger external jugular vein, put a small rolled towel under the shoulders and place the patient in 30° Trendelenburg position, prepare the site antiseptically, and have an assistant compress the vein gently with pressure just above the clavicle to further distend it. Rotation of the head 45–90° away from the side of cannulation and slight extension of the neck and traction of the skin over the vein with one hand will tether the vein into a straighter course to facilitate successful cannulation. The vein is punctured high in its visible course with an angiocatheter attached to a syringe filled with heparinized saline, and with the needle bent upwards 10–20° to facilitate the very flat, superficial angle of incidence necessary to cannulate the vein without puncturing its back wall. With constant, gentle aspiration of the syringe, the vein is entered and catheter advanced into the vein. Short peripheral catheters of the same size as recommended above should be used. A catheter advanced too far into the venous plexus beneath the clavicle will often exhibit resistance to the free, gravity-driven flow of fluid, and traction or withdrawal of the catheter a few millimeters may be necessary. External jugular catheters are often difficult to secure to the skin on the neck, and suturing them in place is recommended. This will enhance stability postoperatively as the patient begins moving. One advantage of using the external jugular vein for a peripheral venous catheter is that it is easily accessible under the surgical drapes, and can be frequently monitored for extravasation or kinking of the catheter, which is more common with this site than with the other commonly used peripheral veins.

Umbilical vein

The umbilical vein in the fetus is a conduit for carrying oxygenated and detoxified blood from the placenta, through the abdominal wall, the liver and patent ductus venosus to the inferior vena cava (IVC) and the right atrium [2] (Fig. 17.1). This vessel can usually be cannulated at the umbilical stump for the first 3–5 days of postnatal life. Passage into the IVC depends on the patency of the ductus venosus, which often exists for the first few days, just as the ductus arteriosus. Sterile technique without a guidewire is used to pass the catheter blindly a premeasured distance. If no resistance to passage is met and free blood return is achieved, the catheter tip is usually in the high IVC or right atrium, and functions as a central venous catheter. Catheter tip position must be determined by radiography as soon as possible to determine if it is through the ductus venosus into the IVC or the right atrium. Often, the ductus venosus is not patent, and the catheter tip passes into branches of the hepatic veins, and is visible in the liver radiographically. In this location, the catheter must not be used except for emergencies. Central venous pressure monitoring is inaccurate in this position, and portal vein thrombosis, liver and intestinal necrosis can occur with the infusion of hyperosmolar or vasoactive drugs such as sodium bicarbonate and dopamine. An alternative site for central access must be chosen.

Percutaneous central venous access

Percutaneous central venous access can be utilized for several indications:

- difficult peripheral venous access or need for prolonged vascular access
- need to monitor central venous pressure, i.e. large fluid shifts or blood loss, or cardiovascular surgery
- need for vasoactive infusions [3].

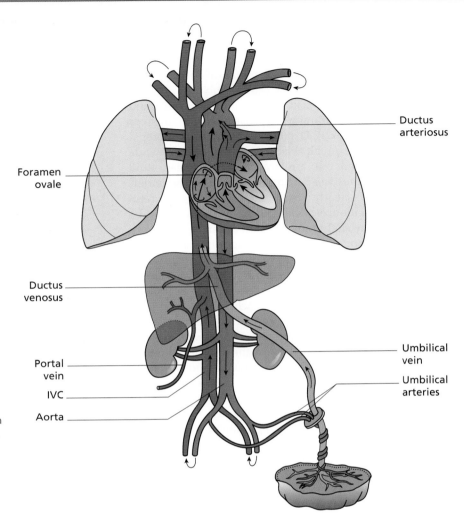

Figure 17.1 The fetal circulation. A catheter placed in the umbilical vein should have its tip through the ductus venosus into the inferior vena cava at or near its junction with the right atrium. The tip of an umbilical artery catheter should lie at the level of the third lumbar vertebral body, between the origin of the renal arteries and the bifurcation of the aorta. Reproduced from Parellada and Guest [2] with permission from Lippincott Williams & Wilkins.

Precise indications will vary according to the practitioner. A double-lumen central catheter of the smallest acceptable size is recommended for percutaneous central venous catheter placement. For all sites, either audio Doppler or two-dimensional ultrasound can be used to facilitate insertion. The larger distal lumen is used for central venous pressure monitoring and drug injection, and the smaller proximal lumen for vasoactive and other infusions. The smallest available double-lumen catheter is currently 4 Fr in size. Superior vena cava (SVC) catheters should be used with caution or not at all in patients weighing less than 4 kg because of the increased risk of thrombosis (see Complications). Recommended sizes and lengths are shown in Table 17.1.

Sterile technique using gown and wide draping leads to a "cleaner" insertion technique with fewer infectious complications [4]. In cardiac patients, the left side SVC lines should generally be avoided. The risk of erosion/perforation is greater, and 5–15% of patients with congenital cardiac disease have a persistent left SVC, which

Table 17.1 Recommended central venous catheter sizes and lengths according to weight

Patient weight	IJ/subclavian vein	Femoral vein
<10 kg	4 Fr, 2 lumen, 8 cm	4 Fr, 2 lumen, 12 cm
10–30 kg	4 Fr, 2 lumen, 12 cm	4 Fr, 2 lumen, 12–15 cm
30–50 kg	5 Fr, 2 lumen, 12–15 cm	5 Fr, 2 lumen, 15 cm
50–70 kg	7 Fr, 2 lumen, 15 cm	7 Fr, 2 lumen, 20 cm
>70 kg	8 Fr, 2 lumen, 16 cm	8 Fr, 2 lumen 20 cm

most often drains either to the coronary sinus or the left atrium, neither of which is a desirable location for a catheter tip. So, if left-sided line placement is contemplated, ascertain by echo/cath report the presence of the left SVC. If this is not known in a patient with congenital heart disease, choose an alternative site, i.e. femoral venous.

The following general discussion of the Seldinger technique in pediatric patients can be applied to all percutaneous vascular access sites, either venous or arterial. The Seldinger technique is used for all percutaneous central venous cannulations. A central line insertion and maintenance "bundle" will reduce infection rates and should be used, including a checklist to ensure all steps are followed [5] (Box 17.1). After wide sterile skin preparation with iodine or chlorhexidine-based solution, wide draping is carried out, preferably with a clear, fluid impermeable adhesive aperture drape so that the underlying anatomy is clearly visible. Slow, controlled, careful needle manipulation, especially in small infants, must be emphasized. The slight movement in or out of only 1 mm or less may be enough to prevent passage of the guidewire. It is very important to have the guidewire prepared to insert and immediately accessible when the vein is entered, so the anesthesiologist does not have to look away from the puncture site to reach for the wire on a distant tray, often resulting in enough movement of the needle to prevent successful guidewire passage.

After the desired vein is entered, the needle position is fixed by stabilizing it against the patient's body with the heel of non-dominant hand, and the guidewire is carefully advanced into the right atrium. The resistance to wire passage should be minimal. Experienced operators learn to recognize the "feel" of a guidewire passing successfully. If any resistance is encountered, the wire must be carefully withdrawn, and another approach made if the needle is still in the vessel, ascertained by free aspiration of blood. Forcing a guidewire in the face of resistance can lead to significant complications.

The electrocardiogram should be carefully observed as the guidewire is slowly advanced. Premature atrial contractions (PAC) are usually observed as the first guidewire-induced dysrhythmia, signifying atrial location. If no PACs are observed, the operator should suspect that the guidewire is not in the atrium. If ventricular extrasystoles are the first observed dysrhythmia, especially if they are multifocal in nature, the wire is very likely in an artery, and the left ventricle has been entered retrograde.

After guidewire passage, a very small skin incision with a #11 scalpel is made. Finally, careful dilation and catheter passage follow. The dilators in the pre-packaged central venous catheter kits are often one size larger than the catheter, i.e. 5 Fr dilator for 4 Fr catheter. This may be undesirable for small infants, and either passage of the catheter without dilation or use of a dilator the same size as the catheter is preferable to make the smallest possible hole in the vein to minimize bleeding and trauma to the vessel wall, both of which may lead to an increased incidence of thrombosis or vascular insufficiency.

Meticulous attention must be paid to blood loss in small infants during catheterization procedures, with

---

Box 17.1 Central line catheter care bundles

Insertion bundle

- Wash hands before the procedure
- For all children aged ≥2 mo, use chlorhexidine gluconate to scrub the insertion site for 30 s for all areas except the groin, which should be scrubbed for 2 min. Scrubbing should be followed by 30 to 60 s of air drying
- No iodine skin prep or ointment is used at the insertion site
- Use a sterilized prepackaged tray with catheter that contains all necessary equipment and supplies including full sterile barriers
- Create an insertion checklist, which empowers staff to stop a nonemergent procedure if it does not follow sterile insertion practices
- Use only polyurethane or Teflon catheters[a]
- Conduct insertion training for all care providers, including sides and video

Maintenance bundle

- Assess daily whether catheter is needed
- Catheter-site care
  - No iodine ointment
  - Use a chlorhexidine gluconate scrub to sites for dressing changes (30-s scrub, 30-s air-dry)
  - Change gauze dressings every 2 d unless they are soiled, dampened, or loosened[a]
  - Change clear dressings every 7 d unless they are soiled, dampened, or loosened[a]
  - Use a prepackaged dressing-change kit or supply area
- Catheter hub, cap, and tubing care
  - Replace administration sets, including add-on devices, no more frequently than every 72 h unless they are soiled or suspected to be infected
  - Replace tubing that is used to administer blood, blood products, or lipids within 24 h of initiating infusion[a]
  - Change caps no more often then 72 h (or according to manufacturer recommendations); however, caps should be replaced when the administration set is changed[a]
  - The prepackaged cap-change kit, or supply area elements to be designated by the local institution

[a]These procedures are according to the CDC recommendations.

---

direct compression of bleeding puncture sites using the heel of the non-dominant hand, while threading dilators, catheters, etc. Use of an assistant may be necessary in difficult catheterizations. After passage of the catheter to the desired depth, it is secured with sutures and a dressing. If more than 1 cm of catheter is outside the patient, additional suturing or catheter holding devices are necessary.

Internal jugular vein

The right internal jugular (IJ) vein is the most common site chosen for central venous access in pediatric cardiac surgery, and is often an excellent choice for other major surgery. It is large, and runs in close proximity superficial to the carotid artery along most of its length. The primary advantage of using the IJ vein is that it provides a direct route to the right atrium, and thus a high rate of optimal catheter positioning if the vessel can be cannulated. Various studies report only a 0–2% incidence of catheter tip outside the thorax, in contrast to 5–10% for the subclavian route [6,7]. The primary disadvantage comes from difficulty in cannulation in small infants, who have large heads and short necks, and thus difficulty in obtaining the shallow angle of approach necessary to access the vessel. Also some series report a 10–15% incidence of carotid artery puncture in infants and ultrasound studies of neck vessel anatomy reveal the partial or complete overlap of the IJ vein anterior to the carotid artery [7]. This site is also not comfortable for some awake infants, and tip migration may be significant with turning the head or flexion/extension of the neck [8]. All insertion techniques involve placing a small roll under the shoulders, using steep Trendelenburg position, and rotating the head no more than 45° to the left. Greater rotation will produce more overlap of the IJ vein and carotid artery, and increase the risk of carotid puncture [9]. Recent studies have demonstrated that liver compression and simulated Valsalva maneuver also increase the diameter of the IJ vein, possibly increasing the success rate of cannulation [10].

There are numerous approaches to the IJ vein, some of which are described here (Fig. 17.2).

- Muscular "triangle" method: puncture at the top of the junction where the sternal and clavicular heads of the sternomastoid muscle meet, lateral to the carotid impulse, directing the needle at the ipsilateral nipple. These landmarks are often not well defined in infants.
- Puncture exactly halfway along a line between the mastoid process and the sternal notch, just lateral to the carotid impulse.
- Use the cricoid ring as a landmark, and puncture just lateral to the carotid impulse.
- Jugular notch technique: puncture just lateral to the carotid impulse, just above the jugular notch on the medial clavicle – a low approach.

An ultrasound technique (see below) should be used to clearly identify the course of the vessel and to detect any significant overlap with the carotid artery. There is no need to use a finder needle for small catheters, where access needle is 20 ga or smaller. Surface landmarks are often inaccurate for estimating the correct depth of insertion for SVC lines, i.e. locating the tip midway between the sternal notch and nipple. See discussion below for a method of ascertaining the correct placement for all sites.

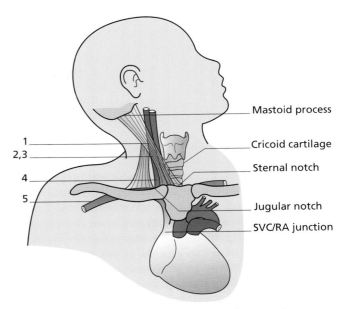

Figure 17.2 Sites for central venous cannulation of the superior vena cava. 1: high approach, midway between mastoid process and sternal notch; 2,3: middle approach using apex of muscular triangle or cricoid cartilage; 4: low approach using jugular notch; 5: lateral approach to subclavian venepuncture. Reproduced from Andropoulos et al [31] with permission from Lippincott Williams & Wilkins.

Subclavian vein

The subclavian vein is positioned immediately behind the medial third of the clavicle [11,12]. Advantages of this route include the subclavian vein's relatively constant position in all ages in reference to surface landmarks, stability and less tip migration with patient movement, and comfort for the awake patient [13,14]. Disadvantages include an incidence of pneumothorax, especially with an inexperienced operator, and an occasional inability to dilate the space between the clavicle and first rib. Also in 5–20% of patients, subclavian catheters will enter the contralateral brachiocephalic vein or ipsilateral internal jugular vein, instead of the SVC [15].

Technique (see Video clip 17.1)
A small rolled towel is positioned vertically between the scapulae, steep Trendelenburg position is used, and the arms are restrained in neutral position at the patient's sides. This position maximizes the length of subclavian vein overlapping the clavicle and moves the vein anterior, bringing it in close proximity to the posterior surface of the clavicle [11]. The right subclavian vein should always be the first choice (see below). Turn the head toward the side being punctured (i.e. toward right for right-sided line). This position will compress the internal jugular vein on that side and prevent the guidewire from entering it, especially in infants [16], which may lead to complications such as dural sinus thrombosis [17]. It will not,

however, prevent the guidewire from crossing the midline and entering the contralateral brachiocephalic vein [16]. The needle is bent upwards in midshaft at a 10–20° angle to insure a very shallow course. In our experience the puncture site that is most successful is 1–2 cm lateral to the midpoint of the clavicle [11], directly lateral from the sternal notch, with the needle directed at the sternal notch.

Contact the clavicle first to insure a shallow angle of incidence to minimize the risk of pneumothorax. Then, the needle is "walked" carefully underneath the clavicle and advanced slowly with constant aspiration until blood return is achieved. Advancing the needle only during expiration is recommended to minimize the risk of pneumothorax. Having an assistant manually ventilate the patient will facilitate this process. If not successful, the needle is withdrawn slowly with gentle aspiration, because about 50% of infant subclavian veins are cannulated during withdrawal due to compression or kinking of the vein during needle advancement. Slow, controlled, careful needle manipulation, especially in small infants, must be emphasized. After the vein is entered, advance the guidewire; there should be no resistance. Look for premature atrial contractions, sometimes only one or two, as a sign that the wire is in the heart. If no dysrhythmias are seen, withdraw the wire, rotate it 90° clockwise, and advance it again until PACs are seen. Use a dilator (be very careful not to advance it too far – only far enough to expand the space between the clavicle and first rib) and pass the catheter to the desired depth using one of the guidelines noted below.

Complications during subclavian catheterization occur when a needle angle of incidence is too cephalad, resulting in arterial puncture, or too posterior, resulting in pneumothorax. If the needle course remains shallow, just underneath the clavicle, and directed straight horizontally at the sternal notch, complications are rare. Advancing the needle too far in infants may result in puncture of the trachea.

External jugular vein

Advantages of this approach are its superficial location and thus low risk of arterial puncture. A disadvantage is that the younger the patient, the less likely it is that the guidewire will pass into the atrium; the success rate is less than 50% if the patient is less than 1 year old and only 59% in patients less than 5 years [18,19]. Positioning is the same as the internal jugular approach – the vein is punctured high in its course and the guidewire is passed. Often it can be observed turning medially toward the SVC. If no resistance is felt and PACs are seen, or the guidewire is visualized on the transesophageal echocardiogram (TEE), then passage has been successful. Because of the low success rate of central cannulation from the

external jugular vein approach, our practice is to use the internal jugular vein first in all patients.

Femoral vein (see Video clip 17.2)

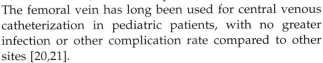

The femoral vein has long been used for central venous catheterization in pediatric patients, with no greater infection or other complication rate compared to other sites [20,21].

Technique

The patient is positioned with a rolled towel under the hips for moderate extension. The puncture site should be 1–2 cm inferior to the inguinal ligament (line from the anterior superior iliac spine to the symphysis pubis) and 0.5–1 cm medial to the femoral artery impulse, with the needle directed at the umbilicus. Ultrasound guidance (see below) is important for the greatest chance for first-pass, atraumatic placement. The guidewire is passed, ensuring no resistance. A vessel dilator is used and then the catheter is passed all the way to the hub to position the tip in the mid inferior vena cava (IVC). It is important to puncture the vessel well below the inguinal ligament, to minimize the risk of unrecognized retroperitoneal bleeding. Bleeding below the inguinal ligament is easily recognized and treated with direct pressure.

Several studies have conclusively demonstrated that in the absence of increased intra-abdominal pressure or IVC obstruction, mean central venous pressure as measured in the IVC below the diaphragm is identical to that measured in the right atrium in patients with and without congenital heart disease [22–26]. The only caveat is in the patient with interrupted IVC with azygous vein continuation into the SVC, a condition commonly encountered in patients with the heterotaxy syndromes. The equivalence of IVC and right atrial pressures under these conditions has not been evaluated, but the catheter can be used as any other central line for infusion of drugs and fluids.

Ascertainment of correct position of central venous catheters

Correct placement of central venous catheters (CVC) is essential to prevent complications (see below), and to give accurate intravascular pressure information. The tip of a central venous catheter should lie in the SVC, parallel to the vein wall, to minimize the perforation risk. Many authorities recommend placement in the upper half of the SVC, where the tip will be above the pericardial reflection in most patients, thus minimizing the risk of tamponade if perforation occurs [27]. In small patients the SVC is often short, i.e. 4–5 cm total length, and the pericardium is usually opened during cardiac surgery in these patients, providing drainage in case of perforation. In addition, the risk of arrhythmias is present with a catheter positioned

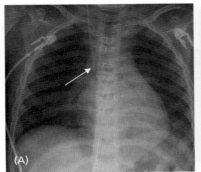
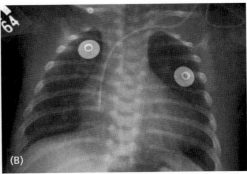

Figure 17.3 (A) Postoperative chest radiograph with the tip of a right internal jugular vein catheter in proper position in the mid-superior vena cava. (B) Tip of catheter malpositioned, deep in the right atrium.

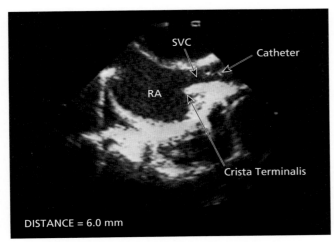

Figure 17.4 Transesophageal echocardiographic image of the superior vena cava (SVC)–right atrial (RA) junction in sagittal plane in an infant. The tip of the right internal jugular catheter is in the SVC, 6 mm above the RA. Reproduced from Andropoulos et al [15] with permission from Lippincott Williams & Wilkins.

in the right atrium. Various methods to determine correct placement are discussed below.

Radiography and echocardiography

The chest radiograph is considered the gold standard for correct placement, but obtaining and processing a chest radiograph is time consuming, costly and usually not necessary in the operating room. A chest radiograph should be obtained immediately postoperatively (Fig. 17.3), position of intravascular catheters ascertained and adjustments made by the anesthesiologist if necessary. It is important to note that an anteroposterior radiograph may miss malposition in one of several ways. The most common is for an SVC catheter to be directed posteriorly down the azygous vein, which may not be detected by anteroposterior radiograph alone. Ideally, the tip of the catheter should be parallel to the SVC wall, in the mid-SVC, but in any case it should be above the SVC–right atrium (RA) junction. The position of the pericardial

reflection is variable in infants and young children, and radiographic landmarks such as the carina above the pericardial reflection are not reliable to ascertain tip placement [28].

If TEE is utilized for cardiac surgery, the tip of the central catheter can usually be visualized in the region of the SVC–RA junction; this is easily done before surgery starts and is a very accurate method of ascertaining correct position [15] (Fig. 17.4).

Electrocardiographically guided placement

The intravascular electrocardiogram (ECG) may be used in children to guide correct CVC placement [29,30]. Either a 0.9% or 3% saline-filled lumen with special ECG adaptor or a guidewire within the lumen attached to a sterile alligator clip and leadwire substituted for the right arm surface ECG lead may be used. Entry of the catheter tip into the right atrium is signified by the sudden appearance of a P atriale, an exaggerated, large, upright P wave. The catheter tip is then pulled back 1–2 cm into the desired position in the SVC. Success rate for proper placement in the reported studies has been 80–90%, but there have been no controlled studies in children comparing this to other methods. This method also requires special equipment which is not always available.

Height- and weight-based formula

A large study of CVC placement in infants and children undergoing congenital heart surgery developed formulas for correct insertion depth based on height and weight [31] (Table 17.2). CVC were inserted in the right internal jugular or subclavian vein and the postoperative radiograph studies were used to determine the tip position in reference to the SVC–RA junction. The length of catheter inside the patient was added to this distance to determine the position of the SVC–RA junction, and formulas developed that would predict placement above the RA, in the SVC 97.5% of the time (95% confidence interval 96–99%). All catheter tips predicted to be in the atrium using these data would be high in the RA within 1 cm of the SVC–RA

Table 17.2 Recommended length of superior vena cava central venous catheter (CVC) insertion in pediatric patients based on weight: right internal jugular or subclavian veins

Patient weight (kg)	Length of CVC insertion (cm)
2–2.9	4
3–4.9	5
5–6.9	6
7–9.9	7
10–12.9	8
13–19.9	9
20–29.9	10
30–39.9	11
40–49.9	12
50–59.9	13
60–69.9	14
70–79.9	15
80 and above	16

junction, minimizing any perforation risk. The formulas are simple and easily implemented because weight and height can be easily measured on all patients undergoing surgery.

For patients with height less than 100 cm:

$$(\text{Height} \div 10) - 1 \, \text{cm}$$

is the correct insertion distance, i.e. a 75 cm patient would have the catheter secured at 6.5 cm for either the right internal jugular or the subclavian route.

For patients with height 100 cm or greater:

$$(\text{Height} \div 10) - 2 \, \text{cm}$$

is the correct distance. The caveats to this seemingly useful technique are that for the internal jugular vein, the puncture site is high, exactly midway between the mastoid process and the sternal notch, and for the subclavian, puncture site is 1–2 cm lateral to the midpoint of the clavicle. If different puncture sites are utilized, the operator must adjust the formulas accordingly. Also, the formulas have not yet been evaluated for accuracy in a prospective fashion.

Percutaneously inserted central catheters

Percutaneously inserted central catheters (PICC) have been utilized in the neonatal nursery for more than a decade, and have become standard practice for ill newborns expected to require prolonged venous access. The complication rate for these catheters is very low, and they are usually relatively easy to insert into the central circulation via the antecubital, saphenous, scalp, hand, axillary or wrist veins, when placed by experienced, skilled personnel. Such personnel include nurses [32] or physicians

placing them at the bedside, or in the interventional radiology suite [33] with ultrasound and fluoroscopic guidance. The key to successful placement is early access, before all large visible superficial veins are injured from attempts at peripheral intravenous placements. For this reason, the PICC line is optimally placed in the critically ill newborn in the first 12–24 h after admission. Like all central venous catheters, they occasionally cause complications such as perforation of the atrium or embolization of a portion of the catheter [34]. The infection rate is very low.

Technique

A suitable vein should be identified. The branches of the basilic vein on the medial half of the antecubital fossa offer the highest success rate because of the large size and direct continuation with the axillary and subclavian veins. The cephalic vein tributaries can also be used, but are less likely to pass into the axillary vein. Other sites, e.g. the saphenous, hand, and scalp veins, are cannulated as for a peripheral intravenous catheter. The site is prepared and draped, and appropriate local anesthesia and/or intravenous analgesia are administered. The vein is entered using a large break-away needle or angiocatheter, and a 2 Fr non-styleted silicone catheter flushed with heparinized saline is passed with forceps a distance measured from the entry site to the SVC–RA junction. Continued easy passage without resistance and continuous ability to aspirate blood signify proper placement. A radiograph, with injection of diluted contrast if needed, should be obtained prior to use. Proper catheter tip position is in the SVC or IVC, not in the right atrium.

Occasionally the PICC line will not pass centrally, i.e. into the intrathoracic portion of the subclavian vein or further, or into the IVC. In this case it should be considered no differently from a peripheral venous line. For central PICC lines, any centrally delivered medication or fluid may be used, i.e. parenteral nutrition, dopamine, CaCl, etc. The 2 Fr PICC lines are too small for rapid fluid boluses or blood products, therefore inadequate as the sole prebypass access for cardiac surgery or for other major surgery. Recently, 3.5–4 Fr soft polyurethane double-lumen PICC lines, with two 22 ga lumens, have become available, which can be placed using modified Seldinger technique, with a central vein placement rate of 66% [35]. Alternatively, 3 Fr PICC lines, placed with the aid of ultrasound and fluoroscopic guidance with a guidewire in the interventional radiology suite, may be used in newborns with caution, especially in the SVC position, because of the risk of thrombosis [36]. In older infants and children, these larger catheters are preferred. Tan et al [37] reported a series of 124 such catheters in cardiac surgical neonates, noting a low thrombosis rate of 1.6% and a low infection rate of 3.6 per 1000 catheter days, with a median onset of 37 days; thus these catheters can be extremely useful in this population.

Arterial access

Tables 17.3 and 17.4 display recommended catheter sizes for arterial access based on site and patient weight.

Radial artery

This is the preferred location in the newborn if an umbilical artery line is not possible or needs to be replaced, and in virtually all other patients. Placement on the same side as an existing or planned systemic to pulmonary artery shunt is avoided, e.g. a right-sided modified Blalock–Taussig shunt.

 Technique (see Video clip 17.3)
The wrist is extended slightly with rolled gauze, the fingers taped loosely to an armboard, with the thumb taped separately in extension to tether skin surface over the radial artery (Fig. 17.5). An angiocatheter flushed with heparinized saline is used as a "liquid stylet" to increase the rapidity of flashback of blood into the hub of the needle after aseptic preparation. The skin is punctured at a 15–20° angle at the proximal wrist crease at the point of maximal impulse of the artery. Palpation is the usual method of identifying the artery, but audio Doppler localization can be helpful if the pulse is weak. Lighter planes of anesthesia provide stronger pulses and increase the success rate of cannulation.

The first attempt, before any hematoma formation or partial dissection of the artery, always yields the greatest chance for success, so the operator should optimize conditions, e.g. positioning, lighting, and identification of the vessel. Puncture of the artery with the needle is signified by brisk flashback. The needle and catheter are then advanced 1–2 mm into the artery and an attempt is made to thread the catheter primarily over the needle its full length into the artery. Threading should have minimal resistance and is signified by the continuing flow of blood

Table 17.3 Recommended arterial catheter sizes: radial, dorsalis pedis, posterior tibial, brachial arteries

Weight	Radial/DP/PT arteries	Brachial artery
<2 kg	24 g	Not recommended
2–5 kg	22 g	24 g
5–30 kg	22 g	22 g
>30 kg	20 g	22 g

DP, dorsalis pedis; PT, posterior tibial.

Table 17.4 Recommended arterial catheter sizes: femoral, axillary arteries

Weight	Femoral/axillary arteries
<10 kg	2.5 Fr, 5 cm long
10–50 kg	3 Fr, 8 cm long
>50 kg	4 Fr, 12 cm long

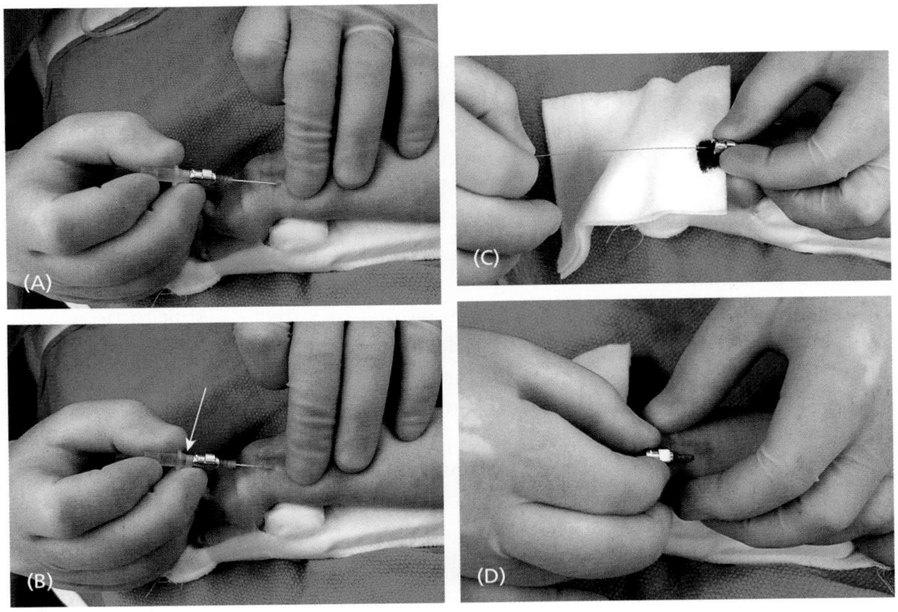

Figure 17.5 Insertion of a radial arterial catheter in an infant. (A) Radial artery is approached with a saline-filled angiocatheter, at the proximal wrist crease. (B) Rapid flashback of arterial blood (*arrow*) is noted with arterial puncture using liquid stylet technique. (C) A 0.015" guidewire is inserted and threaded into the artery. (D) The angiocatheter is threaded over the guidewire.

into hub of needle. If threading is not successful, the needle is replaced carefully in the angiocatheter, and the needle and catheter can be passed through the back wall of artery. Then the needle is removed, and a 0.015″ guidewire with flexible tip can be used to assist threading of catheter. The catheter is pulled back very slowly and when vigorous arterial backflow occurs, the guidewire is passed and the catheter threaded over the guidewire into the artery [38]. Minimal resistance signifies successful threading. If unsuccessful, further attempts may be made at the same site or at slightly more proximal sites to avoid areas of arterial spasm, thrombosis or dissection.

The circulation distal to the catheter should be assessed by inspection of color and capillary refill time of fingertips and nailbeds, and quality of signal from a pulse oximeter probe. A recommended technique for securing the catheter is with a clear adhesive dressing and transparent tape so that the insertion site and hub of the catheter are visible at all times.

Femoral artery

The superficial femoral artery is a large vessel that is easily accessible in almost all patients [39] and is a logical second choice for cardiac surgery when radial arterial access is not available. In infants, especially patients with trisomy 21, transient arterial insufficiency develops in up to 25% of patients after arterial catheterization when 20 ga (3 Fr) catheters are used [39]. For this reason, in the author's institution the smallest commercially available catheter, 2.5 Fr (equal to 21 ga), is used in patients weighing less than 10 kg (see Table 17.4).

Technique

A small towel is placed under the patient's hips to extend the leg slightly to neutral position. Slight external rotation, with the knees restrained by taping to the operating room bed, fixes adequate position. After sterile prep and drape, the course of the superficial femoral artery is palpated and punctured 1–2 cm inferior to the inguinal ligament, to avoid puncturing the artery above the pelvic rim, where a retroperitoneal hematoma could develop. If the pulse is weak, as in the case of aortic arch obstruction, use of audio Doppler effectively identifies the course of the vessel.

The puncture technique varies and may include direct puncture with an angiocatheter or Seldinger technique using the needle in the commercially supplied kit, or a 21 ga butterfly needle with the extension tubing removed. All of the above are flushed with heparinized normal saline to increase the rapidity of flashback. A small flexible guidewire, 0.015″ or 0.018″, is used. It is normally possible to thread a polyethylene catheter over the guidewire without making a skin incision, and under no circumstances is dilating the tract and artery with a dilator recommended, which could cause arterial spasm, dissection or bleeding around the catheter if the puncture site is large. The catheter is secured by suturing around the entry site of catheter and wings around the hub. Distal perfusion is immediately assessed, and a pulse oximeter probe is placed on the foot for continuous monitoring and early warning of arterial perfusion problems.

Brachial artery

The brachial artery has been successfully used for monitoring for cardiac surgery in children, but using this site for arterial monitoring should generally be avoided because it has poor collateral circulation compared to the radial, femoral, and axillary arteries. Theoretically, there should be a higher incidence of arterial insufficiency with this site, but a study by Schindler et al, of 386 brachial artery catheters in infants and children undergoing cardiac surgery, documented no permanent ischemic damage, and only three temporary arterial occlusions, when 22 and 24 ga catheters were used [40]. It should only be used in situations when other options are limited, e.g. a right upper extremity arterial line is required to monitor pressure during cross-clamping for repair of coarctation of the aorta, or during bypass for aortic arch hypoplasia or interruption.

Technique

A 24 ga catheter should be used in patients under 5 kg. The arm is restrained in neutral position on an armboard and the arterial impulse is palpated above the elbow crease, well above the bifurcation into radial and ulnar arteries. Cannulation proceeds as for the radial artery. Meticulous attention must be paid to distal perfusion at all times, and the catheter removed for any signs of ischemia. Pulse oximeter monitoring of distal pulses will provide early detection of perfusion problems. The catheter should be removed or replaced with a catheter in a site with better collateral circulation as soon as possible after the repair.

Axillary artery

The axillary artery is large and well collateralized, and several series in critically ill children have demonstrated this to be a viable option with a low complication rate when other sites are not accessible [41,42]. However, given the potential morbidity of an ischemic arm and hand, and the theoretical problem of intrathoracic bleeding, this puncture site should be considered a last resort when there are limited options.

Technique

The arm is abducted 90° and extended slightly at the shoulder to expose the artery. The artery is palpated high

Table 17.5 Derived hemodynamic parameters

Formula	Normal values		
	Adult	**Infant**	**Child**
$CI = \dfrac{CO}{BSA}$	2.8–4.2 L/min/m²	2–4	3–4
$SVI = \dfrac{SV}{BSA}$	30–65 mL/beat/m²	40–75	40–70
$LVSWI = \dfrac{1.36 \cdot (MAP - PCWP) \cdot SVI}{100}$	45–60 g · m/m²	2–40	30–50
$RVSWI = \dfrac{1.36 \cdot (PAP - CVP) \cdot SI}{100}$	5–10 g · m/m²	5–11	5–10
$SVRI = \dfrac{(MAP - CVP) \cdot 80}{CI}$	1500–2400 dyne · sec · cm⁻⁵ · m²	900–1200	1300–1800
$PVRI = \dfrac{(PAP - PCWP) \cdot 80}{CI}$	250–400 dyne · sec · cm⁻⁵ · m²	<200	<200

BSA, body surface area; CI, cardiac index; CO, thermodilution cardiac output; LVSWI, left ventricular stroke work index; PVRI, pulmonary vascular resistance index; RVSWI, right ventricular stroke work index; SVRI, systemic vascular resistance index; SV, stroke volume; SVI, stroke volume index.

in the axilla and punctured using an angiocatheter, then exchanged over a guidewire for a longer catheter or by primary Seldinger technique. A catheter that is too short (e.g. 22 ga 1″ long) will often be pulled out of the vessel with shoulder extension. Therefore, the shortest recommended catheter is 5 cm long (see Table 17.5). Careful attention must be paid to distal perfusion, as with the brachial artery. Tip position should be ascertained by chest radiograph, and should not lie deeper than the first rib. The proximity to the brachiocephalic vessels makes it imperative that the catheter be flushed very gently by hand after blood draws, and that no air bubbles or clots ever be introduced, because of the risk of retrograde cerebral embolization.

Umbilical artery

The umbilical artery is accessible for the first few days of life and is the site of choice for newborns requiring surgery in the first week of life (see Fig. 17.1). The complication rate is lower with the catheter tip placed in the high position, i.e. above the diaphragm, versus low tip position, i.e. at the level of the third lumbar vertebra [43]. The catheter can be left in place for 7–10 days. A relationship to intestinal ischemia and necrotizing colitis has been demonstrated [44] and enteral feeding with a umbilical arterial catheter (UAC) in place is controversial [45]. Umbilical catheters are most commonly inserted by the neonatal staff in the delivery room or neonatal ICU shortly after birth. Technique involves cutting off the umbilical stump with an umbilical tape encircling the base to provide hemostasis, dilating the umbilical artery, and blindly passing a 3.5 Fr catheter a distance based on weight, then assessing position as soon as possible radio-

graphically. Lower extremity emboli, vascular insufficiency, and renal artery thrombosis have all been described [46]; however, the overall risk is low and this site is highly desirable because it is a large central artery yielding accurate pressure monitoring [47] during all phases of neonatal surgery, and preserves access for future interventions.

Temporal artery

The superficial temporal artery at the level just above the zygomatic arch is large and easily accessible in newborns, particularly the premature infant. It was widely used in the 1970s in neonatal nurseries [48] but rapidly fell out of favor with the realization that significant complications, e.g. retrograde cerebral emboli, were disturbingly common [49,50]. It should only be used when a brachiocephalic pressure must be measured for surgery in the face of an aberrant subclavian artery, so that the only way to measure pressure during cross-clamping or on bypass is via direct aortic pressure or temporal artery pressure. Examples are coarctation of the aorta, aortic arch interruption or hypoplasia, with aberrant right subclavian artery that arises distal to the area of aortic obstruction [51]. The catheter must be used only during the case, blood drawing and flushing should be minimized, and it must be removed as soon as possible after the repair.

Technique

A 24 ga catheter is used for newborns. The artery is palpated just anterosuperior to the tragus of the ear, just superior to the zygomatic arch. A very superficial angle of approach, i.e. 10–15°, is used and the artery is cannulated as described for the radial artery.

Dorsalis pedis/posterior tibial arteries

These arteries are often easily cannulated and quite useful for monitoring and blood sampling during surgery when radial arteries are not available. Superficial foot arteries should not be used for cardiopulmonary bypass cases, because of the well-known peripheral vasoconstriction and vasomotor instability in the early postbypass period, which is more pronounced with these arteries than with the radial artery.

Technique

Dorsalis pedis: the foot is plantarflexed slightly to straighten the course of the artery, which is palpated between the second and third metatarsal. A superficial course is taken and the artery cannulated. *Posterior tibial*: the foot is dorsiflexed to expose the artery between the medial malleolus and the Achilles tendon. The artery is often deep to the puncture site, so a steeper angle of incidence is required.

Ulnar artery

The ulnar artery should only be used as a last resort when other options are not available, because its use is only considered when radial artery attempts have been unsuccessful or thrombosed by past interventions. There is a high risk of ischemia of the hand if both the radial and ulnar artery perfusion is significantly compromised. Despite this, one series of 18 ulnar artery catheters in critically ill infants and children had an ischemia rate not different from radial and femoral artery catheters, of 5.6% [52].

Arterial cutdown

Cutdown of the radial artery is a reliable and often efficient method for establishing access for congenital heart surgery, and other major surgery when other arterial access has failed or is not available. Despite the speed and ease of access for a cutdown, available literature indicates a higher rate of bleeding at the site, infection, failure, distal ischemia, and long-term vessel occlusion compared to percutaneous techniques [53,54].

Technique

The arm is positioned as for percutaneous radial catheterization. After surgical preparation and draping, an incision is made at the proximal wrist crease between the styloid process and the flexor carpi radialis tendon, either parallel or perpendicular to the artery. Sharp and blunt dissection is carried out until the artery is identified, and it is isolated with a heavy silk suture, vessel loop or right angle forceps. It is no longer considered necessary to ligate the artery distally to prevent bleeding, and in fact the artery may remain patent after a cutdown if not ligated distally. The simplest and very effective technique is to cannulate the exposed artery directly with an angi-ocatheter, in the same manner as for percutaneous radial artery catheter placement. The catheter is then sutured to the skin at its hub and the incision closed with nylon sutures on either side of the catheter. Removal entails cutting the suture at the hub of the catheter, removing the catheter, and applying pressure for a few minutes until any bleeding stops. The remaining skin sutures can be removed at a later date.

Percutaneous pulmonary artery catheterization

Percutaneous pulmonary artery (PA) catheterization has a limited role in pediatric anesthesia for several reasons. The small size of many patients precludes placement of adequate sized sheaths and catheters, and many patients in whom PA catheter monitoring would be desirable have intracardiac shunting, invalidating results of standard thermodilution cardiac output measurements and confusing mixed venous oxygen saturation (SvO_2) measurements. In addition, frequent need for right-sided intracardiac surgery makes PA catheterization undesirable. Thus, when pulmonary artery pressure or SvO_2 monitoring is indicated, transthoracic PA lines are the most common method in congenital heart surgery. The availability of continuous central venous oxygen saturation catheters (see below) and the perception that the risk:benefit ratio for PA catheter placement is most often unfavorable limit the indications for this technique.

The most common indications for percutaneous PA catheterization in pediatric anesthesia are in patients over 6 months of age able to accept a 5 or 6 Fr introducer sheath in the femoral or internal jugular vein. Patients having surgery on left heart structures who do not have intracardiac shunting, who are at risk for left ventricular dysfunction or pulmonary hypertension may benefit from the information available. Examples include aortic surgery, aortic valve repair or replacement, subaortic resection or myomectomy for hypertrophic cardiomyopathy, mitral valve repair or replacement. In addition, major surgery, i.e. liver transplant in larger patients, may be an indication for percutaneous PA catheterization.

Technique [55]

An oximetric catheter is recommended. Commercially available models are 5.5 Fr or 8.5 Fr, and thus require a 6 Fr or 9 Fr sheath, respectively. The 5.5 Fr catheter should be used in patients under 50 kg and the 8.5 Fr in patients over 50 kg. The sheath is placed into the internal jugular, femoral or subclavian veins as described above. The preferred sites of insertion are right internal jugular, left subclavian, femoral vein because of the direct path and curvature of the catheter. If an oximetric catheter is used, it is calibrated prior to insertion. The balloon integrity should be tested before insertion by inflating the recommended volume of air or CO_2, and the sterility sleeve is inserted before placement.

The PA and central venous pressure (CVP) ports are connected, flushed, and calibrated before insertion. The PA catheter is inserted 10–15 cm with the balloon deflated, depending on patient size. The balloon is inflated and the catheter advanced slowly toward the tricuspid valve, whose position is indicated by enlarging V waves on the CVP trace. The catheter is advanced through the tricuspid valve by advancing during diastole until the characteristic right ventricular trace is visible, with no dichrotic notch and a diastolic pressure of 0–5 mmHg. Then, the catheter is advanced carefully through the pulmonary valve during systole, until the characteristic PA tracing is visible, with a dichrotic notch and higher diastolic pressure. The catheter is then advanced gently until the pulmonary capillary wedge pressure tracing is obtained, at which time the balloon is deflated so the PA tracing rapidly returns. Difficulty with advancing through the pulmonary valve may be assisted by counterclockwise rotation of the catheter while advancing, positioning the patient right side down and giving a fluid bolus, or by using TEE to visualize the tip and guide subsequent attempts [56]. The catheter must not be left in the wedge position except during brief periods because of the risk of pulmonary artery rupture and lung ischemia distal to the catheter. During bypass, the catheter can be pulled back several centimeters to reduce the risk of perforation on bypass.

Information obtainable with a pulmonary artery catheter

Right atrium, PA, and pulmonary capillary wedge (PCWP) pressures. In the absence of mitral valve stenosis or pulmonary venous or arterial hypertension, PA diastolic ~ PCWP ~ LAP ~ left ventricular end-diastolic pressure, which is proportional to left ventricular end-diastolic volume, the classic measure of preload [57]. Despite the presence of pulmonary hypertension or residual mitral stenosis (diagnosed with postoperative TEE), information from the PA catheter can still be used to direct therapy.

Cardiac index may be measured by standard thermodilution methods, with care taken to input the correct calculation constant into the monitor software according to the catheter size and length, and volume and temperature of injectate. The average of three consecutive injections made in rapid succession at the same point in the respiratory cycle, i.e. expiration, will optimize conditions to achieve an accurate measurement during steady-state conditions. Vascular resistances and stroke volume can also be calculated, using the formulas in Table 17.5 [57,58].

Hemodynamic data represent only half the information available from an oximetric PA catheter. The other half consists of oxygen delivery and consumption measurements and calculations, which may also be used to

Table 17.6 Derived oxygen delivery/consumption parameters

Formula	Normal values		
	Adult	**Infant**	**Child**
Arterial O_2 content $CaO_2 = (1.39 \cdot Hb \cdot SaO_2) + (0.0031 \cdot PaO_2)$	18–20 mL/dL	15–18	16–18
Mixed venous O_2 content $CvO_2 = 1.39 \cdot Hb \cdot SvO_2 + 0.0031 \cdot PvO_2$	13–16 mL/dL	11–14	12–14
Arteriovenous O_2 content difference $avDO_2 = CaO_2 - CvO_2$	4–5.5 mL/dL	4–7	4–6
Pulmonary capillary O_2 content $CcO_2 = 1.39 \cdot Hb \cdot ScO_2 + 0.0031 \cdot PcO_2$	19–21 mL/dL	16–19	17–19
Pulmonary shunt fraction $Q_s/Q_t = 100 \cdot (CcO_2 - CaO_2)/(CcO_2 - CvO_2)$	2–8 percent	2–8	2–8
O_2 delivery index $DO_2I = 10 \cdot CO \cdot CaO_2/BSA$	450–640 mL/min/m²	450–750	450–700
O_2 consumption index $VO_2I = 10 \cdot CO \cdot (CaO_2 - CvO_2)$	85–170 mL/min/m²	150–200	140–190

Hb, hemoglobin; PaO_2, partial pressure of oxygen in arterial blood; PvO_2, partial pressure of oxygen in mixed venous blood; PcO_2, partial pressure of oxygen in pulmonary capillary blood; Qs, pulmonary shunt blood flow; Qt, total pulmonary blood flow; SaO_2, measured arterial oxygen saturation; ScO_2, measured pulmonary capillary oxygen saturation; SvO_2, measured mixed venous oxygen saturation.

guide therapy in the critically ill patient with low cardiac output syndrome [57,58] (Table 17.6). Oxygen consumption/delivery data require either measurement of mixed venous and systemic arterial saturations from blood samples from the tip of the PA catheter and arterial line (measured by co-oximetry, not calculated) or substitution of these values with SvO_2 from the oximetric catheter (a valid assumption if properly calibrated), and pulse oximeter value instead of measured systemic saturation. There are data from the adult and pediatric critical care literature suggesting that the ability to increase and maximize both oxygen delivery and consumption may improve outcome, and is a predictor of survival from critical illness, including postoperative cardiac surgery [59–62].

Ultrasound guidance for vascular access

Numerous studies demonstrate that ultrasound guidance, either two-dimensional visual ultrasound [63] or audio Doppler ultrasound, improves the outcome of central venous cannulation, in both children and adults [64,65]. Use of these methods leads to fewer attempts, decreased insertion time, fewer unintended arterial punctures, and fewer unintended arterial catheter placements. The consensus of many experts in the field of vascular access is that use of these guidance techniques should be considered standard of care.

A 9.2 MHz pencil-thin audio Doppler probe can be gas sterilized and reused. The probe is applied to the site, and the course of the artery and vein is ascertained by their characteristic audio profiles – high-pitched, intermittent, systolic flow for the artery, and a low-pitched, continuous venous hum for the vein. The probe is centered over the loudest signal, perpendicular to the skin surface, and the vessel is punctured exactly in the axis of the center of the probe. A "pop" followed by the continuous sound of blood aspiration can often be heard when the vessel is entered. The guidewire, dilator, and catheter are then passed as above. A variation of the audio Doppler technique is a device with the Doppler probe within the needle [66]. However, these needles are expensive, direct comparison has not shown them to be superior to visual ultrasound for cannulation, and because the lumen of the needle is partially occluded with the Doppler probe, flashback of blood is slow and unreliable.

Two-dimensional echocardiography, in the form of either commercially available devices for CVC cannulation only (Sonosite®) or surface probes on standard echocardiography machines, can be used to image large vessels (Fig. 17.6A). The color Doppler feature on the latter may be particularly useful to identify desired vessels during difficult vascular access. The internal jugular vein (IJV) is the vessel most frequently accessed with ultrasound, and it is visualized superficial to and lateral to the carotid artery. The IJV is also easily compressible with the probe and is gently pulsatile, while the carotid artery is round, difficult to compress with probe pressure, and very pulsatile (Fig. 17.6B). The probe is held directly over the desired vessel, with the goal of puncturing it exactly in the midline. The needle can be seen indenting and then puncturing the vessel during correct placement (Fig. 17.6C).

Visual ultrasound is particularly useful to clarify the anatomy after several previous attempts have been made. One can identify the vessel in the midst of a hematoma that has formed or recognize overlap of the artery and vein. Once the vessel has been punctured and the guidewire passed, the ultrasound can be used to visualize the guidewire in the lumen of the vessel by scanning closer to the heart. Ultrasound methods are described most often for the IJV but are also useful for the

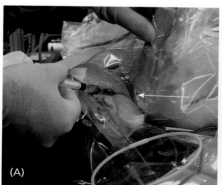
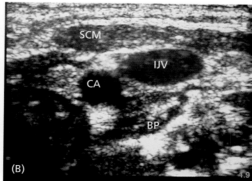
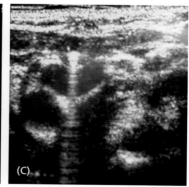

Figure 17.6 (A) Ultrasound-guided puncture of the internal jugular vein in an infant. Arrow denotes 13 MHz pediatric probe. (B) Two-dimensional ultrasound view of the right internal jugular vein and carotid artery in an infant. BP, brachial plexus; CA, carotid artery; IJV, internal jugular vein; SCM, sternocleidomastoid muscle. (C) Needle just prior to puncture of the right IJV.

femoral and subclavian veins. It should also be noted that real-time ultrasonographic visualization of needle insertion, vessel puncture, and guidewire passage of the internal jugular vein in infants results in fewer attempts and faster cannulation than merely marking the skin after ultrasound visualization followed by blind puncture of the vessel [67].

Audio Doppler can be used to assist in the cannulation of any artery, and is particularly useful when pulses are diminished from previous attempts, hypotension or vasospasm. Visual ultrasound can also be used to cannulate radial arteries, and Schwemmer et al found that this technique resulted in a 100% success rate, versus 80% for the traditional palpation method, and also resulted in higher success rate on the first attempt and lower number of attempts [68].

Interpretation of intravascular pressure waveforms

The normal systemic arterial pressure waveform changes with progression distally from the central arterial circulation, e.g. ascending aorta, distally to the abdominal aorta and femoral arteries, and then to the peripheral arteries, such as the radial and dorsalis pedis/posterior tibial arteries [57] (Fig. 17.7). In general, the more central sites

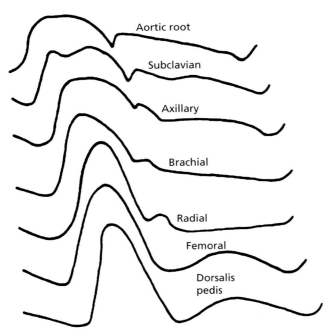

Figure 17.7 Progression of the arterial pressure tracing from the root of the aorta to more peripheral arteries. Pulse wave amplification produces a higher systolic peak and slightly lower diastolic pressure in the smaller distal arteries, especially the dorsalis pedis. Reproduced from Reich et al [57] with permission from Elsevier.

will produce less peaked systolic pressure waves with slightly lower systolic pressure readings. The dicrotic notch is pronounced in the central arteries. With distal progression, pulse wave amplification will produce a higher peaked systolic pressure wave with a slightly higher systolic pressure. This is most pronounced in the arteries of the foot, where the systolic pressure may be 5–15 mmHg higher than the ascending aorta. The mean and diastolic pressures change very little with progression. This concept is very important in interpreting arterial pressure tracings. The postbypass arterial tracing is frequently dampened with catheters in small distal arteries, e.g. radial or foot arteries [69]. This usually resolves within a few minutes after bypass. For particularly long and difficult operations with long bypass and cross-clamp times, or in major non-cardiac cases with substantial blood loss and hemodynamic instability, it may be useful to place catheters in larger arteries, e.g. femoral or umbilical, or to measure the pressure directly in the aortic root immediately after bypass to ascertain an accurate arterial pressure.

The arterial pressure tracing can yield more information than simply the systolic and diastolic blood pressures [70,71]. The slope of the upstroke of the pressure wave may be an indicator of systemic ventricular contractility, i.e. the steeper the upslope, the better the contractility. Significant reductions in contractility flatten the upslope. The position of the dicrotic notch may give an indication of peripheral vascular resistance. In infants, the normal dicrotic notch is in the upper half of the pressure wave. With low peripheral resistance, as in arterial run-off through a patent ductus arteriosus, the dicrotic notch is lower on the descending limb of the waveform, due to diastolic run-off into the pulmonary artery, resulting in a relatively longer period of ventricular systole. The area under the curve of the systolic portion of the arterial tracing increases with increased stroke volume. Finally, a hypovolemic patient will often exhibit more pronounced respiratory variation during positive pressure ventilation, as the stroke volume decreases when positive pressure impedes an already limited venous return (Fig. 17.8). Computerized pulse-contour analysis of the arterial pressure waveform has been used to measure stroke volume (see below under New Techniques in Pediatric Intravascular Monitoring).

Mechanical and electronic components of the intravascular pressure measurement system are important considerations when interpreting waveforms [57]. The shortest possible large-bore, stiff plastic tubing should be used. Minimizing the number of stopcocks and connections will also improve the fidelity of the transmitted pressure wave. Thorough flushing before use to produce a bubble- and clot-free fluid path is critical. Periodic recalibration at the right atrial level is important to account for "drift" in the transducer setting. When ringing or overdamping is recognized, some monitor models offer adjustment of electronic filter frequency. The routine setting should be 12 Hz. If the arterial tracing is underdamped, e.g. overshoot producing an artificially high spike as the systolic pressure, filter frequency may be decreased as low as 3 Hz to compensate. Conversely, if overdamped, the filter frequency may be increased to as high as 40 Hz. Mechanical devices (ROSE®, Accudynamic®) may also be inserted to change the resonance frequency and/or damping factor of the system.

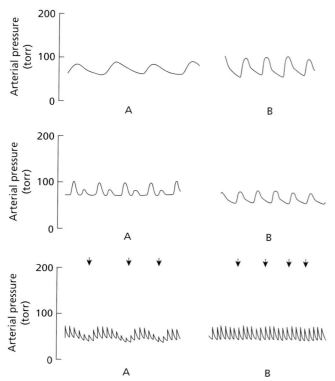

Figure 17.8 (*Top panel*) The arterial pressure tracing with depressed (A) and normal (B) myocardial contractility. (*Middle panel*) Low (A) and normal (B) systemic vascular resistance. (*Lower panel*) Hypovolemia (A) and normovolemia (B) – arrows represent positive pressure ventilations. Reproduced from Gregory [70] with permission from Elsevier.

Under no circumstances should a bubble be intentionally introduced into the system to produce increased damping effect. Appropriateness of resonance frequency may be tested by flushing the system from a pressurized bag of heparinized saline, stopping suddenly, and observing the number and amplitude of oscillations required to return to baseline waveform. Proper damping is signified by one oscillation below and one above the mean before return to normal waveform [72,73].

Failure of arterial pressure monitoring systems is always possible during surgery, due to mechanical problems such as kinking or clotting of the catheter. Spasm of the artery is more common than in adults, and the artery may be compressed, such as aberrant right subclavian compression from a TEE probe or compression of an axillary artery from a sternal retractor. A back-up oscillometric blood pressure cuff should always be present, preferably placed on a different extremity than the arterial catheter.

Central venous, right and left atrial waveforms

Normal atrial (i.e. central venous) pressure waveforms consist of the A, C, and V waves corresponding to atrial contraction, closure of the tricuspid or mitral valves, and ventricular contraction. Normal right atrial A wave pressure is lower than V wave pressure, which is usually less than 10 mmHg. Changes from the normal tracing can give important information about the hemodynamic status and cardiac rhythm of the patient. For example, when atrioventricular synchrony is lost, as in junctional ectopic tachycardia or supraventricular tachycardia, the A wave disappears and the V wave enlarges considerably, reflecting backward transmission of ventricular pressure through an ineffectively emptied atrium (Fig. 17.9). Determining the cardiac rhythm from the ECG is often difficult at rapid heart rates because the P wave of the ECG is indiscernible. The left or right atrial waveform can give crucial added information in this situation, clearly retaining the A wave in cases of sinus tachycardia. Competency of the AV valves can also be assessed from

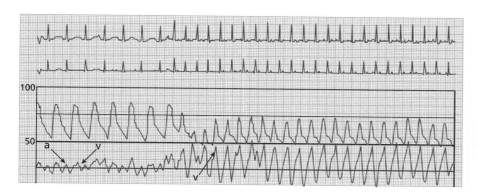

Figure 17.9 ECG demonstrating normal sinus rhythm in the first third of the panel, with onset of supraventricular tachycardia. Note the arterial pressure tracing with a 12–15 torr decrease in systolic pressure, and the loss of the A wave on the central venous pressure tracing, with the appearance of large V waves with a systolic pressure increase from 10 to 16 mmHg.

the atrial tracing. Mitral or tricuspid regurgitation will produce a large V wave on the left atrial tracing. It is often very useful to record the vascular pressure tracings in sinus rhythm at baseline for later comparison.

New techniques in pediatric intravascular monitoring

Cardiac output monitoring

Because traditional percutaneous, balloon-tipped pulmonary artery catheterization is limited in small children and those with intracardiac shunting, several other methods to measure cardiac output and oxygen delivery in patients with congenital heart disease have recently been applied. Lithium dilution cardiac output (LiDCO) uses a standard central line in the SVC or even a peripheral IV catheter, and a special femoral artery catheter equipped with a lithium-detecting electrode. A dilute solution of lithium chloride is injected into the vein and arterial blood is withdrawn into the lithium electrode. The cardiac index is related to the area under the curve of the change of lithium concentration. This method has been demonstrated to have reasonable correlation with thermodilution cardiac output in children after congenital heart surgery. In a study of 48 measurements in 17 patients 2.6–34 kg, correlation between LiDCO and thermodilution cardiac output was good ($r^2 = 0.96$, mean bias -0.1 ± 0.31 L/min) [74].

Transpulmonary thermodilution cardiac output uses a similar principle to LiDCO, with temperature as the indicator instead of lithium concentration. Cold saline is injected into a central venous catheter and, via a thermis-

tor placed in a femoral artery, a time temperature curve is derived, which correlates reasonably well with standard thermodilution cardiac output as measured by a standard pulmonary artery catheter [75]. Both lithium and any thermodilution method are limited to patients without any intracardiac shunting, significantly restricting their use in congenital heart disease.

Yet another newer method is pulse-contour analysis of the arterial waveform (PiCCO), which relates the contour and area under the curve to the stroke volume, and thus the cardiac output. This continuous method is periodically calibrated using the transpulmonary thermodilution cardiac output as described above (again making the method invalid with intracardiac shunting), and demonstrated good correlation with transpulmonary thermodilution in a recent study of 24 pediatric patients after cardiac surgery ($r^2 = 0.86$, mean bias 0.05 ± 0.4 L/min/m^2) [76].

Central venous oxygen saturation monitoring

Monitoring of intravascular oxyhemoglobin saturation using reflectance catheters has been used in the umbilical artery, pulmonary artery, and adult-sized central venous catheters for a number of years, but only recently have standard pediatric sized 4 and 5 Fr, double- and triple-lumen CVCs become available for routine use to measure central venous oxygen saturation (ScvO$_2$) in pediatric patients. In 16 pediatric patients undergoing cardiac surgery, Liakopoulos et al demonstrated good correlation between ScvO$_2$ as measured with the catheter, versus blood co-oximetry ($r^2 = 0.88$, bias $-0.03 \pm 4.72\%$) [77] (Fig. 17.10). The advantage of this method is that it is an

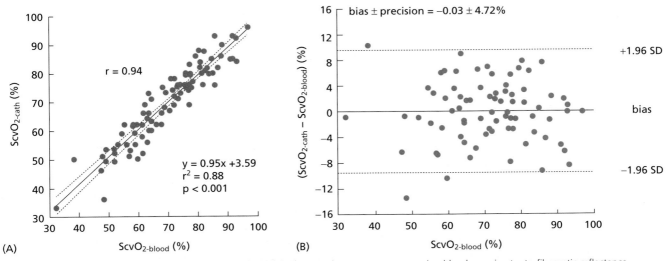

Figure 17.10 Central venous oxyhemoglobin saturation (ScvO$_2$) in the superior vena cava, comparing blood co-oximetry to fiberoptic reflectance spectroscopy. (A) Correlation between catheter (ScvO$_2$-cath %) and blood co-oximetry (ScvO$_2$-blood %). (B) Bland–Altman plot of bias and precision between the two methods. Reproduced from Liakopoulos et al [77] with permission from Lippincott Williams & Wilkins.

accurate measure of oxygen delivery that is independent of intracardiac shunting, and thus may have better utility in the congenital heart disease patient. More outcome data are needed for this technique but it may prove to be a useful adjunct for continuous monitoring of oxygen delivery in major cases.

Emergency vascular access

Intraosseous access to the venous circulation has been described for use during a crisis when no other venous access is available, e.g. during cardiopulmonary resuscitation or shock [78]. Rarely, it may be required for emergency resuscitation in the operating room or intensive care unit, and therefore it is necessary for the pediatric anesthesiologist to be familiar with the technique. Normally this procedure is used only in small children, and the flat surface of the proximal tibia is used. Commercially available 14 or 16 ga intraosseous needles or 16 ga bone marrow aspiration needles may be used. The site is aseptically prepared, the skin is punctured and the outer bony cortex is contacted. With a boring motion, the needle is advanced through the outer cortex into the marrow space, heralded by a sudden loss of resistance. Infants have active marrow production in long bones and when the stylet is removed and the needle aspirated, bone marrow should appear in the hub. Rapid infusion of 10 mL normal saline without extravasation confirms proper placement, and emergency drugs and fluids may be administered. They reach the central circulation via the bone marrow sinusoids, which connect to the emissary veins from the bony cortex and then to the larger veins draining into the central circulation. Drugs injected intraosseously, e.g. epinephrine, reach the heart slightly more slowly than when injected into a central vein, but the peak drug levels are not different [78]. Intraosseous needles should be available for the rare crisis in the operating room or intensive care unit. They should be replaced as soon as possible with conventional peripheral or central venous access.

Complications of vascular access

Thrombosis

Thrombosis is the single most frequent complication, especially among infants. Central venous thrombosis secondary to vascular access develops in 5.8% of neonatal patients, which is ten times that of older patients, and accounts for 40–50% of central venous thromboses after congenital heart surgery [79]. The frequency significantly decreases in patients over 6 months of age. Factors that contribute to the risk of thrombosis include:

- large-bore catheters in small vessels, i.e. larger than 4 Fr in small infants
- duration of cannulation exceeding 7 days

- venous stasis due to extreme fluid restriction or low cardiac output
- infusion of high osmolarity fluids, i.e. concentrated dextrose in parenteral nutrition fluids
- hypercoagulable states [80].

Other risk factors for thrombosis include protein C resistance due to factor V Leiden mutation, prothrombin mutations, and methylenetetrahydrofolate reductase mutations [81], elevated preoperative C-reactive protein [82] and arterial catheterization with the use of vasoconstrictors such as norepinephrine, vasopressin or terlipressin [83]. Immediate consequences of SVC thrombosis include SVC syndrome [84] with increased intracranial pressure, and chylothorax from ineffective drainage of the thoracic duct into the SVC. IVC thrombus leads to ascites, renal and intestinal dysfunction, and edema of the lower abdomen and extremities. The patient must be assessed carefully for signs of thrombosis, and suspicion of thrombosis should be evaluated by ultrasound examination.

Treatment modalities include removing the catheter, heparinization, thrombolytic agents such as tissue plasminogen activator and urokinase [85–87], antithrombin III replacement [88] and surgical thrombectomy. Mortality from SVC thrombosis is reported to be as high as 33% and therefore it is critical to try to prevent this complication, preferably by avoiding SVC catheters in patients under 4 kg. Thrombosis also leads to a higher rate of infection [89,90]. Heparin-bonded catheters may decrease the rate of thrombosis and do not increase risk of bleeding [89,91]. They may also lead to a lower rate of catheter colonization and infection [92]. However, it is currently not possible to bond both heparin and antibiotics to the same catheter. In patients with occlusion of central veins from previous catheters, magnetic resonance venography may be useful in identifying patent veins for future interventions [93].

Thrombosis or dissection of an artery is a serious complication that must be treated immediately. Immediately after arterial catheter placement, it is important to inspect the distal extremity, comparing it to the other extremity, and palpate distal pulses. Placement of a pulse oximeter probe distal to the catheter serves as a continuous monitor and early warning of vascular insufficiency. Transient compromise to perfusion immediately after catheter placement due to arterial spasm or during low output states may be observed. However, when extremity perfusion is significantly compromised, treatment by removal of the catheter, use of vasodilators, warming the extremity, heparin, thrombolytics, surgical consultation for thrombectomy or surgical reconstruction is indicated [94].

Malposition/perforation

Central venous catheter tips should not lie in the right atrium. Adult and pediatric studies have consistently demonstrated a higher rate of heart and great vessel perforation with associated cardiac tamponade when catheter tips are in the atrium [27,95–99]. Perforation is also less common with right-sided lines, e.g. right IJ or subclavian, because the catheter tip is parallel to the vein wall. The catheter tips of left-sided lines are frequently at a 45–90° angle of incidence to the SVC or atrium, and mechanical models demonstrate that this position is more likely to lead to great vessel perforation [100]. Finally, 5–10% of patients with congenital heart disease have a left SVC [99] which most often drains into the coronary sinus or left atrium and both of these sites are undesirable locations for a catheter tip [101]. Thus the ideal position of a CVC is in the mid SVC with the tip parallel to the vein wall (see Fig. 17.3). Soft polyurethane or silicone catheters are also much less likely to perforate than stiffer polyethylene catheters [100].

Perforation is recognized by inability to consistently aspirate blood, an abnormal waveform, and signs and symptoms of pericardial tamponade or hemothorax. Treatment involves aspiration of all the blood possible through the catheter and establishing alternative access, intravascular volume replacement, and drainage of the pericardial or pleural blood, by needle, tube or surgical exploration.

Many authorities recommend positioning the tip of the catheter in the superior half of the SVC, above the pericardial reflection. This recommendation is based on the theoretical concept that if there is a perforation, cardiac tamponade will not be produced, and also the catheter tip will be above the SVC bypass cannula and thus yield accurate CVP measurements on cardiopulmonary bypass [102]. There are several problems with this approach in pediatric anesthesia and surgery, particularly in small patients. First, the SVC is often only 4–5 cm long, leaving little room for error in placement. It is preferable to have the catheter slightly too deep in the SVC, because this will lead to accurate pressure measurements and proper infusions of drugs and fluids. When a multilumen catheter is positioned too high, a proximal port may not be intravascular, leading to extravasation of important or caustic drugs and fluids [103]. In addition, the pericardium is usually opened in congenital heart surgery and drained postoperatively, rendering placement above the pericardial reflection unnecessary. Many series of catheter placements in children document that the IJ route results in tip placement in the SVC or RA 98–100% of the time, whereas the subclavian route has a 5–15% incidence of catheter malposition, i.e. across the midline in the contralateral brachiocephalic vein or up the ipsilateral internal jugular vein.

Despite numerous previous reports of cardiac perforation by central venous catheters, and the publication of studies documenting height- and weight-based formulas for depth of insertion of SVC catheters in infants [31], reports of cardiac perforation resulting in death or necessitating surgical exploration by sternotomy continue to occur [104].

When IVC catheters are used, accurate CVP measurements are obtained whether above or below the diaphragm usually. Umbilical venous catheters (UVC) should be above the level of the diaphragm at the IVC RA junction, but not in the RA [105] to ensure passage through the ductus venosus and parallel position to the IVC wall [106]. In a series of 128 portal vein thromboses in neonates, 73% of them had a UVC and in half of these the UVC was malpositioned; this constituted a major risk factor for poor outcome [107].

A recently described complication of femoral venous catheters is inadvertent placement in the lumbar venous plexus, which may result in paraplegia from epidural hematoma or infusion of vasoconstrictive substances [108,109]. Catheterization of the lumbar venous plexus usually occurs when there is partial or total occlusion of the IVC from previous interventions, and the guidewire passes posteriorly through collateral circulation into the lumbar plexus. This malposition may be suspected during insertion when resistance to catheter passage is encountered or the catheter will not thread its entire length. An anteroposterior radiograph reveals an abnormal catheter course, often appearing to be more lateral than normal. A lateral radiograph will definitely diagnose such malposition where the catheter tip passes posterior to the vertebral bodies. The catheter must be removed immediately and the patient assessed for neurological deficit if this malposition is discovered. Retroperitoneal hematoma from perforation of the femoroiliac vessels from catheter or guidewire can also occur [110].

Inadvertent arterial puncture can nearly always be prevented by the use of an ultrasound guidance system for central venous catheter placement (see above). However, if this complication occurs, the following general principles are useful. After needle puncture, if there is any question about whether the vessel is an artery, remove the needle immediately, elevate the area, and hold firm pressure for 5–10 min. A small-bore needle puncture of the carotid or femoral artery, e.g. 20 ga or smaller, is not usually an indication to cancel surgery. If a larger hole is created in the artery, i.e. a dilator and the catheter have been placed, pressure transduction can be used to confirm location. In this case, a discussion with the surgeon must ensue. Normally, the catheter can be removed, and pressure held without consequences unless a very large catheter was used, e.g. introducer sheath or large-bore CVP catheter, in which case surgical exploration and repair should be undertaken. In most cases of elective cardiac surgery, it is prudent to postpone the case if a large hole has been made in the artery. The case can usually be safely performed 24h later if no bleeding has occurred. In emergency or urgent cases which must proceed despite a large hole in the artery, the neck or groin should be prepped into the field for exploration if excessive bleeding or hematoma formation occur.

Pneumothorax

This complication is most frequent with the subclavian approach, but also may occur with the internal jugular approach, especially with the low puncture sites, e.g. jugular notch approach. To avoid this complication with the subclavian approach, it is important to advance the needle only during expiration. A very shallow approach with the needle directed just posterior to the clavicle and at the sternal notch is also important. For the IJV, a higher puncture site and limiting the caudad advancement of the needle to stop above the clavicle will usually prevent this complication [111].

Continuous aspiration should be performed as the needle is advanced using a saline-filled syringe. If air is aspirated as the needle advances, attempts at venipuncture should stop immediately and careful monitoring for compromise of ventilation and hemodymanics should ensue. A chest radiograph should be obtained if the start of surgery is not imminent to make the diagnosis, and pleural drainage by needle, catheter or tube should be undertaken if indicated. After sternotomy, the pleura can be opened on that side during sternotomy if pneumothorax is diagnosed or suspected.

Infection

Catheter-related sepsis results in significant morbidity, some mortality, prolongation of ICU stay, and increased expense. The incidence of arterial catheter related infection is low. A study of 340 arterial catheters in children revealed a 2.3% incidence of local site infection and 0.6% catheter sepsis [112]. However, central venous catheter-associated bloodstream infection is a major problem. There is strong evidence that several strategies may be employed to reduce this complication [113]. The first is the use of full barrier precautions, e.g. sterile gown, mask, gloves, and careful septic technique during insertion [5]. Second, chlorhexidine has been shown to be superior to other antiseptic solutions. Finally, antibiotic bonding to the resin of the catheter will reduce infection [114]. This can be done in several ways, i.e. antibiotics already embedded in the resin (minocycline/rifampin or chlorhexidine/silver sulfadiazine) or applied at the time of insertion by soaking the outer and inner surfaces of the catheter in a negatively charged antibiotic at 100mg/mL concentration such as vancomycin, cefazolin or other cephalosporins. Antibiotic is slowly released from the catheter, delaying and reducing colonization and reducing the incidence of catheter sepsis. The increased cost per

catheter is about $20 but one episode of catheter sepsis is estimated to cost $14,000 in 1995 dollars [114]. In a study of antibiotic-impregnated catheters in 225 critically ill children, minocyline/rifampin-coated catheters delayed the onset of infection in those patients who were infected to 18 days, from 5 days in non-antibiotic catheters [115]. Central venous catheters indwelling more than 5–7 days have an increased incidence of colonization and sepsis [116] as well as vessel thrombosis.

Suspicion of catheter sepsis should be followed by peripheral blood culture, and blood culture from the central line. The catheter should be removed when possible and the tip cultured. Institute antibiotic therapy empirically tailored to the most common institution-specific pathogens, and provide coverage for *Staph. epidermidis*, which continues to be a common pathogen in catheter-related sepsis. A comprehensive, systematic intervention program to prevent central line-associated bloodstream infections in a very busy cardiac ICU, including insertion, access, and maintenance protocols, and a protocol for timely removal of central lines, reduced the infection rate from 7.8 infections per 1000 catheter days to 2.3 infections per 1000 catheter days [117]. A recommended central line insertion bundle is displayed in Table 17.2.

Arrhythmias

Other complications associated with vascular access procedures include arrhythmias. Ectopic atrial tachycardia, in particular, has been associated with a catheter tip in the right atrium [118,119]. Atrial fibrillation has also been associated with CVC placement [120]. More commonly, arrhythmias occur with the passage of the guidewire [121] and include isolated premature atrial contractions, supraventricular tachycardia and, if the guidewire is advanced into the right ventricle, premature ventricular contractions and even ventricular tachycardia or fibrillation. Complete heart block has also been described during guidewire passage in small infants [122]. Great care must be taken when passing the guidewire to stop advancing it when significant arrhythmias are encountered, and when advancing the catheter over the wire, to retract the wire as the catheter is advanced. Patients particularly at risk for significant arrhythmia are those with known history of arrhythmia and also those with significant right ventricular hypertrophy.

Systemic air embolus

Systemic air embolus is a constant threat for patients with central or peripheral venous catheters and intracardiac shunting [123], particularly two-ventricle patients with right-to-left shunting and single-ventricle patients in infancy who have obligate mixing of systemic and pulmonary venous return in the systemic ventricle. Air may lodge in the coronary arteries (especially the right), pulmonary artery or cerebral vessels, leading to potentially serious complications. Observation of the TEE or transcranial Doppler ultrasound as used for neurological monitoring reveals rapid passage of any introduced systemic venous air into the aorta and cerebral circulation. For this reason, meticulous attention must be paid to prevent introduction of air into the systemic venous circulation as much as possible. Precautions include thorough de-airing of all intravenous infusions before connection to the patient, de-airing of continuous flush central venous lines, air filters on continuous infusions, and careful technique when injecting drugs and fluids. The latter involves holding any syringe upright, flushing fluid from the proximal intravenous tubing into it, and aspirating and tapping the syringe first before injecting so that any air is trapped at the superior aspect of the syringe. Constant vigilance of all infusions, and use of TEE as a monitor for intracardiac air and the transcranial Doppler for systemic arterial air, may reduce the risk of significant air embolus.

Other complications

Thoracic duct injury, chylothorax [124], brachial plexus injury, cervical dural puncture [125], phrenic nerve injury [126], vertebral arteriovenous fistula [127], Horner syndrome [128], and tracheal puncture have also been described. These complications can essentially be eliminated with skilled personnel using ultrasound-guided techniques to accurately identify the location of the vessel.

Finally, embolization of catheter or guidewire fragments sheared off during difficult insertion procedures occurs occasionally [17]. Never withdraw a guidewire or catheter through a needle if any resistance is encountered. If resistance is encountered, the guidewire and needle, or catheter and needle, must be withdrawn completely from the vessel together as a unit.

Respiratory monitoring

The continuous monitoring of ventilation in the anesthetized patient is the standard of care for pediatric anesthesia [129]. Inadequate ventilation is one of the most frequent causes of patient injury in the American Society of Anesthesiologists' Closed Claims database [130], including in pediatric patients. This section will review methods of respiratory monitoring, including inspection and auscultation, pulse oximetry, capnography and anesthetic gas monitoring, and the monitoring of ventilation volumes and pressures.

Inspection and auscultation

Although not often emphasized due to the proliferation of technology to monitor ventilation, inspection of the patient for adequate and symmetrical chest rise, lack of signs of inspiratory or expiratory obstruction, and lack of cyanosis or pallor representing inadequate oxygenation are important monitoring techniques for every anesthetized patient. The precordial or esophageal stethoscope, although used less frequently in recent years [131], still is very useful for continuous auscultatory monitoring of respiration and heart tones, and serves as an adjunct to the electronic devices used for every case. A standard stethoscope is essential equipment to have available at all times to assess ventilation, as equipment failures do occur.

Pulse oximetry

Pulse oximetry uses the unique light absorption characteristics of oxy- and deoxyhemoglobin to estimate the arterial oxygen saturation (SpO_2). In standard pulse oximetry, two wavelengths of 660 and 930 nm are used, transmitted through tissue to a detector that uses an algorithm to measure only the pulsating, arterial portion of oxyhemoglobin and filters out absorption due to non-pulsating capillaries, veins, bone and soft tissue [132]. The widespread clinical availability of pulse oximetry since the mid-1980s has done more to change anesthetic and critical care practice in the past two decades than any other single monitor. Despite the obvious intuitive value of measuring SpO_2 to prevent arterial desaturation episodes, to date there are only four published large controlled trials of pulse oximetry and outcome, all in adults, and although these trials demonstrated reduced incidence of perioperative hypoxemia, they did not demonstrate a difference in outcomes [133].

The utility of pulse oximetry in pediatric anesthesia was conclusively shown by Coté et al in two studies [134,135]. The first was a single-blind study of 152 patients where all had pulse oximetry but in half the data were not available to practitioners, whereas in the other half the monitor and alarms were available. Major desaturation (<85% for >30 sec) occurred more frequently in the blinded group (35 versus 11, p = 0.021). The pulse oximeter diagnosed hypoxemia before cyanosis and bradycardia were evident. In a second single-blind study of pulse oximetry and capnography in 402 patients, 260 ventilation problems were detected in 153 patients; blinding the oximeter data increased the number of patients experiencing major desaturation events (31 versus 12, p = 0.003), blinding the capnograph data had less effect, with only five of 59 major desaturation events first diagnosed by the capnograph, versus 41 by the oximeter and 13 by the anesthesiologist. These studies firmly established the utility of the pulse oximeter in preventing and diagnosing major desaturation events, and were the cornerstone of the current requirement for pulse oximetry in all pediatric anesthetic and sedation cases.

Pitfalls, problems, and artifacts of pulse oximetry

There are a variety of manufacturers of pulse oximeters, and the instructions for each should be followed carefully, particularly the proper disposable or reusable probe size for each patient. In small infants less than 3 kg, it is often desirable to wrap the disposable probe around the hand or foot, as these will allow light transmission but are often more secure than their tiny digits. Bright ambient light should be shielded by covering the probe. Despite the ubiquitous use of pulse oximetry, it should be remembered that there are myriad manufacturers and proprietary algorithms for signal acquisition and averaging, and that in the normal arterial oxygen saturation ranges >90%, pulse oximetry is accurate to ± 2%, with potentially less accuracy at SpO_2 <90% [132].

Cyanotic congenital heart disease (CHD) is common in pediatric anesthesia, and several studies have compared SpO_2 to measured blood arterial oxyhemoglobin saturations in cyanotic CHD using co-oximetry. Schmitt et al [136] studied 56 children with cyanotic CHD undergoing cardiac surgery with two simultaneous steady-state measurements comparing SpO_2 to co-oximeter measured arterial blood oxygen saturation (SaO_2) in each patient. The linear regression between SpO_2 and SaO_2 was 0.91; however, using Bland–Altman analysis, the bias and precision between the two methods were very close when SpO_2 was >80%, but much worse when SpO_2 was <80%, with the pulse oximeter overestimating the measured arterial saturation by 5.8%, and two standard deviations of precision being only 10%. In a more recent study using two modern generation pulse oximeters (see below), Torres et al [137] made 122 paired observations in 46 children with acyanotic and cyanotic CHD after cardiopulmonary bypass, and found that in patients with SpO_2 <90%, the bias was 3–6%, with the oximeter reading higher than the measured blood saturation, with precision 5–6%. Thus, although the pulse oximeter is an excellent trend monitor in cyanotic CHD, it will consistently overestimate the true arterial saturation, especially with SpO_2 <80%.

Poor peripheral perfusion states are common in pediatric anesthesia due to hypothermia, hypovolemia, cardiogenic shock, and many other etiologies. Since pulse oximetry relies on adequate perfusion of the digits so the device can detect oxyhemoglobin saturation in pulsating tissue, vasoconstriction that accompanies the conditions noted above can prevent detection of minimal levels of arterial pulsation and prevent the pulse oximeter from functioning. Villaneuva et al [138] studied 19 children 2–60 kg requiring arterial catheters for surgery, and measured the performance of two older generation pulse oximeters for accuracy and functioning in response to low perfusion states induced by both inflation of a blood pressure cuff and by clinical conditions, using seven perfusion variables (age, weight, core and skin temperature, hemoglobin, pulse pressure, and laser Doppler blood flow). They compared bias in 94 paired measurements between SpO_2 and measured arterial hemoglobin saturation. Overall, bias was within ± 2%. Factors increasing bias included decreased weight, decreased pulse pressure, decreased core temperature, and decreased laser Doppler flow. The strongest predictor of inaccurate readings was skin temperature <30°C. In the six instances of oximeter failure to function, low skin temperature was present in all. Pulse oximetry can also serve as a perfusion monitor in an extremity or digit distal to an arterial catheter, i.e. radial or femoral; if an adequate pulse oximeter plethysmograph signal is present, it is a sign of adequate perfusion.

Intravascular dyes which absorb light in the same range as hemoglobin predictably will affect SpO_2. Among the commonly used dyes, methylene blue produces a significant, short-lived, artifactual desaturation. Indocyanine green produces a less profound desaturation effect, and indigo carmine's effect is even less profound [139]. Although bilirubin light absorption spectrum has some overlap with hemoglobin, hyperbilirubinemia has been shown to have little effect on the accuracy of pulse oximetry [140]. Fetal hemoglobin also has little effect on the accuracy of pulse oximetry [141].

The usual sites for pulse oximetry on the extremities may be unavailable due to burns, trauma, surgery on the extremities or congenital malformations. In these cases, conventional pulse oximeter probes have been placed on the earlobe, bridge of nose, buccal mucosa, tongue, and penis [142–144]. More central locations (buccal mucosa, tongue, nose) will experience desaturation and resaturation changes significantly earlier than the distal sites on the hand or foot [145]. In cases where major vascular structures may be occluded during surgery or where access to the extremities is limited (cardiac surgery), it is often helpful to place two or more pulse oximeter probes on both upper and lower extremities, in case of failure of one site to function.

Newer developments in pulse oximetry

Newer generation pulse oximeters developed over the past 5–10 years (Masimo Signal Extraction and Rainbow Technologies, Masimo Corporation, Mission Viejo, CA, and Nellcor N-395 and N-595, Nellcor-Puritan Bennett Corporation, Pleasanton, CA) have been designed to address some of the limitations of the older technology, and to extend the capabilities of pulse oximetry to measure new parameters, such as total hemoglobin and perfusion by quantifying the plethysmographic signal. The new technologies incorporate more sensitive electronic filtering designed to detect true arterial pulsation during motion or poor peripheral perfusion. In a study of 75 children monitored in the postanesthesia care unit where motion artifact is a frequent problem, Malviya et al [146] compared the new with the old technology and determined that the new technology correctly determined the 27 true desaturation events of SpO_2 <90% 100% of the time, whereas the older technology was successful only 59% of the time. In addition, false alarms were reduced by 50% with the new technology.

The newer technologies use up to eight wavelengths of light and are capable of determining accurate SpO_2 in the presence of abnormal hemoglobins, including carboxyhemoglobin and methemoglobin [147]. With increasing concentrations of either of these abnormal hemoglobins, conventional two-wavelength pulse oximetry reads an SpO_2 that converges toward 85%, the isosbestic point for normal hemoglobin. However, because both of these substances have higher affinity for hemoglobin than oxygen, the true oxygen saturation is significantly lower. The additional wavelengths will detect these abnormal hemoglobins and also measure a true SpO_2, and thus are important additions if the patient is at risk for these conditions.

Despite this technological advance, unless the patient is at risk for CO inhalation, such as after a burn injury, or methemoglobinemia, such as with high-concentration NO inhalation, its utility in routine pediatric anesthesia is limited. Another novel use of the new technology is to measure total hemoglobin; this is proportional to the total absorption of light in the light path, but depends on a constant SpO_2 and blood volume, i.e. changes in the amount of hemoglobin in the light path due to changes in intravascular volume can be confused with changes in absolute hemoglobin concentration. With these caveats, this non-invasive estimation of hemoglobin concentration has reasonable accuracy, and could find clinical utility as a trend monitor [147].

Finally, despite these advances in technology, Robertson & Hoffman [148] found that two different late-generation pulse oximeters performed significantly differently under adverse clinical conditions in terms of rejection of data, and that as SpO_2 decreased, particularly to <70%, there was significant disagreement, with a bias of 3–7% at these low saturations.

Pulse oximetry can serve as a more objective index of peripheral perfusion by converting the pulsatile component of the light absorption signal into an electric signal that represents the plethysmograph at that particular location. Displaying this signal continuously can serve as a useful estimate of tissue perfusion in that location, i.e. a strong beat-to-beat signal variation represents adequate tissue perfusion. In addition, the degree of respiratory variation of arterial pulse pressure with positive pressure variation can be an important measure of fluid status, i.e. the greater the respiratory variation in the pulse pressure, the more the relative hypovolemia; intravascular fluid

administration will often reduce this respiratory variation [149]. Because the plethysmograph derived from pulse oximetry is derived from arterial pulsations, it is now being used as a non-invasive monitor of volume status. The variation in the plethysomographic waveform amplitude of the pulse oximeter has been shown to correlate well with variation in arterial pulse pressure intraoperatively and in the intensive care unit; future study will be required to determine whether this modality could be used clinically.

All of the above cited data suggest that pulse oximeter values, particularly under challenging clinical conditions, should always be interpreted in light of the clinical condition of the patient and other respiratory and circulatory parameters.

Capnography

Monitoring of end-tidal carbon dioxide (CO_2) is a requirement for all general anesthetics, both to confirm the initial correct placement of endotracheal tubes and other airway devices, and also to continuously monitor adequacy of ventilation [129]. Most capnographs utilize infrared light to quantify CO_2 in the exhaled gas, and there are two major configurations: mainstream and sidestream. Mainstream capnography uses an in-line detector in the breathing circuit near the connector of the endotracheal tube. It requires disposable cuvettes and frequent calibration. Advantages are rapid response time and no aspiration of gas from the breathing circuit. Disadvantages include a bulky apparatus that may place tension on the endotracheal tube. Sidestream capnographs aspirate gas from the breathing circuit at the elbow distal to the Y-piece. Advantages include lightweight small-bore tubing for aspiration and automatic calibration. Disadvantages include a relatively slower response time, and potential for aspiration of large volumes of gas up to 200 mL/min, which may be problematic with small infants and low fresh gas flows. Microstream capnography uses lower gas aspiration volumes of 50 mL/min or less [150].

After direct laryngoscopy to visualize an endotracheal tube through the vocal cords into the trachea, capnography is the gold standard to confirm correct placement of the endotracheal tube. However, this method is certainly not foolproof, and false-positive detection of CO_2 with a waveform may be seen with esophageal intubation and detection of CO_2 introduced into the stomach with mask ventilation; this yields low values of end-tidal CO_2 which disappear within 5–6 breaths. A tube sited at or just above the larynx can detect CO_2 but be at risk for dislodgment. Falsely negative CO_2 detection with correct endotracheal tube placement may be seen in cardiac arrest or very low cardiac output states where pulmonary blood flow is insufficient. It may also be seen with severe bronchospasm preventing gas exchange.

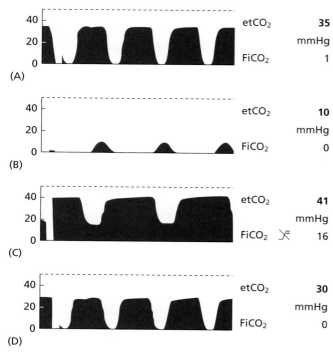

Figure 17.11 Common capnography variants. (A) Normal: note rapid upslope and flat plateau with minimal inspired CO_2. (B) Large leak: causes include large endotracheal tube leak or partial disconnection of sampling line. (C) Rebreathing CO_2: causes include increased anatomical dead space in patient or circuit, exhausted CO_2 absorber, addition of inspired CO_2. (D) Large $ETCO_2$–$PaCO_2$ gap: $PaCO_2$ was 40 mmHg in this patient with cyanotic heart disease.

A normal end-tidal CO_2 tracing has a rapid upslope, a long flat plateau with minimal upslope, rapid return to baseline of zero without rebreathing, and immediate transition into the next inspiration (Fig. 17.11A). Common findings include separation between end-expiratory and the next inspiration with large endotracheal tube leak (Fig. 17.11B). If the exhaled CO_2 does not return to baseline of zero, rebreathing may be occurring, often caused by a faulty expiratory valve or by increased dead space in the breathing system, i.e. by a condenser humidifier too large for the patient's tidal volumes (Fig. 17.11C). A steep expiratory upslope often signifies expiratory obstruction, most often from bronchospasm. Oscillations of the $ETCO_2$ values during the plateau phase usually signify minimal ventilator volumes caused by displacement of the lungs by the cardiac stroke volume.

Besides monitoring the adequacy of ventilation, the purpose of capnography is to estimate, as accurately as possible, the patient's arterial CO_2 tension to avoid hypercapnia and its undesirable effects on pulmonary artery and intracranial pressure, and hypocapnia and its undesirable effects in decreasing cerebral blood flow. The difference between end-tidal and arterial CO_2 in patients with normal heart and lungs, and no increase in anatomical or physiological dead space, is less than 3–5 mmHg. In pediatric anesthesia, the gap is often larger and there are several causes. Dead space in the breathing circuit (an extension of the anatomical dead space where there is flow of gas but no gas exchange, thereby diluting the exhaled CO_2) is a common cause, especially for small patients. The dead space volume in endotracheal tubes, endotracheal tube connectors, condenser humidifiers, Y-pieces and elbows, and mainstream capnographs will often cause a significant underestimation of the arterial CO_2. Generally, the smaller the patient, the greater the effect. Premature infants less than 1.5 kg in weight are especially affected [151]. Using small-volume endotracheal tube connectors, placing condenser humidifiers proximal to the CO_2 sampling line, or special endotracheal tubes with a CO_2 sampling lumen that extends to the tip of the endotracheal tube, have all been used to increase the accuracy of capnography in small patients [152–154] (Fig. 17.12C).

Cyanotic congenital heart disease is another common cause in pediatrics. Right-to-left intracardiac shunting causes blood to bypass the lungs, reducing pulmonary blood flow and thus the volume of blood relinquishing CO_2 to the exhaled gas. The end-tidal to arterial CO_2 gap may be 15–20 mmHg or greater with significant cyanosis [155] (Fig. 17.11D). The relationship varies with each patient but in general, the more cyanotic the patient (greater reduction in pulmonary blood flow), the greater the CO_2 gap. Improving pulmonary blood flow, such as by the placement of a systemic to pulmonary artery shunt, will decrease the end-tidal to arterial gap. Patients with significant pulmonary hypertension with or without intracardiac shunt will often have a large gap. A decreasing end-tidal to arterial CO_2 gap often signifies increased pulmonary blood flow, accompanied by improvement in pulmonary hypertension or cardiac output. Finally, intrapulmonary shunting, such as that caused by lobar consolidation from pneumonia or atelectasis, causes a variable increase in end-tidal to arterial CO_2 difference, depending on the accompanying degree of hypoxic pulmonary vasoconstriction.

Capnography is useful for monitoring of ventilation in patients without an endotracheal tube. Although the dead space is increased under a facemask, capnography is effective in monitoring the adequacy of tidal volumes with spontaneous or assisted mask ventilation. Similarly, the dead space is slightly increased with the larger bore airway of the laryngeal mask airway, but monitoring of CO_2 is essential when this device is used. Finally, monitoring ventilation with a divided, CO_2 sampling nasal cannula during spontaneous ventilation with a natural airway during sedation and monitored anesthesia cases is now common practice and is especially useful when there is not direct proximity to the patient, i.e. MRI scanner [156].

As with any monitor using a mechanical/electrical interface, spurious capnograms and end-tidal CO_2 values can be caused by equipment malfunction or failure. A partially disconnected CO_2 sampling line or cracked connector can entrain room air and artificially lower end-tidal CO_2 values. A CO_2 sampling line occluded by exhaled moisture or secretions will read little or no end-tidal CO_2. Automatic machine calibration at inopportune times, i.e. immediately after intubation, as well as other malfunctions make it necessary to possess adequate clinical skills of auscultation by precordial, esophageal or standard stethoscope.

Anesthetic agent monitoring

Most modern anesthetic gas concentration monitors are sidestream units combined with capnography, and use polychromatic infrared analyzers that detect each of the halogenated agents individually, as well as CO_2, N_2O and O_2. These units are easy to use and calibrate, economical to operate, reliable, and are reasonably accurate. Mass spectroscopy has greater accuracy and also can measure nitrogen concentration, which is important in the diagnosis of pulmonary embolus. However, these units are more expensive and have largely been superseded by the infrared monitors. And although the modern units are fairly accurate, deviations as high as 5–11% relative value are seen with infrared when compared to the gold standard gas chromatography [157]. Thus, although it is important to measure inspired and end-tidal anesthetic concentrations, assessment of the relative anesthetic depth of the individual patient is critical. As with capnography, newer microstream technology which min-

imizes dead space will both improve response times and allow for aspiration of smaller volumes of gas from the breathing circuit for sampling, which is important in the care of small infants [158].

Ventilatory volumes and pressures

Modern anesthesia machines have the capability to measure airway pressures, volumes, and flows using spirometery combined with pneumotachygraph technology; however, in most cases these parameters are not measured at the patient airway but at some point proximal to all the connections of the circle breathing system. This configuration introduces the potential for significant error in measurement of pressures and tidal volumes, particularly in small patients weighing less than 5–10 kg with tidal volumes <100 cc, because of the compression volume of the circle system. In other words, the average plastic disposable circle system has a compliance volume loss of 1–3 mL per cmH$_2$O of pressure during inspiration; as much as 60 mL tidal volume is not delivered to the patient but rather to the circle system, with peak pressures of 20 cmH$_2$O above end-expiratory pressure (Fig. 17.12). Badgwell et al [159] determined that with a standard disposable pediatric circle system and standard adult anesthesia bellows, total compliance volume of the system is about 190 mL with a peak inspiratory pressure of 20.

It is obvious that with small infants, the anesthesia machine readout may be very inaccurate. There are two potential solutions to this problem. First, newer generation modern anesthesia machines can calculate an exact breathing circuit compression volume during a preanesthesia machine check; during volume ventilation additional volume is added to each breath equal to the

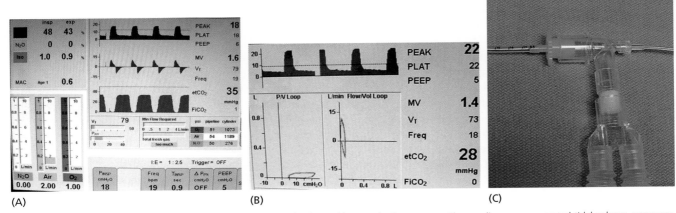

(A) (B) (C)

Figure 17.12 Respiratory monitoring. (A) Standard modern anesthesia machine monitoring screen with compliance-compensated tidal volume, pressures, flows, inspiratory time, anesthetic gas concentration. (B) Respiratory loops: flow–volume and pressure–volume loops. (C) Configuration to minimize dead space: pediatric circle system; small infant condenser humidifier proximal to sampling line; minimum dead space (0.5 mL) connector.

compliance compensation volume [160]. This is only accurate if the circle system configuration is not changed after the machine check, i.e. if a distensible breathing circuit is extended to its full length, the compliance volume changes. Also, some systems will limit the extent of compliance compensation allowed for small tidal volumes less than 100–200 cc as a safety measure, so that sudden large inappropriate tidal volumes are not delivered to small patients in the event of a change in compression volume. The second method of solving this issue is to use a spirometry system attached to the proximal end of the endotracheal tube so that volumes and pressures are measured at the airway; this is possible with a variety of systems whether integrated into the anesthesia delivery system or stand-alone units made for infants.

Temperature monitoring

Accurate monitoring of temperature during general anesthesia is an accepted standard of care in pediatric patients, because changes in body temperature are anticipated in these patients for a variety of reasons. The physiology of maintenance of body temperature, methods of achieving this, and complications of temperature homeostasis are discussed in Chapter 40. Measurement of temperature has been simplified by easy availability of thermocouple stand-alone probes, or esophageal stethoscopes, bladder catheters, skin temperature probes, tympanic membrane probes or pulmonary artery catheters with incorporated thermistors.

Central core temperature is best measured in the esophagus, rectum or nasopharynx. These sites are generally accepted to be the most accurate, and will be equivalent if the probes are placed properly. This means in the mid-esophagus, at least 2–5 cm into the rectum, and in the case of nasopharyngeal temperature, with the probe inserted to a depth equal to the distance from the nares to the tragus of the ear, placing the tip of the probe under the cribriform plate and thus in the closest proximity to the brain. Axillary temperature is often simple and convenient, especially in short pediatric cases, but several minutes may be required for temperature equilibration, and readings will be about 1°C lower. For major intraabdominal, intrathoracic, intracranial cases or surgery in small infants, a core temperature site should be chosen. For monitored anesthesia care or sedation cases, temperature monitoring should be readily available and used if temperature change is anticipated. If the brain is particularly at risk, i.e. intracranial or cardiopulmonary bypass cases, actual brain temperature may be up to 2°C above rectal temperature [161]. Measurement of skin temperature, i.e. sole of the foot, versus core temperature may provide added information to assess the degree of heat loss or peripheral vasoconstriction during major surgery. With thermal homeostasis and adequate peripheral perfusion, skin temperature at the sole of the foot should be no more than 5° below core temperature.

Urinary monitoring

Monitoring of urine output with a bladder catheter is important for major surgery, where significant blood loss, hemodynamic change or fluid shifts are anticipated. Although influenced by a multitude of factors, generally a urine output of 1 cc/kg/h or greater is assumed to indicate adequate intravascular volume status and perfusion to the kidneys. Low or absent urine output can be due to mechanical obstruction of the tubing, hypovolemia or antidiuretic hormone secretion, with hypovolemia by far the most frequent cause. Although possible, measuring urinary sodium and osmolarity is rarely performed intraoperatively. Excessive urine output can be caused by hypervolemia, hyperosmolarity of the urine as seen in hyperglycemia (renal glucose threshold approximately 180 mg/dL in infants and children, may be lower in neonates), osmotic agents such as mannitol or diuretics such as furosemide. The color of the urine may provide important information; hematuria can be seen with hemolysis from cardiopulmonary bypass or a transfusion reaction, tea-colored urine from myoglobinuria during malignant hyperthermia or significant muscle crush injury. Cloudy urine may be from calcium oxalate crystals, proteinuria with concentrated urine or from urinary tract infection.

Blood gas and other point-of-care testing

Rapid point-of-care testing, either in the operating room or in close proximity with rapid turnaround time, has made real-time monitoring of multiple parameters possible, especially for major surgery associated with significant blood loss or unstable patients in whom frequent assessment of blood gas values, hemoglobin, and other parameters is important to guide care. There are a variety of machines available but among the most useful is the point-of-care blood gas machine that also measures electrolytes, hematocrit, glucose, ionized calcium, measured oxygen saturation, and lactate values (Fig. 17.13). Modern machines can make all of these measurements on 0.5 cc or less of heparinized whole blood, with results available in less than 2 min. Temperature correction algorithms and electronic recording of values make these machines suitable for electronic medical records. In cardiac surgery, major trauma, neonatal, spine surgery, thoracic surgery,

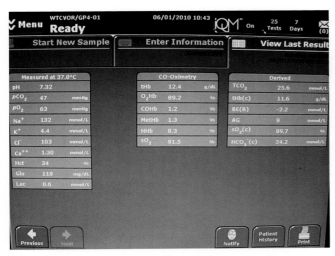

Figure 17.13 Point-of-care monitor for blood gases, electrolytes, hematocrit, ionized calcium, glucose, lactate, co-oximetry. 0.5 mL heparinized blood sample, 80-sec measurement time, temperature correction.

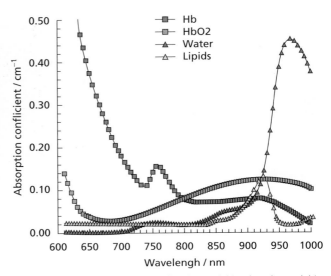

Figure 17.14 Absorption spectrum of oxyhemoglobin, deoxyhemoglobin, water, and lipids. Reproduced by courtesy of Somanetics Corporation.

and other major surgical cases, measuring these parameters at regular intervals may provide rapid early warning of major changes in the patient's condition, e.g. metabolic acidosis, significant anemia or worsening A-aO$_2$ gradient, that are not evident from standard monitoring, and are available significantly sooner than sending the sample out to the hospital's regular clinical laboratories.

Other rapid tests available as point-of-care tests include rapid coagulation assessment with partial thromboplastin time, thromboelastography, or rapid platelet function tests, potentially directing specific therapy to improve coagulation in the individual patient. For all new modalities, an analysis of the cost/ benefit ratio, and careful assessment of the potential to improve outcomes are important. See Chapter 11 for a further discussion of coagulation monitoring.

Neuromuscular transmission monitoring

Accurate assessment of the status of neuromuscular blockade in children is important when non-depolarizing neuromuscular blocking agents are utilized, because simply relying on an estimate of the half-life of the drugs is notoriously inaccurate [162]. Standard nerve-stimulating devices utilize current of 30–80 mA, and the most common method is to utilize the train-of-four scheme. The most common and standard placement for leads is to use small ECG leads, placed over the ulnar nerve, so that the thumb adduction via activation of the adductor pollicis brevis nerve can be observed. Any "fade" in the amplitude of contraction, observed visually, indicates residual neuromuscular blockade. The absence of any contraction

with the train of four, or contraction only after a tetanic stumulus of 50 or 100 MHz, indicates dense neuromuscular blockade, and that reversal with neostigmine or other anticholinesterase agents should not be attempted. Other sites, such as the peroneal nerve or facial nerve, may also be utilized, the latter with caution because direct muscle contraction may be observed, causing an underestimation of the degree of blockade.

Central nervous system monitoring

Near infrared spectroscopy

Near infrared spectroscopy (NIRS) is used to measure both cerebral and somatic oxyhemoglobin saturation. Since its now classic description in 1977 by Jobsis [163], this technology has been the subject of over 1000 publications and, because of its non-invasive, compact, portable nature and potential for measuring tissue oxygenation in the brain and other organ systems during surgery and critical illness, is gaining more widespread clinical use. This section will examine the technical aspects of NIRS, parameters measured and clinical uses in pediatric cardiac and non-cardiac surgery and critical care, evidence for effectiveness in improving clinical outcomes, and pitfalls and complications of usage.

Technical concepts of near infrared spectroscopy

Near infrared spectroscopy (NIRS) is a non-invasive optical technique used to monitor brain tissue oxygenation. Most devices utilize 2–4 wavelengths of infrared light at 700–1000 nm, where oxygenated and deoxygenated hemoglobin have distinct absorption spectra [164–166] (Fig. 17.14). Commercially available devices measure

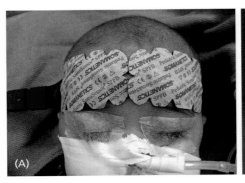

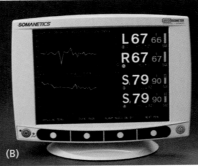

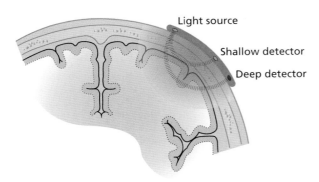

Light source

Shallow detector

Deep detector

Figure 17.16 NIRS method: a light or laser-emitting diode emits light, which passes through the skin, skull, and meninges and into a small portion of the frontal cerebral cortex. Some light is scattered and some is absorbed by oxy- and deoxyhemoglobin, and a portion passes through tissues and is detected by a shallow and deep detectors, 3 and 4 cm from light source. The shallow component is subtracted out, leaving mostly intracranial signal. Reproduced courtesy of Somanetics Corporation.

Figure 17.15 (A) Bilateral NIRS probes on an infant. (B) Four-channel NIRS monitor screen. L and R designate left and right cerebral hemispheres; S3 designates renal saturation with a probe placed on the flank at the T10–11 level; S4 designates mesenteric saturation with a probe placed in the midline between the umbilicus and symphysis pubis. See text for further explanation.

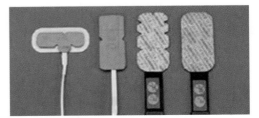

Figure 17.17 Different NIRS probes for neonate cerebral 1–4 kg (*far left*), neonatal somatic 1–4 kg (*second from left*), pediatric cerebral/somatic (4–40 kg) (*second from right*), adult >40 kg (*far right*). Reproduced courtesy of Somanetics Corporation.

the concentration of oxy- and deoxyhemoglobin, using variants of the Beer–Lambert equation:

$$\log\left(\frac{I}{I_0}\right) = \varepsilon_\lambda LC$$

where I_0 is the intensity of light before passing through the tissue, I is the intensity of light after passing through the tissue, and the ratio of I/I_0 is absorption. Absorption of near infrared light depends on the optical path length (L), the concentration of the chromophore in that path (C), and the molar absorptivity of the chromophore at the specific wavelength used (ε_λ).

Cerebral oximetry assumes that 75% of the cerebral blood volume in the light path is venous and 25% arterial. This 75/25 ratio is derived from theoretical anatomical models. Watzman et al [167] attempted to verify this index in children with congenital heart disease by measuring jugular venous bulb saturation and arterial saturation, and comparing it to cerebral saturation measured with frequency-domain NIRS. The actual ratio in patients varied widely, but averaged 85/15.

In the various models of cerebral oximeters currently on the market, the sensor electrode is placed on the forehead (Fig. 17.15A) below the hairline. A light-emitting diode or laser emits infrared light, which passes through a "banana-shaped" tissue volume in the frontal cerebral cortex, to two or three detectors placed 3–5 cm from the emitter. The screen displays regional cerebral oxygen saturation (rSO$_2$) and trend over time (Fig. 17.15B). By using different sensing optodes and multiple wavelengths, extracranial and intracranial hemoglobin absorption can be separated. Narrow arcs of light travel across skin and skull but do not penetrate the cerebral cortex. Deep arcs of light cross skin, skull, dura, and cortex (Fig. 17.16). Subtracting the two absorptions measured, shallow from deep, leaves absorption that is due to intracerebral chromophores, and this processing renders the cerebral specificity of the oximeter (Fig. 17.17). However, the accuracy of NIRS is confounded by the light scattering which alters the optical path length and the available commercial clinical devices solve this problem differently. The depth of light penetration is 2–4 cm.

Three cerebral oximeters are currently widely commercially available: the INVOS 5100, NIRO 200 and the Foresight. Of the three, the Somanetics INVOS system (Somanetics Inc., Troy, MI, USA) is in most common use and has disposable probes, including an adult probe for patients over 40 kg, as well as a pediatric probe designed

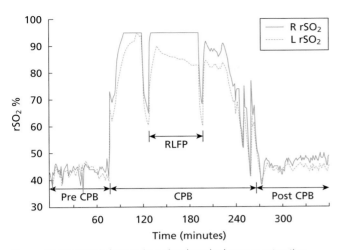

Figure 17.18 Typical changes in regional cerebral oxygen saturation (rSO_2) during cardiac surgery in a neonate with hypoplastic left heart syndrome undergoing Norwood stage I palliation, with cardiopulmonary bypass, regional cerebral low flow perfusion (RLFP), and deep hypothermic circulatory arrest (DHCA). Note precipitous decline at minute 115 with onset of DHCA for atrial septectomy, and again at minute 185 for replacement of aortic cannula.

for patients 4–40 kg which uses a different algorithm that takes into account the thinner skull and extracranial tissues compared to the adult [168]. More recently, a neonatal probe has become available which is easier to apply as it conforms well to the smaller forehead shape. It uses two wavelengths, 730 and 810 nm, and has one light-emitting diode (LED) and two detectors, spaced at 3 cm and 4 cm apart from the emitter, and uses spatially resolved spectroscopy (Fig. 17.18). The distinct absorption coefficients of oxy- and deoxyhemoglobin permit measurement of the relative signals from these compounds in the light path and the INVOS device reports oxyhemoglobin/total hemoglobin (oxy- + deoxyhemoglobin) × 100, as the measured regional cerebral oxygen saturation (rSO_2), in percentage. The rSO_2 is reported as a percentage on a scale from 15% to 95%. A subtraction algorithm based on probe size removes most of the transmitted shallow (3 cm detector) signal, leaving over 85% of the remaining signal derived from brain frontal cortex. This device is United States Food and Drug Administration (FDA) approved for use in children and adults as a trend-only monitor. It is compact, non-invasive, and requires little warm-up. A signal strength indicator displays adequacy of detected signal, and the device does not depend on pulsatility like a pulse oximeter, and operates at all temperatures. Cerebral blood volume index (Crbvi) can also be calculated, representing the total hemoglobin in the light path, which may be used as an estimate of cerebral blood volume. However, this application is not approved by the FDA for clinical use but only for research purposes.

The NIRO 200 (Hamamatsu Photonics, Hamamatsu, Japan) uses three wavelengths of near infrared light (775, 810, and 850 nm) emitted by a laser diode and detected by a photodiode. It uses spatially resolved spectrophotometry, and the three wavelengths allow better determination of light path length according to the Beer–Lambert Law, which allows calculation of absolute concentrations of oxygenated and total hemoglobin. The NIRO 200 reports a tissue oxygenation index (TOI), as well as hemoglobin indices, including changes in total hemoglobin and oxy- and deoxyhemoglobin. The probes are not disposable but are attached with a disposable probe holder. This device may potentially be more accurate than the INVOS system due to the increased number of wavelengths of light, but it is not FDA approved for use in the United States.

A more recent FDA-approved device is the Foresight monitor (Casmed, Branford, CT). This device uses four wavelengths of light: 690, 778, 800, and 850 nm. The purpose of the additional wavelengths is to better discriminate non-hemoglobin sources of infrared absorption, which may lead to a more accurate calculation of oxygenated and total hemoglobin concentrations [169]. The Foresight monitor reports the percentage of oxygenated hemoglobin to total hemoglobin as a cerebral tissue oxygen saturation ($SCTO_2$), and is marketed as an absolute cerebral tissue oxygen saturation. Currently available probes are disposable, and are appropriate only for patients 2.5–8 kg and >40 kg.

Comparison between these commercial devices reveals differences in measured values due to the different numbers of wavelength and subtraction algorithms, thus making direct data comparisons difficult [165]. However, regardless of the device used, it is important to remember that all devices measure combined arterial and venous blood oxygen saturation, and cannot be assumed to be identical to jugular venous bulb oxygen saturation ($SjvO_2$). Maneuvers to increase arterial oxygen saturation, i.e. increasing FiO_2, will increase cerebral oxygenation as measured by these devices, but the $SjvO_2$ may remain unchanged.

The Foresight device is still relatively new and comparison data with the INVOS are not available. However, the Foresight monitor may predict a more accurate value for the true brain saturation compared to the INVOS monitor that will make between-patient comparisons easier.

In an attempt to validate the non-invasive measurement of cerebral oxygen saturation in children with congenital heart disease, $SjvO_2$ and rSO_2 have been compared. In 40 infants and children undergoing congenital heart surgery or cardiac catheterization [170], the correlation for paired measurements was inconclusive except for infants less than 1 year of age. In 30 patients undergoing cardiac catheterization, an improved correlation (r = 0.93) was found [171], and there was a linear correlation between changes in arterial CO_2 and cerebral saturation.

Somatic near infrared oximetry

Using the same principles of unique light absorption spectra of hemoglobin species, NIRS has also been used to measure tissue oxygenation in skeletal muscle, i.e. quadriceps, forearm or thenar eminence muscle, in adults and children [172]. In addition, a probe placed over the flank at the T10–L2 level will measure tissue saturation in skeletal muscle and, in small infants, renal oxygenation due to the small light penetrance distance needed in these patients [173] (Fig. 17.19). Finally, mesenteric saturation has also been measured in infants with a probe placed in the midline between the umbilicus and the symphysis pubis [174].

Parameters monitored with near infrared spectroscopy

To simplify terminology, the term rSO_2, for regional oxygen saturation, will be utilized for the remainder of this chapter, regardless of the device used. Cerebral rSO_2 measurements are an estimate of venous-weighted oxyhemoglobin saturation in the sample volume illuminated by the light path, i.e. the frontal cerebral cortex in most situations. rSO_2 can be altered by any of the factors that affect the cerebral oxygen supply/demand ratio and is especially affected by the unique features of the cerebral circulation, including cerebral autoregulation and alterations in cerebral blood flow according to $PaCO_2$. Any factor that decreases cerebral oxygen consumption will

generally increase rSO_2, and any factor that increases oxygen delivery to the brain will also generally increase rSO2. Box 17.2 lists some of the common alterable clinical factors that can be used to change rSO_2. Since cerebral rSO_2 is influenced by arterial oxygenation, improving this parameter will often increase rSO_2, even if $SjvO_2$ is little altered.

For pediatric patients undergoing congenital heart surgery, baseline rSO_2 varies with cardiac lesion [166]. The baseline cerebral saturation is about 70% in acyanotic patients without large left-to-right intracardiac shunts breathing room air. On room air, rSO_2 for cyanotic patients, or acyanotic patients with large left-to-right intracardiac shunts, is usually 40–60%; hypoplastic left heart syndrome (HLHS) patients receiving <21% FiO_2 preoperatively have lower rSO_2, averaging 53%, versus those receiving FiO_2 0.21 and 3% inspired CO_2, where rSO_2 averages 68% [175].

Taking into account pediatric cardiac surgery outcome data (see below), some practitioners would consider a relative decline from a baseline of 20% or more (e.g. from a baseline of 60% to a nadir of 48%) cause for intervention. The software on most oximeters will continuously calculate this relative difference from baseline. Other practitioners would use an absolute value of rSO_2 of 50% as cause for intervention.

Cerebral oximetry reflects a balance between oxygen delivery and oxygen consumption by the brain ($CMRO_2$).

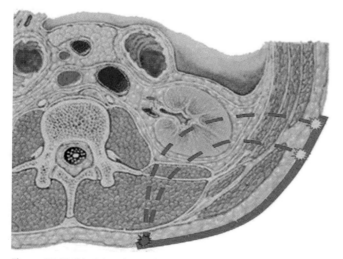

Figure 17.19 Principles of somatic NIRS. In a neonate or small infant, a NIRS probe placed on the flank over the T10–12 area measures the oxyhemoglobin saturation of the tissues in the light path, particularly muscle and renal tissue beds. Reproduced courtesy of George Hoffman MD.

Box 17.2 Factors affecting cerebral oxygen consumption and delivery

Factors decreasing $CMRO_2$ and generally increasing rSO_2

- Hypothermia
- Increasing sedation, anesthesia, analgesia with benzodiazepines, opioids, dexmedetomidine
- Treating seizures

Factors increasing oxygen delivery to brain and generally increasing rSO_2

- Increasing $PaCO_2$
- Increasing hemoglobin
- Increasing cardiac output
- Increasing FiO_2 or other ventilatory maneuvers to increase SpO_2
- Increasing mean arterial pressure (outside limits of autoregulation, i.e. hypotension)
- Increasing CPB flow rate
- Increasing CPP
- Minimizing cerebral venous pressure to increase CPP, i.e. obstructed venous bypass cannula

$CMRO_2$, cerebral metabolic rate for oxygen; CPB, cardiopulmonary bypass; CPP, cerebral perfusion pressure; rSO_2, regional brain oxygen saturation.

The cerebral oxygen content will therefore be affected by both the arterial saturation of hemoglobin and the hemoglobin concentration. There then must exist a cerebral saturation value, or ischemic threshold, below which brain injury is likely due to oxygen deprivation as demand outstrips supply. In a neonatal piglet study using frequency domain NIRS [176], Kurth et al showed that cerebral lactate levels rose at rSO_2 values of 44% or lower; major EEG changes occurred when the cerebral saturation declined to 37%, with reductions in cerebral adenosine triphosphate (ATP) levels when oximetry readings were 33% or lower. This concept was confirmed in another neonatal piglet model using hypoxic gas mixtures for 30 min at normothermia, demonstrating that rSO_2 >40% did not change EEG or brain pathology obtained 72 h later; rSO_2 30–40% produced no EEG changes but at 72 h there were ischemic neuronal changes in the hippocampus, and mitochondrial injury occurred. At rSO_2 <30%, there was circulatory failure, EEG amplitude decreased, and there was vacuolization of neurons and severe mitochondrial injury [177]. Finally, in a similar piglet model, the hypoxic-ischemic cerebral saturation time threshold for brain injury found rSO_2 of 35% for 2 h or more produced brain injury [178]. In general most pediatric clinical studies use either 20% below established baseline or an oximetry reading of 45–50% for the threshold for treatment based on evidence of new MRI lesions or clinical exam that brain injury is more likely to develop under these circumstances [179,180].

In the absence of absolute criteria for intervention to prevent neurological injury (see below under Outcomes), each anesthesiologist must take into account the unique pathophysiology of each patient and the monitoring system used, and decide on criteria for intervention, much like all the other physiological variables measured for surgery and critical care.

Clinical data in pediatric cardiac surgery

Changes in cerebral oxygenation have been characterized during cardiopulmonary bypass in children with or without deep hypothermic circulatory arrest [181]. rSO_2 predictably decreases during deep hypothermic circulatory arrest (DHCA) to a nadir approximately 60–70% below baseline values obtained pre-bypass [181] and the nadir is reached at about 40 min, after which there is no further decrease. At this point it appears that the brain does not continue the uptake of oxygen and interestingly, this time period appears to correlate with clinical and experimental studies suggesting that 40–45 min is the limit for safe duration for circulatory arrest [182,183]. The DHCA initiation at higher temperature results in a faster fall in rSO_2, reaching the nadir sooner [184]. Reperfusion immediately results in an increase in rSO_2 levels seen at full bypass flow before DHCA.

The question often arises whether bilateral cerebral hemisphere NIRS monitoring is necessary. In a study of 20 patients undergoing a special cardiopulmonary bypass technique, antegrade cerebral perfusion, via the right innominate artery, half of the patients had a left/right difference of >10% [185]. In 60 neonates undergoing surgery with conventional bypass, only 10% had greater than 10% difference between left and right sides at baseline, and this difference persisted in only one patient [186]. Based on these data, bilateral monitoring is probably necessary only when special cardiopulmonary bypass (CPB) techniques are used for aortic arch reconstruction or when anatomical variants, i.e. bilateral superior vena cavae or abnormalities of the brachiocephalic vessels, are present.

Treatment of low rSO_2

Whether during adult or pediatric cardiac surgery with CPB, the general approach to treating low rSO_2 is similar and involves increasing oxygen delivery to the brain or decreasing oxygen consumption. One approach to treatment is displayed in Box 17.3.

In critical care medicine, cerebral NIRS has been used to monitor adequacy of cerebral oxygen delivery and as a surrogate for adequacy of global oxygen delivery, in patients after cardiac surgery and those on extracorporeal membrane oxygenation (ECMO) or ventricular assist devices [169,187]. Changes in rSO_2 have a close correlation with changes in mixed venous saturation (SvO_2) in both single- and two-ventricle patients after congenital cardiac surgery [188,189].

Clinical uses of somatic near infrared spectroscopy in pediatric surgery and critical care

Near infrared spectroscopy can be used to measure tissue oxygenation in surgery and critical illness, and because of its non-invasive, continuous nature, has intuitive appeal in conditions where low cardiac output and other causes of shock would benefit from such continuous monitoring.

Somatic NIRS using a probe placed on the flank at T10–L2 has been studied in a series of neonates during and after single-ventricle surgical palliation by Hoffman et al [173]. In nine neonates undergoing CPB with regional cerebral perfusion (RCP), mean cerebral rSO_2 prebypass was 65% and somatic rSO_2 59%, and during RCP cerebral rSO_2 was 81% versus 41% somatic rSO_2, signifying relative tissue hypoxia due to lack of perfusion to subdiaphragmatic organs during this technique. After CPB, cerebral rSO_2 decreased to 53%, but somatic rSO_2 increased to 76% [173]. In 79 postoperative neonates undergoing Norwood Stage I palliation for hypoplastic left heart syndrome, a cerebral–somatic rSO_2 difference of <10% significantly increased the risk for biochemical shock, mortality

Box 17.3 Treatment algorithm for low cerebral oxygen saturation (rSO$_2$)

1. Establish baseline rSO$_2$ on FiO$_2$ 0.21, PaCO$_2$ 40 mmHg, stable baseline hemodynamics, awake before induction of anesthesia, or prebypass if possible
2. Treat decreased rSO$_2$ of >20% relative value below baseline, or <50% absolute value
3. Pre/postbypass (in order of ease/rapidity to institute):
   (a) Increase FiO$_2$
   (b) Increase PaCO$_2$
   (c) Increase cardiac output/O$_2$ delivery with volume infusions, inotropic support, vasodilators, etc.
   (d) Increase depth of anesthesia
   (e) Decrease temperature
   (f) Increase hemoglobin
4. During CPB:
   (a) Increase CPB flow and/or mean arterial pressure
   (b) Increase PaCO$_2$
   (c) Increase FiO$_2$
   (d) Decrease temperature
   (e) Increase hemoglobin
   (f) Check aortic and venous cannula positioning
   (g) Check for aortic dissection

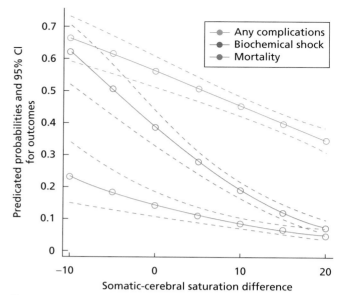

Figure 17.20 Relationship between somatic rSO$_2$–cerebral rSO$_2$ difference and the incidence of complications in 79 patients in the 48h after Norwood stage I palliation for hypoplastic left heart syndrome. Reproduced from Hoffman et al [190] with permission from Lippincott Williams & Wilkins.

or other complications [190] (Fig. 17.20). Mean somatic rSO$_2$ <70% was associated with a significantly increased risk of prolonged ICU stay, shock, and other complications.

Somatic NIRS has also been used to measure mesenteric rSO$_2$ in neonates and infants after cardiac surgery, with a probe placed on the abdomen between the umbilicus and symphysis pubis. In a study of 20 patients, Kaufman et al [191] compared mesenteric NIRS and flank NIRS at T10–L2 to gastric pH measured by tonometry and lactate values. In 122 simultaneous measurements made in the first 48 h after surgery, mesenteric rSO$_2$ correlated significantly with gastric pH (r = 0.79), serum lactate (r = 0.77), and SvO$_2$ (r = 0.89). These correlations were all better than those using flank NIRS. The authors concluded that mesenteric NIRS is a sensitive monitor of splanchnic tissue oxygenation, and may have utility in managing these patients and improving outcomes.

These studies lend credence to the idea that NIRS-directed targeted interventions could be utilized to improve oxygen delivery to tissues and organs, and potentially improve outcomes from surgery, anesthesia and critical illness. To date, there is a lack of such published studies, but the non-invasive continuous nature of NIRS monitoring should make such studies more likely to be performed.

Outcome studies of near infrared spectroscopy

There is increasing evidence from pediatric cardiac surgery studies that prolonged low NIRS values are associated

with adverse short-term neurological outcomes. Dent et al [179] studied 15 neonates undergoing the Norwood operation who underwent preoperative, intraoperative and postoperative rSO$_2$ monitoring. A prolonged low rSO$_2$ (>180 min with rSO$_2$ ≤ 45%) was associated with a higher risk of new ischemic lesions on postoperative MRI when compared to the presurgical study, with a sensitivity of 82%, specificity of 75%, positive predictive value of 90%, and negative predictive value of 60%. Therefore, both the extent of decreased cerebral saturation (ischemic threshold) and the time spent below this ischemic threshold are important in predicting the development of new postoperative brain injury by MRI.

There is additional clinical evidence suggesting that low cerebral saturations correlate with adverse neurological outcome. In a study of 26 infants and children undergoing surgery utilizing DHCA [181], three patients had acute neurological changes – seizures in one and prolonged coma in two – all of whom manifest low rSO$_2$. In these three patients the increase in rSO$_2$ was much less after the onset of CPB and the duration of cooling before DHCA shorter. In a retrospective study of multimodality neurological monitoring in 250 infants and children undergoing cardiac surgery with bypass [180], relative cerebral oxygen desaturation of more than 20% below prebypass baseline resulted in abnormal events in 58%. If left untreated, 26% of these patients had adverse postoperative neurological events.

In a study of 16 patients undergoing neonatal cardiac surgery, with NIRS monitoring and pre- and postoperative brain MRI, six of 16 patients developed a new post-operative brain injury; these patients had a lower rSO₂ during the aortic cross-clamp period than those without new brain injury. (48% versus 57%, p = 0.008) [192]. In a recent study of 44 neonates undergoing the Norwood operation, who were tested at age 4–5 using a visual-motor integration (VMI) test, the first 34 patients did not have NIRS monitoring and the last 10 did have NIRS monitoring with a strict treatment protocol for low rSO₂ values <50%. No patients with NIRS monitoring had a VMI score <85 (normal is 100), versus 6% without NIRS monitoring. Mean rSO₂ in the perioperative period was associated with VMI score, with no patient with mean rSO₂ ≥ 55 having VMI less than 96 [193].

Toet et al [194] studied 20 neonates undergoing the arterial switch operation and monitored rSO₂ for 4–12 h preoperatively, intraoperatively, and for 36 hours postoperatively, without intervention. Seven patients had a mean preoperative rSO₂ ≤35%, and two of these patients had significantly abnormal Bayley Scales of Infant Development Scores at 30–36 months, of 1–2 standard deviations below the normal population mean.

Kussman et al [195] studied 104 infants aged 9 months or less undergoing complete two-ventricle repair of transposition of the great arteries, tetralogy of Fallot or ventricular septal defect. Bilateral NIRS was monitored during the intraoperative period, and for 18 h postoperatively but no intervention was made on the basis of rSO₂ values. The aim of the study was to evaluate changes in rSO₂ and to determine association between low rSO₂ and early postoperative outcomes, including death, stroke, seizures or choreo-athetosis. An rSO₂ threshhold of 45% was chosen as the cut-off for analysis. pH stat blood gas management and hematocrit of 25–35%, along with brief DHCA and some low-flow bypass, was utilized. Eighty-one of 104 patients had no desaturation below 45%, 12 had brief desaturation below 45% for 1–39 min, and 11 had more prolonged desaturation of 60–383 min. Because no patient in the study died or suffered any neurological complication, the relationship between low rSO₂ and early neurological outcome could not be determined. There was also not a relationship between low rSO₂ and postoperative cardiac index, lactate, severity of illness or days ventilated, in the ICU or hospital. Thirty-nine of these patients had a period of DHCA, and important data about the rate of decline of rSO₂ under optimal CPB conditions were reported (Fig. 17.21). The important finding is that brief periods of DHCA <30 min did not result in nadir values of rSO₂, suggesting that this technique does not deplete the brain of oxygen stores and lending more credence to the idea that this practice is safe. The lack of an association between rSO₂ and early gross neurological outcomes is not unexpected, given that these were all two-ventricle patients, completely repaired,

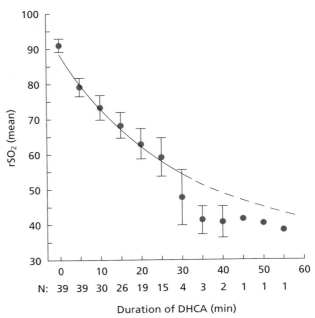

Figure 17.21 Pattern of cerebral rSO₂ during deep hypothermic circulatory arrest (DHCA) in 39 infants with D-transposition of the great arteries who underwent ≥5 min of DHCA. Data are presented as mean ± 1.96 SEM. The number of subjects (N) available for analysis at 5-min intervals of DHCA is shown. The fitted non-linear exponential decay curve (*solid line*) is based on data from 0 to 30 min with higher weight given to mean rSO₂ values calculated with more subjects. The fit is extrapolated beyond 30 min (*dashed line*). Reproduced from Kussman et al [195] with permission from Lippincott Williams & Wilkins.

with normal arterial oxygen saturations postoperatively. The low incidence and severity of cerebral desaturation in this population have been previously described [196] (Fig. 17.22).

Another potential benefit of routine NIRS monitoring is to avert the rare but very real and devastating potential neurological disaster from cannulation problems, where rSO₂ declines dramatically from cannula malposition and cerebral arterial or venous obstruction, yet all other bypass parameters are normal [197,198]. In neonates and infants, it is clear that mixed venous saturation in the bypass circuit bears very poor association with cerebral saturation, emphasizing the point that intracerebral desaturation may go unnoticed [199].

In a systematic review of 56 publications describing 1300 patients using NIRS monitoring for congenital heart disease in the operating room, intensive care unit, and cardiac catheterization laboratory, Hirsch et al [200] concluded that the technology did serve as a reliable, continuous, non-invasive monitor of cerebral oxygenation. However, to date there have not been any published prospective, randomized, controlled studies of NIRS monitoring versus no NIRS monitoring, with short- or long-term follow-up in pediatric patients. Many centers

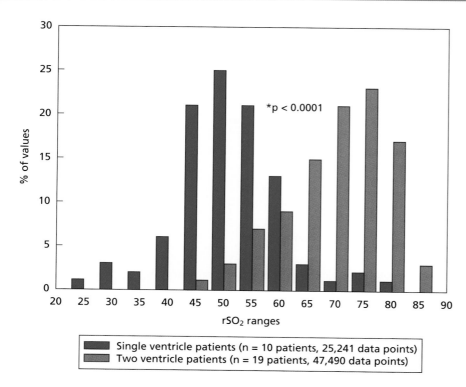

Figure 17.22 Frequency of rSO_2 values recorded at 1-min intervals in the first 48h postoperatively in neonates undergoing repair of hypoplastic left heart syndrome (single-ventricle patients) or D-transposition of the great arteries (two-ventricle patients). Reproduced from Andropoulos et al [196] with permission from Lippincott Williams & Wilkins.

where NIRS is now in routine clinical use will not have sufficient equipoise to conduct such a study.

Transcranial Doppler ultrasound

Transcranial Doppler ultrasound (TCD) is a sensitive, real-time monitor of cerebral blood flow velocity and emboli during congenital heart surgery. Currently available instruments utilize pulsed-wave ultrasound at 2 Mhz frequency, which is range gated, emits a power of 100 mW, and has a sample volume length of up to 15 mm. A display of the frequency spectrum of Doppler signals is easily interpreted, and peak systolic and mean flow velocities, in cm/sec, are displayed, as well as a pulsatility index which is equal to the peak velocity minus the end-diastolic velocity, divided by the mean velocity.

The most consistent and reproducible technique for clinical use in patients of all ages is to monitor the middle cerebral artery (MCA) through the temporal window, which can usually be found just above the zygoma and just anterior to the tragus of the ear [201]. Several transducer probes are available, ranging from very small disk probes suitable for infants and children, to larger, heavier probes for adolescents and adults. The depth of the sample volume and angle of insonation are adjusted until the bifurcation of the MCA and the anterior cerebral artery (ACA) is detected. This is heralded by a maximal antegrade signal (positive deflection, toward the transducer) from the MCA, accompanied by retrograde flow

(negative deflection, away from the transducer) of the same or very similar velocity and waveform, as the MCA flow. The same location should be monitored for an individual patient. Insonation at the MCA–ACA bifurcation also offers the advantage of minimizing interpatient variability. In addition, the MCA supplies the largest volume of tissue of any of the basal cerebral arteries [202]. In infants, an alternative site for monitoring is through the anterior fontanelle, using a hand-held pencil-type probe, placing the probe over the lateral edge of the fontanelle and aiming caudally, at a greater depth than for the temporal window.

Transcranial Doppler has been used extensively in pediatric cardiac surgical research to examine cerebral physiology in response to cardiopulmonary bypass, hypothermia, low-flow bypass, regional low-flow perfusion to the brain and circulatory arrest. Hillier et al [203] used TCD to study cerebrovascular hemodynamics during hypothermic bypass with DHCA in 10 infants, finding that cerebral blood flow velocity did not return to baseline levels after DHCA. Calculated cerebral vascular resistance (mean arterial pressure – central venous pressure/cerebral blood flow velocity (CBFV)) was increased immediately after DHCA, and remained so until the end of bypass. The observed decrease in CBFV during cooling was thought to be due to decreased metabolic demand by the brain and thus less blood flow, although α-stat strategy was used. This could be explained by relative cerebral vasoconstriction during cooling in smaller arterioles downstream to the MCA and ACA, since these large arteries do not change their caliber in response to changes in $PaCO_2$ [204]. TCD of the MCA through the temporal window was used to describe the cerebral pressure–flow velocity relationship during hypothermic bypass in 25 infants less than 9 months old. CBFV was examined over a wide range of cerebral perfusion pressures (varying from 6 to 90 mmHg), and at three temperatures: normothermia (36–37°C), moderate hypothermia (23–25°C), and profound hypothermia (14–20°C). Cerebral pressure flow autoregulation was preserved at normothermia, partially affected at moderate hypothermia, and totally lost at profound hypothermia, results which agree with previous research done using xenon to quantitate cerebral blood flow [205].

Transcranial Doppler has also been utilized to determine the threshold of detectable cerebral perfusion during low-flow cardiopulmonary bypass. Zimmerman et al [206] studied 28 neonates undergoing the arterial switch operation with α-stat pH management. At 14–15°C the pump flow was sequentially reduced to 0 mL/kg/min. All patients had detectable cerebral blood flow down to 20 mL/kg/min, while one had no perfusion at 20 mL/kg/min, and eight had none at 10 mL/kg/min, leading the authors to conclude that 30 mL/kg/min was the minimum acceptable flow in this population. Finally, Andropoulos et al [207] used TCD of the MCA to determine the level of bypass flow necessary during regional low-flow perfusion for neonatal aortic arch reconstruction. They studied 34 neonates undergoing the Norwood operation or aortic arch advancement and established a baseline mean CBFV (22 cm/sec) under full-flow bypass (150 mL/kg/min) using pH stat management at 17–22°C. They then used TCD to determine how much bypass flow was necessary to match this value, finding that a mean of 63 mL/kg/min was necessary.

Cerebral emboli are a frequent threat during open heart surgery in children. Emboli are easily detected by TCD, although this is subject to artifacts such as electrocautery and physical contact with the ultrasound transducer [208]. The number of emboli detected in the carotid artery during pediatric congenital heart surgery did not appear to correlate with acute postoperative neurological deficits [208]. However, acute drops in cerebral blood flow detected by TCD can allow for adjustment of aortic or superior vena cava cannulas, which may avert neurological disaster [209].

Electroencephalographic technologies

The standard electroencephalogram (EEG) employing 2–16 channels has been utilized in congenital heart surgery [180]. It is a rough guide of anesthetic depth and can document electrocerebral silence before DHCA [210].

EEG is affected by several factors including anesthetic agents, temperature, and CPB. Impracticalities of the use of an intraoperative EEG include electrical signal interference, complexity of placement and interpretation. Newer devices using processed EEG technology are more user friendly and have been extensively reviewed [211,212]. The value of perioperative EEG monitoring in congenital heart surgery is unclear. For example, hypoplastic left heart syndrome neonates frequently have a normal perioperative EEG yet frequently demonstrate abnormalities of pre- and postoperative brain MRI suggestive of ischemia [179].

The Bispectral Index (BIS) monitor (Aspect Medical Systems, Nantick, MA) is currently promoted to guide the depth of anesthesia. BIS sensor electrodes are applied to the forehead and temple, producing a frontal-temporal montage, which connects to a processing unit. The device is easy to use, electrodes are easy to place and the monitor requires no calibration or warm-up time. Via a proprietary algorithm of the Aspect Corporation, BIS uses Fourier transformation and bispectral analysis of a one-channel processed EEG pattern to compute a single number, the Bispectral BIS index [213]. This index ranges from 0 (isoelectric EEG) to 100 (awake) with mean awake values in the 90–100 range in adults, infants and children [214]. Depth of sedation is difficult to predict using BIS scores due to significant individual variability and anesthetic agent [215]. For BIS to be effective as a monitor of the depth of anesthesia, one would have to know exact BIS values for each anesthetic administered for an individual patient, thus reducing its value [216]. BIS can be used to recognize EEG burst suppression or electrical silence, which could be useful during deep hypothermic circulatory arrest. The monitor displays a real-time EEG waveform, but is subject to motion artifact, EMG activity and radiofrequency interference from electrical equipment in the operating room. Little or no data exist in children on the use of other EEG devices such as the Physiometrix®, Narcotrend® or Cerebral Function Monitor® [211].

During CPB, hemodilution and hypothermia alter pharmacokinetics and pharmacodynamics, which can lead to awareness under anesthesia. The overall incidence of awareness in adults undergoing cardiac surgery varies from 1.1% [216] to 23% which is more than in general surgical procedures [217,218]. The incidence of awareness under general anesthesia is similar in children [219]. Although there are no documented reports of awareness under anesthesia in children undergoing heart surgery, BIS monitoring may still be useful to detect a level of awareness.

In a cohort of children undergoing open heart surgery with an anesthetic tailored for "fast-tracking," BIS scores increased during rewarming, a period considered at risk for awareness under anesthesia [220]. However, in this study, and in a similar study in infants less than 1 year of age [221], BIS did not correlate with stress hormone levels, a surrogate for light levels of anesthesia, nor with plasma fentanyl levels. At present, there is little evidence to support the use of BIS in neonates and infants undergoing anesthesia and therefore the value of BIS to assess burst suppression during DHCA is in further doubt. This is due to the different sleep arousal patterns in this subset.

Because of the similarities of the full EEG in children over age 12 to the adult EEG, processed EEG monitoring in older children above the age of 12 years will produce similar patterns to those of the adult. Therefore it would appear more logical to use these devices in older patients, and especially under special anesthetic techniques, i.e. total intravenous anesthesia for spine surgery in the adolescent [222,223].

CASE STUDY

A 3-year-old, 14.2 kg, 95 cm tall boy presented for major resection of stage IV Wilms tumor with IVC extension [224]. He presented 3 months before the scheduled surgery with significant right-sided abdominal distension and pain. He did not have any other medical problems, and did not exhibit the phenotype of any genetic syndrome. Initial imaging with MRI revealed unilateral large renal tumor with renal vein and IVC extension to just below the right atrium. Fine needle aspiration with computed tomography guidance revealed Wilms tumor with favorable histology. There were no intracardiac masses, but there were eight pulmonary nodules. Because of the IVC extension near the right atrium, preoperative chemotherapy with vincristine, actinomycin D, and doxorubicin was initiated. Long-term central venous access (Port-a-Cath®) was placed via the left subclavian vein 1 week after diagnosis. Echocardiography the day before surgery revealed normal cardiac anatomy and function, without intracardiac shunting, masses or valvular disease. Tumor mass could be seen in the IVC just below the right atrium. Chest radiograph was clear. Vital signs were: BP 120/85 mmHg, P 125 bpm, R 28/min, T 36.5°C, SpO₂ 98% on room air. Preoperative laboratory studies included normal electrolytes, BUN 16 mg/dL, creatinine 0.6 mg/dL, hemoglobin 10.5 g/dL, white blood cell count 7500/mm³, platelet count 156,000/mm³, and normal prothrombin, partial thromboplastin, international normalized ratio (INR), and liver function tests.

A combined surgical procedure with cardiac and general surgeons was planned, via a right thoracoabdominal incision with cardiopulmonary bypass standby. Four units of irradiated, CMV-safe packed red blood cells (PRBC) were cross-matched. Because of the anticipated large blood loss and plan to leave the trachea intubated postoperatively, epidural analgesia was not used. After premedication with midazolam 2 mg IV, the patient was transported to the operating room where late-generation pulse oximeter, ECG, and automated oscillometric blood pressure cuff were placed. After preoxygenation, anesthesia was induced with propofol 2 mg/kg, fentanyl 3 μg/kg, and vecuronium 0.3 mg/kg. After tracheal intubation with a 4.5 mm cuffed orotracheal tube, a 22 ga right radial arterial catheter was placed. Because of the need to cross-clamp the IVC for tumor resection, a 20 ga IV catheter was placed in the right and 18 ga IV catheter in the left antecubital vein. The patient's blood volume was estimated to be 75 mL/kg or 1065 mL. It was decided that transfusion would be initiated at hematocrit of 25%, so allowable blood loss was calculated as 1065 mL × (32%−25%)/32% = 232 mL. Because of the anticipated large blood loss and fluid shifts, and variation in cardiac output, a continuous central venous oxygen saturation (ScvO₂) catheter was placed in the right internal jugular vein (IJV). Full sterile barrier precautions and ultrasound guidance were used, the IJV was entered first pass and a 4.5 Fr double-lumen ScvO₂ catheter was secured at 8 cm after confirmation of guidewire placement in the vein. A pediatric TEE probe was placed to monitor for intracardiac tumor emboli, and cardiac filling and function. A 10 Fr urinary catheter and rectal temperature probe were placed, a full-body forced air warming blanket placed under the patient, and he was positioned in left lateral decubitus position. Anesthesia was maintained with isoflurane, 0.5–1.5% end-tidal concentration, and intermittent boluses of fentanyl, midazolam, and vecuronium.

The surgical plan was to perform the thoracoabdominal incision, expose the right kidney and tumor with retroperitoneal dissection, and then cross-clamp the IVC to debulk the tumor and prevent emboli. If it was not possible to cross-clamp above the tumor, a short period of cardiopulmonary bypass was planned to remove the IVC and right atrial tumor. The IVC was cross-clamped successfully with retraction of the right lung, after intravascular volume loading with 15 mL/kg 5% albumin resulting in an increase of central venous pressure (CVP) from 5 to 10 mmHg. A large decrease in venous return, accompanied by decrease of CVP to 3 mmHg, decreased blood pressure to 55/35 mmHg, and increase in heart rate to 135 bpm with a decrease in ScvO₂ from 74% baseline (calibrated with a measured oxygen saturation drawn from the CVP catheter) to 44%, ensued. The end-tidal CO_2 also decreased from 37 to 23 mmHg, reflecting decreased cardiac output and pulmonary blood flow, but TEE revealed no evidence of pulmonary embolus.

During the 30 min of IVC cross-clamp, necrotic but non-friable tumor mass was resected from the IVC down as far as possible toward the renal veins. Blood loss was 350 mL during this phase, and was replaced with two units PRBC, with an additional six units ordered at that time. Intermittent boluses of calcium chloride ($CaCl_2$), 10 mg/kg and a low-dose epinephrine infusion of 0.03 µg/kg/min were used during this period to augment cardiac output and vascular tone, because of the intermittent hypotension, and decrease in $ScvO_2$ to 40–50% range. After de-airing, and repair of the IVC incision, the cross-clamp was released and the patient suffered a period of bradycardia to a heart rate of 50 bpm, hypotension to 45/25 mmHg, arterial desaturation to 88%, and decreased $ScvO_2$ to 30%. This responded to two 10 µg/kg boluses of epinephrine, sodium bicarbonate 2 meq/kg, intravascular volume infusion with 5% albumin 10 mL/kg, additional $CaCl_2$, and hyperventilation. Using a point-of-care system in the operating room, arterial blood gases after cross-clamp removal and resuscitation revealed a pH 7.25, $PaCO_2$ 34 mmHg, PaO_2 250 mmHg, base deficit of −13, and lactate of 8.5 mmol/L, with hematocrit of 32%. End-tidal CO_2 had been as low as 18 mmHg, and returned to 32 mmHg after the period of cross-clamp. TEE revealed no tumor emboli during this period, but depressed biventricular function after removal of the cross-clamp. After additional sodium bicarbonate and increasing epinephrine to 0.05 µg/kg/min, biventricular function normalized.

The resection of kidney and tumor, retroperitoneal lymph node dissection, and removal of tumor from renal veins and the remainder of the IVC required 6 additional hours of surgery. Hourly values of vital signs, blood gas values, hematocrit, blood loss, and $ScvO_2$ are listed in Table 17.7. Urine output became bloody 2 h into the resection, and was maintained at 2 mL/kg/h with intravascular volume infusions without adding diuretics. Temperature was maintained at 35.5–36.5°C throughout the case with the forced air warming blanket set at 38°C, warmed intravenous fluids, colloids, and blood, with fluid warmer set at 41°C and room temperature warmed to 25°C, as well as the use of a condenser humidifier.

A tissue factor-activated thromboelastogram (TEG) was sent 4 h into the case and with turnaround time of 20 min,

revealed a significant coagulopathy with prolonged r and K times, reduced α angle, and reduced maximum amplitude. This occurred after a total blood loss of 1000 mL and resulted in infusion of half a pheresis unit of platelets (equivalent to three random single units), one unit of fresh frozen plasma (FFP), and two units of cryoprecipitate, to treat the thrombocytopenia, hypofibrinogenemia, and depleted coagulation factors indicated by the severely abnormal TEG. Five hours into the resection, the serum K+ level was 6.3 mmol/L, presumably secondary to transfusion of the 12 units of PRBC to that time. As serum glucose was 288 mg/dL at the time, the hyperkalemia was treated with regular insulin 3 units, 25% dextrose 0.5 mL/kg, $CaCl_2$, and sodium bicarbonate, and by the next hour K+ was 4.4 mmol/L.

At the end of the case, total blood loss was estimated to be 3250 mL and the patient received 14 units PRBC, four units FFP, eight units cryoprecipitate, and two full pheresis units of platelets. Additional fluids were 300 mL of 5% albumin and 100 mL Plasmalyte®. Urine output total was 250 mL. Total fentanyl dose was 150 µg/kg. TEE during the case revealed no evidence of air or tumor embolus, variable biventricular function and filling, but by the end of the case hemostasis had been achieved, cardiac function was normal, and epinephrine weaned to 0.02 µg/kg/min. The patient was transported with his trachea intubated to the pediatric intensive care unit after loading with 0.3 mg/kg of morphine, and additional midazolam. He was extubated 48 h later and made an excellent recovery without significant end-organ dysfunction, and intact neurological status.

Conclusions

This case illustrates the use of continuous hemodynamic monitoring, including $ScvO_2$, to instantaneously guide treatment during a major tumor resection with wide hemodynamic swings due to massive blood loss, cross-clamping the IVC, and impendence of venous return during IVC compression. In addition, TEE was used to rule out tumor emboli, and hourly rapid point-of-care testing of arterial blood gases, electrolyes, hematocrit, glucose, lactate, and ionized calcium, as well as rapid TEG, used to direct therapy to restore intravascular volume, cardiac output and oxygen delivery, and the coagulation system. End-organ injury was prevented by effective management guided by intensive monitoring.

Table 17.7 Hourly intraoperative values for Wilms tumor case study

Hour	1	2	3	4	5	6	7
BP mmHg	92/52	76/40	82/40	72/32	76/36	66/37	78/47
HR bpm	105	135	125	138	139	142	119
pH	7.36	7.25	7.32	7.30	7.28	7.26	7.34
$PaCO_2$ mmHg	36	34	35	38	36	37	38
PaO_2 mmHg	356	250	345	326	237	178	192
BE calculated mmol/L	−4	−13	−6	−6	−9	−11	−5
Hct%	32	32	26	28	30	31	34
$ScvO_2$%	74%	68%	57%	59%	60%	64%	69%
Ca^{2+} mmol/L	1.15	1.02	0.98	1.05	1.11	1.03	1.13
Glucose mg/dL	115	187	197	235	288	125	110
K+ mmol/L	4.2	4.6	4.9	5.2	6.3	4.4	4.5
Lactate mmol/L	1.8	8.5	8.6	9.0	8.8	8.4	7.6

BE, base excess; BP, blood pressure; Ca^{2+}, serum ionized calcium; Hct%, percentage hematocrit; HR, heart rate; K+, serum ionized potassium; $ScvO_2$, central venous oxygen saturation in superior vena cava.

Annotated references

A full reference list for this chapter is available at:
http://www.wiley.com/go/gregory/andropoulos/pediatricanesthesia

5. Miller MR, Griswold M, Harris JM 2nd et al. Decreasing PICU catheter-associated bloodstream infections: NACHRI's quality transformation efforts. Pediatrics 2010; 125: 206–13. Outlines the evidence base and proper procedures for central catheter placement, and the conclusive evidence that such procedures reduce infections, morbidity, and death.

31. Andropoulos DB, Bent ST, Skjonsby B, Stayer SA. The optimal length of insertion of central venous catheters for pediatric patients. Anesth Analg 2001; 93: 883–6. Provides the basis for correct placement if superior vena cava catheters to prevent cardiac perforation in >500 patients.

63. Verghese ST, McGill WA, Patel RI et al. Ultrasound-guided internal jugular venous cannulation in infants: a prospective comparison with the traditional palpation method. Anesthesiology 1999; 91: 71–7. Provides the evidence that ultrasound guided internal jugular cannulation in infants is superior to traditional landmark palpation methods, with an optimal study design.

135. Cote CJ, Rolf N, Liu LM et al. A single blind study of combined pulse oximetry and capnography in children. Anesthesiology 1991; 74: 980–87. The classic study demonstrating a substantial reduction in critical desaturations and ventilation problems with both methods combined. Provides the major evidence base to require such monitoring.

155. Choudhury M, Kiran U, Choudhary SK et al. Arterial-to-end-tidal carbon dioxide tension difference in children with congenital heart disease. J Cardiothorac Vasc Anesth 2006; 20: 196–201. A careful study of 100 children with cyanotic and acyanotic heart disease, and their predicted to observed arterial to end tidal CO_2 differences before and after surgery. Concludes that there are many variables, making it difficult to predict the difference in an individual patient, but in general the more cyanotic the patient, the larger the difference.

159. Badgwell JM, Swan J, Foster AC. Volume controlled ventilation is made possible in infants by using compliant breathing circuits with large compression volume. Anesth Analg 1996; 82: 719–23. A now classic study defining the problems of adapting adult anesthesia circuits, ventilators, and monitoring to infants and small children. Provided the basis for the design of modern anesthesia ventilators for children.

180. Austin EH III, Edmonds HL Jr, Auden SM. Benefit of neurophysiologic monitoring for pediatric cardiac surgery. J Thorac Cardiovasc Surg 1997; 114: 707–15, 717. To date, the best study, in 250 children, that application of neuromonitoring, including near infrared spectroscopy, with a treatment algorithm, will improve acute neurological outcomes in pediatric cardiac surgery.

190. Hoffman GM, Ghanayem NS, Mussatto KM et al. Postoperative two-site NIRS predicts complications and mortality after stage 1 palliation of hypoplastic left heart syndrome. Anesthesiology 2007; 107: A234. Provides the basis for the use of somatic near infrared spectroscopy to manage neonates after cardiac surgery, using this new non-invasive method to direct treatment.

191. Kaufman J, Almodovar MC, Zuk J, Freisen RH. Correlation of abdominal site near infrared spectroscopy with gastric tonometry in infants following surgery for congenital heart disease. Pediatr Crit Care Med 2008; 9: 62–8. Provides the basis, and data, that near infrared spectroscopy is a valid, viable, non-invasive method to monitor the systemic circulation in major pediatric surgery.

222. Davidson AJ. Monitoring the anaesthetic depth in children – an update. Curr Opin Anaesthesiol 2007; 20(3): 236–43. A recent review of methods for monitoring anesthetic depth in children.

Video clips

This chapter contains the following video clips:

Video clip 17.1 Ultrasound guided internal jugular vein catheterization.
Video clip 17.2 Doppler assisted femoral vein catheterization.
Video clip 17.3 Radial artery catheterization.
They can be accessed at:

http://www.wiley.com/go/gregory/andropoulos/pediatricanesthesia

CHAPTER 18

Pediatric Regional Anesthesia

Claude Ecoffey

Service d'Anesthésie-Réanimation Chirurgicale, Hôpital Pontchaillou, University of Rennes, Rennes, France

Introduction

Pediatric regional anesthesia has attained widespread use internationally because of its efficacy and safety; its use is supported by the extensive data from the international literature underlining the safety and efficacy of this technique [1–3]. Safer drugs and dedicated pediatric tools are the keys to this success. This is so despite the fact that general anesthesia is necessary in most children for the regional block to be performed easily, safely, and effectively. Indeed, the benefit/risk ratio is excellent, especially for peripheral blocks, even when beginners perform these blocks. All the regional blocks require complete knowledge of the anatomical landmarks and underlying nerve anatomy, and specialists in pediatric anesthesiology should supervise trainees closely in order to prevent repeated errors. Despite its well-known benefits, clinical failures can occur during the application of regional anesthetic technique. Neurovascular anatomy is highly vari-able, and currently available nerve localization techniques provide little or no information regarding the anatomical spread of local anesthesia; furthermore, traditional nerve localization techniques (nerve stimulation) rely on anatomical assumptions that may be incorrect.

Recently, ultrasound guidance has been shown to improve block characteristics, resulting in shorter block performance time, higher success rates, shorter onset, longer block duration, reduction in volume of local anesthetic agents required, and better visibility of neuraxial structures.

Embryology and developmental physiology of the peripheral nervous system

The nervous system and the spinal cord are not fully developed at birth, and several morphological

Gregory's Pediatric Anesthesia, Fifth Edition. Edited by George A. Gregory, Dean B. Andropoulos.

particularities must be considered. There are some differences in the anatomy of spinal cord meninges between a neonate and an adult. During the embryonic period, the spinal cord fills the spinal canal but from the fetal period onward, the growth of the spinal canal exceeds that of neural structures; consequently, the caudal end of the spinal cord and the dural sac occur at progressively higher levels. The tip of the spinal cord is at L3 at birth and L1–2 at 1 year. In the same way, the meninges are at S3 at birth and S4–5 at 1 year. In addition, infants and children weighing less than 15 kg have a relatively high volume of cerebrospinal fluid (CSF), 4 mL/kg bodyweight, compared with adult values of 2 mL/kg bodyweight. The contents of the epidural space in infants differ from those of adults. Instead of having mature, densely packed fat lobules, divided by fibrous strands, they have spongy, gelatinous lobules with distinct spaces permitting the wide longitudinal spread of injected solutions.

The spine undergoes significant morphological and structural change throughout childhood and adolescence. At birth, it displays a simple regular flexure throughout, so that any epidural needle with the same orientation can be inserted in any given intervertebral space. With the development of the cervical flexure in the sitting position, i.e. head position sustained upright, and then that of the lumbar lordosis with the development of standing and walking, the orientation of the epidural needle must be modified accordingly. During infancy and early childhood, the vertebrae are cartilaginous; ossification of the vertebrae is a progressive phenomenon. The ossification nucleus can be damaged by incorrect epidural block technique. Due to the late osseous fusion of the sacrum, intervertebral epidural approaches can be performed at all sacral levels throughout childhood.

Myelination begins in cervical neuromeres during the fetal period and continues downward and upward until the 12th year of life [4]. In an infant, the fiber diameter is smaller, the myelin sheath thinner and the internodal distance smaller, so a lower concentration of local anesthetic is needed to achieve the nerve block and to avoid toxic effects. Furthermore, the relative resistance to epidural blockade of the L5–S1 nerve roots observed in adults does not occur in pediatric patients because of the smaller diameter of nerve fibers. The local distribution is excellent due also to the fact that nerve envelopes are loosely attached to underlying nerve structures, which favors the spread of local anesthetics along the nerves and the roots.

There are important differences between infants, small children and adults in the physiological effects of central blocks. It is a constant finding that the incidence of clinically significant hypotension and bradycardia following spinal or epidural anesthesia is lower than in adult patients [5]. Despite the absence of prior intravenous volume loading and the high level of sympathetic blockade, blood pressure and cardiac index are not modified by the block [6]. There is less vasodilation in infants than in older children and adults, and infants respond to high thoracic sympathetic blocade by reflex withdrawal of vagal parasympathetic tone to the heart [7].

Local anesthetics and toxicity

Amide local anesthetics used for regional anesthesia in pediatric patients are potent sodium channel blockers and thus they block impulse conduction in axons. Local anesthetics (LAs) have other actions that may contribute to both local and systemic toxicities and to beneficial systemic actions on inflammatory responses [4] or chronic pain conditions. Amide local anesthetics are potent sodium channel blockers with marked stereospecificity, which consistently influences their action, especially their toxic action on the heart. At toxic concentrations, they induce severe arrhythmias with the potential for cardiac arrest.

The primary local anesthetic agents used in pediatric regional techniques are 2-chloroprocaine, lidocaine, bupivacaine, ropivacaine, mepivacaine, and tetracaine. The pharmacology of local anesthetics in children is similar to that in adults. In neonates and infants, however, the greater total body water volume results in a larger volume of distribution and therefore longer elimination half-life. 2-Chloroprocaine 2% or 3% has a short time to onset of action and a short duration of action. Lidocaine 0.5% to 2% has a short time to onset and medium duration of action. It can be used for peripheral blocks or epidural anesthesia. Bupivacaine 0.1% to 0.5% has a longer onset time and duration of action than lidocaine or 2-chloroprocaine but has a greater potential for severe cardiotoxicity than other agents. It can be used for peripheral blocks, spinal anesthesia, and caudal or epidural anesthesia and analgesia. Tetracaine 1% is used for spinal anesthesia. Mepivacaine is approximately equally potent to lidocaine and can safely be used for peripheral nerve blocks. It can provide a rapid onset of block, with a shorter duration of motor block that may allow for rapid recovery in the postoperative period. Ropivacaine 0.2% to 1% and levobupivacaine 0.25 to 0.5% may replace the racemic mixture of bupivacaine because of their decreased potential for central nervous system toxicity and cardiotoxicity. Ropivacaine differs from bupivacaine in various aspects: it is a pure S-enantiomer and its lipid solubility is markedly lower; these characteristics can significantly improve its safety profile. Levobupivacaine, the S-enantiomer of racemic bupivacaine, is less cardiotoxic while showing similar LA properties and the potency of racemic bupivacaine. Indeed, several cases of central nervous system toxicity have been reported after inadvertent intravascular administration of ropivacaine or levobupivacaine in adults, but only a few cases of cardiovascular toxicity have been reported to date [8,9]. The outcome of these inadvertent intravascular administrations was favorable, even in a neonate [10].

Pharmacokinetic factors

When injected into the body, the pure isomers do not undergo interconversion, meaning that they do not transform into the usual racemic compounds.

Local anesthetics bind to blood components – erythrocytes and serum proteins such as α1-acid glycoprotein (AAG) and albumin [11]. These buffer systems have different levels of importance; the AAG is by far the most important because it is specific. The red blood cells play a lesser role in sequestration of LA, with only 15–22% of bupivacaine molecules bound in erythrocytes at varying total concentrations of the LA [12]. This buffer system may become important when the LA blood concentration is very high beyond the toxic concentrations and with anemia (red blood cells bind less than 15% of molecules of LA when the hematocrit is <30%). Binding of amide LA to serum proteins is more important. Like all weak bases, amides are mainly bound to the AAG and serum albumin [11]. AAG concentration is 50–80 times lower in plasma than is albumin, particularly in infants. The determination of serum albumin LA binding is characterized by a low affinity but a high capacity, while the affinity of binding to the AAG is high but the capacity is low.

The AAG is the main serum protein involved in the binding of LA. Because AAG is a major acute-phase protein, its concentration rapidly increases when inflammatory processes develop, particularly during the first 6 h of the postoperative period [13]. In addition, the affinity of LA increases with the inflammatory processes; acidosis decreases this affinity. Neonates and infants have a lower AAG concentration in serum compared to adults [14] and therefore, their free fraction of LA is increased accordingly (Fig. 18.1). This has important clinical implications since, at least in steady state, the toxic effects of LAs are directly related to the free (unbound) drug concentration. In summary, there are no differences in protein binding between R- and S-enantiomers of bupivacaine, at least when the concentrations, even toxic, are observed in clinical practice [15].

After passing through the bloodstream, the amide LAs are excreted by the liver. This phase involves cytochrome P450. The clearance of bupivacaine, like the clearance of ropivacaine and levobupivacaine, ranges from 3 to 6 mL/kg/min. The renal clearance is low so the main metabolism of these agents is hepatic.

Local anesthetics are metabolized by cytochrome P450 (CYP). The main CYP isoforms involved are CYP3A4 for

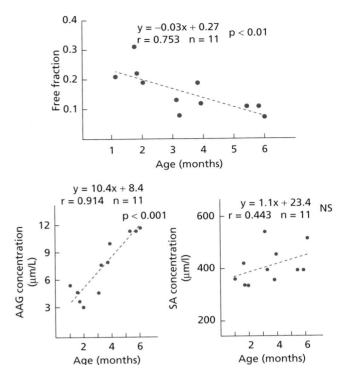

Figure 18.1 The major proteins involved in binding and the relationship between their concentrations and age (AAG, α1-acid glycoprotein, SA, serum albumin) (*bottom*) and the relationship between free fraction of bupivacaine in serum and age (*top*). The free fraction is increased at least until 6 months of life. Reproduced from Mazoit et al [14] with permission from Lippincott Williams and Wilkins.

lidocaine and bupivacaine [16] and CYP1A2 for ropivacaine [17]. CYP3A4 is not mature at birth but is partly replaced by CYP3A7 [18]. At 1 month of age, the intrinsic clearance of bupivacaine is only one-third of that in adults, and two-thirds at 6 months. CYP1A2 is not fully mature before the age of 3 years. Indeed, the clearance of ropivacaine does not reach its maximum before the age of 8 years [19]. However, at birth this clearance is not as low as expected [20], even with levobupivacaine [21], and ropivacaine and levobupivacaine may be used even in younger patients. Finally, the S- and R-enantiomers of LA kinetics are very similar and the slight differences that have been described do not have any clinical consequences.

Pharmacodynamic factors

The R- and S-enantiomers of a LA molecule have different pharmacodynamic effects on the myocardium and the nerve. The physiology of nerve activity is the summation of numerous complex events and interactions. A simple explanation is that in most cases, modulation of impulse frequency and not modulation of amplitude is more important in blocking function of the nerve. Upon the basic background activity is imposed an added impulse, for example a painful stimulus. The effects of LAs can be improved when the signal they are trying to block increases in frequency. Thus, in addition to the basic block (tonic block), there is added a nerve blockade (phasic block) whose intensity will increase with the frequency of nerve discharge or the heart rate, in the case of myocardial toxicity. Purkinje fibers of the myocardium are more sensitive to the blockade of sodium channels by LA than other fibers or myocytes. While heart rate is rather slow (between 40 and 200 beats/min), the frequency of nerve impulses is much faster. Therefore, the nerves, when stimulated, are immediately blocked due to this high fre-

quency of baseline activity, while the intensity of heart block increases with tachycardia. This is the physiological explanation for the preferential nerve block, well before any cardiac toxicity.

The S-enantiomers are unique in that they cause phasic blocks smaller than the R-enantiomers (and therefore than the racemic mixtures). In the nerve, difference is small because sodium channels involved at this level are minimally sensitive to the phasic block, because baseline frequency of nerve discharge is already rapid. In the heart, the difference is more important [22,23]. When the heart rate increases, the S-enantiomers increase the block of the sodium channels they generate much more slowly than the racemic mixtures (the difference between ropivacaine and levobupivacaine remains the same, equal to the difference in power level of the nerve) [22] (Fig. 18.2). However, though there is no intrinsic difference between newborn and adult animals, phasic block (the one that increases with frequency) plays a very important role (Fig. 18.3) [24] and we can well imagine that an infant, whose heart beats at 150 beats/min, is significantly more sensitive than an adult, whose heart beats at 75 beats/min.

The S-enantiomers levobupivacaine and ropivacaine cause moderate vasoconstriction, whatever the concentration range studied.

Adjuvants

The therapeutic index of LAs in infants may be so narrow that the maximum safe infusion rates of the amides are too low to provide sole analgesia for most major surgery in the thorax and abdomen. This would indicate a need

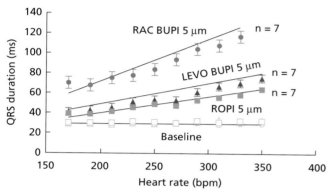

Figure 18.2 Rate dependence of QRS widening. QRS duration was measured at varying frequencies on isolated rabbit heart with bupivacaine, levobupivacaine and ropivacaine. The faster the heart rate, the more rapidly QRS widening occurred. Reproduced from Mazoit et al [22] with permission from Lippincott Williams and Wilkins.

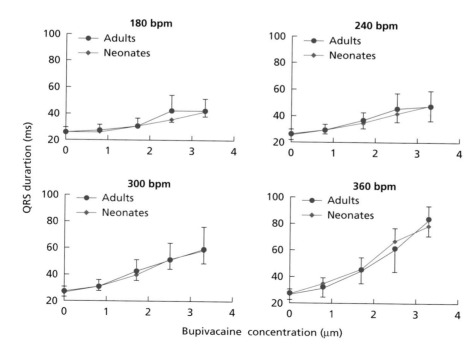

Figure 18.3 QRS widening as a function of bupivacaine concentration in the perfusate. The block is rate dependent, but no difference was found between adult and newborn rabbits. Reproduced from Mazoit et al [24] with permission from Lippincott Williams and Wilkins.

for combining LAs with either opioids or clonidine (or S+ ketamine, not available in some countries) to provide safe synergistic analgesic effects while maintaining safe LA dosing, administering acetaminophen and non-steroidal anti-inflammatory drugs (NSAIDs) to provide an additional systemic analgesic effect, and permiting low-dose intravenous opioids as rescue analgesics.

Intrathecal and epidural opioids were first administered to human subjects in 1979 [25] and since that time they have been proven to provide effective and prolonged analgesia. The presence of high concentrations of opioid receptors in the spinal cord makes it possible to achieve analgesia with small doses of morphine administered in either the intrathecal or epidural spaces. Intrathecal and epidural morphine doses produce more profound and prolonged analgesia than comparable morphine doses administered parenterally, and are capable of relieving both visceral and somatic pain. The use of morphine by the epidural route, either caudal [26] or lumbar [27], gives prolonged analgesia (more than 12h with a single injection of morphine) following abdominal, thoracic and cardiac surgery, and allows respiratory physiotherapy without pain. In addition, intrathecal morphine injection has been used to obtain postoperative analgesia following cardiac surgery or spinal fusion. A systematic review of post-thoracotomy analgesia concluded that a thoracic epidural infusion of LA with an opioid provided the most consistently effective analgesia [27]. The usual doses of epidural morphine range from 30 to 50 μg /kg. For single doses of epidural fentanyl, the dose range is 1–2 μg/kg, and for sufentanil 0.5–0.75 μg/kg. The dose for intrathecal morphine is 0.01–0.02 μg/kg. Continuous epidural infusion of LA can be combined with fentanyl 0.2 μg/kg/h or sufentanil 0.1 μg/kg/h.

This improvement in analgesia has to be balanced against the high incidence of undesirable side-effects which include respiratory depression (which may occur several hours after initial administration), nausea, vomiting, pruritus and urinary retention [28]. When administered for treatment of side-effects after epidural morphine, nalbuphine is better than naloxone for treating pruritus and vomiting/nausea [29]. For peripheral nerve blocks, there is little evidence for any analgesic benefit of using opioid analgesics in brachial plexus block over systemic administration.

Clonidine acts at the dorsal horn level, reducing the release of substance P. It gives an antinociceptive potentiation, prolonging the analgesic effect of bupivacaine or mepivacaine. The sedation provided by clonidine, due to an action at the locus coeruleus level, is dose dependent: sedation does not occur with a dose of 1 μg /kg or less, it is only apparent with a dose of 2 μg/kg or more. Usually, it is not considered a drawback for the pediatric patient (the child is both pain free and quiet) and children are

easily aroused. No side-effects have been described: no respiratory depression or hypotension (only with 5 μg/kg is there moderate hypotension). For continuous epidural infusion, clonidine doses lower than 0.08 μg/kg/h were not associated with any measurable effect, whereas doses of 0.08 μg/kg/h or greater produced both clinically and statistically significant improvements in postoperative analgesia [30]. Because a dose of 0.12 μg/kg/h was sufficient to provide excellent analgesia, higher doses may not be advisable as they produce excessive sedation with no increase in analgesia.

Ketamine is a potent anesthetic whose action is through the antagonism of N-methyl-D-aspartate receptors, present at the spinal level and involved in pain modulation. Older studies have been performed, using the preservative-containing formula on adults and in children. Newer studies performed with preservative-free ketamine, both the racemic and the isomeric drug, show that a dose of S-ketamine ranging between 0.25 and 0.5 mg/kg is optimal for prolonging the pain relief given by local anesthetic [31].

The addition of bicarbonate reduces the pain on injection [32]. This alters the pKa of the solution, making the LA available in the active cationic form. See Chapter 33 for further discussion of pain management.

Systemic toxicity

Recent reports in humans suggest that lipid emulsion (Intralipid®) is an effective therapy for cardiac toxicity from high systemic concentrations of ropivacaine and bupivacaine, even in patients for whom conventional resuscitation is ineffective [33]. The solubility of long-acting local anesthetics in lipid emulsions and the high binding capacity of these emulsions most probably explain their clinical efficacy in cases of toxicity. The long-chain triglyceride emulsion Intralipid® appears to be about 2.5 times more efficacious than the 50/50 medium-chain/long-chain Medialipide® emulsion [34]. No data exist in pediatrics except for a recent case in which a 20% lipid infusion was used to successfully treat a ventricular arrhythmia, after a ropivacaine and lidocaine injection in a psoas compartment block in a healthy 13-year-old child [35]. Indeed, a bolus of 1.5 mL/kg and then an infusion of 0.5–1 mL/kg/min of Intralipid® in combination with usual resuscitation should be useful to treat LA cardiac toxicity in children.

Preferably, lipid rescue is administered via a central venous catheter but in its absence, peripheral veins can also be used. A 20% lipid emulsion bolus over 1 min is recommended with an initial dose of 1.5 mL/kg, immediately followed by 1 mg atropine and small boluses of 10 μg/kg epinephrine in order to limit the increase in heart rate which is deleterious, as discussed above [22]. Chest compressions should not be interrupted. The

Intralipid bolus can be repeated with a maximum of 4 mL/kg/min. The lipid infusion is to be maintained at a rate of 0.5 mL/kg/min until hemodynamic recovery.

Lipid infusions act as an antidote to LA intoxication and should be readily available for emergencies, much in the way that type O-negative blood and dantrolene are now available universally. Intralipid® has a low cost and a shelf-life of up to 1 year. Guidelines for the management of severe LA toxicity provide essential information, which should be available in all hospitals, particularly in units where LA are administered. See Chapter 40 for further details of management of LA toxicity.

Local tissue toxicity

Skeletal muscle toxicity is a rare and uncommon side-effect of LAs, although experimental data show that intra-muscular injections of these agents regularly result in calcified myonecrosis [36]. All LAs that have been examined are myotoxic, in which the extent of muscle damage is dose dependent and worsens with serial or continuous administration. Pathophysiologically, increased intracellular Ca^{2+} levels appear to be the most important element in myocyte injury [37]. Lipophilicity also determines the extent of Ca^{2+} release by local anesthetics, as the effects of racemic bupivacaine and levobupivacaine were significantly more pronounced than those of ropivacaine isomers [38]. Consequently, a rank order of myotoxic potency (ropivacaine < bupivacaine < levobupivacaine) is suggested. The clinical impact of LA-induced myotoxicity is still controversial. Only a few case reports of myotoxic complications after LA administration have been published in adults. In particular, the occurrence of clinically relevant myopathy and myonecrosis has been described after continuous peripheral blocks; some experimental data have shown more toxicity in young animals,[39] so particular care must be taken with prolonged continuous infusion in infants.

Most recently, several studies have revealed that LAs might irreversibly damage chondrocytes in articular cartilage, which may contribute to cartilage degeneration [40]. Bupivacaine especially showed profound chondrotoxic effects in experimental models and although these results cannot be directly extrapolated to the clinical setting, caution should be exercised in the intra-articular use of this agent. Ropivacaine seems to be less chondrotoxic than bupivacaine [41] whereas the chondrotoxic potency of levobupivacaine has yet to be assessed.

Blocks for infants and children

Advantages of regional anesthesia

Regional anesthesia, in combination with light general anesthesia, provides several advantages for the pediatric patient. The most significant advantage, as demonstrated by several authors, is intra- and postoperative pain relief. Regional anesthesia is also useful when general anesthesia is technically difficult or is associated with increased morbidity and mortality, such as in the case of the ex-premature infant with the risk of postanesthetic apnea [42], the child with severe chronic respiratory disease [43] or the child with myopathy [44]. Regional anesthesia may offer an alternative to general anesthesia in children with a history of malignant hyperthermia.

Disadvantages of regional anesthesia

Regional anesthesia requires extra time to perform the block and allow it to become effective. Therefore, the use of an induction room will smooth the operating room work. If general anesthesia is needed to perform the block, an assistant can be helpful in supporting the airway and monitoring the patient during performance of the block. Critics of this combined technique suggest that one may be exposing the child to the risks and complications inherent in both. This fear, however, is more a theoretical consideration than a practical one. However, pediatric anesthesiologists now view regional anesthesia as an adjunct to general anesthesia, in much the same way that a neuromuscular blocking agent or intravenous narcotic supplements general anesthesia with a volatile agent [45].

Choice of regional anesthesia in children

Although blocks which are commonly used in adults are not always suitable for children, some regional blocks are particularly useful for children.

The recent Association of French Speaking Paediatric Anaesthetists (ADARPEF) study has clearly shown a transition in practice from predominantly central blocks to an increased number of peripheral nerve blocks, including catheter techniques (Tables 18.1, 18.2) [3]. The most common extremity blocks were axillary, both lateral and popliteal sciatic, femoral and iliofascial block. Face and trunk blocks represented the largest proportion of peripheral blocks. Trunk blocks were used significantly more often. They are characterized by the emergence of techniques that were not clearly accounted by the first ADARPEF study, i.e. (in order of decreasing frequency) ilio-inguinal, paraumbilical, pudendal, and thoracic and lumbar paravertebral blocks [1]. Facial blocks, not detailed previously, were a new and now widely used practice for facial and reconstructive surgery, particularly in cleft palate repair.

In addition, the recent ADARPEF study has recorded a significant number of catheter placements [3]. They were inserted for central as well in peripheral regional anesthe-

Table 18.1 Different regional block procedures according to patient's age: results from the first published ADARPEFstudy, local procedures excluded (n = 19,103)

Technique		0–30 days premature n = 149	0–30 days full term n = 398	1–6 mo premature n = 641	1–6 mo full term n = 2067	6 mo–3 yr n = 6164	3–12 yr n = 8114	>12 yr n = 1570	Total blocks	%
Central	Caudals	108	300	407	1536	4610	4978	172	12,111	63
	Other epidurals	5	38	30	176	416	1122	612	2396	13
	Spinals	30	25	188	137	50	18	58	506	3
Peripheral	Upper limbs	1	0	0	10	92	478	416	997	5
	Lower limbs	0	0	3	7	30	181	175	396	2
	Trunk, abdomen	5	35	13	201	969	1337	137	2697	14

Source: Giaufré et al [1].

Table 18.2 Different regional block procedures according to patient's age: results from the second published ADARPEFstudy (n = 31,132)

Technique		0–30 days premature n = 121	0–30 days full term n = 475	1–6 mo premature n = 822	1–6 mo full term n = 2442	6 mo–3 yr n = 10,499	3–12 yr n = 12,974	>12 yr n = 3,799	Total blocks	%
Central	Epidurals	82	227	428	1082	4495	3311	473	10,098	32.4
	Spinals	9	9	38	40	43	60	188	387	1.3
	Others central	0	0	0	4	1	23	43	71	0.3
Peripheral	Upper limbs	1	2	5	36	454	1099	484	2081	6.7
	Lower limbs	2	12	14	62	529	1540	1665	3824	12.4
	Trunk, abdomen	22	154	288	1063	4506	6185	612	12,830	41.0
	Face, head	5	71	49	155	471	756	334	1841	5.9

Source: Ecoffey et al [3].

sia, most of them being neuraxial. Indeed, neuraxial continuous epidural analgesia is one of the preferred techniques for obtaining pain relief in children (particularly postoperative pain relief in younger children). Perineural catheters have become a common practice, primarily in hip and foot surgery. Several prospective studies demonstrated the benefits of continuous peripheral nerve blockade after orthopedic procedures in children. Placement of a brachial plexus catheter for pain control is less common in children than in adults. The emergence of peripheral nerve catheter techniques allows provision of postoperative pain relief for the majority orthopedic surgeries using regional anesthesia techniques [46,47] and to treat complex regional pain syndrome in adolescents [48]. The recent ADARPEF study confirmed this emergence of peripheral catheters, mainly axillary and sciatic popliteal, and records slightly fewer neuraxial catheters than the recently published United Kingdom audit, which reported 10,633 epidural catheters (about 2000 per year) [2]. These results confirmed a retrospective report from a single institution (10,929 regional anesthesia procedures performed during a 17-year period) revealing a dramatic decrease in central neuraxial blocks [49]; continuous postoperative analgesia via perineural catheters emerged as routine practice in children in the late 1990s following both peer recommendations and evolution of devices.

Regional blockade with or without general anesthesia

Without general anesthesia

Most children do not like needles or injections. Small, frightened children are unlikely to keep still unless well sedated. Thus LA techniques alone are not usually used in children under about 8–10 years of age. After that age, a co-operative child who has had the procedure explained may tolerate a block for such procedures as suturing lacerations, reduction of a fracture or minor procedures on an extremity. Adequate sedation and/or the presence of a reassuring parent facilitates the procedure. New methods of giving sedatives, opioids, and LAs transdermally will be of great benefit to peripheral LA techniques in the conscious child.

If the use of a nerve stimulator is planned, the child will need to be well sedated. A nerve stimulator will facilitate the use of neural blockade in an anxious child, since motor responses can be obtained without causing discomfort if sedation is adequate. The use of ultrasonography alone is helpful to perform peripheral blocks in an awake child, due to the lack of elicited motor responses.

With general anesthesia

In children, regional anesthesia is often combined with light general anesthesia, but there must be justifiable advantages to the child. Such potential advantages are summarized above. In addition, general anesthesia decreases central nervous system (CNS) toxicity and dysrhythmias caused by LAs [50,51]. The decision to intubate the trachea or to use a laryngeal mask airway should be based on the usual criteria, such as a full stomach, upper abdominal surgery or the need to maintain adequate ventilation. If indicated, the trachea should be intubated before the block is begun.

Techniques for performing regional anesthesia

Patient monitoring

Monitors should be applied and functions tested before the block is performed. In particular, the electrocardiogram should be adjusted so that the P wave, QRS complex, and upright T wave can be seen clearly. Baseline systolic blood pressure and heart rates should be noted.

Skin preparation

Bacterial colonization of epidural and caudal catheters in children occurs at a rate of 6–35%. Gram-positive organisms are most common, though gram-negative colonization may also occur, particularly with caudal catheters. Children under 3 years of age are also most likely to have colonization of caudal catheters. Despite high rates of colonization, serious epidural infections are exceedingly rare. Chlorhexidine may be better than povidone-iodine for reducing the risk of catheter colonization in children [52].

Test dose

While placement of regional blocks under general anesthesia is considered standard practice in children, the search for the ideal "test dose" to reduce the risk of inadvertent intravascular injection continues. The original "test dose" described an increase in heart rate and blood pressure following intravenous administration of epinephrine 0.5 µg/kg, which is equivalent to 0.1 mL/kg IV injection of LA with epinephrine 1:200,000. In children these hemodynamic changes vary with the anesthetic agent used (halothane, sevoflurane or isoflurane) and whether prior atropine has been administered. However, an increase in heart rate of 10 beats per minute above baseline occurring within 1 min of injection of 0.1 mL/kg of LA with 1:200,000 epinephrine is a reasonable predictor of intravascular injection for children anesthetized with sevoflurane. Monitoring the ECG changes, i.e. >25% change in T wave or ST segment changes irrespective of the lead chosen, is considered by some to be more specific and more reliable [53].

These changes have been questioned recently as it seems that similar changes in heart rate, blood pressure, and T wave may be seen following a painful stimulus (surgical incision). The temporal relationship is important and a secondary decrease in pulse rate detected after intravenous epinephrine distinguishes this from the response seen after a painful stimulus [54]. Nonetheless, LA solution should be administered slowly over a period of at least 60–120 sec, irrespective of the type of block, with repeated aspirations.

Sympathetic blockade

A clinically significant decrease in blood pressure related to sympathectomy from central neuraxial blocks is rare in children younger than 8 years of age [5]. Volume loading before such blocks, commonly practiced in adults, is unnecessary in this age group. In older patients, the sympathetic block results in a slight (20–25%) but consistent decrease in blood pressure. Even in adolescents, however, fluids or vasopressors are rarely required to treat the hemodynamic effects of central neuraxial blocks.

Contraindications

Contraindications to central neuraxial blocks are few and similar to those in adults. They include coagulopathy, infection at the insertion site, true LA allergy, and abnormal superficial landmarks or lumbosacral myelomeningocele because of the risk of malposition of the cord or dural sac. Progressive neurological disease is a relative contraindication primarily because of medico-legal concerns. The safety of central neuraxial techniques in the presence of a ventriculoperitoneal shunt has not been studied. Risks and benefits in these patients should be carefully considered on an individual basis.

Though it is rare to encounter opposition to the use of peripheral nerve blocks, certain conditions may call for a judicious avoidance of them. Relative contraindications include local infection, generalized sepsis, coagulopathy, predisposition to compartment syndrome, and parental or child dissent.

Nerve stimulator

Though not a substitute for anatomical knowledge, a nerve stimulator is useful to localize peripheral motor nerves in anesthetized children. In addition, the surface mapping of peripheral nerves with a nerve stimulator is helpful in children [55]. Because paresthesia cannot be elicited in an anesthetized child, the use of a nerve stimulator may decrease the potential for nerve damage. A nerve stimulator capable of delivering low voltage is preferred [56]. The stimulator should deliver electric current in short pulses lasting 50–100 msec of a constant intensity adjusted from 1.5 mA to 0.7 mA (0.5 mA if awake), and emitted at a frequency of 1–2 Hz. The sheathed needle is connected to the negative polarity of the generator, whereas the skin electrode is connected to the anode. Before injection, the appropriate muscular contractions should be obtained for a minimal intensity. An aspiration test should be done preceding each injection. When this has been identified, 1–2 mL of local anesthetic agent is injected. Immediate abolition of muscle movement indicates correct placement of the needle.

Impact of ultrasound on regional anesthesia

A significant problem in regional anesthesia is that a large number of techniques still do not achieve a success rate of close to 100%. Indeed, the key to successful regional anesthesia has always been the accuracy of needle and LA placement in relation to the nerve structures to be blocked. In 1994, Kapral introduced ultrasound guidance into regional anesthesia [57]. About 10 years later, Marhofer introduced this technique into pediatric regional anesthesia practice [58]. Real-time ultrasound guidance allows the demonstration of the target, whether it is nerve, fascial plane or anatomical space, and the monitoring of the distribution of the injected LA. Furthermore, ultrasound guidance allows the anesthesiologist to reposition the needle in the case of maldistribution of the LA.

There is some evidence to support ultrasound for various outcomes in pediatric regional anesthesia (Table 18.3) [59]. More randomized controlled studies with significant outcomes are required to further support these findings and to evaluate the potential for ultrasound to reduce complications of regional anesthesia in children. In addition, there are still two large obstacles to be overcome before this technique can attain the position of "gold standard" for the performance of regional anesthesia in infants and children. First, department heads and hospital managers need to make the necessary funds available to purchase ultrasound equipment. Second, training in the use of ultrasound-guided techniques is not easy. Dedicated efforts must be made to allow at least key individuals to attend focused training, so that these people can start to use and teach these techniques in their own institutions. Although the ultrasound-guided techniques will predominate in the future [60,61], more traditional techniques should not be forgotten.

Central neuraxial blocks

Caudal block

This is the most useful pediatric central block, as it is widely applicable and technically simple. It can provide analgesia for surgery up to and including the umbilicus. This technique can be used successfully in neonatal rectal surgery [62].

Performance of a caudal block (see Video clip 18.1)
The anesthetic agent is injected through the sacral hiatus, which is formed by failure of fusion of the fifth sacral vertebral arch. The hiatus is easily palpated in children as a triangular-shaped depression bounded on either side by the sacral cornua (Fig. 18.4). Following induction of general anesthesia, the child is placed in the lateral position with the knees drawn up, the upper knee being flexed more than the lower. The best approach to the sacral hiatus is found at the apex of an equilateral triangle based on a line drawn between the two posterior superior iliac spines (Fig. 18.5). A short beveled 22 gauge needle is inserted at 45° to the skin. When the needle pierces the sacrococcygeal membrane and enters the sacral canal, a distinct "pop" is felt. Then the needle is advanced an additional 0.5–1 cm, depending on the child's age, on a plane parallel to the spinal axis. After aspiration to exclude bone marrow, dural puncture or venepuncture, incremental doses of LA should be injected.

When there is difficulty identifying the sacral hiatus, the technique of intervertebral sacral blockade has been described in children. The puncture of the ligamentum flavum is performed in the S2–3 interspace, which is easily identified because it is the interspace just below the level of the posterior superior iliac spines.

On the other hand, we do not recommend the use of caudal epidural catheters because of the risk of sepsis due to the proximity of the anus. Therefore, caudal block is a single-shot technique. The lumbar epidural route is preferred if reinjection is needed, or in children weighing more than 20–25 kg to reduce the total amount of LA used. In this group of patients, we may use the lumbar epidural block as a single-shot technique. Moreover, if we

Table 18.3 Statements of evidence and grades of recommendation for the ultrasound guidance regional anesthesia outcomes

Evaluated outcomes	Statements of evidence	Grade of recommandation
Peripheral nerve blockade		
Reduces block performance time		
No evidence found	N/A	N/A
Hastens block onset		
Ultrasound guidance reduces onset of sensory block for upper extremity PNBs	Ib	B
Improves block success		
Ultrasound guidance does not improve block success rates in upper extremity PNBs when compared with nerve situation guidance	Ib	B
Ultrasound guidance improves the intraoperative block success for PNBs at the trunk	Ib	A
Improves block quality		
Ultrasound guidance prolongs analgesia for upper and lower extremity blocks	Ib	A
Ultrasound-guided blocks at the anterior trunk improve early postoperative pain relief for inguinal and umbilical procedures	Ib	B
Reduces local anesthetic dose		
Ultrasound guidance reduces the volume of local anesthetic required for successful perioperative analgesia in PNBs	Ib	A
Ultrasound guidance achieves sufficient intraoperative analgesia using minimal volumes (0.1 mL/kg) of local anesthetic for blocks of the nerves in the anterior trunk	Ib	B
Neuraxial anesthesia		
Clear visibility of landmarks		
Ultrasound enables sufficient visibility of the dura mater and ligamentum flavum in neonates, infants and children	Ib	A
Good prediction of depth to LOR		
Preprocedural ultrasound imaging offers a moderate prediction of the depth to LOR	III	B
Visibility of needle puncture of LOR		
Ultrasound offers visibility of a needle within the epidural space in neonates	III	B
Visibility of catheter (directly or indirectly)		
Ultrasound guidance can directly detect catheters during advancement in some young infants	III	B
Ultrasound guidance can confirm epidural catheter placement via surrogacy during injection of fluid	III	B
Reduces bone contact		
Bone contact can be reduced in most cases in infants and children using real-time ultrasound guidance	III	B

Source: Tsui and Pillay [59]. LOR, loss of resistance; PNB, peripheral nerve block.

want to prolong caudal block and to avoid a lumbar catheter, it is possible to use clonidine.

Local anesthetic dosage
Several dosage regimes have been recommended, but the author prefers the bodyweight method. Thus, 0.25% bupivacaine 0.5 mL/kg for lumbosacral areas (i.e. orthopedic surgery of lower limb) and 1 mL/kg for the thoracolumbar area (i.e. herniorrhaphy and orchidopexy) is administered [63]. Recently, it has been

shown that caudal analgesia with a larger volume of diluted ropivacaine (0.15%), i.e. 1.5 mL/kg, provides better quality and longer duration after discharge than a smaller volume of more concentrated ropivacaine [64].

Use of ultrasound guidance
Ultrasound can be used to identify the sacral hiatus in obese children and can also be used to monitor whether the LA solution is injected in the correct anatomical place. It is also feasible to monitor the cephalad spread of local

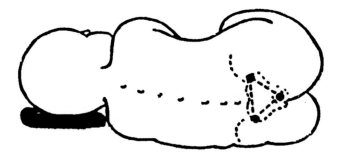

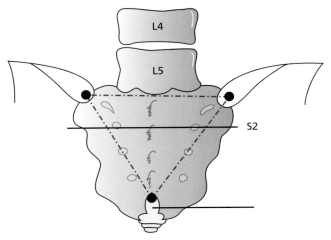

Figure 18.4 Cutaneous landmarks and needle injection for a caudal block. See text for futher details.

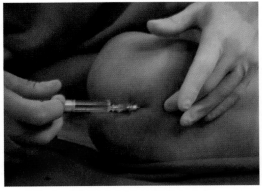

Figure 18.5 Bony landmarks for a caudal block. See text for futher details.

anesthetics within the caudal–epidural space [65]. However, so far there are no published data to suggest that ultrasound assistance does in fact provide any substantial benefits compared with a traditional landmark-based technique. The results of future prospective randomized studies on the possible benefits of ultrasound assistance in this context are awaited with anticipation.

Epidural block

The greatest advantage of epidural block is the long-term analgesia following major surgery of the chest and abdomen and some orthopedic procedures, with continuous LA injection combined with administration of opioids or clonidine [2,66,67].

Performance of an epidural block

As described above with the caudal block, general anesthesia is introduced first. The technique of lumbar epidural anesthesia in children is similar to that in adults. The smaller the patient, the narrower the epidural space, and modifications of equipment are required if the epidural needle and catheter are to be safely placed and dural puncture avoided. The midline approach is preferred. However, the distance between skin and epidural space depends on the age of the child. We use an 18 gauge Tuohy needle (10 cm length) with a 20 gauge epidural catheter in children older than 4 years and a 19 gauge Tuohy needle (5 cm length) with a 21 gauge epidural catheter in children younger than 4 years. The puncture is performed at the L3–4 or L4–5 interspace in order to decrease the potential risk of trauma to the spinal cord. Indeed, in infants the spinal cord may extend lower than the L2–3 interspace. The correct positioning of the Tuohy needle is ascertained by the loss-of-resistance technique with an air-filled syringe instead of saline to avoid diluting the very small volumes of anesthetics used. Nonetheless, a patchy analgesia has been reported with use of a large volume of air [68] and case reports of venous air embolism cause many pediatric anesthesiologists to prefer the saline loss-of-resistance method [69]. The catheter should be threaded with minimal resistance, and the tip should be placed as close as possible to the spinal nerves innervating the area of the surgical field, with no more than 2–4 cm of catheter inserted into the epidural space, as measured from the end of the needle. Tsui and colleagues have developed a novel approach to confirm cephalad advancement of catheters by use of electrical nerve stimulation directly through the catheter [70]. Other groups with an acceptably rapid learning curve should confirm these results. Luer-Lok adapters with bacteriostatic filters are connected to the free end of the catheter.

Thoracic epidural analgesia may be provided for upper abdominal and thoracic surgery, with the catheter tip placed at the level of the spinal dermatome innervating the area of the incision. After induction of general anesthesia and positioning the patient in the lateral decubitus position, the thoracic spine should be extended maximally by drawing knees to chest and flexing the cervical spine with chin to chest (paying attention to airway patency), with an assistant steadying the patient with a hand on the sternum to provide counterpressure during needle placement. Because of the more acute caudad angulation of the spinous processes of the thoracic verte-brae compared to the lumbar vertebrae, a more cephalad angulation of the epidural needle is required to pass between the spinous processes. A midline approach is used, and very careful attention paid to progress of needle excursion in the interspinous ligaments and ligamentum flavum. Because of lack of calcification of these ligaments, especially in younger children, the loss of resistance felt when passing through the ligamentum flavum is not as distinct. These features in younger children, coupled with the small distances involved and the presence of the spinal cord during thoracic epidural anesthesia, make ultrasound guidance potentially a very important technique to improve accuracy of placement [59,60].

Local anesthetic dosage

A dose of 0.5 mL/kg (0.75 mL/kg for infants below 18 months old) is used for initial loading, and 0.25 mL/kg for subsequent "top-up" in order to obtain intraoperative analgesia. After injection into the epidural space, the epidural space seems to protect patients: indeed, absorption into the bloodstream follows a biphasic process. The buffering properties of the epidural space are important and prevent a rapid rise in concentration. Sometimes, in order to have better muscle relaxation, it is possible to use the local anesthetic in combination with intravenous muscle relaxants.

The useful dosage of bupivacaine to obtain pain relief in the postoperative period may be supplied by giving a continuous infusion (0.1–0.125% bupivacaine, 0.3–0.4 mL/kg/h) [71]. The disadvantages of continuous bupivacaine epidural infusion are a high risk of urinary retention and motor block of the legs. The latter can cause anxiety in children between 4 and 8 years old, who may not understand why they cannot move their legs. The use of ropivacaine or levobupivacaine could help to decrease the risk of motor blockade [72].

Use of ultrasound guidance

Willschke and colleagues have investigated the potential usefulness of ultrasound assistance when performing epidural anesthesia in infants and children [73,74]. In addition, they compared epidural catheter placement using either the traditional landmark-based technique or ultrasound assistance and found a reduction in performance time by visualization of the skin–epidural space [75] and fewer episodes of bone contact when using ultrasound. The described technique does, however, require a very skilled assistant handling the ultrasound probe and, apart from the need for a "skilled third arm," there is also interference between the operator and the ultrasound probe. Recently, Karmakar et al reported the use of ultrasound-assisted epidural blockade using a spring-loaded syringe in adults [76]. Such a modification of the technique makes

it possible to for a single operator perform the block (holding the ultrasound probe in one hand and the Touhy needle/spring-loaded syringe in the other). This may represent a modification of this approach that makes ultrasound assistance clinically valuable in the context of epidural blockade, also.

Spinal block

This block is a useful technique in the ex-premature infant scheduled for inguinal herniorrhaphy because it is the only form of pediatric regional anesthesia in which the block is routinely performed and the operation carried out on a conscious patient. It is well known that ex-premature infants are more prone to complications, such as apnea, hypoxia and bradycardia, during the first postoperative hours following general anesthesia [42,77]. Moreover, premature infants with a history of bronchopulmonary dysplasia may be at even further risk of developing postanesthetic complications because of the depressant effects of halogenated agents on intercostal muscles, lung volumes, and chemo- and baroreceptor responses. Avoiding general anesthesia is very useful.

Performance of a spinal block (see Video clip 18.2)

As discussed with epidural block, the subarachnoid puncture should be made caudal to L3 to avoid possible damage to the spinal cord. The puncture is performed with the child turned in the lateral position with lower extremities flexed and the neck extended. Indeed, it has been shown that hypoxemia occurs during lumbar puncture in the sick neonate when the infant's neck was flexed for the spinal tap [78]. A 22-gauge, 3.5 cm styletted (or 25 gauge 1.5 cm) lumbar puncture needle is inserted in a midline position. An unstyletted needle increases the risk of development of an epidermoid tumor. The needle is advanced slowly, and the stylet is frequently removed in order to watch for the free-flowing return of CSF.

Local anesthetic used

Tetracaine 0.5% with 5% dextrose is the most common local anesthetic used: 0.13 mL/kg in infants weighing less than 4 kg and 0.07 mL/kg in infants weighing more than 4 kg [77]. Hyperbaric bupivacaine, isobaric levobupivacaine or ropivacaine can also be used [79,80]. Duration of spinal block is shorter in infants than in adults, probably due to the larger volume of CSF. Indeed, a relationship between duration of motor blockade and age has been reported [5]. In addition, the timing in relation to the baby's feeding requirements is important for two reasons. First of all, the crying of a hungry baby renders a hernia repair much more difficult. Therefore, a pacifier can usually keep the baby quiet and the upper limb should be immobilized. Secondly, hypotension from the sympathetic block following the spinal anesthesia can occur if the fasting is prolonged [81].

In older children, there are few indications for spinal block, due to the short duration of postoperative analgesia. Nonetheless, the child with a full stomach scheduled for a testicular torsion should be a good candidate for a spinal block without sedation. The usual dosage of 1% tetracaine plus 10% glucose is 1 mg per year of age (below 3 years: 0.2 mg/kg). The other LA can also be used in older children.

Use of ultrasound guidance

Recently, caudal anesthesia was shown to be technically less difficult than spinal anesthesia and to have a higher success rate. Its application as an awake regional anesthesia technique in these patients seems more appropriate than spinal anesthesia [82]. However, theoretically, ultrasound could be used to help predict or determine (if using in real time) the depth to reach either the subarachnoid space or some depth within the spinal canal. However, there is no published literature directly related to ultrasound imaging for spinal anesthesia in pediatrics.

Peripheral nerve blocks

Brachial plexus and branches

Fractures of the upper extremity, especially at the elbow and wrist, are common injuries during the summer months when children are outside playing on jungle gyms and skateboards. These patients often present in the late afternoon or early evening, having eaten just prior to the traumatic event. Surgery focuses on reduction and realignment procedures with hardware insertion and casting. Use of sedation may complicate the anesthetic considerations of a full stomach. Brachial plexus blockade may be established with a variety of effective techniques. In addition, ultrasound guidance is very useful [83,84].

Interscalene approach

There are few indications for interscalene brachial plexus blocks in the pediatric population. Blockade of the brachial plexus high in the neck by an interscalene approach is relatively simple in children because of the lack of fat and ease with which the scalenus and medius can be palpated with the index and middle fingers. The groove between these muscles runs parallel to the posterior border of the sternocleidomastoid, and is identified when the palpating fingers fall off the posterior portion of the sternocleidomastoid at the level of the cricoid cartilage. The groove may also be identified at the point where the external jugular vein crosses the sternocleidomastoid. The sheathed needle is inserted between the palpating fingers with the tip directed towards the sternal notch

and angled posteriorly towards the transverse process of the vertebral body and not the vertebral artery. The use of a nerve stimulator may be of assistance in the performance of this block.

Use of ultrasound guidance

Few case reports have been published describing ultrasound-guided interscalene block in children [85]. With the patient positioned supine and head turned slightly to the contralateral side, in a transverse oblique plane at the level of the cricoid, the anechoic compressible internal jugular vein and pulsatile carotid artery are visualized medial to the anterior scalene muscle and deep to the triangular-shaped sternocleidomastoid muscle. The roots of the brachial plexus appear as distinct hypoechoic oval or round bodies arranged in a cephalocaudal orientation in between the bulky anterior and middle scalene muscles (Fig. 18.6).

Periclavicular blocks

The *parascalene approach* to the brachial plexus has been described by Dalens et al and is recommended for elective or emergency surgery of the upper limb when lesions are located above the elbow or when the limb cannot be

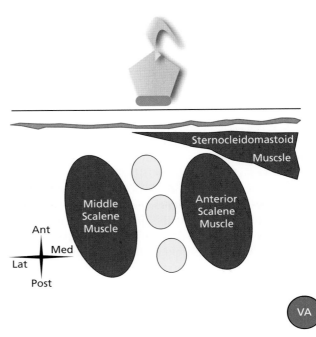

Figure 18.6 Sonoanatomy of interscalene region. The ultrasound probe is depicted at the top of the figure. The roots of the brachial plexus appear as distinct hypoechoic oval or round bodies arranged in a cephalocaudal orientation in between the bulky anterior and middle scalene muscles, depicted here in yellow. VA, vertebral artery. See text for futher details.

moved, either because of severe pain or because of the nature of the lesion itself [86]. Specific contraindications are acute or chronic respiratory insufficiency or whenever the surgery mandates bilateral supraclavicular block, due to the possibility of phrenic block. Some side-effects can occur: stellate ganglion block with a Horner syndrome, risk of damage to the vertebral artery or the large blood vessels of the neck, or pneumothorax.

The patient position is supine with the head turned away from the side to be blocked, the arms extended along the sides of the body, and the shoulders raised with a roll sheet. The anatomical landmarks are the midpoint of the clavicle and Chassaignac's tubercle (anterior tubercle of the transverse process of the sixth cervical vertebra) which is projected on the skin at the intersection of the sternocleidomastoid, with the transverse plane passing through the cricoid cartilage. The point of puncture is situated at the junction of the upper two-thirds and lower one-third of the line joining the midpoint of the clavicle and Chassaignac's tubercle. The sheathed needle is inserted perpendicularly to the skin in an anteroposterior plane, until muscle twitches are elicited. If the needle is too lateral, muscle contractions of the shoulder are seen when the supraclavicular nerve, which lies outside the plexus, is stimulated. If the needle is too medial or too deep, the phrenic nerve may be stimulated, leading to contractions of the diaphragm. In either case, the needle should be withdrawn up to the subcutaneous tissue and redirected correctly.

In contrast to the parascalene and interscalene techniques described above, Winnie's *subclavian perivascular approach* to the brachial plexus is not often used in pediatrics. In the same way, the optimal injection site for the *infraclavicular approach* to the brachial plexus in children is still a subject of debate. Some authors argue that the vertical infraclavicular brachial plexus block, which is very popular in adults, is dangerous in children because of its proximity to the cervical pleura. A more lateral approach was described in 1981 [87]; Kapral et al modified this coracoid block and advocated a vertical variant called the lateral vertical coracoid block [88]. The main advantage of this block is the greater distance between the puncture site and the dome of the cervical pleura. This technique was later reported by Fleischmann et al to be a safe and highly effective approach to the brachial plexus in children when compared with the axillary approach [89].

 Use of ultrasound guidance (see Video clip 18.3)
Because of the high risk of potentially serious side-effects, most anesthesiologists have avoided the supraclavicular and infraclavicular approaches in children, in whom the anatomical relations are even closer than in adults [90]. With the introduction of ultrasound guidance, the supra-

clavicular approach to the brachial plexus is once again becoming popular in children. The probe is first placed in a coronal oblique plane at the lateral end of and just above the upper border of the clavicle. It is then moved medially until an image of the subclavian artery appears on the middle of the screen (Fig. 18.7). At this point, the plexus is located superior and lateral to the artery, and the neurovascular structures are noted to be above the first rib. In the supraclavicular fossa, the divisions of the brachial plexus are visualized as a cluster of hypoechoic nodules immediately cephalad and lateral to the anechoic pulsative subclavian artery and above the first rib. In a prospective, randomized study, Marhofer et al compared ultrasound-guided and nerve stimulator-guided infraclavicular brachial plexus blocks in children with upper extremity fractures [91]. Not only was the ultrasound-guided technique associated with less pain during the performance of the block but it was also found to produce a faster onset time (9 versus 15 min) and a longer duration of the block (384 min versus 310 min). Furthermore, the sensory and motor block characteristics were better in the ultrasound-guided group at 10 min after the completion of the block procedure.

Recently, De José María et al demonstrated that ultrasound-guided supraclavicular plexus block is as effective as an ultrasound-guided infraclavicular plexus block in children aged 5–15 years [92]. However, the supraclavicular plexus block appeared to be associated with

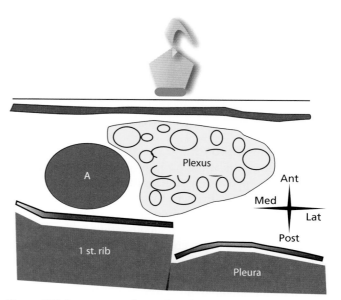

Figure 18.7 Sonoanatomy of supraclavicular region. The ultrasound probe is depicted at the top of the figure. The subclavian artery appears on the middle of the screen. At this location, the plexus is located superior and lateral to the artery, and the neurovascular structures are noted to be above the first rib. A, subclavian artery. See text for futher details.

fewer failed blocks when compared with the infraclavicular approach. These data imply that in experienced hands, a supraclavicular block is a safe and useful alternative for pediatric hand and arm surgery.

Axillary approach

The axillary approach to the brachial plexus was introduced into pediatric regional anesthesia in 1960 and is frequently used because of its low complication rate [93]. The indication for an axillary approach is for elective or emergency surgery on the forearm and hand. The specific contraindications are axillary lymphadenopathy or when the situation requires that the limb be immobile, such as with intense pain or an unstable fracture.

The positioning of the patient is determined by the patient's ability to co-operate, which may be limited by pain or enhanced by a light plane of general anesthesia. The arm should be abducted 45–90° and externally rotated. The correct position is determined by the operator's ability to identify the axillary arterial pulsation and to trace it beneath pectoralis major towards the apex of the axilla. The anatomical landmarks are the axillary artery, major pectoral muscle, and the coracobrachialis muscle. The point of puncture is situated at the intersection where the pectoralis major muscle crosses the coracobrachialis muscle, at the upper border of the axillary artery. The needle is introduced at an angle of 45° at the upper margin of the axillary artery with the needle pointing toward the midpoint of the clavicle. A characteristic pop is felt as the needle enters the periplexus sheath and the axillary artery pulsations are transmitted to the needle. Muscle twitches are seen in the forearm and the hand.

Once the correct position of the needle is confirmed, the injection can begin. At least three major nerves (median,

radial and musculocutaneous) have to be located to obtain a complete forearm and hand block in 90% of the patients within 20–30 min in adults. Only one nerve, median or radial, should be assessed due to the excellent diffusion in the periplexus sheath. Indeed, Carre et al showed in a double-blind, prospective study that a multiple injection technique provides no benefit for children with regard to the quality of sensory and motor block as long as an LA volume of 0.5 mL/kg is used [94]. A volume of 0.3–0.5 mL/kg is used (do not use over 35 mL). If a tourniquet is necessary for the surgical procedure and in order to have good tolerance of it, a subcutaneous infiltration of local anesthetic solution at the puncture point may be needed to block the cutaneous medial nerve. Catheters can be tunneled away from the insertion site if a long implantation is expected, or merely sutured in place and the site covered with a clear plastic dressing to facilitate daily inspections for disconnection, erythema, drainage or other signs of infection. This approach in pediatric patients yields success near 100%, and a high benefit/risk ratio.

Use of ultrasound guidance

There is no original report of ultrasound-guided axillary block in children. The patient is positioned supine with the arm abducted to 90° and flexed at the elbow. With the probe placed perpendicular to the anterior axillary fold, a short-axis view of the neurovascular bundle can be obtained (Fig. 18.8). The nerves are pictured as distinct hypoechoic nodules with internal hyperechoic punctuations typically situated lateral (median nerve), medial (ulnar nerve), and posterior (radial nerve) to the anechoic pulsatile axillary artery. It is noteworthy that the location of these three nerves relative to the axillary artery can be highly variable. This block could be performed with

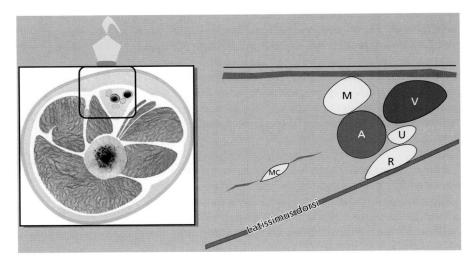

Figure 18.8 Sonoanatomy of axillary region. The ultrasound probe is depicted at the top of the left figure. The right figure is a magnified view. The nerves are pictured as distinct hypoechoic nodules with internal hyperechoic punctuations typically situated lateral (median nerve), medial (ulnar nerve), and posterior (radial nerve) to the anechoic pulsatile axillary artery. A, axillary artery; V, axillary vein; MC, musculocutaneous nerve; M, median nerve; U, ulnar nerve; R, radial nerve. See text for further details.

similar techniques used in adults. Multiple punctures will not be necessary to anesthetize all the relevant nerves for many surgical procedures [95] and possibly musculocutaneous nerves will require separate blockade. In addition, topographic variations of the four main nerves at the axilla were found to be numerous [96,97]; this is a reason to use ultrasound guidance.

Lumbar plexus and branches

The innervation of the skin, muscles, periosteum, and joints of the hip, thigh, and knee make the blockade of the lumbar plexus particularly useful in pediatric patients. Analgesia for lower extremity procedures in children frequently involves areas innervated by branches of the lumbar plexus. Procedures involving joint or bone realignment, especially with insertion of hardware, are common, particularly in disabled children where the ability to sit upright in a wheelchair or to manage transfers from chair to bed and vice versa is vital to reducing their dependence on the family or nursing staff. In those with cerebral palsy, lengthening of muscle and tendons is equally important. Unfortunately, these children may suffer from long periods of muscle spasm and pain following surgery. Due to their disabilities, communication regarding the efficacy of pain relief may be very difficult. Regional techniques, which effectively block the development of muscle spasm, eliminate the need for benzodiazepines and their supposed muscle relaxant effect. A clearer sensorium facilitates care delivery and assessment of pain relief. Congenital hip dislocation, which does not respond to immobilization in plaster, may require open reduction. In this setting, unilateral blockade of the lumbar plexus or bilateral blockade from a central approach makes life easier for all concerned.

Psoas compartment block

Posterior lumbar plexus block represents one of the most challenging techniques in terms of both ultrasound imaging and needle guidance. The use of nerve stimulation in addition to ultrasound imaging is still recommended to confirm correct needle placement. It should therefore only be performed or supervised by experienced clinicians. The clinical value of this technique has not yet been studied systematically. The well-recognized advantage of a posterior approach to lumbar plexus is a reliable block of the femoral nerve, obturator nerve, and lateral cutaneous nerve of the thigh with a single injection.

One concern about this technique is that systemic LA toxicity might occur because of the rapid absorption of large volumes or because of inadvertent injection into one of the large paravertebral blood vessels [35]. Bilateral spread is also a known side-effect of posterior lumbar plexus block.

Femoral block

The area anesthetized by a femoral block will be the quadriceps group of muscles, the periostium of the shaft of femur, skin on the anterior aspect of the thigh, the medial part of the leg and a small portion of the foot. The indications are analgesia in patients with fracture of the femur [98] and surgery on the thigh and analgesia for knee and leg surgery with a sciatic block combined.

The anatomical landmarks in a patient supine with the lower limb abducted, the knee slightly flexed, and the lateral border of the feet in contact with the bed is the inguinal ligament, which extends from the anterosuperior iliac spine to the pubic tubercle and the femoral artery, which can be palpated just below the inguinal ligament. The femoral nerve compartment lies two layers of fascia below the skin, inferior to the inguinal ligament and lateral to the femoral artery pulse. The site of puncture is 0.5–1.0 cm below the inguinal ligament and lateral to the femoral artery. The needle (length 25 mm under 25 kg, 50 mm over 25 kg) is inserted perpendicular to the skin surface or with a slight upward tilt until muscle twitches of the rectus femoris are seen. Sometimes the correct insertion of a short-bevel needle will yield two fascial "pops" as it penetrates the fascia iliaca and fascia lata to enter the nerve compartment. A volume of 0.3–0.5 mL/kg is used (do not use over 35 mL).

Use of ultrasound guidance (see Video clip 18.4)

As when using conventional techniques, the femoral artery is the key landmark when using ultrasound guidance for femoral nerve blockade (Fig. 18.9). With the probe placed perpendicular to the nerve axis (i.e. coronal oblique) at the level of and parallel to the inguinal crease,

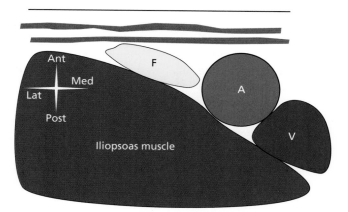

Figure 18.9 Sonoanatomy of femoral region. With the probe placed perpendicular to the nerve axis (i.e. coronal oblique) at the level of and parallel to the inguinal crease, the nerve appears lateral to the large, circular, and anechoic femoral artery. F, femoral nerve; A, femoral artery; V, femoral vein. See text for further details.

the nerve appears lateral to the large, circular, and anechoic femoral artery. When compared with nerve stimulation, Oberndorfer et al showed that ultrasound guidance is associated with a prolonged duration of blockade in children receiving femoral and sciatic nerve blocks [99]. This could also be achieved with smaller volumes of local anesthetics than with the nerve stimulator-guided nerve blocks.

Fascia iliaca compartment block

The fascia iliaca compartment block blocks the femoral nerve in all cases, the lateral cutaneous nerve of the thigh and the obturator nerve (75 % of cases) [100]. The anatomical landmark in a patient supine with a slight abduction of the thigh is the inguinal ligament, which extends from the anterosuperior iliac spine to the pubic tubercle and the femoral artery. The site of puncture is 0.5–1.0 cm below the junction of the lateral one-third and the medial two-thirds of the inguinal ligament lateral to the femoral artery. The needle is introduced at right angles to the skin. A first loss of resistance is felt when the needle pierces the fascia lata, and the second is felt as it penetrates the fascia iliaca. For this block, the use of a nerve stimulator is not needed. In addition, a catheter for continuous infusion of local anesthetic can be used, as with femoral block.

Sciatic nerve

With contributions from the lumbar roots (L4, L5) and the sacral roots (S1, S2, S3), the sciatic nerve is the largest in the body. The indications for sciatic nerve block include analgesia for trauma of the leg and foot. In elective surgery, a sciatic nerve block can be performed for surgery on the foot and with a femoral nerve block combined. Thus, any operations on the lower limb can be performed. In addition, pediatric orthopedic procedures on the lower extremity below the knee relate primarily to congenital deformities such as talipes equino varus and structural imbalances caused by cerebral palsy. Leg length discrepancy may also require prolonged treatment with an external fixator. In this setting, any length, which can be gained early with excellent analgesia from regional blockade, will shorten the hospitalization and reduce the associated expenses.

The *anterior approach* to the sciatic nerve relies on the path of the sciatic nerve between the ischial tuberosity and the greater trochanter of the femur. The patient lies supine with the leg in a neutral position. After a sterile prep and drape, two parallel lines are drawn with a perpendicular dropped between them. The first line follows the inguinal ligament from the anterior superior iliac spine to the pubic tubercle. The perpendicular is drawn from the intersection of the medial one-third and lateral two-thirds of the first line. The second line is drawn from

the greater trochanter parallel to the inguinal ligament until it intersects the perpendicular. At this point, a short-bevel needle is inserted until the surface of the femur is reached. The needle is then withdrawn and redirected to pass behind the lesser trochanter and enters the neurovascular sheath containing the sciatic nerve, the sciatic artery, and the inferior gluteal veins. The use of a nerve stimulator is mandatory in order to achieve dorsiflexion of the foot and eversion (tibial nerve) or plantarflexion of the foot and inversion (common peroneal nerve).

The *posterior approach* to the sciatic nerve identifies the nerve at the same level as the anterior approach described above. In this setting, the patient is placed in the lateral position with the upper leg flexed at the hip. At the midpoint of a line drawn from the ischial tuberosity to the greater trochanter, a short-bevel needle is inserted with a nerve stimulator attached (length 25 mm under 10 kg, 50 mm until 25 kg, 100 mm over 25 kg). The depth at which twitches are seen depends on the age (16–60 mm). When the chosen endpoint is found, the injection of 1 mL of local anesthetic will abolish the stimulation muscle activity, i.e. dorsiflexion of the foot and eversion (tibial nerve) or plantarflexion of the foot and inversion (common peroneal nerve). The volume is 0.5 mL/kg (do not use over 35 mL). When a femoral nerve block is combined with a sciatic nerve block, the total dose is reduced by one-third for each block.

In the *lateral approach* to the sciatic nerve, the patient position is supine with, if possible, the leg lightly rotated externally. The point of puncture is located on the lateral aspect of the thigh (1–2 cm depending on age) below the greater trochanter. The needle is inserted perpendicular to the long axis of the limb in the horizontal plane directed toward the position bordering the femur and the ischial tuberosity. If the needle touches bone, it is withdrawn and reinserted more dorsally, under the femur. The depth at which the sciatic nerve is found depends on age. Lateral sciatic nerve block is simple and the child does not need to be moved.

For the *medial popliteal nerve approach*, the indication is foot surgery except the medial aspect of the thigh that will be blocked with a saphenous nerve block. The patient position is prone in which case the legs are flexed at about 30° with a rolled towel underneath the ankles. The anatomical landmarks are between the tendons of the biceps femoris and the semitendinosus, the intercondylar line, and the bissector of the angle created with the summit of the popliteal fossa. The point of puncture is located 1 cm lateral to the bissector, at the junction of the upper-third and the lower two-thirds of the segment extending from the summit of the popliteal fossa and the intercondylar line. The needle is inserted at right angles to the posterior aspect of the popliteal fossa until muscle twitches are elicited in the flexor muscles of the foot. The volume (0.5 mL/kg) injected should be less than 35 mL and reduced by one-third if combined with a femoral block.

 Use of ultrasound guidance (see Video clip 18.5)
Subgluteal and popliteal approaches are commonly used for sciatic nerve blockade in children with the use of ultrasound guidance. In the subgluteal region, the sciatic nerve appears predominantly hyperechoic and is often elliptical in a short-axis view. On the other hand, a caudal-to-cephalad scan can effectively locate the sciatic nerve in the posterior popliteal fossa at a location where the tibial and common peroneal components have yet to separate. At the popliteal crease, a transversely positioned linear probe captures the tibial and common peroneal nerves, the former located medially and lateral to the adjacent popliteal vessels (Fig. 18.10). The tibial nerve is often located in close proximity to the tibial artery and the tibial vein. The nerves appear round to oval and hyperechoic compared with the surrounding musculature. The hyperechoic border of the femur (condyles) may be apparent. Gray et al published the first report on ultrasound-guided peripheral nerve block in children in 2003, in which they

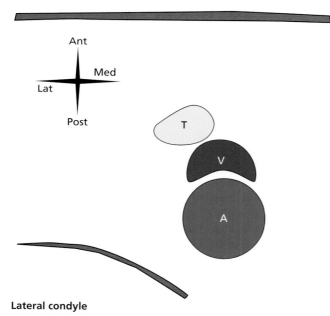

Lateral condyle

Figure 18.10 Sonoanatomy of popliteal sciatic region. At the popliteal crease, a transversely positioned linear probe captures the tibial and common peroneal nerves, the former located medially and lateral to the adjacent popliteal vessels. The tibial nerve is often located in close proximity to the tibial artery and tibial vein. The nerves appear round to oval and hyperechoic compared with the surrounding musculature. The hyperechoic border of the femur (condyles) may be apparent. T, tibial nerve; A, tibial artery, V, tibial vein. See text for futher details.

performed sciatic nerve block in the subgluteal region of a 7 year old [101]. More recently, studies with ultrasound-guided sciatic nerve blockade using a subgluteal approach have been published [99,102].

Continuous peripheral nerve blocks

Single-shot peripheral blocks are widely used in children but they provide analgesia only for a few hours. These blocks are even safer than central ones but few studies describe this technique in children, except recently infraclavicular block [103] and sciatic block [46,103]. The indications for a catheter for continuous peripheral nerve blocks are severe pain, long intraoperative time requiring re-dosing, and pain control necessary for many days. Otherwise, painful rehabilitation and physiotherapy are probably the main indication because good rehabilitation can only be performed if pain is under control. Indeed, in adults, it has become daily clinical practice supported by a large quantity of data, providing effective analgesia and allowing active physiotherapy, essential to achieving optimal functional recovery. Catheters can be maintained in position for several days and even if so far there are only reports from adults being sent home with a catheter infusion, in the future this method will also be applied in children.

A recent study has reported the efficacy of continuous peripheral nerve blocks with elastomeric disposable pumps associated with initial Bier blocks for the treatment of recurrent complex regional pain syndrome in children [104]. All the studies published so far underline the efficacy and safety of analgesia via a peripheral catheter, and no complications or side-effects linked to the long-term infusions have been described, with only a few accidental removals and some drug leakage [105]. They are at least as efficient as epidural analgesia, but produce fewer side-effects [104]. Sometimes a combination of peripheral blocks as a continuous sciatic block with a single shot 3-in-1 block for tourniquet pain and light general anesthesia provides good intraoperative conditions for leg and foot surgery and adequate postoperative pain relief [106]. Additional sedation to minimize the discomfort of a cast may be a consideration in the first 24 h [102].

As continuous regional analgesia is considered a safe and efficacious technique for postoperative pain relief in children after lower limb surgery, the feasibility of patient-controlled regional analgesia in a similar acute pain situation was recently evaluated. Both techniques are efficacious and satisfactory. However, patient-controlled regional analgesia with ropivacaine 0.2% can provide adequate postoperative analgesia for pediatric orthopedic procedures with smaller doses of ropivacaine and lower total plasma concentrations of ropivacaine than with continuous regional analgesia [107].

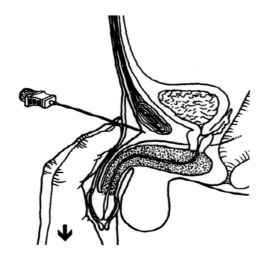

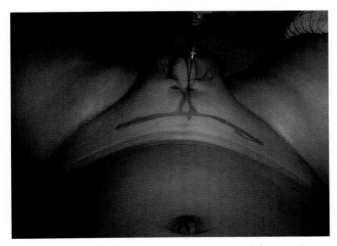

Figure 18.11 Anatomy, landmarks and needle approach for a penile block. The anatomical landmark is the pubic symphysis. After gently pulling the penis downward, the two points are marked just below the pubic symphysis, each pubic ramus about 0.5–1.0 cm on either side of the pubic symphysis. The puncture is performed with a 22 gauge needle, 30 mm in length. See text for futher details.

Other nerve blocks

Penile nerve block

The indication is surgery on the foreskin (phimosis, paraphimosis, circumcision). The anatomical landmark is the pubic symphysis (Fig. 18.11) [108]. The puncture is performed with a 22 gauge needle, 30 mm in length. After gently pulling the penis downward, the two symmetric puncture sites are identified immediately below the pubic symphysis at a distance of 0.5 to 1 cm from the midline. The needle is introduced at the puncture site, perpendicular to the skin. The penetration is stopped in the subpubic space, after distinct elastic recoil is felt, corresponding to the crossing of the deep membranous layer of the super-ficial fascia. The depth of insertion correlates with age (8 mm for a newborn, 30 mm for a young adult). The same procedure is repeated on the opposite side. The volume should be 0.1 mL/kg for each side with 0.5 % ropivacaine or levobupivacaine without epinephrine [109]. Epinephrine is absolutely contraindicated because it can lead to a spasm of the dorsal arteries of the penis, with subsequent ischemia and necrosis of the gland. In addition, the midline puncture, the old technique, can injure the dorsal artery of the penis, leading to a compressive hematoma, possibly resulting in gland necrosis.

Use of ultrasound guidance

By placing a probe sagittally along the shaft of the penis, the subpubic space can be located as a triangle containing the deep penile fascia (inferiorly), the pubic symphysis (superiorly), and the membranous layer of the superficial (Scarpa's) fascia. Ultrasound-guided penile nerve block improved the efficacy of the block in terms of the early postoperative pain [110].

Ilio-inguinal iliohypogastric nerve block (II/IH block)

The main indication is hernia repair. The anatomical landmark is the anterior superior iliac spine. A short-bevel 22 gauge needle is to be inserted just below and medial to the anterior superior iliac spine (ASIS). The medial distance depends on the size of the child, being 0.5 cm in the infant and 2 cm in the adolescent. The needle is slowly advanced until there is a loss of resistance, which occurs as the aponeurosis of the external oblique is being pierced. The needle is then immobilized in this position. A volume of 0.4–0.5 mL/kg with 0.5% levobupivacaine or 0.5% ropivacaine without epinephrine is used.

Use of ultrasound guidance

This peripheral nerve block is one of the best studied with regard to the use of ultrasound guidance [111–115]. After placement of a linear probe or a hockey stick probe along the ASIS with the probe oriented toward the umbilicus, the three layers of the abdominal wall muscles can be recognized. The ilio-inguinal and iliohypogastric nerves are seen as two hypoechoic structures between the internal oblique and transversus abdominis muscles (Fig. 18.12). A short-bevel needle (e.g. 22 gauge, 40 mm with facette tip) is used. Indeed, a reliable endpoint for the inexperienced practitioner of ultrasound-guided II/IH nerve block may be the transversus abdominis/internal oblique plane where the nerves are reported to be found in 100% of cases [114]. By postinjection ultrasonographic control, Weintraud et al were able to show that the use of the classic landmark-based approach resulted in only 14% of the injections being made at the correct anatomical location [113]. Not surprisingly, the overall success rate of

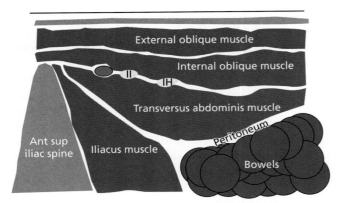

Figure 18.12 Sonoanatomy of abdominal region. After placement of a linear probe or a hockey stick ultrasound probe along the anterior superior iliac spine with the probe oriented toward the umbilicus, the three layers of the abdominal wall muscles can be recognized. The ilio-inguinal and iliohypogastric nerves are seen as two hypoechoic structures between the internal oblique and transversus abdominis muscles. II, ilio-inguinal nerve; IH, iliohypogastric nerve. See text for futher details.

the II/IH nerve block was found to be only 61% in this study.

In a prospective randomized study by Willschke et al, the efficacy of an ultrasound-guided II/IH nerve block was compared with the landmark-based approach [111]. It was clearly demonstrated that use of the ultrasound-guided technique was associated with a significantly higher success rate, as evidenced by a reduced hemodynamic reaction to skin incision (4% versus 24%) and a considerable reduction in the number of patients needing supplemental analgesia in the recovery room (6% versus 40%). In a further study by the same authors, they showed that a substantial reduction in the volume of LA (traditionally recommended volume 0.4–0.5 mL/kg) is possible when using ultrasound guidance. Using a modified up/down technique, they found that an effective II/IH nerve block can be achieved using a volume of LA as low as 0.075 mL/kg when using ultrasound guidance [112].

Weintraud and colleagues have recently published a study in which plasma concentrations following either landmark-based or ultrasound-guided II/IH nerve block was analyzed following the administration of equal volumes and amounts of ropivacaine (0.25 mL/kg of 0.5% ropivacaine) [115]. Somewhat surprisingly, the maximum plasma concentration (C_{max}) was found to be higher and the time to maximum concentration (T_{max}) shorter when ultrasound guidance was used, indicating more rapid absorption when the LA was injected at the correct anatomical position. The most likely explanation for this

unanticipated finding is that when the LA is deposited between the fasciae of the internal oblique and transversus abdominis muscles, the area of absorption will increase substantially compared with when the drug is mainly injected intramuscularly.

Transversus abdominis plane block

The transversus abdominis plane (TAP) block is increasingly being used to provide analgesia after surgery involving the abdominal wall. Rafi introduced this block technique in 2001 as a landmark technique [116]. The block requires injection of LA into a plane between the transversus abdominis and internal oblique muscles. Recently, a cadaver study demonstrated that with an ultrasound-guided single injection of 20 mL of aniline blue dye in the TAP, the ninth thoracic nerve (T9) was not surrounded by the injectate, whereas the segmental nerves T10, T11, T12 and L1 were surrounded by the injected dye in 50%, 100%, 100% and 93% of the cases, respectively [117]. Ultrasound can help the practioner readily visualize the muscle layers at the lateral abdominal wall, though not allowing clear distinction between the individual muscles. Linear and parallel hyperechoic striations are apparent, beneath which lies a hypoechoic-appearing region representing the peritoneum [118]. The external oblique abdominal muscle will lie superficial, overlying the internal oblique and transversus abdominis muscles. As for the rectus sheath and umbilical blocks, the nerves (in this block, the lower thoracic and first lumbar spinal nerves) will not be viewed with clarity because they would appear with similar echogenicity as the muscle layers and travel tangentially to the ultrasound beam axis at this location. A short-bevel needle (e.g. 22 gauge, 80–100 mm with facette tip) is used. Finally, only a few case series of children have been published [119–121]; all other publications deal with the adult use of this block.

Transversus abdominis plane block represents an interesting and effective regional anesthetic technique for the provision of pain relief after abdominal surgery. Future studies should define its risks and benefits, and compare them with epidural techniques, which can be considered the "gold standard" for the provision of abdominal analgesia.

Rectus sheath block and umbilical block

To perform the rectus sheath block, the probe is placed just below the umbilicus (i.e. above the arcuate line). The anterior and posterior aspects of the rectus sheath and the enclosed rectus abdominis muscle are visualized. The sheath appears hyperechoic with multiple linear layers, lying on the anterior and posterior aspects of the rectus muscle. Willschke et al [121] and De José María et al [122] stated that their injection site was situated at the location where an optimal view of the posterior sheath was obtained. A short-bevel needle (e.g. 22 gauge, 40 mm with facette tip) was inserted in an in-plane approach at the inferior edge of a linear probe, using an angle most suitable for the depth of the sheath. The needle tip was placed just inside the rectus sheath near the posterior aspect of the rectus abdominis muscle.

Paravertebral block

Paravertebal block has been used to provide postoperative pain relief for adults and children in a variety of settings [123]. Satisfactory pain relief has been demonstrated for unilateral thoracotomies and urological surgery. The percutaneous insertion can be performed with equipment found in most epidural trays, in a patient placed in the lateral decubitus position. Because of the variation of size in children, the use of a loss-of-resistance technique to find the space is better than judging the location by depth alone. Potential complications are pneumothorax and vascular puncture; hypotension is rare due to the lack of sympathectomy [124].

Use of ultrasound guidance

Ultrasonographically, the transverse process of the thoracic vertebra and rib is identified at the appropriate thoracic level [125]. The transducer is moved cranially until an intercostal ultrasound view is obtained, indicated by visualization of the parietal pleura. An in-plane needle insertion approach from lateral to medial is used, and a total of 0.2–0.3 mL/kg of LA is injected through the needle and a subsequently threaded catheter, while the spread of LA is observed. An ultrasound-guided out-of-plane paravertebral block with the ultrasound probe positioned longitudinally to the paravertebral area has also been described.

Infraorbital nerve block

The infraorbital nerve is the terminal branch of the second division of the trigeminal nerve and is purely sensory. It leaves the skull through the foramen rotundum and enters the pterygopalatine fossa. There it exits the infraorbital foramen, dividing into four branches: inferior palpebral, external nasal, internal nasal, and superior labial. These branches innervate the lower lid, the lateral inferior portion of the nose and its vestibule, the upper lip, the mucosa along the upper lip, and the vermilion border. This block can be used to provide postoperative analgesia

and to favor early feeding resumption after cleft lip repair in infants [126,127]. It can also be used for nasal septal reconstruction, rhinoplasty, and in patients undergoing endoscopic sinus surgery.

Different approaches are used, including intraoral and extraoral; recently a suprazygomatic approach has been described [127]. For the intraoral approach, after palpation of the infraorbital foramen, the upper lip is folded back and a 27 gauge needle is advanced to the infraorbital foramen parallel to the maxillary premolar [126]. By placing a finger at the level of the infraorbital foramen, the cephalad progression of the needle is checked. A volume of 0.5–1 mL of 0.25% levobupivacaine with 1:200,000 epinephrine is injected after careful aspiration.

Complications of blocks and their treatment

Performing a regional block may result in different complications, most of which can be avoided by learning the correct technique, using an appropriate device, and applying the basic safety rules. Despite the fact that most regional anesthetic techniques are performed under sedation or general anesthesia, large prospective and retrospective studies have demonstrated a low complication rate, particularly with peripheral nerve blocks, and fewer long-term sequelae when compared with adults having the same procedure.

Complications related to the device used

Block needles are used blindly and may thus damage a nerve trunk, especially when they are inserted without careful regard for nerve anatomy. Vascular lesions may lead to compressive hematoma and, at spinal levels, definitive paraplegia. If a spinal hematoma is suspected, a diagnosis must be established urgently by magnetic resonance imaging or computed tomography, and surgical treatment must follow immediately. Attempted peripheral nerve blocks can produce other injuries such as arterial wounds and pneumothorax, the presenting symptoms of which can be delayed by several hours.

The technique of determining the nerve/space location may produce complications. These include nerve damage while seeking paresthesias, and complications related to the medium used for the loss-of-resistance technique while locating the epidural space. These include dilution and increase in the injected volume of local anesthetic with saline headache, patchy anesthesia, lumbar compression, multiradicular syndrome, subcutaneous cervical emphysema or venous air embolism. Headache is the most common complication of dural puncture in adults; its occurrence is less common in children. The treatment includes keeping the patient in supine position, hydration with intravenous fluids, analgesia, and an autologous epidural blood patch (0.3 mL/kg) [128] which is not always free of complications. Failure to respond to the blood patch warrants further investigation. The use of caffeine or sumatriptan (5-HT$_{1D}$ receptor agonist) has not been reported in children.

Complications of catheters

Insertion of an epidural catheter can lead to several complications: misplacement, kinking, knotting, rupture (especially if attempts are made to withdraw the catheter through the epidural needle). Secondary migrations into the subarachnoid space, a blood vessel, the subdural space or the paravertebral space are sometimes reported. Leakage around the puncture point occurs in approximately 10% of cases, and inadvertent removal is not infrequent; also, several pediatric cases of catheter infection have been reported. Some complications, such as cutting and knotting, become apparent only on removal of the catheter; in most cases, they are directly related to the length of catheter introduced into the epidural space, which usually should not exceed 2–4 cm. The frequency of catheter-related complications has been noted to be as high as 11% in a pediatric series [129]. Malfunctioning of infusion pumps is not uncommon.

Complications related to faulty technique

Epidural abscess, meningitis, arachnoiditis, radiculopathies, discitis, and vertebral osteitis have been reported following central blocks. Interposed bacterial filters are effective in preventing contamination. Inadvertent dural puncture with subsequent intrathecal injection of an epidural dose of local anesthetic results in total spinal anesthesia, the clinical expression of which is almost immediate respiratory arrest requiring rapid control of ventilation and, in adolescents, cardiovascular collapse. Subdural injection results in a delayed (20 min) and short-duration (60 min) block with an extensive distribution of analgesia (involving cranial nerves up to the fifth pair) but with no or minimal motor and sympathetic blockade. The injection of large volumes may result in excessive spread of the local anesthetic, which can reach distant nerves, or in too high levels of epidural/spinal anesthesia with subsequent respiratory failure due to intercostal muscle paralysis (above T4) or even in diaphragmatic paralysis (C4). Interscalene brachial plexus, lumbar plexus, and intercostal nerve blocks may lead to the same complications.

Complications due to the local anesthetic solution

The use of wrong solutions or additives can lead to definitive neurological damage; a highly effective way to avoid syringe mismatch consists of using a specific cart for regional block procedures. Interruption of blood flow in the artery of Adamkiewicz, due either to the surgical procedure or, hypothetically, to vasoconstriction resulting from the administration of local anesthetics with epinephrine, may result in anterior spinal artery syndrome, which combines definitive loss of lower limb motor function with, at least partially, intact sensory function. Epidural anesthesia has been implicated in the flaring of latent infections (herpes, neuroimmunological diseases such as Guillain–Barré syndrome). Of greater concern is the risk of unmasking latent neurological diseases such as spinal cord compression, cerebral tumors, angiomas or an epidural abscesses. Allergy to aminoamides is rare, and most adverse reactions are related to adrenaline.

Treatment of LA convulsions consists of supplementing the child with oxygen and providing respiratory assistance; if convulsions persist after oxygenation, it is recommended that small intravenous doses of benzodiazepines (diazepam 0.1 mg/kg, midazolam 0.05 mg/kg) or thiopental 4 mg/kg be administered. Persistent convulsions require muscle relaxation (succinylcholine injection 1.5–2 mg/kg), intubation, and assisted pulmonary ventilation to prevent acidosis.

Treatment of LA cardiac arrest: immediate treatment is required, including oxygen supplementation, ventilation and, if appropriate, external cardiac massage, sodium bicarbonate, and inotropic support. Ventricular tachycardia or fibrillation requires electrical defibrillation; 20% Intralipid bolus of 1.5 mL/kg and then an infusion of 0.5–1 mL/kg/min is also indicated. See Chapter 40 for more detailed discussion of treatment of LA toxicity, including cardiac arrest.

Epidemiology of complications

Complications were rare and similar in both ADARPEF studies [1,3]. As reported in the literature, they were more frequent (four times in the recent ADARPEF study) in children aged <6 months than in children aged >6 months. Central regional anesthesia has the highest incidence of complications (seven times higher than peripheral). The incidence was low despite an increase in the use of central neuraxial blockade in the 12 last years. Significant complications are rare, as indicated by results from a UK audit (5 years, 10,633 epidurals performed) reporting permanent residual neurological deficit in a child aged 3 months (1 year follow-up), two epidural abscesses, one case of meningitis, one postdural puncture headache requiring active blood patching, and one drug error resulting in cauda equina syndrome. The UK audit also reported five cases of severe neuropathy/radiculopathy which resolved over a period of 4–10 months using pharmacological therapy in a pain clinic. Thus, in this study the incidence of serious complications was 0.09% [2]. The recent ADARPEF study [3] records a very low overall morbidity, almost six times lower than in central regional anesthesia. This result should encourage anesthesiologists to use peripheral rather than neuraxial (including caudal) blocks as often as possible when appropriate.

The use of catheters does not seem to increase the occurrence of complications, even if cardiac toxicity following a secondary injection through a catheter is due to an inadvertent displacement of the catheter. Some complications (drug error, wrong side, block of the upper limbs due to an extended spinal anesthesia) were avoidable. In the recent ADARPEF study, LA toxicity resulted in one case of convulsions [3] while the UK audit only reported two respiratory arrests and one seizure following central regional anesthesia [2]. None of these complications required lipid rescue treatment. Some other complications (prolonged duration of spinal anesthesia in two premature infants, one drug error, and a case of cardiac toxicity without cardiac arrest) were probably also avoidable. It is thus possible to improve the safety of pediatric regional anesthesia provided basic precautions are followed.

Safety and ultrasound guidance

Despite the theoretical advantages of ultrasound imaging during the performance of nerve blocks, no large prospective studies in pediatrics have so far been published in support of the notion that the use of ultrasound does in fact reduce the incidence of complications compared with alternative nerve blocking techniques. The possibility of visualizing the nerve structures as well as important nearby anatomical structures (e.g. vessels, pleura and peritoneum) most likely reduces the incidence of inadvertent complication due to misplacement of the tip of the blocking needle. The reduced volume of local anesthetic needed to produce an adequate block should also reduce the risk of systemic toxicity due to rapid absorption of local anesthetics from the injection site (Table 18.4). Indeed, using a conventional up/down technique and measuring the cross-sectional area of the ulnar nerve in the proximal part of the forearm [130] and of the sciatic nerve [131] in adults, a 95% median effective dose for an effective ulnar nerve block with 1% mepivacaine can be as low as $0.11\,mL/mm^2$ nerve, corresponding to a total volume of 0.7 mL, and a 99% median effective dose can be $0.10\,mL/mm^2$. Thus, there is good evidence that effective peripheral nerve blocks can be achieved by using considerably smaller volumes of local anesthetics when using ultrasound guidance.

Because serious complications luckily are very rare following peripheral nerve blockade in infants and children [1,3], it is unlikely that even large-scale studies will prove ultrasound guidance to be superior to other approaches with regard to the rate of complications. However, it does not seem reasonable to expect that the use of ultrasound should result in an increased rate of complications.

Conclusions

The goal of regional anesthesia in the pediatric population must always be the provision of effective, safe analgesia with low rates of morbidity and low risk of adverse side-effects. Indeed, safety concerns are prominent because most children coming for surgery and anesthesia are healthy and tolerate systemic opioids with a good safety margin.

Studies have demonstrated a diminished stress response, fewer episodes of hypoxia, greater cardiovascular stability, faster return of gastrointestinal function, a reduced need for postoperative ventilation and a shorter stay in intensive care in children who have had surgery performed under regional anesthesia.

In this era of evidence-based medicine, purists would claim that further prospective studies with larger sample sizes are necessary to demonstrate that regional anesthesia has significant benefits and offers a better outcome than other forms of analgesia in children.

Finally, ultrasound guidance has been shown to improve the block characteristics and probably the safety of regional anesthesia in pediatrics.

Table 18.4 Reduction of local anesthetic volume with ultrasound guidance

Technique	Ultrasound guidance dosages	Landmarks dosages
Supraclavicular block [92]	0.3 mL/kg	0.5 mL/kg
Infraclavicular block [91]	0.2 mL/kg	0.5 mL/kg
Sciatic block [99]	0.2 mL/kg	0.3 mL/kg
Femoral block [99]	0.15 mL/kg	0.3 mL/kg
Rectus sheath block [122]	0.1 mL/kg each side	0.3 mL/kg
Ilio-inguinal block [112]	0.1 mL/kg each side	0.4 mL/kg

CASE STUDY

A 7-year-old child was scheduled for primary, elective, unilateral metatarsal osteotomy which was expected to require a lengthy administration of potent analgesics, and a hospitalization of 4–5 days. The anesthetic procedure was combined general anesthesia and regional anesthesia with continuous popliteal sciatic catheter, on an ambulatory basis. Therefore the parents were required to:

- live within a 1-h drive from the hospital
- be able to contact medical staff or nurses 24 h a day
- be able to return to the hospital quickly if required
- understand a visual analog scale
- provide rescue oral analgesics
- observe the analgesic device (catheter and elastomeric pump) and the skin under the dressing
- screen possible local anesthetic-related complications.

A peripheral nerve catheter was placed in the child under general anesthesia just before surgery. After premedication with oral midazolam, anesthesia was induced and maintained using sevoflurane, oxygen, and nitrous oxygen via a facemask. Intravenous saline solution, at a rate of 5–10 mL/kg/h, was infused throughout the procedure. The child received an antibiotic and antiemetic prophylaxis (0.2 mg/kg dexamethasone). With the child in lateral position, ultrasound-guided placement of a peripheral nerve sciatic catheter was performed. As described by Koscielniak-Nielsen et al [132], we were able to view the catheter exiting the needle tip and during advancement while using long-axis views of the nerves [131].

After confirming the nerve identity using a long-axis plane, the probe was rotated 90° and the needle and catheter were introduced in-plane with a tangential angle. Injection of local anesthetic confirmed the needle tip and catheter location. The catheter was introduced 15 mm beyond the introducer cannula, affixed securely to the skin by a "U" stitch, covered by transparent dressing, and taped onto the thigh. After negative aspiration, 0.2 mL/kg of ropivacaine 5 mg/mL was injected in divided doses via the catheter, with gentle aspiration every 2 mL. During the surgical procedure, if intravenous opioid rescue was required, the blockade was considered ineffective and the catheter would be removed. Since the surgery lasted more than 1 h, an additional injection of 0.1 mL/kg of the same local anesthetic solution was administered hourly.

For the surgical procedure, a tourniquet was applied at the thigh and inflated according to the surgeon's discretion. In the postanesthetic care unit, the sensory and motor blockade of the foot was evaluated. As soon as the child's toe motor function recovered, the sciatic popliteal catheter was connected to a multirate, disposable infusion elastomeric pump (Infusor LV, Baxter, Deerfield, IL, USA), containing 200 mL of 0.2% ropivacaine, with 1.5 μg/mL

clonidine (mainly for its sedative effect in children), giving a fixed infusion rate according to the child's weight (0.1 mL/kg, i.e. 2.5 mL/h; infusor rate possibilities 0.5–5 mL/h). In the hospital, if pain control was considered insufficient, intravenous acetaminophen or opioids was given as rescue. The criteria for discharge from the hospital depended on the presence of a plaster splint (observation day 1 in hospital) and the absence of local postoperative complications. Totally efficient continuous sciatic nerve block, i.e. the ability to ambulate with crutches without assistance or dizziness, and urinary voiding were also required before home discharge.

Before home discharge, nurses gave the parents the following training: extensive explanation about the use of the visual analog scale to diagnose pain, elastomeric device surveillance, and evaluation of sensory and motor blockade, spontaneous mobility, and short delay in capillary refill after pressure on the child's test toes. When the child fulfilled the criteria for discharge, the medical staff checked both the child's and parents' comprehension of the provided instructions. The parents agreed never to leave their child alone, and to record (four times daily, at breakfast, lunch, dinner, and bedtime) the following items: changes in behavior, sleep disturbance, quality of appetite, play activity, the occurrence of any adverse effects and technical problems possibly related to the analgesic technique, temperature, evaluation of the blockade and the integrity of the child's dressing, episodes of pain, and the use of an oral rescue analgesic (acetaminophen twice a day, or a combination of acetaminophen and codeine at bedtime). Instructions were provided regarding protection of the anesthetized limb, signs of local anesthetic toxicity, a direct return to the hospital if needed, and 24-h contact information. The elastomeric pump was filled before discharge. At the end of the procedure, the child returned to hospital and met with the medical staff. The parents shared their feelings and observations about the postoperative period at home, and their overall satisfaction. The catheter was then removed, and its distal portion was sent for bacteriological analysis.

A total of 47 children were treated with this protocol in a recent prospective feasibility study [134]. The main finding of this observational study is that analgesia at home by continuous sciatic nerve block with an infusion elastomeric pump is effective, with pain control rated excellent or good in 89% of patients. It is also feasible and associated with no major complications in this study, and enables children to experience ambulatory or shortened hospital stays [133]. Another interesting point is that parents trained by nurses readily understood the method of pain screening, and managed the analgesic device well.

Annotated references

A full reference list for this chapter is available at:
http://www.wiley.com/go/gregory/andropoulos/pediatricanesthesia

2. Llewellyn N, Moriarty DA. The national pediatric epidural audit. Paediatr Anaesth 2007; 17: 520–33. This study reported the largest clinical use of continuous epidural and possible complications.

3. Ecoffey C, Lacroix F, Giaufré E et al. Epidemiology and morbidity of regional anesthesia in children: a follow-up one-year prospective survey of the French-Language Society of Pediatric Anesthesiologists (ADARPEF). Paediatr Anaesth 2010; 20: 1061–9. The ADARPEF group has conducted a large survey on peripheral and central blocks showing changes in practice and evolution of complications.

11. Mazoit JX, Dalens BJ. Pharmacokinetics of local anaesthetics in infants and children. Clin Pharmacokinet 2004; 43: 17–32. This is a synthetic review of LA pharmocology in pediatrics.

59. Tsui BC, Pillay JJ. Evidence-based medicine: assessment of ultrasound imaging for regional anesthesia in infants, children, and adolescents. Reg Anesth Pain Med 2010; 35(Suppl): S47–54. The first review of evidence-based medicine with ultrasound for regional anesthesia in pediatrics.

60. Tsui BCH, Suresh S. Ultrasound imaging for regional anesthesia in infants, children, and adolescents: a review of current literature and its application in the practice of extremity and trunk blocks. Anesthesiology 2010; 112: 473–92. A comprehensive narrative review of the literature pertaining to techniques described and outcomes evaluated for ultrasound imaging in pediatric peripheral blocks.

61. Tsui BC, Suresh S. Ultrasound imaging for regional anesthesia in infants, children, and adolescents: a review of current literature and its application in the practice of neuraxial blocks. Anesthesiology 2010; 112: 719–28. A comprehensive narrative review of the literature pertaining to techniques described and outcomes evaluated for ultrasound imaging in pediatric neuraxial blocks.

Video clips

This chapter contains the following video clips:

Video clip 18.1 Caudal block.
Video clip 18.2 Spinal block.
Video clip 18.3 Supraclavicular nerve block–ultrasound-guided.
Video clip 18.4 Femoral nerve block–ultrasound-guided.
Video clip 18.5 Sciatic nerve block–ultrasound-guided.
They can be accessed at:

http://www.wiley.com/go/gregory/andropoulos/pediatricanesthesia

CHAPTER 19

Anesthesia for Fetal Intervention and Surgery

Mark D. Rollins & Mark A. Rosen

Department of Anesthesia and Perioperative Care, University of California San Francisco, San Francisco, CA, USA

Introduction

Sir (Albert) William Liley, a New Zealand perinatologist, was the first to demonstrate that fetal diagnosis and treatment were possible when he treated Rh disease-induced fetal hydrops (erythroblastosis fetalis) with intraperitoneal blood transfusion [1]. He had determined the correlation between the severity of rhesus isoimmunization and the bilirubin-induced deviation of the spectral absorption curve of amniotic fluid. Amniocentesis is now a standard procedure in obstetric practice. Others attempted exchange transfusion by directly cannulating fetal vessels through a small uterine incision. Early results were not encouraging and further attempts at fetal surgery were abandoned [2]. A decade later G.C. Liggins, another New Zealand perinatologist, demonstrated the beneficial effects of maternal glucocorticoid administration to augment fetal surfactant production in fetuses at risk for respiratory distress syndrome of prematurity [2]. In the early 1980s, after careful experimentation and practice in sheep [3–5] and monkeys [6], the first successful human fetal surgery was performed at the University of California San Francisco by Michael Harrison to treat lower urinary tract obstruction-induced bilateral hydronephrosis by creating a vesicostomy [7].

Fetal surgery would not have been possible without the improvements in sonographic resolution that occurred in the early 1980s. Curvilinear or convex abdominal transducers that better fit the obstetric abdomen provided wider fields of view at greater distances from the transducer. Improvements in digital signaling processing and extensive use of wide aperture transducers, coherent image processing, and harmonic imaging improved spatial and contrast resolution, background noise reduction, dynamic range, and near and far field visualization. Advances in prenatal diagnosis substantially improved the ability to recognize and more precisely delineate fetal anatomy and anomalies.

Associated with these advances in imaging were advances in amniocentesis that permitted analysis of amniotic fluid for detection of many metabolic disorders and chromosomal abnormalities, assessment of fetal pulmonary maturity, and severity of fetal hemolytic anemia. Advances in fetoscopy have allowed direct visualization of the fetus and the ability to obtain samples from organs and tissue. They also allowed fetal blood sampling, but this was replaced by ultrasound-guided percutaneous umbilical blood sampling (PUBS).

Serial sonographic examinations of fetuses facilitated delineation of the pathophysiology and natural history of

---

congenital diaphragmatic hernia, hydrocephalus, non-immune hydrops, and obstructive hydronephrosis. However, most anatomical malformations diagnosed *in utero* are unsuitable for antenatal intervention and surgery.

Fetal surgery would also not be possible without the information sharing and collective conceptualization among physicians from a wide variety of disciplines who are interested in fetal diagnosis and therapy. This was greatly facilitated by Harrison's early (1981) organization of a symposium with worldwide experts [8]. A registry for fetal interventions was established and ethical guidelines adopted, leading to the creation of the International Fetal Medicine and Surgery Society and subsequently to the journal *Fetal Diagnosis and Therapy*. The pioneering work from a few medical centers spawned the field of fetal medicine worldwide. Fetal treatment centers around the world now rely on the expertise of radiologists, geneticists, perinatologists, pediatric cardiologists, neonatologists, social workers, support staff, and many others, as well as fetal surgeons and anesthesiologists.

Before undertaking fetal surgery, its feasibility, safety, and efficacy must be assured. Fetal surgery requires a normal fetal karyotype and a selected, accurately diagnosed and isolated anomaly that has a high probability of resulting in death, severe disability or irreversible harm before fetal lung maturity occurs, and for which removing the lesion might allow development to proceed relatively normally. Accurate and complete diagnosis is required to avoid interventions that would be futile or when the fetus is so mildly affected that postnatal treatment would be equally effective. There should be a good physiological rationale that was tested in animals and in controlled human trials that established efficacy and safety of the procedure. Family counseling for risks and potential benefits must be comprehensive and must include options for elective termination of pregnancy or continuation of pregnancy without therapy. Consent must also include a discussion that the surgery and potential benefits for the fetus might incur risks for the mother. Maternal risk must be small, and careful preoperative assessment is mandatory to ensure that the risk is acceptably low [9,10].

Fetal surgical interventions are broadly categorized into three different kinds of procedures. "Open procedures" involve maternal laparotomy and hysterotomy and uterine stapling to seal membranes to the endometrium and provide hemostasis. Most myelomeningocele repairs and resections of congenital cystic adenomatoid malformations and saccrococcygeal teratomas are performed "open." Open procedures are technically more complicated and entail the most maternal and fetal risk, particularly for postoperative membrane separation, preterm labor, rupture of membranes, and preterm delivery. Chorio-amniotic membrane separation can cause amniotic bands, umbilical cord strangulation, and fetal demise [11]. Preterm delivery causes significant morbidity and mortality for fetuses that otherwise might benefit from these interventions. Consequently, preoperative, intraoperative, and postoperative tocolysis is crucial. Inadequate postoperative tocolysis and preterm rupture of membranes is a major hindrance to fetal surgery. Fortunately, overall maternal risks are minimal but include blood loss, blood transfusion, infection, placental abruption, and pulmonary edema from tocolysis [12]. Location and orientation of the uterine incision mandates cesarean delivery for this and all subsequent pregnancies after open procedures.

The second type of fetal surgery is "minimally invasive or percutaneous" that involves uterine puncture with needles or trocars to perform endoscopic or sonographically guided procedures. Minimally invasive procedures are less risky than open procedures but preterm rupture of membranes is still a major problem. These techniques are employed for fetal blood sampling, treatment of fetal anemia by intrauterine transfusion, treatment of unbalanced blood flow between monochorionic twins, radiofrequency ablation of umbilical blood flow of a non-viable twin, and tracheal occlusion by endoluminal balloon placement to treat congenital diaphragmatic hernia. The trend in fetal surgery is to develop minimally invasive techniques to avoid open procedures.

The third type of fetal surgical intervention, the *ex utero* intrapartum treatment (EXIT) procedure, is a modification of cesarean section [13]. EXIT procedures provide time to secure a difficult airway by tracheal intubation, bronchoscopy or tracheostomy for conditions that would make newborn tracheal intubation unfeasible or very difficult (e.g. embryonic cervical tumors such as cystic hygromas, cervical teratomas). The EXIT procedure is also used for thoracotomy to treat cystic adenomatoid malformation, transitioning from placental gas exchange to extracorporeal membrane oxygenation (ECMO) for anticipated pulmonary insufficiency or complete resection of a giant cervical teratoma. EXIT preserves placental gas exchange during surgery. This has allowed us to perform several surgical procedures that lasted more than 2.5 h and maintain placental circulation without causing hypercarbia or acidosis at delivery [14].

Fetal surgery: indications, procedures, and outcomes

The following sections summarize the rationale for fetal intervention and provide a description of both surgical and anesthetic considerations for each procedure, and a review of outcome data. Details of anesthetic techniques are presented.

Congenital diaphragmatic hernia

Approximately 1 in 2000–5000 neonates have a congenital diaphragmatic hernia (CDH) [15,16]. Incomplete fetal diaphragm formation allows the abdominal contents to enter the thoracic cavity and produce varying degrees of pulmonary parenchymal and vascular hypoplasia. Pathophysiological changes include decreased alveoli number, thickened interstitial tissue and alveolar walls, decreased surface area for gas exchange, reduced lung compliance, and decreased pulmonary vasculature that has medial hyperplasia and adventitial thickening [17]. After birth, hypoxia, hypercarbia, and acidosis induce further pulmonary vasculature constriction and pulmonary hypertension. This increases right-to-left shunting of blood and causes further hypoxia and acidosis.

The majority of CDHs are left-sided and more than half are associated with other birth defects [18]. The rate of mortality varies by center but is frequently greater than 60%. Mortality is associated with the degree of pulmonary insufficiency and pulmonary hypertension [19,20]. Survival of patients with CDH has improved in tertiary care centers by:

- removing the herniated abdominal contents from the chest and closing the diaphragm defect
- ventilation techniques that cause less barotrauma (high-frequency oscillation)
- administration of surfactant
- ECMO.

Although advanced ventilation techniques and ECMO were not of benefit in randomized prospective trials, centers utilizing these methods report improved outcomes among neonates who have a poor initial prognosis [19,21]. Postnatal CDH survival now occurs in 60–85% of patients, but it is significantly affected by the presence of other defects and by disease severity. Outcomes vary widely among centers [22–24].

It was postulated that correction of CDH *in utero* might improve fetal lung development and significantly reduce the degree of pulmonary hypoplasia present at birth. In controlled trials, fetal lamb models of CDH confirmed the benefit of *in utero* repair in that progression of pulmonary hypoplasia and pulmonary vascular changes were less severe, and newborn survival improved [3]. Although removing the abdominal contents from the chest and repairing the defect is technically feasible, it is difficult in human fetuses, and intervention for those with severe disease had limited success [25]. A lesson learned from these patients was the need to place an abdominal patch to prevent increases in intra-abdominal pressure and the associated compromise of the ductus venosus blood flow. In addition, it was found both thoracic and abdominal incisions were needed to facilitate both removal of the liver from the chest and placement of the diaphragmatic patch. However, replacing the liver

in the abdomen often caused acute and severe decreases in cardiac preload and intraoperative fetal mortality [25]. Problems with blood loss from the uterine incision and amniotic fluid leaks after uterine closure were solved. However, preterm labor remained a significant problem after surgery and caused neonatal morbidity and mortality. Results from a small prospective trial of open fetal surgical intervention comparing *in utero* repair with surgical repair after birth failed to demonstrate that fetal surgical intervention improved outcomes [20].

Given the difficulties encountered with primary repair of CDH *in utero*, another strategy was pursued. It was known that fetal lungs secrete about 125 mL/kg/day of fluid that normally exits the fetal trachea and mouth into the amniotic fluid. Since fetuses with congenital high airway obstruction cannot expel the fluid, they develop hyperplastic lungs [26]. It was reasoned that reversibly obstructing the trachea would cause lung fluid accumulation, lung expansion and growth, and decrease the amount of pulmonary hypoplasia. The concept of "plug the lung until it grows" (PLUG) was tested in fetal lambs and shown to decrease pulmonary hypoplasia and herniation of abdominal contents and to improve neonatal respiratory function [27–29]. Although *in utero* tracheal occlusion decreases much of the pulmonary hypoplasia and hypertension, there are fewer type II pneumocytes and less secreted surfactant. Removing the tracheal obstruction before delivery may reduce this unwanted effect [30,31].

The initial method of creating a reversible, controlled tracheal occlusion during open fetal surgery required both maternal laparotomy and hysterotomy, and involved application of either an internal tracheal plug or external tracheal clip [32]. The large water-impermeable foam plug used initially to block the fetal trachea reduced pulmonary hypoplasia but was difficult to remove and caused tracheal malacia. A smaller plug was easier to remove but did not completely occlude the trachea and failed to improve the fetus' pulmonary status. Next, an external tracheal metallic clip was placed around the trachea after meticulous dissection and attempts to avoid injuring the recurrent laryngeal and vagus nerves. Since the clip or plug had to be removed surgically, the EXIT procedure was developed (see below).

Unfortunately, few patients survived these initial open procedures. Of the first 13 fetuses undergoing this treatment, only 15% survived compared to 38% of fetuses receiving standard postnatal treatment [33]. Preterm labor occurred at 30 ± 0.6 weeks' gestation and was a major cause of mortality in the treated group; the non-treated group was born at 37.5 ± 0.5 weeks. A second series of 15 fetuses with CDH treated with external clips at the Children's Hospital of Philadelphia also had a 30% survival rate [34], but tracheal occlusion did not consistently improve the lung hypoplasia or postnatal pulmonary function.

Improvements in endoscopic and ultrasound imaging techniques allowed refinement of minimally invasive techniques for tracheal occlusion. These video-assisted fetal endoscopic (FETENDO) techniques replaced open surgical procedures for tracheal occlusion. Application of external fetal tracheal clips by FETENDO improved survival to 75% in eight fetuses [33]. To reduce fetal laryngeal nerve and tracheal trauma, a small balloon was placed in the trachea by percutaneous endoscopic endotracheal intubation *in utero* at University of California San Francisco (UCSF). The balloon, which is typically used for endovascular occlusion of intracranial aneurysms, is inflated to occlude the tracheal lumen, detached, and left in place until delivery via EXIT procedure (Figs 19.1, 19.2). The balloon is deflated and removed by endoscopy prior to birth.

A prospective randomized controlled trial (1999–2001) compared fetal tracheal occlusion (n = 11) for intrauterine treatment of severe CDH with repair after birth (n = 13) [35]. Eligibility included 22–28 weeks' gestation, a left-sided CDH, herniation of the liver into the left hemithorax, normal karyotype, and a low lung to head ratio (LHR) <1.4. LHR is the ratio of cross-sectional area of the contralateral lung to the head circumference as determined by two-dimensional ultrasound and is a good indicator of the severity of pulmonary hypoplasia and the likelihood of survival [36]. The trial was stopped due to an unexpectedly high survival rate in the control arm (77% versus 73%). Secondary measures of neonatal mor-

bidity were not different between groups, but premature rupture of membranes and preterm delivery were more common in the fetal treatment group (gestational age 30.8 weeks versus 37.0 weeks) [35]. A reason for the lack of difference in morbidity at 90 days may have been overly broad LHR inclusion criteria. In fetuses with liver herniation into the chest, at 22–28 weeks' gestation LHR predicts fetal survival, which is inversely proportional to LHR [37]. Using a LHR of 1.4 likely allowed inclusion of many fetuses who would survive with standard care. Table 19.1 compares outcomes of expectant and treated fetuses with left-sided CDH and liver herniation.

Minimally invasive fetoscopy for tracheal occlusion and prenatal tracheal balloon removal 24 or more hours before delivery may improve lung growth, minimize effects on type II alveolar cells [38], and potentially avoid morbid EXIT procedures. Comparison of the EXIT procedure to predelivery balloon removal in 24 fetuses with severe CDH (LHR ≤1.0 plus intrathoracic liver) that underwent fetal endoscopic tracheal occlusion (FETO) at 26–28 weeks' gestation demonstrated improved 28-day survival (p = 0.013) in the balloon reversal group (83%) compared to the EXIT group (33%) [39]. There was no maternal hemorrhage, pulmonary edema or infection. This "plug–unplug sequence" may be more ideal in that the cyclical occlusion and release may allow pulmonary structural maturation, pulmonary artery remodeling, and pneumocyte maturation [39]. An ongoing multicenter European study is determining survival of FETO on fetuses with severe left-sided CDH (LHR <1.0) and intrathoracic liver herniation [40]. A detachable tracheal

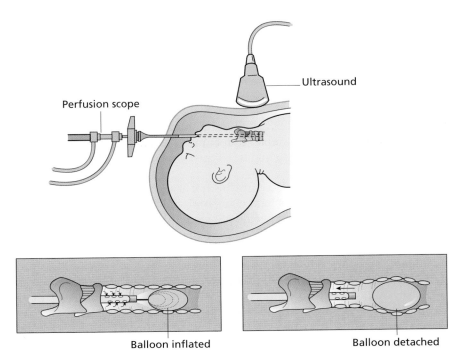

Figure 19.1 Schematic of the FETENDO fetal balloon placement. Courtesy of UCSF Fetal Treatment Center.

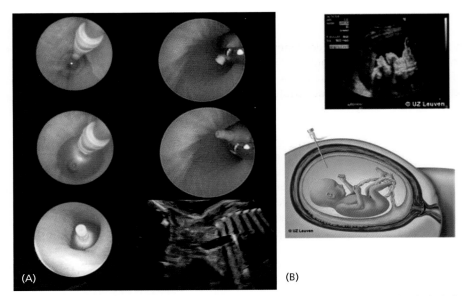

Figure 19.2 (A) Fetoscopic images of tracheal balloon insertion. (*Left column, top to bottom*) The catheter, loaded with the balloon, is inserted, the balloon is inflated between carina and vocal cords and then detached. (*Right column*) The upper two images show the balloon being retrieved by fetoscopic extraction, using a 1 mm forceps. The bottom panel is an ultrasound image of the balloon in place. (B) Schematic drawing of cannula insertion towards the fetal mouth. Above the schematic is the ultrasound image in the direction of the cannula. Reproduced from Gucciardo et al. Best Pract Obstet Gynaecol 2008; 12: 123–38 with permission from Elsevier.

Table 19.1 Postnatal survival rate in fetuses with left-sided CDH and intrathoracic liver herniation based on fetal LHR at 23–29 weeks' gestation

	Expectant management		Fetoscopic tracheal occlusion	
LHR (mm)	n	Survival	n	Survival
0.4–0.5	2	0	6	1 (16.7%)
0.6–0.7	6	0	13	8 (61.5%)
0.8–0.9	19	3 (15.8%)	9	7 (77.8%)
1.0–1.1	23	14 (60.8%)		
1.2–1.3	19	13 (68.4%)		
1.4–1.5	11	8 (72.7%)		
≥1.6	6	5 (83.3%)		
Total	86	43 (50%)	28	16 (57.1%)

CDH, congenital diaphragmatic hernia; LHR, lung-to-head ratio.
Modified from Jani et al [40].

balloon is endoscopically placed in the trachea and is removed prenatally by either fetal endoscopic tracheoscopy or by ultrasound-guided needle puncture. An EXIT procedure is occasionally required. Postnatal therapy includes neonatal tracheal intubation, high-frequency ventilation, and nitric oxide or ECMO if needed. Survival data from this study are displayed in Table 19.1. Patients with severe CDH who underwent FETO showed improved survival compared to those treated with expectant management [40]. An increased LHR was associated with increased survival.

Improvements in occlusion device are needed to allow complete, sustained tracheal occlusion throughout gestation without damaging the trachea or surrounding structures. Further trials are required to determine the optimal timing, duration, and protocol for occlusion to improve fetal survival. Future studies should not only address survival but also morbidity and quality of life for survivors of this treatment.

Ex utero intrapartum treatment procedure

The EXIT procedure was developed to allow adequate time to manage and secure the airway of fetuses at birth who had undergone *in utero* tracheal occlusion or PLUG [13]. The EXIT procedure is widely used for cases in which the neonatal airway may be difficult or impossible to manage, i.e. fetal neck masses and congenital high airway obstruction (CHAOS). It is also used for other surgical procedures, such as a thoracotomy to excise large cystic adenomatoid malformations, for separation of conjoined twins or for transition to ECMO. It is also useful for severe lung hypoplasia (e.g. unilateral pulmonary agenesis) and selected cardiac lesions ("blue babies") for transition to ventilatory support and/or ECMO when resuscitation could otherwise be jeopardized by compromised oxygenation [41,42].

During the EXIT procedure, the neonate is partially delivered by cesarean section and the connection between fetus, placenta, and mother remains intact. This allows gas exchange (including maternally inhaled anesthetic agents) through the placenta rather than the fetal lungs. Uterine relaxation is necessary to prevent uterine contractions, separation of the placenta from the endometrium or the compromise of uterine blood flow. Some EXIT procedures have lasted more than 2.5 h. During this time, placental circulation was adequate, as demonstrated by normal umbilical cord blood gases and absence of fetal acidosis at delivery [14].

For fetal surgery to be successful, a multidisciplinary team of fetal surgeons, anesthesiologists, ultrasonographers, maternal-fetal medicine specialists, and dedicated operating room nurses is needed. Maternal considerations, positioning, induction of anesthesia, and tracheal intubation are similar to those with general anesthesia for cesarean deliveries. (See Anesthesia for open fetal procedures below.)

Often >2 minimum alveolar concentration (MAC) of halogenated vapor is required to maintain profound uterine relaxation and prevent placental separation from the uterine endometrium. In some cases, periodic boluses of intravenous nitroglycerine (50–200 μg) or a continuous infusion of nitroglycerine (1–20 μg/kg/min) are required in addition to or instead of a halogenated vapor to provide adequate uterine relaxation. In certain cases EXIT has been successfully accomplished with neuraxial blockade and nitroglycerine [43]. Although nitroglycerine crosses the placenta, it causes minimal fetal effects because much of the nitroglycerine is metabolized at the placental interface [43,44].

The use of high MAC levels often decreases maternal cardiac output and uteroplacental blood flow and causes vasodilation and hypotension. Close hemodynamic monitoring is, therefore, required. Vasopressors, such as phenylephrine and/or ephedrine, are given as needed and are preferred to volume expansion, which may cause maternal pulmonary edema.

The uterus must be flaccid and atonic for hysterotomy. The location of the placenta and fetus is determined by ultrasound, the uterine incision avoids the placenta, and a stapling device is used to ensure hemostasis [45]. Some early EXIT procedures were terminated for uncontrolled maternal bleeding [46]. Following hysterotomy, the fetal head and upper torso are brought outside the uterus. Keeping part of the fetus *in utero* helps maintain uterine volume and facilitates fetal warmth. A sterile pulse oximeter probe is applied to the fetal hand for monitoring heart rate and oxygen saturation. Occasionally partial delivery of the fetus causes fetal bradycardia from occult umbilical cord compression and full delivery of the fetus is necessary. Partial delivery allows placental–fetal gas exchange to continue while the airway is secured or surgery is performed (Fig. 19.3). Anesthetic is transferred to the fetus via the placenta; muscle relaxant, opioid or resuscitation drugs are given by fetal intramuscular injec-

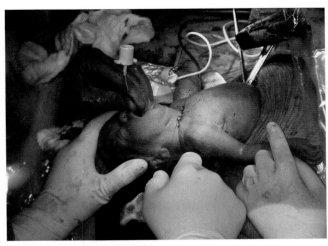

Figure 19.3 Partial delivery during EXIT procedure with airway secured and pulse oximeter monitor placed on left hand and occluded from light with foil. Courtesy of UCSF Fetal Treatment Center.

tion (see Anesthesia for open fetal procedures). Fetal well-being is continuously monitored by pulse oximetry (see Fig. 19.3) and by periodic echocardiography. The mother breathes at least 50% inspired oxygen to improve fetal oxygenation [47]. Typical fetal saturations are 40–60%; 30–40% saturation is considered adequate. Despite maternal PaO_2s >600 mmHg, fetal arterial pO_2s are <60 mmHg due to the nature of placental oxygen transfer [48]. Decreases in fetal heart rate or arterial saturation can result from maternal hypotension, placental abruption, umbilical cord compression or kinking, or from loss of uterine relaxation. Anesthesiologists play a key role in monitoring the fetus and ensuring its safety by maintaining adequate uterine relaxation and appropriate maternal hemodynamics.

When the EXIT procedure is used for delivery of a fetus with CDH after *in utero* tracheal occlusion, fetal bronchoscopy is performed to pierce the tracheal occlusive balloon and retrieve it. Oral tracheal intubation is accomplished by direct laryngoscopy with a 3.0–3.5 tracheal tube. After the trachea is intubated, surfactant is usually administered and the lungs are ventilated with oxygen. Peak inspiratory pressures are monitored with a manometer and maintained at the lowest pressures required for adequate pulmonary ventilation. Typically a positive end-expiratory pressure of 5 cmH₂O is used to increase functional residual volume. Before delivery and termination of "placental support," endotracheal tube placement is confirmed by direct observation, breath sounds, and end-tidal CO_2. Fetal pulmonary ventilation typically increases arterial oxygen saturation to >90%. After the baby's oxygen saturation increases, the cord is clamped, the baby is delivered, and the neonatologists provide further resuscitation as needed.

Failure of fetal arterial oxygen saturation to rise above 90% with pulmonary ventilation has been used to initiate ECMO before delivery [49]. This allows time to insert vascular cannulas and initiate ECMO before the fetus is removed from placental gas exchange. In other cases, fetal ascites or cystic masses can be decompressed before securing the airway; this makes it easier to manipulate the head and upper airway and ventilate the fetal lungs. For longer surgeries or when intravascular fetal volume or red blood cell mass must be increased, a fetal intravenous catheter is inserted into an upper extremity vein.

Immediately after cord clamping and fetal delivery, the halogenated anesthetic is reduced or discontinued and oxytocin is administered to antagonize uterine relaxation and initiate and maintain normal postpartum uterine tone. Other agents, such as methergine, prostaglandin-F2α or prostaglandin-E are used if uterine atony persists. Oxytocin is often continued for 4h postpartum to minimize uterine atony. As the concentration of halogenated anesthetic is reduced or discontinued, intravenous opioids are administered and the concentration of inspired nitrous oxide is increased to provide maternal anesthesia to complete surgery.

Six case series (4–52 patients) of EXIT have determined neonatal outcome [50]. Ninety-seven to 100% of infants were born alive. Average blood loss was 850–1150 mL and the mean time on uteroplacental circulation following hysterotomy was 28–45 min. Long-term outcomes of these neonates depended on the severity of the pathology necessitating the EXIT procedure.

Maternal outcomes after EXIT procedures have been excellent. Whenever possible, low transverse uterine incisions are used to decrease the risk of uterine rupture with subsequent pregnancies. Noah et al compared complications in 34 mothers who underwent EXIT procedures to 52 women who underwent cesarean delivery prior to labor [51], and found small increases in both wound complication rates and estimated blood loss in the EXIT procedure group but no difference in maternal transfusion requirements, postoperative hematocrit levels, and length of hospital stay [51].

Twin–twin transfusion syndrome

The majority of monochorionic twins have abnormal chorionic blood vessel connections in the placenta, which can result in twin–twin transfusion syndrome (TTTS). Normally, the umbilical artery carries deoxygenated blood to the surface of the placenta where it branches, traverses the placental surface, and then descends into capillary divisions where gas and nutrients are exchanged with the maternal circulation. The returning "paired" system consists of a vein that lies directly next to an artery as it returns to the umbilical cord (Fig. 19.4). This vascular configuration is associated with placental cotyledons and represents normal fetal placental vascular anatomy.

In TTTS, a branch from the umbilical artery travels along the surface of the placenta and descends into the cotyledon where, instead of connecting with a paired vein, it connects with an *unpaired* vein that now carries blood to its twin [52] (Fig. 19.5).

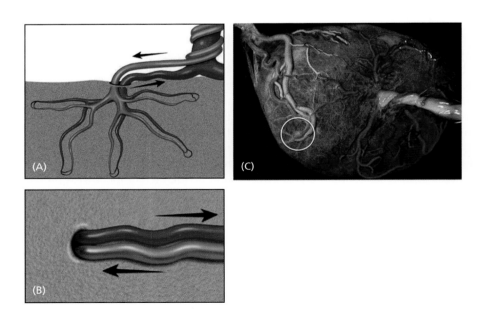

Figure 19.4 (A) Normal angio-architecture (cotyledon). (B) Superficial view of bidirectional flow into and out of a cotyledon. (C) Normal arteriovenous pair on placental pathology specimen. Reproduced from Rand and Lee. Clin Perinatol 2009; 36: 417–30 with permission from Elsevier.

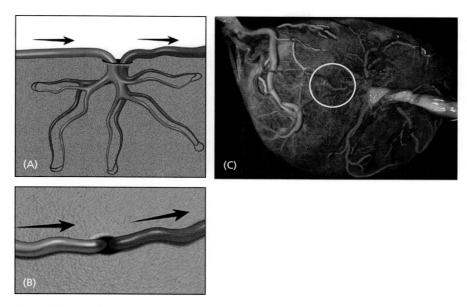

Figure 19.5 (A) Abnormal inter-twin connection: AV anastomosis. (B) Superficial view of unidirectional flow into and out of the cotyledon as a result of the inter-twin AV anastomosis. (C) AV anastomosis seen superficially on placental pathology specimen. Reproduced from Rand and Lee. Clin Perinatol 2009; 36: 417–30 with permission from Elsevier.

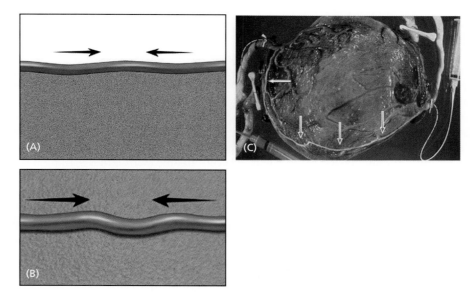

Figure 19.6 (A) AA anastomosis. (B) Superficial view of bidirectional flow in AA anastomosis. (C) Superficial view of AA anastomosis (*arrows*) between cord insertions (both marginal) on placental pathology specimen. Reproduced from Rand and Lee. Clin Perinatol 2009; 36: 417–30 with permission from Elsevier.

In monochorionic twins, blood moves unidirectionally from one twin to the other via this abnormal arterial–venous (AV) connection. Whether the flow goes to or from either fetus depends on which one contributes the arterial vascular connection. These one-way AV connections are common in monochorionic placentas [52], yet only about 10% of monochorionic pregnancies have TTTS, which suggests that the abnormal AV connections and overall blood flow are relatively balanced between most fetuses.

The unequal chronic blood flow distribution between the twins causes the symptoms of TTTS [53]. Artery-to-artery (AA) and vein-to-vein (VV) end-to-end anastomoses also occur in monochorionic placentas (Fig. 19.6).

These connections remain on the placental surface and cause turbulent bidirectional flow. An AA connection protects against TTTS if it equalizes overall resistances and blood flow between the twins. AA anastomoses are associated with nine times less TTTS [54]. Placental sharing, vasoactive mediators, and abnormal cord insertion may also influence the development of TTTS [55]. This syndrome usually presents at 15–26 weeks' gestation [56] in approximately 9–10% of monochorionic twin pregnancies [57]. TTTS results in ≥80% mortality if untreated and a 15–50% risk of morbidity (e.g. cardiac, renal, neurological, gastrointestinal) in survivors [58].

The unbalanced flow of TTTS causes hypovolemia, oliguria, oligohydramnios, and intrauterine growth restriction in the donor twin (often referred to as a "stuck" or "pump" twin). This twin is at risk of developing neonatal renal failure, renal tubular dysgenesis and dysfunction, and high cardiac output-induced hydrops fetalis. Part of the mechanism of TTTS may be hypovolemia-induced upregulation of the renin synthesis system, increased angiotensin II, aldosterone, and antidiuretic hormone, which causes further fetal vasoconstriction and reduction of placental blood flow in the donor fetus [59]. The recipient twin has polycythemia, polyuria, polyhydramnios and hypertrophic cardiomyopathy and is at risk for hydrops fetalis and fetal death.

A major threat to both twins is polyhydramnios-induced preterm rupture of the membranes and preterm labor. For unclear reasons, survivors of TTTS are at risk for CNS white matter lesions and long-term disability. The increased risk of impaired neurodevelopment is associated with higher gestational age at intervention, increased severity stage of TTTS, and lower gestational ages at birth [60]. In the past, the diagnosis of TTTS was based on a ≥20% difference in birthweight and a >5 g/dL difference in cord hemoglobin concentrations. Current diagnostic criteria are based on ultrasound findings, including size discordance, which is not always present and is not necessary for the diagnosis [61]. These ultrasound-based criteria focus on discrepancy between amniotic fluid sac volumes, umbilical cord size, presence of cardiac dysfunction in the recipient twin, abnormal umbilical artery or ductus venosus blood flow velocity, and significant fetal size discordance [55]. In addition, multiple staging systems have been developed that are based on progression of size discordance and abnormal changes in the twins. These staging systems are helpful for prognosis of outcome, treatment options, and communication between physicians and centers [55].

A variety of treatment strategies for TTTS have been devised. Each is intended to decrease morbidity and improve survival of one or both twins. These include serial amnioreduction to control polyhydramnios and decrease preterm labor; surgical microseptostomy of the inter-twin amnion membrane to equalize amniotic pressures; selective fetoscopic laser photocoagulation (SFLP) of selected abnormal inter-twin vascular anastomoses to equalize the resistance and blood flow between the twins; and fetoscopic cord coagulation to selectively terminate the unhealthy recipient twin to improve survival of the donor.

Amnioreduction

Serial amnioreduction was the first treatment utilized for TTTS and was designed to decrease the morbidity from polyhydramnios in the recipient twin. Amnioreduction decreased preterm delivery and improved uteroplacental perfusion by reducing intrauterine pressure [62]. Mari et al used international registry data to examine the effects of amnioreduction on 223 sets of twins diagnosed with TTTS before 28 weeks' gestation [63]. They reported medians of two amnioreductions, 3550 mL of fluid removed, and a gestational age at delivery of 29 weeks. Intrauterine death occurred in 18% of recipients and 26% for donors, with an overall survival rate at birth of 78%. By 4 weeks of age, only 60% of infants were alive; 65% of recipients and 55% of donors survived [63]. Possible complications from amnioreduction included infection, placental abruption, premature rupture of membranes, and preterm labor.

Microseptostomy

Microseptostomy was developed to improve uteroplacental blood flow by equalizing pressures between the two amniotic cavities. Eighty-three percent of 12 patients with TTTS undergoing microseptostomy survived [64]. In a prospective randomized trial, 73 women with TTTS were treated with either serial amnioreduction or septostomy. No difference was found in either overall perinatal survival (64% versus 70%) or survival of at least one infant during pregnancy (78% versus 80%) [65]. Microseptostomy is seldom used today because if a single amniotic cavity is inadvertently created, there is a risk of umbilical cord entanglement.

Selective fetoscopic laser photocoagulation

In utero SFLP is a minimally invasive procedure that coagulates abnormal communicating vessels between the twins. A Nd:YAG or diode laser is introduced through a semi-flexible ≤2.0 mm diameter endoscope. Typically, the fetoscope and laser are inserted percutaneously into the recipient twin's amniotic sac that has polyhydramnios (Fig. 19.7). Neuraxial blockade is commonly employed for anesthesia, but infiltration of local anesthesia into the trocar insertion site in the myometrium is also effective. Fetoscope placement is determined by placental location and is guided by ultrasonography. Vascular anastomoses on the surface of the placenta are directly visualized.

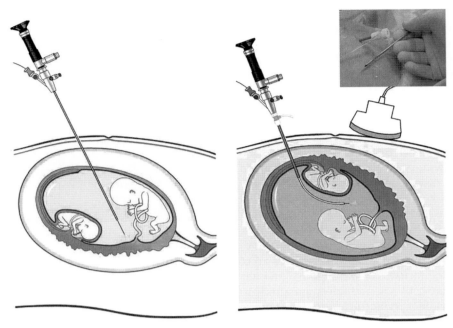

Figure 19.7 Direct insertion of the fetoscope through the sheath – without cannula (*left*). An anterior placenta, with the use of a curved sheath and a flexible cannula (*right*). A photo of flexible cannula in place (*insert*). Use of a cannula allows change of instruments, with only a minimal increase in diameter. Reproduced from Deprest et al. Curr Opin Anaesthesiol 2008; 21: 298–307 with permission from Lippincott Williams and Wilkins.

Identification of the connecting vessels and their oxygen status is possible because the arteries crossing on top of the veins are a darker red color due to oxyhemoglobin desaturation [56]. Using the fetoscope, chorionic plate vessels that cross the membrane separating the amniotic sacs are visually traced to each fetal umbilical cord insertion. Based on their angio-architecture, abnormal vessels are identified [52] and selectively coagulated with laser. Due to the location of the fetuses, placenta, and cord insertions, many procedures require some non-selective coagulation. Non-selective ablation of vessels is associated with higher rates of intrauterine deaths from acute placental insufficiency [66]. Frequently, some of the abnormal twin–twin anastomoses are not visualized and remain intact after laser therapy. Complete obliteration of all connecting vessels is unnecessary for successful outcomes [67,68]. Following laser ablation, an amnioreduction is often done when the fetoscope is removed to reduce the polyhydramniotic sac to a normal or slightly lower volume. Fetal monitoring and periodic ultrasound imaging are performed for 24–48h after surgery.

A multicenter prospective randomized trial compared endoscopic laser surgery to serial amnioreduction for TTTS that was diagnosed before 26 weeks' gestation. The study was stopped early because interim analysis demonstrated a benefit of the laser treatment group [69]. The laser group had a greater likelihood of at least one twin surviving at both 28 days (76% versus 56%, p < 0.01) and 6 months of age (76% versus 51%, p = 0.002) [69]. The laser treatment group also had significantly fewer neurological complications at 6 months of extra-uterine life. Another prospective randomized multicenter trial of amnioreduction and SFLP found no difference in 30-day mortality for either the recipient or donor twin [54]. Fetal "recipient" mortality was increased for SFLP but was offset by an increase in neonatal "recipient" mortality in the amnioreduction group [54]. The hypertensive cardiomyopathy of the "recipient" twin was an important factor in survival, which might be the result of vasoactive hormones (renin-angiotensin system) from the "donor" that compromise the recipient.

A recent meta-analysis of literature from 1997–2007 that compared laser therapy with amnioreduction concluded that fetuses treated with laser therapy were more likely to survive [70]. The same group found a significant difference (p < 0.001) in overall survival rate between donors (60%) and recipients (70%), with no difference in neurological morbidity between groups [71].

The most common complication of laser therapy for TTTS is preterm rupture of membranes, but risks also include transplacental entry of the trocar, spontaneous preterm labor, infection, and hemorrhage.

In summary, randomized controlled trials and meta-analysis suggest that fetoscopic laser ablation is superior to serial amnioreduction and should be considered as treatment for TTTS to improve both neonatal survival and outcome. This conclusion is echoed by a Cochrane review of the subject [72].

Fetoscopic cord coagulation

In cases where salvage of the recipient twin is unlikely, fetoscopic cord coagulation (FCC) or ligation can be used. It attempts to significantly improve the outcome of the remaining fetus by stopping twin–twin blood flow and its associated morbidities. FCC has also been used following SLEP if the laser therapy worsened the fetal condition [54].

Twin reversed arterial perfusion sequence

In monochorionic twin pregnancies, retrograde blood flow through AA anastomoses that allows blood to flow from one twin to the other is known as the twin reversed arterial perfusion (TRAP) sequence. The twin receiving the retrograde flow has a non-functioning heart or acardia. This condition is associated with other lethal anomalies that include acephalus. The acardiac twin receives all of its blood flow from the normal or "pump twin" and has no direct placental connection. Blood flows retrograde to the acardiac twin via the umbilical artery and returns from the acardiac twin via the umbilical vein. Instead of entering the placenta, this blood bypasses the placenta and flows into the normal twin via a VV connection [73]. This puts the normal twin at risk for high-output congestive heart failure, preterm birth, and polyhydramnios [74]. The incidence of TRAP is about 1 in 35,000 livebirths, affecting about 1% of monochorionic twins and 3% of monochorionic triplets [75,76]. The risk of death for the pump twin is >50% if the condition remains untreated and 90% if the acardiac twin is >75% of the size of the normal twin [77]. Additionally, there is a linear relationship between the size ratio of the acardiac-to-pump twin and the risk of mortality in the normal twin [77].

Early diagnosis is beneficial for optimal management. Unfortunately, both twins can have cardiac activity and still have the diagnosis of TRAP if the "acardiac" twin has a malformed cardiac mass without effective pumping. The diagnosis is confirmed by documenting retrograde flow to the acardiac twin by ultrasound Doppler imaging.

The primary goal of treatment is to stop blood flow between the twins by interrupting the connecting vasculature. Initially, this was accomplished by extracting the acardiac twin through an open hysterotomy (Fig. 19.8). Currently, either percutaneous endoscopic laser ablation of placental vascular anastomoses or image-guided percutaneous radiofrequency coagulation of the umbilical cord is employed [78–80]. A retrospective study of 60 TRAP cases (mean gestational age 18.3 weeks) from three European centers which used fetoscopic laser coagulation of the placental vascular anastomoses or of the umbilical cord reported 80% survival rate and a mean gestational age at birth of 37.4 weeks for the pump twin [81].

Radiofrequency ablation (RFA) is used to thermally coagulate the base of the acardiac twin's umbilical cord [79]. At UCSF, RFA is performed by inserting a

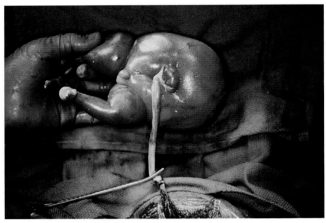

Figure 19.8 Open selective extraction of an acardiac twin. Courtesy of UCSF Fetal Treatment Center.

radiofrequency generator to the acardiac fetal abdominal wall through a 17 gauge needle under ultrasound guidance and coagulating the insertion site of the umbilical cord. As with other minimally invasive techniques, maternal anesthesia can be produced by infiltrating the skin with local anesthetic or by neuraxial blockade and intravenous sedation. RFA endpoints include reaching a predetermined impedance level or temperature. At 110°C, a 2 cm diameter area of tissue coagulation is produced. Absence of flow to the acardiac twin is confirmed by ultrasound color Doppler at the end of the procedure and on postoperative day 1. In a single-institution retrospective review of 26 cases of monochorionic diamniotic twins with TRAP who were treated with RFA, there was 92% survival of the pump twins who on average were born at 35.6 weeks [79].

Myelomeningocele

Open spina bifida or myelomeningocele (MMC) is a nonlethal neural tube defect that occurs early in gestation and results in protrusion and exposure of meninges and spinal cord through a spinal defect. These neural elements may be injured by exposure to amniotic fluid during gestation, making possible early fetal repair attractive. The definitive cause of MMC remains unknown, but is likely multifactorial. Taking folate during pregnancy has decreased the incidence of this lesion to 1 in 2000 livebirths.

Animal studies suggest that part of the ultimate neural damage arises from chemical neurotoxicity and secondary neural destruction by components of amniotic fluid or meconium [82]. In sheep, covering the MMC neural defect decreased neurological morbidity and increased the likelihood of normal anal sphincter function [83]. Using somatosensory evoked potentials, Julia demonstrated decreased neurological sequelae following *in utero* repair of a surgically created MMC in rabbits [84]. Examination of fetuses with MMC early in gestation showed an open but undamaged spinal cord. Examination of stillborn fetuses at later gestations demonstrated recent neural injury and tissue loss [82]. Direct trauma to the exposed cord and mutations in the *PAX3* gene have also been implicated in causing MMC [85].

α-Fetoprotein screening of maternal blood detects MMC during the first trimester and affords the option of pregnancy termination. The 5-year mortality of MMC is about 8% of livebirths [86]. Secondary complications include hydrocephalus, Arnold–Chiari II malformation, motor and sensory nerve deficits (including paraplegia), bowel and bladder incontinence, spinal cord tethering, sexual dysfunction, and cognitive impairment [87]. Approximately 80% of children with MMC require ventriculoperitoneal shunting for the treatment of hydrocephalus [88]. The primary purpose of fetal treatment of MMC is to cover the fetal neural contents early in gestation to prevent additional damage by prolonged exposure to the uterine environment.

Initial attempts at *in utero* repair of MMC were done endoscopically and used a maternal split-thickness skin graft to cover the defect [89]. Unfortunately, the success of these initial attempts was poor [90]. Subsequently, open fetal surgery has been used to correct this lesion *in utero* (Fig. 19.9) using either a primary closure (Fig. 19.10) or a dermal patch (Fig. 19.11), depending on the size of the defect. Investigators at Vanderbilt University compared 26 patients corrected *in utero* to historic controls and reported a significant reduction in hindbrain herniation (4% versus 50%) and a decrease in shunt-dependent hydrocephalus (58% versus 92%) [91]. However, lower extremity motor function closely matched the level of the mean anatomical lesion in both groups. A retrospective chart review of 54 children who underwent *in utero* repair of MMC at the Children's Hospital of Philadelphia found better neonatal neuromotor function of the legs than predicted by prenatal ultrasound [92]. The recent analysis and publication of a randomized unmasked trial comparing outcomes from in utero myelomeningocele repair

versus postnatal repair demonstrated the efficacy of prenatal intervention [218]. The primary outcome measures for the management of myelomeningocele study (MOMS) included a composite of fetal or neonatal death, the need for cerebral spinal fluid shunt placement by 12 months of age, and mental development and motor function assessed at 30 months of age. The study was stopped early for efficacy as it showed fetal surgery significantly reduced the need for shunts as well as improved motor function. However, prenatal intervention was associated with increased risk of preterm birth and uterine dehiscence. Based on these results, it is likely the incidence of open fetal myelomeningocele repair will increase in the future. Specific maternal and fetal considerations for open repair of MMC are detailed in the section on anesthesia for open fetal procedures.

Congenital cystic adenomatoid malformation

Congenital cystic adenomatoid malformation (CCAM) is a discrete pulmonary mass that contains both solid and cystic components that are <1 mm to several cm in diameter. CCAMs have been previously classified by size or by histology [93,94] (see Chapter 24). Recently, they have been classified into two types based on ultrasound imaging and size [95]. Malformations containing single or multiple cysts >5 mm in diameter on ultrasound are

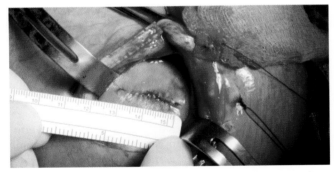

Figure 19.10 Primary closure of fetal myelomeningocele. Courtesy of UCSF Fetal Treatment Center.

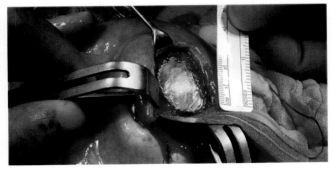

Figure 19.11 Closure of fetal myelomeningocele with dermal patch. Courtesy of UCSF Fetal Treatment Center.

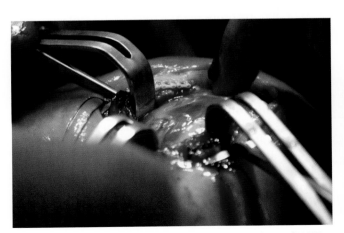

Figure 19.9 Open repair of fetal myelomeningocele. Courtesy of UCSF Fetal Treatment Center.

termed "macrocystic"; they may develop into large solitary cysts of several centimeters in diameter. Smaller lesions with cysts <5mm diameter are termed "microcystic"; they appear as solid images by ultrasound. The incidence of CCAM is estimated to be 1 in 25,000 pregnancies [96]. CCAMs are distinguished from other fetal lung masses based on five histological characteristics: mucosal polypoid projections; more cystic wall smooth muscle and elastic tissue; a lack of cartilage; presence of mucus-secreting cells; and no inflammatory markers [95]. The differential diagnosis of CCAM includes bronchopulmonary sequestration, congenital lobar emphysema, peripheral bronchial atresia, and mixed lesions that include CCAM [97].

The overall fetal outcome depends on CCAM size, tumor growth characteristics, presence of hydrops, and secondary morbidity from large masses that cause a fetal mediastinal shift, pulmonary hypoplasia or polyhydramnios [98,99]. Smaller CCAMs detected *in utero* are resected after birth, usually by excising the affected pulmonary lobe. The CCAM volume ratio (CVR) is the quotient of the calculated CCAM volume and the fetal head circumference normalized for gestational age as determined by ultrasound imaging [100]. A CVR >1.6 is associated with greater risk of fetal hydrops. Bilateral fetal masses or the presence of hydrops are associated with poor outcomes [100,101]. Periodic ultrasound surveillance of these masses is critical since they can grow rapidly and unpredictably.

Possible fetal surgical strategies include aspiration and drainage of cysts, thoracoamniotic shunt placement, percutaneous laser ablation, and resection of the mass during open fetal surgery [102]. Aspiration of cysts may improve the fetus' condition temporarily, but the fluid often reaccumulates. Placement of shunts can produce sustained decompression and resolution of hydrops *in utero*, and allow definitive treatment after birth [103]. Without intervention, large CCAMs may cause significant pleural effusions and pulmonary hypoplasia. Unfortunately, some cystic lesions are compartmentalized and cannot be successfully drained. Thoracoamniotic shunts may be displaced, malfunction or occlude, and may cause fetal hemorrhage, placental abruption, preterm labor, and chorio-amnionitis [100,102]. Administration of betametasone to fetuses with CCAMs and hydrops can improve outcomes [104].

Solid microcystic CCAMs or other large masses not amenable to drainage or shunting can be resected during open fetal surgery (Fig. 19.12). The lobe containing the lesion is resected during a hysterotomy and fetal thoracotomy [105]. Anesthetic considerations are described in the section on anesthesia for open fetal procedures. A retrospective review of 30 fetuses at UCSF who had large CCAMs and hydrops showed a 50% 30-day survival after birth following open surgical resection [106]. Only 3% (1

of 33) of fetuses with similar CCAMs survived without surgical intervention.

Improved selection criteria and the potential for minimally invasive video-assisted thorascopic radiofrequency ablation of the tumor hold promise for improved outcomes [102].

Sacrococcygeal teratoma

Fetuses with sacrococcygeal teratoma (SCT) are typically diagnosed in the second trimester of pregnancy; the incidence of SCT is 1 in 40,000 livebirths [107,108]. The lesions can grow to 500–1000 cubic centimeters [109]. Perinatal mortality is high due to massive tumor enlargement, hydrops, and placentomegaly. The perinatal mortality of 23 fetuses with SCT was 43% [109]. These tumors also cause significant arteriovenous shunting, and the resultant high-output cardiac failure is often the cause of fetal death. Fetal hydrops may be associated with "mirror syndrome" in which the mother develops a hyperdynamic high cardiac output state similar to that of the fetus and has superimposed symptoms of pre-eclampsia [110]. Fetuses with large lesions are at risk for intrapartum dystocia, tumor rupture and hemorrhage, and bladder outlet obstruction. They are born by cesarean section.

Several SCTs have been successfully removed *in utero* with resolution of hydrops noted in the weeks following the procedure [14]. Successful operations for large sacrococcygeal teratomas require catheterization of a fetal hand or umbilical cord vein to allow blood and fluid resuscitation during tumor resection. To date, outcome of hydropic fetuses with SCT has not been improved by surgery. Minimally invasive surgery using RFA and thermocoagulation attempts to reduce the tumor's blood supply and improve outcomes, although it is unclear whether or not this happens [14].

Fetal urinary tract obstruction

Urinary tract obstructions are detected by ultrasound in approximately 1% of pregnancies [111]. The great majority of these abnormalities have no significant clinical consequence. Only 1 in 1000 pregnancies has congenital obstructive uropathy (see Chapter 29) [112]. The clinical morbidity from fetal urinary tract obstruction depends on the location of the obstruction, severity, duration, age at onset, and gender of the fetus [111]. Congenital bilateral hydronephrosis from obstruction of the fetal urethra has a worse prognosis than unilateral upper urinary tract obstructions. Although the exact etiology may vary, posterior urethral valves are often the cause of bilateral hydronephrosis in male fetuses. Other possible causes include obstruction of the ureteropelvic and ureterovesical junctions, ectopic ureter, ureterocele, megacystis megaureter, multicystic kidney or more complex pathologies [113]. These anomalies are easily detected by ultrasonography

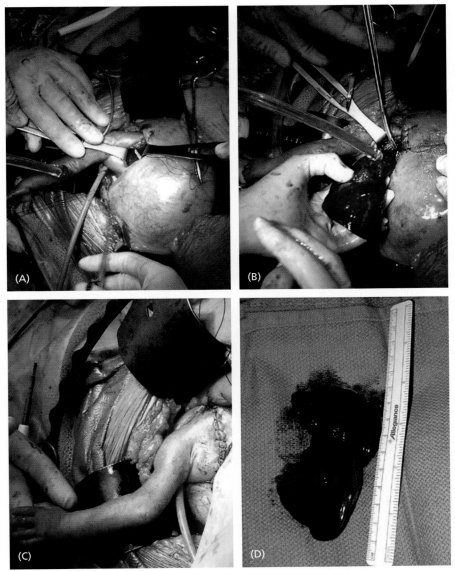

Figure 19.12 (A) Open resection of fetal congenital cystic adenomatoid malformation (CCAM) with fetal thoracotomy shown. (B) Resected CCAM mass. (C) Primary closure of fetal thoracotomy. (D) Pathology specimen of resected CCAM mass. Courtesy of UCSF Fetal Treatment Center.

and commonly result in oligohydramnios. Before 16 weeks' gestation, a transudate of maternal plasma forms the amniotic fluid; after 16 weeks, fetal urine is its primary source. An ultrasound grading system based on fetal renal pelvis anteroposterior diameter is commonly used to assess the severity of prenatal hydronephrosis [114]. Not only should an extensive ultrasound evaluation of the entire urinary tract be done, cardiac or neural tube defects should also be sought because they occur more commonly in fetuses with lower urinary tract obstructions [111]. Occasionally, amnio-infusion of warmed isotonic solution may be needed to improve imaging conditions.

Severe urinary tract obstruction causes oligohydramnios, hydroureteronephrosis, and bladder distension, which in turn cause pulmonary hypoplasia, facial and extremity deformations, renal dysplasia and dysfunction, and deficiencies of abdominal muscle (Fig. 19.13) [115]. These problems significantly reduce postnatal survival, primarily by causing lung hypoplasia.

Placement of a double pigtail catheter between the fetal bladder and amniotic cavity allows decompression and drainage of the bladder *in utero*. This reduces oligohydramnios and its associated morbidities (pulmonary hypoplasia and umbilical cord compression) and improves renal development. The first intervention for congenital hydronephrosis was performed by open hysterotomy at UCSF. The neonate was born at 35 weeks' gestational age and died from lung hypoplasia [115]. Improved selection

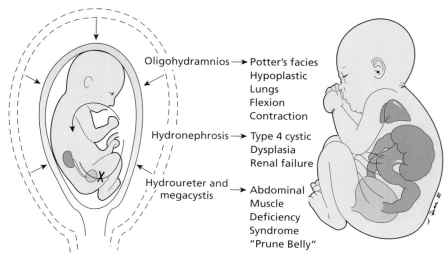

Figure 19.13 Developmental consequences of fetal urethral obstruction. Severe urinary tract obstruction results in significant fetal sequelae that can reduce postnatal survival. Reproduced from Harrison et al [115] with permission from the American Medical Association.

and placement of vesicoamniotic shunts allowed successful treatment of congenital hydronephrosis [7]. An algorithm with specific criteria was proposed to improve fetal candidate selection and outcome [116]. Components of the algorithm included fetal karyotype, an ultrasound examination looking for additional anatomical abnormalities, and fetal urine sampling to determine the amount of renal dysfunction. Fetal intervention requires a male karyotype (females often have more complex urinary abnormalities), absence of other structural abnormalities that affect outcome, and the presence of oligohydramnios or decreasing amniotic fluid volume. Serial sampling of fetal urine on 3–5 occasions, complete bladder drainage, 24–48-h intervals between samples, and assessment of sodium, chloride, calcium, osmolality, protein, and β2-microglobulin improves fetal outcome prediction [111,117]. Increased levels of these components of fetal urine are associated with advanced renal damage and a poor prognosis [118]. Detection of lesions early in gestation, the degree of oligohydramnios, and the presence of additional abnormalities all predict worse outcomes.

Vesicoamniotic catheter shunt placement is often difficult because oligohydramnios compromises ultrasound imaging. Potential complications of catheter insertion include catheter occlusion or displacement, chorioamnionitis, premature rupture of membranes, fetal trauma, abdominal wall defects (gastroschisis), placental separation and hemorrhage, preterm labor, and maternal leakage of amniotic fluid [111]. This minimally invasive intervention requires neuraxial anesthesia or infiltration of local anesthetic into the maternal abdominal wall and uterine musculature. The neonate will require definitive repair of the underlying problem after birth.

A single-institution, retrospective review of 34 vesicoamniotic shunt placements for heterogeneous causes of

obstructive uropathy between 1987 and 1996 reported 50% survival to at least 2 years of age; 43% of survivors had normal renal function [119]. A recent retrospective review of 20 pregnancies with male fetuses with lower urinary tract obstruction reported overall 1-year survival of 90% and only two neonatal deaths from pulmonary hypoplasia [120]. Eight children had normal renal function, 11 had normal bladder function with spontaneous voiding, and eight had respiratory difficulty [120]. Currently, a multicenter randomized controlled trial is comparing survival and renal function in fetuses with lower urinary tract obstruction treated with either vesicoamniotic shunting or conservative therapy [121]. Minimally invasive percutaneous cystoscopy with laser ablation of the posterior urethral valves may reverse pulmonary and renal morbidity, but its efficacy is uncertain at this time [122,123].

Fetal cardiac anomalies

Congenital cardiac anomalies occur in 0.08–0.1% (8–10/1000) of livebirths [124]. About 3.4–4 per 1000 livebirths require surgical or interventional treatment for these anomalies in infancy [125]. Significant improvement in ultrasound imaging allows *in utero* diagnosis of cardiac abnormalities as early as 12–14 weeks' gestation. It also allows better determination of the physiological relevance of the anomaly for the fetus [126]. *In utero* interventional cardiac catheterization has been done in an attempt to reverse detrimental consequences of cardiac lesions before they cause irreversible damage [127].

This technique has been used for aortic and pulmonary valvuloplasty to treat aortic and pulmonary valvular stenoses. Significant aortic stenosis causes fetal blood to flow primarily through the low-resistance foramen ovale, which diminishes left ventricular growth and causes hypoplastic left heart syndrome (HLHS). In severe cases, biventricular cardiac function is so reduced that neonatal palliative univentricular surgery or heart transplantation are the only options [126]. Fetal aortic valvuloplasty for severe aortic stenosis carries a high risk for HLHS, and fetal intervention has been shown to reverse hydrops and heart failure, and improve cardiac hemodynamics [128–130]. Hypoplastic right heart syndrome occurs with severe fetal pulmonary valvular stenosis or atresia. Significant tricuspid regurgitation produces high central venous pressures and hydrops [127]. *In utero* intervention for pulmonary stenosis has had mixed success [127,131,132]. The criteria and optimal gestational age at which *in utero* intervention should occur are uncertain. Guidelines for patient selection for *in utero* aortic vavuloplasty include degree of stenosis, left ventricular length, left-to-right shunting, and reversal of aortic arch flow [133]. Guidelines for *in utero* pulmonary valvuloplasty include biventricular output, degree of stenosis, estimated right ventricular pressures, and presence of hydrops [134].

Open fetal cardiac methods have been used to optimally position the fetus for cardiac catheterization. However, minimally invasive techniques are preferred because they decrease maternal morbidity and premature labor. A small laparotomy may be required when the fetal position is suboptimal, when maternal obesity limits visualization or when an anterior-lying placenta prevents direct needle trajectory [127]. The initial percutaneous approach for aortic valvular repair was described by Maxwell [135]. Currently, ultrasound imaging is used to visualize the fetus while it is positioned with the left chest anterior to allow unobstructed visualization and a cannula path that is parallel with the fetal aortic outflow tract [136]. A small cannula (≤19 gauge) is passed percutaneously through the maternal abdomen and fetal chest wall, into the left ventricle, and through the aortic valve. The valvuloplasty is performed with a high-pressure small (e.g. 2 mm) balloon-tipped catheter. Similar techniques have been used for right heart valvuloplasty and atrial septoplasty [127]. Fetal intervention also has been suggested to treat complete heart block that is unresponsive to other forms of therapy, especially when it is thought that cardiac output is insufficient to sustain fetal life [137].

Infiltration of local anesthetic or neuraxial anesthesia with supplemental intravenous sedation is appropriate for these procedures. Intramuscular narcotics and muscle relaxants are given to the fetus (see Minimally invasive and percutaneous procedures). Fetal resuscitation drugs should be readily available to treat bradycardia or other arrhythmias. Other complications include valvular insufficiency, pericardial effusions, infection, and preterm labor.

Anesthetic management of fetal procedures

Anesthetic management of fetal surgical procedures is similar to anesthesia for non-obstetric surgery during pregnancy. Although the anesthesiologist must optimize fetal well-being and the conditions required for successful surgical and fetal outcomes, the paramount focus must be maternal safety. Consequently, anesthesiologists must participate in determining potential maternal risk compared to potential fetal benefit and exclude women in whom the benefit/risk ratio is low. Pregnancy-induced hormonal changes, mechanical effects of a growing uterus, and, changes in maternal physiology have important implications for administration of anesthesia. To ensure maternal and fetal safety, the anesthesiologist must understand these physiological changes and how they affect anesthetic management, and must take an active role in perioperative management of both patients.

Unlike other surgical procedures performed during pregnancy for maternal indications (e.g. appendectomy) where the fetus is an innocent bystander, fetal surgery involves two surgical patients and the anesthesiologist must balance the needs of both. For fetal procedures, the anesthesiologist must consider the fetus' requirements for anesthesia (see below) and the perioperative control of uterine tone.

Physiological changes of pregnancy and anesthetic implications

During pregnancy, women undergo fundamental changes in anatomy and physiology [138,139]. These changes and the associated morbidities of the fetal procedure place mothers at significantly greater risk for complications during anesthesia than non-pregnant women. A detailed understanding of these changes and their anesthetic implications is required to prepare for and respond immediately to complications such as fetal distress and maternal hemorrhage. Although the physiological changes of pregnancy affect all organ systems, this section only focuses on cardiovascular, respiratory, and gastrointestinal changes and their anesthetic implications in the perioperative period. A more detailed discourse on this subject is found in obstetric anesthesia texts [139].

Maternal cardiovascular system
Hematology
Maternal intravascular volume begins to increase in the first trimester of pregnancy. Larger increases in plasma volume (45%) than in erythrocyte volume (20%) cause physiological (dilutional) anemia of pregnancy. The hemoglobin concentration is normally 11 g/dL or greater during pregnancy [138].

Pregnancy induces a hypercoagulable state. Factors I, VII, VIII, IX, X, and XII increase and factors XI, XIII, and antithrombin III decrease. These changes reduce both prothrombin (PT) and partial thromboplastin time (PTT) by 20%. Platelet levels are normal or reduced by 10%, and the leukocyte count is commonly elevated.

Cardiac output

Cardiac output increases 10% above the pre-pregnant state by 10 weeks' gestation and by 40–50% by the third trimester. Increases in both heart rate (15–25%) and stroke volume (25–30%) are responsible for this rise. During labor, maternal cardiac output increases further. Each uterine contraction autotransfuses 300–500 mL of blood into the maternal central circulation. The greatest increase in cardiac output occurs immediately after delivery, when it is elevated by as much as 80% above predelivery levels. This abrupt increase in cardiac output is secondary to removal of aortocaval compression, autotransfusion from the contracted uterus, and decreased venous pressure in the lower extremities [140]. These changes in cardiac output are a significant risk for patients with major cardiac disease, e.g. fixed valvular lesions or left ventricular outflow tract obstruction.

Aortocaval compression

The gravid uterus may decrease preload, cardiac output, and maternal blood pressure by compressing the vena cava of supine pregnant women, especially at term. Venous blood from the lower extremities is redirected to the heart via the azygos, epidural, and vertebral veins. When supine, significant aortoiliac artery compression occurs in 15–20% of pregnant women. Vena cava compression is universal and often occurs as early as 13–16 weeks of gestation. Approximately 15% of women experience significant hypotension in the supine position late in gestation. In addition, symptoms of nausea, vomiting, diaphoresis, and decreased mental status may accompany the reduction in blood pressure.

Anesthetic implications

The majority of pregnant women experience minimal supine hypotension because they increase systemic vascular resistance to compensate for reduced venous return. Anesthetic interventions that diminish sympathetic tone (e.g. neuraxial blockade, general anesthesia) exacerbate the effects of vena cava compression and hypotension in supine mothers. Compression of the abdominal aorta by the gravid uterus can also produce lower extremity hypotension and reduced uterine and fetal blood flow that may not be reflected by upper extremity maternal blood pressures. Therefore supine positioning is to be avoided during the perioperative period in the second and third trimesters of pregnancy. To help preserve uterine blood flow and fetal circulation, the right hip is elevated 10–15 cm with a wedge or lateral table tilt. A >25% decrease in maternal blood pressure for >10–15 min may cause fetal hypoperfusion and progressive fetal acidosis.

Vena cava compression contributes to lower extremity venous stasis and increases the risk of venous thrombosis and pulmonary embolus. The venous stasis and hypercoagulable state of pregnancy require deep venous thrombosis prophylaxis in the postoperative period (sequential compression devices, low molecular weight heparin, encourage mobility). In addition, vena cava compression causes epidural veins to dilate, and this increases the risk of accidentally placing an epidural catheter in a vein and injecting local anesthetic intravenously. Vascular injection or accidental intrathecal injection of a dose of local anesthetic that is appropriate for epidural anesthesia may have grave maternal and fetal consequences (e.g. seizures, hemodynamic collapse, death). Consequently a "test dose" of 3 mL of 1.5% lidocaine with 1:200,000 epinephrine is injected prior to giving larger (therapeutic) doses of local anesthetic through an epidural catheter. Increases in heart rate and blood pressure in excess of 20% (intravascular injection) or a rapid loss of lower extremity sensation and onset of motor block (intrathecal injection) are evidence of a misplaced epidural catheter.

Maternal airway and pulmonary systems
Upper airway

During pregnancy, the pharynx, larynx, and trachea have increased capillary engorgement and tissue friability, making both laryngoscopy and tracheal intubation more challenging. It is frequently appropriate to use smaller cuffed endotracheal tubes (6.0 and 6.5 mm internal diameter) because the larynx may be edematous and narrowed. Because of increased tissue friability, oropharyngeal suctioning and airway instrumentation may induce bleeding. Routine use of nasogastric tubes is contraindicated.

Ventilation and oxygenation

At term, minute ventilation is increased approximately 50% and oxygen consumption more than 20%; functional residual capacity is decreased 20%. Resting maternal CO_2 decreases from 40 mmHg to 30–32 mmHg in the first trimester of pregnancy. Arterial pH is slightly alkalotic (7.42–7.44) due to decreased concentrations of bicarbonate (compensatory metabolic acidosis)

Anesthetic implications

Airway management by facemask, laryngeal mask or tracheal intubation can be technically difficult in pregnant women because of their increased anteroposterior chest diameter, enlarged breasts, and laryngeal narrowing. The increased oxygen consumption and decreased oxygen reserve allow more rapid oxygen desaturation during hypoventilation, apnea, and general anesthesia. Obesity exacerbates this desaturation. Pregnancy-induced changes in both airway and respiratory physiology make ventilation and tracheal intubation more difficult and increase the potential for complications. During general anesthesia and controlled ventilation for fetal surgery, the maternal arterial CO_2 should be maintained at physiological levels (30–32 mmHg). Alkalosis reduces uterine blood flow and causes fetal acid–base abnormalities. Excessive positive pressure ventilation can increase maternal mean intrathoracic pressure and decrease cardiac preload, cardiac output, and uterine blood flow [141]. Severe hypocapnia shifts the oxyhemoglobin dissociation curve leftward, increasing maternal hemoglobin affinity for oxygen. Lastly, arterial pCO_2 of <20 mmHg can decrease umbilical blood flow [142] and jeopardize the fetus.

Maternal gastrointestinal system
Women beyond 20 weeks' gestation are at risk for regurgitation and aspiration of gastric content during the induction of anesthesia or with deep sedation. The gravid uterus displaces the stomach cephalad and anteriorly and the pylorus cephalad and posteriorly. The normally intra-abdominal portion of the esophagus is elevated into the thorax, decreasing the competence of the esophageal sphincter. Elevated progesterone and estrogen levels during pregnancy reduce esophageal sphincter tone. The gravid uterus increases gastric pressure, and placental gastrin secretion lowers gastric fluid pH. Consequently, maternal symptoms of gastric reflux increase with increasing duration of pregnancy in most pregnant women [143]. Although gastric emptying is not delayed until the onset of labor, systemic or neuraxial boluses of opioids during surgery can delay gastric emptying and further increase the risk of aspiration [144].

Anesthetic implications
Beyond midgestation, or earlier if there are symptoms of gastric reflux, women are at increased risk for pulmonary aspiration of acidic gastric contents. Regardless of when the last ingestion of food occurred, pregnant women should be considered as having a full stomach and assumed to have increased risk for pulmonary aspiration of gastric contents. A non-particulate antacid, such as sodium citrate 30 mL, is used as premedication for all procedures. Rapid-sequence induction of anesthesia and tracheal intubation, utilizing cricoid pressure and a styleted, cuffed tracheal tube, is routinely employed during induction of general anesthesia in pregnant women after midgestation. The risk of aspiration during tracheal extubation is similar to that during induction of anesthesia [145]. Consequently, the trachea is not extu-

bated until protective airway reflexes have returned. Metoclopramide (10 mg IV), when given at least 15 min before the start of anesthesia, decreases the risk of aspiration at both induction of anesthesia and tracheal extubation. However, prior opioid administration reduces the effectiveness of metoclopramide and may cause extrapyramidal signs [146]. H_2 receptor antagonists also effectively increase gastric pH and are recommended by some practitioners [147].

Maternal central nervous system
The MAC of volatile anesthetics decreases 30–40% during pregnancy. In addition, pregnant women are more sensitive to local anesthetics, which decreases the local anesthetic dose requirement for epidural or spinal anesthesia. This increased sensitivity begins in the first trimester, before there is significant aortocaval compression, suggesting a role for biochemical changes (progesterone mediated) [148,149]. Engorgement of epidural veins and the corresponding decrease in the size of the epidural space with advancing gestation may facilitate the spread of local anesthetics.

Anesthetic implications
The decreased MAC in pregnant women increases the possibility of anesthetic overdose. Alveolar concentrations of inhaled anesthetics that may not anesthetize non-pregnant women can produce unconsciousness in pregnant women. This degree of central nervous system depression can impair protective upper airway reflexes and increase the risk of pulmonary aspiration. To obtain a similar level of surgical block, the dose of local anesthetic used for neuraxial blocks should be reduced by approximately one-third of that used for non-pregnant patients.

Uteroplacental and fetal physiology
Uterine blood flow
Uterine blood flow increases from approximately 100 mL/min in the non-pregnant state to about 700 mL/min (about 10% of cardiac output) at term. The placenta receives about 80% of the uterine blood flow (UBF) and the myometrium 20%. Uterine vasculature has limited autoregulation and is essentially maximally dilated throughout pregnancy.

Reduced uterine perfusion pressure or increased arterial resistance reduces maternal UBF. Decreased perfusion pressure results from systemic hypotension (hypovolemia, aortocaval compression) and neuraxial or general anesthesia. Arterial CO_2 below 20 mmHg, stress-induced endogenous catecholamines, and exogenous vasopressors also increase the resistance of the uterine arteries and can decrease UBF.

Placental exchange and fetal circulation

The placenta is the interface between the fetal and maternal circulatory systems. Maternal blood is delivered to the placenta by the uterine arteries. Oxygen-poor fetal blood arrives at the placenta via two umbilical arteries, and oxygen- and nutrient-rich blood returns from the placenta to the fetus through a single umbilical vein.

Oxygen transfer to the fetus depends on a variety of factors including ratio of maternal UBF to fetal umbilical blood flow; oxygen partial pressure gradient; respective hemoglobin concentrations and affinities; placental diffusing capacity; and acid–base status of the fetal and maternal blood (Bohr effect). The fetal oxyhemoglobin dissociation curve is left-shifted (greater oxygen affinity) while the maternal hemoglobin dissociation curve is right-shifted (decreased oxygen affinity). This facilitates oxygen transfer to the fetus. After the first trimester, the fetal-placental blood volume is 120–160 mL/kg, depending on the gestational age [150].

Fetal hypovolemia reduces fetal organ perfusion because the immature sympathetic nervous system and baroreceptor activity are unable to compensate by vasoconstriction. The fetus also has limited capacity to increase cardiac output in response to stresses. Fetuses also become rapidly hypothermic when outside the uterus because of transdermal heat loss and immature thermoregulatory vasoconstriction. They produce their own coagulation factors (which do not cross the placenta). The concentration of these factors increases with gestational age. Despite this increase, fetuses clot less well than adults.

Maternal-fetal exchange of most drugs and other substances of <1000 daltons is principally by diffusion. Transfer of substances across the placenta to the fetus depends on maternal-to-fetal concentration gradients; maternal protein binding; molecular weight of the substance; lipid solubility; and the degree of substance ionization. In most instances, the drug concentration in maternal blood is the major determinant of how much drug ultimately reaches the fetus.

Fetal uptake of substances that cross the placenta is facilitated by the more acidic pH (0.1 unit) of fetal compared to maternal blood. Weakly basic drugs (local anesthetics, opioids) that cross the placenta in the non-ionized form are ionized in the fetal circulation and accumulate against a concentration gradient (ion trapping). Therefore, distressed acidotic fetuses can accumulate high concentrations of local anesthetic. If there is an inadvertent maternal intravascular local anesthetic injection, the fetus often develops bradycardia, ventricular arrhythmia, acidosis, and severe cardiac depression.

The anatomy of the fetal circulation helps decrease fetal exposure to potentially high concentrations of drugs in umbilical venous blood. Approximately 75% of umbilical venous blood initially passes through the fetal liver, which may result in significant drug metabolism before the drug reaches the fetal heart and brain (first-pass metabolism) if the enzymes for metabolism are present (see Chapter 9). Fetal/neonatal enzyme system activities are lower than those of adults, but most drugs can be metabolized. In addition, drugs entering the fetal inferior vena cava via the ductus venosus are initially diluted by drug-free blood returning from the fetal lower extremities and pelvic viscera. These characteristics of the fetal circulation markedly decrease fetal plasma drug concentrations compared to maternal concentrations.

Anesthetic implications

Adequate uterine blood flow and oxygenation are critical to fetal well-being. Because asphyxiated fetuses cannot increase oxygen extraction, they compensate by redistributing blood flow from the periphery to vital organs. Both hypercapnia and hypocapnia reduce uterine blood flow, which causes fetal acidosis. In addition to left uterine displacement, eucarbia for the mother (30 mmHg end-tidal CO_2) should be maintained during general anesthesia. When regional or general anesthesia techniques are used, a FiO_2 of 0.5 or higher is recommended during the procedure. In addition, maintenance of maternal blood pressure near baseline values is critical to fetal well-being. Use of vasopressors and judicious fluid administration are frequently required to maintain normal maternal blood pressure. Despite the historical use of ephedrine as the vasopressor of choice, phenylephrine (α-adrenergic) has proven to be extremely useful for treatment of maternal hypotension that is associated with neuraxial anesthesia [151–153].

Teratogenicity

Many drugs, including anesthetics, are known teratogens in at least one animal species. Organogenesis occurs primarily between 15 and 56 days of gestation in humans. Most fetal procedures are performed well beyond this critical period. At the present time, there is no evidence that any currently used anesthetic administered during pregnancy is teratogenic in humans. However, anesthetics cause neurodegeneration and widespread apoptosis in neonatal animals. A few studies also demonstrate cognitive impairment in adult animals who were exposed to anesthetics as neonates. Unfortunately, these data in animals cannot be extrapolated to humans. Clinical evidence is still scarce and amounts to an associative and not causal relationship [154].

Impact of anesthesia on the fetus

In addition to decreased uterine blood flow and potential fetal compromise, certain anesthetics depress the fetal cardiovascular and central nervous systems or increase the risk of preterm labor and delivery. Anesthetics typically used for induction of anesthesia, such as thiopental (4–6 mg/kg) and propofol (2.0–2.5 mg/kg), are highly lipid soluble, render the pregnant patient unconscious within 30 sec, and have peak concentrations in the fetal circulation within minutes after administration to the mother. Etomidate also has a quick onset of action and rapidly crosses the placenta. Unlike thiopental and propofol, etomidate has minimal cardiovascular effects in the mother but is painful on injection, can cause involuntary muscle tremors, causes significant nausea and vomiting, and can decrease seizure thresholds and increase the risk of seizures. At typical induction doses (0.3 mg/kg), maternal etomidate administration decreases neonatal cortisol production in <6h but the clinical significance of this remains uncertain [155]. Induction of anesthesia with ketamine can increase uterine tone and uterine contractions, and compromise uteroplacental perfusion. Therefore, it is rarely used.

Volatile anesthetics are rapidly transferred across the placenta because they are non-ionized, highly lipid-soluble, low molecular weight substances. By causing some uterine vasodilation and relaxation, modest amounts of maternal hypotension can be compensated for and uterine perfusion maintained. Fetal concentrations of these agents depend directly on the concentration and duration of anesthetic in the mother. Halogenated agents (≥2 MAC) depress fetal myocardium and lead to progressive fetal acidosis [156]. Yet even the high concentrations (2–3 MAC) used with the EXIT procedure appear well tolerated if maternal arterial blood pressure is maintained.

Placental transfer of local anesthetics and opioids is facilitated by their relatively low molecular weights. Most systemic anesthetics and opioids decrease fetal heart rate variability and may have minimal effects on baseline fetal heart rate, but do not cause fetal heart rate decelerations or bradycardia.

Succinylcholine has a low molecular weight, is highly ionized, and does not readily cross the placenta unless it is given in large doses (4 mg/kg) or repeatedly. The high molecular weight and poor lipid solubility of non-depolarizing neuromuscular agents prevent them from entering the fetal circulation in significant quantities. Thus, during general anesthesia for fetal procedures, fetuses remain unparalyzed by muscle relaxants given into the maternal circulation.

Neostigmine, glycopyrrolate, and heparin also have limited placental transfer, but atropine and esmolol easily diffuse into the fetal circulation and cause fetal tachycardia and bradycardia respectively. In general, drugs that readily cross the blood–brain barrier also cross the placenta.

Fetal pain and anesthesia

Whether or when fetuses experience pain and whether they require or benefit from anesthesia for surgical inter-

vention are inadequately understood and controversial. Surgical pain is defined as an unpleasant sensory and emotional response to tissue damage and a subjective experience involving cognition, sensation and affective processes [157]. Although pain is commonly associated with physical noxious stimuli, it is clearly more than nociception or the simple reflex activity of a withdrawal response [158]. Pain is fundamentally a psychological construct that can exist in the absence of physical stimuli (e.g. phantom limb pain). The psychological nature of pain distinguishes it from nociception, which involves activation of nociceptive pathways without the subjective emotional experience of pain. Most definitions of pain suggest that the experience is highly subjective, organized into a conceptual framework, and based on previous painful injuries [157]. While the ability to experience pain must begin at some point and is clearly present in neonates, it is unclear when fetuses actually first feel pain.

Reflex movements and biochemical evidence of a "stress response" can be triggered by a noxious stimulus without involving the cerebral cortex and without conscious pain perception. An example is withdrawal from a noxious stimulus mediated in the spinal cord without conscious perception of pain (Fig. 19.14). This occurs by about 18 weeks' gestation. Peripheral sensory receptor nociception is transmitted by afferent fibers that synapse on interneurons in the spinal cord and then synapse on spinal cord motor neurons. These motor neurons trigger muscle contractions that cause limb flexion and movement. The stress response can be mediated in the spinal cord, brainstem or basal ganglia without cortical involvement (see Chapter 7).

It is generally accepted that experiencing pain requires higher cognitive functioning and cortical recognition that the stimulus is unpleasant. This requires intact neural pathways from the periphery, through the spinal cord, to the thalamus, which relays the stimulus to the primary sensory cortex, the insular cortex, and the anterior cingulated cortex (Fig. 19.15). Peripheral sensory receptor afferents also synapse on spinal cord neurons that project to the thalamus, which relays afferent stimuli to the cerebral cortex and activates many different cortical regions. Sensory receptors and spinal cord synapses required for nociception develop earlier than the thalamocortical pathways required for conscious perception of pain. It is doubtful that fetal perception of pain is possible before there are pathways from the periphery to the brain and before cortical structures develop and become functional. However, the stage of gestation at which fetal pain perception is possible and whether the fetus must be awake or aware of its surroundings to perceive pain is unknown.

Nerve terminals for detection of touch, temperature, and vibration (not pain) are present deep in human skin by 6 weeks of gestation and become more numerous and

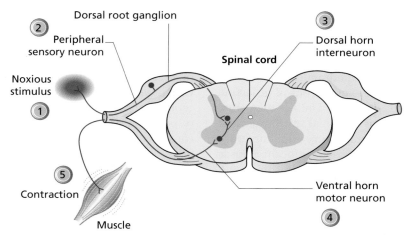

Figure 19.14 Early in development, reflex responses to noxious stimuli occur before thalamocortical circuits are functional; noxious stimuli trigger reflex movement without cortical involvement. Activated by a noxious stimulus (1), a peripheral sensory neuron (2) synapses on a dorsal horn interneuron (3) that in turn synapses on a ventral horn motor neuron (4), leading to reflex muscle contraction and limb withdrawal (5). Reproduced from Lee et al [158] with permission from the American Medical Association.

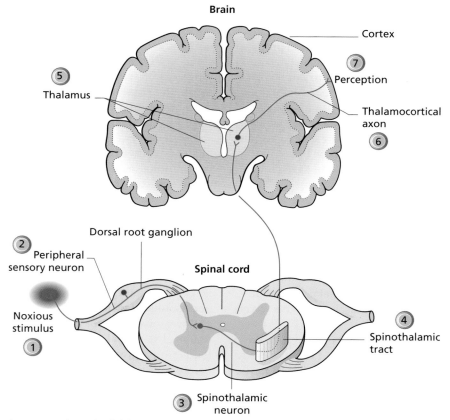

Figure 19.15 Later in development, noxious stimuli (1) activate peripheral sensory neurons (2) that synapse on spinothalamic tract neurons (3), the axons of which extend up the spinal cord as the spinothalamic tract (4) to synapse on neurons of the thalamus (5). From here, thalamocortical axons (6) synapse on cortical neurons, resulting in the conscious perception of pain (7). Reproduced from Lee et al [158] with permission from the American Medical Association.

have extended towards the skin surface by 10 weeks [159]. Immature skin nociceptors are probably present by 10 weeks and definitely present by 17 weeks [160]. Nociceptors develop slightly later in internal organs.

Peripheral nerve fibers that control movement first grow into the spinal cord at about 8 weeks of gestation. When these fibers connect with nociceptors is unknown but in other mammals this is more delayed than other sensory inputs. One human study suggests that nerve fibers from nociceptors do not enter the spinal cord before about 19 weeks [161]. The cerebral cortex develops after the fetal spinal cord and brainstem.

The developing cerebral wall consists of transient fetal zones where neuronal proliferation, cell migration, apoptosis, axonal outgrowth and synaptogenesis occur according to a highly specific timetable. Early in development, the cerebral cortex is a smooth layer without sulci and gyri and, like the thalamus, has no internal cellular organization [159]. The insular cortex starts developing in humans around 15 weeks' gestation, and the cortical subplate develops about 13 weeks. The subplate is a temporary structure located one layer deep to the cortical plate. The subplate recedes after 32–34 weeks' gestation and the cortical plate develops into the six layers of the cerebral cortex [162–164]. The subplate is crucial in cortex development because it serves as a waiting zone for various afferents, including thalamic afferents that are en route to the developing cortex. The subplate is also critical for establishing connections between the thalamus and cortex and for precise organization and laminar relocation of these afferent pathways.

The first fibers from the thalamus reach the subplate by 12 and 18 weeks' gestation and remain in the subplate until maturation of the cortical plate. By 24 weeks, substantial thalamocortical fibers have amassed in the subplate and have grown into the maturing cortex by 24 and 32 weeks. The gestational age at which thalamic pain fibers reach the human cortex can only be estimated from histological studies of other thalamocortical circuits. Thalamic projections reach the visual subplate at 20–22 weeks [163,165], the visual cortex at 23–27 weeks [166], and the auditory cortical plate at about 26–28 weeks' gestation [167]. The subplate thins in the insula and in areas of the brain where cortical folding occurs early. It disappears after a period of rapid relocation of fibers to the cortex at around 34 weeks' gestation. Massive brain growth and maturation occur after 34 weeks' gestation. This results in the typical cortical sulci and gyri and in development of extensive intracortical pathways and pathways from the cortex to the thalamus, midbrain, and spinal cord.

Given the development of pain pathways and interpretation of cortical function, it is unlikely that fetuses experience pain before 24 weeks' gestation (and perhaps significantly later) because the cortex must subsequently undergo considerable development and establish enormously complex and highly integrated neural networking, with dendritic and synaptic rearrangements that occur during late fetal life and infancy and continue into early childhood.

Although development of neural pathways from the periphery to the cortex is important, development of the cortex itself is probably necessary for fetuses to experience pain. The neural networking must also be functional. Although there are no specific electroencephalographic patterns for fetal pain, EEG studies provide some evidence for functionality. Studies at 24 weeks' gestation show the presence of cortical electrical activity only 2% of the time, with bursts that last about 20 sec and inactive periods that last up to 8 min [168]. By 30 weeks, EEG patterns are similar to those of wakefulness and sleep, but they are not continuous and are discordant with fetal behavior. By 34 weeks, electrical activity is present 80% of the time and EEG patterns become more distinct [169–172].

Can the fetus experience pain before there are connections from the periphery to cortex or before there is significant brain electrical activity? Some investigators have postulated that nociceptive information may be transmitted earlier through neurological connections from peripheral tissue through the brainstem and thalamus to the subplate. They argue that the midbrain reticular system is responsible for "consciousness" rather than the thalamocortical system [173]. Although midbrain systems are crucial for the waking state, instincts, orienting, goal-directed control, and purposeful behavior, consciousness is widely regarded as a very complex phenomenon for which the cerebral cortex is indispensable. Awareness and wakefulness are different phenomena.

Preterm neonates who undergo surgery with minimal anesthesia have circulatory, sympathoadrenal, and pituitary adrenal responses that are characteristic of stress. These include release of catecholamines, growth hormone, glucagon, cortisol, aldosterone, and other corticosteroids, as well as decreased insulin secretion [174,175]. Anesthesia blunts the neonatal stress response [176]. Opioids also improve the outcome of preterm neonates by attenuating the stress response [177].

In the human fetus, inserting a needle into the intrahepatic vein for blood transfusion induces the stress response, while needling the insensate umbilical cord does not. This response includes increased plasma β-endorphin and cortisol concentrations and decreased Doppler-determined middle cerebral artery pulsatility index. The latter is consistent with redistribution of blood flow to vital organs, including the brain [178]. The stress response to intrahepatic vein needling is blunted by 10 μg/kg of fentanyl [179]. Human fetuses elaborate pituitary-adrenal, sympathoadrenal, and circulatory stress responses to noxious stimuli as early as 18 weeks' gestation [180–183]. During late gestation, fetuses respond to environmental stimuli (e.g. noises, light, music, pressure, touch, and cold) [184]. However, these physiological stress related responses or reflex responses to external stimuli are not necessarily equivalent to the multidimensional, subjective phenomenon we call pain. Reduction in stress hormones is not necessarily indicative of adequate analgesia [185]. The stress response is largely mediated in the spinal cord, brainstem or basal ganglia, not the cortex.

Two studies used near-infrared spectroscopy to measure changes in cerebral oxygenation over the somatosensory cortex and demonstrated that noxious stimulation of preterm infants caused cortical responses that differed from those of non-noxious stimulation. They concluded that noxious information can be transmitted to the infant cortex from 24 weeks' gestation onward [186,187]. Preterm neonates have cortical evoked potentials after heel lancing [188]. Although these studies provide evidence of functional neural activity in the sensory cortex of 24-week-old preterm neonates, the primary sensory cortex is not the only brain area that mediates painful experiences; continued development and organization of the cortex are likely necessary. These were preterm neonates, not fetuses. *In utero*, the low level of oxygen alone may preclude awareness and the ability to experience pain. Furthermore, endogenous neuroinhibitors produced in the placenta (e.g. adenosine, allopregnanolone, pregnanolone, prostaglandin-D2, various placental peptide inhibitors) sustain fetal sleep and suppress fetal awareness [189]. Late-gestation fetuses oscillate between REM and NREM sleep 95% of the time. Data suggest that the other 5% of the time they are in a form of indeterminate transitional sleep, suggesting that the fetus is always asleep [190]. Unlike neonates, noxious stimuli do not appear to cause cortical arousal to a wakeful state in fetuses. Wakefulness is a state of arousal mediated by the brainstem and thalamus in communication with the cortex. It must be understood that wakefulness does not equal awareness. Thus, the intrauterine environment might keep the fetus from being awake, aware, and from experiencing pain. Maybe awareness is only possible after birth.

Although noxious stimulation might not affect fetal consciousness, it might influence neurological or behavioral development. Circumcision of a non-anesthetized neonate increases the infant's pain response to injections 6 months later, and fetal stress has long-term adverse hormonal effects in young monkeys [191,192]. Consequently, it is possible that noxious stimuli can have adverse long-term neurodevelopmental consequences that could be attenuated or blocked by anesthesia [173]. Of course, these effects later in life do not prove that the causal event was experienced as pain.

Anesthetic implications

Because it is unclear when fetuses feel pain, it seems best to err on the side of providing adequate fetal anesthesia [193]. Altogether, clinical observations of fetal and neonatal behavior, information about the development of mechanisms of pain perception, and studies of fetal and neonatal responses to noxious stimuli provide a compelling physiological and philosophical rationale for providing adequate fetal anesthesia, especially after 24–26 weeks' gestation. Although we do not know whether or when fetuses actually experience pain, noxious stimulation during fetal life causes a stress response, which could have short- and long-term adverse effects on the developing CNS. The link between the stress response and pain is not always predictable, but the threshold for pain relief is reliably well below the threshold for stress response ablation. Furthermore, the stress response to noxious stimulation is clear evidence that the fetal nervous system is reactive [194].

Despite ongoing debate regarding fetal capacity for pain perception, fetal anesthesia and analgesia are warranted for fetal surgical procedures. Evidence of fetal pain is unnecessary to justify providing fetal analgesia or anesthesia because doing so serves other purposes, including inhibition of fetal movement during a procedure; prevention of hormonal stress responses associated with poor surgical outcomes in neonates; prevention of possible adverse effects on long-term neurodevelopment and behavior; and for open procedures, to ensure profound uterine relaxation to prevent contractions and placental separation during open procedures. Anesthesia has been administered to fetuses undergoing *in utero* procedures since the inception of fetal surgery in 1981, and it is now practiced worldwide [195].

Perioperative and procedural considerations

Preoperative assessment and considerations

The anesthesiologist must conduct a thorough preoperative assessment of both the mother and fetus. In addition to a standard preoperative history and physical examination, specific details should be obtained regarding how the pregnancy is affecting this mother. A thorough respiratory and circulatory evaluation should include questions about shortness of breath, episodes of syncope or feeling lightheaded, and severity of gastric reflux. Imaging studies should be reviewed because they provide placental location and anatomical information about the fetal lesion. This information may alter the surgical approach and patient positioning and necessitate modification of the anesthetic plan. In certain circumstances, general anesthesia is chosen over neuraxial or local anesthesia if the maternal position compromises her safety or the duration of the surgery will be protracted. Most minimally invasive procedures can be performed with just a maternal type and screen of blood, while readily available, cross-matched blood is required for open procedures because the risk of hemorrhage is greater. In addition, type O-negative, leukocyte-depleted, irradiated, CMV-negative blood that is cross-matched against the mother should be readily available for fetuses undergoing open procedures. Maternal IgG antibodies cross the placenta.

Risks and benefits

The primary goal of *in utero* surgery is to improve neonatal outcomes over those possible when surgical or medical interventions are performed after preterm or term birth. The intrauterine environment offers quicker wound healing, decreased scar formation, and an ideal postoperative recovery environment because the placental/fetal circulation provides all the fetus' nutritional, metabolic, and oxygen requirements.

Risks to the fetus (renal failure, fetal demise, CNS injuries, postoperative amniotic fluid leaks, membrane separation, preterm rupture of membranes, preterm labor, and preterm delivery) are relatively high. Chorio-amniotic membrane separation can cause amniotic bands, umbilical cord strangulation, and fetal demise. Preterm delivery carries significant morbidity and mortality for fetuses that might otherwise benefit from therapeutic interventions if they were born at term.

Maternal safety must be considered when developing an appropriate fetal management plan. The vast majority of fetal conditions that might benefit from fetal surgery pose no direct risk to the mother, but the procedure itself or medications administered may have risk for her, as does postoperative pain and discomfort. Although the potential for significant maternal morbidity is always present, fortunately maternal morbidity is relatively minimal or uncommon [9,10]. In a retrospective review of 87 hysterotomies performed at UCSF between 1989 and 2003, 28% of mothers had pulmonary edema, 52% had premature rupture of membranes, 13% required blood products, 9% had chorio-amnionitis, and the risk of preterm delivery was high and occurred at a mean gestational age of 30 weeks [9]. These risks include hemorrhage, wound infection or chorio-amnionitis, placental abruption, uterine rupture, and side-effects of tocolytics (including pulmonary edema) [12,196]. In addition, the risks of pulmonary aspiration, difficult ventilation/tracheal intubation, and hemodynamic compromise are increased during pregnancy. Open fetal procedures involve a hysterotomy incision that is away from the uterine segment. This necessitates cesarean delivery of the current and all future pregnancies of patients that have undergone an open fetal procedure. Future reproductive capabilities do not seem to be compromised [197]. Maternal safety and welfare must be balanced against the risk of fetal death or caring for a child with a significant morbidity.

Interdisciplinary team

Perioperative care by a multidisciplinary team is essential for success of fetal surgical procedures and care of the mothers. In addition to the anesthesiologist's preoperative assessment, a typical case requires input from ultrasonographers and radiologists regarding ultrasound and MRI imaging to confirm diagnosis, detail the abnormal anatomy, and rule out other pathological lesions. Maternal-fetal medicine physicians, geneticists, and neonatologists provide patient counseling, fetal karyotyping and information about the likely condition of the newborn with or without *in utero* intervention. Fetal surgeons provide details of the procedure and associated risks and outcome potential to the family, and social workers and nurse co-ordinators address unique family situations, logistics and concerns, and potential psychological issues. Maternal partners must be involved in the process to alleviate potential perceptions of guilt or coercion, depending on the mother's final decision. Regular interdisciplinary meetings with obstetric anesthesiologists, obstetricians, fetal surgeons, neonatologists, maternal-fetal medicine experts, ultrasonographers, operating room staff, nurse co-ordinators, and social workers allow team communication and provide awareness of patient developments by all caregivers. This maximizes the chance of successful outcomes for both mothers and fetuses. Before undertaking any fetal procedure, members of all disciplines should meet to ensure that a complete, detailed, and appropriate plan is in place and the necessary equipment and personnel are available.

General intraoperative and postoperative considerations

Maternal analgesia/anesthesia for fetal surgery can be provided with local infiltration of the skin and uterine wall, intravenous maternal sedation, neuraxial anesthesia, general anesthesia or a combination of techniques.

In addition to the maternal anesthetic plan and the fetal surgical procedure, strategies must be developed for fetal monitoring, fetal analgesia and/or neuromuscular relaxation, management of unanticipated fetal or maternal distress, postoperative fetal and uterine monitoring, and maternal postoperative analgesia. The anesthesiologist must consider the anesthetic requirements of the fetus and appropriate intraoperative fetal monitoring (ultrasound, doptones, fetal oximetry), and the potential need for fetal intravenous access for fluid resuscitation or blood transfusion. Fetal analgesia and anesthesia can be provided by direct intravenous or intramuscular administration of drugs to the fetus, or placental transfer of maternal intravenous agents or general anesthetics. Many anesthetic compounds readily cross the placenta (e.g.

induction agents, halogenated anesthetics, nitrous oxide, opioids, benzodiazepines), but only small amounts of muscle relaxants do so.

Fetal surgery necessitates control of uterine tone and profound uterine relaxation is required for open procedures. Concern for increased uterine tone and initiation of premature labor requires continuous or intermittent postoperative fetal heart rate and uterine activity monitoring, sometimes for days. Maternal postoperative analgesia includes intrathecal narcotics, continuous epidural analgesia, patient-controlled intravenous analgesia (PCA) or oral medications.

Finally, the anesthesiologist should be prepared, if the need arises, for emergency fetal delivery or uterine evacuation. If maternal cardiac arrest is precipitated by local anesthetic overdose, total spinal or severe hemorrhage, and resuscitation cannot be accomplished in 4 min, the fetus should be delivered as an emergency. Emergency cesarean delivery relieves aortocaval compression, improves the effectiveness of resuscitation, and increases the maternal and possibly the fetal chances for survival [198].

The following sections are generic descriptions of anesthetic approaches for both minimally invasive and open fetal procedures, and of postoperative management used at the University of California San Francisco. Our colleagues at other fetal treatment centers in the United States and Europe may employ variations on these techniques. The EXIT procedure is described previously and in the case study at the end of this chapter. Basic anesthetic considerations are similar to those for any woman undergoing surgery during pregnancy [199,200].

Minimally invasive and percutaneous procedures

Amniocentesis, cordocentesis, intrauterine blood transfusion, needle aspiration of cysts, shunt placement into the fetal bladder or thorax, or SFLP for TTTS are typically defined as minimally invasive. These procedures are performed using an ultrasound-guided needle or by inserting a single, small-diameter sheath or cannula that allows insertion of an endoscope. Local anesthetic infiltration of the abdominal wall or neuraxial anesthesia is usually adequate for these procedures. If the procedure involves multiple needle punctures at various locations, large instruments or a mini laparotomy, neuraxial anesthesia often provides better maternal comfort. Choice of anesthesia technique is based on the surgical approach, anticipated duration of the procedure, and need for postoperative analgesia. Typically, the anesthetic is supplemented by conscious sedation. General anesthesia is rarely necessary unless placental location makes uterine exteriorization necessary. General anesthesia provides

maternal comfort and prevents increased uterine tone during uterine manipulation. Before the procedure starts, the mother should be appropriately fasted, receive prophylaxis against aspiration, have adequate intravenous access, and be fully monitored. The technique used is similar to that described in the following section on open fetal procedures.

Use of local or neuraxial anesthesia does not provide fetal analgesia or immobility. Supplemental analgesia (opioids), anxiolysis (midazolam), and sedation (low-dose propofol infusion) provided to the mother will sedate her and may provide minimal fetal immobility and some analgesia following placental transfer. A randomized, blinded, controlled trial demonstrated that remifentanil (0.1 µg/kg/min) resulted in more fetal immobility and better surgical operating conditions [201]. Any maternal sedation regime must assure that the mother remains within a level of "conscious sedation" to minimize maternal respiratory depression, loss of maternal airway reflexes, and pulmonary aspiration.

Fetal immobilization is unnecessary for certain minimally invasive fetal procedures, such as laser surgery of the chorionic plate (e.g. SFLP for TTTS). However, fetal movement may compromise the success of certain procedures by making them technically difficult or impossible. As an example, in the case of intrauterine transfusion or blood sampling, fetal movement may be hazardous because displacement of the needle or catheter may cause trauma, bleeding or compromise of the umbilical circulation and require emergency delivery. If the procedure requires fetal immobility and/or analgesia, muscle relaxants and/or opioids can be administered directly to the fetus. Non-depolarizing neuromuscular blocking agents, such as pancuronium or vecuronium, can be administered to the fetus by ultrasound-guided intramuscular (0.3 mg/kg) or umbilical venous (0.1–0.25 mg/kg) injection [202,203]. Pancuronium might be preferred for its longer duration of action and its vagolytic effect on fetal heart rate. Fetal paralysis with either agent occurs in 2–5 min. Vecuronium is often chosen when only 1–2 h of fetal immobility are desired.

For procedures involving noxious stimulation of the fetus (e.g. shunt catheter placement, cardiac septoplasty), intramuscular or intravascular opioid (e.g. fentanyl 10–25 µg/kg) can be administered to the fetus [179,199]. If general anesthesia is administered to the mother, placental transfer of inhaled anesthetic is sufficient to adequately immobilize and anesthetize the fetus.

A plan should be in place for treatment of fetal distress and should include having available weight-appropriate doses of drugs for fetal resuscitation (e.g. atropine, epinephrine). This plan may range from supportive or palliative therapy to emergency delivery. Cordocentesis occasionally causes prolonged fetal bradycardia, especially if the needle punctures the umbilical artery rather than the umbilical vein. Persistent fetal bradycardia in this situation or during other minimally invasive procedures may require an emergency cesarean section if the gestational age is compatible with extrauterine viability. Consequently, the anesthesiologist must be prepared to emergently provide general anesthesia if it is required.

Open fetal surgical procedures

In utero procedures that require a maternal laparotomy and hysterotomy (e.g. myelomeningocele repair, sacrococcygeal teratoma resection) are typically performed using general anesthesia. In addition to anesthetic considerations required for minimally invasive fetal surgery and for surgery for maternal indications, open fetal procedures have some unique issues. These include the need for profound uterine relaxation; increased potential for significant maternal or fetal blood loss or fluid shifts; intraoperative fetal monitoring, fetal anesthesia, and the potential need for fetal resuscitation; and postoperative maternal analgesia and uterine quiescence. Box 19.1 details specific considerations that must be addressed before undertaking open fetal surgery. The majority of these items are also useful when planning for minimally invasive and EXIT procedures.

A non-particulate antacid is given preoperatively for prophylaxis against aspiration, rectal indometacin is placed for prophylactic tocolysis, and an epidural catheter inserted for postoperative analgesia. Type and cross-matched blood products are obtained for both mother and fetus. Sequential compression devices are placed on the mother's lower extremities to minimize the risk of deep venous thrombosis. Minimal preanesthetic medication (opioids or anxiolytics) is used so as not to increase hypotension when maximal doses of a volatile halogenated agent are administered. Similar to what occurs when any general anesthetic is administered after about 20 weeks of gestation, the patient is positioned with left uterine displacement, is adequately preoxygenated, and rapid-sequence induction and tracheal intubation are performed during cricoid pressure. Prior to incision, anesthesia is typically maintained with low concentrations of volatile agent. During this time, the ultrasonographer determines fetal presentation and placental location, additional large-bore vascular access is obtained, the urinary bladder is catheterized, and prophylactic antibiotics are administered.

For both open and EXIT procedures, 2–3 MAC of volatile anesthetic agent is used to provide maternal and fetal anesthesia and the surgical tocolysis (uterine atony) required for the procedure. Volatile anesthetic agents inhibit myometrial contractility by calcium-sensitive potassium channel modulation [204]. The human uterus has a thick, muscular layer that is sensitive to stimulation

---

Box 19.1 Considerations for open fetal surgery

Preoperative considerations

1. Maternal counseling by multidisciplinary team
2. Complete maternal history and physical exam
3. Imaging studies to define fetal lesion and placental location
4. Complete fetal work-up to exclude other anomalies or karyotype abnormalities
5. Surgical meeting or "time out" with all team members prior to starting
6. Prophylactic premedication: non-particulate antacid (aspiration) and rectal indometacin (tocolysis)
7. Blood products typed and cross-matched for potential maternal and fetal transfusion
8. Epidural catheter placement for postoperative analgesia
9. Sequential compression devices on lower extremities for thrombosis prophylaxis
10. Fetal resuscitation drugs transferred to scrub nurse in unit doses

Intraoperative considerations

1. Left uterine displacement and standard monitors
2. Preoxygenate for 3 min prior to induction
3. Rapid-sequence induction and intubation
4. Maintain maternal FiO_2 at ≥50% and end-tidal CO_2 26–28 mmHg
5. Ultrasonography to determine fetal and placental positioning
6. Urinary catheter placed and additional large-bore intravenous access obtained
7. Administer prophylactic antibiotics
8. Following incision, initiate high concentrations of volatile anesthetics (2–3 MAC)
9. Consider intravenous nitroglycerine if uterine tone remains increased
10. Maintain blood pressure with IV phenylephrine or ephedrine
11. Intramuscular administration of fetal opioid and paralytic with ultrasound guidance or by direct vision
12. Place fetal pulse oximeter and use periodic ultrasound for fetal monitoring
13. Obtain fetal vascular access if significant fetal blood loss expected
14. Restrict maternal maintenance fluids to <2 L to decrease risk of pulmonary edema
15. Administer loading dose of IV magnesium sulfate when uterine closure begins
16. Discontinue halogenated agents after magnesium sulfate bolus complete
17. Activate epidural for conclusion of surgery and postoperative analgesia
18. Administer nitrous oxide and opioids to supplement epidural anesthesia
19. Monitor neuromuscular blockers carefully due to potentiation of magnesium sulfate
20. Extubate trachea when patient fully awake

Early postoperative considerations

1. Continue tocolytic therapy
2. Patient-controlled epidural analgesia
3. Monitor uterine activity and fetal heart rate
4. Ongoing fetal evaluation (ultrasonography, etc.)

or manipulation. Thus, uterine incision and stimulation may produce strong uterine contractions. Halogenated anesthetics cause dose-dependent inhibition of uterine contractions and myometrial tone. Complete uterine relaxation is essential because increased tone compromises uterine perfusion, especially during uterine manipulation, and increases the risk for partial placental separation. High intravenous doses of nitroglycerine may also be used as a supplemental or primary agent for intraoperative uterine relaxation [44].

Prior to hysterotomy, the volatile agent is increased (>2 MAC) and the uterus is assessed for increased tone. Fetal uptake and distribution of maternal anesthetic gases take longer than the mother, but fetal MAC is lower [205]. If increased uterine tone is noted before or after incision, the halogenated agent can be increased (up to 3 MAC) or additional small boluses of IV nitroglycerine can be given (50–200 μg intravenously) or by continuous infusion. If nitroglycerine is used without high concentrations of volatile anesthetic, an infusion of up to 20 μg/kg/min IV may be required. Although nitroglycerine crosses to the fetal circulation, fetal effects are minimal because there is significant metabolism of nitroglycerine by the placenta [44]. Arterial blood pressure is maintained with IV phenylephrine or ephedrine as needed to maintain adequate mean arterial pressures (>65 mmHg). Maternal monitoring by arterial line and central venous catheter is not typically used.

Brief fetal exposure to more than 2–3 MAC of inhaled anesthetic appears to be safe. However, the combined impact of adequate fetal anesthesia with a halogenated agent, intrauterine manipulation, and fetal stress on fetal cardiovascular stability and regional blood flow is unknown. Recent animal studies have demonstrated neuronal apoptosis in the developing brain when a variety of agents are administered to induce and maintain general anesthesia [154,206]. Implications for the fetus and neonate from brief anesthetic exposures are currently unknown, due to lack of human studies and difficulties extrapolating animal study methods to humans. In our experience at the University of California San Francisco, long and deep maternal inhalation anesthesia has not caused fetal hypoxia, hypercarbia or acidosis, even after 2h of exposure. However, others have reported acidosis after only 45min of fetal anesthesia [207].

Cross-matched blood for the mother and O-negative, CMV-negative, leuko-reduced, irradiated blood for fetal transfusion should be readily available in the operating room. For open procedures with the potential for significant fetal blood loss (e.g. sacrococcygeal teratoma resection), close attention to fetal monitoring and estimated fetal blood loss is required. It may be necessary to insert a fetal intravenous catheter to transfuse blood. Vascular access is obtained in a fetal hand or arm vein, or by surgical cut-down on the internal jugular vein.

Intraoperative ultrasound is used to determine placental location and fetal position. Uterine incision is made away from the placenta but in a position that allows for appropriate exposure of the fetal part. A stapling device with absorbable lactomer staples is used to prevent excessive bleeding and seal the membranes to the endometrium [208]. During surgery, the exposed fetus and uterus are bathed with warm fluids and intrauterine temperature monitored.

With ultrasound guidance or direct vision, opioid (e.g. fentanyl 10–25 μg/kg) and muscle relaxant (e.g. pancuronium or vecuronium 0.1–0.3 mg/kg) are administered intramuscularly before the fetal incision [199,209]. However, these agents are seldom required when the mother is anesthetized with a general anesthetic. Drugs for fetal resuscitation (atropine 0.02 mg/kg, epinephrine 1 μg/kg, and crystalloid 10 mL/kg) are sterilely transferred to the scrub nurse for administration (if needed) under direction of the anesthesiologist. Each syringe is prepared with a single, unit weight-based dose and appropriately labeled. Multiple dose syringes should be avoided to reduce the risk of accidental overdosing.

Maternal and fetal anesthesia, uterine incision, fetal manipulation, and surgical stress may adversely affect uteroplacental and fetoplacental circulation by several mechanisms. Maternal hypotension increases uterine activity and causes maternal hyperventilation and hypocarbia, which impair uteroplacental and/or umbilical blood flow. Manipulation of the fetus may affect cardiac output, regional distribution of cardiac output, and/or umbilical blood flow. Direct compression of the umbilical cord, inferior vena cava and/or mediastinum adversely affects fetal circulation. Fetal well-being is assessed by continuous fetal pulse oximetry, periodic fetal heart rate (FHR) monitoring by intraoperative ultrasonography, fetal echocardiography for assessment of ventricular contractility, and/or direct fetal ECG. The predictive value of pulse oximetry may be superior to FHR monitoring. In fetal lambs, bradycardia was found to be a late sign of fetal distress following umbilical cord compression [210]. However, in our experience and that of others [211], bradycardia can precede oxygen desaturation during human fetal surgery. Ultrasonography can assess fetal heart rate by either direct visualization of heart motion or by Doppler assessment of umbilical cord blood flow. Echocardiography can be used to assess fetal cardiac contractility and filling volume. Unfortunately, the sterile transducer cannot be left in position continuously because it interferes with surgery. Under specific circumstances, capillary or umbilical venous blood samples can be obtained for blood gas, pH, electrolyte, and glucose determinations. One significant limitation is the inability to monitor fetal blood pressure easily. In the future, placental vessels might be catheterized for continuous blood pressure monitoring and blood gas determinations. Fetal ECG waveform analysis might also provide additional useful information.

During surgical closure, a loading dose of magnesium sulfate is administered (4–6 g) intravenously over 20 min and is followed by an intravenous infusion of 1–2 g/h to (hopefully) maintain uterine atony and prevent postoperative contractions. Intraoperatively, maternal intravenous fluids are normally restricted to minimize the risk of postoperative pulmonary edema that is associated with the use of tocolytic agents [9,212]. Inspired concentrations of halogenated agents are significantly decreased or discontinued once the magnesium sulfate bolus has been administered. Maternal anesthesia can be maintained with a combination of IV fentanyl, nitrous oxide in oxygen, and activation of epidural anesthesia after first carefully testing for catheter position. Discontinuing the high-dose volatile agent at the beginning of surgical closure allows more time for the elimination of volatile halogenated agent from tissues. This regimen facilitates timely tracheal extubation of a fully awake patient and minimizes the likelihood of coughing or straining and jeopardizing the integrity of the uterine closure. The epidural allows the patient to emerge pain free. If neuromuscular agents are utilized, the absence of neuromuscular blockade should be determined prior to tracheal extubation, since magnesium sulfate potentiates neuromuscular blockade. When utilized, neuromuscular agents must be carefully titrated in anticipation of later administration of magnesium.

Whatever anesthetic technique is used for open fetal surgery, it must ensure adequate uteroplacental perfusion, profound uterine relaxation, maternal hemodynamic stability, fetal anesthesia and immobility, and minimal fetal myocardial depression and compromise.

Postoperative management

Management of postoperative preterm labor has been one of the most difficult aspects of fetal surgery [32], but prevention and treatment of uterine contractions are essential for optimal fetal outcomes. Postoperative tocolysis has included a variety of agents, including magnesium sulfate, β-adrenergics, indometacin, and calcium-entry blockers. Magnesium likely competes with calcium at voltage-operated calcium-sensitive potassium channels by an action similar to volatile anesthetics [204]. Indometacin blocks the synthesis of prostaglandins, and β-adrenergic agents act directly on the uterus by activating adenylate cyclase and thereby reducing intracellular calcium. The relative inefficacy of tocolytic agents and their adverse side-effects have made this aspect of postoperative management challenging. Tocolysis is normally unnecessary after cordocentesis or intrauterine transfusion but for more invasive percutaneous procedures (e.g. shunt catheter placement, endoscopic techniques), postoperative tocolytics are used at most centers.

With open fetal procedures, early postoperative uterine contractions are expected and tocolysis is provided by a continuous infusion of magnesium sulfate for approximately 24 h. This is supplemented with indometacin and occasionally with terbutaline or nifedipine as indicated.

Postoperative analgesia can be provided by several days of continuous epidural analgesia or by intravenous opioids by PCA. Effective analgesia may help prevent preterm labor by decreasing plasma oxytocin levels [213]. In addition to preterm labor, other postoperative concerns include rupture of membranes, infection, and fetal complications that include heart failure, intracranial hemorrhage, indometacin-induced constriction of the ductus arteriosus, and fetal demise. Uterine activity and FHR are monitored closely during the first few postoperative days. The fetus is evaluated daily by ultrasonography and echocardiography, looking for ductal narrowing, cardiac valvular function, and oligohydramnios. In some cases, magnetic resonance imaging is used to determine the presence of intracranial hemorrhage.

Future of fetal therapy and surgery

The future of fetal diagnosis and therapy is bright and provides many opportunities for advances that benefit the fetus and perhaps adults with diseases that originate during fetal development. Fetal tissue engineering may provide perinatal treatment of congenital anomalies. For example, neural stem cells can mediate repair of postnatal spinal cord impairments in experimental animals, suggesting that stem cells might be used to promote fetal spinal cord repair for myelomeningocele [214–216]. Prenatal gene therapy with viral vectors or naked DNA, combined with microbubble-enhanced ultrasound, holds promise for possible treatment of hemophilia disorders, cystic fibrosis, and muscular dystrophy [217].

The future for fetal surgical intervention is that the majority of interventions will be performed percutaneously, using imaging or endoscopic guidance. Further miniaturization of surgical tools and improvements in endoscopes will facilitate this. Although use of minimally invasive techniques will simplify anesthetic management, many issues remain unresolved because research in this area is difficult. Potential neurotoxicity of anesthetic agents in the fetal and neonatal brain, impact of surgical stress on the fetus and/or later in life, and optimal anesthetic techniques are among the many issues that require further evaluation. Future advances in fetal therapy and surgery require careful consideration of potential fetal benefit and fetal risk and, most importantly, maternal risk. Maternal safety remains a paramount concern for the anesthesiologist.

CASE STUDY

Ultrasound diagnosis of a large (>6 cm) fetal neck mass, consistent with a cervical teratoma, was made in a 25-year-old, gravida 1 woman at 32 weeks' gestation. The mother was otherwise healthy, and no other anatomical abnormalities were detected in the fetus. The ultrasound images and patient's history were discussed at the weekly, multidisciplinary fetal treatment conference and it was decided to re-evaluate the fetus in 2 weeks. The delivery strategy was by EXIT procedure at 38 weeks' gestation after confirming fetal lung maturity by amniocentesis. Concern was expressed that it would not be possible to intubate the trachea by laryngoscopy during the EXIT procedure, given the massive size of the lesion. No significant changes occurred in the mother during the ensuing 2 weeks, and she was admitted at 38 weeks' gestation for amniocentesis. Measurement of surfactant phospholipids secreted by the fetal lungs revealed a favorable lecithin/sphingomyelin ratio and presence of phosphatidylglycerol (PG) and gave assurance of lung maturation. The EXIT procedure was scheduled for the following morning. All team members were notified and their availability confirmed by the perinatologists who performed the amniocentesis. The fetal surgery team included pediatric surgeons (fetal surgeons), radiologists (ultrasonographers), neonatologists, anesthesiologists, and nurses.

Before entering the operating room, all team members participated in a pre-procedure conference to ensure the availability and readiness of all necessary equipment and personnel, and to discuss the surgical plan, issues specific to the case, and potential complications that might arise. In preparation for the procedure, the anesthesiologists checked their anesthesia machine, maternal and fetal drugs and their doses, and ensured that a manometer, sterile hand ventilation bag, and separate source of oxygen supply were available for ventilating the fetal lungs once an airway was established. The anesthesiologists had a second pulse oximeter and sterile probe for fetal monitoring. They also prepared a combination of paralytic agent and opioid to administer to the fetus and transferred the sterile "cocktail" to the scrub nurse. Similarly, two doses of atropine and two doses of epinephrine were prepared in labeled, 1 mL syringes for emergency administration to the fetus, if needed. Each labeled 1 mL syringe was prepared by unit weight-based dosing so excessive doses could not be mistakenly given from a multidose syringe during an emergency. The scrub nurse ensured the appropriate surgical equipment was available, as well as sterile laryngoscopes, bronchoscopes, a Jackson-Rees non-rebreathing circuit, endotracheal tubes, cables and sensors for pulse oximetry, including transparent adhesive medical dressing to secure

the oximeter and an opaque cover to shield the oximeter sensor from the surgical lights.

The mother was premedicated with 30 mL of sodium citrate before entering the operating room. A 'time-out" was completed, and an epidural catheter was placed for postoperative pain control. The mother was then positioned supine and left uterine displacement was initiated to prevent aortocaval compression by the gravid uterus; 100% oxygen was administered by tight-fitting facemask while pulse oximeter, arterial blood pressure cuff, and electrocardiogram leads were applied. The fetus was evaluated by ultrasonography and was noted to be in a cephalic presentation; the fetal heart rate was 130 beats per minute with appropriate variability. After denitrogenation of the mother's lungs and application of cricoid pressure, rapid-sequence induction of anesthesia was performed with propofol and succinylcholine and the trachea was rapidly intubated. Once tracheal intubation was confirmed by auscultation and by normal-appearing carbon dioxide end-tidal waveform tracings, sevoflurane was administered. A urinary catheter and a second large-bore intravenous catheter were placed. Prophylactic antibiotics were administered, and the abdomen was prepped and draped. The fetal surgeon, perinatologist, and neonatologist positioned themselves around the surgical table, and the equipment was readied. The neonatologist passed the oxygen supply line to the fetal breathing circuit and an additional catheter for connection to the manometer over the drape to the anesthesiologist. Together, they ensured the integrity and dynamics of the circuit, with a pop-off valve set for 20 cmH$_2$O to avoid iatrogenic pneumothorax when fetal ventilation was initiated. The pulse oximeter cable was passed over the drape and connected to the second oximeter. The sensor was tested to ensure all connections were intact.

Following a Pfannenstiel incision, the sevoflurane concentration was increased, and was 1.9 MAC when the hysterotomy occurred. No vasopressor support was required to maintain the mean arterial pressures above 65 mmHg. The uterus was visualized and palpated to assess tone. Since it was not sufficiently relaxed, the inspired concentration of sevoflurane was increased. The ultrasonographer determined the edges of the placenta so the surgeons could avoid it during hysterotomy. After 5 min, the end-tidal sevoflurane concentration was 2.6 MAC, the mother's vital signs were stable, the fetal heart rate was about 130 beats/min, and the uterus was appropriately soft. A purse-string suture was placed in the uterine wall and an incision was made that was just large enough to insert a uterine stapler to divide the myometrium and membranes and to apply absorbable staples to seal the edges of the hysterotomy and provide hemostatis. Given the somewhat anterior location of the placenta, the hysterotomy was performed towards the uterine fundus using the "classic" uterine incision, which will require all future babies to be delivered by cesarean section without having undergone labor.

Once the uterus was opened, a "cocktail" of 3 mg morphine and 0.4 mg pancuronium was administered into the fetus' left triceps muscle. The fetal head and upper thorax were delivered, and the pulse oximeter was placed across the fetus' left palm and secured with a transparent adhesive dressing and covered with an opaque dressing to shield the sensor from the surgical lights. The pediatric surgeon, neonatologist, and anesthesiologist were unable to visualize airway structures by laryngoscopy and bronchoscopy (Fig. 19.16). Initially, a decision was made to perform a tracheostomy, but this was considered unwise given the size of the neck lesion. Instead, during the next 2h the teratoma was excised while the fetus was maintained on placental support and monitored by pulse oximetry. Peripheral venous access was obtained in the left arm (Fig. 19.17). After the teratoma was resected, it was necessary to perform a tracheostomy. After the airway was secured, positive pressure ventilation was initiated with peak pressures of 20 cmH$_2$O and a positive end-expiratory pressure of 4 cmH$_2$O. The fetal oxygen saturation rapidly rose and when it exceeded 90%, the umbilical cord was clamped and cut, and the newborn was delivered to the awaiting neonatal resuscitation team for further care. Blood gases from a doubly clamped segment of the umbilical cord were normal and showed no evidence of acidosis.

After cord clamping, sevoflurane was discontinued, an infusion of oxytocin (30 units) was started, the mother's lungs were ventilated with 70% nitrous oxide in oxygen, intravenous fentanyl (100 µg) was administered, and a test dose was given through the epidural catheter. When it was determined that the catheter was not in a vein or subarachnoid, epidural lidocaine 2% was administered. The perinatologist closed the uterus and abdomen, and the patient awakened without pain. She received 2 L of crystalloid, no colloid or blood, had 150 mL of urine output, and an estimated blood loss of 650 mL. Fluids were purposely minimized to decrease the risk of pulmonary compromise. Over the first 36 postoperative hours, analgesia was provided with an infusion of bupivacaine 0.1% into the epidural space using patient-controlled epidural analgesia. The mother did well. The pathology confirmed a teratoma, and the neonate did well.

Key points

1. Successful EXIT procedures are a multidisciplinary team effort in which detailed preoperative planning and discussion among all team members are crucial.
2. Detailed anatomical information regarding airway mass and placental position is needed for appropriate patient selection and optimal outcome.
3. Thorough preparation and planning for unanticipated emergency events (e.g. fetal bradycardia, maternal hemorrhage, failed fetal tracheal intubation) are critical to successful outcome.
4. Prolonged exposure to anesthesia does not lead to fetal acidosis.

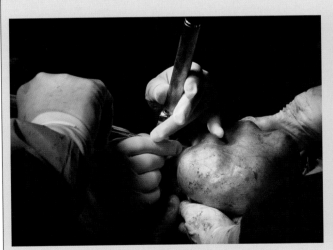

Figure 19.16 Laryngoscopy-assisted bronchoscopy of a fetus with a large neck mass during the EXIT procedure. Courtesy of UCSF Fetal Treatment Center.

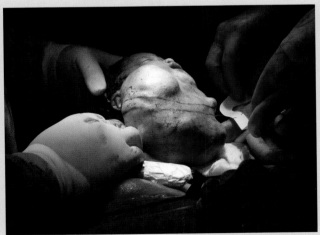

Figure 19.17 Preparation of fetus for neck mass resection. Fetus is maintained on placental support with pulse oximetry monitoring (right hand) and peripheral venous access (left arm). Courtesy of UCSF Fetal Treatment Center.

Annotated references

A full reference list for this chapter is available at:
http://www.wiley.com/go/gregory/andropoulos/pediatricanesthesia

3. Harrison MR, Bressack MA, Churg AM et al. Correction of congenital diaphragmatic hernia *in utero*. II. Simulated correction permits fetal lung growth with survival at birth. Surgery 1980; 88: 260–8. This is one of the earliest studies demonstrating the rationale for fetal surgery. The investigators created a model of a progressively enlarging intrathoracic mass in the sheep fetus using a conical silicone rubber balloon to produce severe pulmonary hypoplasia, simulating the pathophysiology of congenital diaphragmatic hernia. This study demonstrated that simulated correction later in gestation by balloon decompression allowed sufficient lung growth and development to alleviate the respiratory insufficiency and allow neonatal survival. Lambs without simulated correction died. Those with simulated correction had increased lung weight, air capacity, compliance, and area of the pulmonary vascular bed. Efficacy of *in utero* correction of an anatomical defect was confirmed.

6. Harrison MR, Anderson J, Rosen MA et al. Fetal surgery in the primate I. Anesthetic, surgical, and tocolytic management to maximize fetal-neonatal survival. J Pediatr Surg 1982; 17: 115–22. Although fetal surgery had been successful in the ovine and other lower animal models, the gravid uterus of the primate is more sensitive to surgical stimulation and induction of preterm labor. Surgical, anesthetic and tocolytic techniques were refined in monkeys to allow fetal surgery in the late second and early third trimesters without increasing maternal or fetal-neonatal mortality.

7. Harrison MR, Golbus MS, Filly RA et al. Fetal surgery for congenital hydronephrosis. N Engl J Med 1982; 306: 591–3. This is a case report of the first open fetal surgery; bilateral ureterostomies were performed at 21 weeks' gestation for bilateral hydronephrosis.

13. Mychaliska GB, Bealer JF, Graf JL et al. Operating on placental support: the *ex utero* intrapartum treatment procedure. J Pediatr Surg 1997; 32: 227–30; discussion 30–1. To address the clinical problem of neonatal airway obstruction created by temporary tracheal occlusion for treatment of congenital diaphragmatic hernia, the *ex utero* intrapartum treatment (EXIT) procedure was established. EXIT allows fetal treatment to be performed while maintaining the fetoplacental circulation until the neonatal airway is secured. Use of this technique rapidly expanded to include many other causes of prenatally diagnosed airway obstruction.

39. Jani J, Gratacos E, Greenough A et al. Percutaneous fetal endoscopic tracheal occlusion (FETO) for severe left-sided congenital diaphragmatic hernia. Clin Obstet Gynecol 2005; 48: 910–22. These investiga-

tors from Leuven, Belgium, pioneered advances in minimally invasive fetal surgical techniques. This paper reports the evolution of their fetoscopic tracheal occlusion technique for fetuses with severe congenital diaphragmatic hernia. Rather than restoration of airway patency by EXIT, they employed a technique of *in utero* reversal of occlusion (plug–unplug sequence), based on data showing less deterioration of alveolar type II cell counts and to avoid the need for hysterotomy (EXIT).

158. Lee SJ, Ralston HJ, Drey EA et al. Fetal pain: a systematic multidisciplinary review of the evidence. JAMA 2005; 294: 947–54. The human fetus can mount a hormonal stress response to noxious stimulation, but whether the fetus can experience pain remains controversial. This paper reviews the evidence regarding the capacity for fetal pain based on neurodevelopment.

178. Giannakoulopoulos X, Sepulveda W, Kourtis P et al. Fetal plasma cortisol and beta-endorphin response to intrauterine needling. Lancet 1994; 344(8915): 77–81. This landmark study clearly demonstrated that the human fetus has a hormonal stress response to noxious stimulation, raising the possibility that the fetus feels pain *in utero* and may benefit from anesthesia. Cortisol and β-endorphin concentrations increased with prolonged fetal abdominal needling (to access the intrahepatic vein), but not with needling the placental cord insertion, which is not innervated.

179. Fisk NM, Gitau R, Teixeira JM et al. Effect of direct fetal opioid analgesia on fetal hormonal and hemodynamic stress response to intrauterine needling. Anesthesiology 2001; 95: 828–35. In another important study, these investigators demonstrate that the hormonal stress response of the human fetus to abdominal needling can be attenuated by intravenous fentanyl. Whether the fetus can experience pain remains controversial, but this study demonstrates that the hormonal stress response can be modified by fetal anesthetic administration

189. Mellor DJ, Diesch TJ, Gunn AJ et al. The importance of 'awareness' for understanding fetal pain. Brain Res Brain Res Rev 2005; 49: 455–71. Understanding whether the fetus can experience pain based on neurodevelopment alone may be inadequate. This provocative paper examines the role of endogenous neuroinhibitors, such as adenosine and pregnanolone, that are produced by the fetoplacental unit and contribute to fetal sleep states, suppressing fetal awareness.

205. Gregory GA, Wade JG, Beihl DR et al. Fetal anesthetic requirement (MAC) for halothane. Anesth Analg 1983; 62: 9–14. In a novel set of experiments, these investigators demonstrated that the MAC of the sheep fetus was significantly lower than that of the pregnant ewe. This has significant implications for fetal surgery and anesthesia.

CHAPTER 20
Anesthesia for Premature Infants

George A. Gregory

Department of Anesthesia and Perioperative Care, University of California San Francisco, San Francisco, CA, USA

Introduction

Preoperative evaluation of premature neonates is the most important part of anesthesia. During this time the anesthetist determines what abnormalities are present, gathers information from the intensive care nursery (ICN) team, and makes plans to care for the infant during the perioperative period. The following pages provide information about premature infants, preoperative evaluation, and provision of anesthesia. This information is the basis for understanding the physiology and pathophysiology of preterm neonates, which is necessary for effective evaluation of these patients for surgery and for providing appropriate care for them.

Background

Six percent of infants are born prematurely, i.e. <37 weeks' gestation. The more immature they are at birth, the more likely they are to die during the neonatal period and to have serious complications. Great strides have been made in reducing this mortality rate, even in very small infants. It is now expected that at least 60–70% of infants weighing <750 g at birth will survive [1]. With this increased survival has come a host of complications that often require surgery, including patent ductus arteriosus (PDA), retinopathy of prematurity (ROP), necrotizing enterocolitis (NEC), intraventricular hemorrhage (IVH) with hydrocephalus, and inguinal hernias, to name a few.

Most body organs undergo continuous structural and functional development during the last 3 months of gestation. Infants born prematurely have inadequately developed organs that are required to perform functions that may be beyond their capacity. Consequently, preterm infants are less able to maintain their body temperature, suck, swallow, eat, and sustain breathing. Many of them experience asphyxia at or just before birth, predisposing them to central nervous system injury, intraventricular hemorrhage, necrotizing enterocolitis, myocardial dysfunction, and the respiratory distress syndrome (RDS).

Preterm infants can be divided into three groups: borderline premature (36–37 weeks' gestation); moderately premature (31–35 weeks' gestation); and severely premature ("micropremies", 24–30 weeks' gestation). The problems of each group increase in number and severity with decreasing gestational age [2].

Borderline prematurity

Sixteen percent of all livebirths are borderline premature and can usually be cared for in the normal neonatal nursery. However, they do require close observation for the first 12 h of life, because, as a group, they have more difficulty maintaining their body temperature without added external heat, and they may not suck and feed well. If feeding is a problem, gavage feeding may be required for a few days, and they may be slow to regain their birthweight, especially if they have RDS. Eight percent of borderline premature infants born by cesarean section have RDS versus 1% of those born vaginally, probably because those born vaginally more effectively remove water from the lungs [3].

Because they are predisposed to respiratory distress, the respiratory system of near-term infants must be carefully evaluated during the preoperative visit. Intercostal retractions, tachypnea, grunting respirations, and cyanosis suggest RDS but also may be signs of meconium aspiration, pneumothorax or pneumonia in these large preterm infants. Temperature instability and hyperbilirubinemia suggest sepsis but are usually just manifestations of prematurity.

Moderate prematurity

Moderately premature infants (31–36 weeks' gestation) account for 6–7% of all births. The neonatal mortality of infants born at 31 weeks' gestation is below 5% whereas it is nearly zero at 36 weeks' gestation if there are no congenital anomalies. The major causes of death are intracranial hemorrhage, sepsis, and RDS.

Extremely premature infants (micropremies)

Infants of 24–30 weeks' gestation make up about 1% of all liveborn infants. However, they account for more than 70% of neonatal mortality. They also account for a major portion of neurologically damaged infants later in life. The causes of death include birth asphyxia, acidosis, and respiratory failure (congestive heart failure, patent ductus arteriosus, RDS, infections, especially β-streptococcus and listeria), necrotizing enterocolitis, and intracranial hemorrhage. All the problems of prematurity are exaggerated in these very immature infants.

About one out of 200 term infants, one out of 20 moderately premature infants, and one out of two infants weighing less than 1 kg at birth suffer birth asphyxia. Preterm fetuses are more prone to asphyxia than term fetuses because the preterm infant's blood oxygen content is lower (due to lower hemoglobin concentrations) than

that of term infants. Slight degrees of stress lead to anaerobic metabolism and metabolic acidosis, which in turn reduce cardiac output and increase cerebral blood flow. The latter may damage the central nervous system (CNS) if it causes the fragile vessels of the periventricular areas of the brain to bleed [4,5]. Causes of asphyxia include antepartum hemorrhage, intrauterine infections, breech delivery, and RDS. Treatment of birth asphyxia has been described elsewhere [6].

Most severely premature infants are asphyxiated at birth and often require tracheal intubation and assisted ventilation or nasal continuous positive pressure breathing (nCPAP) as part of delivery room resuscitation. It is hoped that early application of nCPAP will avoid some of the complications of tracheal intubation and mechanical ventilation, although this is unproven [7]. However, early nCPAP does reduce the number infants who require mechanical ventilation by approximately 50% [8]. These infants frequently have both metabolic and respiratory acidosis and require mechanical ventilation, blood volume expansion and, if necessary, a slow, cautious infusion of enough sodium bicarbonate or tris(hydroxymethyl)aminomethane (THAM) to correct their pH to 7.3.

During resuscitation, ventilation should be controlled during sodium bicarbonate infusion and should never be infused more rapidly than 1 mEq/kg/min. Rapid infusion of bicarbonate may quickly expand the intravascular volume, raise the arterial blood pressure, and increase the $PaCO_2$, all of which can cause intracranial hemorrhage in premature neonates. Fifty mL of sodium bicarbonate (50 meq) produces 1250 cc of CO_2 when the bicarbonate is fully reacted with hydrogen ions. This is of little consequence if the lungs are normal and can easily excrete the additional CO_2. If the lungs are abnormal, the $PaCO_2$ may rise rapidly and cause IVH or cardiac arrest. Artificial ventilation is one way to prevent these complications. What is considered an "adequate" $PaCO_2$ has changed over the years. Many preterm neonates now undergo "permissive hypercapnia" with $PaCO_2$ as high as 70 mmHg if the pH is 7.2 or above [9]. Compensation for the hypercapnia includes bicarbonate retention and a positive base excess. If the $PaCO_2$ is reduced to normal, the pH increases and cerebral blood flow decreases. This alkalosis may also decrease the ionized calcium concentration, myocardial function, and arterial blood pressure.

In the past, hypoglycemia was partly responsible for the increased incidence of CNS damage in small preterm infants [10]. Fortunately, hypoglycemia is less common today because blood glucose concentrations are maintained between 50 and 90 mg/dL, not 20–40 mg/dL as in the past. Hyperglycemia is also to be avoided because fewer hyperglycemic patients can be resuscitated from a cardiac arrest and those who are resuscitated have more

CNS damage [11]. Hyperglycemia also causes an osmotic diuresis and can cause hypovolemia. Unlike older patients, premature infants spill glucose in their urine with blood sugar concentrations as low as 125 mg/dL.

Common problems associated with prematurity

The following are some problems associated with prematurity. While they are covered more fully in other chapters, they are presented here to give an overview of the problems and to provide a means of organizing one's thoughts when planning anesthesia for a preterm infant.

In general, anesthesia for premature infants is fraught with problems because they often have multisystem disease and respond poorly to anesthesia. To reduce the risk, it is important to garner as much information preoperatively as possible. A common mistake, especially among novice anesthetists, is to ignore the fact that those caring for the infant in the NICU have considered the patient's problems over an extended period of time and have come to a plan of therapy based on an understanding of these problems. It is neither appropriate nor sensible to alter this plan, unless there is an urgent reason to do so, without thorough discussions with the neonatologists.

Temperature regulation

Hypothermia, or even exposure to a cold environment, increases the metabolic rate and oxygen consumption of preterm infants, which can cause hypoxemia, acidosis, apnea or respiratory distress and is a risk factor for infant mortality [12]. The minimal oxygen consumption of preterm infants is 4.3–5.4 cc/kg/min on day 1 and 8–9 cc/kg/min by 2 weeks of age [13]. As the oxygen consumption increases, so do the ventilation and caloric requirements. Body heat is dissipated by conduction, convection, radiation, and evaporation. During mechanical ventilation, heat and liquid are lost from the lungs, especially when dry gases are used in the operating room. This can be avoided by using warmed, humidified gases. The surface/volume ratio of preterm infants is high, and their flaccid, open posture tends to increase heat loss rather than conserve it. The preterm neonate's lack of insulating fat allows more heat loss from the core to the surface.

Evaporative heat loss accounts for approximately 25% of the heat lost in term neonates and adults. Brück [14] showed that preterm neonates can vasoconstrict and increase heat production when exposed to cold, but they still lose heat because they lack insulation and their overall heat production is lower. The rise in metabolic rate in preterm neonates is approximately linear between 28° and 36°C [13]. Extremely low birthweight neonates do not peripherally vasoconstrict, which is a problem in cold operating rooms [15].

Young infants become agitated and move more in response to cold. Serum norepinephrine concentrations increase, which stimulates brown fat metabolism and heat production. The increased heat produced warms the CNS and vital organs [16]. Primitive brown fat cells begin to differentiate from reticular cells at 26–30 weeks' gestation [17] and increase in size and number for 3–6 weeks after birth. Infants born before the cells fully develop have more difficulty maintaining their body temperature when exposed to cold environments, as do hypoglycemic infants and those with CNS damage.

Because small premature infants lose heat and water through their thin, transparent skin, they easily become dehydrated, especially when cared for under a radiant warmer and are fluid restricted. Covering the premature infant's body with clear plastic film, and the head with a cap significantly reduces both heat and water loss, as does warming and fully humidifying the inspired gases to 34–37°C [18,19]. The addition of forced air warming systems, circulating water blankets, and room temperature of 30°C provide maximal efficiency in reducing dry heat loss [20].

The clinical consequences of chilling include periodic breathing or apnea, bradycardia, metabolic acidosis, hyperglycemia, and aspiration of gastric contents. Fewer infants nursed in non-neutral thermal environments survive [21]. Those who survive gain weight more slowly. Maternal anesthesia (general) and neonatal fentanyl analgesia cause hypothermia in some infants, while morphine or conduction anesthesia does not [22].

Respiratory manifestations
Respiratory distress

Respiratory distress is common in preterm infants. It occurs three times more often after cesarean section than after a vaginal birth. The less mature the infant, the more severe the disease tends to be, although some very immature infants escape this affliction, especially if given surfactant shortly after birth or if there was chorio-amnionitis [23]. Survival of preterm infants depends on their size and gestational age. Moderately premature babies (1500–2500 g) with RDS require more support of ventilation and fewer of them survive than their larger counterparts. Despite their small size, more than 95% of the former should survive. Eighty-five percent of those weighing less than 1000 g and about 80% of those weighing less than 750 g now survive. Administration of exogenous pulmonary surfactant at birth has increased survival and decreased serious complications [24,25]. This rapidly improves lung function, which can lead to pulmonary gas leaks and lung injury if ventilation pressures are not decreased appropriately. The increased lung compliance improves oxygenation, which increases the likelihood of both ROP (see below) and inflammatory lung damage. Thus the Fio_2 must also be rapidly reduced to acceptable levels.

In addition to surfactant administration, in recent years ventilation strategies have changed in premature infants with RDS in an attempt to reduce the incidence and severity of bronchopulmonary dysplasia (BPD – see below). Targeting lower SpO_2 of 87–94% instead of 95–98%, employing nCPAP instead of endotracheal intubation, and limiting positive pressure ventilation by allowing permissive hypercapnia have all been demonstrated to reduce the severity of RDS and the incidence of BPD. In contrast, high-frequency oscillatory ventilation does not improve RDS or reduce incidence of BPD. Routine treatment with dexamethasone resulted in a lower severity of lung disease and less BPD; however, it is associated with increased risk of intestinal perforation, cerebral palsy, and neurodevelopmental impairment so its use has greatly diminished in recent years [26]. Finally, inhaled nitric oxide in infants less than 1250 g, when administered for 14 days, resulted in significantly greater BPD-free survival in one large multicenter study, and did not adversely affect long-term neurodevelopmental outcomes [27].

Bronchopulmonary dysplasia

Many preterm infants develop chronic lung disease (BPD) as a result of mechanical ventilation, oxygen administration, infection, inflammation or a combination of these factors [28]. The number of infants with BPD is increasing because more 500–750 g infants now survive [29,30]. Today's BPD differs from that described by Northway et al [31]. Many of today's preterm infants have no oxygen requirement above that of room air and normal lung function for a few days after birth, probably because of prenatal steroids and/or the administration of surface-active material after birth. Lung function then deteriorates, often in association with pulmonary infections [32], and the oxygen requirements increase and respiratory failure develops. The deterioration is made worse if the child has a PDA [33]. Furthermore, the chronic lung disease (CLD) of today's smaller infants has changed [34]. Today's CLD consists of simplified lungs, increased alveolar size, decreased alveolar number, and dysplastic pulmonary vasculature [35]. The end-result of these lung abnormalities is maldistribution of ventilation and perfusion, hypercarbia, hypoxemia, and occasionally the need for prolonged mechanical ventilation. Later in life, if they require surgery, their lung function [36] and gas transfer will be reduced [37]. Positive end-expiratory pressure (PEEP) and furosemide 0.5–1 mg/kg every 6–12 h are frequently used to treat pulmonary edema and improve gas exchange. However, furosemide often causes metabolic

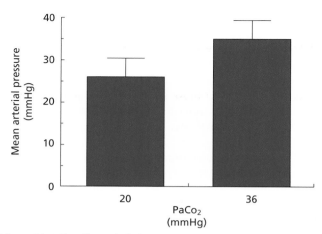

Figure 20.1 The effects of alkalosis on mean arterial pressure in premature infants. Ventilation was maintained constant and CO_2 was added to raise the $PaCO_2$, to normal.

alkalosis, especially if these babies are not given sufficient potassium and chloride. CO_2 is retained to compensate for the alkalosis. Reducing the $PaCO_2$ may cause severe alkalosis, reduced arterial blood pressure, and reduced cerebral blood flow (Fig. 20.1). Some preterm infants require higher ventilator pressures (tidal volumes) and oxygen concentrations during surgery, but many have improved ventilation and reduced oxygen requirements. During surgery, many infants can be ventilated with room air to maintain appropriate oxygen saturations. Although an oxygen saturation of 87–94% is felt (hoped) to be safe, the infant's PaO_2 would be 30–40 mmHg were they still *in utero*.

Apnea

Periodic breathing (cessation of breathing for <15 sec) and apnea (cessation of breathing for >20 sec or <20 sec with a decrease in SaO_2 plus bradycardia) are common in preterm infants, especially after the first week of life [38]. The incidence of apnea is inversely related to postconceptual age [39]. The causes of apnea are multiple and include anemia (hematocrit <30%), hypo- and hyperthermia, hypo- and hyperglycemia, hypo- and hypercalcemia, hypo- and hypervolemia, anemia, decreased functional residual capacity, patent ductus arteriosus, constipation, hypothyroidism, poorly developed control of respiration, excessive handling and stimulation, birth trauma, maternal drugs (narcotics), seizures, infections, and congenital heart disease. However, the primary cause of apnea of prematurity is immaturity of the central nervous system. Repeated apnea increases the likelihood of CNS damage due to repeated episodes of hypoxemia [40]. Infants who had apneic spells in the ICN usually must be ventilated from the time anesthesia is induced. Giving caffeine 5 or 10 mg/kg IV before surgery reduces or prevents postoperative apnea and oxygen desaturation, especially in patients who have had previous apneic spells, a hemoglobin concentration below 10 g/dL or pre-existing CNS injury [41].

Moderately premature infants, especially those recovering from RDS and those requiring mechanical ventilation, may have chronic lung disease. If they do, the $PaCO_2$ is frequently elevated and the PaO_2 or SaO_2 decreased during room air breathing. Care should be taken not to overexpand the lungs of premature infants, as this may lead to severe lung injury [42,43].

Patent ductus arteriosus

Fifty percent of full-term infants close their ductus arteriosus by 24 h of age and almost all of them do so after 72 h [44]. Most preterm infants of 30 weeks' gestation or more close their ductus arteriosus by 96 h of age. However, the ductus arteriosus of smaller preterm infants often remains open [45] and symptoms of a PDA often appear between the third to fifth day after birth [46]. Infants treated with surfactant at or near birth may have a significant PDA within a few hours of birth as the lungs expand and pulmonary vascular resistance decreases. A PDA murmur is usually heard at the left upper sternal border and is often continuous. It is loudest during exhalation or apnea, and its intensity is increased by hyperventilation. Patients with a PDA have bounding pulses and a widened pulse pressure (Fig. 20.2). A gallop rhythm may be present.

As the left-to-right shunt increases, so does the pulmonary blood flow. If the heart cannot keep up with the increased demand for cardiac output, congestive heart failure (CHF), manifested by increased respiratory failure (intercostal retractions, diminished breath sounds, poor air entry, rales), tachycardia, and a gallop rhythm develop. The PaO_2 decreases and the $PaCO_2$ rises. Apnea, increasing requirements for oxygen and mechanical ventilation, and a widened pulse pressure are often the earliest signs of a PDA. Signs of failure often appear before a murmur is heard [47] and if the ductus arteriosus is very large, no murmur is heard. In this case, a PDA is usually detected

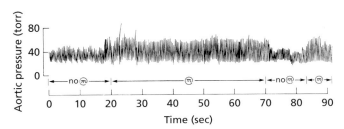

Figure 20.2 Aortic blood pressure of a preterm infant during periods when a PDA was present and was absent. Note the widening of the pulse pressure and elevated arterial pressure when the murmur was present. Courtesy of Dr Joseph A. Kitterman.

by changes in oxygenation, increased need for mechanical ventilation, and an echocardiogram.

The initial treatment of a PDA is medical, which includes fluid restriction [48,49] (occasionally to the point of dehydration) and administration of cyclo-oxygenase inhibitors, indometacin and ibuprofen [50,51] and diuretics. Indometacin has greatly reduced the number of patients requiring surgical closure of a ductus arteriosus, but it has not reduced the incidence of CLD or CNS injury [52].

If fluid restriction prevents adequate calorie intake, surgical ligation of the ductus arteriosus is usually undertaken. Early closure of the ductus arteriosus (either with indometacin or surgically) allows earlier weaning from mechanical ventilation and initiation of feeding within a few days after surgery.

A second reason to close a patent PDA early is to reduce the incidence of necrotizing enterocolitis [53]. A large PDA shunts as much as 80% of the cardiac output away from the systemic circulation and into the lungs, leaving little blood for the remaining body. Because the gut is one of the first organs to be deprived of blood, it is the shock organ in neonates. The use of prostaglandin synthetase inhibitors has not increased the incidence of necrotizing enterocolitis, but early ligation of the PDA may do so.

Central nervous system injury

Premature infants have two predominant forms of CNS injury. The most common in very premature infants is periventricular white matter injury, which is a leading cause of later cerebral palsy. The pathophysiology is incompletely understood, but the immature oligodendrocyte precursors are exquisitely sensitive to a number of common insults, including hypoxemia, hypotension, and inflammation [26]. The arterial supply to these areas is not fully developed, leading to vulnerability to ischemia. In addition, because of the fragile state of the developing vascular supply in the germinal matrix, these vessels are prone to rupture, causing the common complication of intraventricular hemorrhage (IVH). Grade I IVH is confined to the germinal matrix, grade II IVH occurs when bleeding extends to the cerebral ventricles, grade III IVH involves ventricular dilation, and grade IV IVH includes parenchymal extension of the bleed. Grades III and IV IVH may lead to hydrocephalus requiring ventricular-peritoneal shunting, a common procedure in premature neonates. Chapters 7 and 23 discuss pathogenesis and treatment of these disorders in more detail.

Infection

Infections (e.g. pneumonia, sepsis, and meningitis) are common in preterm infants, especially those who are moderately or severely preterm, because both their cellular and tissue immunity are reduced. Although the

Table 20.1 White blood cell count and differential count during the first 2 weeks of life

Age	Leukocytes	Neutrophils					Lymphocytes	Monocytes
		Total	Segs.	Bands	Eosinophils	Basophils		
Birth								
Mean	18,100	11,000	9,400	1,600	400	100	5,500	1,050
Range	9.0–30.0	6.0–26			20–850	0–640	2.0–11.0	0.4–3.1
Mean %	–	61	52	9	2.2	0.6	31	5.8
7 days								
Mean	12,200	5,500	4,700	830	500	50	5,000	1,100
Range	5.0–21.0	1.5–10.0			70–1,100	0–250	2.0–17.0	0.3–2.7
Mean %	–	45	39	6	4.1	0.4	41	9.1
14 days								
Mean	11,400	4,500	3,900	630	350	50	5,500	1,000
Range	5.0–20.0	1.0–9.5			70–1,000	0–230	2.0–17.0	0.2–2.4
Mean %	–	40	34	5.5	3.1	0.4	48	8.8

Reproduced from Avery [55] with permission from Lippincott, Williams & Wilkins.

signs of sepsis are often subtle, sepsis is suspected if the infant is hypo- or hyperthermic (despite a neutral thermal environment), lethargic, mottled, gray or apneic. If despite a constant infusion of glucose, the serum glucose concentration increases, sepsis should be suspected. Laboratory examinations may be helpful but preterm infants are often septic without positive blood cultures, elevated white blood cell (WBC) counts or fevers. In fact, this is more often true than not. The presence of an abnormal WBC count, whether increased or decreased, is diagnostically helpful (Table 20.1). A shift to the left toward neutrophil predominance is also helpful, but this is not always present. Band counts in excess of 15% are abnormal and are a good indicator of infection in preterm infants [54]. Cerebrospinal fluid (CSF) should contain fewer than 1 WBC per 200 red blood cells (RBCs), although an absolute count of 70 WBC/mm^3 may be normal [55]. The concentration of glucose in the CSF should be at least 50–60% of that in the blood. Urine should contain fewer than 5 WBCs per high-power field. A bladder tap urine specimen should be devoid of WBCs.

Preterm infants respond appropriately to antibiotics, although the dosage and interval between doses often must be altered (see Appendix A). Aminoglycosides may cause muscle weakness or paralysis and act synergistically with non-depolarizing muscle relaxants to increase their effect.

Necrotizing enterocolitis

Necrotizing enterocolitis is a common surgical emergency, especially in tiny preterm infants [53,56], and 10–50% of patients with this problem die [57]. The most common associations with NEC are prematurity, feeding per os,

excess feeding, and overgrowth of the bowel with non-normal bacterial flora [58,59]. An infant who suddenly develops abdominal distension, vomiting, bloody stools, reducing substances in the stool, and shock should be suspected of having NEC. Shock occurs because large amounts of fluid are translocated into the peritoneal cavity, gut, and other tissues and because of bacterial toxins. Radiographs of the abdomen demonstrate distended loops of bowel, air in the bowel wall and, if the bowel has perforated (which occurs about one-third of the time), free air in the peritoneal cavity. Such infants are extremely ill (often moribund), hypovolemic, and require fluid resuscitation with blood, colloid, and large volumes of saline or lactated Ringer's solution prior to surgery if they are to survive. Administering the quantity of fluid needed to accomplish volume resuscitation often worsens any respiratory failure and increases their need for mechanical ventilation. Infants with NEC should be started on IV broad-spectrum antibiotics preoperatively. Most survive, although about 10% of those who survive have short gut syndrome [60]. Many infants with NEC have cerebral palsy, severe neurological delay, and mental retardation, which may complicate anesthesia later in life [61].

Hematological manifestations

Preterm infants are frequently anemic because their ability to produce RBCs is reduced and because their caregivers frequently take blood for tests. Compensatory responses include tachycardia, increased cardiac output, and increased extraction of oxygen from blood. If the oxygen demand is unmet, lactic acidosis occurs. Low iron stores and inadequate iron intake worsen the anemia. As long as preterm infants have respiratory or cardiovascular problems, their hemoglobin levels should probably be maintained at or above 10 g/dL by blood transfusions from a limited number of units of packed RBCs and by the administration of epoetin alfa. A hemoglobin concentration of 14–15 g/dL is more likely to reduce the number of apneic spells and the CHF associated with a PDA than a hemoglobin of 8–10 g/dL. One study found that limiting transfusion was associated with higher rates of CNS hemorrhage, periventricular leukomalacia, and apnea [62] but another study failed to find these problems [63]. It is probably unwise to begin surgery for preterm infants if their hemoglobin concentration is <10 g/dL unless forced to do so by an absolute emergency. Transfusion of blood with adult hemoglobin, besides raising the hematocrit, shifts the oxygen dissociation curve to the right, which improves oxygen delivery to the tissues.

The WBC count of normal preterm infants is shown in Table 20.1. At birth, the WBC is higher than at later ages; it decreases over the first week of life. Stress can elevate the WBC count to 40,000–50,000/mm^3. Septic neonates either increase or decrease their WBC.

Erythropoietin (EPO) is produced in the liver and regulates erythropoiesis. Growing fetuses have high levels of erythropoiesis, a relatively high hematocrit, and predominant synthesis of hemoglobin F (fetal hemoglobin). The high concentrations of EPO present at birth decline relatively rapidly. The concentration of hemoglobin decreases over time and causes many preterm infants to be anemic. Phibbs et al [64] showed that giving 100 μg/kg of recombinant human erythropoietin intravenously to anemic preterm infants twice weekly for 6 weeks increased the reticulocyte counts (and RBCs) faster than a placebo and did not suppress subsequent release of endogenous EPO. The need for blood transfusions was reduced.

On rare occasions, premature infants are polycythemic. If the hematocrit exceeds 65%, an exchange transfusion may be required before surgery to prevent occlusion of their renal, portal or cerebral veins, especially if the patient becomes hypovolemic and/or hypotensive during surgery. If it is necessary to operate on a polycythemic child, sufficient fluid must be administered during surgery to maintain a normal or slightly increased intravascular volume. Hypotension must be treated immediately.

Nutrition and growth

Premature infants frequently have difficulty sucking effectively for some time after birth and require intermittent or continuous gavage feedings. While their gastric capacity and gastrointestinal motility are adequate to accept the instilled food, they often have difficulty absorbing their feeds. As a result, intravenous fluids and nutrition are commonly required. Infants who will not be fed

orally for 3 or 4 days after birth usually receive intravenous feedings with glucose 12.5%, protein (amino acids) 2–3 g/kg/day, and lipids 3 g/kg/day within the first few hours of life [65]. From this diet they derive 80–100 kcal/kg/day, depending on the volume of fluid infused, which is usually sufficient to maintain positive nitrogen balance, prevent tissue breakdown, and allow some growth (albeit inadequate). Attempts to feed asphyxiated infants early are often associated with NEC or abdominal distension and regurgitation of gastric contents. When this occurs, oral feedings are usually delayed for 5–6 days. While enough free water is required to maintain normal intra- and extravascular fluid volumes, administering more than 130–150 mL/kg/day increases the likelihood of a PDA, congestive heart failure, and the risk for NEC. Electrolytes (3 mEq/kg sodium, 2 mEq/kg potassium, 200–500 mg/kg calcium gluconate), and vitamins (including vitamin E) should be administered in the maintenance fluids. Because antibiotics kill gut flora, vitamin K 0.2 mg is administered twice weekly as long as the patient is receiving antibiotics [66]. Failure to do this increases the risk of bleeding during surgery.

Serum chemistry determinations
Calcium

During the last trimester of pregnancy, fetal concentrations of calcium exceed those of the mother [67]. At birth, the maternal supply of calcium is withdrawn and the baby's serum calcium concentration decreases, often to 7.5–8.5 mg/dL. If the baby takes in sufficient calcium, the levels increase after several days. Despite the low concentrations of total calcium, ionized calcium concentrations are normal (because serum protein concentrations are lower, at 3–4.5 g/dL). Consequently, total serum calcium concentrations above 7 mg/dL are adequate if ionized calcium concentrations are normal [68]. Phosphate and magnesium concentrations are similar to those of term infants.

If the patient has symptoms of hypocalcemia (e.g. twitching, seizures, hypotension), calcium gluconate 10–30 mg/kg is administered slowly intravenously. Hyperventilation decreases the unbound fraction of calcium, which can lower the seizure threshold. Despite the presence of hypocalcemia, the electrocardiogram (ECG) is usually normal.

Sodium

The serum sodium concentrations of tiny preterm infants are labile. They rise quickly with dehydration and decrease just as quickly with overhydration. Hypernatremia can damage the CNS, and hyponatremia (<120 mEq/L) can cause seizures. Water intoxication is usually associated with persistent hyponatremia.

Hypertonic saline is seldom required to correct hyponatremia; fluid restriction usually suffices.

Glucose

Most neonatologists attempt to maintain the postnatal nutrition of preterm infants at or above their requirements during fetal life in the hope of maintaining normal growth. This goal is seldom met for many reasons [69]. Glucose provides most of the energy for many organs, including the brain. Most non-anesthetized larger preterm infants tolerate an infusion of 5–7 mg/kg/min of glucose without developing hyperglycemia, glucosuria, polyuria or dehydration, but many extremely low birthweight infants (23–25 weeks' gestation) require at least 10 mg/kg/min to maintain normoglycemia and growth. The only way to know the serum glucose concentrations is to measure them frequently, especially in the operating room. Excessively high serum glucose concentrations (>200 mg/dL) can cause an osmotic diuresis, hypovolemia, and possibly CNS injury [70,71]. With adequate nutrition, preterm infants gain 25–30 g/day and increase their head circumference by 0.8–1 cm/wk. It may, however, be difficult to provide sufficient nutrition to achieve this growth for myriad reasons. The level of nutrition and weight gain should be determined carefully before surgery because infants with poor preoperative nutritional states often tolerate anesthesia and surgery less well.

The blood glucose concentrations of many preterm infants are below 40 mg/dL, which constitutes hypoglycemia. If present, hypoglycemia should be corrected with 10–20% dextrose 2–5 mL/kg over 5 min and with a continuous infusion of sufficient dextrose to maintain the glucose concentration between 50 and 90 mg/dL. Many preterm infants have an SaO_2 of 80–90%. However, if they are hypoglycemic and anemic in addition to having their SaO_2 at these low levels, their growth rates are often reduced [72].

Bilirubin

Because they conjugate substances less well, preterm infants often have higher serum bilirubin concentrations, especially those who are bruised, polycythemic or have intracranial, gastrointestinal or pulmonary hemorrhage. The relative hypoproteinemia, the decreased effectiveness of the blood–brain barrier, and the often-present acidemia increase their susceptibility to kernicterus – brain injury secondary to the direct neurotoxic effects of prolonged high serum unconjugated bilirubin concentrations . Even low concentrations of bilirubin (10–15 mg/dL) are sufficient to produce kernicterus in acidotic infants [73,74]. It may be necessary to do a two-volume exchange transfusion before surgery if the patient's indirect bilirubin concentration is elevated and if time permits,

Table 20.2 Serum bilirubin concentrations for exchange transfusion

Birth weight (g)	Serum bilirubin concentrations for exchange transfusion (mg/dL)	
	Norma/infants[†]	Abnormal infants[‡]
<1,000	10.0	10.0[§]
1,001–1,250	13.0	10.0[§]
1,251–1,500	15.0	13.0
1,501–2,000	17.0	15.0
2,001–2,500	18.0	17.0
>2,500	20.0	18.0

* These guidelines have not been validated.
[†] There have been case reports of basal ganglion staining at concentrations considerably lower than 10mg.
[‡] Normal infants are defined for this purpose as having none of the problem listed below.
[§] Abnormal infants have one or more of the following problems: perinatal asphyxia prolonged hypoxemia, acidemia, persistent hypothermia, hypoalbuminemia, hemolysis, sepsis, hyperglycemia, elevated free fatty acids or presence of drugs that compete for bilirubin binding, and signs of clinical or central nervous system deterioration.
Data from American Academy of Pediatrics, Committee on Fetus and Newborns Standards and Recommendations for Hospital Care of Newborn Infants, 6th ed. Evanston, IL, American Academy of Pediatrics, 1977.

because intraoperative hypoxemia and acidosis may prove disastrous (Table 20.2).

Retinopathy of prematurity

Fifty percent of infants weighing 1000–1500 g at birth have some degree of ROP [75]. Seventy-eight percent of those weighing 750–999 g have ROP, and more than 90% of those weighing less than 750 g have some degree of ROP. ROP is rare in term infants. Retinopathy of prematurity is divided into five stages [76].

- Stage 1: a thin white line separates the posterior vascularized portion of the retina from the anterior avascular retina.
- Stage 2: the demarcation line increases in volume and elevates. At this point it is known as the "ridge." The changes found in stage 1 and 2 regress in 80% of patients. Between 5% and 10% of premature infants with stage 1 and 2 disease progress to stage 3 [77].
- Stage 3: tissue proliferation develops from the ridge, usually posteriorly. Stage 3 can be mild, moderate or severe, depending on the volume of the extraretinal tissue [76].
- Stage 4: partial retinal detachment occurs with the macula still attached (stage 4a). The macula is detached in stage 4b.
- Stage 5: total retinal detachment occurs in stages 4 and 5.

Retinopathy of prematurity begins with retinal blood vessel constriction, reduced vascular endothelial growth factor (VEGF), and retinal hypoxia [78]. The retinal hypoxia stimulates VEGF production and vascular proliferation, hemorrhage, and (in the worst cases) retinal detachment. While oxygen is a major contributing factor to the development of ROP, it is not the only factor [61]. It is unknown what levels of oxygenation cause ROP, but a PaO_2 of 150 mmHg for as little as 1–2 h (the length of many surgical procedures) has done so. It is also possible that ROP might develop at considerably lower PaO_2 because the retinas of preterm infants, were they still *in utero*, would be exposed to a PaO_2 of 30–40 mmHg, not 50 mmHg or more, as often occurs after birth. Preterm infants whose SaO_2 was maintained between 80% and 96% for the first several postnatal weeks had less ROP than those with higher SaO_2 [78]. Interestingly, after 31 weeks' gestation, an SaO_2 of 94–99% was required to reduce the risk of further retinal damage. At this age the lower oxygen concentrations and mild hypoxia were adding to the retinal hypoxia. After discussion with the neonatologist, it may be appropriate to maintain higher oxygen saturations in *this specific group* of patients during surgery.

The left-shifted oxygen dissociation curve of fetal hemoglobin (HbF) releases less oxygen to the tissues, which may protect the retina. Transfusion with adult blood may increase the risk of developing ROP because the right-shifted oxygen dissociation curve releases more oxygen. Chorio-amnionitis and neonatal systemic inflammatory disease also increase ROP [79].

Vitamin E and omega-3 fish oils may protect against ROP by their membrane-stabilizing and antioxidant actions [80,81]. While vitamin E concentrations normally decrease rapidly after birth, due to inadequate intake and storage of vitamin E, administering more than physiological amounts of vitamin E to premature infants has little beneficial effect and may increase the incidence of necrotizing enterocolitis and infection [82,83].

Approximately 85% of acute ROP undergoes spontaneous regression [84]. Grades 1 and 2 regress in 2–3 months, while grade 3 regresses in 6 months or more. Most grade 4 and 5 ROP results in blindness or limited vision in approximately 25% in infants who were at high risk for retinal detachment [85].

Patients with ROP come to the anesthetist's attention because they require an eye examination, photocoagulation or scleral buckling under anesthesia. It is unknown if exposure to increased oxygen concentrations during anesthesia worsens pre-existing ROP. Because we do not know, it is better to keep the SaO_2 during anesthesia at the same levels used in the ICN, usually between 87% and 92% [86]. Because many of these patients also have chronic lung disease and maldistribution of ventilation and

perfusion, their SaO_2 can rapidly decrease with the induction of anesthesia. Adding a small amount of PEEP (2–5 cmH_2O) often improves both the match of ventilation-perfusion and oxygenation. Excessive PEEP may overdistend the ventilated portions of the lung and decrease oxygenation. Aoyama et al have published a sensible plan for anesthetizing patients with ROP [87]. They point out that many patients require postoperative mechanical ventilation and ICU care after surgery, even if they did not require them preoperatively. Because the surgeons often inject air into the eye during surgery, it is best to avoid nitrous oxide and use air as the carrier gas for the inhaled anesthetic.

Preoperative preparation

History

During the preoperative visit, the patient's chart must be read, understood, and thoroughly discussed with the physicians and nurses caring for the patient. It is the nurses who stand at the bedside 24 h a day and provide the patient's minute-to-minute care. They know the idiosyncrasies of each patient. For example, the nurses may know that very brief periods of apnea cause severe hypoxemia and cyanosis or that the patient's perfusion decreases when his blood glucose concentration is <40 mg/dL or when the ionized calcium concentration is below 0.9 mmol/L.

Both the fetal and birth histories are important when planning an anesthetic for preterm infants. If the infant was asphyxiated before or at birth, the effects of asphyxia (right ventricular dysfunction, coagulation abnormalities, etc.) may still be present. Autoregulation of the cerebral circulation may be absent [5,88,89]; if so, sudden increases in arterial pressure may rupture fragile cerebral vessels and cause intracranial hemorrhage [90].

Myocardial function may still be depressed and the heart may show signs of hypoxic strain, including insufficiency of the tricuspid valve. Blood flow to the gut may be reduced. Both the blood volume and the hemoglobin concentration may be low if they were not corrected. These abnormalities can persist for several days after birth.

A maternal medication history should be sought in every case because many pregnant women take prescription or non-prescription drugs. A few use illicit drugs, and the baby may be undergoing drug withdrawal at the time of surgery. The symptoms of narcotic withdrawal include agitation, tremors, poor feeding, vomiting, and occasionally seizures. Infants withdrawing from barbiturates, diazepam or methadone may only do so at 5–10 days of age. Fetuses who are repeatedly exposed to cocaine, which causes premature delivery, may also have pulmonary hypertension and bowel perforation. Infants born after maternal ingestion of large doses of aspirin or acetaminophen may have pulmonary hypertension and persistent fetal circulation (PFC) during the first few days of life [91,92]. PFC must be considered in any severely hypoxemic infant.

Systems review and examination
Head, eyes, ears, nose, and throat
Congenital anomalies of the face and mouth are common, either as part of a syndrome or as a lone entity. A cleft palate may be missed when infants are mechanically ventilated from birth. If the anesthetist must reintubate the patient's trachea, a cleft palate may make this more difficult because the tongue cannot be fixed against the palate and flops over the laryngoscope blade, obstructing the anesthetist's view of the glottis. The small mouth and the relatively large tongue of preterm infants frequently obstruct breathing, especially when pressure is applied to the submental triangle while holding an anesthesia mask on the patient's face. Even slight pressure in this area can completely obstruct the airway. Anesthesia masks with large air-filled cuffs are dangerous if they slip off the bridge of the nose and compress the nares while the mouth is being held closed. Most babies are obligatory nasal breathers for several months after birth [93]. A nasogastric tube (NGT) obstructs half of the unintubated infant's upper airway when the mouth is closed. This often increases respiratory work and leads to apnea during the induction of anesthesia. Nasogastric tubes should be removed and reinserted orally if necessary. Atropine, if administered to patients with some types of cataracts or with glaucoma, may increase the intraocular pressure and further damage the eye (see Chapter 31).

Pulmonary system
As stated above, pulmonary dysfunction is common in preterm infants. Therefore, the pulmonary system must be evaluated carefully before anesthesia and surgery. Answers should be sought to the following questions.

- Does the patient now have or is he/she recovering from RDS? If so, how much support of breathing is required? What are the ventilator rates, pressures (peak-inspired and end-expiratory), inspired oxygen concentrations, and inspiratory times? Is the patient breathing spontaneously during mechanical ventilation? Is he/she triggering inspiration by the ventilator? What SaO_2, blood gas, and pH values do spontaneous breathing or the ventilator settings occasion? How labile are the blood gases? Do the blood gases and pH change when the patient is moved from side to side or

onto the back or abdomen[94], when the trachea is suctioned or when the chest is percussed [95]? It may be a problem if the patient must be turned into the lateral position for surgery and this position causes deterioration of the blood gases and pH.

- Has the patient had a pulmonary hemorrhage? If so, has the bleeding stopped?
- Is pneumonia present? Pneumonia may be difficult to differentiate from RDS, pulmonary edema or chronic lung disease on radiograph. A WBC count, a differential WBC count, and a smear of the tracheal secretions may be helpful in making this differentiation. If the infant has pneumonia, the tracheal smear will show both WBCs and bacteria. Either finding alone is seldom significant.
- Is the endotracheal tube (ETT) fixed securely in place? Accidental extubation of the trachea on the way to the operating room is disconcerting. Tape used to hold the ETT in place should not completely encircle the infant's head to prevent brainstem hemorrhage [96].
- Does the infant have intercostal retractions? Most preterm infants have grade 1-of-4 to 2-of-4 retractions because their chest walls are not fully developed. Those with pulmonary disease have grade 3-of-4 to 4-of-4 retractions. Retractions indicate increased work of breathing, decreased lung compliance, increased airway resistance or all three.
- Can rales be heard? Most preterm infants have occasional rales. Moist rales indicate intra-alveolar fluid, usually associated with pulmonary edema or infection. Dry rales are usually associated with atelectasis. Rhonchi are also common, especially after several days of tracheal intubation.
- Are there secretions? White or clear secretions are seldom significant. Yellow, green or brown secretions often indicate infection. Frothy, pink or blood-tinged secretions are usually indicative of pulmonary edema or pulmonary hemorrhage.

Preterm infants normally breathe 30–60 times per minute. However, those with lung disease can have respiratory rates of 150 breaths/min or more, especially when lung compliance is reduced. Babies "choose" to breathe rapidly and shallowly rather than slowly and deeply, probably because the metabolic cost of breathing rapidly and shallowly is less. Rapid respirations help maintain the functional residual capacity by not allowing sufficient time for complete exhalation. Unless PEEP is applied, slow respiratory rates decrease functional residual capacity (Fig. 20.3) [97].

Evaluating blood gas and oxygen saturation data gives important clues to the patient's responses to ventilatory maneuvers. Preterm infants normally have lower PaO_2 than term babies (Tables 20.3, 20.4). Therefore, small changes in PaO_2 cause large changes in oxygen saturation and in oxygen content [98]. Brief periods of apnea lead to hypoxemia. Is the patient having apneic spells (see above)? Apneic spells are often indicative of other problems. If the infant is having or has had apnea, he/she may have postoperative apnea and require mechanical ventilation for a variable amount of time (see Chapter 21). Figure 20.4 shows the chest radiographs of a normal infant and one with hyaline membrane disease.

Cardiovascular system

Many preterm infants have problems with their cardiovascular systems (including patent ductus arteriosus, hypotension, shock) [99,100] but congenital heart disease is less common. Because the bulk of muscle is laid down in the pulmonary arteries during the third trimester of pregnancy, infants born earlier have less muscle and are prone to develop a PDA and increased left-to-right shunting of blood through the ductus arteriosus earlier in life (3–5 days of age) than in term infants (7–14 days of age). The net result is increased pulmonary blood flow, pulmonary edema, congestive heart failure, reduced lung compliance, hypoxemia, and CO_2 retention. Surfactant administration establishes the functional residual capacity (FRC) more quickly, which is associated with a PDA and left-to-right shunting of blood within a few hours after birth.

Congestive heart failure may not be heralded by tachycardia in preterm infants, as it is in older patients. In fact, the heart rate is often monotonously regular and usually within normal limits (120–160 beats/min) (Table 20.5). A third heart sound (gallop) may be present but may be difficult to hear because of the rapid heart rate and

Table 20.3 Normal arterial blood gases

Parameter	Birth	1 hour	5 hours	1 day	5 days	7 days
Pao_2 (mmHg)						
X̄	46.6	63.3	73.7	72.7	72.1	73.1
SD	9.9	11.3	12.0	9.5	10.5	9.7
$Paco_2$ (mmHg)						
X̄	46.1	36.1	35.2	33.4	34.8	35.9
SD	7.0	4.2	3.6	3.1	3.5	3.1
pH						
X̄	7.207	7.332	7.339	7.369	7.371	7.37
SD	0.051	0.031	0.028	0.032	0.031	0.02

X̄, mean; SD, standard deviation.
Reproduced from Koch & Wendel. Biol Neonate 1968; 12: 136, with permission from Karger.

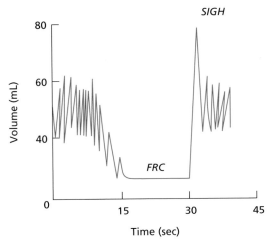

Figure 20.3 Changes in functional residual capacity (FRC) with bradypnea and apnea. Reproduced from Gregory [97] with permission from Lippincott, Williams & Wilkins.

Table 20.4 Arterial blood gases in normal preterm infants

Parameter	Birth	3–5 hours	13–24 hours	5–10 days
Pao_2				
X̄	–	59.5	67.0	80.3
SD	–	7.7	15.2	12.0
$Paco_2$				
X̄	–	47.0	27.2	36.4
SD	–	8.5	8.4	4.2
pH				
X̄	7.32	7.329	7.464	7.378
SD		0.38	0.064	0.043

X̄, mean; SD, standard deviation.
Reproduced from Orzalesi et al. Arch Dis Child 1967; 42: 174, with permission from BMJ Publishing Group Ltd.

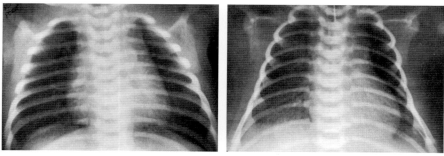

Figure 20.4 Chest x-rays of a normal preterm infant (*left*) and one with respiratory distress syndrome (*right*). Note the air bronchograms, the loss of lung volume and the heart border in the latter. Courtesy of Dr Robert C. Brasch.

RDS   CHF

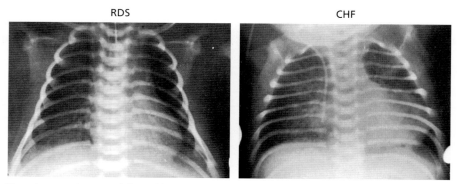

Figure 20.5 Chest x-ray films of a normal preterm infant with respiratory distress syndrome (*left*) and one with a patent ductus arteriosus and congestive heart failure (*right*). Note the enlarged heart, the central fluffiness, and the loss of clear vascular shadows in the latter. Courtesy of Dr Robert C. Brasch.

Table 20.5 Heart rate in preterm infants with patent ductus arteriosus

Condition	Heart rate (bpm)
Normal cardiac function	150 ± 18
Congestive heart failure	148 ± 22
Postligation ductus arteriosus	146 ± 18

environmental noise (e.g. mechanical ventilators, alarms, monitors, people). Murmurs can be difficult to hear for the same reason. Two murmurs are commonly present in preterm infants, that of a PDA and that of tricuspid insufficiency. The PDA murmur is a systolic ejection murmur that is best heard along the upper left sternal border when the ductal flow is small. When it is large, the murmur extends into diastole, is continuous, and is heard throughout the chest. The "machinery murmur" described in older patients is seldom heard. The murmur of tricuspid insufficiency is systolic in nature and is best heard along the right sternal border. It seldom radiates far, and it disappears after several days of life as ventricular function improves.

Congestive heart failure reduces peripheral perfusion and slows capillary filling. The pulses are decreased, except in patients with a PDA. Peripheral edema is common, in part because serum protein concentrations are low (see above). Edema usually appears first in the eyelids. Pitting edema of the feet and shins is uncommon in other than the sickest babies. Puffiness of the feet, however, is common.

The chest radiographs of preterm infants with CHF are frequently difficult to differentiate from those of infants with RDS. The former usually show central fluffiness and slightly larger markings than those of RDS (Fig. 20.5).

The liver size is a good indicator of right-sided heart failure and of CHF in preterm infants because their livers are very distensible. The inferior margin is normally sharp and located 1–2 cm below the right costal margin; with CHF, the liver can quickly distend into the pelvis. Just as quickly, it returns to its normal position with appropriate therapy. Applying excessive pressure when examining the abdomen may push the liver up into the thoracic cavity and make the liver appear smaller than it really is. The position of the liver edge can usually be determined by gently running one's fingertips over the right upper abdomen or by percussing the abdomen. Percussion is especially useful when the abdomen is distended. Enlarged livers often extend across the midline, which may make it difficult to differentiate from the spleen, which also is often enlarged during CHF.

Abdomen

The abdomen of preterm infants is normally protuberant and soft. The venous pattern of the abdominal wall is prominent and is exaggerated with liver disease. Intra-abdominal organs are generally easy to palpate. The spleen is usually palpable below the left costal margin in patients who have erythroblastosis fetalis, systemic infections, liver disease or fluid overload. The ascites of erythroblastotic infants may interfere with ventilation of the lungs and make it necessary to remove some of the fluid by paracentesis to allow adequate ventilation of the infant's lungs. In some cases paracentesis may be required before the induction of anesthesia.

The preterm infant's kidneys are easily palpable as small masses in the retroperitoneum. They may be enlarged by renal vein thromboses or by renal, ureteral or bladder anomalies. The urinary bladder is usually felt as a round mass extending above the pelvic rim. Obstruction of the urethra can cause the bladder to distend above the umbilicus. The ureters are occasionally palpable as cords running longitudinally in the retroperitoneum.

It is often possible to see loops of distended bowel through the abdominal wall. Abdominal distension is seldom a cause of abdominal tenderness unless peritonitis is present. Then the abdomen is tender, rigid, and edematous enough to leave one's fingerprints on the skin. Intraperitoneal fluid often passes through the inguinal canals and distends the scrota. As a consequence, inguinal hernias occur in about 30% of premature male infants. Redness around the umbilicus is often a sign of systemic or intra-abdominal infections.

One should ascertain patency of the anus before the infant undergoes surgery. Occasionally an imperforate anus is missed in very sick infants. Nothing (including thermometers) should be inserted more than 0.5 cm into the rectum to avoid perforating the bowel.

Central nervous system

The incidence of CNS injury increases with increasing degrees of prematurity and asphyxia (see Chapter 23). CNS injury is usually manifested as flaccidity, hypertonia, hypotonia or a difference in tone between the upper and lower or between the right and left sides of the body. Deep tendon reflexes and the grasp reflex are often absent. Normal preterm infants normally have a positive Babinski sign. The back, neck, and sacral area should be examined for evidence of a meningomyelocele. Again, these lesions can be missed preoperatively when very ill infants are placed on their backs and left there for days because of the extent of their illness.

State of hydration

The hydration state of preterm infants should be carefully assessed during the preoperative visit. Their large surface/volume ratio, thin skin, rapid respiratory rates, relatively large minute volumes, and infrared warmers increase water losses [101]. Failure to replace these losses adequately leads to dehydration. Covering the baby with clear plastic film significantly reduces water and heat losses. Reducing fluid intake to less than 130 mL/kg/day to decrease the incidence of PDA in preterm infants occasionally leads to severe fluid and calorie restriction [49]. Restricting fluid and caloric intake may cause infants to be dehydrated and undernourished when they present for surgery. Administration of potent diuretics, such as furosemide, can cause further dehydration. Preterm infants third space fluids more easily than older patients because the preterm infant's capillaries leak easily, serum protein levels are lower and the oncotic pressure is reduced [102,103]. As a consequence, infants with sepsis or shock lose large amounts of fluid into the peritoneal cavity. These patients commonly gain 20–50% of their bodyweight, despite being intravascular volume depleted.

Laboratory findings

Most sick preterm infants undergo a multitude of laboratory tests, the results of which must be reviewed and understood before anesthesia is induced.

Hematology

In well infants, a hemoglobin concentration above 7 g/dL is usually adequate. In infants with cardiorespiratory disease, the concentration of hemoglobin should exceed 9 g/dL to ensure adequate oxygen-carrying capacity. As discussed above, the hemoglobin (Hgb) concentration decreases rapidly after birth, frequently because caregivers extract large volumes of blood for tests.

Besides knowing the PaO_2 and SaO_2, it is important to determine the oxygen content of the patient's blood:

$$([\{1.36 \text{ mL oxygen/g Hgb} \times \text{Hgb g/dL}\} \times SaO_2] + 0.003 \times PaO_2).$$

0.003 is the solubility coefficient of oxygen in plasma. If the hemoglobin concentration were 10 g, the oxygen content would be about 13.1 cc oxygen/100 mL of blood. The entire body extracts about 5 volumes percent of oxygen from the blood. However, the heart extracts 12 volumes percent from blood passing through it. There is barely enough oxygen present to meet cardiac demands. If the Hb concentration were 5 g, the oxygen content of the arterial blood would be about 6.5 cc/100 mL of blood, which is insufficient to meet cardiac demands, unless coronary blood flow increases and cardiac oxygen requirements remain constant or decrease while the oxygen extraction from blood increases. This is a precarious position in which to begin surgery. Infants with low hemoglobin concentrations should be transfused before surgery if possible to normalize their blood oxygen content.

Electrolytes

The concentrations of the serum electrolytes vary more in preterm infants than in older patients because premature infants are affected more severely by small changes in fluid and electrolyte intake, by fluid and electrolyte losses, and by their environment. A single electrolyte value can be misleading; serial values are much more helpful. A rise in serum sodium is usually a result of either dehydration or excessive sodium administration. The latter is associated with peripheral edema. Although hyperkalemia is common, it seldom affects the ECG. Hypokalemia (<3 mEq/L) is also common, especially when preterm infants are given potent diuretics. Inadvertent hyperventilation and alkalosis further reduce the serum potassium concentration when potassium moves into the cells in exchange for hydrogen ions. The serum concentration of chloride is normally higher in preterm infants (105–115 mEq/L) than in older children, which in part accounts for the commonly present metabolic acidosis.

The total calcium concentration is usually lower than that of term infants (see above), but the ionized calcium concentrations of the two groups are similar. Hyperventilation may reduce the ionized calcium concentration to unacceptable levels. The tendency of most neonatologists is to maintain the total serum calcium concentration above 7 mg/dL if the ionized calcium concentrations are normal for age [68].

Coagulation status

At birth, the levels of coagulation factors are approximately 50% of adult values, although babies seldom bleed because of this [104-106]. Their platelet counts are similar to those of normal adults, but their platelets probably function less well. Does the infant have a bleeding diathesis? Infants who are asphyxiated at birth have depression of factors V, VII, and VIII, which return to normal within 3–4 days if the infants are resuscitated quickly [107]. These levels may not return to normal for a week or more if the hypoxia is prolonged. The latter infants are frequently thrombocytopenic, often below 10,000/mm³. Even at these levels, bleeding seldom occurs in the absence of surgery or injury. Therefore, it is seldom necessary to transfuse platelets to premature infants unless they require surgery or their platelet count is below 5000/mm³, especially when their other clotting parameters are normal and there is no evidence of bleeding. When surgery is required, platelets should be transfused to raise their concentration to 50,000/mm³ or greater. If the surgical procedure lasts for several hours, another platelet transfusion may be required. If the patient has not received vitamin K after birth, has been nil per os (NPO) and has received IV antibiotics, vitamin K 0.3 mg/kg should be administered preoperatively to preterm infants [106].

Bleeding disorders, such as disseminated intravascular coagulation (DIC), must be corrected preoperatively with fresh frozen plasma, cryoprecipitate or factor VIIa. If both the clotting factors and the platelets are decreased, the patient will benefit from fresh whole blood because it contains all of the clotting factors, platelets, proteins, and RBCs required.

Preoperative plan

For very ill preterm infants, it is advisable to have the help of a second anesthetist during surgery. It is difficult for one person to ventilate the patient's lungs, give fluids and blood, watch the surgical field and monitors, and keep the anesthesia record at the same time (although automatic record keeping has made this easier – see Chapter 44). In an attempt to prevent hypothermia, the operating room should be warmed to 37°C or above before the patient arrives and a servo-controlled infrared heater should be placed over the operating table. A water-circulated heating blanket should be placed under the sheet covering the table and maintained at 35–37°C. Pressure transducers used to monitor arterial and central venous pressure should be set up and calibrated if needed. Intravenous solutions are made up if they differ from those being infused in the nursery. Patients often receive 5% dextrose in 0.2 normal saline in the ICN. This solution should not be used to replace fluid losses during surgery. Ringer's lactate or normal saline is used for this purpose. Fluid should be warmed and delivered through an infusion pump when possible. If a drip chamber is used, it should never contain more fluid than is safe to give in 1 h. This avoids accidental overhydration if the IV infusion runs wide open.

Before transport to the operating room, an exchange of information between the ICN physician and nurse and the anesthesiologist should occur, summarizing current status and any special concerns the team has. Transporting preterm infants to and from the operating room can be dangerous. During transport, the anesthetist should always accompany sick infants to reduce this risk. The patient is connected to battery-operated arterial blood pressure, ECG, and oxygen saturation monitor during transport. Infusion pumps should continue to infuse fluids and drugs, especially vasoactive drugs. Ventilation is supported during

Table 20.6 Body temperature of preterm infants during transport to and from the operating room

Time	Body temperature (°C)
Preoperative: nursery	36.4 ± 0.5
Preoperative: operating room	35.7 ± 0.7
End of surgery	36.4 ± 1.0
Postoperative: nursery	35.9 ± 1.7

transport, usually with a Jackson-Reese device, and a portable air-oxygen blender. Sufficient oxygen should be administered to keep the oxygen saturation between 87% and 92% [98].

The inspired oxygen concentration should not be 100% during transport or in the operating room unless that concentration of oxygen is needed to maintain the desired oxygen saturation. Otherwise, the FiO_2 should be kept as low as possible while providing appropriate oxygen saturations. Use of an air-oxygen blender is required during transport to the operating room so the Fio_2 can be properly adjusted.

Keeping the patient warm is a major problem during transport. Table 20.6 shows the changes in body temperature of preterm infants being transported to and from the operating room for surgery. Note the loss of nearly a degree of body temperature during this short period. Their body temperature increased to normal in the operating room and decreased again during the trip back to the nursery. These heat losses can usually be prevented by covering the baby's body with clear plastic film and warm blankets, covering the infant's head with a cap, and placing a chemical heating pad under the patient (Porta-Warm, Allegiance Health Care Corp.). Elevators should be waiting for the patient, not vice versa. The operating room should be warm, and the infant should go directly into the operating room and be immediately placed under a servo-controlled radiant warmer.

In most instances, it is better to ligate a PDA, insert a Broviac catheter or treat necrotizing enterocolitis in the NICU rather than transport the child to the operating room. This allows the patient's mechanical ventilator and monitors to be used during surgery. The infection rates of patients undergoing surgery in the ICN are the same as those of patients undergoing surgery in an operating room [108].

Induction of anesthesia

Although preterm infants require anesthesia [109], their requirements are lower than those of older patients [110,111]. Failure to provide adequate anesthesia

predisposes them to hypertension and intracranial hemorrhage if their cerebral vascular autoregulation is absent, which it commonly is [112]. When this occurs, increases or decreases in arterial blood pressure increase or decrease cerebral blood flow. Adequate anesthesia prevents or attenuates these changes in pressure. Because deep anesthesia reduces the arterial blood pressure of infants and children more than it does that of adults [113], arterial blood pressure must be supported with fluid and vasopressors when necessary. Increases in heart rate and arterial blood pressure are usually signs of light anesthesia. However, the heart rate often does not change during hypotension because the baroreceptors of preterm infants are obtunded by even light levels of anesthesia [113]. Seventy percent nitrous oxide reduces the barore-sponse to the same extent as halothane [114]. Fentanyl 10 μg/kg also depresses the baroreceptor reflex significantly [115] though this does not cause hypotension. Anand and associates showed that inadequate anesthesia induces a stress response in preterm infants [109] and that underanesthetized infants have a 10-fold greater complication rate.

Inserting an ETT without anesthesia or analgesia increases arterial and intracranial pressures [116]. Obviously, some patients are too ill to anesthetize before inserting an ETT, but this is uncommon after the immediate neonatal period.

Anesthesia is often induced with inhaled anesthetics (usually sevoflurane) and sufficient oxygen to maintain the desired SaO_2. If controlled ventilation is required during the induction of anesthesia, the anesthetic concentration must be reduced to prevent sudden, severe hypotension [117]. An alternative anesthetic technique employs propofol 1–2 mg/kg or fentanyl 10–30 μg/kg intravenously given over 1–2 min [110]. Once the eyelid reflexes are lost, an ETT can be inserted. If an assistant places a finger in the patient's suprasternal notch, the tip of the ETT can be felt as it encounters the finger. At this point the tube tip is in the mid-trachea and advancement of the tube can be stopped and the tube fixed in place. This reduces inadvertent endobronchial intubation. If necessary, the patient can be paralyzed with pancuronium bromide 0.1 mg/kg or rocuronium 0.3–1.0 mg/kg. Pancuronium is often preferred for premature infants because it increases the heart rate and prevents bradycardia, which better maintains cardiac output.

Maintenance of anesthesia

There are few data on the anesthetic requirements of preterm infants, especially extremely premature infants [111]. However, experience suggests that premature

Table 20.7 Relation between heart rate and systolic blood pressure in preterm infants anesthetized with halothane for ligation of a patent ductus arteriosus

Condition	Heart rate (bpm)	Systolic pressure (mmHg)
Preinduction	146 ± 20	62 ± 16
Before ductal ligation	143 ± 17	48 ± 16
After ductal ligation	145 ± 16	66 ± 15

infants require less anesthesia than their healthy full-term counterparts. The sevoflurane requirement for infants undergoing ligation of PDA is approximately 50–80% of that of term infants. At that dosage, no change occurs in either heart rate or arterial blood pressure with skin incision [111].

Preterm infants anesthetized with inhaled anesthetics are more often hypotensive than older patients [118], probably because there is less response of peripheral vessels to catecholamines [113], myocardial depression, and loss of baroresponse [119]. Because preterm infants depend heavily on tachycardia for cardiac output, loss of baroresponses makes it difficult for them to respond appropriately to hypotension. Table 20.7 shows the heart rate and arterial blood pressures of preterm infants anesthetized with halothane for ligation of a patent ductus arteriosus. Note the heart rate did not increase when the blood pressure decreased or increased, so baroreceptor function was reduced. Similar data are unavailable for sevoflurane, but the changes are almost certainly similar.

To avoid anesthesia-induced hypotension, fentanyl has been used to anesthetize preterm infants [110,120]. Administering 10–30 μg/kg of fentanyl prevents changes in both heart rate and arterial blood pressure with a skin incision. When the blood volume is adequate, fentanyl administration seldom causes hypotension. Patients regularly receiving fentanyl in the NICU may require much higher doses of fentanyl for surgery, often more than 50 μg/kg. As with all drugs, fentanyl should be titrated to the desired clinical effect. Muscle relaxants are often used to prevent movement and to reduce anesthetic requirements. Paralyzed premature infants must, however, be anesthetized! Nitrous oxide, like other anesthetics, can cause hypotension and cardiac arrest in hypovolemic patients.

The lungs of preterm infants should be mechanically ventilated during anesthesia and surgery. Operating room mechanical ventilators are poor substitutes for those used in the ICN, but ICN ventilators cannot deliver inhaled anesthetics. If an ICN ventilator is used, a narcotic-based anesthetic will provide adequate anesthesia. No ventilator adequately compensates for changes in compliance and resistance of the lungs induced by retractors, packs, and hands. Consequently, the lungs of small preterm infants are often ventilated by hand while observing the surgical field and chest expansion. The lowest pressures and tidal volumes possible should be used to *normally* expand the chest and lungs. If the neonate required PEEP in the NICU, he/she will require it during anesthesia and surgery. The initial ventilator settings used during anesthesia should mimic those determined by the physicians, nurses, and respiratory therapists in the NICU to produce the best blood gases and oxygen saturations. These variables can be adjusted as needed. In the operating room, the lungs of premature infants are mechanically ventilated. To avoid administering high oxygen concentration, it must be possible to adjust the FiO_2 between 0.21 to 1.0 during surgery. Administering high oxygen concentrations to preterm infants who do not need them unnecessarily exposes the infants to the risk of ROP (see above).

Actively determining and replacing the premature infant's blood losses with blood and fluid is crucial because the blood volumes of premature infants are small, 85–100 mL/kg. Consequently, in a 1 kg infant a loss of 10 mL of blood is equivalent to a 10% loss of blood volume. It is often difficult to accurately determine blood losses during surgery. Weighing the used sponges is a more accurate method of doing so than merely looking at them and guessing how much blood is in them. A 1 g increase in sponge weight equals 1 mL of blood. Suctioned blood should be collected in small bottles to more accurately determine blood losses. Volumes of flush solutions must be accurately recorded so they can be subtracted from the amount of fluid in the blood collection bottle. The most difficult part of estimating blood loss is determining how much blood is lost into the surgical drapes and into the tissues. Because of these inadequacies in blood loss determinations, it is often necessary to increase the estimated blood loss by 25–50% and to administer that amount of blood or an appropriate volume of crystalloid while monitoring intravascular pressures, heart rate, and determining serial hematocrits. Low hematocrits are corrected with packed RBCs.

The volume of fluid administered depends in great part on the amount of surgical trauma occurring. Abdominal or thoracic procedures are more traumatic than peripheral procedures and therefore require 8–12 mL/kg/h or more of lactated Ringer's solution. Replacing fluid losses with 0.2 or 0.3 normal saline is dangerous because it leads to hyponatremia, water overload, and occasionally death. Infusing approximately 5–7 mg/kg/min of glucose is a good starting dose under anesthesia, unless the patient was receiving higher concentrations of glucose in the ICN. The blood glucose concentration should be

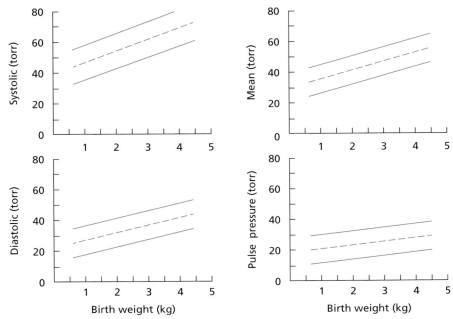

Figure 20.6 Systolic, diastolic, and mean arterial blood pressures and pulse pressures of infants between 610 and 4200 g. Reproduced from Versmold et al [121] with permission from American Pediatrics Association.

Table 20.8 Serum and urine glucose values and urine volume in a 1 kg infant

Assay	Time (h)			
	Baseline	**1**	**2**	**Recovery**
Serum glucose (mg/dL)	45–90	90	175	130
Urine glucose	1+	2+	4+	4+
Fluid intake (mL/kg/h)	4	7	15	12
Glucose infused (mg/h)	400	700	1,500	1,200

measured frequently and maintained between 50 and 90 mg/dL. Giving more glucose may cause hyperglycemia (Tables 20.8–20.10).

Additional fluid should consist of lactated Ringer's solution (without glucose), 5% albumin, blood or a combination of these. Intravenous alimentation fluid is *never* used to replace fluid losses during surgery because doing so causes severe hyperglycemia and possibly CNS damage. Instead, the anesthetist should infuse hyperalimentation fluids at their preoperative rate and provide additional fluid needs with plain lactated Ringer's solution. The blood glucose concentration can be determined during surgery with a glucometer and the infusion rates of dextrose altered as needed.

Adequate replacement of colloid and crystalloid is aided by measuring central venous pressure (CVP), mean arterial pressure (MAP), and urine output. Mean arterial blood pressure is a good indicator of intravascular volume. An arterial blood pressure that is two standard deviations below normal for that age group [121] indicates hypotension and suggests hypovolemia (Fig. 20.6). Infusing adequate fluid usually returns the blood pressure to normal. CVP is also a useful measurement of intravascular volume status. A CVP below 3 cmH$_2$O suggests hypovolemia.

Urine output is also a good indicator of intravascular volume. It should exceed 0.75 mL/kg/h. The urine specific gravity of normal neonates is usually less than 1.005 [122]. A urine specific gravity in excess of 1.009 usually indicates that the patient is conserving fluid (see above). If the skin over the fontanelle is below the inner table of the skull, and the baby is not crying, he is probably hypovolemic.

Body temperature is maintained between 36°C and 37°C to avoid postoperative hypoventilation, delayed awakening from anesthesia, atelectasis, respiratory and metabolic acidosis, infection, poor feeding, and aspiration of gastric contents. The body temperature is maintained in the normal range by warming the operating room and the inspired gases. Intravenous fluids and blood can be warmed using a conventional fluid warmer set to 38–41°C, and leaving only a short length of tubing to the patient's IV catheter, so that the fluid will not cool in a long length of tubing. The short segment of tubing must be visible so air bubbles can be detected and removed. Even small air bubbles (0.1 cc) can be lethal if they lodge in a coronary or cerebral artery

Table 20.9 Blood and urine glucose concentrations in term and preterm infants during surgery (% of patients)

Age	% of Patients by Urine* Results				% of Patients by Blood† Results (mg/dl)		
	Negative	*2+*	*3+*	*4+*	*45–90*	*130–175*	*≥250*
Preterm	50	20	15	15	40	50	10
Term	70	14	10	6	66	20	25

*Labstix.
†Dextrostix.

Table 20.10 Effects of adding glucose to intravenous fluid of infants and children during surgery

Age	Glucose Concentration (mg/dl)			
	Ringer's Lactate		*D-5 Ringer's Lactate*	
	Infants	*Children*	*Infants*	*Children*
Preoperative Anesthesia	78 ± 12	95 ± 13	76 ± 9	87 ± 13
20 min	88 ± 20	122 ± 17	143 ± 18	147 ± 38
60 min	78 ± 12	93 ± 18	201 ± 39	186 ± 37
120 min	81 ± 15	93 ± 12	213 ± 41	158 ± 32

*Glucose was added when the intravenous infusion was started in those receiving glucose. Infants were 1 week to I year of age. Children were 1 to 7 years of age.

because the foramen ovale is patent in most of these neonates.

Recovery from anesthesia

Emergence from anesthesia can be as dangerous as induction of anesthesia. There is often pressure to quickly remove the patient from the operating room so that the next case can start. This pressure must be resisted while careful preparations are made to transport the patient to the recovery area, usually the ICN. Before the patient leaves the operating room, it must be known that the ICN nurses are available and ready to receive and care for the patient. The ICN should be informed of the FiO_2, ventilator settings, body temperature, and planned postoperative pain therapy before the patient leaves the operating room. After transport to the ICN, a complete verbal exchange of information from the anesthesia team and surgeons to the ICN nursing and

physician team is important, to inform them of intraoperative events.

In most instances the lungs of preterm infants should be ventilated on the way to and in the ICN. It can then be decided whether mechanical ventilation is required postoperatively or not. Muscle relaxants must be reversed and adequate spontaneous ventilation established before an ETT is removed.

Many preterm infants who are less than 44 weeks' gestation develop postoperative apnea [123,124]. The incidence of apnea is related inversely to the gestational age at birth [125]. Although the cause of apnea is unknown, it may be due to persistence of small amounts of anesthetic in the CNS that affect the autonomic nervous system [126] or it might be related to an incompletely developed CNS [127]. Most postoperative apnea occurs during the first 4h after surgery but may occur 12 or more hours after surgery [128]. Patients who are <46 weeks' gestation are usually monitored for apnea and SaO_2 in hospital for 12–24h after surgery due to their high risk for apnea. Those with gestational ages of 47–60 weeks' gestation are evaluated carefully for 6h postoperatively. If there is no evidence of apnea, bradycardia or oxygen desaturation, they can be discharged home, all else being normal. Those older than 60 weeks' gestation can be treated as normal term infants and can be discharged home after surgery if there are no other problems. Infants who develop postoperative apnea may require mechanical ventilation for several hours to several days. This possibility usually precludes outpatient surgery for infants who are less than 50 weeks postconceptual age, although one study disputes this conclusion [129].

Welborn and associates found that ex-premature infants whose hematocrit was below 30% had an increased incidence of apnea [130]. Eighty-nine percent of the infants with low hematocrits were apneic after surgery while only 21% of those with a hematocrit of greater than 30% were apneic.

The same authors found less apnea in infants treated with spinal anesthesia than in those anesthetized with general anesthesia [131]. No instances of apnea occurred with spinal anesthesia unless the patients were also sedated. Eight of nine infants premedicated with ketamine had significant apnea while five of 16 had postoperative apnea if not given the drug. Although spinal anesthesia caused fewer instances of postoperative apnea [132], apnea and total spinal anesthesia have occurred [133,134]. Kunst et al found no difference in the rate of apnea in patients who received either form of anesthesia [135]. Patients undergoing general anesthesia were more likely to have oxygen desaturation and bradycardia than those undergoing spinal anesthetic. Tashiro and associates [136] found that gestational age, birthweight, postconceptual age, and use of aminophylline preoperatively were associated with a need for postoperative ventilation. Approximately one-third of the infants undergoing hernia repairs had postoperative apnea [137]. Welborn et al found that IV caffeine 5 mg/kg prevented life-threatening postoperative apnea and eliminated the need for mechanical ventilation [138]. It had no effect on lesser degrees of apnea. By delaying surgery until the patient is more than 44 weeks' postconceptual age, most postoperative apnea can be avoided. Patients who require surgery before 44 weeks' gestation should receive intravenous caffeine.

Anesthesia for micropremies

The marked improvement in the survival of very premature infants ("micropremies," i.e. 400–1000 g at birth) over the past few years has resulted in many surgeries before discharge from hospital. Some of these patients have poor neurological and developmental outcomes. Evidence suggests that only 67–71% of 24–25-week gestation infants are neurologically normal compared to 89% of those born at 26 weeks' gestation (Table 20.11). An additional 22% of 24-week gestation infants have neurological examinations that are suspicious for injury [139,140].

Only 28% of neonates born at 24 weeks' gestation have normal cognitive development at 4.5–7 years of age. Eleven percent of 24–27-week gestation infants had cerebral palsy. The outcome of small infants was significantly improved by delaying their birth until 26 weeks' gestation. Infants with CNS injuries are more likely to have hypotension and bradycardia with anesthesia.

The problems of micropremies are similar to those of larger premature infants, but worse. Because they are so immature, micropremies do not have true alveoli and the distance between their capillaries and their gas exchange units is greater, making oxygenation more difficult. The high surface/volume ratio and the thin fragile skin increase fluid loss and make it more difficult to maintain their body temperature. Removing tape or monitor pads often removes their skin and leaves large weeping abrasions.

To maintain hydration and prevent/treat hypotension, it is often necessary to administer very large volumes of fluid (often >200 mL/kg/day) and vasopressors. Failure to do so results in dehydration and hypotension. However, administering these volumes of fluid may cause a PDA, heart failure, and pulmonary edema.

The normal mean arterial blood pressure for infants of 24–26 weeks' gestation infants is debatable but is grossly the same as the gestational age. Blood pressures measured by non-invasive means are often higher than those measured intravascularly (Table 20.12). Consequently, micropremies may be hypotensive despite having non-invasive mean arterial blood pressures that would be considered normal for gestational age. Determining the state of hydration is more difficult in these patients because they have little or no subcutaneous tissue, their skin is paper thin, and their pulses are frequently difficult to feel. The skin over their fontanelles is level with the outer table of the skull. Their urine output is usually more than 1 mL/kg/h and the specific gravity <1.005.

The anesthesia requirement of micropremies is unknown. However, from previous data it appears that the MAC for halothane is less than 0.55. The dose of sevoflurane is about 60% of that of term infants. Opioids in adequate doses provide anesthesia for these infants; their arterial pressures are more stable than during

Table 20.11 Neurological and developmental outcome of micropremies

	24 Weeks	25 Weeks	26 Weeks
No. of infants followed	18	30	38
Neurologically normal	12 (67%)	22 (73%)	34 (89%)
Neurologically suspicious	4 (22%)	2 (7%)	0
Cerebral palsy	2 (11%)	6 (20%)	4 (11%)
Normal cognitive development	5 (28%)	14 (47%)	27 (71%)
Borderline cognitive development	6 (33%)	7 (23%)	7 (18%)
Deficient cognitive development	7 (39%)	9 (30%)	4 (11%)

*Data are presented as n (%).
†Kruskal-Wallis $\chi^2 = 10.6542$, $p = 0.005$ for cognitive outcome and gestational age.
Reproduced from Piecuch et al [140], with permission from Lippincott, Williams & Wilkins.

Table 20.12 Arterial blood pressures determined non-invasively and from an indwelling arterial catheter: comparison of cuff and intra-arterial pressures

Method	N	MAP	Systolic/diastolic
Cuff	15	32 ± 5	46 ± 5/22 ± 3
Line	15	26 ± 6	38 ± 4/15 ± 3

Table 20.13 Vital signs during fentanyl and halothane anesthesia (23–26 weeks' gestation)

	Halothane				Fentanyl		
	HR	*MAP*	*CVP*		*HR*	*MAP*	*CVP*
Awake	148 ± 17	31 ± 3	4 ± 1	Awake	152 ± 17	31 ± 3	4 ± 1
0.5 MAC	138 ± 26	28 ± 4	5 ± 1	10 µg/kg	148 ± 26	30 ± 4	4 ± 1
1.0	130 ± 28	27 ± 3	5 ± 2	30 µg/kg	147 ± 13	30 ± 3	3 ± 1

inhaled anesthesia (Table 20.13). Since these children are often mechanically ventilated after surgery, muscle paralysis with pancuronium 0.1 mg/kg and anesthesia with fentanyl 10–50 µg/kg provides adequate conditions for any surgery. Although small premature infants have cerebrovascular autoregulation, it is very fragile and easily disrupted. This increases the likelihood of intracranial hemorrhage and central nervous system injury if the anesthesia is inadequate.

Micropremies have high fluid requirements during surgery. Failure to provide the required amount of fluid results in hypotension and/or shock. All fluid should be administered via calibrated pumps when possible to avoid excess fluid administration.

Where should the surgery for micropremies be performed? Many institutions do it in the NICU because it is easier to take nurses, doctors, and technicians to the NICU than it is to take the patients to the operating room. The infection rate is no different whether the patient undergoes surgery in the ICN or the operating room.

Common surgical problems of micropremies are described elsewhere in this book. Patent ductus arteriosus is covered in Chapter 25, thoracotomy for pulmonary resection in Chapter 24, hydrocephalus in Chapter 23, and necrotizing enterocolitis and inguinal hernia in Chapter 28. The following is a case study that illustrates and integrates many of the points discussed above.

CASE STUDY

The infant was 5 days old at the time we were asked to evaluate him for anesthesia and surgery for NEC. He was born after 29 weeks' gestation and weighed 980 g at birth. On the day of surgery his weight was 840 g, a 15% weight loss from birth. He was severely asphyxiated at birth and required immediate tracheal intubation and assisted ventilation.

His initial blood gas values were pH 7.00, PaCO$_2$ 63 mmHg, and PaO$_2$ 43 mmHg (SaO$_2$ 91%) despite ventilation with 100% oxygen. His mean arterial blood pressure was 16 mmHg at 5 min of age. Ventilation was continued, and 10 mL of whole blood were administered over 5 min, which brought his mean arterial blood pressure to 28 mmHg. His blood gases improved following the transfusion. By 25 min of age the PaO$_2$ was 165 mmHg (SaO$_2$ 100%), the PaCO$_2$ 33 mmHg, and the pH 7.34. He was transferred to the NICU after the PaO$_2$ had been reduced to 63 mmHg (SaO$_2$ 97%) by progressively decreasing the FiO$_2$ to 0.67. A chest radiograph demonstrated classic RDS.

During the next 4 days, the RDS improved and the NICU staff reduced the level of assisted ventilation. On day 1 he received 5% dextrose in water, equal to 50 mL/kg/day, plus electrolytes. This rate was increased to 70 mL/kg/day thereafter. He was covered with clear plastic film to reduce evaporative heat loss. The baby was started on ampicillin and gentamicin shortly after birth because it was uncertain if sepsis was present. When the blood, urine, and CSF cultures failed to demonstrate bacteria on day 3, the antibiotics were discontinued. The initial hemoglobin value was 12.5 g/dL. Because of blood sampling, the hemoglobin concentration decreased to 9.5 g/dL. He was transfused to increase it to 11.2 g/dL on the third day of extrauterine life.

On day 5, the infant developed abdominal distension, vomiting, and bloody stools following attempts to feed him with breast milk. His respiratory distress, which had been improving, now worsened. He required higher ventilator rates and pressures and a higher FiO$_2$. An abdominal radiograph showed free air in the peritoneal cavity and a diagnosis of necrotizing enterocolitis was made. At this point, he was scheduled for surgery.

A review of the records and his physical examination demonstrated the following.

Hydration

His skin was pale and mottled and failed to return to its resting position for 8 sec after being tented up. The fontanelle was sunken below the inner table of his skull. It took more than 6 sec for the skin of his fingers and toes to fill with blood after they were blanched. His extremities were cold from the groins and axillae outward. There were no pulses in his feet or wrists and his groin pulses were markedly diminished. The pulse rate was 150 beats per minute (bpm) and the arterial pressure 40/15 mmHg, with a mean pressure of 23 mmHg. There had been no urine output for 6 h and only 2 mL of urine during the 4 h previous to that. The urine specific gravity of his last sample was 1.028.

Chest findings

He had bilateral rales that did not clear when the ETT was suctioned. Air entry into the upper lobes of the lungs was appropriate but was decreased in the bases. An ETT was in place in the mid-trachea and was fixed securely. The PaO_2 was 72 mmHg (SaO_2 98%), the $PaCO_2$ 30 mmHg, and the pH 7.21. His base deficit was −15 mEq/L. He was ventilated 20 times per minute with peak pressures of 30 cmH$_2$O, and PEEP of 5 cmH$_2$O.

Cardiovascular findings

His heart rate was normal (150 bpm) and there was no murmur or gallop. The point of maximal cardiac impulse was in the fourth interspace anteriorly. His pulses were as above.

Abdominal findings

His abdomen was grossly distended. Loops of bowel were visible through the anterior abdominal wall, which was edematous, warm, and tender. Bowel sounds were absent. The liver was not palpable, but it could be percussed 1 cm below the right costal margin.

Laboratory data

His WBC count was 29,300/mm^3 with a shift to the left. Fifteen percent of these cells were bands. His hemoglobin was 14.5 g/dL. His electrolytes showed a sodium concentration of 147 mEq/L, potassium 5.3 mEq/L, chloride 120 mEq/L, and bicarbonate 17 mEq/L. His serum calcium concentration was 6.3 mg/dL and his ionized calcium was 1.0 mmol/L. The total protein concentration was 4.5 mg/dL.

Discussions with the nurses indicated that the infant would become severely cyanotic and his SaO_2 would abruptly decline to 80–88% when the ETT was disconnected for tracheal suctioning. They also pointed out that his body temperature was labile and that he required increasing amounts of exogenous heat to maintain his body temperature in the normal range.

Preoperative preparation

On the basis of the above information, it was clear that the infant was severely intravascular volume depleted, although his bodyweight had not changed over the past

12 h. His peripheral perfusion and arterial blood pressure were decreased. The lack of urine output for 6 h indicated not only that the intravascular volume was decreased but also that he had more than a 70% chance of becoming hypotensive with the induction of anesthesia. The rise in his hemoglobin concentration also indicated intravascular volume depletion. A central venous line was inserted with local anesthesia and was connected to a pressure transducer. The CVP was 0 cmH$_2$O. Lactated Ringer's solution 10 mL/kg was infused over 15 min which increased his CVP to 2 cmH$_2$O. Additional lactated Ringer's solution 10 mL/kg raised the CVP to 5 cmH$_2$O. With this increase, the peripheral perfusion improved and the mean arterial pressure rose to 32 mmHg. His urine output increased to 2 mL/kg/h, and the urine specific gravity decreased to 1.006. He needed less mechanical ventilation because the PaO_2 rose to 123 mmHg (SaO_2 100%) and the $PaCO_2$ decreased to 18 mmHg. His base deficit rose to −5 meq/L without infusing sodium bicarbonate. His blood glucose concentration was now 128 mg/dL. Calcium gluconate 150 mg/kg was administered to treat the hypocalcemia. Repeat electrolyte determinations showed a calcium concentration of 8.1 mg/dL and ionized calcium of 1.02 mmol/L, a sodium concentration of 140 mEq/L, a potassium concentration of 4.5 mEq/L, and a chloride concentration of 115 mEq/L. His hemoglobin concentration had decreased to 11.0 g/dL after rehydration.

After 90 min of preparation, the patient was transported to the operating room while being manually ventilated at the same pressures, rates, and inspired oxygen concentration used in the nursery.

Surgery

The patient was anesthetized and operated on in his intensive care bed. Anesthesia was induced with fentanyl 20 μg/kg, and he was paralyzed with pancuronium 0.1 mg/kg. Surgery began within 5 min of his arrival in the operating room. The inspired oxygen was maintained at a level that kept the PaO_2 between 50 and 70 mmHg (SaO_2 91–96%) by using air as the carrier gas and adding oxygen as needed. Oxygen saturation was measured continuously with a pulse oximeter, and the blood gases and pH were measured intermittently, as was the serum glucose. The total calcium concentration was determined once during the 2-h procedure and was found to be 6.9 mg/dL. The concentration of ionized calcium was 1.01 mmol/L. Calcium gluconate 20 mg was given slowly through the central venous line. A blood loss of 15 mL was replaced with packed RBCs, bringing the hemoglobin to 15 g/dL. His IV fluids included 5% dextrose in lactated Ringer's solution 4 mL/h and lactated Ringer's solution without glucose 6 mL/h, which maintained the blood glucose concentration and the arterial and central venous pressures within normal limits. The bowel

Continued

was resected and an end-to-end anastomosis performed in addition to a diverting colostomy.

His body temperature was maintained within normal limits by wrapping the extremities with sheet wadding, covering his head with a cap, placing a warming pad under him, warming and humidifying the inspired gases to 37°C, warming the infused fluids, and placing him on a forced air warming blanket. At the end of the procedure he was covered with warm blankets and clear plastic film. His ventilation was controlled during transport to the NICU. Mechanical ventilation and paralysis were continued in the postoperative period. Once we were sure that the vital signs and ventilation were adequate, his care was transferred to the NICU staff after a complete report of intraoperative events.

His condition continued to improve over the next week, and he was weaned from mechanical ventilation and fed intravenously through the central venous line. He was discharged from the hospital at 2 months of age neurologically intact and eating well. At 4 months of age, his colostomy was closed, and he has done well since.

Conclusion

This case illustrates how severely dehydrated such premature patients can be and how well they respond to fluid replacement. It also shows how stable they can become once the deficits are replaced.

Annotated references

A full reference list for this chapter is available at:
http://www.wiley.com/go/gregory/andropoulos/pediatricanesthesia

1. Locatelli A, Roncaglia N, Andreoti C et al. Factors affecting survival in infants weighing 750g or less. Eur J Obstet Gynecol Reprod Biol 2005; 123: 52–5. This paper provides a good understanding of what factors affect the survival and outcome of the micropremies who constitute an increasing amount of anesthesia practice.

8. Morley CJ, Davis PG, Doyle LW et al. Nasal CPAP or intubation at birth for very preterm infants. N Engl J Med 2008; 358: 700–8. This paper provides information on the effect of CPAP applied in the delivery room needed to understand the ventilatory care provided to many micropremies.

21. McCall EM, Alderice F, Halliday HL et al. Interventions to prevent hypothermia at birth in preterm and/or low birth-weight infants (review). Cochrane Database Syst Rev 2010; 17: CD004210. This is an excellent review of thermoregulation in preterm infants. Many useful references are provided.

23. Jobe AH. Lung maturation: the survival miracle of very low birth weight infants. Pediatr Neonatol 2010; 51: 7–13. An excellent primer on lung development (or lack thereof) in micropremies.

26. Eichenwald EC, Stark AR. Management and outcomes of very low birth weight. N Engl J Med 2008; 358: 1700–11. A thorough review of care for low birthweight infants.

34. Bancalri E, Claure N, Sosenko IRS. Bronchopulmonary dysplasia: changes in pathogenesis, epidemiology and definition. Semin Neonatol 2003; 8: 63–71. This is a clear description of the "new BPD" and is the first description of the problems we see today with small preterm infants.

36. Jacob SV, Lands LC, Coates AL et al. Exercise ability in survivors of severe bronchopulmonary dysplasia. Am J Respir Crit Care Med

1997; 155: 1925–9. This paper provides useful information on the respiratory and cardiovascular outcome of premature infants.

40. Walther-Larsen S, Rasmusen LS. The former preterm infant and risk of post-operative apnoea: recommendations for management. Acta Anaesthesiol Scand 2006; 50: 888–93. This is a good description of the incidence of postoperative apnea in ex-preterm infants.

42. Bjorklund U, Ingimarsson J, Curstedt T et al. Manual ventilation with a few large breaths at birth compromises the therapeutic effect of subsequent surfactant replacement in immature lambs. Pediatr Res 1997; 42: 348–55. This is one of the most important papers published in neonatology in the past 20 years. It points out the effects of excessive tidal volumes on lung injury. This could also occur when the lungs are overexpanded in the operating room.

44. Clyman RI. Patent ductus arteriosus in the preterm. In: Taeusch HW, Ballard R, Gleason C (eds) Avery's Diseases of the Newborn, 6th edn. Philadelphia: Elsevier-Saunders, 2000. This is a very clear description of PDA by one of the experts in the field. The physiology and pharmacology are well explained.

76. Gole GA, Ellis AL, Katz X et al. The international classification of retinopathy of prematurity revisited: International Committee for the Classification of Retinopathy of Prematurity. Arch Opthamol 2005; 123: 991–9. This paper describes the classification of ROP and its causes.

109. Anand KJS, Sippell WG, Aynsley-Green A. Randomized trial of fentanyl anaesthesia in preterm babies undergoing surgery: effects on the stress response. Lancet 1987; 1(8524): 62–6. This is the first paper to define the chemical and physiological changes associated with inadequate anesthesia in preterm infants.

CHAPTER 21

Anesthesia for the Full-Term and Ex-Premature Infant

Neil S. Morton, Ross Fairgrieve, Anthony Moores & Ewan Wallace
Department of Anaesthesia, Royal Hospital for Sick Children, Glasgow, Scotland, UK

Introduction

More premature babies are surviving and presenting for surgery in early life with residual effects of prematurity, complications of prematurity and neonatal intensive care and co-morbidities. The risk of perioperative apnea has been elucidated and anesthetic techniques with modern volatile agents or using awake regional anesthesia have been developed to try to minimize this risk, particularly for inguinal hernia repair. For more major congenital abnormalities such as tracheo-esophageal fistula (TEF), abdominal wall defects and congenital diaphragmatic hernia, the principles of neonatal anesthesia are described in general, with particular refinements of technique for each of these major lesions described in detail. The dilemma for the anesthesiologist of having to provide anesthesia for a muscle biopsy in an infant is also discussed. The current neonatal resuscitation algorithm is discussed with information from recent trials of techniques aimed at trying to improve outcomes.

Residua and complications of prematurity

With advances in obstetric and neonatal care, a higher proportion of premature babies are surviving and presenting for anesthesia and surgery in early life [1–3]. Often the survivors have one or more residua of prematurity (Box 21.1) or complications of prematurity or neonatal intensive care unit (NICU) management. The incidence and severity of disabilities tend to be in

Box 21.1 Residua or complications of prematurity in the young infant of importance to the pediatric anesthesiologist

- Chronic lung disease
- Airway problems
- Apnea
- Cerebral damage
- Eye problems
- Anemia
- Patent ductus arteriosus (PDA)
- Difficult vascular access
- Altered pain threshold

proportion to the degree of prematurity and length of NICU stay [2,4].

Chronic lung disease

Significant chronic lung disease, or bronchopulmonary dysplasia (BPD), persists in up to 10% of ex-premature infants. The severity and incidence have been ameliorated by antenatal maternal steroid therapy, exogenous surfactant treatment, new ventilatory support strategies to minimize barotrauma and volutrauma and improved monitoring to prevent oxygen toxicity (see Chapter 20). However, because a higher proportion of premature babies are surviving, the number of babies presenting for surgery and anesthesia with some degree of lung disease has tended to increase over the last 10 years.

The mechanisms leading to chronic lung disease are detailed in Chapter 20 but a useful clinical classification of severity of BPD [5] highlights for the anesthesiologist those at particular risk of perioperative pulmonary complications such as pneumothorax, interstitial emphysema, bronchospasm, hypoxemia and pulmonary hypertension. For babies born at less than 32 weeks' gestational age who are assessed at hospital discharge or 36 weeks' postconceptional age as having needed supplemental oxygen for at least 28 days, the severity of BPD is *mild* if the baby is now breathing room air, *moderate* if the baby is now needing less than 30% oxygen and *severe* if the baby now needs 30% oxygen or more and/or positive pressure ventilation or nasal continuous positive airway pressure (CPAP) [5]. To minimize perioperative deterioration in lung function, strategies for the anesthesiologist include use of awake regional anesthesia techniques where feasible (see below) or, for those who need general anesthesia, tracheal intubation with controlled ventilation is usually recommended with administration of the minimum effective inspired oxygen concentration to maintain arterial oxyhemoglobin saturation between 92% and 96%, use of minimum effective peak inspiratory pressures, application of low levels of positive end-expiratory pressure

(PEEP) to minimize airway collapse, permissive hypercapnia and relatively slow ventilatory frequency with shorter inspiratory:expiratory (I:E) ratio to minimize gas trapping and overinflation of lung segments. Bronchodilator medication should be continued on the day of surgery and postoperatively. For severe BPD cases, elective postoperative ventilatory support may well be required, although with good regional analgesia, early extubation may be possible for certain operative procedures.

Airway problems

Subglottic stenosis, tracheal stenosis, tracheomalacia and bronchomalacia may occur in up to 10% of ex-premature babies.

Subglottic stenosis at the level of the cricoid ring is most often due to repeated tracheal intubation, use of too large a tracheal tube or where tracheal intubation has been needed for a very long time. It may also be associated with gastro-esophageal reflux with repeated spillover of acid or bile into the airway. It may well be that in an infant presenting for elective surgery, consideration should be given to therapy for the subglottic stenosis as a higher priority, depending on its severity, but this decision requires careful discussion. Where anesthesia has to be given, a much smaller tracheal tube diameter than expected may be required and elective steroid therapy given prior to extubation to minimize mucosal edema.

Tracheomalacia may be primary or secondary to extrinsic compression (e.g. vascular ring) or prolonged positive pressure ventilation. The tracheal cartilages may be underdeveloped and the membranous part of the trachea posteriorly may be widened. Tracheal collapse typically occurs on expiration, giving expiratory stridor, a seal-like cough and expiratory wheeze. A similar pattern may be seen with *bronchomalacia* which may be primary or secondary to extrinsic compression, for example from a large pulmonary artery or left atrium. Bronchomalacia may lead to unilateral lung collapse or hyperinflation. Care must be exercised on starting positive pressure ventilation to ensure sufficient end-expiratory pressure to splint the collapsible large airways open on expiration to avoid stacking of breaths and gross hyperinflation of the lung. On extubation of the trachea, babies with tracheobronchomalacia benefit from postextubation CPAP or bilevel positive airway pressure (BiPAP) to minimize postoperative lung collapse and respiratory failure.

Apnea

The mechanisms of apnea in the premature and ex-premature infant are described in detail in Chapter 20. Apnea has been recognized as an issue for such babies for over 40 years [6] and soon after this was reported, the use of xanthine derivatives such as aminophylline [7] or theophylline [8,9] and their active metabolite caffeine [8–14] as therapy was elucidated. Anesthesiologists became aware of this work when the problem of postoperative apnea was highlighted by landmark reports during the 1980s [15–20] and key dose-finding studies of caffeine as prophylaxis [21,22]. Around this time, there was also interest in the use of "awake" regional anesthesia as an alternative to general anesthesia for such cases, particularly for inguinal surgery (see below). Comparative trials of general with regional anesthesia were undertaken (see below) and risk factors for postoperative apnea were further elucidated [23–28], most notably in a combined analysis by Coté et al [29]. This made clear that the main risk factors are young postconceptual age, anemia (hematocrit <30%) and nature of the surgery [29]. The importance of this analysis for clinical practice has been immeasurable in helping clarify risks for all ex-premature infants up to 60 weeks' postconceptual age, allowing guidance for monitoring and postoperative care to be developed and helping decision making about day care and time of discharge [29].

In summary, the risk/benefit ratio suggests a default position of considering admission for monitoring of all ex-premature infants who are younger than 60 weeks' postconceptual age as the postoperative apnea risk is around 1 in 200 for non-anemic infants who have not exhibited apnea in the postanesthesia care unit (PACU) until around 55 weeks postconceptional age (PCA) (Fig. 21.1).

For those with co-morbidities, those for more major surgery, who are anemic with hematocrit <30% or who become apneic in the PACU, admission for at least 12h after the last apneic episode, and caffeine 10 mg/kg intravenously are recommended [30,31]. These guidelines apply whatever anesthetic technique has been used, including awake regional anesthesia, although some authors have questioned this recently based on their own local expert practice [32,33] (see below). There have been reports of postoperative apnea in full-term neonates [34–37] and it is prudent therefore to admit and monitor full-term infants of less than 44 weeks PCA who show any respiratory abnormality during recovery from anesthesia for monitoring for at least 12 apnea-free hours.

Cerebral damage

Residual cerebral damage may occur from birth asphyxia, intraventicular hemorrhage, periventricular leukomalacia, hydrocephalus or seizures. The mechanisms of cerebral damage are detailed in Chapter 20. The clinical effects are manifest as cerebral palsy, cognitive and behavioral deficits, hearing loss and visual impairment. Longer term follow-up published in 2005 showed that around 1 in 5 very premature babies had severe disabilities at age 5 years and only 1 in 4 exhibited normal development [38]. More recent analyses [39] suggest that some centers are

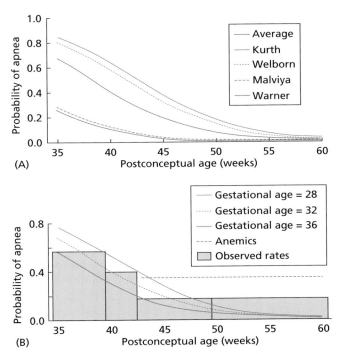

Figure 21.1 (A) Postoperative apnea risk showing variation among centers. (B) Postoperative apnea risk by gestational age and postconceptual age and influence of apnea. Reproduced from Coté et al [29] with permission from Lippincott Williams and Wilkins.

achieving much lower prevalence rates of cerebral palsy (as low as 1.9% in very preterm infants born at 20–27 weeks' gestation) and rates of hearing and vision loss as low as 1% [39].

The anesthesiologist should make a detailed preoperative assessment of residual neurological impairment and document this baseline carefully, noting the pathology underlying the deficit, presence of hydrocephalus and/or a ventriculoperitoneal shunt, seizures and their pattern and frequency, and antiseizure medication. These findings may affect choice of anesthetic agent and technique, use of central regional blockade, need for perioperative antibiotics and decisions about early extubation or elective postoperative ventilatory support. The documentation is also important from a medico-legal perspective to minimize the risk of subsequently being accused of causing neurological damage by anesthetic agents, techniques or procedures. Anesthetic goals should be to maintain a normal range of blood pressure, carbon dioxide levels and arterial oxyhemoglobin saturation in the range 92–96% and in particular to minimize episodes of fluctuation above and below these norms for age.

Eye problems

The mechanisms of retinopathy of prematurity (ROP) are described in Chapter 20. Residual eye problems occur in up to 50% of ex-premature babies [40] and the anesthesiologist needs to be aware of the importance of avoiding hypoxia and hyperoxia and thereby potentially exacerbating the retinal damage. Thus titrating oxygen delivery to maintain stable arterial oxyhemoglobin saturation values of 92–96% and avoiding major fluctuations is recommended [41].

Anemia

The full-term neonate usually has a high hematocrit of 45–55%, depending on the degree of placental autotransfusion at delivery, and this level starts to fall within the first week of life. In response to increased oxygen saturation after birth, the levels of erythropoietin decrease and so replacement of short half-life red blood cells containing fetal hemoglobin with longer half-life cells containing adult hemoglobin is delayed. This results in a low point of hematocrit of 24–30% at around 2–3 months of age. In the premature baby, this low point of hematocrit often occurs earlier (1–2 months of age) and is more profound (21–27%) due to repeated blood sampling and nutritional deficiencies of iron, folic acid and vitamin E. Many neonatal intensive care units (NICU) aim to maintain the hematocrit in the range 36–45%, especially in the sickest infants with severe lung disease, low arterial oxyhemoglobin saturations and low cardiac output states.

A study of preterm babies weighing between 500 and 1300 g showed that restricting blood transfusion resulted in more medical complications (brain hemorrhage, periventricular leukomalacia and apnea) [42]. Use of exogenous erythropoietin as therapy to increase hematocrit levels in the NICU showed initial promise but resulted in an increased incidence of retinopathy of prematurity, although this only occurs when very large doses of erythropoietin are given [43]. For anesthesia, it is important to optimize oxygen delivery. Transfusion with blood containing adult hemoglobin, which releases oxygen to tissues more readily, may be required. There is an important association between the incidence and severity of perioperative apnea and anemia (see above) [24,29]. For individual cases, transfusion triggers will depend on the starting hematocrit, the likelihood of blood losses, the risk of apnea and the presence and severity of co-morbidities such as BPD and cardiac disease [44].

Patent ductus arteriosus

Patent ductus arteriosus (PDA) is common amongst ex-premature babies and the prevalence has increased with improved survival rates and as a concurrent effect of exogenous surfactant therapy. PDA may still be present when an ex-premature baby presents for other surgery, especially emergency surgery. For elective surgery, consideration should be given to closure of the duct first either by medical therapy (e.g. with indometacin or ibu-

profen [45]), transcatheter device closure, thoracoscopic duct ligation/clipping or open duct ligation/clipping, as appropriate. The presence of a PDA adds risks because of left-to-right shunting with increased lung water, decreased lung compliance, pulmonary hypertension, congestive heart failure, potential for shunt reversal and increased risk of hypotension, especially diastolic hypotension due to excessive run-off into the pulmonary circuit. Coronary arterial hypoperfusion with myocardial ischemia can occur. The low diastolic blood pressure can also result in splanchnic hypoperfusion. Cardiac output reserves are also diminished for the ill baby, for example with necrotizing enterocolitis or if bleeding occurs during surgery, and severe hypotension may occur in such cases.

Difficult vascular access

Ex-premature infants may present serious difficulties with peripheral and central venous access and sometimes also arterial access, particularly if they have had a long and complicated NICU stay. Peripheral veins may have been used repeatedly for blood sampling or cannulated for intravenous fluid and drug administration or for central venous access using a peripherally inserted central catheter (PICC). Central veins may have become thrombosed and this often induces collateral venous channels to expand, which can be very difficult to cannulate, catheterize and sustain.

Altered pain perception and responses and tolerance to analgesics and sedatives

Most premature babies are exposed to multiple painful procedures in early life and these can alter sensory perception, including that for pain, and also induce long-term changes in sensory responses and behavior [46–54]. This can manifest clinically as increased sensitivity to pain [46] and increased analgesic requirements or, alternatively, reduced sensitivity to pain [54] so for the anesthesiologist, this emphasizes the importance of individualizing pain assessment and management. In addition, premature babies may have had considerable exposure to sedative and analgesic drugs during their NICU stay and may have developed tolerance with important effects on their individual dose requirements [55–58].

Operating room environment for the neonate

The operating room (OR) environment for the neonate must carry a range of appropriate equipment drugs and fluids and must have appropriate means of maintaining the baby's temperature to minimize heat losses to the environment. The ambient room temperature should be increased to around 23–25°C (80–85°F), anesthetic inspired gases should be warmed and humidified, IV fluids should be delivered via a warming device and a forced warm air delivery device and/or warming blanket used. The exposure of the baby to the ambient environment should be minimized to avoid heat losses.

For awake regional anesthesia, the ambient light level should be lowered and monitor alarm volumes reduced to a minimum. Monitoring equipment should comply with current standards and include electrocardiogram (ECG), stethoscope, arterial blood pressure (BP), temperature, pulse oximetry, anesthetic agent monitor and capnography. Appropriate sizes of pulse oximeter probes and provision to monitor pre- and postductal saturations should be available. The anesthetic machine should be able to deliver air and oxygen to allow titration of inspired oxygen to avoid hypoxia or hyperoxia and should have a ventilator capable of supporting small infants, including delivery of PEEP if needed. Many pediatric anesthesiologists prefer non-rebreathing circuits but circle systems are now being used more widely. Technological advances allow improved gas monitoring, including accurate tidal volume and pressure measurement, which can be very helpful. Invasive pressure monitoring should be readily available. A full range of airway equipment appropriate for small infants must be immediately available including facemasks, oral airways, laryngeal mask airways (LMAs), suction catheters, stylets, tracheal tubes and laryngoscope blades. A full range of anesthetic, analgesic, muscle relaxant and resuscitation drugs and IV fluids (including dextrose 10%) should be immediately available. Peripheral and central venous cannulas of appropriate size and length should be immediately to hand and small size intraosseous needles also. Many ORs will construct a neonatal cart which is checked regularly to ensure all equipment is present in case of an emergency. Where difficult intubation is anticipated, an appropriate sized fiberoptic bronchoscope, videolaryngoscope, and intubation aids such as guidewires and airway exchange catheters should be available.

Postoperative extubation versus postoperative ventilation

For the neonate undergoing surgery under endotracheal general anesthesia, the question of whether to extubate or not at the end of surgery is a common dilemma. For some infants with major co-morbidity undergoing major surgery, the decision may be clear but for others it may be more difficult. Newborn and ex-premature infants differ physiologically from older children with regard to certain aspects of their respiratory physiology and this has some bearing on the decision (see Chapter 20). Minute ventilation and therefore the relative work of breathing

in the neonate is 3–4 times greater than in adults because of much higher oxygen consumption [59]. During normal tidal ventilation, neonatal lungs are close to closing volume [60]. This means more rapid desaturation during apneic episodes. Furthermore, respiratory control mechanisms are not fully mature and hypoxia can result in short periods of hyperventilation followed by apnea [61]. An immature respiratory center is also sensitive to the effects of volatile anesthetics, sedative and opioid drugs. These factors mean that for all but the shortest and non-stimulating procedures, tracheal intubation and controlled ventilation are appropriate.

In general, the attainment of normal physiological parameters is a prerequisite prior to extubation of the ex-premature or term neonate following general anesthesia. The infant should be awake and able to flex the hips and lift the arms. Muscle relaxation should be fully reversed and there should be a regular respiratory pattern with adequate minute ventilation and a satisfactory $PaCO_2$. The infant should also be normothermic as the consequences of hypothermia include delayed drug metabolism, hypoxia and apnea (see above) [6]. Apnea risk is a particularly important factor in those <44 weeks PCA [28] with a lesser but not insignificant risk in those infants born at less than 37 weeks where the risk persists until 60 weeks PCA [29]. Prophylactic respiratory stimulants such as caffeine or theophylline are highly recommended in these groups, particularly if early extubation is being considered [30,31,62]. Anemia in the immediate postoperative period should be corrected as a hemoglobin level of <10 g/dL has also been shown to significantly increase the risk of postoperative apneic episodes [24].

Opioid administration is a factor which must also be considered. The less well-developed neonatal blood–brain barrier allows greater penetration of opioids into the cerebrospinal fluid in the newborn [63]. Moreover, an immature respiratory center is more sensitive to the respiratory depressant effects of opioid drugs [64]. The use of shorter acting opioids such as alfentanil or remifentanil may facilitate extubation but transition to ongoing analgesia can be difficult to manage. Care must be exercised, however, with the use of morphine which has a much longer half-life and its active metabolite morphine-6-glucuronide is excreted renally. Immature renal tubular function in the term and ex-premature infant therefore means that there is reduced clearance of morphine, thus prolonging its effect. For the neonate undergoing surgery, intubation and postoperative ventilation may be mandatory, for example in the case of repair of congenital diaphragmatic hernia or in long-gap esophageal atresia (EA). Significant hypothermia, hypoglycemia, hypocalcemia or other uncorrected biochemical abnormalities are also indications for postoperative ventilation. Similarly, there is rarely reason to consider extubation in the syndromic infant or in the case of major thoracic, abdominal or airway surgery. However, early extubation, either in the operating room or within 3h, has found feasibility in some neonates undergoing cardiac surgery [65]. The advantages are thought to be reduced postoperative complications, a shorter hospital stay and reduced costs. This is only achievable in some centers and with a dedicated and highly involved multidisciplinary team approach.

For infants undergoing some abdominal or thoracic procedures, the choice of anesthetic technique can influence the decision to extubate post procedure. Desflurane, with its low blood/gas and tissues/gas solubility coefficients, has a very rapid offset and while it may be irritant and unsuitable for spontaneous ventilation, it is a very useful agent in the ventilated neonate and is the volatile agent of choice when extubation is required. The addition of local anesthetic techniques to supplement general anesthesia may reduce or eliminate the need for opioids. Inguinal hernia repair, for example, can be achieved easily without opioids by either supplemental ilioinguinal nerve blockade or caudal epidural anesthesia. Epidural techniques (see Chapter 18) are appropriate in many scenarios and often allow a reduction in opioid administration. Caudally sited epidural anesthesia is a straightforward procedure and is useful for both abdominal and thoracic surgery, depending on level. In esophageal atresia repair, it has been shown to reduce the need for postoperative ventilatory support [66].

Because of their size and relative physiological immaturity, neonates and ex-premature infants require careful consideration for postoperative extubation. They are sensitive to many environmental, physiological and pharmacological factors and before the decision to extubate is taken, the anesthesiologist must take all these factors into account.

Inguinal hernia

Inguinal hernias are frequently found in up to one-third of ex-premature neonates [67] and it is recommended that they are repaired surgically in early life because of the risks of incarceration of bowel in the hernia sac (bowel obstruction, bowel infarction) and the risk of testicular infarction. The need for early surgery has to be balanced against the risks of anesthesia, perioperative apnea and medical co-morbidities, including the residual effects of prematurity (see above). The optimal timing of surgery [68] has to be decided on an individual case basis but some need urgent repair, particularly irreducible hernias, those associated with frank signs of bowel obstruction or very large hernias where the testicular blood supply may be compressed or compromised. The decision-making process has been affected by recent concerns about devel-

opmental neurotoxicity of general anesthetic and sedative agents [69–71]. This has led to renewed interest in awake regional anesthesia techniques [72–87]. A large multicenter comparative trial of neurodevelopmental outcome after regional or general anesthesia is in process (GAS study) [69]. Some units now favor delaying repair but the risks of leaving hernias unrepaired are significant in an already vulnerable population [68]. Surgical techniques and attitudes to prophylactic repair of the contralateral side are evolving with the advent of laparoscopy [88,89]. Many centers now undertake these procedures entirely laparoscopically, while others use the technology to inspect the contralateral side. Open repair is still widely practiced and gives good results.

All surgical repair techniques have complications (infection, bleeding, testicular infarction, bowel perforation, hernia recurrence) and opinion is still divided as to whether open surgery or laparoscopy has a lower incidence of these various problems [89]. Often the hernia repair is scheduled towards the end of the baby's hospital stay prior to discharge home from the NICU or specialist children's center, although some babies go home first and are then readmitted at a slightly later stage if the hernias are deemed to be low risk.

The baby should be assessed for residual effects or complications of prematurity or NICU care as noted above and in particular assessed for the known risk factors related to PCA, anemia, co-morbidities [29] and nature of the hernia (elective, emergency, unilateral, bilateral, very large, incarcerated or complex) and surgical technique (open, laparoscopic, open with contralateral inspection) [89]. Whichever anesthetic technique is used, general anesthesia or awake regional anesthesia, the guidance above about monitoring and aftercare should be used. Consider the use of caffeine 10mg/kg IV if the baby is not already receiving it. The choice of anesthetic technique should be discussed in detail with the surgical team and with the parents and informed consent obtained.

Anesthetic and analgesic techniques

There are two main groups of techniques, both with a considerable evidence base behind them, namely awake regional anesthesia and general endotracheal anesthesia (usually with a regional analgesic component).

Awake regional anesthesia

This may be provided by a single-shot spinal (subarachnoid) injection of local anesthetic [32,72–76,83,84,87,90–101], a single-shot caudal (epidural) injection of local anesthetic [20,76,77,84,87,102,103], a combination of these (see Case Study below) or a catheter-based caudal anesthetic (single or multiple shots and/or continuous infusion of local anesthetic) [79,80]. Plain local anesthetic solutions are preferred for ex-premature and term

Table 21.1 Recommended doses of local anesthetic agents for awake regional anesthesia for inguinal hernia repair in neonates

Local anesthetic	Concentration	Dose (mg/kg)	Reference
Spinal anesthesia			
Tetracaine	10 mg/mL hyperbaric	1	[93]
Bupivacaine	5 mg/mL hyperbaric	0.3	[75]
Bupivacaine	5 mg/mL isobaric	1	[109]
Levobupivacaine	5 mg/mL isobaric	1.2	[109]
Ropivacaine	5 mg/mL	1	[101, 109]
Caudal anesthesia			
Bupivacaine	2.5 mg/mL	2	[87]
Levobupivacaine	2.5 mg/mL	2	[110]
Ropivacaine	2 mg/mL	2	[110]

neonates because additives such as clonidine can produce an increased apnea risk [104–108]. However, epinephrine has been shown to prolong spinal anesthesia with tetracaine by about one-third. The local anesthetic agents used include tetracaine [93], bupivacaine [74,75,109], ropivacaine [101,109] and levobupivacaine [109] (see Table 21.1).

Spinal anesthesia has the advantage of quicker onset than a caudal but duration may be shorter and the institution of the block can be technically challenging, with a failure rate of up to 10%. The doses in Table 21.1 typically give a block adequate for inguinal surgery lasting around 1 h but a tetracaine spinal may extend this by a further hour [87]. Supplementation of the spinal block with any sedative or anesthetic agent results in loss of the benefits in terms of reduced apnea. Sucrose analgesia is a useful adjunct and often helps settle a restless baby [111]. Some authors feel that a caudal is more likely to succeed and more anesthesiologists are familiar with caudal blocks so the disadvantage of slow onset is countered by improved reliability and longer duration of action [87].

General anesthesia

General endotracheal anesthesia could be regarded as the standard technique but early study results were confounded by use of older volatile agents such as halothane [93]. With newer volatile agents such as sevoflurane and desflurane showing promise for infant anesthesia in terms of speed of recovery and low incidence of postoperative respiratory complications [112–114], a head-to-head study of spinal with sevoflurane anesthesia for hernia repair in ex-premature infants [97] favored spinal anesthesia in terms of reduced early respiratory adverse events but there were a number of failures to secure a spinal block which gave cause for concern.

So general anesthesia with modern volatile agents, supplemented by local anesthetic infiltration, peripheral nerve block or a caudal is a more reliable and flexible technique and may be essential in certain cases, in particular incarcerated, complex or very large bilateral hernias. With an increasing trend towards laparoscopic repair, it may well be that general anesthesia for such cases will be needed more often in the future.

Abdominal wall defects

Abdominal wall defects are congenital abnormalities that are usually detected antenatally by fetal ultrasonography. Gastroschisis and omphalocele are the most common defects resulting in herniation of viscera through a defect in the upper or lower abdominal wall [115,116]. Although the anesthetic management of these conditions is essentially the same, these two conditions have significant embryological and clinical differences [117].

Gastroschisis

Gastroschisis is a congenital defect of the abdominal wall resulting in herniation of the abdominal contents, most commonly the small and large intestine (Fig. 21.2). The incidence of gastroschisis is approximately 1 in 3000–8000 livebirths. It is more common in mothers aged <20 years, the babies tend to be born prematurely with a low birthweight and in recent years the incidence has been rising, for reasons unknown [118–120]. Specialist antenatal and postnatal care results in a survival rate of over 90%.

The defect is usually on the right side of a normally developed and positioned umbilical cord and the viscera are not enclosed in a peritoneal sac. The vertical opening is approximately 2–5 cm in length, making herniation of other organs, such as the liver, unusual. The herniated intestine often appears dilated, foreshortened, and edematous and is covered in a thick inflammatory fibrin peel, probably due to exposure to amniotic fluid *in utero*. The intestine is often functionally abnormal and this may be complicated by the presence of intestinal atresia, stenosis

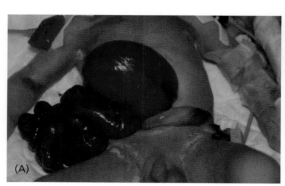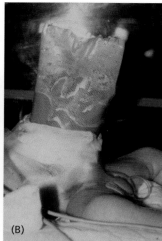

Figure 21.2 (A) Gastroschisis. (B) Silo for gastroschisis.

or malrotation [121]. Associated congenital anomalies are uncommon in gastroschisis, but initial routine investigations should aim to exclude potential cardiac abnormalities. The etiology of gastroschisis is not certain but is thought to involve vascular disruption of either the right umbilical vein or right omphalomesenteric artery. The result is paraumbilical ischemia and atrophy of the layers that form the anterior abdominal wall at the base of the umbilicus [122].

Following delivery, the initial priorities for gastroschisis must focus on ensuring that the newborn has a safe and patent airway, ventilation and oxygenation are not compromised by the defect, the exposed bowel is protected, and that fluid and heat loss are minimized and adequately managed. Reduction of the abdominal contents should take place urgently within hours of delivery to minimize the risk of volvulus, ischemia and infection. A nasogastric tube should be inserted to decompress the bowel, minimizing any splinting of the diaphragm and reducing the risk of regurgitation and aspiration. If signs of respiratory distress are evident or the newborn requires large volumes of fluid resuscitation then endotracheal intubation and ventilation are necessary.

The exposed bowel should be covered and supported using a sterile plastic wrap or a clear polythene bag to cover the lower limbs and abdomen to minimize fluid and heat loss.

The newborn should be dried and then placed under a radiant heater or in a heated incubator. Patients with gastroschisis should be nursed on their right side in a lateral decubitus position to enhance venous return from the gut and avoid vascular compromise. In patients with a large omphalocele, the position of the viscera and liver may compress the inferior vena cava in the supine position and so preferentially these infants should be nursed on their left side. Intravenous access is required early to allow fluid resuscitation, administration of broad-spectrum antibiotics, blood sampling and cross-match if going to surgery. Umbilical vessel catheterization is contraindicated. Third space losses in gastroschisis or ruptured omphalocele can be substantial and require fluid resuscitation with isotonic solutions: 0.9% normal saline, Hartmann solution, 5% albumin, blood or blood products. Boluses of 20 mL/kg should be given and the adequacy of resuscitation regularly monitored. Regular assessment of capillary refill, core–peripheral temperature gradients, heart rate, urine output and evidence of correction of acid–base disturbance will help guide the resuscitation efforts. Insertion of a peripheral arterial line is invaluable for repeated sampling to detect acid–base or electrolyte changes during the resuscitation and perioperative period.

Surgical management of the newborn depends on the size of the defect. Small defects can be closed by primary closure in the OR under general anesthesia or in the NICU without an anesthetic. If the defect is large then concerns arise from the effects of returning the abdominal viscera into a relatively small abdominal cavity, resulting in raised intra-abdominal pressure and abdominal compartment syndrome (ACS). Raised intra-abdominal pressure reduces venous return from compression of the inferior vena cava, decreasing cardiac output. Perfusion of the renal and splanchnic circulation is impaired, potentially leading to renal failure and bowel ischemia, causing intestinal perforation, necrotizing enterocolitis and a metabolic acidosis. Raised intra-abdominal pressure increases tension on the wound, causing dehiscence, and also results in splinting of the diaphragm, causing respiratory failure. The safety of primary closure can be assessed intraoperatively by measurement of intragastric, bladder, and central venous pressures or changes in ventilatory pressures as an indirect way of measuring intra-abdominal pressure. Intragastric or intravesical pressures less than 20 mmHg were found to result in successful primary closure and no ACS in neonates with gastroschisis [123,124]. Peak plateau respiratory pressures should be kept below 25 cmH$_2$O [125]. Gastric tonometry and pulse oximetry have also been used to help predict the onset of ACS [126,127]. If the surgeon is unable to perform a primary closure then a staged reduction is undertaken. The neonate is initially taken to the OR and fitted with a protective silastic silo. This is suspended above the incubator, allowing gravity to ease the viscera back into the abdominal cavity over the next 5–7 days. Each day the silo is gradually reduced in size, minimizing the risk of ACS. Once reduced, the neonate is returned to theater for surgical closure of the abdominal wall defect.

Important anesthetic considerations include the following.

- Ensure the baby is adequately resuscitated and preoperative tests are performed before coming to the OR.
- Actively warm the neonate during transfer to the OR in their incubator and on arrival in the OR with overhead radiant heaters, warm air blankets on the OR table, intravenous fluid warmers and humidified and warmed anesthetic gases. Monitor core and peripheral temperatures perioperatively.
- Aspirate the nasogastric tube preinduction in left and right lateral, prone and supine positions.
- Induction may be a rapid-sequence induction (RSI) or modified RSI. Sevoflurane gas induction may be performed and atracurium or vecuronium used for muscle relaxation prior to intubation.
- Nitrous oxide should be avoided to prevent further intestinal distension.
- Analgesia with morphine or fentanyl and, for smaller defects where early extubation is anticipated, a regional block technique may be used.
- Maintenance fluids (containing 10% dextrose) supplemented with boluses of albumin 5% or other isotonic solutions should be titrated according to the cardiovascular status of the neonate.
- In addition to routine monitoring, intragastric or intravesical pressures and urine output should be measured to assist in deciding whether a primary closure is possible.
- An intra-arterial cannula is useful for regular blood sampling and acid-base monitoring. Central venous cannulation, either conventional via internal jugular or subclavian routes or PICC lines, is necessary for large defects where repeat procedures or prolonged total parenteral nutrition (TPN) are required.

- The majority of neonates are returned to the NICU intubated, ventilated, paralyzed and sedated for further monitoring and ongoing management. They are ventilated until the bowel has settled back into the abdomen. TPN feeds, antibiotics and muscle relaxants are given.

In some centers, reduction may take place in the NICU without general anesthesia. NICU reduction is carried out in newborns who are stable and uncomplicated, i.e. absence of perforations, volvulus, atresias and obstruction [128,129]. The introduction of a spring-loaded silo that can be fitted at the bedside without any sutures or anesthesia has permitted staged closure in the NICU. When the reduction is complete the umbilicus is often used to plug the defect.

Outcome in gastroschisis is generally good unless complicated by intestinal atresia, stenosis, perforation, NEC, volvulus, sepsis, rare associated cardiac abnormalities or problems relating to prematurity (respiratory distress syndrome, intraventricular hemorrhages) [121].

Omphalocele

Omphalocele has an incidence of 1 in 5000 livebirths. It is an abdominal wall defect where the abdominal viscera herniate into the base of the umbilical cord through the umbilical ring. It is thought to result from failure of the midgut to return to the abdominal cavity around week 10 of gestation, causing incomplete closure of the anterior abdominal wall around the umbilicus. Unlike gastroschisis, the viscera are covered by a membrane and the bowel looks normal. Occasionally the peritoneal sac may rupture and can resemble gastroschisis although examination of the intestine helps differentiate these two conditions. The herniation may be a small defect 2–5 cm in diameter (exomphalos minor) or may be large (greater than 10 cm) involving liver and spleen, with poorly developed abdominal and thoracic cavities and pulmonary hypoplasia (exomphalos major) (Fig. 21.3).

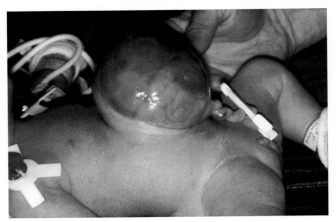

Figure 21.3 Omphalocele (exomphalos major).

Associated congenital abnormalities are much more common than in gastroschisis, with at least 60% of infants born with omphalocele having at least one associated anomaly. These may be cardiac in origin (30–40%), chromosomal abnormalities (trisomy 13, 18 or 21), cloacal or bladder extrophy, or Beckwith–Wiedemann syndrome (macroglossia, organomegaly, hypoglycemia, giantism, and congenital heart disease) [130]. Rarely, omphalocele may be part of the thoraco-abdominal pentalogy of Cantrell with a cleft sternum, anterior diaphragmatic hernia, heart defects and an absent pericardium [131]. Given that associated anomalies are more common in this condition, a thorough preoperative examination with appropriate investigations (chest x-ray, cardiac echo, renal ultrasound and routine blood investigations) should be performed before surgical correction.

Anesthetic management of omphalocele is very similar to that for gastroschisis. Unless the membrane is ruptured, omphalocele repair is less urgent. Defects without rupture of the membranous sac may be allowed to epithelialize on the ward using topical agents (silver sulfadiazine or antibiotic preparations) and a silo, avoiding any surgical intervention in the initial stages. This may take several weeks to months after which the infant will return to surgery for repair of the ventral hernia defect [132]. Care must be taken for cases that come to the OR for reduction or silo fitting if the liver is herniated. Damage to the liver parenchyma or compression of the hepatic veins can result in dramatic periods of cardiovascular instability.

Outcome in omphalocele is mainly dependent on the severity of additional abnormalities and chromosomal defects. Infection, surgical complications, low birthweight, hernia rupture and intestinal obstruction also contribute to mortality rates.

Esophageal atresia and tracheo-esophageal fistula

Esophageal atresia encompasses a group of congenital anomalies in which there is interruption of the continuity of the esophagus. In 86% of cases this co-exists with a distal tracheo-esophageal fistula, while in 7% there is no fistulous connection. In 4% of cases there is a tracheo-esophageal fistula but without esophageal atresia. Esophageal atresia occurs in around 1 in 2500–3000 live-births. In less than half of these, the condition exists in isolation while more than 50% occur in the presence of other congenital anomalies, the most common being one or more of those associated with the VACTERL group of anomalies (vertebral, anorectal, cardiac, tracheo-esophageal, renal and limb defects). The presence of a major cardiac anomaly reduces an almost complete sur-

vival rate to around 80%. Low birthweight is also associated with a survival rate of around 80% while the presence of both of these risk factors together reduces survival to 30–50% [133]. Respiratory insufficiency, however, is the single most significant risk factor affecting outcome [134]. Together, these factors provide a significant challenge to the anesthesiologist.

Clinical features

Two classification systems are in use today, the first being that proposed by Vogt in 1929, later modified by Gross in 1953. These can be summarized as shown in Table 21.2.

The most commonly occurring defect is Gross type C (Vogt 3B) which accounts for 86% of esophageal atresias (Fig. 21.4). These classification systems are, however, not comprehensive and variations other than those described can occur.

Diagnosis

Suspicion may be raised by antenatal ultrasound scan at around 18 weeks' gestation. This may show an absent or small gastric bubble. The incidence of esophageal atresia is also increased in the presence of polyhydramnios. The diagnosis may be confirmed at birth in these babies by failure to pass a nasogastric tube beyond 9–10 cm from the mouth. This is usually confirmed by a plain abdominal and chest radiograph. This may reveal other associ-

Table 21.2 Classification of esophageal atresia and tracheo-esophageal fistula

Gross	Vogt	Description
–	Type I	Esophageal agenesis (not included by Gross). No fistula present
Type A	Type 2	Proximal and distal esophageal stumps with a missing mid segment. No fistula present
Type B	Type 3A	Proximal esophagus meets lower trachea with distal esophageal stump
Type C	Type 3B	Proximal esophageal atresia. Esophagus ends in blind loop superior to sternal angle with the distal esophagus arising from the lower trachea or carina
Type D	Type 3C	Proximal esophagus terminates on lower trachea or carina with distal esophagus arising from carina
Type E (or Type H)		Type D variant where the esophagus is continuous but the presence of a fistula creates the appearance of the letter H
Type F		Esophageal stenosis

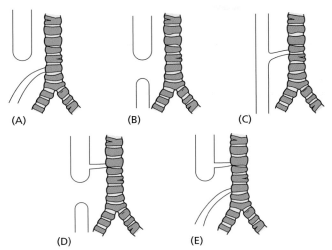

Figure 21.4 Esophageal atresia and tracheo-esophageal fistula variants. (A) The most common arrangement with a blind upper esophageal pouch and a distal TEF (Gross type C, Vogt type 3B). (B) Proximal and distal esophageal stumps with a missing segment and no TEF (Gross type A, Vogt type 2). (C) H-type fistula (Gross type E). (D) Proximal esophagus meets distal trachea with distal esophageal stump (Gross type B, Vogt type 3A). (E) Proximal esophagus terminates on lower trachea with distal esophagus arising from carina (Gross type D, Vogt type 3C).

ated anomalies such as vertebral or rib abnormalities or the "double bubble" associated with duodenal atresia. However, if not suspected prenatally, esophageal atresia may not manifest itself until feeding begins, whereupon the baby may cough, choke and become cyanosed. Failure to recognize the condition swiftly can result in the development of aspiration pneumonitis and dehydration can result due to accumulation of saliva and disturbed swallowing. Initial preoperative surgical management involves the passage of a suction catheter, often a radiopaque double-lumen tube (Replogle tube) into the blind-ending pouch for continuous irrigation and suction.

Preoperative evaluation

The baby with esophageal atresia/tracheo-esophageal fistula presents many challenges for the anesthesiologist. First, due to the large variation in the anatomy of these lesions, correct placement of the endotracheal tube may be difficult. Furthermore, prematurity of 34 weeks' gestation or less is present in 12% of babies with esophageal atresia [135] and may result in moderate-to-severe neonatal respiratory distress syndrome. Associated anomalies may also significantly affect both the difficulty of the anesthetic and the outcome for the patient. Cardiovascular anomalies account for 29% [136] and have been shown to be the single most common mortality-related association in esophageal atresia [137]. Of the other associated anomalies, anorectal defects comprise 14%, genitourinary 14%, gastrointestinal 13%, vertebral/skeletal 10%, respiratory 6%, genetic 4%, and others 11% [136].

Preoperative evaluation of infants with esophageal atresia should include a detailed history of the neonatal course, including delivery. A history of polyhydramnios may also indicate possible renal anomalies and is more common where there are associated chromosomal abnormalities such as Down syndrome or Edwards syndrome. Major neurological anomalies may impair fetal swallowing, also resulting in polyhydramnios. If there is no antenatal suspicion and the infant presents later then a feeding history should be obtained, with special attention being paid to episodes of cyanosis or choking, which may indicate aspiration and the possible development of aspiration pnuemonitis.

Preoperative preparation by this time will have established a blind-ending esophagus, with continual suction and irrigation of the pouch being provided, preferably by a Replogle tube. A full anesthetic history should also be obtained from the parents regarding any significant family reactions to anesthesia. A plain radiograph of the chest and abdomen will confirm the tip of the suction catheter proceeding no further than the upper mediastinum while gas in the stomach is significant in that it confirms the presence of a tracheo-esophageal fistula. Absence of gas suggests an isolated atresia. A clinical examination of the neonate should have established any dysmorphic features and indicated the presence of any major cardiac anomaly; however, cardiac echo is required routinely as a preoperative investigation in these cases. This will define any structural abnormality of the heart but may also reveal a right-sided aortic arch which occurs in 2.5%. This has implications for patient positioning and surgical approach [138] and may also significantly affect ventilation.

A congenital cardiac lesion producing high pulmonary blood flows is unlikely to pose significant physiological problems during the first few days after birth as pulmonary vascular resistance remains high initially. These patients can usually proceed safely for surgical correction. However, patients who have lesions with significant right- or left-sided obstructive components may have either a systemic or pulmonary circulation which is ductus arteriosus dependent. Babies with duct-dependent circulation have been shown to have a significantly increased risk of mortality [139]. In these cases the duct can be kept open with an infusion of prostaglandin E1 and if the baby remains stable and in good condition, surgery may proceed. A small number of patients will present in poor condition with a closed or closing duct. In these cases resuscitation is often required and surgery needs to be delayed. Rarely, such babies will require a palliative shunting procedure or cardiac repair prior to surgery for esophageal atresia [140]. A renal tract ultrasound scan is required due to the associated incidence of genitourinary anomalies. Blood biochemistry and hematology should be ascertained and blood should be cross-matched for surgery. Assessment of the respiratory system is paramount. The presence of respiratory distress is a significant prognostic indicator [134] and has an important bearing on the conduct of anesthesia, in particular with regard to the principle of maintaining low airway pressures. Preoperative oxygen saturation should be measured and increased oxygen requirement noted.

Conduct of general anesthesia

Preparation of the operating environment is as for any other small baby but particular attention needs to be paid to the ambient temperature. This may need to be increased in the case of the premature infant. A heated warming mattress, heated and humidified breathing circuit and warmed intravenous and irrigation fluids will help to prevent heat loss. Intravenous access would ordinarily have been established prior to surgery as these babies are unable to feed. This can be used for maintenance fluids with 5–10% glucose where required. A second IV line is required for replacement therapy, and this should be of sufficient caliber to allow for rapid replacement of blood loss if required. In addition to the application of standard monitoring, invasive arterial pressure monitoring is invaluable as it allows for real-time measurement. This is especially so in the case of aberrant cardiac or great vessel anatomy where surgical access may cause hemodynamic compromise. It also allows for easy blood sampling intra-operatively. This can be particularly useful where significant respiratory compromise exists and allows for rapid and accurate assessment of gas exchange and acid–base status. Central venous access is not usually required but may be necessary in the event of failure to establish adequate peripheral intravenous access.

The major consideration of both anesthetic and surgical management of the neonate with esophageal atresia and tracheo-esophageal fistula is ventilation of the lungs without ventilation of the fistula. Endotracheal tube misplacement can lead to undesirable consequences such as massive gastric distension and resulting respiratory and cardiovascular compromise. Even with a correctly placed endotracheal tube, poorly compliant lungs and a large distal fistula can result in selective passage of anesthetic gases into the gastrointestinal tract, leading to hypoventilation and hypercarbia [141]. The interplay between the variable anatomy of the defect, pre-existing co-morbidity and anesthetic technique may be unpredictable. As a result, techniques have focused on the avoidance of muscle relaxants and positive pressure ventilation until ligation of the fistula is achieved [142]. Traditionally, intubation may have been performed awake but in the preterm neonate, this is associated with an increased risk of intraventricular hemorrhage [143].

One recognized technique is induction of general anesthesia by inhalation with the patient in a semi-supine position. Once adequate depth of anesthesia is achieved and with the patient spontaneously ventilating, laryngoscopy should be performed and the vocal cords sprayed with no more than 3 mg/kg of lidocaine. An appropriately sized endotracheal tube is then passed through the cords and beyond the carina, aiming for endobronchial intubation. This is then confirmed by auscultation and the tube is then withdrawn until ventilation is just heard on both sides. At this point, it is possible to confirm the position of the endotracheal tube by passage of a flexible bronchoscope through it. If all is well then a muscle relaxant may be administered and the patient positioned for surgical repair. This technique is limited, however, by the assumption that the fistula is proximal enough to allow passage of the endotracheal tube beyond it. It also may not be an adequate technique where there is a large fistula. In one series, 11% of fistulae were at or below the carina, with a further 22% being within 1 cm of it [144]. Even with such a lesion, it may be possible to achieve adequate ventilation initially, with problems only being encountered on repositioning of the patient or during surgical manipulation, particularly compression of the right lung. Additionally the patient's condition may preclude spontaneous ventilation, requiring that muscle relaxation be instituted followed by gentle positive pressure ventilation. It is, however, in the preterm neonate with respiratory distress that this is most problematic. Poorly compliant lungs and a large distal fistula can mean an easy egress of ventilatory gases into the stomach with resultant compromise in ventilation [141]. With progressively increasing gastric distension, the stomach may rupture, resulting in a tension pneumoperitoneum which further impairs ventilation [145]. The traditional approach in this instance would be to perform an emergency gastrostomy. However, this often worsens the situation as the sudden reduction in intragastric pressure further facilitates escape of ventilatory gas through the fistula. Resuscitation in this instance is often ineffective until leakage of gas through the esophagus is controlled [146].

Placement of a 2 Fr or 3 Fr Fogarty embolectomy catheter (Baxter Healthcare Corporation, Irvine, CA, USA) through a rigid bronchoscope to occlude the fistula in a neonate with severe respiratory compromise was first described in 1982 [147]. Since then routine rigid bronchoscopy has become standard practice for some as part of the airway management in tracheo-esophageal fistula, with 18% of patients in a retrospective review requiring the insertion of a Fogarty catheter [142]. In this same series, ventilation difficulty was only encountered with a fisutula >3 mm in diameter at or near the carina. Smaller fistulas or those more than 5 mm above the carina were not associated with ventilation problems. Routine preoperative rigid bronchoscopy has also been found to be useful in the diagnosis of abnormal variants and unsuspected findings [134,148]. However, rigid bronchoscopy in the newborn can be technically difficult, often resulting in arterial desaturation, and in those preterm neonates weighing less than 1500 g who have severe respiratory compromise, it may be impossible altogether.

More recently, tracheoscopy-assisted repair of tracheoesophageal fistula has been reported [149]. The technique described involves passage of a narrow-diameter fiberoptic bronchoscope through the endotracheal tube in a neonate who is intubated with established muscle paralysis and low-pressure intermittent positive pressure ventilation (IPPV). The aim is for gentle ventilation with the tip of the endotracheal tube sitting above the fistula so that identification and repair of the fistula take place under direct visual control. In 47 cases over a 10-year period, no adverse events related to the tube being positioned above the fistula occurred. The authors suggest that mandatory positive pressure ventilation with their technique avoids hypercapnia, hypoxia and respiratory acidosis that can result in a potentially disastrous return to fetal circulation. With this technique, unlike rigid bronchoscopy, visualization of the airway can take place at any point during the surgical repair.

In the past, the infant with TEF/EA often underwent an initial surgical gastrostomy, sometimes under local anesthesia, with the thought that this would decompress the stomach and minimize ventilatory problems. The thoracotomy was then performed several days later. However, as noted above, a gastrostomy may allow egress of ventilatory volume through the fistula and out of the gastrostomy. In modern practice the gastrostomy is rarely performed primarily, and usually not at all except in cases of long-gap EA where prolonged healing is required.

In recent years thoracoscopic repair of esophageal atresia with or without TEF has been accomplished. McKinlay described a series of 26 neonates, 20 with TEF/EA and six with isolated EA [150]. Anesthetic technique is described as standard tracheal intubation without bronchial blocker or other special technique. Three thoracoscopic ports are inserted in the right hemithorax with insufflation of CO_2 to a pressure of 6 mmHg, which is often accompanied by hypercarbia and arterial desaturation, requiring adjustment of ventilation as the lung collapses to afford the surgeon a view of the field. The TEF is suture ligated and the esophageal pouches dissected, mobilized, and anastomosed with 5-0 vicryl sutures (Fig. 21.5). The anesthetic techniques were not described in detail, but no severe ventilation problems were apparently encountered. Patient weights were 1.4–3.9 kg and gestational ages 31–41 weeks. There were two early

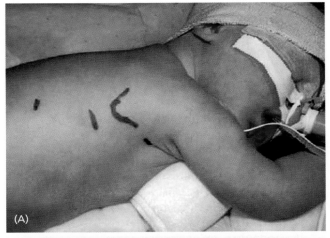

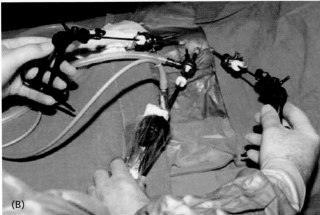

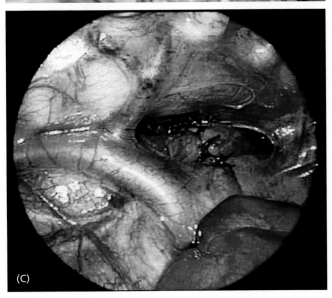

Figure 21.5 (A) Neonate in semi-prone position, with tip of scapula and three port sites for thoracoscopic instruments marked. (B) Port sites and instrument position for surgeon and assistant. (C) Esophageal anastomosis completed with azygous vein intact; note collapsed right lung at lower right quadrant of picture. Reproduced from McKinlay et al [150] with permission from Elsevier.

deaths (one patient with trisomy 18 and another with associated congenital diaphragmatic hernia), and one late death from congenital heart disease. There were seven minor esophageal anastomotic leaks managed conservatively, one recurrent TEF managed thoracoscopically, and nine anastomotic strictures. Further details on the anesthetic management of thoracoscopic surgery are discussed in Chapter 24.

Because of the many different approaches to TEF/EA repair, and even variation within institutions, a thorough preoperative discussion with the surgeon, focusing on airway and ventilation management strategies and contingency plan in case of severe ventilatory compromise, must be held when approaching these patients.

Postoperative anesthetic care

Postoperative ventilation is mandatory in neonates weighing less than 2000 g [59] and in those with respiratory distress or significant cardiac pathology. Repair of the esophageal anastomosis under tension is also an indication for postoperative ventilation, usually for a period of 5 days [133,151]. Furthermore, it has been proposed that safe awake extubation may affect every anastomosis to some degree, whether or not it is a "long-gap" anastomosis under tension, and that emergent reintubation may have catastrophic consequences for an anastomosis [152]. This latter problem leads some institutions to routinely leave the trachea intubated in all these patients, until it is clear that the threat of respiratory insufficiency has passed. Tension at the anastomotic site is recognized to be the most important factor contributing to anastomotic complications, but it is very difficult to assess and measure and should therefore be assumed [153]. Analgesia both intra- and postoperatively can be provided by a long-acting opioid such as morphine. This can be given by intravenous bolus at surgery and continued by infusion in the intensive care unit.

Although postoperative ventilation should be the norm where staffing and facilities exist to provide it, there may be occasion when extubation is planned at the end of surgery. Avoidance of opioids or minimizing their use is desirable although it may be necessary to use a short-acting opioid such as alfentanil or remifentanil. Regional anesthesia may be provided by a caudal catheter technique with insertion to T6–7 level, or supplementary local anesthetic can be injected by the surgeon. If morphine is required postoperatively then it must be used with extreme vigilance.

Congenital diaphragmatic hernia

Congenital diaphragmatic hernia (CDH) occurs with an incidence of approximately 1 in 3000 births and was first described by Bochdalek in 1848. The most common left-sided form bears his name and accounts for approximately 80% of CDH cases. The embryological development of CDH is incompletely understood but it is thought that the defect may result from failure of closure of the pleuroperitoneal canals. Animal studies using rats exposed to the teratogenic herbicide Nitrofen showed that the defect is formed very early in the embryonic period with early ingrowth of the liver through the defect [154]. At a cellular level, there may be abnormalities of epithelial and mesenchymal growth and differentiation which may also have implications for lung development [155]. Further rat studies have suggested that lung hypoplasia as a result of fibroblast growth factor deficiency may precede the development CDH and lend support to the theory of a global mesenchymal embryopathy [156].

Infants presenting with the condition are often born at full term and weigh in excess of 3 kg [157]. Around half of infants with CDH will have other congenital anomalies, with the heart being commonly affected; 4–16% will have chromosomal abnormalities. Survival is often severely affected by the presence of associated anomalies. In the infant with CDH, abdominal viscera, most commonly bowel, herniate through the defect into the thoracic cavity, effectively acting as a space-occupying mass. This is accompanied by abnormal pulmonary development, particularly on the affected side, but mediastinal shift can prevent normal growth and development of the contralateral lung. Despite the apparent simplicity of the anatomical defect, the pathophysiology of the condition is complex. The lungs show a decreased number of bronchopulmonary segments, decreased alveolar surface area and abnormal pulmonary vasculature [158]. There is also a thickening of arteriolar smooth muscle that extends to affect the alveolar capillaries. This impairs pulmonary function further by increasing pulmonary artery pressure that can lead to right-to-left shunting.

Diagnosis

The majority of infants with CDH are discovered at prenatal maternal ultrasound scan. This provides an opportunity to arrange for both delivery of the infant in an appropriate center for management and prenatal counseling for the parents and family. It may also allow fetuses with poor outcome to be identified. Ultrasound is, however, dependent on equipment, expertise and experience and may fail to detect the condition prenatally in up to 50% of cases [159].

Two parameters have been shown to be of some prognostic value. First, if there is herniation of the liver into the thoracic cavity, the likelihood of survival is halved [160]. Second, at 24–26 weeks' gestation it is possible to measure the cross-sectional area of the contralateral lung and to compare it with the head circumference. A lung-to-head ratio (LHR) of >1.4 is associated with no mortality compared to a LHR of <0.8 which carries a 100% mortality rate [161]. With the advent of three-dimensional ultrasound, some centers are now able to assess LHR usefully from 24–34 weeks' gestation. Furthermore, fetal magnetic resonance imaging (MRI) has also been found to be a useful modality in the prenatal assessment of CDH [162].

Following prenatal diagnosis, a birth at or as close to term as possible is preferred as preterm delivery is associated with a worse outcome [163]. The infant born with CDH usually presents with a scaphoid abdomen and an unusually prominent ipsilateral chest with an increased anteroposterior diameter. Breath sounds are diminished on the side of the lesion and heart sounds may be deviated towards the contralateral side. Diagnosis may be confirmed with a plain chest radiograph which demonstrates air-filled intestinal loops in the affected side of the thorax and a paucity of intestine in the abdominal cavity. There may also be mediastinal shift with a resultant deviation of heart sounds (Fig. 21.6).

Postnatal management

At or shortly after birth, the majority of infants will develop signs of respiratory distress. If the defect is large then severe hypoxia and respiratory acidosis will be present and the infant will require immediate resuscitation, including endotracheal intubation and mechanical ventilatory assistance. A naso- or orogastric tube is passed to decompress the gut. Pulmonary hypertension may worsen the situation and can result in a persistent fetal circulation with shunting of blood from right to left through the ductus arteriosus and foramen ovale. This further exacerbates hypoxia and hypercarbia and a decrease in systemic oxygenation results in a metabolic acidosis. However, a small minority of infants are born asymptomatic and remain so for the first day of life. In these cases the defect is small and physiologically much less significant. This group usually has an uneventful course following surgical repair.

In the past CDH was considered a surgical emergency and infants were rushed to the operating room but the last decade has seen a change to preoperative stabilization of the infant prior to surgery [164,165]. In particular, stabilization strategies have been aimed at preserving extrapartum circulation and minimizing acidosis with avoidance of further damage to the lungs. Current practice involves transfer of the infant to an intensive care unit and institution of gentle ventilation aimed at minimizing barotrauma [166,167]. Strategies include permissive hypercapnia to a pCO_2 of no greater than 7.8 kPa (60 mmHg) [168]. However, with the frequent association of pulmonary hypertension, this level of hypercarbia is sometimes not tolerated. An oxygen saturation of no less than 80% on 60% inspired oxygen is considered an indication for alternative forms of ventilation or respiratory support [169].

Typically, the stabilization period may range from 24 h to a number of days, depending on the condition of the child. Current practice may allow for stabilization of the sick infant, thus allowing a potentially less fraught perioperative course. However, in a recent large multi-study review, no difference in outcome was demonstrated when delayed repair after stabilization was compared to both repair within 24 h and repair immediately after birth [170]. The availability of extracorporeal membrane oxygenation (ECMO) has become widespread in line with the advent of delayed surgery in these infants. It has been shown that the overall survival rate for infants requiring ECMO is 52.9% versus 77.3% (p < 0.001) for non-ECMO infants. However, in those who were deemed to have a mortality risk of 80% or more, it is associated with improved outcome. Furthermore, in infants with additional risk factors it may worsen outcome [171]. High-frequency oscillatory ventilation (HFOV) and inhaled nitric oxide (iNO) are also frequently used when failure of conventional ventilatory support occurs. HFOV and iNO are both aimed at improving oxygenation. HFOV achieves improved ventilation with a reduction in barotrauma [172] while iNO is used as a selective pulmonary vasodilator aimed at reducing pulmonary vascular resistance. Neither modality has been shown to have any conclusive effect on outcome in infants with CDH [169]. Surfactant and prenatal steroids have found vogue in

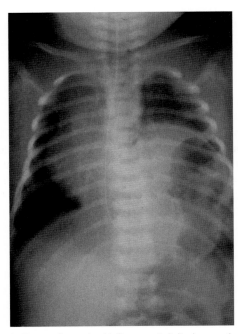

Figure 21.6 Chest radiograph of left congenital diaphragmatic hernia. Note liver and intestines in left hemithorax with heart displaced to right.

recent years. Although steroids are a recognized and valuable treatment for immature lungs, they are of unproven benefit in CDH. Similarly, surfactant has been found to be of little value [169].

Anesthetic care for congential diaphragmatic hernia repair

Immediately after birth, the infant with CDH may be in acute respiratory distress and will need to be intubated as an emergency. Where possible, bag and mask ventilation should be avoided to prevent gaseous distension of the stomach. A naso- or orogastric tube should then be placed to provide intestinal decompression. The infant will then need to be transferred to a NICU for assessment and stabilization.

When it is deemed appropriate to undertake repair, there are several anesthetic concerns. First, pulmonary hypoplasia and the resulting pulmonary hypertension can make the maintenance of adequate oxygenation challenging. Hypoxia, hypercarbia and acidosis all act to increase the pulmonary vascular resistance further [173,174]. Instrumentation of the airway may also result in a dangerous increase in pulmonary vascular resistance [175] and so an opioid such as fentanyl should be given at the beginning of the procedure and can be repeated as necessary. A dose of $25\,\mu g/kg$ has been shown to abolish the stress response to airway instrumentation [176]. The operating room should be prepared as for any neonate requiring major surgery. Standard monitoring is applied. Good venous access is mandatory and central venous access is highly desirable for both the measurement of central venous pressure and the administration of inotropes such as dopamine. Invasive arterial blood pressure monitoring is also required as it provides real-time measurement of intra-arterial pressure. This is particularly useful as surgical access (Fig. 21.7) may result in acute compression of the great vessels, leading to sudden acute

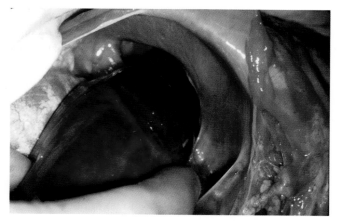

Figure 21.7 Operative appearance of congenital diaphragmatic hernia via left thoracoabdominal incision. Liver is being reduced through large diaphragmatic defect.

hypotension. The surgical approach usually involves a left thoracoabdominal incision, reduction of the intrathoracic intestinal viscera and liver, and repair of the diaphragm, often with a patch made of synthetic material. Furthermore, the changes in pressure that may be seen during the cycling of ventilation can indicate hypovolemia. A urinary catheter is useful to monitor urine output.

The goals of anesthetic management are to provide adequate analgesia and depth of anesthesia with minimal impact on pulmonary vascular resistance and myocardial function. Therefore great care must be exercised with the maintenance of anesthesia. Volatile anesthetic agents are known to attenuate hypoxic pulmonary vasoconstriction [176]. However, they may cause systemic hypotension if not used carefully. For this reason a fentanyl-based anesthetic may be preferable. Nitrous oxide has been shown to have little effect on pulmonary vasculature in infants [177]. However, it should be avoided because of its effect on alveolar PaO_2 and its propensity to worsen bowel distension. Muscle relaxation may be provided by competitive neuromuscular blockade. Vecuronium and rocuronium are appropriate. Pancuronium is best avoided because of its intrinsic sympathomimetic activity. Mechanical ventilatory parameters should be set to allow for adequate oxygenation. A degree of hypercarbia is acceptable as high inflation pressures should be avoided, again being mindful of pulmonary hypertension. If the infant has been stabilized prior to surgery then preoperative PaO_2 and $PaCO_2$ levels serve as a guide to aim for. Throughout the procedure, the anesthesiologist must be prepared to treat a sudden pulmonary hypertensive crisis. In this event, moderate hyperventilation, often manual, may be required with 100% oxygen. The cardiac output may require support and adequate preload should be ensured. Selective pulmonary vasodilators such as inhaled nitric oxide should be available in addition to appropriate inotropic support which may include drugs such as phenylephrine, epinephrine, dopamine, and milrinone. On occasion, it is necessary to repair CDH with the patient supported by either HFOV or ECMO. This makes patient transfer hazardous and in this situation repair is undertaken in the NICU.

Meningomyelocele

Meningomyelocele is a form of neural tube defect occurring in 0.5–1 per 1000 livebirths and is usually diagnosed antenatally. The spinal cord and meninges are exposed to the intrauterine environment and this results in a central sac filled with cerebrospinal fluid, damaged spinal cord, and nerve roots. Invariably this defect is associated with the Arnold–Chiari malformation and hydrocephalus. The cerebellar vermis, fourth ventricle and lower brainstem are herniated downwards below the level of the foramen magnum. Primary closure is usual within the first 2 days to minimize infection. Treatment of hydrocephalus is individualized but a concurrent ventriculoperitoneal (VP) shunt placement may be needed. Fetal repair has been undertaken with reduced need for VP shunting at age 1 year but no improvement in neurological deficits [178].

Problems for the anesthesiologist are positioning for induction, solved by use of pads or a circular gel ring to protect the fragile sac; prone positioning for surgery; awareness of preventing latex allergy by use of a latex-free environment and equipment; the potential for large intraoperative blood losses due to dissection of skin flaps to gain coverage of the defect; and postoperative respiratory problems associated with Arnold–Chiari malformation. These babies may have reduced or absent response to hypoxia and hypercarbia and may have impaired swallowing and gag reflexes [179–181]. See Chapter 23 for further discussion of anesthetic care for patients with this lesion.

Muscle biopsy

Muscle biopsy in an infant usually requires a general anesthetic supplemented by local anesthetic infiltration at the biopsy site. This presents a dilemma for the pediatric anesthesiologist who is being asked to provide anesthesia in a child without a definitive diagnosis and therefore a degree of uncertainty about the individual's response to anesthetic and other drugs. A muscle biopsy is often required for definitive diagnosis of a wide range of disorders (Box 21.2) and supplements information from family history, symptoms and signs, biochemistry, genetic tests and electromyography.

Clinically the infant will usually present with hypotonia or floppiness which may be associated with swallowing difficulties, gastroesophageal reflux and failure to thrive. If reflux is significant, episodes of aspiration may

---

Box 21.2 Indications for muscle biopsy in infants

- Benign congenital hypotonia
- Perinatal asphyxia
- Hypotonic cerebral palsy
- Metabolic disorders
- Spinal cord injury
- Spinal muscular atrophy
- Peripheral nerve disorders
- Congenital myasthenia
- Neonatal myasthenia
- Infantile botulism
- Congenital myopathies
- Muscular dystrophies
- Mitochondrial myopathies
- Glycogen storage disorders

---

have caused significant lung damage. Try to assess the degree and extent of muscle weakness and any evidence of respiratory compromise as these infants often have reduced respiratory reserve and may need postoperative respiratory support even for a short procedure such as muscle biopsy. Avoid sedative premedication and opioids if at all possible. A preoperative ECG and echocardiogram are recommended to check for cardiac involvement, for example in Duchenne muscular dystrophy or mitochondrial myopathy. Avoid prolonged fasting as infants with hypotonia often are prone to hypoglycemia and consider giving IV dextrose from the start of the fluid fast period and continuing intra-and postoperatively. Inhalational anesthesia with sevoflurane with or without tracheal intubation and ventilatory support as appropriate to the individual child are indicated along with local anesthesia of the biopsy site by the surgeon and simple analgesia thereafter with acetaminophen and or non-steroidal anti-inflammatory drugs (NSAIDs). If possible, avoid muscle relaxants and certainly succinylcholine, which can cause dangerous hyperkalemia in some of these disorders. If a non-depolarizing neuromuscular blocking agent is needed, then titrate carefully against neuromuscular monitoring and ensure complete reversal at the end of the procedure. The possibility of malignant hyperthermia is a concern and dantrolene should be available but not administered prophylactically as it can itself exacerbate muscle weakness in some of these disorders. Even after a short procedure, postoperative monitoring should be extended and ventilatory support must be available as required. This may be best carried out in an intensive care setting.

Resuscitation of the newborn

During the transition from intrauterine to extrauterine life, the neonate will undergo a significant and complex physiological change from the fetal circulation to the adult circulation, with a period of time in a transitional circulation. At birth, the neonatal systemic blood pressure increases after the cord is clamped. The first breath of air needs to expand fluid-filled alveoli and for this may require negative intrapleural pressures of up to $70\,cmH_2O$. Oxygen causes the pulmonary vascular resistance to fall because of a reduction in hypoxic pulmonary vasoconstriction and also causes the ductus arteriosus to constrict, thus making the pulmonary artery the route of least resistance from the right ventricle. Flow through the foramen ovale ceases due to the rise in pressures in the left side of the heart. The left ventricle, which is of a similar size at birth, will gradually increase in its function of compliance and contractility.

The World Health Organization estimates that 19% of neonatal deaths worldwide are caused by birth asphyxia

[182]. That equates to nearly 1 million deaths annually. However, the vast majority of newborn infants do not require any form of resuscitation other than drying and being kept warm by being given to their mother, often skin to skin. Approximately 10% of newborns require some assistance to begin breathing at birth, with 1% needing extensive resuscitation [183]. Other studies have estimated that between 5% and 10% of neonates need resuscitation at birth, from simple stimulation to assisted ventilation [184]. Resuscitation of the newborn is commonly managed by the obstetrician or midwife but if there is an anticipated sick neonate, cesarean section or preterm delivery, then neonatologists and occasionally anaesthesiologists are involved.

The following is based on current practice and evidence as well as guidelines produced by the Neonatal Resuscitation Program (NRP) in association with the American Heart Association (AHA) for cardiopulmonary resuscitation (CPR) and emergency cardiovascular care (ECC) of pediatric and neonatal patients [183]. Although neonatologists and pediatricians generally manage newborn resuscitation, the techniques that are set out in the neonatal resuscitation algorithm could be extrapolated to form competencies relevant for any neonatal resuscitation, especially for those patients in their first few weeks of life and those who are preterm. Important trials and studies looking at aspects of neonatal resuscitation have caused recent and significant changes in the therapeutic algorithm. There are also related studies that may change care in the future. These include the use of supplemental oxygen as part of initial resuscitation and therapeutic cooling which aims to decrease the neurological damaged caused by asphyxia at birth. These will be discussed briefly.

Anticipating the need for resuscitation as well as the preparation of appropriate equipment, environment and trained staff are crucial to a successful outcome.

The algorithm shown in Figure 21.8 is taken from guidelines produced by the American Academy of Pediatrics and the AHA. It is divided into four broad categories: A – Assessment and initial care and observations, B – Ventilation, C – Chest compressions, D – Drug and fluid administration. These will be discussed with the emphasis on current significant evidence and recent trials.

Assessment and initial care

Immediate assessment and initial care include drying and stimulating the baby, clearing and positioning the airway, which includes suctioning and positioning the head in the "sniffing" position. Intrapartum suction of meconium has been shown not to improve outcome, so this is no longer recommended by the NRP. There should also be some way of providing a source of warmth during resuscitation and this is normally done under a radiant heat source. Preterm infants and neonates with a very low birthweight

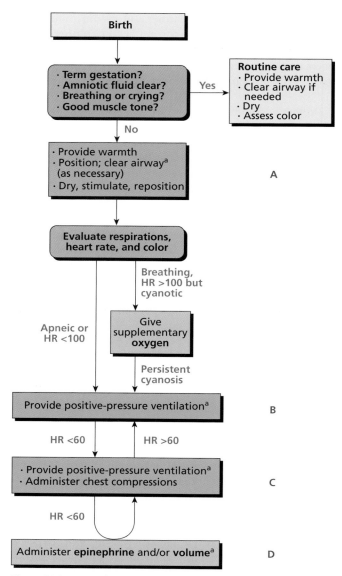

Figure 21.8 Neonatal resuscitation algorithm. [a]Endotracheal intubation may be considered at several steps. Please refer to full guidelines [183] for details. Reproduced from AHA/AAP [183] with permission from the American Heart Association.

(<1500 g) are recommended to have the additional warming technique of being placed in a plastic wrapping, as well as being placed under a radiant heat source. This has been shown to decrease heat loss without hindering ongoing resuscitative measures [183,185,186].

The immediate assessment is of respiratory effort, muscle tone, heart rate, and color. This in practice also includes saturation monitoring. The first major sign of tissue hypoxia in newborns is bradycardia (heart rate <100 as per the guidelines). Bradycardic episodes normally respond well to a brief period of positive pressure ventilation. This is done via a bag and mask, T-piece or manually operated, gas-powered, pressure-regulated resuscitator (Neo-puff™, Fisher and Paykel Healthcare, Auckland, New Zealand). The NRP guidelines then recommend giving supplemental oxygen. There are many studies comparing the risks and benefits of using oxygen to resuscitate neonates.

Oxygen versus air

Firstly, there is evidence linking ventilation of neonates on high concentrations of oxygen, even for short periods of time, to retinopathy of prematurity (ROP), chronic lung disease, oxygen free radical disease of the neonate, infection, and leukemia. Studies comparing initial resuscitation with air and varying concentrations of oxygen are beginning to show some evidence that using air alone can have outcomes comparable to using oxygen supplementation, therefore preventing the risks associated with oxygen therapy. But there is as yet insufficient evidence to resolve all questions [187].

Although some studies have shown that room air may be superior to 100% oxygen as the initial choice for resuscitation [188], it seems standard practice to give 100% oxygen initially during resuscitation. At present, there is insufficient evidence to recommend starting resuscitation with room air over oxygen or oxygen over room air. However, recent changes to the algorithm do state that it is recommended to decrease the oxygen concentration as saturations rise over 95%. It is also stated that it is reasonable practice to start resuscitation with room air if that is the clinician's preference, if there is supplemental oxygen available should it be needed. The AHA guidelines do recommend supplemental oxygen when giving positive pressure ventilation and free flow oxygen to those spontaneously breathing with central cyanosis. Some studies suggest a compromise, aiming for 30–40% oxygen [189]. The use of oxygen blenders with either T-pieces or Neo-puff™ apparatus is recommended.

Temperature control: therapeutic hypothermia

A recent review of literature looking at hypoxic ischemic encephalopathy of newborn infants found that there is now some evidence from trials to show that induced hypothermia helps to improve survival and development at 18 months for, specifically, term babies at risk of brain damage [190]. It should be pointed out that this is not yet a recommended therapeutic intervention as per the NRP guidelines, but is expected to be in the near future. A great deal more research is needed into methods of cooling, whether it is isolated to the head or whole-body therapeutic hypothermia. There is also the difficulty of patient selection. It is unclear which patients would benefit from cooling and also to what temperature and for how long. There are still many important, specific and as yet unanswered questions.

Ventilation

Improving bradycardia is the first sign that effective ventilation is being conducted during resuscitation. Improving color and muscle tone, with a return to spontaneous and regular breathing, normally follows this. Effective ventilation is achieved using a T-piece or self-inflating Ambubag®; however, many centers now use the Neo-puff™ as it has an oxygen blender as part of its design. CO_2 monitoring is the gold standard method of confirming correct placement of the endotracheal tube.

Studies looking at resuscitation of asphyxiated neonates at birth have shown that term babies often require around $30\,cmH_2O$ as an initial inflation pressure [191], with preterm and low-birthweight babies needing higher inflation pressures due to their underdeveloped lungs. Large-volume inflations can cause injury [192] but the inclusion of PEEP has been shown to have a protective effect against lung injury as well as improving lung compliance and gas exchange [193,194].

Chest compressions

Good ventilation strategies are the most effective way of successfully resuscitating a neonate. Chest compressions are only indicated if there is a continuing bradycardia <60 bpm in the face of adequate ventilation and oxygenation. Chest compressions should be started after approximately 1 min of resuscitation as per the algorithm. There should be a period of at least 30 sec where adequate assisted ventilation is delivered before starting chest compressions. The two thumb-encircling hands technique is recommended by the AHA for chest compressions as this should generate higher peak systolic and coronary artery perfusion pressures [182]. The two-finger technique should probably be used if access to the umbilicus is needed for umbilical catheter insertion during resuscitation.

Drugs

If bradycardia persists despite good ventilatory resuscitation with poor perfusion and no improvement in color, muscle tone or saturations then volume expansion and administration of specific drugs, especially epinephrine, are indicated. Emergency umbilical vein access, where the catheter is inserted only 3–5 cm until blood return is obtained, is the preferred route for administration of emergency drugs and fluids [195]. The concentration of epinephrine used is 1:10,000 (0.1 mg/mL).

There is a lack of data on the effectiveness of endotracheal epinephrine but it can be used as a route of access while IV access is being obtained. The dose used for endotracheal epinephrine is 0.1 mg/kg. This is a 10-fold increase in the recommended dose for IV administration. The recommended IV dose is 0.01–0.03 mg/kg per dose. Higher doses are not used as they can cause a paradoxical decrease in myocardial function due to exaggerated hypertensive responses with a subsequent effect of poorer neurological outcome [196]. Other drugs are used during resuscitation but rarely. Naloxone or other narcotic antagonists are not recommended due to a lack of clinical evidence during initial resuscitation and also as they may precipitate withdrawal seizures in newborns of mothers taking regular opioids. The Resuscitation Council (UK) does recommend the administration of sodium bicarbonate when there is no effective cardiac output, or virtually none, prior to a second dose of adrenaline. There are no well-powered studies to support the beneficial effects of sodium bicarbonate use.

CASE STUDY

This case study illustrates the principles of anesthetic management of the ex-premature infant as detailed in this and the previous chapter.

This baby boy weighing 2kg presented for surgical repair of a unilateral large but easily reducible inguinal hernia at 44 weeks' PCA, having been born at 28 weeks PCA by cesarean section after his mother went into premature labor with premature rupture of membranes. The mother had been given predelivery steroids to encourage lung maturation and surfactant production in the baby's lungs but the baby showed signs of *in utero* fetal distress and a decision was made to deliver early. The birthweight was 1kg and the baby required exogenous surfactant therapy, intubation and ventilatory support for 2 weeks using high-frequency oscillation for severe neonatal respiratory distress syndrome complicated by group B streptococcal septicemia. Weaning from ventilatory support was slow and it became evident that the baby had a patent ductus arteriosus. Medical treatment with nasogastric ibuprofen was unsuccessful and the PDA was clipped via a left mini-thoracotomy performed in the NICU. The baby's lung function improved but he continued to require oxygen therapy for several weeks. A right inguinal hernia was noted but was easily reducible.

After discussion with the surgical team and parents and because the baby lived locally, it was agreed to allow him home and readmit at around 44 weeks' PCA when he had grown a bit more and been weaned from oxygen therapy for a number of weeks. He had no residual cerebral damage and echocardiography revealed normal cardiac anatomy with no residual ductal flow. His blood work-up prior to the hernia repair was normal except for a hemoglobin level of 9g/dL.

Thus, this baby presents as an ex-preterm infant of 44 weeks' PCA with mild bronchopulmonary dysplasia and preoperative anemia. He therefore does have a significant risk of postoperative apnea and arrangements were therefore made to admit him after his inguinal herniotomy to the high-dependency area adjacent to the NICU for monitoring overnight even though he was being considered as suitable for an awake regional block technique. The anesthetic options, benefits and risks and postoperative monitoring and analgesia management were discussed with the parents and it was mutually agreed to use a spinal anesthetic supplemented by a single-shot caudal block. The parents were initially concerned that their baby would be upset by being awake in the OR environment but were reassured by discussion about the use of oral sucrose, topical local anesthesia for the spinal injection and IV cannula sites and the use of a quiet warm OR environment.

The possibilities of failure of the technique or the need to supplement with or convert to general anesthesia were covered and the anesthesiologist discussed his personal results for this technique, which were a failure rate of around 5% overall. The parents agreed to this option and to the postoperative plan for overnight admission for monitoring and ongoing pain control with intravenous or oral acetaminophen. The anemia was also discussed as it is an added risk factor for apnea but the parents were not keen on further blood transfusion if this could possibly be avoided. On balance, it was felt that leaving this untreated was an acceptable risk. The anesthesiologist recommended that the baby should be given caffeine intravenously to help further reduce the propensity for apneic spells and this was agreed. The anesthesiologist discussed this plan with the surgeon who was used to operating on these babies under regional blockade and preferred to do open rather than laparoscopic repairs in small infants.

The baby was scheduled as the first case of the morning and the OR was prepared for a neonate with appropriate equipment, drugs and fluids available for a full general anesthetic as well as regional block in case of block failure. The ambient temperature was set to 23°C. A warm air system and warming mattress were set up and the baby was given a breast feed 4h in advance of the scheduled time and a clear fluid drink 2h in advance. Tetracaine gel was applied to the back of each hand and to the lumbar region 30min in advance of the procedure. The baby was brought into the OR and an IV cannula was sited and maintenance fluids were commenced at a rate of 8mL/h. Caffeine 10mg/kg was administered slowly IV. A neonatal pulse oximetry probe was placed on the right hand and ECG leads applied.

The local anesthesia tray was then prepared for a spinal and caudal block and the anesthetic machine and equipment were also made ready for a 2 kg baby, including facemask, oropharyngeal airways, tracheal tubes, anesthetic and muscle relaxant drugs, atropine and intravenous acetaminophen 7.5 mg/kg. For the spinal/caudal block, full aseptic technique was used including surgical scrub, gown, gloves and mask, skin prep and sterile drapes, equipment and drugs. The local anesthetic used was isobaric levobupivacaine 5 mg/mL concentration at a dose of 1 mg/kg (0.2 mL/kg). An additional 0.1 mL was added to allow for the dead space of the needle and its hub. So, for this 2 kg baby that was a volume of 0.4 + 0.1 mL = 0.5 mL drawn into a 1 mL syringe. A 25 G neonatal lumbar puncture needle was used at the L5–S1 interspace with the baby sitting supported by a trained assistant who paid particular attention to supporting the baby's chin to avoid flexion of the head and neck on the trunk which can cause airway obstruction (this baby was too young to have head control) (Fig. 21.9A,B).

After the spinal injection the baby was immediately placed in the left lateral position and a caudal cannula (22 G) inserted via the sacral hiatus (Fig. 21.9C–F). Levobupivacaine at a concentration of 2.5 mg/mL was slowly injected to a dose of 2 mg/kg (0.8 mL/kg) via the sacral hiatus which was a volume of 1.6 mL for this baby. The caudal cannula was then removed and small dressings

applied to the spinal and caudal puncture sites and the electrocautery grounding plate was applied to the baby's back. The baby was then turned supine and a blood pressure cuff was applied to a lower limb and skin temperature probe applied to a toe. A pacifier with dextrose was given to the baby (50% dextrose via a pinhole made in the nipple), who fell asleep (Fig. 21.9G). The legs were straightened out and stayed straight and gentle skin pinch testing showed a block to just above the umbilical level. The room lights were dimmed, noise levels were kept to a minimum and monitor alarm volumes were minimized.

After surgical prep and draping of the operation field, an open herniotomy was performed in conventional fashion via a 1.5 cm skin incision. The baby did not respond to the incision and showed slight signs of arousal during dissection of the hernia sac but settled after sucking further on the pacifier. Oxygen saturation, respiratory rate, pulse and blood pressure were stable throughout. The operation lasted a total of 20 min from prep to dressing. The spinal/caudal took a total of 20 min from patient arrival in the OR to start of skin prep for surgery. The baby was taken straight to the high-dependency unit and monitoring was applied. No apneic episodes were observed overnight and the baby resumed breast feeding 1 h postoperatively. Acetaminophen was administered orally twice before discharge the following day after surgical review. The parents were delighted and felt this had been a very good option for their baby.

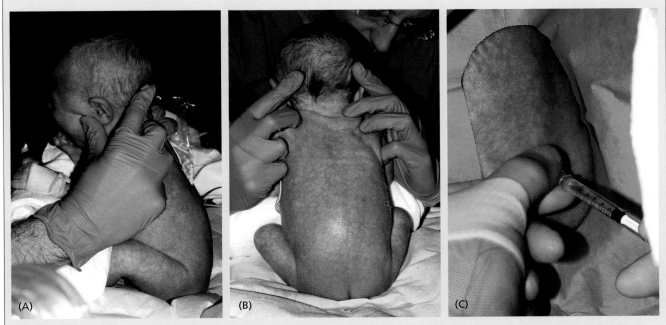

(A)   (B)   (C)

Figure 21.9 Case study sequence of awake spinal-caudal anesthesia. (A) Baby supported in sitting position by trained assistant with head held in neutral position avoiding neck flexion, arms contained and spine curved gently forward to open up the intervertebral spaces. (B) View of the back with the vertebral column in straight alignment. (C) Spinal injection using 25 G needle and 1 mL syringe at L5–S1 interspace. (D) Baby immediately placed in left lateral position for caudal injection. (E) Caudal cannulation using 22 G cannula. (F) Caudal injection of local anesthetic. (G) Pacifier with microdrip feed of 50% dextrose delivered via pinhole in the nipple.

Continued

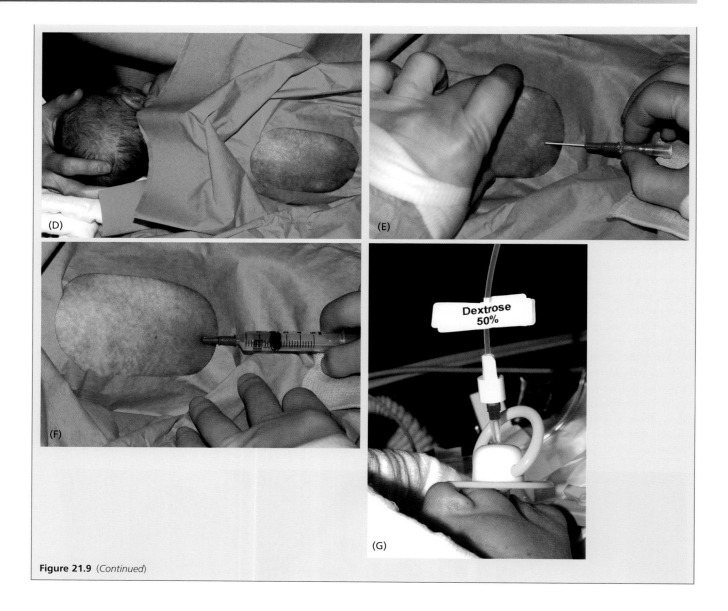

Figure 21.9 (*Continued*)

Annotated references

A full reference list for this chapter is available at:
http://www.wiley.com/go/gregory/andropoulos/pediatricanesthesia

15. Steward DJ. Preterm infants are more prone to complications following minor surgery than are term infants. Anesthesiology 1982; 56: 304–6. The earliest published manuscript describing postanesthetic apnea in ex-premature infants. Gregory described this phenomenon in a textbook chapter in 1981.

21. Welborn LG, de Soto H, Hannallah RS et al. The use of caffeine in the control of post-anesthetic apnea in former premature infants. Anesthesiology 1988; 68: 796–8. The first report of caffeine amelioration of postanesthetic apnea.

29. Coté CJ, Zaslavsky A, Downes JJ et al. Postoperative apnea in former preterm infants after inguinal herniorrhaphy. A combined analysis. Anesthesiology 1995; 82: 809–22. A combination of all pre-

vious data on postanesthetic apnea in former prematures that forms the basis of our understanding of the problem and treatment strategies.

47. Anand KJ. Effects of perinatal pain and stress. Prog Brain Res 2000; 122: 117–29. A comprehensive review of the effects of pain and stress on neurodevelopmental and other outcomes in the perinatal period.

72. Abajian JC, Mellish RW, Browne AF et al. Spinal anesthesia for surgery in the high-risk infant. Anesth Analg 1984; 63: 359–62. An early description of spinal anesthesia alone in the premature and former premature infant.

132. Marven S, Owen A. Contemporary postnatal surgical management strategies for congenital abdominal wall defects. Semin Pediatr Surg 2008; 17: 222–35. A very thorough review of the modern surgical treatment of gastroschisis and omphalocele.

142. Andropoulos DB, Rowe RW, Betts JM. Anaesthetic and surgical airway management during tracheo-oesophageal fistula repair.

Paediatr Anaesth 1998; 8: 313–19. A large retrospective review of airway management techniques and risk factors for adverse ventilatory events in tracheo-esophageal fistula.

169. Brown RA, Bosenberg AT. Evolving management of congenital diaphragmatic hernia. Paediatr Anaesth 2007; 17: 713–19. A thorough contemporary review of treatment options in congenital diaphragmatic hernia.

176. Hickey PR, Hansen DD, Wessel DL et al. Blunting of stress responses in the pulmonary circulation of infants by fentanyl. Anesth Analg 1985; 64: 1137–42. The classic paper describing the cornerstone of treatment and prevention of pulmonary hypertension in high-risk infants.

183. American Heart Association, American Academy of Pediatrics. 2005 American Heart Association (AHA) guidelines for cardiopulmonary resuscitation (CPR) and emergency cardiovascular care (ECC) of pediatric and neonatal patients: neonatal resuscitation guidelines. Pediatrics 2006; 117: e1029–e1038. The latest neonatal resuscitation guidelines.

CHAPTER 22

Anesthesia for the Adolescent and Young Adult Patient

Loren A. Bauman[1], *Joseph R. Tobin*[1] & *Dean B. Andropoulos*[2]

[1]Department of Anesthesiology, Wake Forest University School of Medicine and Wake Forest University Baptist Medical Center, Winston-Salem, NC, USA
[2]Department of Anesthesiology and Pediatrics, Baylor College of Medicine, and Texas Children's Hospital, Houston, TX, USA

Introduction

Adolescence, defined as the time between puberty and adulthood, roughly 13–19 years of age, is a time of significant change for children, even for those without significant health problems. Chronic diseases beginning in infancy and childhood may further complicate the transition to adulthood. The pediatric anesthesiologist cares for patients in both categories and may face a number of challenges in these patients. This chapter first reviews developmental and behavioral issues in adolescents, and then addresses reproductive issues of adolescents as they relate to anesthesia care. Then, common chronic adolescent and young adult illnesses are discussed, including cystic fibrosis, congenital heart disease, cancer, sickle cell anemia, diabetes, inflammatory bowel disease, and developmental disabilities and autism, emphasizing anesthetic care. Finally, obesity and bariatric surgery in the adolescent will be reviewed.

Developmental/behavioral issues in the adolescent

Adolescence, a transitional period between childhood and adulthood, is generally characterized by ongoing cognitive development, greater emotional lability, increased risk-taking behavior, and inconsistencies in behavior modulation [1,2]. Non-compliance with medication administration and other medical treatment regimens, including subspecialty follow-up, is a form of risk-taking behavior. From an evolutionary perspective, while this period prepares the person for independent survival, it also is a period of vulnerability. The social environment is changing. More time is often spent with peers than adult family members. Peer influence is greater and may also influence emotional reactivity. Most of the time these changes are positive but of the 13,000 adolescent deaths in the US annually, about 70% result from risk-taking behavior, including automobile accidents, unintentional trauma, homicide, and suicide.

Several neurobiological hypotheses have been advanced to explain these changes; many have cited increased growth and activity in the prefrontal regions of the brain as the reason for progressively greater cognitive control and affective modulation as a person grows into adulthood. Newer theories implicate the subcortical limbic areas (nucleus accumbens and amygdala) as likely causes of engaging in risky behavior as teenagers, versus adults or younger children. The dopaminergic (DA) system has been linked to reinforcement learning and to high-level cognitive processes and control. The DA system,

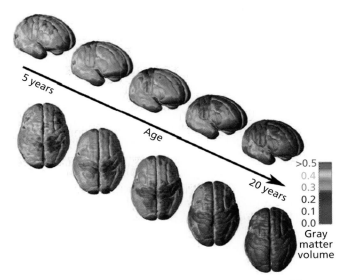

Figure 22.1 Structural changes in gray matter over time derived from serial MRI studies in children, adolescents, and young adults. Right lateral and top views of the dynamic sequence of gray matter maturation over the cortical surface. The side bar shows a color representation in units of gray matter volume. Fifty-two scans from 13 subjects each scanned four times at approximately 2-year intervals. The developmental trajectory of cortical gray matter follows a regionally specific pattern with areas subserving primary functions, such as motor and sensory systems, maturing earliest and higher order association areas, which integrate those primary functions, maturing later. For example, in the temporal lobes the part to reach adult levels latest is the superior temporal gyrus/sulcus which integrates memory, audio-visual input, and object recognition functions. Reproduced from Lenroot and Giedd [3] with permission from Elsevier.

including levels of the neurotransmitter and receptors, undergoes rapid changes during adolescence and some theories postulate that DA activity is greater in the frontal cortex of adolescents, which may result in greater propensity for riskier (and perceived greater reward) behavior. This neurobiological underpinning substantiates the clinical knowledge that, despite their physical size and physiological (i.e. cardiac and pulmonary physiology) similarity to a mature adult and the tendency for healthcare providers to treat them like adults, adolescents have substantial emotional and behavioral differences that may affect anesthetic care [3] (Fig. 22.1).

Substance abuse and "recreational" use of alcohol and drugs (both legal and illegal) is one area of difference between the adolescent and mature adult. Prevalence of alcohol use (any lifetime use) among 10th graders in the US (age 15–16) was estimated at 59.1% in 2009, and any use of illicit drugs, such as marijuana, cocaine, and methamphetamines, was 36.0% [4]. Substance misuse is defined as a maladaptive pattern of use leading to clinically important impairment or distress that is manifested by persistent or recurrent use of the substance despite interference with important functions, such as school,

home life and interpersonal relationships, and issues such as legal problems and use in physically hazardous situations [5]. Substance dependence is much more limited, with daily use of alcohol reported by 1.1% and daily marijuana use by 2.8% of 10th graders [4]. This condition is equivalent to addiction and usually is accompanied by physiological changes related to chronic drug administration, including tolerance, withdrawal, unsuccessful efforts to stop using the drug, interference with important daily activities, and spending a great deal of time and effort obtaining the drug.

Alcohol and drug use and misuse in adolescence have important neurodevelopmental consequences. Functional magnetic resonance imaging (MRI) studies of adults dependent on cocaine have shown abnormal responses in the prefrontal cortex and basal ganglia, including the nucleus accumbens and related structures, and that the clinical effect of cocaine ingestion coincides with rapid saturation of dopamine transporters in the basal ganglia [5]. Other neuroimaging studies have found a smaller prefrontal cortex and hippocampus in young adults who had been dependent on alcohol during adolescence. Large epidemiological studies of US adults found that those who had their first alcoholic drink before age 14 or first drug use before age 15 were three times more likely to develop alcohol or drug dependence than those whose first use was at an older age. Regular use of marijuana before age 15 may be linked with increased risk of subsequent psychosis [5]. As noted above, executive functions are developing in the adolescent and recent research has confirmed associations between poor development of these functions and adolescents who are at high risk of developing alcohol/substance abuse. In addition, there is a familial or genetic component to substance abuse behaviors [6].

Where there is concern that alcohol or substance use may affect the course of the anesthetic, the best course is often to ask the parent or guardian if the anesthesiologist can ask the patient a few questions in private, and then take a history of drug or alcohol use by asking direct questions in a non-threatening, non-accusatory manner, emphasizing that this is necessary to provide the best possible care. In urgent or emergency surgery, where the patient is suspected to be under the influence of alcohol or drugs, it is important to ascertain what drugs were ingested, if possible. Acutely, central nervous system depressants will decrease minimum alveolar concentration (MAC) and other anesthetic requirements, whereas central nervous system (CNS) stimulants often have sympathomimetic effects and increase anesthetic requirements and exaggerate hemodynamic responses, i.e. dangerous hypertension and tachycardia are possible. Chronic use of opioids increases requirements for these drugs, and chronic use of alcohol and other CNS depressants will increase MAC [7–9].

Teen cigarette smoking

Recent US national surveys show that about 20% of 12th graders smoked on at least 1 day in the last month; 8.1% smoked at least 20 days in the last month. This represents a decline of almost 40% since the late 1990s [10]. In the adolescent undergoing anesthesia and surgery, several potential adverse effects of smoking are possible. General anesthesia-related airway and respiratory events are more common in smokers. In a large prospective study of over 26,000 anesthetics, adverse events were compared in 7100 smokers and 19,000 non-smokers, including patients as young as 16 years of age. Respiratory events, including bronchospasm (most frequent event), laryngospasm, hypoxemia, and other events were 2.3 times more common in young smokers [11]. It is well known that carbon monoxide levels in the blood of heavy smokers may exceed 10%, impairing oxygen-carrying capacity and delivery. Cigarettes function as a means to rapidly deliver nicotine to the CNS. Nicotine activates several types of acetylcholine receptors, predominately in the CNS, and is postulated to modulate neurotransmitter release, including dopamine. Despite its potential effects on pain modulation and acute withdrawal of nicotine in the postoperative period, several studies in adults have demonstrated that nicotine withdrawal symptoms are minimal, and thus perhaps this is an opportunity to achieve sustained abstinence from tobacco [12]. An important effect of tobacco smoke exposure is its ability to exacerbate asthma symptoms and to precipitate bronchospasm; since the incidence of asthma is at its peak during adolescence, any teenager with asthma who smokes should be strongly encouraged to quit [13].

Pregnancy/reproductive issues in the adolescent and young adult

Teenage pregnancy testing before anesthesia is a controversial topic but recent data and publications offer some guidance for pediatric anesthesiologists [14,15]. In 2006 in the US, 750,000 women younger than 20 years of age became pregnant. The pregnancy rate was 71.5 pregnancies per 1000 women aged 15–19, meaning pregnancies occurred among about 7% of women in this age group. In general, the teen pregnancy rate has declined for the past 30 years and in 2005, the US teenage pregnancy rate reached its lowest point in more than 30 years (69.5 per 1000), down 41% since its peak in 1990 (116.9). There was a 3% increase in 2006, the first such increase in more than a decade [16]. The teenage birthrate in 2006 was 41.9 births per 1000 women, a total of over 435,000 births. This was 32% lower than the peak rate of 61.8 reached in 1991, but 4% higher than in 2005. From 1986 to 2006, the proportion of teenage pregnancies ending in abortion declined almost one-third, from 46% to 32% of pregnancies among 15–19 year olds. About 18% of the US female population was estimated to become a teen mother in 2006 [17].

These interesting data make the point that teenage pregnancy is not a rare condition, and indicate that the anesthesiologist must consider the possibility that the patient is pregnant when caring for adolescent females. Taking a history about possible pregnancy and missed menstrual periods is known to be inaccurate, so many pediatric anesthesia departments have instituted policies for routine urine human chorionic gonadotropin (HCG) testing in menstruating females before anesthesia. At Texas Children's Hospital (TCH), parents are told that this urine pregnancy testing is routine, but exceptions can be made at the discretion of the anesthesiologist based on medical or cultural grounds. Positive tests are rare, but when pregnancy is detected by serum HCG testing, the surgeon, anesthesiologist, and social worker inform the parent after obtaining permission from the patient. Elective surgery is cancelled because of the potential effects of anesthetics, including benzodiazepines, halogenated anesthetic agents, and nitrous oxide, on early fetal development. Emergency surgery proceeds, but agents that may be implicated in fetal malformations are avoided. At TCH, in 2008–2010, of over 91,000 anesthetics, approximately 9% were performed in menstruating females. During this period, only four of more than 6000 urine HCG tests were positive.

Before implementing a policy concerning preoperative urine pregnancy testing, institutional, local, and state laws and regulations must be consulted. In general, reproductive confidentiality laws mandate that the pregnant teen under the age of 18 has the right to be informed first of a positive test and to decide whether parents are to be notified. In practice, this situation is rare, and the involvement of experts in social work, behavioral health, and adolescent medicine is highly desirable in this complicated situation.

Chronic diseases in the adolescent and young adult, and transition to adult care

Pediatric anesthesiologists care for many patients for procedures caused by chronic diseases that are congenital or start in infancy or early childhood and continue through adolescence, into adulthood. Very often, these patients and their parents are very attached to their caregivers in the pediatric environment and have developed great trust and confidence in them. The expertise in a specialized pediatric field, such as congenital heart disease, is not widely available in the adult care environment, and many of these patients are understandably anxious about changing to providers in an adult setting.

Because over 90% of children with chronic diseases now survive into adolescence and early adulthood, the concept of transition of care to the adult environment has assumed increasing importance in recent years. In a study of 283 patients aged 14–25 years with chronic conditions that spanned a range of subspecialties and had not yet transferred their care to adult healthcare, 50% of patients thought the best age to transfer care was 18–19 years, while 14% felt that 20 years or older was best. Thirty-nine percent of respondents felt that chronological age was the most important factor in deciding when to transfer care, and 34% said that feeling too old to see a pediatric specialist was the most important factor. Only 11% believed that their relationship with the pediatric specialist was a factor, and 3.5% felt that the severity of the chronic disease was important. Barriers to transition included feeling at ease with the pediatric specialist (45%), anxiety because of not knowing the adult specialist (20%), and lack of information about adult services (18%) [18]. This ambivalence on the part of patients, parents, and pediatric caregivers leads to many young adults being cared for in the pediatric setting and to variable policies about age limits for pediatric care, which are often different for different services in the same institution. In a study of 73 pediatric emergency departments (ED) in the US, 79% had age limits for treatment, with 18 and 21 years the most often cited age cut-offs. Those EDs with age limits over 21 years were most often associated with free-standing children's hospitals. There were many subspecialty-specific exceptions to the age policy that allowed older patients to be cared for by pediatricians, with cystic fibrosis (64%), congenital heart disease (56%), and sickle cell disease (53%) the most common. Interestingly, allowing care in the adult environment for patients less than 18 years was most frequent for teen pregnancy (79%), burn patients (50%), and psychiatric patients (40%). Only 18% of institutions had a specific transition of care policy [19].

Recommendations for transition of care for pediatric patients include starting education of the patient and family about transition several years in advance, having the patient acquire increasing age-appropriate information about the disease, and taking increasing responsibility for their own care, i.e. medication administration and insurance information, and having them understand the differences between the adult and pediatric systems [20]. It should also be noted that mentally competent young adult patients (18 years in the US) legally must sign their own consent for treatments.

Several of the most common chronic disease states presenting for anesthesia care occur in the transition period from adolescence to adulthood and will be discussed below.

Cystic fibrosis

Cystic fibrosis (CF) is an autosomal recessive disease that primarily affects the respiratory and gastrointestinal systems. Historically, CF was a uniformly fatal disease of childhood, but has become more a disease of adolescents and adulthood with the mean age of survival now being 37 years. This improvement in mortality is the direct result of more aggressive, standardized treatment involving many disciplines [21–24].

In the past, CF was considered a disease of the Caucasian population. We now know that the incidence of CF in Caucasian, Hispanics, and African American births is 1 in 2500, 1 in 12,000, and 1 in 15,000 respectively. One thousand patients are newly diagnosed with CF each year in the US. The prevalence is growing quickly, due to the increase in median survival age.

The fundamental defect in CF is a gene mutation on the long arm of chromosome 7 that encodes a protein, cystic fibrosis transmembrane receptor (CFTR), in the apical membrane of epithelial cells in submucosal glands. CFTR is important for the regulation of airway surface liquid. The CFTR mutation causes defective chloride secretion and excessive sodium reabsorption that results in loss of airway surface liquid [25,26]. Beyond the problems of regulating surface liquid, a profound inflammatory response is present in patients with CF that is only partially explained by ongoing infection. The cumulative effect of the inflammatory response is persistent progressive symptoms and irreversible lung damage.

More than 1000 known mutations in the CFTR gene have been identified, but genotype and phenotype correlate poorly, especially regarding the severity of lung disease. Certain genotypes are closely tied to development of CF liver disease and portal hypertension (SERPINA1 A allele), while other genotypes increase the risk of developing type 2 diabetes with CF (TCF7L2) or of developing pancreatic insufficiency [27,28].

Pulmonary disease causes 90% of the morbidity and mortality associated with CF. Pulmonary goblet cells exude a thick tenacious mucus that overwhelms mucociliary clearance. Patients develop a severe unremitting cough to try and remove these secretions. The accumulation of secretions leads to airway occlusion, atelectasis, and hypoxemia. Retained viscid mucus is a fertile growth medium for bacteria, especially *Pseudomonas aeruginosa* and *Staphylococcus aureus*. Pulmonary disease begins at a very early age with evidence of lower tract respiratory infections, neutrophilic inflammation, elevated interleukin (IL)-8, and elastase present in infants (median age 3.6 months). *Pseudomonas* can be cultured from over 50% of asymptomatic children. Cough is a poor indicator of

Pseudomonas carriage. Left undetected or untreated, *P. aeruginosa* leads to increased inflammatory cytokine response and poorer clinical status, which are all made worse by the concomitant presence of *Staph. aureus*. In older patients, airway contamination with the fungus *Aspergillus fumigatus* and *Stenotrophomonas maltophilia*, an aerobic motile gram-negative rod of low virulence, develops as a consequence of repeated courses of antibiotics [26]. The infections trigger a neutrophilic inflammatory response that damages airways and eventually causes bronchiectasis and bronchomalacia.

The chest roentgenogram may show hyperinflation and flattened diaphragms, bronchiectasis, and cyst formation. Tram-track radiodensities are parallel lines from advanced peribronchial cuffing and bronchial wall thickening. Computed tomography (CT) scans reveal the extent of pulmonary involvement but may overestimate severity of disease based on exercise tolerance.

Airway reactivity is common and may worsen in adolescence. The response to β-agonist bronchodilators may worsen expiratory flow due to progressive loss of airway cartilaginous support. The airway becomes more dependent on muscle tone for patency, and the airways become floppy and similar to bronchomalacia. Further smooth muscle relaxation by bronchodilators increases airway obstruction.

Pulmonary function tests (PFTs) reveal severe airway obstruction that may be poorly responsive to or worsen with bronchodilators. While PFTs typically demonstrate increased residual volume/total lung volume (RV/TLV) ratios and decreased forced expiratory volume during 25–75% of expiration (FEV_{25-75}), the reduction in forced expiratory volume in 1 sec (FEV_1) correlates with reduced survival [21]. Outcome predictors are rapid loss of pulmonary function, poor nutritional status, presence of *Pseudomonas*, persistent rales on pulmonary examination, and frequent clinical illness from infections [29].

Progressive bronchiectasis and airflow obstruction ultimately lead to hypoxemia and hypercarbia. Destruction of pulmonary architecture and chronic hypoxia cause pulmonary hypertension, right ventricular hypertrophy, and eventually cor pulmonale. Patients may feel better with home oxygen and non-invasive ventilation support with continuous positive airway pressure (CPAP) or bilevel positive airway pressure (BiPAP). These adjuvants may be very helpful during postoperative care.

All mucosal cells are affected by the defective CFTR and the associated generalized mucosal hypertrophy. Nasal mucosal hyperplasia causes chronic sinusitis. Pedunculated nasal polyps are found in nearly half of patients and occur most commonly during adolescence. Although surgical removal of polyps may be necessary, the use of rehydration therapy with hypertonic saline irrigation, topical or inhaled nasal rhDNase, and glucocorticoids may be helpful. The presence of nasal polyposis makes the use of nasopharyngeal airways or nasal tracheal tubes a higher risk than normal.

Pancreatic exocrine function is reduced in 90% of patients. The dysfunctional chloride–bicarbonate exchanger induced by the absent CFTR impairs bicarbonate secretion. Consequently, the volume and pH of pancreatic secretions are reduced. Pancreatic enzymes plug the pancreatic duct; retention of those enzymes causes inflammation and autodigestion of the pancreas.

Antenatal accumulation of viscid secretions causes meconium ileus, a bowel obstruction in neonates that is caused by inspissated secretions derived from the intestinal mucosa glands. Adolescents and adults may have recurrent gastrointestinal obstruction, a meconium ileus equivalent, through a similar mechanism. This condition is better termed distal intestinal obstruction syndrome because it may occur in the colon or the ileum. Advanced pancreatic disease, dehydration, irregular use of pancreatic enzyme supplements, and use of medications that slow intestinal transport are precipitating factors of this condition.

Tenacious secretions obstruct pancreatic exocrine ducts, reducing overall pancreatic secretion of lipase, an enzyme necessary for the hydrolysis and subsequent absorption of fat. Inadequate absorption of fat-soluble vitamins (vitamins A, D, E, and K) worsens the patient's nutritional state and overall quality of life. Vitamin D deficiency leads to fractures due to inadequate calcification of bones. Vitamin K deficiency, caused by either malabsorption or reduced enteral bacterial synthesis of vitamin K synthesis as a result of chronic antibiotic use, causes coagulopathy. Vitamin E deficiency results in ataxia, decreased sensation to vibration, lack of reflexes, and paralysis of eye muscles. A decline in cognitive function is an early sign of vitamin E deficiency, particularly in the preteen years. Vitamin A deficiency causes predominantly eye and skin problems, while excessive supplementation of vitamin A may harm the respiratory and skeletal systems of children. A Cochrane review found no studies that showed that regular vitamin A consumption is beneficial for people with cystic fibrosis [30].

Enteric-coated pancreatic enzyme supplements (Creon®, a delayed release form of pancrelipase, Pancrease (lipase, amylase, and protease)) and fat-soluble vitamin supplements are essential elements of supportive care.

Pancreatic endocrine dysfunction gradually develops from the progressive autodigestion of the pancreas. The loss of islet cell function may trigger diabetes. Curiously, insulin resistance may also be present and further complicate glucose homeostasis. Preparation for intraoperative care requires skilled management of both hyper- and hypoglycemia. Microvascular deterioration of the retina, kidneys, and peripheral nerves is more frequent with prolonged poor glucose management.

The younger the age at diagnosis, the greater is the liver and pancreatic compromise. One-third of patients will have liver dysfunction, fatty infiltration, cirrhosis, and portal hypertension. Death from cirrhosis is the second most common cause of death in patients with CF. This progression typically occurs in specific histocompatibility complex genotypes, with male gender, or when nutrition is poor. If liver disease is suspected from function tests, preoperative evaluations for biliary fibrosis and cirrhosis may be necessary, since they may cause coagulopathy and altered drug metabolism.

Bone demineralization is common in patients with CF. Poor nutritional status, malabsorption of vitamin D, and the administration of steroids are precipitating factors for both fractures and scoliosis. In addition, chronic pulmonary infections increase serum cytokines that stimulate bone resorption. Scoliosis and/or kyphosis is present in 75% of female and over 30% of male patients older than 15 years. Prevention of skeletal degeneration includes aggressive nutritional support, pancreatic enzyme supplements, fat-soluble vitamins, and treatment with growth hormone, calcium, and sex steroids.

Congenital absence of the vas deferens with obstructive azoospermia causes infertility in 95% of males. Menstrual irregularity from chronic disease and thick cervical secretions reduces fertility in females. The natural history of cystic fibrosis is one of progressive deterioration of the condition. It is important to carefully monitor the quality-of-life indicators, the presence of depression, and patients' ability to cope, as these will directly affect a patient's compliance with treatment [31].

Treatment of cystic fibrosis

Inhaled hypertonic saline acutely increases mucociliary clearance and is a safe, inexpensive means of clearing secretions. Chest physiotherapy, employing percussion with exhalation flutter valves or direct chest compression, improves the efficacy of the patient's cough.

Even though used clinically for decades, the effectiveness of inhaled N-acetylcysteine (NAD) (Mucomyst®) has recently been questioned. NAD is thought to reduce mucus viscosity by splitting the disulfide bonds of mucoproteins, but evidence that this improves mucus clearance is absent [32]. However, high-dose oral NAD is thought to modulate inflammation in patients with CF and may counter the intertwined redox and inflammatory imbalances present [33].

Aerosolized antibiotics (i.e. tobramycin, aztreonam) decrease the population of *P. aeruginosa*, thereby reducing hospitalization and the rate of pulmonary deterioration. Even short-term use of inhaled aztreonam improves lung function [34] and quality-of-life indicators.

Oral azithromycin, an acid-stable derivative of the macrolide antibiotic erythromycin, is a recent addition to standardized maintenance therapy for patients with cystic fibrosis. The drug's principal effects appear to be unrelated to its antibiotic effect but acts through modulation of the proinflammation effects of bacterial infection and alteration of the virulence of *Pseudomonas*. Azithromycin interferes with neutrophil recruitment, chemotaxis, and oxidative bursts, all of which injure airways during infections. With protracted use, azithromycin is associated with gradual improvements in FEV_1 and forced vital capacity (FVC). It appears especially useful in patients with persistent *Pseudomonas* infection, an effect that may not be the result of its antibiotic potential. Subinhibitory concentration of azithromycin can be bactericidal to *P. aeruginosa* when exposed for protracted periods [35].

Bacterial growth in biofilms is associated with reduced sensitivity to antibiotics. Biofilm formation is iron dependent, and iron chelation therapy combined with antibiotics reduces biofilm formation and enhances antibiotic susceptibility of *P. aeruginosa* [36].

Deoxyribonuclease I (DNase), a bovine recombinant enzyme, and its recombinant twin rhDNase (Pulmozyme®) catalyze the hydrolytic cleavage of phosphodiester linkages in the DNA in white blood cells that accumulate in the mucus. Hydrolysis of white cell DNA reduces "stickiness" of the mucus, which makes it much easier to clear mucus from the lungs. The net effect is to reduce air trapping, improve FEV_1, and reduce the frequency of clinical infections. Although rhDNase efficaciously reduces atelectasis, hyperinflation, and mediastinal shift over a period of 3 days, its use in the hyperacute setting of the operating room has not been demonstrated. Prolonged use of rhDNase does not reduce pulmonary bacterial colonization, and the timing of its administration to chest percussion is a subject of considerable debate.

A new treatment option is to increase the amount of functioning CFTR at the cell surface. Miglustat (Zavesca®), a drug used for patients with type I Gaucher disease, has a CFTR corrector effect when given by inhalation. Miglustat activates CFTR-dependent chloride transport in mice that have a similar mutation [37]. Another new agent, spiperone, is a psychoactive butyrophenone that activates the specific genetic defect in the chloride channel in airway epithelium. Prolonged use of the long-acting β_2 adrenoreceptor salmeterol acts via the CFTR as a potent chloride secretagogue. Interestingly, it appears to act by reducing the internalization of the β_2 adrenoreceptor, thereby restoring chloride secretion and airway surface liquid [38].

Sinus surgery in cystic fibrosis

The paranasal sinuses become infected before pulmonary contamination and infection begin. As patients age, they are more likely to have infection in both their upper and lower airways. Bacteria spread from the sinuses to the lungs of patients with CF [39]. Because the upper and lower respiratory tracts have the same mucosal lining, improvements in sinus health reduce the frequency and severity of lower tract infections.

Nasal obstruction and chronic rhinosinusitis (CRS) are common otorhinological manifestations of CF. The altered viscoelastic properties of mucus result in impaired ciliary function and obstruction of sinus ostia. Chronic sinusitis and mucosal edema lead to sinonasal polyposis and nasal obstruction in nearly all adolescent and adult patients. Sinonasal disease increases the risks of pneumonia, the bacterial origin of which is the paranasal sinuses [40].

The prevalence of nasal polyposis in children with CF is between 6% and 48% [40]. Nasal polyps begin as an edematous growth of mucosa that is a consequence of inflammatory mucosal reaction in the paranasal sinuses. Polyps are commonly found bilaterally and lead to septal deviation, bulging of the nasal dorsum, and even hypertelorism [41].

Almost all patients with CF have CT abnormalities of their sinuses, but the findings do not correlate well with symptom severity. Surgical intervention for sinus disease is based on management of symptoms, pulmonary status, and frequency of infection. Endoscopic sinus surgery is safe and at least temporarily effective at reducing these complications. Grading the severity of nasal polyposis can help predict the need for future sinus surgery [42].

Chronic high-dose ibuprofen appears to effectively manage nasal polyposis in young adults with CF [43]. Hypertonic saline lavages improve clearance of viscid secretions. Despite aggressive medical management, approximately one-quarter of patients with CF will require sinus surgery. Paranasal sinus surgery in pediatric and young adult patients with CF can be safely performed and improves individual rhinosinusitis symptoms (less facial pain, headache, nasal obstruction, postnasal drip and rhinorrhea). While combined medical and surgical management may yield symptomatic relief, the infections, obstruction, and nasal polyposis can recur because CF is a chronic, unremitting disease.

Intraoperative management of patients with CF undergoing open or endoscopic sinus surgery includes appreciation of the degree of nasal airway obstruction, avoiding instrumentation of nares with tracheal tubes and nasal airways, management of vitamin K-deficient coagulopathy, and having readily available equipment to suction tenacious mucus from the lungs.

Portosystemic shunts

Liver disease occurs in over one-quarter of patients with CF and is the second most common cause of death in these patients [44]. The purported pathophysiological mechanism of liver injury is focal inspissation of bile due to its abnormal viscosity, decreased bile flow, and high concentrations of bile in the liver tissue. Decreased bile flow obstructs small biliary ductules and induces collagen deposition in the portal tracts [45]. The spectrum of clinical liver disease in patients with CF runs from cholestasis to focal biliary cirrhosis to multilobular cirrhosis, and finally to portal hypertension. In its most severe clinical states, portal hypertension occurs in 7% of patients, with a preponderance of male gender. It causes massive splenomegaly, ascites, and bleeding from esophageal varices [46]. Initial management of variceal bleeding may include sclerotherapy, but one of the various forms of portosystemic shunts (Fig. 22.2) is often required to provide more definitive relief of portal hypertension and of its complications [47].

Pulmonary surgery in cystic fibrosis

Pulmonary surgery in patients with CF requires special comment. Surgical treatment of bronchiectasis, whether segmental or diffuse, may be indicated to reduce cough and sputum production, and to decrease formation of new areas of bronchiectasis. Pulmonary function is affected very little by the lung resection, since the area of diseased lung contributes little to respiratory function. Lung resection may reduce the severity of symptoms and improve oxygenation. Even large resections may be tolerated.

In severe or recurring cases of pneumothorax, bleb resection and/or multiple treatments with talc pleurodesis may be necessary. Talc creates an enhanced plural reaction and causes the parietal and visceral pleural surfaces to adhere, thereby reducing the frequency of pneumothorax. This technique is particularly helpful in patients with bleb formation. Unfortunately, future surgical procedures (i.e. lobe resections, lung transplants) are made more difficult by this procedure.

Cystic fibrosis is the third most common indication for pulmonary transplantation in adolescents and adults. The criteria for transplantation are a calculated survival of less than 50%, typically marked by a FEV_1 less than 30%, a PaO_2 of less than 50 mmHg, and a $PaCO_2$ greater than 55 mmHg. The most common precipitating conditions for transplantation are progressive loss of FEV_1 to <30%, severe hypoxemia and hypercarbia, increasing frequency of hospitalization, and hemoptysis. When transplantation is a consideration, bilateral lung transplants are usually required to avoid cross-contamination of the good lung. A review of 9 years of pulmonary transplantation revealed that the

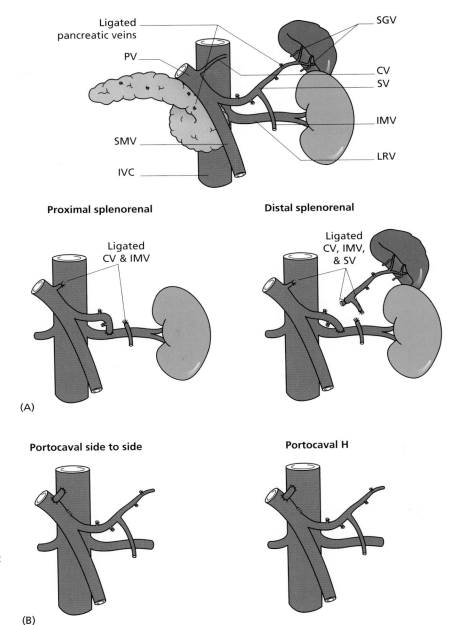

Figure 22.2 The four major types of portocaval shunts. PV, portal vein; CV, cardiac vein; SV, splenic vein; IMV, inferior mesenteric vein; LRV, left renal vein; SMV, superior mesenteric vein; IVC, inferior vena cava; SGV, short gastric veins. Reproduced from Lillegard et al [47] with permission.

cumulative survival of older patients is better than that of younger patients [48]. Older patients have fewer infections, less bronchiolitis obliterans, and fewer graft rejections. Transplantation in patients 6–10 years of age for CF has similar overall survival to patients of the same age being transplanted for other reasons. Evidence-based decision aids help to improve expectations of lung transplantation and prepare patients for the post-transplantation experience [49]. See Chapter 27 for a detailed discussion of the anesthetic management of lung transplantation.

Anesthetic management in cystic fibrosis

Perioperative evaluation depends on the severity of the clinical disease and the extent of the operative intervention planned. Routine chemistries, liver profile, and coagulation assessments are warranted. Exercise tolerance is a good prognostic indicator of the risk for postoperative pulmonary complications. Preoperative arterial blood gases (ABGs) help determine the severity of disease and may help guide postoperative care.

The anesthetic should be designed to facilitate early tracheal extubation and avoid prolonged mechanical ventilation. Volatile agent anesthetics may benefit patients with bronchodilator-responsive bronchospastic disease. Total intravenous anesthesia (TIVA) may be well suited for patients whose degree of airway obstruction worsens with bronchodilators or when vapor diffusion is severely affected by the extent of pulmonary disease.

Propofol normally has 30% first-pass metabolism in the lungs, but clearance of this drug may be substantially increased by the presence of an active inflammatory lung process like cystic fibrosis. Consequently, much larger doses of propofol may be required to achieve adequate anesthesia. Inadequate insulin supply plus resistance to insulin makes intraoperative glucose monitoring imperative. Tracheal tube size should be as large as feasible to facilitate tracheal suctioning. Because of nasal mucosa hypertrophy and the potential for nasal polyps, nasal airway devices should be avoided if possible. Inspired anesthetic gases should be warmed and humidified; frequent airway suctioning, with or without bronchodilators, may be required.

Use of neuromuscular blockade (NMB) may complicate ventilation of patients who rely on muscle tone for airway patency. Avoiding prolonged administration of NMB, particularly in combination with adrenocorticosteroids, is essential to avoid muscle weakness, prolonged ventilation support, and additional pulmonary infections.

Prior to tracheal extubation, tracheal suctioning, with or without aerosolized hypertonic saline, and lung recruitment maneuvers help restore pulmonary function. Patients may need longer periods of observation postoperatively to effectively balance analgesia needs with the need for additional oxygen support.

Non-invasive support of ventilation (CPAP, BiPAP) is helpful postoperatively. Aggressive pulmonary toilet that includes percussion, postural drainage, and flutter valve therapy improves postoperative lung function. Inhaled hypertonic saline or rhDNase may facilitate clearance of secretions and efficaciously treat atelectasis.

Postoperative pain control should not be provided exclusively with opioids because of their effect on intestinal transit and the potential to initiate distal intestinal obstruction syndrome. Acceptable analgesic adjuvants include non-steroidal anti-inflammatory drugs, continuous IV infusion of lidocaine (because of its ability to reduce inflammation), and low-dose ketamine (for modulation of pain via the NMDA receptor). If the procedure and parameters permit, regional or neuroaxial anesthesia may lower the risks of altered drug metabolism and excretion.

Congenital heart disease

Congenital heart disease (CHD) is present in 8 per 1000 births in the US and Europe and is the most common birth defect requiring treatment. Because of improved survival rates (>90%) after neonatal and infant cardiac surgery for complex cardiac lesions, the vast majority of these patients survive into adolescence and adulthood and will present for both cardiac and non-cardiac surgery for the same range of procedures found in patients without CHD. In the US there are approximately 1 million children and 1 million adults over the age of 18 living with CHD. Of these survivors, 55% have simple disease, 30% moderately complex, and 15% complex lesions [50]. In patients with CHD, having current, accurate information about the status of their cardiac condition and repair is crucial. Patients with complex and moderately complex lesions must have a recent evaluation by a cardiologist who has expertise in congenital heart disease, and must have their medical condition optimized for the surgery and anesthetic [51]. Patients with significant potential for cardiovascular instability and need of specialized care should undergo anesthesia whenever possible only in facilities where such expertise is readily available. Infective endocarditis prophylaxis guidelines must be followed [52]. For more detail about the preanesthetic evaluation and anesthetic management of patients with CHD for both cardiac and non-cardiac surgery, see Chapter 25.

Cancer

The most common new cancers diagnosed in the adolescent population, in the 10–14 and 15–19 year age groups, are:

- leukemias (32 and 33 per million)
- lymphomas (25 and 47 per million)
- brain and spinal neoplasms (37 and 43 per million)
- malignant bone tumors (13 and 14 per million)
- soft tissue and other extraosseous sarcomas (13 and 17 per million) [53].

Five-year survival for all cancers in childhood, 1999–2006, is 79.8%, with leukemias and lymphomas having the best survival at 80–90%, and malignant bone and CNS cancer the lowest survival at 60–70% [54].

These adolescent cancer patients require anesthesia for a wide variety of procedures, including primary and secondary tumor resections (sometimes after initial chemotherapy) and metastatic lesions, vascular access procedures, bone marrow aspirations, and many others. The reader is referred to chapters elsewhere in this book for a discussion of anesthetic management of procedures in specific organ systems. Radiation therapy is common in these patients. Emergency radiation therapy in patients with a lymphoma or leukemia and an anterior mediastinal mass and airway obstruction is a rare occurrence, but when present is fraught with the dangers of managing the airway and transporting the patient to a remote location. See Chapter 24 for a discussion of the anesthetic management of the patient with a mediastinal mass.

Many patients require follow-up imaging procedures, including MRI, CT, positron emission tomography/CT (PET/CT), and ultrasound; in the vast majority of adolescent patients, these procedures can be done without anesthesia or sedation.

As with many other congenital and acquired conditions in childhood, survival from childhood cancers has increased dramatically over the past several decades, and many of these patients require anesthesia care for follow-up or treatment of their cancer or for completely unrelated issues. It is important for the anesthesiologist to understand the residual medical and psychological problems that can be present in these adolescents [55]. It also is important to understand the past treatments of these patients, particularly chemotherapy and radiation therapy, which can have severe effects on cardiac and pulmonary function (Table 22.1). For example, anthracycline chemotherapy may cause cardiomyopathy. Consequently, routine follow-up with echocardiography is performed on all these patients. Pulmonary and renal toxicity should also be determined and the anesthetic planned accordingly. Cranial irradiation is used commonly to treat leukemia and CNS tumors. This therapy is associated with a significant incidence of neurodevelopmental disability.

As with many chronic illnesses, survivors of childhood cancer have an increased incidence of psychological problems. In a review of psychological and quality-of-life studies in over 7000 adolescent and young adult cancer survivors, it was found that cancer survivors were 80% more likely to report clinically relevant impairments in mental health, and twice as likely to report emotional distress [56]. Those with particularly high levels of anxiety and depression are patients with CNS tumors, bone tumors, leukemia and lymphoma, and those who have undergone cranial irradiation. Chronic pain may also be an important component of the residual medical problems of cancer survivors.

Sickle cell disease

Sickle cell disease (SCD) is an autosomal dominant condition caused by the substitution of valine for glutamate at the sixth position of the β-globin chain of hemoglobin; this produces hemoglobin S instead of hemoglobin A. Sickle cell anemia is most common in populations whose origins are Africa, South or Central America (especially Panama), Caribbean islands, Mediterranean countries (Turkey, Greece, and Italy), India, and Saudi Arabia. In the US, an estimated 70,000–100,000 children and adults have sickle cell anemia, mainly African Americans. The disease occurs in about 1 out of every 500 African American births and in more than 1 out of every 36,000 Hispanic American births. More than 2 million Americans have sickle cell trait (homozygous hemoglobin AS); this

Table 22.1 Long-term effects of childhood cancer

System	Risk factor	Potential effect
Cardiac	Radiation therapy Anthracyclines	Valvular disease Pericarditis Myocardial infarction Congestive heart failure Sudden death
Pulmonary	Radiation therapy Carmustine/Lomustine Bleomycin	Restrictive lung disease Exercise intolerance

Renal/
urological
	Radiation therapy
	Platinums
	Ifosfamide and
	  cyclophosphamide
	Ciclosporin A
	Nephrectomy
		Atrophy or hypertrophy
		Renal insufficiency or
		  failure
		Hydronephrosis
		Chronic cystitis

Endocrine	Radiation therapy
	Alkylating agents
		Growth failure
		Pituitary, thyroid, and
		  adrenal disease
		Ovarian or testicular
		  failure
		Delayed secondary sex
		  characteristics
		Infertility

Central nervous system	Radiation therapy Intrathecal chemotherapy	Learning disabilities

Psychosocial	Childhood cancer	Post-traumatic stress
		  disorder
		Employment and
		  educational difficulties
		Insurance discrimination
		Adaptation and
		  problem-solving
		  difficulties
		Difficulties with
		  transition to
		  independence

Second malignancies	Radiation therapy Alkylating agents Epipodophyllotoxins Type of primary malignancy	Solid tumors Leukemia Lymphoma Brain tumors

Reproduced from Henderson et al [55] with permission from the American Academy of Pediatrics.

condition occurs in about 1 in 12 African Americans [57]. Homozygous hemoglobin SS causes abnormal aggregation of hemoglobin under conditions of low oxygen tension or acidosis, which results in reduced red cell elasticity and the characteristic sickle shape of erythrocytes

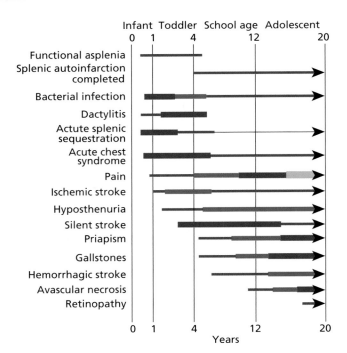

Figure 22.3 Sickle cell disease complications by age. Width and color of arrow shaft signifies the relative incidence of the complication. Reproduced from Redding-Lallinger and Knoll [58] with permission from Elsevier.

seen with homozygous sickle cell disease. This in turn impedes passage of the deformed erythrocytes through capillaries of all organs and results in the myriad problems seen with this disease. (Fig. 22.3). Red cell survival is shortened, which leads to hemolysis and anemia; most patients maintain hemoglobin concentrations of 7–9 g/dL. Homozygous SS patients have hemoglobin S concentrations that exceed 80% and are usually significantly affected by the disease. In the US about two-thirds of sickle cell disease patients have this genotype. Other variants, such as hemoglobin SC disease or hemoglobin S-β-thalassemia, are also frequently encountered. In terms of severity of disease, hemoglobin SS and S-β° thalassemia genotypes generally are most affected, although symptoms are variable. Heterozygous carriers with one copy of the hemoglobin S gene are usually relatively asymptomatic [58].

Problems of particular importance for adolescents with SCD are acute painful crises and chronic pain, strokes, priapism, cholelithiasis, and avascular necrosis of the hip and other joints. Acute chest syndrome episodes that result in pulmonary hypertension are also seen in this age group.

Current therapy for SCD often includes chronic transfusion therapy to maintain higher levels of hemoglobin A and lower levels of hemoglobin S. This therapy has been demonstrated to reduce episodes of painful crisis, stroke, priapism, and acute chest syndrome, and to reduce risk for chronic pain and pulmonary hypertension. However,

it also increases the risk of transfusion reactions. In recent years treatment with hydroxyurea has been shown to increase the percentage of hemoglobin F (fetal hemoglobin) and decrease hemoglobin S. This results in fewer episodes of painful crises and acute chest syndrome. Leukopenia and thrombocytopenia are possible side-effects of hydroxyurea treatment. Packed red blood cell transfusion or exchange transfusion is used for acute problems, such as acute chest syndrome, painful crises, priapism, and acute stroke. Erythrocytes for transfusion should be sickle negative, leukocyte poor, and matched for C, E, c, e and Kell antigens, as well as Rh D and ABO (extended cross-matching or partial phenotypic matching). This reduces the risk of alloantibody sensitization against the many antigens the patient is likely to be exposed to during future transfusion therapy. Hematopoietic stem cell transplantation in children with SCD is 85% effective in curing the disease.

The goal of perioperative anesthetic management in patients with SCD is prevention of excessive sickling of abnormal cells and thus prevention of significant complications, such as acute chest syndrome, painful crises, stroke, and other major problems. The cornerstones of management are avoidance of known precipitating factors for sickling, including hypoxemia, hypovolemia, acidosis, and hypothermia, which induce a vicious cycle of red cell adherence to endothelium, vaso-occlusion, further tissue hypoxia and ischemia, inflammation, activation of coagulation, and further vasoconstriction (Fig. 22.4).

Among the most common surgical procedures that adolescents with SCD require are cholecystectomy for chronic hemolysis-induced cholelithiasis, tonsillectomy, orthopedic procedures for avascular necrosis, and priapism. Case reports and case series of other major procedures, including cardiac surgery with cardiopulmonary bypass, have also been published [59–61]. The most recent consensus guidelines about perioperative management of SCD patients were published in 2002 by the US National Institutes of Health National Heart, Lung, and Blood Institute [62] (Box 22.1). Besides strict attention to preoperative hydration, oxygenation, temperature maintenance with warmed intravenous (IV) fluids, forced-air warming, and avoidance of acidosis and hypovolemia, transfusion to a minimum hemoglobin of 10 g/dL is recommended for all but the simplest procedures. This includes tonsillectomy, open cholecystectomy, major orthopedic procedures, and other major surgery. Laparoscopic cholecystectomy has been performed without problems with hydration alone in one series of 13 patients [61]. Exchange transfusion is indicated only for very severely affected patients or for open heart surgery.

Perioperative analgesia is critically important to prevent severe pain, stress, catecholamine release, and

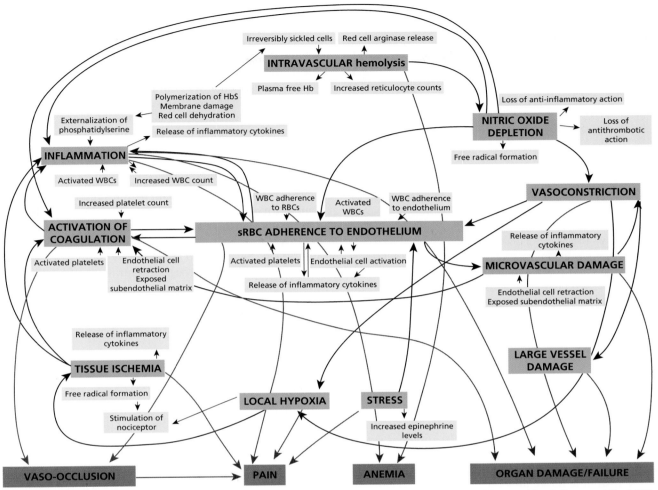

Figure 22.4 Elements of the pathophysiology of sickle cell disease and interactions between them. Reproduced from Redding-Lallinger and Knoll [58] with permission from Elsevier.

precipitation of further acute events. Consequently, provision of intraoperative and postoperative pain relief must be carefully considered. Patient-controlled analgesia is often very effective in the adolescent sickle cell population. It is important to maintain high oxygen saturations with supplemental oxygen in the recovery period. For any sickle cell patient undergoing anesthesia and surgery, consultation with the patient's hematologist for perioperative recommendations is key for providing optimal care and outcomes. See Chapter 11 for more discussion of the perioperative management of patients with sickle cell disease.

Diabetes mellitus

In the adolescent population, diabetes mellitus is usually type 1, although the incidence of type 2 diabetes is increasing in this population (see below under Obesity). Approximately 186,000 children aged 0–19 had a diagno-

sis of diabetes mellitus in 2007 in the US, or 0.2% of this population; 80% of the diabetes was type 1. In the 10–19 year age group, 85% of new diabetes in the non-Hispanic white population in the US was type 1, while in African American and Hispanic populations the proportion of new type 1 versus type 2 cases was 50:50; in the Asian Pacific Islander and Native American populations, new cases are predominantly type 2 [63]. Onset of type 1 diabetes usually occurs during childhood or adolescence and arises from T-cell mediated autoimmune destruction of pancreatic β cells, which causes failure of insulin production, and hyperglycemia.

The incidence of type 1 diabetes is also increasing in many parts of the world. Associated risk factors include genetics, diet, lifestyle, and immune responses to viral infection, with enterovirus most frequently implicated. Insulin therapy is the cornerstone of treatment for type 1 diabetes [64]. Type 2 diabetes is the result of resistance to

Box 22.1 US NHLBI recommendations for perioperative care of the sickle cell disease patient (2002)

- Make sure the operating and anesthesia teams are aware of the diagnosis of a sickle cell syndrome and the need for special attention.
- In patients with SCD-SS and SCD-S β°-thalassemia, simple transfusion to achieve a hemoglobin of 10 g/dL should be performed before all but the lowest-risk procedures.
- For patients with SCD-SC, exchange transfusions may be needed to avoid complications associated with hyperviscosity.
- Alloimmunization should be minimized by giving antigen-matched blood (matched K, C, E, S, Fy, and Jk antigens).
- Patients with SCD, regardless of genotype, should all receive careful attention, with preoperative monitoring of intake and output, hematocrit, peripheral perfusion, and oxygenation status.
- Intraoperative monitoring of blood pressure, cardiac rhythm and rate, and oxygenation should be conducted for all surgical procedures.
- Postoperative care should include attention to hydration, oxygen administration with careful monitoring, and respiratory therapy.

Reproduced from Guidelines for Perioperative Management of Sickle Cell Disease [62] with permission from NHLBI.

the effects of insulin, which causes hyperglycemia. Obesity, particularly adipose tissue deposits in the abdomen and non-alcoholic fatty liver disease, is associated with this disease in adolescents. Treatment is primarily by diet, exercise and, in some cases, oral hypoglycemic drugs, such as metformin, sulfonylureas or thiazolidinediones; insulin is rarely necessary in adolescence [65].

The secondary complications of diabetes, i.e. nephropathy, are rare in adolescents. Most patients with diabetes present for anesthesia because they require the standard surgical procedures seen in patients in this age group. For those who are insulin dependent, there are many insulin types available, ranging from short, medium, to long-acting insulin; dosing occurs one, two or more times per day or on a sliding scale. Insulin pumps that provide continuous basal rates of subcutaneous insulin infusion plus programmable boluses at mealtimes or in response to hyperglycemia are also used [66]. An understanding of the patient's insulin regimen, history of diabetic ketoacidosis or hospitalization, and degree of glycemic control (hemoglobin A1C <7.5%) is important, as is co-ordination with the patient's endocrinologist [67].

Whenever possible, insulin-dependent patients should be scheduled as the first case of the day. Generally, the night before surgery, the patient's normal meal and insulin regimen should be followed. Fasting guidelines are not different from patients without diabetes for a morning case, i.e. nil per os (NPO) for solid food and non-clear liquids for 6 h preoperatively and clear liquids

for up to 2 h preoperatively. For afternoon cases, a light early breakfast may be preferable in those who are insulin dependent. For patients on twice-daily or more frequent insulin administration, the current recommendations are to omit short-acting insulin and to give only 50% of the intermediate insulin dose in the morning. After measuring a baseline blood glucose, an infusion of 5% dextrose in ½ normal saline is begun at maintenance rates 2 h preoperatively or as soon as the patient arrives for an early morning case (1500 mL per 24 h, plus an additional 20 mL/kg/24 h for each kg over 20 kg, maximum 2000 mL/24 h, i.e. 83 mL/h for a 50 kg patient). Also start an insulin infusion with 1 unit regular insulin per 1 mL normal saline, at 0.025–0.1 unit/kg/h, depending on the baseline glucose. Glucose must be measured every hour while receiving an insulin infusion and the insulin rate must be adjusted accordingly with the goal of maintaining blood glucose concentrations of 90–180 mg/dL. Additional boluses of IV regular insulin, of 0.025–0.1 unit/kg, are given for glucose values above 180 mg/dL. Serum electrolytes, i.e. sodium and potassium, are measured at regular intervals and potassium replaced if needed.

After surgery, the glucose and insulin infusion are continued, with the addition of potassium chloride at 20 mEq/L in the IV fluid if the patient remains NPO. If oral intake is allowed, the IV dextrose and insulin can be weaned, and the patient's normal evening meal and insulin regimen can be resumed if glycemic control is adequate. Patients with infusion pumps must be managed in close consultation with the endocrinologist. Pump use may be continued during anesthesia. These recommendations are summarized in Box 22.2. For type 2 diabetes patients on insulin, the guidelines are the same as above. If the patient with type 2 diabetes is taking metformin, discontinue it 24 h before elective surgery. If taking sulfonylureas or thiazolidinediones, these are stopped on the day of surgery.

Adolescent gynecological surgery

Adolescent gynecology is a growing field and because of this, more of these patients are presenting for surgery. Most of these procedures are done laparoscopically. Indications for laparoscopic surgery in females of this age include congenital anomalies, such as Mullerian anomalies and disorders of sex development, which may require diagnosis and treatment. Adnexal masses, such as ovarian torsion, tumors or tubo-ovarian abscess, are also diagnosed and treated with laparoscopy. Other less frequent indications include diagnosis and treatment of endometriosis or pelvic inflammatory disease, and procedures to preserve ovarian function before pelvic irradiation [68,69]. See Chapter 28 for a discussion of the anesthetic management of patients undergoing laparoscopy.

Box 22.2 Guidelines for perioperative management of patients with insulin-dependent diabetes

NPO guidelines	**6 h preoperatively for solid food, non-clear liquids** **2 h preoperatively for clear liquids**
IV fluids	D5 ½ normal saline 2 h preoperatively at 1500 mL/24 h plus 20 mL/kg for every kg over 20 kg, maximum 2000 mL/24 h
Insulin regimen	No change the evening before surgery Omit short-acting AM insulin, give 50% of usual medium-acting insulin dose
Insulin infusion	Start at 0.025–0.1 unit/kg/h depending on baseline glucose
Glucose measurement	Q 1 h during insulin infusion
Glycemic control	Goal: 90–180 mg/dL; increase or decrease insulin infusion accordingly; may give regular insulin IV 0.025–0.1 unit/kg bolus for values >180 mg/dL, or stop insulin infusion briefly for values below 60 mg/dL
Insulin pump patients	Consult endocrinologist for plan
Postoperative treatment	Continue insulin and glucose infusion if NPO; add KCl 20 mEq/L to IV fluids Wean insulin and glucose and resume normal evening meal and insulin regimen if taking food

Inflammatory bowel disease

Inflammatory bowel disease (IBD) is classified as either Crohn's disease or ulcerative colitis, and the overlapping clinical features of these diseases often lead to lack of clarity in diagnosis in adolescents (see Chapter 28) [70]. Twenty to 30% of patients with IBD are less than 20 years of age, and the prevalence of this disease in this age group worldwide has been estimated to be 4–7 per 100,000 [71].

Crohn's disease is a transmural inflammatory disease of the mucosa with episodic progression that can involve any part of the gastrointestinal tract from the mouth to the anus. However, it is often concentrated in the small bowel. Ulcerative colitis is a non-transmural inflammatory disease with episodic progression that is limited to the colon. The clinical features of the IBD depend on its localization and often include diarrhea, abdominal pain, fever, ileus, and the passage of blood and mucus per rectum. Patients with Crohn's disease are less likely to have bloody diarrhea, but rather have abdominal pain or non-specific abdominal symptoms. About 25% have perianal disease. Growth failure is common in both children and adolescents. IBDs are autoimmune diseases that are

associated with susceptibility regions on at least 12 different chromosomes. Other associations include ethnic origin, with northern European descent predominant, lifestyle, and geographic factors. Extraintestinal manifestations include joint and skin involvement (15–25% in Crohn's disease, 2–16% in ulcerative colitis) [72]. Medical treatment of IBD is similar for both Crohn's disease and ulcerative colitis: oral or rectal mesalamine, corticosteroids, purine analogs (6-mercaptopurine, azathioprine), methotrexate in varying combinations, depending on severity of disease and acute relapse status. Newer treatments also include anti-tumor necrosis factor-α antibody drugs (infliximab, adalimumab) or, in severe cases, cyclosporin. In addition, patients with Crohn's disease are usually receiving antibiotics (metronidazole, ciprofloxacin).

Adolescents with IBD often present for surgery for complications of the disease or failed medical management. Indications include bowel perforation/abscess, obstruction, stricture, perianal fistula, toxic megacolon or malignancy. Over 50% of IBD patients ultimately require bowel resection. Recurrence of disease and reoperation are frequent, so bowel conservation is very important for avoiding the complications of short bowel syndrome and long-term dependence on total parenteral nutrition. Ostomy formation may be necessary for more severe cases. Complications after surgery for IBD include wound infection, anastomotic leak, anastomotic stricture, fistula, recurrence of disease, small bowel obstruction, and bleeding; these complications are seen particularly following surgery for Crohn's disease. For ulcerative colitis, total proctocolectomy is curative. The procedure done depends on the clinical status of the patient but usually involves a total colectomy, with or without an ileostomy. Creation of a small bowel reservoir with ileo-anal anastomosis is the definitive procedure. These patients also present frequently for upper and lower gastrointestinal endoscopy for diagnosis and treatment of their disease, and for cancer surveillance that may require sedation or anesthesia provided by the pediatric anesthesiologist.

Preanesthetic evaluation and care must consider nutritional status, chronic pain, medications (including corticosteroids and other immunosuppressant drugs), and history of anesthesia and surgery. Extraintestinal manifestations of the disease must be carefully sought out. As with any chronic disease in the teenage population, psychosocial distress is common in patients with IBD, and anesthetic care must take this into consideration.

Developmental disabilities/autism

Chapter 38 contains an extensive listing of the genetic causes of developmental delay, including autism spectrum disorder. Acquired causes of developmental delay include hypoxic-ischemic brain injury from cardiac or respiratory arrest secondary to a disease state, hypoxemic insults from cardiopulmonary bypass or the perioperative period for congenital heart surgery, trauma, near-drowning, cranial irradiation, toxic exposures, and many other etiologies. Clearly, it is important to understand fully the patient's history and level of functioning and communication; thus the parent or other caregiver is essential in the preoperative evaluation and preparation and approach to the anesthetic. Developmentally delayed adolescents present for a variety of procedures, including dental care, orthopedic procedures, brain imaging, and many others. Having the parent present during IV placement or mask induction of anesthesia may be extremely helpful. Premedication, either oral (benzodiazepines, barbiturates) or intramuscular (ketamine or midazolam), may be necessary to accomplish induction of anesthesia in large, unco-operative, developmentally delayed adolescents.

Obesity in the adolescent

Obesity in children and adolescents is defined in a variety of ways, but one commonly used definition is that of the US Centers for Disease Control: a Body Mass Index (BMI) above the 95th percentile for age, as defined by the 2000 CDC growth charts for normal children [73].

Using this definition, the prevalence of adolescent obesity has increased dramatically in the US between 1976–80 and 2007–08, from 5.0% to 18.1% in patients aged 12–19 years (Fig. 22.5). For boys and girls respectively, this corresponds to a BMI of 24–25 at age 12, 27–28 at age 15, and 29–30 at age 18. Morbid obesity is often defined in adults as a BMI >40. Epidemiological studies suggest that over 90% of cases of adolescent obesity are not accompanied by an underlying medical condition or syndrome but primarily represent excess intake of calories, relative lack of physical activity, and often social/psychological factors, genetic and environmental factors, and possibly a deficiency of the hormone leptin in some cases. About 5% of obese adolescents have an accompanying genetic syndrome, including Prader–Willi and Laurence–Moon–Biedl (a glycogen storage disease), or medical cause such as chronic corticosteroid administration, or physical inactivity, such as accompanies severe muscular dystrophy [74].

Obesity is a complex endocrine state in which the adipose tissue communicates with the brain and peripheral tissues by releasing hormones and cytokines, such as leptin, C-reactive protein (CRP), IL-6, tumor necrosis factor α (TNF-α), lipoproteinlipase, renin, and adiponectin. Significant obesity leads first to insulin resistance and, if well established, to the metabolic syndrome, which

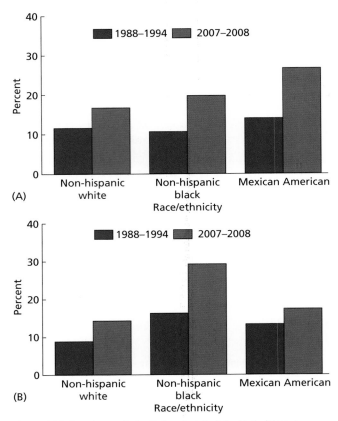

Figure 22.5 Prevalence of obesity by race/ethnicity: United States, 1988–1994 and 2007–2008. (A) Boys aged 12–19 years. (B) Girls aged 12–19 years. Reproduced from National Center for Health Statistics [73] with permission from CDC.

consists of central obesity, hyperinsulinemia, systemic hypertension, and hypertriglyceridemia. Obesity is a chronic inflammatory state. Multisystem complications of obesity include respiratory (asthma, obstructive sleep apnea, atelectasis, hypoxemia), cardiovascular (systemic hypertension, left ventricular hypertrophy, pulmonary hypertension), endocrine (insulin resistance and type 2 diabetes, polycystic ovary syndrome), gastrointestinal (delayed gastric emptying, gastroesophageal reflux, non-alcoholic fatty liver disease), and psychological (depression, poor body image, loss of self-esteem) problems. Diet and behavioral therapy are always attempted, but achieve variable success rates. Drug therapy is sometimes attempted (orlistat to reduce fat absorption). Bariatric surgery is increasingly recommended for morbid obesity in older adolescents after other measures have failed (see below).

Overweight adolescents present for surgery and anesthesia for a range of disorders, including Blount disease or tibia vara and slipped capital femoral epiphysis [75], cholecystectomy from cholesterol-induced cholelithiasis, tonsillectomy for obstructive sleep apnea, and bariatric surgery. Preoperative evaluation must carefully search for co-morbid disease, especially obstructive sleep apnea (OSA). Some adolescents require BiPAP, especially at night.

Obesity is a known significant risk factor for OSA. See Chapter 31 for a detailed discussion of the perioperative patient with OSA. If the patient is managed with BiPAP, BiPAP should be reinstituted in the postanesthesia recovery area if the trachea is extubated, and BiPAP should be maintained until the patient is awake and can maintain a patent airway. Patients with moderate or severe OSA should be admitted to hospital after anesthesia, even after a minor procedure, and may require intensive care unit (ICU) observation [76,77]. Severe pulmonary hypertension merits very careful planning of the anesthetic in consultation with the patient's cardiologist or pulmonologist; ICU admission should be arranged for these patients prior to surgery. See Chapter 25 for anesthetic management of patients with pulmonary hypertension. Airway management may also be complicated by adipose tissue in the tongue, pharynx, and neck, which can collapse with decreased muscle tone and cause airway obstruction. Most often, this can be managed with an oral airway and mask ventilation. In the vast majority of obese teens, mask ventilation, direct laryngoscopy, and tracheal intubation are not difficult. See Chapter 14 for a discussion of management of the difficult airway. Vascular access may be difficult in obese adolescents but it is often possible to place a small peripheral intravenous catheter preoperatively (often in the ventral surface of the wrist) and a larger intravenous catheter after induction of anesthesia. Gastroesophageal reflux disease is common in obese teenagers. Consideration can be given to prophylaxis for gastroesophageal reflux if the patient is not already on therapy, including oral clear antacids, intravenous histamine-2 blocking agents, and gastrointestinal motility agents.

Intravenous drug dosing is problematic and there are no clear data offering definitive guidance on administering drug doses based on actual versus ideal bodyweight; this may be different for lipophilic drugs such as propofol and ionized drugs such as non-depolarizing muscle relaxants. Often the best practice is to start with doses based on ideal bodyweight and titrate additional doses based on the individual patient's pharmacodynamic response (see Chapter 15).

Bariatric surgery in the adolescent

In the mature, morbidly obese adolescent, when diet, exercise programs, and behavioral interventions have failed, there is increasing evidence that bariatric surgery effectively increases weight loss and reverses significant co-morbidities, including type 2 diabetes, OSA, non-alcoholic fatty liver disease, pseudotumor cerebri, quality of life, and depression [78]. Selection criteria for this

Table 22.2 Selection criteria for bariatric surgery in adolescents

BMI (kg/m²)	Co-morbidities
>35	*Serious:* Type 2 diabetes mellitus, moderate or severe obstructive sleep apnea (AHI >15 events/h), pseudotumor cerebri, and severe steatohepatitis
>40	*Other:* Mild obstructive sleep apnea (AHI ≥5 events/h); hypertension, insulin resistance, glucose intolerance, dyslipidemia, impaired quality of life or activities of daily living, among others
Eligibility criteria[a]	
Tanner stage	IV or V (unless severe co-morbidities indicate WLS earlier)
Skeletal maturity	Completed at least 95% of estimated growth (only if planning a diversional or malabsorptive operation, including RYGB)
Lifestyle changes	Demonstrates ability to understand what dietary and physical activity changes will be required for optimal postoperative outcomes
Psychosocial	Evidence for mature decision making, with appropriate understanding of potential risks and benefits of surgery
	Evidence for appropriate social support without evidence of abuse or neglect
	If psychiatric condition (e.g. depression, anxiety, or binge eating disorder) is present, it is under treatment
	Evidence that family and patient have the ability and motivation to comply with recommended treatments pre- and postoperatively, including consistent use of micronutrient supplements. Evidence may include a history of reliable attendance at office visits for weight management and compliance with other medical needs

AHI, apnea-hypopnea index; RYGB, Roux-en-Y gastric bypass; WLS, weight loss surgery.
[a]All of the eligibility criteria must be fulfilled.
Reproduced from Pratt et al [78] with permission from Nature.

surgery are very important, and all must be met before offering bariatric surgery to adolescent patients. (Table 22.2). The most important criteria are BMI >35 with serious co-morbidities, or >40 with milder co-morbidities, skeletal maturity, and stable and mature psychosocial evaluation, with parental support and high likelihood of compliance with diet and medical follow-up regimens. A multidisciplinary team evaluation consisting of gastroenterologists, dieticians, nurse specialists, surgeons, psychologists, and social workers is the standard of care.

Several forms of bariatric surgery have evidence of positive outcomes and low complication rates in adolescents (Fig. 22.6). The first was the Roux-en-Y gastric bypass that was initially performed as an open procedure but is now performed laparoscopically by experienced surgeons. This operation involves creation of a small gastric pouch of 10–30 mL, division of the small intestine and creation of a jejunojenostomy, and finally connection of the gastric pouch to the Roux limb (gastrojejunostomy). Most of the stomach is bypassed, and weight loss occurs mostly through restriction of caloric intake from the small gastric pouch. It is intended as a one-time intervention. In recent adolescent case series, there were no perioperative deaths and fewer complications than in adults. The second operation is the adjustable gastric band, also performed laparoscopically, which involves placing an inflatable silicone band with an inner inflatable balloon around the top of the stomach; this creates a virtual gastric pouch 1–2 cm below the gastroesophageal junction. A catheter leads from the balloon to an implanted subcutaneous pouch, which allows adjustment of balloon size by adding or removing saline. The US Food and Drug Administration has not approved this device for patients under the age of 18. Therefore, any use of the device in adolescent patients should be done in the context of Investigational Device Exemption studies for the purposes of reporting clinical safety and outcomes [79]. In recent adolescent series, complication rates were 6–10%, with no deaths. Reoperation rates, including band removal, were 8–10%. Other operations, such as biliopancreatic diversion, with or without duodenal switch, or laparoscopic sleeve gastrectomy, are not recommended in adolescents.

Conclusion

Adolescence is a time of rapid growth and change, and a number of anesthetic challenges occur that are unique to this age group. Knowledge of physiological and psychosocial development and of the disease processes and procedures common in these patients is important to maximize favorable outcomes. A direct, honest, positive approach to these patients that is distinct from that

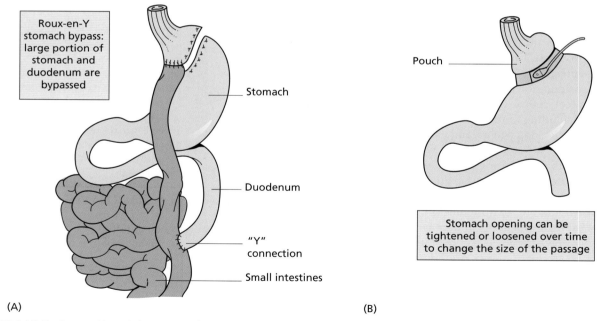

(A)   (B)

Figure 22.6 (A) The Roux-en-Y gastric bypass procedure involves creating a stomach pouch out of a small portion of the stomach and attaching it directly to the small intestine, bypassing a large part of the stomach and duodenum. Not only is the stomach pouch too small to hold large amounts of food, but by skipping the duodenum, fat absorption is substantially reduced. Reproduced from National Library of Medicine [80] with permission from the National Institutes of Health. (B) Adjustable gastric band. Restrictive gastric operations, such as an adjustable gastric banding procedure, serve only to restrict and decrease food intake and do not interfere with the normal digestive process. In this procedure, a hollow band made of special material is placed around the stomach near its upper end, creating the small pouch and a narrow passage into the larger remaining portion of the stomach. This small passage delays the emptying of food from the pouch and causes a feeling of fullness. The band can be tightened or loosened over time to change the size of the passage. Initially, the pouch holds about 1 ounce of food and later expands to 2–3 ounces. Reproduced from National Library of Medicine [81] with permission from the National Institutes of Health.

of the younger child, yet empathetic to the adolescent's developmental stage and disease process, is usually greatly appreciated by these patients and their parents. This approach also facilitates establishing trust with the anesthesiologist in the often brief time for preopera-

tive evaluation and preparation. Transition of patients with chronic pediatric diseases, such as congenital heart disease and cystic fibrosis, to adult care is variable, but the pediatric anesthesiologist should be prepared to care for young adults with these conditions.

CASE STUDY

The patient was a 16-year-old girl presenting for laparoscopic Roux-en-Y gastrojejunostomy. Current BMI was 47.8 (165 cm tall, 130 kg). In reviewing her growth charts, the patient had been above the 99th percentile on the US Centers for Disease Control 2000 growth charts since age 10 and had attempted diet and behavioral therapy for the past 4 years without success. Co-morbidities included type 2 diabetes treated with metformin, gastroesophageal reflux disease treated with pantoprazole, OSA with apnea-hypopnea index of 9 (moderately severe OSA) on sleep study that was treated with BiPAP 10 cm at night by nasal mask. She also had early polycystic ovary syndrome, with facial acne and mild hirsutism. After a full evaluation by the bariatric surgery team, including a psychological evaluation, full explanation of the procedure and follow-up required, and signed contract by the patient and parents to adhere to the follow-up guidelines, the patient was accepted for surgery. She had not had anesthesia or surgery previously, there was no family history of anesthetic problems, and there were no medication allergies. She did not smoke, drink alcohol or use illegal drugs. Menses were irregular, with her last menstrual period occurring 6 weeks prior to surgery.

Physical examination revealed an alert, anxious, morbidly obese teenager. Room air SpO$_2$ was 94% without BiPAP, heart rate 80 beats per minute, respiratory rate 16 breaths per minute, and arterial blood pressure 145/86. Airway examination revealed a Mallampati Class II examination, full range of neck motion, and intact dentition. Lung examination revealed no respiratory distress, distant clear breath sounds, and decreased breath sounds at both bases. Cardiac examination revealed regular rate and rhythm and no murmurs. Peripheral veins were difficult to identify. Preoperative laboratory values included hemoglobin 14 g/dL, hematocrit 42%, white blood cell count 8500/mm^3 with a normal differential white count. Electrolytes were normal, blood urea nitrogen 18 mg/dL, creatinine 1.0 mg/dL, and fasting blood glucose 125 mg/dL. The urine human chorionic gonadotropin test was negative. Chest radiograph revealed mild cardiomegaly and clear lung fields, with the exception of some volume loss at both bases. The patient was informed of the anesthetic procedures and that the plan would be to extubate

her trachea in the operating room when she was awake and able to follow commands and that she would have her BiPAP reinstituted in the postanesthesia care unit (PACU). Furthermore, she was told that she would have patient-controlled analgesia (PCA).

A 20 gauge peripheral IV was started in the dorsum of the left hand on the second attempt. Metformin had been discontinued 2 days preoperatively. Oral sodium citrate and IV metoclopramide and pantoprazole were given in the holding area, along with IV midazolam 2 mg, which provided anxiolysis. The patient was transported to the operating room (OR) where she was positioned on the OR table with a foam wedge under the back and shoulders to optimize airway alignment. Difficult airway adjuncts were available in the OR, including a videolaryngoscope, large adult intubating laryngeal mask airway, and a fiber-optic bronchoscope. After application of standard monitors and preoxygenation for a full 5 min, IV induction of anesthesia was achieved with fentanyl 100 μg and propofol 150 mg IV, which was 2 mg/kg, based on an ideal bodyweight of 75 kg. Her eyelash reflex was lost in 45 sec and mask ventilation was easy once an oral airway was inserted. Rocuronium 80 mg was given to facilitate tracheal intubation, which was accomplished easily using a MacIntosh 3 blade. The view was a grade I Cormack and Lehane view of the larynx. Anesthesia was maintained with desflurane, 6–12% end-tidal concentration. Positive end-expiratory pressure of 8 cmH$_2$O was used to prevent atelectasis, and the patient's lungs were ventilated with tidal volumes of 750 mL and an FIO$_2$ of 0.5. An air-oxygen mixture was used to achieve an SpO$_2$ of 95–98% during the surgery. An 18 g IV was placed after induction of anesthesia.

Laparoscopic Roux-en-Y-gastrojejunostomy proceeded via five separate incisions for ports and instruments, and sufficient CO$_2$ was insufflated to achieve an intraperitoneal pressure of 15–20 cmH$_2$O. The patient was hemodynamically stable throughout the procedure; minute ventilation had to be increased during the CO$_2$ insufflation to achieve end-tidal CO$_2$ of 35–40 mmHg. This was done by increasing the respiratory rate. After 3 h and 15 min of operating time (estimated blood loss 15 mL) and achieving an excellent surgical result and hemostasis, the incisions were closed

Continued

after infiltrating the fascia, subcutaneous tissue, and skin with a total of 30 mL of 0.25% bupivacaine. Ketorolac 30 mg IV, morphine 6 mg IV, and ondansetron 4 mg IV were given during the last hour of the procedure. Neuromuscular blockade was reversed and the patient's respirations were assisted with pressure support ventilation of 15 cmH$_2$O.

When she was awake, following commands, and taking unassisted tidal volume breaths of 500 mL or more, the trachea was extubated with the patient in semi-Fowler position with her head elevated 45°. Ventilation was assisted with facemask CPAP, achieving good tidal volumes and SpO$_2$ of 94–96% without distress. She was then transported to the PACU, where her BiPAP was instituted at end-expiratory pressure of 10 cmH$_2$O, and inspiratory pressures of 15 cmH$_2$O. Patient-controlled analgesia with morphine was instituted in the PACU without a basal rate and with a PCA dose of 1.5 mg morphine with 10 min lockout interval. Ketorolac 30 mg IV Q 6 h × five additional doses, and ondansteron were also ordered. Pneumatic sequential compression stockings for deep vein thrombosis prophylaxis were fitted in the PACU.

After 2 h of monitoring in the PACU, with several visits by the anesthesiologist to ensure satisfactory airway, pulmonary, and pain control status, the patient was transferred to an intermediate care monitored unit. She was mobilized out of bed and into a chair on the night of surgery, and every 4 h during the first postoperative day. Incentive spirometry exercises commenced the first night after surgery. On the second postoperative day, she was assisted out of bed every 4 h and walked around her room. Pain control was adequate, with visual analog scale scores 3–5 on a 10-point scale (10 is maximum), with a total of 22.5 mg morphine used during the first 24 h. Respiratory status was adequate, with no episodes of OSA or oxygen desaturation below an SpO$_2$ of 90%. After 24 h she was able to discontinue the BiPAP while awake, thereafter using it only while sleeping. Clear liquid intake and metformin and pantoprazole were commenced orally on postoperative day 1. Serum glucose was adequately controlled at 120–200 mg/dL. She was discharged to the surgical ward on postoperative day 3, transitioned to oral pain medication with acetaminophen/hydrocodone oral solution, and discharged home on postoperative day 4.

At 6-month follow-up the patient was doing well, had lost 25 kg, and was compliant with her diet regimen and clinic follow-up visits. Her blood pressure had decreased to 130/80 mmHg. Her endocrinologist was considering discontinuing the metformin.

Conclusions

This case illustrates the principles of preanesthetic evaluation of morbidly obese teenage patients and the comorbidities they suffer, including OSA and type 2 diabetes. Careful preoperative preparation for a possible difficult airway, gastrointestinal prophylaxis preoperatively to prevent aspiration of acid gastric contents, and proper patient positioning to facilitate laryngoscopy allowed appropriate airway management. Dosing lipid-soluble induction agents (propofol) based initially on ideal body-weight, maintaining functional residual capacity with positive end-expiratory pressure during laparoscopy and CO$_2$ insufflation, using an insoluble anesthetic gas (desflurane) to minimize uptake by adipose tissue that would delay emergence from anesthesia, minimizing intraoperative opioids, using local anesthesia and non-steroidal anti-inflammatory agent, extubating the trachea with the patient awake, and instituting BiPAP immediately after tracheal extubation helped avoid obstructive apnea and hypoxemia. A pain management regimen of PCA without a basal rate, continued ketorolac administration, and early mobilization and ambulation all aided in avoiding pulmonary and airway morbidity in this patient.

Annotated references

A full reference list for this chapter is available at:
http://www.wiley.com/go/gregory/andropoulos/pediatricanesthesia

21. Huffmyer JL, Littlewood KE, Nemergut EC. Perioperative management of the adult with cystic fibrosis. Anesth Analg 2009; 109: 1949–61. A very well done review that also covers issues with anesthesia in the adolescent cystic fibrosis patient.

51. Warnes CA, Williams RG, Bashore TM et al. ACC/AHA 2008 guidelines for the management of adults with congenital heart disease: a report of the American College of Cardiology/American Heart Association Task Force on Practice Guidelines (Writing Committee to Develop Guidelines on the Management of Adults With Congenital Heart Disease). Developed in collaboration with the American Society of Echocardiography, Heart Rhythm Society, International Society for Adult Congenital Heart Disease, Society for Cardiovascular Angiography and Interventions, and Society of Thoracic Surgeons. J Am Coll Cardiol 2008; 52: e1–121. A very important compendium that includes perioperative and anesthetic management of the adult and adolescent with congenital heart disease for cardiac and non-cardiac surgery.

55. Henderson TO, Friedman DL, Meadows AT. Childhood cancer survivors: transition to adult-focused risk-based care. Pediatrics 2010; 126: 129–36. A very well done review of the sequelae of childhood cancer in the adolescent and young adult.

58. Redding-Lallinger R, Knoll C. Sickle cell disease – pathophysiology and treatment. Curr Probl Pediatr Adolesc Health Care 2006; 36: 347–76. An outstanding review of sickle cell disease in the adolescent.

67. Betts P, Brink S, Silink M et al. Management of children and adolescents with diabetes requiring surgery. Pediatric Diabetes 2009; 10(Suppl. 12): 169–74. The latest published guidelines for insulin, oral

hypoglycemic agents, fluid, and oral intake management in the adolescent with diabetes type 1 or type 2.

71. Kim SC, Ferry GD. Inflammatory bowel diseases in pediatric and adolescent patients: clinical, therapeutic, and psychosocial considerations. Gastroenterology 2004; 126: 1550–60. A comprehensive review of inflammatory bowel disease.

74. Veyckemans F. Child obesity and anaesthetic morbidity. Curr Opin Anaesthesiol 2008; 21: 308–12. An excellent review of anesthetic care of the obese adolescent.

78. Pratt JS, Lenders CM, Dionne EA et al. Best practice updates for pediatric/adolescent weight loss surgery. Obesity 2009; 17: 901–10. A very well done, evidence-based review and best practice update for procedures, indications, evaluation, and care for bariatric surgery in the adolescent.

CHAPTER 23

Anesthesia for Neurosurgical Procedures

Bruno Bissonnette[1], Ken M. Brady[2] & R. Blaine Easley[2]

[1]Department of Anesthesia, University of Toronto, and the Children of the World Anesthesia Foundation, Toronto, Ontario, Canada
[2]Department of Anesthesiology and Pediatrics, Baylor College of Medicine, and Texas Children's Hospital, Houston, TX, USA

Introduction

Anesthesia for neurosurgery presents an interesting challenge to the anesthesiologist [1]. One has little control over the patient's primary lesion, but the selection of anesthetic technique and the recognition of perioperative events and changes may profoundly reduce or prevent significant morbidity. Current neuroanesthetic practice is based on the understanding of cerebral physiology and how it can be manipulated in the presence of intracranial pathology (see Chapter 7). The pediatric neuroanesthesiologist also must contend with the physiological differences in developing children. In addition to the common problems of administering anesthesia to the general pediatric population, special consideration must be given to the effects of anesthesia on the central nervous system (CNS) of children with neurological diseases. This chapter reviews the fundamentals of the clinical management in neurosurgical patients. Discussion of specific neurosurgical conditions and their respective anesthetic management is designed to highlight the common and sometimes unique problems encountered by the pediatric neuroanesthesiologist.

Neuropharmacology

General principles

Evidence from animals suggests that the lethal dose in 50% of the animals (LD50) for many medications is significantly lower in the neonatal and infancy periods than in adults [2]. The sensitivity of the human newborn to most of the sedatives, hypnotics, and opioids is increased, probably owing to increased brain immaturity (incomplete myelination and blood–brain barrier) and to increased permeability for some medications (i.e. the lipid-soluble drugs used in anesthesia) [3]. In addition, the effect of volatile anesthetic agents is influenced by the age of the patient. The minimal alveolar concentration (MAC) in the neonate (0–31 days) is much lower than in infants aged 30–180 days [4]. Although there is an increase in anesthetic requirements in infancy, it must be emphasized that there is a smaller margin of safety between adequate anesthesia and severe cardiopulmonary depression in the infant and child compared with the adult [5]. Therefore, drug dosages must be appropriately calculated and therapeutic effects must be monitored to avoid inadvertent adverse clinical consequences and prolonged effects.

Inhalational anesthetic agents

All currently used inhalational anesthetic agents have variable degrees of cerebrovascular effects. Historically used agents will not be discussed, in favor of focusing on those agents most widely used in current clinical practice.

Isoflurane

Isoflurane is the most popular of the volatile anesthetics for neuroanesthesia. Its popularity is based on the fact that it affects cerebral blood flow less than halothane at equivalent MAC doses [6] and on the belief that isoflurane may provide cerebral protection [7]. Recent studies have suggested multiple synergistic mechanisms by which isoflurane and other volatile agents succeed in providing neuroprotection [8].

Compared to other volatile anesthetics, isoflurane has less effect on cerebral vascular autoregulation [6] and cerebrospinal fluid (CSF) production/resorption [9]. Studies in children suggest that an end-tidal concentration of isoflurane between 0.5 MAC and 1.5 MAC did not change cerebral blood flow velocity and had minimal effects on the cerebrovascular reactivity to CO_2 [10]. Furthermore, there were no time-response effects of 1 MAC isoflurane on cerebral blood flow velocity in anesthetized children [11–13]. Interestingly, despite their dissimilar effects on cerebral blood flow, both isoflurane and halothane have been shown to similarly increase intracranial pressure (ICP) in animal models of brain injury [14].

Sevoflurane

Sevoflurane is similar to isoflurane with regard to its effects on cerebral blood flow, cerebral metabolic rate of O_2 (CMRO$_2$) and ICP in adults [15]. In children, there appears to be no effect on cerebral blood flow during hypo- and normocapnia when 1 MAC concentrations of sevoflurane are used [16]. There was no difference between isoflurane and sevoflurane regarding their relative increases in ICP and reduction in arterial blood pressure resulting in clinically similar reduction in cerebral perfusion pressure [17]. Furthermore, it is suggested that sevoflurane has a protective effect during incomplete ischemia, compared with fentanyl and nitrous oxide techniques in rodents [18].

Desflurane

Desflurane increases cerebral blood flow and decreases CMRO$_2$ in animals. One MAC desflurane has been shown to increase ICP significantly in neurosurgical patients with supratentorial mass lesions, despite hypocapnia [19] although larger studies have not demonstrated this finding [20]. Data in children are limited, though Sponheim et al demonstrated only a modest rise in ICP and a greater reduction in blood pressure which resulted in a decrease in calculated cerebral perfusion pressure compared to isoflurane and sevoflurane [17]. This reduction in mean arterial pressure is perhaps most problematic for managing neurosurgical patients with obvious and subtle issues of increased ICP. Whether this makes intravenous anesthesia a safer option over volatile anesthesia remains a subject of debate [17].

Nitrous oxide

The effect of nitrous oxide (N_2O) on cerebral circulation and its use in neuroanesthesia remain controversial. The reported variability of its effects on cerebral blood flow and ICP is probably due to differences in experimental species, background anesthesia and control of respiration. Subanesthetic doses of N_2O (60–70%) cause excitement, cerebral metabolic stimulation, and increased cerebral blood flow [21]. In infants and children, Leon and Bissonnette showed that 70% N_2O in oxygen with fentanyl-diazepam-caudal epidural anesthesia increased cerebral blood flow significantly compared with an air/O_2 mixture [22]. This increase in cerebral blood flow was not associated with significant changes in mean arterial pressure (MAP), heart rate or cerebrovascular resistance. However, other studies have suggested a direct effect of N_2O on increasing CMRO$_2$ in both animals and humans. Clinically, N_2O has been shown to increase cerebral blood flow and ICP in adults and children [23–25], although the co-administration of intravenous agents (with or without induced hypocapnia) can mitigate these N_2O-induced increases in cerebral blood flow [26,27]. In contrast, volatile agents can further increase cerebral blood flow [28]. Although N_2O is commonly used in neuroanesthesia, it may be prudent to discontinue its administration if the brain is tight. Furthermore, because of its ability to increase CMRO$_2$, it would be unwise to continue N_2O administration when cerebral perfusion is reduced.

Intravenous anesthetic agents
Barbiturates

Barbiturates are a broad class of drugs that bind to the γ-aminobutyric acid (GABA) receptor on the α subunit, creating sedation and amnesia. In addition, barbiturates reduce epileptiform activity, lower ICP, lower cerebral blood flow and reduce CMRO$_2$ in a dose-dependent manner [29,30]. A major problem with barbiturates is that they can significantly reduce myocardial contractility, systemic arterial blood pressure, and cerebral perfusion pressure (CPP) [31]. In non-clinical doses (10–55 mg/kg), thiopental produces an isoelectric EEG and decreases the $CMRO_2$ by 50% [31]. Barbiturates can prevent an increase in ICP [32] during laryngoscopy and tracheal intubation owing to their ability to decrease cerebral blood flow. Cerebral autoregulation and cerebrovascular reactivity to CO_2 are preserved with barbiturates. Production and reabsorption of CSF are not altered [33]. As mentioned, barbiturates are effective in controlling epileptiform activity, except methohexital, which may activate seizure foci in patients [34].

Etomidate

Etomidate is a carboxylated imidazole that binds to the GABA receptors, resulting in hypnosis and amnesia with a reduction of cerebral blood flow (34%) and $CMRO_2$ (45%) [35]. Etomidate appears to directly vasoconstrict the cerebral vasculature, even before the metabolism is suppressed [36]. Thus, administration of etomidate can potentially lower ICP by reducing cerebral blood volume while augmenting or maintaining CPP. Studies of etomidate administration have primarily been undertaken in adults while studies in children are limited. However, the clinical applicability of etomidate was perhaps best illustrated in a small clinical study of intubated pediatric patients with traumatic brain injury with elevated ICP (>20 mmHg for over 5 min). After intravenous etomidate administration, all patients had an increase in MAP from baseline, with a significant lowering of measured ICP and improvement in CPP [37]. Other studies have demonstrated that cerebrovascular reactivity to CO_2 is maintained following administration of etomidate [35].

Although etomidate has a great advantage over other intravenous agents, like barbiturates, because of minimal cardiovascular depression, it has two significant disadavantages that limit its usage outside airway management: suppression of the adrenocortical response to stress, and increased myoclonic activity, especially after prolonged infusion [38].

Propofol

Propofol is a rapidly acting GABA agent that reduces cerebral blood flow and $CMRO_2$ [39]. Although administration of propofol either by bolus or infusion can reduce ICP, the cardiovascular effects of a dose-dependent reduction in MAP may have a net result of lowering CPP in the patient with traumatic brain injury [40]. Although CO_2 cerebrovascular responsiveness is maintained during propofol anesthesia, the observed reduction in cerebral blood flow and cerebral blood volume is not augmented by hyperventilation (end-tidal CO_2 <30 mmHg) in normal children [41]. Although routinely a part of neuroanesthetic management in children and adults, the use of propofol outside the operating room in critically ill pediatric patients is limited by concerns about morbidity and mortality related to propofol infusion syndrome [42].

Benzodiazepines

Benzodiazepines bind to the GABA receptor, resulting in amnesia and anxiolysis. In addition, benzodiazepine administration has been reported to decrease cerebral blood flow by a 25% decrease in $CMRO_2$, reduce ICP, and slow seizure foci [43–45]. However, the sedating effects and relative short duration of action (compared to barbiturates) encourage their widespread usage in patients in both the operating room and intensive care unit. The benzodiazepine antagonist flumazenil has been demonstrated to reverse the beneficial effects of benzodiazepines on cerebral blood flow, $CMRO_2$, and ICP. Consequently, administration of flumazenil should be undertaken with caution in neurological patients with high ICP, abnormal intracranial elastance, and/or a predisposition to seizure [46].

Opioid analgesics

The opioid agents have little or no effect on cerebral blood flow, $CMRO_2$, and ICP [47]. However, if patients are experiencing pain, opioids cause a modest reduction in these variables through indirect effects on the sympathetic nervous system [48]. Fentanyl combined with nitrous oxide decreases cerebral blood flow and $CMRO_2$ by 47% and 18%, respectively [30]. Cerebrovascular reactivity to CO_2 and cerebral autoregulation are preserved with opioids. Finally, fentanyl has no effect on CSF production, but it reduces CSF reabsorption by at least 50% [49]. Fentanyl has no effects on the cerebral circulation of neonatal animals, but alfentanil increases CSF pressure in patients with brain tumors [50]. This effect was less than that observed with sufentanil but greater than that observed with fentanyl. Alfentanil has the greatest effect on MAP and CPP [51]. Some studies reported a decrease in cerebral blood flow and $CMRO_2$ [52] whereas others suggested an increase in cerebral blood flow and ICP [53]. Remifentanil, with an ultra-short elimination half-life, offers the advantage over other opioids of not delaying perioperative neurological assessment [54]. Equipotent infusions of remifentanil and fentanyl were studied in patients undergoing supratentorial tumor surgery in combination with a balanced inhalational anesthetic. Remifentanil appeared to have the same preservative effects as fentanyl on cerebral blood flow (CBF) and cerebrovascular reactivity [55,56].

Ketamine

Ketamine is a mixed N-methyl-D-aspartate (NMDA) receptor agonist/antagonist that causes a dissociative anesthetic state [57]. The effect of ketamine on the cerebral vasculature appears to create potent cerebral vasodilation capable of increasing cerebral blood flow by 60% in normocapnic humans, and thus an increase in ICP [58]. Studies have reported clinical deterioration in patients with increased ICP after ketamine administration [32]. Despite alterations in cerebral tone and CBF, ketamine has a negligible effect on the $CMRO_2$. Although it is suggested that ketamine may have some cerebral protective effects, recent studies in animal models of brain development have shown that it increases neuronal apoptosis even in the absence of brain injury [59]. Regardless, the use of ketamine is generally contraindicated in neuroanesthesia.

Dexmedetomidine

Dexmedetomidine, an α2-adrenergic agonist, causes a unique kind of sedation, acting on the subcortical areas, which resembles natural sleep without respiratory depression. The most common cardiovascular effects are bradycardia and transient hypotension [60]. All effects are typically responsive to slowing the infusion and/or bolusing fluid with or without a vagolytic (i.e. atropine). Experimental data demonstrate both cerebral vasoconstriction and vasodilation, depending on the model and dose studied [61]. In clinically relevant dosages that produce sedation, dexmedetomidine has been shown to reduce CBF in humans and animals unrelated to hemodynamic changes.

In early animal investigations, $CMRO_2$ was unchanged, suggesting the possibility of increasing cerebral vascular resistance [62]. However, additional studies in humans and animals demonstrate that dexmedetomidine maintains a decrease in CBF proportional to its effect on decreasing $CMRO_2$. Further, it appears that CO_2 reactivity of the cerebral vasculature is unaffected by dexmedetomidine. In a study of healthy adults, the relative middle cerebral artery blood flow velocity to CBF and $CMRO_2$ relationship was unchanged following dexmedetomidine administration [63]. Using clinically relevant doses, the authors confirmed that dexmedetomidine decreases CBF and $CMRO_2$ proportionally in healthy humans. In adult patients with brain injury, it appears that dexmedetomidine is more effective than propofol in causing sedation while providing functionality [64].

Clinical experience with dexmedetomidine use in functional neurosurgery is limited to small case series [65]. However, these reports suggest that use of dexmedetomidine does not appear to interfere with electrophysiological monitoring, and have permitted brain mapping during awake craniotomy and microelectrode recording during implantation of deep brain stimulators in adults [66] and children [67]. Studies are under way to investigate the pharmacokinetics and pharmacodynamics of dexmedetomidine in infants and children.

Muscle relaxants

Muscle relaxants have little effect on cerebral circulation.

Succinylcholine

Succinylcholine produces an initial reduction in ICP followed by a rise, especially in patients with decreased intracranial compliance resulting from increased cerebral blood flow [68,69]. The increase in ICP is probably related to cerebral stimulation caused by increases in afferent muscle spindle activity [70]. The increase in ICP and cerebral blood flow with succinylcholine is reduced by prior administration of deep general anesthesia or by precurarization [71]. However, the benefits to pediatric patients with increased ICP from rapid control of the airway and hyperventilation offset the slight increase in ICP caused by succinylcholine. It is important to remember that life-threatening hyperkalemia may occur after administration of succinylcholine to patients with closed head injury even though they do not have conditions classically associated with this adverse effect, including motor deficits, severe cerebral hypoxia [72], subarachnoid hemorrhage [73], cerebrovascular accident with loss of brain substance [74], and paraplegia [75].

Rocuronium

Rocuronium offers an alternative to succinylcholine for rapid-sequence intubation but it does delay the return of spontaneous respiration and neurological assessment provided by succinylcholine [76,77]. However, the availability of sugammadex in some countries, including the European Union and Japan, for reversal of neuromuscular blockade by non-depolarizing agents may make this issue moot [78,79]. Like the other neuromuscular blocking agents, rocuronium has no effect on cerebral blood flow or hemodynamics [80].

Pancuronium, atracurium, and *cis*-atracurium

These agents have no effect on cerebral blood volume, ICP or $CMRO_2$ in the presence of volatile anesthetics [81]. Large doses of *d*-tubocurarine, atracurium or metocurine may release histamine and cause transient cerebrovascular dilation, which could account for a slight increase in ICP. However, a slight decrease in MAP may offset any change in intracerebral blood volume [82]. Use of *cis*-atracurium should not result in histamine release, and has demonstrated improved cardiovascular stability. In addition, the metabolism of the agent by Hoffman degradation allows for its rapid clearance in patients with impaired renal and hepatic function

[83]. Studies in healthy adults have shown that rocuronium and *cis*-atracurium have no effect on cerebral blood flow [80].

Vecuronium

Vecuronium is known for its cardiovascular stability and its relatively short duration of action. In patients with reduced intracranial compliance, vecuronium slightly decreased ICP, probably because there was a concomitant decrease in central venous pressure (CVP) [84].

General anesthetic considerations

The following sections discuss the anesthetic management of pediatric neurosurgical procedures. Topics common to most procedures are reviewed first, followed by discussion of specific considerations and surgical procedures.

Preoperative assessment of the neurosurgical patient

In recent years, increased understanding of cerebral pathophysiology and improved diagnostic imaging techniques have improved the preoperative assessment of neurosurgical patients. However, the cornerstones of assessment of cerebral function are still the history and physical examination. The preoperative anesthetic work-up of the neurosurgical patient includes an assessment of ICP, assessment of the function of vital respiratory and cardiovascular centers that can be affected by neuropathological processes, either in the brainstem or in the spinal cord, and assessment of the specific disturbances in neurological function [85].

Of primary importance is the preoperative recognition of intracranial hypertension and major neurological deficits.

The history and physical findings of intracranial hypertension differ somewhat according to the age group. In general, the clinical presentation of patients with intracranial hypertension varies with the duration of increased ICP. Sudden massive increases in ICP often cause coma. In a less acute case, however, there may be a history of headache on awakening, suggestive of vasodilation caused by sleep-induced hypercapnia and reduced intracranial compliance. Vomiting is a common sign. Neonates and infants often present with a history of increased irritability, poor feeding or lethargy. A bulging anterior fontanelle, dilated scalp veins, cranial enlargement or deformity, and lower extremity motor deficits are also common signs of increased ICP in this age group [86]. Increased ICP in children is frequently caused by a tumor. As ICP reaches critical levels, vomiting, decreased level of consciousness, and evidence of herniation may develop.

Other symptoms include diplopia due to oculomotor or gaze palsies (sunset sign), dysphonia, dysphagia, and/or gait disturbances. Injury to the third cranial nerve may result in ptosis. Injury to the sixth cranial nerve produces a strabismus caused by loss of abduction. Nausea and vomiting usually occur, and older children complain of morning headache. Papilledema and absent venous pulsation of the retinal vessels may be seen on fundoscopy.

Neurogenic pulmonary edema is a syndrome that includes acute hypoxia, pulmonary congestion, pink, frothy, protein-rich pulmonary edema, and radiological evidence of pulmonary infiltrates [87]. It is associated with a variety of intracranial pathological occurrences, including hemorrhage [88], head trauma [89], and seizures [90]. The mechanisms responsible for activating the sympathetic nervous system and the vagal centers, which lead to pulmonary edema, are related to ischemia of the medulla and distortion of the brainstem [91]. Cranial nerve function and the patient's ability to protect the airway must be evaluated. During the preoperative assessment, the possibility of spinal cord dysfunction must be determined. Neurological dysfunction arising from cervical spinal cord injury may affect the respiratory and cardiovascular centers (see below).

Laboratory tests may yield evidence of the syndrome of inappropriate antidiuretic hormone (SIADH) and of electrolyte abnormalities or volume contraction from protracted vomiting. Diabetes insipidus may result in hypernatremia [92]. Disturbances in metabolism, such as hypo- or hyperglycemia, may be present. The preoperative history and chart review may reveal that the patient is receiving steroids to reduce tumor edema. If so, steroids will be required during surgery. Neurosurgical patients may be receiving anticonvulsant medication either to treat seizures or to prevent them. These drugs may have profound effects on the metabolism of other drugs (e.g. barbiturates, narcotics). Patients with suprasellar tumors, such as craniopharyngioma, frequently have pituitary dysfunction and should have a complete endocrine evaluation before surgery.

Skull radiographs, ultrasonography, computed tomography (CT) scan, and magnetic resonance imaging (MRI) aid in the assessment of intracranial hypertension. Skull radiographs may show the "beaten copper sign" and widening of the sagittal sutures in response to chronic increased ICP and universal suture stenosis. In infants and young children, the width of the cranial sutures should not exceed 2mm, and they should not have bridges or closures [93]. Ultrasonography of the brain is useful in premature infants and neonates because it is relatively inexpensive, does not require sedation, and can be performed at the bedside through the fontanelle. The real-time sector scanner can visualize virtually all parts of the brain [94]. The development of CT scan and MRI has revolutionized the investigation of brain disease.

Premedication

The routine use of sedation in pediatric neurosurgical patients is best avoided. If sedatives and opioids are given, the patient must be closely monitored because the drugs may precipitate respiratory depression, hypercarbia, loss of airway integrity, and increased ICP. Exceptions to this rule include patients with intracranial vascular lesions (with no increase in ICP) who may benefit from sedation to reduce the likelihood of precipitating a preoperative hemorrhage. Sedation can be accomplished in small children with pentobarbital 4 mg/kg or chloral hydrate 50 mg/kg administered orally or rectally 1h before surgery. Emotional preparation is essential and is accomplished by the anesthesiologist and the parents working together. In older children, a simple explanation of what to expect before induction of anesthesia will reduce the element of surprise and the incidence of hemodynamic responses in a threatening environment.

Patient positioning

Planning of a successful anesthetic includes the preparation of the operating table with proper equipment to protect the patient after positioning. The anesthesiologist's preoperative visit should provide information on patient positioning during surgery.

Although patient positioning varies according to the neurosurgical procedure, the general principles remain the same. The eyes must be securely taped closed and, if the patient is prone, the face and other vulnerable areas must be padded to prevent localized pressure. Since ventilation may be compromised by incorrect positioning, it is mandatory to ensure that chest excursion remains adequate, especially when the patient is prone. This can be achieved by using suitable bolsters or a frame that allows the abdomen to be pendulous and facilitates respiratory movement during intermittent positive pressure ventilation. The endotracheal tube (ETT) should be taped securely in place; in the prone position, secretions may loosen the tape. A 10° head-up position is usually advisable to improve cerebral venous return and reduce venous congestion. Rotation of the head to one side may kink the jugular veins and reduce venous return. This kinking can be avoided by rotating the trunk to maintain the axial position.

During any surgical procedure, it is important for the anesthesiologist to be able to inspect the ETT and circuit connection and to have access to the ETT for possible endotracheal suctioning. In addition, it is desirable to have a body part, such as a hand or foot, visible during surgery so that peripheral perfusion and color can be readily assessed.

Monitoring

Basic monitoring consists of a precordial/esophageal stethoscope, electrocardiography (ECG), a non-invasive blood pressure measuring device, a temperature probe, a pulse oximeter, and capnometry. In addition, a radial pulse Doppler allows continuous monitoring of peripheral perfusion on a beat-to-beat basis and provides a non-invasive measurement of blood pressure. The Doppler device is especially useful in neonatal anesthesia. A peripheral nerve stimulator for monitoring neuromuscular blockade is desirable. A urinary catheter is required for long surgical procedures and is mandatory if osmotic diuretics are administered.

Induction of anesthesia
General principles

Anesthesia for pediatric neurosurgical procedures often presents a challenge to the anesthesiologist [17]. The anesthetic technique chosen and recognition of perioperative events may have profound effects on morbidity. Pediatric patients range from premature neonates to 18-year-old young adults. Knowledge of normal physiology in these differing age groups is essential. Neonatal anesthesia differs from that in the older child and adult, particularly with regard to the respiratory system, the cardiovascular system, and thermoregulation.

Anesthesia for patients with elevated ICP is fraught with danger. After induction of anesthesia, rapid tracheal intubation and hyperventilation will lower the ICP. The systemic hypertension associated with laryngoscopy may be avoided by giving IV lidocaine at induction of anesthesia. Rapid-sequence induction of anesthesia with thiopental, atropine, lidocaine, and succinylcholine, followed by carefully applied cricoid pressure and manual hyperventilation, is recommended [95]. An alternative is a modified rapid-sequence technique with large-dose rocuronium or vecuronium substituted for succinylcholine. With appropriate cricoid pressure, manual ventilation can be performed without distension of the stomach. Cricoid pressure reduces the likelihood of aspirating gastric contents; delayed gastric emptying is often associated with increased ICP. The rapid rate at which succinylcholine produces satisfactory intubation conditions outweighs the small increase in ICP that it causes. Consequently, succinylcholine is routinely used in pediatric neuroanesthesia. Rocuronium 1–1.2 mg/kg produces intubation conditions comparable to succinylcholine [76]. In patients without ready IV access, anesthesia can be induced via a small butterfly needle, which can be inserted with minimal patient stress or hemodynamic fluctuation. Failing this, it is probably less injurious to children with raised ICP to perform a skillful inhalation induction of anesthesia than it is to subject them to a difficult IV placement. Anesthesia is best maintained with nitrous oxide in oxygen, isoflurane, and a suitable muscle relaxant. Intermittent positive pressure mechanical ventilation is provided. Hypoventilation and hypercarbia are best avoided. An IV opioid can be used in children. Deep levels of anesthesia are not needed and are contraindicated.

Fluid management and intracranial pressure control

Fluid management

Fluid administration to neurosurgical patients depends on the pathology or brain insult being treated. A frequent result of these insults is the development of brain edema, with a resultant increase in ICP. It is essential for the neuroanesthesiologist to understand the principles of fluid movement in the injured brain in order to administer the proper fluid regimen.

Edema formation occurs when there is inequality of net movement of fluid between the intra- and extracellular compartments. Edema is the result of pressure gradients between the hydrostatic, osmotic, and colloid oncotic pressures and the properties of the barrier that separates them. The blood–brain barrier is composed of capillary endothelial cells, which are connected in continuous fashion by tight junctions. This system forms a barrier that excludes polar hydrophilic molecules. The endothelium of the brain differs from that of the rest of the body. In most non-central neural tissue, the tight junction between endothelial cells is 65 angstroms in diameter, whereas it is 7 angstroms in the CNS. In the brain, the size of these junctions is sufficiently small to prevent sodium from traversing them freely. Essential molecules, such as glucose and amino acids, cross the blood–brain barrier by energy-mediated transport systems. Only water freely communicates with both sides of the membrane. This passive movement of water is regulated by oncotic, osmotic, and hydrostatic pressure changes across the barrier. The colloid oncotic pressure is a relatively weak driving force. A reduction of 50% of the colloid oncotic pressure (normal 20 mmHg) results in a pressure gradient across the membrane, which is less than that caused by a transcapillary osmolarity difference of 1 mOsm/L. A reduction in the colloid oncotic pressure of the brain does not have the same impact as that observed in the bowel. This is because the brain's extracellular space is poorly compliant, due to its network of glial cells, and discourages edema formation, even in the presence of a severe colloid oncotic pressure gradient. Administration of Ringer's lactate alone will lead eventually to hemodilution and reduced plasma osmolarity (osmolarity 273 mOsm/L), which would encourage cerebral edema [96].

The choice of fluid must be dictated by the neuropathological process involved. It should maintain an isovo-

lemic, iso-osmolar, and relatively iso-oncotic intravascular volume. For example, a patient with increased ICP and/or a brain mass requires a fluid regimen that balances adequate intravascular volume against efforts to dehydrate the brain mass. In a patient undergoing insertion of a ventricular shunt and/or repair of myelomeningocele, fluid management should replace third-space losses.

An osmolar gradient can be maintained only in areas where the blood–brain barrier is intact. Under normal circumstances, osmotic diuretics and plasma expanders, such as albumin, are excluded. Unfortunately, areas that might benefit the most from dehydration therapy, such as tumor edema, exhibit blood–brain barrier incompetence. Agents of high osmolality move into these tissues and increase the edema.

Efforts to dehydrate the brain are complicated by the need to maintain adequate circulating blood volume. In many neurosurgical procedures, a substantial portion of the blood loss is onto the drapes and is difficult to measure. Furthermore, the use of large amounts of irrigation solution makes it impossible to assess blood loss accurately. The initial phase of any neurosurgical procedure produces blood loss, especially scalp incisions. Infiltration of the scalp with bupivacaine 0.125% with 1:200,000 epinephrine reduces blood loss and reduces hemodynamic responses (increased heart rate and blood pressure) during incision [97]. In all cases, bupivacaine blood levels were within the therapeutic range. Resection of a vascular malformation may require massive volume replacement. Placing large-bore IV catheters and having available sufficient blood products are part of appropriate planning for anesthesia and surgery. Urine output in the face of aggressive diuresis is a misleading indicator of adequate volume replacement. In this instance, CVP monitoring is very useful.

There is no perfect protocol for fluid replacement in neurosurgical patients with increased ICP. However, maintenance of cerebral perfusion should represent the optimal goal of fluid therapy. Most anesthesiologists start osmotic diuretic therapy at the beginning of anesthesia and measure the resulting urine output. As surgery and blood loss progress, volume replacement usually consists of a mixture of crystalloid and colloid solutions to maintain an isovolemic, iso-osmolar, and iso-oncotic intravascular volume. After an initial 20 mL/kg of crystalloid solution, a mixture of normal saline with albumin 5% in a ratio of 3:1 can be given. As described earlier, the brain that has sustained a recent insult (primary lesion) is vulnerable to so-called "secondary insult" (penumbra area) by a minor episode of hypotension, hypoxia or ischemia related to mechanical insult [98], (retraction) [99] or ischemia (hemodynamic instability) [100]. Although rapid administration of normal saline (10 mL/kg) has little effect on cerebral blood volume and ICP, it may reinstitute hemodynamic stability. Blood products should be administered only on the basis of hemodynamic instability and diminished oxygen-carrying capacity.

Solutions containing dextrose are associated with a poorer neurological outcome and are best avoided unless hypoglycemia has been confirmed [101]. Stressed neonates have reduced glycogen stores, and patients from the intensive care unit may have high glucose loads in their parenteral nutrition. Abrupt cessation of high-dextrose solutions can precipitate an insulin-induced hypoglycemia. In these patients, blood glucose levels should be sampled frequently and normoglycemia maintained.

Osmotic and diuretic therapy to reduce intracranial pressure
Hypertonic saline
Some investigators have suggested that extracellular volume dehydration can be accomplished by raising serum osmolality with hypertonic saline (3% saline) [102]. Hypertonic saline solution has been shown to be effective for volume resuscitation, while resulting in less cerebral edema and/or ICP elevation [103]. In children with severe traumatic brain injury, resuscitation with hypertonic saline (sodium 268 mmol/L, 598 mOsm/L) was superior to resuscitation with lactated Ringer's solution (sodium 131 mmol/L, 277 mOsm/L) [104]. Though children treated with the hypertonic saline solution had a shorter ICU stay and fewer ICP interventions, the overall survival rate and duration of hospitalization were no different between groups. In another study of children after traumatic brain injury, 3% hypertonic saline significantly reduced ICP when compared to normal saline resuscitation [105]. Based on these findings and others, there is no difference in recommendation between hypertonic saline or mannitol in the current pediatric brain trauma guidelines [106].

Mannitol
Mannitol (20% solution) remains the most popular diuretic for reducing ICP and providing brain relaxation. Small doses, such as 0.25–0.5 mg/kg, will raise osmolality by 10 mOsm and reduce cerebral edema and ICP [107]. Mannitol's effects begin within 10–15 min of its administration and persist for at least 2 h. Mannitol-induced vasodilation affects intracranial and extracranial vessels and transiently increases cerebral blood volume (CBV) and ICP while simultaneously reducing systemic blood pressure. In particular, some children may show transient hemodynamic instability (during the first 1–2 min) after rapid administration of mannitol [108]. Therefore, the drug should be given at a rate not exceeding 0.5 g/kg over 20–30 min. The initial period of hypotension will be followed by increases in cardiac index, blood volume, and pulmonary capillary wedge pressure, all of which reach peak values 15 min after infusion [109]. The changes in intravascular volume last

for about 30 min and then return to normal levels. Administration of furosemide before administering mannitol may increase venous capacitance, reduce transient increases in intravascular volume, and provide more effective dehydration. There is, however, a danger of producing profound dehydration and severe electrolyte imbalance [110].

Larger doses of mannitol produce a longer duration of action, but there is no scientific evidence that they reduce ICP further. In animal studies, larger doses of mannitol have significantly decreased the rate of CSF formation [111]. In the presence of cerebral ischemia, larger doses of mannitol 2 g/kg can be used with a presumed added benefit of free radical scavenging. In addition, higher mannitol dosages have been shown to increase CBF [112] and cardiac output [113], probably by reducing blood viscosity (rheology) [114] or by acutely increasing intravascular volume. Through the combination of these effects, it has been suggested that mannitol may cause cerebrovascular vasoconstriction and further reduce CBV. Regardless, the net effect is a multifactorial reduction in ICP from mannitol administration that most directly correlates with a reduction in CBV [115].

Loop diuretics
The loop diuretics, such as furosemide and ethacrynic acid, may reduce brain edema by inducing a systemic diuresis, decreasing CSF production [116] and improving cellular water transport [117]. Although furosemide can reduce ICP without increasing cerebral blood volume or blood osmolality, it is not as effective as mannitol [118]. The initial dose of furosemide should be 0.6–1 mg/kg if administered alone, or 0.3–0.4 mg/kg if administered with mannitol to children [119]. It has been suggested that ethacrynic acid reduces secondary brain injury by decreasing glial swelling [120]. Raising serum osmolality above 320 mOsm may precipitate acute renal failure and significant water retention, and create a clinical scenario where negative consequences occur when serum osmolality is decreased during recovery. Periods of aggressive dehydration may be followed by rebound intracranial hypertension during the recovery or normalization period.

Corticosteroids
Corticosteroids are an important part of the therapeutic regimen in neurosurgical patients with raised ICP. They reduce edema around brain tumors, but hours or days may be required to produce an effect. However, the administration of dexamethasone preoperatively or at the induction of anesthesia frequently improves the neurological status before the ICP decreases. It has been suggested that this is in response to a partial restoration of blood–brain barrier function [121].

Temperature homeostasis

In general, extremes of temperature should be avoided and situations of hypothermia and hyperthermia managed aggressively. Often, a normothermic temperature goal of 35.5–36.5°C should be used, with warming measures started below and cooling measures started above these temperature margins. Although hypothermia reduces the $CMRO_2$, it frequently delays drug clearance, slows reversal of muscle relaxants, decreases cardiac output, causes conduction abnormalities, attenuates hypoxic pulmonary vasoconstriction, alters platelet function, causes electrolyte abnormalities, and can induce postoperative shivering [122]. In addition, the intraoperative vasoconstriction produced by hypothermia reverts to vasodilation and redistribution of body heat on rewarming, and the core temperature decreases [123].

Neonates and infants are at greatest risk of hypothermia because of their large surface area relative to body mass. Despite a warm operating room, body temperature falls immediately after induction of anesthesia owing to internal redistribution of body heat from the central compartment to the periphery [124]. As heat loss continues, pediatric patients trigger non-shivering thermogenesis in an attempt to rewarm themselves [125]. In the paralyzed and ventilated patient, body temperature and end-tidal carbon dioxide ($PETCO_2$) concentration may increase at constant minute ventilation [126]. This phenomenon may not be readily apparent owing to cold fluid administration. Temperature monitoring is essential, but the actual site of the probe placement is less important than probe reliability. For this reason, we usually place the probe in the esophagus or rectum. During induction of anesthesia and during placement of IV lines and monitors, a large body surface area is exposed. During these procedures, premature infants and small infants should be placed under a servo-controlled radiant heat lamp. Extremities can be covered with plastic wrap or sheet wadding. Dry inspired gases should be warmed and moisturized with a heat exchanger [127,128]. Although the usefulness of warming blankets has been questioned, they appear to work well as long as they are positioned both above and below the patient. Blood warmers should always be used if substantial fluid replacement is required. Rewarming measures, such as a forced warm air system, can be used in the postoperative period.

Hyperthermia (>38.5°C) in the setting of pediatric traumatic brain injury has been associated with poor outcomes. Studies in both animal models and patients have shown that during and immediately after brain trauma or ischemia, temperature powerfully influences neurological recovery and increases $CMRO_2$ [129]. The association between the development of hyperthermia and increased morbidity and mortality has been described in adult and pediatric patients with ischemic stroke and closed head injury [130]. Based on these data, aggressive cooling strategies with forced air warmers, circulating cooling blankets, cold gastric lavage combined with anti pyretic therapy with acetaminophen and non-steroidal anti-inflammatory agents (NSAIDs) may be required to treat and prevent hyperthermia [131].

Venous air embolism

Venous air embolism is one of the most serious complications of anesthesia and surgery. It may occur whenever the operative site is elevated above the heart, and the risk increases as the height difference increases. Classically, it is associated with posterior fossa surgery in the sitting position, but it is not confined to this procedure. It has been reported in infants and children during procedures involving the skull, such as morcellation of the cranial vault, craniectomy for craniosynostosis, and spinal cord procedures [132]. It has also occurred with the patient in the lateral position [133]. The incidence of venous air embolism has been reduced considerably by use of the prone position for posterior fossa surgery [134] and by use of mechanical ventilation.

Air entrainment occurs when a number of conditions are met, including (1) venous pressure at the operative site that is below atmospheric pressure, (2) a vein that is open to the atmosphere, and (3) a vein that is prevented from collapsing. It most commonly occurs during the first hour of surgery, and the most frequent sites of air entrainment are the cranial diploic veins, the emissary veins, and the intracranial venous sinuses, which are kept open by their dural attachment. Venous air embolism can also occur from veins in muscles and from the puncture site of the multipoint head-holder used in children over 3 years of age [135].

Detection of venous air embolism depends entirely on the sensitivity of the monitors used. The reported incidence of air emboli varies widely [136]. Using highly sensitive precordial Doppler, the reported incidence of air embolus is as high as 58% in adult patients undergoing posterior fossa surgery in a sitting position [137]. Less than half of the cases of detected emboli produce systemic hypotension [138]. In pediatric neurosurgery, the incidence of detectable air emboli is about 33% [139] but systemic complications occur in more than half of the cases. Although children are no more prone to air emboli than adults, they are more susceptible to them. For example, the incidence of air embolism during craniosynostosis repair in supine infants may be as high as 67% [140]. This may explain why, without any obvious reason, some patients experience periods of hypotension. In addition, the increased right-sided pressure may cause air to pass from the right side of the heart to the left via an atrial septal defect, causing paradoxical air embolus (PAE). Anatomically, some 27% of patients have a patent foramen ovale and are potentially at risk for embolization to the left heart. Air also may reach the systemic circulation without the presence of an intracardiac septal defect [141] and may result in cerebral or myocardial infarction.

It is essential to take measures to avoid this potentially disastrous complication. Meticulous avoidance of a pressure gradient between the open tissue and the heart and the routine use of positive pressure ventilation are mandatory. On detecting air entrainment, the anesthesiologist must (1) advise the neurosurgeon to discontinue surgery, flood the surgical field with fluid, and compress the jugular veins and position the operative field lower than the heart to prevent further ingress of air; (2) ventilate the lungs with 100% oxygen; (3) attempt to withdraw air through the central venous catheter; (4) treat any hemodynamic consequences; and (5) if hemodynamic instability persists, turn the patient into a left-side-down position. When venous air is detected during craniotomy in children, air can be successfully aspirated from veins 38–60% of the time [139]. Intravenous fluids [142], appropriate antiarrhythmic and inotropic agents, or vasopressors may be necessary and should be administered as needed. Nitrous oxide must be discontinued because it increases the size of the embolus several-fold, causing further physiological compromise. Some authors have proposed that a positive end-expiratory pressure (PEEP) of $10\,cmH_2O$ might decrease the rate of air entry by increasing venous pressure, but less than $8\,cmH_2O$ pressure is not adequate to do so. It is possible that the use of PEEP may cause paradoxical air embolism [143]. However, $8\,cmH_2O$ PEEP did not raise the right atrial pressure above left atrial pressure [144].

Specific anesthetic considerations

Neuroradiology
Children and infants, unlike adults, frequently require general anesthesia or sedation for neuroradiological diagnostic or interventional therapeutic procedures. Several special problems are related to the administration of anesthesia in this context. Among these is the delivery of care in a remote area away from skilled help, the limitations imposed by cumbersome equipment, the need to be at a distance from the patient during the procedure, and the occasional adverse effects of contrast agents. The principal indication for anesthesia in these circumstances is to provide total immobility for extended periods for young patients who cannot co-operate. The most common procedures are CT scanning, cerebral angiography, lumbar myelography, radiation therapy, and MRI. Specific anesthetic considerations for these procedures depend on the patient's condition and the radiological demands.

Skull abnormalities: craniosynostosis
This is the most common skull anomaly in pediatric anesthesia. Special considerations for patients with craniosynostosis include increased ICP and blood loss.

Children and infants undergoing craniectomy may have increased ICP, and induction of anesthesia should proceed as discussed before. The degree of blood loss is increased in patients with multiple suture synostoses and in those more than 6 months old with thicker bone tables. Most craniosynostosis surgery is performed between 2 and 6 months of age, a period that coincides with physiological anemia. Transfusion may therefore be required to maintain an acceptable hemoglobin level. Simple suture craniectomy in the young child with normal ICP seldom requires arterial line placement. However, adequate IV access for fluid and blood replacement is essential. Children with elevated ICP and those undergoing extensive multiple suture procedures usually require arterial line placement. See Chapter 32 for a more detailed discussion of these procedures.

Hydrocephalus
Hydrocephalus is a congenital or acquired pathological condition with many variations, but it is always characterized by an increase in the amount of CSF that is now or has been under increased pressure (Fig. 23.1). It can

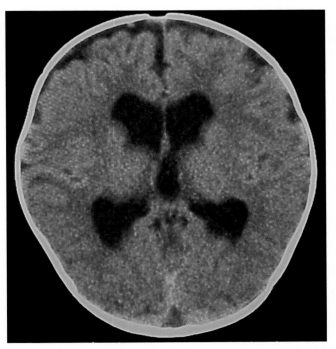

Figure 23.1 This 8-month-old boy was noted to have a recent and rapid head growth and a full anterior fontanelle. This axial CT scan reveals a communicating hydrocephalus. Note the enlarged subarachnoid space over the convexities in addition to the mildly dilated ventricles.

occur at any age. It is caused by one of four basic disease processes: congenital anomalies (e.g. Arnold–Chiari malformation), neoplasms, inflammatory conditions, and overproduction of CSF (choroid plexus papillomas).

Ventricular shunts

Three types of ventricular shunts are in current use: ventriculoperitoneal, ventriculoatrial, and ventriculopleural. Each has its indications and anesthetic implications. Often, as the pediatric patient grows, the shunt must be revised. It must be replaced if it malfunctions or becomes infected. Placement or revision of shunts is common in both severely neurologically impaired children and in otherwise healthy patients. These children may present to the operating room many times and may request a specific anesthesia induction technique. Patients who present for CSF shunting procedures may exhibit a broad spectrum of symptoms and clinical signs, ranging from an apparently healthy child with minimal disability to a seriously ill, comatose patient for whom surgery is urgent.

Considerations

Preanesthetic assessment must include the following.
- *Level of consciousness.* Patients presenting for primary shunting, shunt revision or malfunction may exhibit severe elevations in ICP that require aggressive treatment.
- *Full stomach.* Vomiting or delayed gastric emptying are indications to take precautions against aspiration of gastric contents (e.g. a rapid-sequence induction).
- *Co-existing pathology.* Does the child have evidence of other significant organ system compromise, such as the cerebral palsied child who frequently aspirates?
- *Age-related pathophysiology.* Is the patient likely to have apnea, poor pulmonary compliance or immature renal function?

Monitoring

Routine monitoring has been discussed earlier. Arterial line placement is usually reserved for the patient with uncontrolled ICP and hemodynamic instability.

Preinduction

A shunt scan helps to determine the site of malfunction. In some cases, the increased ICP caused by shunt malfunction can be reduced acutely by tapping the proximal reservoir. Infiltration of the skin with local anesthetic allows the tap to proceed with minimal trauma to the patient. The needle can be left in place to monitor ICP during induction. In the patient at risk for emesis during induction of anesthesia, placement of a nasogastric tube may precipitate coughing and bucking and increase ICP. Severely neurologically compromised children often have gastrostomy tubes, and opening these tubes before induc-

tion of anesthesia is recommended. However, this does not guarantee that the patient will not vomit and aspirate gastric contents.

Induction and intubation

Many patients with hydrocephalus have undergone multiple surgical procedures. If there is no clinical evidence of elevated ICP, anesthesia can be induced by mask or with IV drugs; we usually allow children their preference. On the other hand, children with increased ICP and delayed gastric emptying usually have anesthesia induced with thiopental, atropine, lidocaine, a narcotic, and a nondepolarizing muscle relaxant after preoxygenation. Cricoid pressure is applied and the patient is hyperventilated at low peak inspiratory pressures. Since laryngoscopy is a potent stimulus for increasing ICP, an oral tracheal tube is placed as smoothly as possible.

Maintenance

Patients are placed in a supine position with the head turned, or in a slightly lateral position. Patients with increased ICP should be placed in a 30° head-up position with minimal neck rotation or flexion to improve cerebral venous drainage. Patients whose shunt tubing is placed posteriorly and those who are placed in a lateral position should have an axillary roll placed and all extremities padded.

After the airway is secured, patients with increased ICP are hyperventilated to a $PaCO_2$ of between 25 and 30 mmHg. Patients with normal ICP are maintained at normocapnia. Spontaneous ventilation should be avoided in patients with ventriculopleural shunts to reduce the risk of pneumothorax and in those with ventriculoatrial shunts to avoid air embolism. Also, spontaneous ventilation should be avoided when the cranium is opened. Patients with poor pulmonary compliance and those at risk for apnea should be mechanically ventilated during anesthesia.

Anesthesia is usually maintained with nitrous oxide in oxygen, low concentrations of isoflurane, and minimal narcotic supplementation. Although nitrous oxide increases cerebral blood flow in anesthetized pediatric patients, increases in cerebral blood flow and $CMRO_2$ are effectively blunted by hyperventilation and pretreatment with thiopental. Halogenated anesthetics increase cerebral blood flow, cerebral blood volume, and ICP in a dose-dependent manner, with isoflurane having a less adverse effect than halothane. These agents are therefore either used in low concentrations in patients with elevated ICP or avoided entirely until the CSF is drained. Muscle relaxation is usually maintained with vecuronium or atracurium if the procedure is expected to last a short time.

Ventricular shunt procedures usually are not associated with significant blood loss or third-space losses, and fluid management centers around replacement of intravascular volume associated with emesis or drug-induced diuresis.

The body temperature may decrease during shunt procedures, despite their relatively short duration. Exposure of a large body surface area and cold preparation solution, particularly for ventriculoperitoneal shunting, may cause infants to cool rapidly.

Emergence from anesthesia

Enough time for elimination of the anesthetic agents and adequate reversal of neuromuscular blockade should be ensured before extubation of the trachea. Although it does not provide absolute insurance against regurgitation, the stomach should be suctioned before extubation of the trachea in patients suspected of having increased gastric contents. The patient should be fully awake and have an appropriate gag reflex to protect their airway against emesis. Many patients coming for shunt procedures are severely neurologically impaired and have poor airway control.

Postoperative management

As with any postsurgical patient, supplemental oxygen should be given and the respiratory pattern and adequacy assessed. Neurosurgical patients in general, and preterm infants who are less than 50 weeks' postconceptual age in particular, are likely to have abnormal respiratory patterns or apnea after surgery. Hypothermic patients should be rewarmed before extubation of the trachea.

Analgesics should be used judiciously in neurologically impaired patients. Infiltration of the skin with local anesthetic at the time of surgery substantially reduces the requirement for postoperative analgesia. Patients without preoperative neurological impairment can be given routine postoperative opioid narcotics.

Intracranial tumors

Neoplasms of the CNS account for a major proportion of all solid tumors in children younger than 15 years of age and constitute the second most common cancer in childhood after leukemia. Primary brain tumors are responsible for 20% of all cancers in children and for 20% of childhood cancer deaths. For the year 1991, the incidence for brain tumors in the United States was 3.1 per 100,000 children less than 15 years of age. Unfortunately, treatment of primary malignant brain tumors has not resulted in the same dramatic increase in survival seen with childhood leukemia. However, the survival of children with tumors of the CNS has improved significantly over the last several decades. Despite this improvement, much remains to be accomplished, especially in children less

than 2–3 years of age at the time of diagnosis. From the anesthesiologist's point of view, intracranial brain tumors are divided according to the site of the tumor. The following section describes an anesthetic approach for supratentorial and posterior fossa craniotomies and for surgical excision of craniopharyngiomata.

Supratentorial craniotomy

Supratentorial lesions account for about half of all pediatric brain neoplasms. For reasons related to embryogenesis, pediatric brain tumors often arise from midline structures, including the hypothalamus, epithalamus, and thalamus, and the basal ganglia. These tumors tend to impinge on the ventricular system and cause obstructive hydrocephalus. Hemispheric masses are more common during the first year of life. Their frequency in infants is approximately twice as high as in older children (37% compared with 16–24%). The relative incidence of hemispheric tumors also increases after 8–10 years of age.

Anesthetic considerations

- *Increased intracranial pressure.* The ICP should be estimated. The CT scan and MRI film should be reviewed.
- *Full stomach.* Delayed gastric emptying occurs in the patient with raised ICP.
- *Electrolytes and fluid.* Hydration state and electrolyte balance may be altered in the child with intracranial pathology and SIADH.
- *Age-related pathophysiology.* Anesthetic considerations are identical to those discussed earlier.
- *Positioning.* The head should be elevated not more than 10° from level. It should be confirmed that venous return is not obstructed.

Monitoring

To the routine monitoring previously described, we add an arterial line for hemodynamic monitoring and blood sampling. In patients in whom we expect significant blood loss, hemodynamic instability or air embolism, we insert a central venous catheter. A urinary catheter is inserted because of the duration of the surgical procedure and the use of osmotic diuretics.

Preinduction

Detection of preoperative elevation of ICP in patients undergoing craniotomy is essential. Most patients with large mass lesions, significant tumor edema or obstruction to CSF outflow require an anesthetic approach that aims to reduce ICP. Some children undergo ventriculostomy placement before their definitive surgical procedure, as discussed earlier. Preoperative neurological deficits should be detected and documented. Many patients with intracranial pathology present with SIADH.

Such children have evidence of hyponatremia, low serum osmolality, high urine osmolality, and oliguria. Peripheral edema is rarely present. Preoperative treatment of SIADH usually includes fluid restriction.

Induction of anesthesia and tracheal intubation

Unlike children with normal ICP, induction of anesthesia followed by rapid securing of the airway and hyperventilation are of paramount importance in patients with significantly elevated ICP. Induction of anesthesia generally proceeds as discussed in the section on hydrocephalus and includes IV thiopental, lidocaine, an opioid, and a non-depolarizing muscle relaxant. Cricoid pressure is applied and the patient hyperventilated with low peak inspiratory pressures to avoid inflation of the stomach. Laryngoscopy should proceed as smoothly as possible. Some anesthesiologists prefer nasotracheal intubation for patients in whom postoperative ventilation is expected or to better stabilize the ETTs of small infants.

Maintenance

Patients with increased ICP are generally ventilated to a $PaCO_2$ of 25–30 mmHg. Occasionally, lower levels of $PaCO_2$ are required if the brain is very "tight" and there is uncontrollable intracranial hypertension. Caution must be exercised because extreme hyperventilation may decrease CPP sufficiently to induce cerebral ischemia or to shift blood flow from brain with low flow to areas of brain with impaired autoregulation and high flow. PEEP is generally avoided to facilitate cerebral venous drainage. PEEP may also decrease MAP, which should be considered in patients with decreased CPP. In patients with impaired oxygenation, small amounts of PEEP may correct hypoxia without obstructing venous return.

Pediatric patients are usually placed supine for supratentorial procedures, with the head elevated slightly to facilitate venous drainage. Extremities should be well padded and the eyes protected from injury. Care must be taken to avoid undue flexion, extension or rotation of the neck.

Fluid management can be a problem. Patients with increased ICP are usually dehydrated after receiving mannitol. This increases the potential for hypovolemia and hypotension, especially when there is significant blood loss. CVP monitoring allows early detection of hypovolemia and volume expansion with colloid solutions such as 5% albumin. Simple craniotomy in patients without significantly increased ICP and in procedures with little blood loss frequently requires crystalloid replacement only.

Emergence

The decision to extubate the trachea at the end of the procedure is made on the basis of the success of the surgical intervention, smoothness of the intraoperative course, normalization of ICP, age of the patient, degree of residual neurological deficit, and the presence of factors that affect respiration and airway protection. Patients with inadequate respiratory efforts retain CO_2 and their ICP may therefore be increased. Those without a gag reflex cannot protect their airway. Children who remain sedated and who hyperventilate during the postoperative period should be suspected of having increased ICP. Neonates with poor pulmonary compliance or an immature respiratory drive may require postoperative mechanical ventilation. Barring any of these complications, a child's trachea can be extubated after awakening and after reversal of the neuromuscular blockade and elimination of anesthetic agents.

Postoperative management

As with any postsurgical patient, supplemental oxygen should be administered and the adequacy of respiration assessed. Patients who require postoperative ventilation also require sedation and possibly muscle relaxation, to prevent agitation and increased ICP. Infiltration of local anesthetics into the wound intraoperatively or performance of a cervical superficial plexus block at the end of the procedure can reduce the requirement for postoperative analgesics. A balance between patient comfort and the ability to follow the patient's neurological status must be sought. An obtunded patient must be investigated for increased ICP or other surgically correctible pathology, such as intracranial bleeding. Body temperature should be maintained at a normal level.

The most common cause of increased ICP after surgery is uncontrolled systemic hypertension. When postoperative pain control has been achieved, blood pressure can be controlled with vasodilators. β-Blocking drugs have been used successfully, particularly labetolol, which normally does not cross the blood–brain barrier.

Seizures frequently occur during the immediate postoperative period. Therefore, many surgeons place their patients on anticonvulsants before surgery and continue these drugs postoperatively. Phenobarbital is the most commonly used drug, and phenytoin or other medications are added if the seizures are refractory to treatment.

Craniopharyngioma

Craniopharyngioma is a benign encapsulated tumor of the hypophysis cerebri (Fig. 23.2). Children with this tumor often present with symptoms of endocrine failure, visual disturbances or hydrocephalus, as the tumor grows beyond the sella turcica and compresses the optic chiasm or other midline structures. The trans-sphenoidal approach to this tumor is rarely used in pediatric patients, and most resections are therefore performed through a

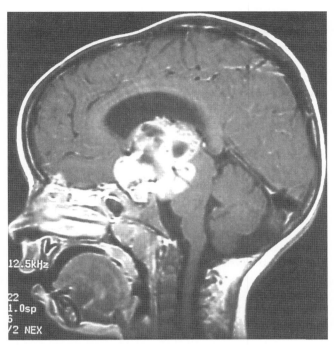

Figure 23.2 Sagittal gadolinium-enhanced T1-weighted MR of a 4-year-old boy with a large craniopharyngioma filing the sella turcica and elevating and distorting the third ventricle.

frontal craniotomy. Anesthesia for craniopharyngioma and hypothalamic tumor surgery is similar to that for supratentorial craniotomy.

Preoperative evaluation of the child with craniopharyngioma focuses on determining the presence of hydrocephalus and on the types of endocrine dysfunction that could affect anesthetic management. Children may present with symptoms of hypothyroidism, growth hormone deficiency, adrenocorticotropic hormone (ACTH) deficiency or diabetes insipidus (DI). Hormone replacement, including thyroid hormone and corticosteroids, may be necessary pre- and postoperatively.

Diabetes insipidus is a complication of pituitary surgery and head injury. It is caused by disruption of antidiuretic hormone (ADH)-secreting cells. It is rarely present preoperatively, but usually begins 4–6 h after surgery, although it occasionally becomes evident intraoperatively. Characteristically, patients produce a large quantity of dilute urine. Their serum osmolality increases and their urine osmolality is low (less than 200 mOsm/L). The urine specific gravity is below 1.002. The patient becomes hypernatremic and hypovolemic. Treatment of DI requires careful determination of the patient's hourly urine output and administration of maintenance fluids plus 75% of the previous hour's urine output. The type of fluid to be administered is determined by the patient's serum electrolyte concentrations. Urine is low in sodium content

and should be replaced with hypotonic solutions, such as D5W half-normal saline. Hyperglycemia and osmotic diuresis may occur if a large volume of D5W is used. Vasopressin or one of its analogs, such as DDAVP (1-deamino-8-D-arginine vasopressin), should be administered at an early stage of DI. When administered intraoperatively, aqueous DDAVP occasionally produces hypertension. Postoperatively, DDAVP is divided into two doses (5–30 μg/day) and given transnasally. If DDAVP is given IV, the dose is one-tenth the intranasal dose, divided into two doses. DDAVP also can be administered by constant infusion at 0.5 milliUnits/kg/h. The rate must be adjusted to achieve the desired degree of antidiuresis.

Postoperative management should include administration of steroids, thyroid, mineralocorticoid, and sex hormone supplements. Insulin-dependent diabetics may have reduced insulin requirements after surgery. Therefore, the amount of glucose in their blood must be closely monitored and their insulin regimens altered as necessary.

Other problems that arise postoperatively include seizures and hyperthermia. Surgical exposure often requires significant retraction of the frontal lobes. Consequently, anticonvulsant prophylaxis may be necessary intraoperatively and should be continued postoperatively. Injury to the hypothalamic thermoregulatory mechanisms may result in hyperthermia. Efforts should be made to maintain normothermia and reduce the risk of hypermetabolic cell injury.

Posterior fossa tumor surgery

Posterior fossa tumors (Fig. 23.3) are more frequent in children than in adults and account for about half of all pediatric brain tumors. The four most common tumors are medulloblastoma (30%), cerebellar astrocytoma (30%), brainstem glioma (30%), and ependymoma (7%). The remaining 3% include acoustic neuroma, meningioma, ganglioglioma, and other much rarer tumors. Cerebellar astrocytomas have no gender predilection but medulloblastoma occurs more frequently in males. Hydrocephalus occurs in 90% of children with medulloblastoma and in virtually all children with cerebellar astrocytoma [145].

The most frequent surgical procedure, other than for tumors, is decompression for Arnold–Chiari malformation with obex occlusion. The Arnold–Chiari malformation is a complex developmental anomaly that characteristically presents with downward displacement of the inferior cerebellar vermis into the upper cervical spinal canal and elongation of the medulla oblongata and the fourth ventricle. Preoperatively, the anesthesiologist should pay particular attention to the neurological symptoms, such as cerebellar dysfunction, upper airway

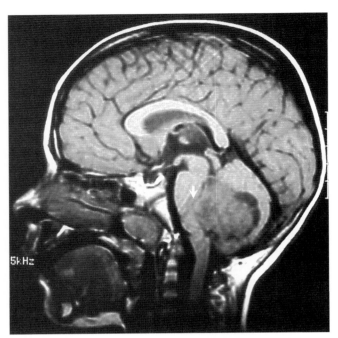

Figure 23.3 Sagittal unenhanced T1-weighted MR of a 4-year-old boy who presented with ataxia, headache and morning vomiting showing probable medulloblastoma with brainstem invasion.

obstruction (inspiratory stridor), cardiovascular instability, and increased intracranial pressure.

Anesthetic considerations

- *Age-related pathophysiology*.
- *Intracranial pressure*. Symptomatic hydrocephalus may require placement of an external ventricular drain (EVD) after induction of anesthesia. Maintenance of cerebral perfusion is essential. Mannitol, furosemide, and corticosteroids may be required.
- *Full stomach*. Pathology in the posterior fossa decreases gastric emptying in children and makes them prone to regurgitation and aspiration of gastric contents with induction of anesthesia.
- *Associated pre-existing problems*. Cardiovascular: some patients may be hypertensive in response to brainstem compression. Pulmonary: recurrent aspiration pneumonia is a common occurrence. Nervous system: central sleep apnea occurs and may persist postoperatively.
- *Air embolism*. See above.
- *Airway management*. Arnold–Chiari malformation or brainstem compression may cause upper airway dysfunction and inspiratory stridor.
- *Fluid and electrolytes*. Preoperative attempts to reduce ICP may cause electrolyte imbalance and contraction of the intravascular volume.
- *Premedication*.

Preoperative evaluation and induction of anesthesia

Preoperative assessment of these patients is similar to that described previously. During the induction of anesthesia, attempts must be made to preserve CPP, to avoid ICP elevations, and to provide an appropriate depth of anesthesia. The choice of anesthetic is not as crucial as the manner in which it is administered. A combination of thiopental, atropine, and a non-depolarizing muscle relaxant associated with a narcotic opioid, such as fentanyl, is common. Succinylcholine can be used safely unless the patient shows signs of severe increased ICP with hemodynamic instability. To minimize the possibility of kinking and obstructing the ETT during positioning, a wire-reinforced armored orotracheal tube can be used. Many neuroanesthesiologists, however, prefer to use a nasotracheal tube for better stability and fixation. Use of an oral tracheal tube with a soft bite block reduces epistaxis and avoids possible nasal mucosal injury and infection.

Maintenance of anesthesia

As with induction of anesthesia, no single anesthetic technique has been shown to be superior, and the maintenance regimen must be tailored to the needs of the patient and the requirement of the surgical procedure. Muscle paralysis is provided with a non-depolarizing muscle relaxant [146], and the ICP is reduced with mannitol and furosemide. The intermittent positive pressure ventilation is adjusted to maintain the $PaCO_2$ between 25 and 28 mmHg.

Patient positioning

Three common patient positions are used for posterior fossa tumor operations. The older literature reported that the prone position is used in 55% of cases, the sitting position in 30%, and the lateral position in 15% [147–149]. In recent years the sitting position has rarely been used in pediatrics because of the increased risk of venous air embolism. It is the anesthesiologist's responsibility to ensure that during positioning the ETT is not advanced into or withdrawn from the trachea, that ventilation is adequate, that pressure points are well padded, and that the neck is not flexed enough to occlude jugular venous drainage. The method of head fixation depends on the age of the patient, the skull thickness, and the surgeon's needs. Horseshoe headrests are useful but the patient's face must be padded carefully and the eyes must be free of compression. After 3 years of age, the multi-pin head-holder is preferable. Infiltration of the pin sites with local anesthetic reduces nociceptive responses.

Monitoring

Monitoring for posterior fossa surgery is basically the same as for supratentorial craniotomy, with one important exception. The precordial Doppler should be used to detect air embolism (see above). Occasionally, sensory-evoked potentials should be obtained during resection of intramedullary or brainstem tumors.

Emergence and recovery from anesthesia

Prompt awakening is mandatory, but it is important to keep the patient hemodynamically stable and unstimulated during tracheal extubation. The pathological process often dictates the appropriate postoperative airway management (e.g. postoperative tracheal intubation is essential after resection of intramedullary tumor). When early tracheal extubation is appropriate, intraoperative administration of narcotics plus lidocaine 0.5–1 mg/kg to infants and children [150] will allow emergence from anesthesia without coughing and straining, which might otherwise lead to a hypertensive episode and intracerebral bleeding. Postoperative pain can usually be managed with morphine 50 µg/kg, with or without acetaminophen. Avoidance of medications that affect the sensorium or the pupils is important.

Myelodysplasia

Hydrocephalus is accompanied by abnormalities in the spinal column and spinal cord in 70% of infants. Myelodysplasia is an abnormality in fusion of the embryological neural groove during the first month of gestation. Failure of neural tube closure results in a sac-like herniation of meninges (meningocele) or a herniation of neural elements (myelomeningocele). The spinal cord is often tethered caudally by the sacral roots, causing orthopedic or urological symptoms in later childhood if the tethered cord is not surgically corrected.

Myelomeningoceles most commonly occur in the lumbosacral region, but they can occur at any level in the neuraxis. Most children with meningomyelocele have an associated Arnold–Chiari type II malformation and hydrocephalus. An encephalocele is most frequently found in the occipital/suboccipital areas or nasally. Anencephaly results from a defect in anterior closure of the neural groove.

Myelodysplasia causes exposure of CNS tissue and places the patient at risk for infection and death. The incidence of infection increases the longer the lesion remains unrepaired but occurs in less than 7% of patients if the defect is repaired within 48 h of birth. Furthermore, delay in closure of the defect increases the likelihood of progressive neural damage and decreased motor function. For these reasons, myelodysplasia is regarded as a surgical emergency, and most neonates present for surgery in the first 24 h of life.

In addition, patients with myelodysplasia have historically had an increased risk for the development of latex allergy. Because of this, routine care of these patients at many centers is to manage them presumptively as having "latex allergy" (see Chapter 40).

Anesthetic considerations

- *Co-existing disease.* Additional pathology may accompany myelodysplasia (Arnold–Chiari, hydrocephalus, congenital heart disease, prematurity).
- *Age-related pathophysiology.*
- *Airway management.* Encephaloceles may be associated with difficulty in control of the airway.
- *Positioning.* Protection of the neuroplaque.
- *Volume status.* High third-space losses from the skin defect.
- *Potential for hypothermia.* Exposure of large body surface area and loss of third-space fluid.

Monitoring

Routine monitoring is necessary. Blood loss can be insidious, especially if the sac is large and significant undermining of skin, relaxing incisions or skin grafting are required for closure of the defect. Blood transfusion may be necessary. Patients with encephaloceles who must undergo craniotomy for repair should have an arterial line placed for blood pressure and hemoglobin measurement. A central venous line may be indicated for repair of a nasal encephalocele when the repair is done in a semi-sitting position.

Preinduction of anesthesia

Infants presenting for repair of meningomyeloceles rarely exhibit increased ICP. The majority of myelodysplastic patients have an associated Arnold–Chiari malformation and most have hydrocephalus, which usually requires ventricular shunt placement. Preoperative assessment of these children reveals a variety of neurological deficits, depending on the level of the lesion. Seventy-five percent of all lesions occur in the lumbosacral region. Lesions above the level of T4 usually result in paraplegia, whereas lesions below S1 allow ambulation. The legs are severely affected by lesions between L4 and S1.

Before induction of anesthesia, the patient's volume status should be assessed. These patients have the potential for large third-space losses from the exposed myelomeningocele.

Induction of anesthesia and tracheal intubation

Anesthesia for patients with lumbosacral or thoracic myelomeningoceles can be induced either in the left lateral position or supine with the sac protected by a cushioned ring. Anesthesia can be induced in a majority of patients with propofol, atropine, and a muscle relaxant. Either a non-depolarizing muscle relaxant or succinylcholine can be used safely [151]. Patients with nasal encephalocele commonly have airway obstruction, and it may be difficult to obtain a good mask fit.

Maintenance of anesthesia

After tracheal intubation, the patient is turned to the prone position. Injury to the exposed neural tissue must be prevented. Chest and hip rolls are placed to ensure that the abdomen is free, to facilitate ventilation and to reduce intra-abdominal pressure and decrease bleeding from the epidural plexus. Since most of these children have an Arnold–Chiari malformation, excessive rotation of the neck should be avoided. The extremities should lie in a relaxed position and be well padded. The lungs are mechanically ventilated. Barotrauma in the immature lung must be prevented. Premature infants (especially those of less than 32 weeks' gestation) are at increased risk for retinopathy of prematurity [152] and lung injury from prolonged exposure to high oxygen concentrations. Anesthesia can be maintained with a variety of agents, but higher-dose opioids and ketamine may cause postoperative apnea. Muscle relaxants are contraindicated during maintenance of anesthesia because nerve stimulation is often required to identify neural structures. The large area of exposed tissue and the liberal use of cold surgical preparation solutions increase the risk of hypothermia in these patients. Care must be taken to prevent drying or thermal injury to the exposed neural tissue by radiant heat lamps.

Myelomeningocele repair is often accomplished with the aid of the surgical microscope, and some surgeons will request that neuromuscular blockade not be used during the repair so that motor response in the lower extremities can be detected.

Emergence

Neonates at risk for apnea after anesthesia, patients with severe central neurological deficits, and those undergoing craniotomy for encephalocele repair should be extubated fully awake. Patients with nasal encephalocele repairs may have residual airway obstruction or blood in the oropharynx, and may require postoperative tracheal intubation.

Basic anesthetic considerations for the postoperative period have been discussed above.

Spinal cord surgery

Common diseases of the spinal cord that require surgery include herniated disks, spondylosis, syringomyelia,

primary or metastatic tumors, hematomas or abscesses, and trauma (Fig. 23.4). In all cases, compression of the spinal cord may produce ischemia, interstitial edema and venous congestion, and may interfere with nerve transmission. Maintaining spinal cord perfusion pressure and reducing spinal cord compression are crucial. Despite apparently optimal surgical and anesthetic management, devastating neurological complications still occur with spinal surgery. Intraoperative monitoring of spinal cord function includes the wake-up test, somatosensory-evoked potentials (SSEPs), and motor-evoked potentials (MEPs). The wake-up test remains the traditional method for assessing spinal cord well-being during corrective procedures on the spinal column. Its main advantage is that it assesses anterior spinal cord (i.e. motor) function, but it does so only at one time. Evoked potential monitors (e.g. SSEP monitoring) generate an electrical potential by stimulation of peripheral nerves (e.g. the median nerve at the wrist or the posterior tibial nerve at the ankle). If nerve transmission is intact, a signal is recorded from the scalp

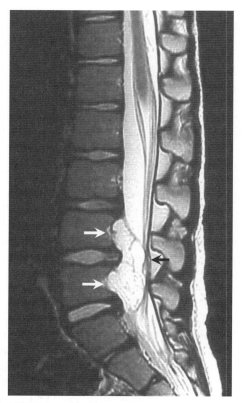

Figure 23.4 This 8-year-old girl presented clinically with bent-over gait and severe back pain. A large extradural lesion was revealed during a sagittal T2-weighted MR. This mass is anterior to the thecal sac with severe compression of the thecal contents (*black arrow*) and scalloping of the posterior vertebral bodies (*white arrows*).

or at various sites along the neural pathway. The electrical signals arise from axonal action potentials and graded postsynaptic potentials as the impulse is propagated from the periphery to the brain. The technique measures only the response of the sensory nervous system. This limitation can be overcome by use of MEPs, in which the motor cortex is stimulated by a transcranial electric current or a pulsed magnetic field generated by a coil placed over the scalp. See Chapter 26 for a more detailed discussion of spinal cord monitoring, and scoliosis surgery.

Head injury

Head trauma is a major cause of morbidity and mortality in the pediatric population. Skull fractures (Fig. 23.5) are found in more than 25% of all children who present at hospitals with head injuries and in more than 50% of fatal cases of childhood head trauma. The incidence of post-traumatic intracranial hematomas varies considerably, but some children with head injuries do require surgical treatment. Failure to recognize the presence of a hematoma may transform an otherwise mild head injury into a fatal or permanently disabling one.

Head injury causes several different pathophysiological events, including intracranial hematomas (epidural, subdural, intracerebral, and brain contusion), brain edema, and systemic effects. Adults suffer more hematomas than children, and children have diffuse cerebral edema more frequently [153].

Epidural hematoma

This lesion is frequently caused by laceration of a middle meningeal artery during a deceleration injury. Children do not necessarily have an overlying skull fracture (Fig. 23.6). Epidural hematomas comprise 25% of all intracranial hematomas in pediatric patients and are a true neurosurgical emergency. In adults there is a lucid interval between the initial loss of consciousness and later neurological deterioration. Children often do not have the initial alteration in the state of consciousness observed in adults. The child who is old enough to talk complains of an increasing headache and then becomes confused or lethargic. Rapid development of hemiparesis, posturing, and pupillary dilation occurs frequently and may confuse

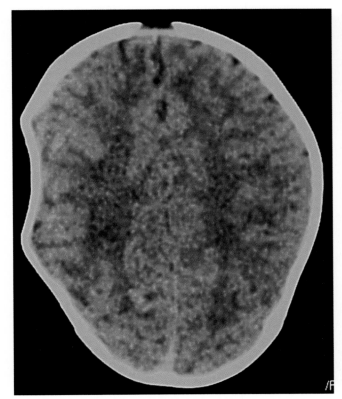

Figure 23.5 Axial non-contrast CT showing no underlying contusion or hematoma in a 4-month-old boy. He suffered no neurological sequelae from this depressed "ping-pong" skull fracture.

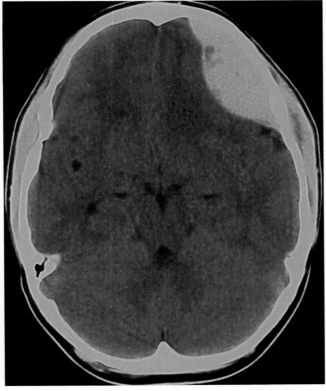

Figure 23.6 This non-enhanced axial CT reveals a typical lens-shaped epidural hematoma. Although the patient presented with a GCS of 14, he quickly became very lethargic.

the diagnosis. Rapid expansion of the hematoma causes herniation of the temporal lobe downward through the tentoria incisura. Anisocoria is an early sign. Herniation eventually leads to rostrocaudal deterioration and is associated with bradycardia, slowed and irregular breathing, and widened pulse pressure (Cushing triad). The relationship between the degree of brain shift and the level of consciousness has been confirmed; the role of uncal herniation in the syndrome has been questioned.

Subdural hematoma

Subdural hematomas are associated with parenchymal contusion, blood vessel laceration, and cortical damage (Fig. 23.7). The mass effect of the contused and edematous brain may prompt surgical removal of the hematoma if the brain region involved is not functionally important. Studies using positron emission tomography have demonstrated that cerebral metabolism and blood flow are reduced by 50% with brain contusion [154]. Severe edema and elevated ICP often lead to persistent neurological deficits.

Intracerebral hematoma

Intracerebral hematomas are rare but carry a poor prognosis. Surgery is usually avoided for fear of damaging viable brain tissue.

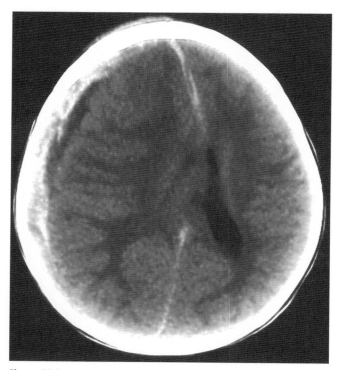

Figure 23.7 A non-contrast axial CT in a 2-year-old comatose boy shows a large right acute subdural hematoma. It is important to notice the tremendous shift of the midline to the left.

Anesthetic considerations

- *Resuscitation and stabilization.* Airway, breathing, and circulation are essential components of the initial clinical assessment. Traumatized patients often have a variety of physiological disturbances, including acid–base and electrolyte imbalances and abnormalities of glucose homeostasis and body temperature control.
- *Neurological status.* The Glasgow Coma Scale provides a means of detecting changes in the patient's condition. Symptoms of raised ICP must be evaluated.
- *Associated injuries.* Pediatric trauma often occurs from high-velocity energy transfer, which leads to injuries to the neck, chest, and abdominal organs.
- *Full stomach.* Vomiting leads to pulmonary aspiration and respiratory complications.
- *Age-related pathophysiology.*

Monitoring

Arterial catheter and central venous line placement is indicated. A urinary catheter should be inserted unless contraindicated by an associated bladder neck injury. Central body temperature should be monitored at all times.

Preinduction of anesthesia

Computed tomography is the procedure of choice for evaluation of head injury during the first 72 h after the accident. Management of an elevated ICP is essential to provide a safe anesthetic. Adequate hemodynamic resuscitation and stabilization must be achieved to maintain a normal CPP and brain tissue oxygenation.

Induction and intubation

Providing a patent airway is an essential part of the management of patients with head injury. Although the airway of an unconscious patient may not be compromised by the injury, tracheal intubation will protect the lungs against aspiration of stomach contents or secretions and allow ventilatory support of patients with increased ICP. The association of head injury and neck injury occurs so often in infants and children that tracheal intubation must be accomplished with minimal manipulation of the neck. The neck should be stabilized by an assistant who applies axial traction. Since a cervical spine fracture is always considered present until proven otherwise in patients with head injury, use of the Sellick maneuver is contraindicated. Patients should be hemodynamically stable before anesthesia is induced. After airway injury has been ruled out, anesthesia should be induced rapidly with atropine, thiopental, lidocaine, and either succinylcholine or a non-depolarizing muscle relaxant such as vecuronium. Ketamine is contraindicated. If the patient is suspected of having a difficult airway, a two-person technique may be required for tracheal intubation. Depending on the age of the patient, the use of a volatile anesthetic and assisted ventilation or the use of neuroleptanesthesia with topicalization of the larynx is recommended.

Maintenance of anesthesia

Anesthetic considerations for maintenance of anesthesia are similar to those previously described for supratentorial surgery. Evacuation of an intracranial hematoma usually requires a craniotomy, which can commonly be done without opening the dura mater. Evacuation of a large hematoma may suddenly decrease ICP and allow upward movement of the brainstem through the tentoria incisura. This may result in transient hemodynamic instability and cardiac arrhythmias.

Emergence and postoperative management

Patients with severe head injury remain intubated after surgery to provide ventilatory support and to control elevated ICP. Transfer to an ICU is indicated for continued care.

Cervical spinal cord injury

Isolated cervical spine injury is uncommon in the pediatric population. However, all children with severe head injury should be treated as though they have a cervical spine injury, until proven otherwise. Injury to the high cervical cord is usually caused by high-velocity injuries to the cranium (Fig. 23.8). Children with cord injury or disruption of the cord often present without respiratory efforts, often in cardiac arrest or with profound hypotension. They frequently die from hypoxic/ischemic encephalopathy and may have serious traumatic brain injury. In one study, all patients with absent vital signs had high cervical cord luxation on a lateral view radiograph of the neck [155]. Physicians caring for such patients might think that the hypotension is related to blood loss from intra-abdominal, pelvic or thoracic injury, or even from devastating cerebral injury and loss of brainstem function.

Anesthetic considerations and management

Some cervical spine injury victims have signs of brain shift and elevated ICP. The anesthetic considerations for these patients include the following.
- Resuscitation and stabilization of cardiopulmonary function, i.e. spinal shock.
- Decreasing ICP and improving cerebral perfusion.
- Stabilization of the cervical spine.
- Correction of metabolic disturbances.
- Treatment of acute respiratory distress syndrome (ARDS).

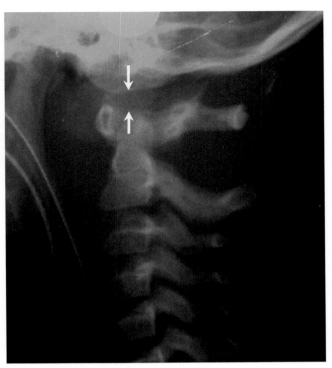

Figure 23.8 Lateral radiograph of the cervical spine of a 6-year-old boy showing a significant separation of the occipital condyles from the arch of C1 (*white arrows*). He presented with a GCS of 3 and no spontaneous respirations.

- Identification of the central rostrocaudal deterioration and uncal herniation.
- Meeting the fluid requirements for trauma victims with iso-osmolar solutions such as normal saline.
- Monitoring arterial pressure, CVP, and urine output.
- Correcting the coagulopathy often caused by brain tissue thromboplastin release.
- Treatment of DI (see craniopharyngioma).
- Treatment of SIADH.
- Controlling the hyperglycemia that frequently occurs in head-injured patients, which is thought to be a good indicator of the severity of the injury and a predictor of outcome. It is advisable to prevent the increase in glucose associated with head injury [156].

Newer procedures in pediatric neurosurgery

There are several recent developments in the neurosurgical procedures performed in the pediatric patient population which require special attention to anesthetic details which affect the outcomes of these procedures.

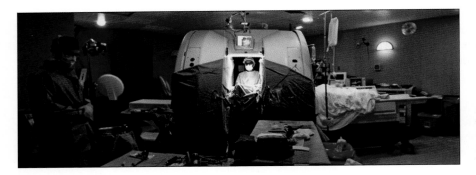

Figure 23.9 The first intraoperative MRI suite was installed at the Brigham and Women's Hospital, Boston, in 1994. Reproduced from Foroglou et al [187] with permission from Taylor & Francis.

Pre-, intra- and postoperative imaging

Computer-assisted navigation is a relatively new surgical tool, designed to improve both neurosurgical safety (through better navigation near critical anatomical structures) and effectiveness (through better localization of pathology). Tumor resection from the brain is made difficult when margins that were distinct on MRI are indistinct to visual inspection. The use of stereotaxy to locate the real-time position of surgical instruments relative to calibrated maps of patient anatomical and functional imaging is the most recent solution to this problem.

Clinical use of stereotaxy was first reported over 50 years ago, and was done by calibrating mechanical frames to atlas data of human anatomy [157]. The next development in neurosurgical stereotaxy was the use of CT scanning to calibrate stereotaxic frames to individual patient anatomy [158]. The technology continued to follow advancements in neuroradiology and engineering. In the last two decades, the technology has incorporated real-time spatial positioning of surgical activity to three-dimensional maps of the patient's intracranial space, eliminating the need for the bulky and uncomfortable frame. These techniques use optical, ultrasonic or electromagnetic signals to track the position in space of surgical instruments relative to fiducial markers placed on the patient scalp at the time of preoperative imaging. The infrared optical devices have, in particular, become popular, and they use a system of cameras, light-emitting diodes, and/or reflective fiducials to track surgical instruments as they pass through the surgical field.

Thus, the science of neuronavigation has gone from frames calibrated to atlas data to real-time position determination in a patient-specific spatial map. The latest advancement in the field is predictable from this progression. The brain is not spatially fixed in time, and moves with position changes and surgical interventions. It has, therefore, become desirable to have not only real-time instrument tracking but also real-time updating of the topographical map of the surgical field. Immediate postoperative MRI of patients after tumor resection is one possible approach, but neurosurgical suites with in-room MRI are becoming a more common approach (Fig. 23.9) [159].

Specific anesthetic considerations for a surgical procedure involving perioperative imaging technologies include the potential for:

- awake patient
- analgesia
- airway maintenance.

Younger or anxious patients unable to co-operate will require general anesthesia, while older children and adults may be appropriate for awake craniotomy techniques.

Anesthetic management of these patients undergoing intraoperative MRI includes previously mentioned considerations inherent to the procedure, plus the added complexity of safely conducting the procedure in the operative environment. This issue involves not only the anesthesia machine and monitoring equipment, but includes all the ancillary equipment including the operating table, warming devices, and surgical equipment, including instrumentation and electrocautery. Thus, the vigilance of the staff for both patient and personnel safety is paramount – this includes limiting OR access and staff proximity to the MRI scanner [160,161].

Awake craniotomy for seizure treatment

Neurosurgical intervention for epilepsy is generally reserved for patients refractory to antiepileptic medications. Three types of surgery for epilepsy may be encountered: resection of a local epileptogenic lesion, such as a cavernous angioma or a focal cortical dysplasia; temporal lobe resection; and placement of a vagal nerve stimulator.

Focal epileptogenic regions of the brain are often delineated by invasive diagnostic mapping procedures. One such example is the placement of a subdural grid. The grids are placed over cortical areas suspected to be epileptogenic. Patients are kept in hospital and taken to an epilepsy observation unit while the grids are monitored for seizure activity. Functional mapping with stimulation of the electrodes is also helpful to define a plan for resection that optimizes seizure reduction and minimizes loss of function. Temporal lobe resection is one of the more common surgical procedures for epilepsy, and can involve varying degrees of resection to include the anterior region of the temporal lobe and underlying hippocampus.

Specific anesthetic considerations for a surgical procedure for treatment of epilepsy include:
- co-operative (awake) patient
- analgesia
- airway maintenance.

Preinduction

The preoperative evaluation must determine the degree of co-operation that can be achieved and if the patient can tolerate an anesthetic/analgesic without difficulty in airway management. Because of these issues, the ability to perform awake mapping is usually limited to older children and adults. Reports of "awake" or "asleep-awake-asleep" (AAA) techniques have been applied in children as young as 4 years of age. However, the majority of children reported in the literature are greater than 11 years old. Anyone experienced in this technique will admit that success is dependent on preparing the parents and the child, establishing realistic expectations and determining if the child is psychologically mature and ready for an awake approach [162]. Patients (whether pediatric or adult) may not be good candidates if they have a movement disorder, poor co-operation with verbal commands or sleep disorders. Sleep apnea and a difficult airway are often considered absolute exclusions from this approach, as additional airway support is difficult given the patient's position during the procedure.

Anesthetic approach

Excision of a seizure focus requires a co-operative though sedated patient, permitting the precise mapping of the surgical site by cortical electroencephalography (ECG) (Fig. 23.10). Those most experienced with this procedure in children advocate a neuroleptic analgesic technique [163]. Historically, this was accomplished with intravenous administration of droperidol and fentanyl with or without a premedication, but newer agents such as dexmedetomidine and propofol are most frequently used. Most will supplement with nitrous oxide/O_2 by facemask to facilitate regional administration of local anesthetic and scalp block for placement of invasive monitoring lines (i.e. arterial and central venous catheters, if needed) and placement of the multi-pin head-holder [97]. Once the holder is in place, vascular access is adequate and patient is positioned, the MAC is provided using a total intravenous anesthetic (TIVA) technique.

Propofol sedation became the first widely used alternative to the classic neuroleptic technique. A variety of

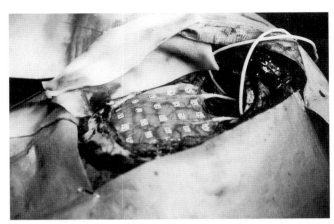

Figure 23.10 Cortical electrode application on the surface of the brain to detect epileptic foci.

approaches have been reported using propofol with and without an opioid (such as fentanyl or remifentanil), and even having propofol dispensed in older children as patient-controlled sedation (PCS) [164,165]. Dexmedetomidine has been utilized in children and adults to facilitate awake craniotomy procedures. Studies evaluating the use of dexmedetomidine for this surgical approach have found successful sedation and reduced needs for supplemental medications for pain or nausea [166].

Electrical currents generated by seizure activity produce magnetic fields that can be measured by magnetoencephalography (MEG). This non-invasive technique is not affected by the soft tissues or bone, and can be integrated with EEG monitoring to improve the accuracy of cortical epileptic foci mapping. Since active seizure activity is required for this technique to be most effective, methohexital (1–1.5 mg/kg) is administered intravenously to increase epileptiform discharges. Note that this should only be done with the appropriate level of monitoring and presence of the anesthesiologist to manage the patient should they become postictal or oversedated.

Hemispherectomy

Children with severe seizure disorders, unresponsive to medical management, may be candidates to undergo resection of the affected cerebral hemisphere, or hemispherectomy [167]. To meet criteria, children typically have a generalizable seizure that comes from a focus in a single hemisphere. This may require prior grid placement with mapping, functional MRI or other imaging prior to the grid removal and hemisphere resection.

Deep brain stimulator placement

Patients with dystonia or refractory seizure acitivty may be candidates for a deep brain stimulator (DBS) [168]. Placement of these devices often requires preoperative imaging for stereotactic guidance followed by an intraoperative phase of the procedure that allows for conducting physiological tasks for improved mapping of the globus pallidus internus (GPI). Similar to an awake craniotomy, an AAA anesthetic can be utilized to facilitate the sometimes lengthy process of imaging followed by awake surgery. In centers that do not have an intraoperative MRI suite, this will require the patient to be imaged under anesthesia in a remote location and then typically transported under anesthesia/sedation and monitoring to the operating room. Once in the OR, the patient can then be emerged, extubated and maintained sedated with MAC using propofol or dexmedetomidine. Neurophysiological monitoring is incorporated to help establish microelectrode recordings to verify and adjust the position of the electrode/lead into the deep target of the brain. Because these procedures tend to be long (6–12h), a general anesthetic for the imaging proportions before the procedure is often required in children [169] while other groups have reported successful completion of the entire procedure in adults with little or no anesthesia (i.e. scalp block only) [170]. Regardless of the technique applied, the goal is to minimize interference with the introperative monitoring while facilitating communication during an often long and drawn-out procedural day, which will include a frame placement and burr-hole drilling [171,172].

Cerebrovascular anomalies

Patients with intracranial vascular malformations such as arteriovenous malformations (AVMs) or cerebral aneurysms are commonly co-managed by the pediatric anesthesiologist in conjunction with neurologists, neurosurgeons and interventional neuroradiology [173]. This may require that one or more anesthetics be provided to facilitate the diagnosis and/or intervention for the lesion. Since congenital and acquired forms of AVMs can be one of the greatest anesthetic challenges throughout life, we will focus on their general management in infants and children.

Arteriovenous malformations and arterial aneurysms can be acquired, but the majority arise from abnormal development of the arteriolar-capillary network that connects the arterial and venous systems. These vascular malformations often consist of large arterial feeding vessels that lead to dilated connecting vessels and then to the venous system. Flow of blood through this low-resistance connection results in progressive distension of the venous structures and increased venous mixed oxygen content from the shunting of blood. Specific AVM scenarios that occur in infants and children involve the posterior cerebral artery and the great vein of Galen (Fig. 23.11). These anomalies often present in the neonatal

period with congestive heart failure (CHF). Alternatively, patients can present with obstructive hydrocephalus from saccular enlargement or dilation of the vein of Galen that directly compresses the aqueduct and prevents drainage of the cerebrospinal fluid.

Outside the neonatal period, many AVMs go undetected until the fourth or fifth decade of life with only 18% reported to be in patients under 15 years of age. Though the incidence is low, when intracranial AVMs occur, neurological injury can result from one or more causes:
- hemorrhage with thrombosis or acute infarction
- compression of adjacent brain tissue or intracranial structures
- parenchymal ischemia created by "steal" of blood flow through the AVM
- congestive heart failure from the shunt
- surgical or interventional injury resulting in disruption or diversion of blood flow from viable brain tissue supplied by the AVM during treatment.

Therefore, families and physicians must balance these potential outcomes when deciding between surgical versus interventional treatment options. Regardless, patients with complex AVM lesions may undergo interventional or stereotactic radiosurgical procedures to control blood flow as definitive or adjunctive therapy. In

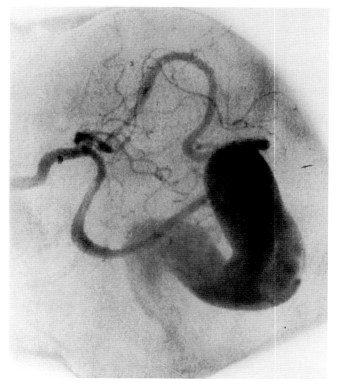

Figure 23.11 Lateral view of an aneurysm of the great vein of Galen. The main arterial contribution is from the anterior cerebral artery. The dilated vein of Galen empties directly into an enlarged straight sinus.

addition, surgical clipping of feeding vessels or removal of aneurysmal tissue may need to be done as either a single or staged procedure, again necessitating clear communication between the anesthesiologist and the various treatment teams to facilitate optimal care.

Anesthetic considerations

Considerations for patients undergoing AVM resection or embolization include the following.

- *Assessment for pre-existing pathophysiology.* Does the patient present with increased ICP or congestive heart failure? Does the patient have additional congenital defects?
- *Age-related pathophysiology.* Will organ system maturity affect the anesthetic technique?
- *Blood loss.* The possibility of massive blood loss is high, especially if pre-resection therapies for embolization were limited.
- *Ventilation pattern.* Hyperventilation to control cerebrovascular tone and reduce inflow is a therapeutic consideration for most AVM treatment.

Monitoring

Routine monitoring is as previously described. Patients undergoing AVM resection should have vascular access via two large-bore peripheral IV catheters that are capable of delivering blood products should hemorrhage occur. Intravenous solutions should be warmed throughout the procedure. Invasive hemodynamic monitoring with an arterial line is essential. CVP monitoring is useful for determining intravascular status, and to facilitate administration of medications. A urinary Foley catheter is essential and should be placed after induction of anesthesia.

Preinduction

Symptoms can vary depending on the age of the patient and the magnitude and size of the AVM [148]. Older children often present with evidence of subarachnoid hemorrhage (SAH) or intraventricular hemorrhage (IVH). Up to 50% of children who present with spontaneous SAH have an AVM as the etiology [174]. In 24% of children, seizure is a common presenting feature. However, the neonatal presentation of AVM is often associated with congestive heart failure and deserves special attention.

The low-resistance pathway of the AVM creates a situation of volume overload and high-output heart failure. The symptoms of congestive heart failure rarely manifest *in utero* because the patency of the ductus arteriosus provides for increased systemic flow through the AVM and reduces the work of the ventricles. However, after birth, with closure of the ductus, the left ventricle alone is left to meet the demands of increased arterial to venous flow. The degree of the arterial to venous shunt will affect the demand on the left ventricle. In addition, in the presence of a low resistance cerebral AVM, a low systemic diastolic pressure results. The low intra-aortic pressure during diastole, combined with increased left end-diastolic pressure and heart rate from the ventricular failure, results in reduced coronary perfusion and worsening myocardial function from ischemia [175]. The cycle of ventricular failure and decreased oxygen delivery to the systemic tissues causes the cascade of adaptive mechanisms, which results in decreased urine output and increased fluid retention [148,149]. Physical examination of the infant shows signs such as tachypnea, pulmonary edema, tachycardia, hepatomegaly, and ECG changes. Echocardiography will often confirm the hyperdynamic nature of the congestive heart failure, and evidence of functional failure of one or both ventricles. Laboratory studies may provide evidence of electrolyte abnormalities from aggressive diuretic management. Some infants may require endotracheal intubation and mechanical ventilation support, and inotropic support, all of which may help reduce the workload of the failing myocardium.

Induction of anesthesia and tracheal intubation

Prevention of hypertension during induction is desirable, given the possible association between AVM bleeding and hypertension. Inhalation or IV induction of anesthesia can be performed if there is no evidence of increased intracranial pressure. This can be accomplished with a variety of anesthetic agents. In the patient with AVM and elevated intracranial pressure, an IV induction is preferable with attention to avoiding hypotension and low cerebral perfusion pressure. In the neonate with AVM and congestive heart failure, special care should be taken to induce anesthesia and maintain cardiac output. Extreme caution should be maintained as many anesthetic agents are myocardial depressants, and could precipitate cardiac arrest. To this end, placement of IV and arterial lines is useful prior to induction. Either oral or nasotracheal intubation is reasonable after induction of anesthesia.

Maintenance of anesthesia

Considerations for maintenance of anesthesia include the following:
- positioning
- ventilation
- anesthetic agents
- blood loss and fluid management
- temperature maintenance.

Positioning for the procedure will be dictated by the site of the AVM. Typically, AVMs receive blood supply from the middle cerebral artery and the majority are approached by a supratentorial craniotomy.

All patients should undergo mechanical ventilation with intended maintenance of normocapnia. Patients with evidence of elevated ICP may require transient hyperventilation to control intracranial pressure, and consideration of ongoing ICP monitoring may be necessary. In general, normocarbia is preferable and hypocarbia should be avoided, as the resultant cerebrovascular vasoconstriction may result in more shunting of blood flow away from normal tissues and into the AVM – potentially contributing to increased cerebral ischemia and increased bleeding from the AVM.

Anesthetic agents used for maintenance are similar to those for any intracranial procedure. If congestive heart failure is absent, then permissive or controlled hypotension can be applied to facilitate control of bleeding from the AVM during ligation. This can be accomplished with infused antihypertensive agents, such as nicardipine, nitroprusside or fenoldepam. Neonates with congestive heart failure undergoing AVM ligation or treatment require inotropic support and are not candidates for permissive hypotensive strategies. In these infants, vasoactive drugs should be readily available and administered through a central venous catheter.

Fluid management in these patients is challenging. Neonates may not tolerated large volume shifts or decreases in hemoglobin concentration, especially if they have elements of cardiac dysfunction. Early efforts to maintain normal intravascular volume and stable hemoglobin content should be the goal. This may necessitate early blood replacement and judicious supplementation with inotropic support.

Maintaining a normal body temperature is important and can be difficult given the fluid losses and sometimes massive transfusion requirements. This usually requires the use of both fluid and convective warming devices that should be adjusted to avoid profound hypothermia and coagulopathy. Though the merits of hypothermia (temperature <35°C) for neuroprotection in neurosurgical procedures are debated, hyperthermia (temperature >38°C) should be avoided as this can worsen ischemic injury by increasing metabolic demands of the brain and the body.

Emergence from anesthesia

Considerations for emergence from anesthesia after AVM treatment include the following.
- Elimination of anesthetic agents.
- Reversal of neuromuscular blockade.
- Assessment of respiration effort and airway patency.
- Assessment of neurological function.

Patients without a history of CHF can be extubated at the end of surgery if they are neurologically appropriate and hemodynamically stable. However, those patients with a history of significant CHF or who are at risk for significant neurological deficits (i.e. required brain resection, significant brain retraction or obvious cerebral edema) should remain sedated and be moved to the intensive care unit with an endotracheal tube in place.

Postoperative management

The basic anesthetic considerations for postoperative care of patients following AVM treatment include the following.
- Cerebral edema.
- Congestive heart failure.
- Hypertension.
- Vasospasm.

Cerebral edema can arise from either the AVM itself or from the therapeutic approach – be it surgical or interventional. Certainly, the interventional procedures for embolization or radiosurgery cause less injury to the tissues getting to the AVM but they can still result in significant edema [176]. In those situations where the edema is anticipated or recognized, leaving the trachea intubated and monitoring the patient in the ICU are indicated. Following resection of a large AVM, it may require several days for the cerebral edema to resolve and the patient's neurological exam and level of consciousness to become appropriate. During this period, supportive care and careful neurological monitoring are of greatest importance.

Despite removal or reduction of the extracardiac shunting of blood, patients with preoperative myocardial dysfunction remain critical in the days following recovery from the surgery and require ICU care. In addition to maintaining an adequate cerebral perfusion pressure, the care team must balance the needs of the myocardium to reduce afterload. Aggressive analgesic and antihypertensive management may be required to prevent sudden increases in arterial blood pressure, which not only stresses the heart but increases the risk of acute intracranial bleeding.

Vasospasm is not a common postoperative complication, but must be a consideration if the patient's neurological status deteriorates or if SAH was present in the perioperative period. The pathogenesis of vasospasm is not completely understood, but early diagnosis and intervention can be beneficial. Transcranial Doppler sonography has been used to guide therapy in adults, but its role in children remains limited. Certainly, these measurements can detect increased blood flow velocities and allow for diagnosis of the condition as well as providing a means of guiding therapy. Treatment is typically with adequate hydration, stable/generous blood pressure, and use of calcium channel blockers [177].

Interventional neuroradiology

Over the past two decades, neuroradiological techniques and expertise in the diagnosis and treatment of diseases of the CNS have undergone significant advances. Interventional neuroradiology (INR), or endovascular neurosurgery, has evolved as a hybrid of traditional neurosurgery and neuroradiology. Though practice varies between institutions, INR has developed a clear role in the management of a variety of neurosurgical conditions, particularly neurovascular diseases (see section on AVMs). INR, like interventional cardiology, can be broadly defined as treatment by endovascular access for the purpose of diagnosis and/or treatment by delivering therapeutic drugs and devices. The number, variety, and complexity of conditions treated using this route are increasing and this creates challenges for the pediatric anesthesiologist [178]. The pediatric anesthesiologist has a crucial role in facilitating neuroradiological procedures, and this requires an understanding of the indication and purpose for the procedures, their potential complications, and the management goals of the neurologists, neurosurgeons and neurointerventionalists, which will vary depending on the individual child.

Though most diagnostic neurological imaging can be accomplished with MRI and CT techniques, the power to both diagnose and intervene makes interventional techniques appealing, though they are often not the first choice for diagnosis [179]. INR procedures can be broadly classified on the basis of treatment goals.

- *Closing or occluding procedures.* Common examples include embolization of aneurysms, AVMs and fistulae of the brain and spine, preoperative embolization of vascular tumors such as meningiomas, temporary or permanent occlusion of intra- or extracranial arteries.
- *Opening procedures.* Common examples include treatment of vasospasm or stenosis by angioplasty and stenting, chemical and mechanical treatment of thrombolysis in stroke.

The most common INR procedures in children are endovascular treatment of aneurysms, AVMs, and preoperative embolization of tumors.

Though specific procedures will have different neurological complications, INR procedures are at higher risk for the following.

- *Hemorrhage.* This can result from vascular injury or dissection of an arterial vessel and/or aneurysmal perforation.
- *Ischemia.* This can result from malpositioning of a catheter or absence of collateral blood flow to a region, thromboembolic complication, displacement of a coil or stent that results in occlusion, and/or vasospasm of the vessel.

Non-neurological complications can also occur and are typical of other interventional procedures; they include contrast reactions, contrast nephropathy, and hematoma/bleeding/hemorrhage at the femoral puncture site.

Anesthetic considerations

At many institutions, the interventional suites are situated remotely from the operating rooms. Because this not only involves multiple floors and distance but sometimes multiple anesthetic locations (i.e. CT angiography pre/post in one location and the INR procedure in a different location), technical support must be co-ordinated for the anesthesia team, patient transport, and potentially remote patient recovery. Other potential problems typical of interventional radiological locations include working in reduced light, limited or poor access to the patient and equipment during the procedure, and concerns about ionizing radiation.

Anesthetic considerations when caring for patients undergoing INR procedures includes maintenance of patient immobility and physiological stability, manipulating systemic and regional blood flow, managing anticoagulation, and treating sudden unexpected complications during the procedure. The medical management of critically ill patients during transport to and from radiology suites and smooth and rapid recovery from anesthesia to facilitate neurological examination are equally important [180,181].

There are no studies demonstrating a clear benefit of one anesthetic management technique over another in the INR suite. Multiple approaches have been reported including general anesthesia, MAC and even sedation and/or awake techniques [179]. Because of the need for immobility in many of these procedures, we favor a general anesthetic with endotracheal intubation. Routine anesthetic monitoring is applied, and arterial blood pressure monitoring can often be obtained from the femoral arterial sheath. If postoperative ICU admission is anticipated with continued hemodynamic control (i.e. permissive hypotension) then a radial arterial catheter should be placed. Vascular access should include two good peripheral IV catheters for fluid and blood product administration. A Foley catheter should be placed to monitor urine output. If vasoactive drugs are to be administered as part of the procedure, a central venous catheter is desirable.

Postoperative considerations

Postanesthetic management of children following diagnostic or mapping neuroradiographic procedures is similar to other interventional cardiology and radiology procedures. Monitored transport to the postanesthetic care unit, with careful monitoring of bleeding complications from the femoral vein and arterial sheath sites, is necessary. In addition, careful neurological monitoring should be performed to assure return to the patient's baseline exam. Any new deficits or decline in neurological status should prompt aggressive assessment by the anesthesiologist and neuroradiologist, as bleeding complications may necessitate imaging, repeat intervention, and/or surgery.

Patients with anticipated swelling, neurological deficit or continued need for hemodynamic monitoring following the procedure should be transferred directly to an intensive care unit with or without tracheal extubation. Management goals should be discussed carefully between the neuroradiologist, neurosurgeons, anesthesiologist and intensivist, so that patient care can be optimized and the risk of ongoing neurological injury minimized. For patients with anticipated swelling and/or deficits, we will often transport the patient to the intensive care unit sedated, intubated and monitored, and then facilitate extubation in the ICU where all concerned parties can examine and agree with the postprocedural neurological examination. This approach can also facilitate any additional neuroimaging, such as CT or MRI, that might be planned or unplanned, prior to admission to the ICU.

Cerebral protection, resuscitation, and outcome

A comprehensive discussion of these topics is beyond the scope of this chapter. See Chapter 7 for a discussion of the physiology of the central nervous system. General principles are presented here for completeness [182].

Cerebral protection

After ischemic injury, the CNS has limited regenerative ability. Brain protection has been defined as the "prevention or amelioration of neuronal damage evidenced by abnormalities in cerebral metabolism, histopathology, or neurologic function occurring after an hypoxic or ischemic event" (i.e. treatment that is instituted before and often sustained throughout the insult) [182]. Brain resuscitation refers to the treatment of the secondary brain injury or simply to therapy given after the primary insult. The secondary consequences of ischemia are those that occur after the cerebral circulation is restored and are usually termed postischemic injury or reperfusion injury. Cell vulnerability differs, depending on the type of neuron. For example, the limbic system, especially the pyramidal cells of the CA1 layer of the hippocampus, Purkinje cells of the cerebellum, and layers 3, 4, and 6 of the cortex, are extremely vulnerable to ischemia; spinal cord cells, on the other hand, seem to tolerate a longer period of oxygen deprivation before they are injured.

Cerebral protection increases oxygen delivery, reduces its demands or ameliorates the pathological process by free radical scavenging or by reducing the effects of excitatory amino acids (glutamate, aspartate) and ionic fluxes. The difficulty with cerebral protection is that these strategies must be instituted before the onset of ischemia. With complete global ischemia, the brain tolerates 4–6 min of oxygen deprivation. The goal of cerebral protection is to delay the onset of irreversible CNS damage. There are no proven methods of cerebral protection except for mild hypothermia in animal models of neurotrama [183–185]. However, recent human trials using hypothermia following neonatal birth asphyxia, cardiac arrest or trauma have demonstrated an unclear benefit to neurological outcome or survival. Whether this variable result relates to the differences in the method and degree of hypothermia administration, variability in clinical practice with the initiation and maintenance of a cooling method, variation in the patient population with co-morbid factors (i.e. renal failure or lung injury), or heterogeneity of the secondary brain injury remains unclear [186]. Therefore, maintaining adequate cerebral perfusion and oxygen delivery, avoiding hyperglycemia and aggressively managing hyperthermia are, at this time, the only means we have to reduce CNS injury.

Cerebral resuscitation

Intracellular events that occur during ischemia or after restoration of circulation and oxygenation contribute to the ultimate neurological damage. Ischemia depolarizes neurons and allows ionic fluxes (Na^+ and Ca^{2+}) into the cells, probably owing to release of glutamate and aspartate and activation of the NMDA receptors. Depletion of adenosine triphosphate (ATP) stores leads to the energy-dependent ion pump's failure to eject Na^+ and Ca^{2+} from the cells. This leads to formation of prostaglandins and oxygen free radicals, to mitochondrial respiratory chain paralysis, acidosis, and finally membrane destruction.

Cerebral outcome

The future of cerebral well-being depends on our level of understanding of the pathophysiology of hypoxic-ischemic injury and our broad-based medical and pharmacological knowledge. Future therapy depends on development of a better understanding of the molecular and cellular processes that cause CNS injury and the development of specific treatments to salvage or protect injured tissue. Ultimately, the goal is to provide effective therapeutic measures that reverse the cascades of cellular events leading to injury.

CASE STUDY

A 2-year-old girl chases a ladybug to her open second-story bedroom window. The window screen is unable to support her weight and she falls two flights, plus an additional half-flight into the basement stairwell, striking the side of her head on a concrete step. Paramedics transport the child from the scene to a prearranged Medivac flight waiting at a nearby school parking lot. She arrives at the trauma bay with generalized tonic-clonic seizure activity and cyanotic lips, with the pulse oximeter registering a heart rate of 80 bpm, and 88% arterial saturation. Her left antecubital region is swollen around the insertion site of an IV that does not run freely, and her last blood pressure recorded on the transport monitor is "timed out."

The trauma team consists of a general pediatric surgeon, pediatric anesthesiologist, pediatric emergency room physician, and three nurses: one from the trauma service, one from the pediatric ICU and one from the pediatric emergency department. Prior to the arrival of the child, the anesthesiologist has chosen, from a shelf of prepackaged, age-dependent trauma supplies, a kit labeled "toddler: 1–3 years; 8–14 kg." The package is unwrapped on the trauma table to reveal the following supplies: size 3 airway mask, laryngoscope handle with Miller 1 and Mac 2 blades and spare bulbs, uncuffed 3.5, 4.0 and 4.5 tracheal tubes and a cuffed 4.5 tracheal tube, sizes 6 and 14 French stylets, sizes 2 and 2.5 laryngeal mask airways, 8 French suction catheters, 60 mm oral airway, sizes 18 and 20 nasal trumpet with lidocaine jelly, tongue blades, an IV start kit with 20 and 22 gauge IV catheters and a 15 gauge interosseous needle.

A pediatric respiratory therapist and a pharmacist have also been paged to the room per rapid response protocol. The pharmacist has a tackle box filled with syringes predrawn and sealed in a sterile hood, including atropine 0.1 mg/mL, epinephrine 100 μg/mL, lidocaine 20 mg/mL, phenylephrine 100 μg/mL, rocuronium 10 mg/mL, succinylcholine 20 mg/mL, pancuronium 1 mg/mL, etomidate 2 mg/mL, fentanyl 50 μg/mL, ketamine 100 mg/mL, midazolam 1 mg/mL, and thiopental 25 mg/mL. The cover of the tackle box is a table of weights and standard doses (in mL) for each of the predrawn medications included.

According to roles predetermined and practiced in a simulator setting, the pediatric anesthesiologist commences with the management and stabilization of the airway and hemodynamics of the patient while the surgeon and ER physician perform the trauma survey. Initial concerns for securing the airway are over-ridden by the more pressing concern for impending herniation, which might be hastened by an uncontrolled and unmedicated laryngoscopy. Bag-mask ventilation is applied to the child with 100% oxygen and jaw thrust while the respiratory therapist holds in-line traction, stabilizing the neck, and cricoid pressure is

held while supporting the back of the neck to avoid posterior displacement in case of C-spine fracture. The anesthesiologist confirms that the lungs of the child are easily ventilated with a mask whereas the trauma surgeon reports a large, minimally responsive left pupil, and the ED physician reports a left hemotympanum. Neurosurgery is called. The ED nurse has transferred the patient monitoring to the overhead monitor, visible to all members of the team, with audible pulse oximeter tone and a blood pressure cuff cycling every minute. The child is still unresponsive with a Glascow Coma Score of 5, no eye opening, no verbal response, and abnormal flexor posturing with stimulation.

The immediate benefits of CO_2 reduction and restoration of normoxia are a reduction in cerebral blood volume and the heart rate rises to 120 bpm. The pulse oximeter reads 100% but the mean blood pressure reads only 45 mmHg. The PICU and trauma nurses are attempting IV placement, which is difficult because of the tonic-clonic seizure activity. The anesthesiologist requests the ED nurse to prepare the interosseous needle, estimates the patient weight at 12 kg, and requests the intramuscular administration of 0.2 mg/kg midazolam to abort the seizure activity. Seizure activity stops within a minute of injection and two IVs are quickly placed. An intravenous bolus of 20 cc/kg of acetate-balanced 2% saline, which is part of the pharmacist tackle kit, is administered. After hypertonic saline administration, the arterial blood pressure is 105/45, mean 65 mmHg, and the heart rate is 105 bpm. Both pupils are now responsive. The anesthesiologist requests drugs for laryngoscopy and intubation. Lidocaine 1 mg/kg and atropine 0.15 mg are given. After 1 min and an additional 20 cc/kg of normal saline, the arterial blood pressure is 100/45, mean 60 mmHg, and the heart rate is now 120 bpm. Thiopental 2 mg/kg (half of the usual induction dose) and rocuronium 1.2 mg/kg are given. The trachea is easily intubated with in-line traction and cricoid pressure still in place. The 4.5 cuffed ETT is secured after confirming placement and ventilation is initiated and titrated to keep the $ETCO_2$ between 30 and 35 mmHg.

The arterial blood pressure after intubation is now 65/25 with a mean of 35 mmHg. Phenylephrine 5 μg/kg is given and the repeat blood pressure is 90/45, mean 55 mmHg. The dose is repeated, along with an additional 10 cc/kg of 2% saline. Repeat blood pressure is 105/55, mean 65 mmHg. The trauma survey is completed and the child is taken to the CT scanner which reveals a large epidural hematoma with midline shift, effacement of cortical sulci and the ipsilateral ventricle, as well as imperceptible basal cisterns.

The child is taken immediately to the operating room for decompression. The anesthesiologists prepare for incision.

Continued

O-positive trauma release blood is requested to the room. An arterial line is started and a second IV is placed. Anesthesia is maintained with intravenous remifentanil and propofol. The child is ventilated without PEEP to an end-tidal CO_2 of 30 mmHg and an arterial blood gas is sent, but the result is not available until the procedure is well under way. Blood pressure is stabilized with phenylephrine infusion titrated to keep systolic blood pressure greater than 90 mmHg and mean arterial blood pressure between 60 and 65 mmHg. Temperature is maintained between 36° and 36.5° without the need for a warming blanket. Mannitol 25 mg/kg is given and a Foley catheter is placed.

Incision is made 50 min after the initial trauma, and the hematoma is evacuated through a craniotomy within 5 min. After evacuation of the hematoma, the heart rate decreased to 65 bpm and the arterial blood pressure decreased to 65/25. Phenylephrine and 10 cc/kg of trauma release blood are immediately given and the pressure responds. An additional 10 cc/kg of saline is required to replace the brisk urine output following mannitol administration.

A parenchymal fiber-optic intracranial pressure monitor is placed upon closure of the dura and skull, reading 12 mmHg with a normal waveform. The child is taken to the ICU with only the remifentanil infusion, as cerebral perfusion pressure is 55 mmHg without phenylephrine. In the ICU, the remifentanil is stopped hourly for neurological checks and within 6 h of admission, the child is opening her eyes and reaching purposefully for the tracheal tube, which is removed. After a night without intracranial pressure elevations at a serum sodium of 145 mg/dL, she is interacting appropriately with her parents at the bedside and her intracranial pressure monitor is removed.

Conclusions

This case illustrates the main anesthetic considerations presented in this chapter in critically ill patients with neurotrauma and increased ICP undergoing emergency procedures, with choices for airway, drug, and hemodynamic management to facilitate successful outcomes.

Annotated references

A full reference list for this chapter is available at:
http://www.wiley.com/go/gregory/andropoulos/pediatricanesthesia

8. Matchett GA, Allard MW, Martin RD et al. Neuroprotective effect of volatile anesthetic agents: molecular mechanisms. Neurol Res 2009; 31: 128–34. A contemporary review of important new data concerning the mechanisms of neuroprotection of volatile anesthetics.

17. Sponheim S, Skraastad O, Helseth E et al. Effects of 0.5 and 1.0 mac isoflurane, sevoflurane and desflurane on intracranial and cerebral perfusion pressures in children. Acta Anaesthesiol Scand 2003; 47: 932–8. A very important modern study establishing the basis for pharmacodynamic responses of the cerebral circulation to common inhaled anesthetics in children.

41. Karsli C, Luginbuehl I, Farrar M et al. Propofol decreases cerebral blood flow velocity in anesthetized children. Can J Anaesth 2002; 49: 830–4. A well done study demonstrating the effects of propofol on cerebral blood flow velocity in children.

54. Abdallah C, Karsli C, Bissonnette B. Fentanyl is more effective than remifentanil at preventing increases in cerebral blood flow velocity during intubation in children. Can J Anaesth 2002; 49: 1070–5. A well done, controlled study comparing two widely used synthetic opioids as to their effects on cerebral blood flow velocity in children during laryngoscopy and tracheal intubation.

67. Ard J, Doyle W, Bekker A. Awake craniotomy with dexmedetomidine in pediatric patients. J Neurosurg Anesthesiol 2003; 15: 263–6.

Description of a novel use of this newer anesthetic agent for awake craniotomy in children.

106. Adelson PD, Bratton SL, Carney NA et al. Guidelines for the acute medical management of severe traumatic brain injury in infants, children, and adolescents. Chapter 11. Use of hyperosmolar therapy in the management of severe pediatric traumatic brain injury. Pediatr Crit Care Med 2003; 4: S40–44. A review of the evidence and treatment strategies for using hyperosmolar therapy in pediatric traumatic brain injury.

131. Adelson PD, Bratton SL, Carney NA et al. Guidelines for the acute medical management of severe traumatic brain injury in infants, children, and adolescents. Chapter 14. The role of temperature control following severe pediatric traumatic brain injury. Pediatr Crit Care Med 2003; 4: S53–5. A review of temperature management of traumatic brain injury and increased intracranial pressure in children.

167. Flack S, Ojemann J, Haberkern C. Cerebral hemispherectomy in infants and young children. Paediatr Anaesth 2008; 18: 967–73. A modern review of the anesthetic care of this extensive and complicated surgery in children.

172. Soriano SG, McCann ME, Laussen PC. Neuroanesthesia. Innovative techniques and monitoring. Anesthesiol Clin North Am 2002; 20: 137–51. A review of monitoring and anesthetic techniques for pediatric neurosurgical procedures.

182. Bissonnette B. Cerebral protection. Paediatr Anaesth 2004; 14: 403–6. An excellent review of the principles and practices of cerebral protection in children.

CHAPTER 24

Anesthesia for Thoracic Surgery

Grant McFadyen[1], Stefan Budac[1], Michael Richards[1] & Lynn D. Martin[2]

[1]Department of Anesthesiology and Pain Medicine, and [2]Pediatrics, Seattle Children's Hospital, and the University of Washington School of Medicine, Seattle, WA, USA

Introduction

Thoracic surgery and anesthesia for thoracic surgery have changed significantly in the pediatric population over the last 15 years with the advent of video-assisted thoracoscopic surgery (VATS) and robotic surgery. While VATS procedures have changed certain aspects of the perioperative and postoperative management of pediatric patients with thoracic disease, thoracotomy continues to be a relatively frequent surgical procedure, particularly in very small infants in whom thoracoscopic equipment is often too large and cumbersome to perform complex procedures. Hence, the pediatric anesthesiologist must have the capacity to manage both surgical approaches within the thoracic cavity.

Certain aspects of anesthetic practice remain common to both thoracoscopic and open procedures, particularly the need for one-lung ventilation (OLV). Indeed, the need to access the thoracic cavity by trocar in VATS (and the inability to pack off the lung) makes OLV even more necessary than during open thoracotomy, where surgeons can use both retraction and packing to facilitate surgical access and visualization without damaging the underlying lung parenchyma. The need for OLV in younger children has led to the development of many devices that allow lung isolation in children in whom the smallest size double-lumen tube (26 Fr) is too large.

Video-assisted thoracoscopic surgery has significantly decreased the requirement for neuroaxial blockade during the intraoperative and postoperative periods due to its less invasive and less painful nature. This has radically decreased the number of inpatient days following complex thoracic procedures [1]; however, due to the continuing need for thoracotomy within the pediatric population, the pediatric anesthesiologist must maintain the ability to provide adequate postoperative analgesia when necessary.

The relatively recent availability of rapid-onset and -offset anesthetic agents, specifically the highly insoluble desflurane and rapidly metabolized remifentanil [2], has allowed anesthesiologists to provide the rapid-onset and profoundly deep anesthesia necessary for thoracic surgery. The effects of these agents are so rapidly reversed at the end of surgery that rapid operating room turnover with alert, awake, compliant postoperative patients has become a reality rather than a pipe dream.

This chapter reviews the pathophysiology of OLV, discusses the anesthetic practice and tools necessary to facilitate the perioperative management of the pediatric thoracic surgery patient, covers analgesia for thoracic

Gregory's Pediatric Anesthesia, Fifth Edition. Edited by George A. Gregory, Dean B. Andropoulos.
© 2012 Blackwell Publishing Ltd. Published 2012 by Blackwell Publishing Ltd.

surgery, and discusses in more detail some of the finer nuances of certain specific thoracic surgical challenges within the pediatric population, namely lobectomy, pneumonectomy, congenital cystic lung disease, anterior mediastinal mass, pectus excavatum, and empyema.

Pathophysiology of one-lung ventilation

During thoracic surgery, several factors have profound effects on the matching of ventilation and perfusion (V/Q). General anesthesia, neuromuscular blockade, mechanical ventilation, the open hemithorax and surgical retraction all affect normal V/Q matching, primarily because of their effects on lung compliance [3]. OLV uncouples V/Q matching in the operative lung, which results in significant hypoxemia if not properly managed [3]. These factors apply equally to children and adults.

The lateral decubitus position

When awake, spontaneously breathing adults with unilateral lung disease are placed in the lateral decubitus position, oxygenation is optimal when the healthy lung is dependent ("down") and the diseased lung is nondependent ("up") [4,5]. Because of the hydrostatic pressure gradient between the two lungs, there is greater perfusion of the dependent, healthy lung than the nondependent, diseased lung, improving V/Q matching.

On the other hand, infants, both those breathing spontaneously and those receiving positive pressure ventilation, behave differently from adults. Oxygenation is improved with the healthy lung "up" and the diseased lung "down" [6,7], in part due to the fact that ventilation may be distributed differently in infants and adults because the soft, more compliant ribcage of infants does not fully support the underlying lung. This results in a functional residual capacity (FRC) that is closer to residual volume, making airway closure more likely in the dependent lung during tidal breathing [8]. In smaller children there is less cephalad displacement of the dependent hemidiaphragm by abdominal organs than in larger subjects. Thus, in accordance with Starling's Law, contraction is less forceful in the dependent hemidiaphragm than in the upper hemidiaphragm, which limits the dependent lung's efficiency of ventilation. Ventilation is therefore distributed preferentially to the non-dependent lung of infants.

The small size of the infant reduces the hydrostatic pressure gradient (present in adults) between the dependent and non-dependent lungs. Consequently, the favorable increase in perfusion of the dependent, ventilated lung, which occurs in adults, is attenuated in infants. It is not known at what age the adult pattern appears. It is suggested that during the postoperative period the child with unilateral lung disease should be nursed supine and in both lateral decubitus positions to determine which position provides optimal gas exchange.

Pulmonary perfusion during one-lung ventilation

Current lung separation techniques have made it easier to deliver the entire tidal volume to the dependent lung. When OLV is initiated, residual oxygen is gradually absorbed from the unventilated alveoli until complete absorption atelectasis occurs. Continued perfusion of the unventilated lung, in addition to positional effects, increases V/Q mismatch or shunt fraction. This right-to-left shunt through the unventilated lung should produce an overall shunt fraction in excess of 50%. Fortunately, observed shunt fractions are much lower. Passive (mechanical) and active (biological) forces account for the lower than expected shunt fraction. Surgical manipulation, the effects of the open or artificial pneumothorax, and physical kinking of pulmonary vessels with lung deflation reduce blood flow to the operative lung. In addition, hypoxic pulmonary vasoconstriction (HPV) increases pulmonary vascular resistance in the unventilated lung, causing a gradual decrease in blood flow and shunt fraction. The true clinical importance of HPV has been questioned [9].

Ventilation during one-lung ventilation

Ventilatory management of patients undergoing OLV has long focused on avoiding hypoxia. Hypoxia, however, is less frequent now because lung isolation is more complete, fiber-optic bronchoscopy permits confirmation of correct bronchial blocker or double-lumen tube position, and the anesthetic agents used have fewer or no detrimental effects on HPV. Recent publications have focused on prevention of acute lung injury (ALI) associated with OLV. ALI occurs after 2.5% of lung resections in adults, but occurs in 7.9% of patients after pneumonectomies. Around 40% of adults with ALI demonstrate morbidity or mortality [10]. Similar outcome data are not available in children. Recommendations for protective lung ventilation (PLV) during OLV include tidal volumes of 6 mL/kg, limiting the plateau airway pressure to <20 cmH$_2$O, and the use of 5–10 cmH$_2$O positive end-expiratory pressure (PEEP) to preserve dependent lung unit aeration, prevent atelectasis and reduce injury from mechanical stress [11]. Continuous positive airway pressure (CPAP) or blow-by oxygen to the operative lung may be required to treat hypoxemia. Resumption of two-lung ventilation with 100% oxygen during surgery may be required if severe or refractory hypoxemia occurs. If this is not possible, the surgeon should consider placing a pulmonary artery clamp on the operative side during pneumonectomy or lung transplant.

Anesthetic requirements for thoracic anesthesia

One-lung ventilation

There are three principal indications for OLV [12].

1. To control the distribution of ventilation: bronchopleural (cutaneous) fistulas, gigantic unilateral lung cysts or bullae, and differential lung ventilation.
2. To avoid spillage of material or contamination: infection, hemorrhage, and unilateral pulmonary lavage.
3. To provide a quiet operative field: thoracoscopy, thoracotomy, and thoracic non-pulmonary surgery.

To facilitate this, there are three basic techniques or devices that are currently widely used to isolate one lung from the other in the pediatric patient.

1. Selective endobronchial intubation with a conventional single-lumen endotracheal tube.
2. A bronchial blocker.
3. A double-lumen tube (DLT).

In the modern era, with widespread availability of the fiber-optic bronchoscope (FOB), clinicians should strive to directly visualize and verify device placement where possible. The choice of device depends on patient age, size, and device availability (Table 24.1, Fig. 24.1).

Endobronchial intubation

The simplest method of isolating one lung and the method most frequently used in the smallest of patients involves advancing a standard endotracheal tube (ETT) past the carina and into the non-operative main bronchus. When passed blindly, the ETT invariably enters the right main bronchus. To selectively intubate the left main bronchus, the ETT is rotated so that the bevel faces the right, the patient's head is rotated to the right and the ETT is advanced [13]. Placement should be confirmed with a

FOB, which requires a good working knowledge of the anatomy of the bronchial tree distal to the carina.

An alternative is to place the ETT in the trachea and pass the FOB into the main bronchus before "railroading" the ETT over it. Unfortunately, the smallest size of FOB available is 2.2 mm in diameter and this is not rigid enough to withstand "railroading" a rigid ETT without potentially causing significant damage to the FOB fibers.

Bronchial blockers
Embolectomy catheter/blocker

Embolectomy catheters effectively achieve lung isolation in the smallest of patients [14]. The blocker can be inserted either through the ETT or alongside it. Fogarty catheters have a central stylet that can be bent to facilitate placing the catheter in either bronchus (Fig. 24.2) whilst being

Table 24.1 Device selection for OLV in children

Age	OLV airway device
Less than 2 years	Selective endobronchial intubation
	Fogarty catheter (4 Fr) as a bronchial blocker
2–6 years	Fogarty catheter (4 Fr or larger) as a bronchial blocker
	Wire-guided endobronchial blocker (5 Fr)
6–10 years	Wire-guided endobronchial blocker (5 Fr or larger)
	Univent tube (3.5 ID)
Over 10 years	Wire-guided endobronchial blocker
	Univent tube
	DLT (26 Fr or larger)

Modified from Choudhry [15].

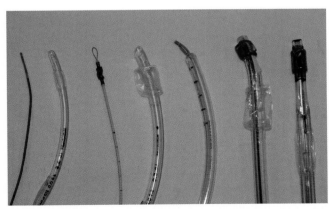

Figure 24.1 The devices available for facilitation of OLV in children. Left to right (smallest to largest): 4 Fr Fogarty catheter, 1.5 ETT (standard), 5 Fr WEB, 5.0 ETT (standard), 3.5 ID Univent tube, 26 Fr (Rusch, Buluth, GA) DLT, 28 Fr (Mallinckrodt Medical, St Louis, MO) DLT.

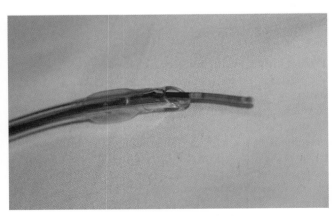

Figure 24.2 4 Fr Fogarty catheter within a standard 3.5 ETT.

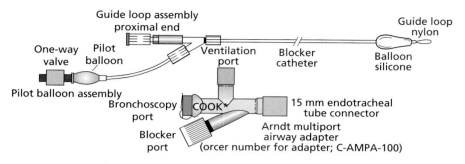

Figure 24.3 labels: Guide loop assembly proximal end; One-way valve; Pilot balloon; Ventilation port; Blocker catheter; Guide loop nylon; Balloon silicone; Pilot balloon assembly; Bronchoscopy port; COOK*; Blocker port; Arndt multiport airway adapter (orcer number for adapter; C-AMPA-100); 15 mm endotracheal tube connector

Figure 24.3 The components of the wire-guided endobronchial blocker (WEB).

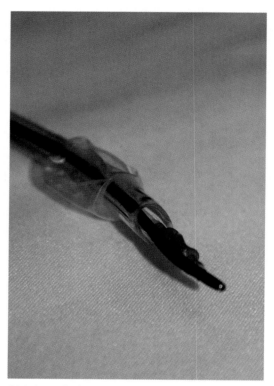

Figure 24.4 A standard 5.0 ETT with FOB and 5 Fr WEB *in situ*.

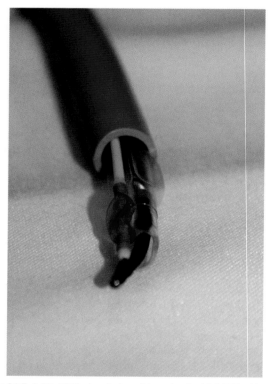

Figure 24.5 A 5 Fr WEB placed alongside a standard 3.5 ETT with the FOB within the ETT.

observed with a FOB through the ETT. The open tip of the catheter allows for lung collapse following isolation and for insufflation of oxygen if necessary.

Wire-guided endobronchial blocker

Wire-guided endobronchial blockers (WEBs) are available in a "pediatric" size – 5 Fr. The blocker is placed through a standard ETT; a guidewire loop attached around the end of a FOB allows direct visualization and placement of the blocker. This device has the benefit of three ports that allow ventilation while the blocker is manipulated into place (Fig. 24.3). The smallest ETT that can be used with the smallest 5 Fr WEB is a 5.0 mm ETT, hence use of this device is limited to children between 2 and 4 years of age (Fig. 24.4).

The blocker can be placed alongside the ETT in smaller patients (Fig. 24.5) when there is insufficient room within the ETT for both blocker and FOB [15].

Univent tube and blocker

The Univent tube (Fuji Systems Corporation, Tokyo, Japan) has a second lumen containing a separate bronchial blocker that is styletted and can be bent to facilitate positioning of the tube (Fig. 24.6). The smallest size Univent tube is 3.5 mm internal diameter; however, the total external diameter is 8 mm, making it comparable in size to a 6.0 mm internal diameter uncuffed ETT. This limits the use of this device to older children (approximately 8 years of age).

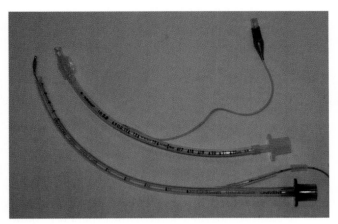

Figure 24.6 The smallest 3.5 ID Univent tube available next to a standard 5.0 ETT.

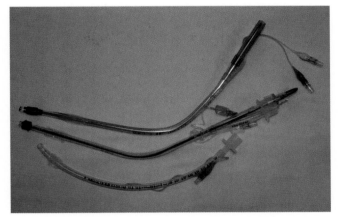

Figure 24.7 Smallest DLTs available. Top to bottom: 28 Fr (Mallinckrodt Medical, St Louis, MO) DLT, 26 Fr (Rusch, Buluth, GA) DLT, 6.0 ETT (standard).

Double-lumen tube

Double-lumen tubes (DLTs) are considered the gold standard for lung isolation in adults; however, the smallest size tubes available are 26 Fr (Rusch, Buluth, GA) and 28 Fr (Mallinckrodt Medical, St Louis, MO) (Fig. 24.7). These tubes can only be utilized in older children (8–10 years of age) and are positioned in the same manner as in adults. Due to the wide variation in the size of pediatric patients, there are no designated depth measurements for the placement of the DLT; hence its location in the bronchus should be confirmed with a FOB.

Anesthetic techniques

Preoperative evaluation and preparation of patients are important and should be as thorough and complete as in all pediatric operative candidates. Some children will be otherwise completely fit and healthy; others may have significant concurrent and severe systemic illness.

Premedication and the anesthesia induction technique are at the discretion of the anesthetic provider and need to be tailored to the individual [16].

Lung isolation, if required, and the postoperative analgesic technique should be planned well in advance. Arterial line placement is recommended for thoracotomy and should be seriously considered for VATS – particularly in small infants and babies in whom the potential for accidental overinflation of the pleural cavity and iatrogenic tension pneumothorax is significant. Lung isolation and deflation should be initiated early, particularly in VATS patients to allow adequate time for the lung to collapse (up to 20 min) and to minimize the need for lung retraction [15]. Once OLV is instituted, the lungs should be ventilated with enough oxygen to achieve oxygen saturations of 94% or above. Nitrous oxide is avoided because it may cause overinflation of tracheal and bronchial balloons and cause airway trauma [17].

There is a perception that isoflurane causes less V/Q mismatch during OLV because it is thought to have less impact on HPV than other volatile agents [18]. Isoflurane's slow offset time makes it less appealing as a primary anesthetic agent. The rapid offset of the more recently developed volatile agents, such as desflurane, particularly after a long case, makes them very appealing for thoracic anesthesia. To minimize inhibition of HPV, we advocate using a maximum of 1 minimum alveolar concentration (MAC) of the chosen volatile anesthetic and adding agents such as propofol and/or opiates that have little impact on HPV to prevent awareness during surgery [19].

When a short-acting volatile agent such as desflurane is combined with the profound μ agonism of remifentanil, regional anesthesia or a non-steroidal anti-inflammatory drug (NSAID) (and where available, intravenous acetaminophen/paracetamol) at the end of the case facilitates rapid emergence from anesthesia and a coherent, relatively pain-free, and interactive patient.

Analgesic requirements for thoracic surgery

Thoracic surgery, especially open thoracotomy and minimally invasive pectus excavatum repair, often results in significant postoperative pain. Thoracotomy is often associated with severe chest wall trauma that includes fractured ribs and peripheral nerve damage. The chest wall must remain in constant motion for effective gas transfer to take place and to clear secretions effectively. This increases the amount of pain. Shallow respirations and a poor cough predispose the child to atelectasis, sputum retention, and postoperative pneumonia. Sensitization of the child to painful stimuli following surgery can cause chronic pain and/or higher pain levels during subsequent surgical procedures. About a third of adult patients suffer from chronic pain after thoracic surgery [20] and the incidence of pain is similar whether the patient undergoes a thoracotomy or VATS [20–22].

Some surgical literature suggests that children should understand "that they are going to have to learn to be comfortable with being uncomfortable" [23]. The authors contest this statement and believe that it is the anesthesiologist's responsibility to their patients to do all they can to prevent/minimize the pain. Suresh asked the question: "If placing a thoracic epidural catheter in adults is considered the 'standard of care' in many institutions across the country, why is the child deprived of the same privilege?" [24]. We agree.

Various pain treatment modalities have been described for the treatment of post-thoracotomy pain, but when the factors influencing the generation of post-thoracotomy pain are considered, regional analgesia is the most logical approach [25]. This is because neurogenic pain, which results from intercostal nerve damage and chest wall trauma, and central nervous system hyperexcitability are poorly responsive to opioids [26,27]. Reliance on these drugs may detrimentally affect respiration and oxygenation [28,29]. To achieve optimal pain relief, it is logical to start the regional analgesic regimen preoperatively [30]. A multimodal analgesic approach that combines an effective afferent nerve block with a NSAID, acetaminophen/paracetamol, and/or low doses of opioids usually achieves an optimal level of postoperative analgesia. Although regional anesthesia is the subject of another chapter (Chapter 18), several regional techniques deserve emphasis in a discussion of anesthesia for thoracic surgery.

Epidural analgesia

In contrast to older children and adults, epidural and subarachnoid blockade in infants and children under the age of about 6 years is characterized by hemodynamic stability, even when the level of the block reaches the upper thoracic dermatomes [31]. Although heart rate variability is lower, heart rate is preserved because the parasympathetic activity modulating heart rate is attenuated in infants [32]. This attenuated vagal tone allows the heart rate to compensate for peripheral vasodilation. Other factors that preserve hemodynamic stability are the relatively small venous capacitance in the lower extremities of infants and the relative lack of resting sympathetic peripheral vascular tone [33].

Thoracic epidural blockade of pain has been shown to improve several measures of respiratory function [34–36]. Evidence suggests that improved postoperative tidal volume and diaphragmatic shortening after thoracic epidural blockade may be due to changes of chest wall con-

formation and diaphragmatic resting length, and to a shift of the workload of breathing from the ribcage to the diaphragm following motor block of intercostal muscles [37].

In infants, thoracic catheter placement can be achieved via the caudal space with cephalad threading of a styletted catheter [38]. Although successful application of this technique has been described in children up to 10 years of age [39], in children over the age of 1 year the chance of the catheter exiting a dural sleeve or becoming knotted or tangled is increased [40,41]. Epidurograms [42], epidural electrocardiography [43], and electrical stimulation [44] have been used to confirm that the catheter tip is positioned at the desired level. With experience, ultrasound (US) has become the modality of choice for visualizing the epidural catheter tip [45–48]. Ultrasound localization is non-invasive, avoids exposure to radiation and contrast medium, and is not affected by the use of neuromuscular blocking drugs or epidural local anesthetics.

Epidural catheter tip placement near the dermatomal level of the surgical incision(s) allows the safest and most effective application of local anesthetics. Thoracic epidural catheters, which may be safely placed in anesthetized infants and children by experienced anesthesiologists [49], have less risk of contamination by stool and urine than caudally placed catheters. A prospective survey of the French-Language Society of Pediatric Anesthesiologists found no complications from thoracic epidurals, whereas there were 0.7 complications per 1000 caudal epidurals. The number of thoracic epidurals was much smaller than caudal epidurals, however (135 versus 15,013) [50].

Paravertebral analgesia

The paravertebral space is wedge shaped. Its boundaries are the superior costotransverse ligament posteriorly; the posterior intercostal membrane laterally; the parietal pleura anteriorly; and the posterolateral aspect of the vertebrae, intervertebral disks, and intervertebral foramen anteriorly. The space contains spinal nerves and dorsal rami, rami communicantes, and the sympathetic chain anteriorly. Injection of local anesthetic into the paravertebral space avoids possible complications of central neuroaxial blockade.

Paravertebral block (PVB) has been employed in children since 1992, when two different techniques were described: Lönnqvist's modification of the original Eason–Wyatt percutaneous catheter technique [51] and Sabanathan's surgical catheter placement during thoracotomy [52]. The main indication for thoracic PVB is unilateral thoracic surgery. Continuous infusion is possible via a catheter placed transcutaneously or surgically via thoracotomy. A rate of 0.25 mL/kg/h is recommended [51,53–55]. The advantage of a PVB is that deposition of local anesthetic into the paravertebral space leads to a unilateral block of one or more adjacent dermatomes. Because all the effects of PVB are unilateral, hypotension, which limits the dose of local anesthetic used in epidural analgesia in children over the age of 6 years, is not a problem. Relatively large doses of drug can therefore be used with consequent improvement in efficacy of the unilateral blockade. The sympathetic chain that is known to be important in pain transmission is reliably blocked by PVB, whereas the central sympathetic blockade produced by epidural and spinal anesthesia leaves this pathway unaffected, thereby allowing central relaying of information (bypassing the blockade) [56]. Confirmation of the lack of provision of high-quality afferent blockade with epidural analgesia is shown by its failure to inhibit somatosensory-evoked potentials and the failure to produce stress inhibition for any surgery more rostral than gynecological or surgery that is more distal [57,58]. There are fewer PVB data for comparison, but PVB abolishes thoracic somatosensory-evoked potentials [59] and inhibits some parameters of the stress response [30,60].

Intercostal analgesia

Intercostal blocks after thoracotomy reduce opioid requirements and improve respiratory function in children with rib fractures [61–63]. The disadvantage of single-shot blocks is their limited duration of action. The development of degradable bupivacaine microspheres, which have a dramatically prolonged duration of action, may increase the usefulness of these blocks in the future [64,65]. Plasma concentrations of local anesthetics after intercostal blocks are greater than those after other regional blocks. Plasma concentrations of the local anesthetic rise faster in children than in adults [66,67].

A continuous infusion of local anesthetic through an extrapleural catheter placed by the surgeon during thoracotomy wound closure can prolong the analgesic effect [62]. The analgesic effect may result from delivering local anesthetic to the paravertebral space [68].

Summary

How can clinicians decide which regional analgesic technique to use in thoracic surgery in children? A meta-analysis of 10 trials that included 520 adult patients concluded that PVB and epidural analgesia provide comparable pain relief after thoracic surgery, but PVB has a better side-effect profile and is associated with a reduction in pulmonary complications [69].

For adult thoracic surgery, the Procedure-Specific Postoperative Pain Management (PROSPECT) Working Group evaluated the available literature comparing various regional analgesic techniques for the management of post-thoracotomy pain [70]. Seventy-four randomized studies in thoracotomy patients were identified

that compared regional analgesic techniques with systemic opioid analgesia or with each other. The authors concluded that evidence supported the use of thoracic paravertebral block as an effective alternative to thoracic epidural local anesthetic (LA) alone, and showed that paravertebral block reduced the incidence of postoperative pulmonary complications compared with systemic analgesia. They suggested that further studies are required to determine whether thoracic paravertebral block provides equivalent pain relief and morbidity to thoracic epidurals when LA is combined with opioids. Apart from thoracic paravertebral block, all other regional analgesic techniques were inferior to thoracic epidural analgesia. In particular, interpleural techniques provide inadequate analgesia. However, if thoracic epidural or paravertebral techniques are not possible or are contraindicated, intercostal nerve block or preoperative intrathecal opioid is recommended.

Thoracoscopy

The field of minimally invasive surgery (MIS) is the fastest growing area of surgical innovation. Each year, as new techniques and tools are developed, more patients benefit from these less invasive surgical procedures. Thoracoscopy has several potential advantages over thoracotomy for resection or repair of intrathoracic abnormalities in children. There is less postprocedure scoliosis, which develops in up to 30% of neonates after thoracotomy [71]. In addition, thoracoscopy is associated with less pain and better pulmonary mechanics postoperatively and with improved cosmesis compared to thoracotomy. Shorter hospital stays, a faster return to normal activity, and a shorter recovery period are just a few of the advantages that MIS offers to pediatric patients.

Originally, VATS was developed to provide biopsy specimens of intrathoracic structures in immunocompromised patients [72]. Although it continues to be used for this purpose in the pediatric population, increasing numbers of pediatric surgical conditions are also being addressed by VATS (Box 24.1).

With the advances in thoracoscopic equipment, including the availability of smaller scopes and improvements in both the fiber-optics and the quality of digital video signals and screen resolution, VATS is being applied to younger and younger children, even to neonates and infants.

Blood loss during thoracoscopic surgery is generally minimal; however, adequate venous access should be secured prior to the start of these procedures because there is the possibility that one of the trocars or an endoscopic instrument will inadvertently injury one of the intrathoracic vascular structures. Access to the

Box 24.1 Thoracoscopic procedures in infants and children

- Diagnostic thoracoscopy
- Lung biopsy
- Pectus repair
- Empyema drainage
- Lung decortication
- Bronchopulmonary sequestration resection
- Cystic adenomatoid malformation resection
- Lobar emphysema resection
- Bronchogenic cyst excision
- Esophageal duplication resection
- Congenital diaphragmatic hernia repair
- Esophageal atresia and tracheo-esophageal fistula repair
- Thymectomy
- Aortopexy
- Vascular ring division
- Patent ductus arteriosus ligation
- Thoracic duct ligation
- Sympathectomy
- Mediastinal mass excision
- Anterior spinal fusion

extremities to obtain additional venous access during the procedure can be limited because these procedures are routinely performed in the lateral decubitus position. Standard perioperative monitoring includes pulse oximetry, electrocardiogram, end-tidal CO_2 and inhaled volatile agent concentration, non-invasive blood pressure measurement, and body temperature.

Routine central venous pressure monitoring offers little additional information that improves or influences anesthetic care of patients with normal cardiovascular function. Central venous access is generally reserved for cases in which adequate peripheral intravenous access is unavailable. Invasive monitoring of arterial blood pressure is not routinely used but its use is guided by the clinical status of the patient.

One-lung ventilation is highly desirable during thoracoscopy because lung deflation improves visualization of thoracic contents and may reduce the risk of retractor-induced lung injury. If OLV cannot be achieved, thoracoscopy can be performed during two-lung ventilation, using CO_2 insufflation and a retractor to displace lung tissue from the operative field [73]. This technique is also useful for improving the surgeon's view when there is inadequate separation of the two lungs and there is overflow ventilation into the operative side. During creation of the artificial pneumothorax, cardiopulmonary function should be monitored closely because displacement of intrathoracic contents and creation of an excessive pneumothorax (caused by either excessive volume or pressure) can decrease venous return or increase left ventricular afterload, which can significantly compromise the cardiovascular system. The effects of the artificial pneumotho-

rax can be minimized by slowly adding the CO_2 (flow rate 1 L/min), limiting the inflating pressure to 4–6 mmHg, and optimizing cardiovascular function, including optimization of myocardial contractility (if required) and restoration of the intravascular status [74].

Another significant risk during creation of an artificial pneumothorax is inadvertent CO_2 embolism [75]. This occurs when the insufflating gas enters the circulation, either by direct injection into the vasculature during insufflation or when gas enters an internal vessel that was damaged during the procedure [76].

Robotic surgery

The field of robotic surgery is progressing exponentially because newer robotic instruments articulate better, which increases the surgeon's dexterity and ability to work in small spaces. Articulated tools and a three-dimensional optical stereoscopic view make the procedure more similar to open procedures for the surgeon. Good preoperative communication with the surgeon is essential to appropriately plan for positioning of the operating room table within the operating room, positioning of the operating robot so the anesthesia provider has good access to the child's airway, and positioning of the child on the operating table. It is of enormous benefit to perform robotic surgery in a dedicated operating room with staff who are experienced in the management of robotic surgery cases.

Lung resection

In developed countries, the age of children undergoing pulmonary resections has steadily decreased over the last decades, reflecting a decline in the number of procedures performed for infectious etiologies. At the same time, there has been a rise in the number of resections performed for congenital malformations. An understanding of normal lung growth in the postnatal period is essential to predict pulmonary function after lung resection in children (see Chapter 6). Alveoli multiply after birth [77] from approximately 20×10^6 at birth (in term infants) to approximately 300×10^6 at 8 years of age. The most rapid increase occurs during the first 3 years of life. After 8 years of age, the alveolar number remains constant. The lung volume doubles between 8 and 25 years of age, which is accounted for by the increased volume of individual alveoli [78].

Lobectomy

While pulmonary resection in adults causes a proportional decrease in lung volume, infants who undergo lung resection have normal pulmonary function and develop normally, live normal lives, and have no physical impairment at rest. McBride et al [79] evaluated the pulmonary function of 15 patients who had undergone lobectomies for congenital lobar emphysema between 1 week and 3 years of age. They found that vital capacity and total lung capacities were within the normal range in the vast majority of these patients 8–30 years after surgery. There was an association between the resected anatomical portion of the lung and the extent of compensatory lung growth. The most vigorous compensatory growth occurred after upper lobectomies. The presence of normal residual volumes in their patients is further evidence that the compensatory growth was consistent with multiplication of alveoli.

Pneumonectomy

Early studies described preserved pulmonary function after pneumonectomies performed during childhood. In 1947, Cournard [80] reported outcomes of four patients who had undergone left pneumonectomies for pulmonary infections between 6 and 16 years of age. The total lung capacity of the remaining lung was greater than would have been predicted for the right lung of an individual without a history of pulmonary resection. In three of the four patients, the vital capacity exceeded the predicted value for a right lung.

Laros and Westermann [81] stratified 130 pneumonectomy patients by age at the time of their operation. Preservation of total lung capacities decreased with increasing age at which the pneumonectomy occurred. The total lung capacity was 96% of the predicted value in patients who were younger than 5 years of age at the time of their pneumonectomy, 85% of predicted in patients between 6 and 20 years of age, but only 70% of predicted in patients between 31 and 40 years of age.

Postpneumonectomy syndrome

The postpneumonectomy syndrome is associated with progressive hyperinflation of the remaining lung and typically leads to progressive dyspnea. It can also lead to bronchomalacia and pulmonary infections. Postpneumonectomy syndrome is most commonly seen after a right pneumonectomy [82] due to counterclockwise rotation of the mediastinal structures and compression of the left mainstem bronchus or left lower lobe bronchus between the aorta and spine posteriorly and the pulmonary artery anteriorly. Postpneumonectomy syndrome can also be encountered after a left pneumonectomy in patients who have a right-sided aortic arch if the airway is compressed between ascending and descending aorta [83]. However, this complication has also been reported in patients after a left pneumonectomy who have a left-sided aortic arch [84]. In this case, the bronchus

intermedius is thought to be compressed between the right pulmonary artery anteriorly and the thoracic spine posteriorly after clockwise rotation of the mediastinal structures into the right pleural cavity.

Early attempts to prevent mediastinal shifts after pneumonectomies in children included thoracoplasties, which were eventually abandoned secondary to the crippling deformities that developed. Other attempts to prevent mediastinal shifts in the past have included instillation of inert substances, such as oil, into the pleural cavity. The principles of treating this syndrome today include a combination of anterior pexy of mediastinal structures, such as the pericardium and pulmonary artery, and an intervention in the postresection pleural cavity to prevent future shifting [85]. For many years, rigid prostheses such as silastic testicular or breast prostheses were placed in the pleural cavities to stabilize the mediastinum [86], but the size of the prosthesis could not be adjusted in a growing child. In 1992, Kosloske and Williamson [87] reported the use of expandable tissue expander prostheses in an effort to address this problem. Finally, placement of endobronchial stents has been reported, mostly in adults.

Thoracic surgical lesions

Thoracic surgery in neonates is done primarily to treat congenital pulmonary anomalies such as congenital cystic lesions, congenital diaphragmatic hernia (CDH), and tracheo-esophageal fistula (TEF). These anomalies often present *in utero* or in the newborn period. Other lesions, such as neoplasms, infectious diseases and musculoskeletal deformities, are found in later childhood. CDH and TEF are described elsewhere (see Chapter 21), but the remainder of these surgical lesions affecting infants and children are reviewed here, along with specific anesthetic considerations.

Congenital cystic lung disease

Of the many types of congenital cystic lesions, the overwhelming majority can be categorized into four groups: congenital cystic adenomatoid malformation (CCAM), bronchopulmonary sequestration (BPS), congenital lobar emphysema (CLE), and bronchogenic cyst (BC). These malformations have distinct features, yet they have significant overlap, suggesting there may be a single pathological mechanism for their development [88]. Of note, CCAM is more correctly termed CPAM (congenital pulmonary airway malformation) since many are neither cystic nor do they have adenoid tissue [89], but will be referred to as CCAM in this text, as is generally found in anesthesia and surgical literature.

Cystic lung lesions are often identified on routine fetal ultrasound at about 20 weeks' gestation [90]. Management in a fetus depends on the lesion itself and on the status of the fetus and mother. Large lesions may compress the esophagus, lung or vena cava and result in polyhydramnios, pulmonary hypoplasia or low-output cardiac failure and fetal hydrops, respectively. When there is evidence of fetal hydrops, intervention options include thoracocentesis, thoracoamniotic shunting, open fetal surgery and resection, *ex utero* intrapartum therapy and resection (EXIT procedure), or early delivery and postnatal resection. For a fetus greater than 32 weeks' gestation, resection during EXIT procedure is recommended. Those less than 32 weeks' gestation have the option of intrauterine surgery [91]. Anesthesia for fetal surgery and EXIT procedure is discussed in Chapter 19.

Small lesions may be asymptomatic or may cause respiratory distress in the newborn period. Initially asymptomatic lesions may develop into infection, pneumothorax or malignant degeneration later in life. Serial imaging has revealed, however, that many large lesions actually decrease in size [92,93]. Postnatal symptoms depend on the size, location and type of lesion, as well as any communication with the gastrointestinal tract or bronchopulmonary tree. Pulmonary hypoplasia can be associated with pulmonary hypertension or respiratory failure and may require extracorporeal membrane oxygenation (ECMO). Many lesions are asymptomatic and remain undiagnosed for years. Almost all patients eventually develop complications, most often as pneumonia unresponsive to medical management.

Patients with prenatally diagnosed lesions should have a computed tomography (CT) scan of the chest after birth. Children with lesions that were not identified prenatally and which cause respiratory distress after birth undergo chest radiography as the first diagnostic test and confirmatory studies, such as CT, afterwards (Figs 24.8, 24.9). Occasionally, magnetic resonance imaging (MRI) and bronchoscopy may be necessary. CCAM, CLE and extralobar BPS are occasionally associated with other congenital anomalies and may necessitate additional preoperative work-up, including echocardiography [88].

While there is consensus that all symptomatic lesions should be resected, there is debate whether asymptomatic lesions should be observed or resected. CCAMs and BPS sometimes resolve spontaneously on fetal ultrasound, but there is no evidence that this occurs after birth. Pulmonary lesions that become undetectable by fetal ultrasound and postnatal radiograph may be visible on CT. Ten percent of asymptomatic CCAMs that were followed conservatively required surgery later [92]. It is therefore still recommended that CCAM, intralobar BPS and BC be resected between 3 and 6 months of age. Extralobar BPS can remain asymptomatic for life but can also cause complica-

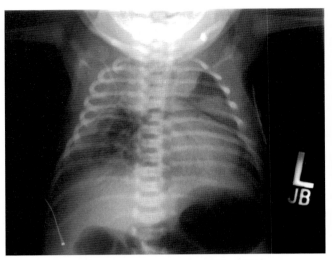

Figure 24.8 Chest radiograph of a newborn with a CCAM.

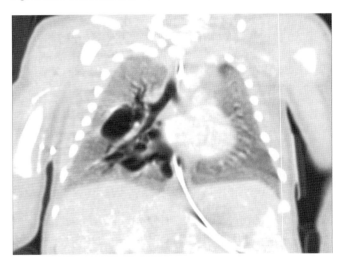

Figure 24.9 Chest CT of a newborn with a CCAM.

tions. A period of observation has been advocated for this lesion [90] and for asymptomatic CLE, which may resolve spontaneously.

When neonates with congenital lung lesions require anesthesia, it must be determined if positive pressure ventilation (PPV) will be tolerated. PPV of the lungs of patients who have lesions with a bronchial connection to abnormal lung parenchyma could develop overdistension of the abnormal lobe and compression of normal lung tissue through a ball-valve effect. This can compromise ventilation, shift the mediastinum, compress the great vessels, and decrease cardiac output. If there is doubt whether there is a bronchial connection to the thoracic lesion, spontaneous ventilation should be maintained during induction and maintenance of anesthesia. Once the affected lung is isolated, PPV and neuromuscular blockade can be safely initiated. Postoperative analgesia can be by intravenous opioids or, preferably, by a thoracic epidural placed directly at the desired level or threaded from the caudal canal. Recently, more congenital lung lesions have been resected using VATS. When VATS is used in the infant population, it is challenging for the anesthetist and surgeon and often results in significantly longer operative times; however, it is safer for the patient and may reduce hospital stay [93,94].

Cystic adenomatoid malformation

A CCAM is a discrete intrapulmonary mass that is either solid or cyst containing, and is typically characterized by increased adenomatous respiratory bronchioles. The cysts can be of various sizes, from 1 mm to over 10 cm. Although the lesion is non-functional, it does communicate with the normal tracheobronchial tree, which can cause air trapping during positive pressure ventilation [91]. CCAM is usually present in only one lung lobe, and occurs in all lobes with equal frequency. When it involves more than one lobe, pneumonectomy may be required. Associated anomalies are uncommon.

Congenital cystic adenomatoid malformations are usually detected *in utero* by ultrasound. They rarely result in pulmonary hypoplasia, hydrops fetalis or fetal demise. Most CCAMs are asymptomatic and are resected electively in the neonatal period. Those that cause cardiac or respiratory distress may necessitate emergency resection, either in the immediate postnatal period or by EXIT procedure [91].

While there is a communication between the lesion and the tracheobronchial tree, CCAMs are usually solid or have small cysts, acting more like solid lesions. Thus it is usually safe to use PPV. Most lesions can be resected without lung isolation, but if necessary OLV is easily accomplished by mainstem intubation. Intraoperative and postoperative pain management is accomplished through an epidural catheter [95].

Bronchopulmonary sequestration

A BPS is a portion of non-functioning lung tissue without a bronchial connection. It typically has an anomalous blood supply, arising from bronchial or aortic vessels, and has systemic, bronchial or azygous venous drainage. BPS is usually found in the lower lobes. The majority of lesions are intralobar (inside lobe pleura) and the rest are extralobar (with their own pleura). BPS can be confused with CCAM and some lesions are considered "hybrid," having features of both BPS and CCAM.

Bronchopulmonary sequestration is frequently diagnosed *in utero*. Detection of a systemic artery from the aorta to fetal lung tissue that is identified by color flow Doppler is pathognomonic for BPS [91]. At birth, most BPSs are asymptomatic and present later in life as antibiotic-resistant pneumonia. Sometimes a large BPS

will compress the lungs and cause respiratory distress. If the blood supply to the lesion is large, high-output cardiac failure may occur. BPS is diagnosed using CT, but a MRI is helpful for mapping the blood supply and drainage before surgical resection.

There are few unique anesthesia concerns for BPS. OLV is helpful for surgical resection, but because there is no connection between a BPS and the bronchial tree, it is safe to use PPV.

Congenital lobar emphysema

Congenital lobar emphysema is an abnormally emphysematous lobe of the lung that communicates with the bronchial tree. It occurs most commonly in the left upper lobe, then the right middle and then left lower lobes and can be distinguished from other cystic pulmonary lesions by ultrasound. It often enlarges before 28 weeks' gestation because fetal lung fluid is trapped within the lesion, similar to the air trapping that occurs postnatally. The lesion may regress and the lung tissue may appear normal at birth [91].

Even though CLE is usually asymptomatic, it is important that patients with CLE are carefully evaluated at birth because of the risk of air trapping in the emphysematous lobe. Overinflation of the lobe may lead to "tension emphysema" and compression of the contralateral lung [96]. At this stage CLE can be confused with a tension pneumothorax and a chest tube may be inappropriately inserted, leading to further respiratory distress. Large lesions may decrease cardiac output and eventually cause cardiac collapse. An emergency thoracotomy with rapid exteriorization of the lobe is required.

The primary concern for anesthetists is avoiding overdistension of the affected lung tissue. PPV may lead to rapid expansion of the lesion, due to a ball-valve effect; an effort should be made to maintain spontaneous ventilation. If PPV is necessary, low inflating pressures should be used. OLV is typically used to isolate the affected lung and once accomplished, it is also safe to use PPV. Nitrous oxide should be avoided throughout the case. At the end of the procedure, two-lung ventilation is instituted to check for gas leaks at the resection site. To reduce the incidence of air leaks, the trachea should be extubated early or, if the trachea remains intubated, the patient should be allowed to breathe spontaneously. The use of VATS is more challenging with CLE than it is with other cystic lung lesions [93]. As with other congenital cystic lesions, pain is well controlled by a thoracic epidural.

Bronchogenic cyst

Bronchogenic cysts are usually mediastinal, solitary unilocular cysts filled with gas, fluid or mucus. They do not communicate with the bronchopulmonary tree and therefore, like bronchopulmonary sequestrations, pose few additional anesthetic concerns. Positive pressure ventilation can be used and some authors have even reported that using nitrous oxide is safe [97].

Anterior mediastinal mass

Anesthetizing children who have anterior mediastinal masses may be associated with a high risk of morbidity and even mortality [98–101] that is caused by cardiovascular and/or respiratory collapse. Fortunately, over the past several decades, as anesthesiologists have become more aware of these risks and as perioperative management has improved, the morbidity and number of fatalities have decreased [102].

Mediastinal masses are located in the anterior, middle or posterior mediastinum, but this designation is somewhat arbitrary and there is overlap between them. Masses in the anterior mediastinum are the lesions that most often cause complications during general anesthesia [103]. Anterior mediastinal masses include several types of tumors, most commonly neuroblastoma in young children and lymphomas (Hodgkin and non-Hodgkin) in adolescents [104]. Other tumors include germ cell tumors, thymoma, bronchogenic cyst, carcinoma, granuloma and cystic hygroma [102]. A tissue biopsy (usually a CT-guided biopsy) is required for diagnosis to guide chemotherapy, radiation therapy and/or surgical resection. Occasionally surgical biopsy through the mediastinum or thorax is necessary.

While most adults with anterior mediastinal masses are asymptomatic, 70% of children have symptoms related to the mass [105]. Typical symptoms include dyspnea, cough, and stridor. Children with these lesions often prefer to sleep in the lateral, semi-erect or even upright position. Symptoms that are associated with increased risk of anesthetic complications include orthopnea, upper body edema or compression of the trachea, bronchus or great vessels [101,104,106,107].

Imaging the mass is mandatory before elective anesthesia is undertaken. Chest radiographs may reveal a widened mediastinum, but CT is needed to demonstrate the size of the mass and the presence and severity of tracheal or great vessel compression (Figs 24.10–24.12). Angiography or echocardiography may be required to further evaluate vascular compression. Obstruction of breathing during induction of anesthesia is associated with 50% or greater compression of the trachea [106]. The tumor size, as defined by mediastinal mass ratios (the maximal width of the mass divided by the maximal width of the thorax), also correlates with tracheal compression and development of airway obstruction [100].

Pulmonary function tests (PFTs) are commonly ordered with the thought that a decreased peak expiratory flow rate (PEFR) or an increased mid-expiratory plateau with

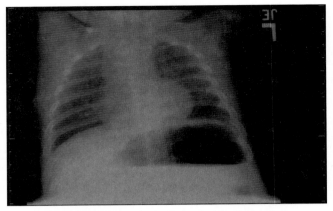

Figure 24.10 Chest radiograph of a 7-month-old patient with an anterior mediastinal mass.

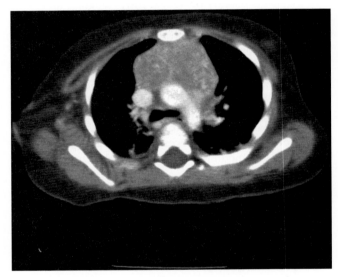

Figure 24.11 Chest CT of a 7-month-old patient with an anterior mediastinal mass, showing compression of the trachea.

changing from the upright to the supine position is indicative of variable intrathoracic airway obstruction and a risk for airway collapse during induction of anesthesia [102,108]. Most studies fail to show any correlation between PFTs and the degree of airway narrowing [106,108,109] or correlation between a decrease in any specific preoperative PFT and postoperative morbidity [110]. Flow-volume studies may, however, demonstrate dynamic compression of the airways that was not identified on CT.

The first consideration when developing an anesthetic plan is whether the proposed procedure is diagnostic or therapeutic. Diagnostic procedures, such as bone marrow biopsy or CT or ultrasound-guided biopsy of peripheral lymph nodes, can be done with local anesthesia or with

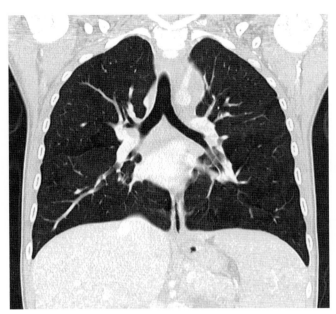

Figure 24.12 Chest CT of a 10-year-old patient with an anterior mediastinal mass. There is no visible compression of the trachea.

minimal sedation in most children. Ketamine (along with an antisialogog) has the advantage of maintaining hemodynamics in patients with cardiovascular compromise. Respiratory complications still occur, however, even when general anesthesia is avoided [104]. Elective procedures requiring general anesthesia should be delayed until chemotherapy and/or radiation therapy has reduced the size of the mediastinal mass. If a tissue diagnosis is necessary prior to chemo/radiation therapy, efforts should be made to obtain the tissue under local anesthesia [111]. Therapeutic procedures obviously necessitate general anesthesia.

Protocols developed for anesthetizing adults who have anterior mediastinal masses [112] use awake, fiber-optic intubations but this is not practical in pediatric patients [113,108] and is dependent on availability of resources, such as cardiopulmonary bypass and radiation therapy. There are, however, anesthetic strategies that can be generally applied in this situation (Fig. 24.13).

Before proceeding with general anesthesia, equipment and personnel should be immediately available to perform rigid bronchoscopy. Spontaneous ventilation should be maintained during induction of general anesthesia. This is usually accomplished by inhalation of a volatile anesthetic. The addition of CPAP may help maintain airway patency and prevent atelectasis. Some patients may require induction of anesthesia in the semi-reclined or upright position. Because loss of airway muscle tone can result in complete airway obstruction, negative thoracic airway pressure should be maintained,

and neuromuscular blocking agents should be avoided. Tracheal intubation should be accomplished while maintaining spontaneous ventilation.

In the event of airway collapse, maneuvers which may help to alleviate the airway obstruction include:
- changing the patient's position to the lateral, recumbent or prone position
- intubating the trachea and advancing the endotracheal tube past the obstruction
- rigid bronchoscopy followed by endotracheal tube placement under direct vision or double-lumen tube placement into the most patent bronchus.

Some institutions advocate having cardiopulmonary bypass on standby. While there are several reports of patients being successfully placed on ECMO or cardiopulmonary bypass, bypass was initiated before the induction of anesthesia [114–118]. We found no published reports of patients successfully placed on bypass after the induction of anesthesia when cardiopulmonary bypass was available only on "standby." Even with a team ready and a pump primed, by the time the vessels are cannulated and circulation is restored, the patient will have likely suffered neurological injury [104]. Therefore cardiopulmonary bypass should not be considered a reasonable salvage plan. If the risk of cardiopulmonary collapse during the induction of anesthesia is high, the patient should be placed on cardiopulmonary bypass before the induction of anesthesia.

Patients presenting for thoracotomy for resection of a mediastinal mass or an open biopsy get excellent postoperative pain relief from a thoracic epidural or paravertebral block, both of which reduce the need for intravenous narcotics and allow the maintenance of spontaneous ventilation [119]. The patient's symptoms may be worse after surgery, particularly after a tumor biopsy in which the adverse effects of anesthesia are present without the benefit of tumor resection [103]. Potential surgical complications include phrenic or recurrent laryngeal nerve damage.

Pectus excavatum

Pectus excavatum is the most common chest wall deformity. It is a congenital defect that results from excessive growth of the costochondral cartilages and inward depression of the sternum. It accounts for 90% of chest wall deformities and has an incidence of approximately 1 in 1000 with a male preponderance of 4:1. Pectus excavatum is sometimes associated with connective tissue disorders such as Ehlers–Danlos and Marfan syndromes. A family history of this deformity is present in as many as 50% of patients with a pectus excavatum [120]. Pectus carinatum (pigeon chest) comprises most of the remaining chest wall deformities.

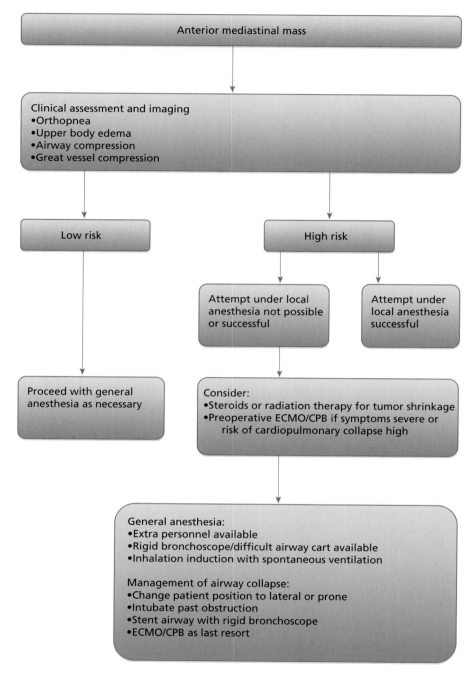

Figure 24.13 Algorithm for management of anterior mediastinal mass.

The severity of the lesion varies widely, from mild asymptomatic to severe deformities that distort the heart and great vessels (Figs 24.14, 24.15). Lesion-induced lung compression can lead to respiratory compromise, chronic airway obstruction, and the need for large negative inspiratory pressures. Compression of the stomach by the depressed chest can cause loss of appetite and impaired weight gain [121]. Most symptoms worsen during ado-lescence and more than half of adults with a pectus have some physical complaints [122]. Psychological complaints are also common [120]. Cardiorespiratory complaints are usually resolved with surgery [123].

Diagnosis of pectus excavatum is made by physical examination. Scoliosis is also present sometimes, particu-larly in female patients. Many patients have a murmur if the chest wall compresses the right ventricle. Characteristic

Table 24.2 Pediatric thoracic lesions

Lesion	Evaluation	Treatment	Anesthetic considerations
Tracheal stenosis			
Acquired	Laryngoscopy/bronchoscopy	Cricoid split	TIVA
Congenital	Laryngoscopy/bronchoscopy	Laryngotracheoplasty	TIVA, postoperative ventilation
Congenital cystic lung disease			
Cystic adenomatoid malformation	CT	VATS versus thoracotomy	Minimize inflating pressure, avoid N_2O
Bronchopulmonary sequestration	CT, MRI	VATS versus thoracotomy	Minimize inflating pressure, avoid N_2O
Congenital lobar emphysema	CT	VATS versus thoracotomy	Spontaneous ventilation, N_2O contraindicated
Bronchogenic cyst	CT	VATS versus thoracotomy	Minimize inflating pressure, avoid N_2O
Congenital diaphragmatic hernia	CXR	Replace abdominal contents, Repair defect	Decrease PVR, minimize inflating pressure, avoid N_2O, may need nitric oxide, HFOV, ECMO
Tracheo-esophageal fistula	CXR	Repair defect	Minimize inflating pressure, occlude fistula with ETT or blocker
Neoplasms			
Mediastinal	CT, MRI, PFTs	Needle or open biopsy, resection	Respiratory and/or cardiovascular collapse, possible OLV
Thoracic	CT, MRI	VATS versus thoracotomy	OLV, effects of chemotherapy and/or radiation therapy
Pectus excavatum	CXR, CT, PFTs, echocardiogram	Nuss versus Ravitch	Postoperative analgesia
Scoliosis	CXR, PFTs	Spinal fusion	Possible OLV with anterior fusion
Empyema	CXR, CT, pleurocentesis	Thoracostomy versus VATS or thoracotomy	Possible OLV

CT, computed tomography; CXR, chest x-ray; ETT, endotracheal tube; MRI, magnetic resonance imaging; OLV, one-lung ventilation; PFT, pulmonary function test; PVR, pulmonary vascular resistance; TIVA, total intravenous anesthesia; VATS, video-assisted thoracoscopic surgery.
Modified from Hammer [16].

ECG findings include a negative P wave in V1, a negative T wave in V1 to V2 or V4, and an incomplete bundle branch block [122].

Surgical repair is typically delayed until late childhood to allow calcification of the sternum and ribs. Techniques for correcting a pectus excavatum include rib resection, external traction, cartilage resection, sternal osteotomy, and internal fixation [124]. The minimally invasive procedure of Nuss inserts a convex steel bar through bilateral thoracic incisions under the sternum and then turns the bar to elevate the sternum. This is the preferred method of repair today [125] because it is associated with shorter operative times, smaller incisions, less dissection, and less blood loss than the traditional Ravitch procedure. The Nuss procedure is successful 92% of the time compared to 70% success with the Ravitch procedure [124]. Pneumothorax is common, but resolves spontaneously in nearly all cases [124,125]. Less common complications of the Nuss procedure include cardiothoracic injuries, dysrhythmias, pleural effusions, hemorrhage, subcutaneous emphysema, and infection of the bar [125,126].

Preoperative concerns include possible heart compression, right ventricular outflow tract obstruction, dysrhythmia, scoliosis and V/Q mismatching. Studies to help delineate the severity of disease include chest radiograph, CT, ECG and possibly echocardiography. Positioning of the patient during surgery can be a challenge. Placing the patient's arms in arthroscopy slings instead of over the head can reduce the incidence of brachial plexus injuries [127]. Continuous arterial blood

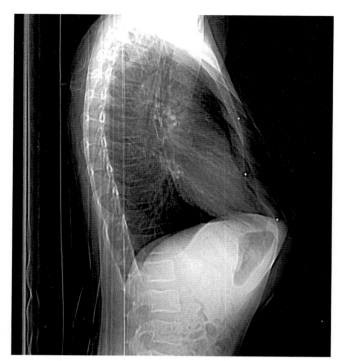

Figure 24.14 Chest radiograph of a 12-year-old patient with pectus excavatum.

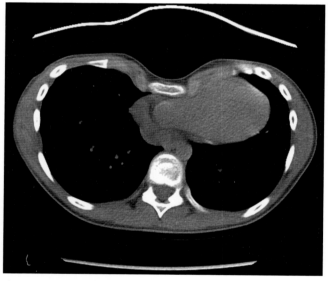

Figure 24.15 Chest CT of a 12-year-old patient with severe pectus excavatum showing cardiac compression.

pressure monitoring may be of benefit during surgery in patients with cardiac disease. Both the Ravitch and Nuss procedures are painful and postoperative pain control can be challenging. Epidural analgesia is both effective [128–130] and superior to patient-controlled analgesia [129,131]. Clonidine is an effective alternative to epidural

opioids, and has fewer side-effects [130]. There may be a role for perioperative hypnosis [132].

Empyema

Empyema or pleural space infection is a complication of bacterial pneumonia. Historically only 0.6% of admissions for pneumonia progressed to empyema [133], but the incidence is rising; more virulent strains of resistant organisms are the cause of this increase [134,135]. Empyema should be considered in any child who has pneumonia. There is neither consensus nor evidence for the best treatment of pleural infections, mostly because there are few prospective randomized controlled studies of the problem [135,136]. Options range from conservative therapy with antibiotics to thoracocentesis, chest tube drainage, fibrinolysis, and finally surgical intervention [135].

Empyema evolves over three stages [137].

1. Exudative, in which fluid is thin with low cellular content and easily aspirated.
2. Fibrinopurulent, in which there is accumulation of leukocytes, fibrin deposition and loculation.
3. Organized, with the formation of a thick fibrous peel that causes lung entrapment.

During this last stage, drainage alone is ineffective in re-expanding the lung. Decortication may be necessary. The exudative stage can be as short as 24 h and the fibrinopurulent stage 2–10 days, while the organizing stage generally lasts 2–4 weeks [138].

Pleural fluid analysis has long been used to stage empyema based on leukocytes, lactate dehydrogenase (LDH), glucose, and pH, but these criteria developed for adult patients have not been validated in the pediatric population [135]. Chest radiographs are not specific for diagnosing or staging of empyema. CT scanning is useful for both diagnosing and evaluating empyema with respect to consolidation, loculation, and pleural thickening (Figs 24.16, 24.17). Ultrasound can estimate the size of the effusion, show pleural thickening or loculi, and guide chest tube insertion. It has the advantage of being portable, which makes it useful for those unable to undergo CT.

Initial treatment for pleural infection is uncontroversial and consists of intravenous antibiotics, analgesics, and antipyretics. Effusions that are enlarging and/or compromising respiratory function should be treated with both antibiotics and drainage. The dilemma is which treatment option should occur next: thoracocentesis, thoracostomy tube drainage without or with fibrinolysis, or surgery. Tube drainage is recommended over repeated pleural taps for larger pleural infections, especially for younger children who seldom tolerate thoracocentesis under local anesthesia alone. Intrapleural fibrinolytics can lyse the fibrinous strands of a loculated empyema, improve pleural drainage, and produce successful outcomes

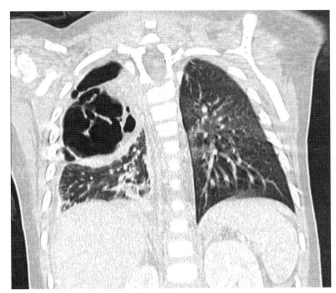

Figure 24.16 Chest CT of a 2-year-old patient with empyema, coronal view.

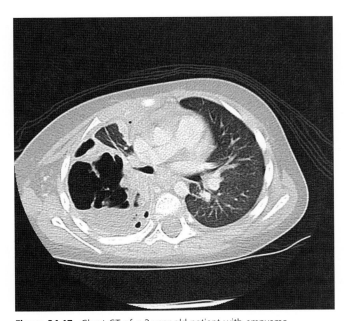

Figure 24.17 Chest CT of a 2-year-old patient with empyema, transverse view.

without surgery in up to 90% of cases [139]. Failure of chest tube drainage, fibrinolytics, and antibiotics should prompt surgical intervention.

Surgical management of empyema consists of VATS, mini-thoracotomy or open thoracotomy. Patients who undergo thoracotomy and debridement have earlier resolution of fever and shorter hospitalization than those treated by chest tube placement alone [135], but thoracotomy and debridement are associated with significant morbidity [140]. The use of VATS to treat empyema is less traumatic than open thoracotomy and has been advocated by many. VATS treatment is usually more effective when used early (within 1 week of diagnosis) in the course of empyema [138]. Only one prospective, randomized trial has compared VATS and thoracostomy drainage [141]. Although a small study (18 patients), it showed that hospital length of stay (LOS), number of days for which a chest tube was required, narcotic use, and the number of radiographic and interventional procedures were fewer in the VATS group. Several meta-analyses have shown that primary operative therapy is associated with shorter hospital stays [142–145] and a lower failure rate (by 11-fold) when compared to non-operative treatment [142]. Patients with necrotizing pneumococcal pneumonia or the need for ICU care before surgery are more likely to have complications and prolonged hospital admissions after thoracoscopy [146].

Patients who are treated conservatively (tube thoracostomy) for an extended period of time may progress to an empyema that, although initially treatable by VATS, becomes organized and only treatable by open thoracotomy. Treatment with VATS should be done early while empyema is still in the fibrinopurulent stage. For this reason many people advocate VATS as initial therapy before tube thoracostomy [147]. There is, however, no clear single therapy strategy for all patients. Each patient must be evaluated based on the stage of their disease and the therapeutic recourses available.

The anesthetic technique for patients with empyema depends on the procedure performed. Many patients tolerate pleurocentesis or tube thoracostomy with local anesthesia and/or minimal sedation. VATS or thoracotomy often necessitates one-lung ventilation. Good postoperative pain control is necessary for adequate lung re-expansion postoperatively. A paravertebral block or a thoracic epidural should be considered in non-septic patients who require a thoracotomy.

Conclusion

This chapter has reviewed the pathophysiology of OLV and the anesthetic practice and equipment necessary to facilitate the perioperative management of the pediatric thoracic surgery patient (including analgesia for thoracic surgery). It has discussed in a little more detail some of the finer nuances of specific thoracic surgical challenges within the pediatric population, namely lobectomy, pneumonectomy, congenital cystic lung disease, anterior mediastinal mass, pectus excavatum, and empyema.

CASE STUDY

A 14-year-old otherwise healthy girl presents for VATS for biopsy of a mediastinal mass.

- What additional information would you want to know at this point? *The additional information should include a detailed history, physical and review of radiological studies with specific emphasis on evaluation of airway and vascular compression.*

The patient presented with a 6-week history of cough, increasing shortness of breath, and wheezing. After failed antibiotic treatment for suspected pneumonia, her symptoms progressed to dyspnea and then orthopnea. A chest radiograph showed an anterior mediastinal mass and CT showed a mass obstructing approximately a third of the distal trachea.

- Would you proceed to surgery? *No. There are alternatives to proceeding with general anesthesia for thoracoscopy. A tissue diagnosis can often be obtained from a lymph node biopsy with local anesthesia. Alternatively, she can receive radiation therapy until the mass is no longer compressing the bronchus and she is asymptomatic. Then the mass can be removed if necessary.*

Lymph node biopsy under local anesthesia was unsuccessful and the oncologist wanted a tissue diagnosis prior to initiating radiation therapy.

- How would you induce anesthesia in this patient? *First, the proper equipment and personnel must be available, including a difficult airway cart, rigid bronchoscope, and personnel trained in its use. We would perform an inhalation induction, maintain spontaneous ventilation, and then place an endotracheal tube under deep inhalational anesthesia while avoiding the use of muscle relaxation.*

- You are having difficulty ventilating the patient's lungs, what would you do next? *The provider would first try to position the patient on her side. If this failed to relieve the obstruction, the endotracheal tube could be advanced in an attempt to stent past the obstruction, even to the point of endobronchial intubation. Finally, the available otolaryngologist could perform rigid bronchoscopy to stent the airway.*

- The obstruction was relieved by advancing the endotracheal tube slightly. What other intraoperative and postoperative factors need to be considered? *Maintenance of spontaneous ventilation for the remainder of the case with judicious use of narcotics would be prudent. The trachea should be extubated awake in the operating room and the patient should be admitted to the pediatric ICU for close postoperative monitoring and early intervention if needed.*

Acknowledgments

We thank Teresa Chapman, MD, Seattle, WA for her assistance in acquiring radiographic images.

Annotated references

A full reference list for this chapter is available at:
http://www.wiley.com/go/gregory/andropoulos/pediatricanesthesia

3. Lohser J. Evidence based management of one lung ventilation. Anesthesiol Clin 2008; 26: 241–72. This is an excellent review of the physiology of OLV. Lohser presents an evidence-based ventilatory strategy for OLV.

15. Choudhry DK. Single-lung ventilation in pediatric anesthesia. Anesthesiol Clin North Am 2005; 23: 693–708. This review article gives an excellent overview of the physiology of single-lung ventilation with a very clear explanation of the ventilation and perfusion changes during the lateral decubitus position. Choudhry also gives a very straightforward approach to device selection to facilitate one-lung ventilation.

16. Hammer GB. Pediatric thoracic anesthesia. Anesthesiol Clin North Am 2002; 20: 153–80. This review article summarizes the main thoracic lesions that present in the pediatric patient, and gives great detail on the strategies available to the pediatric anesthesiologist to provide the best care possible during the management of such surgical cases.

69. Davies RG, Myles S, Graham JM. A comparison of the analgesic efficacy and side-effects of paravertebral vs. epidural blockade for thoracotomy – a systematic review and meta-analysis of randomized trials. Br J Anaesth 2006; 96(4): 418–26. This meta-analysis of 10 trials involving 520 patients found that paravertebral block and epidural analgesia provide comparable pain relief after thoracic surgery, but PVB has a better side-effect profile and is associated with a reduction in pulmonary complications.

70. Joshi GP, Bonnet F et al. A systematic review of randomized trials evaluating regional techniques for post-thoracotomy analgesia. Anesth Analg 2008; 107(30): 1026–40. This systematic review identified 74 studies that compared various regional analgesic techniques with systemic opioid analgesia or with each other. The authors conclude that either thoracic epidural analgesia with LA plus opioid or continuous paravertebral block with local anesthetic can be recommended.

85. Kreisel D, Krupnick AS, Huddleston CB. Outcomes and late complications after pulmonary resections in the pediatric population. Semin Thorac Cardiovasc Surg 2004; 16: 215–19. This informative review discusses surgical outcomes and complications after lung resection.

91. Adzick NS. Management of fetal lung lesions. Clin Perinatol 2009; 36(2): 363–76. This is an excellent and current review of fetal lung lesions by Dr Adzick. It discusses prenatal diagnosis which may lead to intrauterine surgery or EXIT procedures, both new but important procedures that anesthesiologists should be familiar with.

98. Keon TP. Death on induction of anesthesia for cervical node biopsy. Anesthesiology 1981; 55(4): 471–2. This is a case report of a 9 year old with an anterior mediastinal mass who had a cardiac arrest and

died with induction of anesthesia. Published in 1981, it was the first report of anesthetic management of a patient with cardiac tamponade from a mediastinal tumor. It drew to the attention of the anesthesia community the dangers of anesthetizing patients with anterior mediastinal mass.

113. Hammer GB. Anaesthetic management for the child with a mediastinal mass. Paediatr Anaesth 2004; 14(1): 95–7. In this thorough review, Hammer discusses the anesthetic risks of patients with an anterior mediastinal mass and presents an organized algorithm for their evaluation and anesthetic plan.

136. Balfour-Lynn IM. Some consensus but little evidence: guidelines on management of pleural infection in children. Thorax 2005; 60(2): 94–6. There is neither much consensus nor evidence on the best treatment of pleural infections because there are few prospective randomized controlled studies. This article thoroughly discusses the evidence that is available, however, and attempts to develop practical guidelines.

CHAPTER 25
Anesthesia for Congenital Heart Disease

Kirsten C. Odegard, James A. DiNardo & Peter C. Laussen

Cardiac Anesthesia Service, Children's Hospital Boston, and Department of Anesthesia, Harvard Medical School, Boston, MA, USA

Introduction

Among the causes of infant mortality in the United States, congenital anomalies account for the largest diagnostic category [1]. Structural heart disease leads the list of congenital malformations. Over four million children are born each year in the United States and nearly 40,000 of these have some form of congenital heart disease (CHD). Approximately half of these children appear for therapeutic intervention within the first year of life, and the vast majority of them require care by an anesthesiologist.

Initial reports of anesthetic mortality ranging from 3% to 10% in operations for CHD indicated a significant risk of anesthesia in this patient population [2,3]. However, the principles and techniques of pediatric anesthesia presented in this volume allow one to anesthetize CHD patients with minimal anesthetic mortality and morbidity [4–6]. This low anesthetic risk is predicated not only on adherence to these principles but also on an understanding of the pathophysiological circumstance of each patient and the nature of the planned surgical procedure. Implicit in all surgical procedures are potential complications that anesthesiologists, by virtue of their primary role in

Gregory's Pediatric Anesthesia, Fifth Edition. Edited by George A. Gregory, Dean B. Andropoulos.
© 2012 Blackwell Publishing Ltd. Published 2012 by Blackwell Publishing Ltd.

monitoring and maintaining vital functions, are able to identify and treat. For cardiac surgery, knowledge of specific problems related to each type of cardiac repair helps to identify complications during the postbypass and postoperative periods, as well as later complications that affect subsequent anesthesia for non-cardiac procedures. The diagnostic information now available intraoperatively, in the form of intracardiac pressures and oxygen saturations as well as echocardiographic diagnoses, provides the pediatric cardiac anesthesiologist with the opportunity and responsibility to assess the adequacy of surgical intervention and its impact on hemodynamics.

This chapter describes general principles relevant to anesthesia for children with CHD; it does not present "recipes" for individual cardiac defects. The pathophysiology is presented as it relates to principles of management, patient assessment, selection and application of an anesthetic regimen, and specific cardiac lesions and procedures. Knowledge of these principles should permit safe administration of anesthesia to children with CHD undergoing both cardiac and non-cardiac operations. Optimal management will occur when the anesthesiologist regularly becomes involved in the care of these patients and has special insight and rapport with the entire cardiovascular staff, such that care is provided by a cohesive team in a smooth continuum from the preoperative preparation and diagnosis through the postoperative discharge.

Pathophysiology of congenital heart disease

Principles of management

The pathophysiological consequences of CHD are derived primarily from anatomical circumstances that produce abnormalities of flow: outflow obstruction, regurgitant lesions, shunt lesions, and common mixing lesions. Typically in more complex disease, shunts and obstructions may occur in combination. The pathophysiology of the most common purely obstructive lesions occurring outside the neonatal period is comparable to adult disease (e.g. aortic and mitral valve stenosis) and is not extensively reviewed here. Regurgitant lesions rarely exist as pure primary congenital defects except in Ebstein malformation of the tricuspid valve, in which a regurgitant volume flows back through the tricuspid valve and is directed across the patent foramen ovale to produce cyanosis and various degrees of heart failure. However, as a complicating feature of other CHDs, regurgitant lesions produce a volume-overload circulation with progressive ventricular dilation and failure. This is seen most commonly in regurgitation associated with atrioventricular canal defects, semi-lunar valve incompetence as seen in

tetralogy of Fallot with absent pulmonary valve syndrome, in truncal valve regurgitation in truncus arteriosus, or after interventions for aortic stenosis. Much of the remaining pathophysiology of congenital heart disease can be best understood by characterizing lesions with regard to the nature and magnitude of the shunt and the interaction of these shunts with obstructive lesions. Understanding the interactions of the various types of shunts and obstructions simplifies the bewildering variety of congenital heart lesions.

Many congenital heart lesions give rise to some degree of mixing of pulmonary and systemic venous blood, and they alter pulmonary blood flow. Varying degrees of hypoxemia may occur. These pathophysiological mechanisms alter the volume and pressure load of the heart, as well as cardiovascular development. Although such acquired developmental abnormalities may be adaptive, they can also further compound the effects of the original congenital heart defect. The resultant cardiac and pulmonary vascular structural abnormalities may become as important as the original heart defects when the pathophysiology is determined (e.g. severe left ventricular hypertrophy, seen with coarctation of the aorta, and right ventricular hypertrophy with progressive outflow obstruction, seen with tetralogy of Fallot). However, the intracardiac shunting and alterations in pulmonary blood flow comprise the major, unique problems encountered with CHD. These problems complicate the task of administering adequate anesthesia while maintaining normal cardiac output and oxygen transport.

Shunt lesions

Cardiac shunting is the process whereby venous return into one circulatory system is recirculated through the arterial outflow of the same circulatory system. Flow of blood from the systemic venous (right) atrium (RA) to the aorta produces recirculation of systemic venous blood. Flow of blood from the pulmonary venous (left) atrium (LA) to the pulmonary artery (PA) produces recirculation of pulmonary venous blood. Recirculation of blood produces a physiological shunt. Recirculation of pulmonary venous blood produces a physiological left-to-right (L-R) shunt, whereas recirculation of systemic venous blood produces a physiological right-to-left (R-L) shunt. A physiological R-L or L-R shunt commonly is the result of an anatomical R-L or L-R shunt. In an anatomical shunt, blood moves from one circulatory system to the other via a communication (orifice) at the level of the cardiac chambers or great vessels. Physiological shunts can exist in the absence of an anatomical shunt. Transposition physiology is the primary example of this process.

Shunts may occur alone as simple shunts (e.g. a ventricular septal defect (VSD)) or with complicating obstructive lesions in complex shunts such as tetralogy of Fallot.

The direction and magnitude of shunts are variable, both within each cardiac cycle and as a consequence of anesthesia and operative manipulation of the heart, great vessels and lungs, potentially destabilizing the circulation.

The hemodynamics in intracardiac shunts are complex and depend on many factors that determine shunt magnitude and direction (Fig. 25.1). Complete description of the dynamics of a particular shunt requires more data than are usually clinically available. The determinants of shunting may change considerably during anesthesia and operative manipulations without being readily measurable. Nevertheless, the concepts of control of shunting outlined below are useful during the perioperative period when it must be decided which shunts are hemodynamically significant and which are subject to intraoperative change.

Shunt orifice and outflow resistance are the most important determinants of shunting, particularly in ventricular and great vessel shunts. Ventricular compliance may also be important, but primarily as it relates to atrial level shunts. To simplify this discussion, ventricular compliance as a determinant of shunting is not further considered.

Simple shunts

With simple shunts (those without associated obstructive lesions), outflow resistance is equivalent to pulmonary vascular resistance (PVR) on the right and systemic vascular resistance (SVR) on the left (Fig. 25.2). The effects of shunt orifice and vascular resistances on simple shunts are outlined in Table 25.1. Although restrictive shunts are relatively fixed in magnitude by the small shunt orifice, shunt direction and magnitude become more dependent on the ratio of outflow resistances (i.e. the relative resistances of the pulmonary and systemic vascular beds (PVR/SVR)), as the communication becomes larger and non-restrictive (equal to or exceeding the aortic valve area).

When the communication becomes large enough, the two structures effectively become a common chamber and complete mixing occurs. With complete mixing in a common chamber and no outflow obstruction, the amount of pulmonary and systemic blood flow depends on PVR/SVR. Because normal PVR is often much less than SVR (as little as 5% of SVR in older children and adults), pulmonary blood flows can become large with a non-restrictive simple shunt, even during the neonatal period.

Although a number of factors affect PVR/SVR, some are relatively fixed, whereas others are variable and dynamic. Simple shunting can change intraoperatively as dynamic factors change. Thus shunting may be manipulated to variable degrees depending on the size of the communication and the ability to manipulate the dynamic portions of the relative vascular resistance. When shunt orifices are large and non-restrictive, simple shunts are more subject to some manipulation.

Complex shunt lesions

With complex shunts (Fig. 25.3), a fixed outflow obstruction is present at the ventricular outflow, subvalvular, valvular or supravalvular level, or in major vessels such as the pulmonary artery or aorta. The fixed resistance

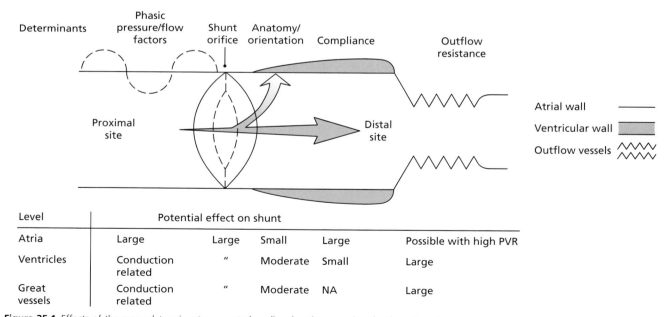

Level	Potential effect on shunt				
Atria	Large	Large	Small	Large	Possible with high PVR
Ventricles	Conduction related	"	Moderate	Small	Large
Great vessels	Conduction related	"	Moderate	NA	Large

Figure 25.1 Effects of the many determinants on central cardiac shunting at various levels. PVR, pulmonary vascular resistance. Reproduced from Berman W. Cardiovascular Shunts: Phylogenetic, Ontogenetic and Clinical Aspects. New York: Raven Press, 1986, with permission from Lippincott, Williams & Wilkins.

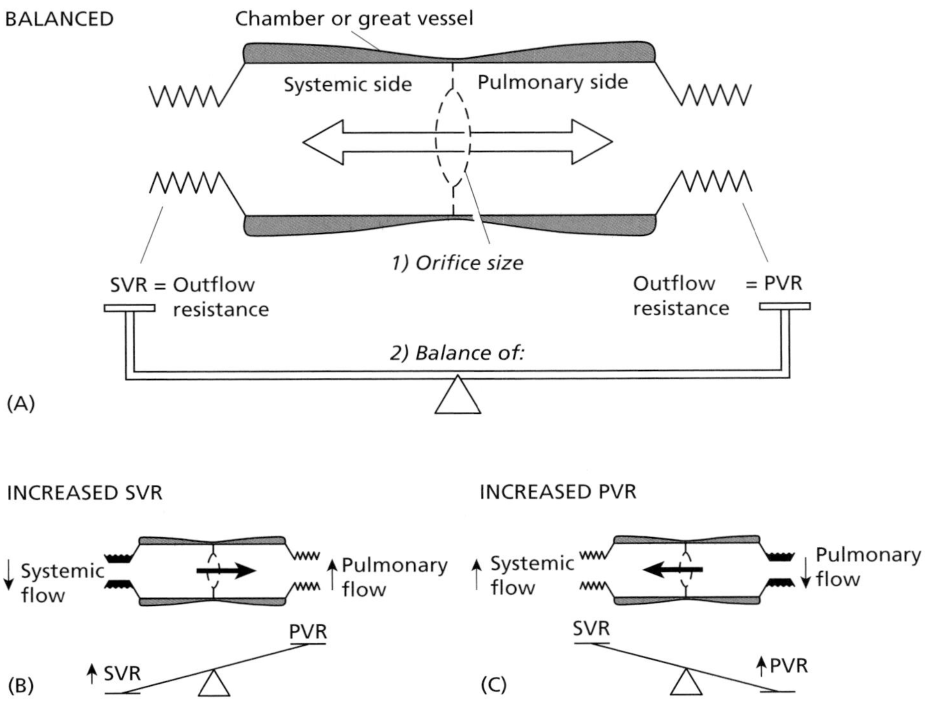

Figure 25.2 Determinants of the magnitude and direction of simple central shunts. (A) Balanced PVR/SVR. (1) Orifice size, generally fixed, is important for determining the magnitude of shunting and the pressure gradient across a shunt. (2) Balance of PVR and SVR is dynamic and determines the direction of shunt and variations in magnitude around the limits fixed by the orifice size. (B) Increased pulmonary flow with increased SVR. (C) Increased systemic flow with increased PVR. Reproduced from Hickey PR, Wessel DL. Anesthesia for treatment of congenital heart disease. In: Kaplan JA (ed) Cardiac Anesthesia. Orlando, FL: Grune and Stratton, 1987 with permission from Elsevier.

Table 25.1 Simple shunts, no obstructive lesions

Restrictive shunts (small communications)	Nonrestrictive shunts (large communications)	Common chambers (complete mixing)
Large pressure gradient	Small pressure gradient	No pressure gradient
Direction and magnitude more *independent* of PVR/SVR	Direction and magnitude more dependent on PVR/SVR	Bidirectional shunting
Less subject to control	More subject to control	Net $\dot{Q}p/\dot{Q}s$ totally depends on PVR/SVR
Examples: small VSD, small PDA, Blalock shunts, small ASD	*Examples:* large VSD, large PDA, large aortopulmonary shunts	*Examples:* single ventricle, truncus arteriosus, single atrium

PDA, patent ductus arteriosus; PVR, pulmonary vascular resistance; $\dot{Q}p$, pulmonary blood flow; $\dot{Q}s$, systemic blood flow; SVR, systemic vascular resistance; VSD, ventricular septal defect.

offered by the obstruction is added to the outflow resistance of the downstream vascular bed, which increases shunting to the opposite side of the circulation. When the fixed resistance is high, the resultant shunting away from the obstructed side is substantially fixed by the high resistance. Therefore, only a portion of a complex shunt is related to the relative resistances in the distal pulmonary and systemic vascular beds, and shunting through any communication is less dependent on PVR/SVR. As the outflow obstruction increases, changes in PVR or SVR become less important for determining flow. This is par-

ticularly true for the right side of the circulation, where normal PVR is low compared with the resistance offered by most right-sided obstructive lesions. For example, in tetralogy of Fallot with severe pulmonic stenosis, a component of the right-to-left shunting across the VSD is fixed by the pulmonary valve stenosis, but an additional, variable component of shunting may be due to variations in PVR or, more commonly, dynamic infundibular obstruction in the right ventricular outflow tract. Dynamic changes in variable portions of the total right-sided outflow obstruction may increase or decrease the total

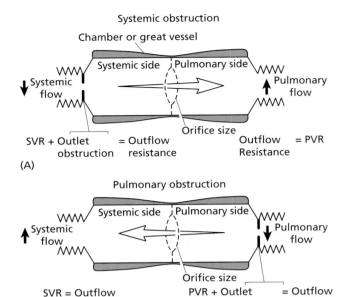

(A)

(B)

Figure 25.3 Determinants of complex shunting with (A) systemic or (B) pulmonary outflow obstruction. Orifice size limits the magnitude of the shunt. Outflow resistances are balanced by outlet obstruction on either side of the circulation and by the systemic vascular resistance (SVR) or pulmonary vascular resistance (PVR). Addition of outlet obstruction increases flow on the opposite side and decreases flow on the same side. Reproduced from Hickey PR, Wessel DL. Anesthesia for treatment of congenital heart disease. In: Kaplan JA (ed) Cardiac Anesthesia. Orlando, FL: Grune and Stratton, 1987 with permission from Elsevier.

amount of right-to-left shunting, thereby increasing or decreasing cyanosis. Right-to-left shunting in the baseline state, when the dynamic obstructive components are minimal, is determined largely by the fixed pulmonary stenosis. These statements presume a constant SVR and cardiac output; large changes in SVR, of course, change shunting by altering the other side of the balance (see Fig. 25.3). Characteristics and examples of complex shunts are listed in Table 25.2.

Complete obstruction and shunts

When obstruction to central outflow of blood becomes complete, as in tricuspid atresia, pulmonary atresia or aortic atresia, shunting across communications proximal to the obstruction becomes total and obligatory. This type of shunting must be associated with another downstream shunt, which provides flow to the obstructed side of the circulation. This associated shunt is exemplified by a patent ductus arteriosus, which provides pulmonary blood flow with pulmonary valvular atresia or provides systemic blood flow with aortic valvular atresia. The downstream shunting is variably dependent on PVR/SVR, depending on the restrictive nature of the shunt orifice.

Table 25.2 Complex shunts (shunt and obstructive lesion)

Partial outflow obstruction	Total outflow obstruction
Shunt magnitude and direction largely fixed by obstructions	Shunt magnitude and direction totally fixed
Shunt depends less on PVR/SVR	All flow goes through shunt
Orifice and obstruction determine pressure gradient	Pressure gradient depends on orifice
Examples: tetralogy of Fallot, VSD and pulmonic stenosis, VSD with coarctation	*Examples:* tricuspid atresia, mitral atresia, pulmonary atresia, aortic atresia

PVR, pulmonary vascular resistance; SVR, systemic vascular resistance.

Manipulation of pulmonary and systemic resistance

Manipulation of PVR/SVR allows some measure of control over shunting, depending on the specific pathophysiology. PVR is particularly important because of the frequency of disturbances of pulmonary blood flow and right-sided defects in CHD. Usually PVR is decreased to improve pulmonary blood flow and right heart function but with some lesions, pulmonary flow may be excessively high at the expense of systemic blood flow and require increases in PVR. Some intraoperative manipulations may increase PVR, a common problem because of the increased reactivity and resistance of the abnormal pulmonary vasculature often found with CHD. These manipulations include sympathetic stimulation, encroachments on lung volumes that produce atelectasis (surgical retraction, pleural and peritoneal collections, abdominal packing), cardiopulmonary bypass (CPB), alveolar hypoxia, and hypoventilation. Ventilation is important because it is subject to control by the anesthesiologist and is crucial for determining PVR via airway pressure, lung volumes, $PaCO_2$, pH, and FIO_2.

Ventilatory control of pulmonary vascular resistance

The PVR can be controlled independently of the SVR by manipulating various aspects of ventilation (Table 25.3), whereas specific or selective pharmacological control of PVR is difficult unless the pulmonary vascular bed is responsive to nitric oxide. Even with selective infusions of rapidly metabolized vasoactive drugs into the pulmonary circulation, systemic drug concentrations and systemic hemodynamic effects can be appreciable [7]. In contrast, high levels of inspired oxygen, especially 100% O_2, decrease elevated PVR in infants without changing (or slightly increasing) SVR, whereas inspired oxygen concentrations of 21% or less increase PVR [8,9]. The effec-

Table 25.3 Manipulations altering pulmonary vascular resistance

Increased PVR	Decreased PVR
Hypoxia	Oxygen
Hypercarbia	Hypocarbia
Acidosis	Alkalosis
Hyperinflation	Normal FRC
Atelectasis	Blocking sympathetic stimulation
High hematocrit	Low hematocrit
Surgical constriction	

PVR, pulmonary vascular resistance; FRC, functional residual capacity.

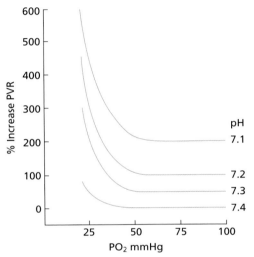

Figure 25.4 Changes in PVR with changes to in PaO_2 and arterial pH. Reproduced from Rudolph & Yuan. J Clin Invest 1966; 45: 399 with permission American Society for Clinical Investigation.

tiveness of oxygen (i.e. hyperoxia) as a pulmonary vasodilator after CPB, however, is unclear [10]. Hypoventilation, with associated acidosis and hypercapnia, also increases PVR [9] (Fig. 25.4). In contrast, hyperventilation to a pH of more than 7.5 reliably decreases PVR in infants with dynamically vasoconstricted small vessels [11,12]. This maneuver increases pulmonary blood flow and decreases right-to-left shunting in neonates, increasing the PaO_2 [13,14]. Some caution is required as prolonged hyperventilation to decrease PVR may in theory cause problems from decreased cerebral blood flow. Recent clinical observations support a link between the extent and duration of hypocapnia and development of white matter injury and subsequent neurobehavioral deficiencies in neonates [15].

The pattern of ventilation and use of positive end-expiratory pressure (PEEP) also can alter PVR. PVR is lowest at normal functional residual capacity (FRC). At low lung volumes (collapsed alveoli), PVR increases [16]. If atelectasis and pulmonary edema are corrected by PEEP, the PVR may in fact decrease. High levels of PEEP, however, may increase PVR, primarily by hyperinflating the alveoli. Different patterns of ventilation may further reduce PVR by stimulating production of prostacyclin in the pulmonary vasculature [17,18].

Anesthetics and pulmonary vascular resistance

The effect of anesthetic agents on PVR for the most part is minimal, although this depends to some extent on the underlying cause of the increase in PVR. Ketamine and nitrous oxide reportedly increase PVR in adults, particularly in patients with mitral stenosis, but do not affect the PVR of infants with normal or elevated PVR when ventilation and FIO_2 are held constant [19–21]. A rise in PVR with ketamine given to sedated children spontaneously breathing room air during cardiac catheterization has been noted [22]. However, in a cohort of patients with pulmonary hypertension spontaneously breathing 0.5% sevoflurane, no change in PVR was seen with ketamine administration [23]. Stress responses in the pulmonary circulation of patients with CHD are of primary concern in some patients during the perioperative period. Large doses of synthetic opioids (e.g. fentanyl) attenuate pulmonary vascular responses to noxious stimuli, such as endotracheal suctioning, in infants, but they do not change the baseline PVR [24,25]. Reactive hypertensive responses in the pulmonary bed are partially mediated by the sympathoadrenal axis and therefore are attenuated by an adequate depth of anesthesia, usually without changing the baseline PVR.

Manipulation of systemic vascular resistance

When deleterious intracardiac shunting cannot be controlled by manipulating PVR, it may be necessary to change SVR. In the presence of a complex shunt with *fixed* pulmonary outflow obstruction and right-to-left shunting (e.g. tetralogy of Fallot), an increase in SVR decreases the right-to-left shunting and increases arterial oxygen saturations [26]. Dynamic increases in infundibular outflow obstruction with tetralogy of Fallot that acutely increase baseline right-to-left shunting and hypercyanotic spells can be treated with IV pressor agents, which are shunted right to left directly into the systemic circulation, thus increasing SVR and decreasing right-to-left shunting. In the presence of a severely restrictive aortopulmonary shunt (e.g. Blalock–Taussig, Waterston) or when coronary perfusion is compromised, increases in systemic arterial pressure with pressor agents may increase pulmonary and coronary blood flow. Use of phenylephrine, norepinephrine or other α-agonists to maintain high systemic perfusion pressure may be beneficial under these circumstances [26]. Alternatively, proximal aortic (or left ventricular) pressure can occasionally be increased by partially occluding the aorta with a clamp to increase SVR.

Pulmonary circulation

Alterations in pulmonary blood flow caused by shunting in patients with CHD may produce several problems: pulmonary vascular obstructive disease, arterial desaturation or an increased volume load on the heart. These alterations are variable because of the changes in PVR that occur during development (Fig. 25.5). Because of these changes, associated problems may appear at different times during development. Dramatic alterations in pulmonary blood flow are seen during the neonatal period at the time of transition to adult-type circulation.

Transitional circulation

The transitional circulation of normal neonates can be viewed as a transient form of CHD. Shunting occurs in either direction through the ductus arteriosus and the foramen ovale until these structures functionally, and later anatomically, close. Initially, high PVR promotes right-to-left shunting through the ductus arteriosus and foramen ovale, which causes hypoxemia (Fig. 25.6; see also Fig. 25.5). Later, as PVR falls, shunting through the ductus reverses and becomes left to right until the ductus closes anatomically (see Figs 25.5, 25.6). When undergoing major non-cardiac surgery, neonates may revert to this transitional circulation despite previous *functional* closure of the ductus arteriosus and foramen ovale. The anesthetic plan should anticipate this possibility, and all neonates should be considered to have potential for intracardiac shunting.

Intraoperatively, hypoxia, acidosis, hypercapnia, hypothermia, sepsis, and prolonged stress favor return to the transitional circulation pattern. This pattern occurs because the degree of hypoxic pulmonary vasoconstriction is much greater in normal newborns than in adults. The resulting high pulmonary artery pressures may exceed aortic pressures and produce intermittent or continuous right-to-left shunting through a patent ductus arteriosus or foramen ovale [27]. Once the period of perioperative stress is over, normal developmental changes modify and functionally eliminate the ductus arteriosus, foramen ovale, and high PVR.

In children with forms of CHD that are "ductus dependent," the transitional circulation serves a palliative role by providing either adequate pulmonary or systemic flow until intervention can establish more normal patterns of flow. In these patients the transitional circulation is actively supported with prostaglandin E1 (see below).

Pulmonary vascular obstructive disease

In the presence of a non-restricted simple shunt (e.g. a large VSD), blood flow into the lungs increases as PVR falls (see Fig. 25.5). However, the pulmonary artery pressure and volume overload resulting from such shunts may, over time, alter pulmonary vascular development and cause pulmonary vascular obstructive disease [28,29] (Fig. 25.7; see also Fig. 25.5) This occurs with large VSDs, atrioventricular canal, transposition of the great arteries, truncus arteriosus, and large patent ductus arteriosus. In lesions such as atrial septal defect (ASD), where only flow is increased and pulmonary artery pressures are initially normal, pulmonary vascular disease takes decades to develop [30]. In contrast, pulmonary vascular disease can occur even during the first year of life in patients with an atrioventricular canal or in the first weeks of life in those

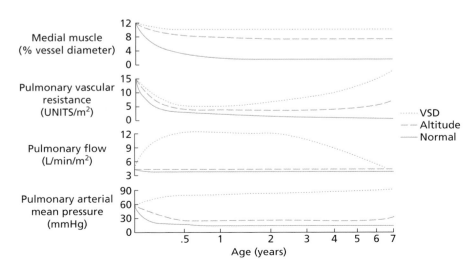

Figure 25.5 Normal and abnormal developmental changes in the pulmonary arterial tree during the first years of life. Pulmonary vascular resistance, arterial smooth muscle (%) and pressure normally decrease during the first year of life. A large, non-restrictive VSD with a large left-to-right shunt results in an immediate increase in flow and a later increase in vascular resistance. Reproduced from Rudolph AM. Congenital Diseases of the Heart. Chicago: Year Book Medical Publishers, 1974, p.79.

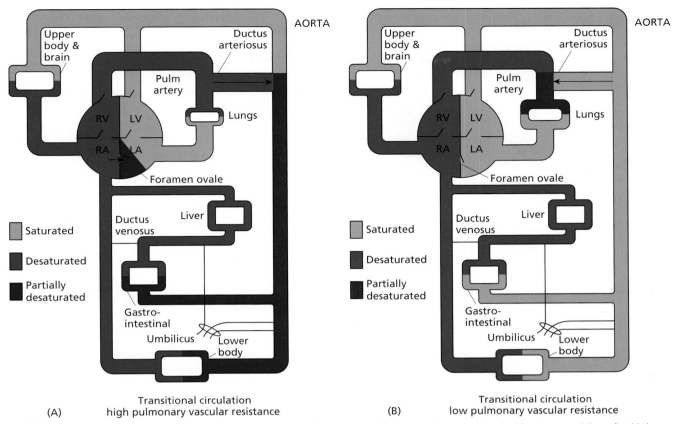

Figure 25.6 Central shunting and blood saturations that occur normally in the transitional circulation during the first few hours and days after birth. (A) During the first few hours, the foramen ovale is widely patent and PVR is high, leading to right-to-left shunting. (B) A second, later stage of transitional circulation occurs when PVR decreases and the ductus arteriosus remains patent, resulting in left-to-right shunting. The foramen ovale is functionally closed. Reproduced from Hickey PR, Crone RK. Cardiovascular physiology and pharmacology in children. In: Ryan J, Todres, D, Cote C, Goudsouzian N (eds) A Practice of Anesthesia for Infants and Children. Orlando, FL: Grune and Stratton, 1986, p.175 with permission from Elsevier.

with transposition of the great arteries and VSD [31]. A progressive rise in PVR may lead to chronic right-to-left shunting and right ventricular failure.

Intraoperatively, the more muscular and less well-arborized pulmonary arterial tree of patients with pulmonary vascular obstructive disease is capable of additional increases in PVR in response to surgical stimuli and stress. Right-to-left shunting may appear or dramatically increase during this time. Minimizing the reactive component of PVR without lowering SVR is often critical in anesthetic management.

Decreased flow in the pulmonary circulation during development can also lead to early significant abnormalities in the pulmonary arterial tree, including hypoplasia in some areas and excessive flow producing vascular obstructive disease in other regions [32]. This is especially true in patients with tetralogy of Fallot and pulmonary atresia, in whom the pulmonary artery anatomy must be addressed early in life.

Arterial desaturation

Systemic arterial desaturation in CHD frequently results from shunting of systemic venous blood into the systemic arterial circulation rather than from pulmonary parenchymal problems. If pulmonary parenchymal disease is also present, it is even more difficult to achieve adequate arterial oxygenation. Shunt-related arterial desaturation can occur whether pulmonary blood flow is greater than, equal to or less than systemic flow. The effects of alterations in pulmonary blood flow on arterial oxygenation in the presence of various shunts are listed in Table 25.4. It is important to realize that an FIO_2 of more than 0.21 has little effect on arterial oxygen tension in the presence of a large right-to-left shunt, but it has more effect as the shunt becomes smaller (Fig. 25.8). This statement presumes no pulmonary parenchymal disease and fully saturated pulmonary venous blood.

Hypoxemia also occurs in situations other than those with a pure right-to-left shunt with decreased pulmonary

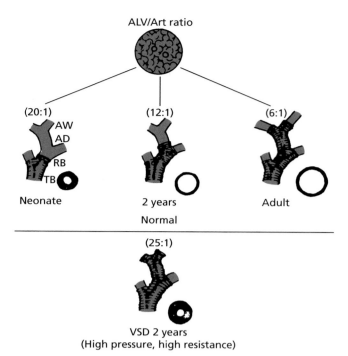

ALV/Art ratio

(20:1)   (12:1)   (6:1)

Neonate   2 years   Adult

Normal

(25:1)

VSD 2 years
(High pressure, high resistance)

Figure 25.7 Developmental changes in the peripheral pulmonary arterial tree in normal infants and in those with a VSD and large left-to-right shunt. The alveolar/arteriolar (ALV/art) ratio decreases with age becasue of extensive arborization of the arterial tree as the arteriolar lumen increases and the muscle layer thins and spreads distally. Pulmonary hypertension and high flow of blood from a left-ro-right shunt in a patient with a VSD cause pulmonary vascular obstructive disease as evidenced by a decreased number of pulmonary arterioles (ALV/art of 25:1), a decrease in vessel lumen, an increase in muscle thickness and a more distal spread of muscle. Letters indicate arterioles from the level of the terminal bronchiolus (TB) to the alveolar wall (AW). RB, respiratory bonchiolus; AD, alveolar duct. Reproduced from Rabinovitch MB, Hawroth SG, Castaneda AR. Lung biopsy in congenital heart disease: a morphometric approach to pulmonary vascular disease. Circulation 1978; 58: 1107 with permission from Lippincott, Williams & Wilkins.

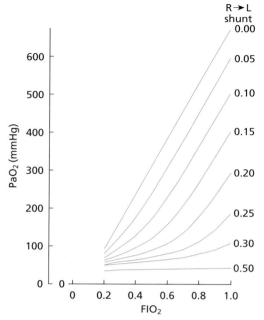

Figure 25.8 Isoshunt graph depicting the relation between inspired FIO_2 and arterial PaO_2, with different amounts of right-to-left shunting. It assumes normal values of pH, $PaCO_2$, pulmonary venous saturation, and mixed venous saturation. Adapted from Lawler P, Nunn J. A reassessment of the validity of the isoshunt graph. Br J Anaesth 1984; 56: 1325 with permission from Oxford University Press.

Table 25.4 Effects of central shunting and pulmonary blood flow on oxygenation

Pulmonary blood flow $\dot{Q}p$	L→R Shunt only	L→R + R→L (mixing)	R→L Shunt only
$\dot{Q}p > \dot{Q}s$	Normoxemia	Hypoxemia*	–
$\dot{Q}p = \dot{Q}s$	–	Hypoxemia	–
$\dot{Q}p < \dot{Q}s$	–	Hypoxemia (severe)	Hypoxemia (severe)

$\dot{Q}p$, pulmonary blood flow; $\dot{Q}s$, systemic blood flow; –, does not occur;
* Normoxemia when $\dot{Q}p/\dot{Q}s \geq 7-10$.

blood flow. If systemic and pulmonary venous blood mix in a vascular chamber, arterial desaturation occurs, even though pulmonary blood flow may be normal or increased (see Table 25.4). Mixing can occur at any anatomical level: right atrium (e.g. total anomalous pulmonary venous connection), left atrium (e.g. tricuspid atresia), ventricle (e.g. single ventricle) or great vessel (e.g. truncus arteriosus). When mixing is complete and pulmonary blood flow is normal or increased, hypoxemia is mild. When mixing is incomplete, hypoxemia may be severe, as occurs with the parallel circulation seen in patients with transposition of the great arteries.

Many poorly understood adaptations occur in patients with severe hypoxemia to allow reasonable levels of oxygen transport and consumption, including polycythemia, increases in 2,3-diphosphoglutarate (2,3-DPG) concentrations, vasodilation with increased blood volume, neovascularization, and alveolar hyperventilation with chronic respiratory alkalosis [33]. These and other poorly defined adaptive mechanisms maintain near-normal levels of mitochondrial oxygen utilization at rest without increase in lactate production. Elevated cardiac output and substantial shifts in the oxyhemoglobin dissociation curve are not essential adaptations in patients with severe hypoxemia [34].

The adaptations, however, may be associated with adverse physiological effects. Polycythemia increases blood viscosity, vascular resistance, and therefore ventricular afterload, especially in the pulmonary circulation [35]. As increasing viscosity elevates afterload, it decreases cardiac output, which opposes the benefit of polycythemia to oxygen-carrying capacity. The net reduction in oxygen *transport* is maladaptive and occurs when the hematocrit exceeds 60%. Such high hematocrits are associated with an appreciable incidence of cerebral and renal thrombosis, which increases with dehydration. This situation makes pre- and postoperative hydration crucial in these patients.

Cyanosis has been implicated in the genesis of coagulation and fibrinolytic defects particularly in patients in whom secondary erythrocytosis produces a hematocrit greater than 60%. The vast majority of studies investigating the effects of cyanosis on hemostasis have been conducted in chronically cyanotic adults and children >1 year old. Thrombocytopenia and qualitative platelet defects are common and are positively correlated with the level of erythrocytosis and arterial oxygen desaturation [36–43]. Defects in bleeding time, clot retraction and platelet aggregation to a variety of mediators have all been described [38,39,44,45]. The importance of erythrocytosis in the genesis of these quantitative and qualitative defects is underscored by the observation that multiple therapeutic phlebotomies using either plasma or isotonic saline to replace whole blood and reduce hematocrit to the 50–60% range result in improvement of platelet count and platelet aggregation [38,40]. In addition, shortened platelet survival time has been reported. Reduced survival time was weakly positively correlated with the level of erythrocytosis and arterial oxygen desaturation [41]. More recently, a baseline deficit in platelet GpIb receptors has been reported in cyanotic children [46]. These receptors play a pivotal role in inducing platelet aggregation and adhesion via von Willebrand factor (vWF). The platelets of cyanotic neonates and infants exhibit a hyporeactive response to thrombin receptor agonist peptides (TRAP) compared to non-cyanotic neonates and infants.

Prolonged prothrombin time (PT), partial thromboplastin time (PTT) and low levels of fibrinogen and factors II, VII, IX, X, XI, and XII have also been reported in association with cyanosis [36,37,39,43,47]. Therapeutic phlebotomies using isotonic saline to replace whole blood and reduce hematocrit to the 50–60% range result in an increase in factor II, VII and V levels [40]. Coagulation factor abnormalities appear to occur with lower frequency than platelet defects but the full extent of coagulation factor abnormalities is unknown because this issue has been incompletely studied.

Chronic disseminated intravascular coagulation (DIC) has been proposed as an additional mechanism leading to a coagulopathic state in cyanotic heart disease [48]. While evidence of accelerated ongoing thrombin generation and fibrinolysis has been detected in cyanotic versus non-cyanotic patients, chronic DIC has not been substantiated [49,50].

Recent evidence documents the overproduction of platelet microparticles in erythrocytotic patients (hematocrit (Hct) >60%) with congenital heart disease [51]. Microparticles are cellular fragments that are the result of exocytotic budding and which contain both cytoplasmic and membrane components. These microparticles express FVa and FXa and are highly procoagulant. Microparticle formation occurs as a result of the high microvascular shear forces which accompany erthrocytosis and can be reduced via hematocrit reduction with therapeutic phelebotomy [51].

Increased pulmonary blood flow

When pulmonary flow is greater than systemic flow (Qp/Qs more than 1), a volume load is imposed on the heart. With pure left-to-right shunts, the additional pulmonary flow does not increase arterial oxygen content. This increased load decreases not only cardiovascular reserve but also pulmonary reserve, because the work of breathing is increased owing to decreased pulmonary compliance and increased airway resistance [52]. These changes are due to increased lung water, compression of bronchi by distended pulmonary vessels at all levels, and general pulmonary vascular congestion. When left-to-right shunts are closed (e.g. ligation of a patent ductus arteriosus), lung compliance improves immediately [53].

Preoperative assessment and preparation

Successful anesthetic management of patients with CHD is based on complete, accurate preoperative assessment and adequate preoperative patient preparation. The clinical and laboratory information routinely available preoperatively (Box 25.1) should be frequently reassessed and integrated with information from continuous monitoring during surgery and the immediate recovery phase. The anesthesiologist must be aware of the physical and laboratory findings that are of particular importance for CHD. Involvement of the anesthesiologist in the preoperative preparation and early postoperative management provides a perspective on the pathophysiology that improves perioperative care.

Physical examination and laboratory data
A complete history and physical examination are required, and when such information is obtained attention should be directed to the extent of cardiopulmonary impairment,

airway abnormalities, and associated extracardiac congenital anomalies. Upper and lower airway problems in patients with Down syndrome, calcium and immunological deficiencies in patients with aortic arch abnormalities, and renal abnormalities in patients with esophageal atresia and CHD are a few of the associated congenital abnormalities with which the anesthesiologist should be familiar. Intercurrent pulmonary infection is a common and significant finding in chronically overcirculated lungs. The presence, degree, and duration of hypoxemia are important details that, in the absence of iron deficiency, are reflected in the hematocrit. The nadir of physiological anemia during infancy may contribute to left-to-right shunting by decreasing the relative PVR [35].

Chest radiography shows heart size, pulmonary vascular congestion, airway compression, and areas of consolidation or atelectasis. The electrocardiogram (ECG) may reveal rhythm disturbances and demonstrate ventricular strain patterns (ST and T wave changes) characteristic of unphysiological pressure or volume burdens on the ventricles. Electrolyte abnormalities caused by congestive heart failure and forced diuresis must also be evaluated preoperatively. Severe hypochloremic metabolic alkalosis may occur in some patients. It is more important to discontinue digoxin preoperatively and to avoid hyperventilation and administration of calcium to these patients during induction of anesthesia. The alkalotic hypokalemic, hypercalcemic, hypotensive, dilated, digoxin-bound myocardium fibrillates with ease.

Echocardiographic and Doppler assessment

Two-dimensional and, recently, real-time three-dimensional echocardiography has revolutionized the field of pediatric cardiology over the last decade. Unlike adults, who may have a limited echocardiographic window, comprehensive cardiac assessment of the pediatric patient is routine. Doppler measurements add greatly to non-invasive diagnostic capabilities. Measurements of pressure gradients across semi-lunar valves and other obstructions are frequently accurate but

may not always correlate with peak systolic ejection gradients measured at catheterization. Nonetheless, most neonates proceed to surgery without catheterization studies. In some instances, catheterization is necessary to clearly delineate coronary or aortopulmonary collateral anatomy or to clarify physiology when other clinical information is ambiguous or contradictory.

Cardiac catheterization

Normal intracardiac pressure and saturation values in children are shown in Figure 25.9.

Shunt localization is usually accomplished using a combination of angiography and measurement of O_2 saturations in the pulmonary veins, superior vena cava (SVC) and inferior vena cava (IVC), right heart chambers, left heart chambers, aorta, and pulmonary artery. Oxygen saturation sampling is used to detect an O_2 saturation step-up in the right heart in the case of a left-to-right shunt or an O_2 saturation step-down in the left heart in the case of a right-to-left shunt. A step-up is defined as >5% increase in the O_2 saturation of blood in a particular location that exceeds the normal variability in that location, whereas a step-down is a >5% decrease in saturation for a given location.

Shunt quantification is based on comparison of systemic and pulmonary blood flows. Systemic (Qs) and pulmonary (Qp) blood flows are calculated by the Fick method.

$$Qp = VO_2 / (PVO_2 \text{ content} - PAO_2 \text{ content})$$

PAO_2 content is the pulmonary arterial O_2 content. PVO_2 content is the pulmonary venous O_2 content. Sampling blood from the left atrium (when the pulmonary veins return to the left atrium) will provide a weighted average of the four pulmonary veins' O_2 content. If a right-to-left atrial-level shunt is present, this sampling site will not provide an accurate assessment of pulmonary vein O_2 content. Each of the four pulmonary veins can be entered and sampled separately to assess for pulmonary sources of venous admixture (e.g. pneumonia, atelectasis or other pulmonary disease). When this is done, segmental areas of intrapulmonary shunt and V/Q mismatch can be detected. The PaO_2 or saturation of pulmonary venous blood from a lung segment with V/Q mismatch will improve with an increase in FIO_2 while there will be no improvement if an intrapulmonary shunt is present.

$$Qs = VO_2 / (SAO_2 \text{ content} - MVO_2 \text{ content})$$

SAO_2 content is systemic arterial O_2 content. MVO_2 content is mixed venous O_2 content. True mixed venous blood is a mixture of desaturated blood from the IVC, SVC and coronary sinus. In a normal heart a mixed

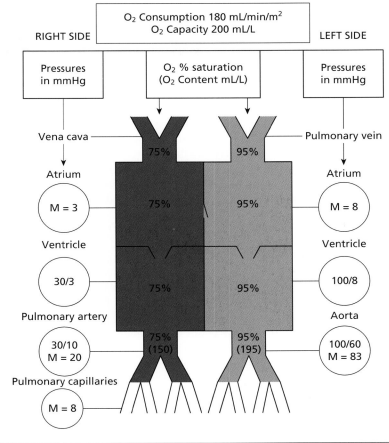

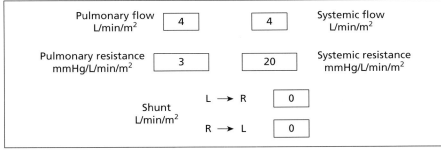

Figure 25.9 Cardiac catheterization findings in a normal child. Numbers in chambers are oxygen saturation (percent) and numbers in parentheses are oxygen content. Pressure in chambers are shown in circles. Note "probe-patent" foramen ovale. M, mean pressure. Reproduced with permission from Nadas AS, Fyler DC. Pediatric Cardiology. Philadelphia: WB Saunders, 1972.

sample of venous blood from these three locations can be obtained from the pulmonary artery. In the presence of an intracardiac left-to-right shunt, PAO_2 saturation will overestimate true MVO_2 saturation because pulmonary arterial blood will be a mixture of mixed venous blood and oxygenated pulmonary venous blood from the left heart. In children, SVC O_2 content is commonly used as a surrogate for MVO_2 content.

After Qp and Qs have been calculated, shunts can be quantified. For an isolated left-to-right shunt, the magnitude of the shunt is Qp – Qs. For an isolated right-to-left shunt, the magnitude of the shunt is Qs – Qp. The ratio Qp/Qs is also useful. It can be calculated from content data alone because the VO_2 terms cancel out:

$$Qp/Qs = \frac{(SAO_2 \text{ content} - MVO_2 \text{ content})}{(PVO_2 \text{ content} - PAO_2 \text{ content})}$$

Furthermore, if the blood is sampled using a low FIO_2, the dissolved O_2 portion of the content equation ($PO_2 \times 0.003$) can be ignored. The hemoglobin $\times$ 1.34 term cancels out and the equation can be simplified to one using just saturation data from the four sites:

$$Qp/Qs = \frac{(SAO_2 \text{ saturation} - MVO_2 \text{ saturation})}{(PVO_2 \text{ saturation} - PAO_2 \text{ saturation})}$$

A $Qp/Qs > 2.0$ constitutes a large shunt, whereas a $Qp/Qs < 1.25–1.5$ constitutes a small shunt. Obviously, a $Qp/Qs < 1.0$ indicates a net right-to-left shunt.

For bidirectional shunts, it is necessary to calculate effective pulmonary blood flow (Qp_{eff}) and effective systemic blood flow (Qs_{eff}). Qp_{eff} is the quantity of desaturated systemic venous blood that traverses the pulmonary capillaries to be oxygenated. Qs_{eff} is the quantity of oxygenated pulmonary venous blood that traverses the systemic capillaries to deliver oxygen to tissue. Qs_{eff} and Qp_{eff} are always equal.

$$Qs_{eff} = Qp_{eff} = VO_2 / (PVO_2 \text{ content} - MVO_2 \text{ content})$$

The left-to-right shunt is defined as $Qp - Qp_{eff}$ while the right-to-left shunt is defined as $Qs - Qs_{eff}$. The net shunt is the difference between these two calculated shunts.

In the presence of a left-to-right shunt and elevated PVR, pressure and saturation measurements are often repeated with the patient breathing 100% oxygen to assess both the reactivity of the pulmonary vascular bed and any contribution of ventilation/perfusion abnormalities to hypoxemia. If breathing 100% oxygen or nitric oxide increases pulmonary blood flow and dramatically increases Qp/Qs (with a fall in PVR), potentially reversible processes such as hypoxic pulmonary vasoconstriction are probably contributing to the elevated PVR. The patient with a high, unresponsive PVR and a small left-to-right shunt despite a large shunt orifice may have extensive pulmonary vascular damage from irreversible obstructive pulmonary vascular disease.

During cardiac catheterization, anatomical abnormalities are identified angiographically. Special angled views provide specific information about the location and extent of congenital defects. Ventricular function is assessed angiographically and physiologically (e.g. by pressure measurements). The calculated size of a cardiac chamber may have an important bearing on its ability to support the circulation of a child with hypoplastic ventricles.

Magnetic resonance and computed tomographic imaging and angiography

Magnetic resonance imaging and angiography (MRI/A) has emerged as an important diagnostic modality in the evaluation of the cardiovascular system following the development of ECG-gated MRI. Image acquisition is triggered to the patient's ECG to counter motion artifacts and to acquire cine sequences that allow imaging of cardiac structures and visualization of blood flow throughout the cardiac cycle. In addition to providing excellent anatomical and three-dimensional images, particularly of the pulmonary veins and thoracic aorta, it is also possible with magnetic resonance angiography (MRA) to qualitatively assess valve and ventricular function, and to quantify flow, ventricular volume, mass and ejection fraction [54,55]. While ferromagnetic implants near the region of interest might produce artifact, sternal wires and vascular clips produce relatively minor disturbances and therefore MRI can be performed in patients who have undergone previous cardiac surgery. Contraindications include patients with pacemakers, recently implanted endovascular or intracardiac implants and aneurysm clips on vessels that will be exposed directly to the magnetic field.

The claustrophobic small bore of the MRI machine and noise during imaging mean that sedation is necessary for most children undergoing cardiac MRI/A procedures. To allow three-dimensional MRA and gradient echo sequences for images of blood flow, breath-hold is necessary during image acquisition, and therefore general anesthesia is frequently required for neonates, infants and young children. As for procedures in the catheterization laboratory, the environment for MRI is often a difficult one in which to administer general anesthesia, and hemodynamic monitoring may be limited [56].

Computed tomographic (CT) imaging and angiography is particularly useful for visualizing extracardiac structures. Its advantages are brief imaging time (< 5 min), therefore minimal or no sedation is often required. Disadvantages are significant radiation exposure; risk: benefit of MRI vs CT are weighed carefully before selecting each modality.

Assessment of patient status and predominant pathophysiology

Frequently, congenital heart defects are complex and can be difficult to categorize or conceptualize. Rather than trying to determine the management for each individual anatomical defect, a physiological approach can be taken. The following questions should be asked.

- How does the systemic venous return reach the systemic arterial circulation to maintain cardiac output? What intracardiac mixing, shunting or outflow obstruction exists?
- Is the circulation in series or parallel? Are the defects amenable to a two-ventricle or single-ventricle repair?
- Is pulmonary blood flow increased or decreased?
- Is there a volume-load or pressure-load on the ventricles?

Appropriate organization of preoperative patient data, preparation of the patient, and decisions about monitoring, anesthetic agents, and postoperative care are best accomplished by focusing on a few major pathophysiological problems, beginning with whether the patient is cyanotic or in congestive heart failure (CHF) (or both).

Most pathophysiological mechanisms in the patient's disease that are pertinent to the anesthetic plan and to optimal preparation of the patient will focus on one of the following major problems: severe hypoxemia, excessive pulmonary blood flow, CHF, obstruction of blood flow from the left heart, and poor ventricular function. Although some patients with CHD present with only one problem, many have multiple inter-related problems.

Severe hypoxemia

Many of the cyanotic forms of CHD present with severe hypoxemia (PaO_2 less than 50 mmHg) during the first few days of life, but without respiratory distress. Infusion of prostaglandin E1 (PGE1) in patients with decreased pulmonary blood flow maintains or re-establishes pulmonary flow through the ductus arteriosus. This may also improve mixing of venous and arterial blood at the atrial level in patients with transposition of the great arteries [57]. Consequently, neonates rarely require surgery while they are severely hypoxemic. During preoperative preparation with PGE1, neurological examination, as well as blood chemistry analysis of renal, hepatic, and hematological function, is necessary to assess the effects of severe hypoxemia on end-organ dysfunction during or after birth.

Cyanotic patients who present for surgery after infancy require adequate pre- and postoperative hydration to prevent the thrombotic problems caused by their high hematocrits. Adequate quantities of blood products for treatment of the coagulopathies are also needed, as outlined above. Premedication must be given cautiously to avoid causing hypoventilation in these patients.

Prostaglandin E1 dilates the ductus arteriosus of the neonate with life-threatening ductus-dependent cardiac lesions and improves the patient's condition before surgery. It can reopen a functionally closed ductus arteriosus for several days after birth, or it can maintain patency of the ductus arteriosus for several months postnatally [57,58]. The common side-effects of PGE1 infusion (apnea, hypotension, fever, central nervous system (CNS) excitation) are easily managed in the neonate when normal therapeutic doses of the drug (0.01–0.1 µg/kg/min) are used [59]. However, PGE1 is a potent vasodilator, so intravascular volume frequently requires augmentation. Patients with intermittent apnea resulting from administration of PGE1 may require mechanical ventilation preoperatively.

Prostaglandin E1 usually improves the arterial oxygenation of hypoxemic neonates who have poor pulmonary perfusion due to obstructed pulmonary flow (critical pulmonic stenosis or pulmonary atresia). By providing pulmonary blood flow from the aorta via the ductus arteriosus, an infusion of PGE1 improves oxygenation and stabilizes the condition of neonates with these lesions. The improved oxygenation reverses the lactic acidosis that may have developed during episodes of severe hypoxia. PGE1 administration for 24 h usually markedly improves the condition of a severely hypoxemic neonate with restricted pulmonary blood flow [60].

Excessive pulmonary blood flow

Excessive pulmonary blood flow is frequently the primary problem of patients with CHD. The anesthesiologist must carefully evaluate the hemodynamic and respiratory impact of left-to-right shunts (see above). Children with left-to-right shunts may have chronic low-grade pulmonary infection and congestion that cannot be eliminated despite optimal preoperative preparation. If so, surgery should not be postponed further. Respiratory syncytial virus infections are particularly prevalent in this population, but improvements in intensive care and palivizumab prophylaxis have markedly improved outcome with this and other viral pneumonias [61].

Aside from the respiratory impairment caused by increased pulmonary blood flow, the left heart must dilate to accept pulmonary venous return that is several times normal. If the body requires more systemic blood flow, the heart responds inefficiently. Most of the increment in cardiac output is recirculated to the lungs. Eventually symptoms of CHF appear.

Children with failing hearts increase endogenous catecholamine production and redistribute cardiac output to favored organs by their increased heart rate and decreased extremity perfusion. In the most severe cases, the evaluation reveals a child whose bodyweight is below the third percentile for age and who is tachypneic, tachycardic, and dusky in room air. The child may have intercostal and substernal retractions and skin that is cool to the touch. Capillary refill may be prolonged. Expiratory wheezes are usually audible (Box 25.2). Medical management with digoxin and diuretics may improve the patient's condition, but the diuretics may induce profound hypochloremic alkalosis and potassium depletion.

These clinical signs and symptoms suggest that profound pathophysiological alterations have occurred. This information, combined with the anatomical description from the two-dimensional echocardiogram and the physiological data from cardiac catheterization, permits accurate assessment of the severity of the illness and formulation of an anesthetic plan. For example, in the sickest patients with respiratory compromise and minimal cardiac reserve, it may be prudent to minimize premedication, begin an IV infusion while the patient is awake, induce anesthesia with an IV opioid while the patient breathes oxygen, and be prepared to support the circulation immediately with inotropic and pressor drugs when necessary. Alternatively, the physical examination may indicate that the patient is only mildly symptomatic and should tolerate a standard premedication

Box 25.2 Symptoms and signs of cardiac failure in a neonate and infant

Failure to thrive

- Poor feeding
- Diaphoresis

Increased respiratory work

- Tachypnea
- Wheezing
- Grunting
- Flaring of ala nasi
- Chest wall retraction

Altered cardiac output

- Tachycardia
- Gallop rhythm
- Cardiomegaly
- Poor extremity perfusion
- Hepatomegaly

and sevoflurane/nitrous oxide inhalation induction of anesthesia for an elective operation.

Obstruction of left heart outflow

Patients who require surgery to relieve obstruction to outflow from the left heart are among the most critically ill children for whom the anesthesiologist must care. These lesions include interruption of the aortic arch, coarctation of the aorta, aortic stenosis, and mitral stenosis or atresia as part of the hypoplastic left heart syndrome. These neonates present with inadequate systemic perfusion and profound metabolic acidosis. The initial pH may be below 7.0 despite a $PaCO_2$ of less than 20 mmHg. Systemic blood flow is largely or completely dependent on blood flow into the aorta from the ductus arteriosus.

Ductal closure in the neonate with these problems causes dramatic worsening of the patient's condition. The patient becomes critically ill or even moribund and requires PGE1 infusion (see above) for survival. PGE1 allows blood flow into the aorta from the pulmonary artery because it maintains the patency of the ductus arteriosus [60,62,63]. In neonates with acidosis, metabolic derangements, and renal failure due to inadequate systemic perfusion, PGE1 infusion improves perfusion and metabolism, and surgery can be deferred until the patient's condition improves. Ventilatory and inotropic support and correction of metabolic acidosis, along with calcium, glucose, and electrolyte abnormalities, are often indicated preoperatively. The stabilization period also

allows assessment of the magnitude of end-organ dysfunction caused by the preceding period of inadequate systemic perfusion. Adequacy of resuscitation, rather than severity of illness at presentation, has an important influence on postoperative outcome [64].

Ventricular dysfunction

Older patients with CHD and poor ventricular function due to chronic ventricular volume overload (aortic or mitral valve regurgitation or long-standing pulmonary-to-systemic arterial shunts) present a different problem. Although patients with large shunts may have complete mixing of systemic and venous blood and only mild-to-moderate hypoxemia as a result of their excessive pulmonary blood flow, the price paid for near-normal arterial oxygen saturation is chronic ventricular dilation and dysfunction as well as pulmonary vascular obstructive disease. Consequently, narrowing of the shunt or a staged approach to single-ventricle repair may be indicated before any other elective surgery can be undertaken.

Assessment should include an estimation of the patient's functional limitation as an indicator of myocardial performance and reserve, quantification of the degree of hypoxia and the amount of pulmonary blood flow, and evaluation of PVR. For patients with increased Qp/Qs, during induction of anesthesia systemic blood flow should be optimized without further augmenting pulmonary flow. However, during maintenance and emergence from anesthesia, retraction of the lung, positional changes, and abdominal distension may increase the hypoxemia and compromise the function of a dilated, poorly contractile ventricle. If this sequence occurs during surgery, the anesthetic management must be altered to improve pulmonary blood flow.

In addition, systolic function of the ventricle may be impaired by intrinsic myopathic abnormalities related to drug toxicity (e.g. adriamycin), inborn enzyme deficiencies or acquired inflammatory or infectious disease. Patients with such dilated cardiomyopathies require optimization of ventricular performance with emphasis on inotropic support and afterload reduction.

Principles of anesthetic management

The diversity of CHD lesions and the variations of severity and pathophysiology of each lesion mandate individualized anesthetic management based on the known effects of anesthetics and other drugs in patients with CHD. Once the critical aspects of the patient's pathophysiology are understood, the anesthetic management plan is formulated, including plans for the surgery, plans for dealing with anticipated problems and complications, and plans for pre- and postoperative care.

General care of patients with congenital heart disease

The patient's condition should be optimal within the limits set by the lesion. Cardiac medications such as antiarrhythmic drugs should be continued preoperatively and anesthetic plans adjusted accordingly. The general preparation for each major pathophysiological problem is outlined above.

Systemic air emboli are a constant threat in children with CHD, regardless of their usual shunting pattern, because of the dynamic nature of shunts during anesthesia and surgery. Air traps are advisable for all IV lines but are not a substitute for meticulous attention and constant vigilance concerning the purging of air bubbles. Direct shunting of micro- and macrobubbles of air into the systemic circulation from multiple IV lines is always possible. Even when shunting patterns are nominally left to right, transient right-to-left shunts may occur during some portions of the cardiac cycle or during straining or coughing in patients with open communications between the left and right sides of the heart when normal transatrial pressure gradients are transiently reversed [65]. Right-to-left shunting may occur even across functionally "closed" communications. A "probe-patent" foramen ovale is common in children, regardless of whether or not they have CHD, and transient right-to-left shunting through the foramen ovale has been documented in a normal child during emergence from anesthesia [66].

Prevention of bacterial endocarditis is an important consideration in patients with CHD undergoing noncardiac surgery [67]. Currently antibiotic prophylaxis is considered reasonable only for those patients deemed at highest risk (Box 25.3) undergoing the following procedures: dental procedures involving manipulation of of gingival tissues, periapical region of teeth, or perforation of oral mucosa; procedures on the respiratory tract; procedures on infected skin, skin structures or musculoskeletal tissue.

The immediate preoperative period is an anxious time for patients and parents. Many patients may have undergone prior surgery or investigational procedures and separation from parents may be difficult. Because many patients are now admitted on the day of surgery, adequate preparation for surgery in the preoperative clinic with a thorough explanation of the planned procedure and conduct of anesthesia, including a plan for induction, is essential. Clear fluids can be administered up to 2h preoperatively, and an extended period of fasting should be avoided where possible, particularly in cyanotic patients.

Given the many types of pathophysiology in CHD patients, no single premedication regimen is recommended. Ideally, one wants a sedated, quiet patient who has adequate ventilation and circulation. Oral midazolam

Box 25.3 Cardiac conditions associated with the highest risk of adverse outcome from endocarditis for which prophylaxis with dental procedures is recommended

- Prosthetic cardiac valve
- Previous IE
- Congenital heart disease (CHD)*
  - Unrepaired cyanotic CHD, including palliative shunts and conduits
  - Completely repaired congenital heart defect with prosthetic material or device, whether placed by surgery or by catheter intervention, during the first 6 months after the procedure[†]
  - Repaired CHD with residual defects at the site or adjacent to the site of a prosthetic patch or prosthetic device (which inhibit endothelialization)
- Cardiac transplantation recipients who develop cardiac valvulopathy

*Except for the conditions listed above, antibiotic prophylaxis is no longer recommended for any other form of CHD.
[†]Prophylaxis is recommended because endothelialization of prosthetic material occurs within 6 months after the procedure.

0.5–1.0 mg/kg is often an effective anxiolytic and, although it may not produce hypnosis, should enable separation from parents. This dose of midazolam in combination with oral ketamine 5–7 mg/kg is a very effective premedicant. An intramuscular premedication with ketamine 4–5 mg/kg, glycopyrrolate 10–20 μg/kg and midazolam 0.1 mg/kg is effective for young children who will separate from their parents in the preoperative holding area, or who have limited hemodynamic reserve and are unsuited for an inhalation induction. However, the effects of premedication on the often fragile circulatory and ventilatory status of these patients must be appreciated, especially as cyanotic patients have decreased hypoxic drive [68].

Induction of anesthesia

Because of the potential for rapid and dramatic hemodynamic changes in young patients with CHD, especially infants, complete preparation of anesthetic and monitoring equipment and required drugs is essential. Adequate assistance should be immediately available during the induction of anesthesia in case problems develop.

The choice of induction technique is influenced by the response to premedication, the parent–child–anesthesiologist relationship, and the anesthetic management plan. In older, non-hypoxemic patients who have minimal compromise of their cardiac reserve, the choice of induction techniques is large. Inhalation, intravenous or intramuscular induction of anesthesia can be accomplished with a variety of drugs with reasonable degrees of safety if individual pathophysiological limitations are understood. For younger, sicker, and less co-operative patients, the choices diminish.

In children with adequate peripheral veins, quick insertion of a small-bore IV needle for induction of anesthesia can be virtually painless. Preoperative use of a topical anesthetic preparation may facilitate IV placement. Co-operative children with an adequate cardiac reserve and difficult IV access or a morbid fear of needles can have anesthesia induced cautiously with inhaled anesthetics, even if they are cyanotic. An IV catheter can then be inserted to facilitate administration of muscle relaxants; these drugs facilitate tracheal intubation and avoid the risk of deep levels of inhalational anesthesia for tracheal intubation in patients whose circulatory systems may have little reserve.

An intravenous induction should be used for all patients with severely limited hemodynamic reserve, particularly those with severe ventricular failure or pulmonary hypertension. In situations where hemodynamic instability during induction is likely, starting an inotrope agent such as dobutamine or dopamine prior to induction should be considered. While the stress of placing an IV may be considerable for some patients, particularly those with difficult IV access following previous procedures, this is preferable to the potential myocardial depression during an inhalation induction with sevoflurane.

Fentanyl 15–25 μg/kg in combination with pancuronium 0.2 mg/kg provides hemodynamic stability and prompt airway control and attenuates the stress-induced increase in PVR associated with intubation. Ketamine 1–3 mg/kg IV is safe and reliable, providing hemodynamic stability and minimal increases in PVR. It is particularly useful in patients with severe CHF and ventricular outflow obstructions. Atropine 20 μg/kg or glycopyrrolate 10 μg/kg is traditionally given concurrently due to increased secretions. If IV access is difficult and stressful in infants, a combination of 4 mg/kg ketamine, glycopyrrolate 10 μg/kg and succinylcholine 2 mg/kg intramuscularly allows prompt induction and airway control.

Propofol can be used in patients with normal ventricular function. Titrated doses are suitable for short procedures such as cardioversion or transesophageal echocardiogram (TEE). Midazolam 0.1–0.2 mg/kg is also a useful adjunct during an opioid induction but may cause hypotension in patients dependent on a high sympathetic drive.

An inhalation induction with sevoflurane is suitable for most infants and children, provided they have stable ventricular function and adequate hemodynamic reserve. This emphasizes the importance of preoperative evaluation when planning the induction technique. Inhalational induction can be used safely in patients with cyanotic heart disease, although uptake may be slower due to the right-to-left shunt [69]. Saturations will generally increase, provided cardiac output is maintained and airway obstruction avoided.

For many younger children, the presence of a parent during inhalation induction may be preferable for both the patient and parent. This is a common technique for normal children undergoing induction of anesthesia for non-cardiac surgery, but careful preoperative preparation and explanation are necessary before this is undertaken in the cardiac operating room.

Maintenance of anesthesia

Anesthesia maintenance techniques depend on the patient's preoperative cardiorespiratory status and pathophysiology of the underlying cardiac defect, the surgical procedure, the conduct of CPB, potential postoperative surgical problems and the anticipated postoperative management. Once induction of anesthesia and control of the airway are accomplished and monitoring is adequate, anesthesia can be maintained with inhaled anesthetics or additional intravenous drugs as dictated by the response of each patient, intraoperative events, and postoperative plans.

Stress responses to pain and other noxious stimuli are profound in even the youngest neonates, regardless of postconceptual age [70–72]. These hormonal and metabolic stress responses can be deleterious [73], particularly in patients with marginal hemodynamic reserve. Intraoperative deterioration in the patient's condition is not always clear, but changes in shunting, surgical manipulation of the heart, lungs or great vessels, and depression of the myocardium by anesthetics are common causes. Decreases in arterial oxygenation or in systemic blood flow and pressure frequently are due to alterations in intracardiac shunting. When circulating blood volume is adequate and anesthesia-related myocardial depression is unlikely, these problems are corrected by appropriately manipulating PVR and SVR. If PVR cannot be altered or is not part of the problem, vasopressor and inotropic drugs are used where indicated to increase SVR and cardiac function.

Choice of anesthetic agents

Use of inhaled anesthetics in children with intracardiac shunting is complicated by differences in uptake and distribution of these agents. A complex computer model suggested that induction of anesthesia is slowed by the presence of central right-to-left shunts, slowed less by mixed shunts, and changed little by pure left-to-right shunts; the changes are proportional to the size of the

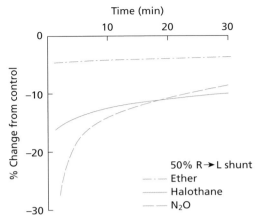

Figure 25.10 Computer-modeled effect of solubility of anesthetic gases on delay of uptake (arterial/inspired gases concentration ratio) in children caused by a 50% right-to-left shunt. Ether is most soluble and thus least affected; nitrous oxide is least soluble. Reproduced from Tanner GE, Angers DG, Barash PG. Effect of left-to-right, mixed left-to-right, and right-to-left shunts on inhalational anesthetic induction in children. Anesth Anag 1985; 64: 101 with permission from Lippincott, Williams & Wilkins.

shunt [69]. These theoretical effects assume a constant cardiac output and are most marked for insoluble gases (e.g. nitrous oxide). Induction of anesthesia with more soluble gases, (e.g. halothane) is less affected (Fig. 25.10). Similar studies comparing the speed of induction with sevoflurane to other potent inhalation agents have not been performed; however, because it is less soluble than halothane, induction with sevoflurane should be expected to be slower in patients with a right-to-left shunt. In children with left-to-right shunts, the speed of inhalation induction is little altered clinically [74]. Data from animals with right-to-left shunts confirm that induction of anesthesia is slowed; data from children with right-to-left shunts are not available [75]. Inhalation induction often seems slower in children with pure right-to-left shunts but this effect is not marked, probably because multiple other variables are affecting uptake. The potentially slow induction of anesthesia in children with pure right-to-left shunts should be remembered when one must rapidly increase the concentration of potent inhaled anesthetics in these patients.

The direct effect of inhaled agents on Qp/Qs appears to be limited. Sevoflurane, halothane, isoflurane, and fentanyl/midazolam do not change Qp/Qs in children with atrial and ventricular septal defects when cautiously administered with 100% oxygen [76].

Potent inhaled anesthetics

The volatile agents most commonly used during pediatric anesthesia are desflurane, isoflurane and sevoflurane.

Halothane is rarely used at present. All three can be used safely to maintain anesthesia in children with cardiac disease, although this depends to some extent on the child's cardiac anomaly and related pathophysiology. Cyanotic children with reasonable functional cardiac reserve can have anesthesia induced with sevoflurane or halothane and oxygen (even 70% nitrous oxide does not significantly decrease arterial oxygen saturation) [77–79]. Nevertheless, it is important that the anesthesiologist has an understanding of the potential effects of these anesthetics in young children with CHD.

Increased sensitivity of the immature cardiovascular system and decreased cardiovascular reserves are more serious problems with potent inhaled anesthetics. Use of these agents may considerably reduce the margin of safety in infants and younger children with severe CHD. Volatile anesthetics depress myocardial function primarily by limiting calcium availability within the myocyte, i.e. by reducing trans-sarcolemmal and sarcoplasmic reticulum calcium flux. The net result is depletion of intracellular calcium stores and, given the immaturity of the neonatal and infant myocardium, the potential for systolic dysfunction in these patients may be increased when volatile agents are used. In addition, diastolic ventricular function may also be impaired because of limited reuptake of calcium into the immature sarcoplasmic reticulum, and dependence upon trans-sarcolemmal sodium–calcium exchange [80].

Therefore, it is not surprising that numerous studies have shown that the immature cardiovascular system of normal infants does not tolerate halothane and isoflurane well; up to 50% of infants with normal cardiovascular systems develop substantial hypotension and bradycardia during induction of anesthesia with these agents unless the cardiovascular system is supported [81,82]. The ventricular function of normal infants declines when anesthesia is induced with isoflurane; stroke volume and ejection fraction decrease by as much as 38% [82]. Somewhat less myocardial depression occurs with halothane in older children [83]. Halothane (1 and 1.5 MAC) depresses cardiac index and contractility in patients with CHD more than comparable levels of sevoflurane, isoflurane, and fentanyl/midazolam anesthesia [84]. In addition, halothane anesthesia may result in more severe hypotension and emergent drug use than sevoflurane anesthesia in infants and children with CHD [85]. Isoflurane causes less direct myocardial depression, is less soluble and therefore has a faster uptake and emergence, has no effect on intracardiac conduction and much less sensitization of the myocardium to catecholamines compared to halothane. As with isoflurane, sevoflurane causes less myocardial depression and has a low risk for arrhythmias in children compared to halothane [86–88]. Sevoflurane anesthesia is associated with prolongation of the QTc interval in infants [89]. Sevoflurane (1 MAC) and fentanyl/midazolam anesthesia have no significant effect on myocardial function in patients with a single ventricle [90].

Nitrous oxide

The use of nitrous oxide in children with CHD and shunts is controversial because of its potential for enlarging systemic air emboli and for increasing PVR. Nitrous oxide may expand intravascular air emboli and exaggerate the effects of other anesthetics on the circulation, even without systemic air embolization [91]. However, neither has been demonstrated to be a clinical problem in patients with CHD.

Nitrous oxide has been reported to decrease cardiac output, systemic arterial pressure, and heart rate in adults, and it increased PVR, especially when the pre-existing PVR is elevated [92,93]. The latter would be detrimental to children with right-to-left shunts, pulmonary hypertension, and decreased pulmonary flow. However, increases in pulmonary artery pressure or PVR in infants given 50% nitrous oxide do not occur, regardless of pre-existing PVR [19]. Mild but significant decreases in cardiac output, systemic arterial pressure, and heart rate were seen in these infants. Furthermore, inhalation induction of anesthesia with 70% nitrous oxide and halothane did not decrease the arterial oxygen saturation of cyanotic children, suggesting that pulmonary blood flow is not decreased and that PVR is not substantially increased by nitrous oxide [77,78]. Although the administration of nitrous oxide prevents the use of 100% oxygen, the arterial oxygen saturation of cyanotic children may not decrease because changes in FIO_2 have little effect on the arterial oxygenation of these patients [94] (see Fig. 25.8). Arterial desaturation that is caused by pulmonary disease is, however, probably a contraindication to the use of nitrous oxide.

Intravenous anesthetics

Some intravenous anesthetics provide a larger margin of safety for induction of anesthesia in the immature and compromised cardiovascular system of neonates and infants with severe cardiac disease. However, very high, transient arterial, cardiac, and brain concentrations of IV agents can occur when normal IV doses of drugs are given as a rapid infusion in children with known right-to-left shunts because mixing, uptake, and metabolism in the pulmonary circulation are bypassed. In dogs with right-to-left shunts, a 1 mg/kg bolus of IV lidocaine resulted in arterial drug concentrations above those reported to cause irreversible myocardial toxicity [95]. Routinely administered bolus doses of lidocaine used for dysrhythmias or intubation, or other drugs such as barbiturates, β-blockers or calcium channel blockers, may be potentially toxic to children with substantial right-to-left shunts.

Ketamine

When IV access or lack of patient co-operation is a problem, intramuscular ketamine (3–5 mg/kg) is well tolerated in sick infants and children with cyanosis or congestive heart failure [96]. Because of the potential effects of ketamine on airways, ventilation, and secretions, it should be given in combination with an antisialagog (e.g. atropine or glycopyrrolate) while the airway and ventilation are carefully maintained, especially in children with decreased oxygen reserves. Ketamine can be mixed with atropine and succinylcholine in the same syringe, the final volume being relatively small, and injection of this mixture allows rapid control of the airway. Small IV doses of ketamine (1–3 mg/kg) are effective for supplemental sedation in unco-operative or apprehensive children who are unwilling to leave their parents. Excessive secretions, airway problems, and apnea do not occur with these doses as they occasionally do with larger IM doses and frequently do with IV doses of ketamine.

Although increased PVR is reported with ketamine in adults, 2 mg/kg IV in premedicated infants and young children usually does not increase pulmonary artery pressure or PVR, even when the baseline PVR is elevated [20,21,23,97]. If hypoventilation or apnea occurs after an IV dose of ketamine, undesirable increases in PVR can occur because of the associated changes in PaO_2 and $PaCO_2$ [20]. Little change in cardiac output, heart rate or arterial pressure is seen after IV ketamine in infants and small children with CHD [20,21]. Despite reports of ketamine having a negative inotropic effect on isolated heart muscle in animal studies (at very high doses), the ejection fraction of children with CHD is well preserved after ketamine. Furthermore, arterial saturation, for the most part, is improved when ketamine is used to induce anesthesia in cyanotic patients. Clinical experience with ketamine as the induction agent has been excellent for sick infants and children with most forms of heart disease, including those with limited pulmonary blood flow and cyanosis. Ketamine alone or in combination with propofol or dexmedetomidine is also useful for sedation and for anesthesia for cardiac catheterization in children with CHD [98].

Opioid anesthesia

High-dose opioid anesthesia provides excellent cardiovascular stability in children with CHD. Morphine (1 mg/kg or more) given slowly over a prolonged period provides reasonable cardiovascular stability in children; however, as in adults, histamine release can occur and cause hypotension. The more potent synthetic opioids, fentanyl (25–75 μg/kg) and sufentanil (5–15 μg/kg), given more slowly, provide better stability of the cardiovascular system on induction of anesthesia when used with pancuronium in very sick infants with CHD [99–103]. Because of its effect on the sympathetic nervous system and duration of action, pancuronium remains the muscle relaxant of choice to use with high-dose synthetic opioids. Shorter acting muscle relaxants such as *cis*-atracurium have a relatively benign hemodynamic profile, but should be administered as a continuous infusion during cardiac surgery because of their short duration of action. The doses of synthetic opioids required to blunt the systemic and pulmonary stress responses in younger and sicker children are generally well tolerated [24,25,71]. Changes in pulmonary and systemic hemodynamics are insignificant in infants with a bolus of fentanyl 15–25 µg/kg. Used with 100% oxygen, these high-dose narcotics are safe and result in increased arterial oxygenation in cyanotic children [100]. Fentanyl doses as low as 10 µg/kg may be sufficient for effective baseline anesthesia in neonates, but larger doses are necessary for prolonged anesthesia [104–106]. A bolus dose of 10–15 µg/kg effectively ameliorates the hemodynamic response to intubation in neonates. For complete suppression of hemodynamic responses to intense stimulation of more vigorous children, supplementation of high-dose opioids with small amounts of inhaled anesthetic may be necessary. Although low doses of fentanyl 2–5 µg/kg facilitate mechanical ventilation and decrease total lung compliance in an awake child, high-dose opioids produce chest wall rigidity and glottic closure in adults and neonates [107,108]. A muscle relaxant is required with rapid infusion of high-dose synthetic opioids.

The high-dose opioid technique is most suitable for sick infants and older children in whom postoperative mechanical ventilation is planned. This technique provides hemodynamic stability, although it does not guarantee suppression of the endocrine response to surgical stimulation. Neonates and infants undergoing deep hypothermic CPB surgery are able to generate a significant stress response [73]. A 17-fold increase in epinephrine and 10-fold increase in norepinephrine levels in infants were seen after 1 h of circulatory arrest at 18°C [109]. Nevertheless, the reported magnitude of the stress response after cardiac surgery is variable, and influenced by patient age, type of anesthesia, level of hypothermia, and the duration of CPB and circulatory arrest [110].

Fentanyl doses of of 50 µg/kg administered prior to CPB, a further 25 µg/kg at the onset of rewarming on CPB, and a further 25 µg/kg after bypass, depending upon hemodynamic stability, are commonly administered. These additional doses or a continuous infusion of potent opioids are necessary for surgery involving CPB, as opioid concentrations decrease markedly during CPB [111]. In a recent study of stress hormone release during infant cardiac surgery and deep hypothermic cardiopulmonary bypass using this fentanyl dosing regimen, the endocrine response was not obtunded, yet there were no adverse outcomes. In addition, no specific relationship between opioid dose, plasma fentanyl level and hormone or metabolic stress response was established [112]. Considering the advances in surgical techniques, conduct of CPB and perioperative management over the past decade that have lead to a significant improvement in patient outcome, a strategy of high-dose opioid anesthesia to blunt the stress response may be less critical.

Remifentanil is a synthetic ultra-short acting opioid, rapidly metabolized by non-specific tissue esterases [113]. It is unique among the currently available opioids because of its extremely short context-sensitive half-time (3–5 min), which is largely independent of the duration of infusion. Remifentanil may cause significant respiratory depression and is usually administered to patients who are mechanically ventilated. It may be useful for patients with limited cardiorespiratory reserve undergoing procedures such as cardiac catheterization or pacemaker placement because intense analgesia is provided without significant hemodynamic complications. It may also be used to maintain anesthesia during mild hypothermic CPB for patients who are extubated immediately after surgery in the operating room, such as after atrial septal defect repair [114]. Patients usually emerge quickly once the infusion has been stopped, and opioid side-effects are reduced because of the short duration of action.

Other intravenous agents

The benzodiazepine derivatives (e.g. midazolam) can be useful when titrated in small doses (0.05–0.1 mg/kg), especially in older patients with CHD. Lack of pain on injection and lack of vascular damage make water-soluble midazolam a more useful benzodiazepine than diazepam, particularly because it has a shorter duration of action. Benzodiazepines are commonly used to ensure adequate hypnosis during opioid-based anesthesia, but may also improve hemodynamic stability. In a study of children with acyanotic heart disease undergoing cardiac surgery, the addition of diazepam to fentanyl-based anesthesia (75 µg/kg) resulted in a more stable hemodynamic profile without an increase in epinephrine levels when compared to an isoflurane-based anesthetic technique [115]. In a study of younger children undergoing correction of tetralogy of Fallot, the combined use of sufentanil and flunitrazepam provided a more stable hemodynamic profile and catecholamine response compared to a sufentanil-based technique alone [116].

Propofol can be used judiciously in patients with CHD. The predominant hemodynamic effect of propofol 1–3 mg/kg is a reduction in SVR with no effect on PVR.

In patients with right-to-left shunting this results in a decrease in pulmonary blood flow and arterial oxygenation saturation [117,118]. The venodilation associated with propofol administration also requires that it be used with caution in patients who have undergone a previous cavopulmonary connection. The resting venous tone is increased in this patient group, and the fall in preload could result in significant hypotension during induction.

Etomidate is an anesthetic induction agent with the advantage of minimal cardiovascular and respiratory depression. An intravenous dose of 0.3 mg/kg induces a rapid loss of consciousness with minimal respiratory depression for a duration of 3–5 min. At this dose it does not substantially alter hemodynamics or either right-to-left or left-to-right shunting in patients with congenital heart disease [119,120]. It may cause pain on injection and is associated with spontaneous movements, hiccoughing and myoclonus. Etomidate may be used as an alternative to the synthetic opioids for induction of patients with limited myocardial reserve. A single dose of etomidate can suppress adrenal steroidogenesis and as a result it is not approved for continuous infusion [121].

Anesthesia for cardiac surgery

Communication between the anesthesia and surgical teams is of utmost importance during surgery for CHD. The manipulations of each team influence the other, and close co-ordination of activities is necessary for optimal patient care. Specific problems occurring with total repair or palliation of specific congenital cardiac lesions are covered later in the chapter. General problems that occur with various types of closed and open cardiac surgical procedures are considered here.

Anesthetic management of closed cardiac procedures

Patent ductus arteriosus, coarctation of the aorta, and repair of vascular rings are the only congenital cardiac anomalies *corrected* with closed procedures. Closed palliative procedures, including systemic-to-pulmonary shunts, pulmonary artery banding, and procedures to improve interatrial mixing (Blalock–Hanlon atrial septectomy), are performed infrequently as the trend to definitively correct the CHD early continues. Anesthesia for closed palliative procedures is in some ways more demanding, because CPB is not available if the patient's hemodynamic status deteriorates. Therefore, monitoring requirements are stringent, and central venous and arterial access are usually mandatory. Pulse oximetry is invaluable in these cases to evaluate the infant's condition and to assess the effectiveness of the closed surgical procedure.

Acid–base and electrolyte balance are meticulously maintained at normal levels throughout closed procedures. When these procedures are done via a thoracotomy, the operative field is rarely visible to the anesthesiologist, and marked deterioration of cardiopulmonary function may result from surgical manipulations. Any deterioration in the infant's condition should be immediately communicated to the surgeon, who has a view of the surgical field and knows what is being done there. Some compromise of ventilation and pulmonary blood flow inevitably occurs during these procedures, occasionally with severe decreases in arterial oxygen saturations.

Mechanical ventilation

Altered lung mechanics and ventilation/perfusion abnormalities are common problems in the immediate postoperative period [122]. Besides preoperative problems secondary to increased Qp/Qs, additional considerations include the surgical incision and lung retraction, increased lung water following CPB, possible pulmonary reperfusion injury, surfactant depletion and restrictive defects from atelectasis and pleural effusions.

In general, neonates and infants with their limited physiological reserve should not be weaned from mechanical ventilation until hemodynamically stable, and factors contributing to an increase in intrapulmonary shunt and altered respiratory mechanics have improved.

Volume-limited ventilation

A traditional approach to mechanical ventilation in children with congenital heart disease has been the use of a volume-limited, time-cycled mode, with large tidal volumes of 15–20 cc/kg and no PEEP. This approach was developed in the early years of congenital heart surgery when older generations of ventilators existed and the monitoring of ventilation was frequently less than ideal. While the peak inspiratory and mean airway pressure are usually increased using large tidal volumes in this mode, changes in compliance and resistance can be readily detected. If there is a sudden change in pulmonary mechanics from atelectasis, pneumothorax or endotracheal tube obstruction, the peak inspiratory pressure alarm limit is reached as the ventilator tries to deliver the preset tidal volume.

However, for neonates and infants, the compressible volume of the ventilator circuit (1–1.5 cc/cmH$_2$O peak inspiratory pressure) means that the delivered tidal volume is less than the preset volume. For older patients receiving larger tidal breaths, the volume lost by compression of gas in the circuit is minimal and rarely affects their tidal ventilation. But for neonates and infants, this compressible volume may be a considerable component of their tidal ventilation. Further, any leak around the endotracheal tube means that a proportion of the delivered tidal volume may also be lost. Inspiratory and expiratory times also need to be closely observed to prevent excessive auto PEEP. Variable time constants, i.e. [compliance× resistance], within regions of the lung are common in children with defects associated with high pulmonary blood flow, as well as following CPB. Using a volume-limited, time-cycled mode, those areas of lung with an increased time constant may be preferentially ventilated and overdistended, contributing to ventilation/perfusion mismatch and potential lung injury.

Pressure-limited ventilation

A pressure-limited, time-cycled mode of ventilation is often appropriate in children less than 10 kg, particularly those with significant alteration in lung compliance and airway resistance. A decelerating flow pattern is used when a breath is delivered to the patient until a preset peak inspiratory pressure is achieved. The delivered tidal volume will vary according to the compliance and resistance of the lung, and therefore from breath to breath. Both the peak inspiratory pressure and the inspiratory time can be manipulated to increase or decrease the delivered tidal volume. A square wave pressure waveform is generated by changing the inspiratory time, which will also alter the mean airway pressure. In general, it is preferable to set a minute ventilation using the lowest possible mean airway pressure. In-line monitoring enabling breath-to-breath assessment of tidal volume and mean airway pressure is essential, with appropriate alarm limits set such that acute changes in compliance and resistance can be detected.

Cardiorespiratory interactions

Cardiorespiratory interactions vary significantly between patients, and it is not possible to provide specific ventilation strategies or protocols that will cover all patients. Rather, the mode of ventilation must be matched to the hemodynamic status of each patient to achieve the appropriate cardiac output and gas exchange. Frequent modifications to the mode and pattern of ventilation may be necessary during recovery after surgery, with attention to changes in lung volume and airway pressure.

Lung volume

Changes in lung volume have a major effect on PVR, which is lowest at FRC, while both hypo- and hyperinflation may result in a significant increase in PVR. At low tidal volumes, alveolar collapse occurs because of reduced interstitial traction on alveolar septae. In addition, radial traction on extra-alveolar vessels such as the branch pulmonary arteries is reduced, thus reducing the cross-sectional diameter. Conversely, hyperinflation of the lung

may cause stretching of the alveolar septae and compression of extra-alveolar vessels.

An increase in PVR increases the afterload or wall stress on the right ventricle (RV), potentially compromising RV function and contributing to decreased left ventricle (LV) compliance secondary to interventricular septal shift. In addition to low cardiac output, signs of RV dysfunction including tricuspid regurgitation, hepatomegaly, ascites, and pleural effusions may be observed.

Intrathoracic pressure

An increase in mean intrathoracic pressure during positive pressure ventilation decreases preload to both pulmonary and systemic ventricles, but has opposite effects on afterload to each ventricle [123].

Right ventricle

The reduction in RV preload that occurs with positive pressure ventilation may reduce cardiac output. Normally the RV diastolic compliance is extremely high and the pulmonary circulation is able to accommodate changes in flow without a large change in pressure. An increase in mean intrathoracic pressure increases the afterload on the RV from direct compression of extra-alveolar and alveolar pulmonary vessels.

Patients with normal RV compliance and without residual volume load or pressure load on the ventricle following surgery usually show little change in RV function from the alteration in preload and afterload that occurs with positive pressure ventilation. However, these effects can be magnified in patients with restrictive RV physiology, in particular neonates who have required a right ventriculotomy for repair of tetralogy of Fallot (TOF), pulmonary atresia or truncus arteriosus. While systolic RV function may be preserved, diastolic dysfunction is common with increased RV end-diastolic pressure and impaired RV filling.

The potential deleterious effects of mechanical ventilation on RV function are important to emphasize. The aim should be to ventilate with a mode that enables the lowest possible mean airway pressure, while maintaining lung volume. While the use of a low peak inspiratory pressure, short inspiratory time, increased intermittent mandatory (IMV) rate and low levels of PEEP has been recommended as one ventilation strategy in patients with restrictive RV physiology, the smaller tidal volumes, e.g. 6–8 cc/kg, during this pattern of ventilation may reduce lung volume and FRC, thereby increasing PVR and afterload on the RV. An alternative strategy in a pressure-limited mode of ventilation is to use larger tidal volumes of 12–15 cc/kg, with a longer inspiratory time of 0.8–1.0 sec, increased peak inspiratory pressure of around 30 cmH$_2$O and low PEEP (i.e. wide ΔP), and slow IMV rate of 12–15 breaths/min. For the same mean airway pressure, RV filling is maintained and RV output augmented by maintaining lung volume and reduced RV afterload.

Left ventricle

Left ventricular preload is also affected by changes in lung volume. Pulmonary blood flow, and therefore preload to the systemic ventricle, may be reduced by an increase or decrease in lung volume secondary to alteration in radial traction on alveoli and extra-alveolar vessels.

The systemic arteries are under higher pressure and not exposed to radial traction effects during inflation or deflation of the lungs. Therefore, changes in lung volume will affect LV preload, but the effect on afterload is dependent upon changes in intrathoracic pressure alone rather than changes in lung volume.

In contrast to the RV, a major effect of positive pressure ventilation on the LV is a reduction in afterload. Using La Place's Law, wall stress is directly proportional to the transmural LV pressure and the radius of curvature of the LV. The transmural pressure across the LV is the difference between the intracavity LV pressure and surrounding intrathoracic pressure. Assuming a constant arterial pressure and ventricular dimension, an increase in intrathoracic pressure, as occurs during positive pressure ventilation, will reduce the transmural gradient and therefore wall stress on the LV [123]. Therefore, positive pressure ventilation and PEEP can have significant beneficial effects in patients with left ventricular failure.

Patients with LV dysfunction and increased end-diastolic volume and pressure can have impaired pulmonary mechanics secondary to increased lung water, decreased lung compliance and increased airway resistance. The work of breathing is increased and neonates can fatigue early because of limited respiratory reserve. A significant proportion of total body oxygen consumption is directed at the increased work of breathing in neonates and infants with LV dysfunction, contributing to poor feeding and failure to thrive. Therefore, positive pressure ventilation has an additional benefit in patients with significant volume overload and systemic ventricular dysfunction by reducing the work of breathing and oxygen demand.

Lung injury

It is important to appreciate that mechanical ventilation may result in significant lung injury, particularly when high tidal volumes are used [124]. Large, rapid changes in tidal volumes may lead to shear stress on the alveolar septae and subsequent alveolar capillary disruption. The same mechanisms that result in air leak may also result in disruption of the microcirculation, causing an increase in total lung water with subsequent increase in airway resistance and reduction in lung compliance.

Lung disease is usually not homogenous, with regions of the lung having different time constants, i.e. the concept of "fast" alveoli and "slow" alveoli. When using a volume-limited strategy, the more compliant alveoli will distend in preference to regions of lung that are collapsed or have slow time constants, thereby resulting in regional alveolar overdistension and trauma. This may be less evident with a pressure-limited strategy, as the more compliant or faster alveoli will distend to the preset pressure limit and then, depending on the inspiratory time, regions of lung with reduced time constants will gradually distend and be recruited.

While a relatively large tidal volume of 12–15 cc/kg is beneficial for many patients following congenital heart surgery for maintaining lung volume at lower PVR, lung injury may occur if a high-volume strategy is continued for a prolonged period (i.e. volutrauma). Using a pressure-limited mode of ventilation will enable a relatively constant tidal volume without a wide swing in peak inspiratory pressure or regional alveolar overdistension. It is essential to continually re-evaluate the mode of ventilation and modify it according to hemodynamic responses. Fortunately, most patients undergoing congenital cardiac surgery do not have parenchymal lung disease and changes in pulmonary mechanics, such as secondary to changes in lung water, are generally resolved following complete surgical repair and diuresis after CPB.

Positive end-expiratory pressure

The use of PEEP in patients with congenital heart disease has been controversial. It was initially perceived not to have a significant effect in terms of improving gas exchange, and there was concern that the increased airway pressure could have a detrimental effect on hemodynamics and contribute to lung injury and air leak.

Nevertheless, PEEP increases FRC, enabling lung recruitment, and redistributes lung water from alveolar septal regions to the more compliant perihilar regions. Both of these effects will improve gas exchange and reduce PVR. However, excessive levels of PEEP may be detrimental by increasing afterload on the RV. Usually 3–5 cmH$_2$O of PEEP will help maintain FRC and redistribute lung water without causing hemodynamic compromise.

Management of cardiopulmonary bypass

Inasmuch as reparative procedures usually entail CPB techniques, the care of these patients must incorporate technical knowledge of CPB issues and take into account the effects of CPB on the function of multiple organ systems. An important component of the improvement in early outcome following congenital heart surgery has been the advances in cardiovascular support, especially cardiopulmonary bypass techniques, myocardial

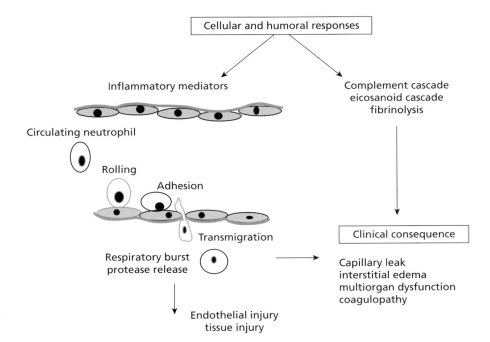

Figure 25.11 Cellular and humoral response to cardiopulmonary bypass.

protection, pharmacological support and mechanical support. It is well recognized that the exposure of blood elements to the non-epithelialized cardiopulmonary bypass circuit, along with ischemic-reperfusion injury, induces a systemic inflammatory response (Fig. 25.11). The effects of the interactions of blood components with the extracorporeal circuit are magnified in children due to the large bypass circuit surface area and priming volume relative to patient blood volume. Humoral responses include activation of complement, kallikrein, eicosanoid and fibrinolytic cascades; cellular responses include platelet activation and an inflammatory response with an adhesion molecule cascade stimulating neutrophil activation and release of proteolytic and vasoactive substances [125].

The clinical consequences include increased interstitial fluid and generalized capillary leak, and potential multiorgan dysfunction. Total lung water is increased with an associated decrease in lung compliance and increase in the alveolar-to-arterial O_2 (A–aO_2) gradient. Myocardial edema results in impaired ventricular systolic and diastolic function. A secondary fall in cardiac output by 20–30% is common in neonates in the first 6–12 h following surgery, contributing to decreased renal function and oliguria. Sternal closure may need to be delayed due to mediastinal edema and associated cardiorespiratory compromise when closure is attempted. Ascites, hepatic ingestion and bowel edema may affect mechanical ventilation, cause a prolonged ileus and delay feeding. A coagulopathy post CPB may contribute to delayed hemostasis.

Over recent years, numerous strategies have evolved to limit the effect of this endothelial injury resulting from the systemic inflammatory response. Of these, the most important strategy is limiting both the time spent on bypass and use of deep hypothermic circulatory arrest (DHCA). This is clearly dependent, however, upon surgical expertise and experience, and in certain situations DHCA is necessary to effect surgical repair. Hypothermia and steroids are important pre-bypass measures to limit activation of the inflammatory response. Attenuating the stress response, the use of antioxidants such as mannitol, altering prime composition to maintain oncotic pressure, and ultrafiltration are also used to limit the clinical consequences of the inflammatory response.

From a practical point of view, the amount of fluid that can be removed by ultrafiltration is limited by the level of blood in the venous reservoir. A number of different ultrafiltration techniques exist in children. Conventional ultrafiltration (CUF) refers to ultrafiltration occurring throughout CPB or during those intervals when venous reservoir volume is sufficient to allow it. This system would be expected to produce hemoconcentration. Modified ultrafiltration (MUF) allows ultrafiltration to continue after weaning from CPB. MUF may be performed utilizing either an arteriovenous or veno-venous system. Blood volume is kept constant as ultrafiltrate is lost by replacing it with blood from the CPB circuit, which passes through the ultrafiltrator before being delivered to the patient. In this way, the CPB circuit can remain primed and the patient's blood, as well as the CPB blood, can be hemoconcentrated. The endpoint for termination of MUF following CPB varies from institution to institution with institutions terminating MUF after a set time interval (15–20 min), a set hematocrit (40%) or a set volume removed (750 mL/m^2). Heparin anticoagulation must be maintained during MUF with protamine reversal of heparin initiated after termination of MUF.

The major advantage of MUF over CUF is that it allows hemoconcentration to continue once CPB has been terminated. As a result, MUF normally allows a greater degree of hemoconcentration than can be obtained with CUF alone, particularly in small children. Some institutions utilize both CUF and MUF as the techniques are not mutually exclusive [126].

Dilutional (DUF) and zero-balance ultrafiltration (ZBUF) utilize the same system as CUF but involve high-volume ultrafiltration during CPB in which crystalloid solution is continuously used to replace the ultrafiltrate in order to maintain reservoir volume. ZBUF utilizes ultrafiltration rates of 200 mL/min/m^2 during rewarming. DUF is performed throughout CPB and utilizes rates of 40–80 mL/kg/h [127,128]. These methods do not result in hemoconcentration but may be beneficial in removing inflammatory mediators. MUF is usually used in conjunction with these techniques to obtain hemoconcentration.

In clinical application, MUF as compared to no ultrafiltration has been demonstrated to reduce total body water, attenuate dilutional anemia and coagulopathy, reduce homologous blood requirements, narrow the A–aO$_2$ gradient, improve LV compliance and systolic function as well as arterial blood pressure, and decrease inotropic requirements in the immediate postfiltration period [129–136]. In a non-randomized, retrospective analysis of cavopulmonary connection procedures (primarily hemi-Fontan and lateral tunnel Fontan), patients in whom MUF was used had a lower incidence of pleural and pericardial effusions and a shorter hospital stay than patients in whom MUF was not used [131]. MUF compared to no ultrafiltration may reduce postoperative ventilatory support times but this has not been a consistent finding despite short-term improvements in pulmonary compliance [129,133,137].

A number of studies have shown MUF to be effective in removing both anti-inflammatory (interleukin 10, interleukin 1 receptor antagonist) and proinflammatory (tumor necrosis factor α, interleukin 1β, interleukin 6, interleukin 8, complement fragments C3a and C5a, and endotoxins) mediators generated during CPB while other studies have not confirmed this efficacy [133,138–144]. In addition, MUF may offer no advantage over CUF in terms of inflammatory mediator removal [140]. The extent to which the beneficial effects of MUF are related to reduction of tissue edema, removal of inflammatory mediators, and hemoconcentration has not been clarified [126].

Zero-balance ultrafiltration in conjunction with MUF or DUF in conjunction with MUF may be a more effective strategy for removal of inflammatory mediators. ZBUF in conjunction with MUF has been shown to be more effective than MUF alone in reducing inflammatory mediator concentrations immediately following filtration [127]. Patients in the ZBUF group also had reduced blood loss, a shorter duration of postoperative ventilatory support and a narrower 24-h A–aO$_2$ gradient [127]. DUF in conjunction with MUF has been shown to be more effective than CUF alone in reducing plasma endothelin 1 and thromboxane B$_2$ levels following CPB and in attenuating postoperative pulmonary hypertension [128,132,145]. In addition, the duration of postoperative ventilatory support and transfusion requirements was reduced in a group of high-risk patients (neonates, patients with pulmonary hypertension, and patients with prolonged CPB times) [132,145]. A recent study demonstrated a modest reduction in interleukin 6, a narrowed A–aO$_2$ gradient, improved pulmonary compliance but no reduction in the length of postoperative ventilatory support with CUF in conjunction with MUF as compared to no ultrafiltration [146]. No advantage in terms of improved postoperative course was demonstrated when CUF combined with MUF was compared to CUF alone, despite the fact that a larger filtrate volume was obtained in the combined group [147,148]. In addition, MUF alone and CUF alone were indistinguishable in their effect on hematocrit, mean arterial pressure, heart rate, and LV shortening fraction when equal filtrate volumes were removed in another trial [149]. Finally, combining DUF and MUF offered no clinical advantage over DUF or MUF alone despite larger filtrate volumes in the combined group [150].

While these techniques are useful to hemoconcentrate and remove total body water immediately after bypass, they do not prevent the inflammatory response. And while it is perhaps modified, this response is nevertheless idiosyncratic; despite all the above maneuvers, some neonates and infants will still manifest significant clinical signs and delayed postoperative recovery. The development of drugs that will prevent the adhesion molecule–endothelial interaction, which is pivotal in the inflammatory response, continues to be pursued in both laboratory and clinical studies. To date, however, no one specific drug or treatment has proven beneficial. This highlights the multifactorial nature of the inflammatory response and that attenuation at multiple levels is important.

Special circumstances exist during management of CPB in patients with CHD that may not apply to adults undergoing correction of acquired heart disease. Venous cannulation in neonates and infants may be single or multiple, depending on the anatomy and bypass technique. Obstruction to venous return is more likely due to the small vessel size and will increase venous pressures, thereby decreasing perfusion pressure to the cerebral and splanchnic circulations. A fall in venous return to bypass circuit, abdominal distension and head suffusion all indicate problems with venous cannulation. Elevated SVC pressures will reduce cerebral blood flow, increase the risk of cerebral edema and reduce the rate of cerebral cooling. Systemic-to-pulmonary shunts and collateral vessels must be controlled when going onto bypass to prevent excessive pulmonary flow with resultant increased blood return to the heart, myocardial distension, systemic hypoperfusion and uneven cooling or rewarming. Most importantly, a high perfusion rate at the pump head does not ensure an equally high systemic flow unless all sources of potential aortopulmonary shunts (e.g. Blalock–Taussig), patent ductus arteriosus or native aortopulmonary collaterals are occluded. If these shunts are not occluded, other indices of the adequacy of the flow should be followed.

There are several bypass management strategies.

- Moderate hypothermia with normal or increased pump flow. Bicaval cannulation is generally used, and the risk of cerebral ischemia is reduced. However, CPB is prolonged and operative conditions may not be ideal. Pump flow rates are generally higher in neonates and infants, reflecting the increased metabolic rate. During bypass, there is no one measure of index that assures adequate perfusion. Generally flow rates of 100–150 mL/kg/min or indexed flows to 2.2–2.5 L/min/m^2 should provide adequate flow at normothermia. Pump perfusion in young patients is regulated primarily by flow rate, so that perfusion pressures of 30 mmHg or less are common in these patients when hemodilution has decreased SVR (low viscosity). A venous oxygen saturation of >75%, even differential temperature cooling, and low lactate levels suggest adequate perfusion [151]. However, these values may be misleading in patients with poor venous drainage, severe hemodilution, malposition of the aortic cannula or in the presence of a large left-to-right shunt. On-line continuous monitoring of blood gas and saturation of oxygen is important to identify trends in oxygen extraction. In addition, these only provide global indices of perfusion, and monitoring regional perfusion would be ideal. While cerebral perfusion can be monitored using transcranial sonography, near infrared spectroscopy and the electroencephalogram (EEG), to date there are no monitors available for routine clinical use to monitor perfusion of other vascular beds.
- Low-flow perfusion in conjuction with deep hypothermia(<18°C). Flow rates of 30–50 mL/kg/min

are often referred to as "low flow" but the optimal flow rates during low-flow bypass are not firmly established.

- Deep hypothermic circulatory arrest (DHCA). This is a technique employed to improve exposure of intracardiac defects and to facilitate aortic arch reconstruction in infants and children. DHCA allows cessation of CPB, venous and arterial cannula removal, and exsanguination of the patient into the venous reservoir of the CPB circuit. There has been substantial refinement of the technique of DHCA since its successful inception in the 1970s. In the current era, DHCA is used selectively and for relatively short intervals (<60 min). It is utilized primarily for the aortic arch reconstruction component of the Norwood procedure, repair of interrupted aortic arch, neonatal repair of total anomalous pulmonary venous connection, and complicated intracardiac repairs in small (<2.5 kg) neonates and infants [152]. Prolonged ischemia to the brain is a major disadvantage and is both time and temperature dependent. Interval durations <40 min are associated with a lower incidence of seizures and fewer neurobehavioral deficiencies than longer intervals [153–156].
- Regional low flow perfusion (RLFP) also known as antegrade cerebral perfusion (ACP). In an effort to prevent the potentially deleterious effects of DHCA on cerebral and somatic perfusion and oxygenation, technical innovations to avoid the use of DHCA for aortic arch reconstruction in children with hypoplastic left heart syndrome undergoing the Norwood procedure and in children with aortic hypoplasia or interruption undergoing biventricular repair have been developed.

A number of techniques to provide ACP via the right innominate artery have been described and are used in conjunction with deep hypothermia [157–160]. These techniques are felt to provide both cerebral and somatic (subdiaphragmatic viscera) perfusion. Somatic perfusion is felt to be the result of the extensive network of arterial collaterals in the neonate which link the supra- and subdiaphragmatic viscera such as the internal thoracic and intercostal arteries. The flow rates necessary to provide optimal cerebral and somatic perfusion during ACP have yet to be determined although rates of 30–70 mL/kg/min are common.

Because of the large body surface area to mass ratio in neonates and infants, a 2–3°C reduction in core temperature is common following induction of anesthesia and prior to bypass. The use of cooling/warming blankets, low ambient temperature and reduced overhead operating light intensity helps maintain a low temperature during bypass and minimizes radiant heating of the myocardium. Surface cooling is aided by placement of ice bags on and around the head and will assist with brain cooling.

Neurological injury is an inherent risk for any patient undergoing cardiac surgery and cardiopulmonary bypass. This has been particularly the case in neonates and infants where DHCA or low-flow techniques have been commonly used. While it is clear that brain maturity, congenital neurological abnormalities, and perinatal injury are important sources of long-term neurobehavioral deficiencies, efforts to improve modifiable sources of neuronal injury are essential [161]. Our current strategies to optimize cerebral protection during deep hypothermic bypass, with or without circulatory arrest, include a longer duration of cooling over 20 min[162–164], the use of a pH-stat strategy of blood gas management during cooling (i.e. additional CO_2 to the oxygenator) [165], a higher hematocrit (approximately 30%) [166], and DHCA intervals <40 min [156].

Weaning from cardiopulmonary bypass

During the rewarming phase, air is vented from the heart before blood is injected into the systemic circulation. Arterial blood gases, electrolytes, and levels of anticoagulation are checked periodically during bypass, but especially during rewarming. Electrolytes, especially ionized calcium, are normalized before separation from bypass is attempted. Adequacy of rewarming is judged by temperature recordings from multiple sites.

The need for vasopressor and inotropic support during weaning from bypass is determined by close observation of the heart during the rewarming phase. Rhythm problems, coronary perfusion problems, and the general state of myocardial contractility can be estimated by directly observing the heart during this period. Separation from bypass is accomplished in concert with the surgical team. Although monitoring of the appropriate intracardiac and intra-arterial pressures and waveforms may accurately indicate both left and right ventricular function, slavish adherence to the monitored values without visual confirmation of the adequacy of cardiac filling and performance can lead to many errors. The small size of the heart and the presence of unsuspected congenital defects sometimes make interpretation of pressures from monitoring lines difficult. When rewarming is complete and cardiac function is judged adequate, weaning from the extracorporeal circulation is accomplished by slowly allowing the heart to fill and eject while ventilation is re-established. Optimal ventricular filling pressures are estimated using filling pressures from preoperative catheterization data, the appearance of the heart, and infusion of small increments of volume while watching filling and systemic arterial pressures. The direct measurement of oxygen saturations from chambers of the heart enables calculations of a residual intracardiac shunt immediately following surgery, and direct pressure measurements across

systemic and pulmonary outflow tracts enable detection of residual significant obstruction. Transesophageal echocardiography has become an important diagnostic method to evaluate ventricular function, as well as assessing atrioventricular and semi-lunar valve competence, outflow obstruction and significant residual intracardiac shunting across the ventricular or atrial septums. If systemic arterial pressure or gas exchange is inadequate, CPB is reinstituted while the problem is analyzed and appropriate corrective measures are taken.

After discontinuing bypass, and despite full rewarming on bypass, mild hypothermia often develops in neonates and infants. Active measures to decrease radiant and evaporative losses are necessary because of the increased metabolic stress, pulmonary vasoreactivity, coagulopathy and potential for dysrhythmias associated with hypothermia. However, hyperthermia must also be actively avoided because of the associated increased metabolic rate and potential for ongoing neurological injury, particularly when myocardial function may be depressed and cerebral autoregulation impaired [167].

Hemostasis may be difficult to obtain if bypass has been prolonged and if there are extensive, high-pressure (often concealed) suture lines. Prompt management and meticulous control of surgical bleeding are essential to prevent the complications associated with a massive transfusion. Besides hemodilution of coagulation factors and platelets, complex surgery with long bypass times increases endothelial injury and exposure to the non-endothelialized surface of the pump circuit, thereby stimulating the intrinsic pathway, and platelet activation and aggregation. Preoperative factors including chronic cyanosis in older patients, and a low CO with tissue hypoperfusion and DIC, hepatic immaturity, and the use of platelet inhibitors such as PGE1 in neonates and infants also contribute to prolonged bleeding after bypass [168,169]. See Chapter 11 for more detailed discussion of the management of hemostasis and blood transfusion.

Sternal closure and tamponade after cardiac operations

Chest closure is a time of particular instability after operations for CHD. The small infant's mediastinum makes compression of the heart and cardiac tamponade ever-present possibilities after chest closure, despite patent drainage tubes. The warning signs of tamponade are frequently not present in small children, even minutes before cardiovascular collapse from tamponade. Any significant deterioration in hemodynamics after chest closure should be first attributed to tamponade if ventilation and cardiac rhythm are adequate. Until the patient is safely transported to the intensive care unit and cardiovascular stability is ensured, continuous attention must be paid to the patient's hemodynamic status after chest closure.

Anesthesia for non-cardiac surgery

The approach to anesthesia for children with CHD outlined above is the same whether the proposed operation is cardiac or non-cardiac. Because non-cardiac surgeons may have less appreciation of the delicate homeostatic balance of the child's cardiac pathophysiology, it is particularly important during non-cardiac surgery that the anesthesiologist understands the pathophysiology of the patient's problem(s). Furthermore, CPB is not immediately available for cardiovascular support if surgery and anesthesia overwhelm the patient's circulatory homeostasis. Because the anesthesiologist must understand and maintain the often fragile circulatory balance during surgery, surgical insults must be anticipated preoperatively and planned for. Familiarity with the child's pathophysiology and the planned non-cardiac procedure should avoid major problems in anesthetic management. Evaluation, preoperative preparation, choice of monitors, induction, maintenance, emergence from anesthesia, and plans for postoperative care are predicated on this familiarity.

An important aspect of the care of children with CHD who are undergoing non-cardiac surgery is a cardiology consultation to delineate the pathological lesion and provide objective assessment of the patient's current hemodynamic status. Most cardiologists have an incomplete appreciation of the physiological stresses that major non-cardiac surgical procedures impose on the cardiopulmonary system. When major blood loss is anticipated, when intrusion into the airway, peritoneal, thoracic or cranial cavity is necessary, or when a prolonged operative procedure is planned, a cardiology consult is often helpful *if* the cardiologist is informed about the anticipated perioperative stresses to homeostasis.

Status of the disease

Children with CHD may present for non-cardiac operations before cardiac surgical treatment, after palliation, or after "repair" of their CHD. Palliated patients still have a distinctly abnormal circulation, and the consequences of CHD (e.g. CHF, hypoxemia, polycythemia, pulmonary vascular disease) may be a problem. It is important to note that even patients whose heart disease has been surgically "corrected" can have significant residual problems. Arrhythmias, ventricular dysfunction, shunts, valvular stenosis or regurgitation, and pulmonary hypertension may remain or develop after surgical "repair" of the CHD. Surgical "corrections" may be classified as

Table 25.5 A classification for congenital cardiac surgical repairs

Type of repair	Outcome

Anatomic
  LV = systemic ventricle
  RV = pulmonary ventricle
  Circulation in series
  Cyanosis corrected
	1. Simple reconstruction: structurally normal after repair (e.g., ASD, VSD, PDA). Late complications unlikely
	2. Complex reconstruction: baffle, conduit, outflow reconstruction or AV valve repair; late complications likely

Physiologic
  Circulation in series
  Cyanosis corrected
	1. Two ventricles:
	  RV = systemic ventricle
	  LV = systemic ventricle (e.g. Senning or Mustard procedure)
	2. Single ventricle:
	  Fontan procedure

RV, right ventricle; LV, left ventricle; ASD, atrial septal defect; VSD, ventricular septal defect; PDA, patent ductus arteriosus; AV, atrioventricular valve.

"anatomical," whereby the circulation is in series and the left ventricle is connected to the aorta, or "physiological," where the circulation is also in series and the patient is no longer cyanosed. However, they may function with the RV as the systemic ventricle or have undergone a single ventricle repair (Table 25.5).

Anesthesia for interventional procedures

Cardiac catheterization laboratory

Adequate sedation and anesthesia during cardiac catheterization are essential to facilitate acquisition of meaningful hemodynamic data and to assist during interventional procedures. For the most part, hemodynamic or diagnostic catheterization procedures can be performed under sedation in all age groups. For many interventional procedures, sedation may be appropriate but for procedures that are associated with significant hemodynamic compromise, or are prolonged, general anesthesia is preferable. Whatever technique is used, it is essential that hemodynamic data be attained in conditions as close to normal as possible. When using sedation, full monitoring is essential to ensure that respiratory depression is avoided. During anesthesia, the effects of inspired oxygen concentration, mechanical ventilation and hemodynamic side-effects of various anesthesia agents must also be appreciated. Postprocedure monitoring in either a recovery room or intensive care unit is mandatory.

Cardiac catheterization laboratories are usually remote from the operating room, and rarely configured to accommodate anesthetic personnel. Relative to patient size, the lateral and anterior-posterior cameras used for imaging are in close proximity to the patient's head and neck, limiting access to the airway. An anesthetic machine and monitors around the patient will further confine the space in which the anesthesiologist may work and limit access to the patient. In addition, the environment is darkened to facilitate viewing of images, and monitoring with capnography and pulse oximetry is mandatory. The environment is also cooler because of computer and cine equipment, and children may become hypothermic from conductive and convective heat loss. In addition, frequent flushing of the catheters and sheaths to prevent clotting or air embolism may also contribute to hypothermia. Unnecessary exposure of the child must be avoided and convective warming blankets used where possible. Care must be taken when positioning a patient on the catheterization table because of the risk of pressure areas and nerve traction injury. In particular, brachial plexus injury may occur when patients have their arms positioned above their heads for a prolonged period of time to make room for the lateral cameras. To facilitate femoral vein and arterial access, the pelvis is commonly elevated from the catheterization table. This may displace abdominal contents cephalad, restricting diaphragm excursion and increasing the risk for respiratory depression in a sedated patient.

In addition to considerations related to the environment, there are a number of potential problems and complications that are inherent to any catheterization procedure, and some related to specific interventions (see below). The minimal monitoring available to all patients in the catheterization laboratory includes automated blood pressure, ECG, pulse oximetry, end-tidal carbon dioxide ($PETCO_2$), and direct observation of the patient's airway and breathing.

Interventional cardiology

Transcatheter treatment of CHD is replacing a number of conventional intraoperative surgical procedures. This experience has a significant impact on the severity and complexity of illness seen in the operating room and in the interventional laboratory. Procedures that are routinely performed in the catheterization laboratory now include balloon valvuloplasty of congenitally stenotic aortic, mitral, and pulmonary valves, angioplasty for pulmonary arterial stenoses and postoperative aortic recoarctation, or angioplasty combined with transcatheter placement of endovascular stents for sustained relief of obstruction in arterial or subarterial (intracardiac) locations, radiofrequency ablation of abnormal conduction pathways, and embolization or device occlusion procedures of systemic-to-pulmonary arterial communications, venous channels, fistulas, muscular VSDs, ASDs or patent ductus arteriosus (PDA). Many procedures (e.g. PDA closure) are performed on an outpatient basis with the full participation of the anesthesiologist [170].

Although many relatively uncomplicated procedures previously performed in the operating room are now performed in the catheterization laboratory, they have been replaced by surgical procedures for previously inoperable patients with more complex disease who have derived benefit from interventional catheterization techniques. These interventions have established an anatomical or physiological circumstance that lends itself to intraoperative repair. Among the best examples are patients with tetralogy of Fallot and pulmonary atresia with hypoplastic pulmonary arteries who are deemed inoperable after an early palliative shunt has failed to provide any meaningful growth of pulmonary arteries. By establishing antegrade flow to the pulmonary artery early in life with a surgically placed homograft from right ventricle to pulmonary artery, the child can undergo serial balloon dilations of the pulmonary arteries with subsequent growth that allows eventual surgical correction with VSD closure. Among patients with single ventricles who have undergone a modified Fontan procedure, high-risk candidates can be assisted during the postoperative period by leaving a communication at the atrial level that allows right-to-left shunting, and hence cardiac output, to be maintained during transient postoperative elevation in pulmonary vascular resistance. This fenestration can subsequently be test-occluded in the catheterization laboratory and permanently occluded with a device if indicated [171].

This collaborative approach to intervention and repair has offered improved results and new futures for patients with many types of serious congenital heart disease. Therefore, the cardiac anesthesiologist is faced with more complex, previously inoperable patients in the operating room, and with more demand for presence in the catheterization laboratory, where the environment is rapidly evolving into a hybrid operating room in need of the skills and balance of the anesthesiologist.

Risks and complications

Placement of catheters in and through the heart increases the risk for dysrhythmias, perforation of the myocardium, damage to valve leaflets and cordae, cerebral vascular accidents and air embolism. The use of radiopaque contrast material may cause an acute allergic reaction (although this is rare in children with non-ionic contrast media), pulmonary hypertension and myocardial depression. Blood loss may be sudden and unexpected when large-bore catheters are used or vessels are ruptured. More insidious blood loss may occur over several hours in heparinized small children or neonates owing to

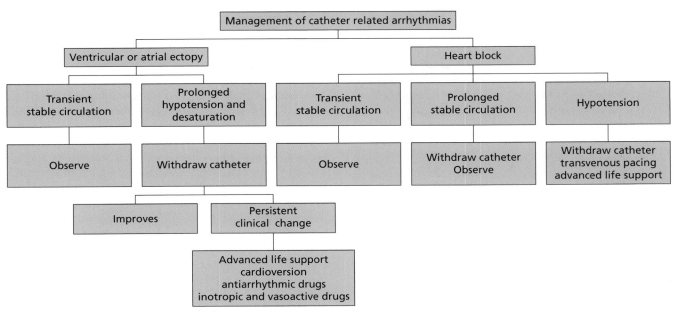

Figure 25.12 Algorithm for treating catheter-induced arrhythmias during cardiac catheterization.

bleeding around the catheter site or multiple aspirations and flushes of catheters. Transfusion requirements and appropriate vascular access should be continually assessed.

Arrhythmias, albeit transient, may be recurrent and fatal if not promptly treated. These include catheter-induced supraventricular tachyarrhythmias, ventricular tachycardia, ventricular fibrillation, and occasionally complete heart block requiring temporary transvenous pacing support. On most occasions, removal of the wire or catheter is sufficient for the arrhythmia to resolve, but when this does not happen, it is important that full resuscitation and cardioversion equipment be available. An algorithm for treating catheter-induced arrhythmias is shown in Figure 25.12.

Complications of various interventional procedures are related in part to the type of procedure, but all share the risks associated with percutaneous vascular access with large catheters that course through the heart and vessels. The specific problems that may occur during various interventional transcatheter procedures are listed in Table 25.6. While the underlying cardiac status or ASA classification of the patient may increase their risk for adverse events during catheterization, in many circumstances complications are sudden, occurring without warning, and reflect the inherent risk for that specific procedure. Many complications are potentially life threatening, and successful treatment of complications depends on prompt action by anesthesiologists co-operating closely with the interventional cardiologists who are manipulating the catheters.

Inadvertent release or detachment of embolic and closure devices results in systemic and pulmonary arterial embolization. Embolization usually occurs immediately after placement, and devices can often be retrieved by use of a variety of retrieval catheters, but in a small minority of cases surgical removal is required. If the device is lodged in the heart or a great vessel, CPB may be required for removal. Device embolization does not usually cause extreme hemodynamic instability or cardiovascular decompensation requiring emergency surgical removal, but an unscheduled surgical procedure is still required. Even after successful transcatheter retrieval, femoral artery and vein reconstruction during anesthesia is occasionally necessary when embolized devices or large dilation balloons are removed through these vessels. Deliberate embolization of aortopulmonary collaterals may decrease pulmonary blood flow excessively, causing severe hypoxemia; general anesthesia and muscle paralysis may be necessary to increase arterial oxygen saturation to acceptable levels by decreasing oxygen consumption while operating room preparations are made.

Balloon dilation of pulmonary arteries
Pulmonary artery balloon dilation and stent placement to relieve stenosis is a common procedure performed in the catheterization laboratory, and complications that may occur during this procedure exemplify many of the potential problems that can occur during any catheterization. Pulmonary artery stenoses may be congenital or acquired lesions. They may be discrete, involving the main or branch pulmonary arteries, or multiple, involving distal

Table 25.6 Complications in the cardiac catheterization laboratory

Procedure	Representative lesion	Complications
Diagnostic catheterization	Congenital heart disease	Blood loss requiring transfusion
		Air embolism
		Cerebral vascular accident
		Myocardial perforation and tamponade
		Femoral vessel occusion
		Arrhythmias; ventricular and supraventricular tachycardia, ventricular fibrillation, complete heart block
Coil embolization	Aortopulmonary collaterals	Fevers
	Blalock–Taussig shunts	Excessive hypoxemia
	Anomalous coronary arteries	Systemic embolization
	Hepatic hemangiomas	Hepatic necrosis
Transcatheter device closure	Patent ductus arteriosus	Air or device embolization
	Atrial septal defect	Blood loss
	Ventricular septal defect	Interference with atrioventricular value function, ventricular arrhythmias, complete heart block
	Baffle leak	
Balloon and stent dilations	Pulmonary artery stenosis	Pulmonary artery tear and bleeding
		Unilateral pulmonary edema
		False aneurysm
		Cardiac arrest (Williams syndrome)
	Blalock–Taussig shunt	Pulmonary artery tear and bleeding
		Thrombosis
		Pulmonary edema
	Pulmonary valve stenosis	Pulmonary insufficiency
	Aortic valve stenosis	Aortic regurgitation
		Ventricular fibrillation (neonate)
	Mitral valve stenosis	Mitral insufficiency
		Pulmonary hypertension
	Coarctation of the aorta	Aortic dissection
		Hypertension
	Right ventricular conduit	False aneurysms
		Stent embolization
Atrial septotomy	Transposition of the great arteries, mitral stenosis (atresia), and restrictive atrial septum	Perforation of the heart and tamponade
Radiofrequency mapping and ablation	Anomalous conduction pathways	Complete heart block
		Supraventricular tachycardia
		Thromboembolus from long sheath and prolonged procedure
Myocardial biopsy	Cardiomyopathy or transplantation	Myocardial perforation
		Complete heart block

segmental vessels. Some factors that determine whether dilation should be performed under sedation or general anesthesia include the extent of balloon dilation, anticipated complications, and the duration of the procedure.

Pulmonary artery disruption is signaled by hemoptysis of various degrees or the appearance of intravascular contrast medium in the pleural space or major lung fissures. In the presence of substantial hemoptysis, immediate endotracheal intubation is indicated for airway control and ventilation. Hypertension and further airway stimulation are avoided. Addition of PEEP may be useful. Heparinization is reversed and blood for transfusion is made immediately available. Intrapulmonary hemorrhage is often self-limited, but hemothorax can be severe and may lead to hypotension and death. Transient unilateral or unilobar pulmonary edema is also seen in the setting of pulmonary artery dilation. This is related to sudden large increases in pulmonary blood flow and distal pulmonary artery pressure after dilation in a previously underperfused pulmonary vascular bed. These two distinct entities, unilateral pulmonary edema and disruption of pulmonary artery integrity, can both occur abruptly, in isolation or together, during pulmonary artery dilation procedures, and both can cause the appearance in the airway of frank blood or blood-tinged edema fluid in substantial quantities. Treatment of both entities starts with endotracheal intubation unless symptoms are minimal.

The function of the right ventricle is critical. At the time of balloon dilation, cardiac output may decrease significantly, causing hypotension, bradycardia, arterial oxygen desaturation and a fall in end-tidal CO_2. As the balloon is only inflated for a few seconds, and provided preload is maintained, the procedure is usually well tolerated and the circulation usually recovers spontaneously. Patients who have a hypertrophied, poorly compliant right ventricle with intraventricular pressures at systemic or suprasystemic levels may not tolerate the sudden increase in afterload associated with balloon dilation, even for a short period. In particular, myocardial ischemia and arrhythmias may occur, causing severe acute RV failure and loss of cardiac output. General anesthesia and controlled ventilation are recommended prior to the intervention in this at-risk group of patients.

Patients who have a dilated right ventricle secondary to a long-standing volume load, such as chronic pulmonary regurgitation, are also at risk for arrhythmias and low output during catheter manipulations and interventions. On most occasions the changes in rhythm are short-lived and settle once the catheters are withdrawn. Nevertheless, anesthesia and airway control are recommended if the circulation is compromised, and a defibrillator and transvenous pacing must be immediately available.

Potential movement at the time of critical balloon dilation or stent placement must be avoided. The dilation of pulmonary arteries is painful and will often cause patients to waken from sedation and move. In addition, dilation of the pulmonary arteries may induce coughing. This is usually not a problem for isolated pulmonary artery dilation but if the patient moves during stent placement, it is possible that lobar or segmental branch pulmonary arteries can be inadvertently obstructed by the stent. Therefore, it is essential that the patient be immobile and additional sedation should be considered immediately prior to stent placement.

Balloon dilation of multiple peripheral pulmonary artery stenoses, such as seen in patients with Williams syndrome, is often a prolonged procedure and associated with significant hemodynamic changes; endotracheal general anesthesia is usually required from the outset. Besides right ventricular hypertension, an additional concern in this group of patients is the risk for pulmonary edema post dilation. This usually occurs immediately following balloon dilation, but can be delayed for up to 24 h. Endotracheal intubation and controlled ventilation are usually necessary until the edema resolves.

Occlusion device insertion

"Umbrella" or "clamshell" device closure of PDA, ASD and VSD is commonly performed in the catheterization laboratory. The placement of a PDA or ASD device is usually associated with minimal hemodynamic disturbance and can be performed in most patients using sedation techniques. General anesthesia may be necessary for airway protection if transesophageal echocardiography is used to guide device placement or if the procedure is prolonged and procedural complications such as device embolization occur.

In contrast to our experience with closure of PDAs or ASDs, transcatheter VSD device closures are prolonged procedures, and often associated with profound hemodynamic instability and blood loss [172]. Intensive care management is frequently required following placement. The indications for VSD device placement include closure of a residual or recurrent septal defect, preoperative closure of defects that may be difficult to reach surgically while on cardiopulmonary bypass and closure of acquired defects such as post myocardial infarction or trauma. While the clinical condition of patients undergoing VSD device placement may therefore vary considerably, the preoperative clinical condition or ASA status is not a predictor of hemodynamic disturbance during device placement. Rather, it is the technique necessary for deploying the occlusion device that results in significant hemodynamic compromise and all patients are therefore susceptible.

Factors contributing to hemodynamic instability include blood loss, arrhythmias from catheter manipulation in the ventricles and across the septum, atrioventricular or aortic valve regurgitation from stenting open of valve leaflets by stiff-walled catheters, and device-related factors such as malposition of the umbrella with arms impinging on valve leaflets or dislodgment from the ventricular septum.

The procedures are often prolonged. Because of the large sheath required for the positioning of the delivery pod and folded umbrella device, and the need for frequent catheter changes through the sheath, considerable blood loss may occur (often concealed by drapes) and the risk for air embolism is also increased. In patients with intracardiac shunts, air embolization may be life threatening. When unoccupied by the device carrier system and collapsed device, the large delivery sheath represents a potential space for air accumulation and subsequent delivery into the heart. In addition, when the entry port of the large delivery sheath is open during removal and reinsertion of various catheters and devices, extreme inspiratory efforts may entrain intracardiac air. Air delivered into the right atrium may be shunted across the ASD even in the presence of nominal left-to-right shunting. Left atrial air embolization during these procedures can be seen with fluoroscopy; it produces ST segment elevation and often hemodynamic changes as it passes into the aorta. The resultant ST segment changes, hypotension, arterial desaturation, and bradycardia generally respond to aspirating and then sealing the entry port, along with administration of atropine, and inotropic and pressor support to maintain coronary perfusion. Meticulous purging of air from the catheter system and sealing of open ports should help to minimize the incidence of air embolism. Use of controlled positive pressure ventilation through an endotracheal tube in an anesthetized, paralyzed patient may also decrease the potential for transcatheter air entrainment during transcatheter closure of intracardiac defects.

Transcatheter radiofrequency ablation

Pediatric patients undergoing radiofrequency ablation vary in age and diagnosis [173]. Ablation may be necessary in the newborn with persistent re-entrant tachycardia or ectopic atrial tachycardia and cardiac failure, as well as in older children with an ectopic focus and otherwise structurally normal heart. An increasing population of patients undergoing ablation are those who have undergone previous surgical repair of congenital heart defects. Patients with persistent volume or pressure load on the right atrium, and those who have required an extensive incision and suture lines within the right atrium, such as following a Mustard, Senning or Fontan procedure, may be at increased risk for supraventricular tachyarrhythmia (SVT) such as atrial flutter and fibrillation. Ventricular tachyarrhythmias may also develop late fol-

lowing repair of certain congenital heart defects, such as RV outflow tract reconstruction for tetralogy of Fallot.

Radiofrequency catheter ablations (RFCA) are usually prolonged procedures. It is difficult for children to lie still for some hours, and therefore endotracheal general anesthesia is preferred. In addition, it is important that patients remain immobile to avoid catheter movement at the time of ablation because sudden patient movement may result in a radiofrequency lesion being created at an incorrect site. For instance, if the focus is close to the AV node, inadvertent movement might displace the catheter and cause permanent AV conduction blockade. On occasion, holding the ventilation either in inspiration or expiration may be necessary to ensure adequate contact of the ablation catheter with the arrhythmic focus.

Although these procedures are prolonged, for the most part they are hemodynamically well tolerated and blood loss is minimal. During mapping, the focus is stimulated and the tachyarrhythmia induced. This may result in hypotension, but this is usually short-lived and can be readily converted via intracardiac pacing. If hypotension is prolonged and intracardiac conversion unsuccessful, transthoracic cardioversion may be necessary and a defibrillator should be immediately available.

Because anesthetic drugs have minimal effects on intrinsic conduction [88,174–177], a range of techniques can be used to maintain general anesthesia during RFCA. However, some tachyarrhythmias, such as ectopic atrial tachycardia, are catecholamine sensitive, and the focus may be difficult to localize after induction of anesthesia. For this reason, it is preferable in these patients to perform the procedure under light sedation or light general anesthesia if necessary.

Cardiac tamponade

Acute myocardial perforation with tamponade occasionally occurs during interventional cardiac catheterization procedures. Prompt support of the circulation with volume infusions and pressor support, along with immediate catheter drainage of the pericardial space, are essential in the event of this complication. Hemopericardium after ventricular puncture is usually self-limited, as the muscular ventricle seals the perforation after the responsible wire or catheter is removed. However, laceration of the more thin-walled atrium may require suture repair under direct vision in the operating room.

Other causes of cardiac tamponade are seen in patients with CHD and treatment frequently requires the assistance of an anesthesiologist. Postoperative tamponade from bleeding immediately after operation, as discussed above, is best handled by facilitation of chest tube drainage or reopening the sternotomy. These patients are usually still anesthetized and mechanically ventilated so that new anesthetic considerations and choices are limited. However, some children develop pericardial effusions at other phases of their illness owing to hydrostatic influences (e.g. patients with modified Fontan operations) or postpericardiotomy syndrome. Fluid in the pericardial space may accumulate under considerable pressure and filling of the heart is impaired. If this problem is left unattended, the transmural pressure in the atria diminishes as the intra-atrial pressures rise and diastolic collapse of the atria can be observed echocardiographically. The patients become symptomatic with a narrow pulse pressure, pulsus paradoxus, tachycardia, respiratory distress, abdominal pain progressing to decreased urine output, hyperkalemia, metabolic acidosis, and hypotension with tremendous endogenous catecholamine response.

When hemodynamics are compromised, draining the fluid is imperative. A percutaneous approach to drainage is preferred when the fluid is accessible through a subxyphoid approach. This may be a formidable task in a frightened, combative child with impending shock. Anesthetic principles guiding sedation for pericardial drainage should focus on maintaining or improving intravascular volume, vascular tone, and the contractile state of the ventricle. Anesthetic agents used for sedation that excessively decrease preload or afterload and transiently impair myocardial function may have disastrous consequences, especially when they are combined with muscle paralysis and positive pressure ventilation, which further impairs ventricular filling. If a child demonstrates serious tamponade symptoms and a large circumferential, percutaneously accessible pericardial effusion is identified echocardiographically, drainage under sedation using a opioid, benzodiazepine or ketamine with local anesthesia is safer than an open surgical procedure with a rapid-sequence induction and positive pressure ventilation.

Pathophysiology and anesthetic management of specific lesions and procedures

A unique feature of managing patients with congenital heart defects is the knowledge, expertise, and technical skills required to manage a heterogeneous population of patients with a wide variety of diagnoses and pathophysiology. The experience at Children's Hospital, Boston, over the past 5 years is shown in Figure 25.13. In addition, there has been a change in management philosophy over the past 20 years towards performing reparative operations on neonates and infants rather than initial palliation and later repair. With the emphasis on early surgical repair, the aim is to promote normal growth and development, and limit the pathophysiological consequences of congenital cardiac defects such as volume overload, pressure overload, and chronic hypoxemia. It is important to note, however, that older children and adults with congenital heart disease are an increasing group of patients

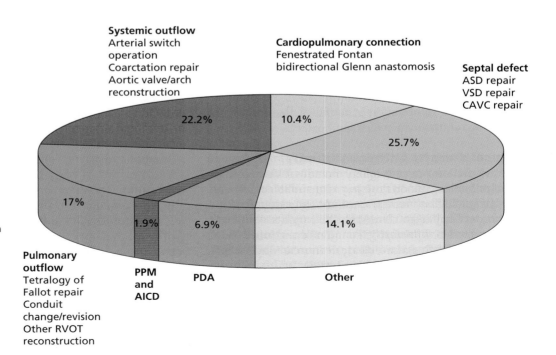

Figure 25.13 Spectrum of congenital cardiac surgical procedures performed at Children's Hospital, Boston, in a typical year. AICD, automated implantable cardioverter-defibrillator; ASD, atrial septal defect: CAVC, complete atrioventricular canal; PDA patent ductus arteriosus; PPM, permanent pacemaker; RVOT, right ventricular outflow tract; VSD, ventricular septal defect.

presenting for cardiac and non-cardiac surgery. This includes patients undergoing a reparative operation, often some years following an initial palliative procedure, and patients who have had previous reparative surgery but subsequently require reintervention because of residual or progressive defects, such as conduit stenosis.

Virtually all congenital cardiac defects are now amenable to either an anatomical or functional repair, but while "corrected," they may not be "cured." However, palliative procedures are often necessary to control pulmonary blood flow prior to repair because of extreme lesion size, anatomical variations or need for maturation before repair. For example, a modified Fontan procedure is the definitive operation for many classes of complex CHD. However, the Fontan procedure requires low PVR and large pulmonary arteries, which are not characteristic of the neonate. Therefore, a shunt may be required to relieve hypoxemia and allow growth of the pulmonary arteries until the child is a few months older. Alternatively, if the pulmonary blood flow is excessive, a pulmonary band is required to minimize the possibility of CHF and to prevent *any* pulmonary vascular obstructive disease from developing until a Fontan repair can be done. Nevertheless, palliative procedures have immediate complications and may seriously compromise subsequent complete surgical repair of the lesion.

This section summarizes the basic pathophysiology of each lesion or procedure as a prelude to discussion of anesthetic management of the lesion. The discussion of anesthetic management before the repair applies equally well to non-cardiac procedures in unrepaired patients and to patients undergoing repair of the CHD but before CPD support is initiated. For some lesions, a separate discussion considers the anesthetic complications that occur after repair. This heading, where appropriate, outlines specific complications and problems that may be encountered months or years after repair of the anomaly. Otherwise, this information is found at the end of the section on anesthetic management.

Surgical shunts: pathophysiology

When the anatomy or physiology includes severe obstruction of pulmonary blood flow and is unsuitable for immediate physiological repair, a shunt is required. This situation is seen most commonly in patients who have tricuspid atresia with restricted pulmonary blood flow, pulmonary atresia, or a single ventricle and severe obstruction to pulmonary blood flow. The surgically created shunt provides sufficient pulmonary blood flow to maintain acceptable arterial oxygen saturation in a circumstance where oxygenated pulmonary venous blood mixes with systemic venous blood. Optimally, the surgical shunt (a simple shunt) provides restrictive flow to the pulmonary circuit, allowing adequate, but not excessive, pulmonary blood flow.

Types of surgical shunts
Aortopulmonary artery shunts

Systemic-to-pulmonary artery shunts are palliative procedures that increase pulmonary blood flow, thereby relieving severe cyanosis, improving functional status and allowing for diffuse growth of small pulmonary arteries. The classic *Blalock–Taussig (B–T) shunt* redirects subclavian artery blood into the branch pulmonary artery on the side opposite the aortic arch [178]. This graft allows some growth during infancy but is unlikely to induce pulmonary vascular disease. Rather than compromise the subclavian artery and upper limb blood flow, a modified B–T shunt is now preferred using a Gore-tex™ synthetic tube graft interposed between the subclavian or innominate artery and the pulmonary artery. Performed either via a thoracotomy or median sternotomy, flow across the shunt is dependent upon the size of the Gore-tex tube (usually 3.5 or 4.0 mm diameter), the length of the tube, and site of take-off from the systemic artery. A shunt arising from the innominate artery is likely to have a higher flow because of a higher perfusion pressure than a more distally placed shunt arising from the subclavian artery. The B–T shunt is associated with low mortality and a low incidence of late postoperative complications. However, distortion of the pulmonary arteries may occur within a few months and seriously affect definitive repair.

The *Potts shunt* (descending aorta to left pulmonary artery) and the *Waterston shunt* (ascending aorta to the right pulmonary artery) are rarely used now because the size of the shunt orifice is difficult to control precisely, they may enlarge substantially with growth, becoming non-restrictive and resulting in excessive pulmonary flow and pulmonary vascular obstructive disease. They produce distortion and stenosis of the branch pulmonary arteries, and also are difficult to dissect and control prior to CPB during subsequent surgery. A *central shunt* between the ascending aorta and main pulmonary artery is occasionally used when branch pulmonary arteries are hypoplastic.

Cavopulmonary artery shunt

The first cavopulmonary artery anastomosis (*Glenn shunt*) was a unidirectional shunt constructed as a palliative procedure for tricuspid atresia. A Glenn shunt provides systemic *venous* blood, instead of systemic arterial blood, to the lungs for gas exchange. The superior vena cava is disconnected from the right atrium and connected directly to the detached right pulmonary artery, i.e. superior vena cava blood perfuses the right lung and flow depends on the pressure gradient between the superior vena cava and left atrial pressures [179]. Therefore, the Glenn shunt is limited to patients with low PVR, which precludes its use in neonates. This shunt is rarely performed today as the pulmonary arteries are not in continuity, and palliation is short-lived because of complications such as thrombosis or occlusion leading to SVC syndrome, and progressive cyanosis secondary to the development of pulmonary arteriovenous collaterals.

An important modification of the Glenn shunt that is now used during staged repair of single-ventricle defects involves the anastomosis of the cephalad portion of the superior vena cava to the right pulmonary artery, as in the original Glenn procedure, except pulmonary artery continuity is maintained and flow is therefore bidirectional through both right and left pulmonary arteries (hence the term bidirectional cavopulmonary anastomosis or bidirectional Glenn (BDG) procedure) [180–182]. It can be performed successfully in children as young as 3–4 months of age, after the PVR has decreased, and has the benefit that effective pulmonary blood flow is increased but with reduced pulmonary artery pressure [183,184]. It avoids imposing the volume load on the ventricle associated with aortopulmonary shunts and minimizes atrial distension and high right atrial pressures inherent in a full Fontan-type operation in a high-risk patient (see below) [185].

Anesthetic management before and during aortopulmonary shunts

Complications of surgical shunts can occur immediately after surgery or years later when another surgical intervention is contemplated. Severe hypoxemia may occur in the operating room during or after creation of the shunt, implying inadequate pulmonary blood flow. Intrapulmonary shunting must always be considered in lungs that are compressed by the surgeons, but mechanical obstruction of flow into the pulmonary artery caused by retraction during surgery or by shunt occlusion (kinking or thrombosis) is the usual cause. An increase in PVR may also reduce flow across the shunt, and inducing an alkalosis by hyperventilation and using a high inspired oxygen concentration may minimize PVR and optimize gas exchange until shunt flow can be improved. As a note of caution, however, an increase in mean intrathoracic pressure and overinflation of the lungs during vigorous mechanical ventilation may further restrict flow across the shunt.

Systemic-to-pulmonary artery shunts are inherently inefficient because they recirculate blood to the lungs without its having reached the systemic circulation. To substantially improve arterial oxygen content, pulmonary blood flow must be several times greater than the systemic flow (Fig. 25.14). However, if the surgically created shunt is not sufficiently restrictive, pulmonary flows become excessive and cause pulmonary edema, wide pulse pressures and, occasionally, inadequate sys-

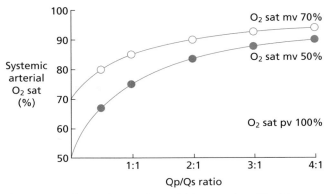

Figure 25.14 Changes in systemic arterial O_2 saturation with mixing lesions as the Qp/Qs (pulmonary/systemic blood flow ratio) changes with different levels of mixed venous (mv) O_2 saturation. It presumes a pulmonary (pv) O_2 saturation of 100%. Reproduced from Rudolph AM. Congenital Diseases of the Heart. Chicago: Year Book Medical Publishers, 1974, p.79.

temic perfusion. Arterial oxygen saturation is relatively high despite complete mixing of systemic and pulmonary venous blood in the left heart. Maneuvers to increase pulmonary vascular resistance (see above) can compensate to a limited degree for excessive pulmonary flow, but shunt revision may be necessary.

Anesthetic considerations after creation of an aortopulmonary shunt

In patients with systemic-to-pulmonary artery shunts, shunt flow is usually restricted by the shunt orifice and the balance between pulmonary and systemic vascular resistance. If the shunt is too large, excessive pulmonary blood flow will be evident by high arterial oxygen saturations, reduced systemic perfusion with increasing metabolic acidosis, low diastolic blood pressure and pulmonary edema. The work of breathing is increased and patients may have difficulty weaning from ventilation. If any shunt is large enough to allow excessive pressure and flow in the pulmonary vascular bed, pulmonary vascular obstructive disease may develop over time.

If the shunt is too small, arterial oxygen saturations will remain low, and pulmonary flow will be dependent on normal or increased systemic arterial pressures. Thus, hypotension seriously compromises arterial oxygenation, particularly as the shunt becomes more restrictive and must be treated aggressively. Other causes of a low oxygen saturation after shunt placement include a low mixed venous oxygen level secondary to a low cardiac output, and reduced oxygen-carrying capacity from relative anemia.

An appropriately sized shunt results in a balanced circulation (Qp/Qs approximately 1:1) with peripheral saturations between 75% and 85% and a normal systolic pressure but a widened pulse pressure. Tachycardia is common initially once the shunt is open, and blood volume replacement is usually necessary. Inotrope support with dopamine may also be necessary as the increased pulmonary blood flow imposes a volume load on the systemic ventricle. The hematocrit should be maintained between 40% and 45%. Afterload reduction with a systemic vasodilator, such as sodium nitroprusside or a phosphodiesterase inhibitor, may be indicated if the patient has poor extremity perfusion, and to improve systemic perfusion if there is a relatively large shunt and excessive pulmonary blood flow. In general, most patients are mechanically ventilated postoperatively until flow is well balanced and adequate systemic perfusion maintained.

Pulmonary artery banding
Pathophysiology
When pulmonary blood flow is excessive and high pressure is communicated from the ventricle to the pulmonary vasculature, surgery may be required to prevent progressive pulmonary vascular obstructive disease or to lessen symptoms of CHF. If total correction of the lesion is not possible, pulmonary blood flow can be reduced by banding the pulmonary artery.

Anesthetic management
With induction of anesthesia for banding of the pulmonary artery, pulmonary vascular resistance occasionally decreases enough to cause massive pulmonary flow and systemic hypotension ("pulmonary steal"). If so, partial occlusion of a branch pulmonary artery with a clamp or ligature reduces pulmonary blood flow and increases peripheral perfusion until the band is applied.

Banding of the pulmonary artery is imprecise, and the hemodynamics after banding are unpredictable. Adequacy of the band is assessed in the operating room by observing a 20–30% increase in systemic blood pressure and a decrease in systemic arterial oxygen saturation. Direct measurement of the pulmonary artery pressure beyond the band may be compared with the systemic arterial pressure. It should be about 50% of the systemic pressure or less. Continuous monitoring of oxygen saturation is helpful for quick assessment of the adequacy of pulmonary blood flow. Saturation by pulse oximeter should be about 80% in common mixing lesions [186]. As hemodynamic criteria are used to assess band tightness, anesthesia is best maintained with high-dose opioids and high concentrations of inhalation agents avoided. If the band is too tight, bradycardia, hypotension and cyanosis will develop, requiring urgent band removal.

The large resistance imposed by banding the pulmonary artery stimulates hypertrophy of the ventricle supplying the banded vessel. Consequently, depression of function of that ventricle quickly reduces pulmonary blood flow, particularly if a VSD or ASD is present, allowing shunting of blood into the systemic circulation. Long-term anatomical hazards of pulmonary artery bands relate to distortion of the anatomy and hypertrophy of the ventricle.

Single ventricle and parallel circulation physiology
Pathophysiology
In patients with a repaired two-ventricle heart, i.e. an "in-series" circulation whereby a separate ventricle ejects blood into the pulmonary artery and the pulmonary venous blood returns to a separate systemic ventricle, systemic oxygenation exclusively represents the efficiency of gas exchange in the lungs; lowering PVR and decreasing right ventricular afterload are important objectives when trying to increase pulmonary blood flow and correct hypoxemia in this situation. However, patients with single-ventricle anatomy represent a unique circumstance that requires physiological interpretation of oxygenation and hemodynamics in light of the "parallel" nature of the circulation. In this circumstance, a single ventricle supplies both pulmonary and systemic blood flow, and lowering pulmonary vascular resistance in these patients may improve oxygenation but adversely affect hemodynamics in some circumstances.

There are many anatomical variations of single-ventricle or univentricular hearts. In general, both AV valves enter a single chamber. Most commonly, a small outflow chamber gives rise to one great artery, usually the aorta. Either AV valve may be atretic; subpulmonary stenosis or atresia is common. Occasionally subaortic stenosis is present at birth or develops subsequently. Therefore, in an infant with a single ventricle the anatomical variations may vary considerably, ranging from tricuspid atresia (a single left ventricle) through double-inlet left ventricle (two AV valves and one single ventricle) to mitral atresia (a single right ventricle, i.e. hypoplastic left heart). Despite the anatomical diagnosis, virtually all patients with effective single-ventricle hearts, as shown in Box 25.4, are amenable to a "physiological" repair, i.e. Fontan procedure.

It is important to note, however, that an effective "parallel" circulation or physiology can exist in patients with two ventricles (see Box 25.4). In these circumstances, the balance between pulmonary and systemic vascular resistance is the critical determinant of systemic perfusion and, therefore, a "balanced" circulation (Qp/Qs = 1). Much of the discussion below regarding maneuvers used to increase or decrease pulmonary blood flow applies in these patients as well prior to surgery. Examples include patients who have a large PDA (left-to-right shunt across the PDA from the aorta to pulmonary artery), common ventricular outflow tract (as in truncus arteriosus), or aortic arch interruption (right-to-left flow from the pulmonary artery to the distal aorta across the PDA to maintain systemic perfusion).

For patients with single ventricle anatomy, there is a common physiological principle, i.e. desaturated systemic venous blood returns to the heart and mixes completely with oxygenated blood returning to the same chamber from the lungs. Common mixing of systemic and pulmonary venous blood means that the aortic O_2 saturation reflects the Qp/Qs. In the absence of lung disease (pulmonary venous desaturation), the pulmonary venous blood with oxygen saturations of 95–100% will drain to the ventricle and mix with systemic venous blood having saturations of 55–60% or less, depending on the amount of oxygen extraction in the periphery. If pulmonary and systemic blood flows are equal (i.e. Qp/

Qs = 1) then the resultant "mixed" O_2 saturation that emerges from the ventricle and is measured in the systemic artery is 75–80%. As the pulmonary blood flow rises in proportion to systemic blood flow, so, too, rises the arterial oxygenation. Consequently, an arterial oxygen saturation of 90% is achieved at the expense of excessive pulmonary blood flow (Qp/Qs >3) and a substantial volume load to the single ventricle, which is required to supply all systemic and pulmonary (three times systemic) blood flow. CHF therefore ensues. If both the pulmonary artery and aorta are anatomically related to the ventricle and unobstructed, then flow to the pulmonary and systemic beds will be partitioned according to the relative resistances of each circuit (i.e. parallel circulations). As the pulmonary vascular resistance falls below SVR during the first few hours of life, pulmonary blood flow increases relative to systemic flow and systemic arterial oxygen saturation rises above 80%. Therefore, systemic oxygen saturation is a convenient marker of Qp/Qs. The effects of alterations of Qp/Qs on systemic arterial oxygen saturation for common mixing lesions are shown in Figure 25.14.

Increased Qp/Qs

The deleterious effects of overcirculated lungs perfused at high pressure and flows, combined with the adverse effects of this volume load, particularly on the neonatal heart which is less capable of increasing stroke volume in response to increasing preload than the mature myocardium, will culminate in a picture of hyperdynamic CHF in which systemic perfusion is compromised and oxygen delivery is impaired despite the elevated arterial oxygen saturation (Fig. 25.15). The myocardium ultimately cannot provide adequate systemic flow as PVR falls and more and more of the stroke volume is inefficiently recirculated to the lungs. Treatment is therefore directed toward raising resistance to blood flow to the lungs, balancing pulmonary and systemic blood flow ratios, and maintaining adequate systemic blood flow (Table 25.7).

Pulmonary vascular resistance can be increased with controlled mechanical hypoventilation to induce a respiratory acidosis, and with a low FIO_2 to induce alveolar hypoxia. Ventilation in room air may suffice, but occasionally a hypoxic gas mixture is necessary. This is achieved by the addition of nitrogen to the inspired gas mixture, reducing the FIO_2 to 0.17–0.19. While these maneuvers are often successful in increasing PVR and reducing pulmonary blood flow, it is important to remember that these patients have limited oxygen reserve and may desaturate suddenly and precipitously. Controlled hypoventilation in effect reduces the functional residual capacity of the lung and therefore oxygen reserve, which is also compromised by the use of a hypoxic inspired gas mixture. Inotropic support is often necessary because of

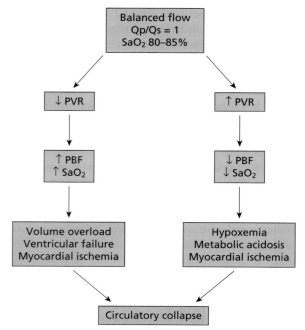

Figure 25.15 Effect of changes in PVR potentially contributing to circulatory collapse in patients with single-ventricle physiology. Qp, pulmonary blood flow; Qs, systemic blood flow; SaO₂, arterial oxygen saturation; PBF, pulmonary blood flow; PVR, pulmonary vascular resistance.

ventricular dysfunction secondary to the increased volume load. Systemic afterload reduction with agents such as phosphodiesterase inhibitors may improve systemic perfusion, although they may also decrease PVR and thus not correct the imbalance of pulmonary and systemic flow. Patients who have continued pulmonary overcirculation with high SaO_2 and reduced systemic perfusion despite the above maneuvers require early surgical intervention to control pulmonary blood flow. At the time of surgery, a snare may be placed around either branch pulmonary artery to effectively limit pulmonary blood flow. Monitoring the SVC O_2 saturation, as a measure of mixed-venous O_2 saturation and therefore cardiac output, is often useful in patients with single-ventricle physiology. For instance, a patient with too much pulmonary blood flow may have an arterial O_2 saturation that is high (i.e. >85%), but a low SVC O_2 saturation (i.e. <50%) if systemic perfusion and cardiac output are reduced. Monitoring changes in the SVC O_2 saturation during treatment is a useful guide to the adequacy of management. In contrast, a patient who is hypoxic with a low arterial O_2 saturation (i.e. <75%) but has a normal arterial-SVC O_2 saturation difference of 25–30% can be assumed to have an adequate cardiac output and other causes for hypoxemia need to be evaluated.

Decreased Qp/Qs

Decreased pulmonary blood flow, i.e. Qp/Qs <1, in patients with a single ventricle and parallel circulation is reflected by hypoxemia with an SaO_2 <80%. Preoperatively this may be due to restricted flow across a small ductus arteriosus, increased PVR secondary to parenchymal lung disease, or increased pulmonary venous pressure secondary to obstructed pulmonary venous drainage or a restrictive atrial septal defect. Initial resuscitation involves maintaining patency of the ductus arteriosus with a PGE1 infusion at a rate of 0.025–0.05 µg/kg/min. Most patients require tracheal intubation and mechanical ventilation either because of apnea secondary to PGE1 or for manipulation of gas exchange to assist balancing pulmonary and systemic flow. Systemic blood pressure, and therefore perfusion pressure across the ductus arteriosus, is maintained with the use of volume and vasopressor agents. Sedation, paralysis, and manipulation of mechanical ventilation to maintain an alkalosis may be effective if PVR is elevated. Nitric oxide as a specific pulmonary vasodilator may also be of use in this situation. Systemic oxygen delivery is maintained by improving cardiac output and red blood cell transfusions are performed to maintain a hematocrit >40%. Interventional cardiac catheterization with balloon septostomy or dilation of a restrictive atrial septal defect may be necessary; however, early surgical intervention and palliation with a systemic-to-pulmonary artery shunt are usually indicated.

Anesthesia considerations

A thorough preoperative assessment is essential to assess the balance of pulmonary and systemic flow, presence of cardiac failure, and possible end-organ injury from reduced systemic perfusion. A spontaneously breathing patient who is well balanced prior to surgery may readily become unbalanced after induction of anesthesia and when mechanically ventilated. The arterial oxygen saturation usually rises once the patient is anesthetized and paralyzed, due to a rise in mixed-venous oxygen saturation from reduced peripheral O_2 extraction, and improved cardiac output secondary to reduced myocardial work and afterload on the ventricle. However, PVR may fall as well, leading to an increase in pulmonary blood flow at the expense of systemic perfusion. Hypotension and a fall in diastolic blood pressure may be evident. In this circumstance, it is important to maintain a low inspired O_2 concentration and ventilate with a low rate and tidal volume to maintain a mild respiratory acidosis. Close monitoring of the arterial blood gas is important, with the ideal being a pH 7.40, PaO_2 40 mmHg and $PaCO_2$ 40 mmHg. If non-invasively monitored, an SaO_2 of 75–85% and end-tidal CO_2 of 40–45 mmHg are usually appropriate.

It is very important that patients be deeply anesthetized to minimize hemodynamic changes, in particular

Table 25.7 Parallel circulation physiology: management considerations

Clinical circumstance	Etiology	Management
Balanced flow SaO$_2$ 80–85% and normotensive	Qp = Qs ~ 1.0	No intervention
Overcirculated SaO$_2$ > 90% and low blood pressure	Qp ≫ Qs Low PVR Large aortopulmonary shunt size (PDA or B-T shunt) **Clinical signs** Wide pulse pressure Poor peripheral perfusion Congestive heart failure Oliguria **Laboratory** Metabolic acidosis Low SvO$_2$ saturation Increased (SaO$_2$–SvO$_2$) difference	**Raise PVR** Controlled hypoventilation Low FiO$_2$ (0.17–0.19) **Increase systemic perfusion** Afterload reduction Inotrope support Treat hypertension **Surgical intervention** Shunt revision
Undercirculated SaO$_2$ < 75% and normal/elevated blood pressure	Qp < Qs High PVR Small or occluded aortopulmonary shunt **Clinical signs** Cyanosis Narrow pulse pressure Myocardial ischemia Loss of murmur (late) **Laboratory** Metabolic acidosis Normal (SaO$_2$–SvO$_2$) difference	**Lower PVR** Controlled hyperventilation Alkalosis Reduce stress response Pulmonary vasodilation **Increase cardiac output** Raise systemic blood pressure Inotrope support **Increase mixed venous O$_2$** Hematocrit > 40% Sedation/anesthesia/paralysis **Surgical intervention** Shunt revision
Low cardiac output SaO$_2$ < 75% and hypotension	Ventricular failure Myocardial ischemia **Clinical signs** Poor peripheral perfusion Oliguria/anuria Narrow pulse pressure **Laboratory** Metabolic acidosis Low SvO$_2$ saturation Increased (SaO$_2$–SvO$_2$) difference	**Ventricular support** Maximize inotrope support Optimize preload Open sternum Minimize stress response **Surgical revision** Aortic arch and coronary anastomosis; transplantation **Mechanical support of the circulation**

Qp , pulmonary blood flow; Qs , systemic blood flow; SaO$_2$, arterial oxygen saturation; SvO$_2$, SVC oxygen saturation; PVR, pulmonary vascular resistance; FiO$_2$, inspired oxygen concentration; PDA, patent ductus arteriosus; B-T, Blalock-Taussig; SVC, superior vena cava.

tachycardia, in response to surgical stimulation. If the patient is overcirculated (i.e. Qp > Qs) and has a low diastolic blood pressure, coronary perfusion may not increase sufficiently to meet the increased demand of myocardial work in response to surgical stress. Myocardial ischemia may therefore occur, usually manifest as ST segment changes on the ECG or sudden onset of dysrhythmias, in particular ventricular fibrillation.

Staged single ventricle repair/Fontan procedure

The "reparative" operation for infants with single ventricles is a modified Fontan procedure. Glenn [179] demonstrated in patients with tricuspid atresia that SVC blood could be directed into the lungs without passing through the heart, and Fontan and associates extended this concept to include blood returning from the inferior vena cava [187,188]. Since the original description, the Fontan procedure and subsequent modifications have been successfully used to treat a wide range of simple and complex single-ventricle congenital heart defects [189]. The repair is "physiological" in that the systemic and pulmonary circulations are separated, or in "series," after directing the systemic venous return directly to the pulmonary artery and patients are no longer cyanosed. However, based on longer-term outcome data, significant problems and complications may develop over time and the repair should perhaps be viewed as palliative rather than curative.

The Fontan procedure has undergone numerous modifications since the first description [189]. The original procedure was described by Fontan in a patient with tricuspid atresia, and involved disconnecting the pulmonary arteries from each other, creating a classic Glenn shunt, connecting the right atrium directly to the left pulmonary artery (PA) using a valved conduit and placing a valve at the IVC–RA junction [187]. It was believed the RA would function as a pumping chamber; however, following the development of echocardiography, it was apparent that the RA functioned primarily as a conduit with little pumping action contributing to pulmonary blood flow, and in the low-pressure venous system, the valves remained opened. Further, this procedure was complicated in the long term by a high risk of pleuro-pericardial effusions and atrial dysrhythmias secondary to the effects of RA hypertension and distension.

An early modification involved the direct anastomosis of the RA appendage to the PA, closing the ASD and patching over the tricuspid valve, if patent [190]. This procedure, however, continued to have a high risk of complications related to RA hypertension.

Over the past 15 years, the total cavopulmonary anastomoses have become the modified Fontan procedure of preference. The SVC is anastomosed directly to the PA and a lateral tunnel created in the RA, baffling IVC flow

to the SVC [191]. This was associated with an improvement in mortality, although morbidity related to baffle hypertension persisted [192–194].

A significant advance was the creation of a fenestration or small hole in the intracardiac baffle, thereby creating an opportunity for a right-to-left atrial shunt. This fenestration is generally "fixed" in size at the time of surgery using a small 4 mm punch [171]. In the event of an increase in RA or PA pressure with reduced flow across the pulmonary vascular bed, and therefore less preload to the systemic ventricle, patients are able to shunt right to left across the fenestration. While patients develop increased cyanosis, cardiac output is maintained. This proved to be very successful and has enabled patients at relatively high risk to undergo a successful modified Fontan procedure [192,195]. While the early mortality has declined further since the introduction of fenestration techniques, the most significant improvement has been in patient morbidity. The incidence of early pleuro-pericardial effusions, ascites (Fig. 25.16) and atrial dysrhythmias has been significantly reduced. The fenestration can be test balloon occluded and easily closed in the cardiac catheterization laboratory with a clamshell device later in the postoperative period.

More recently, the use of an external conduit baffling the IVC to the pulmonary circulation has been reported [196]. A fenestration can be created between the external conduit and RA, if necessary. The major advantage in the immediate postoperative period is that the procedure can be completed on CPB without needing to arrest the heart. In the long term, the risk of atrial dysrhythmias may be reduced because of a lower RA pressure, absence of extensive atrial suture lines and anastomoses that are away from the sinoatrial node arterial supply.

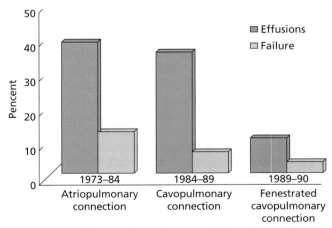

Figure 25.16 Incidence of pleural effusions and failure (i.e. take-down or mortality) during the early surgical evolution of the modified Fontan procedure at Children's Hospital, Boston. Modified from Castaneda AR. From Glenn to Fontan: a continuing evolution. Circulation 1992; 86: 1180 with permission from Lippincott, Williams & Wilkins.

Selection crtieria

Fontan and others originally listed a number of selection criteria that were considered important determinants for a successful early outcome, including age between 4 and 15 years, low PVR (<4 Wood U/m^2), mean pulmonary artery pressure <20 mmHg, systemic ventricle ejection fraction >0.6, normal sinus rhythm, normal atrioventricular valve function, and normal systemic and pulmonary venous drainage [188]. Patients with a diagnosis of tricuspid atresia who meet these criteria had a mortality rate of less than 5% from this procedure [197]. Modifications to these criteria have subsequently been made over the years as experience and surgical techniques have evolved [198,199]. The modified Fontan procedure is now preferably performed in children under 2–4 years of age to enable earlier correction of chronic hypoxemia and to limit the potential longer-term complications associated with prior palliation. The Fontan procedure has also been successfully performed in selected patients greater than 15 years with CHD who have appropriate hemodynamics despite long-term palliation. Unobstructed flow across the pulmonary vascular bed is essential. A mean PA pressure <15 mmHg and a PVR <2 Wood U/m^2 are preferable, as they have been associated with a lower early mortality [200]. Diastolic dysfunction of the ventricle with an elevated end-diastolic pressure (e.g. >12 mmHg) secondary to increased myocardial mass or outflow obstruction is an important consideration which could increase postoperative risk; a higher SVC and PA pressure will be necessary to maintain the transpulmonary gradient and therefore pulmonary blood flow in this situation.

Bidirectional Glenn or cavopulmonary connection

The benefits of a series circuit in patients with single-ventricle physiology include improved systemic oxygenation and a reduction in the obligatory diastolic load borne by the ventricle that is simultaneously asked to fill systemic and pulmonary circuits (parallel circulation). The compensatory ventricular dilation that must occur in a parallel circuit places the ventricle at an unfavorable position on the Starling curve and over time will lead to progressive ventricular dysfunction. As previously noted, the increase in ventricular end-diastolic volume, and eventually end-diastolic pressure, may significantly compromise the Fontan physiology and effective pulmonary blood flow [201]. Therefore, early palliation and relief of any volume-load from the systemic ventricle is an important interim step in the staged management of patients with single-ventricle physiology. For most patients, this can be achieved by performing a bidirectional cavopulmonary connection or bidirectional Glenn (BDG) procedure during infancy, commonly around 3–6 months of age. The volume and pressure load is relieved from the systemic ventricle, but effective pulmonary blood flow is maintained and the chance of a successful conversion to a complete cavopulmonary anastomosis or modified Fontan procedure is improved.

After a bidirectional Glenn procedure, the Qp/Qs is reduced as the source of pulmonary blood flow is from the superior vena cava only. At the time of surgery, the azygous vein is usually ligated to prevent decompression of venous drainage from the SVC to veins below the diaphragm and the inferior vena cava, which could contribute to a lower arterial oxygen saturation. Following the BDG, the arterial oxygen saturation should be in the 80–85% range, and preload to the systemic ventricle maintained by mixing of pulmonary venous blood with systemic venous blood returning via the inferior vena cava to the common atrium. As the volume output of the ventricle must meet only the demands of the systemic circulation, the end-diastolic volume (EDV) is therefore substantially reduced. As the EDV decreases, an alteration in ventricular geometry takes place. In some children, the resulting small, hypertrophic ventricle exhibits diastolic dysfunction that was not present at higher EDV [201,202]. In other children, subaortic obstruction may appear across a bulboventricular foramen that was unobstructed in the preoperative state.

The BDG is usually performed on CPB using mild hypothermia with a beating heart. The complications related to CPB and aortic cross-clamping are therefore minimal, and patients can be weaned and extubated in the early postoperative period [183]. Systemic hypertension is common following the BDG procedure. The etiology remains to be determined, but possible factors include improved contractility and stroke volume after the volume load on the ventricle is removed, and brainstem-mediated mechanisms secondary to the increased systemic and cerebral venous pressure. Treatment with vasodilators may be necessary.

Ideal physiology immediately following the Fontan procedure

The maintenance of effective pulmonary blood flow and cardiac output following the Fontan procedure depends on the pressure gradient between the pulmonary artery and the pulmonary venous atrium. The factors contributing to a successful cavopulmonary connection are shown in Table 25.8. A systemic venous pressure of 10–15 mmHg and a left atrial pressure of 5–10 mmHg, i.e. a transpulmonary gradient of 5–10 mmHg, are ideal.

Intravascular volume must be maintained and hypovolemia treated promptly. Venous capacitance is increased and as patients rewarm and vasodilate following surgery, a significant volume requirement is not unusual. If the stated selection criteria are followed, patients undergoing a modified Fontan procedure will have a low PVR without labile pulmonary hypertension. Therefore,

Table 25.8 Management considerations following a modified Fontan procedure

	Aim	Management
Baffle pressure 10–15 mm Hg	Unobstructed venous return	→ or ↑ Preload
		Low intrathoracic pressure
Pulmonary circulation	PVR < 2 Wood units/m^2 Mean PAp < 15 mmHg Unobstructed pulmonary vessels	Avoid increases in PVR, such as from acidosis, hypo- and hyperinflation of the lung, hypothermia, and excess sympathetic stimulation Early resumption of spontaneous respiration
Left atrium pressure 5–10 mm Hg	Sinus rhythm	Maintain sinus rhythm,
	Competent AV valve	→ or ↑ HR to increase CO
	Ventricle:	→ or ↓ afterload
	Normal diastolic function	→ or ↑ contractility
	Normal systolic function	
	No outflow obstruction	PDE inhibitors useful because of vasodilation, inotropic and lusitropic properties

PVR, pulmonary vuscular resistance; PAp, pulmonary artery pressure; AV, atrioventricular; HR, heart ratio; CO, Cardiac output; PDE, phosphodiesterase; →, maintain/normal; ↑, increase; ↓, decrease.

vigorous hyperventilation and induction of a respiratory and/or metabolic alkalosis to further reduce PVR are often of little benefit in this group of patients; conversely, the increase in mechanical ventilation requirements to induce a respiratory alkalosis may have an adverse effect on pulmonary blood flow. A normal pH and PaCO$_2$ of 40 mmHg should be the goal and, depending on the amount of right-to-left shunt across the fenestration, the arterial oxygen saturation is usually in the 80–90% range. However, PVR may increase following surgery, particularly secondary to an acidosis, hypothermia, atelectasis, hypoventilation, vasoactive drug infusions, and stress response.

Any acidosis must be treated promptly. If the cause is respiratory, ventilation must be adjusted. A metabolic acidosis reflects poor cardiac output, and while correction with bicarbonate may be necessary in the short term to reduce the associated increase in PVR, treatment should be directed at the potential causes, including reduced preload to the systemic ventricle, poor contractility, increased afterload and loss of sinus rhythm.

The beneficial effect of spontaneous ventilation on the hemodynamics of Fontan patients has been largely overstated [203]. While large instantaneous increases in pulmonary blood flow are seen in Fontan patients with normal inspiration, the incremental improvement in flow associated with normal inspiration is quite modest when considered over the entire respiratory cycle. In fact, in adult total cavopulmonary connection (TCPC) patients approximately 30% of systemic venous flow to the pul-

monary arteries is respiratory dependent as compared to 15% in normal two-ventricle patients. Furthermore, while inspiration augments pulmonary flow in TCPC patients, aortic blood flow (cardiac output) is actually higher during expiration. This is identical to the response seen in normal two-ventricle patients. In normal patients this is due to the fact that interventricular dependence results in the inspiratory increase in RV end-diastolic volume and stroke volume, simultaneously reducing LV end-diastolic volume and stroke volume. In TCPC patients in whom interventricular dependence is not a factor, it is due to the pulmonary vasculature serving as a large-volume reservoir.

Given the effects of negative intrathoracic pressure on pulmonary blood flow, the effects of positive pressure ventilation (PPV) on Fontan hemodynamics are of concern. Unfortunately, the effects on Fontan hemodynamics of PPV as compared to spontaneous ventilation have never been systematically evaluated. However, because pulmonary blood flow occurs throughout the respiratory cycle, employing a ventilation strategy that minimizes mean airway pressure is a more rational, physiologically based approach. Available evidence suggests that a near-linear inverse relationship exists between mean airway pressure and cardiac index. The use of PEEP continues to be debated. The beneficial effects of an increase in FRC, maintenance of lung volume and redistribution of lung water need to be balanced against the possible detrimental effect of an increase in mean intrathoracic pressure. A PEEP of 3–5 cmH$_2$0, however, rarely has hemodynamic consequences or substantial effects on effective pulmonary blood flow [204–208].

Non-specific pulmonary vasodilators such as sodium nitroprusside, nitroglycerine, PGE1 and prostacyclin have been used to dilate the pulmonary vasculature in an effort to improve pulmonary blood flow after a Fontan procedure. The results are variable, however. While PVR may fall, pulmonary blood flow could also increase as a result of reduced ventricular end-diastolic pressure and improved ventricular function secondary to the fall in systemic afterload. The response to inhaled NO is also variable and the improvement may relate to changes in ventilation/perfusion matching rather than a direct fall in PVR.

An elevated left atrial pressure may reflect systolic or diastolic ventricular dysfunction, atrioventricular valve regurgitation or stenosis, and loss of sinus rhythm with cannon "a" waves that raise left atrial pressure. Afterload stress is poorly tolerated after a modified Fontan procedure because of the increase in myocardial wall tension and end-diastolic pressure. Although pulmonary blood flow is phasic to a certain extent, a substantial proportion of flow occurs during diastole as well. The diastolic or relaxation characteristics of the ventricle play a significant role in the volume of pulmonary blood flow and, hence, the preload accepted by the ventricle. Therefore, low cardiac output accompanies diastolic dysfunction.

Therapeutic manipulations are not always successful in reversing this dysfunction once it is manifest. The right-sided filling pressure must be increased to maintain the transpulmonary gradient, and treatment with inotropes and vasodilators initiated. Despite the temptation to use them in low cardiac output states, the addition of inotropes may not improve hemodynamics and may actually worsen diastolic relaxation if large doses of drugs such as epinephrine are used. One should scrupulously maintain or augment circulating volume to avoid additional reductions in EDV. The phosphodiesterase inhibitor milrinone is particularly beneficial. Besides being a weak inotrope with pulmonary and systemic vasodilating properties, its lusitropic action will assist by improving diastolic relaxation and lowering ventricular end-diastolic pressure, thereby improving effective pulmonary blood flow and cardiac output. If a severe low output state with acidosis persists, take-down of the modified Fontan operation and conversion to a BDG anastomosis or other palliative procedure are life saving.

Early postoperative complications after the Fontan procedure

Not all patients require a fenestration for a successful, uncomplicated Fontan operation. Those with ideal preoperative hemodynamics often maintain an adequate pulmonary blood flow and cardiac output without requiring a right-to-left shunt across the baffle. Similarly, not all Fontan patients who have received a fenestration will use it to shunt right to left in the immediate postoperative period. These patients are fully saturated following surgery, and may have an elevated right-sided filling pressure, but nevertheless maintain an adequate cardiac output. The problem is predicting which patients are at risk for low cardiac output after a Fontan procedure, and who will benefit from placement of a fenestration; even patients with ideal preoperative hemodynamics may manifest a significant low-output state after surgery. Because of this, essentially all patients have a fenestrated Fontan procedure at Children's Hospital, Boston. Premature closure of the fenestration may occur in the immediate postoperative period, leading to a low cardiac output state with progressive metabolic acidosis and large chest drain losses from high right-sided venous pressures. Patients may respond to volume replacement, inotrope support and vasodilation; however, if hypotension and acidosis persist, cardiac catheterization and removal of thrombus or dilation of the fenestration may need to be urgently undertaken [209] (Table 25.9).

Arterial O_2 saturation levels may vary substantially following a modified Fontan procedure. Common causes of persistent arterial O_2 desaturation <75% include a poor cardiac output with a low mixed-venous O_2, a large right-to-left shunt across the fenestration or additional "leak" in the baffle pathway producing more shunting. An intrapulmonary shunt, and venous admixture from decompressing vessels draining either from the PA to the systemic venous circulation or systemic vein to the pulmonary venous system are additional causes [210]. Re-evaluation with echocardiography and cardiac catheterization may be necessary.

The incidence of recurrent pleural effusions and ascites has decreased since introduction of the fenestrated baffle [211]. Nevertheless, for some patients this remains a major problem with associated respiratory compromise, hypovolemia and possible hypoproteinemia [212]. Usually secondary to persistent elevation of systemic venous pressure, re-evaluation with cardiac catheterization may be indicated.

Atrial flutter and/or fibrillation, heart block, and, less commonly, ventricular dysrhythmia may have a significant impact on immediate recovery, as well as long-term outcome. Sudden loss of sinus rhythm initially causes an increase in left atrial and ventricular end-diastolic pressure, and fall in cardiac output. The SVC or PA pressure must be increased, usually with volume replacement, to maintain the transpulmonary gradient. Prompt treatment with antiarrhythmic drugs, pacing or cardioversion is necessary.

Table 25.9 Circumstances, etiology and treatment strategies for patients with low cardiac output immediately following the Fontan procedure

Circumstance	Etiology	Treatment
Increased TPG:		
Baffle > 20 mm Hg	Inadequate pulmonary blood flow and preload	Volume replacement
LAp < 10 mm Hg	to left atrium:	Reduce PVR
TPG increased >> 10 mm Hg	Increased PVR	Correct acidosis
Clinical state:	Pulmonary artery stenosis	Inotrope support
High SaO$_2$/low SvO$_2$	Pulmonary vein stenosis	Systemic vasodilation
Hypotension/tachycardia	Premature fenestration closure	Catheter or surgical intervention
Poor peripheral perfusion		
SVC syndrome with pleural effusions and		
increased chest tube drainage		
Ascites/hepatomegaly		
Metabolic acidosis		
Normal TPG:		
Baffle > 20 mm Hg	Ventricular failure:	Maintain preload
LAp > 15 mm Hg	Systolic dysfunction	Inotrope support
TPG normal 5–10 mm Hg	Diastolic dysfunction	Systemic vasodilation
Clinical slate:	AV valve regurgitation and/or stenosis	Establish sinus rhythm or AV synchrony
Low SaO$_2$/low SvO$_2$	Loss of sinus rhythm	Correct acidosis
Hypotension/tachycardia	Afterload stress	Mechanical support
Poor peripheral perfusion		Surgical intervention, including takedown to
Metabolic acidosis		BDG and transplantation

LAp, left atrial pressure; TPG, transpulmonary gradient; SaO$_2$, systemic arterial oxygen saturation; SvO$_2$, SVC oxygen saturation; SVC, superior vena cava; PVR, pulmonary vascular resistance; AV, atrioventricular; BDG, bidirectional Glenn anastomosis.

Anesthetic considerations for patients following a Fontan procedure

There are no prospective studies that have evaluated the effects of specific anesthetic techniques and drugs in patients with Fontan physiology. Anesthetic management will vary on a case-by-case basis according to the functional and clinical status of each patient, and the specific complications unique to the Fontan procedure. An increasing hazard function for failure or reintervention, a late decline in functional status and 15-year survival between 60% and 73% have been reported on intermediate-to-late follow-up [213–215]. However, these figures include patients operated upon in the earlier surgical years, and with improved surgical techniques and patient selection, subsequent survival figures have improved [216,217].

Arrhythmias, in particular atrial flutter, sick sinus syndrome and heart block, have been reported in 20% or more of survivors 10 years following the Fontan procedure. The probability of freedom from atrial flutter has been reported as about 40% at 15 years post Fontan procedure, although these data include patients from different surgical eras [218]. Predisposing factors include surgery involving the atrium with extensive suture lines, disrupted sinoatrial node blood supply, and chronic atrial distension. In addition, older age at Fontan operation, longer duration of follow-up, and type of surgical procedure are associated with an increased incidence of atrial flutter after Fontan operation. Patients with recurrent arrhythmias are often treated with long-term antiarrhythmic drugs, present for repeat cardioversions and may undergo radiofrequency ablation of re-entrant flutter pathways [173,219,220]. There are no recommendations at this time for prophylactic antiarrhythmic drugs, such as digoxin or amiodarone, prior to anesthesia for noncardiac surgery but it is important that facilities for immediate external cardiac pacing or cardioversion are readily available in the operating room for these patients.

There is an increased incidence of thromboembolism in patients who have undergone the Fontan procedure, but the routine use of long-term anticoagulation remains controversial. The actual incidence of thromboembolism is difficult to determine because of the heterogeneous patient population. A large retrospective review of 645 patients who underwent the Fontan procedure at Children's Hospital, Boston, over a 15-year period, between 1978 and 1993, described 17 patients (2.6%) who suffered a stroke following the Fontan procedure, presumed secondary to a thromboembolic event [221]. The nature of the Fontan circulation with increased venous pressure and stasis of flow through the right atrial baffle, atrial dysrhythmias, alterations in pro- and anticoagulant factors and possible increased resting venous tone in this population of patients, are all contributing factors [222,223]. The role of prophylactic anticoagulant therapy in congenital heart disease in general, and the Fontan population in particular, is poorly defined. Antiplatelet therapy with aspirin is commonly used in the immediate and early postoperative period, although the benefit of long-term use has not been evaluated. In high-risk patients, and those who have had previous thrombus formation, coumadin therapy for an extended period is recommended. Patients with Fontan physiology may be at increased risk for deep venous thrombosis, or thrombus formation within the Fontan baffle or atrial appendage following non-cardiac surgery. Prophylactic subcutaneous heparin should be considered for older Fontan patients undergoing non-cardiac procedures, and patients should be kept well hydrated and mobilized early after surgery.

Protein-losing enteropathy (PLE) has been reported in 3–14% of Fontan patients on long-term follow-up [224]. Defined as persistent hypoalbuminemia (<3.0 mg/dL) in the absence of liver and renal disease, associated clinical features include abdominal pain, diarrhea, edema and ascites. Patients frequently have limited hemodynamic reserve with increased systemic venous pressure, decreased cardiac index and increased end-diastolic ventricular pressure.

Most patients with stable single-ventricle physiology subjectively report that they are able to lead relatively normal lives with moderate exercise tolerance. Nevertheless, deterioration in function according to New York Heart Association classification has been reported over longer follow-up [225,226]. Objective evaluation with exercise testing demonstrates the limited cardiorespiratory reserve of many Fontan patients [225,226]. The implications of these findings for subsequent anesthetics have not been studied, but the response to exercise testing may be useful for assessing a patient's ability to tolerate the stress of anesthesia and surgery. Compared to normal control subjects, those with Fontan physiology frequently demonstrate a reduced maximal exercise workload, less endurance, take longer to recover after stopping exercise and have a lower anaerobic threshold and maximal oxygen consumption. A fall in arterial oxygen saturation and an increase in arteriovenous oxygen saturation difference is common because of the suboptimal increase in cardiac index [227]. The inability to increase effective pulmonary blood flow and stroke volume during strenuous exercise underscores the importance of the pulmonary vascular bed in determining ventricular filling and the dependence upon heart rate to increase cardiac output.

Intraoperative monitoring during major surgery needs careful planning in patients with Fontan physiology.

Placement of a central venous line into the SVC will enable monitoring of systemic venous return, pulmonary artery pressure and mixed venous oxygen saturation. An important consideration, however, is the risk of thrombosis and obstruction to venous return. Cardiac catheterization may be indicated prior to surgery if there has been a change in symptoms or deterioration in function. In particular, prior to major surgery and if significant fluid shifts are anticipated, performing a hemodynamic study immediately prior to surgery is often beneficial. Besides being able to assess baseline hemodynamics, a balloon-tipped catheter can be wedged in a pulmonary capillary to measure the transpulmonary gradient. Positioning the catheter using pressure waveforms alone is difficult because there is no pulsatile arterial pressure waveform and the balloon may not readily float out to a lung segment. Placement under direct vision using fluoroscopy is preferable. Attempted measurement of cardiac output using thermodilution will also be inaccurate.

Tetralogy of Fallot
Pathophysiology
The four anatomical features of tetralogy of Fallot include a VSD, right ventricular outflow tract obstruction, overriding of the aorta, and right ventricular hypertrophy. In addition, there may also be VSDs of the muscular region of the septum and right-sided obstruction of the pulmonary valve and the main and branch pulmonary arteries.

The resistance to right ventricular outflow forces systemic venous return right to left across the ventricular septal defect (complex shunt) and into the aorta, producing arterial desaturation (Fig. 25.17). Pulmonary blood flow is less than systemic flow. The amount of blood that shunts right to left through the ventricular septal defect varies with the magnitude of the right ventricular outflow tract obstruction and with the SVR. Distal pulmonary vascular resistance is low and has minimal influence on shunting. Systemic vasodilation, in conjunction with increasing dynamic infundibular stenosis, intensifies right-to-left shunting and therefore hypoxemia, producing hypercyanotic "spells." Such spells can occur at any time before surgical correction of the anomalies and can be life threatening. Their treatment is outlined below. Because the morbidity associated with recurrent hypercyanotic spells is significant, many physicians consider recurrent episodes of hypercyanosis to be an indication for corrective surgery at any age.

Anesthetic management
The surgical approach to TOF may involve either an early or delayed repair. The delayed repair in a symptomatic neonate requires early palliation with a systemic-to-pulmonary artery shunt to prevent hypercyanotic episodes,

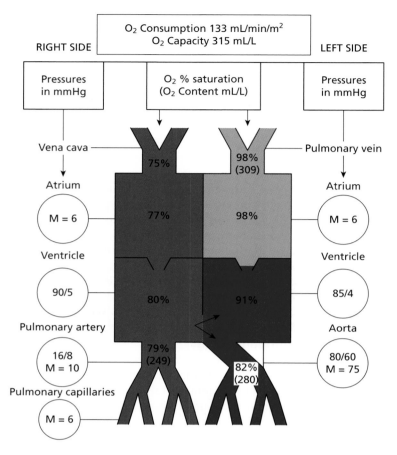

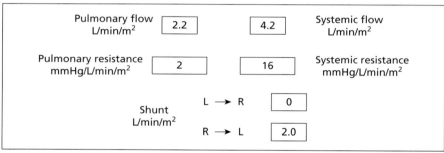

Figure 25.17 Catheterization findings in a patient with tetralogy of Fallot. Reproduced with permission from Nadas AS, Fyler DC. Pediatric Cardiology. Philadelphia: WB Saunders, 1972.

followed by a transatrial and transpulmonary artery repair after 3 months of age [228]. Excellent outcome has been achieved with this approach and the need for a transpulmonary valve annulus outflow patch (transannular patch) at the time of surgery is reduced. More recently, aggressive efforts to preserve the RV outflow tract and pulmonary valve have been used, given the long-term consequences of pulmonary regurgitation and arrhythmogenic scar tissue in the right ventricular outflow tract (RVOT) in this population [229]. Some continue to argue that the risks of cyanosis and complications related to a systemic-to-pulmonary artery shunt argue for an

early complete repair of TOF regardless of symptoms [230]. This may be performed in the neonate or young infant depending upon the degree of obstruction and arterial oxygen saturation level. Complete repair in neonates and young infants more often requires a transventricular approach to close the VSD, with pericardial augmentation of the RVOT. A ventriculotomy is performed in the RVOT and is frequently extended distally through the pulmonary valve annulus and beyond any associated pulmonary artery stenosis. The outflow tract is then enlarged with pericardium or synthetic material, and obstructing muscle bundles are resected to relieve the outflow tract obstruction. Pulmonary regurgitation results after a transannular incision that may compromise ventricular function in the postoperative period. In approximately 8% of patients, abnormalities in the origin and distribution of the coronary arteries preclude placement of the right ventricular outflow patch [231,232], making it necessary to bypass the stenosis by placing an external conduit from the body of the right ventricle to the pulmonary artery.

Anesthetic management of these patients should maintain systemic vascular resistance, minimize pulmonary vascular resistance, and avoid myocardial depression. Hypercyanotic spells in non-anesthetized children are traditionally treated initially with 100% oxygen by facemask, a knee–chest position, and morphine sulfate. This regimen usually causes the dynamic infundibular stenosis to relax while maintaining systemic resistance. Deeply cyanotic and lethargic patients are given IV crystalloid infusions to augment circulating blood volume. Continued severe hypoxemia is treated with a vasopressor (e.g. phenylephrine 1–2 µg/kg) to increase SVR, and sometimes by judicious use of IV propranolol or esmolol to slow the heart rate; the latter allows more filling time and relaxes the infundibulum. If a hypercyanotic spell persists despite treatment, immediate surgical correction of the anomaly is indicated. The child can be anesthetized with IV opioids and an inhalation agent may be beneficial to reduce hyperdynamic outflow tract obstruction. Anesthetic agents that predominantly decrease SVR should be used with caution. The pattern of mechanical ventilation is critical as excessive inspiratory pressure or short expiratory times will increase the mean intrathoracic pressure and further reduce antegrade flow across the RV outflow.

When weaning patients from CPB following tetralogy repair, the aim of therapy is to support right ventricular function and minimize afterload on the RV. This is particularly important following repair in neonates or small infants. While systolic dysfunction of the RV may occur following neonatal ventriculotomy, more commonly the clinical picture is one of a "restrictive physiology" reflecting reduced RV compliance or diastolic function [233,234]. Factors contributing to diastolic dysfunction include ventriculotomy, lung and myocardial edema following CPB, inadequate myocardial protection of the hypertrophied ventricle during aortic cross-clamp, coronary artery injury, residual outflow tract obstruction, volume load on the ventricle from a residual VSD or pulmonary regurgitation and dysrhythmias.

Patients usually separate from CPB with a satisfactory blood pressure and atrial filling pressures <10mmHg on inotrope support, such as dopamine 5–10µg/kg/min. However, in neonates during the first 6–12 h after surgery, a low cardiac output state with increased right-sided filling pressures from diastolic dysfunction is common following a right ventriculotomy, and continued sedation and paralysis are usually necessary for the first 24–48h to minimize the stress response and associated myocardial work. Preload must be maintained, despite elevation of the RA pressure. In addition to high right-sided filling pressures, pleural effusions and/or ascites may develop. Significant inotrope support is often required, and a phosphodiesterase inhibitor, such as amrinone or milrinone, is beneficial because of its lusitropic properties. Because of the restrictive defect, even a relatively small volume load from a residual VSD or pulmonary regurgitation is often poorly tolerated in the early postoperative period, and it may take 2–3 days before RV compliance improves following surgery and cardiac output increases. While the patent foramen ovale or any ASD is usually closed at the time of surgery in older patients, it is beneficial to leave a small atrial communication following neonatal repair. In the face of diastolic dysfunction and increased RV end-diastolic pressure, a right-to-left atrial shunt will maintain preload to the left ventricle and therefore cardiac output. Patients may be desaturated initially following surgery because of this shunting. As RV compliance and function improve, the amount of shunt decreases and both antegrade pulmonary blood flow and arterial oxygen saturation increase.

Arrhythmias following repair include heart block, ventricular ectopy and junctional ectopic tachycardia. It is important to maintain sinus rhythm to avoid additional diastolic dysfunction and an increase in end-diastolic pressure. Atrioventricular pacing may be necessary for heart block. Complete right bundle branch block is typical on the postoperative ECG.

Most patients recover systolic ventricular function postoperatively. However, there is a small group of patients, especially those repaired at older ages, in whom significant ventricular dysfunction remains. Pulmonary valve insufficiency may contribute to residual ventricular systolic dysfunction [235]. The most common cause of systolic dysfunction immediately after repair of CHD is a residual or unrecognized additional VSD [236,237] which causes a volume load on the left ventricle and pressure load on the hypertrophied right ventricle, leading to right ventricular failure and poor cardiac output. A residual VSD combined with a residual right ventricular outflow obstruction is particularly deleterious.

In some patients the distal pulmonary arteries may be so hypoplastic and stenotic that they cannot be satisfactorily corrected. Suprasystemic pressure develops in the right ventricle, which in some cases can be ameliorated by partially opening the VSD to allow an intracardiac right-to-left ventricular shunt. This shunt unloads the compromised right ventricle at the expense of decreased arterial oxygen saturation.

Anesthetic considerations after right ventricle outflow reconstruction

Reconstruction of the RV outflow tract may lead to significant problems that affect RV function and risk for arrhythmias over time. While most of the long-term outcome data pertain to patients following tetralogy of Fallot repair, similar complications and risks are also likely for those who have undergone an extensive RV outflow reconstruction, such as placement of a conduit from the right ventricle to the pulmonary artery for correction of pulmonary atresia, truncus arteriosus and the Rastelli procedure for transposition of the great arteries with pulmonary stenosis.

Complete surgical repair of TOF has been successfully performed for over 40 years, with recent studies reporting a 30–35-year actuarial survival of about 85%. Many patients report leading relatively normal lives, but RV dysfunction may progress after repair and may only be evident on exercise stress testing or echocardiography. A spectrum of problems may develop, ranging from a dilated RV with systolic dysfunction to diastolic dysfunction from a poorly compliant RV, and these need to be thoroughly evaluated preoperatively (Table 25.10). In addition, continued evaluation is necessary because of the increased risk of ventricular dysrhythmias and late sudden death. Factors that may adversely affect long-term survival include older age at initial repair, initial palliative procedures and residual chronic pressure and/or volume load such as from pulmonary insufficiency or stenosis [238,239].

Table 25.10 Long-term follow-up after tetralogy of Fallot repair: right ventricular function

Circumstance	Clinical
Systolic dysfunction: "nonrestrictive"	RV dilation: cardiomegaly
	Significant pulmonary regurgitation
	Volume overload: ↑ RVEDV, ↓ RV ejection fraction
	↓ Maximal exercise capacity and endurance
	↑ Risk for ventricular arrhythmias and possibly sudden death
Diastolic dysfunction: "restrictive"	↓ RV compliance: cardiomegaly less likely
	Limited pulmonary regurgitation
	↑ RVEDP, contractility maintained
	Improved exercise capacity
	Lower risk for ventricular dysrhythmias

RV, right ventricle; RVEDV, right ventricle end-diastolic volume; RVEDP, right ventricle end-diastolic pressure; ↑, increased; ↓, decreased.

Both RV and LV systolic dysfunction secondary to a residual volume load from pulmonary regurgitation (PR) after tetralogy repair are predictors of late morbidity [238,239]. There is also an association between RV dilation from PR and the risk of ventricular tachycardia (VT) and sudden death [240]. The consequences of chronic PR are reflected by cardiomegaly on chest x-ray, an increase in RV end-diastolic volume by echocardiography and on exercise testing as a reduction in anaerobic threshold, maximal exercise performance and endurance [241]. Patients who have significant pulmonary regurgitation and reduced RV function are at potential risk of a fall in cardiac output during anesthesia, particularly as positive pressure ventilation may increase the amount of regurgitation. Once again, it is difficult to predict those patients who are more likely to have instability during anesthesia for non-cardiac surgery; nor is it possible to formulate a "recipe" for anesthesia that will be suited to all patients. Nevertheless, preoperative exercise testing may provide some insight as to hemodynamic reserve.

An important group to distinguish are those patients who have restrictive physiology or diastolic dysfunction secondary to reduced ventricular compliance. They usually do not have cardiomegaly, demonstrate better exercise tolerance and the risk for ventricular dysrhythmias is possibly decreased. Although the RV is hypertrophied, function is generally well preserved on echocardiography with minimal pulmonary regurgitation [233].

The incidence of significant RV outflow obstruction developing over time is low. Residual obstruction contributes to early mortality within the first year after surgery, but is well tolerated in the long term. A gradient more than 40 mmHg across the RV outflow is uncommon and the pressure ratio between the RV and LV is usually less than 0.5. The gradient may become more significant with time, but as the progression is usually slow, RV dysfunction occurs late.

A wide variation in the incidence of ventricular ectopy has been reported in numerous follow-up studies, including up to 15% of patients on routine ECG and up to 75% of patients on Holter monitor. Multiple risk factors including an older age at repair, residual hemodynamic abnormalities, and duration of follow-up have all been considered important [173,220,240]. In common with these factors is probable myocardial injury and fibrosis from chronic pressure and volume overload, and cyanosis. While ventricular ectopy is common in asymptomatic patients during ambulatory ECG Holter monitoring and exercise stress testing, it is often low grade and has not identified those patients at risk for sudden death. Electrophysiological induction of sustained VT, especially when monomorphic, is suggestive of the presence of a re-entrant arrhythmic pathway. Although dependent on the stimulation protocol used to induce VT, the presence of monomorphic VT in a symptomatic patient with syncope and palpitations is significant and indicates treatment with radiofrequency ablation, surgical cryoablation, antiarrhythmic drugs or placement of an implantable cardioversion-defibrillator (ICD) [173,220,242]. The risk for ventricular dysrhythmias during anesthesia is unknown. While preoperative prophylaxis with antiarrhythmic drugs is not recommended, a means of external defibrillation and pacing must be readily available.

Pulmonary atresia
Pathophysiology
Atresia of the pulmonary valve or main pulmonary artery forms a spectrum of cardiac defects, the management of which depends on the extent of atresia, size of the RV and tricuspid valve (TV), presence of a VSD and collateral vessels, surface area of the pulmonary vascular bed and coronary artery anatomy. At birth, pulmonary blood flow is derived either from a PDA or from other aortopulmonary collateral blood vessels. These collaterals, which arise from the descending aorta and supply both lungs, may be extensive. The RV is usually hypertrophied, and a restrictive physiology is common during initial postoperative recovery.

At one end of the spectrum, critical pulmonary stenosis may exist with a variable degree of hypoplasia of the right ventricle, tricuspid valve, and pulmonary artery. There is no VSD. With critical pulmonic stenosis, only a pinhole orifice is present in the pulmonic valve, but the right ventricle is generally less hypoplastic than with pulmonary atresia. A fixed obligatory shunt of all systemic venous return occurs from the right to the left atrium, where blood mixes completely with pulmonary venous blood. Some blood may flow into the right ventricle, but because there is no outlet, blood regurgitates back across the tricuspid valve and eventually reaches the left atrium and left ventricle. Pulmonary blood flow is derived exclusively or predominantly from a PDA. These patients usually do not have extensive aortopulmonary collateral blood flow; consequently, they often become cyanotic when the PDA closes after birth. Critical pulmonary valve stenosis can be effectively treated by balloon dilation in the catheterization laboratory. Antegrade flow across the RV outflow may not improve immediately, but gradually increases over days as RV compliance improves.

Pulmonary valve atresia or short-segment main pulmonary artery atresia, with a VSD (PA/VSD) and normal-sized TV, RV and branch pulmonary arteries, is completely repaired in the neonate, usually involving placement of a pericardial patch to reconstruct the outflow tract. If there is long-segment pulmonary artery atresia, a homograft "conduit" is necessary to reconstruct the RV outflow. Conduits may be extrinsically compressed or kinked at the time of sternal closure, causing partial RV outflow obstruction or direct compression of a coronary artery leading to ischemia.

The intracardiac anatomy of tetralogy of Fallot with pulmonary atresia (TOF/PA) is similar to that of simple tetralogy of Fallot, but the right ventricular outflow tract is atretic. Because of the atretic right ventricular outflow tract, all systemic venous return courses right to left through the VSD. Therefore, complete mixing of pulmonary and systemic venous return occurs in the left ventricle and aorta, producing arterial hypoxemia. Infants with tetralogy of Fallot and associated pulmonary atresia regularly exhibit significant systemic-to-pulmonary collateral flow. If antegrade flow is established from the right ventricle into the main pulmonary artery by a reparative procedure, the left-to-right shunt via collateral flow will impose a diastolic load on the left ventricle. Preoperative occlusion of these collateral vessels can be accomplished by interventional techniques in the cardiac catheterization laboratory but may leave the child precariously cyanotic in the hours before operation. The most effective temporizing therapy is to reduce oxygen consumption (e.g. anesthesia, mechanical ventilation) and to increase the systemic perfusion pressure across other systemic-to-pulmonary communications.

Patients with pulmonary atresia, a ventricular septal defect, but small RV and TV may not tolerate a complete initial repair. The RV may be unable to cope with the entire cardiac output, resulting in a low output state and RV failure (see below). Alternative management strategies therefore include initial palliation with a shunt and/or RV outflow patch to improve pulmonary blood flow, or a repair of the outflow tract with fenestration of the VSD patch to enable a right-to-left shunt at that level. Two-ventricle repair may ultimately be limited by growth of the tricuspid valve. If the right ventricle subsequently grows, the shunt and the patent foramen ovale ASD and VSD can be closed surgically.

Patients with pulmonary atresia and an intact ventricular septum (PA/IVS) usually have a small RV and TV, which in general makes them unsuitable for a two-ventricle repair in the long term. Initial palliation with an aortopulmonary shunt is necessary; reconstruction of the RV outflow with a pericardial patch or conduit may also be considered if the RV is a sufficient size such that a two-ventricle repair could be considered. Prior to surgery, the coronary anatomy should be determined, usually by cardiac catheterization. A large conal branch or aberrant left coronary artery across the RV outflow tract may restrict the size of a ventriculotomy and placement of a patch or conduit. Patients with pulmonary atresia, a hypoplastic RV and intact ventricular septum may have numerous fistulous connections between the small hypertensive RV cavity and the coronary circulation [243,244]. A significant proportion of the myocardium may therefore be dependent upon coronary perfusion directly from the RV. If, in addition, there are proximal coronary artery stenoses restricting coronary perfusion from the aortic root, then decompression of the RV following reconstruction of the RV outflow tract can lead to myocardial infarction.

At the worst end of the spectrum, severe pulmonary atresia may be associated with a hypoplastic RV and diminutive pulmonary arteries that are not suitable for primary repair [245]. A palliative procedure with a B–T or central shunt is usually necessary at first to improve pulmonary blood flow, followed by staged single-ventricle repair (see Managing Fontan physiology).

Multiple aortopulmonary collateral arteries may be present, supplying some or all segments of the lung. They can be associated with a large left-to-right shunt, contributing to volume overload and pulmonary hypertension. Larger collateral vessels supplying significant portions of the lung can be anastomosed or "unifocalized" to the native pulmonary arteries, with the ultimate aim being to establish full antegrade pulmonary blood flow. Smaller vessels to some segments of lung can be coiled in the cardiac catheterization laboratory, provided there is antegrade flow from the native pulmonary arteries to those lung segments.

When the pulmonary arteries are very diminutive it is important to establish early antegrade flow from right ventricle to pulmonary artery, in an effort to promote growth and establish a pathway to the pulmonary arteries for subsequent balloon dilation. A B–T shunt may be necessary to provide sufficient pulmonary blood flow if the pulmonary arteries and right ventricle are small. Initially, the VSD can be left open, and postoperative management of cyanosis or CHF will be determined by the size of and the resistance offered by the pulmonary circuit. The course in these patients can be dynamic and demanding of the most experienced practitioners. When collaterals are occluded in the operating room and RV to diminutive pulmonary artery continuity is established, cyanosis may ensue and therapy is aimed at lowering PVR and/or (re)establishing adequate pulmonary blood flow. On the other hand, if the hemoglobin is fully saturated in the aorta with elevated pulmonary artery oxygen saturation and left atrial pressure, then a left-to-right shunt through the VSD may be developing, which will produce a volume load on the left ventricle and an unstable postoperative course, dictating VSD closure. When the patient is not fully saturated in the aorta but is suffering from a volume-loaded left ventricle with low cardiac output and high left atrial pressure postoperatively, excessive systemic-to-pulmonary collaterals may be the culprits, requiring catheterization laboratory investigation and occlusion or immediate reoperation.

Anesthetic management

Anesthetic management of patients with pulmonary atresia is similar to that for tetralogy of Fallot, except that hypercyanotic spells do not occur in the same fashion. Maintaining the patency of the ductus for the perioperative treatment of neonates with pulmonary atresia and critical pulmonary stenosis is essential. If the right ventricle is sufficiently well developed and the main pulmonary artery is present, it may be possible to perform a pulmonary valvotomy and provide adequate pulmonary blood flow without a supplemental systemic-to-pulmonary artery shunt. The goal of therapy is to improve oxygenation and decrease right ventricular afterload. Because the underdeveloped non-compliant right ventricle requires high filling pressures, consequently, there may be substantial right-to-left shunting through the foramen ovale, making these infants hypoxemic during the immediate postoperative period. With growth and improved compliance of the right ventricle, the right-to-left shunting diminishes and the infant's oxygenation improves substantially. If hypoxemia persists, a PGE1 infusion should be started to increase pulmonary blood flow through the ductus arteriosus while arrangements are made to surgically create a pulmonary artery–systemic artery shunt.

In patients with long-segment pulmonary atresia, the need for a conduit to bridge the gap between the right ventricle and the pulmonary artery complicates the repair. Again, right ventricular failure may occur postoperatively, especially when there is a residual VSD or an outflow obstruction. The conduit may obstruct acutely during chest closure, further elevating pressure in the right ventricle.

After the VSD is closed and blood flow is from the right ventricle to the pulmonary arteries, there may be excessive pulmonary blood flow (Qp/Qs >1) owing to the combined flow into the pulmonary arteries from the right ventricle and from aortopulmonary collaterals described above. If this occurs, the patient develops CHF and requires intraoperative inotropic support of the heart and an extended period of postoperative mechanical ventilation. With large collateral flows, the pulse pressure is large and diastolic pressure low. The patients may require surgery to ligate the collateral vessels or may require embolization.

Anesthetic considerations after repair

Patients with tetralogy of Fallot and pulmonary atresia are subject to the same late problems and complications as patients with tetralogy of Fallot alone. In addition, they may develop progressive conduit obstruction after surgery.

Tricuspid atresia
Pathology
In this condition an imperforate tricuspid valve and hypoplasia of the right ventricle are present, often accompanied by a VSD of variable size and by pulmonic stenosis. A fixed obligatory shunt of all systemic venous return occurs from the right atrium through the patent foramen ovale or ASD into the left atrium, where complete mixing takes place. The degree of hypoxemia depends on the amount of pulmonary blood flow, which is regulated by the severity of the pulmonic stenosis. The common presentation is characterized by significant hypoxemia caused by the decreased pulmonary blood flow induced by either a restrictive VSD or a severe pulmonic stenosis.

Anesthetic management
The reparative operation of choice for tricuspid atresia is a modified Fontan procedure, but a palliative procedure may initially be required to improve pulmonary blood flow. A pulmonary artery band may be needed if the pulmonary blood flow is increased, or a shunt may have to be created for the severely hypoxemic child with decreased pulmonary blood flow. The anesthetic management and complications are those discussed in the sections on shunts, banding, and modified Fontan procedures (see above). Complications of chronic hypoxemia and cyanosis are also present.

Transposition of the great arteries
Pathophysiology
With transposition of the great arteries, the right ventricle gives rise to the aorta (Fig. 25.18). Almost 50% of patients with this anomaly have a VSD, and some of them have a variable degree of subpulmonic stenosis (see Fig. 25.18). Oxygenated pulmonary venous blood returns to the left atrium and is recirculated to the pulmonary artery without reaching the systemic circulation. Similarly, systemic venous blood returns to the right atrium and ventricle and is ejected into the aorta again. Obviously, this arrangement is compatible with life only for a few circulation times unless there is some mixing of pulmonary and systemic venous blood via a patent ductus arteriosus or an opening in the atrial or ventricular septum at birth. The physiological disturbance in these patients is one of inadequate mixing of pulmonary and systemic blood rather than one of inadequate pulmonary blood flow.

Mixing of blood at the atrial level can be improved by balloon atrial septostomy. If dangerous levels of hypoxemia persist after the septostomy and metabolic acidosis ensues, an infusion of PGE1 can maintain the patency of the ductus arteriosus, increase pulmonary blood flow (by increasing left-to-right shunting across the PDA), and thereby increase the volume of oxygenated blood entering the left atrium. The volume-overloaded left atrium is likely to shunt part of its contents into the right atrium and thereby improve the oxygen saturation of aortic blood. Unlike the kinetics with other lesions, increased shunting of blood during anesthesia improves arterial oxygen saturation before correction of the transposition.

Depending on the particular anatomy and the presence of a VSD or pulmonary stenosis, one of three corrective procedures is used. The intraoperative and postoperative problems encountered differ with each type of procedure.

Atrial baffle procedure (Mustard and Senning)
An atrial-level partition is created with baffling to redirect pulmonary venous blood across the tricuspid valve to the right ventricle and thus to the aorta [246]. Systemic venous return is directed across the atrial septum to the mitral valve, into the left ventricle, and out the pulmonary artery. Although the pulmonary and systemic circuits are then connected serially instead of in parallel, this arrangement leaves the patient with a morphological right ventricle and tricuspid valve in continuity with the aorta. This ventricle must therefore work against systemic arterial pressure and resistance.

One problem with atrial baffles is that they can obstruct systemic and pulmonary venous return [247]. When this occurs, the patient manifests signs and symptoms of systemic venous obstruction, as evidenced by superior vena cava syndrome or other signs of systemic venous hypertension. When the pulmonary venous pathway is obstructed, pulmonary venous hypertension may be manifested by respiratory failure, poor gas exchange, and pulmonary edema (seen on chest radiograph). Severe pulmonary venous obstruction is manifested in the operating room by the presence of copious amounts of bloody fluid in the endotracheal tube, low cardiac output, and frequently poor oxygenation. Residual interatrial shunts also may cause intra- or postoperative hypoxemia. Long-term rhythm disturbances, along with limitations of ventricular and atrioventricualr valve function, have made this operation nearly obsolete.

Arterial switch procedure
Because of the complications associated with atrial baffle procedures, Jatene and others explored whether anatomical correction of this lesion, by dividing both great arteries and reattaching them to the opposite, anatomically correct ventricle, would improve survival [248,249]. This procedure is now performed in virtually all patients with straightforward transposition of the great arteries. It requires excision and reimplantation of the coronary arteries to the neo-aorta (formerly the proximal main pulmonary artery).

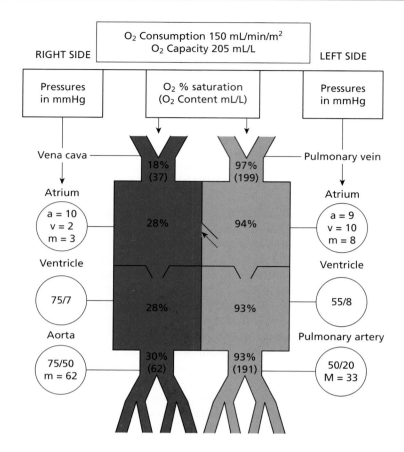

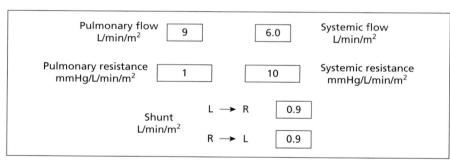

Figure 25.18 Catheterization findings in a patient with *d*-transposition of the great arteries and restricted pulmonary flow. Reproduced with permission from Nadas AS, Fyler DC. Pediatric Cardiology. Philadelphia: WB Saunders, 1972.

The success of the arterial switch procedure depends on adequate preparation of the left ventricle and technical proficiency with the coronary transfer. Anatomical correction of transposition of the great vessels is done during the neonatal period when PVR (left ventricular afterload) and left ventricular pressure have both been high. Left ventricular mass decreases progressively after birth in this lesion, and if the ability of the left ventricle to tolerate the work required is misjudged, the child may develop severe left ventricular failure postoperatively and require inotropic support and afterload reduction to provide normal cardiac output.

Infants with transposition of the great arteries who are more than a few weeks of age and have an intact ventricular septum may have decreased left ventricular pressure and mass. In such cases, the left ventricle may not tolerate the work required to perfuse the systemic vessels. However, if the neonate has a non-restrictive VSD, the left ventricle is accustomed to high pressure and may tolerate the increase in workload at any age. In older patients with an intact ventricular septum, banding the pulmonary artery can prepare the left ventricle to function as a systemic ventricle by increasing its afterload and muscle mass. If the left ventricle is "prepared" by banding the pulmonary artery and augmenting pulmonary blood flow with a modified Blalock–Taussig shunt, then an arterial switch procedure can usually be accomplished 1 week later after hypertrophy and hyperplasia have occurred [250]. However, during this interval these patients are cyanotic, with a volume-loaded right ventricle and a pressure-loaded left ventricle, and they may require considerable pharmacological support [251].

In experienced centers, the incidence of mortality for neonatal repair of transposition of the great arteries is now less than 3% and may be less than 2% for most anatomical arrangements of coronary arteries if the aortic arch is normal [252–254]. Midterm follow-up of these patients shows excellent outcome. Alternative operations are reserved almost exclusively for patients with particularly difficult coronary anatomy or pulmonic (neo-aortic) stenosis.

Myocardial ischemia or infarction may occur after mobilization and reimplantation of the coronary arteries, especially if they are stretched or twisted. Inotropic support, maintenance of coronary perfusion pressures, control of heart rate, and treatment with vasodilators may be particularly useful, as in adult patients with myocardial ischemia. Postoperative bleeding and tamponade occur more commonly with this operation because there are multiple arterial anastomoses.

Ventricular switch (Rastelli procedure)

In patients with a large VSD and severe subpulmonic stenosis, the VSD can be closed obliquely to direct left ventricular flow to the aorta. The pulmonary valve is oversewn and the right ventricle connected to the pulmonary artery with a conduit [255]. Complications of the Rastelli procedure include obstruction of left ventricular outflow due to narrowing of the subaortic region by the VSD patch. The conduit also may obstruct during or after the immediate postoperative period [256,257]. There is a small but significant incidence of heart block in these patients, which can be a difficult postoperative problem.

Anesthetic considerations after repair

Patients who have a morphological right ventricle remaining as the systemic ventricle and the pulmonary ventricle can be regarded as having a physiological or functional two-ventricle repair. Actuarial survival figures at 20 years have been quoted up to 80%, but significant long-term functional deterioration is likely with increasing risk of right heart failure, sudden death and dysrhythmias [258–261]. This situation is evidenced by systemic (right) ventricular dysfunction and tricuspid valve regurgitation long after the repair [262,263].

Unfortunately, late arrhythmias continue to be a problem. There is a progressive loss of sinus rhythm following both the Mustard and Senning operations. Actuarial analysis of several series reveals that by 10 years post operation, only about 60–70% of patients will be in sinus rhythm at rest and by 20 years, this will decrease to 40–50% [264–268]. In one series, only 7% of patients who underwent a Senning procedure for TGV with VSD were in sinus rhythmn at 15 years [258]. The majority of patients not in sinus rhythm will be in a junctional rhythm without the necessity for a pacemaker. Atrial flutter is present in 8% of patients at 5 years and in 27% at 20 years [268]. Late development of atrial flutter/fibrillation may be a surrogate marker for ventricular dysfunction and as such may put the patient at risk for VT and sudden death [269].

The exercise response of patients who have undergone an atrial switch procedure is clearly abnormal, with RV dysfunction, chronotrophic impairment, failure to augment ventricular filling and stroke volume, deconditioning, and impaired lung function all playing a role [270–273]. Asymptomatic children have a normal increase in cardiac output in response to submaximal exercise. However, they clearly have a reduced maximal aerobic capacity and oxygen consumption [272,274–276].

The fact that there is poor direct correlation between RV ejection fraction and exercise capacity emphasizes the mutifactorial nature of this problem [271]. A recent investigation utilizing load-independent measures of RV systolic and diastolic function concluded that the primary limitation to exercise capacity in Mustard patients was not impaired systolic or diastolic function but a limited ability to maintain an increased stroke volume as heart rate increased during exercise [271].

One of the major advances in congenital heart surgery over the past 10–15 years has been the development of the arterial switch operation (ASO) to correct transportation of the great arteries. Long-term survival data are not available as the oldest survivors are only in their teenage years, but based on intermediate-term follow-up data, the risk for reoperation and complications after the arterial switch operation remains small.

Virtually all coronary artery patterns are amenable to the arterial switch operation. Early concerns existed regarding the long-term patency and growth potential of the reimplanted coronary arteries. Fortunately, these problems have not materialized on a large scale. The overwhelming majority (90–97%) of patients have normal-sized, patent coronary arteries as assessed by coronary angiography [277–281]. A recent study of a large cohort demonstrated that survival without coronary events (death from myocardial infarction (MI), sudden death, and reoperation for coronary stenoses) is 92.7 % at 1 year and 88.2% at 15 years [280]. Patients with complex preoperative coronary anatomy are at increased risk of late occlusion [281].

After repair, the "native" pulmonary valve becomes the "neo-aortic" valve. Aortic insufficiency occurs in approximately 10–15% of patients at long-term follow-up with the majority (96%) graded as trivial or mild [252,282]. Time has shown aortic insufficiency to be a rare source of morbidity or indication for reoperation following the ASO [252,253].

In contrast to the atrial switch procedures, electrophysiological abnormalities are uncommon after the ASO. The most common abnormalities noted at midterm and long-term follow-up are rare asymptomatic atrial and ventricular premature beats [282–284].

Supravalvar pulmonary artery stenosis was an early complication, but is now less common with surgical techniques that extensively mobilize, augment and reconstruct the pulmonary arteries. The incidence of supravalvular stenosis severe enough to require reoperation (generally a gradient greater than 50–60 mmHg) is approximately 4–8% [252,253]. There continue to be refinements in surgical technique to further reduce the incidence of this complication [285].

Assessment of myocardial performance using echocardiography, cardiac catheterization and exercise testing following the ASO has demonstrated function identical to age-matched controls [286]. Based upon the currently available clinical, functional and hemodynamic data, a patient who has undergone a previous ASO with no evidence of subsequent problems should be treated as for any patient with a structurally normal heart when presenting for non-cardiac surgery.

Late complications of the Rastelli procedure include progressive conduit obstruction and right ventricular hypertension, residual VSDs and, occasionally, subaortic obstruction from diversion of left ventricular outflow across the VSD to the aorta.

Total anomalous pulmonary venous connection
Pathophysiology
Patients with total anomalous pulmonary venous connection are cyanotic because their pulmonary veins connect to a systemic vein and they have various degrees of pulmonary venous obstruction. The venous connection may be above the level of the heart (e.g. to the superior vena cava, innominate or azygos vein), directly to the right atrium or below the level of the heart and the diaphragm (e.g. to the hepatic veins). Patients with this anomaly must have a patent foramen ovale or an ASD that allows blood flow to the left side of the heart.

This anatomical arrangement provides complete mixing of all systemic and pulmonary venous blood in the right atrium. Unless there is significant stenosis of the pulmonary venous connection, most of this right atrial blood passes through the right ventricle into the pulmonary artery, which increases pulmonary blood flow. If pulmonary venous return is significantly inhibited, there is increased pulmonary venous congestion and decreased pulmonary blood flow.

Anesthetic management
These patients may be very ill, with hypoxemia, severe pulmonary edema, and pulmonary artery hypertension. Resuscitation, including mechanical ventilation, PEEP, and inotropic support of the myocardium, is followed by early surgical intervention to relieve the pulmonary venous obstruction. Although the patients are hypoxemic, their primary pathology is caused by obstructed venous return from the lungs. Therapy that increases pulmonary blood flow (e.g. PGE1) must be avoided. Surgical repair of total anomalous pulmonary venous connection requires attachment or redirection of the pulmonary venous confluence to the left atrium [287].

Intraoperative and postoperative problems are often related to residual or recurrent stenosis of the pulmonary veins. In patients who had severe stenosis and pulmonary venous hypertension preoperatively, the pulmonary vascular bed is highly reactive. This reactivity may produce high pulmonary artery pressures and poor right ventricular function after bypass and during the early postoperative period. Anesthetic management of these patients after completion of the repair should emphasize inotropic support of the right ventricle and avoidance of myocardial depressant drugs, and minimize pulmonary vascular resistance. Early extubation of the trachea is usually not feasible. Mechanical ventilation with hyperventilation and other postoperative therapy to decrease PVR are required. Use of inhaled nitric oxide has been particularly useful in this population.

Anesthetic considerations after repair
Other than the potential for late development of recurrent pulmonary venous obstruction, these patients generally do well and have good cardiovascular reserve once recovery from the surgery is complete [288]. The size of the pulmonary veins at birth may be a predictor of late complications with recurrent pulmonary vein stenosis [289].

Atrial septal defect
Pathophysiology
There are three anatomical varieties of ASD. The most common, ASD secundum, is a deficit in the septum primum, which ordinarily covers the region of the foramen ovale. ASD primum is a deficit of the inferior portion of the atrial septum (endocardial cushion) and is usually accompanied by a cleft in the anterior leaflet of the mitral valve. Sinus venous defects are located near the junction of the right atrium and the superior or inferior

vena cava; they are frequently associated with a partial anomalous pulmonary venous connection.

Left-to-right shunting (simple) occurs at the atrial level, causing a low-pressure volume load to the right ventricle. Pulmonary blood flow is increased, but not enough to make these patients symptomatic during early childhood. However, later in life, as the left ventricle becomes less compliant and the left atrial pressures increase, the left-to-right shunt and volume load increase and symptoms of CHF may occur. In rare patients the long-standing increase in pulmonary blood flows causes pulmonary vascular obstructive disease [30].

Anesthetic management

The defect can be closed directly with sutures or, if it is sufficiently large, with a synthetic patch. Sinus venosus defects associated with partial anomalous pulmonary venous connection require a more extensive patch that also directs the partial anomalous pulmonary venous return into the left atrium.

These patients are among the healthiest encountered. Their anesthesia can be managed in many ways. Early tracheal extubation is usual. Atrial arrhythmias, including atrial flutter and atrial fibrillation, are rarely seen during the postoperative period. Mitral regurgitation may occur in patients who have undergone repair of an ASD primum. Although transient left ventricular failure has been reported, these patients rarely require inotropic support. Residual ASDs are uncommon, but occasionally failure to recognize partial anomalous pulmonary venous return results in a residual left-to-right shunt. Most patients can be extubated during the immediate postoperative period or in the operating room. With the exceptions mentioned above, these patients usually have nearly normal cardiovascular function and reserve after repair. As noted above, many of these defects can be closed in the catheterization laboratory with occlusion devices; only large defects with inadequate atrial borders, multiple defects or those associated with partial anomalous pulmonary venous return are closed surgically.

Ventricular septal defect
Pathophysiology

Defects in the ventricular septum occur at several locations in the muscular partition dividing the ventricles. Simple shunting occurs across the ventricular septum. The magnitude of pulmonary blood flow is determined by the size of the VSD and the PVR [290] (Fig. 25.19). With a non-restrictive defect, high left ventricular flows and pressures are transmitted to the pulmonary artery. Therefore, surgical repair is indicated within the first 2 years of life to prevent the progression of pulmonary vascular obstructive disease [28,32]. In patients with established pulmonary vascular disease, the pulmonary

arteriolar changes may not recede when the defect is closed. In such cases, there may be progressive PVR elevation. The growth and development of the pulmonary vascular bed are significant factors in the patient's ability to normalize pulmonary vascular hemodynamics after surgery [291]. When PVR approaches or exceeds systemic vascular resistance, right-to-left shunting occurs through the VSD and the patients develop progressive hypoxemia (Eisenmenger syndrome) [292]. Closing the VSD in this circumstance adds the risk for acute right heart failure to that of progressive increases in PVR.

Anesthetic management

The defects are closed during CPB. The most common septal defect, the membranous defect, is frequently repaired through a right atriotomy and the tricuspid valve. However, lesions in the inferior apical muscular septum or those high in the ventricular outflow tract may require a left or right ventriculotomy. If so, the postoperative ventricular function may be impaired.

Before repair, measures that decrease PVR may appreciably increase left-to-right shunting in patients with a non-restrictive defect and may increase the degree of CHF. Postoperative right or left ventricular failure may be a manifestation of the preoperative status of the myocardium, a result of the ventriculotomy and CPB, or both. Small infants who fail to thrive, who are malnourished, and who have significant CHF preoperatively may have excessive lung water and may require prolonged mechanical ventilation postoperatively [293]. Such infants may have limited intraoperative tolerance for anesthetics that depress the myocardium or for maneuvers that increase pulmonary blood flow.

Persistent CHF and an audible murmur postoperatively, evidence of low cardiac output or the need for extensive inotropic support intraoperatively suggest that a residual or previously unrecognized VSD is continuing to place a volume and pressure load on the ventricles. When PVR is increased preoperatively, the increase in right ventricular afterload caused by closure of the VSD may be poorly tolerated, leading to the need for inotropic support of the heart and measures to decrease PVR. Occasionally ventricular outflow tract obstruction is caused by placement of the septal patch. Aortic regurgitation caused by prolapse of one of the aortic valve cusps can develop in subaortic or subpulmonic VSDs. In addition, heart block may occur after closure of VSDs with a patch. A pacemaker may be needed to maintain an adequate heart rate and cardiac output.

Anesthetic considerations after repair

In the absence of residual VSDs, outflow obstruction, and heart block, most of these patients regain relatively normal myocardial function, especially if the VSD is

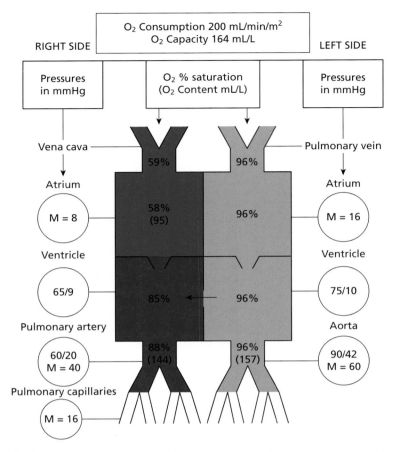

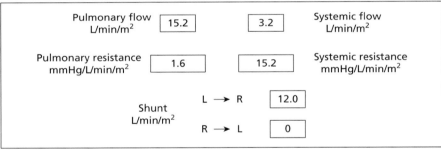

Figure 25.19 Catheterization findings in a patient with a VSD and pulmonary artery hypertension. Reproduced with permission from Nadas AS, Fyler DC. Pediatric Cardiology. Philadelphia: WB Saunders, 1972.

repaired early. However, a small percentage of patients, especially those who have had a large defect repaired late in childhood, continue to have some degree of ventricular dysfunction and also some pulmonary hypertension [294,295].

Atrioventricular canal defects
Pathophysiology
The endocardial cushion defect, complete common atrioventricular (AV) canal, consists of defects in the atrial and ventricular septa and the AV valvular tissue. All four chambers communicate and share a single common AV valve. The atrial and ventricular shunts communicate

volume and systemic pressures to the right ventricle and pulmonary artery. The ventricular shunt orifice is usually non-restrictive (simple shunt); therefore, PVR governs the degree of excess pulmonary blood flow. Mitral regurgitation and direct left ventricular-to-right atrial shunting may further contribute to atrial hypertension and total left-to-right shunting.

Anesthetic management
Surgical repair of this lesion consists of division of the common AV valve and closure of the atrial and ventricular septal defect with a single patch, modified single-patch or two-patch technique [296]. In addition, the mitral

valve (and sometimes the tricuspid valve) requires suture approximation and resuspension of the separated portions.

These patients have large left-to-right shunts. As a result of their high pulmonary blood flows, they have CHF and pulmonary hypertension. Myocardial depressants and therapy that decreases PVR while increasing shunt flow may be poorly tolerated before repair. Some patients, especially older children, may have obstructive pulmonary vascular disease. All of the potential complications of ASD and VSD closures are seen in these patients. In addition, the mitral valve may be regurgitant [297]. Inotropic support for the failing heart, afterload reduction for mitral regurgitation, and measures to decrease pulmonary vascular resistance may be required intra- and postoperatively after repair.

Patients with Down syndrome frequently have an associated complete AV canal. Measures to decrease PVR and the use of prolonged ventilatory support are often necessary because their airways and pulmonary vascular beds are hyper-reactive. The large tongues, upper airway obstruction, and difficult vascular access of these patients pose additional problems. The most frequent postoperative problems in Down syndrome patients are residual VSDs, mitral insufficiency, and pulmonary hypertension [298–300].

Patent ductus arteriosus
Pathophysiology
The ductus arteriosus is a fetal vascular communication between the main pulmonary artery at its bifurcation and the descending aorta below the origin of the left subclavian artery. When patent, it provides a simple shunt between the systemic and pulmonary arteries. The magnitude and direction of flow between the systemic and pulmonary vessels are determined by the relative resistances to flow in the two vascular beds and the diameter (resistance) of the ductus itself. With a large, non-restrictive ductus and low pulmonary vascular resistance, the pulmonary blood flow is excessive and the volume load of the left heart is large. Systolic and diastolic flow away from the aorta may steal blood from vital organs (e.g. pulmonary steal) and compromise end-organ function at many sites. In addition, overcirculated lungs and elevated left atrial pressure increase the work of breathing.

Anesthetic management
Although the patent ductus arteriosus of premature infants can often be closed medically with indomethacin or ibuprofen, contraindications to the use of these agents (e.g. intracranial hemorrhage, renal dysfunction, and hyperbilirubinemia) may require that the defect be closed surgically [301]. Whereas thoracotomy and surgical ligation of the ductus arteriosus are standard in older infants and children, some centers now occlude the ductus with a percutaneously inserted coil or occlusion device [302] or by using video-assisted thoracoscopic surgery (VATS) [303]. Advantages of VATS compared with open thoracotomy include decreased postoperative pain, shorter hospital stay and decreased incidence of chest wall deformity [304].

Healthy asymptomatic patients undergoing surgery can be extubated in the operating room, allowing many options for anesthetic management. However, the fragile premature infant with severe lung disease may require mechanical ventilation for protracted periods after ligation of the ductus arteriosus. Fentanyl, pancuronium, oxygen, and air constitute a common anesthetic regimen for this procedure. Anesthetic management of the premature infant in the operating room requires special considerations of gas exchange, hemodynamic performance, temperature regulation, metabolism, and drug and oxygen toxicity. Thoracotomy and lung retraction usually decrease lung compliance and increase oxygen and ventilatory requirements. A transient rise in systemic blood pressure with ligation of the ductus arteriosus may increase left ventricular afterload or elevate cerebral perfusion pressure to the detriment of a premature patient. Inadvertent ligation of the left pulmonary artery or descending aorta has occurred because the ductus arteriosus is often the same size as the descending aorta.

Ligation of an isolated ductus arteriosus generally results in normal cardiovascular function and reserve several months postoperatively [305].

Truncus arteriosus
Pathophysiology
With truncus arteriosus, the embryonic truncus fails to separate normally into the two great arteries. Indeed, a single great artery leaves the heart and gives rise to the coronary, pulmonary, and systemic circulations. The truncus straddles a large VSD and receives blood from both ventricles.

There is complete mixing of systemic and pulmonary venous blood in the single great artery, which causes mild hypoxemia. One or two pulmonary arteries may originate from the ascending truncus; the pulmonary artery orifice is seldom restrictive. The resulting shunt (simple) produces excessive pulmonary blood flow early in life as the pulmonary vascular resistance decreases. This "pulmonary steal" may elevate the arterial oxygen saturation and decrease the systemic blood flow. In such a case, net systemic oxygen transport decreases and lactic acidosis develops. Children with truncus arteriosus are at risk for developing early pulmonary vascular obstructive disease [306]. Regurgitation of blood through the truncal valve may place an additional volume load on the ventricles.

Anesthetic management

Complete repair of this lesion should be performed early, even in the neonate, before the development of irreversible pulmonary vascular changes [307,308]. The VSD is closed with a synthetic patch and the pulmonary arteries are detached from the truncus. Continuity is established between the right ventricle and the pulmonary arteries with a valved conduit. The truncal valve may require valvuloplasty if a significant amount of blood regurgitates through it.

Anesthetic management centers around control of pulmonary blood flow and ventricular support. Pulmonary blood flow may increase further with anesthetic agents, hyperventilation, alkalosis, and oxygen administration, resulting in hypotension and acute ventricular failure. If measures to *increase* PVR do not decrease pulmonary flow, occlusion of one branch of the pulmonary artery with a tourniquet limits pulmonary flow and restores systemic perfusion pressure until CPB can be instituted. Because these patients are frequently in high-output CHF, myocardial depressants should be used with caution.

Immediately after repair, the combination of persistent pulmonary artery hypertension and right ventricular failure can be fatal. Hence, aggressive measures should be taken to provide normal myocardial function and lower the PVR. A residual VSD adds an additional volume and pressure load on the ventricles and may have a devastating impact on the patient's hemodynamics and oxygenation. A VSD should be suspected in patients who are not doing well postoperatively. Any residual VSD should be repaired if feasible. Truncal valve regurgitation or stenosis may induce left ventricular failure early during the postoperative period.

Anesthetic considerations after repair

Obstruction of the pulmonary conduit and the accompanying right ventricular hypertension may occur early or late during the postoperative course. Usually the conduit is unable to support flow in the growing child after several postoperative years. Late development of truncal (aortic) valve regurgitation is possible. For patients who underwent repair later in childhood, residual persistent pulmonary hypertension may be a problem.

Coarctation of the aorta
Pathophysiology

Patients with coarctation of the aorta have a narrowing of the descending aorta near the insertion of the ductus arteriosus into the aorta. Sometimes coarctation of the aorta is associated with hypoplasia of the aortic isthmus proximal to the coarctation. Aortic and mitral valve abnormalities, as well as VSDs, may also be present.

With severe obstruction to blood flow in the descending aorta of neonates, systemic perfusion is inadequate, causing profound metabolic acidosis. The increase in left ventricular afterload is not well tolerated, and an elevated left ventricular end-diastolic pressure (LVEDP) reflexively causes pulmonary artery hypertension. Flow below the coarctation may then be provided primarily by right-to-left flow from the right ventricle and pulmonary artery through the ductus arteriosus. Maintaining or re-establishing duct flow can be accomplished with PGE1 infusion, which also reduces the left ventricular afterload.

With less severe forms of coarctation, the child may adapt to the obstruction by developing collateral circulation to the lower body and by increasing the left ventricular muscle mass. Upper extremity hypertension may be the only manifestation of the defect.

Anesthetic management

The optimal treatment for neonates, infants and children is currently felt to be complete excision of the area of coarctation and surrounding ductal tissue with end-to-end anastomosis. Alternatively, a reverse subclavian patch repair can be undertaken. In this technique, the left subclavian artery is ligated and transected with the proximal portion of the artery used as a flap to augment the area of coarctation. Following this procedure, left arm pulses will be weak or absent. Dacron patch aortoplasty following resection of the posterior coarctation ridge has also been used, but this technique is associated with late development of hypertension and aneurysm formation as compared to end-to-end anastomosis [309]. All approaches require 10–25 min of aortic cross-clamping above and below the area of coarctation.

Acidosis, hypertension or spinal cord ischemia can occur during this period. Paraplegia is an extremely rare but tragic complication of the procedure. Extreme upper body hypertension may compromise left ventricular function and decrease cardiac output, especially to the lower body, and must be expectantly treated. If the elevated arterial pressure in the head is transmitted to the cerebrospinal fluid (CSF), the CSF pressure may be elevated. If these elevated pressures are transmitted to the CSF below the level of the coarctation, net spinal cord perfusion pressure is decreased [310]. Alternatively, if upper body hypertension is overtreated with vasodilators during cross-clamping of the aorta, the arterial pressure may be inadequate in the vasodilated lower half of the body, which is supplied by collaterals. If this occurs, spinal cord or renal ischemia may result [311].

These complications are not so much related to changes in proximal aortic pressure or distal CSF pressure as they are to distal perfusion pressures, adequacy of arterial collaterals, and duration of cross-clamping [312,313]. Monitoring of arterial pressures in the lower extremities may be helpful but impractical during the cross-clamp period. Hyperthermia to 38°C and 40°C during cross-clamping is associated with an increased incidence of paraplegia and transient renal failure [314]. Therefore, mild hypothermia (32–34°C) is used in some centers during aortic cross-clamping as a possible prophylaxis for these rare but tragic problems.

After the cross-clamp is removed and repair is complete, rebound hypertension may be a problem as the patient emerges from the anesthetic. The etiology of this persistent hypertension is multifactorial. The pulsatility of the postcoarctation descending aorta remains reduced following hemodynamically ideal repair [315]. The geometry of the aortic arch following coarctation and distal aortic arch repair is also a determinant of subsequent upper body vascular responses, pulse wave velocity, and left ventricular mass. Anatomy with a high arch height to width ratio (Gothic arch) is associated with impaired vascular response, increased pulse wave velocity, central aortic stiffness and increased LV mass as compared to anatomy with a lower arch height to width ratio (Crenel and normal Romanesque arch anatomy) [316,317]. Abnormalities in baroreceptor reflexes and in the renin-angiotensin-aldosterone system have also been implicated as factors in persistent hypertension following successful coarctation repair [318]. Recent evidence suggests that abnormalities in cardiovascular reflexes are already present in neonates with coarctation prior to repair [319].

Development of abdominal pain and bowel ischemia during the postoperative period is related to insufficient flow in the mesenteric artery. Better control of postoperative hypertension has diminished the incidence of the severe form of this syndrome. Although propranolol and hydralazine may be useful for treating the moderate forms of postoperative hypertension, the more severe variety is best treated with sodium nitroprusside during the first few hours after surgery. Captopril may be a useful oral agent for treatment of persistent hypertension, and IV forms of enalapril are now available [320].

Anesthetic considerations after repair

Persistent hypertension and left ventricular hypertrophy may be problems for anesthetic management in as many as one-third of patients after adequate repair of coarctation of the aorta [321]. If the left subclavian artery was used for the repair, the left arm cannot be used for accurate blood pressure measurements. Restenosis of the coarctation is routinely balloon dilated in the interventional catheterization laboratory.

Interrupted aortic arch
Pathophysiology

In some patients the aorta is completely interrupted at one or more points along the aortic arch. A patent ductus arteriosus and a VSD are nearly always present, and these supply systemic blood flow below the interrupted arch. In addition, left ventricular outflow obstruction may be present [322].

Flow beyond the interruption is supplied entirely by blood that is shunted right to left through the ductus arteriosus. Ductal closure eliminates blood flow to the lower body and leads to metabolic acidosis. Patency of the ductus arteriosus is re-established with PGE1 [323]. There is a left-to-right shunt through the VSD, which may cause excessive pulmonary blood flow and respiratory insufficiency.

Anesthetic management

Repair of this lesion in neonates consists of a patch closure of the VSD and a direct anastomosis of the descending aorta to the underside of the transverse arch. Alternatively, the pulmonary artery is banded after the graft insertion and the VSD closure is deferred, but this palliative approach is generally discouraged.

The introduction of PGE1 has substantially improved preoperative resuscitation and perioperative morbidity and has simplified anesthetic management. However, the residual effects of protracted poor perfusion may complicate the intra- and postoperative course of these patients. PGE1 infusion should be continued until the onset of CPB. Circulatory problems after CPB that require inotropic support may be caused by a significant residual VSD, by obstruction of blood flow in the aorta or by subaortic stenosis aggravated by the VSD closure and a narrow subaortic region [324].

Late problems are related to obstruction of the descending aorta with subsequent growth of the child. These problems are similar to those seen with coarctation of the aorta. Subaortic stenosis may also develop and presents considerable surgical challenges to adequate relief of obstruction.

Critical aortic stenosis
Pathophysiology

The aortic valves of these patients show thickening and rigidity. They have various degrees of fusion of the valvular commissures. In the newborn the valve appears amorphous. There also may be evidence of endocardial fibroelastosis of the left ventricle and functional or anatomical abnormalities of the mitral valve.

Left ventricular outflow tract obstruction is poorly tolerated in the neonate because it causes left ventricular failure, poor systemic perfusion, hypotension, and pulmonary congestion. Myocardial perfusion is often borderline because the coronary perfusion pressure is relatively low and intraventricular pressure is high. Ventricular fibrillation may occur with surgical manipulation of the heart. In extreme cases, systemic blood flow may be partly supported from the right ventricle by right-to-left flow through the ductus arteriosus, provided that there is atrial septal communication. Stabilization of the patient's condition can be aided by infusion of PGE1 to increase systemic perfusion.

Anesthetic management

The treatment options for this isolated anomaly in the neonate are percutaneous balloon angioplasty and surgical valvotomy [325]. Myocardial depressants and rapid heart rates are poorly tolerated during either procedure. A defibrillator should be available for immediate use. Preoperative resuscitation of the left ventricle is imperative. Inadequate relief of the obstruction and persistence of left ventricular failure can complicate and prolong the postprocedure course. Residual stenosis or other added hemodynamic burdens further reduce myocardial performance. Mitral regurgitation may continue intraoperatively, and aortic regurgitation may occur after the valvotomy. Myocardial ischemia is not generally a problem after valvotomy. If the obstruction is adequately relieved, afterload reduction and inotropic agents may improve the poor myocardial function often evident postoperatively, especially when there is some degree of aortic regurgitation. In some patients, associated hypoplasia of the left ventricle or mitral valve may inhibit recovery and dictate a therapeutic approach to hypoplastic left heart.

Hypoplastic left heart syndrome
Pathophysiology

Few other congenital heart lesions have provoked as much controversy over management as hypoplastic left heart syndrome. It is a uniformly fatal disease if left untreated and debate continues over staged palliation versus neonatal transplantation versus comfort care [326,327]. The results of surgical management vary between institutions, and are clearly dependent upon expertise and experience, as well as the clinical condition of the neonate at presentation, and degree of hypoplasia of left heart structures [328].

This common example of single-ventricle physiology also represents the most severe form of obstructive left heart lesion. An anatomical spectrum of disease is implied for the lesion, but in its most severe and common presentation there is atresia or marked hypoplasia of the aortic and mitral valves with critical underdevelopment of the

left atrium, left ventricle, and ascending aorta. A 1 or 2 mm ascending aorta gives rise to the coronary circulation and the head vessels before converging with the ductus arteriosus, where the aorta becomes larger and supplies the circulation to the lower body. Pulmonary venous return arrives in the diminutive left atrium and cannot cross the atretic mitral valve; therefore, it is directed to the right atrium and right ventricle, where common mixing occurs with the systemic venous return and all blood is ejected into the pulmonary artery. Systemic blood flow is then supplied from the pulmonary artery, right to left, across the PDA. As the PDA constricts in the neonatal period, systemic blood flow decreases and all ventricular output is directed to the lungs. The Qp/Qs ratio approaches infinity as Qs nears zero. Therefore, one has the paradoxical presentation of high PO_2 (70–150 mmHg) in the face of profound metabolic acidosis. When the ductus arteriosus is reopened with PGE1, systemic perfusion is re-established, the acidosis resolves and the PO_2 returns to the 40–60 mmHg range, representative of a Qp/Qs ratio between 1 and 2.

Anesthetic management

Adequate preoperative resuscitation with PGE1 and correction of metabolic acidosis and end-organ dysfunction is crucial to the anesthetic preparation and management of patients with this lesion. Further facilitation of resuscitation can be enhanced by judicious use of inotropic agents, which can optimize cardiac output and blood flow to such organs as the kidneys. However, excessive delay in the timing of surgical intervention will result in a gradual reduction in pulmonary vascular resistance over days, with excessive pulmonary blood flow and inadequate systemic perfusion.

The surgical reconstructive approach to this lesion currently entails three operations, which ultimately aim to provide a 2- or 3-year-old child with a reconstructed aortic arch and a Fontan type of circulation for single-ventricle physiology [329]. In the first stage of the reconstruction (Norwood operation), the pulmonary artery is transected at the bifurcation and an anastomosis is performed to the ascending aorta, which has been surgically incised so that the aortic and pulmonary arterial confluences arise together from the single right ventricle as the neo-aorta, which is extended into the remaining native aorta using homograft material. Pulmonary blood flow is established with either a 3.5 or 4 mm modified Blalock–Taussig shunt or a 5 or 6 mm unvalved RV-to-PA conduit (Sano shunt). The atrial septum is excised to ensure free flow of pulmonary venous return over to the tricuspid valve. In addition to HLHS, the Norwood operation is also used to repair other complex single-ventricle defects with systemic outflow obstruction or hypoplasia [330].

The anesthetic considerations are the same as those outlined in detail for patients with single-ventricle physiology. The intraoperative and postoperative management requires careful manipulation of PVR and SVR to provide adequate but not excessive pulmonary blood flow and oxygen delivery while maintaining sufficient systemic and coronary artery perfusion. The precarious nature of the coronary os, which may be extremely small and closely approximated to the suture lines, means that even small variations in hemodynamics may compromise myocardial blood flow. Myocardial depressants are poorly tolerated, and ventricular failure and tricuspid (systemic) valve regurgitation can inhibit recovery.

The physiology of the modified Blalock–Taussig shunt and of the RV-to-PA conduit as a source of pulmonary blood flow differs in some important aspects. With a modified Blalock–Taussig shunt, blood is distributed to the pulmonary circulation in both systole and diastole after it has entered the systemic arterial tree (from the innominate artery to the pulmonary artery) while with a Sano conduit, blood is distributed to the pulmonary circulation in systole before it has entered the systemic arterial tree (from the RV to the pulmonary artery; much like a double-outlet RV). As a result, for a given cardiac output and Qp/Qs, the pulse pressure is wider and the aortic diastolic blood pressure lower in patients with a modified Blalock–Taussig shunt. The higher diastolic blood pressure obtained with the Sano shunt may provide better cerebral, coronary and splanchnic perfusion. The Sano shunt requires creation of a small right ventriculotomy. The RV is the systemic ventricle and the long-term functional consequences of this ventriculotomy are unknown. The Sano conduit is valveless, resulting in some pulmonary insufficiency. The volume load on the RV induced by this is small and probably offset by the fact that Sano shunt patients have a slightly lower Qp/Qs and volume load than modified Blalock–Taussig shunt patients.

After CPB in the Norwood palliation procedure, the pulmonary vascular resistance may be transiently elevated and the modified Blalock–Taussig or Sano shunt barely adequate to sustain pulmonary blood flow and achieve adequate oxygenation. In this circumstance, hyperventilation with 100% oxygen and alkalosis may be required, with inotropic support of the systemic blood pressure. However, within hours, and sometimes within minutes, pulmonary vascular resistance falls, myocardial function is restored, and the Qp/Qs may become excessive. Hypoventilation with room air and the use of systemic vasodilators are not always effective at reversing the pulmonary steal phenomenon in this circumstance.

More drastic measures, such as ventilation with hypoxic gas mixtures or ventilation with added CO_2, have been advocated by some centers and have been intermittently embraced and abandoned by others over the years [331–333].

The Stage 1 hybrid procedure for HLHS is an alternative to the Norwood Stage 1 procedure with either a modified Blalock–Taussig shunt or a RV-to-PA conduit [334,335]. The hybrid procedure obviates the need for CPB and the associated use of either DHCA or ACP in the neonate. This procedure must be done in a location ("hybrid operating room") that provides full cardiac catheterization infrastructure, including biplane cardioangiography, in a sterile operating room environment. The procedure (Fig. 25.20) involves off-pump placement of a bare metallic stent in the ductus arteriosus, bilateral pulmonary artery banding, and dilation/stenting of the intra-atrial septum. The balloon atrial septostomy is generally performed prior to discharge from the hospital unless there is obstruction of pulmonary venous blood delivery to the right ventricle and pulmonary venous hypertension detected earlier. The physiological burden associated with CPB and DHCA or ACP avoided in the first stage is then incurred at the time of the comprehensive Stage 2 (bidirectional Glenn shunt, Stansel anastomosis, aortic arch reconstruction, and definitive atrial septectomy) performed at 3–6 months of age.

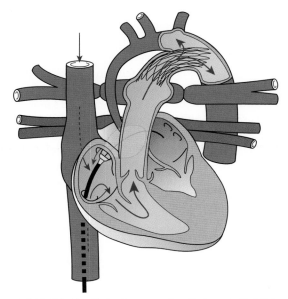

Figure 25.20 Hybrid palliation in a neonate with hypoplastic left heart syndrome. Note stent in the patent ductus arteriosus and bilateral pulmonary artery banding.

CASE STUDY

The patient is a term 3-month-old male weighting 4.0 kg s/p Stage repair on day 3 of life for HLHS with mitral and aortic atresia. He presents now for percutaneous endoscopic gastrostomy tube placement. The parents request that a circumcision be performed during the same anesthetic. The patient is poorly tolerant of oral feeds, has demonstrated poor weight gain and somatic growth (25th percentile for height and weight), and has medically managed gastroesophageal reflux. Oral medications are: 1/2 baby aspirin QD, furosemide 8 mg TID, digoxin 0.02 mg BID, captopril 1 mg TID, and ranitidine 8 mg BID.

Echocardiogram done 1 week ago reveals a patent Damis–Kaye–Stansel (DKS) anastomosis, non-restrictive atrial septum, a patent right modified Blalock–Taussig shunt without pulmonary stenoses, and a narrowed aorta at the junction of the isthmus and descending aorta with a peak Doppler-derived gradient of 30 mmHg without evidence of continuous flow in the abdominal aorta. There is mild-to-moderate tricuspid regurgitation and mild-to-moderate global right ventricular dysfunction.

Blood pressure is 70/30 mm Hg in the left arm, heart rate is 165 bpm in sinus rhythm, and the SaO_2 is 75% on room air. CXR reveals an enlarged cardiac silhouette with some increase in pulmonary vascular markings.

Questions

1. What is your assessment of this child's cardiovascular status? What is the significance of the tricuspid regurgitation and right ventricular dysfunction in the setting of residual arch obstruction? What is the likely mechanism of the tricuspid regurgitation (TR)? Are the increased pulmonary vascular markings due to ventricular dysfunction, a high Qp/Qs or both?
2. Could better medical management of this child's heart failure obviate the need for a feeding tube?
3. Should this infant undergo an arch dilation in the cardiac catheterization laboratory prior to the proposed surgery? Should this patient be considered for an early bidirectional Glenn as a means of decreasing the volume load on his RV and improving the TR?
4. Which A.M. medications will you have the parents give and which if any should be held? Is this infant an appropriate A.M. admission case or should he be admitted the night prior to surgery? Is the ICU necessary postoperatively?
5. What premedication will you administer? How will you induce and maintain anesthesia? What monitoring is necessary?

Induction of anesthesia proceeds smoothly and the anesthesia is maintained with remifentanil 0.5 μg/kg/min and iso-flurane 0.7% in 100% O_2. During introduction of the endoscope ST segment depression is noted in V_5. BP is 60/25 mmHg, HR is 170 bpm, $ETCO_2$ is 35 mmHg, and SaO_2 is 75%.

Questions

6. How will you adjust the ventilator (rate, tidal volume, PEEP, FIO_2)?
7. Is a fluid bolus warranted? Should inotropic support be initiated? Which inotrope?
8. How will you assess the adequacy of systemic oxygen delivery?
9. What is the mechanism of myocardial ischemia?
10. Once hemodynamics are stabilized and the ischemia resolves, should the case continue?

Discussion

The primary goal in the management of patients with single-ventricle physiology is optimization of systemic oxygen delivery and perfusion pressure. This is necessary if end-organ (myocardial, renal, hepatic, splanchnic) dysfunction and failure are to be prevented. This goal is achieved by balancing the systemic and pulmonary circulations. The term "balanced circulation" is used because both laboratory and clinical investigations have demonstrated that maximal systemic oxygen delivery (the product of systemic oxygen content and systemic blood flow) is achieved for a given single-ventricle output when Qp/Qs is at or just below 1/1. This relationship is illustrated in the graphs (Figs 25.21–25.25). Increases in Qp/Qs in excess of 1/1 are associated with a progressive decrease in systemic oxygen delivery because the subsequent increase in systemic oxygen content is more than offset by the progressive decrease in systemic blood flow (Fig. 25.21). Decreases in Qp/Qs just below 1/1 are associated with a precipitous decrease in systemic oxygen delivery because the subsequent increase in systemic blood flow is more than offset by the dramatic decrease in systemic oxygen content.

Since Qp/Qs is not a readily measurable parameter in a clinical setting, pulse oximetry is commonly used as a surrogate method of assessing the extent to which a balanced circulation exists. An arterial saturation of 75–80% is felt to be indicative of a balanced circulation (Fig. 25.22). It is important to point out, however, that an arterial saturation of 75–80% is indicative of a Qp/Qs at or near 1/1 only if the pulmonary venous saturation is 95–100% and the mixed venous (SVC) saturation is 55–60% (Fig. 25.23). In fact, based on these assumptions, the equation used to calculate Qp/Qs in patients with univentricular physiology (SaO_2 –

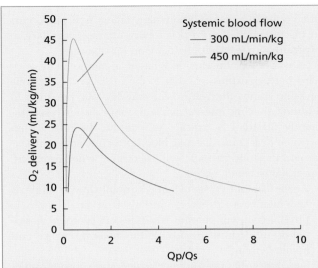

Figure 25.21 Pulmonary/systemic blood flow ratio vs systemic oxygen delivery.

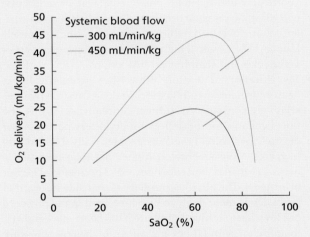

Figure 25.22 Systemic arterial oxygen saturation vs systemic oxygen delivery.

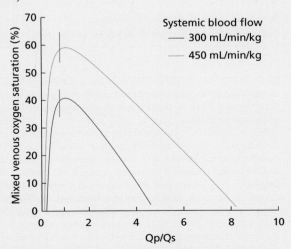

Figure 25.23 Pulmonary/systemic blood flow ratio vs mixed venous oxygen saturation (Ssvc%).

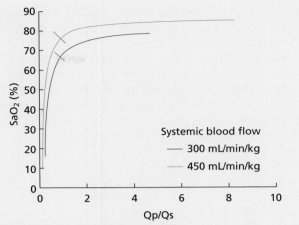

Figure 25.24 Pulmonary/systemic blood flow ratio vs systemic arterial oxygen saturation.

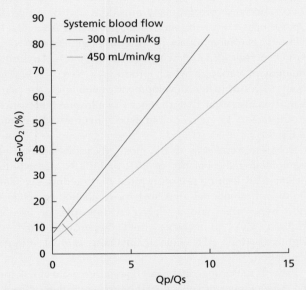

Figure 25.25 Pulmonary/systemic blood flow ratio vs arteriovenous oxygen difference.

$SsvcO_2)/SpvO_2 - SaO_2$) can be simplified to: $25/(95 - SaO_2)$. In this simplified equation, $SpvO_2$ is assumed to be 95% and the AV O_2 saturation difference is assumed to 25%. Use of this simplified equation requires that the FIO_2 be at or near 21% in order that the dissolved O_2 content of the pulmonary venous blood can be ignored and an $SpvO_2$ of 95% used. Unfortunately, an arterial saturation of 75–80% can exist at the extremes of Qp/Qs depending on pulmonary and systemic venous saturation (Fig. 25.24). Specifically, in the presence of a high Qp/Qs it is possible for there to be inadequate systemic oxygen delivery (systemic venous desaturation, a wide AV O_2 difference, metabolic acidosis) in the presence of what is considered to be an adequate arterial saturation of 75–80%. In addition, clinically unrec-

Continued

ognized episodes of pulmonary venous desaturation ($SpvO_2$ <90%) further confound assessment of Qp/Qs based on SaO_2.

Mathematical modeling of univentricular physiology reveals that systemic O_2 delivery is a complex function of cardiac output (CO), pulmonary venous O_2 content, systemic O_2 consumption, and Qp/Qs. In fact, SaO_2 correlates poorly with Qp/Qs and the measurement of $SpvO_2$ and $SsvcO_2$ substantially improves estimation of Qp/Qs. Regression analysis demonstrates that SaO_2 accounts for 8% of the error in estimating Qp/Qs while $SsvcO_2$ and $SpvO_2$ contribute 48% and 44% respectively. The figures illustrate the effect of CO (systemic blood flow 450 versus 300 mL/min/kg) on O_2 delivery, SvO_2, SaO_2, and Sa-vO_2 as Qp/Qs varies with $SpvO_2$ = 95% and O_2 consumption = 9 mL/min/kg. It is clear that while SaO_2 remains satisfactory over a wide range of Qp/Qs, O_2 delivery and $SsvcO_2$ decrease precipitously outside a narrow range of Qp/Qs near 1.0. By the time a SaO_2 of 80% is reached, O_2 delivery is precipitously on the decline. Furthermore, Sa-vO_2 increases linearly with increasing Qp/Qs. Any combination of variables which produces a $SsvcO_2$ <30% is likely to result in the development of anaerobic metabolism. It is also clear that a higher CO allows maintenance of satisfactory O_2 delivery and $SsvcO_2$ over a wider range of Qp/Qs.

Debate continues as to the most efficacious method of manipulating the balance of SVR and PVR. Methods to elevate PVR include use of inspired N_2 to reduce alveolar O_2, use of intentional alveolar hypoventilation to achieve mild hypercarbia and a slightly acidotic pH, or use of inspired CO_2 to achieve mild hypercarbia and a slightly acidotic pH while maintaining normal minute ventilation.

Patients with congenital heart disease are more at risk for the development of subendocardial ischemia than is commonly appreciated. In some congenital lesions abnormalities in the coronary circulation predispose to the development of myocardial ischemia but in many others, ischemia occurs in the presence of normal coronary arteries secondary to myocardial oxygen supply/demand imbalance.

Subendocardial perfusion is largely determined by coronary perfusion pressure that is the mean aortic diastolic pressure minus the ventricular end-diastolic pressure. In addition, the time interval available for perfusion (predominantly diastole) is critical. As a result, the relationship between heart rate, diastolic blood pressure, and ventricular end-diastolic pressure will determine whether subendocardial ischemia occurs.

- Aortic diastolic pressure that is normally low in neonates and infants is further compromised in single-ventricle physiology lesions because these lesions promote diastolic run-off of aortic blood into the lower resistance pulmonary circuit.
- Subendocardial pressure is elevated and subendocardial perfusion is compromised in the presence of an elevated ventricular end-diastolic pressure. Elevated ventricular end-diastolic pressure occurs as the result of the ventricular volume overload, which accompanies single-ventricle lesions, lesions with a high Qp/Qs, and regurgitant atrioventricular and semi-lunar valve lesions.
- The duration of diastole diminishes geometrically as heart rate increases while the duration of systole remains relatively constant. As a direct consequence of this, the time available for diastolic coronary artery perfusion, or diastolic perfusion time, falls geometrically as heart rate increases. Consequently, a higher diastolic pressure is necessary to maintain subendocardial perfusion at higher heart rates. The obvious corollary is that subendocardial perfusion is more likely to be maintained in the presence of a low diastolic blood pressure if the heart rate is slower. In an infant with HLHS and an aortic diastolic pressure of 25 mmHg, a heart rate of 130–140 bpm may well be tolerated without evidence of subendocardial ischemia whereas it is unlikely that a heart rate of 170–180 bpm will be tolerated at the same diastolic pressure.

Annotated references

A full reference list for this chapter is available at:
http://www.wiley.com/go/gregory/andropoulos/pediatricanesthesia

2. Harmel MH, Lamont A. Anesthesia in the surgical treatment of congenital pulmonic stenosis. Anesth Analg 1946; 7: 477. The first account of a series of anesthetics for patients with congenital heart disease.

6. Ramamoorthy C, Haberkern CM, Bhananker SM et al. Anesthesia-related cardiac arrest in children with heart disease: data from the Pediatric Perioperative Cardiac Arrest (POCA) registry. Anesth Analg 2010; 110: 1376–82. A very important contemporary review of the risk factors for cardiac arrest in patients with both congenital and acquired heart disease.

63. Norwood WI, Lang P, Hansen DD. Physiologic repair of aortic atresia-hypoplastic left heart syndrome. N Engl J Med 1983; 308: 23–6. The landmark paper, demonstrating collaboration among cardiac surgery, anesthesiology, and cardiology to produce a therapeutic breakthrough in one of the most common and difficult congenital cardiac lesions.

67. Wilson W, Taubert KA, Gewitz M et al. Prevention of infective endocarditis: guidelines from the American Heart Association: a guideline from the American Heart Association Rheumatic Fever, Endocarditis, and Kawasaki Disease Committee, Council on Cardiovascular Disease in the Young, and the Council on Clinical Cardiology, Council on Cardiovascular Surgery and Anesthesia, and the Quality of Care and Outcomes Research Interdisciplinary Working Group. Circulation 2007; 116: 1736–54. The most recent guidelines for prevention of infective endocarditis. Prophylaxis need has been significantly reduced based on extensive review of the evidence.

73. Anand KJ, Hickey PR. Halothane-morphine compared with high-dose sufentanil for anesthesia and postoperative analgesia in neo-

natal cardiac surgery. N Engl J Med 1992; 326: 1–9. A landmark paper demonstrating that anesthetic technique that limits the stress response for complex neonatal surgery improves mortality and morbidity.

90. Ikemba CM, Su JT, Stayer SA et al. Myocardial performance index with sevoflurane-pancuronium versus fentanyl-midazolam-pancuronium in infants with a functional single ventricle. Anesthesiology 2004; 101: 1298–305. An important modern study demonstrating minimal effect of standard anesthetic regimens on myocardial function in single-ventricle infants.

149. Thompson LD, McElhinney DB, Findlay P et al. A prospective randomized study comparing volume-standardized modified and conventional ultrafiltration in pediatric cardiac surgery. J Thorac Cardiovasc Surg 2001; 122: 220–8. An important, controlled study investigating the utility of either conventional or modified ultrafiltration, demonstrating that either technique will improve clinical outcomes, versus no hemofiltration.

156. Wypij D, Newburger JW, Rappaport LA et al. The effect of duration of deep hypothermic circulatory arrest in infant heart surgery on late neurodevelopment: the Boston Circulatory Arrest Trial. J Thorac Cardiovasc Surg 2003; 126: 1397–403. A landmark study of long-term follow-up of neonates undergoing surgery for the arterial switch operation, demonstrating that deep hypothermic circulatory arrest times greater than 41 min were associated with worsening neurodevelopmental outcomes at age 8 years.

166. Wypij D, Jonas RA, Bellinger DC et al. The effect of hematocrit during hypothermic cardiopulmonary bypass in infant heart surgery: results from the combined Boston hematocrit trials. J Thorac Cardiovasc Surg 2008; 135: 355–60. A very important large modern study demonstrating that hematocrit above 25% on bypass improves neurodevelopmental outcomes in infants.

328. Ohye RG, Sleeper LA, Mahony L et al. Comparison of shunt types in the Norwood procedure for single-ventricle lesions. N Engl J Med 2010; 362: 1980–92. An important multicentered study comparing outcomes of the classic Blalock–Taussig shunt Norwood operation to the right ventricle to pulmonary artery conduit Norwood, demonstrating lower rate of death or transplantation at age 12 months with the RV-PA conduit.

CHAPTER 26
Anesthesia for Spinal Surgery in Children

Joseph D. Tobias

Department of Anesthesiology and Pain Medicine, Nationwide Children's Hospital and The Ohio State University, Columbus, OH, USA

Introduction

Procedures involving the spinal column represent one of the most common of the major orthopedic surgeries in the pediatric-aged patient. Spinal deformities requiring orthopedic surgical intervention may be the result of congenital, acquired or traumatic conditions. They may be related to primary defects of the vertebral column (hemivertebrae), neuromuscular conditions (muscular dystrophy, cerebral palsy), neoplastic, infectious or therapy-related problems (radiation). Regardless of the cause, during surgical procedures to correct spinal deformities, there are several potential factors that may result in morbidity or even mortality, including co-morbid disease processes, patient positioning, blood loss, and neurological damage. In the most recent publication from the Perioperative Cardiac Arrest (POCA) registry, cardiovascular causes of cardiac arrest in the pediatric-aged patient were most common (41%), with hypovolemia from blood loss and hyperkalemia from transfusion being the most common causes of cardiovascular deterioration leading to cardiac arrest [1], the majority of these occurring during either craniofacial reconstruction or spinal surgery [1]. In an attempt to limit perioperative morbidity and mortality during spinal surgery in children, these patients should be approached in a standardized manner which includes a preoperative evaluation for the identification of co-morbid features, the intraoperative anesthetic plan with attention to monitoring, patient positioning, maintenance of normothermia, techniques to limit the need for homologous transfusion, control of coagulation function during large-volume transfusions, and the postoperative regimen with maintenance of hemodynamic and respiratory function as well as the provision of postoperative analgesia.

Surgical procedures on the pediatric spine may involve one or several vertebral levels with an incision at any level of the vertebral column (cervical, thoracic, lumbar, sacral). Further variations include an anterior approach, a posterior approach or, in the case of thoracic and lumbar spine procedures, a combined anterior–posterior (AP) procedure. The majority of the procedures performed in the pediatric-aged patient involve long segment surgery on the thoracic and lumbar spine related to either neuromuscular or idiopathic scoliosis.

This chapter reviews the developmental and gross anatomy of the spine, details the more common surgical procedures, outlines the preoperative assessment, discusses intraoperative anesthetic care, including methods to limit the need for homologous blood transfusion and spinal cord monitoring, and provides options for postoperative care, including pain management.

Developmental and gross anatomy of the spine

Overview

The spine can be divided into four regions corresponding to four natural spinal curves: cervical, thoracic, lumbar, and sacral. These naturally occurring spinal curves are either kyphotic or lordotic. The "normal" spine has thoracic and sacral kyphosis and cervical and lumbar lordosis. The lordosis curvature of the cervical neck and of the lumbar spine develops as a response to weight bearing. As an infant gains strength in the posterior neck muscles, the spine develops with a lordotic curve to support the heavy head. At about 12 months of age, the lumbar spine develops a lordotic curve as a result of walking. Cervical and lumbar lordoses are considered secondary curves due to their dependent development on weight bearing. Their purpose is to keep the spine balanced and to reduce workload on the posterior spinal musculature. The thoracic and sacral kyphosis are considered to be primary curves. Normal cervical lordosis ranges typically from 20° to 40° while lumbar lordosis ranges between 30° and 50°. Acceptable thoracic kyphosis curvature is 20–50°. Medically, there is a broad range of acceptable sacral curvature since S1–5 are fused in a kyphotic angle.

Abnormal curvatures of the spine that this chapter will address are scoliosis and kyphosis [2–4]. Scoliosis is a complex three-dimensional deformity which involves changes in the coronal, sagittal, and axial alignment of the spine. The structural changes include wedging of the vertebral body, rotation of the vertebral body to the convex side of the curve, and deformities of the posterior elements. These structural changes are greatest at the apex of the curve. At this point, the pedicle is shortened and thickened, the lamina heavier, and the spinous process deviated toward the concave aspect of the curve. The vertebral body becomes wedge shaped and thicker on the concave aspect of the curve as a result of the compression forces during spinal growth. On the convex side, the vertebral body becomes thinner since it is expanded. The transverse processes approach the sagittal plane on the convex side and are more towards the concave side in the frontal plane. Additionally, rib prominence is often noticed on the convex side of the curve. This is due to the rotation of the thoracic vertebra. These spinal structural and rib alterations result in an asymmetrical thoracic cavity and may compromise respiratory function, leading to restrictive lung disease.

There are several potential etiologies for scoliosis [2,3]. Congenital scoliosis describes a failure of formation or segmentation of the vertebrae. Neuromuscular scoliosis may be caused by cerebral palsy, muscular dystrophy, myelomeningocele, poliomyelitis, and other disease affecting the muscle or nervous system. Syndromes associated with development of a scoliotic spine include Marfan syndrome, neurofibromatosis, and bone dysphasia. Idiopathic scoliosis is by far the most common of all scoliosis and is classified according to age of development.

Abnormal kyphosis is a spinal deformity that is usually classified as either postural kyphosis, congenital kyphosis or Scheuermann kyphosis. Postural kyphosis, otherwise known as round-back deformity, is a flexible spinal deformity that generally responds to non-operative treatments. Less common but more serious is congenital kyphosis. Surgery is usually recommended with a congenital kyphosis diagnosis given its rapid rate of progression at 5–7° a year and the potential for neurological compromise. Congenital kyphosis, similar to congenital scoliosis, is known to be caused by either a failure of part or all of the vertebral body to form or a failure of segmentation of part or all of the vertebral body.

Scheuermann kyphosis may affect the thoracic, thoracolumbar, and/or lumbar spine. Although several possible etiologies, including hormonal, nutritional, traumatic, vascular, and genetic causes, have been suggested, no definitive etiology for thoracic and thoracolumbar Scheuermann disease has been defined. Trauma is the usual causative factor of lumbar Scheuermann kyphosis. All three Scheuermann kyphosis variations clinically result in rigidity of the affected area. Using a standard radiograph, the diagnostic criteria include ≥5° of wedging in at least three adjacent vertebrae. Additionally, the vertebral endplates are irregular and the disk plates are narrowed. Schmorl nodes, the result of a herniated disk protruding through the weakened endplate, are often visible radiographically. Depending on the symptoms and the degree of curve, treatment includes both non-operative and operative modalities. A curve that is ≥75–80° generally warrants surgical intervention.

Spinal nerves and cord

There are 31 pairs of spinal nerves: eight cervical, 12 thoracic, five lumbar, five sacral, and one coccygeal. The first cervical root exits between the skull and C1 while the eighth cervical nerve root exits between C7 and T1. Thereafter, all nerve roots exit at the same level as their corresponding vertebrae. However, one should note that the nerve roots branch off the spinal cord higher than their actual exit through the intervertebral foramen [4]. Specifically, the spinal nerve must usually travel caudad adjacent to the spinal cord prior to exiting through the vertebral foramen.

Development of these essential nerves is complex. The neural tube is crucial in embryonic development [5] as it becomes the central nervous system and the neural crest forms the majority of the peripheral nervous system. As the neural tube closes, the neural crest migrates between the neural tube and the somite. These neural crest cells form the peripheral nervous system, Schwann cells, and melanocytes. The neural tube becomes the spinal cord, brain, and peripheral afferent nerves and preganglionic fibers of the autonomic nervous system.

While the neural tube closes, the dorsal region separates into two halves, the alar and basal laminae, referred to as the roof and floor plates. The alar plate becomes the sensory pathways, or dorsal columns, whereas the basal plate develops into the motor pathways. The motor pathways or the ventral horn neurons develop axons that form the ventral roots. The axons of the ganglion cells form central processes, which become the dorsal roots and peripheral processes that end in sensory organelles. Motor neurons develop capabilities before sensory nerves, and autonomic nerve function is established last.

Upon gross dissection, one can identify that the motor fibers are located on the anterior side of the spinal cord with the sensory fibers on the posterior side. A group of motor fibers are referred to as ventral roots (anterior roots) while a collection of sensory fibers comprise the dorsal root (posterior root). The sensory nerves have an accumulation of cell bodies outside the spinal cord known as the dorsal root ganglia, which contain the nuclei of the sensory nerves. Directly lateral to the ganglia, the anterior and posterior (ventral and dorsal) nerve roots join to form a common spinal nerve surrounded by a dural sheath. This point is where the peripheral nerve begins. Immediately after formation, the nerve divides into a small dorsal (posterior) ramus and a much larger ventral (anterior) primary ramus. The posterior primary rami serve a column of muscles on either side of the vertebral canal and a narrow strip of overlying skin. All of the other muscle and skin are supplied by the anterior primary rami, which form the cervical, brachial, lumbar, and sacral plexuses and the intercostal nerves.

Additional gross dissection provides a view of the multiple layers of the spinal cord. Protection of the spinal cord is provided by three layers of meninges: dura mater, arachnoid layer, and pia mater. The dura mater, constructed of connective tissue, is the most external layer, gray in color, and is typically easily identified within the spinal canal. A thin subdural space separates the dura mater from the next layer, the arachnoid which provides much of the vascular supply. Between the arachnoid layer and the deepest layer, the pia mater, lies the subarachnoid space. This houses the cerebrospinal fluid, which protects the nerve pathways by providing a fluid as a shock absorber. The pia mater is closely adherent to the spinal cord and the individual nerve roots. Similar to the arachnoid layer, the pia layer is highly vascularized, providing the necessary blood supplies to the neurological structures.

The spinal cord extends from the foramen magnum to L1–4, depending on the age of the patient. With growth and development, the caudal end of the cord moves from its initial position of L3–4 in infancy to its adult level of L1. The end of the spinal cord terminates as the conus medullaris and below this, the thick flexible dural sac contains the spinal nerves collectively known as the cauda equina. Within the cauda equina is the filum terminale, which extends from the conus medullaris to the coccyx. The filum terminale acts as an anchor to keep the lower spinal cord in its normal shape.

Vascular components

Circulation to the spinal cord requires multiple arteries and arteriolar branches [6,7]. The anterior arterial trunk and the two posterior lateral trunks are important suppliers of blood to the cervical, thoracic, and lumbar cord. All of these arteries arise from the vertebral arteries. Radicular arteries of the spinal cord assist these longitudinal arterial pathways. There are up to 17 radicular arteries anteriorly and as many as 25 posteriorly. The thoracic and lumbar radicular arteries are supplied by the aorta whereas the vertebral arteries supply the majority of the radicular arteries in the cervical spine. Additionally, the artery of Adamkiewicz feeds the lumbar section. It is usually on the left side, located at the level of T9–11. It is the largest of the radicular arteries which supply the spinal cord by anastomosing with the anterior (longitudinal) spinal artery. Injury to the artery of Adamkiewicz from trauma or during surgical procedures can result in devastating ischemia of the lower spinal cord and paraplegia. Additionally, the blood supply of the thoracic spine is more tenuous than the cervical or lumbar spine, especially at the T4–9 watershed area, which is more prone to ischemic injury.

A pair of segmental arteries, arising from the aorta, are present at every vertebral level providing blood flow to the extraspinal and intraspinal structures. The segmental arteries divide into many branches at the intervertebral foramen. A second network of segmental arteries lies within the spinal canal in the loose connective tissue of the extradural space. This second anastomotic network provides an alternative pathway for arterial blood flow, ensuring adequate spinal cord circulation after ligation of the segmental arteries during surgery.

Bony components

The surrounding, outer layer of the vertebra consists of cortical bone, which is dense, solid bone tissue made of compact Haversian systems. Within the vertebra lies cancellous bone, a porous, loosely connected bone. Cancellous or trabecular bone is weaker and more susceptible to disease and loss of bone density than cortical bone. Together, these two types of bone (trabecular and cortical) form the vertebral body which is a thin ring with an hourglass shape. The outer cortical bone extends above and below the superior and inferior ends of the vertebrae to form rims. The pedicles, consisting of dense cortical bone surrounding a medullary canal, are two short, rounded processes that extend posteriorly from the lateral margin of the dorsal surface of the vertebral body. The anterior third of the pedicle and the vertebral body together are referred to as an anterior arch.

The posterior arch, which directly attaches laterally to the anterior arch, includes the laminae, the processes (spinous process, transverse process, superior particular process), and the posterior two-thirds of the pedicles. The laminae are two flat plates of bone extending medially from the pedicles to form the posterior wall of the vertebral foramen. The part of the lamina located between the superior and inferior articular processes is called the pars interarticularis. Spondylolysis is a term used to refer to a defect in the pars, most commonly at the L5 level.

The three spinal processes are projections of bony tissue that are the insertion sites for tendons and ligaments. Specifically, two inferior and two superior articular processes extend from the junction of the pedicles and laminae. The inferior articular processes meet with the superior articular processes to form facet joints. The facet joints are surrounded by a capsular membrane containing synovial fluid that, along with the intervertebral disk, provides mobility of the spine. Additionally, two transverse processes (one on each side of the pedicles) extend laterally and provide an attachment point for ligaments and tendons. A single spinous process arises posteriorly from the junction of the two laminae, again providing an attachment point for ligaments and tendons and serving as a lever for motion of the vertebrae.

Additional bony components include the endplate and apophyseal ring. Endplates are located superiorly and inferiorly within the rim of each vertebral body. Each endplate consists of a cartilaginous external layer and a bony internal layer and provides vascular nutrition to the avascular intervertebral disk. These endplates also serve as a growth ring, predominantly in height, for the vertebral body. The endplates are closed by 17–18 years of age. The apophyseal ring of cortical bone surrounds the vertebral body below portions of the endplate. Surgically, it is important to leave as much of the bony endplate intact as possible, thus preventing subsidence of the device into the soft cancellous bone. The endplate is well vascularized, offering an excellent site for a fusion graft. The apophyseal ring is an ideal site for interbody fusion devices.

Surgical procedures on the pediatric spine

Scoliosis is a lateral and rotational deformity of the vertebral column. Its etiology is most commonly idiopathic (60–70%), neuromuscular or related to congenital bony deformities [8–10]. Other less common etiologies include post-traumatic injuries and therapy-related problems (previous surgical procedure or radiation for oncological diseases). Idiopathic scoliosis is more common in females with a female:male ratio of 3–4:1. The timing or need for surgery is based on the Cobb angle. The Cobb angle is calculated by identification of the most affected vertebra in the curve, also known as the apical vertebra (Fig. 26.1A,B). The apical vertebra is the vertebral body that has the greatest rotation and displacement from its ideal alignment. The top and bottom vertebrae of the curved or scoliotic segment are identified. These vertebrae have the most tilt, but the least amount of rotation and displacement. They are located above and below the apical vertebra, respectively.

On the radiograph, a line is drawn along the edge of these two vertebrae and extended out. On the top vertebrae, the line starts on the top, is drawn along the top edge, and slopes downward according to the angle of the vertebra. On the bottom vertebra, the line is drawn along the bottom edge in an upward direction. Perpendicular lines are then drawn from both lines so that they meet each other at the level of the apical vertebra. The Cobb angle is the angle formed by these two intersecting perpendicular lines.

Treatment modalities are based on the Cobb angle. If the angle is ≤15°, follow-up visits are scheduled to monitor the progression of the scoliosis. Bracing is generally indicated for a Cobb angle of 20–40° while surgical intervention is indicated when the Cobb angle is greater than 40° in the lumbar spine or greater than 50° in the thoracic spine. Although some correction of the curve may be feasible, the primary goal of surgical treatment is to stop progression of the curve. Without intervention, progression of the scoliosis will invariably lead to restrictive lung disease and respiratory insufficiency, resulting in severe morbidity (chronic hypoxemia and hypercarbia) and eventual death from cor pulmonale.

Options for surgical treatment include both anterior and posterior procedures. Surgical decision points regarding the approach and surgical therapy include the age of the patient, the underlying cause of the spinal deformity, and the severity of the curve. A patient with neuromuscular scoliosis may be surgically treated with a posterior procedure or may require an anterior spinal release followed by posterior fusion if the deformity is more severe to gain better correction. Although idiopathic scoliosis has been most commonly treated by a posterior approach

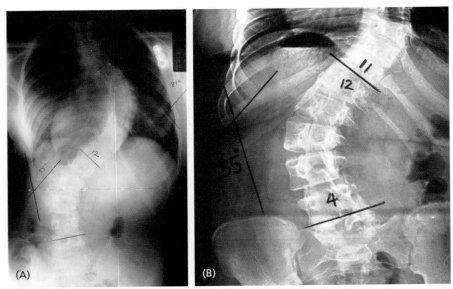

Figure 26.1 Radiographs (A,B) showing the determination of the Cobb angle. The apical vertebra is identified by finding the verbetral body that has the greatest rotation and displacement from its ideal alignment. The top and bottom vertebrae of the curved or scoliotic segment are then identified. These vertebrae have the most tilt but the least amount of rotation and displacement. They are located above and below the apical vertebra, respectively. A line is drawn along the edge of these two vertebrae and extended out. On the top vertebrae, the line is drawn along the top edge and slopes downward according to the angle of the vertebra. On the bottom vertebra, the line is drawn along the bottom edge in an upward direction. Perpendicular lines are then drawn from both lines so that they meet each other at the level of the apical vertebra. The Cobb angle is the angle formed by these two intersecting perpendicular lines.

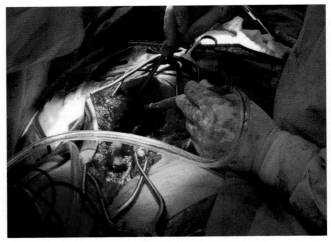

Figure 26.2 Standard long vertical posterior incision for instrumentation and correction of scoliosis.

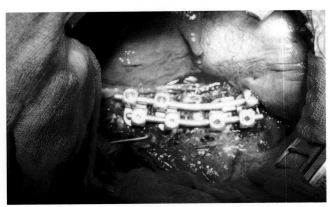

Figure 26.3 Anterior approach for surgical exposure and instrumentation in the treatment of idiopathic scoliosis. With the use of one-lung ventilation, the surgeon's access to the anterolateral aspect of the thoracic and lumbar vertebral bodies can be facilitated.

(Fig. 26.2), in some centers, an anterior approach with instrumentation is being used for idiopathic scoliosis (Fig. 26.3). The underlying diagnosis, the curve magnitude, and the patient's age are all important factors when determining the type of procedure.

One issue that affects the timing of surgery is that the fused segments will no longer grow. As such, complete surgical correction with fusion is undertaken only when spinal growth is nearly complete, generally at ≥12–14 years of age. When surgical treatment is necessary for the juvenile idiopathic scoliosis patient, non-segmental posterior spinal instrumentation without fusion is used (i.e. growing rod). This approach allows correction of the scoliosis without decortications and fusion of numerous vertebral segments. Therefore, normal growth will continue. During the growing rod procedure, specific vertebral levels are decorticated and fused in an attempt to allow for correction of the curvature with normal growth of the remaining spine. In general, the convex sides are decorticated and fused so that the concave sides straighten out with the ensuing growth of the vertebral bodies. Patients undergoing growing rod procedures will require repeated operative intervention at 4–6-month intervals to adjust the growing rods. In most cases, definite posterior spinal fusion with instrumentation is performed once growth of the vertebral column has ceased. This approach is used most commonly in patients with bony congenital anomalies or muscular dystrophies that result in early onset (birth to 10 years of age) of scoliosis.

Anterior surgery for scoliosis

Although idiopathic scoliosis has generally been treated via a posterior approach with posterior spinal fusion, anterior approaches have more recently been developed. Advocates of the anterior approach believe that successful correction of the curve can be achieved while limiting the extent of the fusion, thereby maintaining flexibility and mobility of the spine.

For the anterior approach, the patient is placed in the lateral decubitus position with the operating table flexed. The upper arm is moved forward and rotated away from the posterior portion of the spine. An axillary roll is placed to minimize pressure on the brachial plexus and the vascular structures. Depending on the level of scoliosis (thoracic versus lumbar), entry into the thoracic cavity may be required. When the thoracic cavity is entered, the use of one-lung ventilation may greatly facilitate the surgeon's access to the anterior spine. Following skin incision, access to the spine is achieved through the bed of the convex fifth rib for visualization of T5–12 or via the bed of the 10th rib for access to the thoracolumbar spine. The initial incision extends anteriorly to the lateral border of the rectus sheath with its length determined by the number of levels required to be exposed. The rib to be excised corresponds to the most superior vertebral body requiring exposure. For example, with a T6–12 anterior fusion, the fifth rib is excised. The costal cartilage is split anteriorly which can later serve as a landmark for closure.

Once the spine is exposed, retractors are positioned to protect the lung tissue and peritoneum. The surgeon can now access the vertebral disk or vertebral body with the caveat that segmental vertebral vessels (artery and vein) are present at each level. When necessary, these vessels can be ligated as vascular compromise of the spinal cord

after ligation is uncommon even if several segmental vessels are ligated.

Video-assisted thoracoscopic surgery

Video-assisted thoracoscopic surgical (VATS) techniques have also been incorporated into the surgical treatment of scoliosis. As with other types of VATS procedures, specialized surgical equipment is necessary, including the scope, light sources, cameras, flexible portals, monitors, and specific instrumentation. For the successful completion of such procedures, one-lung ventilation (OLV) is generally mandatory to allow for adequate visualization of the spine (see below). Contraindications to this approach include the inability to tolerate OLV, severe respiratory insufficiency, high airway pressures with positive pressure ventilation, and previous thoracotomy which may result in adhesions, thereby limiting surgical access and the ability to obtain lung deflation during OLV. Positioning and preparation are generally the same as for the open, anterior approach. The surgical landmarks for trocar and instrument placement include the scapular border, 12th rib, and iliac crest.

The first portal is placed at or near the T6–7 interspace in the posterior axillary line. After surgical incision, dissection continues with electrocautery through the intercostal muscle to enter the thoracic cavity. Once adequate lung deflation is ensured, flexible ports are inserted in the intercostal spaces with a trocar. A blunt-tipped needle is placed adjacent to the thoracic spine and a roentgenogram is obtained to confirm the disk spaces intraoperatively. The parietal pleura is completely resected without ligation of the segmental thoracic vessels. The disks and endplates are then removed. After the necessary diskectomies are completed, rib grafts are harvested through the portal sites. Prior to closure, a chest tube is placed through the most posterior inferior portal. The pleura may be closed or left open. The chest tube is connected to a water seal and the anesthesiologist tests for an air leak in the reinflated lung.

Potential perioperative issues include bleeding, damage to the lung tissue, dural tears, lymphatic injury, and sympathetic dysfunction on the operative side. If hemostasis cannot be obtained or visualization is not optimal, conversion to an open anterior approach may be required. Postoperatively, pulmonary problems may occur within the deflated lung, leading to recurrent atelectasis.

Posterior surgery for scoliosis

Over the past 20 years, the surgical approach to scoliosis has changed with advances in segmental posterior spinal instrumentation. As such, correction of both sagittal and coronal plane spinal deformities has improved over older

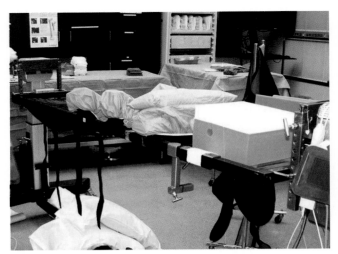

Figure 26.4 Jackson table used for prone positioning of patients during a posterior approach for spinal fusion.

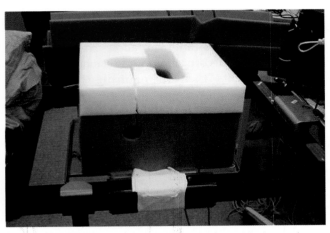

Figure 26.5 Specialized cushion or pillow used for positioning on the Jackson table. When applied appropriately, the pillow should eliminate pressure points on the face and eyes. The endotracheal tube can be brought out through the side hole of the pillow or through the bottom of the pillow and the supporting structure of the Jackson table.

systems such as the Harrington rods. The posterior surgical approach with instrumentation uses the spinous processes, the pedicles, the facets, and the laminae to control the alignment of the vertebral bodies with laminar hooks, pedicle hooks, pedicle screws, facet screws, and wires.

For the classic posterior approach, the patient is placed prone on an appropriate spinal frame with the abdomen hanging freely to avoid compression of the intra-abdominal portion of the inferior vena cava and prevent interference with diaphragmatic movement. Traditionally, a Hall frame or, more recently, a Jackson table is used to support the patient in this position (Fig. 26.4). The patient's face should be well padded without pressure on the eyes (see below for an expanded discussion of postoperative visual compromise) (Fig. 26.5). The patient's back is completely draped with exposure to the entire spine and the iliac crest for harvesting of the bone graft. A midline incision over the spinous processes is made followed by splitting the apophysis and subperiosteal dissection to expose the spine laterally to the transverse processes. Placement of a blunt needle is followed by confirmation of the appropriate vertebral body using either fluoroscopy or plain radiograph. After a facetectomy and wide posterior release at each level, instrumentation is placed. The surgeon inserts pedicle hooks, pedical screws, laminar hooks, and sublaminar wires at the vertebral levels requiring surgical correction of the scoliosis. The first rod is placed on the concave side of the curve and rotated to correct the spinal deformity. This represents a key moment during the instrumentation procedure as alterations in spinal cord perfusion may occur during correction of the curvature. If changes are to be observed with neuromonitoring, it is usually during this portion of the surgery. Once correction is maintained with

the first rod, the second rod is placed. Cross-links are added, allowing an increase in torsional stiffness of the rod's construction. Decortication of the posterior elements prepares the spine for fusion. The placement of bone graft completes the procedure and is followed by a layered closure of the muscles, fascia and skin.

Preoperative and intraoperative care

Preoperative evaluation

The initial step in the perioperative care of pediatric patients presenting for spinal surgery is the preoperative evaluation to identify co-morbid features which may affect their perioperative care and to maximize the patient's preoperative state in the hope of preventing perioperative complications. Of primary importance when evaluating children and adolescents for spine surgery is the impact of the disease process on airway management and cervical spine stability. Cervical spine stability is the spine's ability to resist displacement under normal physiological loads. Patients presenting for cervical spine surgery, especially the trauma patient, should be assumed to have an unstable cervical spine or the potential for subluxation during flexion or extension of the neck which can result in spinal cord compromise [11]. Cervical spine issues and resultant instability may be related to a traumatic event or a congenital syndrome with associated cervical spine involvement such as trisomy 21, achondroplasia or other more uncommon craniofacial syndromes such as Pfeiffer, Apert or Crouzon syndrome [12–15]. Subluxation and upper cervical intervertebral fusions have been reported in 30% of patients with Pfeiffer syndrome and odontoid hypoplasia with the risk of C1–2 subluxation has been reported in patients with Crouzon syndrome and the mucopolysaccharidoses [13,14]. Ligamentous laxity and the potential for cervical subluxation is also present in patients with trisomy 21 [15].

Patients with achondroplasia may have associated stenosis of the foramen magnum which may also affect airway management. Foramen magnum stenosis results from hypertrophy of the bony margins of the foramen magnum and can lead to narrowing of the cervical spinal canal with compression of the cervical spinal cord or medulla. In children with achondroplasia, who manifest neurological or respiratory symptoms related to foramen magnum stenosis, the diameter of the foramen magnum has been shown to be more than three standard deviations smaller than the mean for age-matched controls of normal stature.

Even in the absence of associated syndromes, cervical spine involvement from scoliosis or kyphosis may limit normal cervical spine movement, thereby leading to difficulties with endotracheal intubation. Given these issues, as time permits, an evaluation of the cervical spine for subluxation may be indicated as part of the preoperative work-up in such patients. Preoperative evaluation for cervical spine abnormalities includes a physical examination with an evaluation of neck movement supplemented with radiograph examination (flexion/extension films) or computed tomography scanning. If potential issues are identified during the evaluation process, various approaches to obtaining endotracheal intubation are available which can be performed in the anesthetized, sedated or awake state [11]. During anesthetic induction and airway manipulation, prevention of cervical spine movement can be accomplished by the use of manual in-line stabilization. In older, co-operative patients, awake airway techniques commonly used in the adult population (intravenous sedation with glossopharyngeal nerve and superior laryngeal nerve blockade) followed by direct laryngoscopy or fiber-optic bronchoscopy for endotracheal intubation may be feasible.

Patients with craniofacial syndromes may also have midface anatomical issues that affect airway management, including ease of bag-valve-mask ventilation and endotracheal intubation [12,13]. Common features of many of the craniofacial syndromes include micrognathia, microstoma, midface (maxillary) hypoplasia, and lip/palatal abnormalities. Glossal hypertrophy may be present in neuromuscular conditions or in association with trisomy 21. Although beyond the scope of this chapter, identification of potential difficulties with direct laryngoscopy and endotracheal intubation should prompt alternative approaches to the airway, including indirect video laryngoscopy or fiber-optic techniques. Additionally,

there should be ready access to the equipment required for management of a difficult airway, including various sizes of laryngeal mask airway or a similar type of supraglottic device. See Chapter 14 for detailed discussion of management of the difficult airway.

Another situation faced by the anesthesia provider which affects perioperative airway management is the patient with an *in situ* tracheostomy requiring airway management and prone positioning for spinal surgery. Although there have been some suggestions regarding strategies to manage a tracheostomy in the perioperative period, including use of an existing tracheostomy, change to a cuffed tracheostomy, placement of an endotracheal tube (ETT) through the tracheostomy stoma or use of standard orotracheal intubation [16], there are no definitive consensus guidelines available. Although the presence of a tracheostomy initially may facilitate airway management, positioning and other intraoperative issues may affect airway patency. Most importantly, if a standard tracheostomy tube is used, given its rigidity, traction from the anesthesia circuit may cause posterior displacement of its lumen with occlusion against the tracheal wall [17]. Such problems can generally be avoided by exchanging the tracheostomy for an appropriately sized armored endotracheal tube. Use of the armored tube may avoid positional changes related to traction on the tube due to the weight of the anesthesia circuit. After exchange of the tracheostomy, the armored ETT can be secured in place using a suture to the neck or the anterior chest wall. Given that the tracheostomy site enters the trachea closer to the carina than standard endotracheal intubation techniques, careful placement and auscultation of bilateral breath sounds are necessary to avoid endobronchial intubation. Appropriate positioning of the endotracheal tube should be confirmed in the neutral position and with the neck flexed.

Following evaluation of the airway and cervical spine, the preoperative examination follows a sequential organ system approach. Co-morbidities of the central and peripheral nervous and muscular systems may be a frequent feature in the pediatric patient presenting for spine surgery. Pediatric patients with scoliosis presenting for spinal surgery may have associated cerebral palsy and static encephalopathy or associated neuromuscular conditions. The preoperative assessment and documentation of neurological and neuromuscular function will help in the identification of perioperative injuries related to the surgical procedure or positioning and aid in differentiating these from pre-existing conditions. Patients with cerebral palsy may have an associated seizure disorder with the need for one or more anticonvulsant medications. During the preoperative evaluation, therapeutic serum anticonvulsant concentrations should be documented and the parents instructed to give the usual anticonvulsant medications on the morning of surgery. Although many of the newer medications have long half-lives, perioperative dosing is recommended whenever feasible. Intraoperatively, appropriate conversion to intravenous administration is available for several anticonvulsant medications so that therapeutic levels are maintained perioperatively. Postoperatively, dosing can be converted to the oral route when the patient's status permits or alternative routes of delivery (intravenous or rectal) may be used.

Chronic anticonvulsant therapy leads to the induction of hepatic enzymes, thereby altering the pharmacokinetics and pharmacodynamics of several drugs, including neuromuscular blocking agents (NMBAs). Increasing the intraoperative doses of NMBAs and certain intravenous anesthetic induction agents may be necessary with concomitant anticonvulsant therapy [18–20]. Additionally, a secondary factor affecting dosing of NMBAs is the fact that many anticonvulsant agents have weak neuromuscular blocking properties, leading to the upregulation of acetylcholine receptors. Therefore, increased dosing requirements may be seen even for agents such as *cis*-atracurium which are not dependent on hepatic metabolism for their elimination.

Mental retardation and associated visual and hearing disturbances may present a major challenge in the communication with and assessment of the patient. Some degree of intellectual impairment is noted in 30–50% of patients with Duchenne muscular dystrophy (DMD) and in a greater percentage of patients with cerebral palsy. In addition to limiting preoperative co-operation and understanding, these issues may be particularly problematic during the postoperative period when pain assessment may be difficult (see below).

Depending on the degree of scoliosis and the presence of co-morbid disease processes, there may be some degree of preoperative compromise of respiratory function from restrictive lung disease. Progressive scoliosis results in a restrictive defect with a decrease in the vital capacity, total lung capacity, and forced expiratory volume with no change in residual volume. The decrease is greater in patients with congenital or infantile scoliosis when compared to adolescent scoliosis [21,22]. The severity of respiratory impairment is related to the angle of the scoliosis, the number of vertebral levels involved, the cephalad level of the scoliosis , and the loss of the normal thoracic kyphosis. Respiratory compromise is worse in younger patients and those with infantile or congenital scoliosis. Muirhead and Conner noted that there was a moderate or severe ventilation defect (40–59% predicted for age) in 14 of 41 children with either infantile or congenital scoliosis compared to only four of the 51 adolescents with idiopathic scoliosis [21]. No child with a vital capacity ≥40% predicted for age required postoperative respira-

tory support. Other investigators have demonstrated that the effect of the surgical procedure on lung function is dependent on the surgical approach and the type of surgery. Surgical procedures involving the thorax (anterior spinal fusion) lead to a reduction in lung function at 3 months with a return to preoperative values by 2 years while the standard posterior approach leads to improved respiratory function at both 3 months and 2 years [22,23].

Of even greater concern when providing preoperative care for patients with neuromuscular disorders is the ability to determine the degree of respiratory compromise which is a contraindication to scoliosis surgery. Given its greater impact on respiratory function, this need is greater if an anterior approach is chosen when compared to a standard posterior approach. In the adult population, it has been suggested that prolonged postoperative mechanical ventilation is likely to be required in patients with a reduction of the forced vital capacity (FVC) or the forced expiratory volume in 1 second (FEV_1) to less than 40% predicted. However, as there are generally fewer co-morbid features in children, such as associated cardiac disease when compared with adults, it is likely that the same criteria used to predict postoperative respiratory function in adults should not necessarily be applied to pediatric patients.

The lack of predictive power of preoperative pulmonary function testing in children has been previously demonstrated by Tobias et al in a cohort of pediatric oncology patients requiring repeated thoracotomy for excision of metastatic disease [24]. After 32 thoracotomies in 19 pediatric oncology patients, there was a consistent decrease in pulmonary function test (PFT) values with a decrease in the FVC (% predicted for age) from 68 ± 3.6% to 60 ± 2.4% (p < 0.01) and the FEV_1 from 69 ± 4.2% to 60 ± 3.8% (p < 0.01). There was no permanent morbidity noted even in patients with decreased preoperative respiratory function. Five of the patients had severe preoperative decreases in pulmonary function (≤40% predicted for age). Although the incidence of morbidity, defined as postoperative mechanical ventilation, supplemental oxygen for more than 12h or persistent air leak, was three out of five in this group versus three of 20 in patients with mild or moderate lung disease (PFT 60–80% predicted for age), there was no postoperative mortality and no need for prolonged mechanical ventilation.

Similar data have more recently been reported by Harper et al in a cohort of adolescents with Duchenne muscular dystrophy and compromised respiratory function [25]. In their cohort of 45 patients, 20 had a preoperative FVC ≤30% predicted for age. The authors reported no statistically significant difference in several postoperative variables, including the duration of postoperative endotracheal intubation, duration of bi-level positive airway pressure (BiPAP) support, total time with ventilator assistance, and inpatient stay. However, there were significant cardiorespiratory complications in both groups, demonstrating that this is a high-risk population with the potential for perioperative complications. Five patients (25%) with an FVC ≤30% had complications including acute respiratory distress syndrome (ARDS), respiratory tract infections, and the need for a tracheostomy while four (16%) with a preoperative FVC ≥30% had complications. The one death in the cohort was in a patient with an FVC of 18% who initially had an uncomplicated postoperative course, but went on to develop ARDS.

Although the majority of patients presenting for spinal surgery without co-morbid conditions (idiopathic scoliosis) will not require postoperative mechanical ventilation, factors such as co-morbid conditions, intraoperative blood loss, and surgical duration may mandate providing a short period of postoperative mechanical ventilation to ensure patient safety. In addition to respiratory function, airway issues may necessitate postoperative mechanical ventilation. Prolonged procedures in the prone position may result in airway or lingual edema, thereby necessitating postoperative endotracheal intubation. Almenrader and Patel reviewed their 18-month experience in a cohort of 42 patients with non-idiopathic scoliosis [26]. In their series, 23.8% of patients required postoperative mechanical ventilation. Consistent with the data of Harper et al, they noted that patients with Duchenne muscular dystrophy and those with a preoperative FVC ≤30% were more likely to require postoperative respiratory support (40% in their series). They suggest the use of non-invasive ventilator techniques to ease the transition from mechanical to spontaneous ventilation.

In addition to respiratory issues in patients undergoing scoliosis surgery, perioperative morbidity and mortality may also be related to secondary cardiac involvement. Myocardial dysfunction in this group of patients may be related to the primary disease process such as muscular dystrophy or, less commonly, chronic hypoxemia from restrictive lung disease and associated cor pulmonale. The latter is uncommon as scoliosis is frequently addressed prior to the development of chronic cardiovascular effects. More commonly, various neuromuscular conditions such as the muscular dystrophies or myotonic dystrophies may lead to myocardial involvement with alterations in the contractile function or conduction abnormalities. Of these conditions, Duchenne muscular dystrophy is the most common disorder, with an incidence of 1 in 3300 male births. It is inherited as an X-linked disorder generally presenting as weakness during the first decade of life, usually between 4 and 8 years of age. The genetic defect results in a deficiency of the protein dystrophin in skeletal, cardiac, and smooth muscle. Although skeletal muscle involvement with weakness predominates as the major clinical feature of this disorder, as these patients enter the second and third decades of life, progressive myocardial involvement leads to impaired myocardial contractility, conduction disturbances, and arrhythmias.

The potential impact of this disorder on perioperative morbidity and even mortality cannot be ignored as the literature has demonstrated a significantly increased risk during anesthetic care in these patients [27]. Sethna et al reported intraoperative cardiac arrest and death in two of 25 patients requiring anesthetic care during various surgical procedures [27]. Given the potential for associated myocardial involvement in many patients, some type of preoperative screening to assess myocardial function and conduction disturbances may be indicated. In most cases, this will include transthoracic echocardiography and a 12-lead electrocardiogram (ECG). More recently, it has been suggested that the combination of a preoperative chest radiograph and ECG can be used to screen for the presence of myocardial dysfunction [28]. Although Clendenin et al noted that an abnormality on the chest radiograph (increased cardiac silhouette) and abnormal findings on the ECG were predictive in 81% of their 255 patients, echocardiography remains the gold standard [28].

A second group that tends to be increasing in the spinal surgery population is those with associated congenital heart disease. In this group of patients, especially those with residual lesions or single-ventricle physiology, preoperative assessment is of paramount importance to guide intraoperative care. In these patients or when myocardial dysfunction is identified, additional intraoperative monitoring (transesophageal echocardiography) with consultation from pediatric cardiology may be required. Furthermore, close observation during positioning is suggested as these patients may deteriorate rapidly with the institution of positive pressure ventilation or when turned prone due to changes in venous return or increased intrathoracic pressure.

The preoperative evaluation and preparation of the patient are essential to limit allogeneic blood product use. Simple measures to reduce the need for allogeneic blood products include identification and treatment of anemia prior to elective spinal surgery. In the adult population, age greater than 50 years, preoperative hemoglobin less than 12 g/dL, fusion of more than two levels, and transpedicular osteotomy have been identified as independent risk factors for the need for perioperative transfusion [29]. Routine screening for the identification of preoperative anemia and its treatment are particularly important in patients with poor nutritional status or following menarche. Although treatment with oral iron is generally effective, a more rapid response within 2–3 weeks can be obtained with intravenous iron therapy [30].

More aggressive and more expensive preoperative blood avoidance techniques may include the administration of erythropoietin to augment preoperative autologous donation or the yield of intraoperative isovolemic hemodilution (see below). Issues with erythropoietin include varying reports of its efficacy, with some studies showing no benefit, variations in dosing regimens, and the need for weekly visits with laboratory measurement of hemoglobin and subcutaneous injections, as well as the potential to increase the incidence of postoperative deep vein thrombotic events. In a retrospective analysis of 178 pediatric patients undergoing spinal surgery, Vitale et al reported that homologous transfusions were administered to 30.6% of patients who did not receive erythropoietin versus only 17.5% of those who did (p < 0.05) [31]. In a subgroup analysis of patients with idiopathic scoliosis, the need for homologous transfusion was 3.9% in those receiving erythropoietin versus 23.5% of those who did not (p = 0.006). They also noted a shorter hospital stay in those patients who had received erythropoietin (6.7 versus 9.3 days, p = 0.02). Subsequent work from the same investigators demonstrated no benefit of preoperative erythropoietin in limiting the need for allogeneic transfusion in a cohort of 61 patients with neuromuscular scoliosis [32].

Other investigators have suggested the efficacy of erythropoietin when used in combination with an autologous blood donation strategy [33]. Although such techniques are feasible in the pediatric population, given the need for repeated phlebotomy and laboratory analysis with the inherent time, cost, and pain issues for the patient, there has been a significant decrease in the interest in and use of preoperative autologous blood donation. More recently, the safety of erythropoietin has been questioned. In the adult, population, Stowell et al reported a higher incidence of deep vein thrombosis of 4.7% versus 2.1% in a cohort of 680 adults [34].

Patients presenting for major orthopedic surgery may have chronic medical or nutritional conditions that affect coagulation function. The chronic administration of anticonvulsants including phenytoin and carbamazepime may adversely affect coagulation function. Nutritional issues and poor intake of vitamin K may result in a low levels of vitamin K-dependent coagulation factors, leading to preoperative coagulation dysfunction. Preoperative screening of coagulation function and simple measures such as the administration of vitamin K (oral or intramuscular) may alleviate such problems. Patients with chronic orthopedic problems and pain frequently use non-steroidal anti-inflammatory agents (NSAIDs). Although acetylsalicylic acid irreversibly inhibits cyclo-oxygenase and platelet function for the life of the platelet, NSAIDs cause reversible inhibition of platelet function that is dependent on the plasma concentration and hence the half-life of the NSAID. Discontinuation of most NSAIDs for 2–5 days prior to surgery will result in return of normal platelet function.

Premedication, anesthetic induction, and positioning

Various agents or combinations may be required preoperatively in patients undergoing spinal surgery. Premedication regimens may include:

- high-flow nebulization of albuterol and an anticholinergic agent such as ipratropium in patients with airway reactivity or lidocaine if a fiber-optic intubation is planned due to a difficult airway scenario
- gastrointestinal prophylaxis in patients at risk for aspiration may include agents to increase gastric pH such as H_2-antagonists (ranitidine), proton pump inhibitors or oral non-particulate antacids and motility agents such as metoclopramide
- dexamethasone for patients with airway reactivity and to decrease postoperative nausea and vomiting
- an anticholinergic agent such as glycopyrrolate or atropine to dry secretions, especially if a fiber-optic intubation technique is planned, to blunt cholinergic-mediated airway reactivity and to prevent bradycardia during laryngoscopy and ET intubation
- hydrocortisone if patients are chronically receiving supplementation (chronic corticosteroid therapy is frequently used in patients with Duchenne muscular dystrophy given data suggesting its ability to slow progression of the disease [35])
- an anxiolytic which generally follows the standard practice in pediatric anesthesia including either oral midazolam in patients without intravenous access or intravenous midazolam in those with pre-existing IV access.

Following premedication, the patient is transported to the operating room and routine American Society of Anesthesiologists' monitors are placed. From the start of anesthetic care, attention should be paid to the maintenance of normothermia. Hypothermia is particularly common and may occur rapidly in patients with cerebral palsy and failure to thrive who may have limited body fat. Patients with static encephalopathy and related conditions may have abnormal central control of temperature, thereby placing them at further risk of hypothermia. In addition to other physiological effects, perioperative hypothermia has been shown to be a key factor in increasing intraoperative blood loss during major surgical procedures [36,37]. The maintenance of normothermia includes preoperative warming of the patient using forced air devices, keeping the operating room warmed until the patient is positioned and covered, warming intravenous fluids, blood and blood

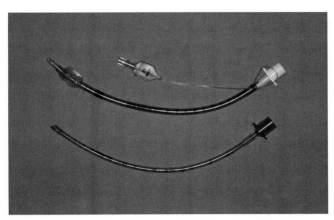

Figure 26.6 Wire-reinforced endotracheal tube to prevent kinking during prone positioning with head flexion.

products, and the intraoperative use of forced air warming devices.

The technique and medications used for the induction of anesthesia are guided by the patient's co-morbid conditions, the assessment of the ease of tracheal intubation, and the patient's preference and/or demographics (age and cognitive function). For anterior or posterior spine surgery, a reinforced endotracheal tube may be used to prevent inadvertent airway occlusion during surgical dissection and/or neck flexion (Fig. 26.6). During prolonged cases with neck flexion, there may be a risk for non-reinforced ETTs to warm, bend, and obstruct if they are held in a flexed position over a protracted period of time. Although the time-honored practice has been to use uncuffed ETTs in patients less than 6–8 years of age, given limited access to the airway during the surgical procedure and the potential need for occlusion of the airway to provide adequate positive pressure ventilation, cuffed ETTs are being used more frequently to provide intraoperative anesthetic care. Once the ETT is secured in place and an esophageal stethoscope placed, a gauze roll is placed in the mouth to prevent biting during motor-evoked potential stimulation (see below).

Several agents are available for the induction and maintenance of anesthesia in patients with stable cardiovascular function. In the absence of IV access, anesthetic induction can be carried out with sevoflurane in oxygen or oxygen and nitrous oxide. In patients with previously established IV access, several of the commonly used IV induction agents are suitable. If there is a plan for extubation in the operating room or immediately postoperatively, propofol may provide a more rapid awakening and a better recovery profile during the immediate postoperative period than induction with barbiturates such as thiopental. Although its effect on adrenal function has led to a re-evaluation of its use during endotracheal intubation

in the critically ill ICU patient, etomidate may still be an appropriate choice for anesthetic induction in patients with diminished myocardial function.

Once adequate bag-mask ventilation has been demonstrated, inhalation or intravenous induction techniques can be followed by the administration of a non-depolarizing NMBA. Succinylcholine is contraindicated in patients with various neurological and myopathic conditions given the potential for rhabdomyolysis, hyperkalemia, and cardiac arrest. Similar problems with succinylcholine may occur in patients within 48–72 h following a spinal cord injury. In the absence of concerns about a difficult airway, endotracheal intubation can be facilitated with an intermediate-acting (vecuronium, rocuronium, *cis*-atracurium, atracurium) or short-acting (mivacurium) non-depolarizing NMBA [38]. The dosing of these agents should be titrated using train-of-four (TOF) monitoring, especially in patients with DMD and other myopathies as even a single dose for endotracheal intubation of an intermediate-acting NMBA may result in a prolonged duration of neuromuscular blockade. When motor-evoked potentials are being used to monitor spinal cord function, a single dose of a non-depolarizing NMBA can be used to facilitate endotracheal intubation with the understanding that repeated dosing will generally not be used once the patient is turned prone.

After the airway is secured, adequate intravenous access and invasive cardiovascular monitoring as indicated are obtained. Several factors may be responsible for hemodynamic changes during spinal surgery in pediatric patients, including co-morbid conditions, positioning on the operating room table, and blood loss. In general, for major spinal surgical procedures, two large-bore peripheral intravenous cannulas are placed for the rapid administration of fluids, blood, and blood products. Additional invasive hemodynamic monitoring with an arterial cannula and central venous access may be obtained, depending on the patient's condition and the surgical expertise. In experienced hands, blood loss is generally minimal in patients with idiopathic scoliosis (400–600 mL), thereby eliminating the need for central venous access. The accuracy of central venous pressure (CVP) monitoring in the prone position has been questioned [39]. In a cohort of 12 pediatric patients undergoing spinal fusion, hemodynamic assessment using CVP monitoring and echocardiography was assessed in the supine positioning and after positioning prone. CVP increased from a mean of 8.7 to 17.7 mm Hg while left ventricular end-diastolic diameter decreased from 37.1 mm to 33.2 mm, thereby leading the authors to conclude that CVP may be a misleading monitor of cardiac volume in scoliosis patients in the prone position.

Once appropriate vascular access and monitoring have been established, the patient is then positioned on the operating room table. Patient positioning will be dependent on the specific type of surgery, with either prone positioning for posterior spinal fusion or lateral positioning if an anterior approach is chosen. If the cervical spine and upper thoracic vertebrae are included in the surgical field, neutral positioning of the head is required. Alternatively, for posterior spinal fusion that does not involve the lower cervical or high thoracic area or isolated lumbar surgery, the patient can be positioned prone and the head turned 90°, thereby limiting the potential for pressure points on the eyes and face. Regardless of the positioning, careful padding of pressure points is needed since many of these procedures can last up to 8 h.

Positioning should also take into account techniques to minimize venous pressure at the surgical site to reduce bleeding. This is done by using rolls under the chest and pelvis to keep the abdomen free and by reverse Trendelenburg positioning. Mild reverse Trendelenburg positioning also helps to limit the development of dependent edema in the face, tongue and upper airway and may also limit the increase in intraocular pressure (IOP) which may occur with prone positioning. Alternatively, specialized frames (e.g. Wilson frame or Jackson table) can be used to position the patient and decrease venous pressure and therefore surgical bleeding (see Fig. 26.4). Use of the Jackson table with longitudinal bolsters has been shown to have the least effect on cardiovascular performance [39,40]. Keeping the abdomen free also facilitates mechanical ventilation by preventing compromise of diaphragmatic movement.

A major concern during surgical procedures in the prone position is the occurrence of postoperative visual impairment or blindness. Increased IOP with prone positioning has been postulated to be one of the contributing factors for this rare but devastating complication of blindness following prone surgical procedures [41–43]. In a cohort of 20 adults undergoing surgery in the prone position, IOP was 19 ± 1 mmHg in the awake state, decreased to 13 ± 1 mmHg in the supine position after the induction of anesthesia, but then increased to 40 ± 2 mmHg after 320 ± 107 min in the prone position. Although various theories have been suggested to explain postoperative visual loss (POVL), no unifying theory (ischemic, thrombotic, oncotic, embolic) has been accepted. Given the devastating consequences and potential medicolegal implications of this phenomenon, the Postoperative Visual Loss Registry was established in 1999 in an attempt to determine factors associated with POVL [44]. In the registry, the authors reviewed 93 voluntarily reported cases of visual disturbances following spine surgery and noted that of the 83 cases of ischemic optic neuropathy, blood loss greater than 1000 mL and surgical duration of greater than 6 h were present in 96% of the cases. Although other etiologies are feasible and appropriate positioning

is mandatory to avoid ocular pressure, the current literature suggests that the majority of factors, including surgical duration and blood loss, are frequently outside the control of the anesthesia provider.

For anterior procedures, the patient will be positioned in the lateral position and a thoracotomy performed to gain access to the vertebral column. Alternatively, there is increasing experience with the use of thoracoscopic approaches for such procedures. Regardless of the approach (open thoracotomy or thoracoscopy), OLV can greatly enhance the surgeon's view of the surgical field.

One-lung ventilation for anterior approaches

Options for OLV include a double-lumen endotracheal tube (DLT), a bronchial blocker or selective mainstem intubation [45–47]. The smallest commercially available DLT is 26 French, which can be used in patients who are 8–10 years of age. Advantages of a DLT include rapid placement, easy separation of the lungs, completion deflation of the operative lung, improved pulmonary toilet with access for suctioning of both lungs, the ability to rapidly switch to two-lung ventilation if needed, and the feasibility of administering continuous positive airway pressure (CPAP) or oxygen insufflation to the operative lung should this become necessary to improve oxygenation. In patients whose size precludes the use of a DLT, the bronchus on the operative side can be occluded with a balloon-tipped catheter that is placed using fiberoptic bronchoscopic guidance. Several different devices can be used as bronchial blockers including a Fogarty embolectomy catheter, atrio-septostomy catheter, pulmonary artery catheter, the Arndt endobronchial blocker (Cook Critical Care, Birmingham, IN), and the Univent endotracheal tube (Fuji Systems, Tokyo, Japan). Devices with a central channel have the advantage of allowing some degree of suctioning through the channel, not to clear the lung of secretions, as the channel is too small for that purpose, but rather to deflate the operative lung and improve surgical visualization or for the insufflation of oxygen and the application of CPAP. Without the central channel, air or gas cannot exit from the lung once the balloon is inflated; therefore the lung may not deflate totally and may obscure surgical visualization.

The final option for lung separation is selective endobronchial intubation. The major disadvantage of this is that it is not possible to quickly change from OLV to two-lung ventilation as this requires repositioning the ETT from the mainstem bronchus into the trachea and vice versa. Additionally, with movement of the ETT, inadvertent extubation may occur which may be particularly problematic for the patient in the lateral decubitus position. Placement into the right mainstem bronchus can generally be accomplished blindly while left-sided placement requires guidance using a fiber-optic bronchoscope because of the different anatomical orientation of the left and right mainstem bronchi. See Chapter 24 for additional discussion of one lung ventilation techniques.

Techniques to limit homologous transfusion

There is a growing body of evidence demonstrating the potential adverse effects of the administration of allogeneic blood products [48–52]. These adverse effects include the transmission of infectious diseases, immunosuppression, transfusion-related acute lung injury, transfusion reactions, and graft-versus-host disease. Of specific concern during the performance of major orthopedic surgical procedures is accumulating data demonstrating the association and potential causative role of allogeneic blood product use and postoperative infectious complications [49,50]. The primary focus on techniques to limit perioperative transfusions remains the appropriate preoperative preparation of the patient as well as attention to basic intraoperative tenets of pediatric anesthesiology such as patient positioning and maintenance of normothermia.

The general perioperative considerations which have a major impact on the perioperative need for allogeneic blood products include optimization of preoperative hemoglobin and coagulation function, including avoidance of NSAIDs preoperatively as well as attention to intraoperative anesthetic technique, including choice of fluid for intraoperative resuscitation and fluid therapy, proper patient positioning, and maintenance of normothermia (see above) [53,54]. As outlined above, the use of preoperative erythropoietin may be costly and time-consuming and is therefore generally reserved for specific circumstances where avoidance of allogeneic transfusions is mandated, such as the Jehovah's Witness patient [55]. A more cost-effective approach is the identification and treatment of preoperative anemia, which may be especially prevalent in girls who have started their menstrual cycle. In most circumstances, treatment of anemia can be accomplished with nothing more than oral iron therapy.

The choice of intraoperative fluid administration may affect coagulation function, thereby affecting blood loss. During acute normovolemic hemodilution (ANH), intraoperative phlebotomy is performed and the blood removed is replaced with crystalloids and/or colloids. Due to the dilution of proteins with anticoagulatory effects, such as antithrombin III, hemodilution results in increased coagulation function [56]. Replacement with albumin or gelatin-based solutions has no effect or may actually improve coagulation function. Because of their effects on von Willebrand factor, either medium or high molecular weight hydroxyethyl starches may adversely affect coagulation function, in particular platelet function, when used in doses exceeding 10–15 mL/kg [57].

As important as the preoperative preparation of the patient is the recognition that there is no universal trigger for the administration of allogeneic blood products [58,59]. In the absence of co-morbid diseases which compromise end-organ oxygenation or limit the compensatory mechanisms for anemia, hemoglobin levels down to 7 g/dL are generally well tolerated. Even in a recent prospective trial in the adult ICU population, with a restrictive strategy for the administration of blood (blood administered only for a hemoglobin less than 7 g/dL), no difference in outcome was noticed when compared to a liberal transfusion protocol (blood administered for a hemoglobin less than 10 g/dL) [59]. In fact, in the less critically ill patients (APACHE score less than 20) and in those less than 55 years of age, there was a statistically significant improvement in 30-day mortality in the restrictive transfusion group.

Additional specialized techniques to limit perioperative allogeneic blood transfusions during spinal surgery may include:
- autologous transfusion therapy including preoperative donation with the use of erythropoietin and intraoperative collection using ANH
- intraoperative and postoperative blood salvage
- pharmacological manipulation of the coagulation cascade with antifibrinolytic agents (ε-aminocaproic acid (EACA), tranexamic acid (TXA), aprotinin) or procoagulant agents including desmopressin (DDAVP) and recombinant factor VIIa (rFVIIa) or
- controlled hypotension.

The goal of performing pediatric spine surgery without the use of allogeneic blood products is best accomplished by combining several of these techniques [60]. The use of these techniques will depend on the co-morbidities of the patient, the type of surgery, and likelihood of the need for allogeneic transfusions. During spinal surgery, factors which increase the likelihood of the need for allogeneic transfusions include the number of vertebral bodies fused and the presence of neuromuscular scoliosis [61,62]

Preoperative donation

Although preoperative donation of autologous blood was first suggested by Fantus in 1937 when he founded the first blood bank in the United States, the technique did not become popular until much later, during the 1980s. Advantages of preoperative donation include reduction of exposure to allogeneic blood, the availability of blood for patients with rare phenotypes, reduction of blood shortages, avoidance of transfusion-induced immunosuppression, and the availability of blood for some patients who refuse transfusions based on religious beliefs [63].

There are no contraindications to the autologous donation based on the patient's weight or age. Patients who weigh more than 50 kilograms can generally donate a standard unit of blood (450 ± 50 mL) whereas patients weighing less than 50 kg will donate proportionately smaller volumes based on their weight and the presenting hemoglobin or hematocrit. Prior to donation, the hematocrit should be more than 33%. All patients enrolled in an autologous donation program should be on replacement iron therapy to augment erythropoiesis. Specific contraindications to autologous blood donation are similar to those for the donation of blood for allogeneic use. In general, patients with end-organ disease or limitations of the compensatory mechanisms which maintain tissue oxygen delivery during anemia are not candidates.

The efficacy of red blood cell production can be augmented by iron supplementation and the administration of erythropoietin [64]. Donations may be made every 3 days, but the usual practice is to donate one unit per week. The last unit should be donated at least 5–7 days prior to surgery to allow plasma proteins to normalize to restore intravascular volume and to allow for adequate erythropoiesis so that the patient does not present to the operating room with anemia. Although this technique has been endorsed by some as the easiest means of avoiding allogeneic transfusions [60], its use has decreased significantly over the past 5–10 years. Concerns regarding the use of autologous blood include the lack of standardized screening of these units for infectious diseases. As such, it is feasible to have an infected unit of blood sitting in the blood bank. Additionally, as the primary factor involved in major complications and death following the administration of allogeneic blood products is a clerical error with the transfusion of the wrong blood product, autologous units can be involved just as easily as allogeneic units. Many of the units of autologous blood are never used and therefore wasted if there is no standardized policy and procedure for their routine screening and subsequent move into the allogeneic pool. Additional limitations include the cost involved, time constraints as patients must return to the hospital several times before their operative procedure, and difficulties with vascular access in infants and children.

Acute normovolemic hemodilution

Perhaps a more cost-effective and safer means of obtaining autologous blood is ANH [65]. The technique involves the intraoperative removal of blood, generally after the induction of anesthesia and prior to the start of the surgical procedure. Blood is removed via a large-bore intravenous cannula, arterial cannula or central line and replaced with an equal volume of colloid or crystalloid in a ratio of 1:3 to maintain normovolemia. The blood is collected in standard CPD-A blood bank bags until they are full (approximately 450–500 mL) or weighed to ensure that the appropriate amount of blood is removed. The amount of blood that can be safely removed is determined by the formula:

$$EBV \times (\text{initial hematocrit} - \text{target hematocrit})/ \\ \text{mean hematocrit}$$

EBV is estimated blood volume, and the mean hematocrit is the average between the initial and the target hematocrit. The removed blood can kept at room temperature for up to 4 h, thus maintaining the efficacy of platelets and clotting factors and providing a significant advantage over allogeneic blood and even predonated autologous blood. Intraoperatively, as needed, the blood is infused in the opposite order that it was withdrawn so that the units with the highest hematocrit are saved until the end of the procedure when there is the least amount of bleeding.

Compensatory physiological mechanisms to maintain oxygen delivery to the tissues despite a decrease in hematocrit include a decrease in blood viscosity resulting in increased venous return, peripheral vasodilation, increased cardiac output, and rightward shift of the oxyhemoglobin dissociation curve. Additionally, as oxygen delivery declines, oxygen extraction at the tissue level can increase to maintain adequate oxygen delivery to tissues. Although not recommended for routine clinical practice, the efficacy of the compensatory mechanisms was demonstrated by the study of Fontana et al which evaluated the effects of extreme ANH in eight adolescents undergoing posterior spinal fusion for idiopathic scoliosis [66]. During hemodilution, the hemoglobin decreased from 10.0 ± 1.6 g/dL to 3.0 ± 0.8 g/dL. Although oxygen delivery decreased from 532.1 ± 138.1 to 262 ± 57.1 mL/min/M^2, the oxygen extraction ration increased from 17.3 ± 6.2% to 44.4 ± 5.9%. There was also an increase in cardiac output and maintenance of a stable heart rate. Although there was a decrease in the mixed venous oxygen saturation from 90.8 ± 5.4% to 72.3 ± 7.8% after ANH, the final value was still clinically acceptable and indicative of adequate tissue oxygenation.

Intraoperative blood salvage

The basic premise of intraoperative blood salvage is that shed blood is collected, anticoagulated, filtered for clots and debris, and then reinfused. There are three different techniques of intraoperative salvage. Semi-continuous flow devices were the first to be introduced and although they are the most complex to use, are still the type used most commonly for intraoperative blood collection and reinfusion. The commercially available equipment consists of an aspiration and anticoagulation assembly, a reservoir (various sizes are available depending on the size of the patient), a centrifuge bowl, a waste bag, and tubing. A double-line aspiration set includes an anticoagulation line that permits either heparin or citrate to combine with the aspirated blood at a controlled rate. The anticoagulated blood is collected into a disposable reservoir containing a filter. The filtered blood is then pumped into a bowl, centrifuged, washed with saline, and pumped into a reinfusion bag. Most of the white blood cells, platelets, clotting factors, free plasma hemoglobin, and anticoagulant are removed in the washing process and eliminated in the waste bag. The process takes approximately 5–10 min, resulting in a blood cell suspension with a hematocrit of 45–60%. Newer pediatric-specific devices are available which now allow the processing of smaller volumes of blood.

The second type of intraoperative salvage, otherwise known as the canister collection technique, uses a rigid canister with a sterile, disposable liner. Blood is aspirated from the wound and anticoagulant added in a manner similar to that of semi-continuous flow devices. The blood is collected in a rigid plastic reservoir containing a disposable liner. The blood can either be washed prior to infusion or reinfused without washing. Functioning platelets and coagulation factors are present if the blood is left unwashed; however, there is an increased risk of adverse effects due to cellular debris, free hemoglobin, and fragmented blood components. This type is rarely used in the perioperative setting.

The third type of collection is a single-use, self-contained rigid plastic reservoir that collects the shed blood. The anticoagulant (citrate) is placed in the container prior to use. This apparatus is most commonly used for postoperative blood collection and reinfusion. The surgical drains are connected to the canister, and every 4 h the canister is replaced and the blood reinfused. Coagulation factors and platelets are present in this blood as well. Adverse effects may occur as a result of cell fragmentation and the release of free hemoglobin.

Suggested indications for perioperative blood salvage include anticipated blood loss exceeding 20% of the patient's blood volume or a procedure during which more than 10% of patients require transfusion. Contraindications include situations in which there may be contamination of the collected blood with infectious or non-infectious agents (amniotic fluid, hemostatic agents such as topical thrombin or protamine). Potential complications include air and fat embolism, hemolysis, pulmonary dysfunction, renal dysfunction, coagulopathy, hypocalcemia, and sepsis [67]. Coagulopathy may occur related to the initiation of disseminated intravascular coagulation (DIC) due to incorrect technique and the infusion of blood cell fragments or the infusion of residual anticoagulant after washing [68]. Hemolysis may occur if the suction level is too high or if the aspiration method causes excessive mixing of air with blood. Free

hemoglobin may be released during salvage and washing because of erythrocyte damage. Free hemoglobin levels exceeding 100–150 mg/dL may lead to hemoglobinuria and acute renal failure, as the binding capacity of haptoglobin is saturated and free hemoglobin is filtered in the renal tubules. Metabolic consequences of cell salvage may also be seen, including a metabolic acidosis and alterations in electrolytes such as magnesium, calcium, and potassium. Despite its potential complications and cost for the initial purchase of the machine and disposable items, it represents an effective means of limiting the need for allogeneic transfusion [69].

Pharmacological manipulation of the coagulation cascade

Various agents have been used as prophylactic measures, even in patients with normal baseline coagulation function, to decrease intraoperative blood loss. Although these agents have been studied in well-designed, prospective trials, the outcomes of the studies are, at times, conflicting. Another issue to consider with the administration of any agent that alters coagulation function is the potential to invoke a prothrombotic state with venous or arterial thrombotic complications.

1-Deamino-8-D-arginine vasopressin (DDAVP) is a synthetic analog of vasopressin initially used in the treatment of diabetes insipidus. Its hemostatic effects result from the release of factor VIII and von Willebrand factor (vWF) from endothelial cells. Factor VIII, a glycoprotein, accelerates the activation of factor X by factor IX while vWF increases platelet adherence to vascular subendothelium, augments the formation of molecular bridges between platelets to increase aggregation, protects factor VIII in the plasma from proteolytic enzymes, and stimulates the synthesis of factor VIII. Although anecdotal reports have demonstrated its efficacy in augmenting coagulation function in various acquired and inherited forms of platelet dysfunction, prospective trials have failed to show an effect on blood loss during spinal surgery in pediatric patients [70].

ε-Aminocaproic acid (EACA) and tranexamic acid (TA) are γ-amino carboxylic acid analogs of lysine that inhibit fibrinolysis by preventing the conversion of plasminogen to plasmin. In the plasma, plasminogen is activated by tissue plasminogen activator to form plasmin which cleaves fibrin, thereby preventing the formation of the fibrin mesh. This fibrinolytic system is a basic defense mechanism that prevents the excessive deposition of fibrin following the activation of the coagulation cascade. Plasmin can also hydrolyze activated factors V and VIII. EACA and TA bind to the lysine group that binds plasminogen and plasmin to fibrinogen, thus displacing these molecules from the fibrinogen surface and inhibiting fibrinolysis.

One of the issues with the use of agents such as EACA and TXA is that various dosing regimens have been reported in the literature and there remains significant variation in current clinical practice [71]. In general, both drugs are administered as a loading dose followed by an infusion during the intraoperative period, with some studies continuing the infusion for a brief period of time into the postoperative course. Dosing regimens for EACA include an intravenous loading dose of 100–150 mg/kg (maximum 5 g) followed by an infusion of 10–15 mg/kg/h (maximum 1 g/h). Ninety percent of EACA is excreted in the urine within 4–6 h of administration. Although TA is generally considered to be pharmacologically 7–10 times as potent as EACA, similar doses have been used clinically during spinal surgery. Adverse effects of EACA or TA may be related to the effect on coagulation function and the route of excretion. Since these agents are cleared by the kidneys, thrombosis of the kidneys, ureters or lower urinary tract may occur if urological bleeding is present. Both EACA and TA may be associated with hypotension during rapid intravenous administration. Given their limited adverse effect profile and general efficacy, these agents are commonly used as a means of limiting intraoperative blood loss during spinal surgery [71].

Florentino-Pineda et al evaluated the efficacy of EACA (100 mg/kg followed by 10 mg/kg/h) in 28 adolescents undergoing postoperative spinal fusion [72]. Patients who received EACA had decreased intraoperative blood loss (988 ± 411 mL versus 1405 ± 670 mL, p = 0.024) and decreased transfusion requirements (1.2 ± 1.1 units versus 2.2 ± 1.3 units, p = 0.003). TXA has been similarly effective in reducing blood loss during spinal fusion in pediatric patients with either idiopathic or neuromuscular scoliosis [73,74].

Aprotinin is a naturally occurring serine protease inhibitor first isolated from bovine lung in 1930. Its effects on coagulation function include both the inhibition of fibrinolysis by inactivating serine proteases including trypsin and plasma kallikrein, which convert plasminogen to plasmin, and the augmentation of platelet adhesion by protecting membrane-bound glycoprotein receptors (vWF receptor) from degradation by plasmin. As with the other antifibrinolytic agents, aprotinin has been shown to decrease blood loss and reduce requirements for allogeneic blood products during spinal surgery in children and adolescents [75].

Following intravenous administration, aprotinin undergoes rapid redistribution into the extracellular fluid, followed by accumulation in renal tubular epithelium with subsequent lysosomal degradation. The dose is expressed as kallikrein-inhibitory units (KIU). Potential adverse effects of aprotinin include allergic reactions and renal toxicity. Anaphylactoid reactions have been reported and are more frequent in patients previously exposed to aprotinin. However, even with previous exposure, the incidence of anaphylaxis is low, at less than 0.1%. The major concern with aprotinin, which led to its withdrawal from the market, is its effects on renal function. Although controversial, its use has been associated with renal failure in the high-risk adult population following cardiac surgery [76]. Renal toxicity is postulated to result from aprotinin's strong affinity for renal tissue and subsequent accumulation in proximal tubular epithelial cells or from its inhibition of serine proteases (kallikrein-kinin system). Histopathological examination of renal tissue reveals obstructed proximal convoluted tubules and swollen tubular epithelial cells. Given these effects, aprotinin has been withdrawn from the market.

Controlled hypotension

Controlled hypotension (deliberate or induced hypotension) may be defined as a deliberate reduction of systolic blood pressure to 80–90 mmHg, a reduction of mean arterial pressure (MAP) to 50–65 mmHg or a 30% reduction of baseline MAP, the latter being relevant for the pediatric-aged patient whose baseline MAP may be within the 50–65 mmHg range to start with. Although the primary premise for the use of controlled hypotension is as a means of limiting intraoperative blood loss, an additional benefit may be improved visualization of the surgical field and thus shorter surgical times.

Advances in drug therapy have provided the clinician with several pharmacological options for controlled hypotension in the pediatric patient [77]. The agents available for controlled hypotension can be divided into those used by themselves (primary agents) and adjunctive or secondary agents which are used to limit the dose requirements and therefore the adverse effects of primary agents. Primary agents include regional anesthetic techniques (spinal and epidural anesthesia), the inhalational anesthetic agents (halothane, isoflurane, sevoflurane), the nitrovasodilators (sodium nitroprusside and nitroglycerin), trimethaphan, prostaglandin E1 (PGE1), and adenosine. The calcium channel blockers and β-adrenergic antagonists have been used as both primary agents and as adjuncts to other agents. The pharmacological agents used primarily as adjuncts or secondary agents include the angiotensin-converting enzyme inhibitors and α-adrenergic agonists such as clonidine. When neurological monitoring is used (see below), the potential impact of the agent used for controlled hypotension must be considered.

Sodium nitroprusside (SNP) is one of the agents most commonly used for controlled hypotension. It is a direct-acting, non-selective peripheral vasodilator that primarily dilates resistance vessels, leading to venous pooling and decreased systemic vascular resistance. It has a rapid onset of action (approximately 30 sec), a peak hypotensive effect within 2 min with a return of blood pressure to baseline values within 3 min of its discontinuation. SNP releases nitric oxide (formerly endothelial-derived relaxant factor), which activates guanylate cyclase, leading to an increase in the intracellular concentration of cyclic guanosine monophosphate (cGMP). cGMP decreases the availability of intracellular calcium through one of two mechanisms: decreased release from the sarcoplasmic reticulum into smooth muscle or increased uptake by the sarcoplasmic reticulum. The net result is decreased free cytosolic calcium and vascular smooth muscle relaxation. Adverse effects include rebound hypertension, coronary steal, increased intracranial pressure, increased intrapulmonary shunt with ablation of hypoxic pulmonary vasoconstriction, platelet dysfunction, and cyanide/thiocyanate toxicity. Direct peripheral vasodilation also results in baroreceptor-mediated sympathetic responses with tachycardia and increased myocardial contractility. The renin-angiotensin system and sympathetic nervous system are also activated. The result is increased cardiac output which may offset the initial drop in MAP. Plasma catecholamine and renin activity may remain elevated after discontinuation of SNP, resulting in rebound hypertension.

Nicardipine is a calcium channel antagonist of the dihyropyridine class that dilates the systemic, cerebral, and coronary vasculature with limited effects on myocardial contractility and stroke volume. Unlike SNP, nicardipine does have some intrinsic negative chronotropic effects which may limit the rebound tachycardia. Like other direct-acting vasodilators, nicardipine and the other calcium channel antagonists may increase intracranial pressure. Studies comparing SNP with nicardipine have demonstrated several potential advantages of nicardipine, including fewer episodes of excessive hypotension, less rebound tachycardia, less activation of the renin-angiontensin and sympathetic nervous systems, and in some studies decreased blood loss [78]. One disadvantage of nicardipine is that its effect is somewhat prolonged (20–30 min) following discontinuation of the infusion. More recently, a new dihydropyridine, clevidipine, has been added to the list of agents which may be used for intraoperative blood pressure control [79]. Although its hemodynamic effects are similar to those of nicardipine, it is metabolized by plasma and tissue esterases, thereby resulting in a half-life of 2–3 min.

Spinal cord monitoring

Without electrophysiological monitoring, the incidence of neurological deficits following surgical procedures on the vertebral column may be as high as 3.7–6.9%. This can be decreased to less than 1% with appropriate monitoring [80]. The American Academy of Neurology, in their guidelines on intraoperative monitoring, concluded that the evidence favors the use of monitoring as a safe and efficacious tool in clinical situations where this is a significant nervous system risk, provided its limitations are appreciated [80]. One of the major limitations is that animal studies have demonstrated a window of opportunity of less than 10 min from the time when changes in monitoring are noted until permanent damage is done. Additionally, when various techniques are used, such as somatosensory or motor-evoked potentials, the anesthetic technique must be modified to facilitate processing of the technique (see below).

There are four techniques of intraoperative monitoring: the ankle clonus test, the wake-up test, somatosensory-evoked potentials (SSEPs), and motor-evoked potentials (MEPs). The ankle clonus test was the first to be used intraoperatively to assess spinal cord integrity [81]. During the normal awake state, descending inhibitory fibers prevent clonus in response to an ankle stretch. Likewise, the reflex is inhibited during deep levels of anesthesia. However, during emergence from anesthesia, inhibition of the central descending pathways allows ankle clonus to be elicited following dorsiflexion of the foot/ankle. If there has been damage to the spinal cord, flaccid paralysis will be present and therefore no spinal reflexes can be elicited. To elicit ankle clonus, neuromuscular blockade must be reversed or absent and the patient is allowed to emerge from general anesthesia as is done with a wake-up test (see below). In most circumstances, the ankle clonus test can be elicited prior to the patient regaining consciousness and therefore at a deeper level of anesthesia than a true wake-up test [81]. The test is both extremely sensitive and specific; however, it does not provide a continuous monitor of spinal cord function and is present only at a specific depth of anesthesia.

The wake-up test was originally reported in the 1970s as a means of monitoring spinal cord integrity. The technique should include a preoperative discussion with the patient regarding what the test entails, its purpose, timing during the procedure, and the fact that there may be some intraoperative recall during the period of time when the test is performed. At the appropriate intraoperative time, neuromuscular blockade is reversed and the depth of anesthesia decreased. The speed with which a patient will respond to verbal stimuli can be increased by the use of short-acting anesthetic agents (desflurane, propofol, and remifentanil). With the use of these agents, responsiveness and a successful wake-up test can generally be accomplished within 10 min of the surgeon's request. The use of reversal agents for opioids and benzodiazepines, although available in clinical practice, is not recommended as they may have prolonged effects which will interfere with the resumption of anesthesia after the wake-up test. The depth of anesthesia and the patient's awakening can also be judged by the use of neurophysiological or depth of anesthesia monitors such as the BIS (Bispectral Index®) monitor (Aspect Medical, Newton, MA). As the depth of anesthesia is decreased, one anesthesia provider stands at the head of the bed with one hand on the patient's head to limit the risk of sudden inadvertent movements. The other hand is used to feel the patient's response to a verbal command. When the patient reaches a light plane of anesthesia, a voluntary movement in the motor groups above the level of surgery (e.g. squeezing one's hand) is requested initially to ensure that the patient is awake enough to follow commands. This is then followed by a request to move the lower extremities to ensure that motor function is still intact. Once a positive response is achieved in the lower extremities, the depth of anesthesia is deepened by the bolus administration of propofol or thiopental. The wake-up test does entail certain risks, including having an awake patient in the prone position on the operating room table. Inadvertent or sudden movements may result in patient injury, dislodgment of venous or arterial cannulas, and hypertension with exacerbation of bleeding. Additionally, like the ankle clonus test, it provides only a single assessment of spinal cord integrity. In most centers, the wake-up test is used only when there are questionable findings on electrophysiological monitoring (see below).

Electophysiological monitors include both SSEPs and MEPs. SSEPs are monitored by stimulation of a distal nerve, generally in the leg (posterior tibial), and measuring the response at the cervical level and the central nervous system via standard EEG electrodes. The pathways involved include the peripheral nerve, the dorsomedial columns (fasciculus gracilis and fasciculus cuneatus) of the spinal cord, and the cerebral cortex. SSEPs do not monitor anterior cord (motor) function. Given the close proximity of the tracts (motor and sensory) in the spinal cord, damage to the motor tracts generally results in damage to the sensory tracts, making SSEPs a fairly reliable measure of motor function. However, given that the dorsomedial tracts and the anterior aspect of the spinal cord do not share the same arterial supply, isolated damage to the motor tract with intact SSEPs has been reported.

Since SSEPs can be affected by anesthetic agents, baseline recordings are performed after an appropriate level of anesthesia has been achieved [82]. The variables measured include both the height of the response (amplitude) and the time it takes the response to travel from the periphery to the central nervous system (latency). Significant changes include a reduction in the amplitude of ≥50% or an increase in the latency of ≥10%. The potent inhalational anesthetic agents and nitrous oxide cause a decrease in the amplitude and an increase in the latency of SSEPs. However, acceptable monitoring can be achieved with 0.5 MAC of isoflurane, sevoflurane or des-

flurane. Although practices vary from center to center, nitrous oxide is generally avoided. Intravenous anesthetic agents have been shown to have less of an effect on SSEPs, making a total intravenous anesthetic technique using propofol or midazolam combined with an opioid an effective option. In generally, either propofol or 0.5 MAC of an inhalational anesthetic agent is combined with a continuous infusion of a potent synthetic opioid, generally either sufentanil or remifentanil. Neuromuscular blocking agents have no effect on SSEPs, but will obviously eliminate the ability to obtain MEPs.

More recently, due to the concern that there can be isolated motor damage with intact SSEPs, many centers have moved to monitoring MEPs along with SSEPs. As with SSEPs, MEPs are affected by the type of anesthetic agent used. Various techniques have been recommended and there is variation from center to center, but the anesthetic technique is generally the same as for SSEP monitoring.

A recent addition to the anesthetic armamentarium is dexmedetomidine (Precedex®, Hospira Worldwide Inc, Lake Forest, IL), the pharmacologically active dextroisomer of medetomidine, which exerts its physiological effects via α_2-adrenergic receptors. Its use in perioperative care continues to increase given its ability to decrease requirements for the inhalational anesthetic agents and propofol as well as its ability to decrease postoperative opioid requirements [83,84]. Of particular note during spinal surgery and neurophysiological monitoring is that provided the depth of anesthesia is maintained, no change in these parameters should be seen with the use of dexmedetomidine as part of the intraoperative anesthetic care [85,86]. With MEP monitoring, the level of neuromuscular blockade must be kept stable with maintenance of one or two twitches of the train-of-four. Alternatively, as is our preference, neuromuscular blockade with a short-acting agent is used only for endotracheal intubation and no neuromuscular blocking agents are used during the case.

Intraoperative anesthetic care

Intraoperative anesthesia is generally best co-ordinated with the physicians and technicians providing intraoperative neurophysiological monitoring as significant variations in preference exist from center to center. The techniques generally combine either a propofol infusion or a low-dose inhalational anesthetic agent (0.5–1 MAC) with a potent synthetic opioid infusion (remifentanil or sufentanil). As mentioned previously, dexmedetomidine may be added to the intraoperative regimen to limit the requirements for either propofol or the inhalational anesthetic agent. We have also found that these agents can be effectively titrated to achieve an acceptable level of blood pressure control to provide controlled hypotension with a limited need for supplemental antihypertensive agents.

In most cases when propofol, remifentanil, and dexmedetomidine infusions are used, controlled hypotension can be maintained with only an occasional need for intermittent doses of labetalol.

Although remifentanil is a frequent component of intraoperative care for spinal surgery, one issue that has been identified with its use is the development of acute opioid tolerance [87]. This may result in an increased opioid requirement during the postoperative period. Crawford et al investigated the effects of remifentanil on postoperative opioid requirements in a cohort of 30 adolescents undergoing posterior spinal fusion for the treatment of idiopathic scoliosis [87]. Thirty adolescents were randomized to receive a continuous infusion of remifentanil or intermittent doses of morphine as part of their intraoperative anesthetic regimen. Cumulative morphine use during the first 24 postoperative hours was 30% greater in the group receiving remifentanil. Despite such observations, the mechanisms responsible for the postoperative hyperalgesia remain undefined. Although it has been attributed to effects of remifentanil at the NMDA receptor, the hyperalgesia is not blocked by the administration of ketamine [88].

Another potential adjunct for the intraoperative anesthetic care of patients during spinal surgery is the inclusion of a magnesium sulfate infusion [89–91]. A magnesium sulfate infusion has been shown to decrease intraoperative anesthetic requirements for propofol, the inhalational anesthetic agents and neuromuscular blocking agents, be an effective agent for controlled hypotension, and even decreased postoperative opioid requirements. In a prospective trial of 61 children with cerebral palsy undergoing spinal fusion, patients were randomized to receive magnesium sulfate (50 mg/kg followed by an infusion of 15 mg/kg/h) or a saline placebo [91]. Postoperative analgesic requirements and pain scores were lower at 24 and 48 h in the group that had received magnesium sulfate.

Additional intraoperative considerations include alterations in care which may affect postoperative surgical site infections (SSI) and the treatment of acute intraoperative events. Although various factors are involved in the genesis of a SSI, recent data have focused on the potential beneficial impact of the intraoperative FIO_2. As oxygen is required for neutrophil killing of bacteria, it has been postulated that increasing the inspired FIO_2 may decrease the incidence of SSIs. In a case–control study, Maragakis et al compared the intraoperative course of 104 patients with SSIs to a randomly selected control group [92].

Given the complexity of the surgical procedure, various unique intraoperative complications may occur. As there is extensive removal of cortical bone and placement of screws, intrahemodynamic instability may occur related to either air, marrow or fat emboli [93]. Early recognition of such events is mandatory as cessation of surgical manipulation and flooding the surgical field with saline may limit the impact on hemodynamic status. In more extreme cases, resuscitation in the prone position may be necessary. Although flipping the patient may be an option, even rapid closure of the surgical wound and flipping can result in the loss of precious minutes of resuscitation. Several case reports and animal studies demonstrate that effective cardiopulmonary resuscitation can performed in the prone position [94]. The technique involves the placement of one hand over each scapula with compressions performed in a perpendicular motion toward the operating room table. If the patient is on a specialized frame, the thoracic supports will generally provide enough counter-pressure for effective changes in intrathoracic pressure.

Postoperative care including pain management

One of the keys to the successful care of the pediatric spine patient is to provide a smooth transition from the operating room to the intensive care unit (ICU). This process begins with the preoperative preparation and education of the patient, preferably with a tour of the pediatric ICU. The patient should also be instructed regarding the correct use of incentive spirometry and patient-controlled analgesia if the use of these devices is planned. In some institutions, direct admission to the pediatric inpatient ward and not the pediatric ICU is feasible following spinal surgery. In such instances, a 2–4-h stay in the postanesthesia care unit is used to ensure cardiorespiratory stability.

At the completion of the procedures, it may be desirable to have an appropriate level of responsiveness so that a neurological examination can be performed to demonstrate adequate upper and lower extremity function. The decision to continue mechanical ventilation into the postoperative period is made on a individual basis. In all patients in whom there is any possibility of the need for postoperative mechanical ventilation, this should be discussed preoperatively with the parents and the patient. The need for mechanical ventilation may be related to either the patient (neuromuscular disorder, preoperative pulmonary dysfunction) or the surgical procedure (blood loss of more than one blood volume). In specific cases, the best option may be to provide 2–4 h of postoperative mechanical ventilation to ensure cardiorespiratory stability, normal coagulation function, and correction of metabolic parameters. Once this is accomplished, the trachea can be extubated in the ICU setting. Given the prolonged prone positioning, lingual edema may be present and result in postoperative upper airway obstruction. Excessive lingual edema may mandate continuing mechanical ventilation into the postoperative period. When the cuff is deflated, an adequate airway leak should be present before tracheal extubation.

Due to the significant length of the surgical incision and the degree of bony and soft tissue dissection required for such procedures, there may be significant postoperative pain. Accordingly, effective analgesia is a key in the provision of a stable postoperative course. Effective analgesia is generally best provided using a multi-modality approach, which includes analgesic agents, anxiolytic agents, and medications to control muscle spasms. Muscle spasms may be particularly problematic in patients with underlying cerebral palsy. Options for the provision of analgesia include the intravenous administration of medications and/or regional anesthetic techniques. For intravenous administration, we prefer the use of patient-controlled analgesia (PCA). Although young patients or those with developmental disabilities may not be able to activate the device, nurse-controlled or parent-controlled analgesia may be provided. By using the device in this manner, the bedside nurse has ready access to a supply of opioid to provide an immediate dose to a patient who is in pain. Prior to instituting PCA, an appropriate level of analgesia must be achieved by the careful titration of opioid. This is generally done in the operating room on completion of the surgical procedure.

Once neurophysiological monitoring is completed, the remifentanil and propofol infusions are discontinued and desflurane or sevoflurane started to maintain the BIS at 50–60. Once spontaneous ventilation begins, incremental doses of either hydromorphone (2–3 μg/kg) or morphine (20 μg/kg) are titrated based on the patient's respiratory rate. Once tracheal extubation is completed, additional complaints of pain are treated with opioid. Once adequate analgesia is achieved, the PCA device is started to maintain analgesia. Given the significant interpatient variability that may occur, it is necessary to use age-appropriate pain scores and titrate the PCA doses up or down based on the patient's response.

To limit the total dose of opioid required and thus opioid-related adverse effects, adjunctive agents can be used. There is still significant controversy regarding the potential adverse effects of NSAIDs on bone formation. Given these concerns, many centers choose not to use these agents following spinal surgery in children. Our preference is to administer a fixed dose of acetaminophen (10 mg/kg either by mouth or per rectum) every 4–6 h around the clock. Given the propensity of these patients to develop muscle spasms and the need, in some patients, to provide anxiolysis, benzodiazepines such as diazepam may be added to the postoperative regimen either on an as-needed basis or at fixed intervals. Alternatively, there may be a role for the α_2-adrenergic agonists to provide anxiolysis as well as relief of muscle

spasms. Dexmedetomidine is a novel α_2-adrenergic agent which currently has FDA approval for the sedation of adult patients in the ICU setting for 24h. Unlike clonidine, it has a half-life of 2–3h, thus allowing its titration by continuous infusion. Given its limited effects on respiratory function and its ability to potentiate opioid-induced analgesia, it may also have a role in the ICU setting to provide anxiolysis following major surgical procedures, including spine surgery. Although our experience is preliminary and anecdotal, a continuous infusion of dexmedetomidine (0.25–0.5 μg/kg/h) may be efficacious in these patients. Despite the need to provide effective analgesia, adverse effects including respiratory depression may occur, especially in patients with co-morbid features. In such patients, close monitoring of respiratory function with continuous pulse oximetry may be indicated.

The other class of agent that has gained popularity as an adjunct to opioid analgesia following spinal surgery is the γ-amino butyric acid analogs such as gabapentin and pregabalin [95–98]. In a prospective study of adult patients undergoing posterior lumbar spinal fusion, van Elstraete et al investigated the dose of gabapentin required to decreased morphine requirements by 30% [95]. Using an up-and-down sequential allocation model, they demonstrated that the median effective pre-emptive dose of gabapentin was 21.7 mg/kg. In a prospective study of 59 patients, 9–18 years of age, undergoing posterior spinal fusion, Rusy et al randomized patients to receive gabapentin (15 mg/kg preoperatively followed by 5 mg/kg by mouth three times a day for 5 days) or placebo [96]. Gabapentin significantly reduced total morphine consumption and pain scores in the PACU and on the first postoperative day. In addition to working during the acute postoperative period, the adult data suggest more prolonged effects of perioperative pregabalin with decreased pain scores and improved functional outcomes 3 months after surgery [97].

Given successes in other surgical procedures, there is also significant interest in the potential use of regional anesthetic techniques as a means of controlling pain following spine surgery in children. Reports in the literature regarding the use of regional anesthesia following spine surgery have included several variations:
- the dose of the medications used
- the route of delivery (intrathecal or epidural)
- the mode of delivery (single dose, intermittent bolus dosing or continuous infusion)
- the number of catheters used (one versus two)
- the medications infused (opioids or local anesthetics or both)
- the opioid used (morphine, fentanyl, hydromorphone)
- analgesic regimen of the control group, if present (intermittent "as-needed" morphine or PCA)

- the type of surgery (short-segment lumbar fusion, short-segment laminectomy for dorsal rhizotomy, posterior spinal fusion, and anterior spinal fusion)
- the surgical approach (open versus thoracoscopic).

The reader is referred to a review of the reports regarding the use of regional anesthetic techniques following spine surgery in pediatric patients and a recent meta-analysis evaluating these techniques [99,100]. The evaluation of the efficacy of regional anesthetic techniques is clouded by the variation in the techniques which has been previously outlined. Future trials are needed to determine the optimal postoperative analgesic regimens for these procedures.

Conclusion

There are many challenges facing the anesthesia provider during spine surgery in pediatric patients. As with any surgical procedure, the care of these patients begins with a thorough preoperative evaluation to identify co-morbid features which are present in many of these patients. Although idiopathic scoliosis is still a common disease, many of these patients will have associated neurological or myopathic conditions which affect anesthetic care. Intraoperative issues include techniques for airway management, vascular access, blood conservation techniques, patient positioning, intraoperative neurological monitoring, the administration of blood and blood products, and the maintenance of fluid and electrolyte homeostasis. There is also a need for a smooth transition to the postoperative period with an ongoing monitor to ensure stable cardiorespiratory function and an aggressive approach to the provision of effective postoperative analgesia.

CASE STUDY

A 14-year-old, 72 kg adolescent presented for posterior spinal fusion in the treatment of idiopathic scoliosis. His past medical history was unremarkable for co-morbid medical conditions or previous anesthetic care. Preoperative preparation included the administration of iron and two subcutaneous doses of erythropoietin. Preoperative coagulation function (PT, PTT and INR) was within normal limits and the hemoglobin was 14.6 g/dL. The patient was held nil per os for 6 h and transported to the operating room where routine American Society of Anesthesiologists' monitors were placed. Following the inhalation of nitrous oxide for 3 min, a large-bore peripheral intravenous cannula was placed followed by intravenous induction with 3 mg/kg of propofol and 5 μ/kg of fentanyl. Tracheal intubation was facilitated by rocuronium (0.4 mg/kg). Core body temperature was monitored using an esophageal stethoscope. A rolled gauze pad was placed in the mouth to prevent lingual damage during neurophysiological monitoring.

Following anesthetic induction, maintenance anesthesia consisted of desflurane (expired concentration 4–5%). A second large-bore peripheral intravenous cannula and a radial arterial cannula were placed. Depth of anesthesia was monitored using a Bispectral Index (BIS). Intraoperative monitoring with both SSEP and MEP monitoring was planned and the appropriate electrodes were placed over the extremities and scalp. During placement of the monitoring electrodes, isovolemic hemodilution was accomplished by the withdrawal of blood from a peripheral intravenous cannula into a standard blood bank bag containing the anticoagulant solution CPD (citrate-phosphate-dextrose). A tetrastarch solution was administered in a ratio of 1:1 for the blood that was withdrawn. A total of 700 mL of whole blood was removed, resulting in a hemoglobin of 11.2 g/dL. The patient was turned prone onto a Jackson table and a pillow was placed to prevent pressure to the eyes and face.

To facilitate SSEP and MEP monitoring, total intravenous anesthesia was provided by a combination of propofol, remifentanil and dexmedetomidine. No additional doses of a neuromuscular blocking agent were administered. The dexmedetomidine was started at 0.5 μg/kg/h without a loading dose. The propofol was started at 120 μg/kg/min and titrated to maintain the BIS at 40–60. The remifentanil was started at 0.1 μg/kg/min and increased as needed to maintain controlled hypotension with a MAP of 50–65 mmHg. Once positioned prone, a forced air heating device was used to maintain normothermia. The antifibrinolytic agent ε-aminocaproic acid was administered as a bolus dose of 100 mg/kg followed by an infusion of 10 mg/kg/h until the wound was closed.

Intraoperatively, during surgical dissection to the vertebral column, the MAP increased to 75–80 mmHg despite a remifentanil infusion at 0.3 μg/kg/min. To provide controlled hypotension, the calcium channel antagonist clevidipine was started at 1 μg/kg/min and increased in increments of 0.5–1 μg/kg/min every 3 min to achieve an MAP of 50–65 mmHg. With the clevidipine infusion at 2.5 μg/kg/min, the MAP was effectively decreased to the target range. The clevidipine infusion was continued until the surgical dissection had been completed. Intraoperatively, the propofol infusion was decreased to 70–80 μg/kg/min based on the BIS number. Intraoperatively, blood salvage with a cell saver from the surgical suction devices was employed. With the total intravenous

Continued

anesthesia (TIVA) technique, effective monitoring of SSEPs and MEPs was achieved. The TIVA technique was titrated to allow for a wake-up test or ankle clonus test should there be changes in neurophysiological monitoring which did not respond to anesthetic manipulation of hemodynamic parameters.

Intraoperative arterial blood gas parameters and hemoglobin values were monitored. As the hemoglobin value decreased to less than 8 g/dL, the 700 mL of blood that had been removed preoperatively by isovolemic hemodilution was administered. The surgical hardware was placed without incident and the wound was closed. During wound closure, 400 mL of intraoperatively salvaged blood was washed and returned to the patient.

Once monitoring of neurophysiological function was no longer indicated, the propofol and remifentanil infusions were discontinued and desflurane was started to maintain the BIS at 40–60. Once there was return of spontaneous ventilation, hydromorphone in incremental bolus doses of 0.1 mg was administered to achieve a respiratory rate of 8–12 breaths/min. The dexmedetomidine was continued at 0.5 μg/kg/h. Ondansetron (4 mg) and dexamethasone (4 mg) were administered to prevent postoperative nausea and vomiting. At the completion of the surgical procedure, the desflurane was discontinued and the patient was turned supine.

Once there was eye opening and appropriate response to verbal commands, the patient's trachea was extubated. The patient was transported to the postanesthesia care unit and then to the pediatric ICU for overnight observation. Postoperative analgesia was provided by a hydromorphone PCA and the dexmedetomidine infusion for 24 h. The hemoglobin value on postoperative day 1 was 13.6 g/dL. The remainder of the hospital course was unremarkable.

This case illustrates several of the basic tenets required for performance of anesthesia during spinal surgery. Of prime importance is tailoring of the anesthetic regimen to allow for effective monitoring of spinal cord function using SSEP and MEP modalities. This generally includes the use of a TIVA technique with propofol and a synthetic opioid such as remifentanil or sufentanil. During neurophysiological monitoring, if changes occur, immediate communication with the surgeon is necessary to allow for the reversal of any surgical intervention which may have resulted in these changes. This may include removal of recently placed hardware. If the neurophysiological changes do not respond to surgical intervention or simple manipulations of the hemodynamic parameters such as increasing the MAP or the hemoglobin, the anesthesia provider must be ready to allow for a wake-up test or ankle clonus test. Both require a rapid decrease in the depth of anesthesia which may be facilitated by the use of short-acting intravenous anesthetic agents. A second component of anesthetic care during spinal surgery is the use of techniques to limit intraoperative blood loss, including basic maneuvers such as effective patient positioning to avoid abdominal compression and distension of epidural veins as well as maintenance of normothermia. Additional techniques may include isovolemic hemodilution, administration of an antifibrinolytic agent, intraoperative blood salvage, and controlled hypotension. The final component is the provision of effective postoperative analgesia with the use of a regional anesthetic technique (epidural or intrathecal opioids) or opioid analgesia administered via PCA. A dexmedetomidine infusion may be added to decrease postoperative opioid requirements.

Annotated references

A full reference list for this chapter is available at:
http://www.wiley.com/go/gregory/andropoulos/pediatricanesthesia

25. Harper CM, Ambler G, Edge G. The prognostic value of preoperative predicted forced vital capacity in corrective spinal surgery for Duchenne's muscular dystrophy. Anaesthesia 2004; 59: 1160–2. In this cohort of 45 patients, 20 patients had a preoperative FVC ≤30% predicted for age. There was no statistically significant difference in several postoperative variables, including the duration of postoperative endotracheal intubation, duration of BiPAP support, total time with ventilator assistance, and inpatient stay. However, there were significant cardiorespiratory complications in both groups, demonstrating that this is a high-risk population with the potential for perioperative complications. Five patients (25%) with an FVC ≤30% had complications including ARDS, respiratory tract infections, and the need for a tracheostomy while four (16%) with a preoperative FVC ≥30% had complications. The one death in the cohort was in a patient with an FVC of 18% who initially had an uncomplicated postoperative course, but went on to develop ARDS.

13. Butler MG, Hayes BG, Hathaway MM et al. Specific genetic diseases at risk for sedation/anesthesia complications. Anesth Analg 2000; 91: 837–55. Review article which addresses various co-morbid genetic conditions and their impact on general anesthesia and procedural sedation with details on associated co-morbid conditions which may affect airway management.

60. Guay J, de Moerloose P, Lasne D. Minimizing perioperative blood loss and transfusions in children. Can J Anaesth 2006; 53: 559–67. Review article outlining factors predictive of the need for allogeneic blood products during various surgical procedures and reviewing techniques to limit intraoperative blood loss.

77. Tobias JD. Controlled hypotension in children undergoing spinal surgery: a critical review of available agents. Paediatr Drugs 2002; 4: 439–53. General review of the pharmacology and use of the various agents available for the induction of controlled hypotension during spinal surgery.

99. Tobias JD. Intrathecal and epidural analgesia following spine surgery in the pediatric population. Anesth Analg 2004; 98: 956–65. Review article of the reports from the literature outlining the various regional anesthetic techniques that have been used for pain management fol-

lowing spinal surgery. These techniques include single-shot intrathecal and epidural analgesia as well as continuous epidural analgesia via an indwelling catheter.

Further reading

Raw DA, Beattied JK, Hunter JM (2003). Anaesthesia for spinal surgery in adults. Br J Anaesth **91**, 886–904. General review article regarding the various perioperative issues involved with caring for adult patients undergoing spinal surgery. The article reviews the preoperative evaluation of these patients, specific intraoperative care, and postoperative care including analgesic techniques.

Soundararajan N, Cunliffe M (2007). Anaesthesia for spinal surgery in children. Br J Anaesth**99**, 86–94. Review article regarding the care of infants and children undergoing spinal surgery. The article reviews the perioperative care of such paitents and also discusses the specific impact of certain co-morbid conditions.

Tobias JD (2004). Strategies for minimizing blood loss in orthopedic surgery. Sem Hematol **41**(suppl), 145–156. Review article regarding the techniques used to minimize the need for allogeneic blood products during major orthopedic surgery including preoperative autologous donation, isovolemic hemodilution, controlled hypotension, and manipulation of the coagulation cascade.

CHAPTER 27
Anesthesia for Transplantation

Stephen A. Stayer[1], Glynn Williams[2] & Dean B. Andropoulos[1]

[1]Department of Anesthesiology and Pediatrics, Baylor College of Medicine, and Texas Children's Hospital, Houston, TX, USA
[2]Pediatric Cardiovascular Anesthesiology, Lucille Packard Children's Hospital at Stanford, and Stanford University School of Medicine, Palo Alto, CA, USA

Introduction

Medical progress has made organ transplantation an accepted therapeutic modality for treating a variety of diseases affecting various organ systems in infants and children. Improvements in immunosuppressive therapy, surgical techniques, and organ preservation have permitted utilization of transplantation in a greater number of patients, and pediatric patients in particular have benefited from the growth of transplantation. The scope and magnitude of various transplant procedures in infants and children with underlying organ system disease will continue to challenge anesthesiologists caring for these patients. In addition, as more children undergo transplantation, anesthesiologists must be prepared to care for them following transplantation, including the management of post-transplant complications and procedures.

Anesthetic management of these procedures requires understanding the physiological implications of organ failure, as well as specific requirements of the transplant procedure [1]. To facilitate this discussion, issues related to the anesthetic care of children undergoing liver, renal, heart, heart-lung, lung, and multivisceral transplantation will be discussed separately. In addition, other chapters describe anesthetic care of infants and children with specific organ dysfunction who require surgery.

Perioperative anesthetic management of solid organ transplant procedures has a number of similarities. Because of the logistic constraints involving donor organ procurement and admission of patients awaiting transplantation, there is limited time available to the anesthesia team for preparation. During this time, the patient must be admitted to the hospital and an updated history and physical examination and laboratory studies must be obtained. The short period of preparation usually limits the duration of nil per os (NPO) status for most children, which has implications for the anesthesiologist. Because several vascular anastomoses are required, there is significant potential for hemorrhage. Adequate vascular access, invasive monitoring, and availability of adequate quantities of blood product are required. Given the severity of underlying diseases, the physiological alterations they cause, and the frequency of intraoperative changes in the patient's condition, arterial blood gas and pH, blood chemistry profiles, and other hematological testing often are required during transplant procedures. When new transplantation programs are established, anesthesia departments should take an active role in defining the requirements and availability of these ancillary services to help in the care of these patients. Because of the urgent or emergency nature of most transplant cases, the resources must be available to the anesthesia team 24-h, 7 days a week basis.

Care of organ donors after neurological death

Once brain death has been established in a donor, and suitability of the donor organs has been confirmed, the emphasis for patient care is directed toward organ preservation by maintaining cardiac output and oxygen delivery. After placement of the organs according to the United Network for Organ Sharing (UNOS) waiting list criteria in the US, co-ordination of the arrival of the harvesting teams is done by the local organ procurement agency, and an operating room time selected. The anesthesia team needs to ensure preservation of oxygen delivery to the harvested organs by maintaining adequate ventilation, cardiac output, hemoglobin, and blood pressure within target ranges. Diabetes insipidus is often present, requiring close attention to urine output and electrolytes, replacement of losses, and desmopressin (DDAVP) administration. Because of loss of sympathetic outflow from the central nervous system, hypotension and cardiovascular compromise are a constant possibility during the preparation for harvest. Close communication with the

surgical team, or teams for multiple organ harvests, will assure optimal organ retrieval.

Brain-dead donors do not experience pain but they may experience hemodynamic changes from spinal cord reflexes with surgical incision and should be treated with inhalational anesthetics or opioids. After wide abdominal exposure, the retrieval team will ask for heparin (200–400 units/kg). Organs are generally removed according to their susceptibility to ischemia, with the heart first and the kidney last. After the heart, great vessels, and lungs are dissected out, the donor aorta is cross-clamped and the heart perfused with a preservation solution such as standard crystalloid cardioplegia or Celsior® to provide both cardioplegia and organ preservation. The organs are then placed in ice for transport at 4°C.

Donation after cardiac death

Because of the ongoing shortage of donors for all organs, the concept of organ donation after cardiac death is advocated. Families may request organ donation after withdrawal of mechanical ventilatory support in patients who are otherwise suitable for donation, with an irreversible neurological injury, who do not have brainstem death.

This condition must be confirmed by the patient's physicians and agreed to by the patient's next of kin. In order to optimize organ retrieval, patients and families are typically taken to the operating room where ventilatory and circulatory support is withdrawn. A physician not involved with the organ procurement determines an irreversible cessation of cardiac and respiratory function, and the organ recovery takes place. As of 1 July 2007 in the US, transplant centers and organ procurement organizations are required to have policies and procedures in place for this process. Donation after cardiac death increased the number of donors by over 600 in 2006 [2].

Immunosuppression for pediatric solid organ transplantation

Review of the history of solid organ transplantation demonstrates that successful outcomes are impossible without effective immunosuppression. The aim of immunotherapy is to minimize the risk of rejection and drug toxicity. Currently, pediatric solid organ transplantation protocols for induction, maintenance and desensitization vary widely between centers. Even single organ transplant groups are far from consensus on the ideal approach to immunosuppression [3]. A general strategy is depicted in Figure 27.1 [3]. Most transplant patients require indefinite maintenance therapy, although about 20% of pediatric

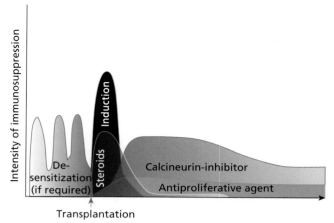

Figure 27.1 Time line showing the different approaches for immunosuppression in relation to the time of transplant. Pretransplant protocols are reserved for patients with specific risk factors (e.g. HLA sensitization or ABO-incompatible transplantation). Depending on the transplanted organ and center, the use of induction may or may not be part of the protocol. Furthermore, low-dose steroids may remain part of the maintenance therapy, supporting a regimen of one or two drugs of different classes. Additional treatments are used for treatment of rejection. Reproduced from Urschel et al [3] with permission from Elsevier.

liver transplant recipients and some kidney recipients have been successfully weaned from immunosuppression late after transplantation [4]. Figure 27.2 illustrates the cellular targets of immunosuppressive drugs, and commonly used drugs are detailed in Table 27.1 [3]. Discussion of individual agents is beyond the scope of this chapter and has been addressed recently [3,5–10].

It is important to monitor drug levels because co-existing disease and drug interactions can result in sub-therapeutic or toxic drug effects. Nephrotoxic agents should be avoided even if renal function is normal. Cystic fibrosis patients have unreliable gastric absorption and hepatic clearance and are at risk of developing acute toxicity from oral medications like cyclosporin. Hepatic enzymes such as cytochrome P450 metabolize commonly used immunosuppressant drugs. Perioperative drugs (e.g. metoclopramide, amiodarone, antibiotics, barbiturates, phenytoin) may induce or inhibit cytochrome P450 and alter drug levels of calcineurin and mammalian target of rapamycin (mTOR) inhibitors. Newer immunosuppressant medications often do not include liquid forms required for young children. Such liquid preparations must be compounded by local pharmacies and may have a short shelf-life, making them difficult to manage for patients not residing near a pediatric medical center. Moreover, absorption and pharmacokinetic data for infants and children often do not exist, making dosing decisions in drugs that may have narrow therapeutic windows challenging [11].

Table 27.1 Immunosuppressive options in pediatric transplantation

Drug name	Mechanism	Comments
Induction therapy		
Polyclonal antibodies		
Rabbit ATG Equine ATG	Antibodies against thymus-derived epitopes	Aim for lymphocyte count of 0.1– 0.3×10^3/mL
Monoclonal antibodies		
Basiliximab Daclizumab	IL-2 receptor (CD25) blocking antibodies Inhibit T-cell activation	Start before transplant Start before transplant
Induction and maintenance therapy		
Steroids		
Methylprednisolone Prednisone	Inhibition of activator protein-1 and nuclear factor κ-B	Can be discontinued in liver, heart and kidney. Usually continue in lung
Maintenance therapy		
Calcineurin inhibitors		
Cyclosporin (CSA) Tacrolimus (TAC)	Inhibit expansion and differentiation of T-cells Inhibit expansion and differentiation of T-cells	Choice and target level of drug depend on type of organ, time after transplant and individual variables (e.g. renal dysfunction)
Antiproliferative drugs		
Mycophenolate mofetil (MMF) Azathioprine	Inhibit *de novo* DNA synthesis	Change from one to other formulation may relieve gastrointestinal problems Avoid MMF/ecMPA use in pregnancy Limit sun exposure on azathioprine
mTOR inhibitors		
Sirolimus Everolimus	Arrest in cell cycle and differentiation	May be protective against coronary allograft vasculopathy

Reproduced from Urschel et al [3] with permission from Elsevier.

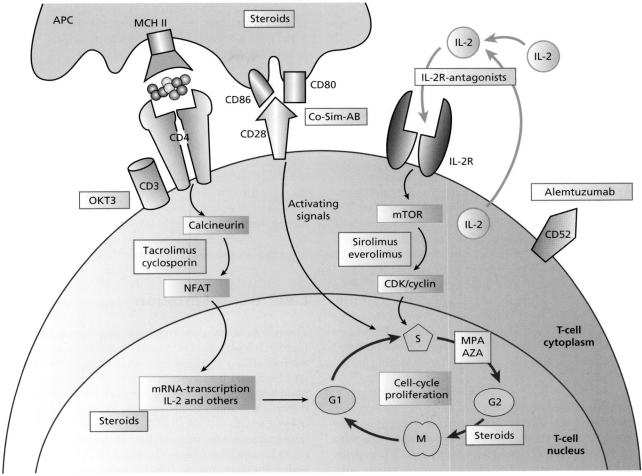

Figure 27.2 T-cell activation and proliferation results from presentation of a peptide fragment of the donor antigen in the major histocompatibility complex class II (MHC II) of the antigen-presenting cell (APC) and a co-signal from interaction from CD80/CD86 and CD28. This mechanism results in activation of calcineurin, which leads to production of interleukin-2 (IL-2). Autocrine stimulation by IL-2 results in cell proliferation by a pathway involving target of rapamycin (mTOR) and cyclin/cyclin-dependent kinase (CDK). Immunosuppressive agents exert their effects at a number of different targets to prevent T-cell proliferation. The CD80/CD86 and CD28 interaction is targeted by specific antibodies (Co-stim-AB) abatacept and belatacept. Basiliximab and daclizumab (IL-2R antagonists) target the receptor for IL-2, required for cell activation via mTOR, which is targeted by sirolimus and everolimus. Tacrolimus and cyclosporin interfere in the signal transduction from the T-cell receptor by inhibiting calcineurin nuclear factor of activated T-cells (NFAT). Mycophenolic acid (MPA), mycophenolate mofetil (MMF) and azathioprine (AZA) interfere in the cell cycle, preventing the T-cell as well as the B-cell from proliferating. Steroids target multiple sites in the interaction. Alemtuzumab (ATM) and muronomab (OKT3) target specific lymphocytic surface structures to induce cytolysis; a similar principle is used for antithymocyte globulins (ATG) but with multiple targets on the surface. Reproduced from Urschel et al [3] with permission from Elsevier.

Induction therapy

Induction immunotherapy is intense immunosuppression in the immediate perioperative phase of organ implantation to reduce the incidence of acute rejection in the early post-transplant phase [4,12,13]. Also, there are longer term benefits because chronic graft failure and decreased long-term survival correlate with the frequency of acute rejection. However, the side-effects of induction agents are significant (polyclonal antibodies, opportunistic infections, post-transplant lymphoproliferative disorder (PTLD), anaphylaxis, monoclonal antibodies, hypersensitivity reactions). Induction therapy allows a delayed and

gentle introduction of maintenance immunotherapy, thereby reducing the potential for harm (e.g. renal damage) from toxic drug concentrations [14,15].

Maintenance therapy
Steroids

Corticosteroids are used in most solid-organ transplant protocols for induction, maintenance and acute rejection. Their side-effects include hypertension, diabetes mellitus, osteopenia, poor wound healing, cataracts, emotional lability, hyperlipidemia, salt and water retention, Cushingoid habitus, weight gain, hirsutism, acne, and growth impairment. Steroid-free maintenance has been successfully achieved in liver, heart and kidney but not lung transplantation [16,17].

Calcineurin inhibitors

Adult data comparing the two calcineurin inhibitors (CNI) indicate that tacrolimus improved graft survival and prevented acute rejection more effectively than cyclosporin. Nephrotoxicity is an adverse side-effect common to both and is a major concern in pediatric solid-organ transplant patients. Acute toxicity is dose dependent and can lead to chronic renal damage and transplantation. Renal-sparing strategies include the use of mycophenolic acid (MPA) and mTOR inhibitors. The side-effect profiles of CNI drugs are similar; generally hirsutism, hypertrichosis, gingival hyperplasia, hypertension, and hyperlipidemia are more likely with cyclosporin and diabetes, tremor, peripheral neuropathy, alopecia, and gastrointestinal symptoms are more common with tacrolimus. The seizures associated with CNI agents seem dose related and are thought to be due to ischemia from cerebral vasoconstriction. Autoimmune hemolytic anemia and leukopenia have been reported with both drugs, but may improve by switching to the other CNI.

Antiproliferative agents

The principal side-effect of azathioprine is bone marrow depression. Other concerns are UV-dependent increase in skin cancers, pancreatitis and hepatotoxicity. Azathioprine has largely been replaced by MPA-containing drugs such as mycophenolate mofetil (MMF) have similar mechanisms of action but are more potent and have better efficacy [18]. The two main side-effects of MPA are gastrointestinal problems and marrow depression.

Mammalian target of rapamycin inhibitors

Mammalian target of rapamycin inhibitors such as sirolimus and everolimus cause an arrest in cell cycle and cell differentiation. Sirolimus inhibits vascular smooth muscle proliferation and hence may have a protective effect against coronary artery vasculopathy in cardiac allografts [19]. Adverse side-effects of mTOR inhibitors include renal dysfunction, hyperlipidemia (typically responds to statins), delayed wound healing, bone marrow suppression, aphthous ulcers and systemic inflammatory response syndrome (e.g. pnuemonitis). The anti-CD20 monoclonal antibody rituximab may be added.

Acute rejection therapy

Usual first-line therapy is steroids, with the addition of polyclonal lymphocyte-depleting antibodies (antithymocyte globulin, ATG) in more severe cases of rejection.

Maintenance immunosuppression might be switched from cyclosporin to tacrolimus. Antibody-mediated rejection is treated with plasmapheresis and IV immunoglobulin.

Newer agents

Normal immune tolerance to self-antigens involves central and peripheral mechanisms that potentially may be manipulated to allow recipient tolerance to alloantigens [20]. Anti-CD52 antibodies cause profound lymphocyte depletion and were thought to hold promise as a tolerance-inducing agent. However, clinical studies to date are discouraging.

Abatacept and belatacept cause co-stimulation blockade of T-cell CD28 receptor binding to CD80/CD86 of the antigen-presenting cell and may allow less nephrotoxic maintenance regimens. Pediatric data are lacking.

Liver transplantation

Thomas E. Starzl performed the first human liver transplant in a 3-year old child with biliary atresia in 1963. The attempt ended in failure from intraoperative hemorrhage, and Dr Starzl performed the first successful liver transplant in a child in 1967. One-year survival after liver transplant remained below 50% until the introduction of cyclosporin in 1979. By 1983, pediatric liver transplantation was deemed the standard of care for hepatic failure or end-stage liver disease [21] and in 2002, the pediatric end-stage liver disease (PELD) and model for end-stage liver disease (MELD) scores were implemented to prioritize organ allocation to the sickest patients, rather than to those with the longest wait time, as had been the case. In addition, the PELD system conferred special status and protection to pediatric organs and recipients. Today pediatric liver transplantation is one of the most successful solid-organ transplants. According to US Organ Procurement and Transplantation Network (OPTN)/ Scientific Registry of Transplant Recipients (SRTR) data, the 1-year patient survival rate is 83–91%, depending on the age at transplant [22]. The number of pediatric liver transplants per year has remained steady in the last 10 years, averaging approximately 600 annually. Currently, pediatric transplants account for about 10% of all liver transplants in the United States, and the majority of these transplants involve children less than 12 years of age. Liver transplantation is now performed on infants less than 3 months of age with graft survival and patient survival that are similar to older patients [23].

Indications for hepatic transplantation

The indications for liver transplant are listed in Table 27.2. Life-threatening complications secondary to hepatic

Table 27.2 Underlying diagnoses of children undergoing liver transplantation

Diagnosis	Frequency (%)
Cholestatic liver disease	48
Biliary atresia (15%)	
Other: Alagille syndrome, sclerosing cholangitis, progressive familial intrahepatic cholestasis	
Fulminant hepatic failure	11
Metabolic liver disease	13
Primary non-hepatic disease: ornithine transcarbamylase deficiency, primary hyperoxaluria type 1, organic acidemia	
Primary hepatic disease: Wilson disease, α1-antitrypsin deficiency, tyrosinemia, cystic fibrosis	
Liver tumors	4
Other	9

Reproduced from Ng et al [24] with permission from the American Academy of Pediatrics.

Table 27.3 Pathophysiology in end-stage liver disease

Organ System	Common Findings
Cardiovascular	Hyperdynamic circulation; increased cardiac output, decreased systemic vascular resistance, increased stroke volume and ejection fraction Expanded plasma volume Arteriovenous shunting
Pulmonary	Restrictive pulmonary function secondary to ascites Hypoxemia secondary to ventilation/perfusion mismatch, impaired hypoxic pulmonary vasoconstriction, intrapulmonary shunting Pulmonary hypertension Hepatopulmonary syndrome
Central nervous system	Encephalopathy Cerebral edema with fulminant hepatic failure
Gastrointestinal	Hepatic dysfunction: synthetic, metabolic, excretory aspects Portal hypertension (esophageal varices, portal hypertensive gastropathy) Delayed gastric emptying
Renal	Renal dysfunction from prerenal azotemia (secondary in diuretics)
Hematologic	Elevated PT Thrombocytopenia Anemia Hypofibrinogenemia, dysfibrinogenemia Fibrinolysis Disseminated intravascular coagulation
Fluids, electrolytes, acid–base status	Intravascular volume depletion (secondary to diuretics) Hypokalemia, hyponatremia Metabolic alkalosis Metabolic acidosis (especially fulminant hepatic failure)

failure or chronic end-stage liver disease are the primary indications for transplantation. Another indication is progressive primary liver disease refractory to maximal medical management, before the development of life-threatening complications. A smaller number of liver transplants are performed for metabolic disease, in which liver replacement is curative, and for unresectable primary liver tumors. Fulminant hepatic failure (FHF) is the indication for liver transplantation in approximately 11% of pediatric cases [24]. These children commonly present with rapidly developing life-threatening complications, and therefore establishment of the underlying diagnosis is not always feasible. Approximately 13% of children undergo liver transplantation because of metabolic diseases [25–28], and these patients generally have excellent outcomes [27,29]. Pediatric patients with liver tumors represent a growing group of transplant recipients. Hepatoblastoma is the most common pediatric primary liver tumor. Resection in combination with systemic chemotherapy is the preferred method of treatment. If the tumor is unresectable after appropriate chemotherapy, transplantation may be offered if there has been a demonstrated response to therapy, even in the face of pulmonary metastases [30–32]

Pathophysiology of end-stage liver disease

Patients with end-stage liver disease that results from many causes manifest similar pathophysiology (Table 27.3). The clinical manifestations from end-stage liver disease develop from the loss of hepatocytes and resulting fibrosis. The loss of hepatocytes results in the development of coagulopathy, hypocholesterolemia, hypoalbuminemia, and encephalopathy. Hepatocellular injury results in fibrosis and destruction of the portal triad with increased resistance to liver blood flow leading to portal hypertension manifest by varices (esophageal, bowel), hemorrhoids, ascites, spontaneous bacterial peritonitis, splenomegaly with thrombocytopenia, and hepatic encephalopathy.

The cardiovascular system undergoes marked changes as the child develops cirrhosis and end-stage liver disease. Patients frequently have a hyperdynamic circulation, decreased systemic vascular resistance, increased cardiac output, and a slightly decreased arterial blood pressure. The pathophysiology producing peripheral vasodilation remains obscure, and the "humoral factor" theory is the most widely accepted explanation [33]. In cirrhosis, increased intrahepatic resistance induces portosystemic collateral formation, allowing gut-derived humoral substances (endocannabinoids and nitric oxide (NO)) to enter the systemic circulation directly without detoxification by the liver. The hyperdynamic circulation of the patient has important implications for the anesthesiologist, including a decreased sensitivity to catecholamines and vasoconstrictors, an increase in mixed venous oxygen saturation, with a decreased arteriovenous oxygen difference. Because of the vasodilated state, anesthetics may cause severe hypotension in this patient population.

Patients with end-stage liver disease also manifest significant changes in the pulmonary system and are frequently hypoxemic. Many patients with chronic liver disease have abnormal pulmonary mechanics and some degree of alveolar hypoventilation. The presence of ascites and increased infra-abdominal pressure alters respiratory mechanics and often reduces functional residual capacity. Atelectasis produces ventilation/perfusion mismatch and is common in patients with ascites, hepatosplenomegaly, and/or pleural effusions. Hepatopulmonary syndrome (HPS) is characterized by hypoxia from intrapulmonary arteriovenous shunting and intrapulmonary vascular dilation [34]. The diagnosis is predicated on either arterial hypoxia (PaO_2 <70 mmHg) or an alveolar-arterial gradient greater than 20 mmHg in the setting of pulmonary vascular dilation. Intrapulmonary vascular dilation can best be demonstrated on echocardiography or by macroaggregated albumin perfusion scan [35]. Again, the most likely explanation for the development of HPS is systemic absorption of nitric oxide from the gut without detoxification in the liver. Supplemental oxygen therapy is the mainstay of supportive therapy and definitive treatment is liver transplantation. A case series of seven children with hepatopulmonary syndrome and severe hypoxemia were successfully transplanted and recovered from hepatopulmonary syndrome on average within 24 weeks of their liver transplant [36].

Portopulmonary hypertension (PPH) is defined as pulmonary artery hypertension (pulmonary systolic pressure ≥25 mmHg) in the setting of normal pulmonary capillary wedge pressure and portal hypertension [37]. The incidence of PPH is 0.2–0.7% in adults with cirrhosis and is present in 3–9% of adults undergoing liver transplantation [38]. The incidence in children is probably lower, and occurrences are limited to case reports and one case series. The signs and symptoms of PPH on presentation include a new heart murmur, dyspnea, and

syncope. Echocardiography can diagnose pulmonary hypertension and is one reason why routine screening of potential liver transplant candidates includes a baseline echocardiogram [39]. The largest retrospective review of 43 adult patients found mean pulmonary artery pressure (MPAP) to be predictive of outcome. Those patients with a MPAP <35 mmHg did not have increased mortality after orthotopic liver transplantation (OLT). In contrast, those with a MPAP = 35–45 mmHg had a mortality of 50%, and those with a MPAP >50 mmHg had 100% mortality [40].

Among children with PPH, early identification is essential. If PPH is suggested by screening echocardiography, a cardiac catheterization should be performed to confirm the diagnosis, measure the pulmonary pressures, and assess the response to NO and epoprostenol. Children who respond to medical management may be candidates for liver transplantation [41]. Severe PPH is generally a contraindication for liver transplantation because of the high mortality.

Hepatic encephalopathy is a significant neurological complication of liver disease that may be acute, as seen in fulminant hepatic failure, or chronic. Table 27.4 presents the staging of hepatic encephalopathy [42]. Cerebral edema is a feature of both acute and chronic encephalopathy; however, it is more severe and happens more rapidly in acute hepatic encephalopathy, commonly leading to increased intracranial pressure (ICP). The pathogenesis is thought to be due to hyperammonemia that more readily crosses the blood–brain barrier and will cause astrocytes to swell, leading to low-grade cerebral edema [43]. Blood

Table 27.4 West Haven criteria for altered mental status in hepatic encephalopathy

Grade 0	Minimal hepatic encephalopathy, lack of detectable changes in personality or behavior; no asterixis
Grade 1	Trivial lack of awareness, shortened attention span, sleep disturbance, altered mood, and slowing the ability to perform mental tasks; asterixis may be present
Grade 2	Lethargy or apathy, disorientation to time, amnesia of recent events, impaired simple computations, inappropriate behavior, and slurred speech; asterixis is present
Grade 3	Somnolence, confusion, disorientation to place, bizarre behavior, clonus, nystagmus, and positive Babinski sign; asterixis usually absent
Grade 4	Coma, lack of verbal, eye, and oral response to stimuli

Reproduced from Zafirova & O'Connor [42] with permission from Lippincott Williams and Wilkins.

ammonia levels develop from catabolism of endogenous protein and gastrointestinal absorption. Ammonia is formed when bacteria in the gut break down nitrogen-containing products, which are then absorbed into the portal circulation. Therefore, blood ammonia levels will increase from increased catabolism due to infection, increased gut absorption from high protein diets, gastrointestinal bleeding, and renal failure. Arterial ammonia levels over 200 µg/dL have been strongly correlated with cerebral herniation and death. Other factors that may contribute to cerebral edema include benzodiazepines, hyponatremia, and inflammatory cytokines. Management typically focuses on reducing gastrointestinal production and absorption of ammonia. Lactulose is often prescribed to create an osmotic diuresis and to acidify the lumen of the gut to trap ammonia and minimize absorption, yet has not been shown to improve survival [42]. Antibiotics (e.g. neomycin and metronidazole) are sometimes used to kill the gastrointestinal bacteria involved in metabolizing nitrogen products to ammonia.

As hepatic encephalopathy progresses, the child's ability to manage the airway should be carefully assessed. Children with grade 3 and 4 disease commonly require endotracheal intubation to protect their airway and to maintain oxygenation and ventilation. Increased ICP occurs in 38–81% of adult patients with fulminant hepatic failure [44] and brain computed tomography is recommended in those with grade 3–4 hepatic encephalopathy. Simple therapeutic measures, which can be performed on all patients, include elevation of the head of the bed to 30° and minimizing stimulation. Acute hyperventilation fails to reduce episodes of cerebral edema, and it does not delay onset of herniation [44]. Intracranial pressure monitors may help to diagnose intracranial hypertension and optimize management, although their use remains controversial [45,46]. Non-randomized trials have shown no survival advantage. Medical management to reduce ICP includes intravenous administration of sodium thiopental or propofol to minimize stimulation and to directly reduce ICP. Mannitol can be administered if ICP remains increased. Hypothermia has also been used to treat increased ICP. In a trial of 14 patients with fulminant hepatic failure, ICP was significantly reduced by mild hypothermia to 32–33°C [45]. Corticosteroids have no role in this setting [47] and OLT remains the definitive treatment.

The gastrointestinal system undergoes many changes when patients have end-stage liver disease, including abnormal synthetic, metabolic, and excretory functions of the liver and portal hypertension. Complications of portal hypertension include (1) altered hepatic and intestinal lymph flow and decreased plasma oncotic pressure, which facilitate the development of ascites, and (2) gastrointestinal bleeding from esophageal and gastric varices or from portal hypertensive gastropathy.

Renal failure commonly complicates acute and chronic liver disease in adults but the incidence in children is considerably lower [48]. Renal insufficiency is common and may be caused by prerenal azotemia, acute tubular necrosis or hepatorenal syndrome. Prerenal azotemia may develop from the use of diuretics, gastrointestinal bleeding, splanchnic pooling, and sepsis. Acute tubular necrosis develops when the kidney becomes ischemic from these same etiologies. Hepatorenal syndrome is characterized by renal insufficiency or failure in the setting of liver failure and portal hypertension.

The pathophysiology of hepatorenal syndrome is thought to be secondary to intense renal vasoconstriction from activation of the renin-angiotensin, arginine vasopressin, and sympathetic nervous systems [49]. Hepatorenal syndrome presents as prerenal azotemia (increased creatinine, decreased urine sodium) but a fluid challenge will not improve renal function. Rapid progression of renal failure from hepatorenal syndrome is classified as type 1, and is characterized by a rapid progression of renal failure with a 100% increase in creatinine in less than 2 weeks. This form usually occurs in acute liver failure. In type 2, renal failure progresses over weeks to months. Dopamine, diuretics, and octreotide have all been used to remove excess volume and optimize renal perfusion; however, OLT remains the definitive therapy because renal failure is reversible if the liver is replaced [50]. Combined liver-kidney transplantation is an option for children with both liver and renal disease.

Hematological abnormalities occur with liver disease because synthesis of fibrinogen and factors II, V, VII, IX, and X decreases [51]. Because of the decreased synthesis of these factors, the prothrombin time (PT) and the partial thromboplastin time (PTT) are increased. Thrombocytopenia is common when patients develop hypersplenism in response to portal hypertension. Also, anticoagulant factors (protein C and S, antithrombin III) are reduced in patients with end-stage liver disease. The altered hemostasis increases the risk of inserting vascular catheters and nasogastric tubes, and increases the potential for excessive bleeding from surgical wounds. Antifibrinolytics such as aprotinin and aminocaproic acid have been reported to reduce blood loss; however, there are insufficient data to recommend their use.

Electrolytes and acid–base balance often are altered in chronic liver disease by renal dysfunction and/or the use of diuretics. Acid–base changes may be due to renal dysfunction or to changes in ventilation. The intravascular volume status may be difficult to assess in patients with liver disease due to the presence of ascites, peripheral edema, and anasarca. The effective plasma volume is often inadequate. Consequently, intraoperative measurement of central filling pressures is required during transplantation.

Anesthetic management

Preoperative evaluation

Most transplant centers utilize a multidisciplinary approach for the evaluation of patients for liver transplantation. Typical laboratory studies include blood typing, blood chemistries, liver and renal function tests, coagulation profiles, and viral serologies. Cardiac and pulmonary systems are assessed through electrocardiogram (ECG), chest x-ray, and echocardiography. A careful neurological examination should be performed to detect any problems present in the preoperative period. Anatomical assessment of the native liver typically includes abdominal ultrasound and/or computed tomography or magnetic resonance imaging. A liver biopsy may be indicated to confirm the diagnosis or severity of the liver disease. Also, an assessment of the psychosocial and financial situation of the child's family is performed. Following the initial evaluation, the patient's history and data are presented to a selection committee, which decides if the patient is a candidate for transplantation. Patients approved for transplantation are then activated on the transplant center's recipient list. In situations of acute hepatic failure or rapid decompensation of chronic liver disease, the evaluation process can be condensed to a few hours.

Referral to the transplant center and acceptance of the child as a transplant candidate allow the transplant center physicians the opportunity to optimize the patient's medical condition while the child awaits transplantation. Medical therapy to control ascites, infection, and encephalopathy is initiated. Nutritional assessment and diet modification are frequently performed. Endoscopy and sclerotherapy may be performed to treat gastrointestinal bleeding. If the patient has cardiopulmonary disease, additional studies, including arterial blood gases, response to inhaled oxygen, and cardiac catheterization, may be indicated (see discussion above). Vitamin K may be administered to improve hemostatic function. Prophylactic dental work or dental extraction and tonsillectomy and adenoidectomy are performed if required prior to transplantation and initiation of immunosuppression.

Perioperative period

In general, patients are admitted from home when a potential donor is identified. Because of the logistical complications associated with scheduling, performing donor surgery, and transporting the donor organ to the transplant center, 8–12 h notice is often provided to the patient, family, and transplant team members.

Upon admission to the hospital, interval history and physical examination are performed to seek evidence of new changes and complications since the original pre-transplant evaluation. Whenever possible, the child is made NPO prior to surgery. In addition to routine blood tests, multiple additional blood samples are obtained for serological studies, and specialized immunotesting. A peripheral intravenous (IV) line is usually started and maintenance fluids administered.

Following arrival of the donor organ at the hospital, final inspection and possible biopsy and frozen section of the liver are performed. Following notification from the transplant surgeon that the liver is appropriate for transplantation, the child is transported to a warm operating room. In some children, especially those who are older, premedication may be required with either intravenous or oral midazolam. Children with hepatic encephalopathy should not receive premedication because midazolam may produce significantly greater central nervous system (CNS) depression among these patients and may potentially increase intracranial pressure. Routine monitors (pulse oximetry, ECG, arterial blood pressure) are applied prior to induction of anesthesia. One hundred percent oxygen is administered by facemask. Because of concerns that these patients have a full stomach and may aspirate gastric contents, cricoid pressure is applied and a rapid-sequence induction of anesthesia is performed for most patients. Those who present for elective transplant to correct a metabolic disease may undergo inhalational induction. Since patients with significant ascites are likely to have a reduced functional residual capacity (FRC), adequate preoxygenation is required. Once the airway is secure, mechanical ventilation with an increased inspired concentration of oxygen and positive end-expiratory pressure (PEEP) is initiated. Cuffed endotracheal tubes are favored because they will make a reliable seal between the tracheal tube and the tracheal mucosa and reduce the risk of inadequate ventilation and monitoring of ventilation from a leak around the endotracheal tube.

Following tracheal intubation, vascular access is obtained and monitoring catheters are inserted. Ideally, two large-bore intravenous lines are placed in the upper extremities (20–22 gauge for infants, 18–20 gauge for a young child, and larger for older children). Adequate venous access is critical during any liver transplant procedure because the anesthesia team must be able to respond rapidly to surgical hemorrhage. The fluid delivery system must allow for sufficient control over the volume and rate of fluid and blood product administration in small children to prevent overhydration. An arterial catheter is inserted, preferably in a radial artery, because the aorta may be cross-clamped during reconstruction of hepatic arterial inflow. A multi-lumen central venous catheter is inserted after induction. One lumen is used for central venous pressure monitoring and the other lumens for infusion of medications and/or volume. The surgical team may decide to insert a tunneled central line if long-term access is likely to be needed in the postoperative period. Measuring pulmonary artery pressures may facilitate the perioperative management of patients with cardiac disease or associated pulmonary hypertension. Except for these rare cases, central venous pressure monitoring is sufficient in infants and children for liver transplant. Many adult centers use transesophageal echocardiography to monitor cardiac function and filling during liver transplantation but this is much less common in the pediatric setting [52].

Particular attention is paid to maintaining normal body temperature during pediatric liver transplantation. Numerous factors facilitate development of unintentional hypothermia: exposure of the abdominal contents to air, duration of surgery, rapid administration of cool intravenous fluids and blood products, and implantation of the cold liver graft and wash-out of the cold storage solution during reperfusion of the organ. Rigorous attention is paid to warming the operating room and to the use of insulated wrapping of exposed extremities, forced-air warming blankets, humidified anesthesia circuit, and warming of all intravenous fluids.

No particular anesthetic regimen has proven superior in liver transplantation. A combination of potent inhaled anesthetic, bolus doses of opioids or an infusion provides a relatively stable intraoperative course during liver transplantation. Higher concentrations of inhaled anesthetics reduce splanchnic blood flow and should probably be avoided. Sevoflurane, isoflurane and desflurane are commonly used with success when added to a balanced anesthetic technique with opioids. Nitrous oxide should not be used in order to avoid bowel distension. A comparison of right ventricular function in adult patients undergoing liver transplantation found no difference between propofol and isoflurane [53]. Even though the primary metabolic pathway for propofol is hepatic, there appears to be extrahepatic metabolism in the lung, kidney, and intestine [54,55].

Intravenous opioids have been used extensively in the anesthetic management of adult and pediatric patients undergoing liver transplant. Although end-stage liver disease is likely to affect the distribution and plasma clearance of opioids, the functioning newly transplanted liver graft will improve opioid clearance. Opioid analgesics undergo hepatic biotransformation via mixed function oxidase (e.g. fentanyl) and glucuronosyltransferase (e.g. morphine). Because the hepatic extraction of morphine and fentanyl is high, plasma clearance is less affected by alterations in hepatic function than by alterations in hepatic blood flow. Morphine, fentanyl, and sufentanil appear to have unchanged plasma clearance and

volumes of distribution in patients with end-stage liver disease, which may reflect the ability of the large volume of distribution to buffer any decrease in drug metabolism. In contrast, alfentanil, with its volume of distribution approximately 25% that of the other opioids, has a decreased plasma clearance and an increased free fraction of drug in patients with cirrhosis. The impact of large changes in and replacement of intravascular volume during the course of a lengthy liver transplant procedure is not known.

Liver disease affects the duration of action of nondepolarizing muscle relaxants. The action of pancuronium is prolonged in patients with liver disease. The duration of action of vecuronium depends on the extent of liver disease and on the dose of vecuronium. Vecuronium in a bolus of 0.1 mg/kg has the same pharmacokinetics in both patients with normal livers and those with liver disease [56]. In more advanced liver disease, a dose of 0.2 mg/kg of vecuronium may have a prolonged duration of action [57,58]. Similarly, rocuronium will have prolonged duration of action after repeated doses despite a normal onset of action for the first dose [59]. Redistribution of the drug within the body may be important for the termination of the drug's effect in patients with liver disease, but when larger doses of drug are administered, reduced hepatic clearance becomes more evident. Studies suggest that the liver graft with normal function rapidly resumes its role of drug metabolism [60,61]. Despite the overall uncertainty of anesthetic drug metabolism in the perioperative period following liver transplantation, delayed recovery from anesthetic drugs and neuromuscular blockade rarely poses a clinical problem.

The timing of extubation of the trachea varies among centers; however, immediate postoperative extubation has gained acceptance and is practiced more commonly. In the author's institutions, tracheal extubation in the OR is performed in over 50% of patients. Most commonly, the decision to extubate the patient early is based on the presence or absence of co-morbidities.

Because of the duration of the procedure and the potential for hypoperfusion of the skin and extremities, positioning is critical to prevent injuries. All extremities should be padded, and all cables and wires need to be wrapped and protected from the skin. The head should be turned and repositioned periodically to prevent pressure sores and alopecia.

Surgical procedure

Liver transplantation is usually divided into four stages: dissection, anhepatic, and reperfusion with biliary anastomosis. During the dissection period, the liver is mobilized via a large bilateral subcostal incision. All perihepatic adhesions are lysed, the suprahepatic vena cava, infrahepatic vena cava, and structures in the porta hepatis (portal vein, hepatic artery, and common bile duct) are identified and mobilized. Lysis of dense adhesions following a Kasai portoenterostomy or other previous surgery usually prolongs the dissection time and increases blood loss during this period. Adequate replacement of blood components during this time is essential.

Prior to implantation, the donor organ is stored in preservation solution, most commonly University of Wisconsin (UW) solution. Because of the high potassium content (120 mEq/L), the donor organ is perfused with a cold crystalloid or colloid solution to remove the preservation solution before the liver is implanted. When the dissection phase is complete in the recipient, the preservation solution is flushed out of the donor liver and it is brought into the operative field. However, flushing the donor liver with large volumes of fluid does not always remove all of the potassium, air, and particulate matter. Consequently, when the donor organ is reperfused, the recipient will receive a bolus of hypothermic solution, and may be subjected to hyperkalemia, thrombotic and air emboli. Bradycardia and increases in pulmonary artery pressure are common, and occasionally, there is a hyperkalemic cardiac arrest at the time the donor organ is reperfused.

The anhepatic stage begins with cross-clamping the suprahepatic vena cava, infrahepatic vena cava, portal vein, and hepatic artery. This surgical approach will significantly reduce preload from cross-clamping the inferior vena cava (IVC). However, patients with chronic cirrhosis develop collateral circulation, and inferior vena cross-clamp is generally well tolerated. Partial clamping of the IVC is used for reduced-size grafts or when IVC cross-clamping produces cardiovascular instability. Using the piggy-back technique [62], the liver is dissected away from the inferior vena cava, the short hepatic veins, portal vein, and left, right, and middle hepatic veins. The infrahepatic vena cava of the donor is oversewn, and the suprahepatic vena cava is anastomosed to the native hepatic veins. In addition, a portocaval shunt can be established for children who do not tolerate clamping of the portal vein. Typically, these recipients have not developed collateral flow secondary to portal hypertension (e.g. metabolic liver disease and acute fulminant hepatic failure). During the anhepatic period, the native liver is completely excised, bleeding is controlled in the retrohepatic area, and the donor liver is sutured in place. The liver is most commonly reperfused with venous inflow, which accounts for approximately 80% of liver blood flow. The anhepatic period ends with restoration of blood flow to the new liver.

Following restoration of blood flow into the new liver, the final stage of the operation, reperfusion, has started. The surgical goals during this time include completion or revision of the hepatic artery anastomoses and establish-

ment of biliary drainage. In infants and children, reconstruction of the hepatic arterial inflow may be more difficult and frequently includes reconstruction via a patch graft from the recipient aorta or donor saphenous vein graft to celiac trunk, hepatic artery or aorta. Biliary drainage may occur via a direct choledochocholedochostomy or, more commonly in children, via a Roux-en-Y choledochojejunostomy. A major goal during the early reperfusion period is control of bleeding. This period requires close communication between surgeons and anesthesiologists to determine the presence of a coagulopathy (common in the early reperfusion period) as opposed to defined surgical bleeding (common following the total hepatectomy of the native liver and multiple vascular anastomoses and following previous abdominal surgery). The operating team uses a variety of clinical observations (color, texture, bile production) and laboratory measurements (PT, metabolic acidosis, ionized calcium, and glucose concentration) to document the status and quality of liver graft function.

Occasionally, infants who have cardiac anomalies and intracardiac shunts require liver transplantation. This is especially dangerous because when the graft is reperfused there is the likelihood of air, clot, and other debris entering the systemic circulation. If this occurs, there is the danger of coronary artery or cerebral artery embolism. One method used to reduce this risk is to leave the vena cava above the liver clamped and to open the vena cava below to allow the initial blood entering the liver from the portal vein to exit the vena cava into the abdomen. This often means that one-fourth to one-third of the blood volume is lost via this route. This period of phlebotomy requires rapid replacement of blood, but is effective in reducing the risk of systemic embolization.

Intraoperative management issues
Hemodynamics

Periods of hemodynamic instability are common during liver transplantation. In the earlier portions of the anesthetic (e.g. during line placement, preparing and draping the skin), the general debilitating effects of end-stage liver disease and the reduced blood volume induced by diuresis may limit the patient's ability to compensate for the hypotensive effects of anesthetics. In response to abdominal incision and dissection around the native liver, surgical stimulation may overcome light levels of anesthesia and produce hypertension and tachycardia.

A more common scenario is development of hypotension at various points during the operation. Massive blood loss must always be entertained in the differential diagnosis for hypotension. Given the site of surgery, the presence of extensive abdominal and retroperitoneal collateral vessels, and scar tissue from previous surgeries, bleeding may be significant during the dissection phase of surgery. It should always be kept in mind that splenic bleeding is a possibility. The changes in hemodynamics during the anhepatic period are frequently the most complicated to understand. With application of the venous clamps to the portal vein and to the infrahepatic and suprahepatic vena cava, there is an abrupt decrease in venous return to the right side of the heart and subsequently to the left side of the heart. Although there may be a brief period of hypotension in response to application of the clamp, infants and children appear to tolerate moderate hypovolemia and maintain normal systemic arterial pressures. Stimulation may produce hypertension and tachycardia if the anesthesia level is light. Reflex tachycardia, reduction in central venous pressure (CVP), dampening of the arterial waveform during positive pressure ventilation, and development of a metabolic acidosis are all consistent with significant hypovolemia. In addition, this same hemodynamic picture may develop from surgical manipulation, resulting in compression of the inferior vena cava or right ventricle.

In adult patients, cardiac index may decrease 30–50% when the venous clamps are applied, but systemic arterial pressure is only slightly decreased because there is a compensatory increase in systemic vascular resistance. Volume administration during the anhepatic period is guided by central venous pressure, systemic arterial pressure, and the arterial pressure waveform. While surgical attention is focused on the vascular anastomoses during the anhepatic period, significant bleeding may continue from areas behind the liver and at other sites of collateral flow. In rare situations, vasopressin (0.1–0.3 units/min IV) may be required to decrease splanchnic blood flow while the anastomoses are being completed. Fluid administration may include crystalloid, colloid or blood products, depending upon the hemoglobin, PT, and preference of the surgeon and anesthesiologist. Colloid solutions may have particular benefit during the anhepatic period and end of the dissection period. Care should be taken not to administer excessive fluid during the anhepatic phase because when the blood is returned to the central circulation with unclamping the inferior vena cava, a high CVP will impair hepatic venous drainage. Typically a CVP of 8–10 mmHg is adequate to maintain arterial pressure at the time of reperfusion with little need for vasopressors.

Because the portal vein is clamped during the anhepatic period, portal venous hypertension develops. Because of the increased venous pressure, there is a tendency toward fluid translocation and bowel edema during the anhepatic period. Administration of colloid solutions during the dissection and anhepatic period may reduce the amount of bowel edema that develops and facilitate closure of the abdomen at the end of the operation. In addition, the extent of bowel edema may influence the duration of impaired intestinal motility following the operation. Because large volumes of hydroxyethyl starch are associated with coagulopathy, albumin solutions are routinely utilized for colloid administration. Patients with persistent hypotension may require cardiovascular support with dopamine or epinephrine during this time.

Infants and children commonly have normal urine outputs during the anhepatic period, apparently because there are other pathways by which venous blood can return to the central circulation. However, low urine output during the anhepatic phase is not an indication for fluid administration because of the potential adverse effects of high CVP and the routine recovery of urine output after removal of the venous cross-clamp. The CVP is a better indicator of hydration status.

Completion of the anhepatic period restores venous return from the lower extremities and splanchnic bed. Despite adequate intravascular volume, hypotension is a common finding following graft reperfusion. Numerous factors are felt to contribute to the hemodynamic changes associated with reperfusion. Immediately upon reperfusion, a combination of hypotension, bradycardia, and supraventricular and ventricular dysrhythmias may develop. Prior to reperfusion, a small bolus of fluids may be administered to optimize ventricular filling. Acid–base status is checked approximately 5–10 min before reperfusion. Sodium bicarbonate and calcium are administered to achieve a high-normal pH and calcium levels prior to cross-clamp release. At the moment of reperfusion, attention must be divided between the cardiac monitor and the surgical field. Evidence of life-threatening hemorrhage requires the immediate infusion of blood products while the surgeons control the bleeding. Inspection of the cardiac monitor will detect ECG changes consistent with profound bradycardia and/or hyperkalemia. Bradycardia may result from the sudden atrial stretch occurring with restoration of normal venous return and/or influx of cold storage flush solution, with profound alterations in pH and electrolyte content. If the heart rate decreases by 30–40%, atropine should be administered, and warm solutions should be instilled into the abdominal cavity.

Electrocardiogram evidence of hyperkalemia includes development of peaked T waves (rare in babies), QRS widening, and sine-wave formation. Inspection of the arterial waveform trace will confirm the loss of mechanical activity. The occurrence of hyperkalemia at the time of reperfusion represents systemic toxicity of organ preservation solution that was not removed when the organ was flushed. Acute interventions for hyperkalemia include administration of calcium and bicarbonate, and circulatory support with closed chest cardiac massage and epinephrine. Because the surge in serum potassium is transient, treatment is directed towards decreasing the concentration of serum potassium and restoring the cardiac rhythm. The potassium concentration increases 0.5–1.5 mEq/L at the time of reperfusion in almost all patients. Because this increase in potassium is expected during reperfusion, care should be taken to prevent increases in potassium concentrations during the dissection and anhepatic periods. Forced diuresis (renal dose dopamine, diuretic administration) can help lower the potassium level. In addition, insulin and glucose administration effectively decreases the serum potassium concentration during the anhepatic period. Following the abrupt increase at reperfusion, potassium concentrations tend to decrease during the remainder of the operation. Urinary losses of potassium account for some of the decrease, while potassium uptake by muscle cells and allograft liver cells also contributes to the decrease in serum potassium. Potassium administration is indicated if the serum potassium concentration decreases and the urine output remains adequate in the postreperfusion period.

Other factors, including transient hypocalcemia, acidosis, and hypothermia, contribute to hypotension following graft reperfusion. Studies in adult transplant patients suggest that approximately 30–40% of patients develop a "post-reperfusion" syndrome consisting of decreased arterial blood pressure and profound vasodilation [63]. A study utilizing transesophageal echocardiography (TEE) found right ventricular dysfunction (paradoxical motion of interventricular septum, right atrial enlargement, right-to-left interatrial deviation) following reperfusion. In addition, the pulmonary circulation is known to be sensitive to acute alterations in temperature and pH. Perfusion of the lungs with ice-cold, hyperkalemic, acidic blood may increase pulmonary vascular resistance and cause right ventricular dysfunction. Embolization of air, clot, and cellular debris can occur at the time of graft reperfusion, as was shown by the TEE study mentioned above.

Perturbations of hemodynamics at reperfusion can affect other organs and systems. The liver graft is sensitive to increased levels of central venous and pulmonary artery pressure. Vascular engorgement of the liver is common following reperfusion of the liver, especially if the CVP was greater than 10 mmHg before the liver was reperfused. Because the arterial blood supply to the liver may still be compromised (e.g. during the hepatic arterial reconstruction), excessive passive engorgement of the liver may deprive some areas of the liver of oxygen and cause poor restoration of graft function. Anesthetic management must attempt to prevent liver graft engorgement. If the systemic arterial pressure is adequate, infusion of nitroglycerin may reduce elevated central blood volumes and graft swelling or engorgement. Specific treatment for pulmonary hypertension includes increased ventilation, correction of acid–base status, and normalizing body temperature.

Hemostasis

Intraoperative hemostasis is a complex issue during orthotopic liver transplantation [51,61]. The hemostatic system is often impaired by intrinsic liver disease and as a result of the transplant procedure. Based upon preoperative diagnosis and coagulation testing, several groups have attempted to predict the risk of intraoperative bleeding during liver transplant [64]. However, a predictive score that indicates a low likelihood of bleeding is not a reason to decrease the level of preparedness. Blood products should be immediately available for transfusion. Low potassium units of blood should be used (less than 2 weeks since collection) or it is prudent to wash units of packed red blood cells to remove the excess potassium. Once the initial extent of dissection and coagulopathy is determined, the need for additional cross-matching of blood and/or preparation of fresh frozen plasma, cryoprecipitate, and platelets can be determined. In the event of significant hemorrhage, the blood bank must be notified of anticipated increased requirements for blood products.

The anesthesia team is responsible for maintaining adequate hemostasis during liver transplant procedures. Central to this role is the ability to rapidly monitor coagulation status intraoperatively. For the monitoring system to be effective, the anesthesiologist must have rapid access to the results of these tests so that the abnormalities can be corrected immediately. Routine coagulation testing should include measurement of PT, activated PTT, platelet count, hemoglobin concentration, and fibrinogen concentration. Thromboelastography (TEG), a specific type of whole-blood viscoelastic coagulation monitoring, has been used successfully by some clinicians during liver transplantation [65]. It is a test of clot strength and requires a 30–60-min recording of clot formation and lysis. The TEG gives an indication of clotting factor activity, platelet function, and fibrinolysis. Since significant fibrinolysis is less common in children, TEG monitoring is not routinely utilized in most centers [52].

Intraoperative management of coagulopathy during liver transplantation includes the administration of blood products and potential pharmacological interventions. The principal blood product administered is fresh frozen plasma (FFP), which will correct clotting factor deficiencies. Because hepatic artery thrombosis is one of the most common causes of graft failure in pediatric patients, FFP is administered to correct and maintain values for PT and PTT close to 1.5 times prolonged from normal, depending on the amount and severity of intraoperative bleeding. Cryoprecipitate is administered when infusing FFP does not correct a low fibrinogen concentration (<80–

100 mg/dL). In the postreperfusion period, intravascular filling pressures may be elevated. Consequently, the decreased volume of cryoprecipitate is better tolerated.

Thrombocytopenia is a common finding during liver transplantation. Many patients have decreased platelet counts because portal hypertension has induced hypersplenism. Intraoperative thrombocytopenia may develop or worsen due to replacement of blood loss during the dissection phase with solutions that do not contain platelets. Platelet counts decrease slightly during the anhepatic period and decrease significantly upon reperfusion of the graft. Platelet entrapment within the grafted liver has been demonstrated in a porcine model of liver transplantation; in addition, platelet activation and consumption increase following reperfusion of the graft. Platelet counts of 50,000–100,000 commonly develop and are not an indication for platelet transfusion in the absence of excess bleeding. Overtransfusion of platelets may also increase the risk of hepatic artery thrombosis. Platelet transfusion is indicated if thrombocytopenia is present and there is a clinical impression of abnormal hemostatic function.

Severe postreperfusion coagulopathy occurs in some patients who undergo liver transplantation, possibly because of the reperfusion-initiated disseminated intravascular coagulation. Studies indicate that primary fibrinolysis may develop during liver transplantation due to changes in the circulating concentration of tissue-type plasminogen activator (t-PA). Both ε-aminocaproic acid (EACA) and aprotinin have been utilized to pharmacologically reduce the severity of fibrinolysis during orthotopic liver transplantation. EACA improves the TEG findings of fibrinolysis during liver transplantation; however, prophylactic use of EACA has not been demonstrated to be of value. Administration of aprotinin, a protease inhibitor of kallikrein, decreases the laboratory abnormalities associated with fibrinolysis and reduces transfusion requirement during liver transplantation [66]. The worldwide marketing of this agent was suspended in 2008 due to complications in the adult cardiac surgery population, including thrombosis, stroke, and renal failure, and it is not available in the US. Children are hypercoagulable after liver transplantation because of a decrease in protein C and antithrombin III [67] and they may be more likely to develop hepatic artery thrombosis or emboli [68–70]. Therefore antifibrinolytics are not routinely used in most pediatric transplant centers.

Hepatic artery thrombosis may result from disorders of the coagulation system and/or technical factors in hepatic arterial reconstruction. Intraoperative and postoperative Doppler ultrasound examinations of the hepatic arterial and portal vein anastomoses are commonly used to assess patency of the anastomoses. Because of the potential for graft loss with vessel thrombosis, a slightly anticoagu-

lated state is maintained in infants and small children following liver transplantation. This includes avoiding fully correcting the heparin effect in the operating room, maintaining a slightly higher prothrombin time, and early administration of aspirin. At Texas Children's Hospital, our practice is to start a heparin infusion in the operating room once hemostasis has been achieved after reperfusion and to continue this infusion for the first few days postoperatively. In addition, hyperviscosity from overtransfusion of red cells should be avoided. Maintaining the hemoglobin between 8 and 10 mg/dL provides adequate oxygen-carrying capacity.

Metabolic control (K$^+$, Ca^{2+}, acid–base, glucose)

Acute changes in acid–base status, potassium concentration, ionized calcium, and glucose are common, both before and during liver transplantation. Concomitant renal dysfunction promotes acid–base changes and exacerbates electrolyte problems. Diuretic therapy can cause electrolyte imbalance (hyponatremia, hypokalemia, hypocalcemia) and prerenal azotemia. A common pattern of electrolyte changes develops in most patients. Consequently, an anticipated treatment plan can be developed. Routine intraoperative monitoring of arterial blood gases, electrolytes, and glucose concentrations will define the need for and further refine intraoperative electrolyte therapy. Because of the multiple factors contributing to hemodynamic instability in these patients, these parameters are more tightly controlled than in other operations.

Many patients who present for surgery have hyponatremia due to prerenal azotemia and the use of diuretics. Care should be taken to avoid a rapid rise in sodium concentrations during surgery from the use of salt-containing solutions, sodium bicarbonate and blood products. Also, both hypo- and hyperkalemia are frequently encountered during surgery (see discussion above).

Patients undergoing liver transplantation are particularly susceptible to the development of ionized hypocalcemia. Although total calcium concentrations are decreased in patients with chronic liver disease, ionized calcium concentrations are normal. Intraoperative administration of blood products decreases ionized calcium and magnesium concentrations because citrate-based anticoagulant solutions used in collection and storage of blood products bind these ions. Citrate usually is metabolized rapidly by the liver. In normal patients, low ionized calcium concentrations only occur following massive and rapid administration of blood products. Patients with end-stage liver disease are particularly sensitive to the administration of citrate-containing blood products, and administration of moderate amounts of FFP can significantly decrease ionized calcium concentrations.

Profoundly low ionized calcium concentrations, particularly during the anhepatic period, may cause myocardial depression and hypotension. Given the potential for dramatic changes in the ionized calcium concentration, direct measurement of ionized calcium is particularly useful during liver transplantation. Calcium replacement therapy during the dissection and anhepatic phases can be achieved with either bolus administration or constant infusion of calcium. Calcium chloride and calcium gluconate are equally effective in increasing the ionized calcium concentration during the anhepatic period [71]. Calcium requirements are expected to increase (often markedly) during the anhepatic period and to quickly decrease following reperfusion of the hepatic allograft. With restoration of blood flow to the liver graft, metabolism of citrate proceeds at a much greater rate than occurred with the native liver or during the anhepatic phases. Reduction in calcium requirement following reperfusion is consistent with adequate hepatic allograft function. As mentioned earlier, normal ionized calcium concentrations at the end of the anhepatic period may protect against the cardiovascular effect of abrupt increases in potassium from the reperfused liver. Measurement of ionized calcium 5 min before graft reperfusion and administration of calcium prior to reperfusion is suggested.

Metabolic acidosis is extremely common during orthotopic liver transplantation. Numerous factors contribute to its development, including tissue hypoperfusion, decreased or absent metabolism of lactate, citrate, and other metabolic acids by the liver, rapid administration of acidic blood products, associated renal impairment, and acidic effluent from the liver allograft. During the dissection period, development of acidosis most commonly reflects global tissue hypoperfusion. Administration of additional intravascular volume and restoration of adequate blood pressure and cardiac output often corrects the acidosis. The anhepatic period in particular is associated with rapid development of acidemia. The contribution of decreased tissue perfusion (caused by the abnormal hemodynamics associated with vena cava and portal vein occlusion) and the absence of hepatic function is unknown. Sodium bicarbonate is used to treat metabolic acidosis during the anhepatic period, and the amount of bicarbonate administered is based on the rapidity and severity of changes in acid–base balance. In general, with base deficits greater than 5–8 mEq/L or pH less than 7.35 ($PaCO_2$ <40 mmHg), bicarbonate should be administered to create a relatively normal pH immediately prior to reperfusion of the graft. Arterial blood gases and pH measurements obtained approximately 5 min prior to reperfusion will determine the amount of bicarbonate required.

Following reperfusion of the liver graft, metabolic acidosis frequently recurs. Treatment of severe metabolic acidosis at this point is indicated when there is concomitant myocardial depression and/or there are signs of persistent hyperkalemia. Normally, the exacerbation of metabolic acidosis quickly abates during the postreperfusion period; this abatement is one of the early signs that the graft is functioning. The liver allograft usually resumes metabolic function rapidly, and hepatic metabolism of lactate and citrate frequently leads to the development of a metabolic alkalosis in the later portions of the operation and in the postoperative period. Resolution of metabolic acidosis (and development of alkalosis) is indicative of adequate allograft function, although the sensitivity and specificity of these findings are not known. The extent of the metabolic alkalosis is related to the amount of intraoperative transfusion, and not to the amount of bicarbonate administered.

Glucose balance is complicated by liver transplantation. Hypoglycemia may be present in patients with fulminant liver failure or severe chronic liver disease and may necessitate preoperative administration of dextrose-containing fluids. It usually is necessary to administer glucose to these patients before the graft is reperfused. In theory, the anhepatic period should pose a greater risk of hypoglycemia because there is no liver in the circulation. Numerous factors are present that help maintain a relatively normal glucose concentration in the blood during the anhepatic period: stress response to surgery, steroid administration, dextrose-containing blood products, and reduced glucose utilization due to hypothermia. Since organ preservation solutions and flush solutions frequently contain dextrose, glucose concentrations commonly increase after reperfusion of the graft. Hyperglycemia in the reperfusion period also has been suggested as a marker for allograft function. Small infants may have markedly decreased glycogen stores when presenting for liver transplantation and are frequently at increased risk for developing hypoglycemia. Preoperative and frequent intraoperative glucose determinations are the best methods of detecting abnormal glucose levels. Dextrose should be administered if hypoglycemia is present. Persistent hyperglycemia, glucose greater than 250 mg/dL, is treated with insulin administration.

Temperature maintenance

Hypothermia is common during liver transplantation, despite utilization of multiple methods to conserve body heat. The long intra-abdominal operation, massive fluid and blood product administration, and implantation of a graft that has a temperature near zero all contribute to the development of hypothermia. There is usually a 1–2°C decrease in body temperature when the ice-cold donor liver is placed in the abdomen. There also may be an abrupt decrease in core temperature of 1–2°C with reperfusion when cold flush solution is infused into the systemic circulation. Profound hypothermia carries significant theoretic risk, including cardiac depression, arrhythmias, abnormalities in clotting function, and decreased renal function. Because of these risks, specific efforts are directed at maintaining core temperature. Heating the operating room is imperative for infants and small children. A forced-air warming blanket is placed beneath the child and the exposed extremities are wrapped. Forced-air warming is useful over the legs and/or upper extremities in larger patients. Intravenous fluids and blood products are warmed prior to their administration. Lowering of fresh gas flows and using a humidifier will reduce the heat loss caused by use of cold dry inspired gases.

Special techniques
Reduced-size grafts (pare-down, split, live donor grafts)

Three advances in surgical technique have improved the number of available grafts for children: dividing the liver and using a reduced-size graft, or even two grafts for two recipients, and living donor transplantation. The surgical technique most commonly used to split the liver is performed while still *in vivo* (in the heart-beating donor) as compared with *ex vivo* (splitting performed after the graft is removed from the donor). This decreases cold ischemia time and facilitates hemostasis of the liver edge. This technique results in improved child and graft survivals [72,73]. The Studies in Pediatric Liver Transplantation (SPLIT) group is an excellent source of data regarding pediatric liver transplantation in North America. This group represents 46 pediatric liver transplant centers across America and Canada and reflects the results of programs with a strong pediatric emphasis. The most recent review of the SPLIT database reveals patient survival rates of 91.4% and 86.5%, at 1 and 5 years following liver transplantation, respectively [74].

Living related transplantation has greatly benefited the pediatric transplant population, particularly in countries in which there is limited availability of deceased donor grafts for cultural or even legal reasons [75]. In this procedure, a left lateral segmentectomy (segments 2 and 3) is performed in the donor and transplanted in a similar fashion to the whole organ. Approximately 300 living donor liver transplants are performed annually and 20% of these are in child recipients [22]. Despite the success of this technique for the recipients, there is considerable risk to the donor. Complications include exposure to blood products, peripheral nerve injuries, biliary leakage, abdominal wall defects, pleural effusions, pneumonia, pulmonary emboli, and death [76,77].

Retransplantation

Hepatic retransplantation is performed to treat primary non-function of the allograft, allograft dysfunction result-ing from thrombosis of the hepatic artery or portal vein, rejection unresponsive to aggressive medical therapy, or recurrent or primary disease in the transplanted liver. Retransplantation rates are 10–20%. Because of the dense adhesions around the transplanted liver, significant hemorrhage may occur during the dissection phase. In addition, if the liver has sustained an ischemic insult, disruption of the vascular anastomoses may occur and produce catastrophic hemorrhage. There must be adequate vascular access to allow massive volume resuscitation. Sufficient blood products must be available in the operating room to rapidly instill one blood volume in the patient. Most reports indicate that patient survival following retransplantation of the liver is worse than it is following the primary transplant. However, a recently published manuscript found graft and patient survival after retransplantation to be similar to primary liver transplantation [78].

Renal transplantation

Indications

Renal transplantation is the optimal therapy for children with chronic renal insufficiency (CRI) and end-stage renal disease (ESRD). Despite the availability of dialysis for children, transplantation is the preferred long-term management for children with ESRD to allow the best chance for normal growth, activity, and development. Also, the risk for death is more than four times higher with dialysis than with renal transplantation [79]. The incidence of ESRD in children 0–19 years of age is between 5 and 12 per million. The incidence increases with age and males are more likely to develop ESRD than females secondary to the higher rate of congenital urological anomalies. The etiologies of ESRD, and therefore the disease processes leading to transplant, differ depending on the age of the patient. For children under 5 years of age, congenital lesions (renal dysplasia/aplasia, obstructive uropathy, complex urogenital malformations, and congenital nephrosis) are responsible for the majority of pediatric transplants. Over 5 years of age, glomerulonephritis (e.g. focal glomerulosclerosis, membranoproliferative glomerulonephritis) and recurrent pyelonephritis are major causes of ESRD. The North America Pediatric Renal Transplant Co-operative Study (NPRTCS) (https://web.emmes.com/study/ped/registry) registry reported that from 1987 to 2008, in 9854 transplants, 47% were over 12 years of age, 33% were 6–12 years of age, 15% were 2–5 years, and only 5% were under 2 years of age.

The outcome of renal transplantation in children is encouraging. The North American Pediatric Renal Transplant Co-operative Study annually reports the overall graft survival rate (Table 27.5).

Table 27.5 Kidney transplant graft survival rates from the North American Pediatric Renal Transplant Co-operative Study

Cohort group	Graft survival rate					
	Living donor			Deceased donor		
	1 yr	3 yr	5 yr	1 yr	3 yr	5 yr
1987–1990	89.4	81.2	74.6	75.2	63.5	54.8
1991–1994	91.8	85.4	80.4	85.2	76.4	69.5
1995–1998	94.0	90.5	85.3	90.6	81.8	73.9
1999–2002	95.9	91.2	85.9	92.7	83.9	79.5
2003–2007	96.1	90.6	–	94.4	81.1	–

Data from the North America Pediatric Renal Transplant Co-operative Study (NPRTCS).

Pathophysiology

A patient's fluid and electrolyte balance is dramatically altered by renal failure. Hypervolemia, hypovolemia (after dialysis), hyponatremia, hyperkalemia, hypocalcemia, hyperphosphatemia, and metabolic acidosis are common. Because the failing kidney may not excrete adequate free water, hypervolemia is frequent and is a cause of hypertension. Hypovolemia can occur after aggressive dialysis. Hyponatremia occurs when water retention exceeds sodium retention, or when there is salt wasting plus an inability to concentrate urine. Hyperkalemia may be a major problem due to its effects on the cardiac conduction system, and it may require treatment before general anesthesia can be safely induced. Hypocalcemia is secondary to the hyperphosphatemia that results from the kidney's inability to excrete phosphates. Metabolic acidosis develops because the failing kidney cannot excrete the body's daily production of metabolic acids.

Many organ systems are affected by ESRD. Hypertension, increased cardiac output, pericarditis, arrhythmias, and cardiomyopathy are manifestations of the altered cardiovascular system. Hypertension occurs secondary to fluid overload or to alterations in the renin-angiotensin-aldosterone system. Patients with anemia compensate for their decreased oxygen-carrying capacity by increasing their cardiac output. The use of recombinant erythropoietin has decreased the incidence of severe anemia in ESRD patients. Congestive heart failure due to hypertension

and volume overload, a uremia-induced cardiomyopathy, and pericardial disease may complicate the management of children with ESRD. Pulmonary edema can develop as a result of fluid overload, hypoproteinemia, and altered pulmonary capillary permeability.

Anemia develops due to decreased erythropoietin production and decreased erythrocyte life span, despite normal reticulocyte counts. Uremic toxins decrease red blood cell (RBC) life span and suppress bone marrow function. The anemia is normocytic and normochromic, despite renal failure- induced deficiencies in folate and vitamin B12. There is an increased concentration of 2,3-diphosphoglycerate (2,3-DPG) which, in conjunction with the metabolic acidosis, shifts the oxygen–hemoglobin dissociation curve to the right. This shift and an increased cardiac output partially compensate for the decreased oxygen-carrying content caused by the anemia. Coagulation is often altered in uremic patients by residual heparinization following dialysis and by abnormal platelet function. Platelets are usually normal in number and life span but have a reversible functional defect secondary to accumulation of guanidinosuccinic acid, which inhibits adenosine diphosphate (ADP)-induced activation of platelet factor III, which is needed for normal platelet adhesion [80].

Renal failure induces numerous neurological effects. Uremic encephalopathy manifests as a global depression that is reversible with dialysis. Uncontrolled hypertension may lead to either focal neurological deficits or seizures; hypertension must be controlled. Seizures may also occur with rapid electrolyte changes (e.g. hyponatremia). Peripheral neuropathies are common in patients with renal failure and usually consist of axonal degeneration with segmental demyelination. The median and common peroneal nerves are frequently involved. Autonomic dysfunction develops in children with ESRD. Baroreceptor activity may be abnormal and lead to hypotension that is unresponsive to intraoperative volume administration.

Nutrition is generally poor in ESRD. Uremia causes anorexia, leading to poor caloric intake and growth retardation. Despite the need for protein and calories, protein intake must be carefully controlled to prevent worsening metabolic acidosis. Renal osteodystrophy, aluminum toxicity, altered somatomedin activity, and insulin and growth hormone resistance are all associated with the growth failure [81]. Delayed gastric emptying is common in children with renal failure. Therefore, patients undergoing a renal transplant may have an increased risk of aspiration of gastric contents regardless of the NPO interval.

Preoperative assessment and preparation

There are two sources of kidneys for transplantation into children: cadaver and living donors. Because living donor transplants are elective operations, there is adequate time to optimize the nutritional, hydration, and metabolic status of the patient.

Evaluation of the fluid and electrolyte status of the patient is of primary importance. If the patient has been recently dialysed, a review of the dialysis records is often helpful. Changes in weight, blood pressure, and electrolyte concentrations before and after dialysis should be noted. The patient's dry weight is the minimum weight not associated with hypotension or cardiovascular instability; the current weight compared to the dry weight will indicate the volume status of the patient. Because there are significant changes in electrolytes (e.g. Na+, K+) after dialysis, serum electrolytes should be determined after dialysis. Hypertension in patients with ESRD is common and frequently indicates hypervolemia. However, many patients also require antihypertensive medications, which should be continued until the time of surgery to avoid intraoperative rebound hypertension.

The physical examination should assess the airway and cardiopulmonary status of the patient and determine if a functioning arteriovenous shunt is present. If so, it must be protected during the operation. Patients with nephrotic syndrome or those who have been on steroids may be edematous, which could make tracheal intubation more challenging. Due to the delayed gastric emptying of patients with ESRD, the use of an antacid or anti-H_2 agent and metoclopramide may be helpful before anesthesia induction.

Surgical technique

Pediatric renal transplantation employs more than one surgical technique. In older children (weighing >20 kg), the standard surgical approach is similar to that of adults, that is, a lower abdominal incision with extraperitoneal placement of the donor kidney in the iliac fossa. Vascular anastomoses are usually to the iliac vein (end-to-side) and iliac or hypogastric arteries (end-to-side or end-to-end). For infants and small children (weighing <20 kg), a midline incision is made and the kidney placed intra-abdominally. The vascular connections are made to the inferior vena cava and the lower abdominal aorta. The aorta and vena cava are cross-clamped while the anastomoses are being completed. In addition, the donor organs for most small children are from older children or adults, with obvious size implications.

Anesthetic management

Premedication with midazolam is usually safe and may allay anxiety if needed. Standard ASA monitors are used, and because of the potential for acute blood loss, large-bore peripheral intravenous access and blood warmer are indicated. Because the patient's volume status is difficult to determine and may vary considerably during the oper-

ation, measurement of the CVP helps guide appropriate fluid management. The CVP catheter can also be used to obtain blood samples for laboratory tests and to administer vasoactive medications into the central circulation. However, preservation of sites for long-term vascular access in patients who may need hemodialysis in the future should be considered, and the subclavian veins are generally avoided for this reason. Larger, older children can usually be adequately managed with peripheral IV access alone. Also, an indwelling arterial catheter is not routinely used for adults or older children, but it may be quite helpful for smaller children, especially if the aorta is to be cross-clamped. One must be careful not to risk the patency of an existing arteriovenous shunt or to compromise future placement of such a shunt.

Anesthesia for renal transplantation is usually induced with intravenous drugs because the patients frequently have an IV catheter already in place. For patients without an IV catheter, inhaled induction of anesthesia is a viable alternative. The pharmacokinetics and pharmacodynamics of anesthetic drugs are altered in patients with ESRD, and this must be taken into account when administering drugs to induce anesthesia. Propofol will produce vasodilation and potentially hypotension in patients who are hypovolemic. Thiopental is normally extensively plasma protein bound. Children with ESRD have decreased plasma protein concentrations. Therefore, the effects of thiopental may be greater than expected, although the greater volume of distribution found in patients with renal failure may offset some of thiopental's increased availability. Ketamine can also be used as an IV induction agent for patients with ESRD, but its sympathomimetic effects may exacerbate pre-existing hypertension. To blunt the autonomic response to laryngoscopy and tracheal intubation, opioids or lidocaine can be given intravenously. As with all sick children, careful titration of anesthetic drugs to the desired effect is always the safest approach.

The choice of muscle relaxant for tracheal intubation continues to generate discussion. Because delayed gastric emptying is common in patients with renal failure, patients undergoing renal transplantation may be at increased risk for regurgitation and possible aspiration of gastric contents. This situation makes a rapid-sequence intravenous induction of anesthesia with an intravenous induction agent, cricoid pressure, and succinylcholine theoretically advantageous. However, the administration of succinylcholine may cause serum potassium concentrations to rise 0.5–0.75 mEq/L, in normal patients [82]. A number of conditions lead to an exaggerated rise of serum potassium and subsequent hyperkalemic arrest. Patients with ESRD are at risk for hyperkalemia if they have uremic neuropathy or if they have not been dialysed recently [83]. An alternative to succinylcholine is to perform a modified rapid-sequence intravenous induction of anesthesia using an intravenous agent, a non-depolarizing muscle relaxant, cricoid pressure, and controlled ventilation. The non-depolarizing muscle relaxant used should not depend on renal pathways of elimination. Two categories that fit this requirement are the atracurium/*cis*-atracurium family, whose elimination is by Hoffman degradation and ester hydrolysis, and the steroid-based muscle relaxants that are predominantly metabolized by the liver. The steroid-based muscle relaxants vecuronium and rocuronium have some dependence on renal excretion, perhaps 10–25%, that will lead to some prolongation of onset and duration of action of the drugs when used in patients with ESRD.

Maintenance of general anesthesia during renal transplantation is usually provided by a combination of potent inhaled anesthetic agents and opioids. Nitrous oxide can be used, but it may distend the intestines and make it more difficult to close the abdomen at the end of the operation. Sevoflurane has the theoretical problem of producing a metabolite, compound A, that has been associated with renal concentrating defects, and although useful for inhaled induction of anesthesia, should probably not be the first choice for maintenance of anesthesia [84]. Fentanyl is the most widely used opioid for renal transplantation. No active metabolites are excreted by the kidneys, and there is extensive experience with its use in children without significant complication. The metabolites of morphine are excreted by the kidney so probably it should not be the first choice for intraoperative analgesia.

If the patient has an arteriovenous shunt, the extremity with the shunt must be positioned so that the shunt is protected and available to allow the anesthesiologist to periodically determine that the shunt is functional. A blood pressure cuff should not be used on that extremity. At the very least, the shunt should be checked both at the beginning and the end of the operation for a thrill or bruit and the presence of either or both should be documented on the anesthetic record.

Fluid management during renal transplantation is challenging owing to reduced preoperative renal function and to blood loss and third space fluid losses during the operation. Preoperative fluid status is discussed above. Interstitial fluid losses (third space) and blood losses are determined in the usual fashion (see Chapters 10, 11 and 17). Fluid administration should be based on estimates of need and clinical criteria, including vital signs and CVP when utilized. It should be recognized that hypovolemia should be avoided and fluid administered to produce normovolemia to hypervolemia with adequate blood pressure to the new organ. An isotonic crystalloid solution is a suitable choice of fluid. Theoretically, lactated Ringer's solution should be avoided due to the potassium

(4 mEq/L) that it contains. On the other hand, normal saline is hypernatremic (154 mEq/L) and can lead to a hypernatremic metabolic acidosis if given in large quantities. Intermittent measurements of the serum electrolyte and glucose concentrations are always suitable to follow the metabolic status of the patient. If a blood transfusion is required, washed or fresh packed red blood cells are preferred due to the small volume and the minimal amount of potassium present after washing. The blood should also be irradiated to minimize graft-versus-host reactions in an immunocompromised host.

The surgeons may request a higher than normal mean arterial pressure (MAP) to ensure adequate perfusion of the new kidney. Whenever a new kidney is placed into a small recipient (<20 kg), it is possible that the aorta will be cross-clamped to perform the arterial anastomosis. When the aorta is subsequently unclamped, the blood pressure may decrease dramatically secondary to reduced afterload and the return of acidotic blood from the lower extremities. Furthermore, a large quantity of blood is diverted to the renal allograft, which will decrease the arterial blood pressure if the intravascular volume is inadequate. The anesthesiologist must be prepared to treat abrupt changes in arterial pressure with fluid and drugs. It must be remembered that these changes occur with patients who usually have baseline hypertension. Vascular thrombosis is a potential cause of graft failure in the smallest of recipients so the outcome may indeed depend on the reperfusion management.

The anesthesiologist will also be involved with the administration of immunosuppressant medications, antibiotics, diuretics, and other drugs during the operation. The surgeon or nephrologist should notify the anesthesiologist of the doses and timing of these medications. It is helpful to determine the common side-effects of these drugs that may affect anesthetic management. Antilymphocyte antibodies include muronab-CD3 (OKT3), alemtuzumab (Campath), antithymocyte globulin (equine – Atgam), and antithymocyte globulin (thymoglobulin). The infusion of these agents causes a cytokine response which can include fever, chills, rigors, and malaise that should be pretreated with acetaminophen, corticosteroids, and diphenhydramine [85,86]. Anti-interleukin-2 antibodies include basiliximab (Simulect) and daclizumab (Zenapax). These medications do not cause a cytokine response. Side-effects from anti-interleukin-2 antibodies are comparable to placebo except for an acute hypersensitivity reaction that can occur with basiliximab [85].

At the end of the operation, it should be determined whether the patient's trachea will be extubated. If so, residual neuromuscular blockade should be antagonized. Prolongation of the action of neuromuscular blockers is matched by prolongation of action of the reversal agents.

The patient should be awake when the trachea is extubated. If there is evidence of pulmonary edema, or a relatively large kidney is placed into the abdomen of a small child, tracheal extubation can be delayed and the patient transported to a pediatric intensive care unit (ICU) and the patient's condition allowed to stabilize.

Postoperative pain control is most commonly achieved by the administration of intravenous opioids. Epidural analgesia can be used, but the association with possible hypotension has tended to limit its widespread use as well as the alterations in coagulation status of patients with ESRD.

Heart transplantation

History

The first pediatric human heart transplant was performed in December 1967 in Brooklyn, New York, by Dr Adrian Kantrowitz and associates [87], only 3 days after the first human heart transplant by Christian Barnard. The recipient was a 17-day-old patient with Ebstein anomaly; the donor was an anencephalic infant. The recipient survived a few hours and died of apparent acute graft dysfunction [88]. Cyclosporin became available in 1978 and the first successful infant cardiac transplant was performed by Cooley and associates at Texas Children's Hospital in 1984 [88,89]. The number of pediatric heart transplants performed worldwide increased throughout the 1980s and early 1990s to the present number of approximately 400 transplants annually, and has remained relatively constant since 1991 [90,91].

Indications for heart transplantation

The three major indications for pediatric heart transplantation are congenital heart disease, end-stage cardiomyopathy, and retransplantation for cardiac graft failure [90]. The relative proportion of each of these indications changes with age, with two-thirds of recipients less than 1 year receiving a transplant for congenital heart disease and approximately one-third for cardiomyopathy. Figure 27.3 shows the diagnosis distribution. In the 1–10-year age group, indications are almost evenly allocated to congenital heart disease and cardiomyopathy, and in patients 11–17 years of age, two-thirds have cardiomyopathy as the indication, with congenital heart disease less frequent and retransplant becoming the indication for 7% of transplants in this age group [90,91]. Figure 27.4 shows the frequency of transplant by age.

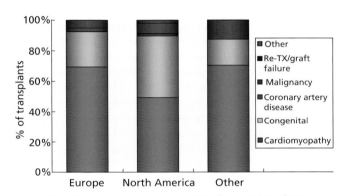

Figure 27.3 Diagnosis distribution by location for transplants from January 2000 through June 2008. Reproduced from Kirk et al [91] with permission from Elsevier.

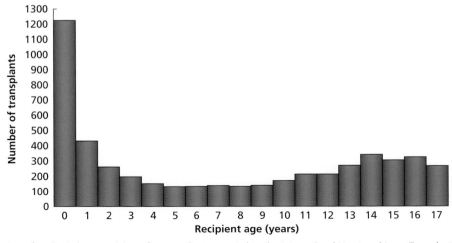

Figure 27.4 Age distribution of pediatric heart recipients for transplants reported to the International Heart and Lung Transplant Registry from January 1996 through June 2008. Reproduced from Kirk et al [91] with permission from Elsevier.

Precise indications vary by institution, but groups such as the American Heart Association have convened panels of experts to consider the evidence base for pediatric heart transplantation and develop recommendations for indications [92]. Because no randomized trials (level A evidence) exist, the recommendations are based on non-randomized studies and registries (level B evidence) and consensus opinions of experts (level C evidence). Class I (general agreement of usefulness and efficacy) and Class IIA (weight of evidence and opinion is in favor of usefulness/efficacy) indications include cardiomyopathy or repaired/unrepaired congenital heart disease with severe systemic ventricular dysfunction despite maximal medical therapy, with associated severe limitation of exercise and activity or growth failure. Additional indications are life-threatening arrhythmias not amenable to drug or defibrillator treatment, restrictive or other cardiomyopathy with reactive pulmonary hypertension reducible to <6 Woods units/m^2, with risk of developing irreversible pulmonary hypertension. In single-ventricle infants, indications for transplant as primary therapy include severe atrioventricular valve or semi-lunar valve insufficiency, stenosis or atresia in proximal coronary arteries, or severe ventricular dysfunction [92]. Other indications include severe cyanosis or protein-losing enteropathy not amenable to medical or surgical therapy. Indications for retransplantation include normal or depressed ventricular function associated with at least moderate coronary artery vasculopathy. Class IIB (no efficacy established) and Class III (contraindicated) contraindications include previous infection with hepatitis B or C virus, or HIV; history of substance abuse; history of significant behavioral, psychological or cognitive disorders, or history of non-compliance or poor family support structure. More absolute contraindications include irreversible multisystem disease, fixed severely elevated pulmonary vascular resistance, or severe hypoplasia of the central branch pulmonary arteries or veins. Contraindications for retransplantation include primary transplant less than 6 months previously, and ongoing acute allograft rejection.

Cardiomyopathies: dilated, hypertrophic, restrictive

Causes of dilated cardiomyopathy include viral myocarditis from agents such as parvovirus or coxsackie virus, mitochondrial myopathies such as central core disease, extensive myocardial infarction from anomalous origin of the left coronary artery from the pulmonary artery, or cardiotoxic chemotherapy from anthracyclines [93]. These etiologies account for approximately 80% of transplants for cardiomyopathy [92]. Hypertrophic cardiomyopathies have a diverse spectrum of etiologies, including inborn errors of metabolism. They account for about 12% of cardiomyopathy transplants. Restrictive cardiomyopa-thies are more rare, and are characterized by diastolic dysfunction with normal ventricular size and wall thickness. These patients have a high incidence of pulmonary hypertension and sudden death, and are not amenable to other surgical or medical therapy, and so have a high rate of listing for transplantation when diagnosed. These patients account for approximately 5% of cardiomyopathy transplants [92].

Congenital heart diseases

In the modern era, virtually all patients with congenital heart disease are offered some form of corrective or palliative surgery; however, some patients will meet the criteria for transplant despite apparent successful surgery or from issues arising perioperatively, i.e. coronary artery or myocardial injury. Approximately a third of these patients are single-ventricle patients with residual poor ventricular function, severe valvar regurgitation or ongoing cyanosis [93] (Table 27.6). Other major causes include transposition of the great vessels, and left or right ventricular outflow tract obstructive lesions.

Retransplantation

Coronary artery vasculopathy, a chronic low-grade rejection phenomenon resulting in gradual vascular occlusion, is seen in 11% of recipients at 5 years, and 17% of recipients at 10 years after transplant [90] and results in listing for retransplantation if ventricular function deteriorates, or significant dysrhythmias or heart block ensue, because of the risk of sudden death. These patients often do not experience angina because of the denervated state of the transplanted heart.

Pretransplant work-up

The decision to list a patient for cardiac transplant is made by a multidisciplinary group led by the medical transplant team, the patient's primary cardiologist, and the surgical transplant team. They assess the patient's and family's capacity to comply with the complicated regimens necessary for ongoing care [94]; recent echocardiographic, cardiac catheterization, and other imaging information; cardiac rhythm; and evidence of pulmonary hypertension. In addition, other organ dysfunction such as neurological disease is reviewed and treatment optimized. Dental status should be assessed, and any caries or other decay treated.

Blood tests required before transplant include ABO/Rh typing, Epstein–Barr virus (EBV), cytomegalovirus (CMV), hepatitis B and C, and HIV status. A panel reactive antibody (PRA) screen is performed to determine the level of antibodies to red blood cell antigens from prior transfusions. High levels of antibodies to specific antigens may prevent transplant from a donor with those antigens, and a "virtual cross-match" is performed for donor and

Table 27.6 Diagnosis in pediatric cardiac transplant recipients with congenital heart disease

Diagnosis	n (N = 488)	%
Single ventricle	176	36%
D-transposition of the great arteries	58	12%
Right ventricular outflow tract lesions	49	10%
Ventricular/atrial septal defect	38	8%
Left ventricular outflow tract lesions	38	8%
L-transposition of the great arteries	39	8%
Complete AV canal	37	8%
Other	53	11%

AV indicates atrioventricular.

Diagnoses of patients >6 months of age with previously repaired or palliated congenital heart disease undergoing cardiac transplant. Data from Cardiac Transplant Research Database and Pediatric Heart Transplant Study Group [93].

recipient red cell antigens before accepting the organ. A strongly positive cross-match for specific antigens may prevent transplantation from a donor with those antigens. Other strategies for patients with high PRA titers include preoperative plasmapheresis, thymoglobulin, and cyclophosphamide treatment to reduce titers [95]. Human leukocyte antigen (HLA) matching is not routinely performed because of time constraints, and limited availability of donor organs.

Once listed for transplant, the patient is designated as status 1A (mechanical circulatory support, mechanical ventilation or high-dose/multiple inotropes, infant with severe reactive pulmonary hypertension, refractory arrhythmias with life expectancy <14 days), 1B (low-dose inotropes, growth failure) or 2 (does not meet status 1A or 1B criteria). Status 7 patients are patients who are temporarily unable to receive a transplant due to a reversible condition such as infection [96]. In the United States, organ donation and allocation are currently overseen by the United Network for Organ Sharing which operates the Organ Procurement and Transplantation Network under contract from the US Department of Health and Human Services, and the Health Resources and Services Administration. These organizations maintain the waiting lists for each type of transplant, and determine the rules for organ allocation, which depend on patient status and to some extent on proximity to the donor. Waiting times depend on age, with the median waiting time for pediatric patients being 60–80 days for those who receive transplants [97]. However, in infants <1 year, the number of donors is only about one-third the number of patients listed for transplantation [5] and the mortality rate while awaiting transplant is as high as 30–40% [98].

Anesthesia for cardiac transplantation

The basic anesthetic considerations for transplantation do not differ from the normal preparation for congenital cardiac surgery. See Chapter 25 for a detailed discussion of pathophysiology. A thorough preoperative evalution and consultation with the patient and family and explanation of the anesthetic procedures are performed, within the time constraints imposed by the timing of organ harvest. The preoperative condition ranges from hospitalized status 1A patients maintained on extracorporeal membrane oxygenation (ECMO) or ventricular assist devices (VAD) to those called in from home. Some patients may have recent oral intake, and are at increased risk for pulmonary aspiration. The timing of entrance into the operating room must be planned and communicated with frequent updates due to difficulties in co-ordinating harvesting teams and donor hospital operating room time. It is preferable to err on the side of having the patient in the OR too early than too late; prolonged ischemic time will affect graft function and possibly long-term outcome. Time to place invasive vascular access lines and other anesthetic preparations must be considered when deciding an OR time.

Prebypass period

Intravenous or oral premedication, often with midazolam, is administered as necessary. Some patients will be maintained in the ICU on mechanical ventilation with inotropic support and some will receive mechanical circulatory support. A co-ordinated operating room transport is required to avoid a disruption of mechanical circulatory support. After arrival in the operating room, immunosuppressive drugs, for example azathioprine and corticosteroids, should be given prior to or soon after induction, as ordered by the transplant team. These critical medications may be easily overlooked in the busy OR environment. Standard non-invasive monitoring is most commonly used for induction, and invasive arterial access obtained after tracheal intubation in small children. However, older patients and those at very high risk of cardiovascular collapse may benefit from placing arterial access prior to induction.

Most pretransplant patients are at significant risk of developing dysrhythmias or cardiac collapse with the induction of anesthesia and positive pressure ventilation. Therefore, methods of resuscitation must be immediately at hand to support the patient. These include resuscitative medications, defibrillator, and the ability to rescue the patient with emergency cardiopulmonary bypass. Intravenous induction can often be accomplished with gradual titration of midazolam 0.05–0.1 mg/kg per dose, and fentanyl 1–5 μg/kg per dose, followed by muscle relaxation. Assisted and then controlled mask ventilation is assumed, with frequent determination of non-invasive blood pressure. Another option for intravenous induction includes etomidate 0.1–0.3mg/kg, which has little or no hemodynamic effect or effect on cardiac contractility [99]. Ketamine 1–2mg/kg IV should be used with caution in patients who are receiving infusions of β-adrenergic agonists, because the direct myocardial depressant effects of ketamine may be unmasked in patients whose endogenous catecholamines are depleted [100,101]. Propofol and thiopental should generally be avoided because of their venous and arterial vasodilating properties.

Tracheal intubation is accomplished after appropriate depth of anesthesia and muscle relaxation are achieved. Some centers prefer nasotracheal intubation in patients less than about 30 kg because of the perceived stability of the airway while transesophageal echocardiography is in use. A cuffed endotracheal tube is recommended for all patients except neonates, to minimize any air leak. And even in the neonatal population, the minimal risk of laryngeal injury from the use of a cuffed tube is greatly outweighed by the risk of an inability to effectively ventilate a patient with pulmonary hypertension. Cardiovascular compromise after induction must be anticipated and rapidly treated with volume expansion or vasopressors. Among patients with pulmonary hypertension, increases in pulmonary arterial pressure can be minimized by the use of larger doses of opioids, 100% oxygen, and mild hyperventilation prior to tracheal intubation. If a pulmonary hypertensive crisis develops, treatment with systemic vasopressors and pulmonary vasodilators, including inhaled nitric oxide, is immediately undertaken.

Invasive arterial access is necessary and is most commonly achieved after induction, being mindful to avoid arteries on the side of previous systemic to pulmonary shunts, thrombosed arteries or other abnormal or aberrant vessels. Normally, right or left radial or femoral arteries are preferred. Brachial or axillary arteries are not recommended for access because of the risk of ischemic complications, and pedal arteries are not reliable; a surgical cutdown is preferred if percutaneous access cannot be obtained in a reasonably short period of time. Double- or triple-lumen central venous access is essential, and may be obtained after induction in the internal jugular, femoral or subclavian veins. Strict sterile placement with full barrier precautions and ultrasound guidance will minimize complications and facilitate rapid insertion [102]. Antibiotic-impregnated catheters may prevent catheter-associated infections, and are important in immunosuppressed patients [102]. Some institutions avoid the right internal jugular vein as it is the access for future myocardial biopsies. Transthoracic intracardiac catheters can be placed for central venous access during rewarming on bypass, but adequate large-bore peripheral venous access must be assured before bypass, especially among repeat

sternotomy patients. Additional monitoring includes transesophageal echocardiography, which is useful to assess post-transplant cardiac function and status of cardiac and great vessel anastomoses. We routinely utilize near infrared spectroscopy (NIRS) measurement of cerebral oxygen saturation because of the high risk of cerebral oxygen desaturation from a low cardiac output state in these patients. Early detection and treatment of cerebral oxygen desaturation may lead to improved neurological outcomes. Although patients with poor cardiac function undergoing transplant are at higher risk for anesthesia awareness, processed EEG monitoring for depth of anesthesia will not reliably prevent this significant problem and is not recommended for use in this situation, particularly in young children [103].

Because many of these patients have undergone previous sternotomies and are at greater risk for intra- and postoperative hemorrhage, antifibrinolytic agents are often utilized. These include ε-aminocaproic acid, tranexamic acid or aprotinin, the latter only after a thorough assessment of the risk/benefit ratio of using the drug (aprotinin is not currently available in the US) [104]. Antibiotic prophylaxis, often cefazolin in uncomplicated transplants, is given 30–60min before incision, repeated after institution of bypass, and every 4h thereafter while in the operating room.

Patient positioning, preparation, draping, and sternotomy are accomplished as efficiently as possible. Mediastinal, heart, and great vessel dissection and preparation are also done quickly in order to minimize donor ischemic time. Prebypass anesthetic management is carried out according to the pathophysiology of the patient's underlying cardiac disease and response to surgical and anesthetic interventions. Maintenance of anesthesia is often achieved with large doses of opioids such as fentanyl, and amnestic agents such as midazolam. Low doses of volatile anesthetic agents are often employed. Although there are few data in children with cardiomyopathy or other causes of poor ventricular function, in congenital heart disease patients, isoflurane preserves cardiac output best of the studied volatile agents, with sevoflurane an acceptable choice due to its slight myocardial depressive effect [105,106].

Cardiopulmonary bypass period

Standard cardiopulmonary bypass (CPB) techniques are used for cardiac transplant, including heparin 300–400 units/kg for anticoagulation, and anticoagulation monitoring with celite activated clotting time (ACT), and heparin level assay or thromboelastography, according to institutional practice. Aorto-bicaval cannulation is utilized. General principles of bypass management used for congenital heart disease are practiced. See Chapter 25 for further details. Recent data suggest that pH stat blood gas management and maintaining higher hematocrits of 30–35% result in better long-term neurological outcomes [107]. Maintaining full flow cardiopulmonary bypass of 150 mL/kg/min for patients under 10 kg, and 2.4–2.8 L/min/m² for those over 10 kg may improve outcomes as well [108]. Moderate hypothermia to 25–28°C is commonly employed and deep hypothermic (<22°C) circulatory arrest (DHCA) is avoided; however, complex reconstruction of pulmonary venous or aortic anatomy may require DHCA. If possible, DHCA periods should be limited to less than 30 min; reperfusing for a short period and then re-instituting DHCA may be required, utilizing cerebral oximetry to guide bypass [109–112]. Ultrafiltration on CPB is very useful to achieve hematocrit goals and remove excess fluid and inflammatory mediators. Alternatively, modified ultrafiltration after CPB can be used to achieve the same goals.

In patients in whom high levels of PRA are measured or in ABO incompatible transplants (see below), an exchange transfusion is performed when CPB is initiated. A double CPB prime volume is prepared, with packed red blood cells and fresh frozen plasma. Upon institution of CPB, the patient's calculated blood volume is drained into a separate collection bag, bypassing the venous reservoir, and discarded. This process will reduce the red cell antibody concentration and limit possibility of acute rejection [113].

Surgical technique consists of orthotopic transplantation [114] where the donor heart is completely excised, except for a cuff of left atrial tissue containing all four pulmonary veins. Donor weight is ideally 80–160% of the recipient's weight. It is important for the surgical team to know the details of the donor's demise (appropriately preserving patient confidentiality), donor cardiac function (ejection fraction) and inotropic support and any donor structural abnormalities such as atrial septal defect (ASD) or patent foramen ovale (PFO). The entire right atrium is removed, leaving superior and inferior vena cavae for anastomosis. After arrival of the donor heart, the ABO and rH type of both the donor and recipient are checked and independently verified by two people, including the transplant surgeon. The donor heart is typically preserved with a solution such as crystalloid cardioplegia or Celsior® and stored on ice at 4°C. The heart is placed in the mediastinum and the left atrial anastomosis is performed first. Then the aortic anastomosis is performed. The aortic cross-clamp is usually removed at this point to minimize the donor heart ischemic time. Under normal circumstances, a limit of 5 h of donor ischemic time is desired, meaning the time from donor heart cross-clamp at harvest until cross-clamp removal. This limits donor organ transport time to 3 ½–4 h. Although transplantation of hearts with longer ischemic times is reported, beyond 5 h of ischemia graft

function worsens and long-term graft function may be compromised [90].

After the aortic cross-clamp is removed, the donor heart commonly experiences ventricular fibrillation due to ischemia and/or electrolyte imbalance, and must be defibrillated (initial energy 2–10 joules) several times, until sinus rhythm is achieved. Lidocaine 2 mg/kg into the CPB circuit is given 5 min before aortic cross-clamp removal, and a repeat dose of 1 mg/kg can be given if more than 1–2 defibrillations are required. Magnesium sulfate 25–50 mg/kg is often helpful, as is a lidocaine infusion at 20–40 μg/kg/min. Rarely, amiodarone 5 mg/kg load, repeated up to two additional doses, may be required. With the cross-clamp removed and the heart beating, the bicaval anastomoses and the pulmonary artery anastomoses are completed. The surgeon must pay particular attention to the anatomy of congenital heart disease recipients. There may be a need for extensive aortic arch reconstruction, requiring a long length of donor aorta in patients with hypoplastic left heart syndrome, or for a long length of donor superior vena cava in single-ventricle patients with cavopulmonary anastomoses.

With establishment of sinus rhythm and completion of the anastomoses, rewarming is accomplished. Additional intravenous anesthetics and muscle relaxants are administered. During this period inotropic support is instituted, according to institutional preference, and taking into account ischemic time, systemic and pulmonary vascular resistance, and appearance of the myocardial function on visual inspection and transesophageal echocardiography. Low-dose epinephrine, 0.03–0.05 μg/kg/min, is a common choice in this setting. Milrinone 0.25–0.75 μg/kg/min, with or without a loading dose of 25–75 μg/kg over 15–30 min, is also useful in this situation for its inotropic, pulmonary and systemic vasodilator properties, as well as low propensity for arrhythmogenicity. Because the denervated heart has limited capacity to alter heart rate, and sinus node discharge of the donor heart often slows with edema, inflammation or hypothermia, an isoproterenol infusion in low doses of 0.01–0.03 μg/kg/min is often very useful to maintain adequate heart rate. Temporary atrial pacing can also be utilized. Recipients with pulmonary hypertension, and situations where the donor is smaller than the recipient (the donor right heart may have insufficient ability to overcome the recipient pulmonary vascular resistance (PVR)), the right heart can be supported with milrinone or inhaled nitric oxide, at 10–40 parts per million (PPM) [115]. In extreme cases a right VAD may be temporarily needed until the right heart is adequately conditioned.

Near the completion of surgery, additional transthoracic monitoring catheters, such as right and left atrial lines, and occasionally pulmonary artery lines, are placed by the surgeon, along with temporary atrial pacing wires, which may be needed to support the denervated heart. Ventilation is commenced with 100% oxygen, designed to produce mild hypocarbia of 32–35 mmHg. Once heart rate and rhythm, hematocrit, ventilation, and electrolytes are optimized, CPB is weaned slowly with gradual volume loading of the heart, using TEE monitoring to assess for intracardiac air, as well as biventricular function. After separation from CPB, cardiac function is assessed with TEE, as is the status of the anastomoses of the aorta, pulmonary artery, vena cava, and left atrium, with particular attention paid to any pulmonary venous obstruction. After ensuring a period of adequate hemodynamics and cardiac function, protamine 1–1.3 mg per mg of heparin in the original dose is administered, to neutralize the anticoagulation. The TEE probe is removed if no longer needed, and surgical hemostasis is achieved. Platelets and cryoprecipitate (rich in fibrinogen) are often required to achieve hemostasis, particularly with repeat sternotomy and complicated great vessel reconstruction [116]. Patients who are supported with ventricular assist devices before heart transplant typically receive intensive anticoagulation to prevent thrombosis and embolization, and this group of patients more commonly develop uncontrollable hemorrhage after bypass. In this situation, recombinant factor VIIA, 90 µg/kg, repeated up to two additional times if bleeding persists, has been very useful to achieve hemostasis when administration of plasma, cryoprecipitate, and platelets has failed to achieve hemostasis [116].

Postbypass period

In a few unstable patients, particularly small infants, the sternum may be left open for a period of 24–48 h to allow bleeding and myocardial performance to improve; these patients must have the sternum closed as soon as possible to reduce the risk of infection in the immunosuppressed patient.

After bypass, attention is directed to the need for additional antibiotic or corticosteroid/immunosuppressive medications. Extubation of pediatric cardiac transplant patients in the operating room is typically avoided, as many patients have an ongoing risk for myocardial dysfunction, arrhythmias, bleeding, and pulmonary hypertension. If the patient is stable, tracheal extubation can often be achieved in 12–24 h after ICU admission. Upon transfer to the ICU, a thorough patient handoff report is given, including the surgical team discussing surgical issues and the anesthesia team giving a complete report to the attending ICU physician and bedside nurses. A standardized handoff note and verbal communication, along with an opportunity to answer any questions, are recommended practice for the effective transfer of care in these complicated patients.

Post-transplant rejection surveillance

The mainstay of post-transplant surveillance for rejection is myocardial biopsy, with the first biopsy often performed 7–10 days after transplant to assess acute rejection. Biopsies are performed most frequently in the first year after transplant, often every 3 months for uncomplicated cases. Thereafter, biopsy every 6 months is often performed, along with thermodilution cardiac output. Coronary angiography is added to the yearly regimen after 1–2 years, to assess the development of coronary artery vasculopathy. Five to seven biopsies of the right ventricle are obtained, and rejection is usually assessed according to the International Society of Heart and Lung Transplantation (ISHLT) scale, 0–3 according to the degree of lymphocytic infiltration and myocyte damage in the specimen [117].

Rejection is classified as either cellular, primarily lymphocyte infiltration, or humoral, a predominance of antibody-antigen and complement complexes, which is often observed in patients with high PRA titers. Signs of acute rejection can range from low-grade fever and malaise, to poor myocardial function, to cardiovascular collapse. Treatment for acute rejection often begins with large doses of corticosteroids and higher doses of maintenance immune suppressants. Other agents such as antithymocyte globulin, antilymphocyte globulin or interleukin-2 receptor antagonists may also be added according to institutional practice. Plasmapheresis may be used for humoral rejection to reduce the antibody titers until immune suppressants have an effect. Rejecting patients may need additional therapy, including inotropic and ventilatory support, or even mechanical circulatory support with ventricular assist devices or ECMO. If all of these measures fail to reverse the rejection, retransplant is the only remaining treatment option.

Morbidity and mortality after cardiac transplant

Survival after cardiac transplant is characterized by significant early mortality in all age groups followed by a slow attrition [90] (Fig. 27.5). Survival since 2000 has improved, primarily because of improved early survival in the first year, with no difference in the survival curves after 1 year [4] (Fig. 27.6). Early mortality is significantly increased for patients on ECMO, those having a congenital diagnosis, those undergoing retransplantation, and those requiring ventilatory support immediately prior to transplant [90] (Table 27.7). The leading causes of death in the first 30 days are graft failure in 35%, infection in 15%, and multi-organ failure and acute rejection 12% each. The leading cause of late mortality is coronary artery vasculopathy, responsible for 30–35% of deaths beyond 3 years after transplant [4]. Retransplantation is most commonly performed because of severe coronary

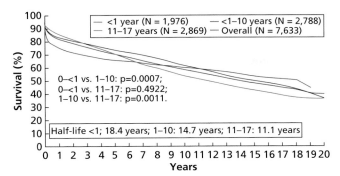

Figure 27.5 Kaplan–Meier survival for transplants from January 1982 through June 2007. Reproduced from Kirk et al [91] with permission from Elsevier.

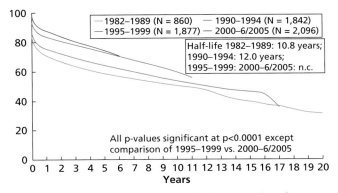

Figure 27.6 Kaplan–Meier survival by era for heart transplants from January 1982 through June 2007. Reproduced from Kirk et al [91] with permission from Elsevier.

artery vasculopathy (CAV) or graft failure, and carries a higher risk of mortality, with a 5-year survival of about 60% in the modern era, versus 75–80% for primary transplantation [118].

Morbidities in cardiac transplant recipients at 5 years after transplant include hypertension in 63% (primarily associated with corticosteroid use), hyperlipidemia in 26%, coronary artery vasculopathy in 11%, and renal dysfunction in 9% [90]. Thus a substantial number of these patients will be taking antihypertensive medications, and some will be taking statins or other cholesterol-lowering drugs. Renal function requires assessment before anesthesia, to avoid or minimize use of agents with primary renal excretion, in appropriate patients. Infection and lymphoma are seen in a very small percentage of pediatric cardiac transplant recipients. Early coronary artery vasculopathy in the first 3 years after transplant is associated with a significantly higher risk of rejection.

Anesthesia for the heart transplant recipient
Endomyocardial biopsy
All cardiac transplant recipients require myocardial biopsy. Access is often gained via the right internal jugular vein, but femoral venous access is also often used and often simplifies the anesthetic and sedation management because the access site is remote from the airway. Some older teenage patients are mature and co-operative enough to receive intravenous sedation and local anesthesia to the access site, and an anesthesiologist is not commonly required. However, many older patients are

Table 27.7 Risk factors for mortality within 1 year for 3756 transplants performed January 1995 through June 2007

Variable	Number	Relative risk	95% Confidence interval	p-value
Congenital diagnosis, age = 0, on ECMO	74	2.70	1.57–4.63	0.0003
Congenital diagnosis, age > 0	893	2.17	1.67–2.83	<0.0001
Retransplant	225	2.09	1.42–3.07	0.0002
On ventilator	706	1.80	1.45–2.23	<0.0001
On dialysis	91	1.62	1.08–2.43	0.0210
Year of transplant: 1995–1996 vs 2001–2002	506	1.55	1.14–2.09	0.0049
Panel reactive antibody ≥10%	344	1.37	1.04–1.79	0.0228
IV drug therapy for infection ≤2 wk HTx	565	1.29	1.03–1.62	0.0267
Donor cause of death = anoxia vs head trauma	863	0.80	0.64–1.00	0.0468
Not ABO identical	843	0.79	0.63–0.99	0.0384
Diagnosis other than congenital, no ECMO, age = 0	295	0.46	0.27–0.78	0.0042

ECMO, extracorporeal membrane oxygenation; HTx, heart transplantation; IV, intravenous.
Note: Reference diagnosis = cardiomyopathy.
Reproduced from Kirk et al [91] with permission from Elsevier.

very anxious due to the lifelong nature of their medical interventions, and require higher doses of sedative medications and associated deeper sedation in order to perform the catherization. In stable outpatients without signs or symptoms of rejection or CAV, moderate or deep IV sedation with a variety of agents can be used, including benzodiazepines, opioids, and propofol. Patients with known or suspected rejection or CAV must be approached with great care. These patients may have significantly compromised cardiac function or very severe CAV with marginal myocardial perfusion. They have very limited reserve if the myocardial oxygen supply–demand balance is upset. Whatever technique is used, these patients should not be subjected to significant reductions in preload or to afterload as myocardial perfusion depends on blood pressure. Agents such as propofol or thiopental should be avoided, blood pressure monitored closely, and hypotension treated immediately. Tachycardia should also be avoided. If general anesthesia is chosen, positive pressure ventilation must be instituted carefully so as not to excessively decrease venous return. General endotracheal anesthesia is often preferred to definitively secure the airway.

Non-cardiac surgery

Cardiac transplant recipients may undergo surgical and diagnostic procedures unrelated to the transplant. In addition to the assessment of cardiac and non-cardiac problems, the anesthesiologist should determine the results of the most recent cardiac biopsy, cardiac output, signs of rejection, and whether there is a suspicion of CAV. Ideally, there should be a cardiology evaluation, including an echocardiogram, within 6 months. The hemodynamic goals noted above for endomyocardial biopsy are the same for non-cardiac surgery. The denervated heart does not respond to vagolytic agents, so bradycardia requires treatment with a direct-acting β1-agonist such as isoproterenol or epinephrine. Infective endocarditis prophylaxis guidelines have been significantly revised, and restrict the need for such prophylaxis to transplant recipients who develop valvulopathy, and only for dental and airway procedures where the respiratory mucosa is incised [119]. Prophylaxis is no longer recommended for gastrointestinal and genitourinary procedures unless there is active infection. Care should be taken with the reversal of non-depolarizing muscle relaxants using neostigmine. Variable parasympathetic reinnervation, along with humoral or cellular rejection, may produce unpredictable responses to neostigmine and glycopyrrolate, which have been reported to produce severe sinus bradycardia and asystole [120]. Stress-dose corticosteroids should be administered as appropriate for significant surgical procedures, where adrenal suppression is suspected.

ABO-incompatible transplantation

As discussed earlier in this chapter, the number of infants listed for cardiac transplantation exceeds the number of donors by approximately 3:1, and there is significant mortality of infants waiting for transplant. Many infant heart transplant recipients who survive the first year after transplant are remarkably free of rejection. In 2001, West and colleagues described a series of infant cardiac transplants in patients up to age 14 months with ABO-incompatible donors [113]. Anesthetic and surgical management of the transplant does not differ, except that an exchange transfusion, as described above, is performed upon institution of cardiopulmonary bypass. In addition, transfused blood products are selected to avoid antibodies to the donor heart. Midterm survival and rejection rates were not different from ABO-compatible transplants, and the waiting list mortality was reduced from 58% to 7% for infant transplants [113]. This technique has been adopted by more institutions, as evidence develops that overall survival of infants listed for transplant improves in the long term [121,122].

Lung transplantation

History

The first human lung transplant was performed on an adult in 1963 by James Hardy at the University of Mississippi [123]. This was followed by adult lobar (Shinoi, 1966) and pediatric heart–lung transplantation (Cooley, 1968) but outcomes were uniformly dismal. Advances over the next decade included the introduction of cyclosporin, better surgical techniques and improved donor organ preservation, leading to the first long-term success with adult heart-lung transplant by Reitz at Stanford in 1981 [124]. Cooper and colleagues in Toronto demonstrated that bronchial omentopexy enhanced the vascularity and integrity of the bronchial anastomosis and subsequently reported the first long-term successful adult (1983) and pediatric (1987) lung transplants [88]. Living donor lobar transplantation was first performed at Stanford by Starnes in 1990.

Data about lung and heart-lung transplantation from many centers around the globe are updated regularly by the ISHLT and can be viewed at its website (www.ishlt.org/registries). The ISHLT Registry 2009 report for the period 1984–2008 included 1278 pediatric lung transplant and 549 pediatric heart-lung transplant procedures [125]. Thirty-six centers reported pediatric lung transplant procedures. Of these, only one (3%) reported between 10 and 19 transplants per year, three centers (8%) reported 5–9 transplants per year, and the remainder (89%) reported <5 transplants per year (Fig. 27.7). Annually, fewer than 100 children received lung transplant surgery. Most

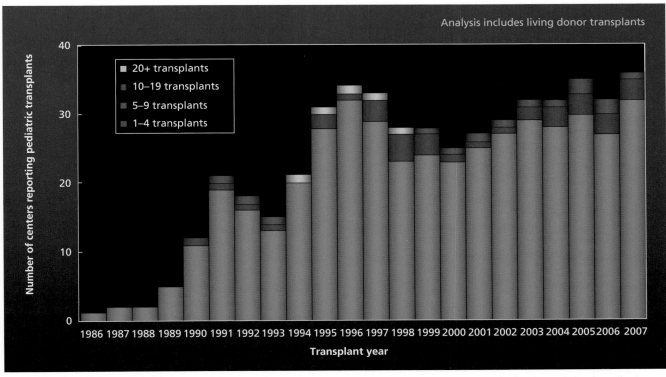

Figure 27.7 Number of centers reporting pediatric lung transplants by center volume. Reproduced from Kirk et al [91] with permission from Elsevier.

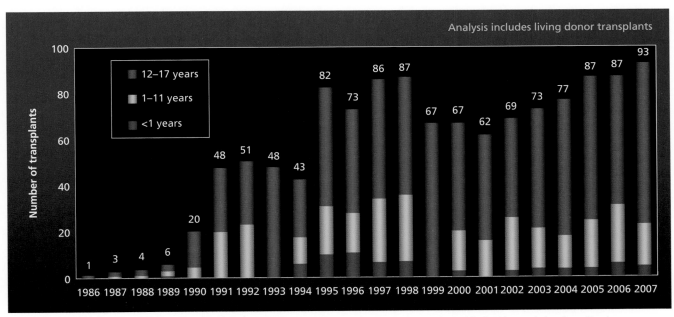

Figure 27.8 Age distribution of pediatric lung recipients by year of transplant. Reproduced from Kirk et al [91] with permission from Elsevier.

patients were adolescents and the number of infant transplants has remained low (Fig. 27.8).

In addition to the specific challenges inherent in caring for children, pediatric lung transplantation has many unique aspects, including a diverse spectrum of pulmonary and non-pulmonary diseases, donor/recipient matching and growth of the transplanted organs. Children receiving transplantation undergo many surgical and diagnostic interventions and frequently require sedation or general anesthesia. Provision of safe perioperative care requires familiarity with the relevant issues, including pulmonary pathophysiology and the conduct and consequences of lung transplantation.

Indications, contraindications, and listing criteria in children

Generally, lung transplant surgery is considered for children with any end-stage lung disease for whom there is no medical treatment [126]. For all children less than 18 years of age, the common primary diagnoses leading to lung transplantation are cystic fibrosis (56%) and pulmonary hypertension, either idiopathic (10%) or related to congenital heart disease (5%) [125], whereas the common primary diagnoses in adults are chronic obstructive pulmonary disease or interstitial lung diseases. Indications for transplantation differ by age (Table 27.8), with cystic fibrosis the predominant indication for children aged 6 years or older.

Cystic fibrosis

Respiratory failure is the most common cause of death in these children. Many variables, such as rate of decline in

FEV_1, elevated pCO_2 (>50 mmHg), falling pO_2 (<55 mmHg), deteriorating nutritional status, frequency of hospitalizations and the 6-minute walk test, are considered before listing the patient for lung transplant [127]. Perioperative management should address non-pulmonary manifestations of cystic fibrosis such as severe malnourishment, chronic infection, pancreatic insufficiency, diabetes mellitus, cholelithiasis, hepatic cirrhosis, distal intestinal obstruction syndrome, sinusitis, nasal polyps, osteoporosis and genitourinary problems [128,129]. Pretransplant mechanical ventilation was predictive of poor 1-year survival after lung transplantation [130]. There are reasonably compelling data documenting the beneficial impact of lung transplantation on functional status, hemodynamics, and quality of life but demonstration of a survival benefit for children remains controversial [131,132].

Pulmonary hypertension

During the Fourth World Symposium on Pulmonary Hypertension held in Dana Point, California, in 2008, a reclassification of pulmonary hypertension based on

Table 27.8 Indications for pediatric lung transplantation, January 1990–June 2008

| Age (years) | <1 y | | 1–5 y | | 6–11 y | | 12–17 y | |
Diagnosis	N	Percent	N	Percent	N	Percent	N	Percent
Cystic fibrosis	2	2.4%	5	5.1%	124	53.0%	547	69.2%
Idiopathic pulmonary arterial hypertension	11	13.4%	22	22.2%	25	10.7%	60	7.6%
Retransplant: obliterative bronchiolitis	–	–	6	6.1%	8	3.4%	25	3.2%
Congenital heart disease	21	25.6%	8	8.1%	4	1.7%	10	1.3%
Idiopathic pulmonary fibrosis	4	4.9%	8	8.1%	10	4.3%	26	3.3%
Obliterative bronchiolitis (not retransplant)	–	–	9	9.1%	10	4.3%	29	3.7%
Retransplant: not obliterative brochiolitis	3	3.7%	2	2.0%	7	3.0%	18	2.3%
Interstitial pneumonitis	6	7.3%	11	11.1%	1	0.4%	5	0.6%
Pulmonary vascular disease	8	9.8%	5	5.1%	7	3.0%	1	0.2%
Eisenmenger syndrome	1	1.2%	5	5.1%	5	2.1%	6	0.8%
Pulmonary fibrosis, other	1	1.2%	1	1.0%	7	3.0%	11	1.4%
Surfactant protein B deficiency	11	13.4%	4	4.0%	–	–	–	–
COPD/emphysema	5	6.1%	2	2.0%	2	0.9%	6	0.8%
Bronchopulmonary dysplasia	2	2.4%	2	2.0%	6	2.6%	–	–
Bronchiectasis	–	–	–	–	4	1.7%	9	1.1%
Other	7	8.5%	9	9.1%	14	6.0%	39	4.9%

COPD, chronic obstructive pulmonary disease.
Reproduced from Kirk et al [91] with permission from Elsevier.

Table 27.9 Recipient survival after lung and heart-lung transplantation (1990–2001)

Time	Survival by diagnosis and type of transplant					
	PPH		ES		Other CHD	
	LT (n = 691)	HLT (n = 302)	LT (n = 196)	HLT (n = 376)	LT (n = 22)	HLT (n = 155)
	(%)	(%)	(%)	(%)	(%)	(%)
3 months	72	72	69	76	79	59
1 year	64	66	58	71	68	45
3 years	54	50	45	57	36	32
5 years	44	41	39	50	36	28
10 years	21	22	29	39	36	7

CHD, congenital heart disease; ES, Eisenmenger syndrome; HLT, heart and lung transplantation; LT, lung transplantation; PPH, primary (idiopathic) pulmonary arterial hypertension.
Reproduced from Klepetko et al [134] with permission from Elsevier.

clinical evolution, histopathology, and response to therapy was proposed. A diagnosis of primary (or idiopathic) pulmonary arterial hypertension is made when no known risk factor is identified. Familial pulmonary arterial hypertension has been linked to mutations in receptors in the transforming growth factor (TGF)-β superfamily, such as BMPR2 (bone morphogenetic protein receptor 2) and in ALK-1 (activin-like kinase 1), which affect vascular intimal proliferation. Pulmonary arterial hypertension associated with congenital heart disease constitutes a heterogenous group of conditions and has been classified based on circulatory pathophysiology [133].

Transplantation options for pulmonary hypertension include lung transplantation, heart-lung transplantation or lung transplantation in combination with repair of the underlying cardiac defect. Survival rates for these strategies have been reviewed (Table 27.9) [134]. In Eisenmenger syndrome secondary to ventricular septal defect, there was a survival benefit of heart-lung over lung transplantation [135]. Transplantation may improve the quality of life of patients with Eisenmenger syndrome but may not improve survival because most unrepaired Eisenmenger patients will survive beyond their 40th birthday [136]. Many children with pulmonary hypertension will be receiving agents such as endothelin receptor antagonists, phosphodiesterase inhibitors, prostacyclin analogs and nitric oxide.

Disorders of surfactant metabolism
Pediatric interstitial lung disease syndrome is an uncommon indication for lung transplantation and includes diseases of surfactant metabolism [137]. Surfactant proteins B, C and ABCA3 transporter are necessary for surfactant homeostasis and mutations in the genes encoding these proteins lead to surfactant dysfunction, giving rise to both lethal and chronic respiratory disease in infants. Patients may require lung transplantation in early infancy because of severe respiratory failure.

Miscellaneous disorders
Lung transplant surgery has been performed in children for a variety of other indications including bronchopulmonary dysplasia, congenital diaphragmatic hernia, hemosiderosis, bronchiolitis obliterans and emphysema.

Criteria for listing and contraindications
The criteria for listing children for lung transplant surgery are based on the natural history of the disease, functional status, and expected improvement in the quality of life. Generally, a clear diagnosis with a life expectancy of less than 2 years is necessary for listing the child for the lung transplant. However, it is hard to develop survival models for relatively rare diseases.

Contraindications to lung transplantation are listed in Table 27.10 [126]. Mechanical ventilation is a risk factor for morbidity and mortality in older children but not infants. Children with cystic fibrosis who are colonized with multidrug-resistant organisms like *Burkholderia cenocepacia* and *B. gladioli* do poorly and most centers consider this a strong contraindication. Children with liver disease secondary to cystic fibrosis may be candidates for combined liver-lung transplant surgery and have good survival rates. Patient and parental psychosocial issues can be particularly challenging and may become a significant contraindication if child and family consistently fail to meet agreed-upon expectations for care and follow-up [11].

Perhaps the most difficult decision for pediatric lung transplant physicians is determining the appropriate time

Table 27.10 Lung transplantation: most commonly agreed-upon contraindications

Absolute	Relative
Active malignancy	Pleurodesis
Sepsis	Renal insufficiency
Active tuberculosis	Markedly abnormal Body Mass Index
Severe neuromuscular disease	Mechanical ventilation
Documented, refractory non-adherence	Scoliosis
Multiple organ dysfunction	Poorly controlled diabetes mellitus
Acquired immunodeficiency syndrome	Osteoporosis
Hepatitis C with histological liver disease	Hepatitis B surface antigen positive
	Fungal infection/colonization
	Chronic airway infection with multiply resistant organisms

Reproduced from Faro et al [126] with permission from Wiley-Blackwell.

to accept organs because there is wide variation in the natural history of the primary diseases (Table 27.11) and the 5-year survival rate after lung transplantation is only about 50%. Most pediatric centers consider multiple factors, including waiting list survival estimates (when available), growth and nutrition status, frequency of hospitalizations, and potential for improvement in overall quality of life, before committing a child to lung transplant.

Donor selection, availability, and the lungs allocation system

Like other organ transplant surgeries, donor availability has been a limiting factor. Only about 15% of the cadaveric donors have lungs that are considered acceptable for transplantation [138]. The Organ Procurement and Transplant Network (OPTN) implemented a new lungs allocation system in 2005 that used medical urgency as the primary determinant of organ allocation and discouraged the use of waiting time [139]. Under this system, a lung allocation score (LAS) is calculated for every patient >12 years of age using multiple variables including age, functional status, forced vital capacity and oxygen requirement. The new policy also mandated that the donor lungs from pediatric donors be preferentially given to pediatric patients. Recent data from adult and pediatric patients suggest that implementation of the LAS system has decreased waiting times and increased the annual number of lung transplant surgeries performed [139].

Table 27.11 Recommendations regarding timing of referral to lung transplant center

Specific disease	Timing of referral
Surfactant deficiencies	Patients with SP-B deficiency and ABCA3 deficiency with refractory respiratory failure should be referred immediately Patients with SP-C deficiency and less severe forms of ABCA3 deficiency may respond to medical therapy and should be referred when unrelenting progression of disease develops
Primary pulmonary hypertension	Patients who present in NYHA class III or IV or have evidence of right heart failure should be referred immediately Patients who fail to respond adequately to vasodilator therapy should also be referred
Eisenmenger syndrome	When the trajectory of pulmonary hypertension appears to be worsening with impaired exercise tolerance and worsening quality of life
Other pulmonary vascular disorders (pulmonary vein stenosis, alveolar capillary dysplasia)	These patients should be referred immediately since they typically do not respond to medical management and are at risk for sudden death
Cystic fibrosis	Patients with percent predicted FEV_1 values less than 30%, frequent hospitalizations, refractory hypoxemia or hypercapnia should be referred for transplant
Bronchopulmonary dysplasia	Patients with recurrent or severe episodes of respiratory failure or evidence for progressive pulmonary hypertension
Diffuse parenchymal lung disease	Patients without evidence for systemic disease that could affect outcome should be referred early

Reproduced from Sweet [11] with permission from the American Thoracic Society.

However, children younger than 12 years of age still received organs based on the waiting time accrued on the transplant list. Recognizing that infants carry the highest waiting list mortality rate among all transplant candidates, the OPTN recently approved proposals to preferentially direct organs from donors under 11 years old to younger children [140].

Donor lungs are selected after thorough medical screening and multiple laboratory tests. In younger children, comparable age and height (<20% discrepancy) are considered acceptable for matching lung volume. Selection criteria are relatively subjective. An ideal donor is younger than 55 years, non-smoker and with no history of cardiopulmonary or significant neurological disease. The donor lungs should produce good gaseous exchange (PaO$_2$ >350 mmHg with FIO$_2$ of 1.0) on moderate amount of ventilatory support. The chest radiography and bronchoscopy should rule out any significant infection, consolidation, and tumor. An expected ischemic time of <6 h is preferred. Optimal donor lung management has been reviewed [141]. To increase the number of potential donors, some centers have advocated acceptance of longer ischemic times and "marginal" donors with reversible mild lung pathology [142]. Biochemical markers in the bronchoalveolar lavage fluid from the donor lungs (e.g. interleukin (IL)-8, IL-6 and IL-1b), are being evaluated as predictors of early and late graft dysfunction [143]. Additionally, using donation after cardiac death lungs is another option that has been considered to alleviate organ shortage [144].

The process of harvest includes systemic heparinization of the donor and infusion of prostaglandin E1 into the main pulmonary artery. A number of preservation solutions have been tried but currently Euro-Collins solution is used by most centers. Lungs are inflated with FIO$_2$ of less than 0.4 to an airway pressure less than 20 cmH$_2$O. Lungs are removed *en bloc* with thoracic aorta, left atrial cuff, and main pulmonary artery [141].

Perioperative management
Preoperative considerations
Candidates for lung transplantation undergo an extensive medical and psychosocial evaluation. Imaging studies of major thoracic systemic and pulmonary vessels may be required for patients with congenital heart disease because abnormal vasculature can alter the conduct of organ harvest and transplantation surgery. Children with pulmonary hypertension undergo a diagnostic cardiac catheterization to quantify hemodynamics and test for reactivity to pulmonary vasodilator therapy. After listing, the child's clinical progress is monitored regularly and an anesthetic consultation obtained. Many children can be living at home with minimal oxygen supplementation while others, especially infants, are on chronic ventilatory or extracorporeal hemodynamic support. Recently, extracorporeal devices that facilitate respiratory exchange have been utilized as a bridge to lung transplant [145,146].

Anesthesia management
Like other solid organ transplants, timing of surgery is unpredictable. Most families are given a hospital pager and have been anticipating the surgery for a long time. Patients are often excited and frightened. Anxiolytics such as midazolam can be safely given to most children but discretion and monitoring are advised because of the potential for compromise to upper airway control, respiratory effort, and hemodynamic stability.

When relevant, the patient and family should be informed preoperatively that surgery may possibly not proceed to transplantation if the donor lungs are deemed unsuitable. Good communication between the donor and recipient teams is vital, with all parties having a clear understanding of the expected time of anesthesia induction and donor organ arrival. Anesthesia preparations are similar to those for pediatric hypothermic open heart surgery. Anesthesiologists often work under considerable time pressure because of concerns about extending the donor organ ischemic time.

Standard NPO guidelines are followed to minimize the risk of aspiration and contamination of the new lungs. The method of anesthesia induction and choice of agents will depend on the patient's clinical and NPO status. The hemodynamic goal is to preserve stability without increasing pulmonary vascular resistance. Both volatile and intravenous anesthetic agents are acceptable. Propofol is safe for hemodynamically stable children (e.g. many cystic fibrosis patients) but ketamine or etomidate may be the preferred drug for patients who have poor cardiac reserve and/or pulmonary hypertension. Anesthetic depth can be maintained with opioids and benzodiazepines and supplemented with inhalational or intravenous agents [147]. Nitrous oxide is best avoided because of concerns about myocardial depression, pulmonary hypertension, air embolism, and the requirement for high concentrations of inspired oxygen. The combination of anesthesia, right ventricular diastolic dysfunction and positive pressure ventilation may unmask a relative intravascular volume deficiency that can be corrected by IV fluid infusion.

Most often, pediatric lung transplants are performed with the assistance of CPB and the airway is secured with a single-lumen endotracheal tube because lung isolation is not required. Frequent toilet of the airway is advised, particularly in patients who have cystic fibrosis. Bronchodilator therapy should be available. Effective oxygenation and carbon dioxide elimination may be difficult during the pre-CPB period, and permissive hypercapnia is acceptable. Ventilation should be adjusted to minimize air trapping because lung hyperinflation can impede venous return to the heart. Strategies to limit airway pressure are advised for patients at increased risk of barotrauma, such as those with restrictive lung disease or chronic obstructive pulmonary disease. Occasionally, especially in infants, a sophisticated pediatric intensive care ventilator may be required in the operating room. Many patients who have end-stage lung disease have a chronic compensatory metabolic alkalosis. Enthusiastic hyperventilation to normal PaCO$_2$ values induces an iatrogenic alkalotic blood pH level that increases cerebral vasoconstriction and leads to relative cerebral ischemia.

Invasive monitoring appropriate for surgery with CPB is established. At many institutions, continuous monitoring of pulmonary pressure with pulmonary artery catheter is limited to adolescents with the pretransplant diagnosis of pulmonary hypertension [148]. The pulmonary artery catheter is introduced through a sheath in the internal jugular vein and advanced to the pulmonary artery after the patient has been weaned from CPB. For smaller children, a transthoracic catheter can be placed directly into the pulmonary artery by the surgeon. Intraoperative transesophageal echocardiography is useful for assessing cardiac anatomy and function, pulmonary hypertension, and to rule out pulmonary venous obstruction [149,150].

Anesthesiologists must ensure that the non-anesthetic drugs such as immunosuppressants and preoperative antibiotics are administered at appropriate times. For children with pulmonary hypertension, selective vasodilators such as nitric oxide and prostacylins must be maintained throughout the prebypass period to avoid rebound pulmonary hypertension.

Children undergoing lung transplantation are at increased risk for perioperative bleeding because of coagulopathies associated with CPB and cyanosis, and bleeding from chest wall adhesions (infections, previous surgery) or abnormal vessels (venovenous or arteriovenous collaterals). Antifibrinolytic prophylaxis with the lysine analogs may help reduce blood loss but there is insufficient information about their efficacy and safety in young children.

The function of the implanted lungs could be adversely affected by donor pathology, ischemia-reperfusion injury, CPB, blood product transfusions, denervation, lymphatic stasis, positive pressure ventilation, oxygen toxicity and hyperacute rejection.

Ischemia-reperfusion injury contributes to primary graft dysfunction (PGD) and can increase the risk of acute and perhaps chronic rejection. Oxygen is readily available to the metabolically active endothelium of lung allografts during the ischemic period and this allows production of free radicals, making lungs more susceptible to graft failure than other solid organs. Reperfusion injury appears to occur in two distinct phases. The first phase, seen immediately after the reperfusion, is initiated by donor macrophages and includes the release of superoxide anions and inflammatory cytokines, with mast cell degranulation and complement activation. These damage the vascular endothelium, causing movement of fluid to the interstitial and alveolar space [151]. The delayed phase of PGD starts a few hours later when the recipient's neutrophils are recruited by cytokines to the injured endothelium. These neutrophils produce reactive super-

oxide anions and greatly amplify the initial injury. Strategies to minimize reperfusion injury include improvements to the lung preservation solution, gentler reperfusion techniques, protective ventilation strategies and inhaled nitric oxide [152]. Ultrafiltration during and after CPB can ameliorate the inflammatory response. However, modified ultrafiltration increases right ventricular volume load and may precipitate right heart failure in the presence of pulmonary hypertension [153].

Before weaning from CPB, a bronchodilator may be administered by metered dose inhalation or nebulization, and the lungs are carefully re-expanded to check for bronchial air leaks and ventilation is resumed. Ventilator parameters are guided by the donor weight. Tidal volume and airway pressures are adjusted so that all atelectatic areas are expanded but not overdistended. Volutrauma caused by overdistension of the new lungs can increase endothelial permeability and potentiate primary graft dysfunction. Typically flexible bronchoscopy is performed to assess the bronchial anastomosis, and to remove blood and secretions from each lung under direct visualization. If possible, inspired oxygen concentrations should be lowered because of concern about oxygen toxicity and free radical damage [154]. Restriction of fluid infusions is advocated because the lung allograft is very sensitive to pulmonary edema but trials substantiating this practice are lacking.

Inhaled selective pulmonary vasodilator therapy (e.g. nitric oxide, epoprostenol) is initiated when pulmonary artery pressures are increased. Some centers routinely administer intravenous prostacyclin or PGE1 to reduce pulmonary artery pressures and preserve right heart function. Pulmonary hypertension must be anticipated and managed carefully [155,156]. Inhaled nitric oxide before and after transplantation may improve allograft function [157]. Right ventricular dysfunction can be supported by intravenous inotropes. Milrinone is a common choice because of its lusitropic and vasodilator effects.

Cardiopulmonary bypass

Although controversial, there is some evidence that CPB is an independent or contributing factor for primary graft dysfunction [158]. Therefore, most adult bilateral lung transplant centers perform lung transplantation using single-lung ventilation through dual-lumen endotracheal tubes. However, most children are physically too small to accommodate a double-lumen tube. Additionally, some children are too tenuous clinically to tolerate a prolonged period of single-lung ventilation. CPB allows the resection of both diseased lungs simultaneously, thus minimizing the risk of cross-contamination of the new lungs. Also, it provides stable hemodynamics during the extensive surgical dissection, greatly simplifies the anesthetic and surgical management, and consequently reduces lung ischemic times. Therefore, most pediatric lung transplants are performed using cardiopulmonary bypass. A large single-center comparison of the incidence of primary graft dysfunction in pediatric and adult lung transplant found no difference, suggesting that CBP did not carry additional risk in children [159].

Surgical technique

Most children undergo bilateral sequential lung transplantation through a trans-sternal, clamshell incision. Very few pediatric single-lung transplants are performed because the primary disease usually affects both lungs. Beating heart CPB with moderate hypothermia (28–32°C) is employed. Aortic cross-clamping and cardioplegia may be necessary if co-existing intracardiac defects require repair. Once CPB is established, both lungs are removed and the recipient's tracheal stump irrigated with an antibiotic solution. Meanwhile, a second surgical team prepares the donor lungs that are then implanted using end-to-end bronchial anastomoses. Since the surgery compromises the bronchial vasculature, peribronchial tissue is sutured loosely around the anastomoses to provide blood flow by new vessel ingrowth. The donor pulmonary artery is attached to the native main pulmonary artery. The pulmonary veins are reconnected to the recipient's left atrium *en bloc*, using the donor's atrial cuff. This method not only reduces the surgical time but also minimizes the risk of developing pulmonary vein stenosis.

Living donor lobar transplant (LDLT) involves two living donors, each providing a lower lobe to the recipient. LDLT has often been used to provide organs rapidly to children with cystic fibrosis who underwent an unexpected rapid progression of their disease. Although outcomes can be comparable to deceased donor transplant [160] and there is some evidence to suggest that the incidence of bronchiolitis obliterans is lower in LDLT recipients [161], the procedure is resource intensive and has ethical implications because 10–20% of donor lobectomy surgeries have serious complications [162,163]. The 2009 ISHLT report noted that the number of LDLT surgeries in pediatric recipients peaked in 1998–1999 and since then has decreased substantially to only three procedures during 2005–2007 [125].

When the recipient's chest is too small to accommodate the donor lungs, the donor lungs can be reduced in size. Options include lobectomy (typically, the right middle lobe or lingula), wedge resection using a linear stapler, single lobe transplant or split lung "bipartitioned" transplant (in which two smaller "lungs" are created from a single deceased donor lung. Reports suggest that outcomes in pediatric recipients of reduced-size organs can be comparable to recipients of full-sized grafts [164].

Early postoperative management

Patients are sedated and on ventilator support when admitted postoperatively for intensive care. Duration of mechanical ventilation has to be individualized for each child but many can be extubated within 12h of the surgery. Infants often have complex clinical problems and are critically ill before surgery; they required ventilation for longer (average 24 days) than older patients with cystic fibrosis (average 3 days) [165].

Some programs elicit the help of pediatric pain service specialists for postoperative pain management. Many centers provide PCA and narcotic infusions. There are no pediatric studies of postoperative analgesia after lung transplantation comparing epidural and intravenous techniques. Regional anesthesia via an epidural catheter has been frequently used in adults and some older children when transplantation was performed without CPB. A recent report of 58 pediatric patients who underwent epidural insertion before surgery and CPB showed no apparent complications from this technique and a median time to extubation of 19h [166]. Epidural analgesia was less effective in adult patients undergoing unilateral and bilateral lung transplantation than in patients undergoing a thoracotomy for other indications, perhaps due to the extensive clamshell incision [167]. A survey of adults found the occurrence of moderate-to-severe persistent pain after lung transplantation was low (5–10%) [168].

Physiological changes and growth of the transplanted lungs

The allograft lungs are denervated but this produces few clinically significant effects on airway reflexes, mucociliary movement and bronchial hyper-reactivity [169]. Lack of afferent stimuli to the respiratory center in transplanted patients results in poor co-ordination between thoracic and abdominal muscles and a subnormal increase in the minute ventilation with carbon dioxide challenge was noted in adult patients [170]. Loss of lymphatic drainage makes the transplanted lungs more susceptible to interstitial edema, increased water content and lower compliance [171].

It is uncertain whether transplanted lungs grow. Although spirometry measurements (i.e. FEV_1 and FVC) after lung transplant may be in the normal range in infants [170] and older children [172], these measurements may indicate increased volume of each alveolar unit rather than alveolar tissue growth or increased surface area for gas exchange. Animal studies demonstrated lung tissue growth and serial imaging studies in humans showed airway growth [173]. The measurement of diffusing capacity for carbon monoxide (DLCO) provides an estimate of gas exchange surface area. A single-center study of the DLCO in pediatric recipients of

Table 27.12 Morbidity at 1 year and 5 years post pediatric lung transplant from April 1994 to June 2008

Outcome	Within 1 year	With 5 years
Hypertension	42.8%	69.2%
Renal dysfunction	10.5%	21.6%
Abnormal creatinine <2.5 mg/dL	7.5%	14.9%
Creatinine >2.5 mg/dL	2.1%	3.7%
Chronic dialysis	0.6%	2.2%
Renal transplant	0.4%	0.7%
Hyperlipidemia	4.8%	11.1%
Diabetes	27.1%	33.1%
Bronchiolitis obliterans syndrome	14.0%	36.6%

Reproduced from Aurora et al [125] with permission from Elsevier.

cadaveric and living donor transplants did not show an appreciable increase in DLCO, suggesting that the increase in lung volume seen after mature lobes is secondary to hyperinflation [174].

Complications of lung transplantation

Common complications are summarized in Table 27.12 [125].

Airway complications

A single-center study involving 470 bronchial anastomoses at risk reported 42 (9%) airway complications (stenosis, n = 36; dehiscence, n = 4; malacia, n = 2) requiring interventions. Most (90%) complications were diagnosed within the first 3 months after transplantation. Associated risk factors were preoperative *Pseudomonas cepacia*, postoperative fungal lung infection, and prolonged mechanical ventilation [175]. Infants are prone to developing tracheobronchomalacia and dynamic airway obstruction. Often the problem resolves without surgical intervention but the patients may need prolonged ventilatory support [176]. Airway stenosis is usually treated successfully with repeated mechanical balloon dilation through a rigid bronchoscope. Stents are generally avoided in children with potential for airway growth; the devices are difficult to remove and can cause problems with exuberant granulation tissue growing through the wire mesh.

Vascular complications

A perfusion scan is typically performed early after surgery to quantify the distribution of pulmonary blood flow. Vascular complications are infrequent, with pulmonary vein obstruction being the most common problem. Cardiac catheterization is indicated if a vascular abnormality is suspected. Any significant obstruction to pulmonary blood flow requires urgent treatment by either surgery or interventional cardiac catheterization [177].

Nerve injuries

Early re-exploration of the chest was performed in 11% of cases in one series, most commonly for bleeding [177]. Phrenic nerve injury (typically the right) occurred in 22% of cases and previous thoracotomy was a risk factor. Hoarseness from left recurrent laryngeal nerve injury was noted in 10% of patients. Most of these nerve injuries resolved in the first several months after transplantation, but some patients required diaphragm plication because of poor respiratory function [177,178]. Injury to the vagus nerve frequently leads to gastropharyngeal reflux and gastric paresis. Gastroesophageal reflux disease and resulting recurrent silent aspiration has been implicated in deteriorating graft function and bronchiolitis obliterans syndrome [179]. The incidence of severe gastroesophageal reflux is high (50%), particularly in the young [180]. Patients with deteriorating pulmonary function have been shown to benefit from surgical treatment of gastro-esophageal reflux [181].

Arrhythmias

Arrhythmias that require therapy include atrial flutter (11% of pediatric transplants), atrial fibrillation and supraventricular tachycardia [182]. Most can be controlled with drug therapy. The left atrial suture line is the presumed source.

Primary graft dysfunction

Primary graft dysfunction (PGD) represents a severe form of acute injury to the allograft and is characterized by patchy pulmonary infiltrates, a low ratio of arterial oxygen to the fraction of inspired oxygen, diminished lung compliance, and pathological findings of diffuse alveolar damage [183,184]. There are many opportunities for lung damage during the processes of donor death, organ harvesting, allograft preservation and transplantation. PGD is the net product of these insults, with ischemic reperfusion injury being a major contributor [185]. Interestingly, primary pulmonary hypertension is a recipient risk factor independently associated with the development of PGD [186], presumably from right ventricle dysfunction. PGD may contribute to nearly half of the short-term mortality after lung transplantation [187]. Survivors of PGD even have increased risk of death extending beyond the first post-transplant year and PGD is associated with the subsequent development of bronchiolitis obliterans syndrome [187,188].

Once PGD develops, patients are managed with aggressive cardiopulmonary support involving mechanical ventilation or non-invasive ventilation in the prone position [189], inotropes and occasionally the use of ECMO. Early use of nitric oxide reduces the early mortality [190]. In most patients PGD resolves over several days. Children who need extracorporeal support have significantly higher mortality.

The preventive strategies used to reduce the incidence of PGD include minimizing reperfusion injury, reducing ischemic time, improving donor management and avoiding volu- and barotrauma. Surgeons routinely allow ejection of a small amount of blood into the pulmonary artery immediately after establishing vascular supply to the first lung. PGE1 and prostacyclin may reduce the incidence and severity of the reperfusion injury [191]. The value of prophylactic nitric oxide is questionable [192].

Rejection
Hyperacute rejection
This rare complication may lead to early graft failure and results from circulating preformed recipient serum antibodies binding to donor tissue antigens and causing complement-mediated graft injury. Endothelial cells lining the blood vessels of the new organ are the principal targets. Preformed antibodies directed at HLA or endothelial antigens are generally attributed to prior blood transfusions, a previous transplant or pregnancy. To evaluate the risk for this complication, testing for PRA is performed during the assessment process. PRAs include a mix of 60–100 different samples that express a wide range of antigens tested with the recipient serum. Sensitized patients with high PRA scores may qualify for specialized therapies such as intra- and postoperative plasmapheresis, thymoglobulin and intravenous immunoglobulins [152].

Acute rejection
Acute cellular rejection is T-cell mediated and is common in the first year after lung transplantation, especially during the first 3 months. Clinically, it may be difficult to differentiate from an acute respiratory infection and the histopathological findings are not always helpful. Often the diagnosis of acute rejection is made on clinical suspicion and confirmed by the response to therapy. Some patients are asymptomatic and the acute rejection is detected by airflow limitation (a 10% decrease from baseline in FEV_1 is considered significant). Others present with dyspnea and hypoxia and have infiltrates on chest radiograph. Infants and toddlers have immature immune systems and a lower incidence of acute rejection compared with older children [193]. Also, patients who receive lung-liver transplants have less acute rejection and bronchiolitis obliterans [194]. A pathological diagnosis of acute cellular rejection is based on the presence of perivascular and interstitial mononuclear cell infiltrates in the lung biopsy samples. Histology is classified as follows: acute rejection (A0–A4); lymphocytic bronchitis (B0–B2R, Bx); obliterative bronchitis (C0–C1) [195]. Lymphocytic bronchiolitis represents airway-directed rejection. In adults, acute rejection and lymphocytic bronchitis have

consistently been identified as strong risk factors for chronic rejection [196] but the evidence is less convincing for pediatric lung transplant recipients [197]. It is unclear to what extent humoral rejection, which is antibody mediated, occurs among lung transplant recipients [195].

Methylprednisolone pulse at 10 mg/kg/dose daily for 3 days followed by augmented oral prednisone is the treatment for acute cellular rejection. Overall, the response to this treatment is improvement of symptoms and pulmonary function test results within several days. Management of steroid-resistant acute rejection is currently controversial. Treatment options for humoral rejection include plasmapheresis for antibody removal and immunoglobulin infusion.

Chronic rejection
Chronic rejection is the primary obstacle to better long-term outcomes after lung transplantation (Fig. 27.9). It manifests as obliterative bronchiolitis which is characterized histologically by fibroproliferative tissue remodeling with extracellular matrix deposition and results in small airway occlusion with sparing of the alveoli. Because the pathology has a patchy distribution, diagnosis by transbronchial biopsy has low sensitivity and specificity. Therefore, a clinical surrogate – the bronchiolitis obliterans syndrome (BOS) – was created and is defined as a progressive deterioration in pulmonary function tests (Table 27.13) [195]. Measurement of lung function in young children can be challenging. Changes in lung function tests are likely late manifestations of obliterative bronchiolitis but other diagnostic modalities, including imaging and exhaled biomarkers, have not proven useful.

The etiology of BOS is unclear. Identified risk factors include late or recurrent refractory acute rejection, lymphocytic bronchiolitis, CMV infection, ischemia reperfusion injury (longer ischemia times), HLA mismatches, infection, and gastroesophageal reflux with aspiration.

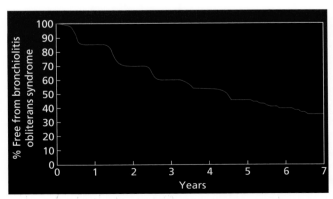

Figure 27.9 Pediatric lung recipients: freedom from bronchiolitis obliterans syndrome (follow-ups: April 1994–June 2008). Reproduced from Kirk et al [91] with permission from Elsevier.

Table 27.13 Classification of bronchiolitis obliterans syndrome

Stage	Definition
BOS 0	$FEV_1 > 90\%$ of baseline and $FEF_{25-75\%} > 75\%$ of baseline
BOS 0-p	$FEV_1 = 81–90\%$ of baseline or $FEF_{25-75\%} \leq 75\%$ of baseline
BOS 1	$FEV_1 = 66–80\%$ of baseline
BOS 2	$FEV_1 = 51–65\%$ of baseline
BOS 3	$FEV_1 \leq 50\%$ of baseline

BOS, bronchiolitis obliterans syndrome; $FEF_{25-75\%}$, forced expiratory flow between 25% and 75% of vital capacity; FEV_1, forced expiratory volume in 1 sec. Baseline: the average of the two highest measurements at least 3 weeks apart after transplantation.
Reproduced from Estenne et al [228] with permission from Elsevier.

Young children, LDLT recipients and liver-lung recipients have a lower risk of BOS.

To date, there is no effective treatment for BOS. Therapies attempted include pulse steroids, methotrexate, cyclophosphamide, cytolytic therapy, inhaled cyclosporin, total lymphoid irradiation, photophoresis and switching to a different immunosuppression protocol [198]. Azithromycin and other macrolides may be useful [199]. Antireflux surgery may reverse the decline in pulmonary function in some patients and statins have beneficial potential because they induce apoptosis in fibroblasts. Retransplantation is considered in relatively few patients; risk of postsurgical death within 1 year is nearly 50% [125].

Immunosuppression

Higher doses of immunosuppressant agents are administered for pediatric lung transplantation than for other solid organ transplantation. Induction immunosuppression is currently used in approximately half of recipients, with about 10% receiving polyclonal antilymphocyte globulin and 40% receiving IL-2 receptor antagonists [125]. Most patients are given triple drug therapy for maintenance immunosuppression. This consists of a calcineurin inhibitor (tacrolimus more commonly than cyclosporin), cell cycle inhibitors like azathioprine or mycophenolate mofetil and prednisone. Sirolimus (target of rapamycin inhibitor) is seldom administered during the first year post transplant, but is more common at 5-year follow-up. Virtually all patients receive long-term maintenance corticosteroids [125].

Infection

Infections occur in 60–90% of recipients. The risk of infection is largely determined by the interaction of three factors: (i) technical/anatomical factors that involve the transplant procedure itself, and the perioperative aspects of care such as the management of vascular access, drains, and the endotracheal tube; (ii) environmental exposure to pathogens; and (iii) the patient's net state of immunosuppression [200]. Bacterial infections are most common but fungal and viral infections result in higher mortality. Hypogammaglobulinemia post transplant was associated with increased infections [201].

Respiratory viral infections are associated with decreased 1-year survival after transplantation [202]. Common pathogens included adenovirus, rhinovirus, respiratory syncytial virus, and parainfluenza virus. Fungal infections were independently associated with a decreased 1-year post-transplant survival [203,204] and most centers routinely administer antifungal prophylaxis. Lung transplant patients are also at increased risk for invasive mold infections [205].

Cytomegalovirus after lung transplantation is a serious infectious complication, especially in CMV-negative recipients receiving CMV-positive donor lungs (i.e. mismatch). Pediatric patients are at increased risk for mismatch because they are more likely to be CMV negative and their incidence of CMV disease was 30% [206]. CMV disease was associated with increased mortality after pediatric lung transplantation. Usually it presents as pneumonitis but can also involve the liver, small bowel, and retina. Antiviral prophylaxis (e.g. ganciclovir) is beneficial although the optimal duration of prophylaxis is uncertain. Surveillance blood testing to measure the viral load is recommended.

Surveillance

Lung transplant recipients are closely monitored for rejection and other complications. Routine monitoring for rejection includes daily home spirometry, regular pulmonary function testing, chest radiographs, bronchopulmonary lavages and transbronchial lung biopsies (a typical biopsy schedule would be at 2 and 6 weeks, and 3, 6, 9 and 12 months after transplant) [152]. Transbronchial biopsies are the mainstay of rejection surveillance in young children because spirometry is not feasible [207]. Infant pulmonary tests (peak expiratory flow rate) using thoracoabdominal compressions can be done but require anesthesia and are not part of the BOS criteria. Sometimes it is difficult to obtain sufficient tissue via transbronchial biopsy in small children and an open lung biopsy may be necessary [11,172,208].

Outcome
Lung transplant

Survival after lung transplantation is similar in children and adult recipients and has improved in recent years. Children transplanted between 2002 and 2007 had a 1-year survival of 83% and a 5-year survival of 50% [125]. These outcomes are inferior to those for other pediatric solid organ transplantation. Children in the 1–10-year age group have better long-term outcomes than infants or

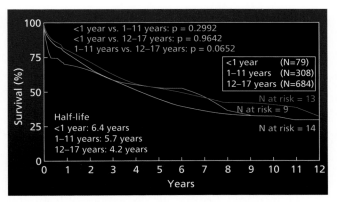

Figure 27.10 Pediatric lung transplantation: Kaplan–Meier survival by age group (transplants: January 1990–June 2007). Reproduced from Kirk et al [91] with permission from Elsevier.

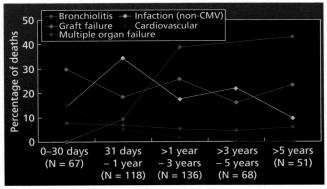

Figure 27.11 Pediatric lung recipients: relative incidence of leading causes of death (deaths: January 1992–June 2008). Reproduced from Kirk et al [91] with permission from Elsevier.

adolescents (Fig. 27.10). Infants have higher early mortality but have better long-term outcome than children above 11 years of age. This may be due in part to the observation that infants and toddlers appear to be more immunologically tolerant of the allograft [193]. Significant risk factors for mortality include preoperative ventilatory support, earlier era of transplant, center volume of <5 pediatric lung transplants per year and adolescent age group. The poor long-term outcome of adolescents is ascribed to the propensity for poor adherence to medical therapies [209]. Children with tetralogy of Fallot and pulmonary atresia had worse outcome after lung transplantation than patients with Eisenmenger syndrome or pulmonary vein stenosis [210]. Graft failure, technical issues, cardiovascular failure and infection are common causes of death in the early post-transplant period, whereas infection, graft failure and BOS are common causes of late death (Fig. 27.11). Children undergoing repeat lung transplant have slightly poorer outcome (41% 5-year survival).

Heart-lung transplant

Fewer than 20 heart-lung transplants are reported per year to the ISHLT [125]. The majority of procedures are for congenital heart disease, primary pulmonary hypertension or cystic fibrosis. A higher proportion of younger children undergo heart-lung transplantation compared with lung transplantation but the majority of procedures are performed in adolescents. Survival after heart-lung transplantation is slowly improving, with 5-year survival of 45% in the most recent era. Infants appear to do worse than older children.

Intestinal, multivisceral, and pancreatic transplantation

Indications

Successful transplantation of liver, kidneys, hearts, and lungs has led transplant surgeons to attempt to treat other illnesses affecting infants and children. In children, the short-gut syndrome, which results from necrotizing enterocolitis, intestinal malrotation and volvulus, or congenital defects (intestinal atresia, abdominal wall defects), leads to dependence on total parenteral nutrition (TPN). The long-term sequelae of TPN include steatotic liver disease and eventual hepatic failure and the complications of long-term venous access. Isolated small bowel transplants, combined small bowel-liver transplants, and extensive multivisceral transplants (liver, pancreas, gastrointestinal tract from stomach to colon) have been performed in an attempt to manage short-gut syndrome. The results of intestinal transplantation have improved over the past decade. Transplantation of the intestine before liver failure improves early outcomes [211]. In 2005, the results of nearly 1000 intestinal transplant procedures (from 62 centers in 19 countries) were summarized in the report of the International Intestinal Transplant Registry (IITR) [212]. The most recent cohort (transplanted after 1998) demonstrated 65% overall 1-year patient survival and over 80% 1-year survival in those recipients who received induction therapy combined with tacrolimus. Recently, a single-center series reported 1- and 5-year patient and graft survival to be 78–85% and 56–61% respectively, despite divergent immunosuppression protocols [213]. More than 80% of transplant recipients who survive attain freedom from parenteral nutrition and resume normal daily activities.

Pancreas transplantation has been utilized most commonly as combined renal and pancreas transplantation for treatment of ESRD in diabetics with other end-organ dysfunction (retinopathy, neuropathy). Because of the interval between development of insulin-dependent diabetes in children and end-organ complications, few reports of pancreas transplantation have been reported in children, apart from the multivisceral procedures described above. The number of pancreas transplants peaked in 2004 and steadily declined through 2008. Even though pancreas transplantation of diabetic patients has stabilized or improved their nephropathy, retinopathy, and neuropathy, immunological failure of the transplant has led to abandonment of isolated pancreas transplant and only combined kidney and pancreas transplants are now performed in children [214].

Anesthetic management

The exact form of intestinal transplantation (i.e. isolated, combined liver-small bowel or multivisceral transplantation) depends upon the cause of intestinal failure and associated extraintestinal organ involvement. Following identification of an appropriate donor, the recipient undergoes a regimen designed to purge and decontaminate the intestinal tract. Routine premedication is avoided, but may be required and administered under appropriate monitoring situations. Rapid-sequence induction of general anesthesia and tracheal intubation is planned. Despite normal or slightly impaired hepatic function, there is a potential for extensive blood loss and hemorrhage in most of these cases. Previous abdominal surgery and extensive dissection and evisceration of the native organs prolong the dissection period and increase blood loss. Venous access sites, particularly around the central circulation, may be limited because of previous TPN catheters. However, central venous access is essential for management. Arterial blood pressure and central venous pressure should be monitored directly. Intraoperative management is similar to liver transplantation: hemodynamic stability may require rapid infusion of crystalloid, colloids or blood products; maintaining metabolic homeostasis requires frequent arterial blood gases and electrolyte concentration determinations.

In multivisceral transplantation and combined pancreatic renal transplantation, particular attention is required to maintain normoglycemia. Tight intraoperative control of the glucose concentration may result in improved pancreatic allograft function. To achieve glucose concentrations of 80–150 mg/dL requires frequent intraoperative determinations of glucose concentration, and titration of a regular insulin infusion. A period of hyperglycemia is common following reperfusion of the pancreatic graft and requires additional insulin administration.

Complications following transplant

Rejection

A common complication associated with all forms of allograft transplantation is rejection of the transplanted tissue by the recipient. Rejection in the early post-transplant period may be a subtle process and difficult to assess by routine physical and laboratory examination. Clinical signs of rejection will vary by the transplanted organ, and are not likely to be specific. Therefore, there is need for early histological evaluation of the organ to diagnose acute rejection. Many transplant centers routinely biopsy the organ at weekly to monthly intervals to search for evidence of acute rejection. This generally requires an invasive procedure requiring anesthesia or sedation in children. Routine immunosuppression is altered in the face of acute rejection. Steroid administration is increased first, and then maintenance immunosuppressive therapy may be increased. See specific discussions of heart and lung rejection and surveillance above.

Infection

Immunosuppression leads to an increased risk of infection. Various forms of infection are more common at different time periods [200,215,216]. In the *first month*, there are three major causes of infection: infection that was present in the recipient before transplant, infection conveyed with a contaminated allograft, and typical postoperative infections also observed in immunocompetent patients, such as surgical wound infections, pneumonia, infected lines or drains.

One to 6 months after transplantation is when more intense immune suppression produces the greatest effect on the risk of infection. During this period, two major classes of infection predominate: chronic viral infections and opportunistic infections. Viral pathogens such as CMV, EBV, human herpes virus 6 (HHV-6), and the hepatitis viruses (B and C) may be acquired from the donor, reactivated in the host, or the patient may become infected with a new strain of these viruses. During this 1–6-month post-transplant period, opportunistic infections are also observed and include organisms such as *Listeria monocytogenes*, *Aspergillus fumigatus*, and *Pneumocystis jiroveci*.

Once patients are *more than 6 months* post transplant, their infectious risk can be broken down into two categories of patients: those with a good result from transplant and a smaller group with a poor graft function. The majority of patients have good graft function, are on maintenance immunosuppression therapy, and are at greatest risk from typical community-acquired infections such as influenza, parainfluenza, and respiratory syncytial virus. The smaller group of patients with acute and chronic immunosuppression, poor allograft function and, often, chronic viral infection remain at high risk for recurrent infections related to mechanical problems from surgery as well as opportunistic infections attributable to organisms like *Pneumocystis jiroveci*, *Listeria monocytogenes*, *Cryptococcus neoformans*, and *Nocardia asteroides*. Infectious risk and outcomes related to lung transplant are discussed above.

Malignancy

The risk of developing cancer after solid organ transplantation is about 5–10-fold more than that of the general population. Children receiving transplants are at high risk of developing a malignancy during their lifetime. The cumulative risk of cancer increases with age and is >50% at 20 years after transplantation.

Post-transplant lymphoproliferative disease (PTLD) is the most common cancer observed in children following solid organ transplantation, accounting for half of all such malignancies [217]. The incidence is about 5–10%. PTLD results from the uncontrolled proliferation of lymphocytes in the immunosuppressed transplant recipient and is a major contributor to long-term morbidity and mortality in this population. Among children, most cases are associated with EBV infection. PTLD is an early event (i.e. within the first 2 years after transplant) in most cases, likely because of more intense immunosuppression used for induction therapy or the exposure of the EBV-naive host to the virus, often from EBV-infected passenger lymphocytes in the allograft. PTLD commonly affects the lung allograft, lymphoid tissues, gastrointestinal tract and liver. Gastrointestinal involvement is associated with increased mortality [218]. Therapy for PTLD includes empiric reduction in immunosuppression, antiviral drugs, monoclonal antibodies specifically targeting the B-lymphocyte antigen CD20 (e.g. rituximab), or chemotherapy, when appropriate.

Renal dysfunction

Renal dysfunction is one of the most common complications following solid organ transplantation. Ojo and colleagues found that the cumulative 5-year risk of chronic renal failure, defined as the need for either chronic dialysis or kidney transplantation, was 6.9–21.3%, depending on type of organ transplanted [219]. This study included more than 69,000 non-renal solid organ transplant recipients who were predominantly adults. The risk of death increased more than fourfold with the onset of chronic renal failure, and the cost of care was dramatically increased [219]. Table 27.14 shows the risk of renal failure related to the type of organ transplant.

There are multiple factors that produce renal dysfunction following solid organ transplantation; however, the calcineurin inhibitors (CNI) cyclosporin and tacrolimus are the major contributing factors. The CNI produce both acute and chronic nephrotoxicity. Acute nephrotoxicity involves afferent arteriolar vasoconstriction and reduced renal plasma flow, and is associated with high trough levels. In contrast, chronic CNI-induced nephrotoxicity is not predicted by individual trough levels, and is characterized by potentially irreversible structural changes including arteriolopathy, tubulointerstitial fibrosis and, eventually, glomerulosclerosis [220]. Strategies for man-

agement of post-transplant renal dysfunction have largely focused on CNI minimization, replacement or avoidance.

Table 27.14 Cumulative Incidence of Chronic Renal Failure According to the Type of Transplanted Organ*

Type of Organ	Cumulative Incidence of Chronic Renal Failure after Transplantation			Relative Risk of Chronic Renal Failure (95% CI)
	12 Mo	36 Mo	60 Mo	
	percentage ± SE			
Heart	1.9 ± 0.1	6.8 ± 0.2	10.9 ± 0.2	0.63 (0.61–0.66)
Heart–lung	1.7 ± 0.5	4.2 ± 0.9	6.9 ± 1.1	0.48 (0.36–0.65)
Intestine	9.6 ± 2.0	14.2 ± 2.4	21.3 ± 3.4	1.36 (1.00–1.86)
Liver	8.0 ± 0.1	13.9 ± 0.2	18.1 ± 0.2	1.00 (reference group)
Lung	2.9 ± 0.2	10.0 ± 0.4	15.8 ± 0.5	0.99 (0.93–1.06)

*CI denotes confidence interval.
Reproduced from Ojo et al [219] with permission from the Massachusetts Medical Society.

Growth and developmental delay

Organ failure frequently leads to a poor nutritional state and growth failure. After organ transplant, most patients demonstrate catch-up growth, yet a large percentage of patients do not reach their predicted adult height and weight. Immunosuppression regimens that limit the use of steroids seem to be well tolerated and allow for better growth; however, the long-term effect of CNI on growth is not well studied and may also contribute to growth failure [221]. Growth hormone can be used but there are theoretical concerns about the risk of triggering rejection [11].

Solid-organ transplant recipients display a wide range of developmental outcomes, from normal development to significant delays. Factors that lead to poor developmental outcome likely include long-term hospitalization, chronic malnutrition in the pretransplant period, and surgical complications. Children who receive heart transplantation may have better cognitive outcomes than expected considering the results of older studies of children with cyanotic congenital heart disease. The cognitive outcomes of liver and kidney transplant recipients may also be improving, but many still require special educational resources. Infants requiring intestine or liver and intestine transplant are probably at the highest risk for cognitive delay, but longitudinal studies that confirm these delays are lacking [221]. In all cases neurological co-morbidities increase the risk of delay. Despite recent

Table 27.15 Incidence of hypertension in pediatric solid organ transplantation

Organ	Prevalence			References
	2 years	**5 years**	**7 years**	
Kidney	75%	70%		North American Pediatric Renal Transplant Cooperative Study
Liver	14.5%/15.7%			Studies in Pediatric liver Transplantation
Heart Lung		71.6%	64.7%	International Society for Heart and lung Transplantation

Reproduced from Dharnidharka et al [222] with permission from Wiley-Blackwell.

advances, a significant proportion of liver and heart recipients have serious developmental delay or neurological injury.

Cardiovascular side-effects

Immunosuppressive agents produce cardiovascular toxicity, causing an increased likelihood of hypertension, hyperlipidemia, hypercholesterolemia, and diabetes mellitus. Hypertension is found in 62–75% of pediatric patients (Table 27.15) [222]. Although both tacrolimus and cyclosporin can cause hypertension, cyclosporin appears to have a greater impact on blood pressure [223].

These side-effects are treated via an alteration of immunosuppressive regimen, or addition of specific medications to address each risk factor or complication. Since steroids and CNI provide the mainstay of immunosuppressive treatments, they generally cannot be eliminated. Steroid withdrawal or reduction as well as the use of tacolimus over cyclosporin may decrease the risk of hypertension, dyslipidemia or diabetes mellitus [220]. All classes of antihypertensive medications have been used and are ideally chosen based on the therapeutic profile. In addition to surveillance of tacrolimus levels, long-term monitoring of cardiac function may also be warranted in high-risk populations.

Post-transplant surgery

Regardless of the transplant procedure, as transplant recipients age, they are likely to acquire diseases or conditions that require additional surgery. Prior to such procedures, the anesthesiologist must assess the function of the transplanted organ, review the status of the patient's immunosuppression, and perform a careful assessment of the other organ systems. Hypertension and chronic renal insufficiency are common findings in patients (see above). Most patients will demonstrate findings of chronic steroid administration.

Quality of life

The functional status of most long-term survivors of solid organ transplantation is good, with greater than 80–90% of 5-year survivors from kidney, liver, heart and lung transplantation reporting no limitations in activity. Despite excellent function, children may experience psychological difficulties and an impaired quality of life [224]. Pediatric studies focusing on quality of life after transplantation remain scarce [223–225]. Research thus far shows improved overall quality of life after kidney, liver, heart and lung transplantation, although the debate continues for cystic fibrosis [132]. The quality of life after small bowel transplantation is probably equal to or better than quality of life on parenteral nutrition, and children report quality of life similar to normal schoolchildren. A study that used qualitative interviews to examine psychosocial issues after lung transplantation in adolescents with cystic fibrosis reported that patients were able to develop long-term goals and had a wish to reclaim control over their lives as much as possible and adjust to a new lifestyle, yet common emotional responses included fear and anxiety over rejection, uncertainty over the future, and frustration with parental overprotectiveness [226].

It has been proposed that quality of life should be included in the assessment of transplantation benefit [227]. Currently, timing of transplantation relies primarily on estimates of survival benefit because comprehensive objective measures of quality of life for pediatric lung transplantation are not available.

Annotated references

A full reference list for this chapter is available at:
http://www.wiley.com/go/gregory/andropoulos/pediatricanesthesia

3. Urschel S, Altamirano-Diaz LA, West LJ. Immunosuppression armamentarium in 2010: mechanistic and clinical considerations. Pediatr Clin North Am 2010; 57: 433–57. A comprehensive review of modern immunosuppression strategies.

11. Sweet SC. Pediatric lung transplantation. Proc Am Thorac Soc 2009; 6: 122–7. An excellent overview of pediatric lung transplantation.

24. Ng VL, Fecteau A, Shepherd R et al. Outcomes of 5-year survivors of pediatric liver transplantation: report on 461 children from a north american multicenter registry. Pediatrics 2008; 122(6): e1128–e1135. A comprehensive review of oucomes of pediatric liver transplantation in the modern era.

42. Zafirova Z, O'Connor M. Hepatic encephalopathy: current management strategies and treatment, including management and monitoring of cerebral edema and intracranial hypertension in fulminant hepatic failure. Curr Opin Anaesthesiol 2010; 23: 121–7. A contemporary review of management of hepatic encephalopathy.

74. Kamath BM, Olthoff KM. Liver transplantation in children: update 2010. Pediatr Clin North Am 2010; 57:401–14. A contemporary review of pediatric liver transplantation.

79. McDonald SP, Craig JC. Long-term survival of children with end-stage renal disease. N Engl J Med 2004; 350: 2654–62. Review of end-stage renal disease in children, including transplantation as therapy.

91. Kirk R, Edwards LB, Aurora P et al. Registry of the International Society for Heart and Lung Transplantation: Twelfth Official Pediatric Heart Transplantation Report 2009. J Heart Lung Transplant 2009; 28: 993–1006. The latest comprehensive annual report for pediatric heart and lung transplantation.

113. West LJ, Pollock-Barziv SM, Dipchand AI et al. ABO-incompatible heart transplantation in infants. N Engl J Med 2001; 344: 793–800. A very important paper describing techniques and outcomes for ABO-incompatible infant heart transplantation, which has significantly changed our approach to these patients.

124. Reitz BA, Wallwork JL, Hunt SA et al. Heart-lung transplantation: successful therapy for patients with pulmonary vascular disease. N Engl J Med 1982; 306: 557–64. The landmark paper describing heart-lung transplantation for pulmonary vascular disease.

193. Elizur A, Faro A, Huddleston CB et al. Lung transplantation in infants and toddlers from 1990 to 2004 at St. Louis Children's Hospital. Am J Transplant 2009; 9: 719–26. An important review from one of the largest and most successful pediatric lung transplant centers.

CHAPTER 28

Anesthesia for Abdominal Surgery

Lena S. Sun[1,2], *Neeta R. Saraiya*[1] & *Philipp J. Houck*[1]

Department of Anesthesiology[1] and Pediatrics[2], Columbia University College of Physicians and Surgeons, New York, NY, USA

ABDOMINAL SURGICAL CONDITIONS

Intussusception

Intussusception is a common cause of intestinal obstruction and abdominal pain. The incidence of this lesion is 1 in 2000 infants and children and it is a true pediatric emergency. Intussusceptions occur when a segment of bowel (the intussusceptum) invaginates into the distal bowel (the intussuscipiens), usually in an antegrade direction. This results in venous congestion and bowel wall edema. If intussusception is not recognized and treated rapidly, bowel necrosis and perforation may result. Overall mortality from intussusception is less than 1%, and the outcome is excellent if the condition is diagnosed early and treated within 24h of onset.

Epidemiology

Intussusception occurs primarily in infants and toddlers, and males are affected twice as often as females. The peak incidence of this abnormality occurs between 5 and 9 months of age; between 10% and 25% of cases occur after 2 years of age [1]. Intussusception rarely occurs in patients younger than 2 months of age, but rare instances have been reported in preterm infants.

Ninety percent of intussusceptions are idiopathic, but lymphoid hyperplasia has been suggested to be the "lead point" in the pathogenesis of some intussusceptions [2]. The incidence of this disease is higher during autumn and spring, suggesting that it might be a sequela of a previous viral infection [3]. Indeed, adenovirus, rotavirus, and human herpesvirus-6 infections have been associated with intussusceptions [4].

After introduction of the oral rotavirus vaccine in 1999, some >3-month-old infants developed intussusception, usually 3–14 days after the first dose of the vaccine was given [5]. This caused the vaccine to be withdrawn from the market [6]. Other common lead points are Meckel diverticulum, intestinal polyps, and lymphoma. Patients with systemic conditions, such as Henoch–Schönlein purpura, Peutz–Jeghers syndrome, familial polyposis, nephrotic syndrome, mesenteric nodes, and inverted appendical stumps, are also prone to developing intussusception [7–9]. Recurrent intussusception is uncommon but has been reported in 1–3% of infants and young

---

children after operative repair and in 10–15% after hydro-static reductions of the lesion [10].

Pathophysiology

Ileocolic intussusception accounts for more than 90% of the cases of intussusception, though it can occur in any segment of the bowel. The intussusceptum and its blood supply are propagated distally along the intestine. Venous congestion and bowel wall edema occur due to compression of the blood vessels by surrounding tissue. As the obstruction progresses, the arterial blood supply can be compromised and intestinal ischemia and bowel infarction may occur [1].

Clinical presentation

Intussusception has both typical and atypical presentations, but many patients present with non-specific signs and symptoms. The classic presentation is a young child with a history of a recent viral illness, vomiting, and/or diarrhea. The classic clinical triad of intermittent abdominal pain, redcurrant jelly stool, and a palpable mass is found in 7.5–40% of affected children. Twenty percent of the children are pain free at initial presentation [11]. Infants younger than 4 months of age have a higher incidence of painless intussusception. Thirty percent of them present with diarrhea and are often misdiagnosed as having gastroenteritis [12].

Vomiting is the most common symptom and is frequently the only clinical finding in infants. Older children may present with colicky abdominal pain and bilious vomiting. Early in the course of the illness, stools are normal. Subsequently they become dark red and mucoid and resemble redcurrant jelly (indicating ischemia or mucosal sloughing).

A palpable right upper quadrant mass is often present on physical examination and is usually sausage shaped and ill defined. The mass may enlarge during episodes of pain. Some patients present with syncope, sepsis, and/or hypovolemic shock.

Diagnosis

No reliable clinical model accurately diagnoses all patients who present with intussusception. Plain abdominal films, ultrasound or a computed tomographic (CT) scan help to confirm the diagnosis.

Management

Management of an intussusception has changed significantly in recent years. Barium, aqueous or air enemas now are used to successfully reduce the intussusception (60–90% for air, and 60–80% for barium/aqueous contrast enemas). When non-operative reduction of the lesion is unsuccessful or is contraindicated, patients undergo surgery to reduce the lesion. Aggressive fluid resuscita-

tion is often required before, during, and after surgery. Antibiotics are also required.

Preoxygenation and rapid-sequence intravenous induction of anesthesia with propofol and a muscle relaxant (succinylcholine or rocuronium) are used to facilitate tracheal intubation and reduce the risk of regurgitation and aspiration of gastric contents. Maintenance of anesthesia is accomplished with isoflurane, sevoflurane or an opioid-based anesthetic in critically ill patients.

Key points

- Intussusception is a common cause of bowel obstruction in young children and has an incidence of 1 in 2000.
- The classic clinical triad of intussusception is intermittent abdominal pain, redcurrant jelly stools, and a palpable abdominal mass.
- A palpable sausage-shaped mass is often present in the right upper quadrant of the abdomen on physical examination.
- Barium, aqueous, and air enemas successfully reduce the intussusception in more than half of the patients; operative reduction is required if this fails.
- Aggressive fluid resuscitation may be required preoperatively to correct hypovolemia.

Biliary atresia

Biliary atresia is defined as the absence of patent extrahepatic bile ducts and is a common cause of jaundice in neonates and infants. If untreated, biliary atresia leads to cirrhosis and liver failure within the first 2 years of life. The incidence of biliary atresia ranges from 1 in 10,000 to 1 in 16,700 livebirths, with a slight female preponderance [13,14]. There are three main types of biliary atresia: type I, atresia at the site of the common bile duct (11.9%); type II, atresia at the site of the hepatic duct (2.5%); type III, atresia at the porta hepatis (84.1%) [15]. Ten to 20% of patients with biliary atresia have other congenital malformations, the most common being poylsplenia [15]. Other anomalies include asplenia, anomalies of the inferior vena cava, bowel atresia, annular pancreas, and genitourinary anomalies [15,16].

Etiology

The exact cause of biliary atresia remains elusive, but there is some association between perinatal viral infections (reovirus type 3, rotavirus, cytomegalovirus, human papillomavirus, respiratory syncytial virus, and Epstein–Barr virus) and biliary atresia [17–21]. There may also be a genetic predisposition to its development. Defects in the immune response, autoimmune disorders, and defects in morphogenesis are other possible causes of biliary atresia.

Pathophysiology

Whatever the cause, the end result is complete obstruction of the lumen of the extrahepatic bile ducts and progressive inflammation of the intrahepatic ducts. The degree of intrahepatic bile duct involvement is responsible for much of the morbidity encountered after hepatic portoenterostomy (Kasai procedure).

Clinical presentation

Most patients present with jaundice, acholic stools, dark urine, and an enlarged, firm liver within several weeks after birth; eventually the child develops cirrhosis and splenomegaly. Coagulopathy and portal hypertension often follow. Malabsorption of fat-soluble vitamins leads to anemia, malnutrition, and failure to thrive. Karrer et al reported a less than 10% 3-year survival of children who do not undergo a definitive biliary drainage procedure [13].

Diagnosis

No single test reliably diagnoses biliary artesia. However, a combination of physical examination, serological evaluation of liver function, ultrasonography, and percutaneous liver biopsy is useful for making the diagnosis. An absolute, definitive diagnosis requires surgical exploration.

Management

Currently biliary atresia is managed in two phases [22].
- *Phase 1:* attempts are made to preserve the infant's liver by performing a Kasai procedure, which involves excising all of the extrahepatic biliary structures from the liver hilus. The denuded hilus is then anastomosed to the jejunal limb of a Roux-en-Y. It is hoped that microscopic biliary structures within the transected fibrous tissue will drain into the intestinal conduit. The Kasai procedure never works in about one-third of infants, it works for several years in another third, and it works for more than 10 years in the remaining third.
- *Phase 2:* if bile flow is not restored by the Kasai procedure or the cirrhosis worsens, the infant becomes a candidate for liver transplantation (see Chapter 27).

Anesthetic management for infants with biliary atresia can be challenging, since they are frequently malnourished and occasionally dehydrated. It is important to note and understand all of the laboratory and other diagnostic studies preoperatively. Blood products should be available because many of these patients are coagulopathic, and have significant potential for intraoperative blood loss during surgery done around major intra-abdominal vascular structures, e.g. the inferior vena cava (IVC) and the

hepatic artery. Depending on the infant's condition and the type of surgery, the procedure may be scheduled as same-day surgery or after admission to hospital prior to surgery. Intravenous (IV) access may be difficult in these patients.

Anesthesia is usually induced with intravenous propofol and fentanyl; muscle paralysis is provided with rocuronium or pancuronium. Anesthesia is often maintained with either isoflurane or sevoflurane. It is preferable to have IV access in the upper extremity in case there is massive bleeding. Having a functioning arterial line during surgery is very helpful. Intraoperative hypotension is common with IVC compression by surgical instruments or with sudden blood loss. All replacement IV and irrigation fluids should be warmed. Plans are made before surgery for postoperative respiratory and pain management.

Some children develop cholangitis after a Kasai procedure and are very ill.

Key points
- Biliary atresia is a common cause of cirrhosis and liver failure during the first 2 years of life.
- Complete obstruction of the lumen of extrahepatic bile ducts and progressive cellular inflammation of the intrahepatic ducts are common.
- These patients present with jaundice, acholic stools, dark urine, and an enlarged firm liver within weeks after birth.
- Biliary atresia is managed in two phases: phase 1 – Kasai procedure, phase 2 – liver transplantation.

Malrotation of the bowel and intestinal atresia

Intestinal obstruction can occur at any age, but the etiology of obstruction varies according to the age of the patient. It is often embryological in origin, especially in children less than 1 year of age. The common congenital causes of bowel obstruction include bowel atresia/stenosis, malrotation of the bowel, Hirschsprung disease, imperforate anus, and meconium ileus. Congenital or acquired small bowel obstructions are more common in children than are large bowel obstructions. Hernias, intramural and extramural intestinal lesions, tumors, inflammatory bowel disease, intestinal volvulus, and adhesions are some of the common causes of pediatric bowel obstruction. Adhesions account for about 60% of all small bowel obstructions [23]. Early diagnosis of intestinal obstruction depends on early recognition of the symptoms, e.g. bilious vomiting, abdominal distension and tenderness, and radiographic findings.

Intestinal atresia

Jejunoileal atresia and stenosis are common causes of neonatal intestinal obstruction. Atresia is a congenital anomaly that completely occludes the intestinal lumen; this accounts for 95% of the cases of obstruction. Stenosis is defined as a partial intraluminal occlusion that incompletely obstructs the intestine. It is responsible for 5% of jejunoileal obstructions. Jejunoileal obstruction occurs in 1 in 330 (USA) to 1 in 400 (Denmark) to 1 in 1500 livebirths. Intrauterine mesenteric vascular compromise is thought to be the etiology of jejunoileal atresia. On the other hand, mucosal atresia is thought to cause duodenal atresia.

Prenatal ultrasound is useful for diagnosing intestinal atresia in babies whose mothers have polyhydramnios. A history of maternal polyhydramnios, neonatal bilious vomiting, abdominal distension, and failure to defecate meconium on the first day of life is the usual clinical presentation [24]. The diagnosis is confirmed by radiographic examination. Thumb-sized intestinal loops and air–fluid levels are highly suggestive of neonatal intestinal obstruction.

Management of intestinal atresia consists of surgical resection of the atretic/stenotic section of bowel. Common postoperative complications include obstruction at the anastomotic site and anastomotic leaks. Factors contributing to the morbidity and mortality of these patients include associated anomalies, respiratory distress, prematurity, and short bowel syndrome.

Malrotation of the bowel

Intestinal malrotation refers to abnormal rotation of the midgut around the superior mesenteric artery and abnormal fixation of the gut within the peritoneal cavity. Several types of malrotation occur and are caused by errors in growth, rotation, and position of the duodenum and the ligament of Treitz. These abnormalities in rotation range from non-rotation to reversed rotation [25]. The most common form of gut malrotation in children is due to incomplete rotation and narrow attachment of the mesentery of the midgut to the posterior abdominal wall, which predisposes to midgut rotation and volvulus. Rotational abnormalities commonly occur with heterotaxia, which in this case refers to abnormal attachments of the body organs. Major, complex cardiac anomalies and other gastrointestinal anomalies (e.g. malposition of the stomach, liver and pancreas, asplenia or polysplenia) are associated with heterotaxia [24].

Epidemiology

The exact incidence of malrotation of the gut is unknown, but it is thought to be about 1 in 500 livebirths [26]. The incidence is high in patients with heterotaxia (40–90%). There is no gender-specific preponderance for this lesion.

Malrotation is also associated with other congenital or acquired lesions of the gastrointestinal tract (e.g. Hirschsprung disease, intussusceptions, and atresia of the jejunum, duodenum, and esophagus) [27]. These abnormal gut rotations and fixations can obstruct and strangulate the gut at any time between 10 weeks of intrauterine life and adulthood. Malrotation of the gut also occurs in patients with abdominal wall defects, e.g. omphalocele, gastroschisis, and diaphragmatic hernias.

Clinical presentation

Sixty percent of patients presenting with malrotation of the gut do so during the first month of life. Twenty percent present between 1 month and 1 year of age and the remainder present later. Some patients are asymptomatic and their lesion is found accidentally. The usual presenting symptoms of neonates are bilious vomiting or signs of midgut volvulus. Beyond the neonatal period, the presenting symptoms vary from vomiting, intermittent colicky abdominal pain, failure to thrive, diarrhea, constipation, gastrointestinal hemorrhage (i.e. hematemesis or bloody stools), and acute intestinal obstruction [28]. Signs of abdominal distension and peritonitis are often found on physical examination.

Diagnosis

Diagnosis of malrotation is radiological. Making the diagnosis may be difficult if there is heterotaxia because the location of the liver, spleen, and stomach is often ambiguous. Plain radiographs of the abdomen are frequently non-diagnostic. Occasionally, however, there is a "double bubble" sign (i.e. two air-filled structures in the upper abdomen – the stomach on the left and the duodenum on the right – with little or no air seen distally). This finding is usually indicative of acute duodenal obstruction. On an upper gastrointestinal series, if the duodenojejunal flexure and loops of jejunum are on the right side of the abdomen and the cecum is above its normal position on a delayed film, this is diagnostic of malrotation. Abdominal ultrasound and CT scans can fail to rule out the diagnosis of malrotation.

Management

Preoperative management of malrotation requires fluid resuscitation with a balanced salt solution to correct vomiting-induced hypovolemia and dehydration. Attaching a nasogastric tube to suction can increase volume loss. Antibiotics should be administered early. Some patients are severely acidotic from both hypovolemia and poor gut blood flow. If the acidosis is not corrected by fluid replacement, partial correction of pH with bicarbonate or tromethamine (THAM) should be considered. Once the patient is normovolemic, a Ladd procedure is done, which includes derotation of the midgut   volvulus, division of bands and adhesions when present, and an appendectomy. The small bowel is then placed in the right side of the abdomen and the colon on the left side.

These patients must be considered to have a full stomach. Before inducing anesthesia, all laboratory and other diagnostic studies should be reviewed and the degree of acid–base imbalance and electrolyte abnormalities corrected. Adequate venous and intra-arterial access is required.

Just before the induction of anesthesia, the stomach is decompressed through an orogastric or nasogastric tube, and the lungs are preoxygenated. Rapid-sequence induction of anesthesia is accomplished with intravenous propofol 2–3 mg/kg or etomidate 0.2–0.3 mg/kg and a non-depolarizing mucscle relaxant, e.g. rocuronium 1–1.2 mg/kg or pancuronium 0.1–0.2 mg/kg, to facilitate rapid intubation. Intraoperatively, the patient's lungs are ventilated with a mixture of air and oxygen and low concentrations of sevoflurane or isoflurane. Intravenous narcotics, e.g. fentanyl, are titrated to effect. The key to a good outcome is fluid resuscitation and replacement of extracellular fluid losses in the perioperative period. Occasionally large volumes of colloids and blood are required. Circulatory support with vasopressors may be required, especially after derotation of the bowel.

These infants frequently require intensive care after surgery. Depending on the stability of the patient, the magnitude of the surgery, and associated co-morbid conditions, some patients require postoperative mechanical ventilation. Delayed return of intestinal function often makes parenteral nutrition necessary for a period of time.

Intestinal pseudo-obstruction

If the surgeons find no cause for the bowel obstruction, the patient may have intestinal pseudo-obstruction, a condition in which the signs and symptoms of intestinal obstruction are present but no mechanical lesion is found. Pseudo-obstruction is myopathic or neuropathic in etiology and is not limited to the small intestine. Box 28.1 lists the causes of intestinal pseudo-obstruction. These patients have recurrent attacks of variable duration and frequency that include nausea, vomiting, abdominal distension, diarrhea, and constipation.

Treatment of intestinal pseudo-obstruction is difficult and is mainly medical. Erythromycin and octreotide have been used with some success to stimulate intestinal motility and contraction. New treatments that target intestinal serotonin receptors (alosetron) are in clinical trials. Surgery is only helpful for patients who have a short segment of intestinal dysmotility.

Box 28.1 Causes of intestinal pseudo-obstruction

Disorders of the nervous system

- Familial autonomic dysfunction
- Neurofibromatosis
- Autoimmune disease
- Paraneoplastic syndrome
- Hirschsprung disease
- Chagas disease

Disease affecting muscles and nerves

- Muscular dystrophy
- Systemic lupus erythematosus
- Amyloidosis
- Ehlers–Danlos syndrome
- Electrolyte disturbances
- Hypokalemia

Disorders of the endocrine system

- Diabetes mellitus
- Hypothyroidism
- Hyperparathyroidism

Medications

- Narcotics
- Laxatives
- Tricyclic antidepressants
- Phenothiazines

Key points

- Jejunoileal atresia and stenosis are major causes of neonatal intestinal obstruction.
- Abnormal intestinal rotation commonly occurs with heterotaxia, i.e. there are abnormal attachments of body organs.
- Neonates with intestinal malrotation present with bilious vomiting or with signs of midgut volvulus.
- Large volumes of crystalloids, colloids, and blood, as well as circulatory support with vasopressors, may be required. Acidosis is common and may necessitate blood volume expansion and alkali to correct it.

Inflammatory bowel disease

Inflammatory bowel disease (IBD) includes two major forms of chronic intestinal inflammation: Crohn disease and ulcerative colitis. Both are associated with significant morbidity. Prompt and accurate diagnosis and appropriate treatment of IBD minimize its short-term and long-term physical and psychological effects.

Epidemiology

The incidence of IBD is steadily increasing. Over 1 million Americans are afflicted with the disease, and 10–25% of them are children [29]. In pediatric patients, the incidence of Crohn disease is 11 per 100,000 per year compared to 2.3 per 100,000 per year for ulcerative colitis [30]. Males and females are equally afflicted. North America and northern Europe have the largest number of patients with IBD. Caucasians, especially in the Ashkenazi Jewish population, have the highest risk for the disease. However, the increased disease prevalence is occurring in diverse rural and urban populations alike and in people of different ethnic backgrounds.

Etiology

The etiology of IBD is unknown, but a number of risk factors appear to play a role in its development. There appears to be a genetic predisposition because having a first-degree relative with IBD increases your risk for this disease by 5–25% [31]. Monozygotic twins are more likely to have IBD than dizygotic twins. Environmental factors, infections, immune system disorders, and psychological stress play a role in the development of IBD.

Pathophysiology

Ulcerative colitis is usually limited to the colon and rectum. However, the extent of the disease differs between children and adults. It is usually more extensive in children and may present as pancolitis. Microscopic changes of ulcerative colitis are limited to the mucosa and are continuous from the rectum upward [32]. Crohn disease, on the other hand, can affect any part of the gastrointestinal tract from the mouth to the anus. Children with Crohn disease usually have extensive lesions of the ileum and colon when first evaluated. The inflammatory lesions are focal, asymmetrical, and patchy in location and severity. In the colon, Crohn disease may be difficult to distinguish from ulcerative colitis. Patients with IBD also have extraintestinal manifestations and a higher than predicted risk of developing colorectal cancer.

Clinical presentation

The classic presentation of Crohn disease is abdominal pain, diarrhea, and weight loss. Bloody, mucoid diarrhea is classic for ulcerative colitis. Extraintestinal manifestations of IBD include anorexia, lethargy, pyrexia, arthralgia, arthritis, erythema nodosum, uveitis/iritis, and growth failure.

Diagnosis

The gold standard for diagnosing IBD is upper endoscopy, colonoscopy, and tissue histology. However, there is no substitute for a complete history and physical examination.

Laboratory screening tests include erythrocyte sedimentation rate (ESR), C-reactive protein (CRP) [33], and examination of the stool for bacteria and parasites. Fecal inflammatory markers are also helpful for screening and monitoring patients with IBD. Fecal markers include proteins released from activated neutrophils in the bowel mucosa (e.g. lactoferrin, calprotectin, PMN-elastase, lysozyme) [34].

Serological biomarkers include anti-*Saccharomyces cerevisiae* (ASCA) IgA and IgG, anti-*E. coli* outer membrane porin C (OmpC), antiperinuclear antineutrophil (pANCA) IgG, anti-*Pseudomonas fluorescens* CD-related protein (I2) IgA, and antiflagellin (C Bir-1). It has been postulated that patients who have immune reactivity to antimicrobial antigens have a more severe form of disease [35]. Higher ASCA levels are associated with younger age at disease onset, structuring of the bowel, penetrating disease, and a need for surgery in both adults and children with Crohn disease.

Radiographic studies, CT scans, ultrasound, magnetic resonance imaging (MRI), and barium enemas are also used to detect disease and complications of the disease (e.g. abscess); however, use of these modalities is limited.

Management

Inflammatory bowel disease is quite debilitating. Therefore, the goals of management include induction and maintenance of disease remission to facilitate normal growth and development and improve the child's quality of life. Medical management consists of a combination of pharmacological agents, including administering corticosteroids for their anti-inflammatory properties to children who have moderate-to-severe active IBD. Sulfaxazine and 5-aminosalicylate are locally active medications that are useful for induction and maintenance of disease remission [36]. Immunomodulators, such as 6-mercaptopurine (6-MP) and azathioprine, are the most commonly prescribed agents for these children. These drugs act by incorporating 6-thioguanine nucleotide metabolites (6-TGNs) of 6-MP in leukocyte DNA [37]. Methotrexate is a second-line immunomodulator that has significant corticosteroid-sparing effects when injected weekly in children with IBD [37]. Cyclosporin and tacrolimus effectively control severe fulminant ulcerative colitis and fistula formation in Crohn disease by blocking production of the potent proinflammatory cytokine interleukin-2 [38,39].

Biological therapy with infliximab, a chimeric monoclonal antibody (IgG1), is directed against tumor necrosis factor-α (TNF-α) and is widely used in children with IBD [40]. Antibiotics/probiotics, especially ciprofloxacin (Cipro) and metronidazole (Flagyl), are used to prevent and treat infection, e.g. pouchitis [41]. Nutritional therapy with an elemental diet or total parenteral nutrition helps maintain nutrition and improve growth, which is important because poor nutrition is a major cause of growth failure in patients with IBD.

Psychological problems are common in children with IBD due to demanding treatment regimes, frequent relapses of their disease, pain, diarrhea, fecal incontinence, and altered physical appearance. These children frequently do not discuss their problem with peers. Multidisciplinary help is often needed for both the children and their families to help them cope with the practical and psychological implications of IBD [42].

Patients with IBD have an increased risk of developing cancer. It is estimated that the risk of cancer in patients with ulcerative colitis increases 1% per year after the first 10 years of the disease [43]. Patients with total colonic disease have the highest risk. After having the disease for 8–10 years, yearly surveillance of the bowel should be done in all patients, regardless of whether they are symptomatic or asymptomatic.

The incidence of surgery in these patients is declining due to better medical and nutritional management. Since surgery does not cure the disease, it is reserved for failures of medical management or for complications of the disease. Emergency surgery is indicated for fulminant disease that is refractory to medical management, including extensive rectal bleeding or toxic megacolon. In the past, proctocolectomy with ileostomy was standard treatment for ulcerative colitis. Since the 1970s restorative proctocolectomy with ileal-anal anastomosis has been practiced. Some patients develop strictures and require surgery to relieve them.

Anesthetic management of patients with IBD begins with a thorough history and physical examination. Particular attention is paid to the patient's fluid and electrolyte status. Optimizing the fluid and electrolyte status before elective surgery is crucial to a good outcome. Prophylactic steroid administration is recommended for patients who have been on long-term steroid therapy. Patients on total parenteral nutrition (TPN) require monitoring of their blood glucose and metabolic states during the perioperative period. Sudden discontinuation of a TPN solution that contains high glucose concentrations may lead to severe hypoglycemia. No one particular anesthetic technique is preferred.

Combined general and epidural anesthesia should be considered for abdominal surgery, since the epidural will provide significant postoperative pain relief. The extent of the surgery determines how much intraoperative monitoring is necessary. If the patient requires extensive colonic resection, arterial and central venous lines are appropriate. Attention to intraoperative fluid replacement, blood loss, and correction of fluid, electrolyte, glucose, and hematological derangements is important. Postoperative pain management can be challenging because many of these patients were receiving narcotics before surgery for their abdominal pain. Intravenous patient-controlled analgesia (PCA) and regional analgesia provide good pain relief and are used routinely.

Anastomotic leaks and abscess formation are the most frequent complications encountered after surgery. Abscess drainage by an interventional radiologist often requires general anesthesia.

Key points
- Ulcerative colitis is usually limited to the colon and rectum.
- Crohn disease can affect the entire gastrointestinal tract from the mouth to the anus.
- Children with IBD and extraintestinal manifestations have a higher risk of developing colorectal cancer.
- The gold standard for diagnosing IBD is upper endoscopy, colonoscopy and tissue histology.
- Goals of IBD management are induction and maintenance of disease remission.
- Medical management combines pharmacological agents, corticosteroids, and anti-inflammatory agents.
- Emergency surgery is indicated for fulminant disease that is refractory to medical management or for extensive rectal bleeding or toxic megacolon.

Abdominal masses: major abdominal and liver tumors, pheochromocytoma

Neuroblastomas, Wilms tumor, and hepatomas are the most common intraabdominal tumors in children. Neonates and infants with these tumors often present with an abdominal mass and abdominal distension. Box 28.2 lists the differential diagnosis of abdominal masses in children.

Laboratory, radiographic and imaging studies are common diagnostic measures used to determine the cause of the child's problem. Box 28.3 lists useful studies for the initial evaluation of patients with an abdominal mass.

Neuroblastomas
Neuroblastomas arise from neural crest tissue. In the abdomen they arise from the adrenal glands and paraspinal sympathetic ganglia. Neuroblastoma is the most common neoplasm in infancy and the most common extracranial solid tumor during childhood. The behavior patterns of neuroblastomas are heterogeneous and range from complete regression to life-threatening progression despite treatment.

Epidemiology
Neuroblastomas account for more than 7% of malignancies in patients less than 15 years of age and around 15%

Box 28.2 Differential diagnosis of abdominal mass in children

Neonates

Neoplastic

- Teratomas
- Liver hemangiomas

Gastrointestinal

- Intestinal duplication
- Mesentery cysts
- Choledochal cysts

Renal

- Polycystic kidney disease
- Hydronephrosis

Ovarian

- Ovarian cysts
- Ovarian teratomas

Infants and older children

Neoplastic

- Hepatocellular carcinomas
- Hepatoblastomas
- Neuroblastoma
- Wilms tumor
- Teratomas
- Retroperitoneal paraganglioma
- Lymphomas
- Rhabdomyosarcoma

Infectious causes

- Hydatid cysts
- Toxic megacolon
- Retroperitoneal/intra-abdominal abscess

Other

- Impacted feces
- Mesenteric cysts
- Intussusception
- Volvulus

Box 28.3 Studies used when evaluating abdominal mass

Laboratory studies

- Complete blood count with differential white count
- Serum chemistry
- Serum electrolyte levels
- Liver function tests
- Plasma catecholamine levels
- Serum β-chorionic gonadotropin
- Serum α-fetoprotein levels
- Urinalysis
- Uric acid and lactate dehydrogenase concentrations
- Urine for vanillylmandelic acid and catecholamine concentrations

Radiographic imaging studies

- Plain abdominal x-ray
- Abdominal sonogram
- CT scan or MRI study of the abdomen
- MIBG scan

of all pediatric oncology deaths [44]. Approximately 40% of cases are diagnosed by 1 year, 75% by 7 years, and 98% by 10 years of age [45]. More than half of the patients are younger than 2 years old when diagnosed. The incidence of neuroblastoma is slightly more common in boys than girls (ratio of 1.2:1.0) [45]. A familial history of neuroblastoma, with an autosomal dominant pattern of inheritance, has been reported in 1–2% of patients. The median age at diagnosis of familial neuroblastoma is 9 months, com-

pared to 18 months for sporadic cases [44]. Maris et al found that 20% of patients with familial neuroblastomas have bilateral or multifocal tumors with evidence for a locus on chromosome 16p12–13 [46]. Approximately 75% of cases of abdominal neuroblastomas have metastasis at diagnosis, the most common sites being lymph nodes, bone marrow, liver, and skin.

Clinical presentation

The clinical presentation of neuroblastomas varies, depending on the site of the primary disease, the extent of metastasis, the size of the tumor, and any associated paraneoplastic syndromes. Patients in the early stage of the disease may have non-specific symptoms, such as pain and generalized malaise. Between 50% and 75% of patients present with an abdominal mass and may have abdominal pain and abdominal distension, weight loss, failure to thrive, fever, and anemia [45]. Tumors producing catecholamine cause hypertension in 25% of patients. Thoracic tumors may be discovered accidentally on a chest radiograph or when the patient shows signs of Horner syndrome (ptosis, miosis, enophthalmos, anhydrosis, and heterochromia of the iris) on the affected side. Patients with metastatic neuroblastomas can present with proptosis and periorbital ecchymosis, often referred to as "raccoon eyes." Infants with neuroblastomas can have hypokalemia and intractable diarrhea with watery, explosive stools. The diarrhea is thought to be the result of tumor-produced vasoactive intestinal polypeptide.

Diagnosis

Neuroblastomas are diagnosed by serological and urine examinations and by radiological and isotope studies.

While there are no specific serum markers for neuroblastoma, high levels of ferritin, neuron-specific enolase, and lactate dehydrogenase are often present [47]; patients occasionally have high levels of serum and urinary catecholamines. Immunological analysis of serum and bone marrow is sensitive for detection of tumor cells. Radiographic examinations include plain x-rays of the abdomen, CT scan, helical (spiral) CT, MRI, and isotope bone scans. Once the diagnosis is made, the disease is staged according to the International Neuroblastoma Staging System (INSS). The INSS score is one of the main clinical variables used to predict outcomes of patients with neuroblastomas.

Management

Surgery, chemotherapy, radiation therapy, and immunotherapy are the main treatment modalities for neuroblastoma. Surgery is beneficial for patients who have localized tumors. However, more than half of children with neuroblastomas present with metastatic, unresectable tumors. When this occurs, they are initially treated with chemotherapy followed by tumor resection. Children with high-risk neuroblastomas undergo multimodal therapy, including induction of chemotherapy, surgical resection of the primary tumor, radiation therapy, and consolidation chemotherapy.

Surgical resection of the tumor

When children with neuroblastoma present for surgery, a complete history and physical examination and preoperative consultation with the patient's primary physician are important. Evaluation of the complete blood count, serum electrolyte concentrations, echocardiography, and radiological studies is also important. Knowledge of the chemotherapeutic drugs and steroids used is important as both therapies can cause complications.

Intraoperative anesthetic management consists of general anesthesia, tracheal intubation, standard monitoring plus intra-arterial and central venous monitoring. Occasionally neuroblastomas behave like pheochromocytomas.

Pheochromocytoma

Pheochromocytomas arise from catecholamine-producing chromaffin cells and are of neuroectodermal origin. These cells are found anywhere in the sympathoadrenal system but arise most commonly from the adrenal medulla. Tumors arising from extra-adrenal sympathetic and parasympathetic paraganglia are classified as extra-adrenal paragangliomas. Pheochromocytomas and *sympathetic* paragangliomas secrete catecholamines, but most *parasympathetic* paragangliomas are non-secretory. Pheochromocytomas secrete large amounts of adrenaline, noradrenaline, and dopamine, plus various peptides and ectopic hormones: enkephalin, somatostatin, calcitonin, oxytocin, vasopressin, insulin and adrenocorticotropic hormones [48]. Data on the etiology, diagnosis and management of pheochromocytoma in children are limited.

Epidemiology

Pheochromocytomas are one-tenth as common in children as in adults (1 in 500,000 children compared to 1 in 50,000 in adults) [49]. Approximately 10% of tumors are bilateral, 10% are extra-adrenal, 10% are malignant, and 10% are familial. In children, 70% of the tumors are bilateral and extra-adrenal, the majority of them benign [50]. Advances in molecular genetics have allowed mutations in germline cells to be identified in 59% of patients presenting at 18 or fewer years of age and in 70% of patients presenting before age 10 years. The inherited predisposition is related to mutation(s) in the von Hippel–Lindau (VHL) gene, which encodes the subunits B and D of succinate dehydrogenase (SDHB and SDHD) and also the RET proto-oncogene that predisposes patients to the development of multiple endocrine neoplasia type 2 (MEN2) or neurofibromatosis type 1 (NF1). The VHL gene is the most commonly mutated gene in children who present with pheochromocytoma [51].

Though rare, pheochromocytomas may present in the neonatal period. However, they present more commonly in older, male children. There is a female preponderance for the disease during the reproductive years, suggesting a hormonal influence.

Clinical presentation

Patients with pheochromocytomas are thin, anorexic, and hypermetabolic. The most common symptoms include headaches, flushing, palpitations, hypertension, and sweating. Central nervous system manifestations include tremors, nervousness, anxiety, visual disturbances, and psychosis. Cardiovascular symptoms include hypertension, ventricular arrhythmias, cardiomyopathy, and cardiac failure. Some patients have symptoms of gastrointestinal disturbances.

Diagnosis

Pheochromocytoma is diagnosed by biochemical testing and imaging studies. Measurement of 24-h urinary vanillylmandelic acid, total metanephrine, and catecholamine concentrations is valuable [52]. Urinary metanephrine levels are increased in 95% of cases, and vanillylmandelic acid and catecholamine levels are increased in approximately 90% of patients [53]. Plasma catecholamine concentrations that exceed 2000 pg/mL during an hypertensive episode are diagnostic of pheochromocytoma. Normal levels are not. Plasma catecholamine levels between 500 and 1000 pg/mL are suggestive of pheochromocytoma, but further work-up is required [54].

Computed tomographic or MRI scans and ^{123}I-labeled metaiodobenzyl guanidine (MIBG) scintigraphy are all also helpful in making the diagnosis [55]. Abnormal neuroectodermal tissue takes up the isotope, which produces a focal area of increased uptake on the scan. These scans help localize extra-adrenal tumors. Positron emission tomography with 18F fluorodeoxyglucose or hydroxyephedrine is also useful for localizing tumors [56].

Management

Surgical excision of the tumor is the definitive treatment, but this requires optimization of the patient's condition medically before surgery. The goals of medical management include normalization of the arterial blood pressure and heart rate, restoration of blood volume, and prevention of a hypertensive crisis and its subsequent consequences.

Preoperative preparation of the patient should begin at least 10–14 days before surgery. Initial treatment includes α-adrenoreceptor blockade to reduce catecholamine-induced vasoconstriction and its sequelae [57]. Phenoxybenzamine is a non-selective α_1 and α_2 non-competitive blocker that is administered orally in doses of 0.5–1 mg/kg twice a day. The dose is adjusted according to the patient's response to the drug. Phentolamine, a competitive non-selective α-adrenergic blocker, is also used as an adjunct. Adequate α-blockade is demonstrated by the presence of normotension or by the presence of side-effects to the drug, such as orthostatic hypotension tachycardia, nasal congestion, and dizziness [57]. The unopposed β-stimulation following α-blockade causes tachycardia and arrhythmias, which are controlled by β-adrenergic receptor-blocking agents, such as propranolol or labetalol. β-Receptor blockade should never be initiated until α-blockade is fully accomplished because a severe hypertensive crisis can occur due to unopposed α-stimulation. Occasionally, α-methyl-para-tyrosine (metyrosine), which competitively inhibits tyrosine hydroxylase, the rate-limiting step in catecholamine biosynthesis, is added [58] to reduce catecholamine stores in the tumor.

Patients with pheochromocytomas are generally intravascular volume depleted and have circulating plasma volumes of about 15% below normal. Once adequate pharmacological blockade is established, volume resuscitation is required.

Anesthetic management of patients with pheochromocytomas consists of providing stable anesthesia and avoiding surges in catecholamines. In spite of optimal medical management, patients can and do have sudden blood pressure fluctuations during induction of anesthesia and tracheal intubation, during surgical manipulation of the tumor, and after ligation of the tumor's venous drainage. Premedication with oral midazolam is often used to treat patient anxiety. General tracheal anesthesia or combined general and epidural anesthesia have been used successfully for intraoperative management of these patients.

Anesthesia is usually induced by mask with sevoflurane or with intravenous propofol or etomidate. Following induction of anesthesia, large-bore intravenous catheters and an arterial line are inserted. Muscle relaxation is achieved with a non-depolarizing muscle relaxant, such as rocuronium, vecuronium or *cis*-atracurium. A central venous catheter is inserted if one is not already in place. Fentanyl, sufentanil or a continuous infusion of remifentanil can be used. Intraoperative hypertension is managed by infusion of sodium nitroprusside, a potent arteriovenodilator. Esmolol is often used to control tachycardia and hypertension.

Hypotension may occur once the adrenal vein is ligated and the tumor is removed. The hypotension usually responds to fluid administration and discontinuation of vasodilators. Occasionally vasopressors, such as phenylephrine or norepinephrine, are required.

After surgery the patients are admitted to the ICU to monitor for and control hypertension, hypotension, and hypoglycemia. Once the tumor is excised, pancreatic β-cell suppression is removed and insulin levels increase, which may cause hypoglycemia. Lipolysis and glycogenolysis cease after tumor removal and α-blockade. Residual adrenergic blockade may mask the signs and symptoms of hypoglycemia. Consequently, blood glucose concentrations should be closely monitored.

If hypertension persists postoperatively, it is likely that there is a second pheochromocytoma. Normalization of catecholamine levels should be confirmed in all patients. Long-term follow-up is required to detect subsequent development of metachronous tumors and to detect tumors at other sites.

Wilms tumor

Wilms tumor (nephroblastoma) is the most common renal neoplasm affecting children. Diagnosis and treatment of Wilms tumor are discussed in Chapter 29.

Liver tumors

Liver tumors account for 1% of all pediatric tumors. Hepatoblastoma and hepatocellular carcinomas are responsible for most hepatic malignancies during childhood. Two-thirds of all liver tumors are hepatoblastomas. Benign liver tumors include vascular tumors, hamartomas, adenomas, and focal nodular hyperplasia. With advances in surgical technique, anesthesia, and chemotherapy, the 5-year survival of patients with hepatoblastoma has improved from 35% three decades ago to 75% at the present time [59]. However, the prognosis for patients with hepatocellular carcinoma remains poor.

Epidemiology

Hepatoblastoma and hepatocellular carcinomas occur more commonly in males and are more common in 0.5–3-year-old children, the median age at diagnosis being 18 months. Only 5% of new hepatoblastomas are diagnosed in children beyond 4 years of age. Other conditions associated with hepatoblastoma include Beckwith–Wiedemann syndrome, familial adenomatous polyposis, hemihypertrophy, and low birthweight. Hepatocellular carcinomas are diagnosed after 10 years of age and commonly occur in patients with underlying liver disease, such as cirrhosis, tyrosinemia, and other inherited metabolic disorders [60]. Genetic aberrations in several chromosomes have been identified that predispose patients to the development of malignant liver tumors.

Clinical presentation

Most children who have liver cancers present with a painless palpable abdominal mass. They may also have abdominal distension, anorexia, weight loss, and fatigue. Occasionally they present with abdominal pain, constipation, jaundice or sexual precocity.

Diagnosis

Laboratory and imaging studies are key to the diagnosis of liver tumors. Laboratory studies include complete blood count, chemistry panel, liver function tests, coagulation profile, and serum α-fetoprotein (AFP) concentrations. AFP concentrations are the most sensitive laboratory test for hepatoblastoma and hepatocellular carcinomas, but this test is non-specific. On occasion, hepatoblastomas secrete β-human chorionic gonadotropin. Imaging studies, such as CT scan of the abdomen, ultrasonography, MRI, and magnetic resonance angiography, are also useful in diagnosing these tumors. The diagnosis is ultimately made, however, by liver biopsy.

Management

Treatment of hepatoblastoma has improved markedly during the past several decades. Primary resection of benign liver tumors and stage I hepatoblastoma is curative. Unresectable tumors are initially treated with vincristine, cisplatin, and fluorouracil before the tumors are resected. If the tumor remains unresectable despite chemotherapy and is not metastatic, orthotopic liver transplantation is considered.

Preoperative assessment determines the extent of the tumor, whether it has metastasized, and if the patient has received chemotherapy. Careful attention should be paid to the patient's laboratory tests, liver function, blood count, coagulation status, and pulmonary, renal, and cardiac function, especially after chemotherapy. Patients should be typed and cross-matched for packed red blood cells and should have fresh frozen plasma and platelets available before and during surgery.

Anesthetic management of patients with liver tumors is challenging. Standard anesthesia induction agents are used. Tracheal intubation is facilitated with muscle relaxants, preferably *cis*-atracurium because its hepatic metabolism is minor. Standard monitors, plus intra-arterial and a central venous pressure monitoring, are usually used. Large-bore peripheral venous access is obtained, preferably in the upper extremities. In the event of major blood loss, perfusion, normothermia, and a normal pH should be aggressively maintained. It is occasionally necessary during surgery to quickly resuscitate patients who undergo acute, rapid hemorrhage. The main source of bleeding during liver resection is from the hepatic vein, which has no valves. High venous pressure increases bleeding. By keeping the CVP below $5\,cmH_2O$ during the dissection phase, blood loss can be reduced. Vasopressors (e.g. norepinephrine or vasopressin) may be required to maintain arterial blood pressure during some phases of surgery. Whether the trachea is extubated in the operating room or the ICU depends on the extent of the liver resection, the amount of intraoperative blood loss, and the need for volume resuscitation. Postoperative pain is easily managed with a PCA.

Key points

- Neuroblastoma, Wilms tumor, and hepatomas are the most common intra-abdominal tumors in children.
- Neuroblastomas account for about 7% of malignancies in patients younger than 15 years of age and 15% of all pediatric oncology deaths.
- Diagnosis of neuroblastoma requires serological and urine examinations and both radiological and isotope studies.
- Measuring 24-h urinary concentrations of vanillylmandelic acid, total metanephrine, and catecholamines makes the diagnosis of pheochromocytoma.
- Preoperative preparation for pheochromocytoma surgery should begin with phenoxybenzamine-induced α-blockade prior to surgery.
- Hepatoblastoma and hepatocellular carcinomas are the most frequent hepatic malignancies of childhood.

Inguinal hernia

An inguinal hernia is a protrusion of intestine through an open processus vaginalis (Fig. 28.1). An incarcerated hernia is an hernia that is irreducible and does not slide back into the abdominal cavity. When bowel entrapment interferes with the vascular supply of the bowel, the hernia is said to be strangulated.

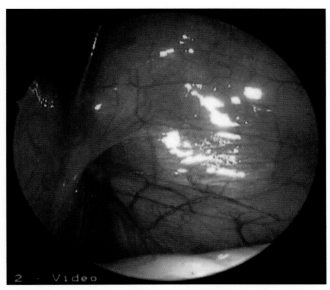

Figure 28.1 Laparoscopic view of a right inguinal hernia in a 2-month-old child.

Table 28.1 Characteristics of inguinal hernias

	Simple	Incarcerated	Strangulated
Hernia sac	Herniates with Valsalva maneuver	Reducible	May or may not be reducible
Pain	No pain	Tender	Tender
Vascular supply	Intact	Intact	Compromised
Urgency	Elective	Within 24–72 h after reduction	Urgent

Epidemiology

Inguinal hernia repair is the most common elective procedure performed in pediatric patients. It occurs in 4.4% of all pediatric patients and is more common in males. Its incidence is 10–30% in premature infants versus 3–5% in full-term neonates [61,62]. Connective tissue disorders and cystic fibrosis also increase the incidence of inguinal hernia. Incarcerated hernias are more frequent in premature babies [63].

Clinical presentation and diagnosis

Inguinal hernias are diagnosed by physical examination when a bulge is felt at the internal or external inguinal ring. Most inguinal hernias are not painful, but large hernias may be. The bulge frequently disappears during sleep or rest. A Valsalva maneuver (e.g. crying) often provokes the bulge. The differential diagnosis of inguinal hernia includes hydrocele, retractable testis, lymphadenopathy, and a neoplastic process. Ultrasound helps diagnose a patent processus vaginalis. Patients with incarcerated hernias present with a tender firm mass in the groin. These children are often inconsolable and may have anorexia. The "silk glove sign" (thickened peritoneum of the patent process vaginalis that can be felt during palpation of the cord) is suggestive of an inguinal hernia [64].

Management

Inguinal hernias do not heal spontaneously, but hydroceles often heal during the first year of life. These hernias require surgical repair to reduce the risk of developing an incarcerated hernia. Incarcerated hernias can usually be manually reduced. Once reduced, the hernia should be repaired during the next 24–48 h to prevent recurrence of the incarceration [65]. If the hernia cannot be reduced, it may progress to strangulation, necrosis, and gangrene of the bowel. Strangulated hernias require immediate surgical correction. General anesthesia and muscle relaxation often make a non-reducible hernia reducible. Some patients with strangulated hernias have necrotic bowel and require bowel resection during herniorrhaphy. Table 28.1 details the characteristics of inguinal hernias.

Children who are <6 months of age are at increased risk for developing strangulated or incarcerated hernias [66]. Consequently, their hernias are usually repaired soon after detection. Whether to operate on the contralateral side is debatable, but 28% of patients with a unilateral, clinically evident hernia early in life subsequently develop a symptomatic contralateral hernia [67]. Fifty percent of <2-year-old children have an open processus vaginalis, which should not be confused with an inguinal hernia. Laparoscopic visualization of the contralateral side is very helpful for determining if a second inguinal hernia exists on this side. This can be done even though the primary repair is done conventionally.

Premature babies often have bilateral inguinal hernias. Because of potential pulmonary complications and the fact that the surgical repair may be more difficult, there is controversy regarding when their hernias should be repaired. The reality is that most preterm neonates undergo hernia repair shortly before discharge home from the NICU for fear they will develop an incarcerated hernia.

Depending on co-morbidity and the surgical requirements, neuroaxial anesthesia, general tracheal, laryngeal mask or facemask anesthesia is appropriate. Laryngeal mask airways (LMAs) should be used with caution in preterm infants. A #1 LMA increases the dead space by approximately 100% and may increase the $PaCO_2$ significantly.

Unless the depth of anesthesia is adequate, laryngospasm may develop during surgical manipulation of the hernia sac. Caudal blocks are often used as an adjunct to general anesthesia. In older patients, ileo-inguinal or ileo-hypogastric nerve blocks can be helpful.

Postoperative apnea occurs in 20–30% of otherwise healthy former preterm infants who undergo inguinal hernia repair [68]. The risk for postoperative apnea decreases with increasing post-conceptional age [69]. Spinal anesthesia is often used for these patients, although doing so does not decrease the incidence of apnea and bradycardia [70]. Ex-premature infants <60 weeks post-conception and full term neonates <45 weeks post-conception are usually admitted to hospital overnight for apnea monitoring.

Long-term outcome
In one study 28% of patients with a unilateral, clinically evident hernia had a symptomatic contralateral hernia later in life. The recurrence rate of an inguinal hernia repaired early in infancy is under 5% [71].

Key points
- Inguinal hernias are common in preterm infants.
- Determine if the hernia is non-incarcerated, incarcerated or strangulated.
- Spinal anesthesia for premature infants does not reduce the incidence of postoperative apnea.

Pyloric stenosis

Epidemiology
The incidence of idiopathic hypertrophic pyloric stenosis (IHPS) is 2–4 per 1000 livebirths, with a female-to-male preponderance of 1:3. Recently, the incidence of IHPS has decreased in some countries. Premature infants develop IHPS later than full-term infants [72].

Etiology
The mechanism for hypertrophy of the pyloric muscle is unknown, but the hypertrophy causes the gastroenteral obstruction (Fig. 28.2). The increased frequency of the condition in males and in first-born infants who have a positive family history for IHPS suggests that the lesion has a genetic predisposition. Feeding-related, environmental factors, duodenal feeding of premature infants, and erythromycin exposure have all been suggested as causes of IHPS. The pyloric muscle fibers are hypertrophic (not increased in number) and are markedly thickened and edematous. After a pyloromyotomy, the pyloric muscle becomes completely normal over time.

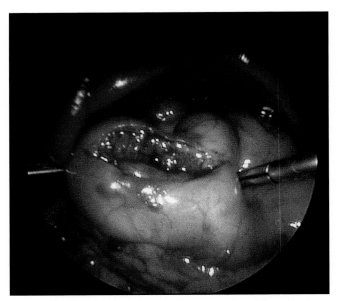

Figure 28.2 Pyloromyotomy. Note that the pyloric muscle has been partially transected and left open to heal. This increases the opening of the pylorus.

Clinical presentation and diagnosis
Between the second and 12th (classically between the third and eighth) weeks of life, most patients with IHPS present with non-bilious, projectile vomiting. The differential diagnosis includes overfeeding, pylorospasm, gastroparesis, gastroesophageal reflux, and duodenal bands. Patients with pyloric stenosis are usually hungry and alert. When dehydration develops, they become lethargic.

The diagnosis of IPHS is usually confirmed by ultrasound. A barium swallow may be indicated if the ultrasound study is inconclusive. The hypertrophic pylorus can often be palpated through the abdominal wall. Careful observation of the child after feeding often reveals a characteristic peristaltic wave moving across the epigastrium. Historically, patients presented at an advanced stage of the disease. Now widespread use of ultrasound and much better understanding of the disease by pediatricians allow the diagnosis to be made earlier. Consequently, fewer patients have severe electrolyte disturbances and dehydration at presentation.

If the diagnosis is made late, patients typically are dehydrated, hypochloremic, hypokalemic, and alkalotic at presentation. They may have lost weight and have gastritis with minor gastrointestinal bleeding. Initially these patients have an alkaline urine and loss of potassium and sodium as renal compensation for their vomiting. Later they secrete acidic urine, which further increases the metabolic alkalosis. This paradoxical aciduria occurs once potassium and sodium are depleted (Fig. 28.3).

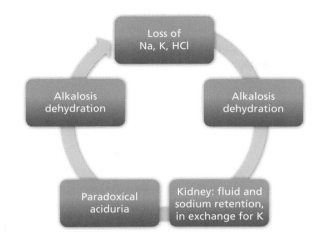

Figure 28.3 Pathophysiology of pyloric stenosis.

Hypocalcemia often accompanies the hyponatremia. If this downward spiral is allowed to continue and additional fluid losses occur, prerenal azotemia, hypovolemic shock, and metabolic acidemia ensue.

Management

Idiopathic hypertrophic pyloric stenosis and concomitant hypovolemia represent a *medical* not a surgical emergency. The hypovolemia, acid–base abnormalities, and electrolyte abnormalities must be corrected prior to the induction of anesthesia. Surgery for IHPS is urgent but is not an emergency. These patients should be made nil per os (NPO) and their stomachs should be decompressed. Intravenous fluid therapy usually includes normal saline (NS), D5–½ NS or ¼ NS at 1.5 times the maintenance fluid requirements. Care should be taken not to give excessive dilute solutions as they may cause seizures and death. Sufficient glucose should be provided to maintain normal blood glucose levels. Once satisfactory urine output is achieved, potassium can be added to the IV fluids. Homeostasis, as reflected by a serum chloride concentration >100 mEq/L and a serum bicarbonate concentration of <30 mEq/L, should be achieved before surgery commences. Urine chloride concentrations >20 mEq/L suggest adequate restoration of intravascular volume, since the kidney retains chloride during volume contraction. An underlying deficiency in glucuronyltransferase is responsible for jaundice in 2% of patients.

Before tracheal intubation, atropine is often given to prevent bradycardia, and the stomach is suctioned while tilting the patient in four different directions to empty the stomach as thoroughly as possible [73]. It is occasionally necessary to lavage the stomach to remove barium or milk curds. The high risk for aspiration of gastric contents warrants intubating the trachea awake or after a rapid-sequence induction or modified rapid-sequence induc-

tion of anesthesia and muscle paralysis with either succinylcholine or a non-depolarizing muscle relaxant. Intraoperatively, air is injected into the stomach through an orogastric catheter to verify the integrity of the duodenal mucosa. Preoperative cerebrospinal fluid alkalosis increases respiratory sensitivity to opioids. Consequently, these drugs are usually avoided because they can slow awakening from anesthesia and cause apnea. Acetaminophen per rectum and infiltration of the wound with local anesthetics are often sufficient for postoperative pain management. Pyloromyotomy can be done open or laparoscopically. The hospital length of stay and postoperative complications are similar with both techniques. Most patients have their trachea extubated at the conclusion of surgery. However, the presence of metabolic alkalosis increases their probability of postoperative apnea. Other common complications of a pyloromyotomy include perforation of the duodenal mucosa (1–2%), wound infection, incisional hernia, incomplete myotomy, and bowel injury [74]. Oral feeds are usually instituted several hours after surgery. Some patients have persistent postoperative vomiting from gastroesophageal reflux or an incomplete myotomy.

In developing countries where access to surgery is inadequate or totally lacking, medical management alone is provided. This consists of fluid and electrolyte replacement and administration of atropine to slow gastrointestinal peristalsis and decrease hypertrophy of the pylorus.

Key points
- Pyloric stenosis is a medical emergency, not a surgical emergency.
- Allow time for adequate preoperative rehydration and correction of electrolytes.
- Tracheal intubation is by rapid-sequence induction or awake.
- Opioids are avoided because they delay awakening from anesthesia and may increase apnea and the need for postoperative mechanical ventilation.

Appendicitis

Epidemiology

Acute appendicitis is the most common abdominal condition requiring surgical intervention. Four out of 1000 patients under 14 years of age will be diagnosed with appendicitis, and their lifetime risk for appendicitis is 7%. No single test, examination or symptom confirms the diagnosis in all cases. About 0.2–0.8% of patients with appendicitis die of complications of the disease. The rate of appendiceal perforation in <4-year-old children is 80–100%, whereas it is 10–20% in children 10–17 years of age. The symptoms of appendicitis in younger children are

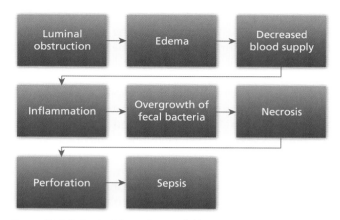

Figure 28.4 Pathophysiology of appendicitis.

often more diffuse [75], which makes the diagnosis more difficult to make. The atypical presentation increases the perforation rate in children [76].

Etiology and pathophysiology

Appendicitis is caused by luminal obstruction of the appendix by edema, inflammation, and overgrowth of fecal bacteria (Fig. 28.4). Lymphoid hyperplasia, a foreign body or fecal matter causes the obstruction. If edema reduces the arterial blood supply, necrosis and perforation of the appendix may occur.

Clinical presentation and diagnosis

The diagnosis of appendicitis is often challenging because the position of the appendix within the abdomen varies. Only half of all patients have the classic symptoms of anorexia and periumbilical pain plus nausea, vomiting, and right lower quadrant pain. About one-third of patients present with atypical symptoms or are unable to describe their symptoms. In children, this leads to a false-negative appendectomy rate of 5–25%. Examinations by CT scan with contrast or ultrasound reduce the false–negative rate. The differential diagnoses include gastroenteritis, tubo-ovarian processes, mesenteric adenitis, cholecystitis, diverticulitis, pelvic inflammatory disease, ureterolithiasis and more. Appendicitis rarely occurs in neonates, and when it does occur the symptoms are virtually indistinguishable from necrotizing enterocolitis [77].

Management

Fluid resuscitation and administration of intravenous broad-spectrum antibiotics that cover enteric organisms are required. Patients with a ruptured appendix require antibiotics until their clinical condition improves. The clinical goal is to perform an appendectomy before the appendix ruptures and to prevent peritonitis, sepsis, and abscess formation. Immediate surgery is not necessary if

the appendix is unruptured and the patient has been appropriately treated with antibiotics [78].

Most appendectomies are done laparoscopically because the incisions are smaller, there are fewer wound infections, and the incidence of ileus is lower. Initial experience with laparoscopic appendectomy suggested a higher incidence of intra-abdominal abscesses, but later studies have not confirmed this.

Anesthetic management

Anesthetic management of children undergoing appendectomy is usually straightforward and usually includes general endotracheal anesthesia. Rapid-sequence induction of anesthesia is used to avoid aspiration of gastric contents. If patients are septic and have a ruptured appendix, aggressive fluid resuscitation is often required. Surgical manipulation of an infected abdomen may induce acute hemodynamic deterioration. Ketorolac plus opioids are usually sufficient for postoperative analgesia after endoscopic surgery. Patient-controlled analgesia is seldom required if the appendix was not ruptured.

Key points

- Rapid-sequence induction of anesthesia is usually required to reduce aspiration of gastric contents.
- Beware of contrast material given as part of the evaluation for appendicitis.
- Patients with a ruptured appendix require additional fluid resuscitation.

SPECIFIC INTERVENTIONAL AND SURGICAL PROCEDURES

Gastrointestinal/endoscopic retrograde cholangiopancreatography/endoscopy procedures

Sedation is adequate for most endoscopic procedures in adults, but children usually require general anesthesia. Since many of the procedures are done in non-operating room locations, it is important that operating room standards be applied when anesthetizing patients in these locations. This includes preoperative evaluation, monitoring, postoperative care, and having help readily available in case a problem arises.

Anesthesiologists must understand the technical aspects of endoscopic procedures, some of which require multiple switching of endoscopes during the procedure for ultrasound examinations, banding varices, obtaining biopsies, and other interventions. Occasionally, the endoscope completely compresses the trachea and/or tracheal tube of an infant and obstructs the airway. Excessive insufflation of gas at high pressures and overdistension of the stomach and bowel may interfere with ventilation. Insufflation pressures should be kept at a minimum, usually 12 cmH$_2$O. At the end of the procedure, the stomach should be suctioned to remove as much gas and secretions as possible. Inserting a rectal tube may aid gas removal. Where multiple instruments are to be inserted through the esophagus or when contrast material or other fluids will be given into the esophagus or stomach during the procedure, it is advisable to intubate the trachea and secure the airway [79].

Esophago-gastro-duodenoscopy

Indications for esophago-gastro-duodenoscopies include gastroesophageal reflux and sclerotherapy for esophageal varices. Most anesthesiologists use inhalational induction of anesthesia if the patient has mild-to-moderate gastro-esophageal reflux disease (GERD). It is usually safer and easier to secure the airway of younger children with a tracheal tube, but some older children can be managed with intravenous anesthesia and a natural airway.

Insertion of the endoscope into the esophagus is the most stimulating part of the procedure and requires the deepest plane of anesthesia when procedures are done with natural airways. Antiflexion of the neck makes insertion of the endoscope easier. The oropharynx can be anesthetized with local anesthetics, but doing so may leave the child without protective airway reflexes after the procedure and increase the likelihood of coughing spells and/or aspiration of fluids.

Most esophago-gastro-duodenoscopies take only a few minutes. If general anesthesia and tracheal intubation are used, it is helpful to avoid the use of muscle relaxants and to administer short-acting opioids, such as remifentanil, for the induction and maintenance of anesthesia. Tracheal intubated patients are usually placed in the supine position for esophago-gastro-duodenoscopies. Patients with eosinophilic esophagitis must undergo repeated esophago-gastro-duodenoscopies. They frequently have multiple food allergies, including to soy and eggs, which contraindicate the use of propofol. They may also have asthma and atopic dermatitis so histamine-releasing drugs should be avoided [80].

Endoscopic retrograde cholangiopancreatography

Endoscopic retrograde cholangiopancreatography (ERCP) is used for patients with choledocholithiasis, for stent placement across malignant or benign strictures, and for tissue sampling [81]. Tracheal intubation is usually required when children undergo ERCP because the procedure can be long, patients are in the semi-prone position, and the use of multiple endoscopes may be required. These patients are often in acute distress from acute cholestasis and cholecystitis; they may also be dehydrated

from prolonged anorexia, nausea, and vomiting. Injection of incremental doses of glucagon may be required during the procedure to increase bile duct motility.

Percutaneous endoscopic gastrostomy

A percutaneous endoscopic gastrostomy (PEG) allows placement of a gastrostomy tube without the need for a laparotomy. PEGs are usually indicated for prolonged nutritional support or decompression of the stomach, although they may not effectively do the latter. Surgical access to the stomach is identical to that used during an esophago-gastro-duodenoscopy; some surgeons verify placement of the gastrostomy by doing a mini-laparoscopy to rule out having produced a gastrocolic fistula.

The underlying disease (cerebral palsy, metabolic disease, congenital malformations) dictates the anesthetic management. Patients who have a PEG in place should have their stomach decompressed prior to and during the induction of inhalational anesthesia. Venting the stomach requires the use of a specific venting tube; the tubes used for feeding do not effectively allow air to escape from the stomach.

Colonoscopies

Colonoscopies are usually done in children who have inflammatory bowel disease or lower intestinal bleeding. Bowel preparation is required and may cause dehydration and electrolyte imbalances. In older children tracheal intubation is often not required for this procedure.

Key points

- Standards for monitoring and patient care in off-site areas should be the same as those used in the OR.
- Secure the airway in smaller children when the esophagus is being instrumented.
- Specific tubes (not feeding tubes) are required to vent gas through a PEG.

Nissen fundoplication and gastrostomy

Gastroesophageal reflux is, to a certain extent, a physiological mechanism. The most common symptoms of this disorder in children are vomiting and regurgitation, pulmonary symptoms, dysphagia, abdominal pain, and hemorrhage [82]. In severe cases, life-threatening aspiration of gastric contents may have occurred.

Fundoplication is indicated for patients who have documented gastroesophageal reflux and fail medical treatment, have recurrent aspiration of gastric contents, intermittent apnea, failure to thrive, and Barrett esophagitis. Infants who have had life-threatening events and gastroesophageal reflux frequently present for a fundoplication after other causes for these problems have been ruled out. In one case series, the life-threatening events resolved in most patients after surgery [83]. Neurologically impaired children who require a gastrostomy tube for feeding may also require fundoplication to prevent aspiration of gastric contents [84].

During a Nissen fundoplication, the fundus of the stomach is plicated 360° around the inferior esophagus to restore lower esophageal sphincter function. Once this is done, the patient cannot vomit. The anterior or Thal fundoplication, on the other hand, uses only a 270° wrap, which maintains the patient's ability to vomit. Intestinal obstruction is common after the open approach [85]. Inability to vomit can cause progressive intestinal distension, bowel ischemia, and death if the bowel obstruction is not quickly relieved.

Typically patients requiring a fundoplication have other underlying diseases, such as cerebral palsy, inborn error of metabolism, trisomy 21 or other neurological impairments. The procedure is done either open or laparoscopically, and if needed, a gastrostomy is placed at same time. If a gastrostomy is placed without doing a fundoplication, the percutaneous approach is usually used.

Management
Symptoms of aspiration pneumonia or asthma may make it difficult to determine when to perform the procedure. One has to balance protecting the lungs from further aspirations with being able to improve the patient's pulmonary status. Rapid-sequence induction of anesthesia is usually warranted. The trachea of most patients can be extubated at the end of the procedure, depending on their preoperative status.

Postoperative issues
The reoperation rate following Nissen fundoplication for recurrent gastroesophageal reflux is high (6–12%) [86].

Key points
- The primary disease often dictates the anesthetic management.
- There is a high risk for aspiration of gastric contents during the induction of anesthesia.
- Patients may present with a suboptimal pulmonary status due to aspiration pneumonia.
- Patients who require a gastrostomy frequently have a Nissen fundoplication to protect against aspiration of gastric contents.

Laparoscopic surgery

Laparoscopic procedures are rapidly replacing many open pediatric surgical procedures (Box 28.4). Some

Box 28.4 Common pediatric laparoscopic procedures

- Appendectomy
- Cholecystectomy
- Gastric banding
- Gastric bypass
- Colectomy
- Inguinal hernia repair
- Nephrectomy
- Pyloromyotomy
- Congenital diaphragmatic hernia
- Nissen fundoplication
- Orchidopexy
- Pyloplasty

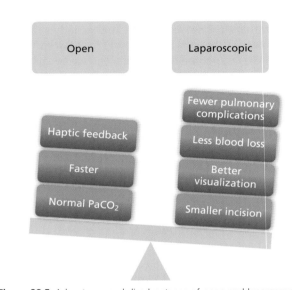

Figure 28.5 Advantages and disadvantages of open and laparoscopic procedures.

advantages of the laparoscopic approach include minimizing the size of the incision and better visualization of the surgical area (Fig. 28.5). The pathophysiological changes associated with a pneumoperitoneum, the longer operating times, mechanical restrictions for the surgeon, and lack of haptic feedback and three-dimensional vision are the main drawbacks of laparoscopic surgery. A number of procedures are done laparoscopically without proof that the outcomes are better than those reported with open procedures.

Laparoscopic abdominal procedures require intraperitoneal access and insufflation of gas, often through the umbilicus. At least one additional incision is required for instrumentation. Various instruments are needed for ligation, stapling, suturing, and manipulation of viscera, but some are impractical for neonatal use because they are too large.

Nissen fundoplication, pyloromyotomy, and repair of tracheo-esophageal fistulas are examples of laparoscopic procedures commonly performed in pediatric patients.

Pathophysiology

The effect of increased intra-abdominal pressure and absorption of the insufflated gas are the two main pathophysiological changes associated with laparoscopic surgery.

Hemodynamic changes

Changes in cardiac output (CO) differ, depending on the patient's position during the procedure.

Patients placed in the reverse Trendelenburg position, e.g. for laparoscopic cholecystectomy, often experience decreased arterial blood pressure, cardiac output, right atrial pressure, and wedge pressure. Pneumoperitoneum often raises the arterial, right atrial, and wedge pressures to their initial levels. Cardiac output also returns to baseline; systemic vascular resistance decreases mildly [87]. The reason why cardiac output normalizes is unclear, but it may be from reduced afterload or activation of the sympathetic nervous system by absorbed carbon dioxide.

In the Trendelenburg position, cardiac output is unchanged or mildly increased from baseline during pneumoperitoneum. The increased intra-abdominal pressure and gravity synergistically reduce cardiac filling.

Changes in arterial blood pressure and pulmonary vascular resistance are independent of the patient's position during laparoscopy. Systemic vascular resistance (SVR) and arterial blood pressure increase. The combination of tachycardia and an elevated SVR raises myocardial oxygen consumption. Insufflation pressures below $10 \text{cmH}_2\text{O}$ have no significant effects on heart rate, arterial blood pressure, oxygen saturation or base excess in children [88].

Absorbed carbon dioxide partially alleviates the effects of the increased intra-abdominal pressure. However, increased intra-abdominal pressure may also produce transient oliguria of the splanchnic and renal vessels. Congestion and stasis of the lower extremities increase the risk for deep vein thrombosis. If there is a patent foramen ovale, the likelihood of paradoxical emboli and air embolism increases when the right atrial pressure rises. Peritoneal stretching may also produce vagally mediated hemodynamic changes.

Absorption of insufflated carbon dioxide

Carbon dioxide is absorbed from the abdominal cavity and causes respiratory acidosis and cardiac arrhythmias (in some patients). The rate of CO_2 absorption is higher when artificial cavities are created (e.g. nephrectomy) [89]. The rate of CO_2 absorption is very high when sub-

cutaneous emphysema is present. Ventilation may increase as much as 400% in response to the CO_2 [90]. Occasionally the increase in ventilation is insufficient to reduce the $PaCO_2$ to acceptable levels. When this occurs, the procedure must be halted and time allowed for return of the $PaCO_2$ to normal. It is rarely necessary to convert to an open procedure because of hypercarbia.

Pulmonary pathophysiology

The usual anesthesia-induced decrease in functional residual capacity and the mismatch of ventilation and perfusion are aggravated by a further decrease in the functional residual capacity as the diaphragm is shifted more cephalad by the pneumoperitoneum. Due to the geometry of the infant's thorax (see Chapter 6), infants rely more on diaphragmatic excursion than on the intercostal muscles for ventilation. Positive end-expiratory pressure counteracts gas-induced pressure on the diaphragm and often improves ventilation and oxygenation. The tip of the tracheal tube can migrate towards the carina and enter a mainstem bronchus when a pneumoperitoneum is present [91].

Despite the negative intraoperative effects of the pneumoperitoneum, there are fewer postoperative pulmonary complications after laparoscopy than with conventional open procedures. On the other hand, the open approach for upper abdominal procedures decreases the vital capacity, FEV_1, and functional residual capacity. These decreases, plus the incisional pain, inhibit coughing and sighing. Laparoscopic cholecystectomy is less often associated with postoperative pneumonia [92,93].

Neuroendocrine effects

Surgical-induced inflammatory and immunosuppression responses are fewer with laparoscopic procedures. The concentrations of interleukin-1 and -6 and tumor necrosis factor α are decreased compared with those found after open procedures. Dysfunction of mononuclear and polymorphonuclear cells, which are part of cell-mediated immunity, appears to be less deranged by laparoscopic procedures. The inflammatory effects are of concern with oncological procedures because tumor spread is a major concern.

Complications

Serious laparoscopy-related complications are rare. CO_2 is the gas used most often because it is more rapidly absorbed if it is inadvertently given intravascularly. Massive CO_2 embolism and venous air embolism produce the same sequelae [94]. Untreated pneumothoraces and pneumomediastina can be disastrous. Subcutaneous emphysema usually requires no treatment. CO_2-induced hypercarbia and acidosis occasionally cause cardiac dysrhythmias. Insertion of a trocar occasionally causes hemorrhage and injures internal organs, especially in thinner infants with more elastic abdominal walls [95].

Key points

- Intravenous access should be obtained above the diaphragm because a pneumoperitoneum can decrease blood flow through the inferior vena cava and delay drug and fluid administration.

- Filling pressures are higher during a pneumoperitoneum because the increased intra-abdominal pressure is transmitted in the thorax. Effective transmural pressures are low to normal.
- Changes in cardiac output in response to a pneumoperitoneum differ, depending on the patient's position.
- Urine output decreases transiently.
- Not all patients tolerate a pneumoperitoneum with high insufflation pressures.

CASE STUDY

An 8-month-old, 10 kg child was brought to the emergency room with a history of loss of appetite, vomiting, irritability, and crying. His mother stated that he had had diarrhea for the last 2 days and that his stools were initially watery but were now mucoid and blood tinged at the last diaper change. Only a minimal amount of urine had been noted during the last 8–12 h. The mother also stated that the child was no longer interactive and had become progressively lethargic during the last 2 days.

The emergency room physician saw the mother and child and obtained the following history. The boy was born at full term by normal vaginal delivery; there were no problems before or after birth. He went to the well baby nursery and was discharged home with the mother 24 h later. At home, the baby was feeding well and received his normal immunizations. He was well until 2 days before admission when he became increasingly irritable and had vomiting and diarrhea.

At admission he was found to be lethargic and had a sunken anterior fontanelle, sunken eyes, and dry oral mucous membranes. His heart rate was 160 beats/min, his arterial blood pressure was 80/40 mmHg and his SaO$_2$ was 99% on room air. His abdomen was distended, and there was abdominal tenderness and guarding. An abdominal mass was palpated.

A peripheral intravenous catheter was inserted and 5% dextrose with 0.45% normal saline was infused at 60 mL/h. Blood was sent for complete blood count and chemistry. Plain radiographs of the abdomen showed a paucity of bowel gas and air–fluid levels.

The white cell count was 18,000 mm^3, the hematocrit 40%, and the platelet count 400,000 mm^3. The serum sodium was 138 mEq/L, serum potassium 4.5 meq/L, serum chloride 100 mEq/L, serum bicarbonate 20 mmol/L, and the blood urea nitrogen and creatinine 20 and 0.5 mg/dL respectively. A surgery consult was obtained and a nasogastric tube was inserted. The surgeon entertained a differential diagnosis of bowel obstruction or intussusception and scheduled the child for an emergency exploratory laparotomy.

The anesthesiologist reviewed the patient's history with the mother and examined the child. The child was lethargic. Fluids were infusing through a peripheral intravenous line. After obtaining informed consent, the child was taken to the operating room.

Rapid-sequence induction of general anesthesia and tracheal intubation were planned. Standard monitors were placed, and suction was applied to the nasogastric tube. After preoxygenation, anesthesia was induced with 2 mg/kg of intravenous propofol and 1.2 mg/kg of intravenous rocuronium. Tracheal intubation was rapidly accomplished. A second peripheral intravenous line, an arterial line, and a Foley catheter were inserted. Anesthesia was maintained with sevoflurane and intravenous fentanyl.

The patient was found to have an ileocolic intussusception, which was easily reduced; however, part of the bowel was ischemic and required resection. Intraoperatively, the patient required additional fluid resuscitation with a crystalloid solution. Blood loss was minimal and no blood transfusion was required. At the end of the surgery, the trachea was extubated and the child was transferred to the intensive care unit. His postoperative pain was controlled with a continuous infusion of morphine and nurse-administered rescue boluses of the drug as needed.

This case illustrates the concepts that were explained in this chapter. Intussusception is a common cause of bowel obstruction in children less than 1 year of age, but the cause of intussusception is unknown in 90% of cases. Prompt diagnosis and treatment decrease the mortality and morbidity associated with intussusception.

Preoperative assessment should include signs of dehydration, such as dry mucosal membranes, sunken fontanelles, sunken eyes, and minimal urine output, which together indicate significant dehydration. Fluid resuscitation should be initiated immediately to replete the intravascular volume. When the volume is repleted, surgery can proceed.

Intraoperatively, the heart rate and arterial blood pressure may not truly reflect the patient's volume status. The urine output should exceed 0.5–1 mL/kg/h; urine output is a useful guide to circulating volume status.

Careful fluid management is essential. The volume of fluid administered equals the sum of hourly maintenance fluid, pre-existing fluid deficits, plus an additional 6–10 mL/kg/h to compensate for the evaporative losses caused by the open abdominal wound.

Hourly fluid maintenance is calculated from the patient's bodyweight (see Chapter 10). For the first 10 kg, it is 4 mL/kg. For 10–20 kg it is 40 mL + 2 mL/kg for every kilogram over 10 kg. If the weight is >20 kg, the requirement is 60 mL + 1 mL/kg for every kilogram above 20 kg.

Careful attention must be paid to blood loss. If significant blood loss is expected, the allowable blood loss should be calculated. Maximum allowable blood loss (MABL) is:

$$\frac{EBV \times (\text{Child's hematocrit} - \text{minimum acceptable hematocrit})}{\text{Child's hematocrit}}$$

The estimated blood volume (EBV) is calculated by:

$$EBV = \text{Weight in kg} \times \text{average blood volume}$$

Estimated blood volume is 95 mL/kg for premature neonates, 85 mL/kg for term neonates, and 65 mL/kg for older children and adults.

The volume of packed red blood cells to be transfused can be determined by the following formula:

$$\frac{EBV \times (\text{desired hematocrit} - \text{present hematocrit})}{\text{Hematocrit of packed red blood cells}}$$

When blood products are used in neonates and infants, they must be filtered and irradiated to prevent emboli and graft-versus-host reactions.

Normothermia is maintained by warming the operating room and the intravenous fluids, using warm irrigation fluids and forced-air convention heating devices. Maintaining normothermia may be difficult during abdominal surgery because the bowels are exposed.

The postoperative decision to extubate the trachea depends on how awake the child is, whether he is breathing spontaneously after the reversal of muscle relaxants, and his core temperature.

Intravenous fluids are continued until oral intake is re-established.

Annotated references

A full reference list for this chapter is available at:
http://www.wiley.com/go/gregory/andropoulos/pediatricanesthesia

2. DiFiore JW. Intussuception. Semin Pediatric Surg 1999; 8: 214–20. This is an excellent review article on intussusceptions, etiology of childhood intussusceptions, and their diagnosis and treatment.

25. Samuel DS. Disorders of intestinal rotation and fixation. In: Grosfeld JL, O'Neill JA Jr, Fonkalsrud EW, Coran AG (eds) Pediatric Surgery. St Louis, MO: Mosby, 2006, pp.1342–57. This book chapter provides excellent illustrations and descriptions of management of malrotation.

42. Mamula P, Markowitz JE, Baldassano RN. Inflammatory bowel disease in early childhood and adolescence: special consideration. Gastroenterol Clin North Am 2003; 32: 967–95. This paper provides special considerations, management, and treatment of inflammatory bowel disease.

44. Maris JM, Hogarty MD, Bagatell R et al. Neuroblastoma. Lancet 2007; 369: 2106–20. This article provides diagnosis, risk stratification and treatment options for neuroblastoma.

65. Lau ST, Lee YH, Caty MG. Current management of hernias and hydroceles. Semin Pediatr Surg 2007; 16: 50–7. This is a very good review of the management of pediatric inguinal hernias and hydroceles.

69. Welborn LG, Rice LJ, Hannallah RS et al. Postoperative apnea in former preterm infants: prospective comparison of spinal and general anesthesia. Anesthesiology 1990; 72: 838–42. A prospective randomized study comparing general anesthesia to spinal anesthesia in former preterm infants.

72. Aspelund G, Langer JC. Current management of hypertrophic pyloric stenosis. Semin Pediatr Surg 2007; 16: 27–33. This review article covers the pathophysiology and management of hypertrophic pyloric stenosis in a clear manner.

84. Novotny NM, Jester AL, Ladd AP. Preoperative prediction of need for fundoplication before gastrostomy tube placement in children. J Pediatr Surg 2009; 44: 173–6; discussion 6–7. This article provides evidence for performing a Nisson fundoplication after a gastrostomy in patients who have cerebral palsy.

92. Putensen-Himmer G, Putensen C, Lammer H et al. Comparison of postoperative respiratory function after laparoscopy or open laparotomy for cholecystectomy. Anesthesiology 1992; 77: 675–80. This randomized study shows that postoperative pulmonary function is less impaired when laparoscopic surgery is done in the upper abdomen.

CHAPTER 29

Anesthesia for Pediatric Urological Procedures

Ira S. Landsman[1], Laura N. Zeigler[1] & Jayant K. Deshpande[2]

[1]Monroe Carell Jr Children's Hospital at Vanderbilt and Department of Anesthesiology, Vanderbilt University Medical Center, Nashville, TN, USA
[2]Department of Pediatrics and Anesthesiology, University of Arkansas for Medical Sciences, Arkansas Children's Hospital, Little Rock, AR, USA

Introduction

Pediatric urological procedures are among the most common encountered by the pediatric anesthesiologist. A thorough understanding of the developmental pathogenesis and surgical procedures of the genitourinary system is important for the anesthesiologist to provide optimized care for these patients. This chapter will review the embryological development of common urogenital anomalies. Then the surgical approach, anesthetic considerations, and anesthetic management of these anomalies, including pain management, will be reviewed.

Development of urological anomalies

Anomalies of the genitourinary system which require surgical procedures under anesthesia often arise from abnormal development *in utero*. A full description of the development of the genitourinary system is beyond the scope of this chapter. See Chapter 8 for further discussion of the development of the genitourinary system. It is helpful to have a brief overview recalling that the urinary and genital systems are closely associated. Normal development is influenced by genetic, hormonal and anatomical factors.

Both the urinary and genital systems develop from intermediate mesoderm at the level of the seventh through the 28th somite [1]. The nephrogenic mass (cord) arises from the dorsal side from a bulge into the coelom called the urogenital ridge, from which the urinary and genital structures are formed. The nephrogenic tissue from the seventh to the 14th somite levels breaks up into four segments: cervical, thoracic, lumbar, and sacral. The cervical nephrotomes eventually give rise to glomeruli. The excretory tubules arise from the thoracic, lumbar and sacral segments. Subsequent development leads to the primitive pronephros. By the fourth week of gestation, the mesonephros is present as an intermediate step in renal development. By around week 10, the mesonephros has receded in females, while evolving into the vas deferens in males. The permanent kidney or metanephros begins to develop early in the fifth week and is functional by the 11th week of development. The metanephric blastema gives rise to nephrons including the Bowman capsule, proximal convoluted tubules, loops of Henle, and distal tubules. The ureters are an outgrowth of the primitive mesonephric duct forming the major and minor calices and collecting ducts. The terminal end of each uereter becomes part of the bladder wall. Each eventually develops a distinct separate entrance into the bladder with time. Normal development of the ureteric bud and the mesonephric blastema is closely dependent on each other.

As the fetus grows, the kidneys migrate from the pelvis to the abdomen. Fetal urine production is critical to normal amniotic fluid circulation. Amniotic fluid is aspirated by the fetus, absorbed into the fetal bloodstream and subsequently excreted into the amniotic sac. Failure to produce adequate amounts of urine can lead to oligohydramnios and associated anomalies. One significant anomaly is pulmonary hypoplasia.

Development of the external genitourinary system occurs in parallel with internal development. The cloaca (Latin for sewer) forms from the caudal end of the hindgut. The allantois and mesonephric ducts open into the cloaca. During weeks 4–7 of development, the cloaca subdivides into the posterior portion, which becomes the anorectal canal, and the anterior portion, which gives rise to the primitive urogenital sinus. The bladder is formed from the upper part of the primitive urogenital sinus. Initially, the bladder is continuous with the allantois; subsequent obliteration of the allantois lumen forms the urachus, which connects the apex of the bladder with the umbilicus. The urachus eventually becomes the median umbilical ligament.

The reproductive system makes its appearance during the fifth and sixth weeks of development. The fetus goes through an indifferent stage in which sex cannot be determined. Eventually, gonads (testes and ovaries) develop from a thickening of the urogenital ridge to form the gonadal ridge and primordial germ cells. Primary sex cords form and grow into the underlying mesenchyme. If the *SRY* gene is present (normal genetic male), differentiation will proceed along the path leading to testes. Absence of the *SRY* gene expression (normal genetic female) will lead to development of ovaries. Development of external genitalia is determined by both genetic and hormonal factors. In the presence of normal testes, androgen production by the adrenal glands is required to stimulate development of mesonephric ducts and produce normal external male genitalia. In the absence of normal androgens, paramesonephric ducts develop and the fetus will develop female external genitalia. External genital development first goes through the indifferent stage with the genital tubercle forming at the upper end of the cloacal membrane. In the male, this tubercle then elongates to form the phallus. Labioscrotal swellings and urogenital folds appear around this time. The cloacal membrane divides to form urogenital and anal openings around the seventh week.

In the male, the phallus elongates to form the penis, pulling the urogenital folds together. When folds start to fuse, they enclose the urethra and the urethral opening moves progressively towards the end of the penis. The labioscrotal swellings fuse to form the scrotum. In the female, the phallus becomes the clitoris. The urogenital folds do not fuse and become the labia minora. The labioscrotal folds fuse only at the ends to form the labia majora.

Anomalies of gonadal development can be divided into anomalies of sex chromosomes, true hermaphrodites, and anomalies of receptors. Conditions that represent anomalies of sex chromosomes include Turner syndrome (45,X), Klinefelter syndrome (47,XXY), and other syndromes with multiple X polyploidy. True hermaphrodites are extremely rare and have both true testes and ovaries. Anomalies of receptors result in testicular feminization syndrome (XY females). Congenital anomalies of the reproductive system in females include ovarian dysgenesis, rudimentary uterus, bifid uterus, septate uterus, and imperforate hymen. Congenital anomalies in males include testicular agenesis, undescended testes, and hypospadias.

Bladder exstrophy

Bladder exstrophy remains one of the most challenging conditions managed by pediatric urologists. It can be likened to the challenges the cardiovascular surgeon faces with repair of the single ventricle. Although rare, this disorder imposes significant physical, functional, social, sexual and psychological burdens on patients and families. For the healthcare system, the multiple, lengthy and complex operative procedures for exstrophy consume resources disproportionate to the small number of affected individuals [2]. The rarity of this condition (2.5 in 100,000 livebirths in the United States) makes it imperative that communication between the anesthesiologist and urologist occurs well before the start of surgery. The correction choices and timing for surgery are continually being modified. While it used to be standard practice to perform surgery in the first several days of life, in some institutions, surgeries are being delayed until the child is 4–6 weeks of age, with no change in the success rate [3].

The goals of reconstructive surgery for bladder exstrophy are to achieve closure of the bladder, obtain urinary continence, preserve renal function, and produce satisfactory appearance and function of the external genitalia. Wound dehiscence, bladder prolapse and multiple attempts at bladder closure have been identified as risk factors for lack of adequate bladder growth and inability to develop urine continence [4].

Classic bladder exstrophy can be conceptualized by visualizing that one blade of a pair of scissors is passing through the urethra into the bladder of a normal person; the other blade is used to cut the layers of the skin, abdominal wall, anterior wall of the bladder, urethra and symphysis pubis, and the cut edges are unfolded laterally as if opening a book (Fig. 29.1) [5].

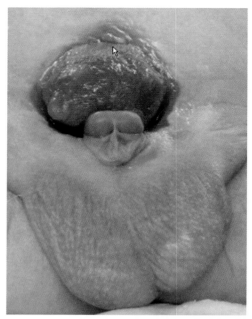

Figure 29.1 Exstrophy of the bladder. Reproduced from Brock and DeMarco [5] with permission from Elsevier.

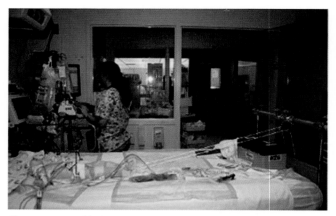

Figure 29.2 Modified Buck traction. The child is positioned with weights maintaining the legs in an extended position parallel to the bed. This figure is available in color online at www.jpedhc.org. Reproduced from Kozlowski [13] with permission from Elsevier.

At birth, classic bladder exstrophy presents with an everted posterior bladder wall of varying size associated with separation of the symphysis pubis. This diastasis causes an outward rotation and eversion of the pubic rami at their junctions with the ischial and iliac bones [5]. Urine may be seen leaking from the inferior margin of the everted posterior bladder wall, but the ureteral orifices are not always obvious. The umbilicus is located on the immediate superior border of the bladder plate, and a small umbilical hernia or an omphalocele is ordinarily seen. The mucosa of the exposed bladder may look normal or thickened. In males, there is complete epispadias with dorsal chordee, and the overall penile length is approximately half of that in unaffected boys. The scrotum is typically separated from the penis and is wide and shallow. Undescended testes and inguinal hernias are common. Females also have epispadias, with separation of the two halves of the clitoris and wide separation of the labia. The anus is displaced anteriorly in both sexes, and there may be rectal prolapse [5,6].

In patients with classic exstrophy of the bladder, anomalous development in other systems is unusual. However, bladder exstrophy can be considered a spectrum of anatomical variants referred to as the exstrophy complex. These variants include bladder exstrophy with imperforate anus and cloacal exstrophy. With extreme cases of classic bladder exstrophy and cloacal exstrophy, omphaloceles are also encountered above the level of the exposed bladder. In cloacal exstrophy, some form of spinal dysraphism, including tethered cord, myelomeningocele or lipomyelomeningocele, is present in nearly all patients, with recent reports ranging from 64% to 100% [7].

Two options have been described for surgical reconstruction: primary single-staged closure of the bladder or a planned staged repair [8–12]. Regardless of the strategy chosen, failure of the initial repair decreases the potential for the later development of continence. Also, in each option pelvic osteotomies are often used to allow approximation of the pubic symphysis. Modified Buck traction is often required after surgery for 4–8 weeks (Fig. 29.2)[13].

Preoperative preparation involves an assessment of all organ systems to ensure that there are no associated anomalies of physiological significance. Preoperative complete blood count, type and cross-match are recommended, especially if pelvic osteotomies are necessary. Appropriate measures are taken to avoid trauma to the exposed bladder mucosa. Antibiotics are administered preoperatively and continued after surgery. The procedure involves long operating times (5–7 h), unpredictable bleeding and fluid shifts after intravenous induction of anesthesia and endotracheal intubation [14]. Therefore, two intravenous catheters should be placed in the upper extremities if possible to avoid the sterile field. Central venous access may be necessary if peripheral venous access is difficult. An arterial line is also placed for both hemodynamic monitoring and measurement of blood gases, hemoglobin, coagulation studies, electrolytes and glucose.

Preoperative placement of an epidural catheter is helpful for intraoperative and postoperative pain management (Fig. 29.3) [4]. The sacrococcygeal ligament is punctured at position 1 (see Fig. 29.3) and an epidural catheter is threaded through the epidural insertion needle to reach a thoracic dermatome level of T10–12. The

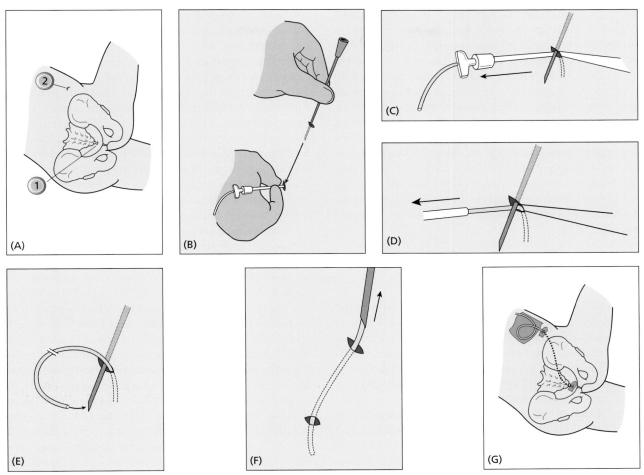

Figure 29.3 Placement of a tunneled caudal epidural catheter is depicted. (A) The sacrococcygeal ligament is punctured at position 1, and then an epidural catheter (approximately 6–10 cm) is threaded through the epidural insertion needle to reach a thoracic dermatomal level of T10–12. (B) The tunneling needle (a 17 or 18 gauge styletted Crawford or Tuohy needle) is inserted on the patient's side, near the posterior superior iliac crest, labeled as position 2. This is the final exit position and should be visible when the child is supine so that the site can be easily inpected. (C) The tunneling needle emerges at the epidural needle insertion (position 1). Note the epidural insertion needle is not removed and is left in place to protect the catheter. An 11 scalpel blade cuts the residual skin and subcutaneous tissue bridge between the two needles. (D) The epidural insertion needle is removed, leaving the catheter in place, depicted as a dashed line. (E) The stylet from the tunneling needle is removed and the distal end of the epidural catheter is threaded into the tunneling needle. (F) The tunneling needle is removed. The subcutaneous portion of the epidural catheter is depicted with a dashed line. (G) The primary insertion site and the final catheter exit site are secured with adhesive strips and covered with a transparent adhesive dressing. A loop is placed in the catheter to prevent accidental dislodgment. Reproduced from Kost-Byerly et al [4] with permission from Elsevier.

tunneling needle (a 17 or 18 gauge styletted Crawford or Tuohy needle) is inserted on the patient's side, near the posterior superior iliac crest, labeled as position 2. This is the final exit position and should be visible when the child is supine so that the site can be easily inspected in the postoperative period. The tunneling needle emerges at the epidural needle insertion (position 1). Note that the epidural insertion needle is not removed and is left in place to protect the catheter. An 11 scalpel blade cuts the residual skin and subcutaneous tissue bridge between the two needles. The epidural insertion needle is removed, leaving the catheter in place, depicted as a dashed line. The stylet from the tunneling needle is removed and the

distal end of the epidural catheter is threaded into the tunneling needle. The tunneling needle is then removed. The subcutaneous portion of the epidural catheter is depicted with a dashed line. The primary insertion site and the final catheter exit site are secured with Steri-Strips and covered with transparent adhesive dressings. A loop is placed in the catheter to prevent accidental dislodgment [4].

At the time of surgery, the patient will have a wide surgical preparation, including the entire body anteriorly and posteriorly below the level of the nipples so that turning the child for surgical orientation does not lead to wound contamination [5]. Timing of the removal of the endotracheal tube after surgery depends on the infant's age, length and complexity of surgery, and amount of fluid and blood the patient received during surgery.

In the postoperative period it is imperative that the baby remain immobilized, sedated, and pain free to prevent movement that would cause distracting forces to compromise the repair. The tunneled epidural catheter is extremely useful in this situation. Epidural infusions through tunneled epidural catheters can provide safe analgesia for up to a month in neonates. Daily communication between pediatric urology, intensive care unit (ICU) staff, the pediatric pain service and experienced nursing staff is the prerequisite to providing analgesia and sedation without undue complications for a neonatal population [4,13].

Posterior urethral valves

The most common cause of severe obstructive uropathy in children is posterior urethral valves (PUV). The urethral valves are tissue leaflets fanning distally from the prostatic urethra to the external urinary sphincter. A slit-like opening usually separates the leaflets. Valves are of unclear embryological origin and cause varying degrees of obstruction. The renal changes range from mild hydronephrosis to severe renal dysplasia; their severity probably depends on the severity of the obstruction and its time of onset during fetal development. As in other cases of obstruction or renal dysplasia, there may be oligohydramnios and pulmonary hypoplasia [15].

If the serum creatinine level remains normal or returns to normal after birth without intervention, treatment consists of transurethral ablation of the valve leaflets, which is performed endoscopically under general anesthesia. If the urethra is too small for transurethral ablation, temporary vesicostomy is preferred, in which the dome of the bladder is exteriorized on the lower abdominal wall. When the child is older, the valves may be ablated and the vesicostomy closed [16].

There are several classifications of this disorder, based on the type and severity of obstruction. The spectrum of abnormalities may represent the different degrees of obstruction, the timing of obstruction, and other genotypical risk factors. Mild obstruction may have a presentation delayed until adolescence. It appears that a partial outlet obstruction can be overcome with bladder wall hypertrophy that generates high voiding pressures [15,16].

An infant with severe PUV may present in the neonatal nursery with anuria and a palpable bladder. The clinical sequelae from PUV result in persistent bilateral hydronephrosis, either from vesicoureteric reflux (VUR) or elevated bladder pressures [16]. When the newborn's condition is especially severe, with associated lung hypoplasia, serial percutaneous needle bladder drainage may be undertaken to decompress the bladder until the newborn is optimized to have surgical repair.

After the diagnosis is established, renal function and the anatomy of the upper urinary tract should be carefully evaluated. In the healthy neonate, a small polyethylene feeding tube (no. 5 or 8 French) is inserted through the urethra into the bladder for several days. Passing the feeding tube may be difficult, because the tube tip may coil in the prostatic urethra, causing urine to drain around the catheter rather than through it. A Foley (balloon) catheter should not be used, because the balloon may cause severe bladder spasm, which may produce severe ureteral obstruction [17].

Posterior urethral valves are now commonly diagnosed in the antenatal period. The ultrasound findings may include bilateral hydronephrosis, a distended thick-walled bladder, and oligohydramnios [16]. The incidence of PUV is 1/5000 livebirths. Of the 500 new cases of PUV each year, 150 will develop end-stage renal disease (ESRD) and require dialysis or transplantation in the first 18 years of life. Some institutions perform *in utero* interventions. Experimental and clinical evidence of the possible benefits of fetal intervention is lacking, and few affected fetuses are candidates. Prenatal diagnosis of PUV, particularly when discovered in the second trimester, is associated with a poorer prognosis than those detected after birth [17]. While antenatal intervention improves pulmonary function and the restoration of amniotic fluid volume, it does not guarantee an improvement in renal insufficiency [15,16].

The appropriate treatment of PUV is determined by examining all contributing factors. These include the overall condition of the infant, renal function, hydration status, and lung maturity [16]. Prophylactic antibiotics are started at birth and the bladder may need decompression. Valve ablation may be undertaken if the creatinine falls to less than 1 mg/dL. When the renal function does not continue to improve, usually a vesicostomy is performed as the initial step to decompress the kidneys. Most boys have a good prognosis if they complete a normal gestation and undergo neonatal valve incision.

These patients may present in the neonatal period for PUV incision and also for circumcision which may decrease the rate of urinary tract infections [16]. In the very small infant where the cystoscope will not pass through the urethra, a vesicostomy may be considered, with delayed valve incisions.

These infants may also have some degree of respiratory compromise, relating to the oliguria [17]. It is thought that the urinary obstruction and lack of urine production *in utero* limits the amount of fluid the fetus then aspirates, which helps to stent open the developing lungs. In turn, this leads to pulmonary hypoplasia and respiratory distress syndrome [18]. An appropriate volume of amniotic fluid, which is produced by the kidneys and then excreted as urine, is necessary for the complete and proper branching of the bronchial tree and alveoli. Physical findings can include poor fetal breathing movements, small chest cavity, ascites, limb deformities from compression, and Potter facies [15]. Potter facies develops *in utero* secondary to the effects of oligohydramnios from any cause. Features include micrognathia, hypertelorism, pulmonary hypoplasia, and spade-like hands [19]. Neonates with pulmonary hypoplasia may require perioperative mechanical ventilation. These patients may require high peak pressures, and permissive hypercapnia must be tolerated. The severe patient may even require an oscillating ventilator, until the lungs mature further.

The preoperative evaluation of a neonate with PUV should include assessment of renal function, including the extent of urinary retention and fluid overload. Appropriate laboratory testing should search for evidence of renal failure. Hyponatremia, azotemia, hypertension, and hyperkalemia must be identified and treated prior to anesthetizing the patient. Patients in renal failure must be treated with appropriate fluid management and judicious use of anesthetic agents affected by renal metabolism.

When PUV cause mild obstruction, the associated complications are also mild or non-existent. The length of surgical intervention is generally less than 1 h and the anesthetic approach includes general anesthesia with endotracheal intubation or laryngeal mask airway (LMA) for airway management. Postoperative pain is minor for cystoscopy and valve ablation.

Circumcision

Circumcision is the most commonly performed surgical procedure in the world. There are very few absolute indications for circumcision, especially in the neonate. The American Academy of Pediatrics does not recommend routine circumcision in otherwise healthy boys. In this age group, if hydronephrosis is present, then a circumcision may help to decrease the likelihood of urinary tract infections [16]. In older children, persistent phimosis and recurrent balanitis are indications for circumcision [16].

Newborn circumcisions are most often done at the bedside or as outpatients with a Plastibell device or Gomco clamp. These procedures are usually performed by the pediatrician or obstetrician while the infant is still in the nursery. Circumcision in older children usually requires freehand sleeve resection performed under general anesthesia. Common surgical complications of circumcision include bleeding, infection, residual redundant skin, meatal stenosis, and skin bridges [20].

When infants and children require general anesthesia, it usually is induced via inhalational induction, a peripheral intravenous line is placed and the airway is secured with an LMA or endotracheal tube. A penile nerve block placed prior to incision is effective in providing intraoperative analgesia and postoperative pain relief [21]. Although caudal epidural anesthesia can be used for analgesia, penile block is usually preferred because less local anesthetic is given and less time is spent performing the block [22].

Hypospadias

Hypospadias is the abnormal ventral opening of the urethral meatus which results from incomplete development of the urethra. This defect may be located anywhere from the corona of the glans to the perineum [22]. Therefore, the extent of surgical dissection and the staging of the repair depend on the complexity of the lesion [23]. Hypospadias is often discovered after a routine neonatal circumcision. Signs of hypospadias include abnormal prepuce, persistent ventral curvature (also known as chordee), and proximally displaced urethral orifice that is rarely obstructive but often stenotic [16]. The meatus is located on the glans or distal shaft in 70–80% of cases and in the middle of the shaft 20–30% of the time [16]. Rarely, the meatus is located in the scrotum or more proximally in the perineum.

Hypospadias can be associated with inguinal hernias, cryptorchidism, and low birthweight. The incidence of hypospadias is higher in patients with affected siblings [24].

Early repair of this defect is important for aesthetic considerations and toilet training, and also for long-term psychosexual adjustment [23]. Skilled pediatric urologists perform this repair in healthy term babies as early as 3 months of age. Delaying the repair past 15 months may increase cognitive, emotional, behavioral, and psychosexual issues. In addition, younger infants may develop less scar tissue and have better wound healing than older children [16].

The goals of repair are straightening the ventral curvature and extending the urethra distally. Historically, these operations were done as staged procedures. Currently, the majority are done as one procedure. Surgery may be staged if the penis has a curvature greater than 30°. A buccal graft may be needed for tubularization of the neourethra during the second stage, which occurs approximately 6 months later [16].

These patients are usually otherwise healthy. General anesthesia with LMA and supplemental caudal anesthesia or a penile block is the most common approach. Postoperative urethral instrumentation must be avoided as catheterization of the newly formed urethra could cause disruption of the repair. These patients often have a urethral catheter left in place postoperatively, to allow passive urine drainage through the neo-urethra for approximately 1 week [16]. The penis is gently compressed with a Telfa® pad and bio-occlusive dressing following the procedure. Complications can include fistulas, meatal stenosis, urethral stricture, dehiscence, and recurrent curvature [16].

Cryptorchidism

Cryptorchidism (undescended testes, UDT) is the most common disorder of sexual differentiation and occurs in approximately 2% of male births [25]. The consequences of cryptorchidism include degeneration of the testes, impaired fertility, and increased risk for germ cell testicular tumors [17]. Despite the significance of this problem, the etiology of UDT in the majority of patients is unknown. It is unclear whether the pathological changes in the cryptorchid testis occur as a result of a primary defect or from secondary changes produced by the higher temperatures imposed on the undescended testis [17].

Two-thirds of patients present with a unilateral abnormality, and the other third present with bilateral abnormalities [16]. When the undescended testicle is unilateral, the right side is more often affected. The incidence ranges from 3.4% to 5.8% in full-term males. The usual timing for testicular descent into the scrotum is during the seventh month of gestation. Spontaneous descent may occur up until the first 6 months of life. A number of risk factors have been implicated as a cause of undescended testicles. These include advanced maternal age, maternal obesity, breech presentation, low parity, preterm birth, low birthweight, and maternal consumption of cola-containing drinks during pregnancy [16,26].

Cryptorchidism may occur as a single isolated abnormality in an otherwise healthy patient or be associated with other congenital anomalies such as prune belly syndrome, PUV, neural tube defects, gastroschisis, and microcephaly [27].

Treatment is focused on prevention of infertility, testicular malignancy, testicular torsion, and the psychological stigma associated with an empty scrotum. The rate of malignancy is approximately 1% in the cryptorchid patient. It is unknown whether this results from the abnormal position of the testis or an abnormality of the testis itself [16]. The rate of infertility is 38% in patients with bilateral cryptorchidism compared to 11% in unilateral cryptorchidism and 6% in normal males.

Treatment includes surgical exploration for the location of the testis. Sixty percent of the time, the testis is located in the inguinal canal or abdomen and 40% of the time, the testis is absent or composed of fibrous tissue. The current method of treatment is orchiopexy, or relocation of the testis into the scrotum. If the location of the testis is not easily determined, the vas deferens and testicular vessels are used to help locate it [22]. Vessel length is the determining factor in deciding whether to undertake the procedure in one or two stages. Small, short spermatic vessels lead to the risk of a non-viable testis if placed into the scrotum without staging. In the first stage, the vessels are dissected and the testicle is brought as close to the scrotum as possible. The second stage 1 or 2 years later moves the testicle the remaining distance into the scrotum. The waiting period allows the blood supply to enlarge and form collateral circulation to supply the testicle.

Hormonal treatments to stimulate testicular descent include human chorionic gonadotropin, gonadotropin-releasing hormone, and luteinizing hormone-releasing hormone. These hormones stimulate the Leydig cells to produce androgens, but the mechanism for testicular descent is unknown [16].

Children who present for orchiopexy are usually otherwise healthy. They require general anesthesia with either an endotracheal tube or LMA for airway management. Caudal epidural block is helpful to minimize postoperative pain. These procedures may be performed with conventional surgical incisions or, if abdominal position of the testes is suspected, laparoscopic surgery is often performed. If the anesthetic level is insufficient, laryngospasm may occur when the testis is manipulated. Otherwise, the postanesthetic course is generally unremarkable.

Testicular torsion

Testicular torsion is a true surgical emergency. The diagnosis is usually made by history, physical examination, and diagnostic imaging studies. There are no definitive diagnostic imaging studies available, although color Doppler, isotope scans, and conventional ultrasound may be useful adjuncts [28]. Testicular torsion is best managed by early exploration, detorsion, and, when the testis is salvageable, fixation. When the testis is not salvageable, the surgeon will proceed with orchiectomy. In either scenario, a contralateral orchiopexy is usually performed [16].

Normally, the tunica vaginalis covers the anterior surface of the testis, epididymis, and spermatic cord, attaching with the gubernaculums and scrotal wall posteriorly, fixing the testis [16]. When these attachments are not secure, torsion may occur, leading to vascular compromise. There is a bimodal distribution in occurrence, with increased frequency during the neonatal period and puberty. During puberty, the rapidly increasing testicular mass increases the chances for rotation. In the neonatal period, the recently descended testis is very motile in the scrotum, increasing the risk of the spermatic cord rotating *en masse* [16].

The patient's history should focus on the age of the patient, association with pain, and history of trauma. The onset and severity of pain may help differentiate torsion from epididymitis. The pain in torsion is acute in onset, severe, and ipsilateral [16]. The patient may also have symptoms of abdominal pain, thigh pain, and nausea and vomiting. The orientation and location of the testis in the scrotum must also be evaluated.

Testicular infarction may occur within a few hours of the torsion. After 8h following the onset of pain, the testicular salvage rate declines precipitously [29]. In addition, studies in rats have confirmed that unilateral torsion can induce bilateral testicular damage and infertility [16]. This may result from reflex vasoconstriction, the formation of autoantibodies or other chemically mediated mechanism [16]. Therefore, surgery under general anesthesia with a rapid-sequence induction should proceed as soon as possible.

Vesicoureteral reflux procedures

Vesicoureteral reflux (VUR) is the retrograde flow of urine across the ureterovesical junction (UVJ). There is a high rate of familial recurrence, suggesting a genetic component. Risk factors for developing this condition include anatomical and functional abnormalities of the UVJ, high intravesical pressures, and impaired ureteral function [16]. If the VUR is severe, renal dysfunction and hypertension may be present preoperatively, although the majority of the presenting patients are healthy.

The unidirectional flow of urine through the normal ureter depends on both active and passive components. It appears that the tunneling path that the ureter travels through the submucosal layers of the bladder wall is inversely related to the rate of VUR. When the submucosal course is short, and therefore perpendicular to the bladder wall, the flap-valve mechanism normally in place to prevent reflux is absent. Additionally, the intravesical pressure must be lower than that in the ureter for there to be flow in the antegrade direction. Common clinical scenarios in which this might occur are in patients with posterior valves, in patients with a neurogenic bladder or when ureteral peristalsis is abnormal [16].

Long-term antibiotic prophylaxis is recommended in these children, especially to the age of 8 years and in those with frequent recurrences [16]. This is continued until the reflux has resolved spontaneously or has been surgically corrected. This prophylaxis has been shown to decrease the amount of renal scarring and renal damage from repeated infections, helping to minimize the progression to chronic renal insufficiency and hypertension.

Management of vesicoureteral reflux may be surgical or medical. The main goal is to prevent pyelonephrosis, which can lead to the above complications. The treatment plan depends on gender, age, grade of reflux, concurrence of urinary tract infections, renal function, and likelihood of resolution [16]. If the reflux is sterile, with no associated urinary tract infection, it is not harmful to the kidneys and has no significant effect on kidney function and can probably be managed medically. Indications for surgical treatment include breakthrough urinary tract infections despite prophylactic antibiotics, VUR associated with congenital anomalies at the UVJ, renal growth retardation and the finding of worsening renal scarring. The endpoint of the surgical treatment is to restore the flap-valve mechanism, thereby preventing the VUR. The gold standard for this remains open surgical repair to establish an adequate submucosal tunnel for the ureter.

There are multiple techniques available for surgical repair, but the main components of each are freeing the ureter for mobilization, submucosal tunnel formation, transferring the ureter through the tunnel, and securing the ureter into the new position [16]. A minimally invasive technique for repair is also available. Using either an extravesical or intravesical approach, laparoscopic reimplantation can be undertaken. Endoscopic injection therapy, most frequently using polytetrafluoro-ethylene (PTFE) or silicone, is introduced submucosally at the 6 o'clock position of the UVJ [16]. By creating a mound at the opening of the UVJ, this narrows the ureteral orifice, thereby decreasing the amount of reflux allowed.

Anesthetic considerations for this case include duration and blood loss, which can be significant during open repair. An epidural catheter or caudal epidural (catheter or single shot) may be placed to supplement anesthesia intra- and postoperatively. Postoperatively, these patients may have significant bladder spasm. This may be effectively treated in a variety of ways, including with belladonna and opium (B and O) suppositories, oral or intravesicular oxybutynin, ketorolac or bupivacaine via epidural or in the bladder [21,20,30].

Ureteropelvic junction obstruction

Ureteropelvic junction (UPJ) obstruction is the most common cause of obstructive uropathy in childhood and usually is caused by intrinsic stenosis. The typical appearance on ultrasonography is grade 3 or 4 hydronephrosis without a dilated ureter. UPJ obstruction most commonly presents on maternal ultrasonography revealing fetal hydronephrosis, as a palpable renal mass in a newborn or infant, as abdominal, flank or back pain, as a febrile urinary tract infection (UTI) or as hematuria after minimal trauma. Approximately 60% of cases occur on the left side, and the male:female ratio is 2:1. In 10% of cases UPJ obstruction is bilateral. In kidneys with UPJ obstruction, renal function may be significantly impaired from pressure atrophy, but approximately half of affected kidneys have relatively normal function [31].

Crossing vessels have been identified in 38–71% of patients with UPJ obstruction and in 19% of patients without UPJ obstruction [32]. Crossing vessels are believed to exacerbate rather than initiate the obstructive process [33]. If not recognized, crossing vessels can cause significant bleeding. These vessels are not excised as part of the repair, but the renal pelvis and ureter are rearranged by dismembered pyeloplasty [34].

The goal of surgery for UPJ obstruction is to preserve renal function by facilitating unobstructed drainage of urine. There are two common techniques: the more popular dismembered pyeloplasty and the flap technique. With the dismembered approach, there is complete severing of the ureter from the pelvis and then reanastomosis. With the flap approach, the renal pelvis is modified with the ureter intact.

The most common surgical approaches are the anterior subcostal, muscle-splitting approach and the dorsal lumbotomy approach. The anterior subcostal approach is performed in a modified supine position with the ipsilateral side at a 15–20° angle. The operating table is flexed at the level of the child's anterior superior iliac spine and a bump placed under the patient. The lumbotomy approach is performed with the child in the prone position.

Pyeloplasty can also be performed by the laparoscopic approach with and without robotics. Potential benefits of the laparoscopic approach include shorter hospital admission, decreased postoperative pain, less superficial scarring and earlier return to normal activity [35]. Because of the small incision used in the open procedure combined with the rapid convalescence of most children, controversy exists about which approach may be advantageous in this age group. The decision is likely left to surgeon preference and experience. Neither approach is responsible for prolonged extreme pain. The mean length of stay for an open procedure is 25h [36].

In most children, the general risk of anesthesia is relatively low. These children are usually healthy, but it is always prudent to search for co-existing diseases. Renal failure is not usually an issue, especially with unilateral disease. Because of positioning and length of surgery, and when a laparoscopic approach is planned, tracheal intubation is usually the safest route. Liberal fluid therapy allows free flow of urine. Regional block with local anesthetic via the caudal route with or without opioids and clonidine provides excellent postoperative pain relief. Because the mean length of hospitalization is about 25h, epidural catheter placement usually is not necessary [20]. Ben-Meir et al demonstrated that a regimen of opioids and non-steroidal anti-inflammatory drugs in children after open pyeloplasty has efficacy similar to that of epidural analgesia [37].

Wilms tumor

Wilms tumor or nephroblastoma is the most common renal tumor of childhood and the seventh most common pediatric malignancy overall, accounting for about 5% of all childhood malignancies [38]. There are approximately 500 new cases of Wilms tumor each year. Most (75%) newly diagnosed patients are under 5 years of age, and usually between 2 and 3 years. Commonly, the tumor presents as a painless mass which is noticed by the parents as an abdominal bulge or a palpated mass. Some patients may exhibit signs and symptoms including malaise, fever, weight loss and frank hypertension. Classic associations with Wilms tumor include crytorchidism or hypospadias, aniridia and/or hemihypertrophy. Box 29.1 lists the characteristics associated with different types of Wilms tumor. The tumor usually involves one kidney but may affect both kidneys in about 5% of cases. As the tumor grows, it may spread by local invasion and in 12% may demonstrate hematogenous spread to the lungs and less commonly to the brain (0.5%) [39]. Children with tumors that are solitary, unilateral and have a low-risk genotype (see below) have an excellent prognosis. Bilateral masses and those with higher risk tumors (by genotype) are associated with significant morbidity and mortality. Common morbidities include recurrence of tumor, complications secondary to chemotherapy or radiation therapy and spread to other organs, particularly the lungs. Recent advances in molecular biology have improved understanding of factors which can affect the outcome of children with Wilms tumor. In particular, the loss of heterozygocity (LOH) of chromosome 1p and/or 16q is associated with anaplastic Wilms tumors, which have a worse prognosis than those without LOH. Older children also are more likely than younger ones to have LOH and therefore a worse prognosis. Patients who exhibit LOH at both the 1p and 16q loci have a significant chance of relapse after therapy and therefore a worse prognosis. Epidemiological and genetic factors have been used to stratify the risk associated with Wilms tumor. These are summarized in Table 29.1.

Children with Wilms tumor may require anesthesia for a variety of conditions, including primary tumor resection, radiological imaging (magnetic resonance imaging,

Table 29.1 Occurrence of characteristic congenital anomalies in Wilms tumor patients according to subgroups of the National Wilms Tumor Study

Subgroup	No. of patients evaluated	Percentage of patients in subgroups with			
		Aniridia	Cryptorchism/hypospadias[a]	Hemihypertrophy	Beckwith–Wiedemann
Unilateral, unicentric	4165	1.3	5.0	2.6	0.5
Unilateral, multicentric	516	1.0	8.6	6.2	2.3
Bilateral at onset	315	1.3	16.8	8.6	1.6
Late bilateral	43	4.7	15.4	4.7	4.7
Familial Wilms tumor	61	1.6	5.1	3.3	0.0
ILNR (±) PLNR	552	2.0	12.2	4.2	2.5
PLNR only	446	0.4	2.3	7.2	1.6
Neither ILNR/PLNR	1748	0.4	3.8	1.8	0.2

[a] Percentage of male patients.
Reproduced from Breslow et al [73] with permission from Wiley-Blackwell.
ILNR, intralobar nephrogenic rests; PLNR, perilobar nephrogenic rests.

Box 29.1 Wilms tumor staging system

I. Tumor limited to kidney and completely excised. The surface of the capsule is intact. Tumor was not ruptured before or during removal. There is no residual tumor apparent beyond the margins of excision.

II. Tumor extends beyond the kidney, but is completely excised. There is regional extension of the tumor, i.e. penetration through the outer surface of the renal capsule into perirenal soft tissues. Vessels outside the kidney substance are infiltrated or contain tumor thrombus. The tumor may have been biopsied or there has been local spillage of tumor contained to the flank. There is no residual tumor apparent at or beyond the margins of excision.

III. Residual non-hematogenous tumor confined to the abdomen. Any one or more of the following occur.
   a. Lymph nodes on biopsy are found to be involved in the hilus, the peri-aortic chains or beyond.
   b. There has been diffuse peritoneal contamination by tumor such as by spillage of tumor beyond the flank before or during surgery, or by tumor growth that has penetrated through the peritoneal surface.
   c. Implants are found on the peritoneal surfaces.
   d. The tumor extends beyond the surgical margins either microscopically or grossly.
   e. The tumor is not completely resectable because of local infiltration into vital structures.

IV. Hematogenous metastases. Deposits beyond stage III, i.e. lung. liver, bone, and brain.

V. Bilateral renal involvement at diagnosis. An attempt should be made to stage each side according to the above criteria on the basis of extent of disease prior to biopsy.

Reproduced from Davidoff [39] with permission from Lippincott Williams and Wilkins.

MRI), diagnostic bone marrow biopsy and lumbar puncture, placement of central lines (percutaneously inserted central catheters, PICC) or radiation therapy. Usually the child will present to the operating room for surgical resection and staging. The main responsibility of the surgeon is to remove the primary tumor completely, without spillage, and to accurately assess the extent to which the tumor has spread, with particular attention to adequately assessing lymph node involvement. There is a difference in approach to the timing of initial surgery between the guidelines of the Children's Oncology Group (COG) in the US and those of the International Society of Pediatric Oncology (SIOP) in Europe. The American practice is to perform primary resection and staging before administering chemotherapy. The SIOP recommends preoperative chemotherapy because the tumor then is easier to resect and may be associated with a decreased incidence of tumor spill and a lower mortality and morbidity rate [39].

Commonly, anesthesia for primary tumor resection is similar to that for any major open laparotomy or radical nephrectomy. Proper preoperative assessment is crucial. The anesthesiologist should be aware of the extent of the tumor and whether it is adherent to surrounding organs. The tumor may involve a good portion of the kidney as well as the inferior vena cava, mesenteric arteries, a portion of the liver or right atrium. Patients with atrial involvement or atrial thrombus may need cardiopulmonary bypass support during the surgical procedure. Bilateral tumors or ones crossing the midline of the abdomen may affect the great vessels, adding a potential risk of significant blood loss. In addition, the anesthesiologist should be aware of any associated anomalies and the nature of any preoperative chemotherapy or radiation therapy. Chemotherapeutic agents such as actinomycin, doxorubicin and vincristine are used for preoperative and postoperative treatment. These drugs may be associated with myelosuppression, cardiotoxicity, pulmonary effects (pleural effusion, pneumonia, and interstitial pneumonitis), hepatotoxicity, and neurotoxicity in children [40]. The incidence varies and may depend on both dose and the patient's individual response to the agent [40–42].

The anesthetic plan depends on the preoperative condition of the patient and the surgical plan. These patients will require endotracheal intubation and general anesthesia with standard monitors. Two intravenous lines are useful, one to provide maintenance IV solutions and the second for rapid infusion of fluids or blood products. If there is intra-atrial involvement or if thoracotomy or cardiopulmonary bypass is required, an arterial line is useful to closely monitor the patient's blood pressure and obtain blood specimens for testing. Central venous access, if not present preoperatively, may be desirable to monitor central pressures and provide longer term venous access. For the abdominal approach, patients are positioned supine and commonly the surgical approach is through a transverse abdominal transperitoneal incision. Epidural analgesia for intraoperative and postoperative pain management may be quite useful. The level of the catheter is determined by the site of the incision. The tip of the catheter is best located at the mid or low thoracic level in order to provide adequate analgesia.

Despite proper planning and execution, up to 12% of cases may have a perioperative complication. Table 29.2 lists some of the possible surgical complications and reported incidence. In addition to these, the anesthesiologist should be mindful of possible injury related to patient positioning and take proper precautions to minimize the risk. Patients may have significant postoperative pain and discomfort depending on the location of the incision and extent of the surgical dissection. Postoperative use of patient- or nurse-controlled epidural analgesia may result in more comfort and rapid return to activity by avoiding the common side-effects of intravenous opioid analgesia. Without surgical complications, patients usually recover from surgery within 3–5 days. Postoperative therapy is determined by the stage of the tumor and risk stratification.

Chronic renal failure and dialysis

Children in acute or chronic renal failure may require peritoneal or hemodialysis. The insertion of the appropri-

Table 29.2 Incidence of surgical complications following surgery for Wilms tumor

Complication	n	%
Bowel obstruction	27	5.1
Extensive hemorrhage	10	1.9
Wound infection	10	1.9
Vascular injury	8	1.5
Splenic injury	6	1.1
Hypotension	3	0.6
Diaphragmatic tear	2	0.4
Liver injury	1	0.2
Chylous ascites	1	0.2
Incisional hernia	1	0.2
Pulmonary embolus	1	0.2
Respiratory failure	1	0.2
Pleural effusion	1	0.2
Pneumothorax	1	0.2
Urinary tract infection	1	0.2
Pancreatitis	1	0.2
Staph. sepsis	1	0.2

Seventy-six complications occurred in 68 of 534 children: 12.7% had at least one complication.
Reproduced from Ritchey M, Shamberger R, Haase G et al. Surgical complications after primary nephrectomy for Wilms' tumor: report from the National Wilms' Tumor Study Group. J Am Coll Surg 2001; 192: 63–8, with permission from Elsevier.

ate catheter in non-critically ill patients is usually performed in the operating room under general anesthesia. The critically ill child may require a procedure in the operating room while undergoing continuous renal replacement therapy (CRRT) in the ICU. This section will describe the types of renal replacement available, the mechanism by which dialysis is performed and finally a discussion of the types of dialysis catheters used for the pediatric patient. The perioperative care of children in renal failure requiring surgery will also be addressed.

Renal replacement therapy (RRT) defines dialysis therapies. However, some authors now refer to dialysis as renal support therapy because only fluid removal and filtering wastes are performed by dialysis and not the endocrine functions [43]. Dialysis employs only two physiologies for solute and fluid movement. Both methods necessitate blood being exposed to a semipermeable membrane against a dialysate solution of different concentration. Regardless of the modality employed, the goal of renal replacement therapy is to precisely control serum electrolytes, clear toxins and provide fluid removal for the patient in renal failure.

Dialysis employs a diffusive clearance while hemofiltration employs convective clearance. Hemodialysis and peritoneal dialysis involve the diffusion of solutes across a concentration gradient from high to low concentration. Dialysate is passed across the semi-permeable membrane countercurrent to blood flow, allowing equilibration of the plasma and dialysate solute concentrations. This process may remove or add solute to the plasma water space, depending upon the composition of dialysate compared to the plasma. Water will also move along a gradient, in effect "following" the solute (ultrafiltration). Diffusive clearance is effective for removal of the small solute, including serum ions and urea, with subsequent fluid removal. In addition, other solutes such as antibiotics, narcotics and other medications will cross the membrane. Diffusion gradients change depending upon blood flow rates, dialysate flow rates and starting concentration gradients. CRRT employing countercurrent dialysate for solute clearance is considered as continuous venovenous hemodialysis (CVVHD) [44].

Hemofiltration uses a pressure gradient for fluid movement instead of solute concentration gradients. It is considered part of the CRRT modalities. A positive hydrostatic pressure drives water across the membrane from the blood side to the filter side and solutes follow water through the membrane. Due to the possibility of large shifts of volume during convective therapies, a filter replacement fluid (FRF) is often utilized to replace fluid lost by convection. In patients undergoing CRRT, bicarbonate is lost in the ultrafiltrate. Therefore, the replacement fluid is usually an isotonic, buffered electrolyte solution. The buffer used in the replacement fluid may be acetate, citrate, lactate or bicarbonate. The use of citrate is becoming more commonplace because it may be used as both a buffer and an anticoagulant to help prevent hemodiafilter clotting [45]. There are many names for the types of hemofiltration performed, including SLEF (slow extended hemofiltration), SCUF (slow continuous ultrafiltration), CVVH (continuous venovenous hemofiltration), and CVVHDF (continuous venovenous hemodiafiltration) [44].

Thresholds for the timing of dialysis in acute renal failure (ARF) are controversial and not well defined [43,46,47]. Indications for renal replacement therapy include volume overload with evidence of hypertension and/or pulmonary edema refractory to diuretic therapy, persistent hyperkalemia, severe metabolic acidosis unresponsive to medical management, neurological symptoms (altered mental status, seizures), and the presence of progressive azotemia. The modulation of inflammatory mediators in ARF with sepsis or multiorgan system failure may be another indication [48]. An additional indication for dialysis is the inability to provide adequate nutritional intake because of the need for severe fluid restriction. In patients with ARF, dialysis support may be necessary for days or weeks [49].

In chronic renal failure, ESRD represents the state in which a patient's renal dysfunction has progressed to the point at which homeostasis and survival can no longer be sustained with native kidney function and maximal medical management. Relative indications for renal replacement therapy include weight loss, malnutrition, persistent nausea and vomiting, refractory metabolic disturbances, refractory hypertension, fluid overload, school performance failure and chronic fatigue. Absolute indications include progressive uremic encephalopathy, bleeding diathesis related to uremia, pericarditis, pulmonary edema, and life-threatening hyperkalemia [43]. The ultimate goal for children with ESRD is successful kidney transplantation because it provides the most normal lifestyle and possibility for rehabilitation for the child and family.

Seventy-five percent of children with ESRD in the US require a period of dialysis before transplantation can be performed. It is recommended that plans for renal replacement therapy be initiated when a child reaches a glomerular filtration rate (GFR) between 29 and 50 (mL/min/1.73 m^2) [49]. The optimal time to actually initiate dialysis, however, is based on a combination of the biochemical and clinical characteristics of the patient, including refractory fluid overload, electrolyte imbalance, acidosis, growth failure or uremic symptoms, fatigue, nausea, and impaired school performance [43]. In general, most nephrologists attempt to initiate dialysis early enough to prevent the development of severe fluid and electrolyte abnormalities, malnutrition, and uremic symptoms. Pre-emptive transplantation before initiation of dialysis is increasingly observed [49]. Management of anesthesia for renal transplantation is discussed in Chapter 27.

The selection of dialysis modality must be individualized to fit the needs of each child. In the United States, two-thirds of children with ESRD are treated with peritoneal dialysis, whereas one-third are treated with hemodialysis. Age is a defining factor in dialysis modality selection; 88% of infants and children from birth to 5 years of age are treated with peritoneal dialysis, whereas 54% of children older than 12 years of age are treated with hemodialysis [50]. In acute renal failure each modality has its indications, contraindications, and challenges (Table 29.3) [46].

Peritoneal dialysis involves the transport of solutes and water across the peritoneum. The blood in the peritoneal capillaries is exposed to the dialysis solution in the peritoneal cavity, which typically contains sodium, chloride, and lactate or bicarbonate along with glucose to make the solution hyperosmolar. During the course of a peritoneal dialysis dwell, three transport processes occur simultaneously: diffusion, ultrafiltration, and absorption. The amount of dialysis achieved and the extent of fluid

Table 29.3 Comparison of the advantages and disadvantages of continuous renal replacement therapies (CRRT), peritoneal dialysis (PD), and intermittent hemodialysis (IHD)

Variable	CRRT	PD	IHD
Continuous therapy	Yes	Yes	No
Hemodynamic stability	Yes	Yes	No
Fluid balance achieved	Yes, pump controlled	Yes/no, variable	Yes, intermittent
Easy to perform	No	Yes	No
Metabolic control	Yes	Yes	Yes, intermittent
Optimal nutrition	Yes	No	No
Continuous toxin removal	Yes	No/yes, depends on the nature of the toxin – larger molecules not well cleared	No
Anticoagulation	Yes, requires continuous anticoagulation	No, anticoagulation not required	Yes/no, intermittent anticoagulation
Rapid poison removal	Yes/no, depending on patient size and dose	No	Yes
Stable intracranial pressure	Yes	Yes/no, less predictable than CRRT	Yes/no, less predictable than CRRT
ICU nursing support	Yes, high level of support	Yes/no, moderate level of support (if frequent, manual cycling can be labor intensive)	No, low level of support
Dialysis nursing support	Yes/no, institution dependent	Yes/no, institution dependent	Yes
Patient mobility	No	Yes, if IPD used	No
Cost	High	Low/moderate. Increases with increased dialysis fluid used	High/moderate
Vascular access required	Yes	No	Yes
Recent abdominal surgery	Yes	No	Yes
VP shunt	Yes	Yes/no, relative contraindication	Yes
Prune belly syndrome	Yes	Yes/no, relative contraindication	Yes
Ultrafiltration control	Yes	Yes/no, variable	Yes, intermittent
PD catheter leakage	No	Yes	No
Infection potential	Yes	Yes	Yes
Use in AKI-associated inborn errors of metabolism	Yes	No	Yes
Use in AKI-associated ingestions	Yes	No	Yes

a Omphalocele, gastroschisis, frequent or extensive abdominal surgery.
Reproduced from Walters et al [46] with permission from Springer.
AKI, acute kidney injury; ICU, intensive care unit; IPD, intermittent peritoneal dialyss; VP, ventriculoperitoneal.

removal depend on the volume of dialysis solution infused (called the dwell), how often this dialysis solution is exchanged, and the concentration of osmotic agent present [51].

Peritoneal dialysis requires less clinical expertise, fewer equipment resources, and decreased cost. It can be used in all pediatric patients including neonates and stable postoperative heart surgery patients. It can be performed in patients with a ventriculoperitoneal shunt and also in patients with prune belly syndrome. Peritoneal dialysis provides gradual solute clearance and ultrafiltration, thus causing less hemodynamic instability. Slow solute clearance and ultrafiltration is an obvious disadvantage for patients with severe fluid overload or severe lactic acidosis requiring precise fluid balance and controlled ultrafiltration that can only be attained with intermittent hemodialysis or continuous renal replacement therapy [46].

Peritoneal dialysis can worsen respiratory distress by limiting diaphragmatic movement. Diaphragm defects are a contraindication to peritoneal dialysis. Because peritoneal dialysis can result in the loss of immunoglobulins, peritonitis is a risk. Catheter malfunction is common, resulting in leaks, hernias, and catheter obstruction.

Intermittent hemodialysis has the clear advantage of rapid ultrafiltration and solute removal when compared to peritoneal dialysis or CRRT. The hemodialysis circuit is composed of the patient's blood compartment access in the form of a surgically placed arteriovenous fistula (AVF) or arteriovenous graft (AVG), or a venous catheter connected to polyethylene tubing through which the patient's blood travels to and from the dialyzer. The dialysate consists of highly purified water into which sodium, potassium, calcium, magnesium, chloride, bicarbonate, and dextrose have been introduced. The low molecular weight waste products that accumulate in uremic blood are absent from the dialysis solution. For this reason, when uremic blood is exposed to dialysis solution, the flux rate of these solutes from blood to dialysate is initially much greater than the back-flux from dialysate to blood. During dialysis, concentration equilibrium is prevented, and the concentration gradient between blood and dialysate is maximized, by continuously refilling the dialysate compartment with fresh dialysis solution and by replacing dialyzed blood with undialyzed blood. Normally, the direction of dialysis solution flow is opposite to the direction of blood flow. The purpose of "countercurrent" flow is to maximize the concentration difference of waste products between blood and dialysate in all parts of the dialyzer [52].

Like peritoneal dialysis, intermittent hemodialysis can be performed outside the ICU. This modality is useful in children with toxic ingestions, tumor lysis syndrome, and inborn errors of metabolism [53,54]. Rapid solute and fluid removal afforded by intermittent hemodialysis can lead to disequilibrium syndrome. Careful dosing and selection of dialysate solution, with judicious use of mannitol are required to prevent dramatic osmolar fluctuation [55,56].

Continual renal replacement therapy refers to any continuous mode of extracorporeal solute or fluid removal. The common denominator to all forms of CRRT is an extracorporeal circuit connected to the patient via an arterial or venous access catheter. A variety of alternative CRRTs have been developed to address many of the problems associated with intermittent hemodialyi-

sis and peritoneal dialyisis discussed above. CRRT provides better metabolic control of azotemia and fluid removal without compromising intravascular volume and facilitates fluid and electrolyte management and nutritional support in critically ill patients. CRRT is an invaluable means of supporting critically ill children with a variety of illnesses, including acute renal failure, drug intoxication, inborn errors of metabolism, liver failure and multiorgan failure. However, the ideal method of applying the technique is unknown [57,58]. On the basis of the successful use of CRRT in patients with ARF, it is now occasionally used to facilitate fluid removal in patients without renal failure but for whom diuretic therapy alone has been unsuccessful or is contraindicated [59].

Dialysis catheter placement in the operating room

For children who do not undergo pre-emptive renal transplantation or who initially present with ESRD, establishment of adequate dialysis access is of paramount importance because it is directly linked to the quality of life and health of the patient. With respect to hemodialysis, all attempts should be made to create a primary arterial venous fistula. For patients without adequate veins, a PTFE graft is required. A native fistula is clearly preferred because of superior patency rates, although this option does require the presence of suitable veins, which excludes infants and small children under 20 kg [52]. Vascular catheters are the predominant vascular access in children. In children with ESRD, renal transplant is the first line of therapy. As an AV graft is recommended for long-term dialysis, such grafts are inappropriate for children who will undergo renal transplantation within a year [60,61].

The National Kidney Foundation Kidney Disease Outcomes Quality Initiative guidelines recommend that the order of vascular access be sequential: the right internal jugular vein, right external jugular vein, the left internal and external jugular veins, subclavian veins, femoral veins, or translumbar access to the inferior vena cava. This order is based on complication rates from lowest to highest [62]. Additionally, these catheters can lead to central venous stenosis and thrombosis, which can make future permanent upper extremity vascular access more difficult to achieve.

Peritoneal dialysis is performed after placement of a Tenckhoff catheter. A double-cuffed peritoneal dialysis catheter is inserted via an open or laparoscopic surgical procedure under general anesthesia. The loop of the catheter is placed in the pelvis. During the procedure, it is important to ascertain that fluid can run freely through the catheter into the abdomen and drain freely as well.

The laparoscopic technique appears to afford no advantage for successful catheter function in the early postoperative period [63]. In addition, other factors that did not influence catheter function include previous peritoneal dialysis (PD) catheter placement, previous abdominal surgery, type of catheter, or location of catheter exit site. However, Argo et al showed that use of the laparoscopic technique was helpful in children with an *in situ* ventriculoperitoneal shunt [64].

The most common cause of catheter failure is occlusion, either from an internal fibrin plug or obstruction by omentum, bowel or other structures. The single controllable factor that was associated with a decreased risk of occlusion was the performance of simultaneous omentectomy. Overall, children weighing less than 10 kg have a higher risk of PD catheter failure than children weighing over 10 kg.

The annualized infection rate decreases with age. Tenckhoff straight and Tenckhoff curled catheters have similar times to first peritonitis infection. Overall, first time peritonitis infection took longer for catheters with two cuffs compared to one, for swan neck tunnels compared to straight tunnels, and for down exit sites compared to up and lateral [50,65].

Children who are scheduled for PD catheter insertion are usually in stable condition with chronic renal failure and are receiving a catheter for RRT in anticipation of renal transplantation. Occasionally, a child in acute renal failure will require surgical insertion of a dialysis catheter, such as the patient with new-onset hemolytic uremic syndrome.

The preoperative evaluation includes a physical exam and review of the patient's metabolic status. The timing of the patient's most recent dialysis session, if any, is very important. Of particular importance are serum potassium concentration, fluid status, and dosing of drugs which undergo predominantly renal clearance. The patient requiring a PD catheter or hemodialysis catheter will require standard ASA monitoring but usually not invasive monitoring. Arterial catheters are normally avoided in these patients, as are blood pressure cuffs on the extremity of an existing AV fistula or graft. Of critical importance is a preoperative discussion with the patient's nephrologist or surgeon about vascular access sites to be avoided. Long-term patency of major veins and arteries is critical to maintain in these patients, who may undergo a number of vascular access procedures over a lifetime. It is also important, when anesthetizing a patient with an existing dialysis fistula, to monitor blood flow during the anesthetic, and maintain blood pressure and intravascular volume status to ensure AV fistula or graft patency. Tracheal intubation is prudent since many children in acute and chronic renal failure have delayed gastric emptying and thus have a pulmonary aspiration

risk. The need for rapid-sequence induction or modified rapid sequence must be determined on an individual patient basis. While succinylcholine may be used for rapid-sequence induction if the serum potassium is at normal levels, rocuronium may be a better choice. Neuromuscular blockade with rocuronium is of similar duration or only slightly prolonged in patients with chronic renal failure (CRF) as compared to patients with normal renal function [66]. Fentanyl and hydromorphone are not metabolized by the kidney and are reasonable choices for perioperative analgesia [67].

Continuous renal replacement therapy in the operating room

Most patients receiving CRRT are critically ill, may be on mechanical ventilator support, and are often receiving myriad vasoactive agents. These patients are challenging because they may have underlying coagulopathies, yet CRRT requires anticoagulation for filter patency. If these children need surgical procedures, in most instances, CRRT treatment can be discontinued while in the operating room. However, in some procedures, for example liver transplantation, CRRT may be used during surgery to optimize fluid and electrolyte management [68].

Most anesthesiologists and OR personnel are not familiar with CRRT or the equipment needed to provide the therapy. It is imperative that a meaningful discussion occur among the intensivists, nephrologists, and surgeons involved in the procedure, in order to outline the operative care of the patient. In our institution, a technician familiar with the CRRT device manages the apparatus in the operating room. Careful monitoring of arterial blood gases and electrolytes is essential to ensure normal acid–base balance [59].

Priapism

Ischemic (veno-occlusive, low-flow) priapism is a nonsexual, persistent erection causing a compartmental syndrome that is a medical, and sometimes surgical, emergency in any episode lasting greater than 4 h. Patients typically report associated pain. In children, the etiologies include sickle cell disease, oncological disease, and neuroleptic drugs. Unlike normal erections which involve engorgement of the corpora cavernosa and the corporus spongiosum, priapism only involves engorgement of the corpora cavernosa.

Trazodone is a triazolopyridine derivative that holds considerable appeal for treatment of depressive illness and adjunct for chronic pain because it has little anticholinergic activity and few cardiovascular side-effects.

However, it possesses significant α-blocking activity, which appears to be a likely explanation for the pathogenesis of priapism in our patient in the Case Study (see below). Trazodone-induced priapism resembles priapism due to sickle cell hemoglobinopathy [69].

In general, since ischemic priapism of more than 4 h in duration irrespective of etiology implies a compartment syndrome, decompression of the corpora cavernosa is recommended for counteracting and preventing ischemic injury. Definitive first-line treatment consists of evacuation of blood and irrigation of the corpora cavernosa along with intracavernous injection of an α-adrenergic sympathomimetic agent. A dorsal nerve block or local penile shaft block is generally performed prior to penile maneuvers. Priapism resolution employing aspiration with or without irrigation is approximately 30%.

Sympathomimetic agents can be expected to exert contractile effects on the cavernous tissue and thus facilitate detumescence. Among these, phenylephrine, as an α_1-selective adrenergic agonist, is the preferred drug for this application since it minimizes the risk of cardiovascular side-effects compared with other sympathomimetic agents having β-adrenergic effects as well. Evacuation of stagnant intracorporal blood may be required for the medication to be most effective [70,71].

In patients with an underlying etiological disorder, intracavernous treatment of ischemic priapism should be provided concurrent with appropriate systemic treatment. This recommendation applies to priapism associated with sickle cell disease as well as that associated with other hematological diseases, metastatic neoplasia or other causes having standard treatments. Support for this recommendation is provided by a literature review showing that ischemic priapism resolved in 37% or less of patients with sickle cell disease managed with systemic medical treatments, whereas much better resolution rates were achieved with therapies directed at the penis [70]. Thus, for priapism related to sickle cell disease, conventionally recommended medical therapies such as analgesia, hydration, oxygenation, alkalinization, and even transfusion may be performed, but these interventions should not lead to delays in intracavernous treatment if prolonged periods of ischemia have occurred [71].

The surgeon may proceed with surgical intervention once it is apparent that intracavernous treatment has failed [70]. A surgical shunt has the objective of facilitating blood drainage from the corpora cavernosa, bypassing the veno-occlusive mechanism of these structures [71]. Surgical correction involves connecting the engorged cavernosal tissue with the glans, corpus spongiosum or dorsal or saphenous vein. This surgically created fistula will allow blood to drain from the corpora cavernosa until the pathological process has resolved. Ideally, the surgically created fistula will spontaneously close after the factors causing the priapism have resolved [72].

CASE STUDY

The patient is an 11-year-old male who has a history of Asperger syndrome and epilepsy. Chronic insomnia had been treated with trazodone for approximately 1 month. On the morning of surgery, he awoke at 9 a.m. with a rigid and painful erection which persisted throughout the day. There was no history of pelvic trauma or sickle cell disease. That evening, he was instructed to proceed immediately to the emergency department. After initial evaluation, the pediatric urologist aspirated his corporal bodies and attempted to irrigate with saline. This did not result in detumescence. Diluted phenylephrine was then injected as per protocol (Fig. 29.4) for the next 1 h [70]. The treatment was unsuccessful and the child was taken to the operating room for a distal shunt after his 15th hour of experiencing priapism.

The patient underwent a modified rapid-sequence induction with rocuronium and propofol. The trachea was intubated and general anesthesia was maintained with an inhalational agent. A caudal epidural block was performed with an appropriate dose of 0.25% bupivacaine for postoperative analgesia and the child was placed in the supine position. A 14 French Foley catheter was placed in the bladder to allow for continuous urine flow. At this point, his erection still remained very rigid. An incision was made approximately 4 mm distal to the coronal collar on the glans and dissected down to the corporal bodies. The corporal bodies were exposed bilaterally and they appeared very dusky; an ellipse of tissue was excised from the tunica albuginea from just above the tips of the corporal bodies bilaterally, resulting in immediate tumescence. Four weeks later, on follow-up outpatient visit, the patient was doing well and able to have spontaneous erections without problems. He is no longer treated with trazodone.

Continued

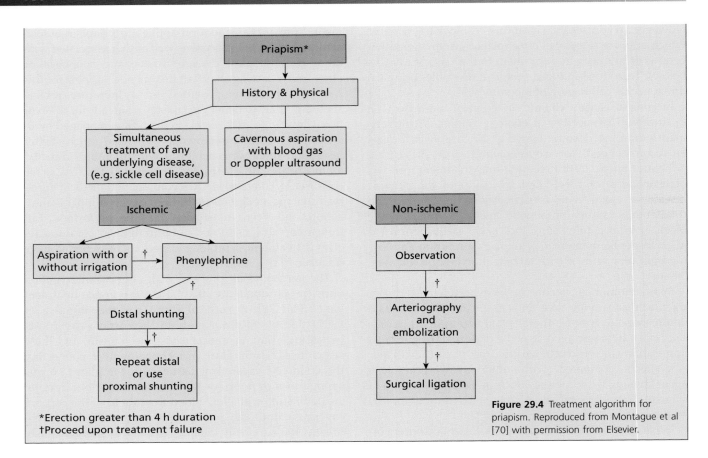

Figure 29.4 Treatment algorithm for priapism. Reproduced from Montague et al [70] with permission from Elsevier.

Annotated references

A full reference list for this chapter is available at:
http://www.wiley.com/go/gregory/andropoulos/pediatricanesthesia

4. Kost-Byerly S, Jackson EV, Yaster M et al. Perioperative anesthetic and analgesic management of newborn bladder exstrophy repair. J Pediatr Urol 2008; 4: 280–5. A comprehensive review article on modern management principles of neonatal bladder exstrophy.

12. Kibar Y, Roth CC, Frimberger D, Kropp BP. Our initial experience with the technique of complete primary repair for bladder exstrophy. J Pediatr Urol 2009; 5: 186–9. A modern series of complete one-stage repair of bladder exstrophy.

35. Tanaka ST, Grantham JA, Thomas JC et al. A comparison of open vs laparoscopic pediatric pyeloplasty using the pediatric health information system database – do benefits of laparoscopic approach recede at younger ages? J Urol 2008; 180: 1479–85. An interesting modern comparison of traditional open pyeloplasty versus a laparoscopic approach.

39. Davidoff AM. Wilms' tumor. Curr Opin Pediatr 2009; 21: 357–64. An excellent contemporary review of Wilms tumor in children.

46. Walters S, Porter C, Brophy P. Dialysis and pediatric acute kidney injury: choice of renal support modality. Pediatr Nephrol 2009; 24: 37–48. A modern review of the etiology of acute renal injury and decision making about choice of renal replacement therapy.

CHAPTER 30
Anesthesia for Orthopedic Surgery

Cathy Lammers & Cecile Wyckaert
Pediatric Anesthesiology, UC Davis Children's Hospital, and University of California, Davis, CA, USA

Clubfoot

Clubfeet or congenital talipes equinovarus are classified as being positional or rigid (Fig. 30.1). Rigid abnormalities are either flexible or resistant. The incidence of clubfoot (CF) is 1/1000 livebirths in the United States but may be higher in certain ethnicities (i.e. Polynesian islanders). Males are twice as affected as females. There is bilateral involvement in 30–50% of cases. Parents of a child with clubfoot have a 10% chance of having another child with clubfoot [1]. The etiology of CF is unknown. Most infants have no identifiable genetic syndrome or extrinsic cause. Extrinsic causes include oligohydramnios, congenital concentric rings, and teratogenic agents. Pathophysiological theories include arrest of fetal development, defective cartilage production, changes in innervation leading to paresis, increased fibrous tissue in muscles and ligaments, abnormal tendon insertion, and possible prenatal polio-like condition; the latter is based on changes in the motor neuron of the anterior horn in the spinal cord [2].

On physical examination, the foot is supinated in the varus position and adducted. Dorsiflexion is limited. The navicular, cuboid, and anterior aspects of the calcaneus are displaced medially [3]. There are contractures of the medial plantar soft tissues. The heel is small and empty. The medial malleolus is difficult to palpate and is often in contact with the navicular bone. The tibia is often internally rotated. The leg muscles are frequently atrophied, especially the peroneal muscle group. Although the number of muscle fibers is normal, they are smaller in size. The calf is often small and remains small even after successful correction of the lesion [4].

The goal of therapy is to correct the deformity early and maintain alignment of the foot until growth ceases [5]. The Pirani scoring system is used to identify the severity of the clubfoot and is based on the curvature of the lateral border, medial crease, uncovering of the lateral head of the talus, posterior crease, emptiness of the heel and degree of dorsiflexion [6]. Non-operative treatment (splinting and casting) begins 2–3 days after birth with forefoot adduction, followed by forefoot supination, and then correction of the equinus [7]. Gentle manipulation of the foot is needed to avoid producing a rocker-bottom foot. If splinting and casting are unsuccessful, surgery is indicated, usually at 6 months of age when the anatomy is more identifiable. In children younger than 5 years of age, soft tissue procedures are indicated. In children older than 5 years, bony reshaping or osteotomy of the calcaneum may be needed. Lateral wedge tarsectomy or triple fusion is required in children older than 10 years [8]. Complications of surgical correction are wound breakdown, infection, avascular necrosis, stiffness, and residual deformity.

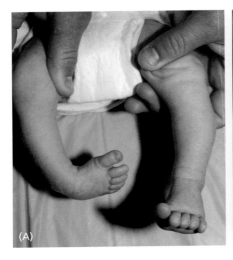
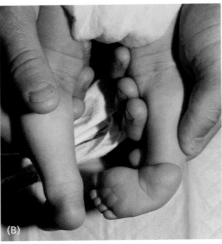

Figure 30.1 Clubfoot. (A) Anterior view of a baby with clubfoot. (B) Posterior view of the same child.

Preoperatively, one looks for co-morbid conditions (e.g. arthrogryposis, myelomeningocele) that include cardiovascular, respiratory, hematological and neurological problems that have their own anesthetic implications. Although both general and regional anesthesia may be performed for clubfoot surgery, peripheral nerve blocks like posterior sciatic and femoral nerve blocks are generally avoided because the surgeons must examine the patient for postoperative neurological changes and for possible compartment syndrome with casting. While spinal and epidural anesthesia have been used for clubfoot surgery, there was no significant decrease in postoperative opiate use [9]. Tourniquets must be used cautiously in patients who have fragile bones. Postoperatively, pain is minimal and amenable to standard doses of narcotics and acetaminophen.

Hip dysplasias/dislocations

Hip dysplasia refers to a hip that can be dislocated from or relocated into the acetabulum. Hip dislocation describes a non-reducible hip that is associated with shortening, decreased abduction, and asymmetry of skinfolds. The normal hip joint consists of a femoral head and the acetabulum which develop from the same primitive mesenchymal cells. In the 11th week of fetal life, the hip joint is fully formed and may begin to dislocate if predisposed to do so [10]. Subluxation of the hip occurs in 1% of newborn infants. Patients with dysplasia or dislocation of the hip do not have the normal tight fit between the femoral head and the acetabulum. The majority of abnormalities in developmental hip dysplasia or dislocation are on the acetabular side. Acetabular shape is determined by 8 years of age in most children. Growth of the acetabulum is affected by abnormal acetabular cartilage which is influenced by several factors, including the presence of a spherical femoral head, interstitial growth within the acetabular head, appositional growth under the perichondrium, and growth of adjacent bones (ileum, ischium and pubis). The dysplastic hip has a ridge (the limbus) in the superior, posterior, and inferior aspects of the acetabulum that is made of cellular hyaline cartilage. The limbus is a hypertrophied labrum [11].

Increased risk for abnormalities of the hips is indicated by female gender, first born, breech delivery, oligohydramnios, a positive family history for hip dysplasia, persistent hip asymmetry, torticollis, and lower limb deformity. All newborns are now screened for hip dysplasia and dislocation with the Ortolani and Barlow signs [12]. The Ortolani sign is positive when the hip is abducted, the trochanter is elevated, and the femoral head glides back into the acetabulum with a characteristic click. The Barlow sign is positive when the femoral head exits the acetabulum with the hip flexed and adducted. Ultrasonography helps to confirm the diagnosis and identify more subtle forms of dysplasia or dislocation. This should be performed in suspected cases at 4–6 weeks of age. If the diagnosis is missed at birth, there are four possible outcomes. The hip may become normal, subluxate or develop partial contact, completely dislocate or remain located in the hip with dysplastic features. Physical findings of late diagnosis include shortened limb, asymmetry of gluteal, thigh or labial skinfolds, and limited hip abduction. Patients with bilateral involvement have a waddling gait and hyperlordosis.

The Pavlik harness is the treatment of choice for infants and neonates with developmental hip dysplasia or dislocation. This device consists of a chest strap, shoulder straps, and anterior and posterior stirrup straps that maintain the hips in flexion and abduction while restricting extension and adduction [13] (Figs 30.2, 30.3).

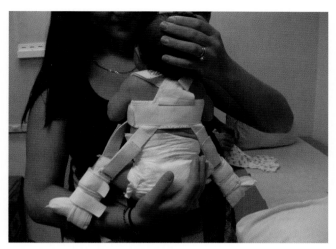

Figure 30.2 Pavlik harness: posterior.

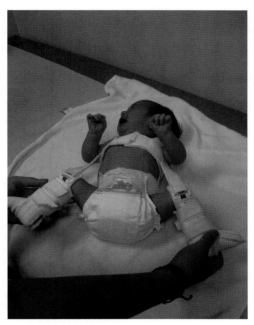

Figure 30.3 Pavlik harness: anterior.

Contraindications to the Pavlik harness include major muscle imbalance (e.g. myelomeningocele), major stiffness (e.g. arthrogryposis), ligamentous laxity (e.g. Ehlers–Danlos), patients older than 10 months of age, and lack of family support and care. The harness is worn until there are no positive findings on clinical, ultrasonographic or radiographic examinations. If the hip remains unstable with use of a Pavlik harness, a hip abduction brace is recommended. Complications of the harness include inferior dislocation, femoral nerve palsy, and avascular necrosis of the hip from excessive hip flexion [14].

An abduction orthotic is an alternative for infants who are more than 9 months of age. This maintains abduction while allowing the child to walk. Skin traction is recommended for older infants who have a dislocated hip and have failed to improve with a Pavlik harness or for children greater than 9 months old. Skin traction is followed by adductor tenotomy, closed reduction of the abnormality, and spica cast application (see below) [15]. Children greater than 2 years old are treated with primary femoral shortening, open reduction of the hip, capsulorrhaphy (suture of capsule tear in order to prevent dislocation) and pelvic osteotomy [16,17]. The decision to perform open reduction of the hip is made in the operating room after arthrography and failed closed hip reduction [18].

Preoperatively, it is important to identify co-morbid conditions or underlying bone pathology that may affect the overall anesthetic. Baseline laboratory studies, such as complete blood count, chemistry, and coagulation studies, are not necessary for healthy children but will help identify abnormalities if co-morbidity exists. Both general and regional anesthesia can be used during correction of hip pathology, if no contraindications exist. Spinal or epidural anesthesia may help with postoperative pain control in inpatients. If an epidural catheter is placed, care must be taken to cut a hole in the spica cast so that the catheter can be removed from the patient. While the child is being placed in a spica cast under anesthesia, care must be taken during cast application to insure that the arms are supported and head and neck are in alignment to prevent injury to major nerves. Postoperatively, oral pain medication can include acetaminophen, opioids, and short-term non-steroidal anti-inflammatory drugs.

Spica cast

Spica casts create stability and immobilize femoral fractures or hip abnormalities (Figs 30.4, 30.5). Contraindications to these devices include unacceptable shortening or angulation of the lower extremities, open fractures, thoracic or intra-abdominal trauma, and large or obese children [19]. Anesthesia is usually required to apply a spica cast. Fluoroscopy is used to determine optimal position, i.e. the affected limb or hip is placed in mild abduction. Too much abduction results in lateral bowing of the femur due to pull of adductors. The degree of hip flexion, hip adduction, and external rotation depends on the location of the femoral fracture or hip abnormality [20]. A folded towel is placed on the anterior thorax and abdomen and padding and casting material are placed over the towel. This creates space between the cast and the thorax/abdomen, allowing for free breathing after the towel is removed. Two layers of stockinette are

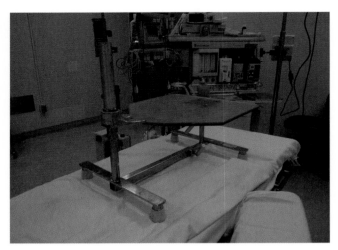

Figure 30.4 Spica cast table.

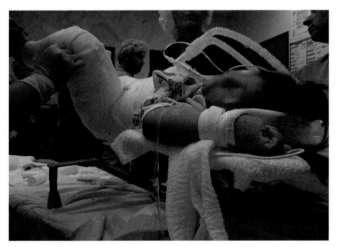

Figure 30.5 Spica cast: child on table.

placed to ensure that the cast padding can be pulled over the edges of the cast. Gore-tex™ soft wrap is often applied prior to applying a thick felt belt across chest, sacrum, posterior superior iliac spine, and anterior superior iliac spine. The casting material is often placed over the non-affected side for stability. A wooden stick is placed between both legs and covered in cast material. This reinforces the cast and prevents breakdown of the cast at the hip joint. In small children, spica casts are applied while the child is on a portable elevated narrow table that provides very little head support.

The goals of anesthesia during cast placement include hemodynamic stability, appropriate amnesia and analgesia, and safe positioning of the patient. The choice of anesthetic technique is dictated by the patient's health status and by any co-existing disease. With elevation of the patient off the operating room table, vigilance is required to assure that the upper extremities and neck are in alignment with the long axis of the body to prevent further nerve injury and paralysis.

Blount disease

Blount disease is a growth disorder of the medial aspect of the tibia in children. It causes the legs to bow outwards below the knees [21]. Normal infants have a small amount of physiological bowing that usually resolves by 2 years of age. In Blount disease the legs remain bowed, and the inner surface of the legs bulge outward just below the knee. A metaphyseal-diaphyseal angle greater than 11° is more indicative of Blount disease [21]. The toes also begin to point inwards as internal tibial rotation and asymmetrical leg shortening develop. Most patients are healthy, without congenital abnormalities, and may not experience much pain. If pain is present, it is usually related to the knee joints.

Blount disease usually affects children younger than 4 years old, in which case it is called infantile tibia vara. Adolescent tibia vara occurs after 4 years of age. Blount disease is more common in Africa, West Indies, and Finland. Sixty to 70% of cases are bilateral and symmetrical [22]. Risk factors for Blount disease include female sex, African-American race, obesity, early age at walking, and a positive family history for this problem. The cause of Blount disease is unknown but may be related to a combination of genetic, environmental, and mechanical factors [23]. The medial aspect of the growth plate fails to develop properly, while the lateral aspect grows normally. This results in deviated growth of the tibia. If untreated, the disease results in the onset of osteo-arthritis in the third decade of life. In the US, estimated prevalence of infantile Blount disease is less than 1% and adolescent disease is 2.5%. The disease is non-existent in non-ambulatory people. Adolescent tibia varus differs from Blount disease in that patients with varus complain more about knee pain, have unilateral involvement in 80% of cases, have shortened leg length, and may be obese [24–26].

Under 2 years of age, observation of the patient and follow-up with an orthopedic surgeon are recommended to distinguish physiological bowing from abnormal bowing. If bowing persists during ages 2–4, orthotic braces from the top of the thigh to the tips of the toes are recommended [27]. In children with severe bowing or who are more than 4 years of age, osteotomies of the tibia and occasionally the fibulae are most commonly performed to correct the misalignment [28]. Other operative treatments include removing the epiphysis to stop abnormal growth or an osteotomy followed by external fixation [29,30]. If treated early, patients develop fully functioning lower limbs and have no limitations of movement. Complications of treatment include loss of alignment of lower extremities, vascular impairment, pathological fractures, and wound infection.

Preoperatively, the anesthetic implications of existing co-morbidities must be considered. Concurrent obesity may lead to airway difficulties, respiratory problems, obstructive sleep apnea, increased risk of aspiration, and difficulty inserting an intravenous catheter. A detailed history and directed physical examination are needed to identify any major organ or airway dysfunction. Intraoperatively, both general and regional anesthesia can be utilized if they are not contraindicated. Fat or venous air embolism must always be suspected if acute decompensation in the patient's condition occurs during surgery. Presenting symptoms of fat embolism under general anesthesia may include hypoxia, petechial rash, and hypotension. Presenting symptoms of venous air embolism under general anesthesia may include decreased end-tidal carbon dioxide and hypotension. Surgical blood loss is usually minimal. Postoperatively, it is important to perform a neurovascular examination to make sure that no important vascular or neural structures were damaged during corrective repair. Pain control is managed easily with intravenous patient-controlled analgesia (PCA) or oral medications, such as acetaminophen and narcotics.

Slipped capital femoral epiphysis

Slipped capital femoral epiphysis (SCFE) consists of a defect of the proximal femoral growth plate, which causes instability of the femoral head. The femoral head is displaced posteriorly and inferiorly from the femoral neck. SCFE presents with hip, medial thigh, and knee pain. The range of motion of the hip is limited and causes a limp. The incidence of SCFE is 10.8/100,000 children. Higher rates of prevalence exist in males, African-Americans, Hispanics, and people who live in the west and north-east of the United States [31]. The average age of occurrence of SCFE is between 10 and 16 years. Twenty percent of patients have bilateral involvement. High-risk patients include those with obesity, hypothyroidism, low concentrations of growth hormone, pituitary tumors, craniopharyngioma, Down syndrome, renal osteodystrophy and adiposogenital syndrome [32–34]. The left hip is affected more commonly than the right. Familial involvement is present in 5–7% of patients with SCFE. In patients younger than 10 years of age, SCFE is associated with metabolic endocrine disorders. Unstable SCFE produces a non-ambulatory patient and has a higher risk of avascular necrosis [35]. On physical examination, internal rotation of the affected leg is very painful.

Emergency treatment is necessary. If surgical correction is performed within 24h of onset, the risk of avascular necrosis decreases. Immediate internal fixation with a screw is the treatment of choice [36]. Repair of SCFE permits early stabilization of slippage, prevention of further slippage, increased physeal closure and improvement of symptoms [37]. The fixation may require revision if the child outgrows the screw. Prophylactic fixation of unaffected hips should only occur if patients have endocrinological or metabolic conditions and are outside the usual age group of 10–16 years [38,39]. Osteotomy of the proximal femur may be required to reposition the femoral head and improve functional range of motion. Bone graft epiphysiodesis and internal fixation can be performed but may result in avascular necrosis, chondrolysis, poor initial fixation, prolonged operative time, increased intraoperative blood loss and loss of epiphyseal position [40].

Preoperatively, a thorough history and physical examination elucidate significant co-morbidities that may affect anesthetic technique. Given that obesity has a high association with SCFE, one must evaluate and prepare for an obstructed airway, restrictive lung disease, and a difficult airway. Some obese patients also have type 2 diabetes. In rare cases hypothyroidism and renal osteodystrophy may also be present. Preoperative studies should include baseline hematocrit, serum electrolytes, and a type and screen for blood.

Intraoperatively, the patient may be placed supine or in lateral position. During positioning of the patient, care must be taken to avoid nerve compression or injury, especially in obese patients. The Chick fracture table (Fig. 30.6) is often used and requires careful

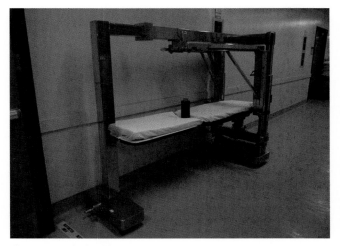

Figure 30.6 Chick table.

padding and securing of the patient to the table. Access to the airway during surgery can be limited. Tracheal intubation is usually done prior to transfer to the fracture table.

The choice of anesthetic technique is influenced by the patient's baseline health status and co-morbidities. General anesthesia, in conjunction with regional anesthesia, may be performed if there are no contraindications to regional anesthesia. A one-time caudal injection of local anesthetic can be helpful; inserting caudal catheters is usually unnecessary. If the patient is obese or has a difficult airway, a modified rapid-sequence induction (RSI) may be considered. Third space fluid losses are usually 3–6 mL/kg/h. Blood loss is typically minimal. Postoperative pain is usually controlled with opioids and acetaminophen. Short-term non-steroidal anti-inflammatory drugs may also be helpful and have not been shown to significantly affect epiphyseal growth.

Hand surgery

Many different types of disorders that require hand surgery exist in childhood (Box 30.1). These include, but are not limited to, extra fingers (polydactyly), webbed fingers (syndactyly), missing fingers (symbrachydactyly – hand or arm deficiency), abnormal thumbs, stiff joints, nerve and skeletal injuries [41,42]. The abnormalities range from mild to severe in their presentations. Given

the complexity and variation of each deformity, only a few of them will be described in detail in this text. Although most hand malformations cause little functional deficit, surgery is usually performed within the first 2 years of life to improve growth and scarring, and reduce psychological trauma. Early surgery also improves adaptation to the use of the newly formed part [43].

Syndactyly surgery is performed after a child is 2 years old and growth of the hand has slowed [44]. Syndactyly is twice as common in boys as in girls and occurs in 1/2000 livebirths. It commonly affects the long and ring fingers [45]. Skin grafts may be required to close the defects caused by separation of the digits. About half of treated children return for surgery during adolescence for further cosmesis once the hand reaches full size [46]. Symbrachydactyly is a condition in which a child is born with small or missing fingers, a short forearm or a missing hand. It is the most common form of hand or arm deficiency [47]. The cause is unknown and is not attributed to genetic inheritance. It is usually unilateral; muscular abnormalities may be present on the ipsilateral side. Although surgery is often not required, it can help to deepen the webs between the fingers and to stabilize the fingers when bone grafts are used. Thumb polydactyly has varying forms, ranging from a broad fingernail to complete double thumbs [48]. Reconstructive surgery sometimes combines parts of the two different thumbs to create one functional thumb. Surgery is usually delayed until the thumb is large enough to allow the surgeon to reconstruct the nerves, ligaments, and bone.

Trigger thumb occurs when a nodule on the tendon causes the thumb to jump or lock into a bent position with movement. This condition develops after birth and is present at 1 year in 3.3/1000 livebirths. Hand surgeons must evaluate and treat this condition promptly to prevent contracture, but 30% of these lesions resolve spontaneously. Treatment involves surgery to enlarge the tendon sheath and allow the tendon to move more smoothly. This is performed usually between the ages of 1 and 3 years.

Radial club hand (RCH) is a deficiency of the radius in the forearm. It occurs 1/30,000–100,000 livebirths and includes absent or an incomplete radius, absent or incomplete thumb, deviation of wrist toward the radial side, and some degree of neuromuscular deficiency. The cause of RCH is unknown, but it has been suggested that irradiation or environmental and nutritional factors may be involved. Radial club hand may be associated with other genetic syndromes such as VACTER (V vertebrae, A anus, C cardiovascular, TE tracheo-esophageal fistula, R renal system), Holt–Oram syndrome (heart and hand syndrome), TAR (thrombocytopenia with absent radius) syndrome and Fanconi anemia [49]. Therefore a thorough investigation of other possible organ abnormalities must

---

Box 30.1 Hand malformations

- Cerebral palsy contractures
- Arthrogryposis contractures
- Juvenile arthritis
- Madelung's deformity – malformed wrist bones
- Ulnar longitudinal deficiency
- Bite wounds
- Retained foreign objects
- Ganglion cysts
- Hemangiomas
- Lipomas
- Vascular malformations
- Amputations
- Crush injury
- Nailbed injury
- Mallet finger – damage to extensor tendon
- Rugger jersey finger – damage to flexor tendon
- Burn wound and scar management
- Polydactyly
- Symbrachydactyly
- Syndactyly

be undertaken. Treatment of radial club hand starts with splinting, casting, and non-surgical manipulation of the hand. If needed, surgery is typically performed between 6 months and 1 year of age. The procedure is called centralization/radialization of carpus on ulnar epiphysis, which relocates the hand over the ulna [50]. The affected limb is usually shorter than the contralateral limb after this repair. If too severe, a procedure can be done between 6 and 8 years of age to lengthen the extremity. If the thumb is absent or underdeveloped, the hand surgeon can also make the index finger into a thumb ("pollicization") to allow grasping.

Preoperative evaluation consists of gathering information about other possible co-morbidities and evaluating the child's maturity and social environment. All may affect the type of anesthesia chosen. For example, it must be determined if children with congenital hand deformities have associated heart, lung, kidney or airway problems that must be addressed. If there are vascular malformations of the hand, one must be suspicious that there are other vascular malformations (e.g. oropharyngeal) and that the child may have a high output state and heart failure. In trauma, full stomach aspiration risks need to be addressed. The child's maturity will also dictate whether a procedure should be performed with sedation or local anesthesia, with or without general anesthesia. If the surgery is elective or semi-urgent, laboratory tests should determine if anemia or coagulopathy is present. If other co-morbidities exist, an electrocardiogram and chest x-ray should be considered if indicated. A baseline neurovascular examination should be performed to evaluate sensation and perfusion to the affected hand. The findings of the examination should be documented in the anesthetic record.

Combined regional and general anesthesia has been shown to improve postoperative recovery and decrease the need for postoperative analgesics. Most children who undergo surgery require general anesthesia. Small cases, such as distal fingertip amputation, can be performed with local anesthesia and sedation if the child is co-operative. More extensive cases are amenable to using a combined regional and general anesthetic if there are no contraindications. Contraindications to peripheral blocks include hand infection, generalized sepsis, coagulopathy, predisposition to compartment syndrome, parental/child dissent, or the surgeon's need to perform an immediate postoperative examination of the extremity [51].

The nerve supply to the hand includes three major branches of the brachial plexus. The median nerve originates from the lateral and medial cords of the brachial plexus (C5–T1). It innervates the muscles involved in pinching and grasping (i.e. flexor carpi radialis, palmaris longus, flexor digitorum superficialis, flexor pollicis longus, flexor digitorum profundus, and pronator quad-

ratus). It provides sensation to the lateral aspect of the palm, including the thenar eminence and the distal ends of the first three and a half fingers dorsally. The ulnar nerve originates from the medial cord of the brachial plexus (C8–T1). Motor branches innervate the flexor carpi ulnaris, flexor digitorum profundus, and the hypothenar muscles. This nerve provides sensation to the medial dorsal aspect of the hand and to the last one and a half fingers. The radial nerve originates from the posterior cord of the brachial plexus (C6–8) and innervates the wrist extensors and provides sensation to the lateral dorsal aspect of the hand and proximal portion of the first three and a half fingers.

Regional anesthetic techniques appropriate for hand surgery include Bier block (intravenous local anesthetic), axillary block (Fig. 30.7), infraclavicular block, wrist block, elbow block and digital block [51]. Of these, the infraclavicular block is best suited to catheter placement because the area is generally cleaner, and it is easier to secure the catheter. Intravenous regional anesthesia is useful in trauma patients who have a full stomach if the patient can be safely sedated. Regional anesthesia is relatively contraindicated in children less than 1 year old due to systemic local anesthetic toxicity. It may also be contraindicated in children susceptible to tourniquet injury (i.e. osteogenesis imperfecta). Most hand surgery requires use of a tourniquet, which is associated with hyper/hypotension and respiratory and lactic acidosis from repeated inflation and deflation of the tourniquet. If not properly applied, tourniquets can lead to paralysis, sensory loss, excessive edema, skin problems and muscle damage.

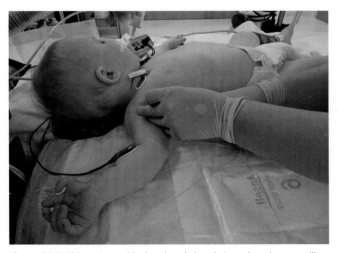

Figure 30.7 This patient with thumb polydactyly is undergoing an axillary nerve block.

Postoperatively, it is important to determine if there are new or worse neurovascular deficits. Pain can be controlled with residual regional anesthetic, intravenous PCA and oral medication. Although not much is known regarding the long-term use of tramadol in children, some studies in healthy children suggest that it can be used safely for 7–30 days and provides good pain control. There was no significant increase in the incidence of side-effects [52,53].

Supracondylar femur fractures

A supracondylar fracture represents 12% of femoral fractures in children and is the most common cause of femur fracture in infants less than 1 year old, often due to child abuse [54]. Although the incidence is slightly less, it is still very common at ages 1–4 years. The American Academy of Orthopedic Surgeons recommends screening children younger than 36 months of age with femoral shaft fracture for child abuse. In adolescents, motor vehicle accidents (cars, bicycles) are the leading cause of femoral shaft fractures. Other causes of femoral shaft fracture include falling hard on the playground and contact sports. Fractures are described by location, shape of fractured ends, and number of fractured parts [55].

Non-surgical treatment of some femoral fractures includes closed reduction, a Pavlik harness or spica casting (see above) [56]. Pathological bone is often treated with closed methods, due to abnormal bone fragility. Closed reductions are often done under sedation, but the child may require general anesthesia if they are uncooperative or the defect is extreme. Pavlik harnesses are soft restraints that go around the patient's shoulders and body and hold the hips in a flexed position. Spica casts typically begin at or below the nipple line of the chest and extend to slightly beyond the fracture or defect [57]. They hold the broken bone in alignment while it heals. The broken bones should not overlap by more than 2 cm when in the cast. Increased growth of the damaged femur will overcome the initial shortening caused by the overlap [58]. If casting causes greater than 3 cm shortening or misalignment of the bones, traction may help to align the bones properly. Children who are older, large or obese and have multiple trauma, head injury, and/or soft tissue damage usually require operative fixation of the bones.

Recently, there has been a trend towards more surgical stabilization than in previous years, due to earlier mobilization, faster rehabilitation, and less time spent in hospital [59]. Flexible intramedullary nails are used in 6–10-year-old children [60]. If the bone is broken into many pieces (comminuted), other options include a plate

with screws to bridge the fracture, an external fixator, or prolonged traction with a temporary pin in the femur [61]. Once skeletal maturity is achieved (about 11 years of age), there is less risk of vascular compromise to the growth plate. Treatment options at this point include flexible or rigid locked intramedullary nails. Rigid locked intramedullary nails allow walking immediately. Most children with femoral shaft fractures will heal, regain normal function, and have legs of equal length. The intramedullary nails may need to be removed after healing if skin or tissue irritation occurs [62]. If there is significant leg length discrepancy, angulation or rotation of the leg, or if infection or non-union persist, further surgical intervention will be required [63].

Preoperatively, it is important to note the mechanism of injury, as this may provide clues to other associated injuries (i.e. neck or skull injury). Conditions associated with bone fragility require care in positioning the patient, care in the use of non-invasive versus invasive blood pressure monitoring, and care in the use of a tourniquet. In addition to thorough airway, respiratory, and cardiovascular examinations, it is important to perform and document a neurovascular examination that will provide the baseline for evaluating postoperative changes. A preoperative hematocrit and a type and cross-match of blood should be obtained because hemorrhage can occur into the thigh with femur fractures.

Intraoperatively, either general or regional anesthesia may be used to provide anesthesia. Spinal anesthesia works well in older, co-operative children if there are concerns for a full stomach or a difficult airway. Peripheral nerve blocks plus general anesthesia work well, but a thorough discussion with the surgeon should take place beforehand, as there is a high risk of compartment syndrome (which can be masked by a nerve block) and coagulopathy. Adequate intravenous access must be present for infusing fluid and blood products. Depending on the location of the fracture and the size of the patient, a tourniquet may be used to limit the amount of blood loss. The anesthesiologist must be prepared for the hemodynamic changes that are sometimes associated with using a tourniquet. Fat and venous air embolism from bone manipulation may also cause adverse hemodynamic effects. Postoperatively, patients are typically placed into casts to stabilize the fracture site. Narcotics and acetaminophen are usually adequate for pain control.

Septic arthritis

Septic arthritis usually occurs in the first 3 years of life or during teenage years (gonoccocal infections). Septic arthritis is a true clinical emergency because it can have serious implications for future joint mobility and organ dysfunction [64]. Pain with passive motion is the most common finding on physical examination. Prior to the introduction of antibiotics, septic arthritis was often severely incapacitating and/or fatal [65]. *Haemophilus influenzae* type b (Hib) was previously the most common causative organism associated with septic arthritis but since the institution of Hib vaccination in the 1970s, *Staphylococcus aureus* is now the foremost culprit [66,67]. Other less common pathogens include *Streptococcus* species, *Pseudomonas aeruginosa*, pneumococci, *Neisseria meningitidis*, *Escherichia coli*, *Klebsiella* species, and Enterobacter. Newborns can acquire *Neisseria gonorrhoeae* from an infected birth canal. *Kingella kingae*, a fastidious aerobic gram-negative micro-organism, has rapidly become a formidable pathogen that is difficult to grow in culture but must be suspected and treated, if present, in children aged 3 and younger [68].

Septic arthritis may develop after a penetrating wound or from trauma, surgery or adjacent cellulitis. However, the most common cause is hematogenous spread from transient bacteremia. Usually in healthy individuals, the bacteremia is quickly eliminated by intrinsic immune defense mechanisms. In immunocompromised and extremely young patients (neonates), the defense mechanisms are too overwhelmed or immature to eliminate the infection. Developing pediatric bone has vascular loops that provide nutrients to the metaphyseal side of the growth plate. The blood supply to this area is relatively slow, and the growth plate is not well covered by the reticuloendothelial system. This leaves the area vulnerable to infection. From 0 to 18 months of age, an abscess in the metaphyseal area may spread into the epiphysis through blood vessels that cross the cartilaginous physis and enter the joint. Those blood vessels disappear after 18 months of age. An abscess in the metaphyseal area will only cause septic arthritis in the areas where the joint capsule is attached to the metaphyses, such as the hip, shoulder, ankle, and elbow joints [65].

Once in the joint, the pathogens and the counteracting leukocytes release proteolytic enzymes that degrade the articular cartilage. Damage can occur in as little as 8h. The synovial membrane becomes edematous and hypertrophied and produces increased amounts of exudative fluid and pus. Increased pressure within the joint can interrupt the blood supply to the epiphysis. This causes bone destruction, loss of adjacent growth plate, dislocated joints, and injury to the capsule ligament. Rupture of the synovium can lead to extracapsular infections, such as myositis, soft tissue abscesses and bacteremia.

Presenting symptoms that should make one suspicious of septic arthritis include fever, malaise, erythema, swelling, and tenderness of the joint. Pain with passive motion

of the joint is the most common finding. As in the hip, the child will hold flexion, abduction, and external rotation to diminish pain and increase intracapsular volume. Refusal to move the affected joint is called pseudoparalysis, which can be mistaken for a neurological problem. Differential diagnosis of septic arthritis includes, but is not limited to, juvenile rheumatoid arthritis (more gradual onset), Legg–Calvé–Perthes disease (avascular necrosis of the proximal femoral head), Lyme disease, mycobacterial or fungal infections, abscess of the psoas muscle (presents with bladder irritability or a femoral nerve neuropraxia [69]), or transient synovitis from a self-limiting viral infection, mostly involving the hip [70]. A high index of suspicion must be present for neonates and immunocompromised patients, as they can have multiple sites affected without fever and without an elevated white blood cell count [71].

Septic arthritis is a true surgical and/or procedural emergency. Aspiration of the joint in the emergency room, interventional radiology suite or operating room must be accomplished quickly to insure prompt diagnosis and appropriate therapy. Typically these cases are completed within several hours of being scheduled. Frequently it is necessary to keep the child anesthetized while a gram stain and initial pathological evaluation of the aspirated fluid are performed. Treatment includes appropriate antibiotic therapy and drainage of the affected joint to prevent degradation of joint and bone. Open drainage of the joint is more effective than percutaneous aspiration and is indicated if the hip, shoulder, and peripheral joints fail to respond to percutaneous aspiration. Open drainage is also indicated for patients with systemic illness, *Staphylococcus aureus* and gram-negative bacteria that produce cartilage-destroying enzymes. Patients with pus in fascial layers have a high mortality rate as these pockets of infection can lead to venous thrombosis.

During the preoperative assessment it is important to find out if any co-morbidities exist. Hematogenous spread of bacteria can cause lung involvement that manifests as pleural effusion, pneumatoceles (lung abscesses), pneumothorax, wheezing, inflammation and edema-induced stridor. If respiratory symptoms present, a chest x-ray may help to identify the problem. Cardiac involvement includes pericardial effusion, myocarditis, endocarditis, and pericarditis, which can all limit cardiac function. An echocardiogram is recommended for patients with congenital defects, unresolved fever or prolonged bacteremia without a known source. Renal function may be affected through hematogenous spread of infection, decreased intravascular volume or medication-induced injury. Baseline laboratory studies and a coagulation profile are helpful as they can be adversely affected by infection. Chronically ill anemic patients may require blood transfusions. Platelets and coagulation factors may be decreased. Disseminated intravascular coagulation is a major complication of dispersed infection so blood products should be available prior to surgery and administered if needed. Adequate venous access must be available for giving volume support, blood products, and inotropes if necessary.

Shoulder or neck septic arthritis may cause cervical ligamentous laxity that can cause C1–2 subluxation during tracheal intubation. Intravascular volume must be repleted prior to induction of anesthesia to avoid hypotension. Chronic illness-induced decreased concentrations of intrinsic catecholamines may also cause acute decompensation of vital signs with induction of anesthesia. Intraoperative manipulation of the infected joint during surgery may release pathogens and their toxins into the bloodstream and produce acute hemodynamic changes. General anesthesia is typically required for these types of surgeries because regional anesthesia may obscure a possible compartment syndrome or lead to a new infectious point of entry/spread or a hematoma if coagulation abnormalities exist. Although positive pressure ventilation may predispose to pneumothorax and decreased venous return, it is still preferred over spontaneous ventilation, which may be associated with breath holding, laryngospasm, and bronchospasm.

Choice of anesthetic drugs can vary. Ketamine should be avoided for induction of anesthesia if catecholamine stores are depleted or are suspected to be depleted, as this can cause hypotension after induction of anesthesia. Succinylcholine should also be avoided if renal dysfunction and chronic illness exist because hyperkalemia can lead to significant injury and/or death.

Postoperatively most patients improve quickly after drainage and removal of infectious material. Fluid, blood products and inotropes should be continued if needed. Pain is controlled with narcotics and acetaminophen. NSAIDS are avoided when renal dysfunction or abnormal coagulation status is present. Although chronic NSAID use has been suggested to inhibit osteogenesis, new evidence indicates that perioperative use of these drugs for 48 h use may not significantly affect osteoblasts and bone formation. This should be addressed with the surgeon on a case-by-case basis.

Osteogenesis imperfecta

Osteogenesis imperfecta (OI), also called brittle bone disease, blue sclera syndrome, fragile bone disease, and Lobstein disease, is a relatively common skeletal dysplasia (Fig. 30.8). It has long been documented in human history and was found in a partially mummified infant's skeleton from Egypt. Oral historians believe that a Viking chieftain named Ivan the Boneless (865 AD) may also have had the disease.

Osteogenesis imperfecta is most commonly identified by three characteristics: blue sclerae, bone fragility, and hearing loss. Less common symptoms include triangular facies, macrocephaly, defective dentition, barrel chest, scoliosis, joint laxity, growth retardation, constipation, and sweating. Type 1 collagen is an important component of bone, ligament, dentin, and sclera. In OI, there is a decrease in either quality or quantity of type 1 collagen. Most cases of OI are autosomal dominant mutations of the genes encoding type 1 collagen [72]. Quantitative defects typically cause mild clinical disease, while qualitative defects cause severe clinical disease.

Osteogenesis imperfecta (types 1–4) occurs in 1/20,000 births. There is no predilection for OI by race, gender or age. More severe forms present at a younger age [73]. Types I and IV have milder clinical presentations, while types II and III are more severe.

- Type I presents with blue sclera, normal birthweight, moderate bone deformity, and variable degrees of bone fragility. Fractures occur when the child begins to walk and diminish after puberty. Twenty percent have scoliosis, and some may have dentinogenesis imperfecta.
- Type II presents with dwarfism, blue sclera, and bowed limbs at birth. Multiple fractures exist at birth, and the disease is usually fatal during or shortly after birth.

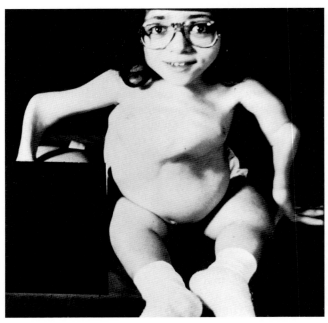

Figure 30.8 Child with osteogenesis imperfecta. Note abnormal chest and extremities.

- Type III presents with severe fragility and bone fractures at birth and frequently requires orthopedic surgery. Blue sclerae become white in adulthood. Dentinogenesis imperfecta is common. The chest and rib cage are spared from involvement in this type of OI. Children usually have bowed limbs and are wheelchair bound and non-ambulatory. They are often of short stature and have a mild pectus carinatum.
- Type IV presents with white sclerae. Patients have moderate bone fragility. Kyphoscoliosis is common.

Recently bisphosphonates have been used to increase bone mass and strength. Intravenous pamidronate, a synthetic analog of pyrophosphate, inhibits osteoclast-mediated bone resorption on the endosteal surface of bone by binding to hydroxyapatite. This allows unopposed osteoblastic new bone formation on the periosteal surface and increases cortical bone thickness. Bisphosphonates decrease the number of fractures by increasing bone mineral density [74]. This decreases bone pain and increases height. Physiotherapy, in conjunction with bisphosphonate therapy, promotes gross motor development and maximizes function. Adverse effects of bisphosphonate therapy include acute febrile reaction, leukopenia, a transient increase in bone pain, mild hypocalcemia, and scleritis. Other medical therapies under investigation include growth hormone, a recombinant human form of parathyroid hormone, bone marrow transplantation, and gene therapy.

Orthopedic goals for osteogenesis imperfecta include improving strength and preventing fractures. The aim of surgical intervention is to improve function [75]. Release of lower limb contractures improves mobility. Bony deformities and fractures are treated with intramedullary stabilization with or without corrective osteotomies [76]. Rods, pins, and wires are preferable to nails, plates, and screws as the former are less frequently associated with bone fractures. Complications of rods include breakage, rotational deformities, and migration. With the use of bisphosphonates, non-extendable rods are being used more often than extendable rods [77]. Posterior spinal arthrodesis is preferable to ineffective bracing for scoliosis. Arthrodesis is done in mild OI patients with greater than 45° curvature or in severe OI with greater than 35° curvature.

Preoperatively, it is important to identify the type of OI and the severity of clinical symptoms. Often the patient has required previous medical care. Lung function may be restricted due to chest wall deformities. A chest x-ray and pulmonary function tests, although not required, may help predict postoperative respiratory failure. Airway examination includes neck mobility, dentition, and mouth opening, as there may be a high likelihood of difficult tracheal intubation due to a short neck, macro-cephaly, macroglossia, and fragile dentition. Ventral brainstem compression by an invaginating clivus-odontoid complex may further make tracheal intubation difficult. Therefore, evaluation of the patient for symptoms of upper cervical cord compression and x-rays of the craniovertebral junction may help prevent injury. Cardiovascular abnormalities, although not significantly increased in comparison to healthy individuals, are usually related (when present) to aortic insufficiency caused by aortic root dilation. If a murmur is present or suspicion of aortic insufficiency is high, echocardiography is indicated. Patients with OI do have an increased risk for bleeding diathesis. The abnormal collagen on platelet–endothelial cell interaction results in increased capillary fragility, defective contraction of small blood vessels, and defective platelet aggregation. Typical coagulation studies (prothrombin time (PT) and partial thromboplastin time (PTT)) will be normal but platelet function will be abnormal. Patients at risk should avoid non-steroidal anti-inflammatory drugs for at least 7 days preoperatively.

Intraoperatively, care must be taken to position and pad the patient so no further fractures occur. Non-invasive blood pressure monitoring may cause fractures [78] so less frequent monitoring or invasive arterial blood pressure monitoring is preferred. Tourniquets may produce fractures and should be placed on top of a soft material such as Kerlex or Coban. Facemasks may damage fragile mandibles and maxillae. Laryngeal mask airways have been used successfully in lieu of facemasks to prevent facial fractures. Tooth guards are used when patients have fragile dentition. The increased incidence of difficult tracheal intubation warrants having a wide variety of airway equipment immediately available, including multiple sizes of tracheal tubes, multiple laryngoscope blades, gum elastic bougies, laryngeal mask airways, video laryngoscopy, and fiber-optic laryngoscopes.

Hyperthermia and lactic acidosis have occurred in patients with OI, possibly from an increased metabolic rate or associated hyperthyroidism, but not from malignant hyperthermia. There is no respiratory acidosis or muscular rigidity with OI. Hyperthermia is more often associated with the administration of anticholinergic drugs and with inhaled anesthetics. A cooling blanket should be used to treat hyperthermia. Succinylcholine is avoided due to the theoretical risk of fasciculation-induced fractures.

Postoperatively, patients may also have febrile responses from the increased metabolic rate or hyperthyroidism. Because these patients suffer from chronic pain, they should be treated with their baseline narcotic plus adjuvant pain medications, as needed. The patient's respiratory status should be carefully evaluated postoperatively to detect obstruction that is caused by residual anesthesia or by decreased hypercapneic-hypoxic respiratory drive from restrictive lung disease. Caution must be exercised during transfer from one bed to another to prevent additional fractures occurring.

Arthrogryposis

Arthrogryposis multiplex congenita presents at birth with multiple contractures throughout the body. It is present in 1/3000 livebirths and is more common in isolated populations such as Finland and the Bedouin community in Israel [79]. Males and females are affected equally. Thirty percent of cases have a genetic abnormality [80].

The major cause of arthrogryposis is fetal akinesia (decreased fetal movement *in utero*) [81]. The etiologies of arthrogryposis are many and include neurogenic, muscular, connective tissue abnormalities, mechanical limitations or maternal factors such as infection, drugs, trauma, and other illnesses. Malformations of the central and peripheral nervous systems are the most common cause of arthrogryposis [82]. Decreased fetal movement can also cause polyhydramnios, pulmonary hypoplasia, micrognathia, ocular hypertelorism and short umbilical cord. Lack of fetal movement results in the development of extra connective tissue around the joints, which limits joint movement and fixes it in a contracted state [83]. Half of patients with associated CNS abnormalities die within the first year. Infants born to mothers with myotonic dystrophy, myasthenia gravis or multiple sclerosis are at high risk for developing resistant contractures. Exposure of mothers to hyperthermia, such as hot tubs or prolonged hot baths, can cause abnormal nerve growth and decreased fetal movement.

Patients with arthrogryposis have cylindrical extremities, decreased subcutaneous tissue, and absent skin creases. Defects are symmetrical and are more severe distally in the hands and feet. Joint dislocation may occur in the hips and knees [84]. Sensation is present but deep tendon reflexes may be decreased or absent. Limb malformations include deletion anomalies, radio-ulnar synostosis, syndactyly and short digits. Deformities associated with fetal akinesia include intrauterine growth retardation, pulmonary hypoplasia, short gut syndrome, scoliosis, genital deformities, and hernias (both inguinal and umbilical). Congenital cardiac anomalies and cardiomyopathy may be present. The genitourinary system may have structural abnormalities. Musculoskeletal abnormalities include decreased muscle mass, soft muscle texture, fibrous bands, and abnormal tendon attachments. The skin is often soft, doughy and thick with webs and dimples over affected joints.

Goals of treatment for arthrogryposis are lower limb alignment, stability for ambulation, and upper limb function for self-care [85]. Early gentle manipulation of the contractures after birth helps passive and active range of motion [86]. Physical therapy is indicated for most forms of arthrogryposis but recurrence of the contractures can be high following stretching, necessitating surgery. Soft tissue surgery should be undertaken early and osteotomies performed when growth plates have fused. The most common deformity in the foot is a rigid talipes equinovarus deformity. The goal is to make the foot plantigrade and braceable. Casting often fails early on and typically the patient has to undergo an extensive medial and lateral release of ankle tendons with postoperative bracing. Recurrence of talipes equinovarus is common and other procedures, such as lateral column shortening (distal calcaneal resection), may be required. In an older child in whom the bone is skeletally mature, a triple arthrodesis (fusion of talocalcaneal and talonavicular and calcaneocuboid joints) is performed. In the knees, flexion deformities are more common than fixed knee deformities and are more resistant to treatment. Moderate contractures of between 20 and 60° require soft tissue release with posterior capsulotomies. Severe contractures of greater than 60° may require femoral shortening in addition to soft tissue release. Older children with severe deformity may require a knee disarticulation. Extension deformities, if unresponsive to physical therapy, will need quadricepsplasty if the child is younger than 6 months of age.

Hip deformities should be addressed after foot and knee deformities have been corrected [87]. Intervention to improve the hip should take place before 1 year of age to make ambulation easier. Hip flexion greater than 35° requires soft tissue release. Bilateral hip dislocations that exceed 35° and the presence of a flexion contracture should be treated with soft tissue release but no reduction [88]. Unilateral hip dislocation requires reduction to avoid the development of scoliosis and pelvic deformity. Upper extremity surgery should be done when the patient is older than 5–6 years. With elbow contractures, the goal is to make possible arm flexion for feeding and extension for hygiene needs. Extension is corrected with either a capsulotomy or capsulotomy plus triceps or pectoralis major transfer. Wrist deformities are usually flexed with ulnar deviation [89]. A severe deformity requires proximal row carpectomy with or without fusion. For severe finger deformities, soft tissue releases and proximal interphalangeal fusions are done. In scoliotic spines, curvatures greater than 35° are treated with spinal fusion.

Preoperatively, any co-morbid conditions that would affect an anesthetic must be identified.

- Cardiac function must be evaluated because congenital abnormalities and cardiomyopathy may be present.

- Respiratory function must also be evaluated as scoliosis may restrict lung function. A weak or hypoplastic diaphragm will also decrease lung function.
- Craniofacial deformities include limited jaw motion, flat nasal bridge, hemangioma, micrognathia, small eyes, corneal opacities, craniosynostosis, and high cleft palate.
- Laryngeal and tracheal clefts/stenoses, as well as hemangiomas, must be detected beforehand because they may cause difficulty with tracheal intubation. A thorough airway examination is required because some patients have limited jaw opening and micrognathia.
- Skin can be doughy and thick, making IV access difficult. Cold and blue distal limbs can be evidence of abnormal skin vasculature.
- There may be vertebral instability secondary to decreased muscle mass and high cervical hypoplasia.
- Renal abnormalities may affect anesthetic drugs that are metabolized or excreted by the kidneys. Structural abnormalities of the genitourinary system may be present.
- Neuromuscular junctions will have upregulation due to decreased muscle mass and increased sensitivity to non-depolarizing medications and a hyperkalemic response to succinylcholine.

Intraoperatively, care with positioning and tourniquet use is needed, as these children have osseous hypoplasia and are prone to fractures. Intraoperative hyperthermia is usually caused by hypermetabolism, not malignant hyperthermia unless there is an underlying predisposing neuromuscular disorder like King–Denborough. Hyperthermia occurs regardless of the type of anesthetic used. A cooling blanket should always be available. A wide array of laryngoscopes, tracheal tubes, laryngeal mask airways, video laryngoscopy, and fiber-optic scopes should readily available, given the high likelihood of difficult intubation.

Choice of anesthetic agent depends on co-morbid conditions. Ventilation may be affected by scoliosis-induced restrictive lung disease. Pneumothorax, either spontaneous or mechanical ventilation induced, may be the result of pulmonary hypoplasia. Postoperatively, there is an increased risk of aspiration when the cause of arthrogryposis is neurogenic or muscular. Therefore, full return of baseline neuromuscular function and ability to protect the airway before emergence from anesthesia and tracheal extubation is required. Patients will be in casts postoperatively for approximately 6 weeks. Preoperative pain medication should be continued into the postoperative period and enough pain medication added to treat surgical pain. This helps prevent narcotic withdrawal and a wind-up phenomenon.

Cerebral palsy

Cerebral palsy (CP) describes the movement and posture disorder that is the result of a motor deficit caused by brain injury *in utero*, at birth or postnatally. It is present in approximately 2 per 1000 births [90]. The clinical features of CP are classified by the number of extremities with motor deficits (mono-, di-, tri- or quadri-). Involvement of one side of the body is hemiparesis. Spastic quadriparesis is the most common form of CP, requiring multiple surgeries. The causes of CP are many, but the exact etiology is often difficult to define in any given infant. The functional limitations from paresis include hypotonia or hypertonia and occasionally extrapyramidal symptoms. Function can frequently be improved by multiple surgical procedures that address the extremities. Surgeries to straighten the spine help maintain posture and lung volumes. Anesthesia is often required to inject medications to treat spasticity and contractures (e.g. botulinium toxin-A or baclofen) [91].

Preoperative assessment and medical optimization should occur ahead of the surgery, since the majority of surgeries are elective.

Anesthetic challenges include appropriate communication with children who can have either normal cognitive abilities or severe developmental delay. A particularly challenging group of CP patients are cognitively intact, non-verbal patients. Patients with hypotonic CP often have the most severe developmental delay. Preoperative discussions with the family should include estimation of the child's developmental level and the best means of communicating with them. Ideally a pain scale is identified that will be used postoperatively so the child and family can become familiar with its use.

Patients with CP may also have epilepsy. Their scheduled antiepileptic drugs are administered, despite preoperative fasting. A history of recent seizure patterns and frequency is obtained. Many of the antiseizure medications affect P450 degradation pathways. Drugs utilizing these pathways for elimination (e.g. non-depolarizing neuromuscular relaxants) will benefit from train-of-four monitoring and more frequent dosing to achieve the desired effects [92].

Pulmonary pathology includes the usual incidence of childhood diseases (e.g. reactive airway disease), and they may be exacerbated by anatomically scoliosis-induced restricted airways. Feeding discoordination increases the risk of aspiration and recurrent respiratory infections. Gastroesophageal reflux is common, difficult to control medically, and often requires fundoplication. Respiratory muscle strength may also be compromised.

Poor oropharyngeal function often causes excessive drooling. This is controlled with antisialogogs or salivary gland surgery. Premedication with glycopyrrolate facilitates tracheal intubation and decreases pooling of secretions intraoperatively.

Patients with severe CP may be chronically underhydrated, since most of them are tube fed and empirically hydrated. Preoperative rehydration may be required. Complete blood count (CBC) and coagulation studies are indicated for potentially bloody procedures because there is an increased incidence of prolonged PT/PTT in this patient group.

Scoliosis surgery is covered in Chapter 26. Other orthopedic procedures often required include extremity surgeries to address contractures and gait abnormalities. Historically these have been done serially as the child grows and movement is evaluated. Some centers are now undertaking elaborate gait and movement studies preoperatively to plan and perform a single operation that addresses multiple extremities simultaneously. The advantage of doing this is that the child can be mobilized more quickly and there is one recovery process instead of several. An important component of this approach is close co-ordination with a pediatric acute pain service to optimize pain management postoperatively, often with regional analgesia.

Clubfoot and hip dislocations are common acquired deformities in CP and often require surgery. They are described in detail above. Heel cord lengthening, adductor myotomy, and hamstring lengthening are the most common surgeries needed.

For clubfoot, the foot is rotated inward, the back of the heel is moved up, and the forefoot deviates medially. During the newborn period the heel cord is cut under local anesthesia and is serially casted. For surgical correction of clubfoot, general anesthesia, with or without caudal block, is usually used. Acquired clubfoot is the result of the paralysis associated with CP.

Contracture releases are performed to facilitate patient comfort, positioning, and mobility. Ober fasciotomy is done for flexion at the hip that is abducted and externally rotated (frog leg in appearance). Incision is anterolateral and just distal to the iliac crest. The fascial attachments are loosened to obtain neutral extension.

The iliotibial (IT) band may be tight, causing flexion of the knee. In the Yount procedure, a distal midlateral longitudinal incision is made above the knee, and a segment of the IT band and lateral intermuscular septum is removed and not repaired.

Tendon lengthening/transfer is done to release contractures. Tendon transfers are done to change the direction of muscle force to compensate for paralysis or paresis of muscle groups.

Intraoperative considerations for CP include maintaining warmth, since these patients tend to be hypothermic. Using warm blankets and forced-air warming devices in the preoperative area facilitates venous cannulation.

Non-depolarizing neuromuscular relaxants are less potent in patients with CP, with or without the presence of chronic anticonvulsants. Contractures present positioning problems and make vessel cannulation difficult.

The use of succinylcholine is controversial and best avoided in CP patients. There are anecdotal reports of succinylcholine-induced cardiac arrest in CP patients [93]. Moreover, Theroux et al reported increased sensitivity of CP patients to succinylcholine due to CP patients having a lower effective dose (ED50) [94]. The relative immobility of CP patients may also upregulate their acetylcholine receptors [95]. However, Dierdorf did report normal plasma potassium concentrations before and after succinylcholine administration in CP patients as well as normal controls [93]. Muscle biopsies demonstrate variable neuromuscular junctions in CP patients undergoing spinal fusion, with about 30% of them having abnormal apposition of the acetylcholine receptor compared to normal control patients undergoing spinal fusion [96]. When the risk for aspiration is increased, sufficient rocuronium can be used to safely allow a modified RSI of anesthesia and tracheal intubation considering the potential risk of hyperkalemia.

Postoperative concerns include resumption of all preoperative medications, with close attention paid to the dosing of antiseizure medication and to spasticity regimens. Serum drug levels may be indicated if medications were discontinued for a prolonged period. Postoperative spasms can be painful and may require acute and chronic pharmacological therapy. Current oral regimens include diazepam, baclofen, tizanidine, and dantrolene. Intrathecal pumps are used to deliver baclofen for chronic spasticity. Baclofen overdosing or underdosing can be life threatening, particularly with abrupt withdrawal of the drug. Regional anesthesia supplementation decreases spasms in some instances.

Neuromuscular diseases

Perhaps one of the most common dilemmas in pediatric anesthesia is the anesthetic choice for a patient with neuromuscular disease, including those with hypotonia of unknown etiology [97]. The potential for anesthethic complications, based on choice of anesthetic technique, is present and yet the recommendations are still varied and controversial. Each technique carries its own risk profile. Furthermore, regardless of anesthetic technique, these patients have a higher incidence of cardiomyopathy and arrhythmias from disease effects on the heart muscle. Respiratory function can also be compromised, due to both decreased respiratory muscle strength and to restrictive function associated with advanced spine and rib cage deformity induced by the diseases.

Neuromuscular diseases can be divided into muscular dystrophy (progressive and congenital), developmental myopathy, and metabolic myopathy.

Progressive muscular dystrophies (Duchenne and Becker)

Progressive muscular dystrophies include the dystrophinopathies (absent or deficient dystrophin such as Duchenne muscular dystrophy (DMD) and Becker muscular dystrophy (BMD)), limb girdle muscular dystrophies, fascio-scapulo-humeral muscular dystrophy, and oculopharyngeal muscular dystrophy. Most expert opinions now agree that there is not an increased risk of malignant hyperthermia (MH), but life-threatening rhabdomyolysis (RHA) can occur. Frail muscle membranes break down with exposure to halogenated volatile agents. Thus, in clinical practice many providers still choose to deliver a trigger-free anesthetic (i.e. avoidance of succinylcholine and volatile anesthetics). The risk of RHA is highest in young children with more muscle mass. As the child ages and the disease progresses, muscle mass decreases and is replaced with fibrosis. An elevated creatine kinase (CK) is common in this group of patients.

Duchenne muscular dystrophy (DMD) usually presents as a toddler or early school-age boy with delayed walking or global motor delay. The incidence is approximately 30 per 100,000 births [98]. They have progressive lower extremity weakness, pseudohypertrophy of the calves, and markedly elevated CK levels. A waddling gait and proximal muscle weakness are hallmark signs. Gower sign is common and describes the process of using the arms to rise from the floor. Approximately one-third will develop cardiomyopathy and or arrhythmias by 14–18 years of age, and cardiac disease does not necessarily follow the severity of skeletal muscle disease. Patients typically die in mid-adulthood from either cardiomyopathy or ventilatory failure.

Becker muscular dystrophy (BMD) is similar to DMD in its clinical presentation but presents in the adolescent years and progresses more slowly, due to a partial loss of dystrophin. It is less common, with an incidence of 3–6 per 100,000 births. Cardiomyopathy generally presents about age 30 with most patients surviving to 30–60 years of age.

Anesthetic risks for progressive muscular dystrophy, in addition to succinylcholine-induced hyperkalemia and RHA, are related to the degree of cardiac and respiratory compromise. Preoperative preparation includes an annual cardiac assessment for cardiomyopathy and/or arrhythmias and pulmonary function tests. Cardiac condition should be medically optimized prior to anesthesia and surgery. Postoperative planning should include longer observation times after surgery and the possible need for ventilatory assistance in an intensive care setting.

Congenital muscular dystrophies

These are characterized by early infancy presentation and slow progression that are sometimes associated with CNS anomalies. The incidence is only about 4 per 100,000 births; thus much less is known and/or written about preferred anesthesia techniques for patients with congenital muscular dystrophy. Creatine kinase levels are usually elevated. There is a case report of an undiagnosed hypermetabolic response with volatile agent use and a report of rhabdomyolysis.

Congenital myopathies (central core disease and core-rod myopathies)

These infants primarily have contractures with decreased muscle strength; diagnosis is based on the histology of a muscle biopsy. The CK level is normal or only mildly increased, and the disease progresses slowly. Central core disease and core-rod myopathy patients are at high risk for MH. Other congenital myopathy patients have milder or no association with MH. However, given the difficulty for the anesthesiologist to track down and interpret specific genetic testing, a trigger-free anesthetic is prudent in the known or suspected congenital myopathy patient.

Myotonias

There are several variants, both autosomal dominant and recessive, and they are divided into dystrophic and non-dystrophic forms. Myotonia congenita is a non-dystrophic form. The primary symptom for all myotonia patients is impaired muscle relaxation following sudden contraction. Succinylcholine can result in total-body sustained contraction and/or masseter muscle rigidity and should be avoided. Anticholinesterase drugs have also been reported to cause sustained contraction so careful titration of short-acting non-depolarizing muscle relaxant is advised only when clinically necessary. Halogenated agents have been used safely in these patients, but there are also some case reports of hypermetabolic reactions.

King–Denborough syndrome

This rare autosomal dominant disease has a high association with MH, so succinylcholine and halogenated agents are avoided. Muscle disease is non-specific and mild. These patients are characterized by short stature, pectus carinatum, kyphosis, cleft palate, low-set ears, ptosis, down-slanting palpebral fissures, and delayed motor development.

Metabolic myopathy (mitochondrial and carnitine disorders)

Mitochondrial diseases interact either with the energy supply to the muscle (ATP synthesis) or with ion channels involved in the process of contraction and relaxation. These patients develop progressive dysfunction in organs with high-energy requirements such as brain and muscle. All anesthetic agents interfere with mitochondrial function so there is no ideal anesthetic for these patients. However, many anesthetics have been conducted safely with all anesthetic agents. There is increasing evidence that propofol infusion syndrome (PRIS) results from mitochondrial dysfunction and thus propofol should be avoided or used cautiously [99] in patients with mitochondrial disease. These patients do not have a clear genetic or clinical association with MH, though there are two case reports of possible MH [100,101]. One suggested anesthetic technique is to use ketamine and a low-dose volatile agent and avoid using propofol. Dexmedetomidine can also be added as another adjuvant agent when titrated carefully with prolonged postoperative observation. Ketamine, midazolam and dexmedetomidine used together for muscle biopsies can be titrated to a depth sufficient to allow muscle biopsy without volatile agent.

Carnitine deficiency or any problem with its transport makes patients dependent on glucose for energy needs. The most common of these rare disorders is carnitine-palmitoyl transferase II deficiency that also has been associated with RHA following stress, exercise or anesthesia. There is one case report of MH.

Other forms of metabolic myopathy include potassium-related periodic paralysis, glycogenoses, and lipid myopathies.

Undiagnosed hypotonia

Clinical experience and a recent retrospective study suggest that a cerebral cause for hypotonia is far more frequent than a peripheral neuromuscular cause in a neonate or infant with undiagnosed hypotonia who is presenting for muscle biopsy [102,103]. Since many infants/small children who present for muscle biopsy are not diagnosed, the best anesthetic choice is difficult to determine [104,105]. Taking a careful family history and reviewing genetic or neurological consultations, as well as lab results, are critical. An elevated CK may represent the presence of an undiagnosed progressive muscular dystrophy, such as DMD or BMD. A recent review article recommends that all children with motor delay and who are not walking at 18 months of age should undergo neurological evaluation and/or genetic evaluation prior to elective general anesthesia or sedation [106]. An elevated serum lactate concentration may be indicative of metabolic myopathies such as mitochondrial diseases. Discussion with the infant or child's pediatrician or neu-

rologist, in addition to obtaining CK and lactate levels, may help elucidate a more exact clinical suspicion or diagnosis to help guide anesthetic planning for diagnostic examinations and elective surgeries.

Anesthetic complications associated with neuromuscular diseases (Box 30.2)

- Succinylcholine-induced hyperkalemic cardiac arrest following succinylcholine administration to patients who have neuromuscular disease still occurs despite the FDA black box warning initiated in 1992. The hyperkalemic response is proportional to the upregulation of the nicotinic acetylcholine receptors (AChRs). Pretreatment with a non-depolarizing neuromuscular relaxant does not prevent succinylcholine-induced hyperkalemia. Thus succinylcholine is avoided for any patient with a known condition associated with upregulation and patients who have weakness and/or hypotonia without a diagnosis.
- Acute RHA occurs due to the breakdown of the muscle surface membrane and causes the release of myoglobin, potassium, and CK. This can be life threatening and difficult to differentiate from malignant hyperthermia.
- Hypermetabolic response with unexplained fever can mimic MH but is distinguished by the absence of acidosis and the presence of a normal CK. This condition has been described during anesthesia in both primary

---

Box 30.2 Severe anesthetic complications associated with neuromuscular and orthopedic diseases

Succinylcholine-induced hyperkalemic cardiac arrest (upregulation of nAChR)

- muscular dystrophy
- acute burn patients
- denervation
- muscle atrophy

Neuromuscular conditions associated with rhabdomyolysis

- Duchenne and Becker muscular dystrophies
- dystrophinopathies (absent or deficient)

Hypermetabolic response with unexplained fever but no acidosis or increase in CK

- Duchenne muscular dystrophy
- osteogenesis imperfecta
- arthrogryposis

Neuromuscular diseases highly associated with MH

- central core disease (and core-rod myopathies)
- King–Denborough

neuromuscular conditions and orthopedic syndromes such as osteogenesis imperfecta and arthrogryposis.

- Malignant hyperthermia (see Chapter 40) has been associated with most neuromuscular diseases but most experts now classify only central core disease and King–Denborough as being high risk for MH.

Juvenile rheumatoid arthritis

Juvenile rheumatoid arthritis (JRA) (also known as Still disease) is diagnosed approximately three times per 100,000 children under the age of 15, and approximately 70% of these patients are female [107]. In addition to the usual childhood surgeries, JRA patients require general anesthesia for surgery on multiple affected joints as well as diagnostic examinations. Intra-articular corticosteroid injection in very young children may also require general anesthesia.

The usual age for presentation of JRA is 2–4 years of age. It is a systemic condition that is characterized by fever, rash, joint redness, leukocytosis, and increased erythrocyte sedimentation rate. It affects collagen and the connective tissues of joints and organs. About 36% of JRA patients have cardiac involvement, with pericarditis being the most common cardiovascular presentation. Severe disease may also include splenomegaly, lymphadenitis, and polyarthritis. JRA is an autoimmune disease that causes deposition of autoantibodies (antinuclear antibodies (ANA) and rheumatoid factor (RF)) in the affected joints. Reactive lysosomal enzymes are released and ultimately damage the joints.

Preoperative preparation includes careful assessment of the airway with regard to neck and jaw mobility because temporomandibular ankylosis, mandibular hypoplasia, and cricoarytenoid arthritis can be present. Fiber-optic intubation of the trachea may be indicated. JRA patients may have atlantoaxial or low cervical subluxation, so extension of the neck should be limited or avoided. Anemia is also common. Children may be on multiple medical therapies, including steroids, non-steroidal anti-inflammatory drugs, and methotrexate.

Postoperative analgesia can be challenging due to the pre-existing chronic pain. Continuous regional anesthesia has been used to provide acute pain relief for larger surgeries, such as hip arthroplasty.

Genetic syndromes and orthopedic surgery

There are many syndromes with accompanying orthopedic problems. Table 30.1 contains a listing of these syndromes. The reader is referred to Chapter 38 for a discussion of the anesthetic approach to patients with these conditions.

Table 30.1 Orthopedic syndromes with potential anesthetic implications

Syndrome	Potential anesthetic implications
Achondroplasia	Chronic respiratory infection, hydrocephalus, long narrow mouth with high arched palate, limited head extension, prominent mandible and forehead, constrictive thoracic cage, cyanotic and apneic episodes, dwarfism
Apert	Facial, limb and cardiac anomalies, hydrocephalus, choanal atresia, craniosynostosis
Arnold–Chiari	Vocal cord paralysis, stridor, respiratory distress, apnea, abnormal swallowing, recurrent aspiration pneumonia, possible ↑ intracranial pressure, unstable blood pressure, weakness → paralysis
Cri du chat	Microcephaly, micrognathia, facial asymmetry, high vaulted palate, cleft lip/palate, feeding and swallowing difficulties with chronic aspiration, congenital heart defects, seizures, severe retardation
Crouzon	Facial and ocular anomalies, upper airway obstruction, choanal atresia, seizures, craniosynostosis, mental retardation
Cornelia de Lange	Facial and cardiac anomalies, micrognathia, seizures, choanal atresia, contractures, hypertonia
Ehlers–Danlos	Joint laxity, fragile blood vessels, cardiac valvular prolapse, glaucoma
Ellis-van Creveld	Facial and cardiac anomalies, small thorax
Freeman–Sheldon	"Whistling facies" with microstomia, ↑ muscle tone, vertebral anomalies, myotonia
Goldenhar	Laryngeal, ocular, cardiac and renal anomalies, cervical spine fusion, hemifacial micrognathia, glaucoma, encephalocele

(Continued)

Table 30.1 (*Continued*)

Syndrome	Potential anesthetic implications
Holt–Oram	Cardiac, vertebral and upper limb and shoulder girdle anomalies, hypoplasia of distal blood vessels
Hurler	Facial anomalies, macroglossia, chronic respiratory infections, growth and mental deficiencies, joint stiffness, cardiac failure, hydrocephalus
Lesch–Nyhan	Self-mutilation, airway distortion 2 degrees to scarification, mental retardation, spasticity, choreo-athetosis, seizures, contractures, hypertension, aspiration pneumonia
Marfan	Joint laxity, vertebral and ocular anomalies, mitral valve prolapse, dilatation or dissection of ascending aorta with aortic valve insufficiency
Möbius	Microstomia, micrognathia, limb and brain anomalies, cranial nerve palsies
Morquio	Odontoid hypoplasia, vertebral anomalies, growth deficiency, aortic value insufficiency, joint contractures
Neurofibromatosis	Brain, vertebral, dermal and cardiac anomalies, subcutaneous tumor with tendency to malignancy, mental deficiency, kyphoscoliosis
Noonan	Facial, vertebral and cardiac anomalies, micrognathia, mental deficiency, pectus evacatium
Radial aplasia-thrombocytopenia (Tar)	Facial, vertebral, cardiac and renal anomalies, micrognathia, severe thrombocytopenia, anemia, intracranial hemorrhage
Robin (Pierre–Robin)	Severe micrognathia, cleft palate, laryngeal anomalies, mandibular growth improves with age during infancy
Treacher Collins	Severe micrognathia (not improving during infancy), facial, auricular and cardiac anomalies, choanal atresia, microstomia, airway hypoplasia
Trisomy 21 (Down)	Odontoid hypoplasia, macroglossia, cardiac defects, joint laxity, mild mental deficiency
Turner (XO)	Micrognathia, short neck, growth retardation, cardiac anomalies
VATER association	Vertebral, cardia, renal and limb anomalies, TE fistula, esophageal atresia, congenital scoliosis, imperforate anus

Modified from Benumof JL. Anesthesia and Uncommon Diseases. 4th edn. Philadelphia, WB Sounders Company; and Katz J, Stewart DJ. Anesthesia and Uncommon Pediatric Disease. 2nd edn. Philadelphia, WB Saunders Company, 1993, with permission.

CASE STUDY

An 8-year-old boy with a history of osteogenesis imperfecta and mild asthma is admitted to the hospital for a mechanical breakage of one of the non-extendable rods in his left femur. He was playing on his crutches at school after lunch with other children when he felt a distinct pop and a sharp pain in his left thigh. In the emergency room, he is crying and slightly wheezing. His vital signs remain stable, his weight is 30 kg, and his height is 50 inches (127 cm). Mother states that he has osteogenesis imperfecta type III with mild deafness. His weight was normal at birth, and he had three fractures. During two previous procedures he had rods placed in both femurs. There is no history of mandibular or maxillary bone fragility. Mother denies any complications with anesthesia but does state that he had a high temperature after his last surgery. The fever dissipated with cooling blankets. A flow murmur was diagnosed at age 2, but no further work-up was done to evaluate this, and the patient has been asymptomatic. He currently requires crutches to ambulate and has not had fainting spells or decreased appetite. His wheezing notably increases with cold air, exercise, and stress. He uses his inhaler approximately three times a month. He has never been hospitalized for his asthma and has never had formal pulmonary function testing done. He was previously on bisphosphonate therapy for 4 years but had some leukopenia and stopped the drug at age 6. Currently his medications include a fentanyl patch and ibuprofen for breakthrough pain.

On physical examination the patient appears well nourished with adequate capillary refill and moist mucous membranes. He has varus deformities on both ankles and slight bowing of both legs with greater deformity on the left. His temperature is 36.9°C. His blood pressure is 109/64, heart rate 117/min, and his respirations are 18 breaths per minute. He has triangular facies, with blue-white sclerae bilaterally; his mouth opening is adequate. He has some limited range of motion of his neck secondary to the occurrence of tingling in the fingers bilaterally when he moves his head. There is macroglossia. His neck is short and his thyromental distance is adequate. There are several small filed-down teeth. Two teeth are missing from the upper jaw. There is mild expiratory wheezing throughout all lung fields as well as mild scoliosis and a pectus carinatum. Cardiovascular examination reveals a mild systolic murmur that is best heard at the left sternal border. The murmur diminishes with inspiration. The left leg is swollen with macular purpura on its lateral aspect. Laboratory data demonstrate a normal hemoglobin concentration and platelet count and a normal chemistry panel. Standard coagulation studies are normal. Chest x-ray shows mild hyperinflation bilaterally and mild scoliosis but normal size cardiac silhouette. Electrocardiogram shows mild left atrial enlargement and occasional premature ventricular contractions. An echocardiogram is not performed due to lack of symptoms and the innocent quality of the murmur (i.e. systolic in nature, diminishes with respiration, non-radiating).

Review of his previous anesthetic records indicates that his airway was abnormally anterior, he had fragile dentition, and two attempts were required to intubate the trachea. The estimated blood loss during the last intramedullary stabilization was 10 mL/kg. No blood products were given at that time. Currently the patient is calm in his mother's arms and allows an intravenous catheter to be placed. It has been 4h since the injury and the last ingestion of solids. He is given 0.1 mg/kg of midazolam intravenously prior to transfer to the operating room. His fentanyl patch is identified and maintained in place. In the operating room, a cooling/warming blanket is placed on the operating table. Careful transfer of the patient results in atraumatic placement on the operating table. All pressure points are padded. A variety of airway equipment is readily available in the operating room. The patient prefers to hold the facemask to his face. All standard ASA monitors are placed, including a non-invasive blood pressure cuff that is set to cycle every 5 min.

Given that the patient has a full stomach and a possibly difficult airway, a modified RSI is planned. The patient is given nebulized albuterol and tooth guards are placed prior to induction of anesthesia. After two full minutes of preoxygenation, remifentanil 1 μg/kg is administered prior to propofol 2 mg/kg. Use of these two agents decreases the sympathetic response and produces a relatively immobile patient for a short period of time without affecting neuromuscular junctions. This provides optimal intubating conditions. If unsuccessful, succinylcholine can still be used

with caution, since there is a risk for a fasciculation-induced fracture. The risk of a lost airway and aspiration of gastric contents must be weighed against the risk of iatrogenic fractures. The head and neck are stabilized with in-line stabilization, and video laryngoscopy is used to visualize the airway. Although there is an anterior, grade 3 view with external pressure, a 5.0 cuffed tracheal tube is placed under direct visualization. General anesthesia is maintained with a total intravenous technique using both propofol and fentanyl infusions with intermittent doses of vecuronium. The intravenous anesthetic technique is chosen to decrease the likelihood of hyperthermia. After establishing hemodynamic stability post induction of anesthesia, the non-invasive arterial blood pressure cuff continues to cycle every 5 min and is changed to a different extremity to avoid iatrogenic fractures. The surgeons then remove the broken non-extendable rod and replace it with a new one. This particular surgery is not amenable to a tourniquet, so none is used. The patient's temperature slowly increases from 36.9°C to 37.4°C. The cooling blanket is used to keep his temperature between 36.5°C and 37.0°C. Bleeding is a little greater than 15 mL/kg, therefore an invasive arterial line is placed to allow blood draws to evaluate for anemia and lactic acidosis, and to provide arterial blood pressure monitoring. The non-invasive blood pressure cuff is stopped.

With evidence of bleeding, relative hypotension and hemoglobin of 7 g, the patient is given 20 mL/kg of packed red blood cells with a good increase in arterial blood pressure and hemoglobin concentration. Despite the transfusion, the surgeon states that there is still oozing in the surgical field. Due to the capillary fragility and qualitative platelet dysfunction present in osteogenesis imperfecta, desmopressin is discussed as a possible treatment. Desmospressin works by increasing plasma concentrations of factor VIII, von Willebrand factor, and tissue plasminogen activator and by increasing platelet adhesiveness. The adverse effects of desmopressin include facial flushing, headache, hypotension, tachycardia, and thrombosis. There also have been a few rare case reports of hyponatremia and seizures in children. The use of desmopressin in patients with osteogenesis imperfecta has not been fully evaluated as an effective method to stop perioperative oozing [108]. Therefore in this instance, given that the bleeding has slowed over time and the risk of causing the aforementioned side-effects, desmopressin is not given.

At the end of surgery, the patient's pH is 7.25 and there is evidence of mild respiratory acidosis, which is attributed to the patient's asthma and pectus carinatum. He is given 10 puffs of albuterol from a metered-dose inhaler and improves. It is deemed appropriate, given his recent PO status, evidence of macroglossia, and a history of difficult tracheal intubation, to extubate his trachea when the patient is fully awake. This assures his airway reflexes will

Continued

be intact. Upon tracheal extubation, the patient has mild wheezing and inspiratory stridor. This resolves with nebulized racemic epinephrine. Postoperatively, he is watched closely in the recovery room for signs of respiratory failure. His temperature remains between 37.0°C and 37.4°C. The cooling blanket is turned off but kept nearby in case his temperature increases. His baseline fentanyl patch is continued, and a morphine PCA is used for breakthrough pain.

His mother is advised to avoid non-steroidal anti-inflammatory medication in the future due to potential bleeding from platelet dysfunction.

With close attention to issues such as fragile bones, restrictive lung physiology, limited cervical neck motion, platelet dysfunction, and chronic pain, one can prevent injury and deliver a safe and effective anesthetic to patients with osteogenesis imperfecta.

Annotated references

A full reference list for this chapter is available at:
http://www.wiley.com/go/gregory/andropoulos/pediatricanesthesia

7. Ponseti IV. Clubfoot management. J Pediatr Orthop 2000; 20: 699–700. The Ponseti method of correcting clubfoot is discussed in detail, and an overview of possible complications of correction is presented.

10. Weinstein SL, Mubarak SJ, Wenger DR. Developmental hip dysplasia and dislocation. Part I. J Bone Joint Surg Am 2003; 85: 1823–32. This article discusses treatment modalities such as Pavlik harness, spica cast, and osteotomies for correction of hip dysplasia. It also provides a thorough overview of the formation of the hip joint and of developmental defects.

23. DeOrio MJ, DeOrio JK. Blount disease: treatment. http://emedicine.medscape.com/article/1250420. This website provides an overview of causative factors and treatment modalities of Blount Disease.

37. Gholve PA, Cameron DB, Millis MB. Slipped capital femoral epiphysis update. Curr Opin Pediatr 2009; 21: 39–45. The authors provide an overview of presenting symptoms, at-risk populations, and treatment outcomes of slipped capital femoral epiphysis.

50. Netscher DT, Baumholtz MA. Treatment of congenital upper extremity problems. Plast Reconstr Surg 2007; 119: 101e–129e. Discusses different congenital hand malformations, appropriate age for surgical intervention, and methods of correction.

54. Loder RT, O'Donnell PW, Feinber JR. Epidemiology and mechanism of femur fractures in children. J Pediatr Orthop 2006; 26: 561–6. Discusses the most likely etiologies of femur fractures in children and their prevalence in the different pediatric populations.

56. Anglen J, Choi L. Treatment options in pediatric femoral shaft fractures. J Orthop Trauma 2005; 19: 724–33. Different surgical orthopedic treatment options are discussed including external fixators, intramedullary nails and spica casts.

57. Epps HR, Molenaar E, O'Connor DP. Immediate single-leg spica cast for pediatric femoral diaphysis fractures. J Pediatr Orthop 2006; 26: 491–6. Evaluates the benefits of immediate spica casting and discusses the complications of delayed treatment in femoral fractures.

65. Frank G, Mahoney HM, Eppes SC. Musculoskeletal infections in children. Pediatr Clin North Am 2005; 52: 1083–6. Helpful overview of different etiologies of septic arthritis and its prevalence in the general pediatric population.

72. Baujat G, Lebre AS, Cormier-Daire V, Le Merrer M. Osteogenesis imperfecta, diagnosis information (clinical and genetic classification). Arch Pediatr 2008; 15: 789–91. Provides details about the different clinical types of osteogenesis imperfecta and diagnostic methodology.

78. Burnett YL, Brennan MP, Klowden AJ et al. Pulse oximetry and blood pressure monitoring: effect of automatic tourniquets and automatic noninvasive blood pressure devices on inducing fractures in pediatric patients with osteogenesis imperfecta. Anesthesiology 1994; 81(3A): A508. Discusses the perils of frequent non-invasive monitoring and tourniquets and provides techniques for limiting iatrogenic fractures in patients with osteogenesis imperfecta.

84. Bamshad M, van Heest AE, Pleasure D. Arthrogryposis: a review and update. J Bone Joint Surg Am 2009; 91 Suppl 4: 40–6. Thorough recent overview of arthrogryposis. Delineates the different types of arthrogryposis and many different etiologies including neurological and muscular disorders.

98. Laugel V, Cossee M, Matis J et al. Diagnostic approach to neonatal hyptonia: retrospective study on 144 neonates. Eur J Pediatr 2008; 167: 517–23. The authors reviewed 144 infants with clinical hypotonia and found 60% to have central causes versus peripheral causes in 28%. They present a diagnostic algorithm to help determine central versus peripheral neuropathy. This article provides practical information for the anesthesiologist caring for hypotonic infants.

CHAPTER 31

Eyes, Ears, Nose, and Throat Surgery

Olutoyin A. Olutoye & Mehernoor F. Watcha

Department of Anesthesiology and Pediatrics, Baylor College of Medicine, and Texas Children's Hospital, Houston, TX, USA

Introduction

Ear, nose, throat, airway, eye, and dental surgery are among the most frequent procedures requiring anesthesia in children. These cases range from very simple brief anesthetics in healthy children to very complex airway procedures in patients with multisystem disease, requiring a significant amount of preoperative planning and communication with the surgeon. This chapter will begin with a discussion of an approach to the child with an upper respiratory tract infection. Then, we will consider the anesthetic management of specific ear, nose, throat, and airway surgery, followed by a discussion of eye surgery. Finally, anesthesia for dental surgery in children will be presented.

Approach to the child with an upper respiratory tract infection

Many children scheduled for surgery including procedures involving the eyes, ears, nose and throat areas present with nasal discharge that may represent either allergic rhinitis or an upper respiratory infection (URI). It is important to differentiate between the two conditions, as URI predisposes to respiratory complications such as breath-holding episodes, laryngospasm, bronchospasm and occasionally stridor [1,2]. Tait et al described a point system to help differentiate between the two conditions, but others have noted that parental reports are just as accurate [3,4].

The anesthesiologist is faced with a dilemma about proceeding or postponing the procedure in a child with URI. The increased risk for laryngospasm, bronchospasm, oxygen desaturation, and postintubation croup with anesthesia during URI should be balanced with the fact that these risks will not be significantly reduced without waiting 4–6 weeks or longer, by which time the child will frequently have another URI [5]. Emergency procedures should be performed even in the presence of significant medical problems. However, elective procedures should be undertaken cautiously in the presence of a URI. Most anesthesiologists would postpone elective surgery in a child presenting with purulent secretions and fever. A number of risk factors for adverse respiratory events in children with URI undergoing surgery have been described, including the age of the child, exposure to second-hand smoke [6], prior history of respiratory disorders such as asthma, cystic fibrosis, bronchopulmonary dysplasia, presence of copious secretions, nasal congestion and surgery involving the airway, along with the choice of anesthetic agents and devices to maintain airway patency. Tait and Malviya have described a reasonable algorithm for managing children with URI, where the decision to proceed or postpone the procedure is based on the urgency, site of the operation (with higher risk for airway surgery), clinical severity of URI symptoms, presence of co-morbid conditions and whether tracheal intubation is planned [7].

Although the term "URI" implies an upper airway infection, the lower airway may also be affected with peripheral airway abnormalities and airway hyper-reactivity. Decreased diffusion capacity, increased closing volumes, abnormal frequency dependence of compliance and increased airway resistance have been reported in patients with URI [8–11]. This may explain why anesthetized children with a URI demonstrated a more rapid decrease in their oxygen saturation to 95% during apnea [12]. Decreased functional residual capacity (FRC) and closing volumes have been noted during spirometry in awake children with URI [13].

Bronchospasm is a major and potentially life-threatening intraoperative event that occurs more frequently in children with URI, including those without a prior history of asthma. Increased airway reactivity may represent immunological and inflammatory mediator release responses to viral infection. Epithelial damage from viral infections may result in airway receptor sensitization and abnormal neural responses to tachykinins such as substance P. The contractile effects of both substance P and capsaicin were enhanced in bronchial ring segments taken from guinea pigs infected with parainfluenza 3. Pretreatment with histamine-1 and -2 (H1, H2), muscarinic, serotonergic, and α-adrenergic blockers did not obliterate the effect of substance P [14]. This non-cholinergic bronchospasm may explain why albuterol pretreatment did not decrease bronchospasm in children with URI [15]. Acetylcholine-related bronchospasm from increased vagal reactivity can be inhibited by atropine [16] which blocks the effect of acetylcholine on the smooth muscle, but also increases the release of acetylcholine from the vagus nerve endings [17]. A better strategy would be to use a more selective drug to block the muscarinic-3 (M3) receptor (stimulation of which causes bronchoconstriction) but not the muscarinic-2 (M2) receptor (which inhibits acetylcholine release at nerve terminals).

Viruses can produce other substances that result in hyper-reactivity of the airway during a URI. Parainfluenza and influenza viruses contain an enzyme, neuraminidase, which cleaves sialic acid residues present on the M2 muscarinic receptor agonist binding sites. Inhibition of the M2 inhibitory site increases acetylcholine release. Studies in guinea pigs have demonstrated alteration of high-affinity agonist binding (carbachol) in lung membrane preparations in response to either neuraminidase or parainfluenza virus. In addition, a neuraminidase blocking agent inhibited viral-induced changes [18].

In children with URI, more respiratory events occur in those who received general anesthesia with endotracheal intubation [1,19,20]. Tracheal intubation elicits a potent airway reflex that enhances the decrease in FRC following induction of general anesthesia [21].

The intense physical and pharmacological stimulation of the airway that occurs during endotracheal intubation results in significant airway hyper-reactivity, particularly in patients with asthma. However, even patients without underlying bronchospastic disease may develop a temporary increase in airway reactivity during viral infections.

Children with URI presenting for minor surgery which does not require instrumentation of the airway are not at increased risk of complications following general anesthesia [3,22]. In contrast, there is a twofold increase in the incidence of laryngospasm in patients with URI symptoms undergoing airway surgery [23]. Rolf & Cote also reported a higher frequency of minor desaturation episodes and an increased risk of bronchospasm following tracheal intubation in children with URIs [19]. The use of a laryngeal mask airway (LMA) in preference to an endotracheal tube when providing anesthesia for children with recent or active URI may cause less tracheal stimulation and respiratory complications from increased airway reactivity [20]. Nevertheless, some studies have shown an association between LMA use and respiratory complications, especially in children with recent (within past 2 weeks) or active URIs [24,25]. Randomized controlled trials are required to determine a true cause-and-effect relationship between the use of LMA and the incidence of respiratory complications [26].

Increased airway reactivity associated with a URI has been stated to last approximately 4–6 weeks. Empey demonstrated a 200% increase in airway resistance after inhaled histamine in adults who had a URI, compared with a 30% increase in controls [27]. The increased airway reactivity persisted as long as 6 weeks after the URI ended. Nandwani studied the upper airway reflex sensitivity of non-smoking, healthy adult patients who inhaled ammonia vapor [28]. Airway reactivity was 2–2.5 times higher than normal, but had returned to baseline 2 weeks after the URI ended. However, many children have at least 6–10 URIs per year, making it difficult to time the procedure for a period when airway reactivity has returned to normal. In addition, it has not been consistently shown that waiting for 6 weeks reliably decreases the incidence of respiratory complications with general anesthesia [5]. In these circumstances, surgery may have to be performed and the anesthesiologist should be prepared to treat bronchospasm aggressively, deliver supplemental oxygen to patients during transport from the operating room to the recovery room, and carefully monitor breathing patterns and oxygen saturation in the recovery room to ensure adequate ventilation and oxygenation before discharge home or to the ward. The anesthesiologist should also consider the preferential use of drugs known to be associated with decreased airway irritability, e.g. sevoflurane rather than desflurane, propofol rather than thiopental.

Although "URI" is considered a single disease process, often with a common set of presenting symptoms, there may be enormous variability in the pathophysiological effects and clinical manifestations of a particular virus, depending on the stage of the illness (e.g. initial symptoms, height of symptoms, recovery phase). Therefore, there will always be a need for subjective interpretation of a particular patient's clinical signs, symptoms, and past history when surgery is proposed.

Anesthesia for specific surgical procedures

Surgery around the head and neck involves sharing of the workspace and airway between the surgeon and anesthesiologist, making close communication between the two imperative for good patient management. A preoperative discussion is useful in determining the factors necessary for optimal operative conditions, and should include a focus on the steps involved in the procedure, patient positioning, intraoperative movement of the tracheal tube, the potential effect of neuromuscular blockade on nerve integrity monitoring, and a need for additional precautions to avoid airway fires. The most common pediatric conditions requiring surgical intervention in the head and neck region include:

- myringotomy and pressure equalization tube insertion for treatment of chronic otitis media infection
- middle ear surgery
- tonsillectomy and adenoidectomy for relief of obstructive sleep apnea or for the management of recurrent streptococcal pharyngitis
- airway surgery for evaluation of subglottic stenosis and resection of laryngeal papillomas
- removal of foreign bodies.

Myringotomy and insertion of pressure equalization (ventilation) tympanostomy tubes (grommets)

Otitis media is one of the most frequent diagnoses made in pediatric patients. It is an inflammation of the middle ear that often accompanies viral or bacterial upper respiratory tract infections. It may be accompanied by a collection of fluid in the middle ear which becomes thick and glue-like and results in conductive hearing loss if left untreated. Failure of antibiotic therapy to resolve these symptoms warrants surgical drainage of the middle ear fluid. A simple myringotomy will create an opening in the tympanic membrane for drainage of accumulated fluid but the drainage path created eventually heals, leading to a recurrence of symptoms. Placement of a ventilating tube in the ear drum provides stenting of the middle ear and allows for drainage of fluid till the tubes are naturally extruded in 6–12 months.

The procedure of myringotomy and/or placement of ventilating tubes can be completed in 5–10 min in most cases, usually requiring only inhalation anesthesia delivered via facemask However, the procedure may be more surgically challenging in children with narrow ear canals as seen in some syndromes (e.g. Down, Apert syndrome). In this situation, the use of an LMA may be considered during maintenance of anesthesia, as it is associated with fewer hypoxemic episodes and better perioperative working conditions for the surgeons during myringotomy tube placement when compared to the use of a facemask and oral airway [29]. Children with cleft palates frequently develop otitis media due to abnormalities in the cartilage and muscles surrounding the eustachian tubes and procedures in these children may last longer than a routine myringotomy tube insertion, but can usually be managed with a facemask.

Anesthetic management for myringotomy tube placement involves a brief inhalation of potent inhalation agents (commonly sevoflurane) and nitrous oxide in oxygen. However, maintenance of airway patency and adequate ventilation is essential, and an oral airway is often placed to alleviate airway obstruction under anesthesia. Assisted ventilation may be required if the depth of anesthesia exceeds the apneic threshold. Most practitioners do not establish vascular access in healthy patients undergoing these short procedures, but do so in children with significant underlying medical conditions. Nevertheless, an intravenous fluid set-up should be readily available in the operating room in case it is required for urgent drug treatment of laryngospasm (see below).

A variety of management strategies exist for the mild postoperative pain associated with myringotomy tube placement, with the predominant therapy based on institutional or anesthesia practitioner preference. Preoperative oral acetaminophen (15–20 mg/kg) or intraoperative acetaminophen suppositories (40–45 mg/kg) are often used, but acetaminophen (10 mg/kg) with codeine (20 mg/kg) has been found to be superior to oral acetaminophen [30]. The intraoperative administration of ketorolac, intranasal butorphanol or fentanyl (2 µg/kg) reduces rescue analgesic requirements [31–33]. This patient population is at high risk for emergence agitation following sevoflurane anesthesia and the administration of intranasal fentanyl has been found to reduce the incidence [34]. Patients receiving an intraoperative nerve block of the auricular branch of the vagus nerve had similar pain scores in the postoperative period to patients who received intranasal fentanyl with less postoperative emesis [35]. Intramuscular morphine at a dose of 0.1 mg/kg has also been administered for analgesia in these patients.

Middle ear and mastoid surgery

Myringotomy tubes are usually extruded spontaneously, but on occasion need to be removed. While the procedure can be performed in an office, small children may not co-operate and removal under general anesthesia may be required in a few cases. The myringotomy opening in the ear drum usually heals spontaneously, but occasionally the insertion of a paper patch or a fat graft may be required for persistent tympanic membrane perforation.

Anesthetic management for insertion of a fat graft differs slightly from a routine myringotomy as the administration of nitrous oxide should be discontinued or limited to 50% maximum prior to the insertion of the tympanic membrane graft in order to prevent pressure-related displacement of the graft. Nitrous oxide diffuses along a concentration gradient into air-filled middle ear spaces more than nitrogen moves out because nitrous oxide has increased solubility in blood (34 times that of nitrogen). While normal passive venting of the eustachian tube occurs at 20–30 cmH$_2$0, nitrous oxide increases pressure such that the ability of the eustachian tube to vent the middle ear within 5 min is exceeded, thereby resulting in pressure build-up, pain and potential graft displacement [36]. Repeated middle ear infections can result in extension to the mastoid area and large perforations in the tympanic membrane which may not be amenable to transcanal repair only and require posterior auricular exposure. The skin over the outer surface of the ear drum can start to grow through the perforation and into the middle ear, forming a destructive and expanding growth called a cholesteatoma. These problems require surgery.

Routine anesthetic management usually requires inhalational agents with opioid administration. Endotracheal intubation is facilitated by intravenous propofol and/or laryngotracheal application of lidocaine. Following endotracheal intubation, the operating table is usually turned 90° or 180° away from the anesthesia machine with the patient's head positioned on a soft headrest below the height of the operating table. In addition, the surgeons may request extreme lateral rotation of the oper-

ating room table to view the ear structures. The anesthesiologist and surgeon must be vigilant to ensure that nerves, muscles and bony structures are properly padded and not injured during positioning, and to prevent accidental dislodgment of the endotracheal tube. The use of extra-long anesthesia circuits could also be considered if the head of the patient is positioned some distance from the anesthetic machine. The surgical drapes should be placed to allow easy access to the patient and endotracheal tube. Careful head positioning is particularly important in children with Down syndrome as well as in achondroplasia as 15–31% of these children are prone to develop atlantoaxial (C1–2) subluxation [37,38]. The facial nerve is in close proximity to the surgical field during middle ear and mastoid surgery and monitoring of nerve integrity will require the avoidance of neuromuscular blockade or demonstration of a return of the neuromuscular response to 70% of baseline.

Bleeding during middle ear surgery should be minimal as the operative site is visualized through a microscope. Concentrated epinephrine is injected around the area of the tympanic vessels to produce vasoconstriction. Close attention should be paid to the concentration and amount of epinephrine injected in order to avoid arrhythmias and wide variations in blood pressure. Relative hypotension (mean arterial pressure ≤25% from baseline) may decrease the degree of bleeding intraoperatively.

The use of nitrous oxide during these cases can result in an increased volume of gas in the air-filled cavities of the middle ear and sinuses. Subsequent discontinuation of nitrous oxide results in immediate absorption and negative pressure in the middle ear with displacement of any patch placed on the tympanum. Disarticulation of the stapes, one of the ossicles in the middle ear, can occur, with a hearing impairment, which may last for up to 6 weeks postoperatively. In addition, nitrous oxide contributes to the high incidence of postoperative nausea and vomiting in children following middle ear surgery. The negative pressure caused by reabsorption of nitrous oxide stimulates the vestibular system by producing traction on the round window. The relatively compliant walls of the eustachian tubes then collapse and prevent re-equilibration with atmospheric pressure [39]. Older children (greater than 8 years of age) appear to have less compliant eustachian tubes and therefore do not suffer effects of negative middle ear pressure contributing to postoperative nausea and vomiting. While all children are predisposed to developing postoperative nausea and vomiting, children under 8 years of age seem to be most affected. Prophylactic administration of antiemetics like dexamethasone and ondansetron is helpful in this patient population. Postoperative opioid requirements and postoperative nausea and vomiting (PONV) were reduced by approximately 66% following great auricular nerve blockade.

However, analgesic requirements were similar in those receiving the nerve block prior to skin incision or 1 hour before the end of surgery [40,41].

A smooth emergence from anesthesia is preferred in these children. Extubation of the trachea while deeply anesthetized can be easily performed if the children are allowed to breathe spontaneously toward the end of surgery and opioids are gradually titrated as tolerated so the patients can emerge with minimal pain. Administration of intravenous lidocaine (1–1.5 mg/kg) in children older than 1 year of age and gentle suctioning of the oropharynx when the patient is awake can minimize or prevent coughing following extubation.

Cochlear implants

Early insertion of cochlear implants is rapidly gaining acceptance as a method of rehabilitation of profoundly hearing impaired children, as this allows an opportunity for better auditory, speech and language skills. These children are more easily mainstreamed with their peers when they receive cochlear implants early in life. Children as young as 6 months can receive cochlear implants as long as special attention is paid to the physiological and anatomical differences in this age group. Surgical placement of cochlear implants involves meticulous soft tissue dissection, hemostasis and bone drilling as bleeding from the bone marrow may be very difficult to control. The cochlear implant stimulates the auditory nerve to enable hearing and intraoperative limits of implant stimulation are set by evoked stapedius reflex thresholds (ESRT) as well as evoked compound action potentials. The latter measurement has not been found to be affected by anesthetics; however, volatile anesthetics abolish the stapedius reflex in more than 50% of children [42] and cause a dose-dependent increase in the ESRT. This results in ESRT levels that overestimate a child's comfort level and can lead to difficulty adjusting to the implant postoperatively. Propofol does not affect the ESRT; therefore the use of volatile anesthetics during this phase of the surgery is discouraged. Other anesthetic considerations are similar to those for middle ear surgery. Appropriate communication with the surgeon ensures the successful outcome of these procedures.

Adenoidectomy and tonsillectomy

Adenoidectomy can be performed alone although it is commonly performed in conjunction with tonsillectomy and/or myringotomy and tube insertion. The indications for adenoidectomy alone include chronic otitis media with effusion secondary to adenoid hyperplasia, chronic sinusitis and chronic or recurrent purulent adenoiditis. Severe adenoid hyperplasia results in nasopharyngeal obstruction, obligate mouth breathing, failure to thrive, and speech disorders. Long-standing nasal obstruction due to adenoid hyperplasia may result in orofacial abnormalities including narrowing of the upper airway and dental abnormalities ("adenoidal facies").

Tonsillectomy with or without adenoidectomy is one of the most common ambulatory pediatric surgery procedures performed in the United States [43]. The most common indications include recurrent or chronic tonsillitis refractory to medical therapy and obstructive adenotonsillar hyperplasia. The association of tonsillitis with peritonsillar abscess or airway obstruction is also an indication for surgical removal of the tonsils. Hypertrophic tonsils may result in chronic airway obstruction, failure to thrive, dysphagia and speech abnormalities, halitosis, cervical pharyngitis and persistent pharyngitis. Children with cardiac valvular disease are predisposed to developing endocarditis due to recurrent streptococcal bacteremia as a result of infected tonsils. Severe airway obstruction can result in carbon dioxide retention, cor pulmonale, and cardiac failure.

Preoperative assessment

Children less than 3 years of age presenting for this surgery require special attention as this age group has the highest respiratory morbidity following adenotonsillectomy [44,45]. The indication for adenotonsillectomy in this age group is obstructive sleep apnea, which has different features in children compared to adults, with a peak age of 2–6 years, equal male/female distribution and an excellent response to adenotonsillectomy. Obstructive sleep apnea (OSA) is at the end of a spectrum of sleep-disordered breathing which starts from normal respiration and includes snoring, upper airway resistance syndrome, obstructive hypopnea and obstructive sleep apnea. Obstructive sleep apnea occurs during rapid eye movement (REM) sleep and is characterized by snoring with continuous partial upper airway obstruction during sleep, resulting in paradoxical respiratory effort, ineffective ventilation, hypercarbia, and hypoxemia [46]. In severe cases, the patient can develop respiratory acidosis and vasoconstriction of the pulmonary vasculature with accompanying right ventricular hypertrophy. Children with severe obstructive sleep apnea are occasionally admitted to the hospital preoperatively for oxygen treatment via non-invasive nasal continuous positive pressure which stents the airway open, prevents airway collapse and improves functional residual capacity. Bilevel positive airway pressure ventilation (BiPAP) may also be instituted; this provides airway pressure that decreases during exhalation and has been found to improve pulmonary hypertension, decrease the postoperative complication rate and may be beneficial in some pediatric patients [47,48].

While snoring, breath-holding or apneic spells, failure to thrive and repeated respiratory infections are

Table 31.1 Respiratory events that may occur during polysomnography

Event	Definition
Central apnea	Pause in airflow with absent respiratory effort, scored when >20 sec or two missed breaths and >3% decrease in oxygen saturation
Obstructive apnea	>90% reduction in air flow despite continuing respiratory effort, scored when event lasts at least 2 missed breaths in children
Obstructive hypopnea	>50% reduction in airflow despite continuing respiratory effort, scored when event lasts at least 2 missed breaths in children and >3% decrease in oxygen saturation or arousal
Mixed apnea	≥90% reduction in air flow, lasting at least 2 missed breaths, and containing absent respiratory effort initially (central apneic pause), followed by resumption of respiratory effort without resumption of airflow (obstructive apnea)
Obstructive hypoventilation	End-tidal CO_2 >50 mmHg for >25% of total sleep time with paradoxical respirations, snoring and no baseline lung disease

Adapted from Schwengel et al [49] with permission from Lippincott Williams and Wilkins.

Table 31.2 Severity ranking system based on polysomnography [56]

	Apnea–hypopnea index	Oxygen saturation nadir
Normal	0–1	>92%
Mild OSA	2–4	
Moderate OSA	5–9	
Severe OSA	>10	<80%

OSA, obstructive sleep apnea.

Peak end-tidal CO_2 ($EtCO_2$) and duration of time spent with $EtCO_2$ >50 mmHg should be considered when assessing severity of OSA.

Adapted from Schwengel et al [49] with permission from Lippincott Williams and Wilkins.

suggestive of obstructive sleep apnea, the gold standard of diagnosis is overnight sleep polysomnography. Table 31.1 lists the respiratory events that may occur during polysomnography.

The number of hypopnea-obstructive episodes that occur during a sleep study is usually combined to give an apnea-hypopnea index (AHI) which is defined as the number of discrete obstructive events per hour that occur. However, this number usually includes central apnea which is a normal occurrence in children and is not associated with any impaired respiration. True documentation of obstructive sleep apnea in children should be based only on obstructive episodes associated with respiratory impairment as normal children tend to have more central apnea episodes and this feature cannot be used to diagnose OSA in children [50,51]. Many sleep laboratories will report an AHI or a respiratory disturbance index (RDI) that includes the total number of respiratory events, including central apnea, that occur per hour. OSA is considered to be severe if the AHI ≥10/h and the oxygen saturation nadir is ≤80% (Table 31.2). The severity of obstructive sleep apnea is usually based on a number of factors: the patient's total clinical picture, frequency and severity of oxygen desaturation during the apneic episodes, duration of elevated carbon dioxide, and the number of obstructive events per hour [52–55].

Special problems

A number of special problems may be encountered in some children who present for adenotonsillectomy. These include patients with craniofacial disorders, Down syndrome, sickle cell disease, and known bleeding disorders. The risks of general anesthesia in these patient populations are discussed in Chapters 11, 14, 32, and 38.

The anesthesiologist should be prepared for potential difficulties in establishing airway patency and tracheal intubation and maintaining ventilation, particularly in patients with craniofacial disorders who present for adenotonsillectomy. For example, patients with mucopolysaccharidosis I (Hurler syndrome) and II (Hunter syndrome) have diffuse infiltration of the upper airway and larynx with abnormal mucopolysaccharidoses which predisposes them to upper airway obstruction and difficult endotracheal intubation. In addition, patients with Hurler syndrome may have cardiac involvement, resulting in valvular, myocardial involvement as well as coronary artery disease which may occur at an early age. Patients with Hunter syndrome may also have severe kyphoscoliosis which may affect positioning for endotracheal intubation.

Patients with trisomy 21 (Down syndrome) also have craniofacial anomalies which may affect intraoperative management during adenotonsillectomy. These patients have a baseline midface hypoplasia characterized by narrow oral and nasal passages and glossoptosis. In addition, these children have hypopharyngeal hypotonia leading to hypopharyngeal collapse during induction of anesthesia. Mask ventilation may be difficult, requiring oral and/or nasal airway. Some of these patients also develop hypertrophy of lingual tonsils, which are located posterior to the tongue and are not easily appreciated on oral examination [57] (Fig. 31.1). Lingual tonsil hypertrophy can be responsible for persistent obstructive sleep apnea following adenotonsillectomy in this group of

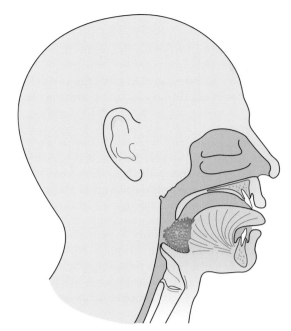

Figure 31.1 Hypertrophied lingual tonsil, difficult to appreciate on oral examination. Reproduced from Olutoye et al [57] with permission from Lippincott Williams and Wilkins.

patients [58]. While these tonsils are not appreciated on oral examination even in their hypertrophied state, the anesthesiologist should be alerted to this condition as it may result in a "cannot ventilate-cannot intubate" clinical scenario [57,59,60].

Patients with sickle cell disease who have recurrent tonsillitis are predisposed to developing sepsis. In addition, hypoxemia in sickle cell patients with OSA may precipitate a sickling crisis. Therefore frequent episodes of tonsillitis (>6 episodes per year) or adenoid hypertrophy resulting in upper airway obstruction are treated very aggressively in this subset of patients. Sickle cell patients undergo special perioperative evaluation and management, depending on the preference of the hematologist at each individual institution. The main goals of these regimens include prevention of perioperative hypoxemia, adequate hydration to decrease blood viscosity and subsequent concentration of sickle cells, increase in hemoglobin level to 10 g/dL via simple blood transfusion and decrease in hemoglobin S concentration by aggressive blood transfusion. There are differences in opinion regarding the trigger hemoglobin value for preoperative blood transfusion in sickle cell patients undergoing minor surgical procedures. Many centers have firm policies for management of sickle cell patients undergoing routine surgery, including temperature maintenance, hydration, oxygen therapy and pain man-

agement. The evidence that these measures are useful has not been well established for minor surgical procedures [61–66]. Patients with sickle cell disease may require an increased amount of analgesia postoperatively [67] and this may pose a challenge as moderate amounts of opioid administration may result in shallow respirations and ultimately hypoxemia, which is avoided in these patients. Preoperative consultation with the hematology service is essential before these surgeries (see Chapter 11).

Coagulation status

The adenotonsillectomy procedure differs from other operations in that a large raw surface (tonsillar bed) is left open and the edges are not apposed for hemostasis. It is therefore very important to obtain a history suggestive of bleeding tendencies, and discontinue medications which interfere with coagulation such as aspirin, nonsteroidal anti-inflammatory drugs and valproic acid prior to surgery. However, discontinuing such medications perioperatively may be problematic as in the case of children with congenital heart disease taking aspirin in order to maintain patency of a Blalock–Taussig shunt. The risks of bleeding need to be balanced against the risks of a clot developing in the shunt. Preoperative consultation with the patient's cardiologist should be obtained. In children with a history suggestive of bleeding disorders, preoperative consultation with a hematologist may be indicated as well. Appropriate laboratory tests include prothrombin time to test the extrinsic and common coagulation pathway, activated partial thromboplastin time (aPTT) to test the intrinsic and common pathway, as well as bleeding times and studies of platelet function.

Von Willebrand disease is a hereditary disorder characterized by a deficiency of von Willebrand factor and prolonged bleeding time while hemophilia A or B is characterized by deficiency of clotting factors VIII and IX respectively. Adequate consultation with the hematology service to determine the dose and time of administration of specific factors to correct the coagulation defect is indicated prior to surgery (see Chapter 11).

Intraoperative management

The duration for adenotonsillectomy is usually 15–30 min and surgery is performed in a variety of ways, including guillotine and snare, cold and hot dissection, ultrasound coblation and electrocautery. Many combinations of inhaled and intravenous agents have been used to provide satisfactory anesthesia for the procedure, but anesthesia usually involves mask induction, establishment of vascular access and tracheal intubation with a preformed curved Ring–Adair–Elwyn (RAE) tube. The use of a preformed oral RAE tube allows for easy positioning of the

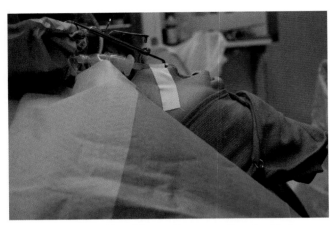

Figure 31.2 Child positioned for tonsillectomy and/or adenoidectomy. The endotracheal tube is secured along the mandible away from the operative field. It is imperative to ensure that the endotracheal tube is not kinked or occluded by the retractor.

self-retaining mouth gag used by the surgeons. In addition, the preformed bend allows the anesthesia circuit to be connected at a location away from the site of surgery (Fig. 31.2). However, many practitioners have been successful with regular oral endotracheal tubes and in some institutions the LMA is routinely used for adenotonsillectomy. A non-depolarizing muscle relaxant may be used to facilitate tracheal intubation but many anesthesiologists will intubate the trachea without muscle relaxants, after an inhalation induction and deepening the anesthetic with propofol 1–2 mg/kg IV, assuming no contraindications. This technique has the advantage of avoiding the need to reverse the muscle relaxant in the case of a very fast surgery, and allows easier resumption of spontaneous ventilation if the plan is to extubate the trachea with deep anesthesia.

Some anesthesiologists recommend the routine use of a cuffed endotracheal tube based on the premise of a reduced leak of anesthetic gases, thereby permitting reduced inspired oxygen concentrations and decreasing the risk of airway fires. Adenotonsillectomy is considered a high-risk procedure in which an ignition source (electrocautery) is in close proximity to an oxidizer-enriched environment (the presence of oxygen in a concentration above that of room air, and/or the presence of nitrous oxide) and combustible tissue, thus completing the triad necessary for the development of an operating room fire [68]. After securing the airway, FIO_2 should be reduced to the lowest practical level, i.e. 0.21–0.30, to minimize the risk of airway fire. The use of cuffed endotracheal tubes limits the number of repeated laryngoscopy attempts, allows for the use of low-flow anesthesia and also decreases the amount of detectable anesthetic gas concentration in the operating room, as well as limiting the oxygen concentration in the orophar-

ynx, reducing the risk of airway fires [69]. There is no existing randomized, controlled trial to determine which method of securing the airway for this procedure is safest.

The trachea can be extubated with the patient awake or deeply anesthetized provided the patient is breathing comfortably without episodes of breath holding. There is no evidence that any one method is associated with increased risks of adverse respiratory events; most randomized trials on this subject have not been sufficiently powered to demonstrate any benefit of one technique versus the other. Some anesthesiologists are reluctant to extubate the trachea under deep anesthesia when a child with OSA has undergone adenotonsillectomy because of the risks of adverse respiratory events when intraoperative opioids have been administered. If the decision is made to extubate the trachea under deep anesthesia, personnel and systems must be in place to detect and treat airway complications (airway obstruction, apnea, laryngospasm) as the patient emerges from anesthesia in the postanesthetic care unit (PACU) after the anesthesiologist has turned over patient care. The anesthetic setting is important in this regard. Extubation decisions may differ in an outpatient surgery setting with no anesthesiologist available for back-up and recovery nurses with limited pediatric experience versus a large children's hospital operating room with readily available personnel and highly experienced pediatric recovery nurses who can respond rapidly and skillfully to airway problems. See below for a discussion of airway emergencies.

Intraoperative pain management resulting in a comfortable patient postoperatively, without episodes of respiratory obstruction, continues to be a challenge for the anesthesiologist. Opioids are the mainstay of analgesic treatment in this patient population. However, children with a history of obstructive sleep apnea may be more sensitive to the effect of opioids and reduced doses may be required to prevent postoperative respiratory depression [70]. In patients with severe OSA, small doses of opioids are titrated to effect in the PACU only after the patient is awake.

Non-steroidal agents (NSAIDs) are not associated with postoperative respiratory depression but concern for their effects on hemostasis has limited their use [71]. A recent Cochrane systematic review of studies failed to show increased bleeding in tonsillectomy patients who received NSAIDs [72]. Different combinations involving opioid and non-steroidal agents have been used in the search for the optimal analgesic regimen [73,74]. This has included the use of acetaminophen administered orally, rectally and more recently in an intravenous form. Rectal doses should be higher (40–45 mg/kg) compared to the oral route (15–20 mg/kg) to achieve satisfactory blood levels.

Intraoperative infiltration of local anesthetics has also been utilized by some surgeons in an attempt to decrease postoperative morbidity in this patient population following surgery [75–77].

The introduction of the α2-agonist dexmedetomidine, with effects of mild analgesia without respiratory depression, has provided a plausible agent for analgesia in adenotonsillectomy patients. It reduces postoperative opioid consumption in adults undergoing major inpatient surgery [78]. In children undergoing adenotonsillectomy, doses of 1 μg/kg and 0.75 μg/kg of dexmedetomidine increased the time to requirement of postoperative opioid medication but the total amount of postoperative morphine consumed by the patients was the same when compared to those who received morphine intraoperatively [79].

Different surgical techniques have also been explored to try to determine which provides the least postoperative morbidity due to pain [80–83].

Intraoperative dexamethasone has been used in these patients to reduce postoperative pain and edema and to prevent nausea and vomiting. The minimum dose for reducing opioid consumption was 0.5 mg/kg, but parents reported reduced pain scores with 1 mg/kg of dexamethasone [84]. More recently, there has been considerable discussion about a report of increased bleeding in this patient population when dexamethasone was used [85]. However, this study has been criticized for the high incidence of primary hemorrhage and need to return to the operating room on the day of operation. Dexamethasone is useful as an antiemetic and its combination with an antiserotonin drug such as ondansetron is recommended for this procedure.

Postoperative complications

Postoperative or secondary hemorrhage and respiratory impairment are the most frequently observed complications following adenotonsillectomy; the incidences of these are significantly dependent on age. Postoperative hemorrhage is more common in children older than 10 years of age [86] while respiratory complications such as supraglottic obstruction, breath holding and need for airway rescue maneuvers are more common in children younger than 3 years of age [52,87,88]. In many institutions, children less than 3 years of age are observed at least overnight in the hospital following adenotonsillectomy, particularly if they have co-morbid conditions (e.g. Down syndrome, developmental delay, OSA). Other complications following adenotonsillectomy which are rare in incidence include uvular edema, uvula amputation, velopharyngeal insufficiency and nasopharyngeal stenosis. Throat pain, otalgia and poor oral intake are also common complications following discharge.

Post-tonsillectomy hemorrhage

This is the most common complication that results in children presenting to the operating room for re-exploration, within the first hour after surgery or more commonly within 2 weeks after the initial surgery. Dislodging of the eschar on the surgical site with exposure of raw mucosal surfaces is usually responsible for hemorrhage that occurs a few days after surgery. This condition requires surgical exploration and cauterization of the bleeding surface. The incidence of post-tonsillectomy hemorrhage is higher in older children. Usually children have been swallowing the blood and therefore should be treated as having a full stomach when they present to the operating room. The degree of bleeding can be assessed clinically by the degree of dehydration observed on clinical examination. Severe dehydration is characterized by dry mucous membranes, sunken orbits, and decreased skin turgor.

Intravenous access may be difficult to obtain in severe cases and the use of an intraosseous catheter may be necessary. Alternatively, large-bore intravenous access should be secured as crystalloid and colloid replacement will be required. Preparation for induction of these children should include having two available suction catheters, preferably firm suction catheters (Yankauer) and drugs for a rapid-sequence induction. Preoxygenation should be followed with rapid sequence induction with the surgeon holding one suction catheter and the other within easy reach of the anesthesiologist. In cases of severe bleeding, the vocal cords may not be visible; in this case the anesthesiologist should direct the endotracheal tube (ETT) at the site where air bubbles are seen escaping from the glottic opening when an assistant presses on the chest wall to produce a forced exhalation. Careful laryngoscopy is recommended as the process of laryngoscopy itself may scrape the tonsillar bed and also precipitate bleeding. Cuffed endotracheal tubes are recommended in the presence of a full stomach. Significant anemia may be present from blood loss so a perioperative hemoglobin level should be obtained and adequate preparation should be made for blood transfusion. Prompt identification of the bleeding sites usually occurs so surgery for cauterization of the tonsillectomy bed lasts only about 20 min. Blood may be transfused intraoperatively or in the recovery room as time permits.

Endoscopic sinus surgery

Chronic sinusitis is characterized by inflammation and occlusion of the sinus ostia which allow drainage from the sinuses into the nose. In some patients adenoidectomy can relieve symptoms, but endoscopic sinus surgery (ESS) has become the mainstay of surgical treatment for chronic sinusitis refractory to antibiotics and adenoidectomy. The operation involves direct telescopic visualization of the nasal mucus membranes with the aid of sharp, biting instruments or the use of a microdebrider to relieve areas of obstruction and improve ventilation through the sinuses, while leaving the mucous membranes intact.

Cystic fibrosis is a common underlying disease in children presenting for this surgery as the associated impaired mucociliary function predisposes them to infection. The anesthesiologist should ensure that these patients are medically optimized prior to surgery.

Bleeding can make surgical visualization difficult, and therefore the nasal cavity is packed with pledgets soaked in one of a number of different vasoconstricting solutions. The most common vasoconstricting solutions which may be used include oxymetazoline 0.025% to 0.05%, phenylephrine 0.25 to 1%, cocaine 4% to 10% and 2% lidocaine with epinephrine 1:100,000 or epinephrine 1:200,000. The anesthesiologist should be aware of the type and dose of vasoconstrictive agent being used and ensure that the maximum allowable concentration/amount has not been exceeded as rapid absorption occurs from raw mucosal surfaces, leading to changes in heart rate (tachycardia or bradycardia) or hypertensive episodes [89,90]. This may occur especially if intraoperative anticholinergics have been administered. Intraoperative hypertension usually is transient and resolves spontaneously without aggressive treatment. In children, the recommended dose of phenylephrine should not exceed 20 μg/kg. Cocaine has been reported to result in myocardial infarction in otherwise healthy individuals [91]. The spread of anesthetic effects of cocaine may also cause blockade of the nasociliary ganglion, resulting in transient anisocoria postoperatively [92].

Intraoperative management for ESS involves endotracheal intubation with the use of an oral RAE tube which is securely fixed along the mandible, allowing easy surgical access to the maxilla and sinuses. The use of cuffed endotracheal tubes prevents fogging of the endoscopic equipment and also prevents excessive gas leak around the tube. Throat packs are almost always utilized during this surgery to prevent escape of gas into the environment from around the endotracheal tube. The anesthesiologist must confirm removal of the throat pack at the conclusion of surgery prior to extubation of the patient as this may be a cause of airway obstruction or emergence agitation postoperatively. Intravenous corticosteroids are warranted during this surgery in order to prevent postoperative swelling.

Frequently, at the end of this surgery, some stenting material is left in the sinuses by the surgeon. This may cause discomfort or a perception of difficult breathing by the patient upon emergence. Therefore, an anesthetic technique that provides adequate analgesia and quick emergence is desired.

A second endoscopic procedure is usually required approximately 6 weeks following the initial surgery in order to remove the existing packs (if non-absorbable packs were used) and to examine the surgical site. This procedure is usually quick and the use of a laryngeal mask airway may be considered.

Airway complications and pathology

Laryngospasm

Laryngospasm is a life-threatening event in which either the true vocal cords or both the true and false vocal cords appose in the midline, resulting in an involuntary closure of the glottis by the intrinsic laryngeal muscles and inability to exchange gas [93]. The primary muscles involved in laryngospasm are the lateral cricoarytenoid, the thyroarytenoid muscles (adductors of the glottis) as well as the cricothyroid muscles which are tensors of the vocal cords. Laryngospasm is the most frequently reported respiratory complication associated with upper respiratory tract infections, particularly in younger children undergoing airway surgery and in those cared for by less experienced anesthesiologists [23]. While most patients who develop laryngospasm have otherwise normal airway anatomy, airway anomalies have been found to have an increased association with laryngospasm [25].

Laryngospasm is most commonly associated with airway manipulation (e.g. intubation or extubation of the trachea), foreign material in the larynx (e.g. secretions) or with light anesthesia in a non-intubated patient. The clinical scenario of laryngospasm may be preceded by an irregular breathing pattern or noisy airway sounds that vary in intensity and tone but usually resemble a high-pitched squeak indicating partial airway obstruction. Airway obstruction as a result of laryngospasm may be partial or total, resulting in an absence of spontaneous ventilation or inability to manually ventilate the patient. In the mildest form, this scenario is usually relieved by airway manipulation such as a jaw thrust or application of continuous positive airway pressure (CPAP) of 10–20 cmH$_2$O for 30–45 sec. If the scenario of partial airway obstruction without arterial desaturation persists, small subhypnotic doses of propofol, 0.5–1 mg/kg, may alleviate symptoms [94,95]. If the condition does not resolve following these interventions, marked oxygen desaturation typically ensues and the administration of a muscle relaxant may become necessary in order to break the laryngospasm and allow ventilation with 100% oxygen. A small dose of intravenous succinylcholine, 0.1–0.3 mg/kg is effective. However, if the child is hypoxemic, administering succinylcholine may precipitate profound bradycardia and further worsen oxygen delivery. If succinylcholine is to be given to a hypoxemic child or if the initial dose is not effective, atropine 20 μg/kg should also be administered prior to the next dose. In situations where laryngospasm occurs prior to placement of an intravenous line, succinycholine may be administered via a number of alternative routes: intramuscular (4 mg/kg), intralingual (1.1 mg/kg), submental or via the intraosseous route [96]. Intravenous lidocaine (2 mg/kg) has been found to control or prevent laryngospasm in both children and adults [97,98]. Aerosolized lidocaine also alleviates symptoms of postextubation laryngospasm [99]. Topical lidocaine is thought to effectively decrease the incidence of laryngospasm by suppressing laryngeal mucosal neuroreceptors without affecting central neural reflex.

In piglets, topical lidocaine decreased both the laryngeal chemoreflex and mechanoreflex without decreasing the superior laryngeal nerve adductor reflex [100]. However, intravenous lidocaine had no effect on laryngeal mucosal reflexes [97]. The increased depth of anesthesia provided by lidocaine appears to decrease the occurrence of laryngospasm.

Whatever the final treatment strategy, early recognition of laryngospasm is essential, particularly in infants and young children in whom oxygen consumption is high and arterial desaturation is very rapid. There is no substitute for well-developed airway management skills.

The LMA provides an alternative to endotracheal intubation for a variety of procedures. Some authors have proposed that this device may reduce airway complications in patients who have a URI as instrumentation of an irritable airway (due to a URI) is avoided. However, in one study, LMAs were associated with a similar incidence of cough, breath holding, excessive secretions, and laryngospasm as occurred with endotracheal tubes [20]. Patients whose airways were managed with an LMA had a lower incidence of mild bronchospasm and a lower incidence of oxygen desaturation during placement of the airway than those treated with an endotracheal tube. Treatment of bronchospasm and laryngospasm that developed during use of an LMA was not addressed in this study. Both may be more difficult to treat because high peak airway pressures cannot be delivered through an LMA.

The lower blood : gas partition coefficient of desflurane of 0.45 allows for rapid emergence from anesthesia. Despite the theoretical advantages, children receiving desflurane have a higher incidence of laryngospasm, breath holding and coughing following either endotracheal extubation or removal of the laryngeal mask airway [101,102]. In general, laryngospasm is unlikely if the anesthetic depth is sufficiently deep to permit tracheal stimulation during intubation and extubation. However, careful vigilance of the anesthesia care provider is essential for rapid management of laryngospasm.

Total airway obstruction following laryngospasm may result in acute pulmonary edema [103,104]. The pathogenesis of this edema is akin to that which occurs following acute obstruction due to trauma, masses [105], croup and epiglottitis [106]. An attempt at ventilation against a closed glottis generates an intrapleural pressure of approximately 30–60 cmH$_2$O. In concert with the catecholamine surge, the intrapleural pressure causes acute pulmonary capillary hypertension and permeability exacerbated by acute hypoxemia. This process, followed by an immediate decrease in airway pressure that occurs with the relief or treatment of laryngospasm, induces pulmonary edema [106]. The increased negative intrapleural pressure and increased venous return (i.e. increased preload) may both result in injury to the microvasculature (i.e. increased permeability). The combination of the preload and the increased vascular permeability allows fluid movement out of the vasculature and produces interstitial edema and pulmonary edema. In addition, negative intrathoracic pressure increases left ventricular transmural pressure (i.e. afterload) [107] and affects cardiac performance. A third process, mechanical stress at the alveolar–capillary membrane, is thought to be responsible for both pulmonary edema as well as frank alveolar hemorrhage. While pulmonary hemorrhage may occur in children as a result of acute airway obstruction [108], other etiologies of pulmonary hemorrhage should be initially ruled out when this complication develops in association with laryngospasm [109].

Laryngospasm-induced pulmonary edema is most effectively managed by prompt tracheal intubation and application of continuous positive airway pressure or positive end-expiratory pressure with positive pressure ventilation. Diuretics, morphine, and sedatives are also effective adjuncts. If the patient has no underlying cardiorespiratory problems, the pulmonary edema resolves quickly, allowing the trachea to be extubated within several hours.

Stridor

Stridor is noisy breathing caused by turbulent flow through the narrowed lumen of an airway. It may be appreciated on inspiration or expiration, depending on the location of the obstruction. Inspiratory stridor occurs as a result of anomalies that narrow the airway above the thoracic inlet (e.g. cysts or masses, laryngomalacia, vocal cord paralysis, hemangiomas, laryngoceles, papillomas), adenotonsillar hypertrophy, midfacial hypoplasia, and croup. Expiratory stridor is most commonly associated with airway obstruction below the thoracic inlet (e.g. cysts, hemangiomas, vascular rings, foreign bodies) [107,110]. Biphasic stridor is common and is characteristic of midtracheal abnormalities secondary to tracheomalacia and tracheal stenosis. Diagnostic laryngoscopy and fiber-optic and/or rigid bronchoscopy and a variety of imaging procedures are often required to determine the etiology of stridor. To accomplish these procedures, deep sedation or general anesthesia usually is required. Therefore, the anesthesiologist should understand the physiology and clinical implications of stridor.

Inspiration through a partially obstructed extrathoracic airway reduces the intraluminal pressure of the extrathoracic airway below atmospheric pressure. The transluminal pressure gradient narrows the lumen further, increasing the stridor. During expiration, the extrathoracic intraluminal pressure is positive and greater than atmospheric, dilating the lumen and decreasing stridor. In contrast, inspiration through a partially obstructed intrathoracic airway reduces extraluminal pressure below intraluminal pressure and dilates the airway. During expiration, the reverse occurs and the expiratory noise (wheezing) worsens [107,110].

A careful medical history covering the severity and duration of symptoms, age and acuteness of onset, as well as a history of previous tracheal intubation, is important. For example, the newborn with severe stridor is likely to have a congenital anomaly of the airway as the etiology. A 3 year old with sudden onset of severe stridor is more likely to have a foreign body or an infectious etiology as the cause. The child in the recovery room or intensive care unit who develops stridor following tracheal extubation is likely to have airway edema as the cause. The severity and rapidity of progression of the symptoms define the diagnostic and treatment plan.

Approximately 45–60% of stridor (except postextubation stridor) in the young infant is due to laryngomalacia [110,111]. Symptoms of laryngomalacia generally are present from birth and must be differentiated from other congenital anomalies that cause stridor. Babies with laryngomalacia usually do not have feeding difficulties, but children with glottic or oropharyngeal lesions or a tracheo-esophageal fistula commonly do have these symptoms. The noise is usually worse in these babies when they are agitated or positioned supine. An occasional improvement in symptoms may occur when these babies are placed in the prone position. Although many of these infants do well and improve as they grow, their stridor often persists for 4–5 years [111].

Although infants and children with laryngomalacia do not have a higher incidence of upper or lower respiratory tract infections, their upper airway obstruction often worsens in the presence of an upper respiratory infection [111]. A child with laryngomalacia and an upper respiratory tract infection presenting for anything but emergency surgery should be carefully evaluated and surgery should proceed cautiously, especially if it will involve general anesthesia with endotracheal intubation. If the surgery is emergency, an endotracheal tube that allows an audible air leak when a positive pressure of 20–25 cmH$_2$O is generated should be used. In addition, the patient should be monitored postoperatively in a pediatric intensive care unit (PICU), where prompt ventilatory support can be provided.

Although uncommon, neurological abnormalities in an infant may present with stridor. Laryngeal nerve paralysis may be caused by birth trauma, cardiac malformations that affect the left recurrent laryngeal nerve or as a postoperative complication following ligation of a patent ductus arteriosus. Frequently, the etiology of the injury is unclear. Unilateral vocal cord paralysis commonly is the result of a peripheral nerve lesion and often improves with growth. Infants with unilateral cord paralysis commonly have stridor or hoarseness and feeding difficulties. Infants with bilateral vocal cord paralysis often have central nervous system disease (e.g. hydrocephalus, Arnold–Chiari malformation, Dandy–Walker cyst, encephalocele, posterior fossa hematomas or child abuse) [112–116]. Some authors relate the stridor to vocal cord paralysis that is caused by stretching the vagus nerve over the jugular foramen. However, it is often unclear why stridor occurs and why it persists after the increased intracranial pressure is normalized. Children who have bilateral vocal cord paralysis and serious respiratory obstruction or recurrent aspiration pneumonia often require a tracheostomy.

Anesthetic considerations for children who are stridorous are similar, regardless of the etiology of the obstruction. Maintaining continuous positive airway pressure during spontaneous ventilation via a facemask can reverse the upper airway pressure gradient and decrease or eliminate the obstruction. It is vital to have a wide range of endotracheal tubes available for intubation as some lesions, such as cricoid ring stenosis, webs, cysts, hemangiomas, epiglottitis and croup, will usually necessitate the use of a smaller than normal endotracheal tube. Lesions such as vocal cord paralysis which may also cause stridor do not narrow the airway. It is important to ensure that the endotracheal tube used for intubation has a leak at approximately 20–25 cmH$_2$O airway pressure in order to prevent further injury to the trachea.

Postextubation stridor is a significant problem in children receiving mechanical ventilation for prolonged periods of time, resulting in laryngeal/tracheal edema, airway narrowing, and stridor. It may also occur in children who have undergone airway surgery or even those who have been intubated for surgery. The use of cuffed endotracheal tubes for general anesthesia in children, previously thought to contribute to the occurrence of postextubation croup, has been found not to result in the development of this condition [117]. The mucosa of the subglottic area in children is vascular and consists of loose areolar tissue and the cricoid cartilage is the narrowest area in the airway of a child less than 5 years of age. Therefore swelling caused by a tight-fitting endotracheal tube, burns or other trauma results in inflammation and narrowing of the internal diameter of the airway, because the cartilage of the trachea prevents edema from being displaced outward. Consequently, this area of the trachea is prone to edema.

Inhaled racemic epinephrine, heliox (79%, 70% or 60% helium in 21%, 30% or 40% oxygen) and occasionally steroids have been utilized to treat stridor. Racemic epinephrine (0.5 mL of 2.25% solution nebulized in 2.5 mL of normal saline) can be administered repeatedly at 5-min intervals to decrease edema if the heart rate is less than 200 beats/minute. Oxygen saturation should be monitored during treatment and if multiple treatments are required, an arterial blood gas should be obtained to ensure that ventilation is adequate. This is important particularly if increased work of breathing is observed in the child.

Heliox may also be used to facilitate ventilation in patients with stridor. The decreased density of heliox compared to oxygen and air provides more laminar flow in obstructed airways and decreases the work of breathing. In order to avoid hypoxia, however, heliox should not be used in children with a high oxygen requirement.

Steroids may be used in the management algorithm for stridor. However, the possible effect of delayed wound healing should be balanced against the possible benefit of steroids on the airway. In instances of failure to wean a patient from mechanical ventilation, without other obvious reasons, a 48-h trial of steroid therapy may lessen airway edema and allow successful extubation.

Supraglottitis

Acute supraglottitis (previously known as epiglottitis) (Fig. 31.3) is a life-threatening infection characterized by

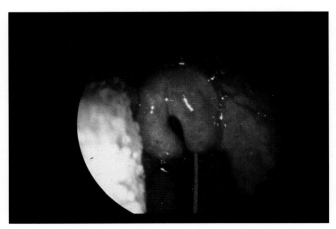

Figure 31.3 Edematous epiglottis in a case of acute epiglottitis. Courtesy of Deidre Larrier MD.

severe edema of the supraglottic structures with a potential risk for upper airway obstruction. Children usually present with complaints of upper respiratory infection (rhinorrhea, cough) followed by severe sore throat and fever. As symptoms progress, the child constantly drools and may prefer to lean forward to improve their breathing pattern. Prior to the routine immunization of children with the *Haemophilus influenzae* type B (Hib) polysaccharide vaccine, many of the invasive cases of acute supraglottitis in children between the ages of 2 and 6 years occurred due to infection with *Haemophilus influenzae* type B. The frequency of this infection and disease process has since diminished in children [118,119] and other causative agents have been implicated, namely group A streptococcus infection [120], *Neisseria meningitides* [121] and *Candida albicans* [122]. Supraglottitis has a fulminant onset and therefore has a characteristic history and presentation; nevertheless, the differential diagnosis for this disease includes laryngotracheobronchitis (croup) and tracheitis (Table 31.3). Tracheitis can present with symptoms similar to those of supraglottitis.

The patient with suspected supraglottitis is at risk for sudden and complete airway obstruction so a multidisciplinary team is generally involved in managing these patients from the time of initial presentation to an emergency room or clinic. It is essential to have this co-ordinated approach established and all services available immediately. When the diagnosis of supraglottitis is made or strongly suspected, the goal is to secure the airway in a controlled, calm manner as soon as possible. Endotracheal intubation is the preferred method of supportive airway care as it is a safe and efficacious alternative to tracheostomy. The following approach is consistent with that reported in other centers [123].

A pediatrician, an anesthesiologist skilled in pediatric airway problems, and a surgeon skilled in placing a tracheostomy in an infant or child should be notified and be present when, or shortly after, the child arrives in the emergency room. A thorough, rapid cardiopulmonary history and assessment are made. Examination of the airway is limited to noting respiratory rate, observing the pattern of breathing, and assessing the work of breathing and level of respiratory distress. At most, the heart and lungs should be examined. Any maneuver that may result in the child becoming agitated should be reserved for the operating room setting; this includes manipulation or examination of the mouth or oropharynx, intravenous catheter placement, venepuncture or arterial blood gas sampling. Instead, the child should remain sitting up on a parent's (or other familiar caretaker's) lap and receive supplemental oxygen. Oxygen saturation is monitored with a pulse oximeter, while the child is observed closely by the medical personnel.

Table 31.3 Supraglottitis, laryngotracheobronchitis, tracheitis

Characteristic	Supraglottitis	Laryngotracheobronchitis	Tracheitis
Age	2–6 years	2 months – 3 years	2–6 years
Onset	Fulminant	Gradual	Gradual
Etiology	Bacterial	Viral	Bacterial
Presentation			
Voice	Muffled	Bark	Bark
Secretions	Drooling	Drooling	None
Fever	>38.5°C	37–38°C	>38.5°C
Distress	Anxious, sitting up	Normal	Toxic appearing, sitting up

In the absence of respiratory distress, obtaining a single lateral radiograph of the neck to confirm the diagnosis may be considered. In this case, the child must receive supplemental oxygen while being transported sitting up to the radiography suite. They must be accompanied by someone who can intubate the trachea instantly if necessary although the ideal place for this to occur is the operating room. If the child is in significant respiratory distress or the diagnosis is made clinically, the child should be promptly transported, sitting up, to the operating room while receiving oxygen and being monitored. Radiological confirmation will be omitted in this urgent scenario. The patient must be accompanied by personnel skilled in pediatric airway management and cardiopulmonary resuscitation (CPR).

The tracheostomy tray should be open with the surgeon present when the patient arrives in the operating room. A smooth induction of anesthesia with sevoflurane in 100% oxygen, with the child sitting on the caretaker's lap, will allow for minimal airway irritation [124]. Halothane was previously used and traditionally allowed for a smooth inhalation induction in this situation. The appropriateness of parental or other caregiver presence during induction of anesthesia needs to be assessed for each patient.

With the onset of anesthesia, the patient is placed in the supine or semi-sitting position, often while continuous positive pressure is applied via facemask to overcome upper airway obstruction. Intravenous catheter placement may commence once an adequate depth of anesthesia has been achieved. Carefully evaluating the depth of anesthesia is vital to avoid precipitating laryngospasm during laryngoscopy and endotracheal intubation. The endotracheal tube should be approximately 0.5–1.0 mm smaller in diameter than is appropriate for the age and size of the patient. An initial orotracheal intubation may subsequently be changed to a nasotracheal tube by some anesthesiologists as the child often remains intubated for a number of days afterwards and a nasotracheal tube is more secure and better tolerated by the patient.

Blood and laryngeal cultures should be obtained during anesthesia, and appropriate antibiotics should be administered intravenously. The selection and dose of antibiotic will vary depending on the organisms seen in a specific geographic area and in a specific patient (e.g. immuno-compromised, HIV infection). If the diagnosis of supraglottitis is ruled out when the upper airway is examined, and if the diagnosis is thought to be bacterial tracheitis, the antibiotic of preference may differ from that chosen to treat supraglottitis. Consulting with the pediatric infectious disease specialist is appropriate. The morbidity from 24–48h of tracheal intubation is minimal with excellent nursing care. Most otolaryngologists prefer the use of an endotracheal tube over performing a tracheostomy to treat airway obstruction. The patient can return to the operating room (OR) for an endoscopic examination of the airway once a leak (indicating resolution of the airway edema) has developed around the tube.

Although supraglottitis is rare in the modern era, the above general approach can be used for any form of acute severe upper airway obstruction.

Endoscopy of the larynx, trachea, and bronchial tree

The major challenge of endoscopy of the respiratory tract is that the anesthesiologist must share the airway with the endoscopist and maintain adequate alveolar ventilation, oxygenation, a quiet surgical field and also provide a clear view in a patient with some degree of upper or lower airway compromise. Communication is essential and best achieved in the preoperative period by a discussion between the entire OR team so that all members are aware of the aims and steps in the procedure, equipment required and any special precautions, e.g. need for spontaneous respiration, potential fire hazards and method of ventilation during the procedure.

Lesions commonly diagnosed endoscopically include laryngomalacia or tracheomalacia, vascular anomalies causing tracheobronchial compression, congenital or acquired subglottic stenosis, vocal cord palsies, papillomas, hemangiomas, cysts, granulomas, and foreign bodies [110,125]. Therapeutic bronchoscopy is performed for extraction of foreign bodies or to selectively aspirate thick, tenacious plugs from the bronchi in order to resolve atelectasis, as occurs in cystic fibrosis [126].

Preoperative evaluation of the airway requires a careful history of the degree of airway obstruction that occurs during sleeping, crying or feeding. It is also important to determine the degree of accompanying respiratory distress (use of accessory muscles of respiration, tachypnea) and which positions or manuevers aggravate or alleviate the symptoms. The anesthesiologist should examine any available chest radiographs, head and neck computed tomographic scans, magnetic resonance imaging scans, pulmonary function tests or arterial blood gas determinations to obtain a complete view of the clinical situation [127,128].

Fiber-optic direct laryngoscopy and bronchoscopy

In rare situations, this procedure can be accomplished with only topical anesthesia and mild sedation in infants or older children. More commonly, general anesthesia is required for an adequate endoscopic examination of the tracheobronchial tree. Preoperative sedatives and opiates should be administered with caution in any child with accompanying airway compromise, and then only with appropriate monitoring and by a person who is skilled in advanced airway management. Some experts recommend an anti-sialogogue to minimize secretions [129–131]. Sedation/anesthesia can be induced with midazolam, propofol or inhaled anesthetics, usually sevoflurane which is less irritating to the airway than desflurane, in an inspired oxygen concentration (FIO_2) of 1.0. The larynx and trachea may also be anesthetized with local anesthetics (2–4% lidocaine, 3–5 mg/kg (total dose)) typically sprayed onto the vocal cords by the endoscopist. This allows for the use of lower concentrations of inhalation agents so spontaneous ventilation can be maintained during observation of vocal cord movement, while providing adequate jaw relaxation and satisfactory conditions for initial airway endoscopy [132]. Propofol infusions, at rates of 150–200 µg/kg/min, along with inhalation agents, also provide adequate conditions for laryngoscopy. Spontaneous ventilation may be maintained throughout the whole procedure. In rare cases, intermittent doses of non-depolarizing neuromuscular blocking agents, such as rocuronium or vecuronium, may be used after the status of the airway is known. Few pediatric anesthesiologists will use succinylcholine in this setting, particularly in light of the recent black box warning (severe contraindication warning by the US

Food and Drug Administration) for succinylcholine [133]. The goal at the end of the procedure is to have a patient with spontaneous ventilation through a natural airway so muscle relaxants must be utilized judiciously, if at all.

Jet ventilation, without an endotracheal tube

Since the late 1960s, jet ventilation through the side-arm of a bronchoscope or directly into the trachea via a specially adapted laryngoscope has been used to ventilate the lungs of patients during endoscopy when the surgeon requires a totally unobstructed view of the upper airway. The Sanders device delivers oxygen through a 14–16 gauge cannula at 50 psi down an open bronchoscope. The Venturi effect created entrains sufficient gas during delivery of the jet of oxygen at high pressure to provide ventilation. The system depends on gas escaping through an open glottis during an unobstructed expiratory phase of respiration. If expiration is obstructed, gas trapping and barotrauma can occur. Dangerously high inflation pressures may be present when the 3 and 4 mm bronchoscopes are used. Pediatric patients are less likely to have a significant gas leak around the bronchoscope, particularly very small patients, and higher inflation pressures may develop [130]. A variety of modifications of the Sanders device have been introduced, which attempt to reduce the incidence of barotrauma during endoscopy procedures while maintaining adequate ventilation. Other complications that may occur include tumor, such as papillomas, other tissue or blood being forced into the airway.

Jet ventilation does not allow precise control of FIO_2 nor does it allow measurement of end-tidal carbon dioxide, or peak or end-expiratory airway pressure. FIO_2 of 1.0 is usually administered, since entrainment of air by the Venturi jet dilutes the oxygen. The volume of air entrained may be 10–20 times that delivered by the jet itself. In order to be effective, the jet ventilation laryngoscope must be aligned carefully with the glottic opening. If this does not occur, poor ventilation, inadequate oxygenation, and/or gastric dilation may result. The use of pulse oximetry does not obviate the need for clinical vigilance, and the anesthesiologist must have a clear view of the patient's chest at all times to ensure that appropriate chest wall movement occurs with each breath.

Miyasaka et al [129] reported that in 6-month to 3-year-old children, maximal inflation pressures and the volume of ventilation are vulnerable to small alterations in variables such as the size of the jet and the bronchoscope, length and angle of the jet, shape of the bronchoscope (tapered or straight), and the introduction of a suction cannula. Tidal volumes in excess of 10 mL/kg were achieved with driving pressures of 24–45 psi. However, the results of this study are applicable only when the

Sanders No. 19 adapter is used. Any modifications should be carefully assessed [129].

Patients with underlying pulmonary disease and poor lung or chest wall compliance are not ideal candidates for jet ventilation as they are particularly susceptible to barotrauma.

Total intravenous anesthesia is commonly administered for jet ventilation via a laryngoscope or bronchoscope and opioids such as fentanyl or remifentanil in combination with propofol or thiopental may be administered to blunt airway reflexes. Muscle relaxants are also frequently administered in order to prevent coughing during the procedure which may lead to severe complications. However, jet ventilation is rarely, if ever, used in small children.

Rigid bronchoscope

The rigid pediatric ventilating bronchoscope is equipped with an optical telescope and a fiber-optic light source. An optical telescope, when used with the Storz® pediatric bronchoscope (Karl Storz-Endoskope, Tuttlingen, Germany), gives superior resolution and magnification, and a wide-angle view [126]. Miniaturized grasping or biopsy forceps can be manipulated through the instrument channel. An advantage of this system is that a closed system is maintained, permitting ventilation while the viewing telescope is in place [126,131]. A forceps may be placed through the main channel of the scope for retrieval of foreign bodies, if the telescope magnification is removed. A side-arm port also makes it possible to attach the ventilating bronchoscope to any anesthetic system to maintain anesthesia and oxygenation, and to assist or control manual ventilation (Fig. 31.4).

The optical telescope used with these systems occupies nearly the entire internal lumen of the smaller bronchoscopes. This reduces the area for gas flow, markedly increases airflow resistance, and retards passive expiration, potentially resulting in hyperinflation and hypoventilation [134]. A persistent increase in intrathoracic

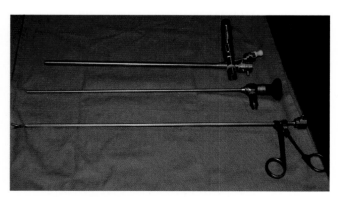

Figure 31.4 Ventilating bronchoscope, optical telescope and foreign body forceps

pressure increases the risk of barotrauma and cardiac output can be impaired [134]. Maintaining adequate expiratory time is essential to allow complete expiration. A 2.8 mm telescope in a 3.5 mm bronchoscope allows adequate exhalation and prevents hyperinflation of the lungs, even during positive pressure ventilation [131]. When smaller scopes are used intermittently, the endoscopist can remove the telescope and occlude the orifice of the scope, thereby allowing the anesthesiologist to deliver brief periods of unobstructed manual hyperventilation [134]. For bronchoscopic examinations of longer duration, intermittent determinations of $PaCO_2$ can confirm the adequacy of ventilation. When evaluating the airway of small infants using a 2.5 mm bronchoscope, the surgeons must remove the telescope more frequently to permit adequate ventilation and complete passive exhalation.

Any rapid deterioration of cardiac function during bronchoscopy should make one highly suspicious of the possible development of a tension pneumothorax [135]. Clinical findings of a pneumothorax alone justify thoracostomy before obtaining a chest radiograph. Vocal cord movement may be evaluated by laryngoscopy as the patient awakens from anesthesia. Care must be taken to avoid inducing laryngospasm during this time.

Airway foreign bodies

Foreign body aspiration

Aspiration of foreign bodies, including organic food items, toy parts, batteries, pin caps, etc. (Fig. 31.5), is a major source of morbidity and mortality in children below 5 years, with a peak incidence between the ages of 1 and 2 years [136–140]. Depending on the nature and location of the aspirated object, removal can be life saving. A detailed discussion with the anesthesia and nursing team to co-ordinate the procedure is mandatory for a smooth procedure and this should occur before the child is brought into the operating room.

A thorough history is pertinent to the diagnosis of foreign body aspiration. Some parents may report witnessing a choking episode which may have been short-lived such that they did not consider it significant at the time. This results in delayed presentation and diagnosis. The presenting symptoms of foreign body aspiration vary depending on the location, size, and duration of aspiration of the object. Acutely, a child may present with hoarseness, stridor, dyspnea, and unilateral decreased air entry or wheezing on auscultation [141–144]. Acute airway distress occurs especially if the object is lodged at or near the glottic inlet. However, normal auscultation or physical examination cannot eliminate the possibility of an aspirated foreign body as 14–45% of patients with an

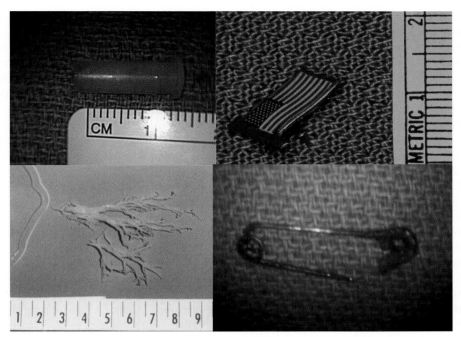

Figure 31.5 A variety of foreign bodies retrieved from the airway, clockwise from top left: plastic tube, toy flag, safety pin and bubble gum. Courtesy of Ellen Friedman MD.

abnormal bronchoscopic finding including foreign bodies have a normal physical examination preoperatively [145–147]. Objects located in the larynx or trachea can be associated with mortality as high as 45% [148]. According to one study, the diagnosis of laryngotracheal foreign body was made within the first 24 h of aspiration in only slightly more than one half the patients. The remaining patients were diagnosed following failure of medical management for croup or reactive airway disease, usually within 1 week of aspiration. Children diagnosed late either did not respond to therapy or their condition deteriorated despite appropriate medical therapy [143,149]. Partial obstruction by smaller objects may go unrecognized for weeks [148] and such children may present with recurrent or chronic pneumonias or bronchiectasis [150]. Some episodes of choking are not witnessed but a high index of suspicion should be raised when a toddler/child presents with respiratory distress in the absence of a prior history of infection or trauma. Chronic abnormalities on chest radiography should be suspicious for pneumonia due to an aspirated foreign object.

A variety of objects can be aspirated (see Fig. 31.5). Radiopaque objects are more easily appreciated on chest radiograph and some plastic toys contain radiopaque markers for easy detection on chest x-ray. Unfortunately, the most frequently aspirated items (food) are radiolucent and are unlikely to be detected by radiography. In such instances, lateral decubitus views can confirm the presence of lower airway obstruction due to the presence of

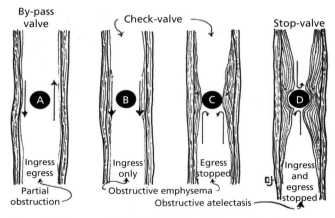

Figure 31.6 Patterns of foreign body-induced airway obstruction. Courtesy of Ellen Friedman MD.

an aspirated foreign body. Four major patterns of airway obstruction have been described [151,152]: bypass valve obstruction, check valve obstruction, ball valve obstruction and stop valve obstruction.

- Bypass valve obstruction involves both phases of respiration and the chest radiograph is usually normal because aeration occurs beyond the point of obstruction although it is somewhat diminished (Fig.31.6A).
- Check valve obstruction is characterized by normal inhalation of air and impedance of exhalation resulting in hyperinflation of the ipsilateral affected lung field.

To appreciate this effect, inspiratory and expiratory radiographic films are required. As expiratory films may be difficult to obtain in children, lateral decubitus films are obtained. When a foreign body has been aspirated, a mediastinal shift should occur toward the normal side if the difference in volume is significant. On a left lateral decubitus film, the mediastinum/heart structures should shift to the left, while on a right lateral decubitus film, the mediastinum should shift to the right. If there is an obstructing foreign body on the right main bronchus, the ipsilateral lung field (right) will remain aerated and inflated on a right lateral decubitus film (Fig. 31.6B, C).

- Ball valve obstruction is characterized by a partial obstruction which intermittently prolapses and obstructs the affected bronchus. A chest radiograph in this instance will notably have a mediastinal shift toward the involved side with decreased air entry leading to early atelectasis and collapse.
- Stop valve obstruction denotes a complete bronchial obstruction with impedance to air flow during both inspiration and expiration. A consolidation of the involved bronchopulmonary segment occurs with subsequent collapse (Fig. 31.6D).

The urgency to proceed with anesthesia and bronchoscopic removal of a foreign body is dictated by the severity of respiratory distress, and the location and nature of the aspirated material. Foreign bodies can move from one part of the airway to another and cause sudden complete airway occlusion. Ideally, the foreign body is removed very shortly after aspiration to minimize the occurrence of pneumonia or other complications. When possible, removal of the object should be done as an urgent, not emergency, procedure in a well-prepared patient [141,153,154]. Bronchoscopic removal of a foreign object is successful 95–98% of the time, but a small number of patients may need repeated bronchoscopies because the foreign body either was not found or it was removed incompletely [141,154]. Rarely, thoracotomy may be necessary [154,155].

A variety of methods have been successfully utilized to anesthetize children for bronchoscopy and retrieval of a foreign body [156,157]. The exact anesthetic technique, however, depends on a number of factors, namely the condition of the patient, suspected location of the foreign body and personal preference of the anesthesiologist or surgeon. The presence of an intravenous catheter before proceeding with surgery allows for administration of an anticholinergic to dry up secretions, prevent a vagal response from insertion of the bronchoscope and attenuate cholinergic-mediated bronchoconstriction during airway manipulation as well as permitting steroid administration to decrease airway swelling. Administration of preoperative sedatives may be controversial as sedation may exacerbate upper airway obstruction.

Inhalation induction allows the anesthesiologist to avoid positive pressure ventilation and the possibility of moving the foreign body distally in the airway and making it more difficult to extract. However, if the child has a "full stomach," spontaneous ventilation will not offer any protection from aspiration of gastric contents. Few anesthesiologists would advocate a rapid-sequence induction of anesthesia in an infant if there is respiratory distress and no absolute delineation of the current location of a foreign body. Routine fasting guidelines should apply if the patient's ventilatory status is stable.

Once anesthesia has been induced, the head of the table should be rotated 90° away from the anesthesiologist with the patient's head to the anesthesiologist's right, and the airway is managed from the patient's left side by the anesthesiologist or by the surgeon who is positioned at the head of the bed. The gums (in an edentulous infant) or teeth are protected from injury with the use of moist gauze or with a plastic guard. A laryngoscope is inserted, topical local anesthetic sprayed on the glottis with an atomizer, and the laryngoscope is reinserted and suspended in the vallecula to expose the epiglottis, arytenoids and vocal folds which are then inspected for any mucosal abrasion or presence of foreign body. A bronchoscope is then inserted to visualize the distal airway. Once the ventilating scope is inserted in the subglottic area, the anesthesia circuit is connected to allow oxygen delivery and positive pressure ventilation if necessary.

For maintenance of anesthesia, most anesthesiologists would follow a "middle course," allowing a child to breathe oxygen and a potent inhalation anesthetic until it can be established that gentle positive pressure ventilation adequately expands the chest. At this point, a decision can be made about muscle relaxation. If the decision is made to avoid muscle relaxants, a deep level of anesthesia is required to permit bronchoscopy without coughing. The addition of topical anesthesia is also helpful in attenuating airway reflexes. Regardless of the method of ventilation chosen, the child's airway is exposed to the atmosphere multiple times during the procedure (when the surgeon removes the bronchoscope or optical eyepiece). For this reason, total intravenous anesthesia is preferred to decrease airway pollution from inhalational agents and also to provide an uninterrupted source of general anesthesia to the patient.

Ideally, spontaneous ventilation should be preserved at least until the nature and location of the foreign body have been identified by bronchoscopy, especially if the object could not be localized radiographically. Even if the position of the foreign body was detected by radiographic studies, the anesthesiologist must always be aware that its position may change intraoperatively.

The use of nitrous oxide during this procedure is contraindicated in most cases because it reduces the inspired concentration of oxygen. Also, if significant air trapping is present, nitrous oxide could increase the gas volume and pressure in the affected lung. Rapid bronchoscopy usually allows rapid removal of the foreign body. On occasion, the bronchoscope may dislodge a tracheal foreign body and push it peripherally into a mainstem bronchus with improvement in ventilation and relief of the immediate crisis.

Occasionally, the size of the foreign body exceeds the internal diameter (ID) of the bronchoscope. When this occurs, the foreign body, the forceps, and bronchoscope must be removed together through immobile vocal cords [153]. Administering a small dose of a short-acting non-depolarizing muscle relaxant allows adequate, brief relaxation to permit removal of the bronchoscope and foreign body. If the foreign body is lost during its attempted removal, the pharynx should be immediately inspected. If the object is not found, the bronchoscope should be reintroduced, and the larynx or trachea re-examined. If tracheal obstruction occurs and the object cannot be immediately removed, it may be necessary to push the object back to its original location to allow ventilation of the lungs. If possible, the foreign body should be returned to the affected lung and not to the unaffected lung because placing it in the unaffected lung could result in unreliable ventilation of either lung. Following removal of the foreign body, the endoscopist must re-examine the airway to look for additional multiple or fragmented foreign bodies and to remove secretions that are distal to the obstruction.

The bronchoscope often must be reinserted several times before the foreign body and secretions are successfully removed. This may produce mucosal edema and respiratory distress after bronchoscopy. Administration of steroids, humidified oxygen, nebulized racemic epinephrine and, rarely, tracheal reintubation for 1 or 2 days may be required until the edema subsides [158]. Initial doses of 0.5–1.5 mg/kg dexamethasone (and smaller doses for 2–3 days) may minimize the subglottic swelling caused by repeated insertion of the bronchoscope. Racemic epinephrine (2.25%) may be given in a 1:6 to 1:10 dilution through a nebulizer and clear plastic facemask for 10-min periods while monitoring the electrocardiogram (ECG). Treatment is repeated as necessary every 2 h [158]. Some patients treated with racemic epinephrine develop "rebound" edema so patients who respond to racemic epinephrine should be monitored carefully for at least 3–4 h after each dose of the drug to determine if "rebound" edema occurs.

Aspirated vegetable matter like peanuts occasionally become fragmented during removal and pose a significant challenge during bronchoscopy. Larger aspirated material may acutely occlude both mainstem bronchi and a thoracotomy by a surgeon skilled in pediatric thoracic surgery would be required for retrieval of the material. A Fogarty No. 3 embolectomy balloon catheter may also help dislodge impacted foreign bodies [126,153].

Although prompt removal of a foreign body through an open rigid bronchoscope is the mainstay of treatment of a tracheal foreign body, diagnostic flexible bronchoscopy also may have a role [159–161]. When foreign body aspiration is not clearly evident by history, physical examinations, and radiography, some surgeons may perform diagnostic flexible bronchoscopy under local anesthesia and sedation instead of a rigid bronchoscopy as this is less traumatic to the patient and their airway [160]. If a foreign body is subsequently identified, the patient then undergoes rigid bronchoscopy. Flexible bronchoscopy is not recommended when respiratory distress is present. The decision to utilize fiber-optic bronchoscopy for diagnostic evaluation for foreign body aspiration depends on the skills and services available at each medical center. The risks of possibly having to undergo two procedures should also be carefully considered.

Esophageal foreign bodies

Endotracheal intubation and airway protection should precede foreign body extraction from the esophagus. Inadvertently dropping an esophageal foreign body into an unprotected larynx can cause a disaster [149]. Endoscopic removal of foreign bodies from the upper gastrointestinal inlet is successful in greater than 98% of cases [161]. It is necessary to perform an immediate second look after removal of the foreign body to ensure there has been no trauma from the attempt and to rule out the presence of more than one foreign body, or a congenital defect (e.g. pouch, esophageal stenosis) that can increase the risk of subsequent impaction of food or other foreign bodies. Frequently, foreign bodies that have passed through the gastric outlet into the small and large intestines pass through the gastrointestinal tract spontaneously and surgical intervention is rarely needed [162]. As with chronic airway foreign bodies, retained esophageal foreign bodies can be treacherous. Complications include bronchoesophageal fistula, aortoesophageal fistula, mediastinitis, esophageal diverticulum, and lobar atelectasis. These retained foreign bodies may require a thoracotomy to remove them [163].

Laser microlaryngeal surgery

The most common indication for laser microlaryngeal surgery is recurrent laryngeal papillomas or juvenile

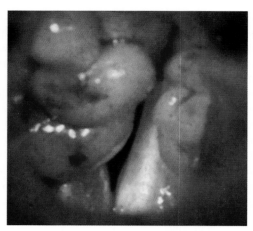

Figure 31.7 Papillomas on the vocal cord. Courtesy of Deidre Larrier MD.

laryngeal papillomatosis which is the most common airway tumor found in children. It is a chronic, debilitating and frequently life-threatening condition. Laryngeal tumors occur as a result of human papillomavirus (HPV) infection which is transmitted from the mother to the child during pregnancy. These tumors are typically located on the vocal cords, epiglottis, and in the larynx or trachea (Fig. 31.7). They are usually symptomatic and result in aphonia, hoarseness, stridor and respiratory distress. When a large number of these tumors are present on a chronic basis, symptoms of right ventricular hypertrophy or cor pulmonale may develop.

Surgical excision and ablation of these lesions, the current mode of management, is possible using carbon dioxide (CO_2) laser through an operating microscope. The CO_2 laser's light waves are absorbed by all biological tissues and rapidly vaporize intracellular water present in tissue, leading to a rapid increase in temperature and denaturation of protein in the targeted tissue. Minimal bleeding occurs as the thermal energy of the laser beam cauterizes capillaries as it vaporizes tissues and very little postoperative edema occurs. The benefit of CO_2 laser treatment is that the surrounding tissues are unaffected. The CO_2 laser has been used with excellent results for treating such lesions as papillomas of the nose, oral cavity or larynx, subglottic stenosis, subglottic hemangioma, glottic webs, choanal atresia, postintubation granuloma, vocal cord nodules, and lymphangiomas [154,164]. It has the advantage of providing excellent hemostasis, with minimal postoperative edema and scarring, rapid healing and preservation of the quality of voice [165,166]. It is the preferred mode of surgical treatment of laryngeal papillomas, even though laser resection does not cure this condition.

In a recent survey of the practices of pediatric otolaryngologists, about 50% of practitioners now use the laryngeal microdebrider rather than CO_2 laser removal for laryngeal papillomas [167]. The microdebrider device uses suction and rotating cold blade excision for more precise removal of papillomas. It has a slightly angulated tip that sucks mobile papilloma tissue into the cutting blade and leaves firmer underlying native tissue intact. A prospective comparison of the microdebrider and the CO_2 laser revealed that the microdebrider resulted in equivalent postoperative pain with greater improvements in voice quality, shorter procedure times and overall lower cost [168].

Adjuvant medical therapy for laryngeal papillomas is also on the rise with the use of cidofovir and interferon which have been beneficial in some children. Cidofovir is, however, reserved for severe cases (requiring four or more surgical treatments per year) due to its carcinogenic potential and lack of supportive data for its use [169]. The newly available HPV vaccine may have an effect on the incidence and severity of laryngeal papillomatosis but to date this has not been studied.

Surgical requirements for suspension laryngoscopy using the CO_2 laser include hyperextension of the neck and a motionless surgical field (i.e. relaxed vocal cords) so that the lesion may be ablated without injury to the surrounding healthy tissue. Prompt recovery of consciousness and protective airway reflexes must be present at the conclusion of surgery.

Anesthesia for laser microlaryngeal surgery

Children with recurrent laryngeal papillomas present frequently for therapy due to the recurrent nature of the tumors. The mainstay of an effective treatment program to keep the airway free is by repeated endoscopic and laser excision of the papillomas until puberty, when they tend to regress [170].

Perioperative anxiety is therefore fairly common in children requiring repeated surgeries. The judicious use of sedatives and, most importantly, a reassuring preoperative visit by the anesthesiologist help to allay fears. A child with significant airway obstruction should only receive preoperative sedation while being monitored and when oxygen, positive pressure ventilation, and suction are available. An anesthesiologist or surgeon skilled in advanced airway intervention must be present at all times. The perioperative care of children with laryngeal papillomas can be very challenging, depending on the location of the lesions. Pedunculated papillomas may obstruct the airway, causing a ball valve obstruction in certain positions. It is prudent therefore to avoid initial administration of muscle relaxants and maintain spontaneous respiration till the surgeon has adequately examined the airway and determined the location of the lesions. These children should be approached in a similar manner to those with anticipated severe airway obstruction, with a slow inhalation induction with sevoflurane in 100% oxygen without stimulation in order to avoid agitation and potential obstruction during induction. It is often helpful to maintain 5–10 cm of positive end-expiratory pressure in the anesthetic system to distend the hypopharynx and to facilitate mask ventilation. Muscle relaxants should be used only after positive-pressure ventilation by mask can be demonstrated.

Laser surgery may be performed during anesthesia with spontaneous, apneic or jet ventilation or with the use of laser-safe endotracheal tubes. However, the use of such tubes is declining, with only 10% of otolaryngologists stating this as their preferred mode of anesthesia in a recent survey [167].

Spontaneous ventilation without intubation allows the surgeon to work without interruption (of intermittent placement of the endotracheal tube to deliver positive pressure ventilation). A deep anesthetic plane achieved with total intravenous anesthesia (TIVA) using propofol (200–300 µg/kg/min) plus intermittent opioid administration (morphine 0.05 mg/kg, fentanyl 2–3 µg/kg or remifentanil infusion 0.1–0.25 µg/kg/min). Aerosolized lidocaine helps decrease airway irritability and intravenous dexamethasone administration helps prevent postoperative swelling. Intermittent mask ventilation may be required to treat periods of hypoxemia; alternatively the patient may be briefly intubated by the surgeon for brief periods of manual ventilation to increase the patient's saturations.

Jet ventilation with intermittent apnea technique is also utilized in some institutions. The operating laryngoscope may be fitted with a catheter through which air is entrained and the lungs are intermittently ventilated by the jet. Jet ventilation also offers a quiet surgical field as there is no movement from large excursions of the diaphragm and it also offers uninterrupted surgery. However, there is some concern about the use of jet ventilation and the possibility of papillomas being forced into the tracheobronchial tree. In addition, this technique may not provide effective ventilation in children with small airway disease. The inability to measure expired carbon dioxide and the possibility of barotrauma are also possible complications. (See Jet ventilation above.)

In an effort to improve existing Venturi jet techniques, Brooker et al developed a subglottic ventilation anesthesia system [171]. The Hunsaker Mon-Jet tube is a laser-safe subglottic jet tube that allows monitoring of tracheal pressure and end-tidal CO_2. The device aligns the jet away from the tracheal mucosa to prevent injecting gas into the submucosa. The device also uses an automatic jet ventilator with an adjustable rate, inspiratory to expiratory (I:E) ratio, and flow rate. Peak inspiratory and peak end-expiratory airway pressures are monitored and the device shuts off if the limits are exceeded.

When there is significant obstruction or depending on the surgeon's or anesthesiologist's preference, the trachea may be intubated after induction of anesthesia with sevoflurane in oxygen. Suspicion has been cast on the possibility of distal tracheal papillomas being spread with intermittent instrumentation of the airway during surgery [167]. Difficulty ventilating the lungs after intubating the trachea may occur if a papilloma is released into the trachea or obstructs the endotracheal tube. An endotracheal tube several sizes smaller than the one appropriate for the child's age is chosen as there usually is scarring from repeated laser therapies and it is important to maintain an adequate view for the surgeon to visualize lesions that need to be treated. The use of an endotracheal tube during laser surgery increases the risk of this surgery as regular polyvinyl chloride (PVC) endotracheal tubes are flammable and can be ignited and vaporized by a laser beam. Red rubber endotracheal tubes wrapped with metallic tape deflect the laser beam but the segment of the tube beyond the vocal cords cannot be covered with metallic tape and is still vulnerable to the laser beam and vaporization. Some non-latex endotracheal tubes have been manufactured specifically for laser surgery but they tend to be more expensive and also have larger outer diameters than their regular PVC endotracheal tube counterparts, especially in the small sizes. There are therefore not adequate for use in small children or children with an airway markedly narrowed by papillomas.

At the conclusion of surgery, an endotracheal tube may be inserted and secured till the child is completely awake or if spontaneous ventilation was maintained during surgery, inhalation agents can be discontinued and the patient transported to the recovery room with blow-by oxygen until the patient finally awakens in the recovery room. Racemic epinephrine for stridor may be required postoperatively.

Safety precautions during laser airway surgery

Laser radiation increases the temperature of absorbent material so flammable material such as surgical drapes must not be in the path of the laser beam. Minimal surgical drapes should be used during laser surgery. Burning of surgical drapes can result in burns to the patient and also produces significant smoke which may result in smoke inhalation injury to the patient and operating room staff [172]. The face, neck and shoulder surfaces should be covered with wet towels which absorb laser energy and prevent burns from deflection of the laser beams during surgery.

In contrast to the argon laser and the neodymium:yttrium-aluminum garnet (Nd:YAG) laser, the CO_2 laser does not penetrate the cornea. Nevertheless, to prevent thermal injury to the cornea or retina from the laser beam, operating room personnel must wear protective eyewear (regular eyewear will suffice for individuals with prescription eye glasses) and the patient's eyes must be protected with moist gauze pads or protective goggles. Argon and Nd:YAG lasers are used primarily in ophthalmological surgery and to treat gastrointestinal bleeding or for excision of endobronchial lesions, respectively. These devices can penetrate the cornea and damage the retina. They also penetrate glass so glass windows in the OR should be covered with appropriate material.

Vital structures some distance from the operative site can be injured by overshoot of the laser beam or by reflection of the beam off a polished instrument. This has caused tracheal laceration in a child undergoing resection of recurrent laryngeal papillomas. The tracheal tear became evident in the recovery room with the development of bilateral pneumothoraces and subcutaneous emphysema. Constant vigilance by recovery room nurses is important to observe and detect laser-induced pneumothorax [173].

In institutions where foil-wrapped endotracheal tubes are used for laser surgery, the foil can be covered with a moist sponge layer to absorb any heat generated. This outside sponge layer also provides a smooth surface that minimizes trauma to the airway. While the shaft of the endotracheal tube can be covered with protective material, the endotracheal tube cuff is vulnerable to the effects of laser radiation and filling the cuff with saline rather than air is recommended. Placement of saline-soaked pledgets above the endotracheal tube cuff during laser surgery has also been recommended.

In addition to the risk of combustion, foil-wrapped tubes may kink, irritate the tracheal mucosa, obstruct the airway if the foil separates from the tube and, on occasion, permit the laser beam to penetrate and ignite unprotected portions of the tube [164,166,174,175].

The mixture of gases delivered into the endotracheal tube may affect the risk of combustion during general anesthesia and laser surgery of the airway. Although helium impedes combustion during carbon dioxide laser surgery, the differences between nitrogen and helium effects on combustibility are not clinically significant [176]. In a previous study, nitrous oxide and oxygen were shown to be additive in their ability to sustain combustion [177]. FIO_2 should be reduced to as low as possible, i.e. 0.21–0.30, with an air-oxygen mixture; N_2O must not be used during laser surgery.

The different methods of airway management during laser surgery have the common goal of preventing airway fires but each method has its own set of problems. If, despite all precautions, ignition of the endotracheal tube should occur, the flow of oxygen should be discontinued immediately and the endotracheal tube should be disconnected from the gas source and immediately removed.

Most materials do not readily burn in air [166]. The anesthesiologist must have direct access to the tube at all times and ensure that the entire tube has been removed from the airway. A chest radiograph should be obtained and bronchoscopy should be performed to reveal the extent of the injury to the lung and trachea caused by direct burn, smoke inhalation or retention of a foreign body. Complications are treated according to the severity of the injury and may include steroids, humidification of inspired gases, tracheostomy, and assisted ventilation. Tracheal stenosis can be a late complication [166].

Other tracheal surgery

Recent studies show that the use of early continuous positive airway pressure (CPAP) in early preterm infants results in shorter periods of intubation and a decrease in the incidence of bronchopulmonary dysplasia [178]. However, with the improved capability of ventilatory support for preterm infants, prolonged periods of tracheal intubation have occurred, resulting in increased survival but accompanied by laryngotracheal injury in as many as 2.5% of neonatal patients [179]. Glottic or subglottic compromise ensues, with the latter being more frequent and serious than the former [180]. The exact location of injury is detected by careful endoscopic evaluation of the airway [179]. Subglottic stenosis may also occur in older children following laryngeal injury. In these instances symptoms such as progressive hoarseness, dyspnea, stridor or feeding difficulties may occur approximately 2–4 weeks following injury. In addition, these children may present with repeated upper respiratory tract infections.

Congenital anomalies of the larynx or trachea may also occur in neonates. For example, some children are born with laryngeal atresia or congenital high airway obstruction in which a large portion of the larynx is absent at term. In these children, an initial life-saving tracheostomy is placed during delivery while the baby is still on placental bypass during *ex utero* intrapartum therapy (EXIT procedure) [181] (see Chapter 19).

Treatment options for subglottic stenosis include tracheostomy or tracheal reconstruction, including the anterior cricoid split and laryngeal reconstruction. The extent or severity of the stenosis determines the nature of surgical repair. The degree of stenosis may be assessed by soft tissue radiographic images of neck and computed tomography with three-dimensional image reconstruction, in which the length of the stenotic segment can be appreciated and precisely measured. In addition, direct inspection of the airway under general anesthesia in the operating room provides valuable information. Depending on the degree of stenosis, a rigid or flexible bronchoscope is utilized to visualize the larynx and trachea beyond the stenotic area. The trachea is usually intubated intraoperatively in order to "size" the trachea. The size of endotracheal tube that can be easily inserted with an audible leak provides information on the degree of stenosis. The most mild instances of subglottic stenosis can be managed by endoscopic dilation or CO_2 laser endoscopic scar excision with or without application of mitomycin, an antimitotic agent designed to prevent reapposition of the raw submucosal edges [182]. A tracheostomy is required for about 50% of patients with congenital subglottic stenosis and for an even higher percentage of patients with severe acquired subglottic stenosis [183] (see Chapter 14). The advent of procedures such as anterior cricoid split may prevent some infants from developing severe subglottic stenosis or may reduce the number of patients requiring a tracheostomy.

Tracheostomy significantly changes the quality of life and although often life-saving, it can be associated with a significant risk of morbidity and mortality. This has led to the development of reconstructive operative therapy such as the anterior cricoid split procedure and external laryngeal reconstruction to allow early decannulation of the trachea at the youngest age possible so speech and language development are not impaired [184].

Anterior cricoid split procedure

The goal is to decompress the area of the subglottic space enclosed by the cricoid ring, the only complete cartilaginous ring of the airway. This procedure is performed over the largest endotracheal tube that can be inserted into the trachea via the nose. A midline vertical cartilaginous incision is made 2mm from the thyroid notch inferiorly through the second tracheal ring (Fig. 31.8) [185]. Stay

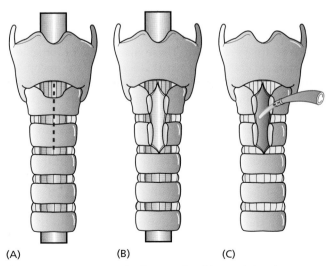

(A)   (B)   (C)

Figure 31.8 Anterior cricoid split. Reproduced from Zalzal and Cotton [185] with permission from Elsevier: www.Expertconsultbook.com.

sutures are placed through the cricoid ring as in a tracheostomy, and the skin incision is closed. The endotracheal tube often is left in place for approximately 1–2 weeks to temporarily stent the incision open as it allows fibrous ingrowth and prevents airway obliteration with granulation tissue. It also allows the mucosal swelling to subside and provides time for the split cricoid to heal. After this period, tracheal extubation is attempted after treatment with steroids.

Laryngeal reconstruction

Positioning for this procedure involves placement of a shoulder roll and hyperextension of the head. Either inhalation or intravenous anesthesia may be used for induction and maintenance during surgery. The existing tracheostomy is replaced with an endotracheal tube; initially an oral RAE tube is inserted through the stoma as this can be easily anchored. The tip of the oral RAE tube may need to be cut in order to prevent endobronchial intubation. Laryngotracheoplasty is performed through a horizontal skin incision with midline dissection from the cartilage of the thyroid notch superiorly to the third or fourth tracheal rings inferiorly (Fig. 31.9) [183]. A vertical median anterior incision is made into the stenotic lumen. Posterior subglottic or posterior commissure stenoses may require a midline posterior cartilaginous incision to increase the posterior lumen. Sculpted segments of harvested costal cartilage are then sutured into the midline incisions, thereby increasing the airway lumen. A solid stent may be necessary to provide support during the postoperative period. This stent may be wired to the tracheostomy tube.

After allowing an appropriate period for stable healing of the grafts, the stents may be removed and the intraluminal granulation tissue excised. Further operative procedures may be required to remove granulation tissue and to allow the epithelium to cover the grafts and operative sites. Decannulation occurs when an adequate airway lumen has been obtained.

Partial cricoid resection with primary thyrotracheal anastomosis was initially performed in adults with significant subglottic stenosis. Previous concerns about performing the procedure when the larynx is still growing have not been confirmed and there are now several reports of a high success rate of approximately 97% in children with subsequent normal laryngotracheal growth following this procedure [186–189]. Since this surgery seems to have no significant effect on the laryngeal growth of young children, this mode of treatment of subglottic stenosis may provide earlier and less traumatic decannulation from tracheostomy.

The anesthetic challenges of these procedures include sharing the airway with the surgeon and repeated removal of the existing airway during the procedure to allow for

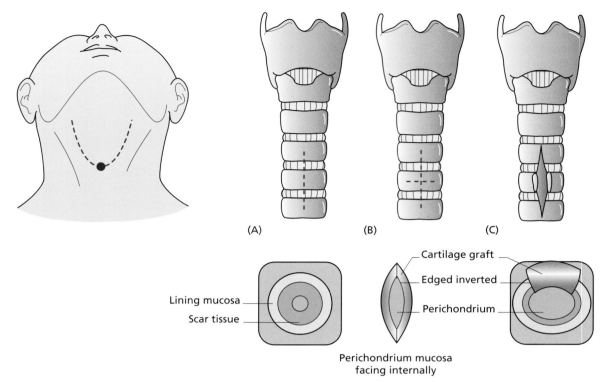

Figure 31.9 Laryngotracheoplasty. Horizontal skin incision incorporating the superior aspect of the tracheostomy stoma. (A) A vertical incision is made in the thyroid cartilage from a point immediately below the anterior commissure through the upper tracheal rings, with care to remain in the midline. (B) The intraluminal scar and lining mucosa are incised along the length of the stenotic segment. (C) The costal cartilage graft is then shaped into an ellipse and placed in position with the lining perichondrium facing internally. Reproduced from Cotton and Myer [183] with permission from Elsevier.

surgical access and stent placement. A quiet surgical field is also essential and postoperatively, adequate sedation and relaxation are mandatory during transport to the intensive care unit.

Eye surgery

Unlike in adults, most pediatric ophthalmological procedures are extraocular rather than intraocular. Extraocular conditions that require operations include the management of nasolacrimal duct obstruction and strabismus. Intraocular conditions that may require a surgical approach in children include glaucoma, cataracts, retinoblastoma and retinopathy of prematurity. Several medical problems are associated with congenital and acquired eye anomalies and pathology. The anesthesiologist must have a good understanding of the associated medical entities as well as the many anesthetic drugs and procedures that profoundly affect ocular physiology (Table 31.4). A basic understanding of intraocular pressure and its control, along with the pharmacology of drugs used by the ophthalmologist and the potential for drug interactions with anesthetics, is necessary to provide adequate anesthesia care for pediatric patients during eye surgery.

Extraocular procedures
Nasolacrimal duct obstruction

Up to 6% of healthy neonates have congenital nasolacrimal duct obstruction, presenting with epiphora or continuous tearing. In the absence of infection, a conservative approach is appropriate for a few months to see if the tear duct opens with time. However, if nasolacrimal duct stenosis persists, a series of procedures with increasing invasiveness are performed. These start with probing and irrigation of the nasolacrimal duct. With the increased safety of general anesthetics, this brief procedure is performed in an operating room. A standard mask induction and maintenance of anesthesia with inhalation agents can provide satisfactory operative conditions. Some anesthesiologists would place an LMA to secure the airway. Instillation of fluorescein dye to test patency of the duct and the possibility of some bleeding potentially increase the risk of laryngospasm with mask or LMA. If simple probing and irrigation are not enough to resolve the condition, the child is brought back for balloon dilation and/or silastic stent placement. The anesthetic management should be the same as for tear duct probing. In a very small percentage of patients the obstruction persists for a while and may result in infections of the tear sac.

Table 31.4 Anesthetic effects of commonly used ophthalmological drugs

Drug	mg/drop	Ophthalmological effect	Anesthetic implications
Atropine (1%)	0.5	Mydriasis, cycloplegia	Tachycardia, flushing
Cocaine (1%)	0.5	Vasoconstriction	Hypertension, dysrhythmia,
Cyclopentolate (1%)	0.5	Mydriasis, cycloplegia	Hyperthermia
			Convulsions – not common
Echothiophate (0.25%)	0.1	Antiglaucoma	Anticholinesterase, long acting
Epinephrine (0.25%)	0.1	Antiglaucoma	Hypertension, dysrhythmias
Phenylephrine (2.5%)	1.2	Mydriasis, vasoconstriction, decongestion	Hypertension
Scopolamine (0.5%)	0.25	Mydriasis, cycloplegia	CNS excitement
Timolol (0.25%)	0.1	Antiglaucoma	β-Blockade, non-selective

CNS, central nervous system.

This may require a more invasive and longer procedure such as dacryocystorhinostomy. The anesthetic management should include securing the airway with tracheal intubation as access to the airway will be unavailable during the operation. Analgesic drugs should also be used. These procedures are performed on an outpatient basis unless the child has some other concomitant medical condition.

Anesthesia for strabismus surgery

Strabismus, a misalignment of the visual axes, can be congenital or acquired and it occurs in 2–7% of children. Strabismus correction is one of the most common surgical procedures in ophthalmology. The congenital form may occur as a result of abnormal innervation while the acquired form may occur following traumatic nerve palsies. Strabismus can also occur in association with congenital myopathies as well as meningomyelocele. The outcome of this surgery is excellent when performed early in life.

The primary considerations for anesthesiologists caring for children having strabismus surgery are cardiovascular effects of medications placed in the eye, the oculocardiac reflex and and postoperative nausea and vomiting. In the past, patients with strabismus were thought to be susceptible to malignant hyperthermia (MH) as most patients with MH had associated musculoskeletal disorders, including strabismus and ptosis. A subsequent review of 2500 patients tested for MH susceptibility did not show any association with strabismus surgery. Malignant hyperthermia is no longer considered to be a risk for children with strabismus and these children are now routinely anesthetized with inhalational anesthetics without an observed increase in the incidence of MH [190,191].

Masseter muscle spasm (MMS) has also been associated with strabismus surgery, particularly in patients who received halothane and succinylcholine [192] although

another study contradicted this finding [193]. The increase in jaw tension initially observed following succinycholine adminstration in addition to an inability to displace the mandible from the maxilla to facilitate insertion of an oral airway is now thought to represent a normal clinical state following succinylcholine administration [190,191].

In summary, it seems the association between strabismus and MH is no longer an issue [194] but if masseter muscle spasm is suspected, it is important to recognize that this patient may be susceptible to developing MH [190,195]. The importance of a detailed anesthetic family history also cannot be overemphasized.

Phenylephrine is placed in the eye(s) to produce mydriasis and hemostasis. However, absorption of the phenylephrine can cause profound systemic vasoconstriction and hypertension. To prevent systemic hypertension, only 1.0–2.5% (not 10%) phenylephrine should be used and only one drop should be instilled into each eye [196,197]. Other agents (0.5% cyclopentolate, 0.5% tropicamide) may be used to induce mydriasis without causing hypertension.

Surgery for strabismus often requires traction on the extraocular muscles, which produces vagal stimulation via the trigemino-vagal reflex (oculocardiac reflex); this reflex can usually be prevented by a delicate surgical technique. A retrobulbar block may trigger the oculocardiac reflex if moderate pressure is applied to the eye but when the block takes effect, it can prevent the oculocardiac reflex by blocking the afferent limb of the trigemino-vagal reflex. This reflex is common during strabismus surgery or any surgery in which there is traction on the rectus muscles or eyelid. It may also be elicited by pressure on the eyeball or empty globe. The afferent pathway of this reflex involves the trigeminal nerve and the efferent limb is the vagus nerve. This trigemino-vagal reflex (or oculocardiac reflex) may result in a variety of dysrhythmias including sinus or junctional bradycardia, atrioventricular block, bigeminy, multifocal premature ventricular contractions, ventricular tachycardia or sinoatrial arrest [192]. The oculocardiac reflex may also occur following a retrobulbar block, enucleation and endoscopic sinus surgery if pressure is applied to ocular muscles and the reflex is not abolished by the administration of local anesthetics. Alerting the surgeons and subsequent alleviation of traction on the rectus muscles or pressure on the eye usually dissipates symptoms. The changes in rhythm may decrease during the surgery, since the reflex may fatigue or diminish with continued intermittent traction. Medical therapy may be required which includes the administration of anticholinergic agents. Administration of glycopyrrolate or atropine 10–20 μg/kg shortly after intubation for eye surgery helps decrease the frequency, intensity, and duration of this reflex.

The LMA provides an effective alternative to endotracheal intubation in normal children scheduled for elective strabismus surgery [198]. In the absence of gastroesophageal reflux, the LMA provides an excellent airway for patients who can sustain spontaneous ventilation for the duration of eye muscle surgery. Hypercarbia may exacerbate the oculocardiac reflex [199] so in order to treat or prevent hypercarbia during anesthesia with an LMA, the anesthesiologist may consider mechanical ventilation with positive inspiratory pressure not exceeding 20–25 mmHg.

Strabismus and postoperative nausea and vomiting

Nausea and vomiting occur in 50–80% of patients following strabismus surgery and may delay discharge from the hospital following surgery. A recent review revealed postoperative nausea and vomiting as the reason for 50% of unplanned overnight hospital admissions following strabismus surgery [200]. The exact mechanism of increased predisposition to nausea and vomiting following strabismus surgery is not known but may be related to altered visual perception and a different afferent input postoperatively or it may be secondary to an oculoemetic reflex, which is analogous to the oculocardiac reflex. Prevention of the oculocardiac reflex during strabismus surgery by prophylactic treatment with anticholinergic agents (atropine or glycopyrrolate) did not reduce the incidence of nausea and/or vomiting [201]. A large number of studies have examined the management of postoperative nausea and vomiting (PONV) in general. Prophylactic antiemetics are clearly indicated with more than one drug according to the consensus statement of the Society for Ambulatory Anesthesia [202]. However, no single agent, combination of agents or anesthetic technique has completely eliminated this problem.

Propofol has contributed to the decline in the incidence of PONV [203] and studies have shown that it offers some protective qualities against developing PONV following strabismus surgery [204–207]. Droperidol and metoclopramide, both antidopaminergic drugs, reduce nausea and vomiting by their action on dopaminergic sites [208,209]. Droperidol was favored in the past as an antiemetic as it was cheaper than its counterpart serotonin antagonist agents. However, it was associated with occasionally prolonged periods of sedation. Furthermore, the recent FDA black box warning against the use of droperidol, citing serious cardiac arrhythmias due to prolongation of the QTc interval and recommendations of 12-lead ECG monitoring 1 h before and 2–3 h postoperatively, has resulted in a drastic decline in the use of this agent [210,211]. In addition, cost considerations are no longer a concern with the availability of generic versions of ondansetron.

Metoclopramide has also been used for many years to treat PONV. However, when compared to ondansetron, a serotonin antagonist, metoclopramide decreased nausea and vomiting to a much lesser degree in patients following strabismus surgery [212,213]. Strategies to decrease PONV in strabismus patients currently revolve around serotonin antagonists. These drugs are frequently administered in conjunction with dexamethasone 50 μg/kg, which was found to be just as effective as doses as high as 250 μg/kg [214]. Nitrous oxide and the use of opioids have been implicated in the development of PONV. Therefore avoidance of nitrous oxide as a maintenance agent and administration of non-steroidal agents such as ketorolac will help decrease the incidence of PONV following strabismus surgery. High-risk patients such as those undergoing strabismus correction surgery will benefit from combination antiemetic therapy [215,216].

Intraocular procedures
Intraocular pressure and its control

Aqueous humor is present in both the anterior and posterior chambers of the eye. The majority of the aqueous humor is produced in the posterior chamber by active secretion, filtration, and diffusion from the blood supply to the ciliary body (Fig. 31.10). Aqueous humor passes from the posterior chamber through the ciliary body behind the iris to the front of the lens, then through the pupil into the anterior chamber. The most lateral portion of the anterior chamber, called the angle, contains a meshwork of tissue that filters the aqueous humor before it reaches the canal of Schlemm and eventually drains into the episcleral veins (Fig. 31.11). This fluid contains no blood cells and only 1% of the concentration of protein found in plasma. Thus, the aqueous humor is clear and allows transmission of light to the retina [217].

Normal intraocular pressure (IOP) is maintained between 10 and 21 mmHg by a balance between the production and drainage of aqueous humor, choroidal blood volume, extraocular muscle pressure, and vitreous humor volume [218]. Sudden increase in IOP may result in acute glaucoma. If this occurs in the presence of an open globe, prolapse of the iris or lens and/or hemorrhage from blood vessels may occur. Therefore it is imperative that the anesthesiologist maintains normal IOP during eye surgery.

Laryngoscopy and intubation of the trachea, coughing, vomiting or straining during induction or emergence from anesthesia can dramatically increase intraocular pressure to values as high as 40 mmHg [219]. Although the effect of laryngoscopy is transient and is of no serious consequence in the patient with normal intraocular physiology, this increase in pressure may be very significant for patients with glaucoma or other eye pathology. Administration of intravenous lidocaine prior to intuba-

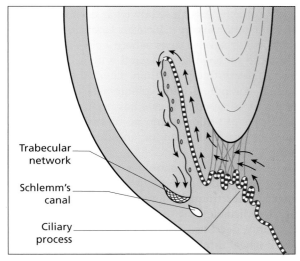

Figure 31.10 Magnified view of ciliary body showing aqueous humor production and flow pattern.

tion has been found to prevent an increase in IOP [220,221]. Intraocular pressure changes with LMA insertion are less than those following tracheal intubation [222]. Coughing causes venous hypertension which increases the intraocular blood volume and has a dramatic effect on intraocular pressure. Several metabolic or acid–base derangements may occur during general anesthesia which can affect IOP. Hypoxia and hypercarbia cause retinal venodilation and can increase IOP [223]. Mild hypo- or hypercarbia produces clinically insignificant effects [224]. Hypothermia decreases IOP by decreasing the rate of aqueous humor production. Arterial pressure changes have little effect on IOP [218].

Intraocular pressure and anesthetics

In general, hypnotic agents, inhalation agents, and opioids tend to decrease IOP, with the exception of ketamine [218]. Earlier reports on the use of ketamine and IOP determined by Schiotz tonometry, which measures corneal compressibility, indicated that it resulted in an elevation of IOP [225], IOP is now routinely measured with applanation tonometry, a method believed to be more accurate. While ketamine does not lower IOP, the IOP measured following ketamine administration may be more reflective of the awake measurement. The use of ketamine may actually be preferable to other agents when an accurate measurement of IOP is necessary as is the case of children with suspected glaucoma in which accurate measurements of the IOP can only be obtained under anesthesia [226,227]. Nystagmus and blepharospasm associated with ketamine may, however, contraindicate its use in children with an open globe injury.

Non-depolarizing muscle relaxants decrease pressure on the globe and may decrease IOP [218]. Succinylcholine, a depolarizing muscle relaxant, increases IOP by inducing tonic extraocular muscle contracture, choroidal

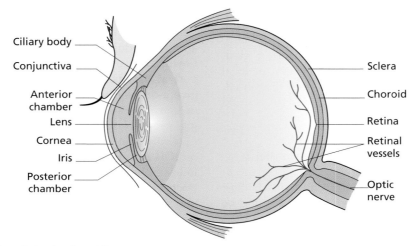

Figure 31.11 Anatomy of the anterior chamber of the eye.

vascular dilation and relaxation of orbital smooth muscle. In normal eyes, an increase in IOP of about 7 mmHg has been observed [228]. This modest increase is transient and of little consequence in a patient with normal IOP. However, if a patient has high IOP, the increase following succinylcholine may be greater and any rise may be significant. In the case of an open globe, an increase in pressure could result in loss of vitreous humor. Despite reports to the contrary, no one method has been shown to prevent the intraocular hypertension observed with the administration of intravenous succinylcholine [229,230]. While some reports state that there are no adverse events following the use of succinycholine for anesthesia in a child with an open globe injury [231], caution should be exercised when using this drug in the presence of an open globe injury. High-dose rocuronium provides a viable option for rapid-sequence induction in this subset of children who present for emergency surgery.

Glaucoma

If outflow of aqueous humor is obstructed for any reason, IOP increases and causes glaucoma. As with cataracts, glaucoma can be an isolated primary congenital disorder or it can be part of a syndrome (e.g. Sturge–Weber syndrome, mesodermal dysgenesis). A late or juvenile form of congenital glaucoma presents after 6 years of age, often in families with a strong history of open-angle glaucoma.

Successful surgical treatment of infantile glaucoma requires early recognition of the problem. Confirming the diagnosis in infants who present with a history of excessive tearing, photophobia, irritability, and buphthalmos usually requires measuring the IOP during a general anesthetic. The eye examination and pressure measurement can be followed by surgery if the diagnosis is confirmed. The initial surgery usually consists of goniotomy or trabeculotomy to create a route for the exit of aqueous humor via Schlemm's canal. If unsuccessful, cryotherapy is sometimes used to destroy the ciliary body and decrease aqueous humor production.

Anesthetic considerations for patients during glaucoma surgery include awareness of associated medical problems, especially if a syndrome has been diagnosed, as well as knowledge of how to manage IOP (see section on Intraocular pressure and its control, above).

Anesthesia for open globe injuries in a patient with a "full stomach"

Traumatic eye injuries are common in children. The best chance of salvaging the eye requires that the wound be surgically explored to remove foreign material and the laceration closed within several hours of the injury. After penetrating trauma, the pressure inside the eye is atmos-

pheric. External pressure on the eye or an increase in internal pressure can prolapse the lens, iris or vitreous and markedly reduce the chance of recovery of vision. The goal preoperatively and during the induction of anesthesia is to prevent coughing, crying, and vomiting because these activities increase intraocular venous blood volume. Increasing intraocular venous blood volume and IOP may cause the ocular contents to extrude.

Preventing an increase in IOP is important but difficult to accomplish. Preoperatively, the child should remain flat and quiet, and the eyes should be patched to minimize eye movements (which can be frightening and confusing to young children). Sedating the child before patching the eyes is essential if the child is too young to co-operate and cannot understand a careful, gentle explanation of the procedure. Giving a young child oral midazolam (0.5–0.75 mg/kg) or diazepam (0.2 mg/kg) may provide sufficient sedation to allow insertion of an IV catheter. After a sedative has been administered, EMLA (eutectic mixture of local anesthetics) cream should be applied to several sites where veins are visible (or likely to be present) and covered with a clear occlusive dressing. Forty-five to 60 min later, the skin should be numb enough to allow painless insertion of an IV catheter. Once vascular access has been achieved, subsequent doses of sedatives can be titrated to effect, and a rapid-sequence induction of anesthesia can be easily accomplished.

The anesthesiologist should assume that all children who present with a penetrating eye injury have a full stomach. After trauma, stomach emptying is so erratic and unpredictable that delaying surgery for 6–8 h does not reliably decrease the risk of aspirating gastric contents. Tracheal intubation should not be attempted until paralysis is complete. This prevents coughing and its potentially catastrophic effect on IOP.

In the presence of an open eye injury, the anesthesiologist must carefully preoxygenate the patient, being careful not to allow the mask to press on the injured eye. Preoxygenation is followed by injection of an anesthetic and a non-depolarizing muscle relaxant into a rapidly flowing IV catheter, preferably directly into an injection port at the site of the catheter. Some anesthesiologists give a dose of lidocaine (2 mg/kg), fentanyl (2–3 μg/kg) or morphine sulfate (0.05–0.1 mg/kg) before administering propofol (2 mg/kg) or thiopental (4–6 mg/kg), to minimize the effects of laryngoscopy and intubation on IOP. Administration of the anesthetic is immediately followed by a dose of a non-depolarizing muscle relaxant (rocuronium 0.8–1.5 mg/kg, vecuronium 0.15–0.2 mg/kg, pancuronium 0.1 mg/kg). These doses of muscle relaxants allow tracheal intubation to be accomplished within 45–60 sec. Rocuronium (0.8–1.5 mg/kg) offers advantages over atracurium, vecuronium, pancuronium and succinylcholine because it provides rapid onset of neuromuscular blockade and a decrease in IOP without side-effects.

Neuromuscular blockade should be monitored during the induction of anesthesia to ensure that paralysis is complete before laryngoscopy is attempted. Sufficient cricoid pressure should be applied to occlude the esophagus and prevent passive regurgitation of stomach contents into the lungs; this pressure should be maintained until the airway is secured. The application of cricoid pressure also may decrease the likelihood of stomach dilation if gentle positive pressure ventilation is required before the trachea is intubated.

For the normal, chubby toddler who has no visible veins, the risk of crying, struggling, and raising IOP while an IV catheter is being inserted may be greater than that of aspiration during induction of anesthesia with inhaled anesthetics and cricoid pressure. Such a toddler could benefit from oral premedication with midazolam. The α2-agonist dexmedetomidine also shows promise as an effective oral premedication [232]. It also is effective as a premedication when administered intranasally [233,234]. Dexmedetomidine is not painful when administered nasally, in contrast to intranasal midazolam which may cause crying and agitation and should therefore be avoided in this setting. Administration of dexmedetomidine has also been found to attenuate the increase in IOP associated with succinylcholine administration [235].

Cataracts

Cataracts in children may be congenital or acquired. Congenital cataracts are of two types: idiopathic and those associated with syndromes. Several syndromes (e.g. Stickle, Hallermann–Steiff, Laurence–Moon–Biedl, Lowe, Conrad cerebrotendinous xanthomatosis, Marfan) are associated with a high incidence of cataracts (see Chapter 38). Metabolic disease states such as galactosemia and chromosomal abnormalities such as trisomy 21 are also associated with the presence of cataracts. Cataracts may be acquired as a complication of radiation therapy for retinoblastoma.

Cataract surgery in otherwise healthy children or in those with minimal associated medical co-morbidities is performed on an outpatient basis. General anesthesia is routinely administered for cataract surgery. One study showed that general anesthesia supplemented with a regional block (subtenon block) resulted in less postoperative pain and fewer requirements for postoperative rescue medication [236]. As with all general anesthetics, associated co-morbidities or medical conditions must be taken into account when administering anesthesia for cataract surgery. A deep plane of anesthesia is required for all patients to minimize the chance of coughing or straining and loss of vitreous humor or other intraocular contents after the globe is incised. If a patient's cardiovascular system cannot tolerate a deep plane of anesthesia, neuromuscular blockade should be established. Succinylcholine should not be administered after the globe is incised, because contraction of the extraocular muscles for 15–20 min can potentially increase IOP sufficiently to extrude the ocular contents through the surgical incision.

Ideally, the patient who has had cataract surgery should not cry excessively or struggle postoperatively. Extubation of the trachea or LMA removal while the patient is still deeply anesthetized will help achieve this goal.

Retinoblastoma

Radiation is the primary treatment for retinoblastoma, a congenital malignancy that usually is diagnosed and treated during the first 3 years of life. Radiation therapy is administered over a 4–6-week period, often 4–5 times per week. During each session, the head must remain absolutely motionless for 45–90 sec. Patients are unattended during the treatment to avoid exposing medical personnel to excessive radiation. Postanesthesia sedation should be minimal to avoid disrupting the infant's feeding and sleeping schedules, so that he or she continues to grow and develop normally during these 4–6 weeks. Propofol bolus (1–2 mg/kg), followed by an infusion usually accomplishes satisfactory anesthesia for these procedures.

These children frequently return to the operating room for examination under anesthesia to monitor tumor growth or resolution. This examination is usually very brief. Smooth inhalation induction of anesthesia with insertion of an LMA and anticholinergic prophylaxis for oculocardiac reflex with or without acetaminophen (oral or rectal) suffices for anesthetic management.

Retinopathy of prematurity

Retinopathy of prematurity (ROP), formerly known as retrolental fibroplasia, is a vasoproliferative disorder of premature infants that may result in blindness. The first stage of this disease is characterized by suppression of vascular endothelial growth factor by hyperoxia, resulting in an arrest of normal retinal vascularization. The second phase is characterized by vascular proliferation induced by hypoxia-triggered stimulation of vascular endothelial growth factor. Hence both hyperoxia and hypoxia play a role in the pathogenesis of ROP [237]. The practice of decreasing the concentration of supplemental oxygen with a corresponding reduction in acceptable baseline oxygen saturations levels to 95% in neonates has reduced the incidence of ROP. This has led to an advocacy of maintaining oxygen saturations at or around 95% in premature infants having surgery. Nevertheless, with the increased survival of low-birthweight infants, more premature babies develop ROP.

Rapidly progressing ROP can lead to blindness and retinal detachment within 1–2 weeks. Hence early intervention with laser photocoagulation or cryotherapy is advocated and these cases are often scheduled as urgent cases in the late afternoon, after ROP is diagnosed upon routine followup eye exam. Laser therapy has been found to result in better visual acuity compared to cryotherapy and is the most widely used treatment for ROP [238,239]. For late-stage retinopathy in which retinal detachment has already occurred, buckling or vitrectomy is performed but these procedures usually fail to provide useful vision [240].

The anesthetic management of these children is challenging as multiple medical co-morbidities exist in this patient population, including apnea of prematurity, bronchopulmonary dysplasia, which may be associated with oxygen requirements, and congenital cardiac anomalies. While general anesthesia with mechanical ventilation is commonly administered for these procedures, the laryngeal mask airway is a viable alternative in the occasional premature infant with mild-to-moderate lung disease who did not require tracheal intubation in the past. Intravenous sedatives, analgesics and topical anesthesia have also been utilized in neonates who are ventilated mechanically or spontaneously breathing [241–243].

The goal is to provide a comfortable patient with minimal cardiorespiratory compromise and a quiet surgical field. While the procedure is not very stimulating, manipulation of the globe may be painful [244]. Opioids must be cautiously administered if pain is suspected during the procedure. Co-existing apnea may be exacerbated by the general anesthetic, and extubation of the trachea should occur only when a regular respiratory pattern without apnea is achieved; caffeine citrate 10 mg/kg IV may be effective in ameliorating significant apnea. These infants may need mechanical ventilation for 12–24h after the procedure, especially if any opioid is required for pain management.

There is some institutional variation in the location where these procedures occur. Laser surgery may be performed in the operating room if the neonate's pulmonary status will allow for transportation. In some institutions, operations are undertaken in the intensive care unit which allows for seamless postintervention monitoring [245]. Patients with ROP are at increased susceptibility to develop strabismus, cataracts and glaucoma and should have yearly examinations to help prevent and treat these conditions.

Dental procedures

Dental procedures in children are routinely performed in the dentist's office with local anesthesia with or without sedation. General anesthesia may be required to facilitate dental work in children with behavioral disturbances such as severe autism and severe developmental delay, or in children with multiple medical problems, and those requiring extensive dental restoration. General anesthesia allows the dentist to complete the restoration in a timely fashion without the use of excessive amounts of local anesthetic or without approaching the limits of sedation they are comfortable with in the dental office.

Sedation versus anesthesia

The use of sedation is occasionally complicated with serious morbidity and mortality in children, with the most serious adverse events relating to respiratory complications [246]. Adverse events usually occur when combinations of drugs include opioids [247,248] or when relatively higher than usual doses of local anesthetics, sedatives or analgesics, including opioids, are administered with inadequate monitoring or insufficiently skilled personnel available [249]. The increase in prevalence of childhood obesity also poses a challenge for the pediatric dentist with regard to administration of sedatives. Administration of sedatives based on the total body-weight may result in oversedation, which in an obese patient can easily result in airway obstruction. In contrast, administration of sedatives based on the lean body mass may result in undersedation and decreased duration of sedative effects [250]. An increase in adverse events following sedation [251,252] and an observed increase in mortality in office-based procedures [253] strengthen the case for improved monitoring during sedation for outpatient procedures in general [254]. A revised recommendation by the Committee on Drugs (COD), Section on Anesthesiology, of the American Academy of Pediatrics, [255] states specifically that:

1. the patient must undergo a documented presedation medical evaluation including a focused airway examination
2. there should be an appropriate interval of fasting before sedation
3. children should not receive sedative or anxiolytic medications without supervision by skilled medical personnel (i.e. medication should not be administered at home or by a technician without medical supervision)
4. sedative and anxiolytic medications should only be administered by or in the presence of individuals skilled in airway management and cardiopulmonary resuscitation
5. age- and size-appropriate equipment and appropriate medications to sustain life should be checked before and be immediately available
6. all patients sedated for a procedure must be continuously monitored with pulse oximetry
7. an individual must be specifically assigned to monitor the patient's cardiorespiratory status during and after the procedure: for deeply sedated patients, that

individual should have no other responsibilities and should record vital signs at least every 5 min

8. specific discharge criteria must be used.

An area of controversy that exists is the exact definition of conscious sedation provided in outpatient settings. Conscious sedation is defined as a state of sedation that "permits appropriate response by the patient to physical stimulation or verbal command, e.g. 'open your eyes'." This implies that the patient retains the capability to interact with the medical care team. Purely reflexive activity, such as the gag reflex, simple withdrawal from pain or making inarticulate noises, does not constitute an appropriate response for the purpose of this definition. A sedated child who displays only reflex activity of this sort is in a state of deep sedation, not a state of conscious sedation. The Committee on Drugs recommends that it is more appropriate to recognize the most current terminology of the American Society of Anesthesiologists [256] and replace the term "conscious sedation" with "moderate sedation."

Considerations for dental surgery

Existing co-morbidities should be considered when planning the anesthetic management for this group of children. Many of them have underlying cardiac anomalies and may require systemic bacterial endocarditis (SBE) prophylaxis (see Chapter 25). The facial and airway structure of some patients may make direct laryngoscopy challenging and may require the use of special equipment to intubate the trachea. Patients with developmental delay or serious behavioral disturbances can pose difficulties because of poor motor control and involuntary movements, spasticity, and aggressive behavior (screaming, biting, kicking), particularly when they are frightened by a strange environment. This behavior may result in difficulty placing and securing an intravenous catheter or in performing an inhalational induction of anesthesia. Intramuscular ketamine 3–5 mg/kg mixed with atropine (10–20 μg/kg) has been useful for the induction of anesthesia in some of these patients [257,258]. After injection of this mixture of drugs, sedation or a "catatonic state" will develop, and the patient can be moved, intravenous access obtained, general anesthesia induced, the patient's trachea intubated, and anesthesia maintained with a technique of choice. Many patients in this category have seizure disorders and should receive their anticonvulsant medications on the day of the procedure. Ketamine can be employed in patients with seizure disorders without precipitating seizures.

Dental anesthesia

Extensive dental restoration is best managed with endotracheal intubation. Most anesthesiologists and dental surgeons prefer nasotracheal rather than orotracheal intubation for dental procedures. The tube can be secured around the patient's head with a fabric tube holder; it should not be taped to the skin. In some patients, however, nasotracheal intubation is not practical. In patients with previous cleft palate repair or epidermolysis bullosa, for example, inserting an endotracheal tube through the nose may cause significant damage. A nasotracheal tube may damage previous repair lines in patients who have undergone palate repair and it may induce blister formation in response to pressure, friction or minor trauma of the mucosa in patients with epidermolysis bullosa. In these cases, an oral RAE tube may be placed instead. The stability of an oral tube is potentially a problem and requires constant attention to prevent the tube from being accidentally removed. Securing and maintaining an orotracheal tube during dental anesthesia requires uncompromising vigilance. Oral tubes are usually secured to one side of the mouth and then carefully secured on the other side when necessary during the procedure.

Following inhalation induction, oxymetazoline drops are applied to both nares to provide mucosal vasoconstriction which helps decrease bleeding during insertion of the endotracheal tube. Graduated sizes of lubricated nasopharyngeal airways may also be placed, to assist in dilation of the nares in preparation for nasotracheal intubation. Placement of the nasotracheal tube in warm water prior to its use helps to decrease the stiffness of the polyvinylchloride tube, and consequently decreases the incidence of epistaxis following nasotracheal intubation. A cuffed endotracheal tube should be inserted when possible. Limiting the number of attempts at nasotracheal intubation may decrease the incidence of epistaxis. Epistaxis can make nasotracheal intubation more difficult because it severely limits visualization of the larynx.

In most children, the endotracheal tube can be inserted under direct vision without difficulty following inhalation induction and propofol 2–3 mg/kg, without muscle relaxant. The vocal cords usually can be visualized easily and the endotracheal tube can be directed through the vocal cords, with or without the use of Magill forceps. The nasal RAE tube is commonly used for dental surgery as it allows the surgeon to use a rubber dam if preferred [259]. The preformed, fixed bend helps stabilize the endotracheal tube, decreases the likelihood of kinking of the tube, and allows a low profile for maximum surgical convenience when the bend is situated at the opening of the nares. The preformed bend also offers some challenges as the distance from the bend to the distal end of the tube is fixed. This may result in endobronchial intubation in children who are shorter than expected for age, while in others the tip of the tube barely extends below the vocal cords. In addition, the presence of the bend makes suctioning difficult.

A gauze throat pack is usually inserted prior to the beginning of surgery to prevent aspiration of blood or extracted teeth. Patients may remain spontaneously ventilating or may be mechanically ventilated during surgery. Because multiple teeth are normally restored, local anesthetic is used infrequently in young children by the dentist because of concerns of a toxic drug dose. Therefore, intraoperative analgesia with fentanyl 1–2 μg/kg, morphine 0.05–0.1 mg/kg, and rectal or IV acetaminophen is often effective for postoperative analgesia. If there is pain in the PACU, morphine 0.05 mg/kg IV, repeated once if needed 20 min after the first dose, is usually sufficient. NSAIDs, i.e. ketorolac, are normally not recommended because inhibition of platelet function may increase gum and mucosal bleeding.

The postoperative period may be characterized by emergence delirium and postoperative nausea and vomiting. Most patients have the procedure performed on an outpatient basis.

CASE STUDY

A 13-year-old obese male, a resident of a home for children with special needs who has a history of severe developmental delay and occasional violent behavior, is scheduled for bilateral strabismus surgery. Other pertinent medical history includes obstructive sleep apnea for which the patient's pediatrician has prescribed a CPAP machine but the patient has been non-compliant with its utilization.

Preoperative considerations

If possible, it will be helpful to obtain information about the severity of the patient's OSA (see Table 31.2) as this will be helpful in planning the anesthetic (may influence administration of intraoperative opioids). The immediate challenge with the care of this patient is how to easily separate the child from his parents or caretaker in order to proceed into the operating room. The patient is unlikely to go back to the operating room with the anesthesia care provider. If he is accompanied by one of the staff of the resident home and has a special rapport with this person, or is accompanied by a parent, the presence of this individual during induction could be encouraged, depending on the institutional practice. An alternative which would eliminate concerns for respiratory difficulty would be administration of intramuscular (IM) ketamine together with IM midazolam and glycopyrrolate to counteract hallucinations and excessive drooling respectively, both due to ketamine administration. Another alternative is the administration of an oral premedication of midazolam 0.5–1 mg/kg. A lower dose would be preferable in this obese child with a history of OSA. Some practitioners would even administer a much lower dose of 0.25 mg/kg PO.

Intraoperative considerations

Administration of IM ketamine (which results in dissociative anesthesia) with a small amount of propofol supplementation may suffice for the insertion of an LMA. Strabismus surgery is typically of short duration (approximately 45 min), especially if only one muscle per eye will be operated on. The patient's obesity and history of sleep apnea, however, may preclude the use of an LMA as relaxation of the hypopharyngeal soft tissue may result in ineffective spontaneous ventilation under anesthesia. The patient may be placed on pressure control ventilation with the pressure not exceeding 20–25 mmHg in order to avoid gastric distension and possible aspiration of gastric contents.

Considering the co-morbid conditions of obesity and sleep apnea, the best option for securing the airway may be endotracheal intubation which provides a protected airway. This child may receive a muscle relaxant of short duration. Desflurane with its low blood:gas solubility would be the ideal inhalation agent for maintenance of anesthesia in this obese patient. Gentle titration of intraoperative opioids of the anesthesia practitioner's choice should be administered, preferably when the patient develops spontaneous ventilation under anesthesia, in which case, the opioids can be titrated to a respiratory rate of 16–20 breaths per minute. For patients with severe OSA, intraoperative opioid administration should be minimized and the gentle titration of opioids following extubation, when the patient is awake, is recommended.

Intraoperatively, the heart rate is observed to decrease to 60 from 110. There is concern that the oculocardiac reflex is being triggered.

This reflex is most commonly elicited by traction on the medial rectus muscle. Administration of IV glycopyrrolate (0.01 mg/kg) and informing the surgeons to gently release traction on the eye muscles during surgery can result in resolution of bradycardia.

At the conclusion of surgery, neuromuscular blockade should be fully reversed and the trachea should be extubated with the patient awake in a semi-sitting or lateral/non-supine position.

Postoperative considerations

This patient should remain in the semi-upright, lateral or other non-supine position throughout recovery in order to decrease the incidence of airway obstruction. Strabismus surgery alone is an outpatient procedure. For this patient with associated co-morbidities, however, the course in the PACU will determine whether or not he should be discharged to the resident home. The degree of care available in the resident home should also be considered (i.e. availability of a nurse on site and the degree of supervision/care the patient will have). Some hospitals have policies regarding the duration of PACU stay for patients with a history of OSA and in fact recommendations by the American Society of Anesthesiology regarding the postoperative management of these patients include postoperative observation in the recovery room for 2–3h longer than those who do not have OSA [49,260]. The recovery of these children from anesthesia occasionally depends on the amount of opioids they have received. If necessary, the administration of oral acetaminophen with codeine or other non-steroidal analgesics should be considered to alleviate additional pain symptoms in the recovery room. Familiar caretakers should be readily allowed into the recovery room to prevent or decrease postanesthetic emergence anxiety.

Despite awake tracheal extubation, the patient cannot be weaned off oxygen, with oxygen saturations intermittently decreasing to (85–88%) for approximately 10 sec. The use of a shoulder roll and oral airway is also required to prevent airway obstruction.

The patient appears to have an oxygen requirement and is experiencing airway obstruction despite normal maneuvers to alleviate the problem, i.e. placement of oral airway and shoulder roll to prevent flexion of the head and obstruction of the airway. A respiratory therapist should be called to fit the patient for a CPAP mask. Hopefully, the patient will be receptive to this while still recovering from anesthesia. Depending on the institution's practice, a consultation with the intensive care unit or step-down unit physician will be warranted to accommodate the use of the CPAP machine and to monitor the patient postoperatively. There is no consensus regarding postoperative disposition of patients with OSA within the hospital setting, i.e. observation postoperatively in the intensive care unit or step-down unit. There is agreement, however, that these patients be observed in a monitored postoperative setting which includes pulse oximetry monitoring [260].

Annotated references

A full reference list for this chapter is available at:
http://www.wiley.com/go/gregory/andropoulos/pediatricanesthesia

7. Tait AR, Malviya S. Anesthesia for the child with an upper respiratory tract infection: still a dilemma? Anesth Analg 2005; 100: 59–65. An excellent contemporary review of the problem of URI and anesthesia in children by authors of several seminal studies in this area.

25. Flick RP, Wilder RT, Pieper SF et al. Risk factors for laryngospasm in children during general anesthesia. Paediatr Anaesth 2008; 18: 289–96. An excellent study of risk factors and treatment of laryngospasm in children.

49. Schwengel DA, Sterni LM, Tunkel DE, Heitmiller ES. Perioperative management of children with obstructive sleep apnea. Anesth Analg 2009; 109: 60–75. An outstanding contemporary review of the problem of obstructive sleep apnea in children, and principles of perioperative and anesthetic management.

68. American Society of Anesthesiologists Task Force on Operating Room Fires, Caplan RA, Barker SJ et al. Practice advisory for the prevention and management of operating room fires. Anesthesiology 2008; 108: 786–801. An excellent review and guideline for prevention and management of airway fires, important because of the frequency of laser usage in pediatric otolaryngological surgery.

96. Al-Alami AA, Zestos MM, Baraka AS. Pediatric laryngospasm: prevention and treatment. Curr Opin Anaesthesiol 2009; 22: 388–95. A modern review of laryngospasm in pediatric anesthesia, and the evidence base for prevention and treatment.

152. Zur KB, Litman RS. Pediatric airway foreign body retrieval: surgical and anesthetic perspectives. Paediatr Anaesth 2009; 19: 109–17. An excellent, modern, combined review of surgical and anesthetic considerations for airway foreign body in children.

169. Johnson K, Derkay C. Palliative aspects of recurrent respiratory papillomatosis. Otolaryngol Clin North Am 2009; 42: 57–70, viii. A thorough, contemporary review of evaluation and treatment of laryngeal papillomatosis.

185. Zalzal GH, Cotton RT. Glottic and subglottic stenosis. In: Flint PW, Haughey BH, Lund VJ et al (eds) Cummings Otolaryngology Head and Neck Surger, 5th edn. Maryland Heights, MO: Elsevier, 2010. A comprehensive reference addressing the management of glottis and subglottic stenosis.

202. Gan TJ, Meyer TA, Apfel CC et al. Society for Ambulatory Anesthesia guidelines for the management of postoperative nausea and vomiting. Anesth Analg 2007; 105: 1615–28. A comprehensive review of management of postoperative nausea and vomiting in children and adults.

216. Kovac AL. Management of postoperative nausea and vomiting in children. Paediatr Drugs 2007; 9: 47–69. A modern review of the management of perioperative nausea and vomiting in children.

CHAPTER 32
Anesthesia for Plastic and Craniofacial Surgery

Ehrenfried Schindler[1], Markus Martini[2] & Martina Messing-Jünger[3]

Departments of [1]Pediatric Anesthesiology and [3]Pediatric Neurosurgery, Asklepios Klinik Sankt Augustin, Sankt Augustin, Germany
[2]Department of Maxillo-Facial Surgery, University Hospital Bonn, Bonn, Germany

Introduction

General anesthesia has allowed surgeons to correct disfiguring lesions in infants and children since the introduction of anesthesia in the middle of the 19th century. Cleft lip and palate reconstruction was among the earliest surgical procedures for which general anesthesia was used for pediatric patients [1]. John Snow published the first report of giving an ether anesthetic to a 7-year-old boy for cleft lip reconstruction in *The Lancet* in 1847. He subsequently administered chloroform for lip reconstruction 147 times between 1847 and 1858, mostly to infants between 3 and 6 weeks of age. Cleft lip and palate repairs have also been an impetus for other innovations in anesthesia care for infants. This includes Ivan Magill's first use of endotracheal anesthesia for an infant in 1924 and Philip Ayre's introduction of the T-piece circuit in 1937 [2]. Modern developments in anesthesia and plastic surgery have permitted increasingly complex reconstruction of disfigured infants and children. The past decade has seen major advances in the understanding of anomalous development and the evolution of diagnostic and therapeutic technology. This chapter focuses on the anesthetic challenges encountered in major craniofacial reconstruction, including cleft lip and palate repair.

Craniofacial embryology

Normal development

The basic structures of the fetus are formed during the embryonic period of gestation, i.e. between postconceptual weeks 2 and 8. The skeleton of the head is composed of the neurocranium (calvaria or cranial vault), the viscerocranium (facial skeleton), and the cranial base. These structures are highly integrated, and their formation and development are closely interwoven. The cranial base is the foundation of the skull, and its formation and development greatly influence the morphology of the other components. Embryologically, the cranial base and facial complex are derived from neural crest tissues; the neurocranium arises from mesoderm [3,4].

The neural tube closes by the third week of gestation. Its dorsal crests are composed of multipotent tissue that migrates widely into adjacent mesenchyme between the diencephalon and the cardiac swelling. Translocated neural crest cells undergo differentiation into a wide variety of cell types and form cartilage, bone, ligaments, muscles, and arteries of the cranial base and facial regions.

Cranial base

The cranial base extends from the foramen magnum to the frontonasal junction and consists of the sphenoid, petrous portion of the temporal bone, and cranial surfaces of the ethmoid bones. The pars basilaris of the clivus and the occipital bone are also part of the base. Phylogenetically, it is the oldest portion of the skull, and its development appears to be genetically determined. The bony structure is preceded by a cartilaginous structure, the chondrocranium, which first appears in the 6th week of gestation. Before chondrification, blood vessels, cranial nerves, and the spinal cord are established between the brain and extracranial sites. Centers of ossification appear during the 8th week of gestation. In contrast to the largely intramembranous bone of the cranial vault, which originates by direct ossification of mesenchyme, the osteogenic membrane, the cranial base is endochondral bone and formed from a cartilaginous prototype. Its sutures are cartilaginous joints (synchondroses), which grow by chondrocyte mitosis. The spheno-occipital synchondrosis is the principal site of growth in the cranial base during childhood.

The cranial base is an important shared junction between the cranial vault and face. Its inner surface relates to the brain and its outer surface relates to the nasopharynx and facial complex. Its shape and size strongly influence final calvarial morphology. The primary stimulus for growth of the cranial base is growth of the brain. The ventral parts of the frontal and temporal lobes determine the size and alignment of the floor of the cranial base, namely the anterior and middle cranial fossae [5]. The cranial base is, in turn, the template on which the upper face develops. Various junctures between the cranial base and facial bones, especially in the nasomaxillary complex, determine the influence of the cranial base on facial growth. The anterior cranial fossa is spatially related to the nasomaxillary complex. The middle cranial fossa is also related to the pharyngeal space and airway. The interposition of three sets of space-occupying sense organs complicates the attachment of these two skull components to each other and influences the growth of the facial skeleton in particular. These interactions become obvious in most craniofacial pathologies, e.g. in hyper- or hypotelorism, are associated with cranial vault or cranial base malformations or plagiocephaly with unilateral coronal synostosis with facial scoliosis.

Cranial vault

The cranial vault consists of the frontal, parietal, temporal, and occipital bones. The mesenchyme that precedes the cranial vault or neurocranium is derived from paraxial mesoderm and is at first arranged as a capsular membrane around the developing brain. Ossification of intramembranous calvarial bones requires the presence of the brain. According to the functional matrix concept, bone growth occurs in response to functional demands. The sutures of the calvaria can be considered interosseous ligaments that connect opposing bone surfaces. The bones of the calvaria are displaced outward by the expanding brain and deposit new bone at the contact edges of the sutures [5]. The ultimate size and shape of the cranial vault are therefore determined by internal hydrostatic pressures that the expanding brain and cerebrospinal fluid (CSF) pulsation waves exert on the cranial sutures. This stimulates compensatory sutural bone growth.

Face

Development of the head and face occurs between the 4th and 10th weeks of gestation by fusion of five facial swellings: the single frontal prominence and paired maxillary and mandibular prominences (Fig. 32.1). This depends upon the inductive activities of the prosencephalic and rhombencepahlic organizing centers, which are regulated by the expression of the sonic hedgehog gene as a signaling protein in the neural floor plate cells [6,7]. The rostral prosencephalic center induces the visual and inner ear apparatus, the upper third of the face, and the neurocranium. The caudal rhombencephalic center is responsible for the viscerofacial skeleton (i.e. middle and lower thirds of the face). Gradients of chemical and physical properties emanating from the organizing centers regulate the process of craniofacial formation [8]. The five facial swellings surround a central depression, which is the stomodeum or future mouth.

The frontal prominence encloses the forebrain from which pairs of thickened ectodermal surface placodes (nasal and optic) are derived. The nasal placodes invaginate to form the nasal passages. The surface ridges or nasomedial and nasolateral processes give rise to the nose, the philtrum of the upper lip, and the primary palate. The nasal complex is formed when the frontal prominence merges with the nasal capsule, which is part of the cranial base. The nasal capsule surrounds the olfactory organs and forms the cartilages of the nostrils and the nasal septum. Septal cartilage intervenes between the

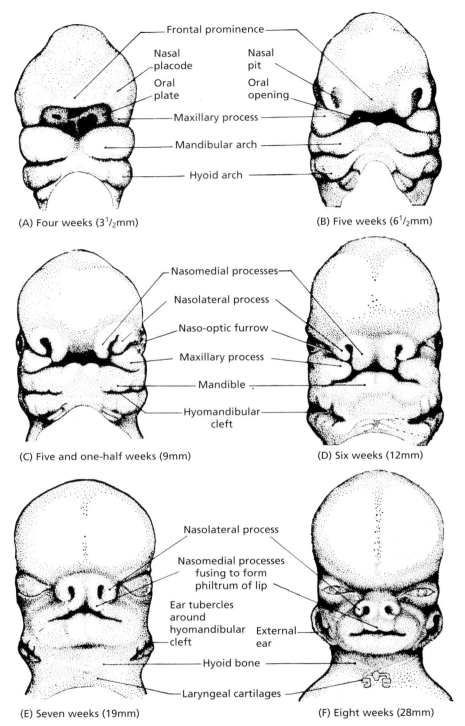

Figure 32.1 Stages in the embryonic development of the face. The median and paramedian structures from upper lip to forehead derive from the frontal prominence. The maxillary and mandibular regions, the ear, and the pharyngeal and laryngeal structures, derive from the branchial arches. Reproduced from Patten BM. Human Embryology, 3rd edn. New York: McGraw-Hill, 1968, p.346 with permission of the McGraw-Hill Companies.

cranial base above and the palate below and plays a major role in subsequent growth of the midface. The optic placodes, which ultimately develop into eyes, are induced by lateral optic diverticula from the forebrain. Expansion of the cerebral hemispheres produces medial migration to a frontal position.

The maxillary and mandibular prominences are derived from the first branchial arch. The branchial arches are five segmented bilateral swellings of the pharyngeal foregut, consisting of a mesodermal core surrounded by neural crest tissue. The arches are separated by branchial grooves externally and pharyngeal pouches internally. The cartilaginous skeleton of the first arch, Meckel's cartilage, provides a template for development of the mandible. The ear and auditory apparatus are derived from the first and second arches and from the first groove and pouch. The external ear components migrate from an initial cervical location. The internal ear components arise from the otic placode, which is induced by the vestibulocochlear nerve. The rest of the branchial arches, grooves, and pouches form various parts of the pharynx and laryngeal apparatus.

The facial prominences and their skeletal cartilage, mesenchyme, and neurovascular bundles undergo cell proliferation, swelling, migration, and fusion in a critically timed series of events. Fusion of the paired mandibular prominences in the midline provides continuity of the lower jaw and lip. Fusion of the maxillary and mandible prominences laterally creates the commissures of the mouth. Fusion of the nasomedial processes and maxillary prominences provides continuity of the upper jaw and lip and separation of the stomodeal chamber into separate oral and nasal cavities. Fusion of the nasomedial processes in the midline forms the central upper lip, the tip of the nose, and the primary palate (see Fig. 32.1).

During the 6th week of development, the secondary palate is formed from palatine shelves that initially grow inferiorly from the maxillary prominences downward into the stomodeum and lateral to the tongue. Initially, these palatal shelves are widely separated from the primary palate owing to their vertical orientation on either side of the tongue. During the 7th–8th week of gestation, coincident with longitudinal growth and straightening of the embryo and withdrawal of the tongue from between the shelves, the lateral palatal shelves rotate to a horizontal position and fuse with each other. The palatal mesenchyme then differentiates into bony and muscular elements that correlate with the position of the hard and soft palate, respectively. In addition to fusing in the midline, the secondary palate fuses with the primary palate and the nasal septum. These fusion processes are complete by the 10th week of embryogenesis; development of the mammalian secondary palate thereby divides the oronasal space into separate oral and nasal

cavities, allowing mastication and respiration to take place simultaneously [9]. The nature of the "intrinsic shelf force" responsible for this reorientation is unknown, although mouth-opening reflexes, which involve withdrawal of the face from against the heart prominence, have been implicated in the withdrawal of the tongue from between the vertical palatal shelves.

The neural crest tissue gives rise to the facial skeleton, and the mesoderm will form the facial muscles. Current studies demonstrate the influence of the cranial base as it adjusts to its broader structural context and provides added support for the developmental and structural integration of the cranial base with both the cranial vault and face [10]. During facial development, cells are monitored by genetically determined pathways and adjust their rates of accumulation, apoptosis, and hyperplasia to produce organs of predetermined size [11]. Forward growth of the mandible relocates the tongue more anteriorly. Successful fusion of the components of the palate by the 12th week requires a complicated synchronization of shelf movements with withdrawal of the tongue and growth of the mandible. By this time the face takes on a human appearance.

Anomalous development

Various genetic and environmental factors cause anomalous craniofacial development [12]. The etiology of craniofacial syndromes and craniosynostosis is heterogeneous and multifactorial. Genetically based malformations may be caused by single-gene deficiencies or by chromosomal aberrations. Genes for several autosomal dominant craniofacial malformations have recently been defined: mutations in genes regulating fibrous growth factor receptors (FGFR-1, FGFR-2, FGFR-3, FGFR-4) and transforming growth factors (TGF-1, TGF-2, TGF-3) as well as *MSX2* and *TWIST* genes [13–15].

The identified gene loci associated with cleft lip and palate include regions on chromosomes 1, 2, 4, 6, 14, 17, 19 and X chromosome (*MHFR, TGFA, D4S175, F13A1, TGFB3, D17S250*) with gene products, e.g. TGFA, TGFβ3, MSX1, IRF6, TBX22, GSTM1 [16,17]. Currently, there are no specific tests available for genetic susceptibility to orofacial clefts. Environmental factors include congenital infections, irradiation, and exposure to chemical teratogens, such as phenytoin, vitamin A analogs, and alcohol. For many malformations, the etiology is unknown.

Maldevelopment can occur through several mechanisms. Malformations that develop during the embryonic period are distinct from deformations that occur later in the fetal period and may be self-correcting with postnatal catch-up growth [6]. Fetal or postnatal head restraint can also cause premature fusion of cranial sutures [15]. Malformations can originate in anomalies of neural crest cells that may be deficient in number, may not complete migration, or may fail to cytodifferentiate. Neural crest tissues also form much of the cardiac conotruncal septum, and there is an association between craniofacial and cardiovascular malformations in syndromes in which neural crest defects play a role [18,19]. Examples include retinoic acid syndrome, DiGeorge syndrome, the CHARGE association, and some variants of hemifacial microsomia. Malformations can also be caused by intrauterine compression of the embryo early in gestation. For example, in the amnion rupture sequence, early rupture of the amnion leads to defective morphogenesis secondary to compression of the embryo. In addition, adherence of amniotic bands to developing embryonic structures may interfere with normal development and result in simple to bizarre malformations that are not associated with embryological lines of fusion.

Malformations may result from intrauterine vascular accidents. For example, a shift in the blood supply of the face from the internal to the external carotid artery occurs during the 7th week of gestation when the normal stapedial artery atrophies. This shift occurs at a critical time of midface and palate development and has the potential to cause deficient blood supply and defects of the midface, upper lip, and palate. Malformations can also be secondary to defects in brain development because all components of the skull depend on the brain development [12–15,20,21]. Several syndromes are described below.

Craniosynostosis

Precocious brain development is reflected by rapid head enlargement, beginning in early gestation and continuing through the first postnatal year. Craniosynostosis, or premature closure of the cranial sutures, arrests skull growth in the related region. Isolated synostosis produces characteristic skull distortions as growth is redirected toward patent sutures (Table 32.1). The degree of skull deformity depends on the number of sutures involved and the time at which premature fusion begins. The earlier the synostosis, the greater the deformity and this may result in reduced intracranial volume. Due to the expanding cerebral structures and reduced intracranial volume, intracranial hypertension can develop later on.

Several different mechanisms are responsible for craniosynostosis [12–15]. Intrauterine constraint of the fetal head, e.g. in multiple pregnancies, can cause isolated nonfamilial craniosynostosis. A genetic defect is responsible for familial simple craniosynostosis and for most craniosynostosis syndromes with known genesis. Ninety different disorders with craniosynostosis have been described. Several specific genetic defects have recently been identified (Table 32.2). Crouzon, Apert, Pfeiffer, and Jackson–Weiss syndromes, once thought to be separate but overlapping entities, are now known to result from different mutations of the same genes [23]. In syndromic

Table 32.1 Nomenclature of craniosynostosis

Affected suture	Traditional name	Literal translation
Sagittal	Scaphocephaly	Boat skull
Metopic	Trigonocephaly	Triangle skull
Unilateral coronal	Plagiocephaly*	Oblique skull
Bicoronal	Brachycephaly	Short skull
Multiple sutures	Acrocephaly[†]	Topmost skull
	Turricephaly[†]	Tower skull
	Oxycephaly	Sharp skull
	Kleeblattschadel	Cloverleaf skull

*Plagiocephaly is not necessarily synonymous with unilateral coronal synostosis.
[†]Some authors use acrocephaly and/or turricephaly synonymously with brachycephaly to indicate bicoronal synostosis.
Adapted from Marsh JL. Comprehensive Care for Craniofacial Deformities. St Louis: CV Mosby, 1985, p 123, with permission from Elsevier.

Table 32.2 Craniosynostosis syndromes

Syndrome	Chromosome localization	Gene
Apert syndrome	10q25.3-q26	FGFR2
Crouzon syndrome	10q25.3-q26	FGFR2
Jackson–Weiss syndrome	10q25.3-q26	FGFR2
Beare–Stevenson cutis gyrata syndrome	10q25.3-q26	FGFR2
Pfeiffer syndrome	10q25.3-q26	FGFR2
	8p11.2-p12	FGFR1
Thanatophoric dysplasia	4pl6	FGFR3
Crouzonodermoskeletal syndrome	4pl6	FGFR3
Muenke craniosynostosis	4pl6	FGFR3
Craniosynostosis, Boston type	5qter	MSX2
Saethre–Chotzen syndrome	7p21-p22	TWIST

Courtesy of M.M. Cohen, Jr.

families, some members have normal phenotypes but different sutures can be affected in different individuals. Syndromes with Mendelian genetic patterns are also described with no molecular genetic evidence so far. Craniosynostosis can also be caused by metabolic and hematological disorders and by microcephaly that is caused by defective brain growth (Box 32.1). Known teratogens that cause craniosynostosis are diphenylhydantoin, aminopterin and methotrexate, retinoic acid, oxymetazoline, and valproic acid.

Craniosynostosis may be an isolated deformation or part of a malformation syndrome. Isolated non-syndromic craniosynostosis occurs in six in every 10,000 births [12]. Sagittal synostosis is most common (57%), coronal synostosis is less frequent (18–29%), and metopic and lambdoidal synostoses are the least frequent, although recently

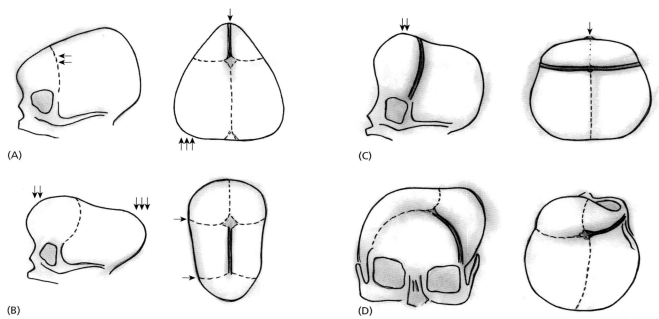

Figure32.2 Single-suture craniosynostosis results in specific cranial deformities. (A) Trigonocephaly is the result of premature closure of the metopic suture and typical features are a frontal keel (↑), anterior displacement of the coronal sutures (↑↑), and compensatory bulging of the parietal squamae (↑↑↑). (B) Scaphocephaly is characterized by bitemporal or biparietal narrowing (↑), frontal (↑↑) and occipital (↑↑↑) compensatory bossing. The shape of the skull resembles the keel of a boat or a saddle. (C) Brachycephaly means short skull and is the result of bicoronal craniosynostosis. The frontal region is flattened (↑) and some cases show early compensatory oxycephalic deformity (↑↑). (D) Anterior plagiocephaly results from unilateral coronal synostosis and causes asymmetrical and rotational deformity of the fronto-orbital region with additional midface and skull deformities.

Box 32.1 Secondary craniosynostosis

Storage disorders

- Hurler
- Morquio

Metabolic disorders

- Rickets
- Hyperthyrioidism

Hematologic disorders

- Polycythemia vera
- Thalassemia

---

there has been a marked rise in the incidence of trigono-cephaly in non-syndromic cases [24]. Calvarial synostosis may also be part of a widespread craniofacial malformation that involves the cranial base and face.

Single suture craniosynostosis

The typical skull deformities following single suture craniosynostosis result from compensatory growth (Fig. 32.2). The cephalic index (maximum biparietal diameter multiplied with 100 divided by maximum anteroposterior diameter) was introduced by the Swedish anatomist

Anders Retzius and is used to measure the extent of deformity as well as for follow-up of later head development. Not all premature craniosynostoses lead to an obvious skull deformity. Typical anthropomorphic skull types are dolichocephalic (long headed), brachycephalic (broad headed) and mesocephalic (moderate head form).

Sagittal craniosynostosis

This is the most frequent form of craniosynostosis and presents the typical scaphocephalic form of skull with an elongated anteroposterior diameter and a narrowed biparietal diameter. The fused sagittal suture often forms a bony ridge and resembles the keel of a boat. The biparietal region is particularly narrow and sometimes lowered (Fig. 32.3). Frontal and/or occipital bossing can be very prominent and result from compensatory skull growth. The head circumference is generally increased, and the head is dolichocephalic. In 11% of cases, additional morphological brain changes were found on MRI studies.

Unicoronal craniosynostosis

The unilateral supraorbital ridge is retruded and the contralateral side sometimes compensates for the lack of growth and protrudes. In most cases, there is facial scoliosis that is caused by unilateral midface involvement. The deformity is described as anterior plagiocephaly. Patients may squint and have a compensatory head tilt (Fig. 32.4).

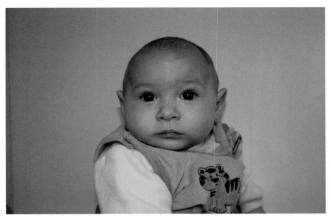

Figure 32.3 Scaphocephalic child with typical biparietal narrowing and resulting flattened head.

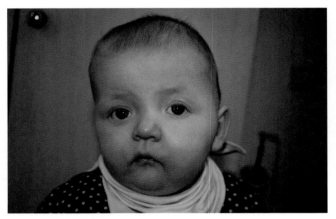

Figure 32.4 Facial scoliosis in a child with anterior plagiocephaly.

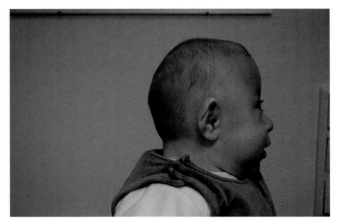

Figure 32.5 Brachycephalic head caused by bicoronal craniosynostosis.

Bicoronal craniosynostosis

This entity can be syndromic and a genetic work-up is indicated. The head circumference is decreasing, due mainly to a marked flattening of the forehead (Fig. 32.5). The orbits and both temporal squamae protrude.

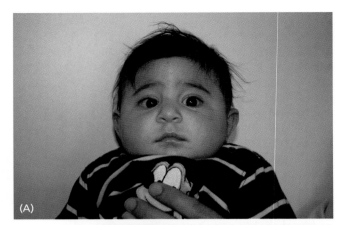

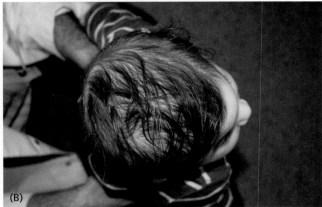

Figure 32.6 (A) Hypotelorism in metopic synostosis. (B) Frontal keel.

Additional turricephalic compensation can occur. This is the typical picture of a brachycephalic head. Early surgery is sometimes necessary to treat elevated intracranial pressure. The midface is often also involved.

Metopic craniosynostosis

The skull deformity with metopic craniosynostosis varies from a frontal ridge to severe trigonocephaly with narrowing of the frontal region and a keel-shaped forehead with hypotelorism and epicanthal folds (Fig. 32.6). It can be associated with genetic syndromes such as Opitz C syndrome or trisomy 11. The head circumference is usually decreased.

Lambdoidal craniosynostosis

Isolated lambdoidal craniosynostis is rare and accounts for only 3% of all premature synostoses. Most of the clinical forms of posterior plagiocephaly are positional deformities and do not require surgical correction. In true lambdoidal craniosynostosis, the contralateral forehead bulges forward. In cases that are caused by position, there is ipsilateral bossing.

Syndromic craniosynostosis
Acrocephalosyndactylies
Craniosynostosis syndromes that are also associated with hand and feet abnormalities are described as acrocephalosyndactylies.

Apert syndrome
Apert syndrome is the most severe of several craniosynostosis syndromes that involves all the craniofacial structures: calvaria, cranial base, and face. Apert syndrome occurs in approximately 1 per 55,000 births due to mutations in the FGFR-2 gene on chromosome 10 [22]. Although the mode of transmission can be autosomal dominant, most cases are sporadic. Apert syndrome is characterized by craniosynostosis, midface hypoplasia and retrusion plus symmetrical syndactyly of the hands and feet (Fig. 32.7A,B). The dysmorphic features are listed in Box 32.2.

In Apert syndrome the craniosynostosis involves multiple cranial sutures, but most commonly involves the coronal sutures and causes brachycephaly. The occiput is usually flattened. The cranial base has a broad, flat, short contour with premature synostosis. The anterior cranial fossa is markedly shortened, which constrains development of the nasomaxillary complex. The nasal cavity, palate, and maxilla are shortened, narrowed, and retropositioned. The midface hypoplasia and brachycephaly result in proptosis because the orbits are too shallow to house the globe. The middle cranial fossa is rotated to a more vertical position than normal, which secondarily diminishes the dimensions of the pharynx. The interorbital space is always large, and the orbits may be misaligned. The shortened cranial base results in a vaulted cranium and a deep forehead. Platybasia, Chiari malformation, and hydrocephalus are relatively common. Severe dental malocclusion is typical. Lateral skull base deformities are responsible for a high rate of hearing disorders. A significant number of patients are mentally retarded; most of the children have IQs below 80.

Saethre–Chotzen syndrome
Phenotypically variable, the relatively common Saethre–Chotzen syndrome is often misdiagnosed. Because mild forms may not be recognized, the true incidence is unclear.

Typical features are brachy- and acrocephalic deformities, mostly due to bicoronal abnormalities and plagiocephaly (Fig. 32.8). The hairline is low and the facial appearance broad, flat, and asymmetrical. The nose is beaked, and there may be ptosis of the eyelids. The inheritance pattern is autosomal dominant.

Pfeiffer syndrome
The clinical phenotype of Pfeiffer syndrome is variable. Patients typically show a turribrachycephalic deformity that is mostly due to abnormal bicoronal sutures. Cloverleaf heads have also been reported. Hypertelorism, proptosis, maxillary hypoplasia, mandibular prognathism and malocclusion occur as well. Ankylotic joints are typical skeletal findings. Severe skull base anomalies are associated with platybasia and Chiari malformation and also with spinal malformations and vertebral fusion. The incidence of this syndrome is about one in 210,000; its inheritance is autosomal dominant. Early surgical correction of the constraining skull structures can lead to normal neurocognitive development if brain growth is not impaired.

Crouzon syndrome
The phenotype of this syndrome is characterized by brachycephaly caused by bicoronal synostosis,

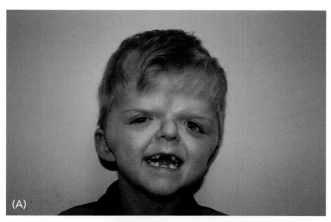

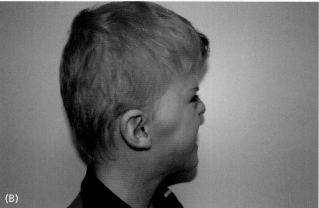

Figure 32.7 Six-year-old boy with typical features of Apert syndrome. (A) Downslanting palpebral fissures, depressed nasal bridge, dental malocclusion. (B) Flat facies due to midface hypoplasia.

Box 32.2 Features of Apert syndrome

Craniofacial dysmorphology

- Craniosynostosis
  - Coronal synostosis most common
  - Steep full forehead (frontal bossing)
  - Flat occiput
  - ± Hydrocephalus
- Maxillary retrusion (midface hypoplasia)
  - Flat facies
- Shallow orbits
  - Exorbitism or proptosis
- Relative mandibular prognathism
- Variable facial asymmetry
- Supraorbital horizontal groove
- Hypertelorism
- Down-slanting palpebral fissures
- Strabismus
- Parrot-beaked nose
- Depressed nasal bridge
- Cleft palate or bifid uvula
- Trapeziodal-shaped (cupid's) lips
- High arched palate
- V-shaped maxillary dental arch
- Severe tooth crowding
- Dental malocclusion
- Reduced nasopharyneal dimensions

Limb dysmorphology

- Syndactyly
  - Osseous and/or cutaneous
  - Fingers and toes

  - Digits 2, 3, 4 always
  - Symmetric
- Thumb and great toe malformations

Occasional abnormalities

- Cardiovascular
  - Atrial septal defect
  - Overriding aorta
  - Ventricular septal defect
  - Pulmonic stenosis
  - Coarctation of aorta
  - Endocardial fibroelastosis
  - Pulmonary artery atrophy
- Skeletal
  - Aplasia or ankylosis of joints
  - Synostosis of radius and humerus
  - Short humerus
  - Cervical spine fusion
- Pulmonary
  - Pulmonary aplasia
  - Cartilaginous anomalies
  - Tracheoesophageal fistula
- Gastrointestinal
  - Pyloric stenosis
  - Ectopic anus
- Renal
  - Polycystic kidney
  - Hydronephrosis
- CNS
  - Mental retardation
  - Hearing deficit

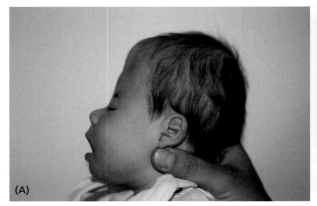
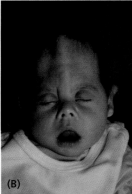

Figure 32.8 Infant with Saethre–Chotzen syndrome. (A) Brachycephaly. (B) Metopic ridge due to premature synostosis and turricephaly.

maxillary hypoplasia, and shallow orbits that lead to ocular proptosis and a beaked nose. Besides coronal synostosis, scaphocephaly, trigonocephaly, and cloverleaf skull may also exist. Skull base abnormalities with platybasia and Chiari malformations are also found. Due to the midfacial deformities, nasopharyngeal airway obstruction is common and may lead to sleep apnea and impaired nose breathing.

The prevalence of Crouzon syndrome is one per 25,000 livebirths, with about two-thirds of cases being familial (autosomal dominant) and one-third sporadic. Neuro-cognitive development is rarely affected.

Cloverleaf skull (Kleeblattschädel)

The cloverleaf skull deformity is the most severe form of craniostenosis and is most often associated with Pfeiffer syndrome. All major sutures and the skull base are involved which produces marked constriction of intracranial structures, including the rapidly developing brain and its vessels, especially important venous structures. Early surgery is mandatory to protect the brain. Chiari malformation and hydrocephalus are common accompaniments of this lesion and need to be treated early as well. Other deformities are hypertelorism, orbital proptosis with visual impairment, and a hypoplastic skull base and midface structures that produce upper airway problems.

Other relatively common craniofacial syndromes are Jackson–Weiss and Carpenter or Antler–Bixler syndrome.

Facial anomalies

Branchial arch malformations

Branchial arch anomalies are symptom complexes caused by deficient development of the branchial arches. They are etiologically and pathogenetically heterogeneous [12] with wide variability in expression. External ear deficiencies, auricular tags, and persistent branchial clefts or cysts are common branchial arch anomalies. Micro- or macrostomia results from abnormal merging of the maxillary and mandibular prominences. These abnormalities are examples of severe first arch anomalies. Micrognathia, also a first arch anomaly, is the result of retarded mandibular development by any mechanism; it may be an intrinsic malformation or a deformation by the chin being compressed against the chest late in gestation.

Treacher Collins syndrome (mandibulofacial dysostosis)

Treacher Collins syndrome (TCS) occurs with an incidence of one in 50,000 livebirths and involves structures derived from the first and second branchial arches [12]. The major facial features include midface hypoplasia, micrognathia, microtia, conductive hearing loss, and a cleft palate that is caused by deficiencies of maxillary and branchial arch mesenchyme. The syndrome can be an autosomal dominant disorder with variable expressivity, but over 50% of cases are new mutations. The gene responsible for this syndrome has been mapped to chromosome 5q31.3–32. The mutation causes aberrant expression of a nucleolar protein named treacle. The abnormalities are bilateral, usually symmetrical, and con-

---

Box 32.3 Features of Treacher Collins syndrome

Facial dysmorphia

- Skeletal hypoplasia/aplasia
  - Malar and zygomatic bones
  - Supraorbital ridges
  - Mandible
- Facial muscle hypoplasia/hypotonia
- Eye
  - Lower lid coloboma or notching
  - Partial absence of lower eyelashes
  - Antimongoloid slant to palpebral fissures
- Ears
  - Auricle malformation, misplacement
  - Ear canal defects, conductive deafness
  - Inner ear malformations
  - Nonpneumatized mastoid
- Pharyngeal hypoplasia
- Dental malocclusion
- High arched palate
- Projection of scalp hair onto lateral cheek
- Bind fistulas, dimples, or tags between the ears and angle of the mouth

Occasional abnormalities

- Macrostomia
- Microstomia
- Cleft palate
- Velopharyngeal incompetence
- Upper eyelid coloboma
- Choanal atresia
- Microphthalmia
- Absence of parotid gland
- Congenital heart disease
- Mental deficiency not common

---

fined to the craniofacial complex (Box 32.3; Fig. 32.9). Besides the facial features, the patients often have choanal atresia, microphthalmia, absence of the parotid gland(s), and congenital heart disease. Mental deficiency is not common.

The characteristic facial appearance is the product of an abnormal cranial base and a dysmorphic mandible and maxillary-malar complex [26]. The face is narrow, with down-sloping palpebral fissures, depressed cheekbones, and a large down-turned mouth. The cranial base angle (nasion-sella-basion angle) is reduced, which positions the posterior pharynx forward. The pharyngeal dimensions are reduced in all dimensions by several hypoplastic skeletal elements [26–28]. Some patients also exhibit a discrete area of constriction near the base of the tongue, such as occurred in an 11-year-old patient whose pharyngeal lumen was 5mm wide [27]. Little correlation exists between the degree of pharyngeal hypoplasia and the

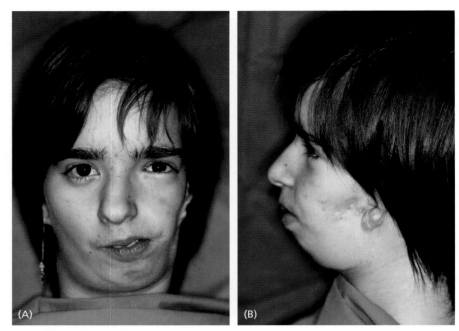

Figure 32.9 Fifteen-year-old girl with mandibulofacial dysostosis. She has no mental but has malar deficiencies, auricle malformation, microtia and retrognathic mandible.

severity of the facial deformity. The malar (cheek) bone is hypoplastic and the orbital wall is deficient. The mandible is disfigured in all dimensions.

Nager and Miller syndromes are characterized by facial features that are similar to those of Treacher Collins plus limb deformities.

Robin sequence
The Pierre Robin sequence (PRS – MIM 261800) is a well-defined subgroup of the CL/P (cleft lip and/or palate) population with an unknown etiology of the branchial arch. PRS is characterized by cleft palate, micrognathia and respiratory difficulties (due to glossoptosis) in the early neonatal period, and is often observed as a part of other mendelian syndromes such as Stickler syndrome, velocardiofacial syndrome and Marshall syndrome or fetal alcohol syndromes [29,30]. PRS is also a part of campomelic dysplasia (CD – MIM 114290), consisting of bowing of the long bones, malformation of the pelvis and spine, rib anomalies, club feet, hypoplastic scapulae, micrognathia, and cleft palate [31]. In a "sequence," some anomalies are secondary to a primary anomaly, whereas in a syndrome, multiple anomalies have a single pathogenesis. The PRS may be the result of deregulation of *SOX9* and *KCNJ2* [32]. The pathogenesis of the Robin sequence is diverse, but the common feature is failure of mandibular development and secondary failure of the tongue to descend from between the palatal shelves. When this is an isolated finding, the deformity may be due to intrauterine mandibular constraint. The mandible is intrinsically normal and will undergo catch-up growth postnatally [6]. If the Robin sequence is associated with a syndrome that includes intrinsic mandibular hypoplasia, the mandible remains small.

Oculo-auriculovertebral spectrum: Goldenhar syndrome and hemifacial microsomia
The oculo-auriculovertebral spectrum (OAVS) is also known as the first and second branchial arch syndrome, hemifacial microsomia, Goldenhar syndrome or facio-auriculovertebral syndrome. This condition is caused by maldevelopment of the first and second branchial arches and is complex and heterogeneous. There is defective facial development involving the ear, eye, zygomatic bone, mandible, parotid gland, tongue, and facial muscles. Maldevelopment is not limited to facial structures: cardiac (tetralogy of Fallot, ventricular septal defect), pulmonary (hypoplasia or aplasia of lung), renal, skeletal (vertebral anomalies, commonly cervical), central structures (cranial nerve anomalies) and other anomalies, including laryngeal anomalies, also occur. The abnormalities present in various combinations, tend to be asymmetrical and are unilateral in 70% of cases [20]. Malformations of the external ear or microtia are mandatory features of the OAVS and occur as an isolated malformation (population frequency of 0.03%), or in association with other anomalies such as mandible hypoplasia, epibulbar dermoids, and spinal vertebral defects. The constellation of anomalies

suggests that they originate at approximately 30–45 days of gestation.

It has been suggested that disturbances in the branchial arches or in neural crest cells impede development of adjacent tissues. A vascular pathogenesis caused by hematoma formation at the time the stapedial artery system develops has been demonstrated in animals [33]. In this model, focal hemorrhage and an expanding hematoma destroy tissues in the ear and jaw areas. Three unrelated children have been reported with similar unilateral craniofacial defects and other structural abnormalities that had a known disruptive vascular pathogenesis [34]. The frequency of occurrence is estimated to be one in 3000–5000 births. The condition is usually sporadic, although familial instances have been reported. Several chromosomal anomalies have been associated with this condition, and it has occurred in infants born to mothers who had taken thalidomide, primidone or retinoic acid. It is usually discordant in monozygotic twins.

Maxillary, mandibular, and auricular hypoplasia is the primary feature of this syndrome. Macrostomia is the result of a lateral facial cleft from the commissure of the mouth. Mandibular condyle deformities, present in all patients, range from slight hypoplasia to complete absence of the condyle with agenesis of the ascending ramus. When accompanied by epibulbar dermoid and vertebral anomalies, it is called the Goldenhar syndrome, and when it occurs predominantly unilaterally it is called hemifacial microsomia. Most of these patients have normal intelligence.

Hypertelorism and orbital malposition

Orbital malposition may occur in any direction and may involve different directions in each orbit. The bones and sutures making up the walls of the orbits may be primarily involved. The malposition may also be the result of craniosynostosis or craniofacial clefting. It may be associated with encephalocele, tumor, or other cranio-orbital malformations. Other cranio-orbital malformations include encephaloceles that involve craniofacial structures; frontoethmoidal or sincipital and basal subtypes (nasofrontal, nasoethmoidal, naso-orbital and transethmoidal) [35]. These malformations lead to significant naso-orbital deformities (Figs 32.10, 32.11). One of the most disfiguring tumors of the orbital region is the plexiform neurofibroma that is associated with neurofibromatosis type 1. Isolated orbital hypertelorism is a skeletal deformity that consists of lateralization of the bony orbit and enlarged ethmoid sinuses. The nose may be slightly involved or severely distorted, and the nasal deformity may be difficult to correct. Dysfunction of the upper eyelid, extraocular muscles, and lacrimal system frequently occurs. Orbital hypotelorism is uncommon

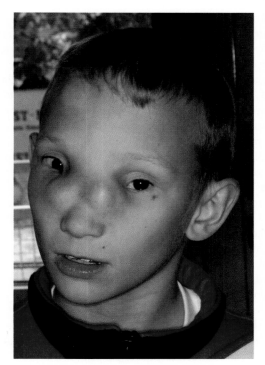

Figure 32.10 Twelve-year-old boy with frontoethmoidal encephalocele with maxillary involvement and hypertelorism.

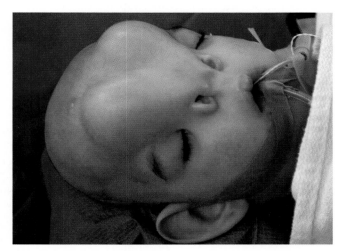

Figure 32.11 Infant with frontonasal cleft and related encephaloceles and hypertelorism.

and is seldom present as an isolated anomaly. It is often seen in metopic craniosynostosis.

Facial clefts

Facial clefting occurs when the skeleton or soft tissues are interrupted. Clefts develop when the facial prominences fail to merge. Clefts that cannot be explained embryologically may be caused by disruptive factors [12]. The causes of most clefts are unknown, and the majority occur sporadically. Skeletal and soft tissue hypo- or aplasia are the anatomical defects of craniofacial clefts. Any part of the cranium or face may be involved. Various combinations of eye, ear, and central nervous system (CNS) deformities are associated with clefts.

Tessier devised an anatomical and descriptive classification that correlates clinical appearance with surgical anatomical findings [36]. This system designates 15 locations (numbered 0 through 14) for clefts and describes their respective courses through bone and soft tissue (Fig. 32.12). Many syndromes that include hypoplastic facial dysmorphology are categorized as clefts. Treacher Collins syndrome includes clefts 6, 7, and 8 in its complete form (see Fig. 32.9) and cleft 6 in its incomplete form. Cleft 6 accounts for the eyelid coloboma, cleft 7 the absence of the zygomatic arch, anterior displacement of the scalp hair, and mandible deformities, and cleft 8 the defects in the lateral orbital rim. The oculo-auriculovertebral spectrum (hemifacial microsomia, Goldenhar) is cleft 7.

Cleft lip and palate

Cleft lip and/or palate are the most frequent congenital craniofacial malformations. They occur in one in 700 births in the United States, and there is a marked racial predilection. The highest incidence is found in parts of Latin America and Asia (China, Japan), the lowest in Israel, South Africa, and southern Europe. Rates of isolated cleft palate are high in Canada and parts of northern Europe and low in parts of Latin America and South Africa [9]. Clefts may be isolated, familial or part of a syndrome. More than 400 syndromes are associated with facial clefts [12]. Cleft lip, cleft palate or both can be part of a syndrome, but more syndromes are associated with cleft palate than with cleft lip. They constitute a heterogeneous group of malformations with great variability in the degree of cleft formation (Fig. 32.13). A cleft lip may be complete, incomplete or only a microform with a small

vermillion notch. Osseous defects in the alveolus and the palate of patients with complete labial clefts contribute to instability of the dental arch; sometimes there is collapse of the lateral segments of the arch. For cleft classification, Kriens proposed the LAHSHAL code to represent clefts of the left and right (L)ip, (A)lveolus, as well as (H)ard

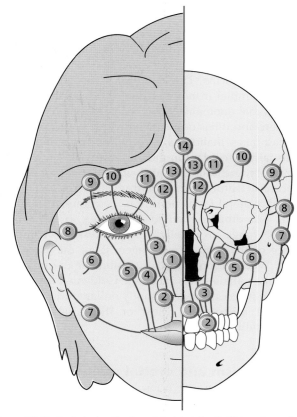

Figure 32.12 Tessier's classification of facial clefts. (*Left*) Locations of clefts on the face. (*Right*) Skeletal pathways.

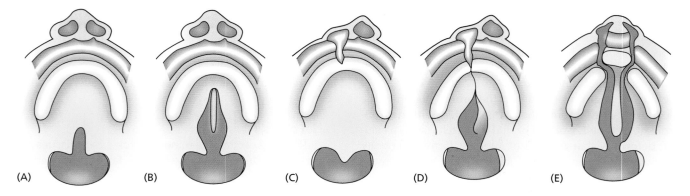

Figure 32.13 Various degrees of cleft palate and lip. (A) Cleft soft palate. (B) Cleft hard and soft palate. (C) Cleft lip and alveolus. (D) Complete unilateral. (E) Complete bilateral.

and (S)oft palate based on the anatomical structures involved [37].

The etiology of clefting is multifactorial and has both genetic and environmental influences. The genes associated with orofacial clefting identified to date are those for non-syndromic cleft lip/palate *MSX1* (chromosome 4p16.1), and *TBX22* (chromosome Xq12-q21). Cleft palate genes are located on chromosome 14 and a locus for cleft lip (IRF6) on chromosome 1q [38,39]. Development of the upper lip and the palate is completed by postconceptional weeks 7 and 9. Maternal smoking during this time increases the risk of clefting by approximately 1.3 times.

The risk for oral clefting may be as high as 20% in some subgroups with maternal smoking (e.g. American Indians/Alaskan natives). Alcohol consumption, poor nutrition (folic acid and vitamin A deficiency), viral infection, medical drugs (e.g. anticonvulsant drugs; diazepam, phenytoin, phenobarbital, carbamazepine; retinoids; systemic corticosteroids), diabetes mellitus, and teratogenic agents (organic solvents, agricultural chemicals) also increase the risk of clefting [40].

Clefting of the upper lip and nostril is the result of failure of the nasomedial process to merge with the maxillary prominences (lateral cleft lip, either uni- or bilateral) or from failure of the two-nasomedial processes to merge (rare median cleft lip or bifid nose). Hypoplasia of the palatal shelves or mistiming of palatal shelf elevation results in cleft palate. Failure to remove the tongue from between the shelves and problems with shelf elevation and contact probably account for most human cleft palates [19]. There may be a critical time in gestation beyond which the palatal shelves cannot meet and fuse. If movement of the palatal shelves from vertical to horizontal is delayed and the head continues to grow, a widening gap is produced between the shelves, and they cannot meet. Clefting of the palate may or may not be associated with a cleft upper lip because the two conditions are separate developmental entities. However, failure of lip fusion may impair subsequent closure of the palatal shelves.

Physiological sequelae of craniofacial malformations

Hydrocephalus and intracranial pressure

In a retrospective review of 1727 patients treated over 20 years, hydrocephalus occurred in patients with non-syndromic craniosynostosis (1447 patients) with similar frequency to that observed in the normal population (0.3%) [41]. In patients with syndromic craniosynostosis, the frequency was 12%. Patients with Kleeblattschädel deformity and Crouzon syndrome were more likely to

have hydrocephalus than those with other syndromes. Jugular foramen stenosis and crowding of the posterior fossa are two primary factors responsible for hydrocephalus in syndromic craniosynostosis [41]. Fusion of cranial base synchondroses produces alterations in the skull base and stenosis of the jugular foramen. The resulting venous hypertension increases the CSF hydrostatic pressure. If major calvarial sutures are open, the head will progressively enlarge and the ventricles and subarachnoid spaces will dilate. If the calvarial sutures are fused, intracranial pressure will increase but ventriculomegaly may not occur until after the synostosis is surgically released. When the posterior fossa is small and crowded, especially if the lambdoidal suture is fused, cerebellar tonsillar herniation or compression of the basal cistern may produce obstructive hydrocephalus.

Intracranial pressure may be elevated without hydrocephalus in patients with craniosynostosis. Presumably, a restrictive cranium is a factor. Renier [42] monitored intracranial pressure during sleep in 350 non-hydrocephalic patients with unoperated craniosynostosis (Table 32.3). The patients ranged in age from 6 weeks to 15 years, and 44% were less than 1 year old. The overall rate of intracranial hypertension was 23% but the proportion varied by type of craniosynostosis and age. For single sagittal synostoses (trigono- and scaphocephaly), the rates were 6% and 8%, respectively. The rate was 12% for single synostoses of a coronal suture (anterior plagiocephaly). Other authors have also reported elevated intracranial pressure with single-suture synostosis, which, in addition to cosmetics, provides a rationale for surgical correction [43,44].

In Renier's study, 26% of patients with synostoses of both coronal sutures (brachycephaly, excluding Apert

Table 32.3 Intracranial pressure before surgery

	Total no. of patients	Baseline ICP (mmHg)		
		≤10	11–15	>15
Trigonocephaly	31	21	8	2
Scaphocephaly	118	76	33	9
Plagiocephaly	65	40	17	8
Brachycephaly	34	17	8	9
Oxycephaly	66	23	7	36
Crouzon syndrome	9	3	0	6
Apert syndrome	16	3	6	7

Modified from Renier D. Intracranial pressure in craniosynostosis: pre- and postoperative recordings-correlation with functional results. In Persing JA, Edgerton MT, Jane JA (eds). Scientific Foundations and Surgical Treatment of Craniosynostosis. Baltimore: Williams & Wilkins, 1989, p 264, with permission.

and Crouzon syndromes) had intracranial hypertension. In extensive synostoses, usually involving both coronal and sagittal sutures (oxycephaly), intracranial hypertension occurred in 54% of patients. In Renier's study, the incidence of intracranial hypertension also increased with age. After 1 year of age, the incidence was four times greater for scaphocephaly and double for plagiocephaly. With brachycephaly, intracranial hypertension was more precocious: 22% of children below 1 year of age had intracranial hypertension compared with 31% over 1 year of age. Oxycephaly is usually not seen before 3 years of age, but can also be seen in very young infants, e.g. in syndromic forms. Eighty-five percent of children with oxycephaly had intracranial hypertension. However, clinical signs and symptoms of elevated intracranial pressure were uncommon. Intracranial volume measurements calculated from computed tomography (CT) scans were not a reliable indication of intracranial pressure (ICP), although markedly reduced intracranial volume did increase the likelihood of intracranial hypertension [43]. Raised intracranial pressure is also of concern after surgical correction and consecutive inappropriate skull growth and should be monitored in patients and followed up by regular ophthalmological examinations to rule out papilledema at least until 8–10 years of age. Papilledema may not be present despite significantly elevated ICP. In children without papilledema, ICP measurements may be indicated to rule out intracranial hypertension. These older children often complain of chronic headache.

In non-syndromic forms of craniosynostosis where the abnormality is confined to the calvarium, the effects of cranial vault expansion are predictable. In complex craniosynostosis, however, the effects are less certain. In Renier's series, 54 patients had postoperative ICP measurements. Before surgery the ICP was elevated in 74% and borderline in 11% of patients. After surgery 7% had elevated and 20% had borderline ICP. In another series 22 patients had their ICP monitored postoperatively. The ICP was elevated in 45% and borderline in 32% [45]. In this series, 34 patients with complex craniosynostosis were evaluated with magnetic resonance imaging (MRI) up to 8 years after surgery. Cerebellar tonsillar herniation was found in 52% and hydrocephalus in 41% percent of patients, over half of whom developed the hydrocephalus after surgery. During follow-up, tonsillar herniation or Chiari malformation can develop as sequelae of insufficient intracranial space. Another report covering a 20-year period noted that the incidence of postoperative hydrocephalus was 45% for patients with syndromes and 4% for patients with isolated craniosynostosis. The incidence of shunt placement was 22% and 1% respectively [46,47].

Upper airway obstruction

Severe malformations involving the face and cranial base are at high risk for upper airway obstruction and undetected obstructive sleep apnea (OSA). Almost 50% of patients with craniofacial dysostosis develop OSA and require airway intervention at some time [48–50]. OSA can be treated pharmacologically, non-surgically (CPAP, nasopharyngeal tube) or surgically, depending on its severity and cause [17,51]. Fifty percent of patients with craniofacial dysostosis are treated with tracheostomy, but nearly 7% in the early and 5% in the late postoperative phase have complications [52–56]. Beside a high incidence of tracheal cartilaginous sleeve, laryngomalacia, tracheomalacia and bronchomalacia, a reduced cranial base angle positions the pharyngeal wall forward and produces anteroposterior shortening of the nasal and oral airway [28]. In addition, the temporomandibular joint may be drawn posteriorly so that the mandible is positioned retrusively [29]. When the mandible is small and retrognathic (e.g. Pierre Robin sequence), the tongue is positioned posteriorly and impinges on the oro- and hypopharynx [26]. Midface hypoplasia and reposition also diminish the dimensions of the nasal airway. Neurological dysfunction, such as pharyngeal hypotonia or inco-ordination, worsens airway obstruction in children with abnormal anatomy [57]. Other skeletal abnormalities, such as turbinate hypertrophy, septal deviation, and choanal narrowing or atresia (e.g. CHARGE syndrome), contribute to upper airway obstruction.

Obstructive sleep apnea is common in craniofacial syndromes [27,28,58–61]. Sher and colleagues [58] used flexible fiber-optic nasopharyngoscopy to identify the mechanisms of pharyngeal obstruction in patients with OSA. Four mechanisms were identified.

1. Posterior movement of the tongue against the posterior pharyngeal wall (Fig. 32.14).
2. Posterior movement of the tongue with compression of the soft palate or cleft palatal tags posteriorly against the posterior pharyngeal wall; the tongue, velum, and posterior pharyngeal wall meet in the upper oropharynx.
3. Movement of the lateral pharyngeal walls medially to appose each other.
4. Pharyngeal constriction in a circular or sphincteric manner.

Sleep apnea may occur from brainstem compression in children with Chiari malformation.

Some patients are successfully managed with nasal continuous positive airway pressure (nCPAP) during sleep [60]. Others with severe airway obstruction may require tracheostomy. Of 251 patients with craniofacial anomalies who underwent surgery over a 5-year period, 20% required tracheostomy to relieve chronic airway obstruction or to

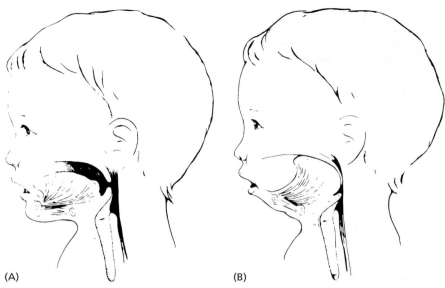

(A)   (B)

Figure 32.14 Anatomical features of the larynx. (A) Normal child. (B) Child with mandibular hypoplasia. Posterior placement of tongue makes the larynx appear to be more anteriorly situated than normal. Reproduced from Handler SD et al. Ann Otol Rhinol Laryngol 1993; 92: 401 with permission from Annals Publishing Company.

manage the airway in the perioperative period [62]. Patients with craniofacial synostosis (Crouzon, Pfeiffer or Apert syndromes) had the highest rate of tracheostomy (48%). Those with mandibular facial dysostosis (Treacher Collins or Nager syndromes) had the next highest rate (41%). Twenty-two percent of patients with oculo-auriculovertebral sequence (Goldenhar and hemifacial microsomia) required tracheostomy. The mean duration of cannulation in infancy or in early childhood was 4 years. Patients who had tracheostomy after 4 years of age required cannulation for less than 6 months, and 60% underwent decannulation 1 week after tracheostomy.

Ear, nose and throat consultation is recommended to determine if an adenoidectomy or tonsillectomy is required prior to craniofacial surgery. Some cases of sleep apnea are effectively treated by adenotonsillectomy.

Patients with Robin sequence, especially non-syndromic patients, who have airway obstruction that is unresponsive to prone or lateral positioning alone respond to nasopharyngeal/nasotracheal intubation or glossopexy (tongue-lip adhesion, TLA). These procedures often relieve airway obstruction during the first months of life while the mandible grows and the airway expands [57,63,64]. In some syndromes (e.g. Treacher Collins and Apert), the anatomical inter-relationships become progressively distorted and the obstruction may worsen, not improve [26,58,65]. To minimize morbidity, the least invasive treatment should be used first. If conservative treatment, including wearing a soft palate plaque (e.g. Tübinger type) [66], does not resolve the problem, further management should be based on the oxygen saturation,

feeding difficulties, and endoscopic findings. A more aggressive approach is the TLA or a perimandibular fixed extension device. Distraction osteogenesis can be used in older children [67]. Finally, if all else fails, a tracheostomy might be indicated.

Associated anomalies

With syndromic craniofacial anomalies, many systems may be malformed, particularly the CNS, the cardiac, and pulmonary systems. Cranial sensory and speech organs can also be malformed, and hearing, vision, and speech may be impaired. Cervical spine anomalies, including intervertebral fusion, occur commonly in Goldenhar syndrome and with craniosynostosis syndromes such as Crouzon, Apert, and Pfeiffer [68–70].

Craniofacial reconstruction: surgical procedures

Paul Tessier introduced major craniofacial surgery in Paris in 1967. He developed the first craniofacial dysjunction procedures that cleaved the face away from the base of the cranium by using both an intracranial and an extracranial approach [71,72]. Over the past 40 years, these techniques have been used to treat a variety of complex congenital and acquired deformities of the face and cranium, including traumatic and neoplastic entities [73]. A co-ordinated interdisciplinary approach is required for this surgery to succeed. There are many reasons for doing the surgery, including improving neurological,

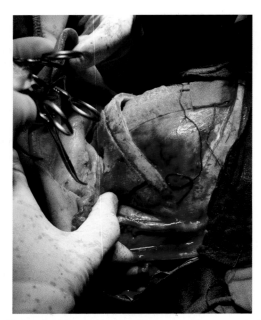

Figure 32.15 After bicoronal incision for intracranial upper and midface procedures, the face is peeled back for wide exposure of the facial skeleton bone.

ocular, nasal, dental and auditory functions as well as improving cosmetic appearance and psychological function [74]. The basic objective of craniofacial surgery is to correct skeletal deformity first and soft tissue afterwards. The basic treatment of the deformed skeleton comprises cutting, disjoining, mobilizing, repositioning, augmenting, and fixing the involved bony structures. Wide exposure of the skeleton is required. Therefore, the soft tissues, including the orbital contents, are extensively dissected and mobilized away from their bony attachments. Intracranial and extracranial approaches are utilized and scalp, pre-auricular, and intraoral incisions are made to avoid producing scars on the face. For intracranial and for upper and midface procedures, the surgical approach is through a bicoronal scalp incision that extends from ear to ear and from which the soft tissues of the scalp and face are reflected forward over the facial mass (Fig. 32.15). This provides wide exposure of the facial skeleton down to the maxillary alveolus. A craniotomy is done, the frontal lobes of the brain are retracted, and the anterior cranial base is exposed. To effectively provide anesthesia for major craniofacial surgery, the anesthesiologist must clearly understand both the lesion and the proposed surgical procedure.

Cranial and facial remodeling

Surgery for cranial and facial remodeling is performed with the goal of normalizing the child's appearance, ensuring sufficient head size and growth, and establishing normal function of the skull structures and related

organs. In most cases, these aims cannot be fully met but significant improvement is possible. In the past, surgical techniques were employed that often did not take into account the substantial variations in the underlying pathology, the patient's age, and the skill of the surgical team. The first technique employed was to open the fused suture, with the hope that this would allow normal skull growth. In the past this method was not successful but recently Jimenez has had success with the procedure [75]. Since it became evident that cranial growth follows intrinsic pathways rather than mechanical rules, the entire cranial vault, including the skull base structures, have been addressed surgically. Whenever the fronto-orbital region is involved, additional maneuvers, such as fronto-orbital advancement, have been used to improve facial appearance and enlarge the intracranial and orbital cavity. In multisuture craniosynostosis, restricted skull growth and potential brain and orbital constriction are the major reasons for early surgery. In addition to fronto-orbital advancement and cranial vault remodeling, posterior distraction surgery can be an option.

In principle, the main surgical goals for these patients comprise three steps: opening of the cranial vault to allow the brain to expand, fronto-orbital advancement to ensure frontal brain expansion and eye protection, and midface advancement to improve nasopharyngeal pathways and dental alignment. Additional procedures may be necessary for orbital malposition and facial clefts.

The typical skin opening for cranial or craniofacial remodeling is a coronal incision. The incision can be straight, curved or zigzag to prevent visible scarring. Attempts should be made to minimize unnecessary blood loss when dividing the galea [76].

Timing and general preparation for surgery

Timing of craniofacial repair is often controversial. As long as there is sufficient head growth, as occurs in most single-suture craniosynostoses and other craniofacial disorders that do not involve the cranial vault, surgery is scheduled in the second half of the first year, usually between 6 and 8 months of age. At that time, the hematological status is stabilized and the bony structures are firmer and easier to remodel than at younger ages. All systemic functions are checked to minimize the overall risk.

Multisuture craniosynostoses can lead to severe skull constriction and require early or even emergency procedures to relieve ICP; elevated ICP significantly increases the risks of surgery and anesthesia. These patients require early evaluation for cardiac, kidney, airway, and hematological disorders.

Parents must be informed about all aspects of craniofacial surgery, including early and late changes in the esthetic appearance of their child, potential surgical risks (mainly blood loss and the need for transfusion of blood and coagulation factors), and the possibility of infection. They should be prepared for significant facial swelling during the first postoperative days, but should also be assured that brain damage and severe complications are rare despite the extent of the surgical procedure. Long-term follow-up is important to detect late intracranial hypertension or recurrent deformity, both of which may require reoperation.

Craniectomy

The principle of craniectomy is to remove a piece of the cranial vault to permit directional skull expansion. Several forms of craniectomy have been used from simple suturectomy, to strip craniectomies, to wide vertex craniectomies in scaphocephalic patients. Barrel stave incisions and lateral strip craniectomies have been utilized to promote lateral skull expansion. Total removal of the cranial vault has been performed, with acceptable outcomes in some cases. Since craniectomies require spontaneous bone regeneration to reshape the skull and protect the brain, these techniques are not recommended in children older than 8–10 months of age.

Strip craniectomy improves craniofacial contour only for isolated sagittal synostosis. For other synostoses, removing, reshaping, and repositioning bone accomplish cranial remodeling. Cranial remodeling may involve any part of the cranium or the entire cranial vault. For complex craniosynostoses that involve the cranial base and face, the sutures involved are commonly those of the anterior cranial vault (coronal, sagittal or metopic sutures) as well as the anterior cranial base (frontosphenoidal, frontoethmoidal, and sphenozygomatic sutures). The surgery releases sutures and advances the upper part of the face forward (fronto-obital advancement) away from the cranial base (Fig 32.16). The principal functional objectives of the surgery are to open the cranium to allow normal brain expansion, to open the nasopharyngeal airway, to provide greater support and protection for the eyes, and to achieve proper alignment of the upper and lower dental arches. This surgery usually requires at least two steps: (1) frontocranial remodeling, with release of the synostosis and advancement of the frontal-supraorbital area, and (2) midface advancement. The segments are fixed in place with wires or resorbable/non-resorbable miniplates, and bone grafts are used to fill gaps. In some cases the forehead is left "floating" with a wide osseous defect.

Cranial vault reconstruction

Total or partial reconstruction of the cranial vault is the method of choice when reshaping and stability of the skull are the aim of the operation. Vault craniotomies are performed and the bony plates are remodeled and transposed to reshape the skull. Stable fixation of bone with wire loops, stitches or miniplates (either titanium or lactic acid polymer) is necessary. Titanium miniplates tend to grow inwards and must be removed after 3 months. Cranial expansion is another surgical aim of total cranial vault reconstruction. Again, cranial plates are excised, transposed, and refixed, leaving substantial gaps in between the bone edges, but the intracranial cavity is enlarged [77]. This technique is indicated for children with multisuture involvement or secondary intracranial hypertension, e.g. after scaphocephaly correction. Larger bone defects (>2 cm) will not close spontaneously after the second year of life, making it necessary to do this surgery before that time. Defects in the calvarium can be filled with autologous grafts, e.g. calvarian split grafts. Children with severe occipital deformity or flattening, e.g. in brachyturricephalic heads, undergo occipital advancement, including a suboccipital bone flap. For mechanical reasons a rigid fixation is necessary.

Fronto-orbital advancement

For anterior skull expansion and correction of the orbital portion, the fronto-orbital advancement has been the standard technique since first described by Tessier and modified by Marchac [78,79]. First a bifrontal flap is excised and removed, then the fronto-orbital bandeau, cutting the edges in a tongue-and-groove fashion. In trigonocephaly or anterior plagiocephaly, the bandeau and the frontal bones are reshaped and sometimes rotated to create the desired fronto-orbital shape. Refixation of bone may be with wire loops, miniplates or tight stitches in older children. In multisuture synostoses, when the primary goal is to enlarge the cranial cavity, fronto-orbital advancement is combined with total vault reconstruction. Shallow orbits are always enlarged to protect the eyes (Fig. 32.17).

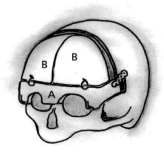

Figure 32.16 Fronto-orbital advancement. Both frontal bone flaps (B) or a coherent bifrontal flap are displaced forward together with the fronto-orbital bandeau (A). Rigid fixation with miniplates or wire loops or tight suturing keeps the bone segments in place.

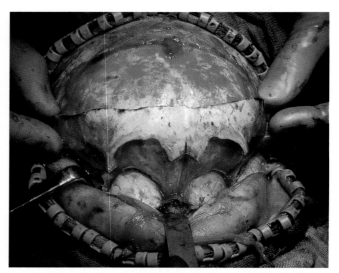

Figure 32.17 During fronto-orbital advancement, the primary goal is the enlargement of the cranial cavity which is combined with total vault reconstruction. After that both orbits are exposed.

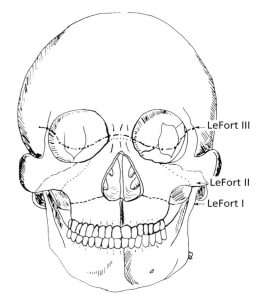

Figure 32.18 Le Fort I, II, and III osteotomies.

Distraction osteosynthesis

Another method of enlarging the volume of the skull is based on the Ilizarov principle of bone distraction. For midface and mandibular correction, distraction osteosynthesis has become standard. The application of distracting devices to transected vault sutures or parts of bone flaps for dynamic skull expansion is less well established.

Additional neurosurgical procedures

Hydrocephalus is relatively common in multisuture or syndromic craniosynostosis and contributes to the elevated intracranial pressure. Ventriculoperitoneal shunting is the procedure of choice in these cases, but interferes with keeping cranial sutures or newly created gaps open as long as possible after cranioplasty procedures. Alternatively, an endoscopic third ventriculostomy can be done in selected cases.

As a consequence of insufficient skull growth, the expanding brain moves downward and causes a Chiari malformation with brainstem compression and secondary hydrocephalus. In some of the affected children, a craniocervical decompression (Gardner decompression) becomes necessary.

Midface advancement

Craniofacial dysjunction and midface advancement are delayed until the patient is at least 4 or 5 years of age. Certain indications or personal preferences lead surgeons to select a specific operative procedure, which usually includes a Le Fort osteotomy (Fig. 32.18). At the begin-

ning of the 20th century, a French surgeon, René le Fort, found that the maxilla, naso-orbital complex, and zygoma fracture in predictable ways at weak points, i.e. the linea minoris resistentiae [80]. These fracture lines are used to produce controlled osteotomies for the correction of skeletal anomalies.

The Le Fort 1 osteotomy is the most common and most useful midface osteotomy (Fig. 32.19). Malocclusion of the teeth is always present and is treated by an interdisciplinary team of maxillofacial surgeons and orthodontists. Surgery is performed through an intraoral incision. Horizontal cuts are made across the nasal floor, the anterior maxilla, and through the pterygomaxillary junction. The maxilla is mobilized downward, advanced, and fixed. The occlusion is secured by arch bars and by a dental splint. Because of the intraoperative intermaxillary fixation, nasotracheal intubation is required. Bone grafts can be used to fill the spaces.

Le Fort II osteotomy is done less often and is used to advance the lower maxilla and entire nose forward (Fig. 32.20). Normally a bicoronal scalp incision and soft tissue reflection are combined with an intraoral incision to expose the midface. There are many variations of midface osteotomies. The osteotomy crosses the nasal bridge and then goes bilaterally down the lateral nasal bones through the inferior orbital rim and across the maxilla to the pterygomaxillary junction. The segment is mobilized and advanced. Bone defects are filled with bone grafts, and the entire segment is fixed with rigid miniplates or wires. Intermaxillary fixation is not really needed when rigid internal fixation plates are used.

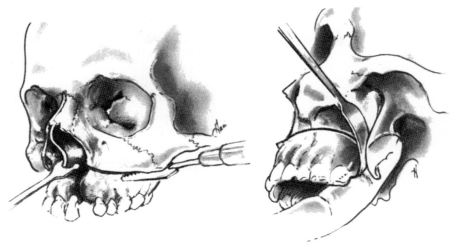

Figure 32.19 Le Fort I osteotomies. Reproduced from Bardach J, Salyer KE. Surgical Techniques in Cleft Lip and Palate, 2nd edn. St Louis: Mosby Year Book, 1991, p.251 with permission.

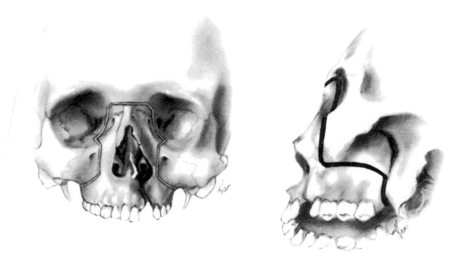

Figure 32.20 Le Fort II osteotomies. Reproduced from Bardach J, Salyer KE. Surgical Techniques in Cleft Lip and Palate, 2nd edn. St Louis: Mosby Year Book, 1991, p.255 with permission.

Midface hypoplasia typically results in an Angle class III malocclusion (a relative mandibular prognathia) with an anterior overbite. A Le Fort III osteotomy is indicated, but an additional Le Fort I osteotomy is often necessary to achieve an intermaxillary relationship that enables stable occlusion. Le Fort III osteotomy (Fig. 32.21) is used for complete underdevelopment of the midface, typical of Apert, Crouzon, Pfeiffer and similar syndromes. It permits the nose, maxilla, and orbits to be advanced after dysjunction of the entire midface. A bicoronal scalp incision is made, the soft tissues are reflected forward over the midface, and the orbital contents are dissected free. The basic osteotomy starts at the frontozygomatic suture and then passes through the orbits below the supraorbital

rim and across the nasal bridge. The pterygomaxillary junctions are separated, and the nasal septum is separated from the skull base. The facial block is advanced after down-fracture and side-to-side and rotary manipulations (see Fig. 32.21). The spaces are filled with bone grafts and the bones are fixed in place. The use of rigid internal fixation plates precludes the need for intermaxillary fixation.

Monoblock frontofacial advancement moves the frontal and orbitofacial blocks forward simultaneously. While the early functional results are good, the complication rate is high and the poor postoperative midface growth makes a reoperation more difficult [81]. The supraorbital area and the facial mass are mobilized *en bloc* and

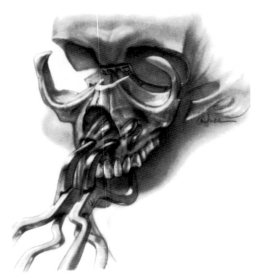

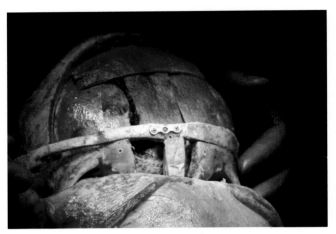

Figure 32.22 After osteotomies and removal of a central block of bone, the orbits are shifted medially. Orbits can be considered as boxes containing the eye. Each orbit can be moved in any plane.

Figure 32.21 Le Fort III osteotomy. Rowe disimpaction forceps are used to "down fracture" the posterior maxillary wall and allow advancement of the midface. Reproduced from Persing JA et al. Surgical treatment of craniosynostosis. In: Persing JA, Jane JA (eds) Scientific Foundations and Surgical Treatment of Craniosynostosis. Baltimore: Williams and Wilkins, 1989, p.229 with permission.

advanced. The frontal bone flap is remodeled when necessary, e.g. exorbitism.

Various combinations and modifications of these osteotomies are performed either simultaneously or in stages. The transverse maxillary osteotomies (Le Fort 1 and II) are usually delayed until adolescence to avoid disruption of the permanent dentition.

Pediatric temporomandibular joint (TMJ) dysfunction from soft tissue or skeletal disorders may be congenital or acquired. The diagnosis and classification of TMJ disorders determine treatment options [82]. In cases of TMJ reconstruction or discontinuity defects of the mandible after trauma, hemimandibulectomy for tumor excision, condylar damage with juvenile idiopathic arthritis or congenital diseases (e.g. hemifacial dysplasia), the goal is to maximize function and cosmesis, preserve quality of life, and restore mastication, speech, and appearance [83]. Treatment includes autogenous bony, cartilage, and condylar grafts, free vascularized flaps, or alloplastic TMJ prosthesis until the skeleton matures [84–87]. A variety of donor sites have been used for this purpose, including the iliac crest, radius, scapula, and fibula. TMJ diseases occurring during growth result in dentofacial deformity and require reconstruction of the occlusion plane. Surgical correction with total joint prostheses can be performed in a single-stage operation with a mono- or bimaxillary orthognathic osteotomy [88]. During surgery the occlusion has to be checked.

Surgical correction of hypertelorism and orbital malposition

Surgical correction of orbital malposition is performed to facilitate correction of strabismus, to normalize facial appearance, and to possibly achieve binocular vision. Surgery is usually performed at about 5 years of age unless there are mitigating circumstances. The orbit can be thought of as a box housing the eye. To correct hypertelorism or other orbital malposition, the box is freed from contiguous bone and repositioned (Fig. 32.22). In moderate and severe degrees of hypertelorism, an intracranial approach is employed: a bicoronal scalp incision is made; soft tissues, including orbital contents and nasal mucosa, are reflected down to midface; a frontal craniotomy is performed; and the frontal lobes of the brain are retracted to expose the anterior cranial fossa. Intra- and extraorbital osteotomies convert the anterior orbit into a mobile box (see Fig. 32.22). A central block of bone (frontal, nasal, ethmoidal) is removed from between the orbits. The orbits, with the globe and other soft tissues, are then moved medially and fixed in place (Fig. 32.23). Bone grafts are inserted into the gaps created at the lateral orbital walls. The nose is rebuilt with bone grafts if necessary. For minor degrees of hypertelorism, an extracranial approach is possible; this eliminates the frontal craniotomy and brain retraction. Extensive soft tissue dissection is still required, but the osteotomies are less extensive. There is also danger of piercing the cribriform plate and causing CSF leakage.

Reconstruction of facial clefts: major facial and mandibular malformations

The anatomical defects of the major facial and mandibular malformation syndromes are skeletal and soft

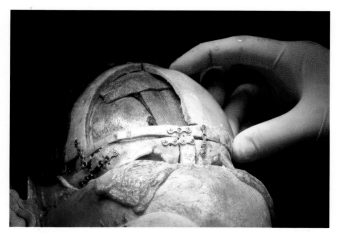

Figure 32.23 Orbits after medial shift and fixation with miniplates.

tissue hypoplasias. Hypoplasia may involve any part of the face and cranium. Reconstruction of these lesions often requires multiple staged surgical procedures. The skeleton must be normalized, the soft tissues augmented, ears and nose reconstructed, and sometimes the face must be reanimated. For the hypoplastic skeleton, displacement osteotomies, repositioning of bones into more normal positions, and calvarial bone grafts are used to augment surfaces and fill spaces.

Soft tissue hypoplasia can involve skin, subcutaneous tissue, cartilage, and the muscles of mastication and facial expression. Various approaches can be taken to augment and restructure soft tissues. Skin and mucosal flaps from local or distant sites may be used. To add bulk and appropriate contours, dermis fat grafts from the groin can be placed subcutaneously. Contour can also be improved with inlay bone grafts. Temporal muscle transfers to the face also add bulk. These procedures may require extensive dissection of soft tissue. Facial nerve palsy can be compensated for with nerve transfer from the motor branch of cranial nerve V; if the malformation is unilateral, cross-face nerve grafts, facial-hypoglossal nerve anastomosis, and microneuromuscle transfers can be attempted.

Traditionally, mandibular reconstruction has followed the same principles as other craniofacial procedures: cut, mobilize, reposition, augment, and fix. In the past the mandible was mobilized through an intraoral incision with bilateral sagittal osteotomies and rotated and advanced into a normal position. Distraction osteogenesis is now replacing the traditional method in many cases (see below). New mandibular parts are constructed from costochondral rib grafts or split cranial grafts. This surgery is usually done before eruption of the permanent teeth.

Distraction osteogenesis

Patients with severe craniofacial dysostosis who require early surgical correction of their deformity before skeletal maturity have clearly benefited from distraction osteogenesis (DO) compared to conventional osteotomy [89]. Distraction osteogenesis is done by producing a bone callus (by osteotomy) and then distracting the proximal and distal ends of the callus. It has been used by some orthopedic surgeons for years to lengthen limbs but did not gain widespread acceptance because of the associated morbidity. In 1988, Ilizarov, a Russian orthopedic surgeon, described using distraction osteogenesis that required only corticotomy and minimal disruption of the periosteum and endosteum; this reduced the incidence of complications and allowed wider application of the technique [90].

Rosenthal first described distraction osteogenesis for widening the mandible in 1930 [91]. Its principal application in craniofacial surgery is for mandibular lengthening [92]. The technique consists of percutaneous insertion of pins into the mandible that are proximal and distal to a corticotomy. The pins are attached to an external fixator-lengthening device, and the mandible is lengthened 1 mm/day by turning a bolt. The authors reported mandibular lengthening of 18–24 mm.

The procedure is considered minimally invasive and achieves an approximately 2–3-fold advancement compared to the conventional procedure. Using conventional osteotomy beyond the age of skeletal maturity has the advantage of a shorter treatment period and greater patient comfort. Distraction is often associated with less blood loss, less tissue exposure, and no need for bone grafting. With DO the postoperative morbidity is decreased, the operation time is reduced, and the procedure can be performed on younger children. Several authors believe that mandibular distraction also induces facial soft tissue growth [93–95]. The disadvantage of this technique is the need for high patient compliance and the high psychological impact [96]. The major complication of extraoral devices is the development of hypertrophic scars when the pins migrate through the skin

Since the original description, mandibular distraction has become increasingly popular for the treatment of mandibular hypoplasia and asymmetry [95,96,97]. Enoral (internal) distracters eliminate facial scars and are less likely to loosen or dislodge. Mandibular distraction has also been used to successfully alleviate the symptoms of respiratory distress and obstructive sleep apnea. A tracheostomy (if in place) can be removed. Mandibular distraction has been applied to infants as young as 14 weeks of age [98]. Both internal and external lengthening devices are being applied to distract the midface [96].

Patients with cleft lip and palate often have severe maxillary hypoplasia in the vertical, horizontal, and transverse dimensions. Traditional protocols rely on combined surgical–orthodontic treatment, including Le Fort I maxillary advancement, maxillary and alveolar bone grafting, and rigid internal fixation. Long-term results of this approach have been disappointing because relapse occurs in more than 20% of the cases. Trans-sinusoidal (TS-MD) placement of a distracter is a possible alternative for patients with cleft lip and palate. The major part of the TS-MD is done within the maxillary sinus and does not interfere with function during distraction and retention or with the patient's social life. Compared with headframe-based extraoral devices for midface distraction, TS-MD is easier for the patient and does not leave extraoral scars after removal of the device. Three-dimensional planning enables the surgeons to plan the distraction vector in three dimensions, but a correction of the vector by distraction is not possible, as it is with the headframe device (Fig. 32.24).

Cleft lip and cleft palate reconstruction

Surgical reconstruction of a cleft lip, palate, and/or nose is undertaken for cosmetic, psychological, and functional purposes. Functional goals are to separate the nasal and oral cavities, to improve speech and swallowing, to prevent middle ear disease, to improve hearing, and to provide normal dental occlusion (Fig. 32.25).

The treatment of children with cleft lip and palate starts during the first weeks after birth with preoperative orthopedics, such as presurgical nasal alveolar molding (PNAM). The PNAM appliance differs from traditional intraoral alveolar molding devices by having nasal prongs as part of the device [98]. An orthodontist adjusts the acrylic appliance by adding and removing material from the leading edge of the maxillary segments weekly. Despite the lack of long-term outcome studies, PNAM is used by many multidisciplinary cleft teams to reduce the width of the alveolar cleft and the corresponding soft tissues of the cleft lip [99].

Primary cleft lip repair is usually performed at 3–6 months of age and often includes a primary rhinoplasty. Cleft palate reconstruction is done at 12–20 months of age before speech develops. There are many ways to close the lip that have excellent results, each with its own advantages and disadvantages. The final result depends on the degree of primary dysmorphology, scarring (surgical technique), the experience of the surgeon, and the time schedule [100]. Tissue deficiency and displacement contribute to anatomical defects. Surgical reconstruction involves dissecting and freeing anatomical elements, undermining the tissue, repositioning the involved muscles in a correct anatomical position, and creating flaps for rotation and advancement of the lip. Reconstruction of the bony palate requires creating bone or mucoperiosteal flaps and also bone grafting. For example, mucoperiosteal flaps can be made from the

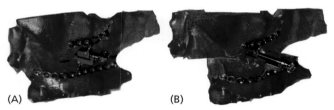

(A)   (B)

Figure 32.24 The TS-MD on a stereolithographic model of the midface. (A) Before and (B) after distraction.

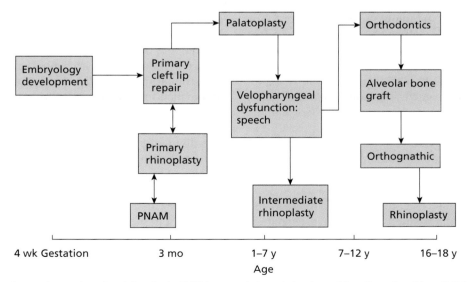

Figure 32.25 Timing and general procedures for cleft patients. PNAM, presurgical nasal alveolar molding. Reproduced from Tollefson et al [98] with permission from the American Medical Association.

palatal shelves and positioned medially to fill the cleft or they can be turned off the vomer and joined to the edge of the bony cleft to close it. If the cleft is sufficiently narrow, paring of the medial palatal edges and elevation of nasal and palatal mucosa may allow closure. Free bone grafting is required traditionally after orthodontic palatal expansion (8–11years of age) of the alveolar ridge. This occurs when 30–60% of the canine tooth roots have developed but before eruption of the tooth into the cleft void. Bone is generally taken from the iliac crest.

Pharyngeal flap

Velopharyngeal incompetence is failure of the velum (soft palate) and posterior pharynx to close or contact appropriately during speech and swallowing. It occurs in 10–30% of patients after cleft palate repair. It can also occur if there is any anatomical or neuromuscular abnormality of the palate or pharynx [101]. Velopharyngeal incompetence causes hypernasal, misarticulated speech. Nasal regurgitation of food and liquid occurs with swallowing.

Diagnosis of velopharyngeal incompetence has greatly improved with videofluoroscopy and nasal endoscopy, which provide a dynamic view of the velopharynx. Direct visualization can identify the closure pattern and contributions of the velum, the lateral and posterior pharyngeal walls, and Passavant ridge to speech [102]. Surgical correction of this defect is commonly attempted by creating a pharyngeal flap in which flaps of mucosa and muscle are raised from the posterior pharynx and attached to the velum (Fig. 32.26). This results in a permanent midline connection between the palate and posterior pharynx. Alternatively, a sphincter pharyngoplasty is performed, in which small lateral pharyngeal flaps are tucked under a wide medial flap to create a bulky transverse roll in the posterior pharynx, which narrows the pharynx and allows contact with the velum.

The result of these procedures is a narrowed nasopharyngeal vault and the potential for obstructed nasal airflow. Obstructive sleep apnea is not uncommon after a pharyngeal flap is created, especially with the Robin sequence [103–105]. Velocardiofacial syndrome is the most common syndrome causing palatal clefting and velopharyngeal insufficiency. It is associated with medially displaced carotid arteries that increase the risk of pharyngoplasty [106]. Velopharyngeal insufficiency can be identified by nasoendoscopy but not with endoral examination. Blind nasal tracheal intubation or insertion of a nasogastric tube should not be attempted in patients who have a pharyngeal flap. However, Kopp reported performing nasotracheal intubation in patients with a pharyngeal flap by first passing a flexible suction catheter to determine the patency of each naris and to identify the pharyngeal flap passages [107]. When the catheter

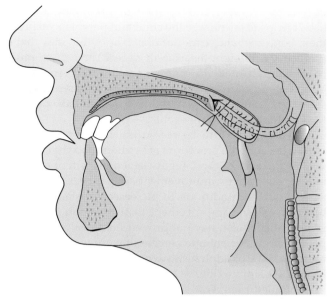

Figure 32.26 Pharyngeal flap. A flap of mucosa and muscle is raised from the posterior pharyngeal wall and attached to the soft palate. Reproduced from Shprintzen RJ et al. Cleft Palate J 1979; 16: 50 with permission from the American Cleft-Craniofacial Association.

emerges through the ostium created by the flap, it is grasped with a clamp and the endotracheal tube gently passed over it.

Anesthesia for craniofacial reconstruction

Preoperative evaluation

Many factors influence the emotional state of patients and families who face major craniofacial surgery [108–11]. Pediatric patients with craniofacial anomalies often have behavioral problems, poor self-image, anxiety, introversion, and negative social experiences. These problems are rarely profound and represent limitations rather than severe psychopathology [111]. Most children with craniofacial anomalies make social and psychological adjustments to their appearance without functioning in a psychosocially deviant range. Surgery is stressful for the patient and parents [112]. They have fear of pain and of physical jeopardy because the surgery is extensive and potentially life threatening. Older children may also fear loss of identity because of the impending changes in their appearance. Parents may be very protective. Many patients undergo multiple surgical procedures over many years, and the child and family have invested great emotion in the process.

It is important to establish rapport and gain the confidence and acceptance of the patient and parents. One can be sensitive yet open and candid in discussing the anomalies. It helps to encourage the child and parents to express their concerns and expectations. The child may have problems with sight, hearing or speech, and these must be accommodated during preoperative preparation. Various hospital activities such as puppet plays, movies, storybooks, and other play therapy may help to prepare the child for the coming events.

It is appropriate to be reassuring to the patient and family, because the procedure offers hope and the surgical results are usually good. Eighty-seven percent of patients report subjective improvement in appearance after surgery [113]. In addition to increased satisfaction with body image and improvement in their emotional state, some patients also have improved behavior and school performance. Ninety-one percent of parents of small children and 77% of adolescents would undergo the surgery again [109,114].

A complete preoperative medical evaluation is required. There are potential differences between craniofacial and isolated orofacial procedures. Patients undergoing craniofacial surgery should have preoperative evaluation, including sleep studies. The possible need for ICP monitoring should be discussed with the parents preoperatively. Patients with craniofacial anomalies often have syndromes and have anomalies of other systems. Relevant and comprehensive information about rare diseases is available on the internet (www.orpha.net). Associated CNS pulmonary and cardiac anomalies are especially noteworthy. Because of the nature and extent of the surgery, a careful history of bleeding tendencies should be obtained. Twenty to 37% of patients undergoing major craniofacial surgery have airway problems [115,116]. Sixty-five percent of patients with mandibular dysostosis (Treacher Collins, Goldenhar or hemifacial microsomal syndrome) and 53% of patients with craniofacial synostosis have problems with their airways.

It is important to evaluate thoroughly and comprehensively the airway because not all airway abnormities are readily apparent. Patients often undergo multiple procedures, so a history of airway problems during previous procedures and how they were managed should be reviewed. If airway management is expected to be difficult and a tracheostomy may be required, this should be discussed with the patient and parents before surgery.

Certain facial, upper airway and neck anomalies make airway management by mask and tracheal intubation difficult. It is difficult to get a good mask fit and seal when there is facial asymmetry, malar hypoplasia or nasal deformities. Anatomical anomalies, such as choanal atresia or stenosis, macroglossia, micrognathia, and diminished nasopharyngeal space, may cause airway obstruction. Secretions or adenoidal hypertrophy may further obstruct small air passages. Awake patients may have signs of airway obstruction, e.g. mouth breathing. Other signs, such as snoring, noisy breathing, and apnea, may be present only during sleep. Snoring with frequent sleep arousals, abnormal movements during sleep, daytime somnolence, nocturnal enuresis, and morning headaches are signs of sleep apnea. A history of sleep apnea can be elicited by asking whether the child snores and holds his or her breath between snores. Poor attention spans and school performance and/or personality and behavioral changes are also symptoms of obstructive sleep apnea. In severe cases, the child may be underweight and have pulmonary artery hypertension or cor pulmonale. Patients with upper airway obstruction during sleep may have airway obstruction during premedication-induced somnolence, during mask induction of anesthesia, and after extubation of the trachea.

Airway anomalies may render direct visualization of the larynx difficult or impossible. Mandibular hypoplasia or micrognathia, microstomia, macroglossia, trismus, and restriction of TMJ movement may make laryngoscopy difficult. Certain anatomical features should be carefully studied, including shape, size, and symmetry of the mandible, anteroposterior distance from the chin to the hyoid bone, tongue size, shape of the palate, movement of temporomandibular joints during mouth opening and during anterior displacement of the jaw, and mouth size when open (interincisor distance). Range of motion of the neck, especially extension, should be determined. Vertebral anomalies, such as cervical vertebral fusion in patients with Goldenhar, Apert, Crouzon, and other craniosynostosis syndromes, may limit neck motion [117]. During endotracheal intubation, retroflexion of the head may be necessary. Patients with Chiari malformation may have brainstem compression during flexion or severe extension of the head. Discussion should take place with the family and surgeon preoperatively about possible consequences of intubation maneuvers. It may be better to accomplish tracheal intubation with a fiber-optic bronchoscope without moving the head from a neutral position.

Laboratory evaluation

When large blood loss is expected, the minimal laboratory testing required in otherwise healthy children usually consists of hemoglobin or hematocrit and type and cross-matching of blood. Tests of coagulation (e.g. prothrombin and partial thromboplastin times, platelet count, and bleeding time) should be considered, especially in young infants. Other laboratory evaluations, such as chest x-ray, electrocardiography (ECG), pulmonary function tests, arterial blood gases, and serum electrolytes, may be required, depending on co-existing conditions.

Preoperative medication

Preoperative medication can be used to augment but not to substitute for psychological preparation. The use of preoperative medication must take into account the need for sedation and the presence of co-existing conditions and airway anomalies. For example, patients with increased intracranial pressure or potential airway obstruction may not safely tolerate respiratory depressants. Optimal sedation should smooth the induction process. Oral benzodiazepines are generally well tolerated for this purpose. Benzodiazepines, pentobarbital, and chloral hydrate can be administered orally or rectally. Fentanyl can be administered in a transmucosal form. Painful intramuscular injections should be avoided when possible. A local anesthetic cream patch (2.5% lidocaine and 2.5% prilocaine) placed above a vein can minimize the pain of inserting a venous catheter. The patch is usually removed 1 h prior to puncture. Antisialagogs can be included with oral premedication but should be used with care because they may cause a dry mouth and fever after the procedure.

Intraoperative anesthetic management

Successful anesthetic management requires close communication between the surgeon and anesthesiologist, especially when the surgeon is working near the airway or when rapid blood loss occurs. Anesthesia management is influenced by the patient's co-existing conditions, airway anomalies, and by particular features of the craniofacial procedure. In general, standard operating procedures (SOP) written by anesthesiologists and surgeons help standardize the intraoperative management of the patient and assure optimal quality of care.

Associated conditions

Associated respiratory, cardiac, and neurological anomalies or disorders will influence anesthetic management. The presence of cervical vertebral anomalies can influence head positioning or the procedure being done. If the patient has complex craniosynostosis, consideration must be given to the possibility for raised ICP, as previously discussed. Signs and symptoms of elevated ICP are uncommon. Even when the ICP is normal, intracranial complications may occur in some areas if the cranial vault inadequately accommodates the brain in all dimensions. Anesthetic induction and maintenance techniques and agents should decrease not increase the ICP of these patients.

Airway anomalies

Unexpected airway obstruction may occur during the induction of anesthesia. Physical appearance is not always a reliable indication of potential airway obstruction, and a past uneventful anesthetic course does not preclude the occurrence of airway problems this time, especially when a cleft palate has been repaired or pharyngeal flap procedure has been done in the interim. When difficulty with the airway is anticipated, a general plan of how to deal with the problem should be formulated ahead of time – no single technique is foolproof. The plan should include provision for several alternative techniques, and the availability of a variety of equipment, especially laryngeal mask airways and small tracheal tubes. It is advisable to proceed cautiously with the anesthesia induction. Spontaneous ventilation offers a margin of safety. Airway catastrophes can be avoided by allowing the patient to breathe spontaneously until it is verified that controlled ventilation is possible and easy to establish.

Difficulty with the facemask fit can be overcome by building up the face with gauze, applying a large mask over the entire face, and by using high gas flows. Clear masks with moldable air cushions often fit best, but care should be taken to assure that the cushion does not impinge on the eyes or obstruct the nares. Some patients develop upper airway obstruction during light levels of anesthesia. This can be prevented or attenuated by clearing the nasal passages of secretions before the induction of anesthesia and by maintaining the "sniffing" position, opening the mouth, applying gentle positive airway pressure (5–10 cmH$_2$O), and employing a "jaw thrust" when the patient is sufficiently anesthetized to tolerate it. Nasopharyngeal and oral airways may also be useful.

With mandibular hypoplasia and other oral and cervical malformations, direct laryngoscopy may be impossible or possible only with unconventional maneuvers. The larynx of these patients is often described as being "anteriorly placed." The larynx is actually in normal position with respect to other cervical structures but the tongue, which is attached to the hypoplastic mandible, is more posterior than normal and overhangs the larynx, giving the impression that the larynx is anteriorly placed [118]. It is often impossible to open the mouth adequately and displace the tongue sufficiently to allow visualization of the larynx.

Laryngeal mask airway (LMA) and fiber-optic bronchoscopy are important tools for airway management of patients with craniofacial malformations. The LMA can be inserted in awake infants (with topical anesthesia) or after induction of anesthesia in infants and children to aid blind or fiber-optic guided tracheal intubation. A mobile "difficult airway" cart, including all devices for unexpected or expected airway difficulties, is recommended (see Chapter 14) [119–121].

Many reports describe difficulty with airway management in patients with craniofacial malformations. Before LMA and fiber-optic bronchoscopy were available, some unconventional maneuvers for obtaining an airway

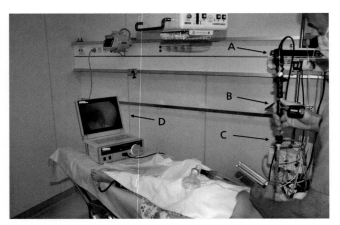

Figure 32.27 Single-handed usage of a Bonfils rigid optical scope for tracheal intubation in a difficult airway situation of a 3-year old child. (A) Optical unit. (B) LED light source. (C) Tube connector with oxygen insufflation. (D) Monitor.

were described, such as forcefully pulling the tongue out with a suture, forceps or custom-made retractors or using a Jackson anterior commissure laryngoscope with an "optical stylet." Blind or tactile tracheal intubation, with and without lighted guides, has also been described [122–125]. Video-assisted rigid endoscopes are now available to facilitate tracheal intubation of patients with a difficult airway. Oxygen is insufflated via the connector tube to prevent hypoxemia during video-assisted tracheal intubation. It is also helpful to use a laryngoscope to open the airway before inserting the rigid scope (Fig. 32.27).

Some patients require a tracheostomy for airway management. In some centers elective tracheostomy is performed when extensive facial osteotomies are planned in small children or when the airway would be difficult to manage if intraoperative reintubation were necessary [126]. When rigid internal fixation with plates is used rather than using intermaxillary ligation, tracheostomy can sometimes be avoided. Some patients already have a tracheostomy in place to treat severe respiratory obstruction. The complications and hazards of tracheostomy in pediatric patients include accidental decannulation of the trachea, tube obstruction, hemorrhage, and air leaks (pneumothorax, pneumomediastinum, and subcutaneous emphysema).

Features of the craniofacial procedure

Several features of craniofacial surgical procedures will influence anesthetic management: the procedure may be long with extensive tissue exposure; massive blood loss may occur; the procedure may be intracranial; and the airway may be in the surgical field.

Long procedure with wide tissue exposure

Major craniofacial procedures average 4–5 h but can last for more than 12 h. Operating time is reduced with an experienced surgical team [127,128]. Meticulous attention must be paid to protecting the anesthetized patient during prolonged surgeries. This includes proper positioning with the joints comfortably flexed, peripheral nerves protected, and pressure points, including the head, adequately padded. The patient may be in a supine, prone or modified prone position for the surgery (Fig. 32.28).

During a long period of wide tissue exposure, large amounts of body heat are lost. Temperature homeostasis is maintained by employing measures to conserve and provide heat, including minimizing the amount of time the patient is exposed to cold air before draping, warming the room to 23–24°C, and using a heat lamp before draping. A warming blanket or forced-air warming device should be used, along with passive insulation (plastic or cloth covers) around the body. Irrigation and intravenous fluids and blood should be warmed, and airway gases should be heated and humidified. When large portions of the cranium are exposed, the skull should be repeatedly bathed in warm irrigation fluid. Corticosteroids are often administered before craniofacial surgery to reduce postoperative facial swelling, but there is little evidence to support doing so.

Excessive blood loss

The magnitude of blood loss is related to the extent and duration of the surgical procedure and may equal multiples of the patient's blood volume for major craniofacial surgery. Blood loss reportedly decreases with greater experience of the team [127,128]. In one study, patients undergoing craniosynostosis repair had a mean estimated red cell volume loss of 91% of total estimated volume (range, 5–400%) [129]. The amount of red cell volume loss was greater for infants less than 6 months of age, for complex versus simple synostosis, and for complex vault remodeling compared to forehead reconstruction and strip craniectomy. Infants who underwent strip craniectomy lost about 60% of their blood volume [130].

Bleeding from the osseous venous plexus is generally continuous and may be quite brisk during osteotomy and bone mobilization. Rapid loss of large volumes of blood can occur with uncontrolled arterial bleeding or inadvertent opening of a dural sinus. For example, the internal maxillary artery may be divided during mandibular osteotomy, and the palatine artery may be cut during a Le Fort 1 procedure. The severed artery may be difficult to identify and clamp if it retracts into an inaccessible location. Irregularities on the internal surface of the cranium (e.g. bone spurs invaginating the dural sinuses) cause dural sinus tears and hemorrhage that often cannot be controlled rapidly. Other sources of major bleeding are

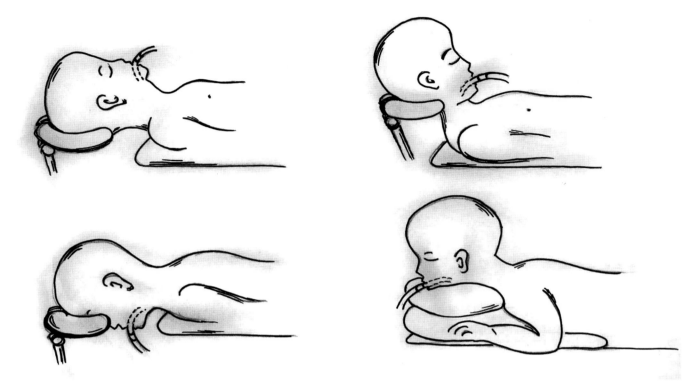

Figure 32.28 Positions in craniosynostosis surgery. (A) Supine position for frontal, frontoparietal and orbitofacial lesions. (B) Supine with head inclination for frontal and parietal and frontobasal lesions. (C) Prone position for parieto-occipital and suboccipital lesions. (D) Prone position with head reclination for total cranial vault exposure.

the major extradural and pharyngeal veins. Scarring and adhesions increase persistent bleeding and make major arterial, sinus, and venous bleeding more likely during repeat operations [131–134].

Blood loss should be aggressively replaced milliliter for milliliter in infants. It is unwise to fall behind in blood replacement as sudden, rapid blood loss may occur. For larger children and adolescents, initial blood loss replacement can be with appropriate volumes of crystalloid or colloid solutions until a reasonable level of hemodilution is achieved. Much of the blood loss is unmeasurable because it is hidden in the surgical field and drapes. Close communication with the surgeon about the pace of bleeding and close monitoring of the patient's intravascular volume are necessary. Normovolemia should be maintained with a combination of packed red blood cells and fresh frozen plasma. Because the child's blood volume is small, serial blood gas analyses should be made and include hematocrit and the level of lactic acidosis to detect decreased tissue perfusion.

Blood and blood components should be available in the operating room. At least two relatively large-bore intravenous (IV) catheters should be in place to permit swift infusion of blood. Blood transfusion may be rapid and

massive and have all the attendant problems (e.g. hypocalcemia, hyperkalemia, and coagulopathy). When blood replacement exceeds one blood volume, coagulation factors, especially platelets, may need replenishment. Osteotomies, especially of the maxilla, may continue to ooze after surgery, so the child's hematocrit should be adequate when he or she leaves the operating room. Induced hypotension is used to limit blood loss and create a drier surgical field, but there is no consensus on its utility and no objective data to support its use in cranial surgery.

Both induced hypotension and hyperventilation can cause cerebral hypoxia [135,136]. Therefore, it is probably unwise to combine the two. Regional brain ischemia may occur even when global perfusion is normal (e.g. when the frontal lobes are retracted). For these reasons, deliberate hypotension may be better suited to extracranial rather than intracranial procedures, although it has been used for both. Nowadays these techniques are seldom used. Other techniques that have been used to reduce or eliminate homologous blood transfusion during craniofacial surgery include preoperative administration of erythropoietin and intraoperative autologous blood salvage [137]. The cost of erythropoietin treatment makes its routine use prohibitive. The usefulness of intraoperative autologous blood salvage in small children is limited because transfusion is usually required before sufficient autologous blood can be collected. Further miniaturization of the available devices may make this technique more attractive.

For many years, antifibrinolytic agents such as aprotinin and tranexamic acid were used to decrease intraoperative blood loss [138]. Since the withdrawal of aprotinin from the market, only tranexamic acid (TXA) is available for this purpose. The optimal dose for intraoperative use has not been defined. Recent evidence from pediatric scoliosis or cardiac surgery recommends 100 mg/kg as a bolus plus 10 mg/kg/h with a maximum dose of 2 g [139]. These doses are very high and care must be taken because of seizures or convulsion which could be seen after administration of TXA in children as well as in adults. Recent recommendations exclude children <1 year of age from therapy with TXA. In our institution we have significantly decreased the dosage of TXA down to 10 mg/kg as a bolus followed by 3 mg/kg/h. If there is excessive bleeding, recombinant factor VIIa (rFVIIa) can be administered. rFVIIa is not approved for intraoperative use in coagulation disorders but is frequently used off label. It is an interesting substance that has promising effects on refractory non-surgical bleeding [140].

Intracranial procedures

Anesthetic techniques that decrease intracranial volume should be employed for intracranial procedures. Fronto-orbital procedures require brain manipulation and retraction to allow adequate exposure of the anterior cranial fossa and facial bones. Reducing the brain bulk decreases the amount of brain retraction necessary. Therefore, anesthetic agents such as halothane, enflurane, and ketamine, which increase intracranial volume, should be avoided. Narcotics, benzodiazepines, thiopental, propofol, isoflurane, sevoflurane, and desflurane, in combination with mild hyperventilation (end-expiratory measured CO_2 between 30 and 35 mmHg) are preferred. Other measures used to decrease intracranial volume include 20–30° head-up positioning and use of diuretics (mannitol and furosemide) [141,142]. The respiratory pattern during mechanical ventilation should not inhibit intracranial CSF and venous drainage. Therefore, positive end-expiratory pressure (PEEP) should be avoided, and mean airway pressure should be maintained as low as is consistent with adequate oxygenation by using a long expiratory time, if possible.

Potential hazards during intracranial procedures include dural sinus tears, cerebral edema, and venous air embolism. Dural sinus tears may produce rapid, massive blood loss. Manipulation and retraction of the brain may cause cerebral injury and edema. Air embolism occurs through open venous channels because the open cranium is usually positioned above the central circulation [142–

144]. Meticulous surgical technique may prevent this complication.

Intraoperative airway management

During a Le Fort midface advancement, the surgeon must work around the airway. With maxillary osteotomy and down-fracturing maneuvers, the nasotracheal tube may be lacerated, transected, or dislodged from the trachea. Pilot tubes for endotracheal tube cuffs are easily cut. A plan should be formulated ahead of time between the surgeon and anesthesiologist for how an endotracheal tube will be replaced should this become necessary. Usually, the surgical field is quickly covered with sterile drapes, and the anesthesiologist is allowed access to the airway. Replacement tubes, catheter guides, and other appropriate equipment for reintubation must be readily available.

When the tracheal tube is in the surgical field, care must be taken to ensure an adequate airway despite lack of access to the face. The anesthesia circuit should be lightweight and all connectors should be well secured. The head of the operating table may be turned 180° from the anesthesia machine. Consequently the airway circuit must have adequate length to allow this. If the surgeon will move the head during the procedure, it must be determined that the endotracheal tube and circuit are unencumbered. Care must be taken when initially positioning the endotracheal tube to avoid either tracheal extubation when the neck is extended or when the maxilla is advanced or endobronchial intubation when the neck is flexed. The maxilla or mandible can be advanced by as much as 3 cm. The tracheal tube should be secured with wires or sutures tied around teeth, nasal septum, mandible, or alveolar ridge. Nasotracheal intubation is required when the procedure is intraoral or when intermaxillary fixation is required. Armor tubes prevent compression of the airway by surgical manipulation. Close communication between surgeon and anesthesiologist is required prior to tracheal intubation to determine the best position for the tracheal tube. Care must be taken to prevent nasal necrosis when a nasotracheal tube will be in place for hours. The hypopharynx should be packed to prevent intraoperative aspiration of blood, bone chips, and tissue. At the end of the procedure, the nose, mouth, and pharynx should be cleared and the stomach aspirated of gas, blood, and other material.

Postoperative swelling of the face and scalp may be severe. The swelling after bilateral midface and mandibular osteotomies may dictate that the tracheal tube remain in place for 12–48 h. This is especially true when intermaxillary fixation and occlusive intraoral prostheses limit access to the airway. Persistent oropharyngeal bleeding, cerebral edema, or pulmonary disease may also delay tracheal extubation. Tracheal extubation should occur when the patient is fully awake, has intact airway reflexes and an empty stomach, and is able to follow commands. Provisions should be made for immediately re-establishing an artificial airway (including wire cutters to release intermaxillary fixation wires) should this become necessary.

Other anesthetic considerations

Anesthetic drugs should be chosen on the basis of the preceding considerations. Depth of anesthesia can be balanced with muscle relaxation to prevent coughing, bucking, or patient movement with erratic surgical stimuli. Preferably, the patient should be awake and comfortable at the end of the procedure so that neurological assessment can be made. This can be accomplished by using a potent narcotic or "balanced" technique or by titrating narcotic when the patient is emerging from anesthesia. Extracranial bone graft sites (rib or iliac crest) may cause more postoperative pain than the cranial sites.

Fluids should provide maintenance requirements, replace interstitial and evaporative losses, and maintain urine output above 0.5 mL/kg/h. The exact amount of fluid required to accomplish these goals will depend on the extent of tissue dissection and exposure. For small infants, electrolyte solutions, like Ringer-acetate with 1% of glucose, provides optimal maintenance of fluids and blood glucose concentrations. A urinary bladder catheter should be placed to prevent bladder distension and for intravascular volume monitoring. Serial blood analyses of arterial pH and blood gases, hemoglobin, electrolytes, ionized calcium, glucose, and coagulation parameters are made.

A high level of physiological monitoring is required. Routine anesthesia monitors, such as ECG, pulse oximeter, temperature, and airway gas and pressure monitors, are used. In addition, an intra-arterial catheter is placed to allow direct blood pressure monitoring and blood sampling. Central venous oxygen saturation can be used to estimate cardiac output in children. A central venous oxygen saturation of <50–60% should prompt detailed evaluation of the patients circulatory condition. Arterial blood pressure and waveform are good indicators of intravascular volume. A broad-based pressure wave, with the dichrotic notch in the upper half of the downslope of the curve and little or no variation with respiration, is a good indicator of normovolemia. A central venous catheter is useful for monitoring intravascular volume and for rapidly infusing drugs and fluids. During intracranial procedures, evidence of venous air embolism should be sought with a capnograph and a precordial Doppler because the open cranium is generally above the central circulation. A central venous catheter may occasionally allow aspiration of entrained air, although early detection and prevention of further entrainment are more important than trying to aspirate the gas.

Perioperative hazards and complications

Although large series of major craniofacial surgery attest to its relative safety, significant morbidity and mortality can occur [145]. Intraoperative death has occurred with massive blood loss and air embolism. Postoperative death has resulted from cerebral, respiratory, and circulatory causes (e.g. cerebral edema, massive extradural hemorrhage, respiratory arrest, respiratory obstruction or tracheal extubation, tracheostomy blockage, and hemorrhage) [146–148]. A recent study analyzed 8101 major craniofacial procedures and determined the mortality rates and major morbiditiy. The authors found that serious complications have significantly decreased and suggested that protocols for airway management, blood salvage and replacement, age-appropriate deep venous prophylaxis, and timing of subcranial midfacial advancements might further reduce the mortality rate [149].

Other reported intraoperative complications include cardiac arrest from severe blood loss, air embolism, and pneumoperitoneum (a complication of tracheostomy), pneumothorax during rib graft procurement, subdural hematoma, and bradycardia from the oculocardiac reflex [150–152]. Stimulation of any sensory branch of the 5th cranial nerve (maxillary, mandibular, ophthalmic) can cause reflex bradycardia and asystole. Reflex bradycardia and asystole have also been noted during maxillofacial and temporomandibular surgery [152]. Ocular pressure should be avoided because it too can cause severe bradycardia.

Several complications related to the endotracheal tube have been reported, including intraoperative tracheal extubation (usually during midface advancement), endotracheal tube blockage by kinking (also during midface advancement), and endotracheal tube laceration [118]. Pilot tubes for cuffed endotracheal tubes have also been lacerated. There are several reports of emergency endotracheal tube replacement intraoperatively. Complications of tracheostomy have included tube kinking, laceration of the posterior tracheal wall, esophageal perforation, and cardiac arrest from pneumoperitoneum [118,153,154]. Subgaleal or epidural drains require special care, especially when placed next to venous sinuses. The vacuum used for drains is related to the size of the used subgaleal or epidural drains. Rapid opening of the suction can cause significant blood loss. Non-fatal postoperative complications have included respiratory obstruction after tracheal extubation, pulmonary edema, cerebral edema, extradural hematoma, subgaleal hemorrhage, seizures, infection, blindness, CSF leaks, facial nerve damage, bone resorption, and hydrocephalus [155].

Anesthesia for cleft lip and cleft palate reconstruction

Preoperative evaluation

The anesthesiologist's approach to patients with a cleft lip and palate is similar to that described in the preceding section for patients with other craniofacial deformities. In this case, however, the surgical procedure is less extensive. By the time the infant with cleft lip comes for surgery at 3 months of age, the parents have usually overcome their initial reactions to their malformed infant and are hopeful that surgery will restore normal appearance and function. Preoperative preparation must accommodate the older child with a cleft palate who may have communication problems due to poor speech and hearing. Many children require multiple procedures. Every effort should be expended to ensure that the anesthetic experience is not unpleasant for either the parent or child.

A complete medical evaluation should be made, with special attention to the presence of other anomalies and syndromes. All patients with a cleft palate have eustachian tube dysfunction and usually have chronic serous otitis with clear rhinorrhea. Acute otic infections should be resolved before surgery. Preoperative sedation is appropriate for children who have no airway compromise.

Intraoperative management of anesthesia

Induction

Most patients with an isolated cleft lip or palate present no difficulty with airway management. Only 3% of 800 patients undergoing repair of cleft lip and palate had difficult laryngoscopy [156]. Those with a difficult airway had retrognathia and/or were less than 6 months of age [157]. The protruding premaxilla associated with extensive bilateral clefts of the lip and alveolus sometimes prevents visualization of the larynx. While the incidence of failed intubation is low [154], it does occur. Therefore, it may be wise to induce anesthesia while the patient is spontaneously breathing. It is useful to have a second anesthesiologist to help with the airway management. The ability to manage the airway should be assessed before the patient is rendered apneic. Airway obstruction may occur if the tongue is impacted in a palatal cleft. This is easily remedied when recognized. Care must be taken to avoid injuring a protruding premaxilla during laryngoscopy. Antisialagog drugs are useful for oral procedures. Inserting a preformed, curved tracheal tube (RAE tube) that lies flat against the face minimizes the potential for tube kinking and dislodgment. A stylet can be used to facilitate tracheal tube insertion when necessary. The tube should be fixed in the midline, with the lip immobile and not distorted (Fig. 32.29).

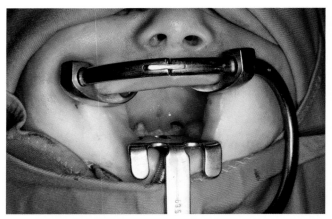

Figure 32.29 "Kilner Dott" mouth gag in place for cleft palate repair in a patient with Pierre Robin sequence (bifid uvula). The metal armored tube is safely secured under the lower part of the mouth gag.

Maintenance

There are several intraoperative special anesthetic considerations for cleft lip and palate reconstruction procedures. The first is that the airway is shared with the surgeon. Thus, the tracheal tube must be well secured to prevent inadvertent dislodgment. Adequacy of the airway should be continuously assessed, especially after patient positioning and placement of a mouth gag or pharyngeal packs. For palate and pharyngeal procedures, correct positioning may require exaggerated neck extension, which may bring the endotracheal tube up and out of the trachea. A mouth gag provides surgical exposure and stabilizes the ET tube, but it may also occlude the tracheal tube (see Fig. 32.29). Pharyngeal packs are placed to prevent aspiration of blood. Compression or kinking of the ET tube may occur with these maneuvers.

Other anesthesia considerations are routine. Fluid and temperature homeostasis must be maintained. Blood loss is rarely sufficient to require transfusion, although it is occasionally necessary in palate and pharyngeal procedures. Inhalation anesthesia is commonly used, but the choice of anesthetic agent is not crucial as long as the considerations outlined here are accommodated.

Postoperative management

The most common acute postoperative problems are bleeding and airway obstruction. At the conclusion of palate and pharyngeal surgery, the pharynx must be inspected for bleeding and the presence of pharyngeal packs. Leaving a pharyngeal pack in place can be lethal when the endotracheal tube is removed. Placing the infant or child in the lateral position permits drainage of blood and secretions from the pharynx. Extubation of the trachea should be delayed until the patient is fully awake and has regained normal neuromuscular function to minimize potential airway obstruction from either anatomical causes or from bleeding. Applying a mask or artificial airways may damage a lip or nose repair, so it is advisable to delay extubation until the patient can maintain a patent airway without assistance. After lip procedures, infants are restrained with arm boards to prevent them from disrupting the repair.

After a palatoplasty or pharyngoplasty, the infant or child awakens from anesthesia with an altered upper airway. The presence of constricting flaps and nasopharyngeal edema compromises the nasal airway and may abruptly convert the child to a mouth-breather. This problem is magnified in patients who have Pierre Robin complex. After pharyngoplasty, 10% or more of patients experience temporary obstructive sleep apnea [157]. Sleep apnea is completely eliminated when the surgical technique is modified and a nasopharyngeal airway is kept in place for the first 48h after surgery. Fifty-seven percent of patients are predominantly or exclusively mouth-breathers after palatoplasty or pharyngoplasty [158]. Up to 72% of patients develop sleep apnea after pharyngoplasty.

Pharyngeal anomalies are common with craniofacial syndromes and place the patients at high risk for airway obstruction, especially after pharyngoplasty [158]. The anomalies may be structural (pharyngeal narrowing related to malformation of the basicranium (Treacher Collins syndrome)) or mandibular (Robin sequence). They may also be functional, e.g. the pharyngeal hypotonia of the velocardiofacial syndrome. One patient died 4 weeks after surgery [159].

Acute postoperative airway obstruction caused by massive lingual swelling has also been reported after palatoplasty. The mouth and tongue should be carefully inspected before tracheal extubation, particularly if the mouth gag has been in place for more than 2h. If the mouth gag must be up for 2h, it should be let down for a few minutes to allow the tongue to be perfused. The lingual swelling is often the result of a reperfusion injury.

Infiltration of local anesthetic will decrease the need for postoperative analgesia. Non-narcotic analgesics are preferred, but when narcotics are required, they should be titrated to effect. Infraorbital nerve blocks can be performed while the patient is asleep to prevent pain after cleft lip surgery [160,161]. Postoperative pain therapy can be guided by using pain scales [162–164].

CASE STUDY

Introduction
A 4-year-old, 11.5kg, 85-cm-tall, boy was scheduled for repeat craniofacial surgery to treat his dysostosis craniofacialis (Crouzon-Syndrome). Crouzon syndrome is characterized by premature closure of calvarial, cranial base, orbit and maxillary complex (craniosynostosis) sutures. His medical history included mild mental and linguistic development retardation. The child had a small mouth, a hypoplastic maxilla, and relative mandibular prognathism. Consequently, it was suspected that pulmonary ventilation and tracheal intubation might be difficult, although during previous surgery he could be ventilated with a bag-and-facemask and it was possible to insert a laryngeal mask airway (LMA). A recent routine diagnostic ophthalmologic consultation showed evidence of residual chronic, subacute elevated intracranial pressure in the fundus of his eyes, papilledema, and beginning optic atrophy.

A sleep study was postponed until after surgery. Routine preoperative laboratory test were within normal limits (Table 32.4).

Considerations for anesthesia
Blood and blood products
Because it was suspected that a large amount of blood might be lost during surgery, packed red blood cells (PRBC) and fresh frozen plasma (FFP) were available for the patient preoperatively. Use of an antifibrinolytic agent, e.g. Tranexamic acid (TXA), (initial dose 10mg/kg BW by bolus followed by 3mg/kg/h) was considered but rejected because of the patient's history of seizures. The anesthesiologist and surgeons decided to administer blood and blood components (FFP) early in the case to prevent abnormally low hemoglobin concentrations (Hb) and maintain normal oxygen carrying capacity in this child who had increased intracranial pressures. It was felt this also would prevent hypovolemia, hypoperfusion, and dangerous levels of lactic acidosis. The decision to administer blood products at the start of surgery was based on the expected level of blood loss and on the retrospective history of blood loss and the need for transfusion of similar patients at our institution.

Induction and maintenance of anesthesia
Anesthesia was induced with propofol (2.5mg /kg) and remifentanil (1μg/kg) with oxygen. The lungs were ventilated to maintain a normal $PaCO_2$. Fiberoptic tracheal intubation was facilitated by administering rocuronium (1mg/kg). No further muscle relaxation was needed during the case. Salivation was prevented by slowly administering atropine sulfate (0.5mg) 30min before the induction of anesthesia. A nasogastric tube and a urinary catheter and

Continued

temperature probe were placed into the urinary bladder after induction of anesthesia. Sevoflurane and remifentanil (5–20 μg/kg/h) were used to maintain anesthesia. Sufficient oxygen was administered to maintain a normal SaO_2. Thirty minutes before the end of anesthesia, a longer acting opioid and a nonsteroidal anti-inflammatory agent (NSAID) was administered.

Cardiovascular monitoring

A double lumen 5 French central venous catheter was inserted in to the right subclavian vein. The left radial artery was cannulated with a 24-gauge catheter for on-line arterial blood pressure monitoring and blood sampling. Monitoring in the perioperative period consisted of continuous measurement of arterial and central venous pressures, temperature (via the urinary catheter), oxygen saturation by pulse oximetry, end-expired CO_2, and urine output. Blood gases, pH, electrolytes, and glucose and lactate concentrations were measured every 1h or more frequently, as required. Central venous oxygen saturation was determined from central venous blood samples and used to estimate cardiac output and blood volume status.

Airway management

Preoperatively it was suspected that oral tracheal intubation might be difficult because of the patient's hypoplastic maxilla and prognathic mandible. His mouth opening was also limited. Consequently, equipment for fiberoptic tracheal intubation was available in the operating room before anesthesia was induced. Because it was known from his previous surgeries that bag-and-mask ventilation was possible and that a laryngeal mask could be inserted and used to ventilate the lungs, general anesthesia was induced before attempting fiberoptic tracheal intubation. If this information had not been available, we would have considered doing fiberoptic tracheal intubation with the patient sedated but with spontaneous ventilation. Because the patient would be in the prone position and it would be necessary to recline the neck during surgery, an armored oral tracheal tube was inserted. Care was taken to fix the tracheal tube securely with wires to the teeth to avoid accidental tracheal extubation during surgery. Because surgery would last several hours, great care was taken to prevent compression of soft facial tissues (eyes, nose) when the patient was placed in the prone position (see Fig. 32.27).

Body temperature

Care was taken to prevent intra-operative hypothermia for several reasons. First, to prevent inhibition of the coagulation system; second, to prevent hypoperfusion and local ischemia (e.g. metabolic acidosis and lactate production); and third to prevent hypoventilation and respiratory acidosis once spontaneous ventilation returned and the trachea was extubated. Prevention of hypothermia would also avoid the negative effects of shivering and cardiovascular depression after surgery.

Intraoperative management

After induction of anesthesia and insertion of the tracheal tube, the surgeons and anesthesiologists together, positioned the patient for surgery. Maintenance fluid consisted of Ringer's solution with 1% dextrose added (4mL/kg/h) to maintain a normal glucose concentration. Volume losses were initially replaced with 4mL/kg/h of Ringer's solution without dextrose as needed. During reflection of the scalp, which was difficult because of adhesions that formed after the earlier surgery, packed red blood cells and fresh frozen plasma (5mL/kg each) were administered. Once the scalp and bone were reflected and surgical coagulation was accomplished, PRCBs and FFP were given as needed to maintain a normal hemoglobin concentration and prevent bleeding. Despite prophylactic administration of PRBCs, Hb/Hct concentrations decreased below initial values (Table 32.4). The estimated blood loss during surgery was 340mL, about 40% of his blood volume. These losses were initially replaced with Ringer's solution and then with PRBCs and FFP. Heat loss was prevented by wrapping the patient's extremities with sheet wadding and by actively warming him with a thermal blanket and warmed-humidified inspired gases. Despite this he initially lost about 1°C in body temperature. Anesthesia was maintained with a combination of sevoflurane and remifentanil, as described above. Because the intraoperative period was uneventful and because spontaneous ventilation returned and was adequate, the trachea was extubated in the operating room once the child was awake. He was transferred to the PICU to monitor for bleeding and for signs of elevated intracranial pressure. Postoperative blood loss was 75mL, which was replaced with PRBCs. Tracheal extubation occurred at the end of surgery because it was felt that it would be easier to monitor for signs of increased intracranial pressure if the patient was awake and spontaneously breathing. Postoperative fluid administration was restricted to that which maintained about 1mL of urine output/kg/hr. This (fluid restriction) was done to reduce the likelihood of increasing intracranial pressure and of causing pulmonary edema. The day after surgery all monitoring lines were removed, and the patient was transferred to the ward in good condition. He was discharged home several days later and has done well.

Conclusions

This case demonstrates several important points.
- Patients with Crouzon abnormalities often have some degree of increased intracranial pressure, which this

child had (papilledema and beginning optic atrophy). Because of the intracranial hypertension, the arterial blood pressure and $ETCO_2$ were maintained within normal preoperative limits to prevent unwanted increases in intracranial pressure and reduced cerebral blood flow.

- The oxygen content of the blood needs to be maintained throughout surgery. Blood loss is common in these cases, especially when there has been previous surgery. This child lost 340 mL of blood during the case despite an infusion of PRBCs and plasma at the beginning of the case and attempts to maintain normal clotting. Adequate fluid and blood products were administered to maintain normal arterial and central blood pressures and to prevent metabolic acidosis.

- It is important to take measures to maintain a normal body temperature during surgery, especially when one wants to extubate the trachea at the end of the surgery. Hypothermia may cause hypoventilation, increased $PaCO_2$, and increased intracranial pressure. If the case lasts long enough, hypothermia may cause clotting abnormalities and increase intraoperative bleeding. Maintaining a normal body temperature must be bal-

anced against the fact that a $1-2^0$ reduction in brain temperature is neuroprotective (see Chapter 7).

- Many children with Crouzon abnormalities have a difficult airway. This child had a small mouth, a hypoplastic maxilla, and prognathism, all of which can be associated with a difficult airway. At times the facemask does not fit the face due to the mid-face hypoplasia. As a result it is difficult to ventilate the lungs with a bag-and-facemask. If the mid-face hypoplasia occludes the nostrils, closing the mouth during attempted bag-and-mask ventilation may completely obstruct the airway. If this occurs, an oral airway should be inserted to keep the mouth and airway open. Knowing that the lungs could be ventilated with a bag-and-mask during previous surgeries was very helpful in this case.

- Measuring intravascular pressures and urine output during surgery helped determine the adequacy of fluid and blood products replacement. Urine glucose concentrations were measured several times during the case because high concentrations of glucose in the blood may cause an osmotic diuresis that gives the false impression of normal urine flow, even in hypovolemic patients.

Table 32.4 Laboratory values determined before and each hour during craniofacial surgery in a patient with Crouzon syndrome.

	Pre-op	1 h	2 h	3 h	End of operation	PICU
Hemoglobin (mg/dL)	11.2	10.4	9.9	10.4	10.1	10.0
PaO_2 (mm Hg)	78.3	89.3	99.1	79.5	91.3	430
$PaCO_2$ (mm Hg)	44.1	43.2	39.8	42.1	49.3	41.5
SaO_2 (%)	99	99	98	98	98	100
pH	7.39	7.41	7.40	7.39	7.29	7.35
BE (meq/L)	0.9	1.0	0	0	−3.6	−2.0
International Normalized Ratio (INR)	1.0	1.2	1.5	1.2	1.2	1.0
Prothrombin time (PT) (sec)	12.0	13.3	16.5	13.4	13.2	13.1
Activated prothrombin time (PTT) (sec)	36.2	40.1	43.2	41.0	40.9	37.2
Platelets (times 10^9/L)	352	205	168	210	289	301
Lactate (mmol/L)	0.9	0.9	1.0	1.2	0.9	0.9
Body core temperature (° C)	36.5	35.5	35.9	36.1	36.4	36.3
PRBC transfused (mL)	–	50	40	50	20	40
FFP (mL)	–	25	25	25	20	20

BE, base excess; PRBC, packed red cells; FFP, fresh frozen plasma; PICU, Pediatric Intensive Care Unit.

Annotated references

A full reference list for this chapter is available at:
http://www.wiley.com/go/gregory/andropoulos/pediatricanesthesia

23. Cohen MM Jr. Perspectives on craniosynostosis: sutural biology, some well-known syndromes, and some unusual syndromes. J Craniofac Surg 2009; 20: 646–51. Recent insights into the biology of suture pathologies.

35. Suwanwela C, Suwanwela N. Amorphological classification of sincipital encephalomeningoceles. J Neurosurg 1972; 36: 201–11. Standard classification of encephaloceles.

36. Tessier P. Anatomical classification of facial, cranio-facial and laterofacial clefts. J Maxillofac Surg 1976; 4: 69–92. Excellent paper on facial cleft classification.

77. Marchac D, Renier D. Craniofacial Surgery for Craniosynostosis. Boston: Little, Brown, 1982. Book written by the pioneers of craniosynostosis surgery.

78. Tessier P. The definitive plastic surgical treatment of the severe facial deformities of craniofacial synostosis: Crouzon's and Apert's diseases. Plast Reconstr Surg 1971; 48: 419–42. Important surgical publication about the treatment of syndromic facial deformities with synostosis involvment.

119. Fiadjoe J, Stricker P. Pediatric difficult airway management: current devices and techniques. Anesthesiol Clin 2009; 27: 185–95. Recent compilation of devices and techniques for pediatric airway management.

138. Schouten ES, van de Pol A, Schouten AN et al. The effect of aprotinin, tranexamic acid, and aminocaproic acid on blood loss and use of blood products in major pediatric surgery: a meta-analysis. Pediatr Crit Care Med 2009; 10: 182–90. This meta-analysis gives an up-to-date overview about indications and problems associated with antifibrinolytic substances and their use in pediatric patients.

146. Hasan RA, Nikolis A, Dutta S, Jackson I. Clinical outcome of perioperative airway and ventilatory management in children undergoing craniofacial surgery. J Craniofac Surg 2004; 15: 655–61. This study demonstrates that when performing complex craniofacial procedures in children, a team approach before surgery and continuous communication between specialists during the perioperative period are imperative.

154. Infosino A. Pediatric upper airway and congenital anomalies. Anesthesiol Clin North Am 2002; 20: 747–66. Pediatric airway management is sometimes challenging. Methods and equipment are well described in this article.

Further reading

Rath GP, Bithal P, Chaturvedi A, Dash H. Complications related to positioning in posterior fossa craniectomy. J Clin Neurosci 2007; 14: 520–5. This retrospective study is an example of how positioning is influencing neurosurgical operations.

CHAPTER 33
Pain Management in Children

Charles Berde & Christine Greco

Department of Anesthesiology, Perioperative and Pain Medicine, Children's Hospital Boston, and Harvard Medical School, Boston, MA, USA

Introduction

The management of pain and related symptoms is part of the daily practice of pediatrics, pediatric anesthesiology, and pediatric intensive care. In this chapter, we will outline some aspects of how the experience of pain changes with age, how analgesics act at different ages, and how to treat some common acute and chronic pain conditions in pediatrics.

Developmental neurophysiology of pain

Studies by Fitzgerald and others have shown that there is considerable maturation of peripheral, spinal, and supraspinal neurological pathways necessary for nociception by late in the second trimester of human gestation [1]. Although the general architecture of the sensory nervous system is established by midgestation, there are some differences in preterm and term neonates compared to older infants as patterns of connections and functions mature over the first months of life. Peripheral sensory fibers involved in nociception have larger, more overlapping, receptive fields and lower thresholds for impulse activation in infant animals, com-pared to mature animals [2]. Descending pain inhibitory pathways, such as the dorsolateral funiculus [3], tend to develop postnatally. This has been interpreted as suggesting that neonates and young infants may perceive pain more intensely or have hyper-responsiveness to pain compared to older infants and children with a more mature nervous system.

Many of these initial studies emphasized maturation of peripheral and spinal mechanisms and simple withdrawal reflexes. More recently, attention has focused on cortical representation of responses to injury in neonates and young infants [4]. Studies of brain activation using near-infrared spectroscopy have shown that a noxious stimulus to the heel of a neonate evokes increased signals overlying the contralateral cerebral cortex [4]. This implies that a specific pattern of activation occurs in response to a noxious stimulus as opposed to the global, non-specific pattern of activation seen with autonomic arousal. This and other evidence suggests that painful stimuli reach the cerebral cortex in infants although this evidence does not establish that pain is perceived as a conscious experience or as suffering in neonates. Despite the delay in the development of spinal descending pathways and neurotransmitters, α-adrenergic agonists and opioids administered via epidural or spinal routes exert analgesic effects in newborn animals [5,6] and humans [7,8].

Several studies have been interpreted as providing evidence that infants are able to form implicit memory of pain and that there are potentially negative behavioral consequences of untreated pain in infants. Taddio showed that infants who were circumcised with little or no analgesia had significantly increased pain behaviors at their 2-, 4-, and 6-month immunizations when compared to infants who were uncircumcised or who had received adequate analgesia [9]. Studies of adult rats who had received persistent inflammatory stimuli as neonates showed long-term changes in the dorsal horn synaptic organization and nociceptive functioning [10]. When newborns undergoing major surgeries were randomized to relatively light versus relatively deep anesthetic techniques they showed better suppression of stress responses with deeper anesthetic techniques, as well as some reductions in postoperative morbidities [11–14]. Conversely, studies of critically ill newborns undergoing mechanical ventilation have not shown a clear benefit from routine administration of morphine infusions, compared to controls who just received intermittent morphine prior to suctioning or other painful procedures [15].

Pain assessment in infants and children

Assessing pain in infants and children is a fundamental aspect of pediatric care and serves as the foundation for treating pain. Most pain assessment tools for infants, toddlers, and preschool children are based on the developmental age of the child and often combine behavioral and physiological parameters, since self-report measures may not be possible in preverbal children or accurate in hospitalized young children. Readers interested in this topic are referred to a consensus statement on pediatric pain measurement [16]. Studies indicate that healthcare providers tend to underestimate pain using observational measures compared to parents' or children's own ratings. Children who are ill, hospitalized and confronted with strangers may not co-operate with self-report measures; pain assessment tools designed for younger children may be more useful in these cases.

Pain assessment in infants and preterm babies is particularly challenging. Infants rely on caregivers to interpret their behavior and other signs in determining whether they have pain. Numerous studies have examined pain responses in infants and have shown that infants exhibit predictable response patterns with respect to stress hormone levels, behavior patterns, and changes in heart rate, oxygen saturation, blood pressure, and other physiological patterns. Neonates who are subjected to repeated heel lancing for blood analyses consistently swipe at the affected foot, indicating their ability to local-ize to the site of pain. Infants display gradations in heart rate, blood pressure, and oxygen saturation in response to varying intensities of pain, indicating their ability to discriminate severity of pain. Nevertheless, physiological parameters are non-specific indicators of pain and can reflect fear, hunger, anxiety and emotional distress as well as pain [17].

As a result of these studies and others, pain assessment tools in infants are typically composite pain scores that combine observed distress behaviors such as facial grimacing, sleep–wake cycles, and body posture with physiological parameters, including heart rate, oxygenation, and blood pressure measurements. Behavioral responses to pain in premature infants may be much more subtle than those observed in full-term infants. In addition, behavioral and physiological pain scales are not applicable in critically ill infants who may be septic, hemodynamically unstable or mechanically ventilated. The Premature Infant Pain Profile (PIPP) (Table 33.1) is a pain assessment tool for procedural pain that has been validated in premature and full-term infants [18]. The PIPP is unique in that gestational age is included in the scoring system in addition to distress behaviors, heart rate, and oxygen saturation. The Faces, Legs, Activity, Cry, Consolability (FLACC) scale combines five types of pain behaviors, including facial expression, leg movement, activity, cry, and consolability, and has been shown to have good inter-rater reliability and validity in children (Fig. 33.1) [19]. It is widely used because it is quick, versatile, and can be applied to infants and older children, including those with developmental disabilities [20].

Concrete thinking and variations in cognitive and language development in toddlers and preschool age children can make pain assessment challenging in this age group. Preschool age children are often able to give simple measures of self-report such as location of pain but cannot provide more abstract details such as quality of pain. It is generally useful to involve parents or other familiar caregivers when questioning young children about their pain.

A variety of pain assessment tools have been developed for young children. Studies indicate that many children tend to prefer faces scales where pictorial representations of faces are used to denote varying degrees of pain. Young children are able to differentiate pain intensity when presented with facial expressions although more than five choices seems to interfere with the child's ability to reliably indicate pain. The Oucher scale (Fig. 33.2), the Wong–Baker scale (Fig. 33.3), and the Bieri faces scale are examples of faces scales that have been validated for use in children as young as 4 years of age. The Oucher scale, developed for use with children of all ethnicities, uses actual photographs of children and is available in several versions, each tailored to child ethnicity. Among

Categories	Scoring		
	0	**1**	**2**
Face	No particular expression or smile	Occasional grimace or frown, withdrawn, disinterested	Frequent to constant quivering chin, clenched jaw
Legs	Normal position or relaxed	Uneasy, restless, tense	Kicking, or legs drawn up
Activity	Lying quietly, normal position, moves easily	Squirming, shifting back and forth, tense	Arched, rigid or jerking
Cry	No cry (awake or asleep)	Moans or whimpers; occasional complaint	Crying steadily, screams or sobs, frequent complaints
Consolability	Content, relaxed	Reassured by occasional touching, hugging or being talked to, distractable	Difficult to console or comfort
Each of the five categories (F) Face; (L) Legs; (A) Activity; (C) Cry; (C) Consolability is scored from 0–2, which results in a total score between zero and ten.			

Figure 33.1 Faces, Legs, Activity, Cry, Consolability (FLACC) scale.

Table 33.1 Premature Infant Pain Profile (PIPP)

Indicators	0	1	2	3
GA in weeks	≥36 weeks	32 to 35 weeks and 6 days	28 to 31 weeks and 6 days	<28 weeks
Observe the NB for 15 sec				
Alertness	Active	Quiet	Active	Quiet
	Awake	Awake	Sleep	Sleeping
	Opened eyes	Opened eyes	Closed eyes	Closed eyes
	Facial movements present	No facial movements	Facial movements present	No facial movements
Record HR and SpO$_2$				
Maximal HR	↑ 0 to 4 bpm	↑ 5 to 14 bpm	↑ 15 to 24 bpm	↑ ≥ 25 bpm
Minimal Saturation	↓ 0 to 2.4%	↓ 2.5 to 4.9%	↓ 5 to 7.4%	↓ ≥ 7.5%
Observe NB for 30 sec				
Frowned forehead	Absent	Minimal	Moderate	Maximal
Eyes squeezed	Absent	Minimal	Moderate	Maximal
Nasolabial furrow	Absent	Minimal	Moderate	Maximal

Absent is defined as 0 to 9% of the observation time; minimal, 10% to 39% of the time; moderate, 40% to 69% of the time; and maximal as 70% or more of the observation time. In this scale, scores vary from zero to 21 points. Scores equal or lower than 6 indicate absence of pain or minimal pain; scores above 12 indicate the presence of moderate to severe pain.
GA, gestational age; NB, newborn.

the different faces scales, in our view there are some psychometric advantages to the Faces Pain Scale – Revised version by Hicks et al (Fig. 33.4) [21].

Parental responses can affect a child's levels of observed behavioral distress; increased parental anxiety tends to correlate with increased levels of self-report pain scores in children undergoing painful procedures. Older school-age children and adolescents have the emotional and cog-

nitive maturity as well as the language development to use self-report scales. Self-report is sometimes not accurate in this age range due to issues regarding behavioral control and self-esteem. Illness, hospitalization, and separation from parents may cause some older children and adolescents to regress emotionally, making pain scales designed for younger children more applicable. The meaning that pain has for a child also can influence their self-report. The Color Analog Pain Scale (Fig. 33.5) is a slide-rule device where gradations of color are used to denote degree of pain which has been validated for use in children as young as 5 years [22].

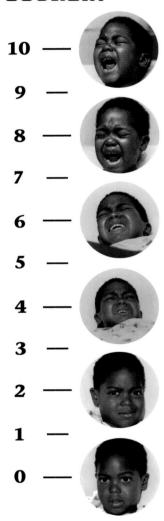

Figure 33.2 Oucher pain scale.

Pain assessment should be part of everyday practice in caring for hospitalized children. A successful, hospital-wide pain assessment program requires a committed, multidisciplinary team of healthcare providers, standard protocols of assessment methods and documentation, staff and parental education programs, and protocols for reassessment after pain treatment interventions. Essential to pain assessment is the use of validated, age-appropriate pain assessment tools as well as consideration of the child's developmental level, presence of fear and anxiety, parental factors, and the context of the child's pain.

Principles of developmental analgesic pharmacology in infants and children

A number of pharmacokinetic and pharmacodynamic factors produce age-related differences in response to analgesics [23]. Neonates and young infants have immature hepatic enzyme systems involved in conjugation, glucuronidation, and sulfation of analgesics such as opioids and amide local anesthetics, causing prolongation of elimination half-life and increasing the risk of drug accumulation. Rates of maturation of individual enzyme functions vary but for most analgesics, metabolism has matured by around age 6 months. Glomerular filtration and renal tubular secretion are reduced in the first several weeks of life. Along with slower elimination of some native drugs that depend primarily on renal clearance, renal immaturity also results in slower elimination of glucuronides of morphine and hydromorphone (which produce analgesia, sedation, respiratory depression, and excitatory reactions) and slow elimination of MEGX, a principal metabolite of lidocaine, which can cause seizures.

Neonates and young infants have reduced levels of α1-acid glycoprotein and albumin, leading to decreased plasma protein binding for many drugs and increased concentrations of free, pharmacologically active, unbound drug. Infants have immature ventilatory reflexes in response to hypoxia [24,25] and hypercarbia [26]. The increased risk of hypoventilation in response to

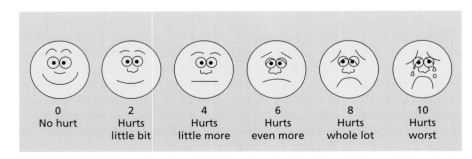

Figure 33.3 Faces (Wong–Baker pain scale).

0 2 4 6 8 10

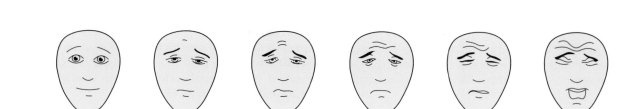

Figure 33.4 Faces Pain Scale   Revised (FPS–R) version.

In the following instructions, say "hurt" or "pain", whichever seems right for a particular child.

"These faces show how much something can hurt. This face [point to left-most face] shows no pain. The faces show more and more pain [point to each from left to right] up to this one [point to right-most face] – it shows very much pain. Point to the face that shows how much you hurt [right now]."

Score the chosen face 0, 2, 4, 6, 8, or 10, counting left to right, so '0' = 'no pain' and '10' = 'very much pain'. Do not use words like 'happy' and 'sad'. This scale is intended to measure how children feel inside, not how their face looks.

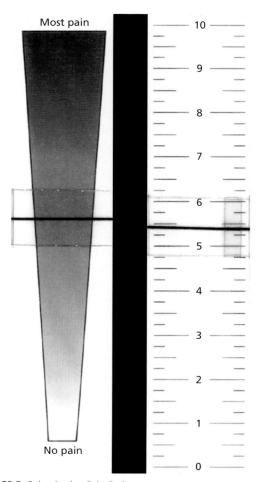

Figure 33.5 Color Analog Pain Scale.

opioids in infants observed in clinical case series [27] probably reflects a combined effect of pharmacokinetic and pharmacodynamic immaturity, as well as the impact of disease states that are over-represented in hospitalized infants.

Non-opioid analgesics

Non-opioid analgesics include acetaminophen, aspirin, the non-steroidal anti-inflammatory drugs (NSAIDs), and the selective cyclo-oxygenase 2 (COX-2) inhibitors. COX enzymes convert arachidonic acid to various prostaglandins that have diverse physiological roles, contributing to pain, hypersensitivity, inflammation, thermoregulation, vasodilation, and protection of gastric mucosal integrity. The cyclo-oxygenase iso-enzymes differ in their distribution and function in a variety of peripheral tissues and in the central nervous system. Aspirin and NSAIDs act on a broad spectrum of COX enzymes. Aspirin's irreversible inhibition of COX-1 in platelets contrasts with the reversible action of NSAIDs; this accounts for the much longer duration of aspirin's antihemostatic actions. The COX-2 inhibitors were developed to specifically inhibit the COX isoenzyme subtype 2, which is expressed preferentially in leukocytes and other cell types involved in inflammation, as well as in neurons and glial cells in the peripheral and central nervous systems. While these drugs are commonly regarded as "peripheral" analgesics, analgesia from all of these drugs involves a combination of peripheral and central actions [28].

Ontogeny of prostanoid biosynthesis and cyclo-oxygenases

Studies by Ririe and co-workers have shown that administration of a COX-1 inhibitor does not reduce hypersensitivity to mechanical stimuli in infant rats. This lack of efficacy of COX-1 inhibitors in infant rats appears to be a result of developmental differences in the COX-1 expression in the spinal cord [29]. These data raise the question of whether commonly used analgesics acting on COX isoforms might be ineffective in infants due to delayed maturation of COX-mediated processes in spinal microglia.

Acetaminophen

Acetaminophen is one of the most widely used analgesics and has a good safety record for use in pediatric patients. It is often combined with opioids for additional analgesic effect. Acetaminophen is also sometimes dosed alternating with ibuprofen, although there are no clinical trials examining the effectiveness of this approach. Although the actual mechanism of analgesic and antipyretic action is somewhat controversial, acetaminophen seems to have effect at the COX-3 isoenzyme, on endogenous cannabinoid receptors, and on TRPV1 receptors [160]. CB1 and TRPV1 receptors are involved in pain and thermoregulatory pathways. Acetaminophen's analgesic actions appear to occur largely via sites within the central nervous system, though there is controversy regarding the importance of central COX-3 inhibition in acetaminophen's analgesic effects [30].

When compared to NSAIDs, acetaminophen exerts minimal peripheral anti-inflammatory effects and is associated with significantly less gastropathy, platelet dysfunction, and anti-inflammatory effect. Approximately 90% of acetaminophen undergoes sulfation and glucuronidation to water-soluble products, which are then eliminated by the kidneys. A small percentage of acetaminophen is metabolized by the CYP450 system to a toxic metabolite that binds to glutathione to form a non-toxic conjugate. Inadvertent dosing errors have led to fulminant hepatic necrosis and failure in infants and children when large doses overwhelm the binding capacity of existing hepatic glutathione stores. Therapeutic oral doses of 10–15 mg/kg result in peak plasma concentrations at 2–3 h. Rectal dosing can be used in anesthetized children or those unable to tolerate oral administration. Peak drug levels generally occur at 70 min but can vary considerably with rectal dosing due to variable absorption. Because rectal absorption is so inefficient, some studies have recommended much higher dosing than traditionally prescribed; rectal dosing with a first dose of 30–45 mg/kg followed by 20 mg/kg every 6–8 h produced generally therapeutic blood concentrations in several studies [31]. Even though the overall bio-availability of rectal acetaminophen is roughly half that of oral formulations, previous American Academy of Pediatrics (AAP) recommendations have listed the same daily maximum doses for oral and rectal acetaminophen.

The analgesic efficacy of acetaminophen in newborns has not been established. It remains unclear whether these negative results reflect a true lack of efficacy due to delayed maturation of the analgesic targets of acetaminophen, inadequate sensitivity of the pain models used, insensitivity of the pain measures used or wash-out of treatment effects by the choice of an overly generous rescue analgesic regimen [32].

Non-steroidal anti-inflammatory drugs

The NSAIDs are widely prescribed as antipyretics, analgesics, and anti-inflammatory agents in children and, considering their widespread use, have a very good safety margin. They are often combined with opioids for improved analgesic effect and to reduce opioid use and side-effects. They are often first-line therapy for inflammatory pain. They produce their anti-inflammatory effect by reversibly inhibiting COX-1 and COX-2 isoenzymes and inhibiting the conversion of arachidonic acid to prostanoids. The clearances of several NSAIDs are slower in neonates and infants but more rapid in young children aged 3–10 years when compared to adults [33]. In postsurgical patients randomly assigned to receive an NSAID or placebo, with parenteral opioids as rescue analgesics, the NSAID groups typically show both lower pain scores and a 30–40% reduction in opioid use. Other studies have shown that standard doses of NSAIDs produce more effective analgesia than 30–60 mg of codeine in adults following surgery [34].

The incidence of serious side-effects from NSAIDs is very low in children 6 months and older, particularly with short-term use. A large-scale study in young children less than the age of 2 years receiving ibuprofen showed a very low incidence of serious side-effects [35]. There are few efficacy data on the use of NSAIDs in neonates. Much of the pharmacokinetic and safety data for use in neonates come from the use of ibuprofen and indometacin in treating patent ductus arteriosus; ibuprofen appears to have less renal toxicity and less risk of hyponatremia than indometacin in this age group. Much of the safety data for long-term use of NSAIDS are based on experience in treating juvenile rheumatoid arthritis [36]. Although children frequently complain of mild gastrointestinal upset with long-term NSAID use, serious gastropathy, gastrointestinal bleeding, and renal toxicity appear to be less common in children than adults. The risk of NSAID-induced renal toxicity can be increased in states of dehydration, with concomitant use of other nephrotoxic drugs, use in pre-existing renal disease, and hypotension.

The use of NSAIDs in children undergoing tonsillectomy remains controversial. NSAIDs are an attractive choice in patients with obstructive sleep apnea who are at risk for airway obstruction and hypoventilation with opioids after a tonsillectomy. Moreover, in a large number of analgesic trials for tonsillectomy, NSAIDs do provide good analgesia. However, since life-threatening immediate and delayed postsurgical bleeding can occur after a tonsillectomy, there has been concern that use of NSAIDs in this setting will increase the risk of bleeding via inhibition of platelet aggregation and prolongation of bleeding time. Various studies in patients having tonsillectomies have shown that NSAIDs provide good analgesia and a reduction in nausea and vomiting after tonsillectomy. Three meta-analyses which examined the use of NSAIDs in children having tonsillectomies produced conflicting results [37–39]. One meta-analysis found that the use of NSAIDs did not result in increased perioperative bleeding and did reduce the incidence of nausea and vomiting compared to other analgesics. Another meta-analysis found a threefold increase in the incidence of serious bleeding with NSAID use. Because of conflicting results among clinical trials and meta-analyses, the practice at our institution is to avoid the use of NSAIDs perioperatively in patients undergoing tonsillectomy, although there are many other centers that consider this practice safe and effective. COX-2 inhibitors for tonsillectomy are reviewed in a subsequent section.

Another controversy surrounding the use of NSAIDs is the concern about bone healing in postsurgical patients who require active bone formation, such as children with scoliosis who have undergone posterior spinal fusion and instrumentation. NSAIDs and COX-2 inhibitors clearly do provide good analgesia and reduced opioid requirements for several types of orthopedic surgery [40]. NSAIDs are thought to interfere with bone healing, since prostanoids produced by osteoblasts are associated with new bone formation and are involved in the balance between bone formation and bone resorption. Recent meta-analyses of case–control and cohort studies have suggested that the effects of short-term use of NSAIDs in most patient groups are clinically minor [39]. Reviews of heterotopic bone formation in adult patients after hip replacement have suggested a higher frequency of non-union; however, patient groups were small and other risks for non-union may have been present. A meta-analysis of the effects of NSAIDs in adult patients with spinal fusions showed that short-term use of normal-dose NSAIDs appeared to be safe after spine fusion but high-dose ketorolac increased the risk of non-union, implying that the risk may be partly dose dependent [40]. In general, children seem much less likely than adults to have impaired bone healing after surgery.

Our recommendation is to adopt a middle course pending more specific data on clinical outcomes and risks. For children at high risk for non-union or impaired bony fusion, NSAIDs probably should be avoided. Conversely, for children who are at comparatively low risk of non-union, who have had severe and difficult-to-control side-effects from opioids or who have significantly increased risks from opioids, an NSAID or COX-2 inhibitor is administered for 1–2 days postoperatively. Some studies suggest that selective COX-2 inhibitors are less likely to inhibit bone formation than traditional NSAIDs.

Ketorolac is a commonly prescribed parenteral NSAID often used as an adjuvant to opioids in the postoperative period. Despite the common belief regarding the "magic" of a parenteral route, ketorolac provides no stronger analgesia than other NSAIDs when given in recommended or equitoxic doses. Typical doses are 0.25 mg/kg every 6 h for a maximum of approximately 5 days. The recommended duration of 5 days is based on the pivotal adult studies used to obtain FDA approval for postoperative use and because of an impression that more prolonged use further increases the risks of adverse events, especially gastropathy. In a randomized controlled trial of infants and children undergoing cardiac surgery, ketorolac did not increase the risk of surgical bleeding or gastrointestinal bleeding [41]. Small case series have not reported harm with use after surgeries in neonates and young infants [42,43], though larger prospective studies are needed to better define the risks of NSAIDs in those age groups.

Prostanoids produced by COX-1 isoenzymes are associated with protection of gastric muscosa and platelet aggregation. Randomized controlled trials in adult patients show that COX-2 inhibitors provide the anti-inflammatory effects of traditional NSAIDs but with lower incidence of gastrointestinal symptoms and bleeding. Anti-inflammatory effects, analgesic efficacy, and incidence of renal toxicity with COX-2 inhibitors are comparable to other NSAIDs. NSAIDs and COX-2 inhibitors both alter the balance of pro- and antithrombotic products of arachidonic acid. For adults with risk factors for coronary artery disease, peripheral vascular disease, and carotid artery disease, COX-2 inhibitors appear to increase risks of cardiovascular events. Rofecoxib and valdecoxib were withdrawn from the market due to reports of cardiovascular complications in adult patients; celecoxib and meloxicam remain available in the US but with warnings regarding these potential risks.

With a few exceptions (e.g. children with genetically based hypercoagulability, children with Moya Moya disease), there is little basis to anticipate significant cardiovascular risks from COX-2 inhibitors in children [36]. We consider them to have a potentially favorable risk/benefit ratio for selected children with inflammatory pain who have severe gastrointestinal side-effects with traditional NSAIDs or those with underlying bleeding disorders, such as children with hemophilia. Certain modified non-acetylating salicylates with relatively mild gastric effects, including salsalate, diflunisal or choline-magnesium salicylate, may also be considered in children who have gastrointestinal side-effects with NSAIDs. Since COX-2 inhibitors have minimal antiplatelet/antihemostatic effects, they should in principle be ideal analgesics for children undergoing tonsillectomy. Available data on the efficacy of COX-2 inhibitors are mixed; some trials found COX-2 inhibitors equal to NSAID comparators and better than placebo [44] while other trials found COX-2 inhibitors either inferior to an NSAID or not distinguishable from placebo [45,46]. Overall numbers of subjects in these trials were small, and there is the potential for failing to identify analgesic effects due to type II error, or for washing out of treatment effects by scheduled use of other analgesics. We could not identify a meta-analysis to assign a confidence interval for their odds ratio for post-tonsillectomy bleeding.

Table 33.2 shows dosing guidelines for commonly used non-opioid analgesics.

Opioids

Opioids are widely used for the treatment of moderate-to-severe pain in infants and children. Safe and effective administration of opioids requires careful patient selection, knowledge of age-related differences in metabolism, dose titration, and aggressive treatment of opioid side-effects. Historically, pediatric patients, particularly infants and young children, received inadequate doses of opioids, partly because of a lack of understanding of how opioids are metabolized and limitations in the ability to assess pain in children. A greater understanding of the pharmacokinetics of opioids, developmental neuroanatomy, and validated pain scores has led to more appropriate dosing and the widespread use of opioids for pain management in infants and children.

Table 33.2 Dosing guidelines for non-opioid analgesics

	Dose <60 kg	Dose >60 kg
Acetaminophen	10–15 mg/kg q 4 h PO	650 mg q 4 h PO
Naproxen	5 mg/kg q 12 h PO	250–500 mg q 12 h PO
Ibuprofen	6–10 mg/kg q 6–8 h PO	400–600 q 6 h PO
Celecoxib	2–4 mg/kg q 12 h PO	100–200 mg q 12 h PO
Ketorolac	0.5 mg/kg q 6–8 h IV, not for >5 d	30 mg q 6–8 h IV, not for >5 d

Dosing guidelines listed herein refer to children >1 year of age.
Further modifications in dosing are required for use of these agents in term and preterm neonates in infants. Modifications are detailed in the text.
PO, orally; q; every.

Ontogeny of opioid actions

Opioid receptors are present by midgestation in a widespread distribution in forebrain, brainstem, and spinal cord. Functional maturation occurs gradually in prenatal and postnatal life. For example, while the infant rat (postnatal day 5) has an extensive complement of opioid receptors in brainstem and forebrain distributions, coupling to Gi/o proteins, as assayed by the ratio of GTP binding to DAMGO binding in brain striosomal preparations, is less than 5% of that seen in adult rat brain preparations [47].

There is an extensive series of animal studies of the effects of acute or chronic opioid administration on subsequent development. For example, chronic opioid exposure in prenatal and early postnatal life in the rat can lead to reductions in brain size, neuronal packing density, and dendritic development, with corresponding functional impairments in learning and locomotion [48]. Chronic opioid exposure in infant rats produces tolerance, withdrawal syndromes, and opioid-induced hyperalgesia [49].

The effects of opioids, ketamine, and other drugs on the developing animal are also modified by the presence of pain, injury, and/or inflammation. In some models, there are apparent long-term benefits of administering opioids prior to injury or inflammation [50]. Thus, extrapolations from animal studies regarding either benefit or harm of analgesics for newborns undergoing intensive care should be very cautious, in part because most animal models do not fully simulate all the types of perturbations seen with prolonged intensive care in humans.

Newborns undergoing intensive care are subjected to a large number of noxious procedures and mechanical ventilation, which *per se* produces stress and distress. Several studies have examined analgesia, side-effects and potential long-term consequences of opioids for ventilated newborns, given either on schedule or around specific noxious procedures. In the NEOPAIN trial, infants receiving chronic morphine infusions did not show more long-term neurological impairments compared to controls, but there was essentially no evidence of benefit on distress measures, and increased open-label episodic morphine administration for distress was associated with worse outcomes [51]. Moreover, morphine has only mild effect on behavioral indices of distress during painful procedures in preterm neonates [52]. At present, there is very little consensus regarding either benefit or harm from opioids or sedatives in critically ill neonates. A recent summary of these issues can be found in Durrmeyer et al [53]. A review by Anand and co-workers of opioid tolerance and dependence in neonatal and pediatric intensive care was recently published [54].

The specific choice of opioids depends on numerous factors including the ability to tolerate oral intake and gut absorption, side-effects, severity of pain, and whether pain is escalating. Oral routes are preferred for mild-to-moderate pain in children who are able to tolerate oral intake and who have adequate gastrointestinal absorption. Intravenous (IV) routes should be used for children who have severe pain that needs to be rapidly controlled, for rapidly escalating pain, and for those who cannot tolerate oral opioids.

Codeine is considered a weak opioid and is often combined with acetaminophen to improve analgesia. It is also used as an antitussive agent. Compared to other opioids, codeine seems to be associated with a higher risk of nausea. Analgesic effect is through the hepatic metabolism of codeine to morphine by CYP2D6 although there is significant variability in both the pharmacokinetics and pharmacodynamics of codeine. In a British cohort of children coming for surgery, 47% had reduced CYP2D6 enzyme concentrations and 36% had no detectable levels of morphine or metabolites after a parenteral dose of 1.5 mg/kg of codeine [55]. In children who lack or have significantly reduced enzyme levels, codeine is essentially inactive and provides no analgesia. Conversely, for patients with CYP2D6 gene duplication or with an ultra-rapid metabolizing allele, codeine may cause respiratory depression or death [56]. It is for these reasons that we discourage the use of codeine.

Oxycodone is an oral opioid frequently used for children with mild-to-moderate pain and is often used in the postoperative setting of converting from parenteral to enteral opioids. While historically oxycodone was used for moderate pain in relatively fixed doses, studies in adults showed that the dose of oxycodone, like morphine, can be escalated for moderate-to-severe pain. Oxycodone undergoes hepatic metabolism to oxymorphone, an active metabolite that is renally eliminated. A pharmacokinetic study of oxycodone in infants showed great variability in both clearance and in the elimination half-life, especially in neonates [57]. Oxycodone is available as an elixir for children unable to swallow pills and as a controlled-release preparation for a small subset of older children with severe or prolonged postoperative pain, e.g. for pain due to cancer or other serious illnesses. Dosing for immediate release is 0.1–0.2 mg/kg/dose every 4h as needed.

Morphine is generally considered the first-line opioid for parenteral use. Metabolism occurs in the liver, primarily through glucuronidation to morphine-3-glucuronide, which has neuroexcitatory actions, and morphine-6-glucuronide, which has analgesic, sedative, and respiratory depressant actions. Both glucuronides are renally eliminated and can accumulate in patients with renal failure, which accounts for the prolonged response and increased side-effects seen in patients with renal failure. Accumulation of morphine-3-glucuronide can contribute to delirium, myoclonus, agitation, and seizures. There is some evidence that morphine is preferentially metabo-lized in neonates to morphine-3-glucuronide and has an increased risk of seizures in this age group [58]. The elimination half-life of morphine in neonates and young infants is more than twice that of older children and is even more prolonged in premature infants [58]. Clearance of morphine in premature infants is less than half that measured in adults.

Studies of morphine efficacy in neonates have yielded mixed results, with some studies showing no apparent analgesic effect of morphine infusion in ventilated neonates in response to endotracheal suctioning. Because of the significant variation in pharmacokinetics of morphine among patients, dosing should be based on age, weight, side-effects, and careful dose titration [58]. Erythema and local urticaria at the site of IV administration are sometimes seen and do not imply an allergy to morphine. Morphine is generally well tolerated with minimal hemodynamic changes during infusions in blinded studies [59] but rapid bolus dosing can be associated with hypotension. Morphine and other opioids produce dose-dependent depression of ventilation by decreasing the brainstem response to hypoxia and hypercarbia and by interfering with central ventilatory centers. Morphine reduces the sense of air hunger in children with cancer and end-stage lung disease and can be given sublingually in this setting for ease of administration and for more rapid onset than enteral dosing. Dosing guidelines for morphine can be found in Table 33.3.

Hydromorphone has similar duration of action to morphine and is frequently used in patient-controlled analgasia (PCA) and epidural analgesia. Like morphine, it is commonly given orally and intravenously, although there is no long-acting preparation available. It differs from morphine in that it is slightly more lipid soluble and approximately five times more potent in steady state when given intravenously [60]. Like morphine, it is metabolized principally by glucuronidation. Hydromorphone is often prescribed for patients with renal insufficiency but this practice is not evidence based. Excitatory effects of either morphine or hydromorphone in patients with renal insufficiency correlate poorly with plasma concentrations of glucuronides [61]. While individual patients may report differences in analgesia or side-effects between morphine and hydromorphone, randomized blinded comparisons have found few clinically meaningful differences in the frequency of side-effects [62].

Methadone is a long-acting opioid that is supplied as a racemic mixture of d- and l-isomers. It has a prolonged elimination half-life, resulting in a long duration of analgesia. There is, however, wide variation in elimination half-life, ranging from 6 to 30h. The bio-availability is quite high, approximately 70–90%. Because of these unique properties, methadone can be dosed intermittently, either orally or intravenously, and can provide

Table 33.3 Initial dosing guidelines for opioids

Drug	Equi-analgesic doses		Usual starting intravenous or subcutaneous doses and intervals		Parenteral Oral dose	Usual starting oral doses and intervals	
	Parenteral	Oral	Child <50kg	Child >50kg	Ratio	Child <50kg	Child >50kg
Codeine	120mg	200mg	NR	NR	1:2	0.5–1.0mg/kg every 3–4h	30–60mg every 3–4h
Morphine	10mg	30mg (long-term) 60mg (single dose)	Bolus: 0.1mg/kg every 2–4h Infusion: 0.03mg/kg/h	Bolus: 5–8mg every 2–4h Infusion: 1.5mg/h	1:3 (long-term) 1:6 (single dose)	Immediate release: 0.3mg/kg every 3–4h Sustained release: 20–35kg 10–15mg every 8–12h 35–50kg; 15–30mg every 8–12h	Immediate release: 15–20mg every 3–4h Sustained release: 30–45mg every 8–12h
Oxycodone	NA	15–20mg	NA	NA	NA	0.1–0.2mg/kg every 3–4h	5–10mg every 3–4h
Methadone[a]	10mg	10–20mg	0.1mg/kg every 4–8h	5–8mg every 4–8h	1:2	0.1–0.2mg/kg every 4–8h	5–10mg every 4–8h
Fentanyl	100μg (0.1mg)	NA	Bolus: 0.5–1.0μg/kg every 1–2h Infusion: 0.5–2.0μg/kg/h	Bolus: 25–50μg every 1–2h Infusion: 25–100μg/h	NA	NA	NA
Hydromorphone	1.5–2mg	6–8mg	Bolus: 0.02mg every 2–4h Infusion: 0.006mg/kg/h	Bolus: 1mg every 2–4h Infusion: 0.3mg/h	1:4	0.04–0.08mg/kg every 3–4h	2–4mg every 3–4h
Meperidine[b]	75–100mg	300mg	Bolus: 0.5–1.0mg/kg every 2–3h	Bolus: 50–75mg every 2–3h	1:4	2–3mg/kg every 3–4h	100–150mg every 3–4h

Doses are for patients over 6 months of age. In infants under 6 months, initial per kilogram doses should begin at roughly 25% of the per kilogram doses recommended here. Higher doses are often required for patients receiving mechanical ventilation. All doses are approximate and should be adjusted according to clinical circumstances. Recommendations are adapted from previous summary tables, including those of a consensus statement from the World Health Organization and the International Association for the Study of Pain.

[a] Methadone requires additional vigilance because it can accumulate and produce delayed sedation. If sedation occurs, doses should be withheld until sedation resolves. Thereafter, doses should be substantially reduced, the interval between doses should be extended to 3 to 12 hours, or both.

[b] The use of meperidine should generally be avoided if other opioids are available, especially with long-term use, because its metabolite can cause seizures.

Adapted from Berde CB, Sethna NF. Analgesics for the treatment of pain in children. N Engl J Med 2002; 347: 1094–103.

NA, not applicable; NR, not recommended.

prolonged, steady-state analgesia similar to a continuous infusion or controlled-release preparations of other opioids.

The l-isomer of methadone acts as a μ opioid; the d-isomer acts as a non-competitive antagonist at the N-methyl-D-aspartate (NMDA) subgroup of excitatory amino acids receptors in the brain, spinal cord, and peripheral nerves. NMDA receptor antagonism results in analgesia, reduction in hyperalgesia, and partial reversing of tolerance to μ opioids [63]. Methadone's combined effect of μ receptor agonism and NMDA antagonism results in incomplete cross-tolerance so that dose conversion between methadone and other opioids depends, in part, on the patient's degree of opioid tolerance [64]. In opioid-naïve patients, the average daily requirement of IV methadone is approximately 30% of the corresponding IV morphine requirement. However, in opioid-tolerant patients, the average daily methadone requirement may be as little as 10% of the total daily morphine dose. This is especially relevant when converting from morphine to methadone in children who are opioid tolerant and when weaning non-ventilated infants and children from prolonged opioid therapy [65].

Because of incomplete cross-tolerance, slow and unpredictable elimination half-life, and variability in plasma concentrations, methadone dosing requires careful titration and frequent assessment for respiratory depression. Methadone has been associated with prolongation of the QT interval, especially when combined with other drugs known to cause prolonged QT. For patients showing oversedation or mild hypoventilation, it may be necessary to hold multiple doses rather than make small incremental changes due to the prolonged duration of action.

For opioid-naïve patients in the postoperative period, our practice is to dose methadone on a "sliding scale" every 4h where patients receive 0.075mg/kg for severe pain, 0.05mg/kg for moderate pain, and 0.025 for mild pain. After 24h of this dosing regimen, patients are then placed on a more regular dosing schedule, with shorter-acting opioids such as morphine or hydromorphone offered for rescue therapy.

Methadone is particularly useful in children with cancer who have nociceptive as well as neuropathic pain. It can be dosed in small children with chronic pain who are unable to swallow sustained-release pills.

Fentanyl is highly lipophilic, that is 70–100 times more potent than morphine in single-dose administration and 30–50 times more potent when given as a continuous intravenous infusion. Because fentanyl has a rapid onset and brief duration, it is often used for brief painful procedures, such as lumbar punctures, bone marrow biopsies, and dressing changes, either by itself or in combination with benzodiazepines or general anesthesia.

Doses of 0.5–1µg/kg, titrated every 1–3min generally provide good analgesia for brief painful procedures in non-ventilated patients. Fentanyl primarily undergoes conversion in the liver to inactive metabolites, making it useful in patients with renal failure. The effect of a single dose of fentanyl is terminated in large measure by rapid redistribution [66,67]. However, with repeated doses or continuous infusion, termination of the fentanyl effect is more determined by elimination rather than redistribution, resulting in prolonged duration of action. The context-sensitive half-life of fentanyl is particularly prolonged in neonates receiving continuous infusions [68]. Rapid administration may cause glottic and chest wall rigidity; treatment can consist of neuromuscular blockade, assisted ventilation, and in some cases administration of naloxone.

Oral transmucosal fentanyl is also used for brief painful procedures [69] and for children with cancer breakthrough pain. The oral transmucosal dose is partially absorbed through the buccal mucosa and partially swallowed so that the overall bio-availability is approximately 50%. The peak analgesic effect occurs at 30–45min. Most children tolerate oral transmucosal fentanyl well, although almost 90% experience facial pruritus.

Transdermal fentanyl is used in selected children with cancer pain [70]. It is also used for a very small number of children with chronic pain who require regular dosing of opioids and have a better side-effects profile with fentanyl than other opioids. Transdermal fentanyl is also used for patients who have difficulty with oral opioids or who have limited intravenous access. Following initial application or with dose escalation, approximately 12–24h are required to reach steady-state plasma levels because of depot accumulation of fentanyl in the skin; this also accounts for continued absorption of the drug at a declining rate after the transdermal fentanyl is removed. Because of these properties, it is not useful in patients with acutely fluctuating pain. Additional short-acting opioids are required with initial application and dose escalation. Drug uptake can be influenced by a number of patient factors, including skin temperature, thickness, adiposity, and inflammation. Transdermal fentanyl should be used only in patients who are opioid tolerant and who have fairly constant pain. Adverse events, including deaths, have been reported among opioid-naïve adult and pediatric patients who were treated with transdermal fentanyl for acute postsurgical pain.

Meperidine is approximately 10 times less potent than morphine. It is metabolized in the liver through hydrolysis and N-demethylation to normeperidine, a metabolite that is renally eliminated. The elimination half-life is 3–4h. Accumulation of normeperidine can cause hyperreflexia, agitation, delirium, and seizures. Life-threatening events have occurred with the use of meperidine in patients taking monoamine oxidase inhibitors and in those with untreated hypothyroidism. Doing so has resulted in metabolic and hemodynamic changes, excitability, seizures, and death. Meperidine is unique among opioids in that it reduces rigors associated with general anesthesia and the administration of blood products. Beyond its use in low doses for rigors or shivering, we generally recommend against use of meperidine for analgesia in children.

Table 33.3 shows initial dosing guidelines for opioid analgesics.

Methods of opioid administration
Intermittent opioid bolus dosing
Intermittent parenteral dosing of opioids can be useful for episodic pain or for initial loading doses in the treatment of acute pain. Particularly with longer dosing intervals, this approach results in wide fluctuations in plasma opioid concentrations and fluctuations in side-effects and pain intensity. Continuous infusions and patient- (or nurse-) controlled analgesia are often used instead of intermittent parenteral bolus dosing to avoid fluctuations in plasma opioid concentration, analgesia, and opioid side-effects.

Continuous opioid infusions
Continuous opioid infusions are useful for maintaining steady-state plasma opioid concentrations [58,71,72]. This approach is often used in intensive care units for ventilated patients who have relatively constant levels of pain; intermittent boluses of opioids are administered for any increases in pain, such as endotracheal tube suctioning. Although continuous infusions achieve steady-state plasma opioid levels and near-constant levels of analgesia, patients who have fluctuations in pain, such as with coughing, chest physiotherapy or getting out of bed, may have increased levels of pain which are not readily relieved by a continuous infusion of drug. In this setting, additional opioid boluses are required. Typical starting dose for continuous infusions of morphine is 0.025 mg/kg/h. Because of patient variations in opioid metabolism and pain intensity, effective starting doses vary considerably. Neonates and young infants require lower starting doses, ranging from 0.005 mg/kg/h in preterm neonates to 0.015 mg/kg/h in young infants aged 2–6 months.

Patient- and nurse-controlled analgesia
Patient-controlled analgesia (PCA) takes into account individual variations in opioid pharmacokinetics and individual fluctuations in pain intensity that cannot be treated by intermittent opioid bolus dosing or continuous infusions [73–76]. PCA involves a delivery system that administers a small preset dose of opioid, usually intra-venously, when the patient depresses a button. There is a preset lock-out time during which no additional boluses can be administered, even if the button is depressed. PCA can also administer a continuous opioid infusion in addition to the intermittent boluses.

Patient-controlled analgesia has been shown to be safe and effective in children aged 7 years and older. Some children as young as 4 or 5 years are able to effectively use PCA. However, there is a higher incidence of failure in younger children because of their inability to understand the causal relationship between depressing the button and obtaining medication for pain relief. PCA is widely used for a variety of painful conditions such as postoperative pain, painful vaso-occlusive crises, and cancer pain. There are conflicting data comparing PCA to continuous opioid infusions. Some studies indicate that PCA use tends to reduce patients' overall opioid use, with fewer opioid side-effects and similar or lower pain scores. Other studies did not find lower total opioid use with PCA compared to continuous opioid infusions.

Nurse-controlled analgesia (NCA) is commonly used for infants and children who are unable to push the PCA button, either due to lack of cognitive abilities or due to physical limitations. Outcome studies indicate that nurse-controlled analgesia is generally safe and effective in children, with good patient, nurse, and parent satisfaction [75,76]. NCA is commonly used in pediatric hospitals for opioid administration to young children following surgery.

Parent-controlled analgesia is widely accepted for use in children with advanced cancer pain and in palliative care, in both home and hospital settings. There is, however, controversy surrounding parent-controlled analgesia for opioid-naive children or in the setting of acute postoperative pain. Advocates of parent-controlled analgesia point out that parents know their children best, especially children with developmental or physical disabilities. The counter-argument is that parents, unlike nurses, do not have the training or expertise to effectively assess risks of opioid dosing or impending respiratory depression. There have been several serious adverse events, including deaths, with the use of parent-controlled analgesia by well-meaning parents. Our view is that parent-controlled analgesia for opioid-naive patients should be restricted to hospitals that have formal education parent programs, protocols for close nurse observation and assessment, and electronic cardiorespiratory monitoring [76].

Opioids commonly used for PCA include morphine, hydromorphone, and fentanyl. Some studies have shown that adding a basal infusion at night for postsurgical patients improves sleep and pain scores. Other studies have shown that basal infusions with PCA increase the risk of desaturation episodes, especially at night. Whether to add a basal infusion depends on a number of factors, including severity of pain, tolerance to opioids, and underlying patient condition that may increase risk of hypoventilation or airway obstruction. In general, patients with mild-to-moderate pain experience good analgesia with demand-only PCA. Our practice is to use PCA bolus dosing without a background basal infusion for children who have received a peripheral nerve block intraoperatively, who have increased risks of respiratory compromise, and for those who are expected to have mild-to-moderate but not severe surgical pain. We do tend to include a basal infusion for children who have cancer pain or pain from vaso-occlusive crises. For these patients, we tend to provide approximately 40–50% of their daily opioid dosing through basal infusions to provide effective analgesia without the need for frequent demand boluses. We often add a basal infusion for 1–2 days postoperatively for patients who have had surgeries expected to result in severe postoperative pain, such as scoliosis surgery or major hip surgery. When fentanyl is chosen for PCA, such as for patients who have had reactions to other opioids, a basal rate is often used because fentanyl is shorter acting than morphine or hydromorphone. Typical starting doses for PCA (and NCA) are listed in Table 33.4.

Opioid side-effects and treatment

Opioids are associated with a range of side-effects, including nausea, vomiting, constipation, urinary retention, pruritus, sedation, and respiratory depression. Although some children may experience different side-effect profiles with different opioids, there are few data to suggest that side-effects differ greatly among commonly used opioids. To many children, severe opioid side-effects, such as relentless nausea or pruritus, may be as distressing as pain. Opioid-sparing approaches to postoperative analgesia, including the use of NSAIDs, should be considered to avoid the complications of opioids on postoperative recovery [77].

Opioid side-effects occur by actions at both peripheral and central sites [78]. For example, opioid-induced nausea and vomiting involve agonist activity at receptors in the chemoreceptor trigger zone as well as in the gastrointestinal tract. Some opioids produce pruritus by peripheral release of histamine; however, small doses of intrathecal morphine are associated with profound pruritus, implying a more central cause of signaling and neurotransmission in the spinal dorsal horn and nucleus caudalis.

Opioid side-effects should be anticipated and treated aggressively. A proactive program with protocols for side-effect management allows for rapid implementation of treatment. The evaluation of the patient with opioid side-effects should include assessment of the severity of side-effect, the degree of patient distress, the expected duration of opioid therapy, and careful consideration of other factors that may masquerade as opioid side-effects. For example, severe itching may be a result of opioids but may also be due to an allergic reaction to other medications.

Constipation is nearly universal among patients receiving opioids, even with short-term use. Stimulant laxatives should be routinely used for all patients anticipated to require more than 1–2 doses of opioids. Methylnaltrexone has decreased ability to cross the blood–brain barrier and acts as a peripheral opioid antagonist [78]. It has been used for opioid-induced constipation that is refractory to laxatives. Doses of methylnaltrexone for children are extrapolated from adult studies.

Opioid-induced pruritus can be relentless and as distressing as pain to some patients. Pruritus occurs in approximately 13% of patients receiving parenteral opioids and 20–80% of patients receiving intrathecal or epidural opioids. Opioid-induced pruritus is thought to occur through activation of opioid receptors in the brain and substantia gelatinosa. Although antihistamines have traditionally been used to treat pruritus, there is good evidence for use of μ receptor antagonists such as naloxone infusions for both opioid-induced pruritus and opioid-induced nausea. In addition, antihistamines can exacerbate sedation, constipation, and urinary retention caused by opioids. In a prospective, randomized trial of 46 children receiving low-dose naloxone infusion (0.25 μg/kg/h) and morphine PCA postoperatively, the incidence and severity of opioid-induced pruritus and nausea were significantly reduced [79]. There was no increase in pain scores or increase in morphine use with the administration of low-dose naloxone. Ultra-low dose naloxone infusions show differential binding to opioid receptors coupled to G-stimulatory versus G-inhibitory proteins so that analgesia is not reversed. Nalbuphine is a widely used μ receptor antagonist used for opioid-induced nausea and vomiting although there are conflicting efficacy data among pediatric patients [80].

Nausea and vomiting are a major source of distress for patients, especially in the postoperative period. There is a strong relationship between postoperative nausea and

Table 33.4 Typical starting doses for patient-controlled (nurse-controlled) analgesia

Drug	Bolus dose (μg/kg)	Continuous rate (μg/kg/h)	4-h limit (μg/kg)
Morphine	20	4–15	300
Hydromorphone	5	1–3	60
Fentanyl	0.25	0.15	4

vomiting and the amount of opioids used postoperatively [81] but other causes should also be considered such as electrolyte abnormalities or impaired kidney function. Ondansetron is a selective 5HT3 receptor antagonist often used in the treatment of nausea and vomiting. Pheno-thiazines, butyrophenones, and metoclopramide have traditionally been used but have the associated risk of extrapyramidal reactions. There is good evidence to support the use of low-dose naloxone infusions in the treatment of nausea and vomiting associated with opioids. The typical dose of low-dose naloxone used in the treatment of opioid-induced pruritus and nausea is 0.25 µg/kg/h.

Children with advanced cancer often experience fatigue and somnolence, and opioid use often exacerbates these symptoms. Other treatable causes of fatigue should be considered, such as anemia, sleep disturbances, and depression. A cross-sectional study of the parents of 141 children who died of cancer reported that 96% of children had fatigue and nearly 50% experienced significant suf-fering from fatigue [82]. Only 13% of children with fatigue received directed treatment. More aggressive treatment of pain with opioids may further exacerbate fatigue and somnolence [83]. Methylphenidate is a stimulant that acts as an adrenergic receptor agonist to indirectly increase the release of dopamine and norepinephrine. Studies in adults support the use of methyphenidate to antagonize opioid-associated sedation and fatigue. Methylphenidate can also provide additional analgesic and antidepressant effects, which can be particularly beneficial for children with advanced cancer.

Please see Table 33.5 for management of common opioid-induced side-effects.

Local anesthetics and regional anesthesia

Developmental pharmacology of local anesthetics

The amino amide local anesthetics, including lidocaine, bupivacaine, levo-bupivacaine, and ropivacaine, undergo

Table 33.5 Management of common opioid side-effects

Side-effect	Comments	Drug dosage
Nausea	Consider switching to different opioid	Ondansetron 10–30 kg: 1–2 mg IV q 8h
	Use antimetics	>30 kg: 2–4 mg IV q 8h
	Exclude other processes (e.g. bowel obstruction)	Naloxone infusion 0.25–1 µg/kg/h
		Metoclopramide 0.1–0.2 mg/kg PO/IV q 6h
Pruritus	Exclude other causes (e.g. drug allergy)	
	Consider switching to different opioid	Nalbuphine 10–20 µg/kg/dose IV q 6h
	Use antipruritics	Naloxone infusion 0.25–1 µg /kg/h
		Diphenhydramine 0.25–0.5 mg/kg PO/IV q 6h
Sedation	Add non-sedating analgesic (eg, ketorolac) and reduce opioid dose	Methylphenidate 0.05–0.2 mg/kg PO bid (morning and mid-day dosing)
	Consider switching to different opioid	Dextroamphetamine 2.5–10 mg every day
Constipation	Regular use of stimulant and stool softener laxatives	Naloxone infusion 0.25–1 µg/kg/h
		Ducosate
		Child: 10–40 mg PO daily
		Adult: 50–200 mg PO daily
		Dulcolax
		Child: 5 mg PO/PR daily
		Adult: 10 mg PO/PR daily
		Methylnaltrexone, alvimopam dosing is extra from adults

bid, twice a day; PO, orally; PR, rectally; q, every.

hepatic metabolism more slowly in neonates and young infants, and weight-scaled clearances reach mature values generally around 6 months of age [84]. In addition, reduced renal clearance of metabolites (e.g. MEGX, the primary metabolite of lidocaine) can contribute to the risk of seizures in neonates. Although plasma esterases involved in metabolism of amino ester local anesthetics are present in reduced amounts in neonates, chloroprocaine clearance occurs quite rapidly in neonates [85]. Local anesthetics have somewhat larger volumes of distribution and reduced protein binding in neonates [84]. The plasma concentrations that produce cardiotoxicity or risk of seizures in human neonates, infants, and children are extrapolated from case reports, adult case series, and adult preclinical toxicological studies [86]. Infant rats tolerate a higher weight-scaled dose of either bupivacaine or ropivacaine (higher LD50) than adult rats [87].

In our view, it seems prudent to conclude that the maximum systemically safe single dose of bupivacaine, levo-bupivacaine, ropivacaine or lidocaine scales directly with bodyweight, and that the hourly maximum infusion rates in neonates and infants less than 3–5 months of age should be reduced by about 50% relative to the recommended rates for older infants and children.

Topical anesthetics

Topical anesthetics are widely used in children for pain associated with immunizations, venepunctures, accessing indwelling central venous ports, and other types of needle pain [88,89]. The stratum corneum of the epidermis is a relatively impermeable barrier to local anesthetics and a variety of strategies have been developed to permit uptake of local anesthetics across this barrier.

EMLA

Eutectic mixture of local anesthetics (EMLA) (lidocaine and prilocaine) was one of the first topical anesthetics commercially available for use on intact skin and has been extensively used and studied [90,91]. The physicochemical feature of this type of mixture is that it permits a higher aqueous solubility of the uncharged forms. This permits a higher effective concentration at the stratum corneum and increases the rate of uptake. A meta-analysis of controlled trials in children and adults showed that EMLA reduced pain associated with venepunctures in 85% of patients.

Applying a thicker layer and increasing the duration of application to 90–120 min can increase its effectiveness. Applying a thin layer (0.5 mm) compared to a thick layer (2 mm) resulted in significantly less pain relief with venepunctures. Even with longer duration of application, absorption into the epidermis was limited to no more than 6 mm. Application times of less than 45 min result in

high failure rates and with short application times, tetracaine gel appears more effective than EMLA [91]. Blanching is commonly seen with EMLA and is due to vasoconstriction of superficial capillaries.

Clinical trials have shown effectiveness of EMLA in reducing the pain or distress of a number of common pediatric procedures, including venous cannulation, venepuncture, circumcision, urethral meatotomy, immunizations, allergy testing, accessing implanted central venous access ports, and laceration repair.

S-Caine patch

The S-Caine patch (Synera™) is drug delivery device consisting of a eutectic mixture of lidocaine (70 mg) and tetracaine (70 mg) integrated with an oxygen-activated heating element. The heating element enhances the delivery of the local anesthetics across the epidermis. When removed from its storage pouch, the heating element becomes activated and the patch begins to heat, warming the skin after application. Controlled trials in children and adults showed that application of the patch for 20 min produced good skin analgesia for venous cannulation [92]. A randomized placebo-controlled trial of the S-Caine patch showed that the majority of patients had good pain relief with vascular access procedures. The most common side-effects were local transient skin reactions, such as localized pruritus and erythema. Unlike EMLA, Synera is associated with mild vasodilation due to the vasodilating properties of lidocaine and mild heating of the skin.

Jet propulsion injectors

Jet propulsion injectors (J-tip system and Powerject) are needleless syringe devices that utilize compressed gas, typically carbon dioxide, to rapidly propel a predetermined amount of local anesthetic through the stratum corneum. These types of devices are attractive in that the local anesthetic effect occurs within several minutes and it is a needleless system. However, efficacy data are somewhat mixed. A randomized trial in adult patients showed that subcutaneous lidocaine infiltration was significantly more effective at reducing pain from venous cannulation. Other randomized studies in adults have found a failure rate of approximately 10%, and 17% of patients had mild bleeding at the site. A study comparing the J-tip system to EMLA in children found that the J-tip system provided better analgesia than EMLA for IV cannulation [93].

Iontophoresis

Iontophoresis employs an electrical field to drive local anesthetics in their charged ionic form across the stratum corneum. Iontophoresis produces cutaneous anesthesia in a much shorter time. The most common anesthetic used by this route is 2% lidocaine with 1:100,000 epinephrine. Skin analgesia occurs within 10–15 min and typically lasts for 15 min. Iontophoresis appears to result in deeper levels of dermal anesthesia and may penetrate deeply enough to numb both skin and veins, allowing for less painful venous cannulation. Randomized prospective studies in children comparing EMLA with iontophoresis of 2% lidocaine and 1:100,000 epinephrine found no significant differences in pain relief with venous cannulation. Superficial and partial-thickness burns have been reported with lidocaine iontophoresis when placed over areas with skin defects or when high currents have been used. A mild tingling sensation often occurs during drug delivery. It is recommended that the system be removed if pain rather than tingling is experienced. Longer application times are needed when lower currents are used, but the tingling sensation can be made almost undetectable.

Epidural analgesia

Epidural analgesia can provide excellent postoperative analgesia for infants and children undergoing a variety of surgical procedures including thoracic, perineal, lower extremity, and abdominal procedures. (Detailed discussion of peripheral nerve blocks can be found in Chapter 18.) Epidural analgesia is also used for certain chronic pain conditions such as complex regional pain syndrome (CRPS) (Fig. 33.6), especially when used as part of a rehabilitation program that emphasizes active mobilization.

An inherent difference between epidural catheter placement in adults and children is that, unlike for adults [94],

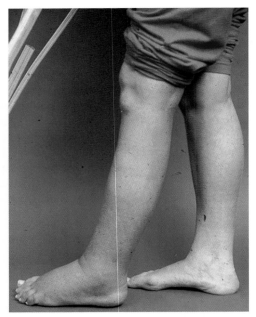

Figure 33.6 Complex regional pain syndrome (CRPS) presentation.

most epidural catheters in children are placed while anesthetized. Most pediatric anesthesia providers agree on the safety of placing a lumbar epidural catheter in an anesthetized rather than an awake, moving child. However, there is somewhat more controversy surrounding the safety of direct needle placement in the thoracic region, particularly in infants, due to concerns about neurological complications. Published case series and prospective clinical outcome studies showed generally good safety, though from available data it is difficult to ascribe confidence intervals on the specific risk for anesthetized thoracic needle puncture in different age groups [95,96]. To avoid the potentially increased risk, an alternative method is to advance catheters from the caudal region cephalad to thoracic dermatomes. This may be performed blindly or with additional guidance by fluoroscopy, ultrasound [97], nerve stimulation guidance [98] or by electrocardiography [99]. Several reports in infants show that these techniques can be safe alternatives to direct needle placement, with success rates of roughly 80–98%. Failure rates with blind placement are greater for infants larger than 5 kg. Infants clear amide local anesthetics more slowly than older children so that lower infusion rates are necessary and repeated local anesthetic dosing is more likely to produce systemic accumulation of drug and toxicity.

Because of the limitations of using safe local anesthetic infusion rates, it is crucial in infants and young children to place epidural catheter tips in the correct surgical dermatome. When placing epidural catheters directly in a thoracic dermatome or when advancing epidural catheters cephalad to the thoracic region, our practice is to obtain confirmation of proper placement radiographically, through ultrasound or by electrical stimulation. Blind advancement of catheters from lumbar to thoracic levels has a failure rate of approximately 30%. One method of radiographic confirmation of proper epidural catheter tip placement is an epidurogram in which a small amount (0.5–1 mL) of radiocontrast dye is injected through the epidural catheter that can be detected on a plain radiograph (Fig. 33.7). Catheters can also be advanced from lumbar or caudal routes under fluoroscopic guidance, and catheter tip positions can be confirmed by a contrast epidurogram.

In our experience, lumbar-to-thoracic placement of catheters is more successful if placement occurs at L1–2 rather than lower levels, and with the epidural needle angled in a cephalad direction, rather than perpendicular to the spine. It is important to note that the distance from skin to epidural space is much shorter at T12–L1 and L1–2 interspaces than at L3–4 or L4–5 which may predispose to inadvertent dural puncture. In our own practice, we make extensive use of electrical stimulation of epidural catheters [100], for confirming placement in the epidural space, for advancing lumbar and caudal catheters to tho-

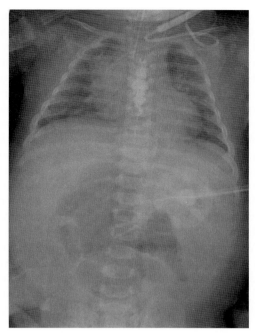

Figure 33.7 Epidurogram following placement of an epidural catheter. Note dye in the thoracic area.

racic dermatomes, and for confirming that the catheter is not wrong-sided (directed contralateral to the side of surgery). In this method, a small amount of electrical current is applied to a saline-filled, wire-wrapped epidural catheter as it is advanced cephalad in the epidural space. Twitches can be observed at the myotomal level of the catheter tip in a current range usually between 2 and 15 mA. Characteristic response patterns indicating epidural, vascular, intrathecal or dural placement can be observed as the catheter is advanced. This technique can also provide information on the sidedness of the epidural catheter so that for a unilateral surgical procedure, predominant myotomal twitching on the non-operative side can be detected and the catheter repositioned. Technical success rates of 98% and analgesic success rates of 85% have been described using this method. Even in older adolescents and adults who may undergo regional anesthesia awake or under light sedation, we find that nerve stimulation is tolerated with minimal distress, provided the current is increased gradually.

It is sometimes necessary to confirm proper position of an epidural catheter postoperatively, for example, in the setting of continued pain despite adequate dosing of epidural infusions. Our common practice is to use a chloroprocaine loading dose, particularly for infants and non-verbal children. Chloroprocaine is an ester local anesthetic that is metabolized by plasma cholinesterases. Although infants have reduced levels of plasma cholinesterases, chloroprocaine is nevertheless rapidly

metabolized. Because of concerns about toxicity due to accumulation of amide local anesthetics in infants and young children, we prefer to use chloroprocaine in place of lidocaine or other amide local anesthetics to check epidural catheter placement. Since most patients will have received infusions of amide local anesthetics intraoperatively, administering a bolus of chloroprocaine avoids the possibility of reaching toxic plasma levels through additional boluses of amide local anesthetics. We inject a loading dose of 3% chloroprocaine incrementally over roughly 2 min through the epidural catheter. For this loading dose, infants receive larger weight-scaled volumes than adolescents. For example, an 8 kg infant might receive a total loading volume of 5 mL (0.62 mL/kg), while a 30 kg 7 year old might receive a total loading volume of 12 mL (0.4 mL/kg), and patients >50 kg get a total loading volume of 15 mL. With these loading volumes, there should be clear clinical signs of sensory and motor block if the catheter is correctly positioned within the epidural space. Behavioral measures of pain relief such as relaxed posture and ceasing of crying are helpful in determining whether preverbal patients are experiencing relief, but objective measures should also be present, such as a motor block and a return of vital signs to baseline values.

Selection of drugs for epidural injection should be individualized and will vary with site of surgery, location of epidural catheter tip, and patient-specific risk factors. For most postoperative children, we recommend infusions of local anesthetics in combination with opioids, clonidine or both rather than local anesthetics alone because of the synergistic effect of combining local anesthetics with adjuvants. Bupivacaine is an amide local anesthetic commonly used in epidural local anesthetic infusions because it has a prolonged duration of action and produces more sensory than motor block. As previously discussed, the clearance of bupivacaine and other amide local anesthetics is reduced in neonates and young infants. Pharmacokinetic studies measuring unbound, pharmacologically active bupivacaine in infants receiving continuous epidural bupivacaine infusions showed that plasma bupivacaine levels rise after the first 48 h and some infants will have plasma bupivacaine levels nearing or exceeding safe limits. Although most infants had an increase in their serum α1-acid glycoprotein concentrations after surgery, the increase did not fully buffer the unbound bupivacaine fraction. Based on these studies, epidural bupivacaine infusion rates in neonates and infants younger than 4 months of age should be limited to 0.2 mg/kg/h. Even at this low infusion rate, accumulation and drug toxicity are possible for infusions lasting more than 72 h [101]. Epidural bupivacaine infusion rates of 0.4 mg/kg/h appear to be safe for children over the age of 6 months.

Ropivacaine is an amide local anesthetic that in adult studies was found to be safer and more sensory selective than bupivacaine. Studies of IV ropivacaine in adult volunteers showed less central nervous system and cardiovascular toxicity than bupivacaine. In double-blind comparisons, ropivacaine and levo-bupivacaine both produced similar analgesic effects as racemic bupivacaine but less extensive motor block [102]. Pharmacokinetic data in infants and children show that the clearance of bupivacaine is slightly more than the clearance of ropivacaine in all ages but as with bupivacaine, clearance of ropivacaine is reduced in neonates and young infants compared to older children [103–105]. Our practice is to use ropivacaine infusion rates up to 0.3 mg/kg/h in infants younger than 6 months and up to 0.5 mg/kg/h for older children.

Lidocaine is used as an epidural local anesthetic for neonates and infants in some centers [106] because of the relative ease of monitoring lidocaine blood concentrations and because of reduced cardiotoxicity relative to bupivacaine. Note that even with lidocaine concentrations in a safe range, there is the potential for seizures due to accumulation of MEGX [107].

Epidural infusion rates of amide local anesthetics are limited in young infants because of the increased risk of toxicity, as detailed above. Chloroprocaine infusions have been used as an alternative to continuous amide local anesthetic infusions to allow for sufficient epidural infusion rates without the associated toxicity concerns of amide local anesthetics. Studies of continuous epidural infusions of chloroprocaine showed good surgical anesthesia without neurotoxicity [85]. Higher weight-scaled infusion rates of chloroprocaine are necessary to achieve a similar extent of sensory block to that seen with bupivacaine and ropivacaine. Our practice is to use 1.5% chloroprocaine at a rate of 0.5 mL/kg/h for mid-thoracic epidural catheters and 0.6–0.7 mL/kg/h for lumbar and low thoracic catheter solutions in neonates and young infants who are monitored in the intensive care unit.

Because of weight-based scaling constraints of local anesthetic infusion rates, one rationale for combining opioids, clonidine or both along with epidural local anesthetic infusions is to provide a stronger analgesic effect while remaining in a safe local anesthetic dosing range. Addition of opioids, either neuraxially or systemically, will intensify the analgesia but increase the frequency of side-effects. Hydromorphone and fentanyl are the most commonly used epidurally administered opioids. In studies in adults, hydromorphone produces analgesia similar to morphine, but with less pruritus. The hydrophilic property of hydromorphone results in more cephalad spread, which can be effective for extensive surgeries that cover multiple dermatomes. However, the cephalad spread of hydromorphone does increase the risk of respiratory depression and we tend to restrict the use of hydromorphone in epidural infusions to infants older than 4 months, infants who are opioid tolerant or those who require ventilatory support for a period of time postoperatively. For older children, we favor hydromorphone over other additives, especially for extensive and painful surgery, for patients who have pre-existing chronic pain and hyperalgesia, and for most cancer surgeries. Fentanyl is used in epidural infusions in infants less than 4 months of age and in children whose surgery does not involve multiple dermatomes or is associated with relatively less pain intensity. In general, slightly lower starting infusion rates should be used when epidural catheter tips are located in the thoracic region or when using hydrophilic opioids.

All neuraxial opioids cause similar opioid side-effects, which are treated in much the same way as side-effects caused by systemically administered opioids. Pruritus is one of the most common side-effects of neuraxial opioids. It is most likely the result of modulation of neurotransmission in the dorsal horn and the trigeminal nucleus caudalis. Low-dose naloxone infusions in doses of 0.25 μg/kg/h are effective at treating opioid-induced pruritus and nausea without reversing analgesia or precipitating withdrawal symptoms.

Clonidine enhances and prolongs the analgesic effect of local anesthetics without contributing to respiratory depression, nausea, urinary retention, pruritus and other opioid-related side-effects. We tend to employ clonidine most commonly for patients who have persistent epidural opioid side-effects despite standard treatments. Hypotension can occur, particularly in adolescents or in patients with inadequate blood and volume replacement.

Please see Table 33.6 for recommended epidural infusion rates.

Acute pain services

Over the past 20 years, there has been much focus on the development of acute pain services, in part because of recognition of the undertreatment of postoperative pain, particularly in children. The Joint Commission has mandated specific hospital-wide standards for the treatment of pain and related symptoms in healthcare settings. There is evidence that acute pain services (APS) reduce patient reports of pain intensity and reduce delays in relieving severe pain. However, the effect of APS on other outcomes, such as incidence of side-effects, critical events and length of hospital stay, is equivocal. Other studies did not consistently show similar outcomes.

The specific organization of pain management programs varies depending on numerous factors including

Table 33.6 Recommended epidural infusion rates (mL/kg/h)*

Solution	<1 month	1–4 months	>4 months**
Bupivacaine 0.1% +/– Fentanyl 2 µg/mL +/– Clonidine 0.4 µg/mL	Rarely used	0.2	0.4
Ropivacaine 0.1% +/– Fentanyl 2 µg/mL +/– Clonidine 0.4 µg/mL	Rarely used	0.3	0.4–0.5
Bupivacaine 0.1% + Hydromorphone 10 µg/mL	Rarely used	Rarely used	0.3–0.4
Ropivacaine 0.1% + Hydromorphone 10 µg/mL	Rarely used	Rarely used	0.3–0.4
Chloroprocaine 1.5% + Fentanyl 0.2 µg/mL +/– Clonidine 0.04 µg/mL	0.5 (mid-thoracic) 0.6–0.7 (lumbar and low thoracic)	0.5 (mid-thoracic) 0.6–0.7 (lumbar and low thoracic)	Rarely used Rarely used

* Infusion rates and solutions should be modified according to clinical circumstances. Little information is available on how best to adjust these rates based on degrees of prematurity. Rates shown reflect upper end of usual infusion rates, based largely on both systemic accumulation of local anesthetics and on expected extent of sensory and/or motor blockade. Solutions containing hydrophilic opioids such as hydromorphone may pose a higher risk for delayed respiratory depression, so appropriate frequency of observation and continuous electronic monitoring is recommended. Higher concentrations of opioids may be considered for selected patients who are opioid tolerant.

** Weight-scaled infusion rates should plateau at values recommended for patients weighing around 45 kg, i.e. maximum infusion rates for larger patients should rarely exceed 15 mL/h.

the average number of postoperative patients, the type of surgical procedures performed, and availability of subspecialists. Although the particular model of pain management program is unique to each hospital, there are common features that should be considered in the organization of acute pain services.

- Multidisciplinary group of clinicians dedicated to pain management, including anesthesiologists, nurses, surgeons, pediatricians, and pharmacists.
- Designated personnel to provide 24-h pain management services.
- Hospital-wide protocols or algorithms for pain assessment, analgesic therapy, monitoring of pain and vital signs, treatment of side-effects, and documentation of pain-related information.
- Hospital-wide standards for management of more specialized analgesic treatments such as epidural catheters, PCA, spinal catheters, peripheral nerve catheters, baclofen pumps, and implanted spinal/epidural ports.
- Education program for clinicians (including pre and post tests).
- Education program for parents and children about risks, benefits, and treatment options.
- Quality assurance program and outcome tracking system.
- Ongoing review of pain management practices.

Formal measures of pain intensity should be assessed at regular intervals and recorded, as is routine for vital signs measurement. Specific pain assessment tools are chosen based on patient's age and cognitive and emotional ability as detailed above in the section on pain assessment in infants and children. In general, a visual analog scale or numerical rating scale is used for children aged 7 years and older. Faces scales, such as the Bieri or Wong–Baker faces, are appropriate for younger children aged 3–7. Ideally, education regarding the use of appropriate pain assessment tools should be reviewed with children and their parents at the preoperative visit. Composite pain scales that include behavioral observations, such as the FLACC Scale, are used for toddlers and non-verbal children. The FLACC and the PIPP are commonly used pain scales for infants and for preterm newborns, respectively.

Protocols for pain and symptom management are the foundation of a comprehensive pain management program. Depending on the type of surgery, patients' medical condition, and the degree of postoperative pain, most postoperative pain is treated by combinations of NSAIDs, opioids, and regional analgesia. For mild postoperative pain, short-acting opioids such as oxycodone alternating with doses of NSAIDs generally provide good pain relief. Oral dosing is preferred when patients are able to tolerate oral intake postoperatively. Parenteral opioids are used in patients with more severe pain or when patients are restricted in their oral intake. PCA or NCA is widely used for infants and children with acute postoperative pain who require parenteral opioids. Regional analgesia including peripheral nerve catheter infusions and epidural infusions can provide excellent postoperative analgesia with opioid sparing and subsequent decrease in opioid side-effects. Protocols for analgesic administration include standardized PCA, epidural, and peripheral nerve catheter ordersets so that range-dosing of opioids and local anesthetics solutions is standardized and somewhat independent of prescriber. Nevertheless, dosing parameters and choice of specific opioid or combined local anesthetic/opioid solutions should be individualized and based on patients' prior opioid use and side-effect profile, severity of pain, location of surgical pain, medical condition, and psychological state. Inherent in pain management protocols are algorithms and ordersets for treatment of side-effects so that patients do not experience delays in receiving treatment for common side-effects, such as pruritus, nausea, and vomiting.

All patients receiving opioids, either systemically or through regional catheters combined with local anesthetics, should be assessed for signs of respiratory depression. Protocols for monitoring level of consciousness and respiratory depression should involve nursing assessment and documentation of levels of sedation at regular intervals. Our practice is to provide electronic cardiorespiratory monitoring for all patients who have a basal rate added to their PCA, patients with risk factors for respiratory depression with opioids, such as those with certain airway diseases or neurological impairments, and young infants who are at risk for apnea with opioids. There have been reports of hypoventilation and critical events among healthy patients receiving epidural analgesia postoperatively, even when fentanyl was used as the opioid in the epidural infusion. We routinely place all patients receiving epidural infusions on cardiorespiratory monitors. While oximetry may be imperfect in detecting hypoventilation, especially when supplemental oxygen is administered, it probably facilitates rescue before serious harm occurs in many cases [108]. Other routine nursing assessment and documentation should include regular assessment of side-effects, extent of sensory and motor block for patients with regional catheters, and total daily amounts of opioids administered so that day-to-day comparisons can be made.

Hospitals with acute pain services need to have a system of immediate response to critical events. The structure of the immediate response system varies among hospitals but it is essential to have clinicians involved who have expertise in pediatric airway management and

who are knowledgeable about the pharmacology of local anesthetics, opioids, and sedatives.

Quality assurance programs should analyze data pertaining to clinical practice, including general outcome measures of PCA, epidural, and other regional techniques. Data concerning adverse events should also be analyzed at regular intervals. Based on analyses of data, quality assurance programs can review institutional policies and practices and make practice guideline recommendations for improvement in safety and patient satisfaction.

Painful conditions in infants and children

Cancer pain

Children with cancer experience a variety of types of pain related to their disease process and cancer treatments [109]. Studies of cancer pain in children have shown that as successful treatment protocols evolve, pain related to cancer treatments is the more predominant source of pain and suffering, including painful mucositis, postamputation pain, and peripheral neuropathies [110]. Repeated needle procedures, such as bone marrow biopsies, lumbar punctures, and repeated venous access, are particularly distressing for children. Tumor-related pain is often present at the time of the initial diagnosis and also results from disease progression with tumor spread to bone, spinal cord, and nerve plexuses. Children with hematological malignancies often present with bone pain from bone marrow infiltration and abdominal pain from capsular stretch of liver and spleen; those who show a good response to induction chemotherapy generally experience resolution of pain. However, a subgroup of children will continue to experience somatic, visceral and neuropathic pain.

Children undergoing treatment of cancer frequently need diagnostic imaging studies, radiation therapy, and brief needle procedures. Aggressive and proactive management will help decrease pain and anxiety associated with these procedures. Cognitive behavioral therapies, such as guided imagery, are useful for children with procedural pain. Topical analgesics should be routinely used for minor needle procedures such as accessing implanted vascular ports or intravenous line insertions. Depending on age, associated medical problems, and severity of pain and other symptoms, general anesthesia or conscious sedation is generally used for more invasive needle procedures, such as bone marrow biopsies and lumbar punctures. Safe sedation protocols have been established by the American Academy of Pediatrics and serve as guidelines for procedural sedation by oncologists and other subspecialists. Children with risk factors for conscious sedation or those who fail prior attempts at conscious sedation require consultation by pediatric anesthesiologists. Daily radiation therapy or diagnostic imaging, such as magnetic resonance imaging (MRI), is not typically painful but do require children to be immobile and brief general anesthesia is usually required.

Mucositis is painful inflammation of the mucosa caused by chemotherapy or radiation. It is a common side-effect in children receiving chemotherapy and is especially intense and prolonged with bone marrow transplantation. Topical agents are often used for symptomatic relief in mild mucositis, but there are limited data showing efficacy. Parenteral opioids given through PCA or NCA are generally used for moderate-to-severe pain from mucositis. Oral opioids are not typically used initially since most children experience painful swallowing from mouth and esophageal involvement. Since many children experience significant pain from mucositis for weeks, our practice is to provide approximately 60% of the total daily opioid dose through a basal rate to provide sustained analgesia without requiring the patient to use the PCA button repeatedly throughout the day and night. For patients with mucositis whose pain is poorly controlled with standard PCA or NCA opioids, a recent trial supports addition of low-dose ketamine to the mixture [111].

Nearly all children who have had amputations experience phantom sensations and many experience phantom pain [112]. Postamputation pain occurs more often in children who have had amputations due to cancer rather than trauma, and administration of chemotherapy may be a risk factor in the development of phantom pain. Regional analgesia, including epidural and peripheral nerve catheters, can provide very effective postoperative analgesia after limb amputations. Although severity of early postamputation pain correlates with likelihood of longer-term pain, studies of pre-emptive actions of several regional anesthetic approaches have yielded mixed outcomes. Treatment with antidepressants, anticonvulsants, NMDA-antagonistic drugs, gabapentin, opioids, and clonidine has shown some success but there are limited data from large, controlled clinical trials. Mirror box therapy and other forms of visual feedback therapies have been used with some success in the treatment of postamputation pain [113]. A mirror is positioned so that it reflects movement of the limb as if the amputated limb is intact.

A stepwise program of analgesic therapy proposed by the World Health Organization can provide good treatment of pain in adults with advanced cancer without intolerable side-effects in a large majority of patients. A similar stepwise analgesic approach has been advocated for the treatment of children with cancer pain where NSAIDs, acetaminophen, and low-dose opioids, such as oxycodone, are initially used for the treatment of mild pain. Morphine, hydromorphone and other opioids are titrated to effect as pain escalates. The use of oral opioids is recommended when possible. For patients with persistent pain, an effective opioid regimen includes the use of long-acting opioids, such as methadone or sustained-release formulations of morphine or oxycodone. Short-acting morphine, oxycodone, hydromorphone or other opioids are added for breakthrough pain. Oral methadone is useful as a long-acting elixir for children who are unable to swallow pills. Conversion from morphine and other short-acting opioids to methadone requires individualization and close observation because of the incomplete cross-tolerance mentioned above. A rough guide for conversion can be found at www.globalrph.net/narcoticconverter. Several sustained-release opioid preparations contain microbeads and it is common practice to open the capsule and sprinkle the microbeads into food just prior to use. However, if the microbeads are chewed or left in contact with food for an extended period of time, they release their contents. Not only does this reverse the sustained-release property, it can also increase the risk of overdose. Parenteral opioids are used when pain is rapidly escalating and oral opioids are not effective or when patients are unable to tolerate oral opioids due to nausea, vomiting, gastrointestinal processes or the inability to swallow. In this setting, PCA or NCA is used, generally with a basal rate. Opioid side-effects should be aggressively treated and in cases of intolerable side-effects, opioid rotation can be helpful.

Although standard dosing of opioids adequately treats cancer pain in most children, a subgroup of children with cancer will have persistent, severe pain despite enormous escalation of opioid dosing (for example 500 mg/kg/h) [114]. Refractory pain despite massive opioid doses is typically seen with tumor metastases to spinal cord and major nerves, causing unrelenting neuropathic pain. Many children with severe cancer pain who are resistant to opioids can be made comfortable through the use of regional anesthetic techniques, such as implanted intrathecal or epidural catheters or ports [115]. The choice of drugs should be individualized and depends on a number of factors, such as location and nature of pain, bowel and bladder function, and level of alertness. In most cases, dilute solutions of local anesthetics and opioids provide good pain relief, although other agents are sometimes added, such as clonidine or ketamine. Our general preference is use intrathecal rather than epidural placement in most cases, because this permits versatile dosing as pain escalates over time, and because over time epidural dosing of local anesthetics is limited by tachyphylaxis and systemic toxicity. We generally prefer placement of ports to facilitate skin care, reduce the risk of infection, and reduce the chance of catheter dislodgment at home. These procedures are performed under general anesthesia and with fluoroscopic guidance. There are a number of technical and management issues involved, and clinicians are encouraged to consult with the authors or with others with experience in this area, since many aspects are not readily extrapolated from either perioperative regional anesthesia or adult chronic pain management.

For a very small percentage of children with advanced disease and refractory pain or terminal dyspnea, there may be a role for administration of sedative infusions. However, in our view, use of sedatives near the end of life should never become routine, and efforts should be made whenever possible to preserve clarity of sensorium and interactiveness [116]. The ethical principle of double effect is commonly invoked to guide prescribing of opioids and sedatives at the end of life. While this principle has become nearly universally accepted, critics have pointed out some difficulties with its justification and application [117].

In addition to pain, children with cancer experience a range of other symptoms, such as fatigue, somnolence, and depressed mood. Some data suggest that the prevalence of symptoms is higher among children who are undergoing chemotherapy, who are hospitalized, and who have solid tumors compared to those with hematological malignancies. A recent study suggested that, as pain is treated more aggressively with opioids, the likelihood of fatigue and somnolence is increased [83]. Studies in adults support the use of stimulants, such as methylphenidate, to counteract somnolence from opioids.

Sickle cell vaso-occlusive episodes

Painful vaso-occlusive episodes are the most common cause of pain in children with sickle hemoglobinopathies [118]. Other acute processes can also present with pain, such as pneumonia, stroke, priapism, acute cholecystitis, splenic sequestration, and avascular necrosis. Fever can be associated with an uncomplicated pain episode or may be a sign of pneumonia, appendicitis or other infection. The pain from vaso-occlusive crises can be unpredictable in severity, location, and frequency, ranging from occasional, mild episodes to frequent, severe and prolonged episodes requiring repeated hospitalizations. Approximately 5% of children with sickle cell disease account for over 30% of hospitalizations and patients with the highest rate of painful episodes and hospitalizations have higher mortality rates [119]. Painful vaso-occlusive crises can occur in children as young as 6 months of age as the protective effects of fetal hemoglobin decrease. Dactylitis is a painful episode involving the hands and feet and is more common in younger children. Adolescents tend to experience back, limb, and chest pain, although the location can be variable. Priapism is caused by sickling of hemoglobin in the sinusoids of the penis and causes prolonged, painful erection.

Children with occasional mild-to-moderate painful episodes are typically managed at home with NSAIDs and oral opioids. Severe, escalating pain is generally managed in the hospital with NSAIDs and a PCA with basal infusions. Opioids should be titrated to effect with close observation for hypoventilation and signs of excessive sedation. Surveys suggest that even with generous PCA dosing, pain scores remain quite high and a considerable percentage of hospitalized patients with vaso-occlusive episodes experience pain on a regular basis [120]. For some patients with severe chest pain, the high doses of opioids necessary to treat pain can result in somnolence, hypoventilation and inability for effective coughing and incentive spirometry, leading to worsening hypoxemia and further pulmonary decline. In selected cases, continuous epidural analgesia may provide improved analgesia and reduce the need for further systemic opioids and reduce opioid-induced somnolence.

Cystic fibrosis

Patients with cystic fibrosis (CF) experience a spectrum of recurrent or persistent pain, particularly chest pain and headaches in the final year of life [121]. Other common types of pain include recurrent limb pains that are sometimes associated with arthritis, and back pain, which is multifactorial. Chest pain is typically the most commonly reported pain in patients with CF, regardless of severity of lung disease. Coughing and chest wall muscle strain from increased work of breathing lead to chronic musculoskeletal chest pain. Severe coughing can result in rib fractures or periosteal tears that produce pinpoint tenderness on exam and severe pleuritic chest pain.

Headaches may be due to a range of causes, including musculoskeletal strain, chronic sinusitis, migraine, hypoxia, and hypercarbia. Over 50% of patients with CF report chronic headaches. Headaches due to muscular contraction and strain are very common and are worsened by excessive coughing and increased use of accessory muscles of respiration. Sinus disease is found in the majority of patients with CF and can contribute to headache pain. In some cases, surgery can reduce pain from sinus-associated headaches. Migraines can be intractable and particularly difficult to treat in patients with CF; many patients do not experience good relief with typical abortive migraine treatments, such as NSAIDs or 5HT1 receptor-specific agonists. With disease progression and worsening of pulmonary function, hypercarbia and hypoxia play a more predominant causative role.

Patients with CF experience a number of other musculoskeletal chronic pain conditions. Chronic back pain is generally a result of chronic muscle strain from severe coughing; however, thoracic and lumbar compression fractures can occur and are often under-recognized. The incidence of CF-associated episodic arthritis in children seems to be similar to that seen in older patients with CF, while hypertrophic pulmonary osteo-arthrophy is more prevalent in adult patients.

Treatment of children with chronic pain from CF depends in part on location and severity of pain, severity of lung disease, the degree to which pain interferes with good pulmonary toilet and response to opioids. There are no controlled clinical trials of non-pharmacological therapies in children with CF, but many patients find acupuncture, biofeedback and other cognitive behavioral therapies helpful. NSAIDs are often used either alone or combined with opioids without contributing to respiratory depression, somnolence or constipation, and may allow for opioid-sparing effects. There may be a role for COX-2 inhibitors for patients who experience GI side-effects with traditional NSAIDs and may be less likely to contribute to hemoptysis. If patients with CF receive opioids postoperatively, there is a very high incidence of constipation; aggressive and pre-emptive use of stimulant laxatives should be considered.

The indications for chronic opioid therapy for children and adults with CF are a subject of controversy. CF is now associated with a median survival that exceeds 40 years of age in many centers, so chronic opioid administration should be undertaken with consideration of long-term consequences. We commonly employ thoracic epidural analgesia for major thoracic and abdominal surgery in patients with CF, especially those undergoing lung transplantation. Patients with CF may benefit from thoracic epidural analgesia in two additional situations: severe chest pain due to rib fractures or a chest tube, and impending bowel obstruction associated with meconium ileus equivalent. For CF patients with meconium ileus, a thoracic epidural infusion of local anesthetic has several benefits: it relieves pain and reduces the requirement for opioids, which further slow the bowel, and it provides thoracic sympathectomy, which directly accelerates bowel motility. Many patients undergoing lung transplantation have had chronic, severe chest pain prior to transplantation, and we have found that infusing higher concentrations of local anesthetics (e.g. ropivacaine 0.2%) in combination with hydromorphone is sometimes necessary to achieve adequate analgesia.

Neuropathic pain

Neuropathic pain refers to pain associated with injury or altered excitability within the peripheral or central nervous system [122]. Unlike nociceptive pain, neuropathic pain can persist independent of ongoing tissue injury or inflammation. A-δ and C-fibers can become activated through a range of mechanisms, including infection, inflammation, ischemia, and transection. Other causes include tumor involvement of nerves, metabolic disorders and chemotherapeutic drugs such as vincristine. Neuronal reorganization and central sensitization occur through sustained C-fiber discharge and "wind-up" in the dorsal horn. An array of complex mechanisms induces central neural changes, including ectopic firing of dorsal root ganglion, decreases in magnesium blockade of NMDA receptors, and changes in afferent A-δ fibers that facilitate pain [122]. Pathways containing opioid receptors and endogenous opioids, serotonin, and norepinephrine project to the rostral ventromedial medulla and spinal dorsal horn. Input from the hypothalamus, amygdala, anterior cingulate area, and insular cortex modulates the pathways and can facilitate or inhibit transmission of pain signals.

Many adult neuropathic pain conditions such as diabetic neuropathy, central post-stroke pain, and trigeminal neuralgia are quite rare in children. There may be an age dependence to the nervous system's responses to several types of nerve injury. For example, while traumatic brachial plexus injury commonly produces severe pain in adults, perinatal brachial plexus injury in human neonates rarely appears painful, except for a subset of infants who subsequently undergo nerve grafting procedures [123]. In two models of painful peripheral nerve injury, infant rats show markedly reduced allodynia and other pain behaviors compared to older rats [124]. The age dependence of neuropathic pain may be related in part to the ontogeny of microglial inflammatory responses to nerve injury [125].

The classic description of neuropathic pain in adults of burning, shooting or pins and needles pain is sometimes seen in children but younger children often have difficulty describing their pain. A thorough neurological examination should help detect underlying disease and should assess whether there are dermatomal deficits. Characteristic physical exam findings include allodynia and hyperalgesia. Allodynia refers to previously non-painful stimuli, such as light touch of the skin, causing pain. The presence of allodynia implies abnormal sensory processing and is an important clinical sign of neuropathic pain. Hyperalgesia refers to normally noxious stimuli, such as light pinprick, producing abnormally exaggerated pain. History and physical examination should guide any additional studies such as testing for thyroid dysfunction, B12 deficiency or heavy metal toxicity. Electromyography can detect signs of denervation in muscles, and nerve conduction studies are useful for objectively assessing function of myelinated large nerve fibers, but these do not measure function of smaller C- and A-fibers commonly involved in neuropathic pain.

Neuropathic pain may occur in a range of static or progressive neurological disorders in childhood, including mitochondrial disorders. Heterozygous Fabry disease can produce painful small-fiber neuropathies that may begin during late childhood or adolescence [126]. Quantitative sensory testing is a non-invasive method of assessing the function of small as well as large sensory nerve fibers. Unlike nerve conduction studies, quantitative sensory testing is well tolerated by children and does not require sedation.

Adults with neuropathic pain are commonly treated with anticonvulsants and antidepressants. While randomized trials show efficacy for conditions such as postherpetic neuralgia and diabetic neuropathy, it should be noted that effect sizes (based on changes in pain scores) are comparatively small, and benefit is often achieved at doses that would be expected to cause significant somnolence or impaired cognition in many patients [127]. Despite the widespread prescribing of drugs such as gabapentin, pregabalin, and duloxetine, there is very little empirical basis for regarding these drugs as either safer or more effective than older drugs, such as tricyclic antidepressants.

The use of drugs for the treatment of neuropathic pain in children is extrapolated from adult studies since there are very few pediatric prospective trials. For children and adolescents with neuropathic pain, we generally use tricylics and anticonvulsants as first-line drugs. Tricyclics are among the most established analgesics in the treatment of diabetic neuropathy, postherpetic neuralgia, and central post-stroke pain in adult patients. Tricyclics can also be helpful in promoting sleep in patients with sleep disorders due to pain. Nortriptyline and amitriptyline are most commonly used, often in twice-daily dosing with a larger portion of the dose give at bedtime. A baseline electrocardiogram is recommended prior to initiation of these drugs. A typical starting dose for nortriptyline is 0.2 mg/kg with dose titration every 3–5 days. Common side-effects are related to anticholinergic effects, including dry mouth, sedation, tachycardia, constipation, and urinary retention. There is less robust evidence for the use of selective serotonin reuptake inhibitors (SSRIs) in the treatment of neuropathic pain in children, but they are often used as an adjuvant in the treatment of associated mood disorders. Overall, antidepressants, including SSRIs, appear less effective for treatment of major depressive disorders in children compared to adults. In randomized trials, placebo responses are common and substantial; effect sizes relative to placebo are relatively small, and numbers needed to treat (NNTs) average 8 or greater [128]. NNTs are somewhat better (lower) for treatment of anxiety disorders in children [128].

Gabapentin and pregabalin are widely prescribed, in part because of historical concerns about risks of antidepressants exacerbating suicidal ideation or attempts. However, meta-analyses of clinical trials of anticonvulsants suggest that multiple anticonvulsants also may increase these risks, even in patients without epilepsy or known severe mood disorders [129]. Parenthetically, anesthesiologists should note that lipid emulsions, which are used to treat bupivacaine cardiotoxicity, also appear to be effective in reversing cardiotoxic effects of several classes of antidepressants and anticonvulsants [130]. While the overall excess risk of severe mood or behavioral changes from antidepressants or anticonvulsants appears relatively low, in our view, clinicians should titrate these medications gradually, should alert parents to report any concerning changes in behavior or affect, and should employ a system of phone and clinic-based follow-up to detect adverse effects of these medications.

Lidocaine 5% transdermal patches are widely prescribed for neuropathic pain and for other forms of pain. Plasma concentrations of lidocaine are quite low. While these formulations appear quite safe, and there are studies supporting efficacy for several types of neuropathic pain in adults, in our view there is a high likelihood that placebo responses contribute substantially to their reported benefits for many patients.

The use of opioids in the treatment of non-cancer related neuropathic pain remains controversial. Opioid prescribing for chronic pain in adults has increased enormously over the past 20 years, with a concomitant increase in deaths in adults and adolescents due to apparent misuse or diversion of prescribed opioids. Diversion of prescribed opioids has increased rapidly as a problem among adolescents [131]. In adult studies for chronic non-cancer pain, evidence for long-term benefit of opioids on pain scores is limited, and most studies show no benefit for measures of functioning or disability. For children and adolescents with non-life limiting chronic pain conditions, there are additional concerns. First, as noted above, opioid tolerance is probably more rapidly achieved in childhood compared to in adults. Second, adolescence appears to be a time of unique vulnerability to addiction to multiple classes of substances. Long-term opioid prescribing for children is relatively infrequent [132]. Due to its NMDA antagonist action, methadone may play a role for select patients with neuropathic pain.

Complex regional pain syndrome type 1 (CRPS1) is characterized by neuropathic limb pain with associated sensory characteristics and neurovascular and sudomotor findings. The term CRPS1 overlaps with what was previously called reflex sympathetic dystrophy or reflex neurovascular dystrophy [133]. Diagnostic criteria for clinical and research purposes have undergone refinement [134]. The classic clinical presentation is burning pain in an arm or leg with allodynia, hyperalgesia, mottling, coolness, swelling and abnormal sweating, although the clinical presentation can vary widely. Various motor findings can also occur such as tremors, fasciculations and dystonia. CRPS 2 refers to this pattern of clinical findings with signs of specific peripheral nerve injury; this is similar to what was traditionally called causalgia. In our view, although there may be important roles for peripheral and autonomic mechanisms, it is useful to view CRPS as being maintained at least in part by abnormal information processing in the brain. These functional brain abnormalities are not purely sensory, but also involve pain modulation [135] and motor representation [136].

Complex regional pain syndrome has unique epidemiological features in children. Multiple case series have found a high female-to-male ratio (approximately 5–8:1) and a preponderance of lower extremity involvement (75–90%) [133,137,138]. The peak age of onset is 10–12 years. It is rarely seen in children less than the age of 6 years. Twenty percent of children have a remote or contralateral limb affected. About 90% of patients recall an inciting trauma but it is usually vague and minor. Some children can present as extremely disabled, have significant school absences and are unable to ambulate independently, but the degree of disability seems to vary widely. Functional MRI (fMRI) has been used to study CNS activation in children with CRPS [139,140]. Some functional and structural changes normalize after the pain from CRPS has resolved, while other changes are persistent [139,140].

Retrospective case series and prospective studies [141] have indicated that the majority of children with CRPS will have improvement in both function and pain through an aggressive rehabilitative approach without the use of nerve blocks or pharmacological agents. The frequency of recurrent episodes may range from 20% to 50% of cases, although most recurrences of symptoms appear to be milder than the initial episode and more readily responsive to reinstitution of aggressive physical therapy, occupational therapy, and cognitive-behavioral therapies. Our practice in treating children with CRPS involves a rehabilitation program with intense physical therapy, occupational therapy, and cognitive-behavioral therapies. A significant aspect of the approach involves patient and parent education about the non-protective nature of neuropathic pain and recognizing factors that reinforce disability and fear of pain. Physical and occupational therapies are directed at active mobilization of the affected limb, resuming independent weight-bearing and aggressive desensitization techniques. For some children, this program can be accomplished as an outpatient but those who fail will need an inpatient or partial hospitalization program. Epidural analgesia or peripheral nerve blocks are used for a comparatively small subgroup of patients

who fail to make good progress with good rehabilitation efforts or for those with severe limb swelling or dystonia that persists after an active multidisciplinary treatment program. If the distribution of pain, allodynia and autonomic abnormality is appropriately limited, there are advantages to the use of peripheral or plexus catheters. Our practice is to use an indwelling catheter technique for several days rather than repeated single injections. We tend to place continuous popliteal-sciatic catheters for lower extremity CRPS and either supraclavicular or infraclavicular catheters for upper extremity CRPS. Patients are then hospitalized and receive continuous local anesthetic infusions of ropivacaine, sometime with the addition of clonidine. During their 3–5-day hospital stay, they receive intense rehabilitation with twice-daily physical therapy and cognitive-behavioral therapy. One case series reported excellent outcomes using primarily popliteal-sciatic catheters maintained at home in children with "stocking-distribution" CRPS [142].

Back pain

Back pain in adults is a major cause of suffering as well as economic loss due to work-related disability. Non-disabling episodic back pain is relatively common in children and adolescents, but daily persistent back pain is overall much less common than in adults [143]. Since persistent severe back pain is relatively less common in younger children, it is appropriate to evaluate for specific serious causes including infections (osteomyelitis, diskitis, pyelonephritis), tumors, benign abnormalities such as osteoid osteoma, and congenital abnormalities, such as tethered cord and diastematomyelia.

Back pain in our referral practice is more commonly seen in adolescents who are competitive athletes, such as gymnasts, dancers, and cheerleaders. A thorough neurological and musculoskeletal exam is necessary to determine likelihood of conditions such as lumbar disk disease, spondylolysis, spondylolisthesis, sacroiliitis, and muscular strain. Patients with muscular pain without evidence of radiculopathy are treated with an exercise program of core strengthening and reducing repetitive stress and trauma to the spine. With proper patient selection, fluoroscopically guided epidural steroid injections appear to provide intermediate-term benefit in adults with lumbar radiculopathy. Our recent review of experience with fluoroscopically guided epidural steroid injections for children and adolescents with lumbar radiculopathy showed that the majority of patients reported significant reductions in pain with an excellent safety profile. In 2–5-year follow-up, fewer than 40% of patients required diskectomy [144].

In adults, extension-related back pain is commonly associated with facet arthropathy. In adolescents, this pattern of pain is commonly seen with spondylolysis and spondylolisthesis. These conditions are commonly treated with a trial of bracing. Adults with cervical or lumbar facet disease commonly receive median branch blocks and, if they provide short-term benefit, radiofrequency denervation procedures [145]. In our practice, we do perform some of these injections using local anesthetic and low doses of steroids. To date, we have been reluctant to perform radiofrequency denervation procedures on patients with a developing spine except in extraordinary circumstances.

Functional abdominal pain (FAP) is a term that has generally been used for recurrent episodic abdominal pain occurring among children and adolescents who are otherwise medically well and who show no evidence for a structural or inflammatory origin of pain [146]. FAP presents in distinct patterns, as codified subsequently by three consensus processes known as the Rome I, II, and III classifications; these have been developed for both adults and children [147]. These conditions account for a high frequency of pediatric office visits, and may account for up to 20% of school days missed due to illness in the US. Most children who present in this manner remain medically well and few eventually are found to have an identifiable structural or inflammatory disorder.

There are common features of functional abdominal pain with respect to clinical characteristics. Most children are between the ages of 4 and 16 years and report episodic, periumbilical pain. Children younger than 4 years should receive further investigation into underlying causes. Children are otherwise generally medically well without systemic signs of disease. Rarely do children report that pain awakens them at night. The diagnostic approach in primary care should be guided by a careful history and physical examination and should avoid unfocused laboratory testing beyond basic studies, such as a complete blood count, urinalysis, and, as appropriate, stool examination. A psychosocial history is important for identifying reinforcing pain behaviors and other behaviors that suggest disability. In general, extensive testing is not helpful and may heighten parental and patient anxiety. Routine radiographic studies without findings on history or physical exam are typically of low yield. For children who have fevers, weight loss, family history of inflammatory bowel disease, and pain that is not periumbilical, these are concerning signs and warrant further evaluation. Abnormalities on physical examination or initial screening tests should also guide additional investigation.

Treatment of functional abdominal pain depends in part on the pattern of clinical presentation and the degree of distress or disability involved. As guided by the history and examination, some clinicians favor empiric trials of treatment of constipation, lactose avoidance or lactose enzyme supplementation, dietary alterations or acid sup-

pression. Education of parents and patients should include discussion about the non-protective character of the pain, and should discourage catastrophizing and overmedicalizing. Cognitive-behavioral interventions are supported by evidence and should be used more widely [148]. In our view, medications form only a part of the management, and should not be used in lieu of lifestyle change, rehabilitative interventions, and cognitive-behavioral interventions. Controlled trials of medications such as amitriptyline have yielded both positive [149] and negative [150] results. Many medications are commonly prescribed based on uncontrolled pediatric case series or extrapolation from adult studies [151].

Episodic headaches are also common in children and adolescents. The frequency of both migraine and tension-type headaches increases through childhood. Prior to adolescence, boys and girls are similarly affected. With the onset of adolescence, the prevalence increases more in girls than in boys, particularly with migraine. Patients and parents are often worried that headache is associated with serious conditions, such as tumors. As with abdominal pain and chest pain, diagnostic evaluation should emphasize the history, including a psychosocial history, and physical examination, including a systematic neurological examination. Practice parameters on imaging for recurrent headaches in childhood have been published [152]. In the absence of features of the clinical presentation that suggest higher risk, imaging studies are generally of low yield [153] or they identify incidental findings [154] that further increase worry but are of generally limited clinical significance.

While recurrent tension-type headaches or episodic migraine are common, for the majority of children in the general population, they do not dramatically impair daily functioning. The subgroup of children who may be referred to pediatric neurologists or pediatric pain physicians tends to be those with more frequent or more severe headaches, or those who have pathological but not readily "fixable" headaches. Examples of the latter include headaches following head trauma or following multiple ventricular shunt procedures with slit ventricles. The occurrence of more disabling recurrent headaches [155] or chronic daily [156] headaches is more prevalent with certain lifestyles, including obesity, smoking, and lack of physical exercise, with some psychological co-morbidities, including anxiety and depression, and with overuse of analgesic medications.

For children with relatively infrequent migraine episodes, there is evidence to support episodic use of NSAIDs and several triptans for abortive treatment [157]. For children and adolescents with disabling recurrent or chronic daily headaches, in our view, treatment should begin with identification of triggering factors, lifestyle modifications, and avoidance of overly frequent use of acetaminophen and NSAIDs. A number of approaches to cognitive-behavioral therapy show strong evidence of efficacy for both migraine and tension-type headaches, and they should be used widely [148].

The use of prophylactic medications for pediatric migraine is often based on custom and on extrapolation from adult studies. For example, cyproheptadine is widely used, despite absence of controlled trials. While several anticonvulsants are widely used, evidence for efficacy is sparse for most anticonvulsants [158]. There is some support for topiramate in recent placebo-controlled pediatric migraine prophylaxis trials [159]. There are positive trials for amitriptyline, trazodone, and several calcium channel blockers, and trials of propranolol have yielded mixed results [157].

Conclusion

The management of acute, recurrent, and chronic pain in children has made considerable progress over the past 30 years. While pain assessment is more challenging in infants and preverbal children, pragmatic measures are now available for all age groups. Treatment should be individualized and may involve combinations of pharmacological, regional, rehabilitative and cognitive-behavioral interventions. Multicenter clinical trials will be helpful for conducting adequately powered clinical trials for many forms of acute and chronic pain in pediatrics.

CASE STUDY

You are working in a pediatric chronic pain clinic when you are paged by one of the emergency room (ER) physicians who asks if you would urgently evaluate a patient who has severe foot pain and is currently being seen in the ER. You agree to see the patient who then shortly arrives in your office. The patient is an 11-year-old competitive gymnast who is accompanied by her mother. The child has an 8-week history of left foot pain, which she attributes to tripping over a gymnastic mat; this event produced a small laceration of her foot and a sprain. An orthopedic surgeon evaluated her after the fall. Her plain radiographs did not show an obvious fracture, but she did wear an aircast boot for 4 weeks without significant improvement. A recent bone scan showed osteopenia of the affected limb. An MRI did not show significant findings. Her pain is significantly worse this morning since falling last night after her left foot "gave out" as she was walking up stairs. She reports that her foot often "gives out" and feels like she has no strength in it. She is otherwise medically well. She describes her pain as a numb, burning sensation over the lateral aspect of her left foot with shooting pains into her calf. She has noticed occasional swelling and redness over the painful area and has also noticed that her foot seems to shake involuntarily. She has difficulty falling asleep due to pain and is unable to have the blankets touch her painful foot.

She and her mother are tearful as she explains how she will miss the state competitions in 1 month if she cannot participate fully. Her mother explains how difficult this has been for the entire family and how she has not been able to work at her job since the onset of her daughter's pain 2 months ago. She does describe how supportive the teachers at her child's school have been by allowing her to attend classes only when she is able to make it.

On examination, she is a small-appearing female who is ambulating with the use of crutches. The lateral aspect of her left foot has a 3 × 3 cm area of slight ecchymosis and edema, which the patient reports comes and goes. Her foot has a mottled appearance. When you lightly touch her foot, she withdraws, begins to cry, and explains that it feels like an intense burning and pins and needles sensation. Her foot and leg feel cool to touch up to the midcalf. She has noticeable atrophy of her gastrocnemius. She refuses to bear weight on her foot during the examination.

You explain to the patient and her mother that her history and physical examination findings are most consistent with a diagnosis of complex regional pain syndrome (CRPS.) Her allodynia and pain in a non-dermatomal distribution are typically seen in CRPS. Neurovascular and motor findings such as edema, intermittent color and temperature changes, and involuntary spasms and tremors are also consistent with CRPS. A bone scan and MRI have ruled out other worrisome conditions such as osteomyelitis or an occult fracture.

Your discussion with the patient and her mother involves extensive education about CRPS and treatment options. CRPS is rare before the age of 8 and peaks around the age of 12–13 years. Girls are six times more likely than boys to have CRPS and the lower extremity is much more commonly involved than an upper extremity by a ratio of 8:1. Twenty percent of children experience spread of their symptoms to a contralateral or remote limb, which is presumably due to central sensitization. The majority of children report an antecedent injury, although in most cases, the injury seems vague and minor, such as the injury that occurred in this patient. Many children with CRPS are involved in highly competitive, individualized sports, such

Continued

as ballet and gymnastics. Studies have shown that children with CRPS have similar scores on depression and anxiety testing compared to other children with chronic pain conditions. Plain radiograph findings in children with CRPS are variable and can show diffuse osteopenia or appear normal, even with long-standing CRPS. Bone scans also show variable results and have little to no predictive value in CRPS but, as in our patient, can exclude other pathology such as infection.

Although CRPS is a clinical diagnosis, quantitative sensory testing (QST) has been used in children to provide more objective evidence of sensory abnormalities. It is used to assess function of cutaneous somatic small fibers and is particularly applicable to children since it is painless and does not require sedation.

In discussing various treatment options, you explain that studies of children with CRPS show that the majority will show a good improvement of function and of pain scores through a multidisciplinary approach of active physical therapy, occupational therapy, and cognitive-behavioral therapy. You explain that in some cases a nerve block is indicated so that patients are able to participate in physical therapy or if you are concerned about limb perfusion. Although the patient's mother wants a medication such as Percocet that will alleviate her daughter's pain quickly so that she can participate in the state gymnastics competition, you explain that data showing efficacy of medications are lacking and there is no "quick fix." However, since the patient is having difficulty with sleep, you do prescribe 10 mg of nortriptyline at night. You order a baseline ECG to detect any underlying dysrhythmia that would place her at additional risk in taking a tricyclic antidepressant. You explain that in general, you do not prescribe opioids routinely for patients with CRPS. You emphasize to the patient and her mother that cognitive-behavioral techniques such as biofeedback are important to her overall recovery and that therapy will be directed at improving her coping skills, maintaining regular school attendance, and normalizing behavioral responses to pain. She will need to have active participation in physical therapy, particularly in attempting to ambulate without the use of assistive devices and in desensitization techniques. You discuss the non-protective nature of neuropathic pain in that, unlike nociceptive pain, which is protective, neuropathic pain is abnormal processing of nerves and pain does not imply tissue injury. If outpatient therapy is not effective, you discuss the possibility of an inpatient or partial hospitalization program for intense rehabilitation.

The patient and her mother return for a follow-up visit in 3 weeks after an outpatient trial of physical therapy and cognitive-behavioral therapy. She has made very little progress in physical therapy. She is very reluctant to be actively involved in physical therapy because of her severe

pain. In fact, she is using a wheelchair almost exclusively now and will not allow anyone or anything to touch her foot, even to examine it. She is tearful throughout the evaluation and keeps her knee flexed to protect her foot. Her foot and calf have a more dusky appearance than before with worsening of muscle atrophy. She reports that she is also experiencing similar pain and color changes in the contralateral foot and ankle. Because of her severe neurovascular findings and her lack of progression in physical therapy due to pain, you offer the patient a nerve block with which the patient and her mother agree. You explain that since her pain is bilateral, you recommend placing an epidural catheter.

Under general anesthesia, she has a lumbar epidural catheter placed guided by fluoroscopy. Using contrast, you are able to visualize the catheter midline in the epidural space with the tip of the epidural at T12–L1. After a negative test dose of lidocaine with epinephrine, you inject 7 mL of 0.25% bupivacaine, which results in bilateral motor and sensory response. She is taken to the recovery room where a continuous epidural infusion of 0.1% bupivacaine with 0.04 µg/mL of clonidine is started at 8 mL/h, which is 0.2 mL/kg/h. She is admitted for an anticipated 4–5-day hospital stay. During her hospitalization she will receive twice-daily physical therapy and daily cognitive-behavioral therapy. She will have a strict schedule each day consisting of physical therapy, psychology therapy, "home" exercises, and school tutoring. She will have to dress each morning in regular clothes and wear her shoes and socks.

She progresses well during the hospitalization and actively participates in all of her therapies and activities. No new medications are started. During the course of her psychology sessions in the hospital, it becomes apparent that the demands of school and competitive gymnastics have been very stressful for her but she does not want to disappoint her parents by reducing her level of gymnastics. The psychologist feels that pain perhaps served as an excuse for her to reduce some of the stressful demands in her life.

On hospital day 5, the catheter is removed. She continues to experience allodynia and neurovascular symptoms, but feels that overall her symptoms have improved to where she could continue her therapy as an outpatient. She is discharged home with physical therapy and psychology follow-up.

At her 4-week follow-up appointment, she walks into the office without the use of assistive devices. She is also wearing her shoes and socks. She and her mother feel that her symptoms have improved by approximately 50%. She is participating in physical therapy three times per week and is compliant with her daily home exercise program. Through family therapy with the psychologist, it has been decided that she will still participate in gymnastics but not at a competitive level. Results of neuropsychological testing indicate that she has a mild learning disability and appropriate accommodations have been provided for her in school. Since she is progressing well as an outpatient, you decide not to pursue a hospital rehabilitative program.

In further follow-up at 3 months, her symptoms are almost entirely resolved and she is attending school on a regular basis.

Teaching points

1. In evaluating children with painful conditions, it is important to perform a thorough history and physical examination to detect underlying or sometimes overlooked causes of pain. For example, other causes of pain in this patient include an isolated nerve injury resulting from her fall or osteomyelitis, since she had erythema, pain, and swelling associated with an open laceration and a presumed fracture. Most children with allodynia in a non-dermatomal pattern associated with motor and neurovascular changes will have CRPS. However, an underlying malignant tumor causing nerve compression can also cause exquisite neuropathic pain and a careful history and physical examination with attention to neurological signs, lymphadenopathy, and distribution of pain will help to clarify possible etiologies.

2. Evidence shows that the majority of children with CRPS will show good response to a conservative approach of intense physical therapy and cognitive-behavioral therapy and many children will never require a nerve block. Nevertheless, treatment must be individualized for each patient. The 11-year-old girl described in this case had a brief trial of outpatient physical therapy and cognitive-behavioral therapy. It was apparent at her follow-up visit that she was unable to actively engage in the physical therapy and cognitive-behavioral therapy necessary to recover. It was therefore decided to pursue a nerve block and initiate aggressive physical therapy and cognitive-behavioral therapy in the hospital.

3. There are numerous classes of drugs used in the treatment of chronic pain, including tricyclic antidepressants, anticonvulsants, and serotonin reuptake inhibitors. It is necessary to understand the wide range of side-effects of these medications and possible interactions as different classes are combined, and medical conditions that may increase risk with a particular drug. Our practice is not to routinely use opioids for chronic, non-malignant pain but occasionally, short courses of opioids can be helpful, particularly when patients have severe pain and are initiating physical therapy.

Annotated references

A full reference list for this chapter is available at:
http://www.wiley.com/go/gregory/andropoulos/pediatricanesthesia

4. Slater R, Boyd S, Meek J, Fitzgerald M. Cortical pain responses in the infant brain. Pain 2006; 123: 332. Changes in cerebral oxygenation over the contralateral somatosensory cortex were measured in infants in response to noxious stimulation. Clear cortical response patterns were produced by noxious stimulation, highlighting the potential for both high-level pain processing and pain-induced plasticity in the human brain from a very early age.

27. Morton NS, Errera A. APA national audit of pediatric opioid infusions. Paediatr Anaesth 2010; 20: 119–25. A prospective audit was conducted to assess serious clinical events in pediatric patients receiving continuous opioid infusions, patient-controlled and nurse-controlled analgesia. The overall incidence of serious events was 1:10,000. Avoidable risk factors were identified such as pump programming errors and concurrent use of sedatives or opioids.

35. Lesko S, Mitchell A. An assessment of the safety of pediatric ibuprofen. A practitioner-based randomized clinical trial. JAMA 1995; 273: 929–33. This randomized double-blind controlled trial demonstrated that the risk of hospitalization for gastrointestinal bleeding, renal failure or anaphylaxis was not increased following short-term use of ibuprofen in children relative to acetaminophen.

55. Williams DG, Patel A, Howard RF. Pharmacogenetics of codeine metabolism in an urban population of children and its implications for analgesic reliability. Br J Anaesth 2002; 89: 839–45. In this randomized, double-blinded study, genetic analysis of the cytochrome P450 enzyme CYP2D6 was performed in 96 children. CYP2D6 is the predominant enzyme involved in codeine metabolism. Forty-six percent of children were found to have genotypes associated with reduced enzyme activity; 36% of children given codeine had no detectable levels of morphine or its metabolites, indicating that codeine would be ineffective in these patients.

75. Howard RF, Lloyd-Thomas A, Thomas M et al. Nurse-controlled analgesia (NCA) following major surgery in 10,000 patients in a children's hospital. Paediatr Anaesth 2010; 20: 126–34. Ten thousand infants and children receiving nurse-controlled morphine were prospectively studied to determine effectiveness, morphine requirements, incidence of side-effects, and serious adverse events. The study demonstrated that NCA morphine is an acceptable, safe, and effective method of postoperative analgesia. Serious adverse events were uncommon but the incidence was greatest in neonates.

97. Tsui BC, Suresh S. Ultrasound imaging for regional anesthesia in infants, children, and adolescents: a review of current literature and its application in the practice of neuraxial blocks. Anesthesiology 2010; 112: 719–28. This study is a prospective case series using electrical stimulation instead of radiographic imaging to guide the advancement of an epidural catheter from the caudal space to thoracic dermatomes. Eighteen of 20 children had satisfactory postoperative epidural analgesia.

101. Larsson BA, Lonnqvist PA, Olsson GL. Plasma concentrations of bupivacaine in neonates after continuous epidural infusion. Anesth Analg 1997; 84: 501–5. In this study of plasma bupivacaine concentrations in neonates, 1.8 mg/kg of bupivacaine was administered in the epidural catheter followed by a continuous infusion of 0.2 mg/kg/h. Although no adverse events occurred, a substantial number of neonates continued to have increasing plasma bupivacaine levels at 48 h, raising concerns about the safety of using epidural bupivacaine infusions longer than 48 h in neonates.

114. Collins JJ, Grier HE, Kinney HC, Berde CB. Control of severe pain in children with terminal malignancy. J Pediatr 1995; 126: 653–7. This retrospective review of 199 children who died of cancer showed that most patients had adequate pain control with standard opioid dosing but a significant group required more extensive management. Patients with a solid tumor metastatic to spine and nerves tended to require more extensive management.

141. Lee BH, Scharff L, Sethna NF et al. Physical therapy and cognitive-behavioral treatment for complex regional pain syndromes. J Pediatr 2002; 141: 135–40. This prospective, randomized trial of physical therapy and cognitive-behavioral therapy for children and adolescents with CRPS demonstrated that most patients experienced reduced pain and improved function with a non-invasive rehabilitative treatment approach.

148. Palermo TM, Eccleston C, Lewandowski AS, Williams AC, Morley S. Randomized controlled trials of psychological therapies for management of chronic pain in children and adolescents: an updated meta-analytic review. Pain 2010; 148: 387–97. This meta-analysis of randomized controlled trials demonstrated improvement in pain relief in children with headache, abdominal pain, and fibromyalgia through the use of psychological therapies.

CHAPTER 34

Outpatient Anesthesia

Joseph A. Scattoloni, Olubukola O. Nafiu & Shobha Malviya

Division of Pediatric Anesthesiology, University of Michigan Health System, Ann Arbor, MI, USA

Introduction

One of the most significant changes in medical practice over the past two decades has been the rapid and enormous expansion of outpatient surgery. This growth has been largely fueled by escalating healthcare costs and an imperative need for efficient utilization of shrinking healthcare resources. Recognition of the numerous benefits of outpatient surgery, including less disruption of family schedules, decreased inconvenience to patients, less psychological disturbance, decreased exposure to nosocomial infections and greater patient satisfaction, has further driven the shift toward performing surgery in the ambulatory setting. This change in practice has affected both adults and children. Indeed, in 2006, over 2.3 million ambulatory anesthetic procedures were performed in children under 15 years of age in the United States alone, which translates to 38 procedures per 1000 children and represents an approximately 50% increase over procedures performed in 1996 [1].

Historically, the practice of outpatient surgery was first reported in 1909 [2], and the first outpatient surgical center was established in Sioux City, Iowa, in 1918 [3]. However, it was not until 1984 that outpatient anesthesia became recognized as a specialty and the Society of Ambulatory Anesthesia was formed.

The growth of the specialty of ambulatory anesthesia was accompanied by significant advances in anesthetic techniques, including the availability of better anesthetic agents that enabled patients to recover faster. Improved analgesic agents and the use of regional analgesia techniques allowed patients to be discharged home in reasonable comfort, or with mild-to-moderate pain that could be adequately managed at home. Such advances, coupled with improvements in surgical techniques, including minimally invasive procedures, made it possible to move procedures from the inpatient to the ambulatory setting. These developments have also resulted in patients with more complex co-morbidities being considered for ambulatory surgery. The ongoing challenge is to provide efficient, high-quality, and safe perioperative care to patients with complex medical histories for a large variety of surgical procedures in diverse venues. Continuous scrutiny of existing systems, along with critical ongoing evaluation of outcomes, is necessary to provide a framework that will guide care that is safe, effective, patient centered, and efficient in the ambulatory surgery setting.

Design and setting for outpatient surgery

Outpatient surgery may be performed safely and efficiently in the pediatric population in a variety of settings. Such environments include hospital-associated ambulatory care facilities, such as operating room suites within hospitals or satellite surgery centers, unaffiliated free-standing facilities, and individual physicians' offices. One of the most significant reasons for implementing outpatient or day surgery is to maximize efficiencies while decreasing costs. Previous investigators have suggested that the ambulatory surgery center (ASC) model, by virtue of its bias toward high volume, provides more efficient, higher quality care at a lower cost compared to hospital-based facilities [4]. The Institute of Medicine has described high-quality care as care that is safe, effective, patient centered, timely, efficient and equitable [5]. These goals may be achieved by focusing on a select population with as few complicating factors as possible.

To ensure the most efficient operation, facilities and personnel should be dedicated solely to pediatric patients, as well as outpatient or day surgery. Administrative and medical personnel at such a center are able to provide a uniquely effective care plan that is perhaps hindered, disadvantaged or even unobtainable when such children are mixed with adults or a more complicated inpatient pediatric patient population. Resource and space constraints may nevertheless force the co-mingling of various patient groups in a single surgical environment. In such cases, special consideration should be given to the needs of pediatric patients and parents. The separation of inpatient (hospital setting) and outpatient waiting and recovery areas is highly desirable. Likewise, where children and adult patients are mixed, special attention should include the incorporation of child-life experts, playroom facilities, changing stations, feeding considerations, and progressive care into the pre- and postoperative setting.

Generally speaking, outpatient surgery requires the same anesthetic and recovery equipment that would be required for any in-hospital patient. At autonomous surgical sites or physicians' offices, certain other minimum capabilities should be available on site: basic laboratory functions, processing facilities for equipment sterility and maintenance, and an informatics system to accommodate medical record utilization. Standard resuscitation equipment specific to pediatric patients of all ages must be available. A fully stocked difficult airway cart should also

be available, and should minimally include some form of video or fiber-optic equipment, as well as materials for an emergency cricothyrotomy. Finally, clearly delineated plans and prearrangements must be conceived and implemented to accommodate any patient who develops complications requiring more extensive care, including emergency transportation and hospital admission [6].

Appropriate procedures

Outpatient or day surgery should be restricted to procedures that combine expeditious and efficient throughput with patient safety that obviates the need for lengthy observation or involved inpatient care. Such procedures must meet minimal criteria [7–9] that would:
- include a relatively limited duration (usually less than 4 h but this may vary from state to state or institution to institution)
- comprise a low hazard of surgical or anesthetic complication
- encompass minimal or easily regulated physiological derangements (including minimal blood loss)
- involve minimal or moderate postoperative pain that is easily treated and managed with oral analgesics (necessitating the ability to resume oral fluids or nutrition in the immediate postoperative period).

By and large, the majority of common pediatric surgeries fit the described ambulatory surgery parameters (Box 34.1). It should be noted that, whereas most adults do not, children do require significant sedation or anesthesia plus comprehensive monitoring for certain brief examinations and minor or rather superficial procedures. As such, myringotomies, circumcisions, cystoscopies, biopsies, and ophthalmological examinations, among others, are often scheduled as outpatient procedures. The fact that the most recent data [1] regarding free-standing ambulatory surgery centers reveal the top three pediatric procedures to be tonsillectomy, adenoidectomy, and myringotomy and tubes only confirms the shift in thought when considering appropriate procedures for the ambulatory setting.

Ear, nose and throat procedures
Historically, pediatric ear, nose and throat (ENT) surgery (most commonly adenotonsillectomy) required overnight hospital admission due to concerns about the occurrence of hemorrhage and airway compromise. Hence, day surgery was previously practiced on a relatively limited population of older, healthy American Society of Anesthesiologists (ASA) I and II patients without obstructive sleep apnea (OSA). Today, despite the fact that OSA has become a primary indicator for these procedures, the push to attain advantages in efficiency, cost containment,

Box 34.1 Commonly performed outpatient surgical procedures

Otolaryngology

- Myringotomy and insertion of tubes
- Adenoidectomy
- T&A (unless contraindicated)
- Frenulectomy
- Laryngoscopy
- Closed reduction of nasal fracture
- Foreign body removal
- Brachial cleft cysts
- Endoscopic sinus surgery
- EUA incl. some DL/bronchoscopies

Ophthalmology

- EUA
- Eye muscle surgery (strabismus)
- Nasolacrimal duct probing
- Excision of chalazion
- Insertion of lens or prosthesis
- Trabeculectomy

Dentistry

- Extraction
- Restoration

Orthopedics

- Cast change
- Arthroscopy
- Closed reduction of fracture
- Manipulation
- Hardware removal
- Percutaneous tenotomies
- Arthrograms

Urology

- Cystoscopy
- Meatotomy
- Orchiopexy
- Circumcision
- Hydrocelectomy
- Testicular biopsy
- Hypospadias repair

General surgery

- Hernia repair
- Excision of cyst
- Ganglion
- Skin lesion
- Suture of lacerations
- Removal of sutures
- Dressing change
- Muscle biopsy
- Sigmoidoscopy
- Bronchoscopy
- Esophagoscopy
- I&D abscess
- Proctological and vaginal procedures

Plastic surgery

- Otoplasty
- Septorhinoplasty
- Scar revision
- Cleft lip and some cleft palate repairs
- Placement of tissue expanders

DL, direct laryngoscopy; EUA, examination under anesthesia; I&D, incision and drainage; T&A, tonsillectomy and adenoidectomy.

and better resource utilization has made outpatient surgery much more appealing [10,11].

Recent studies have substantiated the general safety of performing adenotonsillar procedures in children 4 years and older as outpatients [11,12]. An analysis of national data for pediatric ambulatory ENT surgery confirms the relative safety of such procedures, with minor complications occurring at rates of approximately 1%; however, complication rates for patients younger than 4 years were significantly higher, with 2.5% of patients ($p < 0.001$) returning to the surgery center and 9.3% ($p < 0.011$) having an unplanned hospital admission [13]. Likewise, a systematic literature review noted a statistically significant increase in both complication rates (odds ratio 1.64) and unplanned admissions (odds ratio 1.71) in children younger than 3 years of age [11].

Children with OSA comprise a growing portion of the ENT practice, and these patients have augmented risks (see subsequent discussion). For predisposed patients, tonsil or adenoid surgery inherently creates the potential for worsened airway obstruction or pulmonary complication in the postoperative period. Data suggest that OSA may markedly accentuate the risk; however, it is difficult to independently separate this effect from the more clearly substantiated age effects. Regardless, the literature supports hospital admission for children 3 years old and younger in whom tonsillectomy and adenoidectomy (T&A) is indicated for OSA [14]. Indeed, outpatient T&A is less cost-effective than planned hospital admission for children in this age range [15].

Presenting indications for scheduled ENT surgery may include pathologies that increase risks. Whether suffering from OSA, obesity, central sleep apnea, facial or oral dysmorphism, or even recurrent or continual upper respiratory infections (URIs), each patient must be evaluated individually when considering their selection for day surgery, especially in a free-standing ASC. Those patients under 4 years old or possessing multiple co-morbidities should be seen at a hospital-centered practice to allow for the possibility of lengthier observation or admission.

Patient selection

To accomplish the workflow goals implicit in the outpatient surgery process, patient selection (and preparation) is paramount. Generally healthy ASA class I and II children are excellent surgical candidates who can go home soon after surgery. Initially, ambulatory practices focused on these patients. However, with the evolution of healthcare practice (medications, equipment, interventions), ASA III children with stable systemic disease may also now be cared for in the ambulatory setting. Even more than other patients, these children should be rigorously screened and ought to have prior approval from their surgeon specialist and anesthesiologist to undergo outpatient surgery.

The focal point of the outpatient or ambulatory facility centers on resource allocation. Even a single patient who requires increased attention or unplanned efforts may compromise the overall flow or function of the unit. Such a patient might be a normally healthy child with a history of asthma and a new URI who is more prone to laryngospasm and postoperative bronchospasm, or an otherwise healthy child with micrognathia and previously difficult intubation, or an obese child with known OSA who might need prolonged postoperative monitoring or even positive pressure ventilation. It is not that such patients cannot be safely cared for; it is that their care may be more easily accommodated when their condition is better optimized or at a larger center possessing greater resources and facilities for readily available admission. It is crucial to recognize and triage these patients before they arrive at an ambulatory practice setting.

Preoperative evaluation/screening

While there are specific conditions or pathologies that would seemingly be in conflict with ambulatory procedures, creating a definitive list is debatable. Much depends on the specific environment in which the procedure is to be done – ASC or physician office versus hospital or tertiary care setting. Likewise, such decisions must take into account the comfort level of the assigned staff or anesthesia provider. The conditions listed in Box 34.2 warrant careful preoperative evaluation and screening to determine appropriateness for ambulatory surgery. They provide a framework from which medical directors may develop guidelines appropriate for their site.

Box 34.2 Patient co-morbidities that require special considerations for ambulatory surgery

- Prematurity/exprematurity
- Obstructive sleep apnea
- Obesity
- Uncorrected or hemodynamically significant congenital heart disease
- Known difficult intubation, airway obstruction
- Myopathy
- Inborn errors of metabolism
- History of malignant hyperthermia
- Down syndrome
- Known coagulation disorders
- Sickle cell disease
- Diabetes mellitus

There are clearly conditions that should generally be avoided in such center, e.g. a patient with a previously difficult airway or one with a coagulopathy that previously required considerable blood products or a patient with unstable congenital heart disease. However, even patients with such conditions may appear on a spectrum. There are two basic areas of concern when evaluating such patients. The first and most important is patient safety. For example, if the ASC or outpatient site does not possess the capability to procure or administer blood products, then the hemophiliac or brittle sickle cell anemia patient should probably not be operated on there.

As noted above, after patient safety, the goal of the ambulatory practice is to optimize throughput and efficiency. Any patient's condition that increases the probable perioperative complexity also increases the potential drain on the ambulatory unit's resources. A severely autistic or developmentally delayed child often requires greater resources or attention in the pre- and postoperative setting and thus impedes unit throughput. The difficulty is deciding at what point the potential for unanticipated problems outweighs the benefit of caring for such a patient in the ambulatory setting.

Apnea in the infant

Patient age is generally not regarded as the limiting factor for outpatient procedures; however, term neonates in the first 4–6 weeks of life require special consideration due to concerns stemming from the transition from fetal and neonatal physiology to a more mature homeostatic state. Most significantly, those infants whose brainstem regulation of breathing remains immature are at increased risk of apnea after anesthesia.

With improvements in neonatal intensive care, a greater number of premature infants (less than 37 weeks) now survive through the neonatal period, and a proportionally larger number present for surgery in early infancy. Studies clearly demonstrate an increased risk of postanesthetic apnea in ex-premature infants related to postconceptual age (PCA). The most significant analysis combined eight prospective studies and demonstrated that a PCA of 56 weeks was required to reduce the postanesthetic risk of apnea to less than 1% (95% statistical confidence) in infants with a gestational age of 32 weeks. For those with a gestational age of 35 weeks, the required PCA was 54 weeks [16]. Despite the suggestion that regional techniques might reduce or eliminate this risk [17–19], there have been published case reports of apnea after spinal anesthesia [20,21] and, in fact, a Cochrane review of this topic determined that there was no reliable evidence to demonstrate a reduction in postoperative risk of apnea with spinal versus general anesthesia in former premature infants [22]. There are no data that determine the incidence of apnea in infants born at less than 28 weeks' gestation. This accounts for an increasing number of patients who are ex-premature infants.

Even the healthy full-term infant may have periods of apnea [23]; hence, it is prudent to delay outpatient procedures in such patients. Most institutions set a 4–6-week age requirement for term infants. Alternatively, scheduling such patients early in the day allows for an extended observation period if indicated. The recommended cutoff postconceptual age for outpatient surgery in ex-premature infants varies from 46 to 60 weeks [7,24,25]. Of course, any complicating medical conditions must be considered, and the more premature the infant, the lower the threshold for admission. Likewise, if apnea is documented during the recovery period, the patient should be admitted to hospital for observation. These patients are not candidates for surgery at free-standing centers, due to their need for hospital admission and continuous cardiorespiratory monitoring for apnea.

Obstructive sleep apnea

Beyond its significance as the primary indication for T&A (see above), OSA and its associated risks must be appreciated and understood in the greater context of all pediatric procedures. Peak prevalence of OSA occurs in 3–6 year olds, but rates are on the rise due to the rapid rise in pediatric obesity. OSA is also more prevalent in children with respiratory disease, prematurity, craniofacial anomalies, hypotonia, myelomeningocele, cerebral palsy and other disorders, such as Down syndrome and Arnold–Chiari malformation. Among its most significant manifestations are neurocognitive and behavioral dysfunction, as well as cardiopulmonary sequelae, including pulmonary hypertension and cor pulmonale [26].

Children with OSA are clearly at increased risk during the perioperative period, and those with severe OSA must be assessed closely before proceeding. American Academy of Pediatrics clinical practice guidelines describe risk factors for respiratory complications in children with OSA undergoing T&A. These include age <3 years, severe OSA on polysomnography, cardiac complications of OSA such as right ventricular hypertrophy, failure to thrive, obesity, prematurity, recent respiratory infection, craniofacial anomalies, and neuromuscular disorders [27]. These guidelines also recommend T&A as the first-line treatment for children with severe OSA, although they do not define the exact polysomnography criteria that are indicative of high risk. Finally, these guidelines recommend that patients deemed as high risk be monitored as inpatients following T&A.

Polysomnography is the recognized gold standard to diagnose and quantify the severity of OSA; however, it cannot predict postoperative clinical outcomes. In one study, its positive predictive value for respiratory complications was only 25% [28]. Postoperative complications in children with OSA include laryngospasm, apnea, pulmonary edema, pulmonary hypertension, and pneumonia [29]. Just the incidence of respiratory complications in such children is significantly higher than the general pediatric population (21% versus 1–2%)[28].

Studies have also shown that children with moderate-to-severe OSA (SpO_2 nadir <85%) have increased sensitivity to opioids and are more prone to postoperative apnea [30]. While these patients should be considered on a case-by-case basis, significant or severe OSA should be considered a contraindication to outpatient surgery for all procedures, not just ENT cases.

Obesity

Sixteen percent of children are obese, and obesity is a significant risk in pediatric ambulatory procedures [31,32]. Compared to non-obese patients, obese children are significantly more predisposed to complicating co-morbidities, including asthma, hypertension, gastric reflux, type 2 diabetes, and OSA. More importantly, obesity is associated with an increased incidence of adverse perioperative respiratory events, including difficult mask ventilation, airway obstruction, bronchospasm, significant oxygen desaturation, and overall critical events [33]. Various studies have demonstrated similar perioperative risks, and obesity has been identified as an independent predictor for the likelihood of admission after T&A [34]. Keeping these concerns in mind, the obese patient with any co-morbidity must be evaluated carefully before scheduling for outpatient surgery. Indeed, before being considered for procedures at free-standing ambulatory centers, such patients should be evaluated and approved by the anesthesiologist or the medical director of the center.

Malignant hyperthermia

Children with suspected or confirmed susceptibility to malignant hyperthermia (MH) present special challenges for outpatient anesthesia. Undoubtedly, these children should receive a trigger-free anesthetic, and their temperature and end-tidal carbon dioxide should be monitored continuously. Arterial blood gas monitoring and dantrolene must be available for management of the rare case of MH. Additionally, children with MH susceptibility may require extended monitoring of temperature and heart rate in the postanesthesia care unit (PACU). In the ambulatory setting, an important question is whether the child with MH susceptibility should be routinely admitted for overnight monitoring following a trigger-free anesthetic. A retrospective study of 285 MH-susceptible children undergoing 406 procedures reported no cases of intraoperative pyrexia [35]. The sample included 25 children with biopsy-proven MH. While none of the children developed pyrexia, six had received routine preoperative dantrolene. Of 10 children who developed postoperative pyrexia, none were believed to be experiencing an MH reaction and none was treated with dantrolene, although four of them had received dantrolene prophylactically.

These data suggest that it may be safe to discharge children with MH susceptibility home following a trigger-free anesthetic. However, the facility must be prepared to monitor them for 4h or more and have the ability to transfer the child to an inpatient setting in the rare but unexpected case of a MH reaction. It remains questionable whether the surgical care of these patients is best handled in a hospital-based facility or a free-standing ASC, given the potential hurdle in the throughput goals at the site.

Upper respiratory infection

Among the most difficult scenarios confronting the anesthesia provider in the ambulatory setting is the otherwise healthy child who presents with a new URI. Benign, recurrent viral illnesses may be ubiquitous in the pre- and primary school population and should not necessarily delay surgery. However, more severe symptoms, including fever, lethargy, purulent secretions, a productive cough, or pulmonary involvement, should cause the procedure to be postponed for a minimum of 4 weeks. Likewise, patients with a suspected bacterial infection who are treated with antibiotics should have their condition optimized by their primary care physician before returning for surgery. The difficulty resides in those patients with a URI who fall in between the toxic-appearing child and the bright, interactive child.

These infections, whether viral or bacterial, may increase airway inflammation, irritability, and respiratory tract secretions that may persist for up to 6 weeks. This airway hyper-reactivity during anesthesia can lead to adverse respiratory events, a protracted recovery time, or even hospital admission. Indeed, much of the literature on this topic confirms that an active or even recent URI increases the risk of perioperative complications, including atelectasis, hypoxemia, laryngospasm, and bronchospasm in the pediatric population [36–40]. Furthermore, tracheal intubation, a history of prematurity or reactive airway disease, airway surgery, the presence of copious secretions, nasal congestion, and passive smoking may further increase the risk for patients who have an URI [38,39]. Despite such increased risk, there is little evidence of long-term sequelae; the vast majority of adverse events are manageable with the judicious care of experienced practitioners.

Decisions regarding whether to proceed with elective surgery in a child harboring a URI should be based on findings from a detailed history and physical examination. Parents are often clear in differentiating their child's condition from her or his "typical runny nose" or "allergic symptoms." They should be able to provide lucid differentiation between chronic symptoms and an acute illness. Indeed, confirmation of a URI by the parent was a more reliable predictor of laryngospasm than symptom criteria alone [41]. A 3 year old with recurrent ear infections presenting for myringotomy and tube placement may exhibit symptoms such as fever and congestion. Waiting for an asymptomatic window in such a child may be unrealistic, given the waxing/waning course of the patient's pathology (e.g. otitis media) and the fact that most young children have a new URI about six times a year. With a detailed history regarding the frequency of the symptoms and in the absence of findings on auscultation, it may be reasonable to proceed with surgery in this case. If persistent concerns remain, such patients should be referred to a hospital-based center with greater flexibility for observation and admission.

Preoperative evaluations or phone interviews may help identify patients with an URI in whom it is prudent to delay elective surgery. Postponement of such cases before they arrive in the hospital or ASC avoids a wasted trip for the family and prevents interruptions in the surgical schedule at the ambulatory facility. Elective surgery is usually delayed 2–4 weeks for simple nasopharyngitis, 4 weeks for more severe infections, including those treated with antibiotic, and a minimum of 4–6 weeks, including a follow-up with a primary care physician (before rescheduling), for any URI that includes a lower respiratory tract component (bronchitis, pneumonia, asthma exacerbation, etc.). Ultimately, each of these patients must be evaluated on an individual basis, keeping in mind the severity of their symptoms, the urgency of the scheduled procedure, the presence of identifiable risk factors, and finally the comfort level and experience of the anesthesia provider.

For children in whom it is difficult to make a diagnosis due to the ambiguity of their presentation or the existence of multiple risk factors, a more conservative approach should be taken when considering proceeding at a free-standing surgery site or physician's office.

Asthma

Asthma afflicts approximately 9% of children in the US and is the most common serious childhood illness and the leading cause of school absenteeism. In its severe form, it carries substantial morbidity and mortality. In 2004, it accounted for 3% of all pediatric hospital admissions and emergency department visits [42]. Despite its associated hazards, in the absence of active wheezing and with appropriate patient evaluation, preparation, and perioperative management, children with asthma may be safely anesthetized in an ambulatory setting.

Patient history is crucial when evaluating asthmatic patients. The severity of their condition is based on a spectrum. How frequent and/or severe are their wheezing episodes or exacerbations? How often do they visit the emergency department? Have they ever required admission to the intensive care unit? What is their current medication regimen and has it been stable? Only patients with well-controlled mild-to-moderate reactive airway disease should be considered for outpatient surgery.

Children with mild or intermittent symptoms who do not require continuous medications and who may only require sporadic rescue treatments are usually excellent candidates for surgery. The patient with moderate asthma who requires regular medications to manage their symptoms must continue these medications or treatments through the morning of their procedure. Inhaled steroids and other treatments (e.g. leukotriene inhibitors or cromolyn) necessitate continual use to be effective. A short course of systemic steroids starting the day before the planned procedure may be appropriate for those patients who have required systemic steroids previously. Preoperative prophylactic treatment with a β-agonist may attenuate increases in airway resistance associated with tracheal intubation.

Due to the isolated nature of the free-standing ASC or physician office, a conservative approach is advocated for those patients with asthma who appear well but have evidence of suboptimal disease control: hospitalization for asthma within 3 months of the scheduled procedure; an exacerbation of their asthma within 1 month; wheezing during exercise; more than three wheezing episodes in the past 12 months; the need for systemic steroids within 1 month; a room air O_2 saturation of <96% [7,40]. Caution should be exercised for those patients who are actively wheezing, especially in conjunction with a URI or other respiratory symptoms (e.g. cough or tachypnea). Elective surgery in these patients should be postponed

and rescheduled for a time when they are symptom free and their condition is fully optimized. Severe asthmatic patients (baseline wheezing) are at increased risk, despite optimization of their condition by consultants and assertive preoperative treatments, including systemic steroids and increased bronchodilator therapy. Even with aggressive perioperative management, they should only be scheduled at a hospital-based practice in the event that an exacerbation occurs and they require hospital admission.

Preoperative preparation

The prospect and actual process of any surgical procedure are inherently stressful and anxiety provoking for children and families. Ambulatory surgery may in fact diminish this trauma by minimizing the separation time between parents and children, as well as avoiding a disruptive hospital stay. And yet, the ambulatory model's very emphasis on efficiency and throughput may limit the time and effort allowed for preparation, understanding, and acceptance of the prospective perioperative experience. Fast-tracking patients through outpatient surgical settings restricts the ability to address each patient's psychological needs, needs that may be pronounced in younger children. Ultimately, consideration of these varying child/family requirements (the basis for family-centered care) is integral to the success of the ambulatory model. Ignorance, anxiety, and uncertainty in the preoperative holding area may lead to confusion, patient agitation, delays, and/or staff interventions that strain the surgery center's resources. Moreover, there is evidence that pediatric preoperative patient anxiety is related to emergence delirium (agitation) [43,44] increased pain (hence, opioid requirements with attendant side-effects), and postoperative behavioral problems [45,46]. These outcomes may postpone discharge and further stress the ASC's timetable and resources.

Among the most cited methods for ameliorating surgery's attendant anxieties are the use of sedative premedications, parental presence at induction of anesthesia, and specific presurgery preparation programs for children as well as their parents.

Premedication

In most circumstances sedative premedication effectively reduces preoperative anxiety, and it may reduce perioperative recall and postoperative agitation or maladaptive behavior. Oral midazolam is the most commonly used agent and benefits from a relatively rapid onset and reliable effect. A dose of 0.25–0.5 mg/kg should be administered 20–30 min prior to taking the child to the operating room (the lower dosing requires a longer interval to be effective). Establishing protocols and maintaining communication between the preoperative area and the operating room should allow for timely administration of medication and mitigate possible delays in anesthetic induction due to premedication. A particular concern in the ambulatory setting is the possibility of an extended sedative effect delaying patient discharge. There are studies indicating protracted sedation with the higher dosing regimen but most studies have failed to demonstrate an effect that significantly delays patient discharge [47,48]. In any case, most parents and anesthesia providers will accept the infrequent short to moderate psychological trauma.

Alternative agents are available. Oral ketamine (5 mg/kg) or fentanyl (15–20 μg/kg) may be given, although these are sometimes associated with prolonged recovery (ketamine) and nausea, vomiting, and pruritus (fentanyl). For patients unable to co-operate with oral drug administration, midazolam may be given via intranasal or intramuscular (0.2 mg/kg) routes; the onset of action is more rapid (5–10 min). In the exceptionally unco-operative patient, ketamine (3–4 mg/kg), often combined with midazolam and glycopyrrolate, may be given by intramuscular injection. The resultant nystagmus caused by ketamine may not be a good option for patients undergoing strabismus surgeries. The intramuscular route, however, should be reserved for situations when all other measures have failed since most children have an inherent phobia for needles. Involvement of a child-life specialist and use of distraction techniques may permit children with a high degree of anxiety to co-operate.

Parental presence at induction

Much of the parents' and child's anxiety centers on the separation that occurs when the child departs to the operating room. Indeed, sedative premedication is administered in part to facilitate this separation. Intuitively, allowing parents to be present during the induction of anesthesia should help calm the child while simultaneously allaying parental uncertainty and fear. It may also increase co-operation and parental satisfaction with the entire perioperative experience. This approach, while still somewhat controversial, has garnered a great deal of support and has been implemented in many institutions and surgery centers.

Nevertheless, most current evidence does not support parental presence at induction of anesthesia [47,49] because it does not reliably alleviate the anxiety of either the children or parents. In those instances where parental presence did seem to benefit the participants, sedative premedication was shown to be similarly efficacious.

There are clearly cases where parental presence can and is beneficial; however, this depends on an accurate assessment of individual personalities, as well as interpersonal dynamics between patients, parents, and caregivers. Experienced anesthesia providers quickly evaluate and build rapport with patient and parents, but the limited preoperative interaction necessitated by day surgery scheduling certainly militates against clearly or effectively appraising such complex interactions and advocating for or against parental presence. Notwithstanding, children who may benefit are older, less impulsive or active in temperament, and typically have calmer parents who value preparation and coping skills in stressful situations [50].

Preoperative preparation programs

The increased focus on family-centered care often includes preoperative preparation programs that incorporate a variety of techniques and activities designed to allay child anxiety and assuage parental concern. Among those activities for the children are non-medical play, medical play, tours of the operating rooms and PACU, videos or movies relating to the perioperative course, and teaching of relaxation or coping techniques. Parental involvement is encouraged throughout and may additionally involve parental tours, presence at induction of anesthesia, and early admittance to the PACU to be with their child.

Feeling inadequately prepared leads to increased parental anxiety [51], and there appears to be a relationship between parental anxiety and an increased risk for postoperative agitation and maladaptive behavior by the child [45]. Hence, methods of mitigating parental concerns, such as preoperative preparation programs, may expedite and facilitate patient care and the ambulatory process. Furthermore, ancillary benefits may be attained by integrating such programs into an ambulatory process that already requires preoperative evaluation, education, and attaining the records and financial/insurance information prior to the day of surgery.

Due to increased interest in the family-centered care model, many institutions and pediatric-centered facilities have initiated varying forms of these preparation programs. While there are indications that such programs can make a substantial difference in the overall experience of patients and families, and by association ease the workflow and productivity of the ASC, it is still unclear how effective they are at addressing patient anxiety and subsequent sequelae. Study results are mixed when assessing the efficacy of various measures. Yet even when patient anxiety is reduced, there is evidence that preoperative benefits fail to translate to the induction or postoperative recovery period [52]. This may be due to the unstructured and piecemeal implementation of many plans that rely on specific or unco-ordinated measures.

Recent evidence demonstrated that a highly integrated and evolved preoperative program could successfully reduce preoperative anxiety (significantly reduced when compared to control and parental presence cohorts; similar when compared to a premedication cohort), and improve postoperative outcomes (decreased analgesic consumption, decreased emergence delirium, decreased time to discharge) [46]. Such a fully developed program, however, requires significant resources in staffing and expertise and thus would be very expensive to implement and run. Likewise, to be effective it would require parental enrollment and a large commitment of time. These constraints may limit the application of such programs to larger, hospital-centered practices that have more resources and a patient census benefiting from economies of scale.

Anesthetic agents and techniques

Apart from the economic advantages of ambulatory surgery and anesthesia, there are psychosocial benefits to a child recuperating from surgery at home. Hospital admission is associated with behavioral problems that are possibly due to separation from parents and disruption of family life [53]. To this end, rapid- and short-acting drugs for induction and maintenance of anesthesia have been developed to facilitate early recovery following day case surgery. The ideal anesthetic agent for ambulatory surgery should provide smooth and rapid induction and prompt recovery from general anesthesia, have minimal side-effects, have analgesic properties, and be free of postoperative nausea and vomiting (PONV). Such an agent does not exist. Since induction of anesthesia is a very important component of the overall ambulatory surgery experience, it is important to use the most acceptable and least distressing technique for the child. Induction of anesthesia is most commonly achieved via the inhaled or the intravenous (IV) routes, and maintenance of anesthesia is often exclusively by the inhalational method. In some centers outside the US, rectal administration of drugs is sometimes used to produce sedation or induce anesthesia [54].

Monitoring
American Society of Anesthesiologists monitoring standards must be applied to all children undergoing an anesthetic regardless of the setting in which the surgery is performed, including office-based settings.

Induction technique
Inhalational induction of general anesthesia is the most common technique used by pediatric anesthetists in North America. What constitutes the "gentlest" induction method for children remains unclear [55]. Very often, the method of anesthesia induction is guided by the personal preference of anesthesia providers, institutional practice,

and cultural factors. For example, because of prevailing needle phobia in many children, anesthesia practitioners in the US often avoid IV induction [56]. However, in many other parts of the world, including Europe, IV induction of anesthesia appears to be more favored [57]. Very few investigators have compared the induction characteristics of IV and inhalational techniques. Some investigators contend that because inhalational induction is not always "smooth," it may be associated with long-term negative memories for children and may be a source of severe stress for parents [55]. Still others claim that IV induction can be a pleasant experience for the child provided topical anesthetic cream is applied to the venepuncture site and the cannulation is performed by a skilled practitioner [53].

Inhalational agents
The ideal inhalational agent should have many of the following desirable characteristics: it should be pleasant to inhale (permitting a smooth induction and emergence from anesthesia), potent (allowing the concomitant administration of high fractional oxygen concentration), produce rapid induction and emergence from anesthesia (low solubility), and it should be easy to administer and analyze (infra-red). Such an agent should also be stable in storage, should have minimal to no reaction with soda lime and should not be significantly biotransformed in the body. It should have little or no cardiac or respiratory irritant or depressant effects and should possess some analgesic properties. With the almost total withdrawal of halothane from clinical anesthesia in developed countries, sevoflurane has become the prototype inhalational agent.

Sevoflurane
Sevoflurane, by virtue of its non-pungent smell and relative lack of airway irritant properties, has become the agent of choice for induction of anesthesia via the inhaled route in children. Because of sevoflurane's low blood gas solubility, induction of anesthesia is rapid, as is recovery. This makes it particularly suitable for the ambulatory setting. Other advantages of sevoflurane include its lack of major side-effects, ability to induce and maintain anesthesia with one drug, better conditions for laryngeal mask airway (LMA) insertion, and ability to induce anesthesia without IV access. Notable disadvantages of sevoflurane-based anesthesia, however, include possible pollution of the operating room with anesthetics and excitatory movements during anesthetic induction [58]. A recent meta-analysis comparing the induction characteristics of sevoflurane with propofol concluded that the two drugs had similar efficacy for anesthetic induction, but sevoflurane use was associated with a higher incidence of PONV [58]. Use of sevoflurane for induction and main-

tenance of anesthesia is also associated with excitatory motor movements during induction and emergence [59]. These side-effects may be distressing to parents and may potentially delay discharge from the PACU.

The practice at our institution is to induce anesthesia with sevoflurane and change to isoflurane for the maintenance of anesthesia. In many cases, we begin inhalational induction with a N_2O/O_2 mixture and gradually introduce sevoflurane into the gas mixture. This practice has been shown to dampen the fairly strong odor of sevoflurane and may reduce some of the anxiety and excitement associated with inhalational induction of anesthesia [60].

Isoflurane

Isoflurane has a pungent odor and causes considerable airway irritation, making it a poor choice for anesthesia induction via the inhaled route. Indeed, previous investigators have reported a higher incidence of coughing, breath holding, excessive salivation, and laryngospasm in children who underwent anesthesia induction with isoflurane compared to those who underwent anesthesia induction with halothane for myringotomy and tube placement [61]. Isoflurane is excreted predominantly in the lungs; there is very little hepatic biotransformation of the drug. It is a popular inhalational agent for anesthesia maintenance due to its lower cost compared to sevoflurane.

Desflurane

Due to its low blood gas solubility (about 0.42, which is lower than all currently available volatile anesthetics, and slightly lower than nitrous oxide), recovery from desflurane anesthesia is rapid with prompt return of protective airway reflexes [62]. However, the rapid emergence and recovery from general anesthesia with desflurane is associated with a higher incidence of emergence agitation in children [63,64]. In some patients emergence agitation may be severe enough to require the use of supplemental analgesic or sedative medications in the PACU. Use of these medications and the need for additional observation prolong and complicate PACU care and delay discharge home. Some investigators have determined that administration of $2.5\,\mu g/kg$ of fentanyl, given after induction of anesthesia, successfully reduced the incidence of severe agitation associated with desflurane anesthesia in children without delaying emergence from anesthesia [65].

Recent data indicating that desflurane use is associated with faster return of protective airway reflexes in otherwise healthy overweight and obese adults [66] may make desflurane useful in overweight and obese children. Data indicating rapid wash-out of desflurane compared with sevoflurane in morbidly obese patients have also been published [67]. Studies comparing the emergence characteristics of desflurane between obese and normal weight children are warranted.

Due to its pungent odor and associated airway irritability, however, desflurane is unsuitable for inhalational induction of anesthesia. Several pediatric studies [68–70] have demonstrated a high incidence of airway irritation and/or reactivity, including breath holding, coughing, excessive secretions, and laryngospasm.

Intravenous agents

Although inhalational induction is more popular with outpatient anesthesia, IV induction and (less commonly) maintenance of anesthesia is sometimes preferred or indicated. There is a smooth, rapid loss of consciousness and emergence is rapid with currently available agents.

Propofol

This has rapidly become the most popular IV induction agent because it has many of the properties of an ideal IV agent. Induction of anesthesia is smooth and recovery is rapid, even after prolonged infusion, making it suitable for total intravenous anesthesia (TIVA). Propofol is also becoming the agent of choice for most procedural sedation, especially with recurrent procedures such as radiation therapy or chemotherapy. It is a good antiemetic agent (another desirable characteristic in ambulatory anesthesia) and very often some clinicians may opt for propofol TIVA in patients with a strong history of PONV. It is important to keep in mind that due to their large central volume of distribution and rapid clearance of propofol, children have a higher dose requirement for anesthesia induction with TIVA than adults. The typical induction dose of propofol in children is 2.5–3.5 mg/kg.

Perhaps the biggest drawback to the use of propofol is the fact that up to 70% of patients have pain on injection of the drug [71]. Various techniques have been tried to reduce this rather distressing side-effect. We commonly co-administer lidocaine (1 mg to 1 cc of propofol) and inject the mixture very slowly.

Methohexital

This agent is used for rapid induction and rapid emergence from anesthesia. Typically, a dose of 1.5–2 mg/kg is particularly useful for outpatient dental and other minor procedures like punch biopsies, pulse dye laser therapy, etc. A recent large database analysis of oral maxillofacial surgical (OMS) procedures concluded that although its use was safe for ambulatory OMS procedures, methohexital was associated with more frequent complications [72]. The main drawbacks to its use are pain on injection and a high incidence of excitatory phenomena, which may be quite distressing if parents are present when anesthesia is induced.

Methohexital is also associated with a high incidence of PONV. Rectal methohexital is sometimes used for brief sedation for computed tomography (CT) scan and other non-invasive procedures. It is administered as a 10% solution at a dose of 20–30 mg/kg. Patients should be closely monitored for the occurrence of respiratory depression [73].

Pain management

The strategy for postoperative pain management is an integral part of any anesthetic plan. However, pain management becomes particularly important in children undergoing outpatient surgery to ensure that parents are able to manage their child's analgesia effectively at home. The intraoperative analgesic regimen should, under ideal circumstances, allow the child to emerge from anesthesia in reasonable comfort since it is easier to maintain analgesia in a pain-free child than to achieve analgesia in one with severe pain. Effective analgesia is best achieved using multimodal therapies, including non-opioid and opioid analgesics, as well as appropriate regional techniques based on the surgical procedure and the child's co-morbidities. Education of parents and caregivers regarding assessment of their child's pain and analgesic needs following discharge, in addition to detailed instructions regarding the timing and dosage of prescribed analgesics, are important facets of care for children undergoing outpatient surgery.

Non-opioid analgesics may be used alone for the treatment of mild pain or as important adjuncts in combination with opioids or regional techniques for the multimodal treatment of moderate-to-severe pain. Non-opioid analgesics produce dose-dependent responses but are limited by a ceiling effect, i.e. a concentration is reached above which no additional analgesia is achieved. Therefore, moderate-to-severe pain is rarely managed with these drugs alone.

Acetaminophen

Acetaminophen is the most common analgesic and antipyretic used in children. The recommended dose for oral administration is 10–15 mg/kg every 4 h. An oral loading dose of 30 mg/kg that is followed by a maintenance dose of 10–15 mg/kg may result in an earlier onset of drug action. Rectal administration of acetaminophen results in unpredictable absorption of the drug with variable peak blood concentrations being achieved in 60–180 min [74–76]. One study reported a greater morphine-sparing effect with a less frequent need for additional rescue analgesics for 24 h in children who received 40 mg/kg or 60 mg/kg of rectal acetaminophen, compared to those who received 20 mg/kg or placebo during outpatient surgery [77].

Intravenous formulations of paracetamol (acetaminophen) and its prodrug propacetamol have been available in Europe and Australia for several years. Onset of action following IV administration of paracetamol occurs in 15 min and antipyresis occurs in 30 min [78,79]. One controlled randomized trial reported good analgesia for the first 6 h after surgery in children undergoing T&A who received either rectal acetaminophen 40 mg/kg or IV acetaminophen 15 mg/kg after induction of general anesthesia [80]. However, children who received acetaminophen rectally required rescue analgesics later than those who received the drug IV. The IV formulation of acetaminophen was recently approved by the Food and Drug Administration for use in the United States.

The maximum daily dose of acetaminophen via any route should not exceed 75 mg/kg for infants and children; with a maximum dose of 4 g/day for adolescents. Oral acetaminophen is available in a wide variety of over-the-counter and prescription formulations. These include cold remedies and opioid combination products that place children who may inadvertently receive more than one such formulation at risk of an overdose. Careful review of medications and parental education are needed to minimize this risk.

Non-steroidal anti-inflammatory drugs

Non-steroidal anti-inflammatory drugs provide excellent analgesia for mild-to-moderate pain caused by surgery, injury, and disease. Ibuprofen, one of the oldest orally administered NSAIDs, has been used extensively to treat fever and pain derived from a variety of etiologies including surgery, trauma, and arthritis. The recommended dose of ibuprofen is 10–15 mg/kg every 6 h. Diclofenac 1 mg/kg every 8 h per os (PO), per rectum (PR) or IV also provides effective analgesia after minor surgical procedures in children. In the US, it is only available as an oral tablet; rectal and injectable formulations are available in other countries. Previous studies have reported that children who received diclofenac during inguinal hernia repair experienced comparable analgesia to those who received caudal bupivacaine or IV ketorolac [81–83]. Diclofenac yielded better analgesia, less need for supplemental opioids, less nausea and vomiting, and earlier resumption of oral intake compared to acetaminophen in children undergoing tonsillectomy and/or adenoidectomy [84,85]. However, use of diclofenac has been associated with above-average bleeding in children during tonsillectomy [86].

Ketorolac provides postoperative analgesia in children of all ages that is comparable to opioids. Its lack of opioid side-effects, including respiratory depression, sedation, nausea and pruritus, make it a very attractive choice for the treatment of postoperative pain, especially in the ambulatory setting. However, like other NSAIDs, it does carry the risks of platelet dysfunction, gastrointestinal bleeding, and renal dysfunction.

Some studies of ketorolac in children undergoing tonsillectomy reported a 2–5-fold increase in bleeding complications, including measured blood loss, ease of achieving hemostasis, and bleeding episodes in the PACU, that necessitated re-exploration and hospital admission in some cases [87–90]. Two studies were terminated early when preliminary analysis found an unacceptably greater risk of bleeding in children who had received ketorolac [89,90]. A systematic review of the literature included 25 studies related to the use of NSAIDs for T&A and found that compared with opioids, NSAIDs were equi-analgesic, caused significantly less nausea and vomiting, and were associated with more frequent reoperation for bleeding [91]. This study found that the use of NSAIDs would avoid PONV and its attendant complications in 11/100 patients, but 2/100 would be exposed to the risk of postoperative bleeding and reoperation. A Cochrane review involving 13 studies related to the use of NSAIDs and peritonsillectomy bleeding found no statistically significant increase in the risk of bleeding but reported a significant decrease in the incidence of PONV in children who received NSAIDs compared to other analgesics [92]. Taken together, these data suggest that until further data become available, it may be prudent to avoid the use of NSAIDs during or after tonsillectomy and to use alternative analgesics such as acetaminophen and tramadol to reduce opioid requirements.

Steroids

The role of dexamethasone as a co-analgesic is becoming increasingly recognized in both adults and children [93]. Dexamethasone provides the added benefit of antiemesis, which is highly desirable in ambulatory surgery. The mechanism of steroid-based analgesia appears to be related to its powerful anti-inflammatory effects and reduction of prostaglandins at sites of tissue injuries [94].

Opioid analgesics

Opioids play a fundamental role in the management of postoperative pain. Unfortunately, their use is associated with a number of side-effects, including nausea, vomiting, pruritus, sedation, and respiratory depression (particularly undesirable in ambulatory surgery). The high incidence of PONV and concern about respiratory depression prompt many clinicians to avoid using opioids or to use them sparingly [95].

Oral opioids are suitable for children experiencing mild-to-moderate pain, those who undergo outpatient surgery or as adjuncts to a regional anesthetic technique. In fact, administering an oral opioid upon awakening in the PACU before a regional block wears off may provide a virtually pain-free recovery period. If dosed appropri-

ately and at regular intervals, reasonably constant blood levels can be achieved with oral opioids. In most cases, oral opioids are better tolerated after resumption of oral intake. Codeine and oxycodone, two of the most commonly prescribed oral opioids, are available in liquid form, making them easy to prescribe for infants and young children. While codeine is the most common opioid prescribed for outpatients, it is a weak analgesic and being a prodrug, it requires conversion to morphine to be effective. Developmental and pharmacogenetic variations in this conversion commonly result in ineffective conversion and occasionally in overdose. At higher doses, side-effects such as nausea, vomiting, constipation, and dysphoria are common. Oxycodone causes significantly less nausea and vomiting and appears to be better tolerated by the postoperative child just resuming oral intake.

Children who wake up in moderate-to-severe pain may require IV opioids such as fentanyl or morphine to achieve rapid and effective pain relief. However, careful titration of dosing and frequent assessment of the child are required to ensure adequate analgesia without excessive opioid side-effects, such as respiratory depression, excessive sedation or PONV, that may prolong the PACU stay and delay discharge. Children with OSA have documented increased sensitivity to opioids and investigators have recommended a 50% reduction in morphine doses for children undergoing T&A who had a pulse oximetry nadir to <85% on preoperative sleep studies [30].

Regional blockade

Regional blocks with long-acting local anesthetics provide excellent postoperative analgesia, particularly for genitourinary and orthopedic procedures performed in the outpatient setting. Both peripheral nerve blocks and central neuraxial blocks (caudal or lumbar epidural) may be used. The techniques are discussed in detail in Chapter 18. Peripheral nerve and plexus blocks provide relatively long periods of analgesia lasting for 8–12h in most cases and sometimes exceeding 24h. Depending on the nature of the surgery, this may permit the child to transition to non-opioid analgesics at the time the block wears off, thereby eliminating or reducing the use of opioids and their potential untoward effects. However, appropriate analgesic plans must be made for the parents to follow at home to ensure comfort of the child once the block wears off.

The optimal time to place the block remains a subject of debate; however, there are several purported advantages to placing the block before the onset of surgery [96]. In addition to the potential benefit of pre-emptive analgesia, the effectiveness of a block placed after induction of anesthesia can be assessed during the procedure so that the block can be repeated at the end of the procedure if ineffective. An effective block may decrease general anesthetic requirements and facilitate faster recovery. On the other hand, placing the block at the end of the procedure requires a deeper level of anesthesia to permit block placement, which would delay awakening. Lastly, a block placed at the end of surgery may require some time to become effective, causing the patient to wake up in pain. A single caudal injection of local anesthetic prior to incision does not shorten the duration of postoperative analgesia after procedures lasting 1h or less. Times from recovery until the first request for analgesics in children undergoing inguinal herniorrhaphy who had caudal blocks placed before incision or after surgery were similar [97]. For prolonged procedures, a second caudal block using half the original volume of local anesthetic may be placed prior to emergence. Central neuraxial blocks can be done in the setting of outpatient surgery with dilute concentrations of local anesthetic (0.1–0.15%), since they provide effective postoperative analgesia while avoiding motor blockade and urinary retention. Additives such as clonidine have also been shown in some studies, but not in others, to prolong the action of "single-shot" central neuraxis and some peripheral blocks.

Ilioinguinal-iliohypogastric nerve blocks provide excellent postoperative analgesia for genitourinary procedures, such as inguinal herniorrhaphy and orchidopexy. They are technically easy to perform (see Chapter 18), and the duration (4h) and efficacy of the block appear similar to caudal blocks when bupivacaine with epinephrine is used. A randomized, blinded study found that an ilioinguinal nerve block was as effective as caudal blockade to the T10 level in children undergoing orchidopexy [98]. However, procedures that involve considerable manipulation and traction on the spermatic cord and testis may be better managed with caudal blockade. While a penile block is effective for both circumcision and distal, simple hypospadias repair, a caudal block provides more effective analgesia for more extensive procedures on the penis, such as repair of penile-scrotal hypospadias [99]. Infiltration of the incision site with local anesthetic provides effective analgesia for 4–6h after surgery and should be used at the end of virtually every operation [100,101].

Postoperative nausea and vomiting

Postoperative nausea and vomiting (PONV) is a major concern in pediatric outpatient surgery because it may increase patient discomfort, increase the incidence of wound dehiscence, delay patient discharge, and increase the cost of patient care [102]. PONV, the most common cause for delayed discharge from the PACU, is a source of frustration to parents/caregivers and is a frequent cause of unplanned hospital admission or an early postoperative visit to the emergency department secondary to dehydration and electrolyte derangements [103]. Many adult patients rank PONV as the number one complication of surgery they wish to avoid [104].

Young children often have difficulty describing the occurrence or severity of nausea and for this reason, many investigators use vomiting as their endpoint [105]. Older children may be instructed preoperatively to report any nausea experienced in the postoperative period, but it is not clear whether these "suggestions" increase the reported incidence of nausea in children who may simply answer the way the investigators want. Despite these limitations, the incidence of postoperative vomiting (POV) in children is between 8.9% and 42%, approximately twice the incidence for both nausea and vomiting after surgery in adults [106]. PONV rates may be as high as 50–89% following tonsillectomy, possibly due to swallowed blood, pharyngeal stimulation, and the use of opioids [107].

Risk factors for PONV may be broadly grouped thus: patient factors, surgical factors, and anesthetic factors. Patient factors include age greater than 3 years, gender (female > male), previous history of PONV, family history of PONV, and motion sickness [106,107]. Commonly described surgical factors include type of surgery (strabismus surgery, tonsillectomy, laparoscopic surgery and certain urological procedures) and prolonged surgery [108]. Anesthetic factors, though well described, are controversial and include use of nitrous oxide, difficult mask ventilation, use of opioid medications and reversal of neuromuscular blockade [109]. Many investigators agree that a propofol-based anesthetic is associated with the lowest incidence of PONV [58,110]. A simplified risk score for POV in children is presented in Figure 34.1 [111].

Management of PONV is based on primary prevention and pharmacotherapy. Primary prevention includes a careful history to identify risk factors and tailoring the anesthetic technique to patient and surgical risk factors. Ensuring adequate hydration and nasogastric suctioning following tonsillectomy and/or adenoidectomy are other non-pharmacological techniques that have been employed to reduce the incidence of PONV.

Pharmacotherapy

This may be divided into prophylactic or rescue therapy. It is presently unresolved whether routine prophylaxis is warranted in all patients undergoing general anesthesia or whether prophylaxis should be based on risk stratification. Very often, economic considerations and risk/benefit analysis determine the choice and use of prophylactic PONV medications [112]. An international panel of experts compiled comprehensive evidence-based guidelines for the management of PONV under the auspices of the Society for Ambulatory Anesthesia (SAMBA) [111]. These guidelines suggest that the use of prophylactic antiemetics should be based on valid assessment of risk

Risk factors	Points
Surgery ≥ 30 min.	1
Age ≥ 3 years	1
Strabismus surgery	1
History of POV or PONV in relatives	1
Sum =	0...4

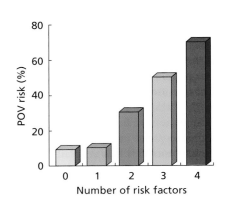

Figure 34.1 Risk factors for POV in children. Simplified risk score to predict the risk for POV in children. When 0, 1, 2, 3 or 4 of the depicted independent predictors are present, the corresponding risk for PONV is approximately 10%, 10%, 30%, 55%, and 70%. Reproduced from Gan et al [111] with permission from Lippincott Williams and Wilkins.

factors for POV as detailed in the algorithm in Figure 34.2. These guidelines recommend that children deemed to be at moderate-to-high risk for POV should receive combination therapy with two or three prophylactic drugs from different classes. Additionally, patients who experience POV despite prophylaxis should receive additional antiemetics from a pharmacological class different from the prophylactic drug, since repeating the same drug within 6 h of the original dose does not confer any benefit.

Commonly used medications include serotonin (5HT3) receptor antagonists (ondansetron, granisetron, and dolasetron), steroids (dexamethasone), antihistamines (promethazine, benadryl), metoclopramide, and droperidol. A systematic review reported good evidence that dexamethasone and the serotonin receptor antagonists ondansetron, granisetron and tropisetron were clinically effective for PONV prohylaxis in children undergoing tonsillectomy with or without adenoidectomy [113]. Furthermore, this review found that dimenhydrinate, perphenazine, droperidol, gastric aspiration and acupuncture were not efficacious in reducing PONV in this population. The 5HT3 receptor antagonists are rapidly becoming the most frequently prescribed agents for both prophylaxis and treatment of PONV [107]. Recent data indicate that ondansetron (0.1 mg/kg, up to 4 mg) was effective in preventing early and delayed PONV in children undergoing various types of surgeries [114]. Due to its efficacy and safety profile, ondansetron has become the most commonly prescribed antiemetic for prophylaxis and treatment of PONV. Despite its established safety record, it is important to be aware of some of the fortunately rare but serious side-effects of ondansetron, which may cause a lethal outcome. Recent data indicate that it may cause QT prolongation leading to ventricular tachycardia [115]. Rarely, it may be associated with sero-

tonin syndrome [116] and malignant hyperthermia reaction in patients with muscular dystrophies [117,118].

Two novel antiemetic agents are now available that will likely have an increasing role in the treatment of PONV. Palonosetron, a second-generation 5HT3 antagonist, was approved by the FDA in 2003. Due to its unique binding properties and greater binding affinity for the receptor, it has a substantially longer half-life of approximately 40 h. A study of adult patients undergoing outpatient laparoscopic surgery with two or more risk factors for PONV found that a single IV dose of 0.075 mg of palonosetron prior to induction of anesthesia significantly increased the complete response rate, i.e. no emetic episodes and no rescue medication compared with placebo [119]. Furthermore, patients who received palonosetron reported less severity of nausea and less interference in their postoperative function due to PONV. Pediatric data with the use of palonosetron are limited to its use for chemotherapy-induced nausea and vomiting. A study that compared children who received ondansetron before the administration of chemotherapy and every 8 h through the hospitalization with those who received a single dose of palonosetron prior to chemotherapy reported significantly reduced intensity of nausea and a significant reduction of emetic events for 3 days of treatment, with some benefits for up to 7 days, in the palonosteron group [120]. No data are available that evaluate the use of palonosetron for PONV in children. Its long duration of action makes it an excellent choice for patients undergoing outpatient surgery, and further studies are needed to evaluate its benefits in this setting.

Aprepitant is a neurokinin-1 (NK1) receptor antagonist that crosses the blood–brain barrier and blocks the emetic effects of substance P [121]. Studies in adults have reported that it reduces PONV following joint arthroplasty and

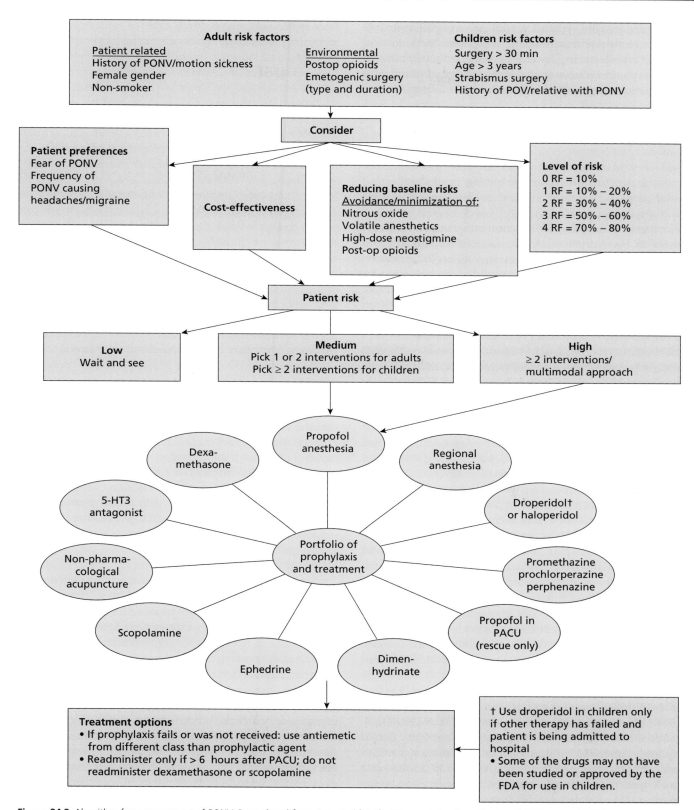

Adult risk factors

Patient related
History of PONV/motion sickness
Female gender
Non-smoker

Environmental
Postop opioids
Emetogenic surgery
(type and duration)

Children risk factors
Surgery > 30 min
Age > 3 years
Strabismus surgery
History of POV/relative with PONV

Consider

Patient preferences
Fear of PONV
Frequency of
PONV causing
headaches/migraine

Cost-effectiveness

Reducing baseline risks
Avoidance/minimization of:
Nitrous oxide
Volatile anesthetics
High-dose neostigmine
Post-op opioids

Level of risk
0 RF = 10%
1 RF = 10% – 20%
2 RF = 30% – 40%
3 RF = 50% – 60%
4 RF = 70% – 80%

Patient risk

Low
Wait and see

Medium
Pick 1 or 2 interventions for adults
Pick ≥ 2 interventions for children

High
≥ 2 interventions/
multimodal approach

Propofol
anesthesia

Dexa-
methasone

Regional
anesthesia

5-HT3
antagonist

Droperidol†
or haloperidol

Non-pharma-
cological
acupuncture

Portfolio of
prophylaxis
and treatment

Promethazine
prochlorperazine
perphenazine

Scopolamine

Propofol in
PACU
(rescue only)

Ephedrine

Dimen-
hydrinate

Treatment options
• If prophylaxis fails or was not received: use antiemetic
  from different class than prophylactic agent
• Readminister only if > 6 hours after PACU; do not
  readminister dexamethasone or scopolamine

† Use droperidol in children only
if other therapy has failed and
patient is being admitted to
hospital
• Some of the drugs may not have
  been studied or approved by the
  FDA for use in children.

Figure 34.2 Algorithm for management of PONV. Reproduced from Gan et al [111] with permission from Lippincott Williams and Wilkins.

abdominal surgery [122,123]. However, no pediatric data are available for this indication. A single oral dose of 40 mg 1 h prior to surgery is recommended for adults. An IV formulation is now available, but its only indication is for chemotherapy-induced nausea and vomiting.

Recovery and discharge

Recovery from anesthesia is a complex process encompassing several outcomes including normalization of physiological endpoints, return to baseline sensorium and activity, and emotional and psychological recovery. For the patient undergoing ambulatory surgery, assessment of recovery has largely focused on a return of acceptable physiological parameters, ability to ambulate, and recovery of consciousness to allow the patient to be safely discharged home. To that end, a number of simple clinical scoring systems that assess recovery have been developed and tested [124–128]. The most widely used scoring system is the score that Aldrete first described in 1970 [124]. The original Aldrete score was a 0–10-point scale comprising five recovery parameters, each of which was scored 0–2, similar to the Apgar Score. Subsequently a number of modifications of this score were made that incorporate fast-track criteria, oxygen saturation rather than observation of color to identify hypoxemia, and consideration of developmental stages in children [125,127,129]. Table 34.1 describes a modified version of the Aldrete score suitable for use in children.

Another score that is easy to use and is well suited for use in children is the Steward Postanesthetic Recovery Score that incorporates three recovery parameters and is scored 0–2 with a maximum achievable score of 6 (Table 34.2) [126]. In addition to monitoring of physiological variables, such as vital signs, oxygen saturation, and level of consciousness, a standardized recovery score should be calculated for each patient on admission, at appropriate intervals during the PACU stay, and on discharge. Each facility must select the recovery score that works best in their setting, taking into consideration the psychometric as well as pragmatic qualities of the scoring system to facilitate its repeated use.

Recently, the limitations of such scoring systems in evaluating the broader and potentially long-term impact of anesthesia and surgery have been recognized [130,131]. In attempts to assess early and long-term recovery across multiple domains, including cognition, emotional recovery and activities of daily living, studies in adults have evaluated the reliability, validity, precision, and pragmatic qualities of instruments that measure postoperative recovery outcomes at various time periods after surgery [130–133]. Most of these instruments would not be suitable for use in children. The Post-Hospital Behavior

Table 34.1 Modified Aldrete score for children

Variable		Score
Airway	Coughing on command or crying	2
	Maintaining good airway	1
	Airway requires maintenance	0
Vital signs	Stable and appropriate for age	2
	Stable but inappropriate for age	1
	Unstable	0
Motor activity	Moving limbs purposefully	2
	Non-purposeful movements	1
	Not moving	0
Consciousness	Awake	2
	Responding to stimuli	1
	Not responding	0
SpO$_2$ on room air	>95	2
	90–94	1
	<90	0

Score ≥9 considered suitable for discharge.
Reproduced from Patel et al [129] with permission from Springer.

Questionnaire (PHBQ) comprises 27 items across six categories of anxiety, including general anxiety, separation anxiety, sleep anxiety, eating disturbances, aggression against authority, and apathy/withdrawal (Box 34.3) [134]. This instrument was designed specifically to evaluate maladaptive and negative behavioral changes in children and has been widely used to assess postoperative behavior changes in the pediatric surgical population [45,135,136].

Discharge criteria

The ASA practice guidelines recommend that each patient care facility should develop suitable recovery and discharge criteria and provide guidance for development of such criteria (Box 34.4) [137]. Box 34.5 summarizes the ASA stance on specific discharge criteria that have been traditionally mandated in some settings, such as requiring that patients void or tolerate oral liquids prior to discharge. These practices prolong recovery stay and evidence to support their benefits in reducing adverse outcomes is insufficient. Indeed, a previous study reported a lower incidence of vomiting and a shorter stay in the day surgery unit in children who were allowed to drink electively compared to those who were required to drink prior to discharge [138]. No child in either group required readmission for vomiting or dehydration. However, the intravenous fluid regimen was liberalized to supply a calculated 8 h deficit in addition to maintenance fluids and intraoperative losses. Adequate intravenous hydra-

Table 34.2 Steward postanesthetic recovery score

Patient sign	Criterion	Score
Consciousness	Awake	2
	Responding to stimuli	1
	Not responding	0
Airway	Coughing on command or crying	2
	Maintaining good airway	1
	Airway requiring maintenance	0
Movement	Moving limbs purposefully	2
	Moving limbs non-purposefully	1
	Not moving	0

Source: Steward [126].

Table 34.3 Criteria for fast-tracking children

Criterion		Score
Level of consciousness	Awake and oriented	2
	Arousable with minimal stimulation	1
	Responsive only to tactic stimulation	0
Physical activity	Appropriate for age and development	2
	Weak for age and development	1
	Unable to move extremities	0
Hemodynamics	BP <15% of baseline MAP	2
	BP 15–30% of baseline MAP	1
	BP >30% below baseline MAP	0
Respiratory stability	Coughing, crying, deep breaths	2
	Hoarseness with crying or coughing	1
	Stridor, dyspnea, wheezing	0
SpO$_2$	>95% on room air	2
	90–95% on room air	1
	<90% on room air	0
Pain	None/mild discomfort	2
	Moderate to severe controlled with IV analgesics	1
	Persistent severe pain	0

A minimum score of 10 (with no score <1 in any individual category) is required for fast-tracking children.
BP, blood pressure; IV, intravenous; MAP, mean arterial pressure.
Reproduced from Patel et al [129] with permission from Springer.

Box 34.3 Items included in the Post-Hospital Behavior Questionnaire (PHBQ)

I. Does your child need a pacifier?
Does your child seem to be afraid of leaving the house with you?
Is your child uninterested in what goes on around him (or her)?
Does your child bite his (or her) fingernails?
Does your child seem to avoid or be afraid of new things?
Does your child have difficulty making up his (or her) mind?
Is your child irregular in his (or her) bowel movements?
Does your child suck his (or her) fingers or thumbs?

II. Does your child get upset when you leave him (or her) alone for a few minutes?
Does your child seem to get upset when someone mentions doctors or hospitals?
Does your child follow you everywhere around the house?
Does your child spend time trying to get or hold your attention?
Does your child have bad dreams at night or wake up and cry?

III. Does your child make a fuss about going to bed at night?
Is your child afraid of the dark?
Does your child have trouble getting to sleep at night?

IV. Does your child make a fuss about eating?
Does your child spend time just sitting or lying and doing nothing?
Does your child have a poor appetite?

V. Does your child have temper tantrums?
Does your child tend to disobey you?

VI. Does your child wet the bed at night?
Does your child need a lot of help doing things?
Is it difficult to get your child interested in activities (like playing games, with toys, and so on)?
Is it difficult to get your child to talk to you?
Does your child seem to be shy or afraid around strangers?
Does your child break toys or other objects?

Source: Vernon et al [134].

tion and correction of fluid deficits prior to discharge may be prudent in children who refuse oral fluids in the PACU.

Discharge before voiding has also not been found to result in readmission for urinary retention. In one study, 30/1719 ambulatory patients who were unable to void but met other discharge criteria were discharged home and followed by a home care nurse [139]. Three of these patients required catheterization at home, and all three had undergone rectal or inguinal surgery under spinal anesthesia. Risk factors for postoperative urinary retention in children include a history of urinary retention or urethral surgery. In the absence of these risk factors, children may be discharged before voiding with instructions to the caregivers to call if they have not voided within a given timeframe.

Box 34.4 Summary of recovery and discharge criteria

General principles

- Medical supervision of recovery and discharge is the responsibility of the supervising practitioner.
- The recovery area should be equipped with appropriate personnel and monitoring and resuscitation equipment.
- Patients should be monitored until appropriate discharge criteria are satisfied.
- Level of consciousness, vital signs, and oxygenation should be recorded at regular intervals.
- A nurse or other individual trained to monitor patients and recognize complications should be in attendance until discharge criteria are fulfilled.
- An individual capable of managing complications should be immediately available until discharge criteria are fulfilled.

Guidelines for discharge

- Patients should be alert and oriented. Patients whose mental status was initially abnormal should have returned to their baseline.
- Vital signs should be stable and within acceptable limits.
- Discharge should occur after patients have met specified criteria
- Use of scoring systems may assist in documentation of fitness for discharge.
- Outpatients should be discharged to a responsible adult who will accompany them home and be able to report any postprocedure complications.
- Outpatients should be provided with written instructions regarding postprocedure diet, medications, activities, and a phone number to be called in case of emergency.

Source: Practice Guidelines for Postanesthetic Care [137].

Box 34.5 Summary of recommendations for discharge

Requiring that patients urinate before discharge

- The requirement for urination before discharge should not be part of a routine discharge protocol and may only be necessary for selected patients.

Requiring that patients drink clear fluids without vomiting before discharge

- The demonstrated ability to drink and retain clear fluids should not be part of a routine discharge protocol but may be appropriate for selected patients. Replacement intravenous hydration is recommended.

Requiring that patients have a responsible individual accompany them home

- As part of a discharge protocol, patients should routinely be required to have a responsible individual to accompany them home and to monitor for complications.

Requiring a minimum mandatory stay in recovery

- A mandatory minimum stay should not be required. Patients should be observed until they are no longer at increased risk for cardiorespiratory depression. Discharge criteria should be designed to minimize the risk of central nervous system or cardiorespiratory depression after discharge.

Source: Practice Guidelines for Postanesthetic Care [137].

Sample discharge criteria are presented in Box 34.6. In the US, all patients who are to be discharged from the PACU must be evaluated for discharge readiness by an anesthesiologist in accordance with Centers for Medicare and Medicaid Services (CMS) guidelines [140].

Fast-tracking

Fast-tracking is the process of bypassing the PACU and transferring the patient who has met specific criteria directly to the step-down or phase II recovery unit. The goal of fast-tracking is to improve efficiency without compromising patient safety or satisfaction. Table 34.3 describes criteria for fast-tracking for children that take into consideration the adequacy of pain relief [129]. A randomized study found a 20 min shorter recovery time for children who were fast-tracked when compared to those who were sent to the PACU, even though both groups met fast-track criteria in the operating room [129]. Children in the fast-track group were less likely to be

given analgesics postoperatively (41% versus 62%) and were more likely to be restless in the phase II recovery unit (31% versus 16%) compared to the children who were sent to the PACU. No child in either group experienced a clinically significant adverse event. A previous study that included patients >12 years of age found that ASA III compared to ASA I, age <60 years and general surgery (compared to orthopedics and ophthalmology) were risk factors for fast-track ineligibility [141]. Consideration of such factors, in addition to standard criteria, may enhance efficient and cost-effective utilization of PACU resources. As stated in the American Society of PeriAnesthesia Nurses standards, "Phase II is a level of care, not a physical place. The decision to fast-track a patient should be based on patient needs, clinical assessments, and desired patient outcomes" [142].

Complications of outpatient anesthesia

Adverse postoperative outcomes are usually multifactorial in origin and are the result of the patient's underlying

Box 34.6 Sample PACU discharge criteria

Criteria for discharge to general care inpatient units

- Stable respiratory status (patent airway, adequate respiratory function, adequate oxygen saturation)
- Stable vital signs within an acceptable range for patient's age, condition and preoperative status
- Awake or easily arousable. Level of consciousness appropriate for preoperative developmental age/status
- Operative area without evidence of significant bleeding
- Adequate analgesia so that comfort needs can be easily managed by resources available at the discharge location
- Normothermic or core temperature that is minimally 36°C or temperature within an acceptable range of preoperative status
- Patients who have received spinal or epidural anesthesia must demonstrate maximum sensory block at the T12 dermatome level and be free of orthostatic hypotension.
- Patients who receive racemic epinephrine will be admitted or monitored for at least 8 h

Criteria for discharge to home

- Tolerate oral fluids with minimal nausea or vomiting or have received adequate intravenous fluid replacement to deter dehydration
- Parents or caregivers have adequate understanding of discharge instructions and are able to provide postoperative care
- Patients who have received spinal or epidural anesthesia must be able to transfer with assistance
- Patients who receive regional anesthesia will be instructed to call the PACU or Surgical Service if they have not voided within 6 h

co-morbidities, anesthetic techniques or the surgical procedure itself. Fortunately, major morbidity and mortality are extremely rare after ambulatory anesthesia. The reported death rate is approximately two per 100,000 procedures [143,144]. However, minor sequelae, such as drowsiness, uncontrolled PONV, unrelieved pain, bleeding, and respiratory complications, may delay discharge and lead to unplanned hospital admission or readmission following discharge.

The most common symptom reported by parents following discharge of their child is unrelieved pain, which was present in 25–91% of patients [145–151]. One study found that tonsillectomy was a predictor for postoperative pain and that the pain lasted for 7 days or longer in 33% of children. Twelve percent of parents believed that postoperative instructions for pain management at home were inadequate [146]. The incidence of PONV following discharge is reportedly 5.9–59% [145–149,152]. Predictors for PONV include emetic symptoms in the hospital, pain at home, age >5 years, and administration of postoperative opioids [146]. Other postdischarge symptoms include drowsiness, headache, dizziness, fever, hoarseness, mild croup, and difficulty voiding. Adequate preparation of

the family/caregivers with individualized discharge education regarding the potential occurrence of complications and symptoms may alleviate parental postdischarge anxiety and promote satisfaction.

Unplanned admission

Unplanned hospital admission for the ambulatory surgery patient increases utilization of resources, is inconvenient for patients and their families, and is a measure of outcome and quality of care. Previous investigators have reported that approximately 2% of children scheduled for outpatient surgery require hospital admission [153–155]. Another study reported that almost 4% of children undergoing ambulatory surgery required a >3 h PACU stay and 1.9% required hospital admission [153]. Prolonged PACU stay occurred most frequently due to PONV (19%) or respiratory complications (16%), including bronchospasm, oxygen desaturation, stridor, and apnea. Respiratory complications and surgical problems, including more extensive surgery than was originally planned, were the most common reasons for unplanned hospital admission. Other investigators reported a 1.8% unplanned admission rate that was commonly due to PONV, postoperative bleeding, or unexpected difficulty with the procedure [155]. Another study reported a 2.2% incidence of unplanned hospital admission in children due to uncontrolled pain, surgical complications, need for extensive surgery, and bleeding [154]. In this study, anesthesia-related causes of unplanned hospital admission included PONV, oxygen desaturation, bronchospasm, and somnolence; social causes including surgery ending late in the day; and medical causes included underlying medical problems or undiagnosed medical disease. Notably, in the latter two studies, orchidopexy was the most common surgical procedure that resulted in unplanned admission. Taken together, these data suggest a need for careful and frequent re-evaluation of selection criteria for outpatient surgery and vigilant monitoring for potential complications in the PACU.

Given the increasing complexity of procedures performed in the ambulatory setting, the diverse settings in which such procedures are performed, and the expanded patient selection criteria, investigators have attempted to identify risk factors for hospital admission following ambulatory surgery. The Outpatient Surgery Admission Index (OSAI) assigns 1 point each for age >65 years, operating time >120 min, cardiac diagnoses, peripheral vascular disease, cerebrovascular disease, malignancy, HIV-positive status, and use of regional anesthesia techniques, and two points are assigned for general anesthesia [156]. The OSAI shows a good correlation between the odds of requiring hospital admission and increasing OSAI score. Most of the conditions used in the OSAI are more prevalent in adults; similar methods for risk assessment in children are needed to enable appropriate allocation of resources and increase the efficiency of ambulatory surgery in this population.

Conclusion

In this era of healthcare reform, it is inevitable that there will be increasing pressure to provide low-cost, efficient, high-quality surgical care. The practice of ambulatory surgery will likely expand further and at a more rapid pace than it has over the past 20 years. The need for development of innovative delivery systems that capitalize upon low-cost organizational structures and prudent management of resources will require resourcefulness of healthcare professionals and administrators alike. In the ambulatory surgery setting, it will be increasingly necessary to prevent such pressures from constraining clinical judgment regarding the safest and most appropriate patient care.

CASE STUDY

A 22-month-old male child presented for hypospadias repair as an outpatient.

History
He had been healthy since birth and had been followed regularly for his well child visits. His immunizations were up to date, and his growth and development had been normal. The parents reported a history of a "cold" with a runny nose and cough that started 7 days prior to the scheduled surgery. His skin was warm to touch, and he had decreased appetite and activity on the first day of his symptoms. Most of his symptoms had resolved without any treatment, but he continued to have an occasional cough. This was his second upper respiratory infection after beginning daycare 6 months ago.

His review of symptoms was otherwise negative, he was on no medications and he had not undergone surgery previously.

He was born at 41 weeks' gestation by emergency cesarean section for fetal bradycardia. His neonatal course was complicated by hyperbilirubinemia that was treated with phototherapy. This caused him to stay one extra day in the newborn nursery.

His family history was negative for anesthesia-related problems. His mother received an uneventful epidural anesthetic for his birth, and his father underwent an uneventful tonsillectomy (to the best of his knowledge) as a child.

Physical examination
The child was active and alert, playing with toys in the surgical waiting room until he was being examined, when he started crying and clinging to his mother. His vital signs were normal for age and his weight was 13.2 kg. He had no dysmorphic features. While it was impossible to perform a detailed airway examination, his neck mobility and anatomy were normal, and his mouth opening was adequate. His breath sounds were initially coarse but cleared when he was distracted and stopped crying. He had normal heart sounds and no murmurs, extra sounds or clicks.

Anesthetic management
The child was fearful of strangers and resisted changing into a hospital gown. Because his mother was concerned that he would not co-operate with mask induction of anesthesia, he was premedicated with 7 mg of midazolam orally. He also received 200 mg of acetaminophen suspension orally for pre-emptive analgesia. Within 15 min, the child appeared visibly calmer. However, he resisted being carried by the anesthesia team but did not resist being wheeled into the operating room in a wagon. Anesthesia was induced with sevoflurane, and intravenous access was obtained after induction of anesthesia. Due to the potential for airway hyper-reactivity from his recent URI, an LMA was placed and anesthesia was maintained with oxygen, nitrous oxide, and sevoflurane. After induction of anesthesia, a caudal block was placed using 7 mL of 0.125% bupivacaine with 1:200,000 epinephrine. The surgery was completed uneventfully and the LMA was removed in the operating room prior to transfer to the PACU.

Postoperative management
The child was asleep but readily arousable on arrival in the PACU. He had stable vital signs and his oxygen saturation was 98% on blow-by oxygen. The oxygen was discontinued and his SaO_2 remained >95% breathing room air. His pain score on awakening was 3/10 by the FLACC Scale. Since 4 h had elapsed from his initial dose of acetaminophen, an additional 150 mg of oral acetaminophen was given. He was reunited with his parents in the PACU. After drinking apple juice, the child had two episodes of emesis in the PACU. He was given 2 mg of ondansetron and no further emesis occurred. The child refused additional fluids but was able

to void in the PACU. He had complete return of motor function and was able to stand prior to discharge. When he met institutional discharge criteria, he was discharged home with a prescription for oxycodone suspension. Telephone follow-up the next day revealed that the child had an uneventful recovery at home and had required one dose of oxycodone upon awakening the morning after the surgery.

Summary

This case describes the perioperative care of a child undergoing a common urological procedure. It illustrates the effective use of a sedative premedication to facilitate separation from the parent. The use of a regional block allowed the child to awaken with minimal pain and significantly reduced his need for opioids.

Annotated references

A full reference list for this chapter is available at:
http://www.wiley.com/go/gregory/andropoulos/pediatricanesthesia

11. Brigger MT, Brietzke SE. Outpatient tonsillectomy in children: a systematic review. Otolaryngol Head Neck Surg 2006; 135: 1–7. All 17 articles included in this systematic review suggested that outpatient pediatric tonsillectomy was safe. Pooled data analysis found a complication rate of 8.8% and an unplanned hospital admission rate of 8%. Children under 4 years of age had a higher risk for complications.

26. Lerman JA. Disquisition on sleep-disordered breathing in children. Paediatr Anaesth 2009; 19: 100–8. This authoritative reference provides a succinct yet complete review of sleep-disordered breathing in children.

33. Tait AR, Voepel-Lewis T, Burke C et al. Incidence and risk factors for perioperative adverse respiratory events in children who are obese. Anesthesiology 2008; 108: 375–80. This large prospective observational study found that obese children had a significantly higher prevalence of co-morbidities and were at higher risk for perioperative adverse respiratory events than non-obese children.

40. Von Ungern-Sternberg BS, Boda K, Chambers NA et al. Risk assessment for respiratory complications in paediatric anaesthesia: a prospective cohort study. Lancet 2010; 376: 773–83. This large prospective study identified risk factors for perioperative respiratory complications, including cold symptoms in the preceding 2 weeks, wheezing during exercise, more than three wheezing episodes in the past year, nocturnal dry cough, passive smoking, eczema, and hay fever. The use of intravenous inductions, noninvasive airway device, cuffed endotracheal tubes (versus uncuffed), propofol maintenance, a consultant anesthetist, and avoidance of topical lidocaine and desflurane protected against respiratory complications.

95. Howard RF. Current status of pain management in children. JAMA 2003; 290: 2464–9. This is arguably one of the best reviews of pediatric pain management. The author details the available options and challenges to optimal perioperative analgesia in children.

105. Olutoye O, Watcha MF. Management of postoperative vomiting in pediatric patients. Int Anesthesiol Clin 2003; 41: 99–117. This is a comprehensive review of the literature on pediatric postoperative nausea and vomiting. The authors chose a clinically relevant approach to their discussion.

112. Hill RP, Lubarsky DA, Phillips-Bute B et al. Cost-effectiveness of prophylactic antiemetic therapy with ondansetron, droperidol, or placebo. Anesthesiology 2000; 92: 958–67. These authors detailed the economic consequences of PONV in high-risk adult patients. Similar models, though difficult to extend to pediatrics, may prove useful. Economic consequences in children could include lost school days and readmission for dehydration due to PONV.

118. Gener B, Burns JM, Griffin S, Boyer EW. Administration of ondansetron is associated with lethal outcome. Pediatrics 2010; 125: e1514. This case report of rare but lethal complication of ondansetron is well written and clinically relevant. Due to the widespread use of ondansetron for both prophylaxis and treatment of PONV, clinicians should be aware of some of the rare but very serious complications of ondansetron.

130. Royse CF, Newman S, Chung F et al. Development and feasibility of a scale to assess postoperative recovery: the post-operative quality recovery scale. Anesthesiology 2010; 113: 892–905. This study evaluated the reliabilty and validity of an instrument designed to assess long-term postoperative recovery across multiple domains, inclduing cognition, emotional recovery, and activities of daily living.

156. Fleisher LA, Pasternak LR, Lyles A. A novel index of elevated risk of inpatient hospital admission immediately following outpatient surgery. Arch Surg 2007; 142: 263–8. These investigators identified factors associated with increased risk for hospital admission in patients undergoing ambulatory surgery. These factors were then compiled into a risk assessment score, the Outpatient Surgery Admission Index (OSAI). This study found that the odds of requiring hospital admission increased significantly with an increasing OSAI score.

CHAPTER 35

Anesthesia for Burns and Trauma

Patrick J. Guffey[1] *& Dean B. Andropoulos*[2]

[1]Department of Anesthesiology, University of Colorado School of Medicine, and Children's Hospital Colorado, Aurora, CO, USA
[2]Department of Anesthesiology and Pediatrics, Baylor College of Medicine, and Texas Children's Hospital, Houston, TX, USA

Introduction

Burns and trauma remain a leading cause of hospitalization and need for anesthesia and critical care in the pediatric population. This chapter discusses anesthesia care of burned children by reviewing the epidemiology, pathophysiology, acute resuscitation and management, and anesthetic care of both initial burn procedures and longer-term reconstructive surgery. Next, anesthesia care for children who have suffered other types of trauma will be reviewed and etiology, acute assessment and management during trauma resuscitation, and trauma anesthesia management in the operating room will be discussed.

Burns

Burns are a significant cause of death and disability in children. In 2007, almost 500 children under the age of 14 died from unintentional fires or burns, making burns the second highest cause of death for children 5–9 years of age, and placing burns in the top six causes of death for all other age groups [1]. Approximately 15,000 children are hospitalized per year for burn injuries, and 1100 succumb to this injury [2,3]. Table 35.1 illustrates the top three causes of burn injuries for five age groups [4–7]. As illustrated, the majority of pediatric burns are from a thermal source, with scalds predominating until age 5, after which direct contact with fire or flame becomes the leading cause until adulthood. Approximately 30% of burned children suffer inhalation injury with flames, superheated air, toxic gas or smoke [8]. Though children are less likely than adults to suffer from inhalational injury, those with inhalation burns have a significantly higher degree of morbidity and mortality, i.e. 3–10% without inhalational injury and 20–30% with it [9–11]. Burns may also be caused by electricity, chemicals, and radiation. High-voltage electrical burns are particularly problematic, as outward appearance does not accurately portray the extent of damage to tissues and organs.

The fatality rate associated with burns has decreased over time, most likely secondary to the more consistent use of specialized burn centers [12]. In the US, underrepresented minority groups are burned more frequently than the general population and may represent an opportunity for targeted burn prevention education [4].

Burns are classified both by the percent of total body surface area (TBSA) affected and by the depth of the injury. An estimate of the BSA involved is most often made from charts devised by Lund and Browder, which adjust surface area proportions for age (Fig. 35.1). The head is relatively larger and the limbs relatively smaller in children than in teenagers and adults, accounting for the difference in surface area. Burn depth is classified as shown in Table 35.2.

Superficial burns (first degree) involve only the outer epidermal layer. Although the area is erythematous, there is minimal tissue damage and the protective barrier functions of the skin remain intact. Because the nerves are also intact, these burns are often very painful. Partial-thickness (second-degree) burns involve the entire epidermis and variable portions of the dermis. There is blistering, weeping of transudated fluids, and severe pain. A superficial second-degree burn involves only the upper part of the dermis. Burns of this type heal rapidly with minimal scarring; the dermis is repopulated with epithelial cells that reside in hair follicles, sweat glands, and other skin appendages anchored in the deep dermis. A deep second-degree burn extends further into the dermis; few viable epidermal cells remain. Re-epithelialization is very slow, and scarring occurs if the wound is not grafted. The local response to burn injury involves not only direct coagulation of burned tissue but also microvascular reactions in the surrounding dermis, and progressive vasoconstriction and thrombosis. Survival of the surrounding dermis and epidermal appendages is dependent on the presence of optimal conditions. Residual heat, mechanical trauma,

Table 35.1 National Burn Repository (2010) – burn etiology [4]

Age group	Etiology – top 3	Cases
Birth – 0.9 years	Scald	2422
	Contact with a hot object	1012
	Fire/flame	244
1–1.9 years	Scald	4636
	Contact with a hot object	2253
	Fire/Flame	444
2–4.9 years	Scald	4401
	Fire/flame	1462
	Contact with a hot object	1330
5–15.9 years	Fire/flame	5763
	Scald	3813
	Contact with a hot object	1036
16–19.9 years	Fire/flame	3348
	Scald	1469
	Other, non-burn	668

Table 35.2 Depth of burn injury

Classification	Skin and tissue layers involved
First degree (superficial)	Epidermis
Second degree (partial thickness)	
Superficial second degree	Epidermis and superficial dermis
Deep second degree	Epidermis and deep dermis
Third degree (full thickness)	Epidermis and full-thickness dermis
Fourth degree (full thickness)	Fascia, muscle, and bone

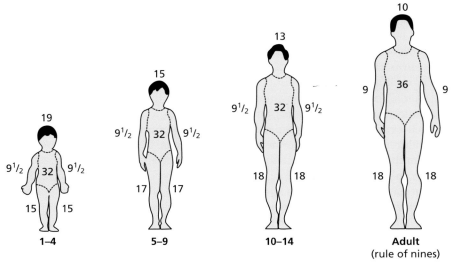

Figure 35.1 Burn assessment chart with body surface areas according to age. Numbers beneath the figures indicate age in years; other numbers indicate percent body surface area indicated by adjacent areas enclosed in dotted lines. Reproduced from Carvahal [94] with permission from Elsevier.

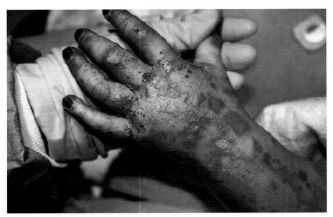

Figure 35.2 Deep partial-thickness burn (deep second degree) in a toddler; this would be considered a major burn because of its location involving the hand. Reproduced from Fabia and Groner [48] with permission from Elsevier.

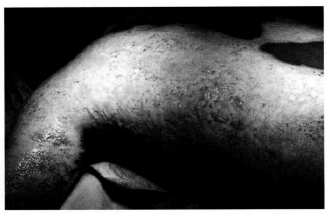

Figure 35.3 Full-thickness (third-degree) scald burn of the back and arm of a toddler. Reproduced from Fabia and Groner [48] with permission from Elsevier.

vasoactive mediators, and dehydration may lead to progressive dermal ischemia [13]. Fluid losses and the metabolic effects of deep dermal burns are similar to those of full-thickness burns.

Third-degree burns involve destruction of the entire epidermis and dermis, leaving no residual epidermal cells to repopulate the burned area. The burned skin takes on a dry, leathery, firm consistency with charring or pearly white discoloration [13]. The tissue is avascular and a zone of ischemia exists between the dead tissue above and deeper living tissue below. Survival of this marginally viable tissue is also dependent on there being optimal conditions. Preventing conversion of viable tissue to eschar is a major goal during the resuscitation period. A fourth-degree burn involves all of the skin structures plus the fascia, muscle or bone underneath (Figs 35.2, 35.3).

Major burn injuries warrant special consideration and referral to specialized burn centers that have expertise in caring for pediatric patients. Major burns are defined as third-degree burns of greater than 10% TBSA or a 20–25% second-degree burn (15–20% in infants); burns involving face, hands, feet or perineum; inhalational burn injuries; chemical or electrical burns; burns associated with trauma; circumferential burns, especially of torso; and burns in children with co-existing medical diseases [14]. It must be emphasized that initial classification of burn injury, both in TBSA and depth, is often revised in the first several days following initial surgical excision of burned tissue; therefore it is best to err on the side of caution during initial assessment when deciding whether or not to refer the patient to a burn center (Box 35.1).

Morbidity and mortality from burn injury increase with increasing size and depth of the burn and in younger

---

Box 35.1 Criteria for definition of major burn injury

- Greater than 10% TBSA third-degree burns
- Greater than 20–25% second-degree burns in children and teenagers
- Greater than 15–20% second-degree burns in neonates and infants
- Burns involving face, hands, feet or perineum
- Chemical or electrical burns
- Burns associated with trauma
- Inhalational burn injuries
- Circumferential burns, especially of the torso
- Burns in children with co-existing medical disease

---

children. These survival rates have improved in recent years with advances in the care of burned children. These improvements were spurred on by better understanding of resuscitation, support during the hypermetabolic phase, wound coverage, infection control, and treatment of inhalational injury [15–21]. Thirteen-to-eighteen year olds have the highest survival rates. Reports from the 1960s to the 1980s indicated 50% survival with 70% TBSA burns in this age group, and only 20% survival for children below 3 years of age with similar degrees of burn [22]. A report from the 1990s indicates that 84% of 11–18 year olds, 72% of 3–10 year olds, and 43% of children under the age of 2 years survived after >85% TBSA burns. Recent reports from the year 2000 and later indicate that survival of 80% TBSA burns in young children is now >60% [23] and survival of 99% TBSA burns in children over age 14 is 50% [24].

Pathophysiology of burn injury

The major function of the skin is to provide a barrier to infection and to reduce heat and fluid losses. Major burn injury disrupts these protective functions. Heat loss ensues when the ability of the peripheral vasculature to vasoconstrict and reduce blood flow is disrupted; this allows heat to be lost from the skin. In addition, disruption of capillaries, arterioles and venules causes significant transudation of massive amounts of fluid and electrolytes. Major burn injury also initiates an enormous inflammatory response to the tissue injury that results in release of both local and systemic inflammatory mediators. Local mediators include leukotrienes, prostaglandins, bradykinin, histamine, nitric oxide, and oxygen free radicals. Systemic inflammatory mediators include interleukins (IL)-1, -6, -8, and -10 and tumor necrosis factor (TNF) [14]. This milieu of proinflammatory cytokines is accompanied by activation of the stress hormone system and release of catecholamines and adrenocortical steroids. This results in a hypermetabolic state which usually occurs 3–5 days after injury, normally lasts until wounds are covered and healing, and slowly subsides over weeks to months. All organs are affected by the inflammatory response and hypermetabolic state. Consequently, anesthesiologists caring for these patients must carefully evaluate them for these changes and be prepared to treat any organ-specific derangements.

During the acute phase these patients may develop decreased tissue perfusion and hypovolemic shock from loss of fluid from both the burn injury site and the inflammation-induced capillary leak. In addition, there may be hemoconcentration and increased blood viscosity, inflammatory mediator-induced myocardial dysfunction, and increased systemic vascular resistance that are the result of increased catecholamine release. Ventricular failure is possible in severe burns [14,25]. Responses to both endogenous and exogenous catecholamines are attenuated in this phase, presumably because myocardial and vascular adrenergic receptors are either maximally stimulated or desensitized by direct effects of the inflammatory mediators. Following the acute effects, which last from a few hours to several days, a hypermetabolic, catecholamine-driven response replaces the cardiovascular depression. Heart rate and cardiac output increase, and often hypertension is present.

The pulmonary system may be affected directly by the burn itself and/or indirectly by the inflammatory response. Inhalation of smoke, flames, toxic gases or carbon monoxide can cause thermal damage and chemical irritation from the products of combustion; these products may cause direct mucosal edema and tissue sloughing, impaired mucociliary clearance, formation of endobronchial casts, inactivation of surfactant, and interstitial edema [14]. Unless superheated gases or particulate matter are involved, only the upper airways are affected by this direct injury. Laryngospasm, bronchospasm, tracheobronchitis and pneumonia, ventilation-perfusion mismatch, and decreased respiratory compliance may develop. Patients with circumferential chest burns often have a restrictive respiratory physiology and decreased total respiratory compliance. Systemic inflammatory response-induced capillary leak may be exacerbated by large volume fluid resuscitation and cause a condition similar to adult respiratory distress syndrome (ARDS). Carbon monoxide (CO) inhalation is more common when fires occur in enclosed spaces. CO inhalation is dangerous because CO binds to hemoglobin with affinity that is >200 times that for oxygen. CO levels that exceed 10–20% are associated with inadequate tissue oxygen delivery. Fires involving nitrogen-containing plastics can cause cyanide toxicity.

A major burn injury is often associated with profound endocrine and metabolic changes that may persist for 9–12 months after the injury and are characterized by release of catecholamines, antidiuretic hormone, renin, angiotensin, aldosterone, cortisol, and glucagon. Basal energy expenditure is increased, core temperature is elevated (38–38.5°C is often the new "normal" temperature), lipolysis, muscle catabolism and glycolysis occur, and insulin resistance develops. The degree of hypermetabolism is proportional to the size of the burn injury. In addition, thyroid (T3 and T4) and parathyroid hormone levels decrease; the latter can depress vitamin D levels.

Renal function may be adversely affected by burn shock and exacerbated by inadequate fluid resuscitation, elevated concentrations of catecholamines resulting in decreased renal blood flow, decreased glomerular filtration rate (GFR), and decreased urine production. Patients with burn-induced electrical injuries, or those with crush injuries, may have extensive muscle damage and myoglobin-induced renal dysfunction or failure. GFR is normal or supernormal during the hypermetabolic phase. Late renal dysfunction or failure can occur from systemic sepsis or from the acute or cumulative effects of nephrotoxic drugs, such as aminoglycoside antibiotics.

Both hypoperfusion and the circulating inflammatory mediators affect the gastrointestinal system early in major burns. Consequently, intestinal ischemia and increased permeability to bacteria and endotoxins may be present. If so, the patient often develops sepsis, ileus, and stress ulceration. A massive capillary leak may lead to ascites and abdominal compartment syndrome. Hepatic dysfunction can occur from liver hypoperfusion, ischemia reperfusion, and circulating inflammatory mediators. Liver injury is diagnosed by the presence of elevated liver enzymes and bilirubin concentrations and by decreased functional liver protein production as evidenced by an elevated prothrombin time. Early enteral feeding with adequate calories is required to meet the needs of the hypermetabolic state and for the rapid growth of young children. Failure to provide these calories affects wound healing.

The hematological system is affected in the acute phase of a major burn. Hemoconcentration from loss of circulating plasma volume is often the first manifestation. Patients are often anemic after the initial resuscitation and treatment phase due to chronic illness and to suppression of erythrocyte production, blood loss associated with frequent debridements, and hemolysis of heat-damaged red blood cells (RBC). The half-life of heat-damaged RBCs is decreased from approximately 21 to 7 days; an ongoing autoimmune hemolytic anemia may also be present. Due to sequestration, the platelet count often decreases to thrombocytopenic levels in the first week following a burn injury. Thereafter, it returns to normal or supernormal levels; in the late phase of the burn injury, thrombocytopenia may be an early indicator of sepsis. Prothrombin (PT) and partial thromboplastin (PTT) times may initially be elevated by liver dysfunction and early derangement of the extrinsic coagulation system, but they return to normal during the ensuing weeks. Fibrin split products are initially elevated, and fibrinogen is decreased for the first several days after a burn, but both return to normal after the initial period; fibrinogen and factor V and VIII levels are then elevated above normal. A hypercoagulable state is often present during the later phases of burn injury. The white blood cell (WBC) count is typically elevated in burn patients, although applying wound dressings that contain silver sulfadiazine may cause leukopenia.

The central nervous system (CNS) of burned patients can be affected by several mechanisms, including hypoxia caused by respiratory injury or CO poisoning. Hypoxia can cause severe CNS injury if it leads to cerebral edema, increased intracranial pressure, coma, and seizures. Burn encephalopathy, which occurs in 14% of burn patients, includes hallucinations, delirium, personality change, seizures, and coma. Hypertensive encephalopathy with seizures occurs in about 7% of hypertensive pediatric burn patients. Electrical burns can directly injure the spinal cord or brain, depending on the entry and exit sites of the current.

Loss of skin, infected burn wounds, tracheal or tracheostomy tubes, and increased gut permeability to bacteria and endotoxins are sources of infection for burned patients. In addition, indwelling foreign devices (central, bladder, and intravenous catheters) are portals for entry of infective organisms. Burn injury depresses immune function, which increases the likelihood of infections. The temperatures and WBC counts of burned patients are persistently elevated and are not reliable indicators of infection in these patients. Feeding intolerance and decreasing platelet count often herald the onset of an infection. Culturing wounds, blood, and the respiratory and urinary tracts and comparing the culture results to earlier cultures is a common means of detecting early infection. Table 35.3 summarizes the changes in organ systems with major burn injury.

Initial evaluation and resuscitation of the burn-injured child

Airway and pulmonary management

Anesthesiologists are frequently involved in the initial resuscitation and management of children with major burn injuries in the emergency department or trauma and burn center. Focus on the airway, breathing, and circulation is the first priority. Respiratory or cardiac arrest mandates immediate tracheal intubation. A history of major burn, smoke inhalation, facial burns, stridor, soot in the nares or pharynx, respiratory distress (wheezing, dyspnea, cough, tachypnea, rales, rhonchi), low SpO_2 indicates a high likelihood of respiratory involvement. Strong consideration should be given to early tracheal intubation, even if gas exchange appears to be adequate on initial presentation, because ensuing swelling of the pharynx, tongue, epiglottis, larynx, and trachea often makes conventional tracheal intubation much more difficult or impossible later on. Oral intubation with a cuffed endotracheal tube (ETT) is recommended. A cuffed tube permits ventilation with higher pressures and minimal gas leak if required to treat significant lung injury. Use of a cuffed tube does not result in more subglottic injury than an uncuffed ETT in critically ill children. Also, initial use of a cuffed tube obviates the potential problems associated with changing an uncuffed to a cuffed ETT if the child develops worse respiratory failure [8,26–27] (Figs 35.4, 35.5).

Both the presumed full stomach and the hemodynamic status of the child must be taken into account when choosing an induction regimen for tracheal intubation of acutely burned children. During the initial phases of burn injury, succinylcholine may be used safely. Other neuromuscular blocking agents can also be used, but higher doses of drug may be required. Drugs used for tracheal intubation should have minimal acute hemodynamic effects, especially in the hypovolemic child. Consequently, it may be preferable to avoid using propofol or thiopental, especially in large doses. Ketamine, etomidate, fentanyl, and midazolam are usually excellent choices for securing the airway. In practice, conventional tracheal intubation is not difficult in the very early burn phase because significant airway edema is absent. Hours or days later when significant edema and airway obstruction are present, special intubation techniques, including video laryngoscopy, laryngeal mask airways, fiber-optic bronchoscopy, cricothyrotomy, and the ability to place a surgical airway, will be required. See Chapter 14 for a

Table 35.3 Major organ system pathophysiological changes with major burn injury

Organ system	Early (acute) manifestations first 3–5 days after injury	Late (hypermetabolic) Until major wounds covered, may persist 9–12 months
Cardiovascular	Decreased CO: myocardial dysfunction Hypovolemia Increased SVR	Increased CO Tachycardia Systemic hypertension
Pulmonary	Airway obstruction and edema Carbon monoxide poisoning Laryngospasm and bronchospasm Tracheitis and pneumonia Adult respiratory distress syndrome	Tracheal stenosis Chest wall restriction Infection: pneumonia and tracheitis
Endocrine and metabolic	Increased catecholamines	Increased metabolic rate Increased core temperature (38–38.5°C) Increased protein catabolism Increased lipolysis Increased glucolysis Insulin resistance Decreased thyroid function Decreased parathyroid function
Renal	Decreased GFR Myoglobinuria	Increased GFR Tubular dysfunction from sepsis or nephrotoxins
Gastrointestinal/hepatic	Ischemia from decreased perfusion Stress ulcers, mucosal injury Ileus Endotoxemia Increased liver function tests, decreased prothrombin time	Stress ulcers Ileus
Hematological	Hemoconcentration Hemolysis Thrombocytopenia Elevated PT, PTT, fibrin split products Decreased fibrinogen	Anemia Elevated WBC Hypercoagulable state: elevated factor V, VIII, platelet count, fibrinogen
Central nervous system	Coma Seizures Cerebral edema Increased intracranial pressure	Hallucination Delirium Personality change Seizures Coma
Infection/immunity	Endotoxemia	Chronic immune dysfunction Burn wound infection Respiratory infection Bloodstream infection Urinary tract infection Endotoxemia Antibiotic-associated enterocolitis Infection with antibiotic-resistant organisms

CO, cardiac output; GFR, glomerular filtration rate; PT, prothrombin time; PTT, partial thromboplastin time; SVR, systemic vascular resistance; WBC, white blood cell count.

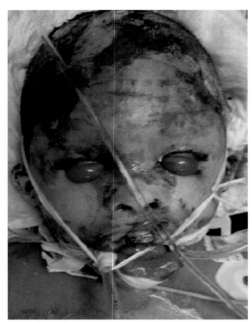

Figure 35.4 Early massive facial burn injury. Note significant facial swelling, but also that this patient's trachea was intubated without problems. Reproduced from Fidkowski et al [8] with permission from Wiley-Blackwell.

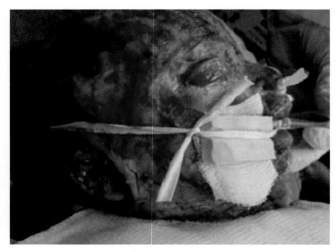

Figure 35.5 Same patient after initial debridement. Reproduced from Fidkowski et al [8] with permission from Wiley-Blackwell.

discussion on managing the difficult airway. Special measures for securing the ETT, such as wiring it to the maxilla or securing it with an umbilical tape and tying the tape behind the head, may be required. Some patients with severe airway or facial burns require tracheostomy.

Suspicion of airway burn or smoke inhalation should prompt rapid assessment and securing of the airway. CO poisoning is a potentially treatable problem that is detected by arterial blood co-oximetry or by some new-generation pulse oximeters (Massimo Rainbow SET, Massimo Corp., Irvine, CA, USA) that measure arterial CO levels [28–31]. One hundred percent oxygen should be administered immediately to patients suspected of having CO poisoning, as this significantly reduces CO's half-life in blood. Patients with CO levels of <20% generally present with milder symptoms, such as light-headedness, nausea, and headache. Their true SaO_2 is >80%. Children with CO levels of 20–40% are confused, disoriented and/or lethargic. Those with CO levels above 40% will have coma, seizures, cardiopulmonary arrest, and death if the CO level is not rapidly reduced. When the FIO_2 is 0.21, the half-life of CO exceeds 4h; when the FIO_2 is 1.0, the half-life is 40–80min. Treatment of severe CO poisoning with hyperbaric oxygen is controversial but may be indicated if this treatment can be initiated quickly. The half-life of CO is only 20min with an FIO_2 of 1.0 and 2.5–3 atmospheres of pressure [8,32]. Bedside fiber-optic or rigid bronchoscopy may further elucidate the extent of the airway injury. These modalities allow bronchoalveolar lavage and suctioning of the airway to clear them of soot, debris or sloughed mucosa. High-resolution computed tomography (CT) scanning may also be useful for assessing the degree of injury [33]. However, care must be taken to assure adequate ventilation and oxygenation during the procedure.

Pulmonary toilet, consisting of suctioning, saline lavage, and inhaled bronchodilators, should be aggressively pursued in an attempt to limit pulmonary compromise. The principles of mechanical ventilation, as they apply to respiratory failure in general, should be used – see Chapter 37 for an extensive discussion of ventilatory management [34]. Although decreased surfactant production occurs with significant airway injury, surfactant replacement has not been reported to improve the lung function of these patients.

Fluid resuscitation

Following recognition that large quantities of saline-containing fluids are required for resuscitation, major improvements in the outcomes of burn-resuscitated patients occurred [35]. After a major burn, there is a rapid reduction of plasma volume, increased microvascular permeability, impaired cell membrane function, cell swelling, and increased tissue osmotic pressure, all of which cause interstitial fluid accumulation [36,37]. Non-burned tissues also become edematous due to endothelial injury and hypoproteinemia. Loss of plasma volume is greatest during the first 4–6h post injury and decreases substantially by 18–24 h if adequate tissue perfusion is maintained. Protein loss is greatest during the first 8 post-burn hours. Smaller amounts of protein continue to be lost until the wounds are completely grafted. Adequate initial volume resuscitation is critical for survival of the patient and to prevent conversion of viable ischemic deep thermal burns to non-viable eschar [38].

Controversy still exists as to the appropriate quantity and composition of fluids required in pediatric patients. In children, adult fluid resuscitation formulae do not work well. Overzealous attempts at restoring blood volume may cause excessive burn edema and serious morbidity. Massive burn wound edema may increase the ischemic insult by impairing cell oxygen availability. The goal of fluid resuscitation is to restore and maintain perfusion and tissue oxygen delivery at optimal levels to protect the zone of ischemia in burned tissue [38]. Restoration of plasma volume should be accomplished without overloading the circulation, preferably over a 24-h period. Formulas for fluid replacement, such as the Parkland formula or the modified Brooke formula, use single calculations based on burn size (e.g. 4 mL/kg/% TBSA burn) that tend to underhydrate pediatric patients. Better estimates of fluid requirements for children are made by calculating burn-related and maintenance requirements separately.

The Parkland formula can be used for the first 24 h by giving lactated Ringer's solution in amounts equal to maintenance requirements PLUS burn requirements of 4 mL/kg/% TBSA burn [39]. When using the Brooke formula, it has been recommended to administer mainte-nance fluids plus an additional 2–3 mL/kg/% TBSA burn for children less than 20 kg [16]. The Galveston formula is the only one developed specifically for chil-dren, which uses BSA for both burn and maintenance fluid calculations [40,41]. The rationale for this approach is that burn-related fluid losses are proportional to burn edema and evaporative fluid losses, both of which are proportional to the surface area burned. This approach avoids underhydration of small children and overhydra-tion of larger children [42]. With the Galveston formula, total fluid requirements for the first day are estimated at 5000 mL/m^2 of burned tissue (burn-related losses) plus 2000 mL/m^2 total BSA (maintenance fluids). Half of the 24-h fluid allowance is administered during the first 8 h and the other half is given during the subsequent 16 h. An isotonic glucose-containing solution with added albumin is used for the first 24 h. This solution consists of 50 mL of 25% human serum albumin added to 950 mL of 5% dextrose in lactated Ringer's solution. For infants less than 1 year of age, the concentration of sodium is lowered and no potassium is added during the first 12–24 h after the burn, or before normal renal function has been demonstrated.

Addition of colloid to the initial hydrating solutions is controversial because of concerns that doing so during the first 24 h after a burn may increase protein accumula-tion in the interstitium and accentuate and prolong edema. The transient systemic endothelial injury and cap-illary leakage after major burns are mediated by proin-flammatory cytokines, complement, arachidonic acid metabolites, and oxygen free radicals [43]. Thus, edema occurring in non-burned tissues does not appear to be the result of altered protein permeability but rather the severe hypoproteinemic state of burned patients [44]. After the first several days, fluid losses are primarily due to burn exudates and evaporation from denuded areas. Maximal weight gain and edema occur 2–3 days after the burn. Thereafter a dieresis ensues, and the patients returns to their preburn weight after approximately 14 days [45]. Since the fluid requirements decrease 24 h after a burn, the Galveston program advocates reducing the fluid requirements to 3750 mL/m^2/TBSA burned plus 1500 mL/m^2/TBSA per day for maintenance fluids. Table 35.4 summarizes the recommendations for fluid resuscitation.

The response of each patient to the burn injury is unique and so is the amount of fluid required to maintain tissue oxygen delivery. Common clinical methods such as vital signs, examination of the extremities for pulses and perfusion, palpation of the liver edge to judge central venous pressure, and urine output are not reliable in the early phase of burn injury, because the area being evaluated is in burned tissue or is obscured or, as in the case of urine output, is greatly affected by hormonal response to the burn. Arterial blood gases and serum lactate concentration should be measured often; an increasing negative base deficit or high serum lactate concentration is suggestive of hypovolemia. Pulmonary artery catheters, which are helpful for determining thermodilution cardiac output and for measuring mixed venous oxygen saturation, have been used during acute burn resuscitation but are technically difficult to place and may distract from the most important task, which is providing adequate fluid resuscitation. Continuous measurement of central venous oxygen saturation ($ScvO_2$) may be useful during resuscitation of these patients, espe-cially since many of them will require central venous access [46,47].

Early burn wound excision and grafting

Early excision and grafting of burn wounds improve sur-vival of children and shorten their length of hospital stay [48–50]. Consequently, this should be done as soon as the patient's condition is deemed stable. For the first several weeks after a serious burn, it is often difficult to deter-mine when the patient's condition is appropriate to undergo surgery. Massive fluid shifts, critical airways,

Table 35.4 Parkland, Brooke, modified Brooke, and Galveston formulas with pediatric supplementation

	First 24 h	Second 24 h	Pediatric supplementation for children less than 20 kg
Parkland	4 mL LR × TBSA × wt (kg)	Colloid at 20–60% plasma volume	LR at calculated maintenance
Brooke	1.5 mL LR + 0.5 mL colloid × TBSA × wt (kg)	0.5 mL LR + 0.25 mL colloid × TBSA × wt (kg)	LR at calculated maintenance
Modified Brooke	2 mL LR × TBSA × wt (kg)	0.3–0.5 mL colloid × TBSA × wt (kg)	LR at 2–3 mL × TBSA × wt (kg) + LR at calculated maintenance
Galveston	5000 mL/m² burned (burn-related losses) PLUS 2000 mL/m² TBSA (maintenance fluids) 50 mL of 25% human serum albumin, mixed with 950 mL of 5% dextrose in D5LR (50% of total in first 8 h, remainder in last 16 h)	3750 mL/m²/TBSA burned (burn-related losses) PLUS 1500 mL/m²/TBSA (maintenance fluids)	NA

and concomitant pulmonary injury, as well as other traumatic injuries, must be carefully considered when making the decision. Mixed distributions of burn depth and the indeterminate depth of many burn injuries add to the challenge. Most authorities agree that burn wounds should be excised and covered to reduce the risk of scarring or infection and if it is estimated that the wounds will not heal within 14 days of the injury.

Two types of excisions are possible: tangential and fascial. With tangential excision, the eschar is sequentially shaved in thin slices until a bleeding, viable matrix is reached so a graft can be placed. Tangential excision is associated with significant blood loss and is generally limited to 15% TBSA or less in very young children. Excision to the muscle fascial plane is faster and is associated with significantly less blood loss; however, because fat and lymphatics are removed, the cosmetic results are less favorable. Consequently, fascial excision is usually reserved for patients with burn wound sepsis and for those in whom it is desirable to limit operating time and blood loss (i.e. when the area to be excised is very large, the patient's condition is unstable, or he/she is otherwise at risk for operative complications) [51,52]. For large burns, total fascial excision can be done early or serial tangential excisions can be done every 3–7 days.

The wound is closed with autogenous skin grafts whenever possible. For large burn wounds, where insufficient autologous skin is available to cover the wound, allografts or xenografts can be used to temporarily cover the wounds; these grafts are immunologically rejected within several weeks and are unsuitable for long-term burn coverage. A number of tissue-engineered or cultured epithelial cell products are available. The method used for skin coverage following tissue excision is highly institution dependent [48] (Figs 35.6, 35.7).

Burn wound dressing changes

Dressing of burn wounds and changing the dressings to assess the wound or to perform further debridement is a daily process in many burned patients. Many dressing materials and regimens are available to promote healing and to prevent infection; the exact protocols used are institution dependent. However, the regularity with which these dressings are changed and the predictable pain and psychological distress this causes pediatric patients are a challenge for the patient and the pediatric anesthesiologist. An interesting recent development has been the application of wound vacuum technology to help close burn wounds. Negative pressure is induced over the wound, which promotes movement of blood, lymph, and interstitial fluid and reduces peripheral edema and bacterial load. Movement of these fluids increases granulation tissue formation and causes epidermal migration [53]. Other dressings and substances that are designed to reduce the frequency of dressing changes, pain, and psychological distress, while producing the same beneficial wound results in children, have recently become available.

Long-term burn wound reconstruction

Patients with significant burns anywhere or burns in critical areas, such as the face, neck, hands, feet, or perineum, will of necessity return many times for reconstructive surgery to improve functionality or cosmesis, once the original burn wound has been treated and healed. These patients often require dozens of anesthetics in a relatively

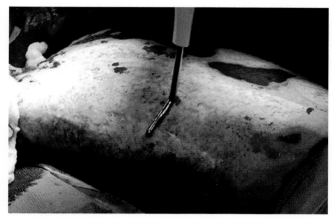

Figure 35.6 Debridement of the burn in Figure 35.3 with hydrosurgery. Reproduced from Fabia and Groner [48] with permission from Elsevier.

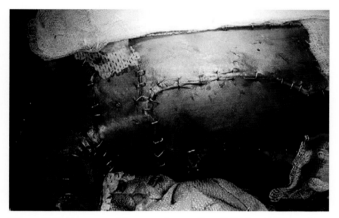

Figure 35.7 Coverage of the same burn with split-thickness skin graft. Reproduced from Fabia and Groner [48] with permission from Elsevier.

short period of time. Careful evaluation and anesthetic planning and discussion with the surgeon, particularly when the airway is involved, are essential for these patients.

Preoperative evaluation of the burn patient

Thorough preoperative evaluation of burn patients is essential when preparing for their anesthetic care. These cases can range from a first-time surgical encounter in a severely burned patient to a patient who is undergoing long-term burn reconstruction and has been anesthetized dozens of times. For the acutely burned patient, attention to the airway and its stability is paramount. If difficult tracheal intubation or reintubation is anticipated, appropriate equipment and surgical back-up must be available. Attention to both the pulmonary and cardiovascular

status and oxygen delivery is equally important. Chest radiographs, CT scans, ventilator settings, and blood gases and pH should be reviewed so the extent of the pulmonary injury can be determined. Vascular access is assessed, including the need to insert additional catheters. The most recent laboratory studies, including hematological, coagulation, electrolytes, renal function, hepatic function, and arterial blood gases, should be reviewed. A thorough physical examination is important for understanding the degree of edema, the unburned areas available for monitoring and catheter placement, and the need for ongoing medications and opioids. Review of the past medical, surgical, and anesthetic history is important, as is determining the presence of drug or latex allergies.

A discussion with the burn surgeon is vital to understand the goals of the surgery, the anticipated blood loss, the sites that will be used to obtain skin grafts, and the plan for positioning of the patient. It is important to understand the patient's current nutritional status and method of feeding, i.e. enteral or parenteral (or both), and to minimize interruptions in feeding by timing nil per os (NPO) orders appropriately. Finally, a discussion with the parent and patient (when appropriate) is necessary for understanding past anesthetic issues, for informing them of the anesthetic procedures, for treatment of postoperative pain, and for answering their questions.

Because many of these patients have had multiple anesthetics for dressing changes, tissue excision, and grafting, it is important to involve a child-life or behavioral specialist in the preoperative preparation of these patients. It is good practice to listen to the child and parent and to understand their preferences for issues such as premedication and the induction of anesthesia.

Intraoperative management of the burn patient

Anxious patients should be given liberal amounts of premedication before transfer from the burn unit or holding area, if possible. Intravenous or oral agents, such as midazolam or ketamine, are effective by either route [54]. Intranasal dexmedetomidine $2\,\mu g/kg$ is effective when given 30–45 min before the procedure. In one study intranasal dexmedetomidine was as efficacious as oral midazolam, 0.5 mg/kg. Both agents produced acceptable separation from parents, induction and emergence conditions, and postoperative pain scores [55]. Parental presence for induction of anesthesia certainly is advocated where available and appropriate. If the patient is receiving continuous infusions of sedatives and/or analgesics, they should be continued during transport of critically ill patients. Careful monitoring of patients receiving these drug infusions is necessary during transport. Strict aseptic technique should be maintained in all aspects of care.

Burned patients may have few areas of non-burned skin for placement of ECG leads, pulse oximeters, and blood pressure cuffs. The anesthesiologist may have to be creative when finding acceptable monitoring sites [14]. Certainly before placing any monitor or catheter in a non-burned area, it is important to ask the surgeon if it is a site he/she plans to use to obtain skin for grafting. For major burn excision and grafting procedures, or for very unstable patients, invasive arterial and central venous monitoring are preferable because they allow beat-to-beat monitoring of blood pressure, blood sampling, measurement of central venous pressure, and reliable vascular access for administration of large amounts of fluids and blood or vasoactive drugs. The femoral area is often unburned and available for central venous or arterial access; however, these areas are often the only ones available for harvesting skin for grafting. Urine output should be measured during major procedures as another means of determining intravascular volume. Given the propensity for hypothermia from large exposed burn surfaces and large fluid volume administration, temperature must also be measured continuously.

The greatest challenges during major excision and grafting procedures are heat conservation and blood loss. Ongoing communication between the surgeon and the anesthesiologist about these issues is essential. Exposure of denuded tissue rapidly leads to hypothermia if no measures are taken to prevent it. Thermoregulation is blocked by general anesthetics and by denervation of burned areas. The slight increase in heat production during the operative period is more than counterbalanced by increased heat loss. Burn patients have a higher than normal core temperature (38–39°C) and are most comfortable in an ambient temperature of 30–31°C [56]. The operating room should be as warm as can be tolerated by surgeons and other personnel and should be draft free. Servo-controlled radiant warmers can be placed above the patient. A warming blanket, forced-air warmer, or a plastic or cloth cover should be placed around non-operative sites. All fluids that come into contact with the patient, including IV and irrigation fluids and blood products, should be warmed. The inspired gases should be warmed and humidified, or at the very least a condenser humidifier should be used. Operative time should be minimized by a well co-ordinated team effort. For example, one surgical team can excise eschar while another harvests grafts. This allows wounds to be covered as expeditiously as possible and limits most procedures to approximately 1.5h of operating time.

Blood loss is rapid and massive for all but the most limited excisions. It is commonly estimated that 3.5–5% of the blood volume is lost for every 1% of the body surface excised [15]. Excising the scalp is a particularly bloody procedure. For small children, blood replacement with warmed, fresh whole blood should be started as soon as the blood loss begins. Unfortunately, whole blood is increasingly difficult to obtain because of blood bank regulations. Because blood loss is difficult to estimate, arterial and central venous pressure should be measured to help assess intravascular volume. Several measures can be taken to reduce bleeding, including applying dilute epinephrine (1:10,000) soaked sponges, spray-on thrombin, or collagen pads to the wound. Tourniquets can be used in some circumstances. The volume of tissue excised should not exceed 10–15% of TBSA at one procedure.

The complications and consequences of massive transfusion must be anticipated, especially acute citrate intoxication and hyperkalemia. Burned patients are chronically hypocalcemic. Consequently, they commonly develop hypotension with rapid infusion of citrate-containing blood products because the excess citrate reduces the concentration of ionized calcium. Simultaneous administration of $CaCl_2$ 5–10mg/kg through a central venous catheter reliably blunts this response [57]. Hyperkalemia can occur with rapid transfusion of multiple units of packed RBCs, especially in small children. Thus, frequent measurement of serum potassium concentrations is desirable. Fresh or washed RBCs or measuring the potassium level in each unit before infusion and not infusing units that have K^+ levels >8mMol/L effectively prevent hyperkalemia. Treatment of hyperkalemia with dextrose, calcium, and insulin, and with alkalization with sodium bicarbonate and hyperventilation plus stopping the surgery may be necessary in extreme cases. Massive transfusion affects coagulation parameters, especially the platelet count. Clotting factors, in the form of fresh frozen plasma, platelets or cryoprecipitate, may also be required. All blood products should be warmed with a properly designed fluid warmer; the ability to rapidly infuse blood products should be available. See Chapter 11 for a more extensive discussion of intraoperative bleeding and administration of blood products. Because bleeding and hypothermia are inter-related, it may be best to abbreviate the procedure if the anesthesiologist is unable to adequately compensate for massive hematological changes. It is preferable to return another day, once resuscitation is complete, rather than risk causing the patient harm.

Because of the hypermetabolic state, there is a need for increased alveolar ventilation. The patient's trachea is usually intubated and ventilation is controlled for all but very short and limited procedures. If the patient has a pulmonary injury and ARDS, a modern anesthesia ventilator is required to deliver adequate inspiratory flows, peak pressures, tidal volumes, and positive end-expiratory pressure. If one is not available, the patient's ICU ventilator should be used [58].

Maintenance fluid requirements are higher than normal in burned patients and these volumes plus additional fluid for intraoperative losses should be administered during the operative period. Surgeons often infiltrate copious amounts of normal saline subcutaneously to facilitate harvesting skin for grafting. This amount of fluid must be compensated for by decreased IV fluid administration. If the patient is receiving parenteral alimentation that contains high concentrations of glucose, similar amounts of glucose (mg/kg/min) should be delivered in the operating room to prevent hypoglycemia. Serum glucose concentrations should be monitored frequently during surgery to detect hyperglycemia and prevent hyperosmolar dehydration.

Pharmacokinetics of drugs in burned patients

Major burn injuries induce many physiological changes that produce profound alterations in the pharmacokinetics of many drugs [59–61]. In the acute phase, cardiac output and tissue blood flow are diminished. This delays clearance and metabolism of many drugs. Later, during the hypermetabolic phase, the reverse is true. Neural and hormonal mechanisms and other circulating mediators also affect drug deposition and action. The principle of titrating drugs and anesthetics to the patient's needs is never more appropriate than in patients with major burns.

Perhaps the most profound pharmacological changes involve muscle relaxants. Burned patients are supersensitive to succinylcholine after the acute burn phase and insensitive to non-depolarizing muscle relaxants [62]. The use of succinlycholine after the resuscitative phase is contraindicated because it may cause lethal hyperkalemia. The hyperkalemia is related to both the dose and time elapsed from the initial burn injury. The exact time of onset is unknown. The response may last as long as 2 years. Consequently, it has been recommended that the use of succinlycholine be avoided for at least several months after complete wound healing has occurred. Succinlycholine is seldom used today except for airway emergencies. Resistance to non-depolarizing muscle relaxants develops about 1 week after injury and is also related to the magnitude of the burn [63]. If the burn exceeds 20% of the BSA, the dose required to produce an appropriate block is often 2–5-fold greater than normal. This phenomenon also occurs in children, and although the exact duration of this effect is unknown, resistance to non-depolarizing muscle relaxants was documented in a child more than 1 year after complete healing of his burn wounds [64].

The mechanism for these alterations is believed to be a denervation-like phenomenon in which the number of acetycholine receptors is increased and the receptors are located at extrajunctional sites in the muscle membrane. This results in a greatly increased number of binding sites, which increases the dose requirement [62]. Drugs that antagonize muscle relaxants should be used in normal doses.

Cardiovascular responses to adrenergic agents are greatly diminished during the hypermetabolic phase. Topical application of epinephrine during wound excision is well tolerated and causes minimal cardiovascular changes and infrequent arrhythmias [60]. After burn injury, myocardial β-adrenergic receptors have a decreased affinity for ligands, impaired receptor-mediated signal transduction, and decreased adenolate cyclase activity, which results in decreased cAMP production [65,66]. Responses to administered cathecholamines, such as epinephrine and dopamine, are also diminished.

Ketamine and inhaled anesthetic agents have been extensively used in burned patients. Repeated administration of these agents has proven to be safe. Total IV anesthesia with propofol and alfentanil has also been reported [67]. Dose requirements for thiopental are increased to 7–8 mg/kg in burned children for at least 1 year after the initial injury [68].

Opioids are the most commonly administered form of analgesia, but the dose requirements for these drugs are high in burned patients [69]. In acutely burned children, the volume of distribution and the elimination half-life of morphine are markedly reduced, and clearance is increased [69]. Many of these children have received long-term infusions or doses of opioids, benzodiazepines or ketamine and have increased requirements for these agents [70]. A recent report indicated that pediatric burn patients who were inadequately sedated with conventional agents were adequately sedated for 11 days with infusions of 0.5 μg/kg/h of dexmedetomidine. Tachyphylaxis or respiratory depression did not occur [71].

Pain in the burn patient

Pain associated with burns is severe, increases with size and depth of the burn, and persists at least until the wounds are well healed [72]. Experimentally induced cutaneous burn injury produced local inflammatory changes that manifest as redness, lowered pain thresholds (allodynia), and enhanced pain response to noxious stimuli (hyperalgesia) [73,74]. Hyperalgesia may be caused by changes in C-polymodal nociceptors that develop a decreased discharge threshold and increased rate of firing [75]. Intense C-fiber stimulation also induces a state of central hypersensitivity in spinal cord dorsal horn neurons [76].

Burn-associated pain can be clinically differentiated into background (constant) and procedural (dressing changes and wound debridement) pain. Successful management of background pain has been reported with acetaminophen and with oral or IV morphine administered every 4h by the clock [72]. Patient-controlled analgesia with morphine is ideal for patients who are able to participate. Opioid tolerance and escalating opioid requirements often develop [77]. See Chapter 33 for a comprehensive discussion of the management of chronic pain and opioid tolerance.

Wound debridement and frequent dressing changes are required for proper wound healing. The procedural pain associated with these activities is often excruciating. Ketamine, opioids, and benzodiazepines are commonly used for sedation and analgesia for these procedures. Light-to-moderate sedation, deep sedation, and general anesthesia may be required. Ketamine is commonly used because it provides intense analgesia with minimal respiratory depression when given IV or orally. A long-acting opioid, such as morphine, may provide adequate analgesia during a dressing change but may cause excessive sedation after the painful stimulus is gone and the patient has returned to the ward. A combination of ketamine and an opioid provides intense analgesia for the surgical event while reducing the opioid dose and its side-effects. Due to its potency and short half-life, fentanyl is a useful drug for burn patients. During the convalescent phase, oral transmucosal fentanyl (10 µg/kg) has been used successfully to manage the pain associated with care of smaller burns [72]. Oral or IV midazolam or lorazepam are important adjuncts for allaying anxiety and producing at least partial amnesia for these events.

Outcome of major burn injury in children

Over the past several decades more pediatric patients with burns have survived due to remarkable advances in early resuscitative care, later intensive care, and burn wound treatment. Consequently, younger and younger severely burned patients are surviving, including those with burns of greater than 80% of their TBSA. As a result, skin and lung injury may have less influence on survival.

During a 10-year review of 3005 admissions to a specialized pediatric burn unit from 1992 to 2001, there were 72 deaths, 71 of which had a complete autopsy [23]. The characteristics of survivors and non-survivors were compared, and important differences were noted. The overall mortality rate was 2.4%. Those who died had a mean burn TBSA of 66%, versus 26% for those who survived (60% versus 14% for third-degree burns). Also, 60% of patients who died and only 16% of survivors had inhalational burns. The ages and weights of the survivors and non-survivors were similar. Diffuse alveolar lung damage was the primary cause of death in 25% of patients. Hypovolemia/inadequate resuscitation was the primary cause of death in 16% of patients. Loss of airway/pulmonary aspiration was primary in 15%. Pneumonia and burn wound sepsis each caused 13% of the deaths, and cerebral anoxia caused 10%. The reviewers felt that approximately one-third of all deaths could have been prevented had some deficiency of care not occurred.

The long-term physical, psychological, and quality of life problems of young adults who had burns involving 30% or more of their body were recently determined [24,78]. Eighty to 90% of them had scores within normal limits for most of the domains of physical strength, dexterity, mobility, and activities of daily living. However, more than 50% qualified for a psychiatric diagnosis, especially anxiety disorder. These people rated their quality of life as significantly lower than that of the reference group. The domains of material well-being, physical well-being, and extramarital relationships were particularly affected. The psychological and physical effects of a major burn cannot be overstated.

Trauma

Trauma is a major cause of hospitalization in pediatric patients, and the leading cause of death in children over the age of 1 year [79]. In the year 2000 approximately $20 billion dollars were spent treating trauma that occurred in 0–19-year-old pediatric patients . The leading cause of injury-induced death in patients under the age of 1 year is unintentional suffocation due to choking or strangulation; motor vehicle accidents are the leading cause of death for children 1–19 years old. In the 1–11 year age group, drowning is the second leading cause of death; in the 12–19 year olds, homicide is the second leading cause of death, with the majority of deaths involving use of firearms. The statistics for non-fatal injuries parallel these causes.

This section will review anesthesia care for major trauma in children.

Organization of trauma services

In the US, the American College of Surgeons (ACS) designates trauma centers as levels I–III. Pediatric trauma centers are either level I or level II [80]. These designations are determined by ACS site visits and also by state or local governing bodies. Pediatric trauma care may take place in a specialized pediatric hospital or in a larger general hospital with an organized trauma service with pediatric specialists as part of the team. For a level I trauma center designation, a qualified trauma surgeon and anesthesiologist, as well as immediate operating room (OR) availability, must be present in the hospital 24h a day. To be designated a level I trauma center, at least 200 pediatric trauma patients less than 15 years of age must be admitted annually. For a pediatric level II designation, these services must be "promptly available" on a 24-h basis, with at least 100 pediatric patients admitted annually. Other requirements include rapid availability of neurosurgery services, radiology, and blood bank support, as well as a defined program manager, database, and quality and outcomes program.

The exact role of the anesthesiologist varies by institution, but in general he/she is responsible for assessing and managing the airway and for assisting with the resuscitation of severe trauma patients, as well as providing sedation, analgesia, and anesthesia for diagnostic and therapeutic procedures during trauma evaluation and initial therapy. An anesthesia trauma tackle box that contains the necessary drugs and equipment for airway management, including laryngoscopes and blades, oral airways, and a wide range of endotracheal tubes and emergency airway management devices, such as laryngeal mask airways and cricothyrotomy kits, should be readily available and restocked immediately after each use. The anesthesiologist may not be called for all trauma evaluations and initial resuscitations. Most institutions have two or more designations for level of trauma activation that are based on a triage system that takes into account the mechanism of injury and the likelihood of requiring airway intervention. Lower level trauma activation may involve emergency physicians or surgeons only.

Initial trauma evaluation

Evaluation of major trauma begins with obtaining a history from the emergency first responders that includes mechanism of injury (motor vehicle accident, fall, drowning), time from injury to treatment, extent of injury, vital signs, and interventions, including vascular access, IV fluids administered, bag and mask ventilation or insertion of a laryngeal or pharyngeal airway or a tracheal tube. Neurological status is assessed and communicated. Time from injury to arrival at the hospital is conveyed, and the trauma system is activated at the level specified by the local institutional policy. Maximal activation usually includes the emergency physician, trauma surgeons, nurses, respiratory therapists, anesthesiologist, and possibly other specialists, such as intensive care medicine specialists. It is important for one physician, usually the trauma surgeon, to lead the evaluation and resuscitation.

Initial evaluation begins with the primary survey of airway, breathing, and circulatory status [81]. Cardiopulmonary resuscitation (CPR) is started or continued in the worst case scenario, with the recognition that the cause of the arrest may be massive hemorrhage from trauma. Chapter 12 presents the principles of CPR in children. The patient's color, respiratory effort and distress, oxygen saturation, pulses, and arterial blood pressure are quickly evaluated, as is the status of vascular access and evidence of ongoing hemorrhage. The neurological system is quickly evaluated using the Glasgow Coma Scale that has been modified for Pediatrics (Box 35.2). After the primary survey and initiation of treatment, the secondary survey is done, which includes a head-to-toe examination that includes the face, head, and neck, focusing on cervical spine injury. Careful removal of a cervical collar is necessary for complete CNS assessment, as is removal of clothing for examination of chest, abdomen, back and spine, extremities, perineum, and rectum. Initial laboratory examination, including complete blood count, arterial or venous blood gases and pH (if indicated), serum electrolytes, blood urea nitrogen, creatinine, glucose, and blood for type and crossmatch, is conducted. Additional vascular access is provided, the bladder is catheterized, and radiographs, including chest, abdomen and extremities, are ordered if indicated. Bedside ultrasound (see below) is a valuable diagnostic tool for initial trauma evaluation. CT scanning is ordered as indicated.

Airway management in the trauma patient

The anesthesiologist is often the one called upon to evaluate and manage the airway and overall patient status to determine if the trauma patient needs emergency tracheal intubation. Indications for tracheal intubation include significant respiratory distress from airway or thoracic trauma, including rib fractures, pneumothorax, and flail chest. Retractions, grunting, hypoxemia, and unequal breath sounds all indicate that emergency tracheal intubation is required. In addition, tracheal intubation and mechanical ventilation may be required to provide adequate gas exchange and adequate oxygen delivery to the brain of patients with CNS trauma or an altered mental status (Glasgow Coma Score (GCS) ≤8), which may indicate significant brain injury. The laryngeal reflexes of these patients are often absent and they cannot protect their airway from aspiration of gastric contents. CT scanning and transport to the scanner are thought to be safer when the airway is controlled. Significant cardiovascular instability from traumatic hemorrhage is often an indication for controlled ventilation. For lesser levels of respiratory distress and depressed consciousness or cardiovascular compromise, it may be sufficient to provide high-flow 100% oxygen by facemask and continuously monitor the SaO_2 and respiratory status. Because modern CT scanning is so rapid, additional sedation that might mandate tracheal intubation may not be required.

Box 35.2 Glasgow Coma Scale modified for pediatric patients

	Response	Score
Eye opening	Spontaneous	4
	To speech	3
	To pain	2
	None	1
Verbal	Coos, babbles	5
	Irritable	4
	Cries to pain	3
	Moans to pain	2
	None	1
Motor	Normal spontaneous movements	6
	Withdraws to touch	5
	Withdraws to pain	4
	Abnormal flexion (decorticate)	3
	Abnormal extension (decerebrate)	2
	Flaccid	1

The condition of patients requiring tracheal intubation ranges from full cardiac or respiratory arrest, in which case no additional sedation or muscle relaxation is needed, to combative patients with vigorous cardiac function who require significant doses of induction agents, analgesics, and muscle relaxants. In the absence of suspected CNS trauma, the cardiovascular status and possible intravascular volume deficit are of paramount importance. Patients with hypovolemia are usually given a bolus of isotonic fluid, such as lactated Ringer's solution or Plasmalyte® 10–20 mL/kg, rapidly while the anesthesiologist is preparing for tracheal intubation. The airway is evaluated for potentially difficult facemask ventilation or tracheal intubation; if difficulty is anticipated, back-up methods, such as a video laryngoscope and surgical airway, must be available. The complexity, time, and limited view with blood in the airway often makes flexible fiber-optic endoscopic intubation impractical in emergency trauma situations. Preoxygenation and assisted facemask ventilation, if needed, are provided. Large-bore suction should be readily available.

Intravenous induction drugs that preserve myocardial contractility, blood pressure, and intravascular volume are preferable. Hypovolemic trauma patients often tolerate etomidate 0.2–0.4 mg/kg or ketamine 1–2 mg/kg IV better than thiopental or propofol because these drugs may cause venodilation and hypotension. Muscle relaxation is frequently needed, and emergency trauma intubation is an indication for the use of succinylcholine. If the anesthesiologist is reasonably certain that tracheal intuba-

tion will be straightforward, non-depolarizing muscle relaxants that have few cardiovascular effects are given in sufficient doses to facilitate muscle relaxation. Rocuronium 1.2–2 mg/kg or vecuronium 0.2–0.4 mg/kg is often used.

It should be assumed that the patient has a full stomach, and gentle cricoid pressure should be applied (see Chapter 14). If a cervical collar is present, it should be temporarily removed for airway management. In-line stabilization (not traction) of the cervical spine is provided by an assistant. Because it may take 1–2 min for adequate muscle relaxation to occur with non-depolarizing drugs, even when large doses are given, gentle, shallow mask ventilation should be initiated rather than allowing the patient to have a prolonged period of apnea before tracheal intubation. After gentle laryngoscopy and tracheal intubation, careful positive pressure ventilation is commenced while closely monitoring the cardiovascular status, since positive pressure ventilation may compromise venous return and cause hypotension in hypovolemic patients. Use of a styletted, cuffed tracheal tube is preferred to minimize difficulty with intubation and gas leaks. Exhaled CO_2 detection is mandatory following tracheal intubation; if no CO_2 is detected, a quick laryngoscopy will determine if the tracheal tube is in the esophagus. If not, it is possible that cardiac output and pulmonary blood flow are so severely compromised that little CO_2 is being presented to the lungs. During or shortly after giving the induction drugs, additional opioids and/or sedative agents are titrated to produce the desired effect.

Tracheal intubation of patients with suspected or actual CNS trauma deserves special attention. Ketamine is contraindicated in this situation because it increases cerebral blood flow and intracranial pressure (ICP). If CNS trauma is isolated and arterial blood pressure and the intravascular volume status are stable, drugs such as thiopental, propofol or etomidate are preferable because they tend to preserve or decrease ICP, cerebral blood flow, and cerebral metabolic rate for oxygen. Adequate depth of anesthesia helps prevent unwanted increases in ICP. Also, it is important to prevent coughing by providing adequate muscle relaxation before attempting laryngoscopy. Pretreatment with IV lidocaine may also mitigate any increases in ICP.

Airway trauma

Blunt or penetrating trauma to the face and neck should increase suspicion of injury to the pharynx, larynx, trachea, and bronchi. Possible injuries include mucosal edema of the pharynx, glottis, and vocal cords. Laryngeal lacerations, arytenoid cartilage dislocation, cricothyroid disruption, and vocal cord paralysis also occur. Although laryngeal fractures are less common in children than soft tissue injuries, they do occur and may involve any part of the laryngeal skeleton. The degree of injury can range from simple, non-displaced fractures to comminuted fractures with loss of cartilage [82]. Laryngotracheal separation is a particularly serious injury that is more common in younger children because their intercartilaginous membranes are less well developed than those of older children. Trauma of the face or neck that is associated with respiratory distress or subcutaneous emphysema suggests disruption of the aerodigestive system.

Should immediate tracheal intubation be required for airway obstruction or severe distress, it must be determined how successful direct laryngoscopy will be. One should proceed with caution before inducing anesthesia and giving muscle relaxation to avoid the "cannot ventilate-cannot intubate" scenario. Large-bore suction must be available for clearing blood from the airway. Videolaryngoscopy and surgical back-up for cricothyrotomy or emergency tracheostomy must be immediately available. If the patient does not require an emergency airway, CT evaluation or fiber-optic rigid laryngoscopy and bronchoscopy by an otolaryngology or trauma surgeon is indicated. Further surgical management, including repair of the injury via thoracotomy, is done as indicated. It is important for the anesthesiologist to maintain constant vigilance for possible further airway compromise.

Vascular access

Adequate large-bore peripheral IV access with at least two catheters should be provided as quickly as possible in patients with major trauma. Any peripheral vein can be used. However, if possible, access should be sought in non-traumatized extremities. In addition, it is preferable to obtain upper extremity access in major abdominal trauma or lower extremity access in major thoracic, upper extremity, neck or facial trauma. In the absence of accessible peripheral veins, insertion of an intraosseous needle into the flat surface of the upper tibia will allow essentially any fluid, blood product or medication to be infused [81]. Generally, the time and difficulty of placing central venous catheters preclude their use during initial trauma resuscitation. During this time, the focus should be on obtaining peripheral IV access and on the rapid evaluation and early treatment of trauma injury. Similarly, arterial catheters are not generally inserted during the acute resuscitation but are placed later after initial evaluation and stabilization. See Chapter 17 for a discussion of the details of vascular access.

Central nervous system trauma

Brain trauma is the leading cause of death among injured children and is responsible for 80% of all trauma deaths.

Each year, almost 30,000 children <19 years of age suffer permanent disability from traumatic brain injury (TBI). Children <13 years of age have 475,000 hospital visits, 37,000 hospitalizations, and nearly 3000 deaths each year related to TBI. Falls account for approximately 40% of pediatric brain injuries, and motor vehicle accidents (MVAs) account for 11%. Pedestrian injuries account for 17% and falls from bicycles 10%. Infants and toddlers are more prone to falls from either a low height or from windows of one or more stories. School-age children are more likely to have sports-related injuries and MVAs. All ages are subject to the sequelae of non-accidental trauma. The teenage population is increasingly affected by penetrating brain trauma from firearms [81].

Head injuries in children range from minor scalp trauma and simple skull fractures to cerebral contusion with cerebral edema. They also include acute subdural, epidural or intracerebral hemorrhage and penetrating brain trauma.

The basic principles of initial evaluation include pupillary examination and determination of the GCS. Signs of serious brain injury and increased intracranial pressure include full fontanelles (when present) and split cranial sutures, depressed level of consciousness, irritability, and "sun-setting sign" (persistent inferior deviation of pupils). Irritability and seizures may also be seen. In older children, headache, neck pain, photophobia, vomiting, decreased levels of consciousness and seizures are also observed. Signs of impending brainstem herniation include Cushing triad (hypertension, bradycardia, irregular respirations) and unequal pupils. Rapid clinical assessment, airway management, immediate CT scanning, and rapid progression to the operating room are the most important principles in managing significant head injury when there is a space-occupying intracranial hematoma.

Maintenance of cerebral blood flow and oxygen delivery to the brain, especially in watershed areas and areas with an intracranial hematoma or edema, is the major goal of managing significant head trauma. The goal is to minimize necrotic death of neurons and astrocytes and to maximize functional outcome. Cerebral perfusion pressure (CPP) (mean arterial pressure minus intracranial pressure) must be maintained at adequate levels, although the normal CPPs of normal children are not known. Because cerebral autoregulation is altered and because every patient is different, and because we do not know the lower limit of cerebral autoregulation, arterial blood pressure should be maintained in the high-normal range for the patient's age. Recent guidelines recommend a CPP of 40 mmHg in the youngest children and 65 mmHg in teenagers. However, because the ICP of a given patient is not known in the acute setting, it is probably better to maintain a mean arterial pressure (MAP) of 60 in young children and 85 in teenagers. To do this may require fluid boluses and/or vasopressors [83,84]. The former practice of hyperventilation to reduce cerebral blood flow, intracranial volume, and intracranial pressure has been demonstrated to produce cerebral ischemia in watershed areas. The goal is to maintain appropriate oxygenation and sufficient ventilation to produce a $PaCO_2$ of 35–40 mmHg. Only with impending brainstem herniation (unequal or unreactive pupils, decorticate or decerebrate posturing) is hyperventilation indicated, and then only until craniotomy for evacuation of the hematoma can be accomplished.

Other principles of management include providing adequate analgesia, sedation, and muscle relaxation to prevent increases in ICP; often opioids such as fentanyl, benzodiazepines such as midazolam, and nondepolarizing muscle relaxants are used in trauma resuscitation and transport to CT scan and the operating room. Figure 35.8 presents the principles of management of increased ICP in acutely brain-injured patients [85]. These agents are used during the initial craniotomy; isoflurane can be used because it provides a favorable cerebral blood flow : cerebral metabolic rate of O_2 ratio. Other principles of management of acute head trauma include using isotonic IV fluids, and not giving excessive amounts because doing so increases cerebral edema. Avoiding hyperglycemia and hyperthermia is also critically important. In the presence of significant cerebral edema or impending herniation, osmotic agents, such as mannitol or hypertonic (3%) saline, can also be given. Surgical management includes craniotomy for evacuation of epidural, subdural or intracerebral hematomas, placement of ICP monitors or ventricular drains or, in severe cases, decompressive craniectomy. See Chapter 23 for a thorough discussion of these procedures and for a more complete discussion of intracranial pathophysiology (Fig. 35.9).

Spinal cord injury is dramatically different in the pediatric population than in adults. Approximately 1100 pediatric patients sustain spinal cord injury each year in the US, which represents less than 10% of all such injuries. Sixty to 80% of the injuries occur in the cervical spine. Spinal cord injury without radiographic abnormality occurs in 30–40% of pediatric patients with spinal cord injuries. Cervical spine injures are rare in patients under 3 years of age, with only 0.66% of blunt trauma patients suffering such injuries in a recent registry report of over 12,000 patients [86].

Patients under 2 years of age are prone to have cord injuries without evidence of bony injury on plain radiographs [81]. Radiographic evaluation includes plain radiographs in the trauma resuscitation room, CT scanning for more accurate diagnosis of bony and soft tissue injuries, and MRI scanning in the subacute setting.

Although actual cervical spine injury is relatively uncommon in young pediatric patients, it must always be ruled out when there is evidence of head injury; most patients will have a cervical collar in place upon transfer to the trauma resuscitation area. As noted above, airway management proceeds with caution in known or suspected cervical spine injury. If the cervical collar is removed temporarily for access to the airway, flexion or extension of the spine must be avoided. Following successful tracheal intubation, the cervical collar is immediately replaced and radiographic evaluation proceeds. In the case of quadriplegia or paraplegia from high thoracic spinal cord injury, loss of sympathetic nerve tone in the arterial system may cause spinal shock, which requires treatment with fluid boluses and vasopressors. High-dose methylprednisolone (30 mg/kg plus 5.4 mg/kg/h for 23 h) is used in many centers in the face of significant spinal cord injury, but this is controversial [87,88].

Thoracic and cardiac trauma

Approximately 85% of major pediatric trauma is blunt trauma. Rib fractures and pulmonary contusion are seen in about 50% of thoracic trauma patients [81]. Twenty percent of patients have a pneumothorax and 10% have a hemothorax. Evaluation of these injuries is by plain radiography and CT scanning; treatment is by thoracostomy tube. Thoracotomy is rarely indicated in the acute trauma setting. A tension pneumothorax that is accompanied by severe respiratory distress, hypotension, and greatly diminished or absent breath sounds on the affected side is treated acutely by inserting a needle through the second anterior intercostal space. This is followed by insertion of a thoracostomy tube.

Cardiac and great vessel trauma is relatively rare and accounts for less than 5% of thoracic trauma cases. However, the sequelae of these injuries are severe and cannot be overlooked in major blunt trauma or penetrating chest trauma in children. In pediatric patients with cardiac trauma (myocardial contusion, coronary artery injury, aortic dissection), almost 90% have evidence of injury to other organs [89]. Premature ventricular contractions, ECG changes (such as ST segment elevation), and hypotension and shock (due to myocardial dysfunction) may be present. Plain radiography and standard CT scans may not make the diagnosis of cardiac trauma. A diagnosis of cardiac tamponade or myocardial dysfunction can be made quickly at the bedside by echocardiography. Trauma-induced cardiac tamponade is rare in children, but when it is present it is heralded by hypotension and pulsus paradoxus. These patients require emergency pericardiocentesis followed by surgical drainage and repair of the cardiac injury.

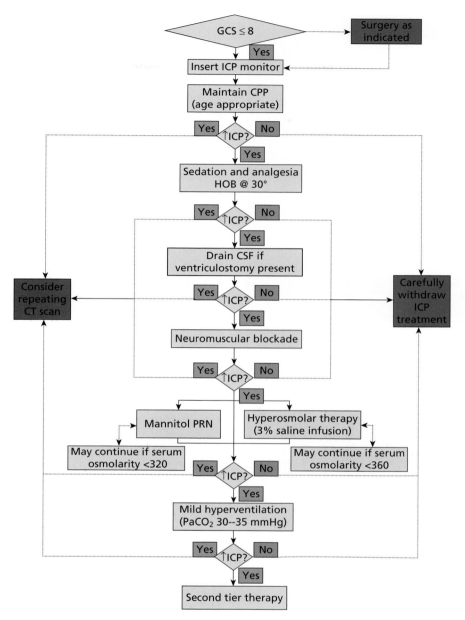

Figure 35.8 Critical pathway for the treatment of intracranial hypertension in children following brain trauma. GCS, Glasgow Coma Scale; ICP, intracranial pressure; CPP, cerebral perfusion pressure; HOB, head of bed; CSF, cerebrospinal fluid; CT computed tomography. Reproduced from Adelson et al [85] with permission from Lippincott Williams and Wilkins.

Myocardial enzymes, such as troponin I and creatine phosphokinase myocardial band, are useful for following the progress of a myocardial injury. Thoracic CT scanning with contrast material is necessary to diagnose aortic injuries, such as dissection. Patients with cardiac trauma who require emergency non-cardiac surgery require extreme vigilance to detect and treat their myocardial dysfunction.

Abdominal trauma

Abdominal injuries occur in 10–15% of major trauma cases in children. Blunt trauma accounts for 85% of abdominal injuries and MVAs account for half of the blunt trauma [81]. The spleen accounts for about 45% of intra-abominal injuries in children [90]. Other injuries include liver contusion or laceration, stomach or intestinal perforation, renal, ureteral or bladder trauma, and

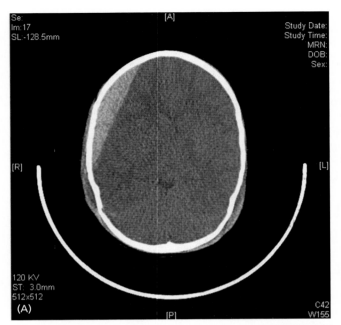

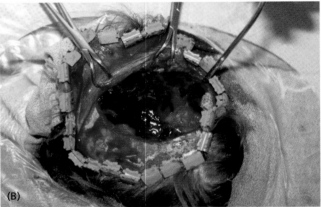

Figure 35.9 (A) Brain CT scan of acute epidural hematoma in a 3 year old after a fall from a second-story window. Note the signs of cerebral edema with effacement of the lateral ventricles, and lack of gray–white matter distinction. (B) Epidural hematoma after craniotomy and reflection of the dura in the same patient.

retroperitoneal hematoma. Abdominal pain is often diffuse, making localization of the injury difficult in pediatric patients. Plain radiography has limited utility in these patients. Bedside portable ultrasound examination using the FAST protocol (focused abdominal sonography for trauma) allows rapid scanning of all four abdominal quadrants looking for free fluid, which, if found, is evidence of major trauma, i.e. splenic rupture or liver laceration. Unfortunately, this protocol does not have adequate sensitivity and specificity, nor has its use been able to reliably guide surgical decisions in children. CT scanning of the abdomen with IV contrast material is the gold standard for diagnosing intra-abdominal trauma and

must be done as rapidly as possible if there is suspicion of significant injury. Oral contrast material is often not used in the acute situation because of delays in administration and movement of the material into the entire gastrointestinal tract.

Non-operative management is the norm for intra-abdominal injury in children, including most injuries to the spleen and liver. Ninety to 95% of patients are successfully treated expectantly, and it is rare to require either operative intervention or blood transfusion for isolated grade I or II injuries (a subcapsular hematoma of ≤50% of surface area or a capsular tear of ≤3 cm that does not involve a major vessel) [91]. Angio-embolization may be attempted in some cases, but it has had limited success in pediatric patients. Laparoscopy is often used instead of a full laparotomy in some abdominal trauma patients [92]. It may be necessary to do an open laparotomy to control major hemorrhage from vascular disruption, or for gastrointestinal perforation or other trauma not amenable to conservative treatment. If this is required, preparations should be made for major blood loss. Surgeons attempt to preserve organ function as much as possible and rarely do a splenectomy, liver resection or nephrectomy.

Extremity trauma

Trauma to the extremities can involve both bones and soft tissue and is often present in pediatric patients with multiple trauma. Although not the focus of the initial trauma survey and treatment of life-threatening problems, extremity trauma should not be overlooked. Therefore, radiographic evaluation of affected extremities is performed as soon as practical after initial evaluation and stabilization of the patient's condition. Compartment syndrome from crush injuries is a major problem that may require fasciotomies to preserve as much viable tissue as possible. In addition, release of myoglobin from crush injuries may cause renal failure. In larger patients, the possibility of a fat or air embolus should be entertained. Significant blood loss from femoral and pelvic fractures is often concealed, and the anesthesiologist must consider this fact when caring for patients with these injuries, especially if the patient is hypotensive. See Chapter 30 for further discussion of management of orthopedic injuries.

The multiple trauma patient

Major or multiple trauma is a systemic disease. Consequently, there is a systemic response that is separate from injury to the brain, chest, abdomen or bone. Initially, a neuroendocrine stress response helps preserve blood flow to vital organs, such as heart and brain. This response may last for several days. A more prolonged inflammatory response follows and causes a syndrome that is similar or identical to the systemic inflammatory response syndrome. Manifestations of this syndrome include capillary leak, edema, multiorgan dysfunction, ARDS, disseminated intravascular coagulation, and myocardial dysfunction. When caring for trauma patients, the anesthesiologist must carefully evaluate the patient during and after the initial resuscitation and treatment to determine if these secondary problems exist. Priorities in the initial management of patients with multiple trauma include control of the airway, restoration of intravascular volume and hemoglobin to assure adequate cardiac output and tissue oxygen delivery, and operative management of life-threatening hemorrhage or intracranial pathology. Afterwards, patients can often be stabilized in the ICU, where further diagnostic evaluations are done, and/or they can be returned to the operating room for more definitive treatment [93]. See Chapter 37 for a presentation of the critical care management of multiple organ dysfunction.

Intraoperative management of the trauma patient

The majority of pediatric patients who suffer major trauma do not require immediate anesthesia and surgery. Rather, the most frequent type of care required of anesthesiologists is airway management during the initial evaluation and treatment in the trauma resuscitation room and transport to the scanner for a 5–10-min CT scan of the brain and abdomen. Then the patient is often transported to the ICU, where further monitoring and evaluation are done and care is planned. The most common reason for immediate operative treatment is evacuation of an epidural or subdural hematoma. The next most common reason is laparotomy for major abdominal trauma. In children, simultaneous laparotomy and craniotomy are rare, as is penetrating trauma to the chest. Patients frequently present to the operating room at a later time for treatment of fractures or soft tissue injury, or for secondary surgery following initial trauma resuscitation.

Major pediatric trauma centers can evaluate, treat, and transport a patient to an operating room for surgery within 30 min of presentation to the center. It is highly desirable for the anesthesiologist to have the help of many people. Consequently, one should not hesitate to enlist surgeons, emergency room or ICU personnel to help in the OR if additional anesthesiologists are not available. The OR must be completely set up at all times with appropriate airway equipment, IV catheters, fluids, and warming devices for a variety of patients from infants to adult-sized teenagers. Pressure infusers that deliver 500 mL per minute must be available. Catheters and transducers for monitoring invasive arterial and central venous pressures must also be available. Proximity to a blood bank that has adequate personnel and can rapidly provide large amounts of packed RBCs, fresh frozen plasma, platelets, and cryoprecipitate is mandatory. If there is insufficient time to fully cross-match blood, type-specific uncross-matched blood is preferable and can be issued within 10–15 min in most centers. In an emergency situation when blood products are required in less time, O negative uncross-matched blood is used. Massive transfusion in a pediatric patient is often defined as transfusion of more than one blood volume over a 24-h period, but a more practical definition in the acute trauma setting is transfusion of 50% of the estimated blood volume in 3 h. If massive transfusion with O negative blood is commenced, the anesthesiologist should continue with the O negative blood even after the patient's blood type is known, because there is always a risk that the anti-A and anti-B antibodies found in some O negative blood will cause hemolytic anemia. Some massive transfusion protocols advocate using a 1:1:1 ratio of packed RBCs, fresh frozen plasma and random donor platelets after identifying massive hemorrhage. See Chapter 11 for an extensive discussion of transfusion therapy.

The anesthesiologist's focus when providing care during acute trauma surgery should be to maintain adequate oxygen delivery to the tissues, particularly the vital organs, by maintaining adequate intravascular volume, hemoglobin concentration, cardiac output, oxygenation, and ventilation. An arterial catheter is often helpful in this setting, but precious time should not be taken to insert one of these catheters if doing so delays definitive surgical treatment, e.g. evacuation of an intracranial hematoma. Obtaining adequate large-bore peripheral IV access is a major priority. If an extremity is accessible after draping for surgery, the anesthesiologist may be able to obtain arterial access but this should not distract from the vital monitoring and treatment of hemorrhage and hemodynamic compromise. Central venous access is obtained when there is time to do so, often after the initial care. When possible, frequent point-of-care determinations of blood gases, hemoglobin, coagulation, electrolytes, ionized calcium, and lactate concentration are very valuable in guiding therapy.

A frequent question asked is what anesthetic should be used in what doses for anesthetizing the unstable hypovolemic major trauma patients. An unconscious patient with head trauma is not at risk for intraoperative awareness; resuscitation to restore adequate hemodynamic status should be the main priority. In general, synthetic opioids such as fentanyl are well tolerated by trauma patients. Providing 25–100 μg/kg of fentanyl for major trauma is not unusual. If there is brain injury, ketamine should not be used. However, ketamine is quite useful for producing analgesia and amnesia in patients with multiple trauma who have no evidence of CNS injury. Small doses of benzodiazepines, such as midazolam, will often provide amnesia. Nitrous oxide should be avoided in trauma patients because they may have encapsulated air in the chest, abdomen or cranium that might be expanded by N₂O. Isoflurane, sevoflurane, and desflurane may be used in small doses, while paying careful attention to decreases in systemic vascular resistance. Scopolamine is an amnestic agent often used in critically unstable trauma patients. Muscle relaxation during trauma surgery is essential; non-depolarizing agents that have minimal cardiovascular effects, such as rocuronium, vecuronium or cis-atracurium, are preferred.

Exposure, infusion of large volumes of IV fluids, and transport to scanners and performing a scan in cool environments often make trauma patients hypothermic. Consequently, the anesthesiologist must measure core temperature and warm the OR and IV fluids, use forced-air warming, humidify and warm the inspired gases, and use radiant warming devices when needed to maintain normothermia. Coagulopathy, increased systemic vascular resistance, and slow awakening from anesthesia are some of the unwanted effects of hypothermia. Every effort should be made to maintain the patient's core temperature above 35°C. Hyperthermia is also potentially dangerous to these patients because it increases oxygen demand in vital organs, particularly the brain, where it may cause hypoxia and extend the zone of infarction in watershed areas and in areas that surround injured tissue. Box 35.3 reviews the major priorities in anesthetic care of the pediatric major trauma patient.

Outcomes of trauma care in children

As noted earlier, pediatric trauma is the leading cause of death in 1–19-year-old patients despite major efforts over the past several decades to reduce the incidence of trauma. The key to attaining optimal outcomes of major pediatric trauma is to use the multidisciplinary approach espoused by the American College of Surgeons. Formal data collection, reporting of adverse events and outcomes of trauma patients are an important part of pediatric trauma care. Fostering a culture of patient safety by measuring outcomes, rapidly studying systems and intervening when problems arise, and having regular quality improvement meetings of the entire trauma team are important for optimizing outcomes. See Chapter 45 for a discussion of multidisciplinary communication, safety, and outcomes programs.

Acknowledgments

Portions of this chapter were previously published as "Anesthesia for plastic surgery," authors Barbara W. Palmisano and Lynn M Rusy, in *Pediatric Anesthesia*, 4th edn, edited by George A. Gregory, published by Churchill Livingstone, New York, 2002, pp. 732–41.

Box 35.3 Priorities for anesthesia care for major pediatric trauma

Airway

- Rapid assessment
- Intubate trachea for GCS ≤8 or respiratory compromise, or need for significant sedation for diagnostic studies
- Rapid or modified rapid sequence with cricoid pressure
- Use small cuffed endotracheal tube
- Remove cervical collar and use in-line stabilization for suspected cervical spine injury
- Use CO₂ detection and auscultation to confirm placement
- Initiate positive pressure ventilation cautiously to minimize compromising venous return
- For trauma: have suction, surgical airway back-up; evaluation with CT or bronchoscopy

Central nervous system

- Manage airway pre-emptively to ensure adequate oxygenation and ventilation
- Hyperventilate only for impending herniation
- Maintain CPP (MAP – ICP) of 40–65 using volume infusion and pressors if necessary

Spinal cord injury

- In-line stabilization (not traction) for airway manipulation
- Anticipate and treat spinal shock: IV volume, pressors
- High-dose methylprednisolone per institutional protocol

Thoracic trauma

- Emergency airway intervention for significant distress
- Tube or needle thoracostomy for tension pneumothorax
- Tube thoracostomy for hemothorax
- Cardiac tamponade: pulsus paradoxus, pericardial effusion by echo – drain emergently
- Cardiac contusion or coronary injury: PVCs, ST elevation, myocardial dysfunction
- Aortic dissection: rapid CT scan with contrast and transport to OR

Abdominal trauma

- Evaluation by CT, non-operative management is the norm
- Prepare for massive transfusion if operative treatment necessary

Extremity trauma

- Compartment syndrome, myoglobinuria and renal failure in crush injury

Multiple trauma

- Neuroendocrine response
- Systemic inflammatory response syndrome:
- Capillary leak
- ARDS
- Multiorgan dysfunction
- Myocardial dysfunction
- Disseminated intravascular coagulation

ARDS, acute respiratory distress syndrome; CPP, cerebral perfusion pressure; CT, computed tomography; GCS, Glasgow Coma SCale; ICP, intracranial pressure; MAP, mean arterial pressure; OR, operating room; PVC, premature ventricular contractions.

CASE STUDY

A 3-year-old boy fell from a second-story window and was found by his mother to be moaning weakly and unresponsive. He had obvious trauma to the left side of his head. Paramedics arrived within 5 min and reported regular respirations, a heart rate (HR) of 140 beats per minute (bpm), an arterial blood pressure (BP) of 75/45 mmHg, and a GCS of 6. His SpO_2 was 100%. They obtained 22 G IV access in the saphenous vein, placed the patient on a backboard with a cervical collar, and transported him to the hospital with facemask oxygen. A high-level trauma activation was initiated, and the patient arrived in the trauma resuscitation area of the emergency department within 15 min of injury. The pediatric anesthesia attending and fellow responded and brought with them the trauma tackle box that contained all airway supplies and drugs required.

Upon initial assessment, the GCS remained at 6. The HR was now 160 bpm, BP 65/40 mmHg, respirations irregular, SpO_2 98% breathing 100% oxygen, and the abdomen was slightly distended. The left pupil was now larger than the right. The trauma surgeon and anesthesiologist agreed that the trachea should be intubated immediately. The neurosurgeon on call arrived shortly thereafter. Quick assessment revealed that the airway would not be difficult to manage. They rapidly administered a bolus of normal saline 150 mL (based on estimated weight of 15 kg) and began preoxygenation with assisted bag and mask respiration. The anesthesiologist gave lidocaine 15 mg, etomidate 3 mg, rocuronium 30 mg, and fentanyl 15 µg IV in rapid succession. The cervical collar was removed and the head and neck stabilized by the neurosurgery resident. Cricoid pressure and gentle rapid mask ventilations were applied. Automated blood pressure measurement was set on the stat mode, and the ECG was continuously monitored. After about 1 min, the pediatric anesthesia fellow quickly intubated the trachea on the first attempt with a styletted, 4.5 mm cuffed endotracheal tube. End-tidal CO_2 was detected, breath sounds were equal, the tube was secured, and the cervical collar was replaced. The blood pressure decreased to 60/30 mmHg and an additional 150 mL of normal saline plus phenylephrine 10 µg were given to increase the blood pressure, which quickly rose to 85/40 mmHg. Positive pressure ventilation was gently instituted. Because of the impending brainstem herniation, hyperventilation was commenced. The primary survey also revealed a contusion on the left flank over the costal margin and no other apparent injury. A second 22 G IV was started in the left hand, and blood was sent for type and cross-match and complete blood count. A Foley catheter was inserted; the urine was clear. Fifteen minutes after arrival, the patient was transported to the CT scanner and

was found to have a large left-sided epidural hematoma with significant midline shift and surrounding cerebral contusion and edema. Because of the abdominal trauma, a rapid CT scan of the abdomen with contrast was done, which revealed a grade II splenic laceration and subcapsular hematoma. Total time in the CT scanner was 10 min.

The patient was then transferred directly to the trauma OR, which was already set up and ready. The OR nursing trauma team was opening equipment for a craniotomy. The patient was turned and positioned, and the neurosurgeon made an incision 35 min after the patient arrived in the emergency department. A 20 G peripheral intravenous catheter was placed in the other saphenous vein during prepping and draping for surgery. Craniotomy commenced and revealed a parietal skull fracture and laceration of the middle meningeal artery. The clot was rapidly evacuated. The estimated blood loss was 500 mL, about half of his blood volume. Cerebral contusion and edema were found in the area adjacent to the epidural hematoma. For this reason, the neurosurgeon had asked that mannitol 0.5 g/kg be given, but this was deferred until the patient's hemodynamic status could be stabilized.

The initial hemoglobin concentration was 10 g/dL. The anesthesiologist ordered 4 units of type-specific blood, which arrived in the OR at the same time as the patient. Two units of packed RBCs (PRBCs) were infused rapidly into the 20 G IV via a warmed pressure infuser. Two doses of calcium gluconate, 30 mg/kg, were given during the transfusion. The lowest blood pressure was 55/25 mmHg at the time of maximum hemorrhage; additional 15 µg boluses of phenylephrine were given twice during the surgery. Hemorrhage was controlled and an additional unit of PRBCs was given to account for the presumed ongoing splenic bleeding. The blood pressure returned to 90/60 mmHg and the HR was 120 bpm. Despite the team's efforts, the patient became hypothermic (esophageal temperature of 34.2°C). For anesthesia, the patient received fentanyl 35 µg/kg, midazolam 0.2 mg/kg, and low-dose isoflurane after his hemodynamics were stable. Forced-air warming was used during the entire case.

Because there was significant cerebral contusion and edema, the neurosurgeon placed an intraventricular drain to both measure ICP and to drain cerebrospinal fluid if needed. The patient's pupils were equal at 3 mm and sluggishly reactive at the end of surgery. After hemodynamic stability was established, mannitol was given. The fellow placed a 22 G right radial artery catheter and the attending inserted a 5 Fr triple-lumen femoral central venous catheter at the end of the surgery. The trauma surgery team, which was present in the OR, decided not to operate for the splenic

Continued

trauma at that time. The initial ICP was 15 mmHg with the patient's head positioned in the midline and elevated 30°. He was then transported to the ICU. Dopamine 5 μg/kg/min was begun just before leaving the OR.

The patient's ICU course was initially difficult. He had ICPs of 25–30 mmHg despite osmolar therapy, continuous sedation, neuromuscular blockade, moderate hyperventilation, and maintaining MAPs of 80–85 mmHg with dopamine. The hemoglobin concentration was stable at 11–13 g/dL. Because the initial platelet count was 85,000 μL and the prothrombin time was 17 sec, two units of platelets and 15 mL/kg of fresh frozen plasma were given. This normalized the clotting parameters. After the neurosurgeon removed CSF to lower ICP, a CT scan revealed no new hemorrhage, but showed significant cerebral contusion plus edema in the left cerebral hemisphere, slit-like ventricles, and a significant midline shift. Because the left pupil began to dilate, the child was returned to the OR 12 h after the initial craniotomy for a decompressive craniectomy, duraplasty, and debridement of some non-viable brain tissue. The ICP decreased to 15–18 mmHg. He was returned to the ICU for intensive management of his ICP, which was successful over the ensuing 5 days. However, he developed ARDS and required positive end-expiratory pressure (PEEP) as high as 8 cmH$_2$O, an FIO$_2$ as high as 0.70, and ventilator rates as high as 30 breaths per minute to maintain a PaCO$_2$ of 35–40 mmHg.

Repeat CT scan of the abdomen 3 days after the injury revealed no progression of the laceration or bleeding, and conservative management was continued. After 7 days, ICP was well controlled and the neuromuscular blockade was discontinued without any change in ICP. The ventriculostomy was removed on day 10. The lungs gradually improved, the patient was weaned from the ventilator; and the trachea was extubated on day 15. He was left with a right hemiparesis. However, he appeared to recognize his mother and reach for familiar objects with his left hand. The patient had no seizures and was transferred to the inpatient rehabilitation unit on day 19.

This case study illustrates the rapid co-ordinated team response at a level I pediatric trauma center, the principles of early airway management, preserving CPP during acute brain injury, rapid diagnosis by CT scanning and transfer to a prepared OR, and prioritizing maintenance of cardiac output and oxygen delivery during significant hemorrhage that occurred in the OR. Further principles of ICP management included dopamine to maintain CPP, mannitol to reduce cerebral edema, ventriculostomy to measure and treat elevated ICP, and early decompressive craniectomy to preserve as much viable brain tissue as possible. The conservative non-operative management of significant splenic trauma is illustrated. After a nearly 3-week ICU stay, the patient had a good neurological outcome given the severity of the injury. With inpatient and outpatient rehabilitation, the prognosis for a good functional neurological outcome is optimistic.

Annotated references

A full reference list for this chapter is available at:
http://www.wiley.com/go/gregory/andropoulos/pediatricanesthesia

8. Fidkowski CW, Fuzaylov G, Sheridan RL, Cote CJ. Inhalational burn injury in children. Paediatr Anaesth 2009; 19: 147–54. An excellent modern review of inhalational injuries in children.

14. Fuzaylov G, Fidkowski CW. Anesthetic considerations for major burn injury in pediatric patients. Paediatr Anaesth 2009; 19: 202–11. A very well-written contemporary review of anesthetic care of the child with major burns.

41. Ansermino JM, Vandebeek CA, Myers D. An allometric model to estimate fluid requirements in children following burn injury. Paediatr Anaesth 2010; 20: 305–12. A very well done comparison of several fluid resuscitation schemes for severely burned children.

48. Fabia R, Groner JI. Advances in the care of children with burns. Adv Pediatr 2009; 56: 219–48. A very comprehensive overview of modern burn care in pediatric patients.

50. Tenenhaus M, Rennekampff HO. Burn surgery. Clin Plast Surg 2007; 34: 697–715. A well done review of the surgical procedures practiced today in burn patients.

81. Avarello JT, Cantor RM. Pediatric major trauma: an approach to evaluation and management. Emerg Med Clin North Am 2007; 25; 803–36. An excellent comprehensive review of trauma in the pediatric patient.

83. Huh JW, Raghupathi R. New concepts in treatment of pediatric traumatic brain injury. Anesthesiol Clin 2009; 27: 213–40. A review of modern advances in the treatment of pediatric brain trauma.

85. Adelson PD, Bratton SL, Carney NA et al. Guidelines for the acute medical management of severe traumatic brain injury in infants, children, and adolescents. Chapter 17. Critical pathway for the treatment of established intracranial hypertension in pediatric traumatic brain injury. Pediatr Crit Care Med 2003; 4: S65–7. An important clinical guideline for the treatment of increased intracranial pressure in the brain-injured pediatric patient.

89. Baum VC. Cardiac trauma in children. Paediatr Anaesth 2002; 12: 110–17. A comprehensive review of cardiac trauma.

91. Gaines BA. Intra-abdominal solid organ injury in children: diagnosis and treatment. J Trauma 2009; 67: S135–9. A concise review of abdominal trauma in children, discussing the modern emphasis on non-interventional approaches.

93. Wetzel RC, Burns RC. Multiple trauma in children: critical care overview. Crit Care Med 2002; 30: S468–77. A very well-written comprehensive overview of the multisystem nature and management of multiple trauma.

CHAPTER 36

Anesthesia and Sedation Outside the Operating Room

Robert S. Holzman & Keira P. Mason

Department of Anesthesiology, Perioperative and Pain Medicine, Children's Hospital Boston, and Harvard Medical School, Boston, MA, USA

Introduction

In the past 18 years, as operating room cases have increased by 250% at the Children's Hospital Boston, anesthesia services outside the operating room have increased by almost 350%, to over 7000 cases annually (Table 36.1). Sedation and anesthesia services for children have accompanied technological advances such as surgical procedures guided by intraoperative magnetic resonance imaging (MRI) or computed tomography (CT). Functional MRI studies can now localize specific areas of the brain responsible for particular actions or behaviors. Although the majority of procedures are accomplished in the radiology suite, they are now complemented by anesthesiology support in gastroenterology, pulmonology, radiation therapy and the oncology clinic (Box 36.1). Anesthesiologists have been leaders in establishing guidelines and recommendations for sedation and anesthesia services provided by both anesthesiologists and non-anesthesiologists [1–4]. In this chapter we will explore the special considerations for providing anesthesia and sedation services in various clinical areas outside the operating room and will review common organizational, equipment and personnel considerations and strategies.

Specific extramural sites

Diagnostic radiology
Computed tomography scan
In the late 1970s, computed tomography (CT) was introduced into clinical practice, with the Nobel Prize awarded to its inventors in 1979. CT differentiates between high-density (calcium, iron, bone, contrast-enhanced vascular and cerebrospinal fluid (CSF) spaces) and low-density (oxygen, nitrogen, carbon in air, fat, CSF, muscle, white matter, gray matter, and water-containing lesions) structures. Because the scan time is quick, CT may be preferable for patients who are medically unstable and in need

Gregory's Pediatric Anesthesia, Fifth Edition. Edited by George A. Gregory, Dean B. Andropoulos.
© 2012 Blackwell Publishing Ltd. Published 2012 by Blackwell Publishing Ltd.

Table 36.1 Anesthetics outside the operating room, Children's Hospital Boston

Year	1992	2008
Total anesthetic cases	13,679	34,311
Radiology: sedation	0	2465
Cardiac cath lab	900	1908
Radiology: general anesthesia	346	1664
GI endoscopy	0	918
Oncology clinic	0	528
Radiation therapy	1065	248
Total outside OR	2311	7731

GI, gastrointestinal; OR, operating room.

Box 36.1 Multidisciplinary programs involving the Department of Anesthesiology, Children's Hospital Boston

- **Advanced Fetal Care Center:** Anesthesia, Cardiology, General Surgery, Genetics, Medicine, Neurology, Neurosurgery, Newborn Medicine, Otorhinolaryngology, Plastic Surgery, Radiology, Urology
- **Brain Injury Program:** Anesthesia, General Surgery, Neurology, Neurosurgery, Orthopedic Surgery, Psychiatry/Psychology, Sports Medicine
- **Center for AeroDigestive Disorders (CADD):** Anesthesia, Gastroenterology, Otorhinolaryngology Pulmonary Program
- **Cleft Lip and Palate Program:** Anesthesia, Audiology, Dentistry, General Surgery, Genetics, Nursing, Oral and Maxillofacial Surgery, Otorhinolaryngology, Pathology, Plastic Surgery, Psychiatry/Psychology, Social Work
- **Craniofacial Anomalies Program:** Anesthesia, Audiology, Dentistry, Genetics, Neurosurery, Nursing, Oral and Maxillofacial Surgery, Otorhinolaryngology, Pathology, Plastic Surgery, Psychiatry/Psychology, Social Work
- **Heart Transplant Program:** Anesthesia, Cardiac Surgery, Cardiology, Cardiovascular Program, General Surgery, Nutrition, Physical Therapy, Pathology, Radiology
- **Intestine and Multivisceral Transplant Program:** Anesthesia, Gastroenterology, General Surgery, Nutrition
- **Liver Transplantation:** General Surgery, Gastroenterology, Nutrition Center, Psychiatry
- **Lung Transplant Program:** Anesthesia, Cardiac Surgery, Cardiology, General Surgery, Psychiatry/Psychology, Respiratory Diseases
- **Pain Treatment Service:** Anesthesia, Physical and Occupational Therapy, Psychiatry, Rheumatology
- **Trauma Program:** Anesthesia, Critical Care Medicine, Emergency Medicine, General Surgery, Neurosurgery, Orthopaedic Surgery, Psychiatry/Psychology, Radiology
- **Vascular Anomalies Center:** Anesthesia, Cardiology, Cardiovascular Program, Dermatology, Endocrinology, General Surgery, Hematology, Medicine, Neurology, Neurosurgery, Nursing, Oncology, Oral and Maxillofacial Surgery, Otorhinolaryngology, Orthopaedic Surgery, Pathology

of rapid diagnosis, for example, the child being evaluated for abuse, altered mental status, an intracranial hemorrhage or abdominal or thoracic mass. These emergency situations usually necessitate a rapid-sequence induction with tracheal intubation.

Computed tomography scans for visualizing the sinuses, ears, inner auditory canal, and temporomandibular bones (e.g. for choanal atresia or craniofacial abnormalities) may require direct coronal imaging with extreme head extension or absolute immobility for three-dimensional (3-D) reconstruction. The more common studies involving 3-D reconstruction are cardiac, craniofacial and pulmonary (larynx, trachea, bronchi and pulmonary parenchyma) imaging. Paired inspiratory and expiratory multidetector computed tomography (MDCT) performed with general anesthesia is a relatively new technique which enables inspiratory and expiratory breath holding to evaluate tracheobronchomalacia (TBM) [5–7].

The cardiac studies are often done in collaboration with cardiologists and radiologists who are able to make structural and functional assessments of the heart. These scans can also be challenging because adenosine is often requested in order to briefly pause heart function so that image quality is maximized [8,9].

Any patient who is at risk for cervical instability should be properly screened prior to neck extension, such as children with Down syndrome, who are at risk for atlantoaxial instability. The incidence of instability varies from 12% to 32% [10]. Many children with Down syndrome require cervical spine radiographs prior to entering grade school or participating in Special Olympics. Usually, the parents are well aware of the radiological findings. The cervical spine films, however, do not predict the risk of dislocation [11]. Rather, neurological signs or symptoms such as abnormal gait, increased clumsiness, fatigue with ambulation or a new preference for sitting games are predictors of risk. The asymptomatic Down syndrome child with radiological evidence of instability may be approved for procedural sedation but unnecessary neck movement should be avoided. Any child who displays neurological signs or symptoms should not be sedated by either a nurse or an anesthesiologist until neurosurgical or orthopedic consultation is obtained.

Radiologists employ gastrografin (diatrizoate meglumine and diatrizoate sodium) when evaluating abdominal masses. Gastrografin diluted to 1.5% is usually considered a clear liquid but the volume administered orally is not insignificant: newborns less than 1 month of age receive 60–90 mL, infants between 1 month and 1 year of age may receive up to 240 mL and children between the ages of 1 and 5 years receive 240–360 mL. Because sedation or anesthesia should usually be accomplished within a window of 1–2h after ingestion of the contrast, most "elective" nil per os (NPO) guidelines would be violated, yet the scan must be completed while the gastrografin is still in the gastrointestinal tract. There are no published data to guide optimal induction or sedation techniques as they relate to aspiration risk in these circumstances. Full-strength (3%) gastrografin is hyperosmolar and hypertonic. All gastrografin should be diluted to an isosmolar and isotonic 1.5% concentration of neutral pH. There is one case report of 1.5% gastrografin aspiration in a child [12] with no adverse sequelae; therefore, the risk of using a 1.5% concentration of gastrografin seems low [13].

Magnetic resonance imaging

The first commercial MRI scanner was introduced in 1990. Over the past two decades MRI has evolved beyond a diagnostic tool for neoplasms, vascular malformations, masses and lesions to encompass a broader role as an aid to diagnosing and evaluating obstructive sleep apnea, developmental delay, behavioral disorders, seizures, failure to thrive, apnea/cyanosis, hypotonia, and mitochondrial/metabolic disorders. Magnetic resonance angiography and venography (MRA and MRV) evaluate vascular flow and can sometimes replace invasive catheterization studies for follow-up or initial evaluations of vascular malformations, interventional treatment or radiotherapy [14].

Functional MRI (fMRI) is an evolving technology which measures the hemodynamic or metabolic response related to neural activity in the brain or spinal cord. fMRI is often able to localize sites of brain activation and is now dominating brain mapping techniques due to its low invasiveness and lack of radiation exposure [15,16]. Some fMRI studies require cognitive facility and are typically interactive with a conscious and responsive patient. fMRI which requires patient responsiveness is generally performed in unsedated children with the aid of distraction techniques and most recently with the use of video goggles (Resonance Technology, Northridge, CA, USA). These goggles are designed specifically for fMRI and are approved for the 1.5 and 3 T environment. They are able to deliver audio and visual stimulation, measure patient response through the use of patient input devices, and track eye movement. fMRI study of sedated children is a relatively new field and those who provide sedation describe propofol and dexmedetomidine infusions as agents which can maintain spontaneous ventilation and immobility while also enabling the child to respond to verbal, tactile or auditory stimulation. fMRI studies on children who require sedation to maintain immobility will be a challenge facing anesthesiologists as we move through this decade.

Three-dimensional studies utilizing MRI have evolved in concert with CT studies. Cardiac studies, vascular imaging and airway examinations have benefited from 3-D technology. The airway studies, in particular, provide a means of diagnosing areas of airway compromise and collapse which were not identified on bronchoscopy and fluoroscopy. These studies have specific anesthetic management implications as they require that the trachea remain un-intubated and the patient breathe spontaneously in order to be able to visualize areas of collapse. The use of intravenous dexmedetomidine, among other techniques, will allow immobility, simulation of natural sleep and maintenance of spontaneous ventilation. As these children present with obstructive sleep apnea, however, the anesthesiologist must anticipate that airway obstruction can occur under sedation as it does during natural sleep [17].

Surgical procedures guided by MRI, commonly referred to as magnetic resonance therapy (MRT), have evolved over the past decade and enable surgeons to benefit from MR imaging intraoperatively. The logistical challenges with creating a surgical suite that is equipped with a MRI scanner are considerable. In addition to the routine precautions that must be taken in a typical diagnostic MRI suite, all surgical supplies and equipment must be MR safe or conditional. In general, access to this surgical suite is restricted to personnel fluent in MR safety procedure and guidelines. MRT is currently being used for neurosurgery to guide the resection of tumors, seizure foci and vascular malformations [18]. Additional applications have extended its use to otolaryngological, general surgery and orthopedic procedures [19].

The MRI environment is unique because of its strong static magnetic field, high-frequency electromagnetic (radiofrequency, RF) waves and a pulsed magnetic field. Magnetic field strengths are measured in units of gauss (G) and tesla (T). One tesla is equal to 10,000 gauss. The main magnetic field of a 1.5 T magnet is about 30,000 times the strength of the earth's magnetic field. The main magnetic field of a 3 T system is 60,000 times the earth's magnet field. To put this into context, the strength of electromagnets used to pick up cars in salvage yards is equivalent to the strength of a 1.5–2.0T magnet. This field strength is able to transform static oxygen cylinders into flying projectiles which can travel at speeds approaching 40 miles per hour. The American College of Radiology established guidelines to minimize the risk of MRI-related mishaps [20] but did not directly address anesthesiologists' unique needs. In 2008 the American Society of Anesthesiologists (ASA) assembled a task force composed of anesthesiologists, a radiologist with MRI expertise, and two methodologists; a Practice Advisory on Anesthetic Care for Magnetic Resonance Imaging followed [21]. This document establishes important recommendations for safe practice as well as consistency of anesthesia care in the MRI environment. In 2008, the Joint Commission recognized the existing and potential hazards of the MRI environment when they published a Sentinel Event Alert [22] specifically identifying eight types of possible injury (Box 36.2).

Box 36.2 The Joint Commission Sentinel Event Alert. Preventing accidents and injuries in the MRI suite

1. "Missile effect" or "projectile" injury in which ferromagnetic objects (those having magnetic properties) such as ink pens, wheelchairs, and oxygen canisters are pulled into the MRI scanner at rapid velocity.
2. Injury related to dislodged ferromagnetic implants such as aneurysm clips, pins in joints, and drug infusion devices.
3. Burns from objects that may heat during the MRI process, such as wires (including lead wires for both implants and external devices) and surgical staples, or from the patient's body touching the inside walls (the bore) of the MRI scanner during the scan.
4. Injury or complication related to equipment or device malfunction or failure caused by the magnetic field. For example, battery-powered devices (laryngoscopes, microinfusion pumps, monitors, etc.) can suddenly fail to operate; some programmable infusion pumps may perform erratically; and pacemakers and implantable defibrillators may not behave as programmed.
5. Injury or complication due to failure to attend to patient support systems during the MRI. This is especially true for patient sedation or anesthesia in MRI arenas. For example, oxygen canisters or infusion pumps run out and staff must either leave the MRI area to retrieve a replacement or move the patient to an area where a replacement can be found.
6. Acoustic injury from the loud knocking noise that the MRI scanner makes.
7. Adverse events related to the administration of MRI contrast agents.
8. Adverse events related to cryogen handling, storage or inadvertent release in superconducting MRI system sites.

Source: The Joint Commission. Preventing accidents and injuries in the MRI suite. 2008. www.jointcommission.org/SentinelEvents/SentinelEventAlert/sea_38.htm.

Box 36.3 MRI safety zones

Zone I: This region includes all areas that are freely accessible to the general public. This area is typically outside the MR environment itself and is the area through which patients, healthcare personnel, and other employees of the MR site access the MR environment. *Access*: General public.

Zone II: This area is the interface between the publicly accessible uncontrolled zone I and the strictly controlled zone III (see below). Typically, the patients are greeted in zone II and are not free to move throughout zone II at will, but rather are under the supervision of MR personnel. It is in zone II that patient histories, answers to medical insurance questions, and answers to MRI screening questions are typically obtained. *Access*: Unscreened MRI patients.

Zone III: This area is the region in which free access by unscreened non-MR personnel or ferromagnetic objects or equipment can result in serious injury or death as a result of interactions between the individuals or equipment and the MR scanner's particular environment. These interactions include, but are not limited to, those with the MR scanner's static and time-varying magnetic fields. All access to zone III is to be strictly restricted, with access to regions within it (including zone IV; see below) controlled by, and entirely under the supervision of, MR personnel. *Access:* Screened MRI patients and personnel.

Zone IV: This area is the MR scanner magnet room. Zone IV, by definition, will always be located within zone III because it is the MR magnet and its associated magnetic field which generate the existence of zone III. *Access:* Screened MRI patients under constant direct supervision of trained MR personnel.

Source: Kanal et al [20].

As technology has advanced, 1.5 T magnets have been supplanted by 3 T magnets. The field strength and magnetic force generated by a 3 T MRI scanner are unforgiving to the careless or accidental introduction of a ferrous object into the environment. Placing a magnet outside the MRI scanner is a crude, helpful and sometimes inaccurate way to test objects. If the object is not attracted to the magnet, this is not an absolute indication that there is no ferrous material present. A positive attraction, however, will provide critical information to the anesthesiologist. Some unusual objects which have found their way into the MRI suite in order to become projectiles include a metal fan, pulse oximeter, shrapnel, wheelchair, cigarette lighter, stethoscope, pager, hearing aid, vacuum cleaner, calculator, hair pin, oxygen tank, prosthetic limb, pencil, insulin infusion pump, keys, watches, and steel-tipped/heeled shoes [23]. Small objects can usually be easily removed from the magnet; large objects may have so much attractive force with the MRI scanner that they are impossible to remove by manual force. In these circumstances, quenching the magnet may be the only way

to release the object. This process is not without substantial risk: as helium gas is vented, condensation and considerable noise fill the suite. All personnel are required to vacate the suite during a quench as there is a risk of hypoxic conditions should the helium accidentally enter the room. The establishment of safety zones in the MRI environment addresses restrictions to access of the MRI environment [20] (Box 36.3). Because the 3 T and 1.5 T scanners have different magnetic field strengths, an object which is safe in a 1.5 T magnet is not necessarily safe in a 3 T magnet. MRI safety labeling is specific for magnetic field strength.

As advances have been made in MRI technology as well as clinical experience, there has been a parallel evolution in labeling practices from the initial standards established by the Food and Drug Administration in 1997 to the current standard for labeling equipment established by the American Society for Testing and Materials (ASTM) International in 2005 [24] (Table 36.2).

Personal risks in the MRI environment apply to anesthesiologists and patients. Anesthesiologists must be aware

Table 36.2 Current terminology used to label implants and devices

	Old terminology (1997)	New terminology (2005)	Icon label
	Food & Drug Administration	**American Society for Testing and Materials (ASTM) International**	
MR safe	The device, when used in the MRI environment, has been demonstrated to present no additional risk to the patient or other individual, but may affect the quality of the diagnostic information. The MRI conditions in which the device was tested should be specified in conjunction with the term MR safe since a device which is safe under one set of conditions may not be found to be so under more extreme MRI conditions	An item that poses no known hazards in all MRI environments. Using the new terminology, "MR safe" items include non-conducting, non-metallic, non-magnetic items such as a plastic Petri dish. An item may be determined to be MR safe by providing a scientifically based rationale rather than test data.	'MR' in green in a white square with a green border, or the letters 'MR' in white within a green square.
MR compatible	A device shall be considered "MR compatible" if it is MR safe and the device, when used in the MRI environment, has been demonstrated to neither significantly affect the quality of the diagnostic information nor have its operations affected by the MR system. The MRI conditions in which the device was tested should be specified in conjunction with the term MR safe since a device which is safe under one set of conditions may not be found to be so under more extreme MR conditions. Using this terminology, MRI testing of an implant or object involved assessments of magnetic field interactions, heating, and, in some cases, induced electrical currents while MR compatibility testing required all of these as well as characterization of artifacts	No longer applies	
MR conditional		An item that has been demonstrated to pose no known hazards in a specified MRI environment with specified conditions of use. Field conditions that define the MRI environment include static magnetic field strength, spatial gradient, dB/dt (time-varying magnetic fields), radiofrequency (RF) fields, and specific absorption rate (SAR). Additional conditions, including specific configurations of the item (e.g. the routing of leads used for a neurostimulation system), may be required. In particular, testing for items that may be placed in the MRI environment should address magnetically induced displacement force and torque, and RF heating. Other possible safety issues include, but are not limited to, thermal injury, induced currents/voltages, electromagnetic compatibility, neurostimulation, acoustic noise, interaction among devices, and the safe functioning of the item and the safe operation of the MR system	'MR' in black inside a yellow triangle with a black border. Item labeling must include results of testing sufficient to characterize the behavior of the item in the MRI environment.
MR unsafe		An item that is known to pose hazards in all MRI environments. MR unsafe items include magnetic items such as a pair of ferromagnetic scissors	MR' in black on a white field inside a red circle with a diagonal red band

of many personal items taken for granted – clipboards, pens, watches, scissors, clamps, credit cards, eyeglasses, paper clips, etc. [25–27]. MRI safety issues include implanted objects (i.e. cardiac pacemakers), ferromagnetic attraction creating "missiles," noise, biological effects of the magnetic field, thermal effects, equipment issues, and claustrophobia. Some stainless steel may contain ferritic, austenitic, and martensitic components [28–30]. Martensitic alloys contain fractions of a crystal phase known as martensite, which has a body-centered cubic structure, is prone to stress corrosion failure and is ferromagnetic. Austenite is formed in the hardening process of low carbon and alloyed steels, and has ferromagnetic properties. Iron, nickel, and cobalt are also ferromagnetic. For this reason, the components of any implanted device should be carefully researched prior to entering the magnet. Stainless steel or surgical stainless objects interacting with an external magnetic field may produce translational (attractive) and rotational (torque) forces. Intracranial aneurysm clips, cochlear and stapedial implants, shrapnel, intraorbital metallic bodies, and prosthetic limbs may move and potentially dislodge. Special precautions should be taken with cochlear implants in the 3 T environment as those non-removable magnets may suffer demagnetization in the scanner [31]. Some eye make-up and tattoos may contain metallic dyes and therefore cause ocular, periorbital and skin irritation [32,33]. Some tissue expanders employed in reconstructive surgery have a magnetic port to help identify the location for intermittent injections of saline [34]. Bivona® tracheostomy tubes (Smiths Medical, Kent, United Kingdom) usually contain ferrous material (although not specified in the package insert) and should be replaced with a Shiley® tracheostomy tube (Covidien-Nellcor, Boulder, CO, USA) prior to entering the MRI environment. Recognizing the unique hazard posed by the MRI environment, in 2008 the Joint Commission issued a Sentinel Event Alert [22].

Cardiac pacemakers present a special hazard in and around the MRI scanner, especially in patients who are pacemaker dependent. Most pacemakers have a reed relay switch that can be activated when exposed to a magnet of sufficient strength [35]. This activation could convert the pacemaker to the asynchronous mode. There are at least two known cases of patients with pacemakers who died from cardiac arrest while in an MRI scanner. The autopsy of one patient determined that the death was the result of an interruption of the pacemaker in the magnetic environment [36]. In addition to the risk of pacemaker malfunction, there is also the chance that torque on the pacer or pacing leads may create a disconnect or microshock [37]. Recent studies demonstrate that with careful preparation, select patients with permanent pacemakers and implantable cardioverter-defibrillators may

safely undergo imaging in the 1.5 T environment without any inhibition or activation of their device [38]. Patients with implanted cardiac pacemakers or cardioverter-defibrillators should only be scanned in locations staffed with radiologists and cardiologists of appropriate expertise [20]. In general, MRI should not be performed on patients with implanted electronic devices. When MRI is considered essential by the referring physician and consulting radiologist, a plan for managing these patients during the scan should be developed in collaboration with the ordering/referring physician, medical director or on-site radiologist and other appropriate consultants (e.g. the patient's pacemaker specialist or cardiologist, or device manufacturer). For implanted pacemakers and implantable cardioverter-defibrillators, it is anticipated that the cardiologist will be physically available during the scan in case the device malfunctions [21]. Following the MRI, a cardiologist should confirm function of the device and recheck it within 1–6 weeks.

The biological effect of MRI should be considered when offering parent-present induction to a parent who is pregnant. To date, there is no evidence to support the risk of MRI-caused chromosomal aberrations in humans. Studies in amphibians demonstrate that exposure to a 4 T magnetic field does not cause any defects in embryological development [33]. Most institutions do not routinely allow pregnant women to accompany their children into the MRI scanner. MRI scans during pregnancy are discouraged by the American College of Radiology during the first and second trimesters, unless fetal imaging is required or the MRI is necessary for emergency medical care [39].

Some patients experience claustrophobia and have difficulty co-operating during the study. Anxiety reactions [40] are estimated to occur in 4–30% of patients [41]. Patients with extreme skeletal abnormalities such as advanced scoliosis or flexion contractures, although motivated, may be unable to lie motionless or supine on the solid, uncushioned MRI table for the extended duration of a spine MRI. These patients may require general anesthesia for positioning and comfort or may need adjunctive pain medication.

Current advances in physiological monitors and anesthesia machines for the MRI environment have optimized the ability of the anesthesia care provider to provide safe care in the MRI suite. Remote monitor displays make it unnecessary for the anesthesiologist to remain in the scan room during most of the procedure; only during breath-holding procedures or contrast injection is it necessary for the anesthesiologist to enter the scanner room during the imaging procedure. The Dräger Fabius® anesthesia machine (Dräger Medical AG, Lubeck, Germany) was designed for use with MRI and approved by the FDA in 2008 for use within both a 1.5 T and 3 T magnetic field up to field strength of 400 gauss (Fig. 36.1). The Fabius, equipped with two vaporizers, has an electronically controlled ventilator capable of delivering multiple modes of ventilation in the MRI suite.

Advances in physiological monitoring now offer the ability to monitor electrocardiogram and pulse oximetry in a 1.5 T and 3 T MRI scanner via wireless, fiber-optic communication (Invivo Precess®, Invivo, Orlando, FL and Medrad Veris® Monitor, Indianola, PA) (Fig. 36.2). Conventional electrocardiogram (ECG) monitoring is not possible because as the lead wires traverse the magnetic

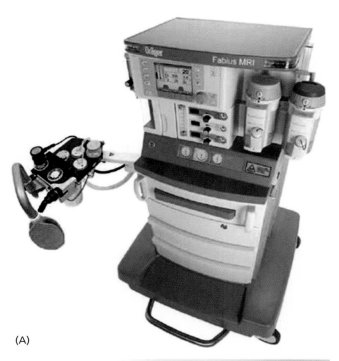

(A)

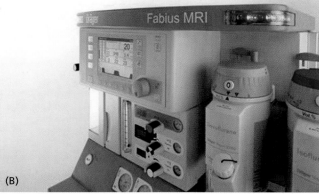

(B)

Figure 36.1 (A) Modern MRI-compatible anesthesia machine, with two vaporizers and ventilator capable of multiple ventilation modes. This system is certified for function in 1.5 and 3 T MRI systems. The machine must be situated outside the 400 gauss magnetic field radius for proper functioning. (B) Close-up view of the magnetic field detection alarms; system alarms when in a magnetic field of 400 gauss or more. Courtesy of Drager Medical Inc., Telford, PA, USA.

fields, image degradation occurs and, most important, the ECG leads will heat and cause patient burns. Fiber-optic ECG monitoring is necessary to minimize the risk of patient burn. Even with fiber-optic cables, it is important to recognize that the connections between the ECG pads and the telemetry box are still hard-wired, and careful attention must be paid to prevent frays, overlap, exposed wires and knots in the cables [42]. It is advisable to provide an interface between the patient's skin and the ECG leads (face cloth). There have been reports of burns from the ECG leads as a result of a current generated between the leads and the patient's sweat. Pulse oximeters are also fiber-optic. Failure to remove the conventional pulse oximeter probe/adhesive has resulted in second- and third-degree burns [42,43]. Respiratory and anesthetic gas monitoring has advanced to the point that complete monitoring, as would occur in the operating room, is now routine with MRI-compatible equipment. For patients with a natural airway, a divided nasal cannula, both to administer supplemental oxygen and to monitor end-tidal CO_2 to detect airway obstruction and to ensure optimal ventilation, is important [44].

Despite the advancing technology in physiological monitors and anesthesia equipment, the MRI environment continues to pose some limitations for anesthesia care. Core temperature monitoring cannot be monitored in the MRI scanner – surface (skin) temperature monitoring cables are available but axillary temperature may not be an adequate substitute for rectal or esophageal temperatures. There are no MRI-conditional nor safe fiber-optic bronchoscopes; difficult airway management must occur outside the MRI scanner room at a safe distance from the magnet.

The advent of special MRI-compatible infusion pumps for agents such as propofol allows the pump to be deployed in the scan room itself, with short tubing lengths to allow accurate delivery of the intended drug or fluid dose. These pumps include the MRIdium® (iRadimed Corp., Winter Park, FL, USA), and Medrad Continuum Infusion System® (Warrendale, PA, USA) (Fig. 36.3). These pumps have remote consoles so that the infusion rates can be changed from the MRI control room via wireless communication algorithms. Although some conventional infusion pumps (Medfusion® 3500 syringe pump, Smiths Medical, Kent, United Kingdom) claim safety in an MRI environment beyond specified distances from the magnet, depending on magnet strength, it is not recommended that these devices be used in the scanner room. Besides the MRI safety aspect, the magnetic and radiofrequency fields can cause pump malfunction in standard systems. An alternative is to utilize standard infusion pumps just outside the door of the scanner room, with multiple lengths of infusion tubing threaded under the door, reaching inside the bore of the scanner to the patient.

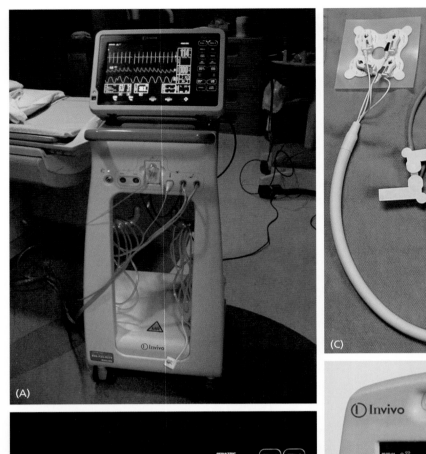

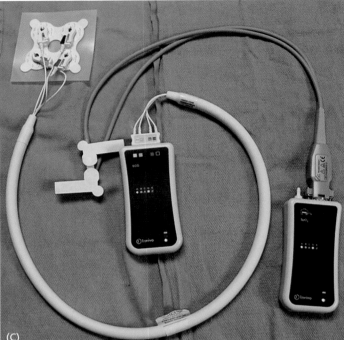

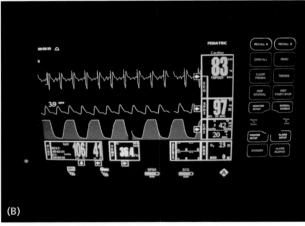

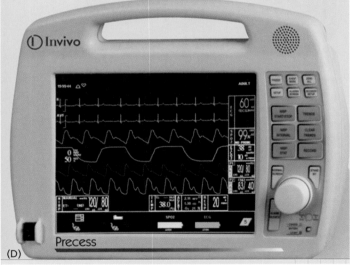

Figure 36.2 Modern MRI-compatible monitor, situated in MRI scanner room. These monitors are capable of monitoring ECG, SpO$_2$, oscillometric blood pressure, end-tidal CO$_2$ via nasal cannula, endotracheal tube, or laryngeal mask airway, anesthetic gases, temperature, and two invasive blood pressures. (B) Remote display in control room. (C) Wireless technology for ECG and SpO$_2$ which minimizes artifacts and allows accurate signal transmission. (D) Close-up of monitor screen with all parameters displayed. Courtesy Invivo Corp., Orlando, FL, USA.

This is commonly used for patients receiving vasoactive infusions requiring very accurate microinfusion pumps. Problems with this approach include increased resistance through the long tubing causing pump malfunction.

The magnetic field may also affect the ECG. The changes in the T-wave are not due to biological effects of the magnetic field but rather to superimposed induced voltages. This effect of the magnetic field on the T-wave is not related to cardiac depolarization, since no changes to the P, Q, R or S wave have ever been observed in patients exposed to fields up to 2 T. There are no reports of MRI affecting heart rate [45], ECG recording [46], cardiac contractility [47] or blood pressure [48]. One study, however, found that humans exposed to a 2 T magnet for 10 min developed a 17% increase in the cardiac cycle length (CCL, the duration of the R-R interval). The CCL reverted

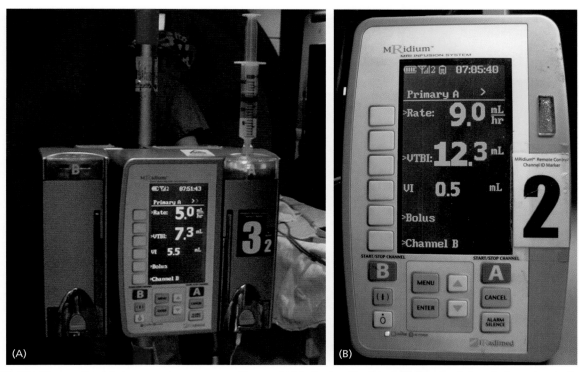

Figure 36.3 (A) MRI-compatible infusion pump in scan room, with propofol infusing in a 7 kg infant. (B) Remote wireless display and controller.

to pre-exposure length within 10 min of removing the patient from the magnetic field [49]. The implications of this finding are unclear. While this change in patients with normal hearts may be of no consequence, the implications of this finding in patients with fragile dysrhythmias or sick sinus syndrome have yet to be determined.

Average noise levels of 95 decibels (dBA) have been measured in a 1.5 T MRI, comparable to noise levels of very heavy traffic (92 dBA) or light road work (90–110 dBA). Exposure to this level of noise has not been considered hazardous if limited to less than 2 h per day [50]. There are case reports, however, of both temporary [51] and permanent [52] hearing loss after an MRI scan. 3 T magnets offer the advantage of less image degradation and improved neuro- and musculoskeletal imaging. However, as the field strength increases, so does the noise [53]. In fact, the peak sound pressure level of a 3 T magnet exceeds 99 dBA, the level approved by the International Electrotechnical Commission. Ear protection is required for all patients undergoing MRI studies for research purposes [20]. Earplugs or MRI-compatible headphones are strongly encouraged for all patients and personnel (family members included) who remain in the 3 T magnet during imaging. fMRI provides additional challenges in the 3 T environment: the noise of the 3 T can interfere with the acoustic stimulation generated for purposes of obtaining the fMRI [54,55].

Although studies in mice [56] and dogs [57] suggest that exposure to magnetic fields may increase body temperature, it is unlikely that static magnetic fields up to 1.5 T have any effect on core body temperature in adult humans [58]. This may be of greater concern in infants and small children, for example in cardiac MRI studies which require a long time [59]. The specific absorption rate (SAR) is measured in watts/kg and is used to follow the effects of radiofrequency heating. The FDA allows a SAR of 0.4 W/kg averaged over the whole body [60]. *Ex vivo* exposure of large metal prostheses to fields over six times that experienced in MRI have not revealed any appreciable heating [61]. So far, there has been no conclusive evidence that RF is a significant clinical issue in magnets up to 3 T. Conversely, the need for a cool room to ensure functioning of the MRI scanner and the lack of MRI-compatible forced-air warming systems, combined with the frequent need for small infants to undergo MRI scanning, frequently results in hypothermia. Often the best prevention is to swaddle the infant in warmed blankets before the procedure to minimize heat loss, and utilize a condenser humidifier if an endotracheal tube or laryngeal mask airway (LMA) is used to manage the airway.

Intravenous gadopentetate dimeglumine (gadolinium) is used to enhance MRI images. With an elimination half-life of 1.3–1.6 h, gadolinium is excreted via the kidneys after forming a complex with chelating agents

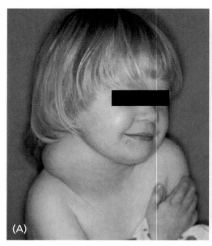
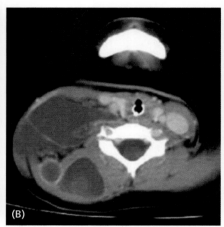
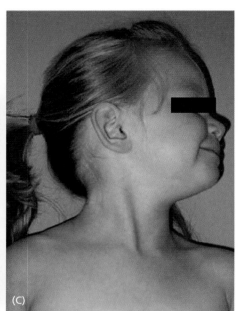

Figure 36.4 Macrocystic lymphatic malformation of the neck and right upper extremity, treated with direct injection of ethanol and then four sessions of OK-432 injection. The ethanol injections were ineffective, but the OK-432 resulted in complete regression of the mass. (A) Clinical photograph before OK-432 sclerotherapy shows a large focal right neck mass. (B) Axial CT scan after intravenous contrast medium injection shows macrocysts in the right neck. The thick-walled cyst was previously injected with ethanol. (C) Clinical photograph taken 1 year after four injections of OK-432 shows complete regression of the right neck mass. Reproduced from Burrows and Mason [214] with permission from Lippincott Williams and Wilkins.

[62]. Adults and children have similar elimination half-lives with 95% excreted within 72 h [63]. Because gadolinium does not contain iodine, it does not produce an osmotic load [64]. Important warnings from the FDA suggest that patients with advanced kidney failure are at risk of developing nephrogenic systemic fibrosis (NSF) or nephrogenic fibrosing dermopathy (NFD) after gadolinium-based MR contrast agents. The FDA first notified healthcare professionals and the public about this risk in June 2006. The American Society of Anesthesiologists MRI Advisory Panel concluded that the anesthesiologist should not administer gadolinium to patients with acute or severe renal insufficiency because of the elevated risk of nephrogenic systemic fibrosis. Rather, the need for and actual administration of gadolinium contrast in this patient group should be the responsibility of the radiologist, nephrologist, and other appropriate consultants [21].

Interventional radiology and angiography

Interventional techniques include non-vascular and vascular intervention [65]. Embolization and sclerotherapy are utilized for treating vascular malformations, aneurysms, fistulas, and hemorrhage as well as accomplishing renal ablation and presurgical embolization of hypervascular masses. Percutaneous transluminal angioplasty and

fibrinolytic therapy are emerging techniques in pediatric institutions. Even in the smallest babies, great success is being reported, and the important contribution that adequate sedation and analgesia can make to ultimate outcome has been recognized [66].

Vascular malformations are congenital aberrant connections between blood vessels and may be composed of lymphatic, arterial, and venous connections (Fig. 36.4). These lesions, present at birth, are often discrete and not clearly visible, although they may expand rapidly, growing with the child. This rapid proliferative phase may occur in response to hormonal changes (pregnancy, puberty), trauma, or other stimuli [67]. Moreover, they may be high-flow or low-flow lesions, depending on which vessels are involved. High-flow lesions include arteriovenous fistulas, some large hemangiomas, and arteriovenous malformations. High-output cardiac failure and congestive heart failure with possible pulmonary edema should be anticipated, especially with high-flow lesions. Low-flow lesions consist of venous, intramuscular venous, and lymphatic malformations.

Because vascular malformations enlarge over time, even asymptomatic lesions may require intervention. Symptomatic patients may suffer from pain, tissue ulceration, disfigurement, airway or cardiovascular compromise, impairment of limb function, coagulopathy, claudication, hemorrhage, and progressive nerve degeneration or palsy. Because large vascular lesions require multiple embolizations, parents and patients are often comforted by seeing familiar faces, another benefit of having a team of anesthesiologists staffing the radiology suites. Vascular embolization can be used as a bridge to surgical resection.

Large hemangiomas may be associated with the coagulopathy of Kasabach–Merritt syndrome. In this condition, the hemangioma traps and destroys platelets and other coagulation factors, resulting in thrombocytopenia and an increased risk of bleeding. As the hemangioma involutes, the coagulation status improves [68]. A condition described as systemic intravascular coagulation (SIC) can occur after the embolization of extensive vascular malformations. This condition is marked by an elevated prothrombin time (PT) with a decrease in coagulation factors and platelets.

When embolizing vascular malformations, radiologists often aim to cut off not only the feeding vessels but also the central confluence (nidus) where much of the arterial shunting occurs. Embolic agents include stainless steel mini-coils, absorbable gelatin pledgets and powder, detachable silicone balloons, polyvinyl alcohol foam, cyanoacrylate glue, and ethanol. The choice of agent depends on the clinical situation and the size of the blood vessel. When permanent occlusion is the goal, polyvinyl alcohol foam and ethanol are often employed. Both occlude at the level of the arterioles and capillaries. Medium to small-sized arteries may be occluded with coils, which are the equivalent of surgical ligation. Particularly in trauma situations, when only temporary (days) occlusion is the goal, absorbable gelatin pledgets or powder are used [69].

Absolute ethanol is injected into vascular malformations to promote sclerosis. Sclerotherapy or embolization with absolute (99.9%) ethanol increases the risk of developing a postprocedure coagulopathy [70] marked by positive d-dimers, elevated PT and decreased platelets. Ethanol causes thrombosis because it injures the vascular endothelium [71]. It also denatures blood proteins. Extensive ethanol injections can cause hematuria and urinary catheters should be inserted to monitor urine output, diuresis, and hematuria. Liberal intravenous fluid replacement will ensure that the hematuria clears prior to discharge. Ethanol can cause neuropathy and tissue necrosis if not injected selectively. Finally, ethanol can also produce significant serum alcohol levels (Fig. 36.5). Up to 1 mL/kg of ethanol can be administered; blood ethanol levels have been greater than the intoxication level of 0.008 mg/dL [72]. Patients with high serum ethanol levels are either sedated or extremely agitated, depending on their individual response to intoxication.

Embolization or balloon occlusion of arterial venous malformations (AVM), vascular tumors, intracranial

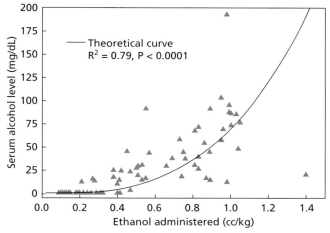

Figure 36.5 Graph shows the positive relationship between serum ethanol level and amount of ethanol administered. Solid line indicates the theoretic curve, where x is the amount of ethanol administered, and y is the predicted serum ethanol level. Triangles represent empirical values. Reproduced from Mason et al [72] with permission from the Radiological Society of North America.

aneurysms and fistula carries considerable risk of catastrophic results. Such risks include a sudden intracranial hemorrhage, acute cerebral ischemia, or catheter or balloon migration. If sedated, the patient may require urgent airway management. Very long cases require a urinary catheter, especially if contrast material is utilized. AVMs involving the head and neck frequently require cannulation of the external carotid artery branches and the thyrocervical trunk. All patients scheduled for embolization should be typed and cross-matched for blood. Those patients who undergo embolization of AVMs of the head and neck are at risk for stroke, cranial nerve palsies, skin necrosis, blindness, infection, and pulmonary embolism [73]. It is important to assess and document the full return of baseline neurological status after the patient is extubated.

Recent advances over the past decade have involved the use of provocative testing during cerebral imaging in order to identify and protect targeted areas of the brain prior to embolization. Provocative or superselective Wada testing has become an important part of endovascular management of numerous extracranial and intracranial vascular conditions. It can be used with neurophysiological monitoring in cases in which patient co-operation and steadiness are important [74]. Nevertheless, the value of awake neurological assessment (wake-up test) cannot be overestimated when neurophysiological monitoring responses are equivocal. Barbiturates, etomidate and, most recently, propofol have been described as agents able to maintain sedation while still preserving the patient's ability to respond [75–79].

Cerebral angiography requires motionlessness as well as exquisite control of ventilation. Anesthetic technique, in choice of agent as well as in control of arterial CO_2 tension, may affect cerebral blood flow and volume and hence the quality of the scan. Cerebral angiography in children may be performed for the diagnosis or follow-up of moya moya disease and the anesthetic technique should minimize the risk of transient ischemic attacks (TIA) and stroke during the procedure [80]. Other considerations include controlled ventilation to facilitate access to and visualization of the vasculature for the radiologist. In the event of vasospasm or difficult access, the radiologist's direct administration of nitroglycerin in small doses (25–50 µg) may facilitate visualization and access. Occlusion of the venous portion of the AVM without complete occlusion of the arterial inflow vessels could result in acute swelling and bleeding. Vascularity reduction through occlusion of major feeder vessels is the goal of embolizing large AVMs prior to planned surgical excision. This may be accomplished as a staged procedure over several days, involving repeat anesthetics.

Angiographic imaging may be enhanced through the use of glucagon. Glucagon is effective for digital subtraction angiography, visceral angiography and selective arterial injection in the viscera. When needed, glucagon is administered in divided doses of 0.25 mg to a maximum of 1.0 mg intravenously. Risks include glucagon-induced hyperglycemia, vomiting (particularly when given rapidly), gastric hypotonia, and provocation signs of pheochromocytoma [81–83]. Children who receive glucagon should routinely receive prophylactic antiemetics.

Ultrasound-directed procedures

Needle biopsies and drainage procedures (kidney, liver, lung, muscle, unknown mass, unknown fluid) are directed with ultrasound guidance. Ultrasound is useful for placement of difficult central catheters (CVL) and peripherally inserted central catheters (PICC lines). The requirement for general anesthesia versus sedation for ultrasound-guided procedures depends in part on the duration of the procedure, the location involved, the risks associated with the procedure and any procedural requirements. The need for controlled ventilation with breath holding may require an endotracheal tube and general anesthesia. Associated secondary effects of the end-organ disease must be kept in mind in the overall anesthetic care plan.

Nuclear medicine

Nuclear medicine is one of the oldest functional imaging disciplines. These scans are useful for identification of epileptic foci in refractory epilepsy, evaluation of cerebrovascular (moya moya) disease and cognitive and behavior disorders [84]. Anesthesiologists become involved when the child's medical history suggests that procedural sedation would not be appropriate. In order to complete these scans, the child must remain motionless for at least 1 h.

The two most common nuclear medicine studies that require the administration of an anesthetic are single photon emission computed tomography (SPECT) and positron emission tomography (PET) scans. SPECT scans use single photon γ-emitting radio-isotopes and rotating γ-cameras to produce three-dimensional brain images. SPECT scans involve the use of radiolabeled technetium-99 (half-life, 6 h), which has a high rate of first-pass extraction as well as intracellular trapping in proportion to regional cerebral blood flow [85]. This scan is ideal when seeking seizure foci, and often precedes surgical resection of the identified focus. The technetium radionuclide is ideal because it remains intracellular and can be visualized on scan hours after a seizure has occurred. Ideally, the child should be scanned within 1–6 h of the seizure. The radionuclides are physiologically harmless and non-allergenic. Caretakers should, however, wear gloves to minimize contact with radiation-containing secretions.

Positron emission tomography scans use PET and radionuclide tracers of metabolic activity such as oxygen or glucose metabolism [86,87]. Unlike SPECT scans, PET scans should be performed during the seizure itself. Because of the short half-life of the glucose tracer (110 min), the scan is best completed during the seizure or within 1 h thereafter.

In addition to using PET scans for diagnostic purposes, nuclear imaging is also being used as an intraoperative adjunct to identify neoplasms, in much the same way that MR imaging has been incorporated into the surgical suite. Surgical suites are currently being equipped with PET scanners [88]. The anesthetic implications of the nuclear medicine environment involve largely the safety precautions that must be implemented with respect to the radio-active nuclide. All bodily fluids (includes saliva, sweat, urine) must be handled with radiation safety precautions.

Radiation oncology

Radiation oncologists use ionizing photons to destroy lymphomas, acute leukemias, Wilms tumor, retinoblastomas and tumors of the central nervous system in children. Repeat sessions are typical, requiring reliable motionlessness in order to precisely aim the beam at malignant cells while sparing healthy cells. A planning session in a simulator is often scheduled prior to the initiation of radiation therapy so that fields to be irradiated can be plotted and marked.

Radiation therapy is usually very brief and non-painful. The key issue is the anesthesiologist's limited access to the patient. Remote video monitoring as well as ECG and pulse oximeter use are crucial. Two or in some locations three video cameras are used to look at the monitors, the chest, and the face of the patient. Central access in young children helps immensely. It is important to remember that babies undergoing radiation therapy following a prolonged fast are at risk for hypoglycemia; delayed awakening or tremulousness should prompt a glucose determination.

Fractionated radiation therapy divides the total radiation therapy course into discrete daily sessions, allowing normal tissue repair between sessions while the tumor burden is lessened or destroyed. Hyperfractionated or multiple-session daily radiation therapy is a modality reported primarily in adults for head and neck cancer. The rationale for twice-daily fractionation in children is that fractionation to growing bone in rats reduces the growth deficit by 25–30%; the hope is that other normal tissues may be similarly spared during growth [89,90]. While one successful approach has been to give infants an initial formula feed 6 h before their first treatment and keep them NPO until recovery from their second anesthetic 6 h after the first [91], with the current liberalization of NPO guidelines we prefer to give children clear liquids during their recovery from the first anesthetic and keep them NPO thereafter for 4 h prior to the second anesthetic.

Stereotactic radiosurgery (γ-knife) is a major advance in the treatment of selected intracranial AVMs and tumors in children [92]. A focused single large fraction of radiation is used instead of smaller, daily fractions. Stereotactic radiosurgery uses relatively weak intensity γ-rays produced by 201 cobalt-60 (60Co) sources which intersect at a single point where all 201 beams converge to destroy tumors, vascular malformations or abnormal tissue sites within the brain. Normal brain tissue surrounding the abnormality is therefore relatively protected from radiation effects. For optimal results, tumor volume ideally has to be small ($\leq 14\,cm^3$) [93].

The stereotactic procedure begins with a CT scan or MRI, followed by computer calculations for dose and the three-dimensional co-ordinates for the beam. The child is placed in a stereotactic head frame which is screwed into the cranium. Most adults are able to tolerate the entire procedure with local anesthesia or sedation. Adults and older children who tolerate this procedure with sedation alone may vomit as a result of the anxiety, the headache or the location of the tumor itself. Once the calculations are complete, the patient is transferred to the radiosurgery suite. Following the irradiation, the patient is allowed to emerge from the anesthetic [92]. The most common perioperative problem is nausea and vomiting, probably due to radiation sensitivity of the chemoreceptor trigger zone. Because the head frame is heavy and cumbersome, it is difficult for the vomiting patient to turn his or her head in order to protect his or her airway. Children (including most adolescents) typically require a general anesthetic. General anesthesia with tracheal intubation is induced prior to placement of the head frame. The key for removal of the head frame is taped to the frame itself. A nasogastric tube is placed for the day's anesthetic.

Stereotactic radiation therapy is more precise localization of the fractionated radiation dose over the same duration of time as conventional radiation therapy, with the adjunctive use of a head frame. Considerations for the head frame include ease of application, reliability, ability to deliver supplemental oxygen and support the airway with a facemask if needed, and rapid removal of the facial restraint should it become necessary.

Total body irradiation (TBI) is generally performed twice a day over a 6-week period, usually in preparation for a bone marrow transplant. As these patients progress with their TBI treatment and become more immunocompromised, there is an increased risk of acquiring an illness during the course of treatment. Vomiting, respiratory illness, poor nutrition or hypovolemia are all possible. Cancellation of a TBI treatment because of an associated illness is discouraged because it disrupts the course of treatment and could compromise the patient's overall prognosis. Ondansetron in combination with dexamethasone or propofol has been found to be beneficial as a prophylactic for nausea and vomiting in children undergoing TBI and should be considered for first-line antiemetic therapy [94]. Although anesthesiologists are wary of the risks of aspiration, both sedation and general endotracheal anesthesia have been found to decrease the incidence of vomiting with TBI [95,96].

Clinic and office procedures

Endoscopy

Gastrointestinal endoscopy constitutes the bulk of procedures performed by a pediatric gastroenterologist [97]. Depending upon the patient and the type of procedure contemplated (therapeutic versus diagnostic), children may require no sedation, minimal to moderately deep sedation or general anesthesia. Over the past 15 years, the volume of endoscopic procedures has increased by 2–4-fold in the adult community, and has most likely increased at a similar rate in children [98].

Although some recommend that deep sedation be limited to anesthesiologist delivery only [99–105], gastroenterologists have reported that they too are able to safely administer and/or supervise sedation [106]. The American Society of Anesthesiologists' Statement on Safe Use of

Propofol makes the point that when it is not possible to have an anesthesiologist involved in the care of every patient then "non-anesthesia personnel who administer propofol should be qualified to rescue patients whose level of sedation becomes deeper than initially intended and who enter, if briefly, a state of general anesthesia" [107]. It is estimated that one-quarter of all adult endoscopies are performed with propofol sedation [98] although there is a wide variation in pediatric practice [108]. Children with more complex medical problems, anticipated airway difficulties, morbid obesity or behavioral problems can undergo their procedure in the operating room. Regardless of the site of the procedure, all patients scheduled for endoscopy should be evaluated beforehand to confirm that they are appropriate candidates. In addition, the anesthetic technique depends on the procedure, the patient and the skill of the endoscopist as well as the limitations and capabilities of the endoscopy suite.

Esophagogastroduodenoscopy

Access to the airway is limited once a transoral endoscope is in place. It is important to maintain spontaneous ventilation during deep sedation because any airway intervention needed typically requires the removal of the endoscope. The two most stimulating portions of the esophagogastroduodenoscopy (EGD) are transoral and transpyloric passage of the endoscope. A smooth endoscope insertion can be aided by topical spray of local anesthesia to the oropharynx to help eliminate coughing and gagging.

Most endoscopy-related respiratory complications occur during EGD, especially in infants and younger children, when compared to colonoscopy. A combination of factors may contribute, including the large size of the endoscope, partial airway obstruction, and abdominal distension due to air introduced into the stomach as well as sedation, leading to hypoventilation. This has lead several groups to select 6 months of age as the time prior to which general anesthesia with endotracheal intubation is required for the procedure, due to the higher respiratory complication rate in this age group [103,105]. Targeted controlled intravenous infusions (TCI) of propofol, with or without dexmedetomidine, have been used effectively in children (3–10 years) who underwent EGD with spontaneous ventilation without endotracheal intubation. In the presence of dexmedetomidine, the dose–response curve of propofol appeared unaffected [109].

Colonoscopy

Access to the airway is unimpeded during a colonoscopy. Deep sedation can be achieved more readily and if respiratory problems occur, airway interventions are straightforward to manage. Patients undergoing colonoscopy will experience increased stimulation during certain parts of the procedure such as traversing the colon to the splenic flexure and the ileocecal valve. At times, abdominal pressure is applied to help advance the colonoscope. The depth of the anesthetic should be adjusted accordingly.

Endoscopic retrograde cannulation of the pancreas

Many institutions report success of procedural sedation in pediatric patients undergoing endoscopic retrograde cannulation of the pancreas (ERCP) [110,111] but general anesthesia with endotracheal intubation may make the procedure easier to perform, especially if it is of long duration, the patient has significant co-morbid diseases or the procedure is performed with the patient in the prone position.

Psychiatric interviews

Intravenous sodium amobarbital has a long history as an adjunct to psychotherapy, having found its peak use during World War II and immediately thereafter in aiding soldiers to deal with the stresses of combat [112]. This technique has enjoyed a resurgence for diagnostic and therapeutic interventions in adults, although pediatric reports are rare. Weller et al reported success for diagnosis and treatment of prepubertal children and emphasized the "back-up" of an anesthesiologist [113]. The induction of a tranquil state until signs of sedation occur, such as slurred speech, a sense of fatigue, difficulty counting backwards, and "basal" vital signs, is not unlike our daily efforts at anxiolysis during monitored anesthesia care. A bispectral index (BIS®, Aspect Medical Systems, Norwood, MA) monitor may prove to be a useful adjunct as well [114]. The psychiatric interview process under these conditions is fascinating to participate in, if only as an observer. Memory retrieval, for instance the uncovering of relationships between current psychopathology and earlier traumatic life events, or symptom removal via therapeutic suggestions are examples of interventions facilitated by the pharmacologically induced relaxed state made possible by the anesthesiologist during the interview.

Anesthetic management of extramural procedures

In the several decades since the initial guidelines for pediatric sedation outside the operating room were published [115], not only have numerous organizations taken it upon themselves to fashion standards of practice, they have variously acknowledged and in many cases overtly approved the practice of non-anesthesiologist adminis-

Box 36.4 Documents from various societies about sedation services

- State regulations for nurses in all 50 states: www.sedationfacts.org/ sedation-standards/nursing-sedation-regulations
- Practice guidelines from the American College of Gastroenterology (ACG): www.acg.gi.org/physicians/clinicalupdates.asp#guidelines
- American Gastroenterological Association: www.gastro.org/ wmspage.cfm?parm1=4453
- Endoscopic Sedation (8/07) (Medical Position Statement)
- Endoscopic Sedation, Administration of Propofol by a GI, Nonanesthesiologist (4/10) (Medical Position Statement)
- AGA Institute Review of Endoscopic Sedation. Gastroenterology 2007; 133: 675–701
- American Gastroenterological Association. Standards for office-based gastrointestinal endoscopy services. Gastroenterology 2001; 121: 440–3
- American Society for Gastrointestinal Endoscopy (ASGE). Practice Guidelines
- Guideline for sedation and anesthesia in GI endoscopy. Gastrointest Endosc 2008; 68: 815–26
- Position statement: nonanesthesiologist administration of propofol for GI endoscopy. Gastrointest Endosc 2009; 70: 1053–9
- Society of Gastroenterology Nurses and Associates. Position Statement: Statement on the Use of Sedation and Analgesia in the Gastrointestinal Endoscopy Setting (2007)
- ADA House of Delegates. Guidelines for the Use of Sedation and General Anesthesia by Dentists (2007)
- American College of Emergency Physicians. Clinical policy for procedural sedation and analgesia in the emergency department. Ann Emerg Med 1998; 31: 663–77
- Pediatric Committee of the American College of Emergency Physicians. Pediatric analgesia and sedation. Ann Emerg Med 1994; 23: 237–50
- Joint Commission. Moderate Sedation Medication and Patient Monitoring: www.jointcommission.org/AccreditationPrograms/ AmbulatoryCare/Standards/09_FAQs/PC/Moderate_Sedation_ Medication.htm
- American College of Cardiology. Clinical expert consensus document on cardiac catheterization laboratory. J Am Coll Cardiol 2001; 37: 2170–214
- American College of Radiology. Practice Guideline for Pediatric Sedation/Analgesia. Revised 2005 (Res. 42)
- American College of Surgeons. Statement on patient safety principles for office-based surgery utilizing moderate sedation/analgesia, deep sedation/analgesia, or general anesthesia. Bull Am Coll Surg 2004; 89(4): 32–4.

tered sedation and analgesia medications, creating their own standards, guidelines, and policy statements, sometimes reinforced by citing relevant peer-reviewed literature in journals. Furthermore, the regulatory environment is different for every state (Box 36.4). As experts in the continuum of sedation and anesthesiology, we sometimes find ourselves in a cognitively, clinically and diplomatically tense and uncertain situation, which ultimately can only be answered through education, collaboration and consistency of policy, at least at the institutional level. The breadth of these regulations, nevertheless, is staggering.

Standards

Until the 1990s, sedation in the United States was limited predominantly to delivery by anesthesiologists, radiologists, dental medicine and emergency medicine physicians. It now encompasses other specialties which include gastroenterology, intensive care medicine, hospital medicine, pediatric medicine and nursing [116–118]. Worldwide, however, the majority of pediatric sedation is still administered by anesthesiologists. The challenge facing sedation care providers is the lack of consensus on sedation standards with respect to skills, training, qualifications, sedatives, physiological monitoring, NPO guidelines, routes of delivery, and emergency preparedness. A global look at sedation guidelines reveals that there is lack of consistency not only between the specialties within a single continent, but also between the continents. Different specialty societies as well as institutions in the United States and worldwide have published guidelines, policies and recommendations, many of which do not agree [119]. In the United States, in response to the deaths of dental patients after sedation with midazolam, the National Institutes of Health and the American Academy of Pediatrics published two nearly identical consensus documents on sedation in 1985 [120–123]. Depth of sedation was introduced as a continuum, consisting of three levels: conscious sedation, deep sedation, and general anesthesia. Recently the terminology has evolved to include four depths (minimal, moderate, deep sedation and general anesthesia) and eliminate the term conscious sedation [3,124,125]. This terminology has been adopted by the Joint Commission and specialty societies worldwide. Limitations of the sedation continuum have been recognized, particularly the subjective determinants of using patient response to verbal and tactile stimulation in order to determine the sedation depths. Future efforts should be made to identify objective criteria in order to determine depth of sedation and, more important, the risk of adverse events [126].

Organization

At a minimum, safe patient care requires appropriate anesthesia equipment and monitors and adequate space and experienced ancillary providers who are knowledgeable and practiced in providing assistance if needed. Each off-site area has its own needs, goals, and guidelines. It is ideal to designate a team of anesthesiologists committed to providing extramural anesthesia care and troubleshooting the logistical challenges in the various locations. Each member should rotate regularly through the different extramural sites in order to maintain familiarity with the procedures, to foster a relationship with the physicians and ancillary personnel and to understand the anesthesia demands unique to each site, including ongoing advances. Technological advances are expanding in the field of radiology, and complicated imaging studies challenge the anesthesiologist to have an understanding of the unique conditions which the study requires.

In the past, extramural locations were not designed with the anesthesiologist in mind. The need for anesthesia had not been anticipated when off-site locations were planned. It is only within the past two decades that the demand for anesthesia services in these sites has substantially expanded. Thus, most off-site locations have not been configured to support an anesthetic. Ideally, anesthesiologists should be involved in the early stages of site design to ensure that minimum standards for anesthesia delivery are met and to troubleshoot engineering issues and advocate for adequate space for anesthetic induction and emergence [114,127]. Physical plant considerations for MRI site planning have been previously described [128]. When anesthesia services are requested, these sites may not meet minimum standards [129] and will require re-engineering to meet minimum requirements of the ASA. The anesthesia machine should be equipped with back-up supplies of E cylinders filled with oxygen and nitrous oxide. If pipeline oxygen is not available, then oxygen should be supplied from H cylinders (6600 L) rather than the smaller E tanks (659 L). For MRI locations in particular, induction of anesthesia or sedation is often best accomplished in an induction area, immediately outside the scanner room, to allow full access to the patient and use of non-MRI compatible equipment such as laryngoscopes. Issues such as airway obstruction, emergence or need for resuscitation are best addressed in such a location and not in the scanner room.

Scavenging systems should be carefully evaluated in the extramural location. Unlike the OR, passive scavenging systems may not always be possible. A safe means of active scavenging may be provided by the vacuum at the wall or wall suction canisters. A scavenging system should be dedicated solely to waste gases. Many MRI scanners do not have wall suction because MRI-compatible wall suction is not widely available. If the suction is located outside the MRI suite, then a mouse-sized hole may be created in the suite's wall to allow suction tubing to be passed inside [128]. A standard anesthesia cart at each anesthetizing location should be fully stocked with essential medications, necessary additional equipment, a spare self-inflating (Ambu®) bag, endotracheal tubes, LMAs, suction catheters, intravenous supplies, laryngoscope handles and blades, and a variety of oral and nasopharyngeal airways [129].

Electrical circuitry and lighting in extramural locations may not be up to operating room standards even if the outlets are grounded and up to hospital grade. Although some extramural locations carry minimal risk of electrical shock or electrocution, these sites do not have line-isolation monitors (LIM) and will not warn of excess leakage of current. Supplemental lighting for record keeping, label verification, establishment of IV access, and visualization of the patient is critical. Even under the best circumstances, for example, lighting is dim in the MRI scanner and monitoring by simple clinical observation can be limited. Anesthesia personnel may not always remain and video monitoring or hardwiring through reinforced walls can allow remote video display of the patient and physiological monitors within.

A storage area large enough to stock anesthesia equipment and supplies must be easily and quickly accessible. This area should be routinely checked, restocked and kept locked when anesthesia services are not required. The need for redundancy of non-disposable supplies is a matter of philosophy. Are two laryngoscopes enough or should there be a third? Is one ECG monitor enough or should there be a battery-operated monitor for back-up and transport? Drugs should be checked per the usual operating room routine and expired medications replaced. Gas cylinder supplies must be reliable, especially in areas without piped oxygen. A code cart should be conveniently located in an area known to all physicians and ancillary personnel. This cart should be routinely checked and restocked. With larger volumes of patients making these significantly sized critical care areas, strong consideration should be given to having a difficult airway cart available at extramural locations.

Finally, extramural anesthetizing locations are often distant from the operating room. Patients may need to remain anesthetized during transport to or from the extramural location. For these circumstances, assured elevator access with key-controlled emergency over-rides is a must. All anesthesiologists who deliver extramural services should be familiar with their surroundings. Checklists are invaluable to guarantee consistent patient care, anesthesia monitoring, equipment, documentation, and back-up assistance.

Practitioners

Interdisciplinary skepticism is abundant and the need for leadership remains crucial; a director of anesthesia and sedation at an extramural location can orchestrate, facilitate and co-ordinate these services as well as educate all clinical stakeholders and the public. Specific guidance is provided in several standards (Box 36.5) from the ASA, especially "Statement on Granting Privileges for Administration of Moderate Sedation to Practitioners Who Are Not Anesthesia Professionals" and further in "Continuum of Depth of Sedation: Definition of General Anesthesia and Levels of Sedation/Analgesia" (Table

Box 36.5 American Society of Anesthesiologists: relevant guidelines for extramural sedation and anesthesia

Statement on Granting Privileges for Administration of Moderate Sedation to Practitioners who are not Anethesia Professionals	Approved by the ASA House of Delegates on 25 October 2005, and amended on 18 October 2006
Continuum of Depth of Sedation: Definition of General Anesthesia and Levels of Sedation/Analgesia	Approved by the ASA House of Delegates on 27 October 2004, and amended on 21 October 2009
Guidelines for Ambulatory Anesthesia and Surgery	Approved by the ASA House of Delegates on 15 October 2003, and last amended on 22 October 2008
Guidelines for Office-Based Anesthesia	Approved by the ASA House of Delegates on 13 October 1999, and last affirmed on 21 October 2009)
Statement on Granting Privileges to Non-anesthesiologists Practitioners for Personally Administering Deep Sedation or Supervising Deep Sedation by Individuals who are not Anesthesia Professionals	Approved by the ASA House of Delegates on 18 October 2006
Statement on Non-operating Room Anesthetizing Locations	Approved by the ASA House of Delegates on 15 October 2003 and amended on 22 October 2008
Statement on Respiratory Monitoring During Endoscopic Procedures	Approved by the ASA House of Delegates on 21 October 2009
Statement on Safe Use of Propofol	Approved by the ASA House of Delegates on 27 October 2004, and amended on 21 October 2009

36.3). By being available to answer questions, provide on-site consultation, examine patients and provide support or emergency airway expertise, the anesthesiologist can also guide a nurse-administered sedation program. Nurses who provide sedation under the supervision of the ordering physician should be Pediatric Advanced Life Support (PALS) and Basic Life Support (BLS) certified. The Joint Commission requires that individuals who administer sedation are able to rescue patients from whatever level of sedation or anesthesia is achieved, whether intentional or unintentional [22]. This is the context within which the ASA documents were created. Attention to the sedation continuum and a paean for translating subjective assessments to more consist-

ently measureable physiological endpoints has recently been published [126].

As recommended by the Joint Commission, sedation-related policies and procedures should be part of a quality assurance initiative which should accompany all sedation programs. Ideally, adverse events such as failed or prolonged sedations, paradoxical reactions, hypoxia, emesis, unscheduled admission, cardiac or respiratory events should be identified and entered into a computerized database. In addition, the extramural nurse should call all patients and families within 24 h in order to follow up on patient outcome and identify any delayed adverse events.

Scheduling and preparation of patients

Appropriate planning for an anesthetic begins with familiarity with the procedure. The requesting service (i.e. neurology, surgery) orders the procedure and then leaves the logistics of scheduling to the extramural service (radiology, anesthesiology). Radiologists recognize that the administration of an anesthetic will lengthen their total time commitment to a patient and potentially limit the number of procedures accomplished in a day [130,131]. A well co-ordinated system for screening patients on the day of the procedure is important. Experienced personnel, ideally a certified pediatric nurse practitioner (CPNP), should be designated to take initial vital signs, review recent medical history, begin IVs if necessary and familiarize the family with the upcoming procedure, including anesthesia.

Screening patients for extramural procedures may be challenging and time consuming. Many children are chronically ill, nutritionally impaired, and medically complicated. These issues must be carefully addressed through attention to the patient's history, physical examination, old medical records, outside consultations and close communication with other medical colleagues. Several consultants may need to confer in order to fully understand the patient's current state of health. Not every procedure is elective. Urgent procedures may be required despite an upper respiratory tract infection (URI), ongoing pneumonia, deteriorating physical status, untreated gastroesophageal reflux, sepsis or hemodynamic instability. In these situations, consultation between the anesthesiologist, the requesting physician and the radiologist should confirm urgency. Anesthesia plans should be adjusted to accommodate the requirements of the procedure (e.g. breath holding for chest CT scan) and the patient's medical condition.

It is not always possible for an anesthesiologist to provide sedation and anesthesia for all children when there is a large volume of cases. A structured nursing sedation program can provide safe and effective sedation. In many hospitals the requesting department "outsources" responsibility for sedation to another

Table 36.3 Continuum of depth of sedation: definition of general anesthesia and levels of sedation/analgesia*

	Minimal sedation (anxiolysis)	Moderate sedation/analgesia ("conscious sedation")	Deep sedation/analgesia	General anesthesia
Responsiveness	Normal response to verbal stimulation	Purposeful** response to verbal or tactile stimulation	Purposeful** response following repeated or painful stimulation	Unrouseable even with painful stimulus
Airway	Unaffected	No intervention required	Intervention may be required	Intervention often required
Spontaneous ventilation	Unaffected	Adequate	May be inadequate	Frequently inadequate
Cardiovascular function	Unaffected	Usually maintained	Usually maintained	May be impaired

Minimal sedation (anxiolysis) is a drug-induced state during which patients respond normally to verbal commands. Although cognitive function and physical co-ordination may be impaired, airway reflexes, and ventilatory and cardiovascular functions are unaffected.

Moderate sedation/analgesia ("conscious sedation") is a drug-induced depression of consciousness during which patients respond purposefully** to verbal commands, either alone or accompanied by light tactile stimulation. No interventions are required to maintain a patent airway, and spontaneous ventilation is adequate. Cardiovascular function is usually maintained.

Deep sedation/analgesia is a drug-induced depression of consciousness during which patients cannot be easily aroused but respond purposefully** following repeated or painful stimulation. The ability to independently maintain ventilatory function may be impaired. Patients may require assistance in maintaining a patent airway, and spontaneous ventilation may be inadequate. Cardiovascular function is usually maintained.

General anesthesia is a drug-induced loss of consciousness during which patients are not arousable, even by painful stimulation. The ability to independently maintain ventilatory function is often impaired. Patients often require assistance in maintaining a patent airway, and positive pressure ventilation may be required because of depressed spontaneous ventilation or drug-induced depression of neuromuscular function. Cardiovascular function may be impaired.

* Monitored anesthesia care does not describe the continuum of depth of sedation, rather it describes "a specific anesthesia service in which an anesthesiologist has been requested to participate in the care of a patient undergoing a diagnostic or therapeutic procedure."

** Reflex withdrawal from a painful stimulus is NOT considered a purposeful response.

*** Rescue of a patient from a deeper level of sedation than intended is an intervention by a practitioner proficient in airway management and advanced life support. The qualified practitioner corrects adverse physiologic consequences of the deeper-than-intended level of sedation (such as hypoventilation, hypoxia and hypotension) and returns the patient to the originally intended level of sedation. It is not appropriate to continue the procedure at an unintended level of sedation.

Because sedation is a continuum, it is not always possible to predict how an individual patient will respond. Hence, practitioners intending to produce a given level of sedation should be able to rescue*** patients whose level of sedation becomes deeper than initially intended. Individuals administering moderate sedation/analgesia ("conscious sedation") should be able to rescue*** patients who enter a state of deep sedation/analgesia, while those administering deep sedation/analgesia should be able to rescue*** patients who enter a state of general anesthesia.

department which could include pediatrics, hospital medicine, anesthesiology, intensive care or emergency medicine. After patient screening, an appropriate referral for either general anesthesia or procedural sedation is the usual result. Because MRI is a unique environment, it is more efficient to have the MRI nurses screen the patient prior to and on the day of the procedure. To ensure consistent decision making, the departments of anesthesiology and radiology should develop a set of guidelines and easily identifiable "red flags" (Box 36.6) to help in this triaging process. If there are any questions or need for additional medical history or studies, the nurse and anesthesiologist must confer before making the final decision regarding general anesthesia or procedural sedation. In addition, chronically ill children often have electrolyte disturbances, coagulation and hematological abnormalities and hemodynamic instability. A consent for the administration of general anesthesia or procedural sedation must be obtained, in line with policies established for anesthesia in the operating room.

Because gastroesophageal regurgitation is common in infants, a detailed clinical history should be taken with regard to the incidence and timing of the regurgitation. If the reflux is predictable (i.e. only associated with mealtimes or soon thereafter), children are usually approved for procedural sedation. NPO guidelines are adjusted to minimize the risk of reflux. For example, if the baby refluxes within 2h of solid feeds but never after 3h, then the NPO guidelines for this infant may be extended to 6h for solids.

Postanesthesia care

Recovery criteria and the postanesthesia care unit (PACU) environment in an extramural location must be no different from the postanesthesia care delivered to children following an operative procedure. Each site must have sources of supplemental oxygen, the ability to deliver positive pressure ventilation, the availability of suction and monitoring equipment and a nursing staff trained in postanesthesia care. Discharge criteria should be estab-

Box 36.6 "Red flags" for sedation

1. **Apnea.** If documented by sleep study, strong clinical history or routine use of an apnea monitor, with significant likelihood of respiratory risk; availability of ICU must be considered.

2. **Unstable cardiac disease.** If cyanotic, depressed myocardial function, significant stenotic or regurgitant lesions, will likely require substantial planning, often in co-ordination with a cardiologist or cardiac anesthesiologist, and availability of ICU.

3. **Respiratory compromise.** Recent (<8 weeks) pneumonia, bronchitis, asthma, respiratory infection; if necessary to proceed, may require general endotracheal anesthesia to control coughing, and availability of ICU.

4. **Craniofacial defect.** Potential for airway difficulty; availability of difficult airway equipment or airway procedures (intubation and extubation) in the OR.

5. **History of a difficult airway.** Potential for airway difficulty; availability of difficult airway equipment or airway procedures (intubation and extubation) in the OR.

6. **Active gastroesophageal reflux or vomiting.** If in poor control, with or without medical or surgical treatment, may require general endotracheal anesthesia with a rapid-sequence induction.

7. **Hypotonia and lack of head control.** If patient is unable to maintain their own airway without assistance, appropriate perioperative planning must include airway support and ICU. Patients with underlying muscular or mitochondrial disorders may have specific anesthetic risks.

8. **Allergies to barbiturates.** Usually the mainstay of a sedation protocol; cross-allergies must be considered.

9. **Prior failed sedation.** Previously unable to be sedated or unsuccessful imaging study because of excessive movement; may require general anesthesia for an optimal study.

10. **Tremors.** Unlikely to be ablated with sedation; may require general anesthesia for an optimal study.

lished by an anesthesiologist in conjunction with the extramural service and its nursing staff.

Analgesic requirements post procedure are extremely variable. While groin puncture may be only mildly annoying for adults, the inability to move about and the ache of blood dissecting subcutaneously causes considerable discomfort in children. Following angiography, all children require a minimum PACU stay of 4 h to ensure that the puncture site does not bleed or develop a hematoma. Ideally, the patient should be pain free and resting supine and motionless in order to minimize the risk of a groin puncture bleed or hematoma. Experienced nursing staff will be able to recognize, manage and call for extra help when they encounter unexpected agitation, delirium or an unanticipated/undesired change in mental status.

Following embolization procedures, patients frequently experience pain or swelling, the severity depending upon the extent of embolization, the agent used for embolization, postembolic swelling and amount of tissue necrosis. A variety of analgesic techniques are available, and the use of steroids perioperatively, while not directly decreas-

ing pain, may be of benefit in reducing edema and postembolic neuritis. Postembolic swelling will influence perioperative airway management for procedures in the head and neck. Pediatric patients may need to remain intubated following such procedures, particularly when edema in the floor of the mouth, tongue, hypo- or oropharynx or anterior neck could compromise the airway.

Nausea or vomiting may increase venous blood pressure because of the Valsalva maneuver, which can aggravate bleeding and swelling in puncture sites or following head and neck procedures. Hypothermia is a risk at some extramural locations because the MRI, CT and interventional radiology equipment require a cool environment. Heating lamps and forced-air heaters may be utilized when safe and appropriate. Finally, with the use of iodine-containing radiocontrast media, sclerosing and embolizing agents, consideration must be given to adequate volume resuscitation and the risk of a contrast reaction as well as bladder catheterization for detection of oliguria, polyuria or hematuria.

Resuscitation

Each extramural anesthetizing location is unique with regard to conducting resuscitation. Redundancy of monitoring devices and equipment is important; one should not be limited to a single item that could malfunction at the time of resuscitation. Patients with multiple allergies, shellfish allergies or atopic disease are at increased risk of exhibiting anaphylaxis to iodine-containing contrast. These patients may benefit from pretreatment with steroids and antihistamines. Areas with restricted access, MRI in particular, should have designated adjacent locations to perform full resuscitation. These areas should be equipped with wall oxygen, suction and full monitoring and resuscitation capability. A self-inflating silicone bag (no ferromagnetic working parts) or non-ferrous Jackson Rees circuit should always be kept inside the MRI suite.

The physicians, nurses, anesthesiologists, technologists and support personnel must know the location of a readily accessible code cart. In addition, a hard board to be placed under the patient during resuscitation should be available. Mock codes should be performed regularly to ensure adequate flow, teamwork and delineation of responsibilities in the event of an emergency. The MRI scanner poses a special problem in the event of cardiorespiratory arrest. Currently, there is no defibrillator which has met FDA approval for entering the MRI environment. Rather, the ASA Task Force on Anesthetic Care for MRI Practice advises that resuscitation be initiated in the MRI scanner as the patient is being removed from the MRI environment to an adjacent area equipped with a defibrillator, physiological monitor and code cart [21].

Protracted resuscitation should never be conducted in the scanner because as support personnel rush inside to assist, unremoved ferrous materials will become projectiles and create an even more hazardous situation. Quenching a magnet should not be an alternative, because it requires a minimum of 3 min to eliminate the magnetic field. In addition, inadequate exhaust during a quench has been known to produce hypoxic conditions in the scanner and has resulted in a patient death. A "black quench" (loss of liquid coolant with resulting coil meltdown) could require replacement of the scanner, a costly and time-consuming undertaking.

Difficult airway management in extramural sites

If a child with a known difficult airway requires endotracheal intubation in order to complete the scheduled procedure, then it is wise to perform the anesthetic induction in the OR, an area where access to difficult airway equipment and extra help is readily available. Regardless of an anesthesiologist's comfort level and familiarity with extramural environments, the same depth of back-up coverage is simply not available.

The unanticipated difficult airway is problematic in a remote location. Therefore it is important to have LMAs stocked in all extramural anesthesia carts. If the trachea cannot be intubated and the lungs cannot be ventilated with a mask, LMAs can provide a successful alternative. Case reports describe the successful use of LMAs in children with difficult craniofacial anomalies, such as Goldenhar syndrome [132,133] and even Pierre Robin sequence [134]. Similarly, a lightwand may facilitate endotracheal intubation in the child with a difficult airway [135]. Recently introduced rigid laryngoscopes with video (e.g. Glidescope®), in infant through pediatric sizes, should be strongly considered for availability in offsite locations.

It is important to recognize that the airway that had not been difficult on induction may become difficult on emergence following sclerotherapy with alcohol and subsequent tissue edema, particularly at the base of the tongue, the neck or the mediastinum [136–138]. These patients will often require several days of airway support and ongoing evaluation in the intensive care unit until tissue swelling and airway compromise are no longer a concern.

Blood loss management outside the operating room

Transfusion requirements are rare in extramural locations, yet preprocedural anemia, accidental perforation of vascular structures or medical transfusion requirements such as sickle cell disease or prematurity may require transfusion therapy. Equipment familiar to the anesthesiologist and identical to that available in the operating room is a welcome sight in a life-threatening emergency. Calling for additional help, establishing additional vascular access and co-ordinating with the blood bank are crucial. Having a runner available may be critical when there is no equivalent to a circulating nurse. It may become necessary to involve a surgeon urgently and transport the patient to the operating room, in which case another anesthesia team setting up the OR while the patient is being prepared for transport would be optimal.

Selection of anesthetic technique and agents

The selection of an anesthetic technique, as in any circumstance, depends on the patient's underlying medical condition, age, drug tolerance and anticipated procedure. The assistance of the department of anesthesiology is often sought when prior sedation has failed [139] and therefore the expectation is set that an anesthetic or deep sedation administered by an anesthesiologist will provide ideal conditions and guarantee successful completion of the procedure. The anesthetic care plan will ultimately be a product of institutional expectations, the patient's comorbidities and the anesthesiologist's preference.

Preparation of the stomach and aspiration prophylaxis are of particular concern for urgently scheduled cases (outside NPO guidelines) or when the medical history suggests aspiration risk. If using H2 receptor antagonists, bronchospasm may occur in asthmatic patients because of the relative increased availability of H1 receptors. H2 blockers may also inhibit metabolism of other concurrently administered medications. Metoclopramide accelerates gastric emptying and increases tone in the lower esophageal sphincter, but is associated with a significant incidence of extrapyramidal side-effects in children. Ondansetron works synergistically with other agents through its vagal blocking actions in the gastrointestinal tract as well as through its inhibition of the chemoreceptor trigger zone via serotonin receptor antagonism, particularly for patients undergoing radiation therapy with pulses of chemotherapy [140,141].

The airway management may be influenced by the procedure itself as well as anticipated postprocedure requirements. Access to the patient's airway in locations outside the operating room is often limited – MRI scanners have a long bore with the patient out of the line of sight of the anesthesiologist, radiation therapy accelerators and total body irradiation are sited within a locked room, interventional procedures are often performed so that the patient can be imaged with biplane fluoroscopy and therefore the physical plant is designed to accommodate the imaging equipment and not the needs of the anesthesiologist. Airway obstruction, laryngospasm, and the presence of secretions may all be difficult to determine. Hypoventilation and apnea are difficult or impossible to determine by direct observation. As long as an appropriate plan is chosen and appropriate monitoring used, there is no evidence to support a specific standard for airway management.

Barbiturates may be useful as a sole method of providing sedation. Pentobarbital (Nembutal), for example, has the advantage of providing sedation, causing minimal respiratory and circulatory depression and is rarely associated with adverse events [142]. Barbiturates have no analgesic properties and can produce paradoxical reactions, especially in children. Furthermore, no antagonist to barbiturates is available, so dosing should be carefully titrated. Intravenous pentobarbital by titration has been used successfully by radiologists while monitoring oral and nasal air flow, oxygen saturation with a pulse oximeter (SpO_2), end-tidal carbon dioxide and cardiac rate and rhythm. Transient decreases in SpO_2 in up to 7.5% of patients have been reported; interventions have included stimulation and head repositioning [143,144]. Other studies have described the use of pentobarbital in both the oral and intravenous form [69,145]. For infants less than 1 year of age, oral pentobarbital is more successful and carries a lower rate of adverse events compared to chloral hydrate [145]. The long half-life of pentobarbital (approximately 24 h) requires careful and conservative recovery and discharge guidelines. The dosage of pentobarbital is 2–6 mg/kg po, up to 9 mg/kg in patients who are receiving barbiturate therapy.

Sodium thiopental in a mean induction dose of 6 mg/kg and a mean total dose of 8.5 ± 3 mg/kg has been used successfully as the sole anesthetic for CT/MRI in 200 children from 1 month to 12 years of age [146]. Methohexital has a shorter recovery time than thiopental and is more effective than oral chloral hydrate [147]. Methohexital-induced seizures in patients with temporal lobe epilepsy have been reported. Thiopental and pentobarbital are alternatives for these patients [148]. For patients taking barbiturate-containing anticonvulsant medications, a higher dose limit is generally more successful. Methohexital has also been used intramuscularly (IM) for radiotherapy, in doses of 8–10 mg/kg. The onset time via this route is often twice or three times longer than rectally administered methohexital [149].

Propofol (2,6-di-isopropylphenol) is an intravenous hypnotic agent which is approved by the FDA in the United States for the induction and maintenance of anesthesia. Its package insert specifies that it "be administered only by persons trained in the administration of general anesthesia" [150]. Although propofol does not

have a labeled indication for children less than 3 years of age, it has been used extensively in this age group as a means of providing sedation or anesthesia. Propofol sedation by bolus or continuous infusion for brain MRI can provide successful imaging conditions but with the risk of need for airway intervention and respiratory compromise [151]. A recent comparison of dexmedetomidine with propofol in children with and without obstructive sleep apnea suggests that dexmedetomidine offers the benefit of preserved respiratory drive, less need for artificial airway support and fewer incidences of airway compromise [17,152].

There is a rare, fatal complication known as propofol infusion syndrome (PRIS) with prolonged propofol administration (>48 h) at high doses (>4 mg/kg/h). PRIS is characterized by metabolic acidosis, rhabdomyolysis of skeletal and cardiac muscle, arrhythmias (bradycardia, atrial fibrillation, ventricular and supraventricular tachycardia, bundle branch block and asystole), myocardial failure, renal failure, hepatomegaly and death [153–158]. Sixty-one patients with PRIS have been recorded in the literature, with deaths in 20 pediatric and 18 adult patients. Seven of these patients (four pediatric and three adult) developed PRIS during anesthesia [159–161]. A fatal case of PRIS at a low infusion rate (67 μg/kg/h) has been reported [161]. In 1992 the deaths of five children who had received long-term, high-dose propofol infusions were reported. These children died from myocardial-related causes, presumed to be related to propofol, in conjunction with lipemic plasma, a metabolic acidosis and an enlarged or fatty liver [153]. Propofol should be used with caution for sedation in critically ill children and adults, as well as for long-term anesthesia in otherwise healthy patients, and doses exceeding 4–5 mg/kg/h for long periods (>48 h) should be avoided [162–164].

Fospropofol (Lusedra®) is a recently introduced, class IV water-soluble phosphorylated prodrug of propofol which is hydrolyzed *in vivo* to release active propofol, formaldehyde, and phosphate. It is an appealing alternative to propofol because of the lack of pain with injection, a decreased potential for hyperlipidemia with long-term administration and less tendency for bacterial infection. Its use by non-anesthesiologists, however, has generated some concern because its lower (and more slowly achieved) peak levels could prompt repeat dosing in an effort to enhance its onset of effect, in comparison with an equipotent dose of propofol. In addition, its clinical effect is longer in duration. So far, only adult studies have been published. Fospropofol carries the same FDA labeling as propofol insofar as it is only to be administered by a trained anesthesia provider [165].

Opiates reduce anesthetic and pre- and postprocedure analgesic requirements. They are reversible with naloxone. While opioids may be unnecessary for purely non-painful diagnostic procedures, they may be very useful for therapeutic interventions, especially for those patients with postprocedural pain. They are also useful following anthracycline chemotherapy, when patients have documented impaired myocardial function [166]. Because opioids depress the ventilatory response to CO_2, this respiratory depression may be of particular concern for children with increased intracranial pressure. Opioids may also worsen pre-existing nausea and vomiting, particularly common for children undergoing cancer treatment.

Benzodiazepines have the advantage of anxiolysis with minimal vomiting and cardiorespiratory depression. Diazepam (Valium®) is painful during intravenous injection and may lead to thrombophlebitis; midazolam (Versed®) is water soluble and therefore may be more suitable intravenously or intramuscularly. The elimination half-life of midazolam averages 2.5h, compared to 20–70h for diazepam [167,168]. Young patients or patients with significant liver disease may have prolonged duration and exaggerated effect from benzodiazepines.

Ketamine has enjoyed great popularity during the past 30 years for sedation, analgesia or anesthesia outside the operating room due to its support of the cardiovascular and respiratory systems. Ketamine-induced nightmares, hallucinations, delusions and agitation are rare in children [169,170]. Ketamine sedation programs, administered by registered nurses and supervised by interventional radiologists, have been developed by anesthesiologists for selected patients and procedures [142,171]. This protocol has allowed painful procedures, and even organ biopsies, to be tolerated by patients who previously would have required general anesthesia [142,172].

Dexmedetomidine (Precedex®, Hospira, Lake Forest, IL, USA) is an α2-adrenergic agonist that was initially approved by the FDA in 1999 for up to 24h of IV administration to intubated adults. In October 2008, it received additional approval for procedural sedation of adults in areas outside the intensive care unit setting. It is still awaiting approval for clinical usage in most European countries. It is not FDA approved for pediatric use. Despite the lack of labeling, dexmedetomidine administration has been described via a variety of routes for sedation, anxiolysis, analgesia and as an anesthetic adjunct. Dexmedetomidine is unique in that it produces a state which resembles natural sleep. Animal model studies demonstrated that sedation mimics the endogenous sleep pathway, stimulating the locus coeruleus [173]. Studies in children suggest that the endogenous sleep pathway may be similarly stimulated in the pediatric population. The electroencephalograms (EEG) of children sedated with dexmedetomidine have been shown to resemble those of natural non-REM sleep [174]. Particularly for pediatric sedation for radiological imaging studies, dexmedetomidine alone can, in high doses, achieve immobility for MRI

and CT examinations [175–177]. While it appears to have minimal effects on respiratory drive and the CO_2 response curve, dexmedetomidine administration may be accompanied by bradycardia, hypotension, and hypertension [175,176,178].

With dexmedetomidine administered at induction doses of 2–3 mg/kg/min over 10 min followed by an infusion of 1.5–2 mg/kg/min, up to a 97.6% success rate for MRI scans has been reported. In this dose range, the incidence of bradycardia was 16%, with a mean arterial pressure within 20% of age-adjusted normal ranges [176]. Although the bradycardia may be disconcerting to pediatric anesthesiologists, there are no reports of cardiac arrest or need for cardiopulmonary resuscitation. Moreover, the use of glycopyrrolate to treat the bradycardia is discouraged, as it may result in extreme hypertension [179].

Some patients will require general anesthesia because of previous sedation failures, the need for a secure airway or procedural logistics. Newer, less soluble anesthetic agents such as sevoflurane and desflurane have pharmacokinetic profiles that compare favorably with propofol in adults [180]; there seems little reason to think that would not be the case with children, although pediatric anesthesiologists often avoid using desflurane because of its pungency and associated airway irritability. Since its introduction to clinical practice in the mid-1990s, sevoflurane has become the volatile anesthetic of choice in children. Its lack of airway irritability and its ability to provide children with stable hemodynamic function coupled with its rapid onset and offset make sevoflurane a useful agent [136].

Volatile agent vaporizer performance in the MRI suite has been studied. The output of a Fortec II® vaporizer (Fraser Harlake, Orchard Park, NY) was variable according to the vaporizer's location and the orientation of the bimetallic strip within the magnetic field [181]. The movements of the bimetallic ferromagnetic temperature compensator within the MRI magnetic field altered vaporizer output by as much as 91% of the dialed output concentration. Several other vaporizers examined (Ohio Forane®, Ohio Medical Products, Madison, WI; Ohmeda Isotec IV® vaporizer, Ohmeda, Steeton, England, and the Forane Vapor 19.1®, Dragerwerk AG, Lubeck, Germany) were incompatible with the MRI environment because of stronger ferromagnetic internal component content or the location of a ferromagnetic spring within the temperature compensator. Measuring inspired and end-tidal levels of volatile agents when delivering a general anesthetic in the MRI environment, may provide reassurance. Modern MRI-compatible anesthesia systems have magnetic field detector systems that inform the anesthesiologist when the machine is within a magnetic field strong enough to affect vaporizer and machine performance. In general, situating the machine and vaporizers as far from the magnet as practically possible within the scan room, and following the manufacturer's instructions as to machine operation, will optimize conditions and ensure accurate volatile anesthetic delivery.

Regional anesthesia, rarely administered outside the pediatric operating room, nevertheless remains a valid choice in some circumstances. Intercostal nerve blocks may be very useful for lung or rib biopsies, chest tubes, biliary or subphrenic drainage procedures, and insertion of biliary stents. Nerve block of the brachial plexus by the axillary, interscalene or supraclavicular route has been reported for the brachial approach to catheterization [182,183] and neuraxial block of the lower extremities for femoral catheterizations and percutaneous approaches to the kidney [184]. Spinal anesthesia has been successfully used for repeat painful radiotherapy on lower extremities, in conjunction with regional hyperthermia and limb exsanguination [185].

Indwelling central catheters are implanted in the majority of radiotherapy patients and can be utilized for induction and maintenance of anesthesia, blood draws, intravenous fluid administration and chemotherapy. Dressing changes are often accomplished in conjunction with the sedation or anesthesia. Antiseptic preparation of all injection sites is critical. At the end of the session the catheter should be carefully flushed with heparinized saline. An alternative to central lines is the use of a heparin lock peripheral IV, changed weekly, with careful parental instruction. Smoothness of emergence is particularly important following angiographic procedures because of the risk of dislodging a clot or bleeding at the puncture site. Some of these patients have been heparinized without protamine reversal. Unlike adults, sandbags and weights are not routinely applied to angiographic cannulation sites of children.

Finally, on occasion, the loss of self-control with sedation results in dysphoria, and some patients fare better when completely awake. Minimal medication may be preferable in patients with complicated and unstable medical conditions who may not tolerate the anesthesia or sedation. Some procedures (unilateral carotid barbiturate injection, or Wada test) may require conversation, interaction and responsiveness of the patient. In these situations, no sedation may be the best alternative.

Safety issues for patients and their anesthesiologists

As anesthesiologists find themselves participating in the care of patients requiring increasingly sophisticated imaging technology, it is appropriate to examine the risks for patients and staff exposed to the types of high energies and contrast agents used.

Ionizing radiation

Radiation exposure is directly proportional to the duration of the procedure and inversely proportional to the square of the distance from the source. Henderson et al monitored the radiation exposure of 16 pediatric anesthesia fellows during a 2-month period [186]. Fellows assigned to the cardiac catheterization lab had fluoroscopy exposure time of 14–85 min per case, typically for 2–3 cases per day. For these anesthesiologists, badge readings ranged from 20 to 180 mrem/month. All non-cardiac anesthesia fellows had undetectable (<10 mrem/month) levels. All fellows wore lead aprons, 50% wore a thyroid shield and one stepped at least 10 feet away from the source during every exposure; this latter fellow had a reading of 30 mrem, despite having spent 26 h in the cath lab. The annual maximum permissible dose (MPD) for non-radiation workers (including anesthesiologists) is 100 mrem or 1 mSievert (mSv, SI unit). For comparison, the MPD for radiation workers is 50 mSv annually and 10 mSv times age cumulatively. MPD during pregnancy for radiation workers (per gestation) is 5 mSv. Safety precautions for all anesthesia practitioners include strict requirements to wear lead aprons and thyroid shields in fluoroscopy areas, to wear radiation detection badges and have them measured at regular intervals, step as far away and out of the direct line of radiation as possible, and use mobile transparent, lead-impregnated plastic "walls" as an extra source of protection (Fig. 36.6).

The American College of Radiology has raised public and professional awareness about the risks of ionizing radiation and the importance of tailoring the dosing to the needs of the child. The Society of Pediatric Radiology established the Image Gently campaign to seek alternative methods of lowering radiation exposure to children during imaging studies (www.imagegently.org). This has expanded from radiation during CT imaging to include procedures in interventional radiology [187–189]. Web-based training and education have been developed to offer a quality improvement module for CT safety in children [190].

High-intensity magnetic fields

Magnetic resonance imaging exposes the patient (and the healthcare workers surrounding the patient) to a static magnetic field, a rapid switched spatial gradient magnetic field and radiofrequency magnetic fields. The static magnetic field, which causes alignment of unpaired tissue protons, may cause movement of ferromagnetic devices such as vascular clips, ventricular shunt connectors, casings for pacemakers, and control devices for pacemakers. Metallic devices in other areas, particularly when invested with fibrous tissue, are less problematic [42,191]. As mentioned previously, tissue expanders may have magnetic ports to facilitate identification of the injection site. Despite their low mass, such ports have a potential for

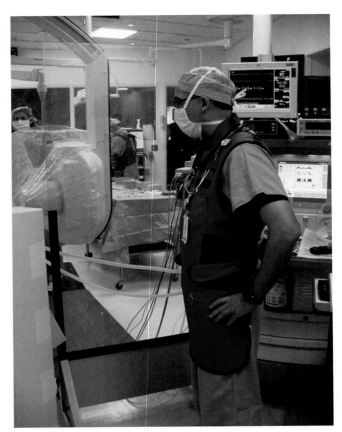

Figure 36.6 Anesthesiologist with proper ionized radiation shielding and safety precautions in a cardiac catheterization laboratory. Note full lead apron with thyroid shield, radiation detection badge, lead-impregnated plastic wall. He is also standing at some distance away from the cameras, and not in the direct line of radiation emission.

torque and movement in the presence of a strong magnetic field so the specific type of tissue expander should be identified prior to patient evaluation in an MRI [34]. Assessment of risk in patients with implants or other possibly ferromagnetic devices or objects consists of a careful history including penetrating wounds, physical examination to look for scars and possibly a plain radiograph of the region in question [192]. Other concerns have been increased blood pressure, cardiac arrhythmias, and impaired mental function. While described or theorized on an experimental basis, little clinical documentation is available.

The magnetic field generates an electrical current 2–3 orders of magnitude less than a defibrillator ($10\,mA/M^2$, compared to 1000–$10,000\,mA/M^2$). This current strength may nevertheless reprogram a programmable pacemaker and interfere with its function [37]. Exposure to a strong external magnetic or electromagnetic field can lead to conversion of a demand pulse generator from synchronous to asynchronous mode, damage to the reed switch (which activates the fixed rate pulse generator), repro-

gramming of pacemaker parameters, induction of currents in the electrode wires, or to displacement of the generator itself. Indeed, it is the sensitivity of some reed switches that has determined the "safety boundary" of magnetic resonance devices as being 5 gauss (5×10^4 T). Patients with implantable defibrillators-cardioverters, implantable infusion (e.g. insulin) pumps, cochlear implants and neurostimulators, are all at risk for having the implant device reprogrammed upon exposure to the magnetic field. Defibrillator failure has been reported in the MRI environment [193].

Radiofrequency (RF) pulses cause heat production in metallic implants and coiled wires such as ECG cables or pulse oximeter cables if looped and lying on the patient's skin. Patients with compromised thermoregulatory abilities, such as those with cardiac problems, fever or taking certain drugs, may be at particular risk. Included in this group are infants, whose SAR is greater than that of adults because of the greater ratio of body surface area to body mass, and whose thermoregulatory abilities may be interfered with during a general anesthetic [58]. SAR refers to the energy absorption (e.g. increasing body temperature) with an increase in the total amount of RF energy absorbed [194].

Increased reports of vertigo, nausea and a metallic taste have been found in a study on human exposure to a 4 T magnetic field (whole-body scanner) [195]. Fertilized frog embryos exposed to a 4 T magnetic field did not demonstrate any adverse effects on early development [33]. An increase in cardiac cycle length of 17% was found in healthy volunteers in a 2 T environment after 10 min of exposure, causing speculation about the effect of the 2 T environment on the sinus node [49]. This may be of particular concern in patients with a pre-existing arrhythmia history. Of more significant concern in pediatric patients is the potential for hypothermia because of the air flow directed through the scanner cavity and the inability to control room temperature or use radiant warmers. The use of warm IV fluid bags, thermal packs, and blankets can decrease heat loss. Excellent reviews of monitoring considerations and equipment choices in the MRI environment as well as patient safety principles are available [26,52,192,194,196,197] and the American College of Radiology (with a representative from the ASA) has published a recent White Paper on magnetic resonance safety [20].

Magnetic resonance imaging and spectroscopy do not employ ionizing radiation. However, secondary harmful effects, such as magnetic objects becoming projectiles within the magnetic field as they approach the bore of the magnet and potentially causing injury, are a consideration [198,199]. Patients (and anesthesiologists) with metallic implants such as vascular clamps, hemostatic clips, dental devices, heart valve prostheses, intravascular coils, filters and stents, ocular implants, orthopedic implants, otological implants, shrapnel, penile implants, and vascular access ports must be individually evaluated for their risk in the MRI environment [200,201].

Use of intravascular contrast media

In a comprehensive review, Goldberg noted that approximately 5% of radiological exams with radiocontrast media (RCM) are complicated by adverse reactions, with one-third of these being severe and requiring immediate treatment [202]. Anaphylaxis during anesthesia has recently been the subject of several consensus conferences [203–205]. Reactions occur most commonly in patients between 20 and 50 years of age and are relatively rare in children. The male:female ratio is about 1:2.5, not dissimilar to the gender distribution of other allergies such as latex, aspirin and neuromuscular blocking agents. With a history of atopy or allergy, the risk of a reaction is increased from 1.5–10-fold. Reactions vary from mild, subjective sensations of restlessness, nausea and vomiting to a rapidly evolving, angioedema-like picture accompanied by respiratory distress, bronchospasm, arrhythmias and cardiac arrest. Because of the high molar concentration of contrast media (often >1000mOsm and sometimes >2000mOsm), caution should be exercised with patients who have a limited cardiovascular reserve such as patients in congestive heart failure or those with cardiomyopathy. In addition, volume-depleted young children (NPO for prolonged intervals, bowel preps) should be prehydrated prior to RCM administration. Because contrast agents are hypertonic, the initial hypertensive response is usually followed by equilibration with the extracellular fluid compartment within 10min, heralded by the onset of diuresis.

Special attention should be paid when administering iodine RCM to any child with a history of congestive heart failure. Patients with hepatic or renal dysfunction should be observed closely for signs of impaired excretion of the RCM. In sickle cell disease, the increase in blood osmolarity may precipitate shrinkage, clumping, and, ultimately, sickling of erythrocytes and vascular occlusion. Sickled cells are known to align with external magnetic fields to which they are exposed; it is unknown how this theoretical concern compares, for example, with the normal forces of deformation imposed on red cells of patients with sickle cell disease in their normal course through the vascular tree [52]. Those patients dependent on a full intravascular volume status (patients with sickle cell disease, cyanotic congenital heart disease with a restricted pulmonary circuit volume, patients with arteriovenous shunts, etc.) should be monitored carefully for an initial rise in filling pressures and intravascular volume and subsequent diuresis following an osmolar load.

Patients with impaired excretory mechanisms, such as those in renal failure, must be monitored closely follow-

ing high osmolar loads. Low osmolar RCM are relatively safe with regard to life-threatening reactions, but moderate non-life threatening reactions requiring some treatment occur 0.2–0.4% of the time and a severe life-threatening reaction can occur in 0.04% of patients [206]. The risk of contrast reaction to non-ionic contrast media is rare. A recent review of 12,494 patients reported overall a 0.46% incidence of contrast reaction, all being mild or moderate and none classified as severe [207].

Gadolinium diethylene triamine penta-acetic acid (DTPA) is a low osmolar ionic contrast medium used for MRI, with a slower clearance in neonates and young infants than adults, yielding longer windows for imaging [208]. Free gadolinium has a biological half-life of several weeks with uptake and excretion taking place in the kidneys and liver. Unfortunately, free gadolinium is quite toxic and is therefore chelated to another structure that restricts the ion and decreases its toxicity. The most common adverse reactions are nausea, vomiting, hives, and headache. Local injection site symptoms include irritation, focal burning or a cool sensation. Transient elevations in serum bilirubin (3–4% of patients) have been reported and a transient elevation in iron for Magnevist® and Omniscan® (15–30% of patients) occurs, which tends to reverse spontaneously within 24–48h [209]. Anaphylactoid reactions occur in the order of 1:100,000 to 1:500,000 and are more rare (<1:100,000 doses) in children.

The older literature states that patients who have had anaphylactic reactions to shellfish are at increased risk of anaphylactoid reaction to RCM. The irony of the statement is that it may be correct but for non-obvious reasons. The original rationale was that shellfish contain high quantities of iodine and therefore it was assumed that there would be a risk of cross-reactivity. However, neither shellfish allergy nor RCM reactions are due to iodine. Atopy *per se* is a risk factor; therefore, the association between atopy and anaphylactic reactions to shellfish and a possible predisposition to a RCM reaction may indeed be valid.

The treatment of severe allergic reactions, whether anaphylactoid or anaphylactic, is no different than for any other allergic reaction. Epinephrine, aminophylline, atropine, diphenhydramine, and steroids have all been employed in order to control varying degrees of adverse reactions. A patient who requires RCM administration and who has had a previous reaction to RCM has an increased (35–60%) risk for a reaction on re-exposure. Pretreatment of these high-risk patients with prednisone and diphenhydramine 1h before RCM administration reduces the risk of reactions to 9%; the addition of ephedrine 1h before RCM administration further reduces the rate to 3.1% [210–212].

Allergic reactions rarely occur with oral agents. The incidence of severe anaphylactoid reactions to gastrointestinally administered agents is approximately 0.004:10,000 and the causes remain unknown. Gastrointestinal complications include nausea, vomiting, and diarrhea. One of the factors that may protect against having an allergic reaction is the poor absorption of oral iodinated contrast agents. Indeed, disruption of the gastrointestinal mucosa is recognized as causing an increase in absorption of oral contrast, and the urinary excretion of contrast in a gastrointestinal study is a well-recognized sign. Yet rarely they will be associated with bronchospasm, flushing, periorbital edema, pruritus, rash, rhinitis, and urticaria.

Conclusion

The demand for anesthesia and sedation services in sites distant from the operating room is continuing to increase. At the Children's Hospital Boston we now have more than 50 multidisciplinary centers focused on specific, complex disorders, often with multiple co-morbidities. Many of these patients require multiple diagnostic and/ or imaging studies for complete evaluation, even if they never are scheduled for surgical repair. Providing patient services in locations remote from the operating room can be challenging and poses risks that may not exist in the operating room. Sedation, monitored anesthesia care, and general anesthesia are all choices which carry risks. Historically, we have considered that avoidance of general anesthesia would minimize the risk of adverse outcome. Closed claims analysis has shown, in adults, that monitored anesthesia care poses risks equal to general anesthesia with respect to severity of injury, death, and permanent brain damage. Furthermore, 24% of all monitored anesthesia care claims involve oversedation and respiratory depression [213]. All stakeholders in the provision of extramural sedation and anesthesia services must recognize that as the demand for these services grows, so also should their ability to understand the specific environment and to perform careful risk analysis when selecting patients and formulating an individual as well as an institutional plan of care.

CASE STUDY

An 18-month-old, 18 kg boy, is scheduled for an MRI of the brain to evaluate new onset of grand mal seizures, photophobia, and increasing irritability. He has been well previously. He is currently on phenobarbital and phenytoin.

This rather large toddler's preanesthetic evaluation has to consider the efficacy of his anticonvulsant therapy because he is on two medications. Grand mal seizures of the tonic-clonic variety are usually the easiest to control, particularly if they originate from a single seizure focus, but generalized tonic-clonic seizures associated with a progressive metabolic disease, or complex partial seizures, are more difficult to control. Multimodal therapy is often required in these circumstances. The history is important here because seizure thresholds may be affected by the administration of or withdrawal from a general anesthetic, in the first case raising the threshold and in the second case lowering it. Therefore, during emergence, the patient may be at increased risk for a seizure.

Many induction plans are acceptable. Intravenous access may be more diffcult prior to induction due to the size of the patient (18 kg at 18 months of age, approximately the size of an average 4 year old), multiple attempts, and the increased stress. Crying and aerophagia would be expected. If a general anesthetic was required we would be inclined to proceed with a parent-present mask induction. If it seemed like deep sedation would be a good strategy and easy intravenous access likely, we would probably plan on using pentobarbital sedation rather than dexmedetomi-

dine, the other alternative we commonly use. The effect of dexmedetomidine on seizure threshold is controversial; some (early) studies indicated that it may lower the seizure threshold, although in these studies enflurane and sevoflurane were used as part of the anesthetic technique. Pentobarbital, on the other hand, would raise the seizure threshhold and perhaps provide a greater margin of safety for this poorly controlled toddler.

With this plan, airway management would likely consist of a natural airway with supplemental oxygen, without any adjunctive devices. Use of a divided nasal cannula capable of end-tidal CO_2 monitoring is an important technique in these patients for early detection of airway obstruction, when the anesthesiologist does not have access to the patient's airway. Video camera monitoring of the patient in the bore of the scanner is often useful to detect inadequate sedation or airway obstruction. Minimal obstruction of the natural airway with preservation of pharyngeal muscle tone will allow the procedure to continue with this level of sedation. If significant upper airway obstruction occurs, the rocking motion of the head, neck, and chest may interfere with the quality of the scan, and therefore the anesthetic plan would need to be modified because the study requires a motionless patient. Total intravenous anesthesia might produce this condition with spontaneous breathing, but flexibility needs to be preserved so that the option exists to progress to a general anesthetic with a laryngeal mask or endotracheal tube.

Safety concerns in the environment of the magnet are critical. Ferrous-containing elements of the anesthetic equipment have to be eliminated for the sake of patient safety as well as the test results. Iron-containing materials become missiles in the MRI scanner, depending on iron content and mass, but magnetic attraction obeys the inverse square law such that the closer it gets to the bore of the magnet, the greater the attraction becomes. Oxygen tanks, tables, and anesthesia machines have been "sucked into" the bore of the magnet. For the anesthesiologist and other medical personnel, anything containing iron in pockets can become projectiles as well, such as stethoscopes, scissors, etc. In addition, personal identification cards such as hospital ID cards and credit cards can have their information rendered useless; beepers and telephones will also have their RF chips scrambled to the point of uselessness.

The duration of PACU stay will depend on how many seizures the patient ordinarily has per day, the competence of the parents in dealing with these seizures, and to some extent the risks of driving home (e.g. distance home, distance to closest hospital, etc.). We would probably keep the patient for 4–6 seizure-free hours in the PACU, with the resumption of his previous PO medications, consultation with his neurologist, and postoperative blood levels, which should be easy to obtain. We would restart his anticonvulsants following the scan. The half-lives are drawn out enough and the onset is long enough that his level will neither decline nor be increased drastically if he resumes his usual PO schedule a few hours later. It will probably be unnecessary to give him any intravenous equivalent doses of his phenobarbital or phenytoin.

Annotated references

A full reference list for this chapter is available at:
http://www.wiley.com/go/gregory/andropoulos/pediatricanesthesia

1. Coté C, Wilson S, Work Group on Sedation, American Academy of Pediatrics, American Academy of Pediatric Dentistry. Guidelines for monitoring and management of pediatric patients during and after sedation for diagnostic and therapeutic procedures: an update. Paediatr Anaesth 2008; 18: 9–10. A recent update on the sedation guidelines for procedural sedation.

3. American Society of Anesthesiologists Task Force on Sedation and Analgesia by Non-anesthesiologists. Practice guidelines for sedation and analgesia by non-anesthesiologists. Anesthesiology 2002; 96: 1004–17. An important document recommending standards for sedation by non-anesthesiologists.

21. American Society of Anesthesiologists Task Force on Anesthetic Care for Magnetic Resonance Imaging. Practice advisory on anesthetic care for magnetic resonance imaging. Anesthesiology 2009; 110: 459–79. An excellent modern comprehensive review on providing anesthetic care for patients undergoing MRI scanning, including a comprehensive discussion of MRI safety.

116. Cravero J. Risk and safety of pediatric sedation/anesthesia for procedures outside the operating room. Curr Opin Anaesth 2009; 22: 509–13. An excellent contemporary review of risks and safety of procedural sedation in children.

117. Cravero J, Beach M, Blike G et al. The incidence and nature of adverse events during pediatric sedation/anesthesia with propofol for procedures outside the operating room: a report from the Pediatric Sedation Research Consortium. Anesth Analg 2009; 108: 795–804. An excellent overview of a large number of sedations with propofol by both anesthesiologists and non-anesthesiologists.

118. Mason K. Sedation trends in the 21st century: the transition to dexmedetomidine for radiological imaging studies. Paediatr Anaesth 2009; 20: 265–72. A modern review of the use of dexmedetomidine in pediatric radiology sedation.

126. Green S, Mason K. Reformulation of the sedation continuum. JAMA 2010; 303: 876–7. An important editorial arguing for a rethinking of the definition of sedation levels, including use of ventilatory monitoring with end-tidal CO_2.

142. Karian V, Burrows P, Zurakowski D et al. The development of a pediatric radiology sedation program. Pediatr Radiol 2002; 32: 348–53. An excellent review of the development of a comprehensive pediatric sedation program at a leading children's hospital.

176. Mason K, Zurakowski D, Zgleszewski S et al. High dose dexmedetomidine as the sole sedative for pediatric MRI. Paediatr Anaesth 2008; 18: 403–11. An important study describing dexmedetomidine as a sole agent for MRI sedation.

188. Sidhu M, Coley B, Goske M et al. Image Gently, Step Lightly: increasing radiation dose awareness in pediatric interventional radiology. Pediatr Radiol 2009; 39: 1135–8. A description of an important initiative to reduce radiation exposure in pediatric patients.

CHAPTER 37
Pediatric Intensive Care

Patrick A. Ross, Robert Bart III & Randall C. Wetzel

Department of Anesthesiology Critical Care Medicine, Children's Hospital Los Angeles, University of Southern California, Keck School of Medicine, Los Angeles, CA, USA

How pediatric intensive care units function

Pediatric intensive care units (PICUs) are quintessentially multidisciplinary units that care for patients of other physicians and must integrate all stakeholders, including the families and child, into the care delivery process. It is obvious that they provide life-saving support for children with a broad spectrum of diseases and thus must not only be multidisciplinary across health professions but also among medical specialists. Indeed, the necessity to care for all aspects of a child's critical illness and integrate the knowledge, wisdom, care, and focus of many providers is the key difference between critical care and other spe-

cialties. The need to work closely with nurses, respiratory therapists and others at the bedside to "create" critical care necessitates integration of these services and the running of the unit in a fashion unique to critical care medicine. Intensivists must manage the critical care environment, all aspects of it, in a manner often unfamiliar to physicians who admit patients to the hospital inpatient unit. The intensivists must have oversight of unit-specific functioning, from design of the facility to the personnel and systems that are required to optimize its performance. The hallmark of an excellent ICU is that the unit's personnel work at their best at all times, and do not merely coalesce around crises in a reactive fashion. The care children receive should be guided by their medical

Gregory's Pediatric Anesthesia, Fifth Edition. Edited by George A. Gregory, Dean B. Andropoulos.
© 2012 Blackwell Publishing Ltd. Published 2012 by Blackwell Publishing Ltd.

condition, the needs of the child and family and the knowledge of the intensivists to avoid "surprises." Ideally, no arrest or death should be a surprise in the ICU. A frantic resuscitation occurring in the ICU often indicates poor systems and a failure of recognition and response in a timely fashion [1,2].

The role of the PICU is, put simply, to provide life support. Thus ICUs must provide everything necessary for this function. First, the facility must meet local, state and federal architectural requirements and contain the hardware of life support: ventilators, extracorporeal membrane oxygenation (ECMO) machines, dialysis machines, monitors, picture archiving communication (PACs) systems, computer records, databases, and appropriate beds. The PICU must be staffed appropriately for its function. Clearly, a cardiothoracic ICU will be staffed with nurses and doctors with different expertise from those a medical PICU – but intensivists, nurses, respiratory therapists, social workers, and multiple medical specialists are necessary and should be tailored to meet the needs of the institution. Just as an ICU cannot exist without the proper equipment, it cannot exist merely with the presence of an intensivist and some critical care nurses – intensive care is by necessity a team endeavor. People and place are important but they are suboptimal without process. The protocols and systems around providing every child in every bed at all times with the appropriate and safe care require intentional organization. The existence of multidisciplinary rounds, mortality and morbidity reviews as well as a robust and unit-specific continuous process improvement system is essential to assure outstanding care. An excellent pediatric critical care unit goes further – it inculcates a culture of positive continual change targeted at improving the care it delivers and innovation around that care.

Relationship between the intensive care unit and the operating room

Intensive care grew from anesthesiology and while there is a lot in common between the two specialties, they have different mindsets. Intensivists manage multiple patients, all aspects of both the patient's care and the care-providing team, and provide care for prolonged periods of time. Very commonly, the continuum of the child's care bridges anesthesiology and the ICU. Communication needs to be excellent between ICU and operating room clinicians, ensuring a seamless transition of care. Our institution has a policy supporting attending handoff between critical care and anesthesia for each case. This communication occurs in both the preanesthetic and postanesthetic setting. Information regarding current ICU management and therapeutic response can simplify a potentially dif-

ficult anesthetic. Similarly, information on the operative and anesthetic course will frame and potentially guide the next several days of management. A complete sign-out regarding an anesthetic includes induction agents, ease of mask ventilation, ease of intubation, decisions regarding extubation, fluid totals, blood and blood products, inotropic agents, medications delivered including timing of antibiotics, complications, laboratory values, most recent blood gas, venous and arterial access, and allergies. Although this information may be available in the anesthetic record, few intensivists are trained to read them, they are frequently not available at transfer, and a short verbal summary by the anesthesiologist provides a greater amount of practical detail.

Family-centered care in the pediatric intensive care unit

Over time, recognition of the role of the family in the PICU has evolved and the decisions made with regard to how best to serve the family of a critically ill child have changed. The inclusion of the family in the care of their child and the care of the family as a unit have been recognized as an important part of critical care and it is often said that the "family is the patient." These efforts have taken place over the last decade and will continue to grow. Currently, at many children's hospitals, parents are invited to participate in multidisciplinary rounds with the nurses, respiratory therapists and physicians working with their child. Our own experience and the literature suggest that family-centered rounds do not take any more time than that allotted for traditional rounds, and do not compromise teaching [3]. Further, the issues of privacy can be dealt with even in an open bed environment. Satisfaction with this model has been reported by families and care providers in the unit. More ICUs may move to this model over time and in each case there is a short learning curve.

Parents of critically ill children undergo severe emotional distress, no matter how routine the process may seem to caregivers; an ICU is a unique and often terrifying experience for families and children. The need for multiple caregivers, changing shifts, endless physicians (residents, students, fellows, multi-specialists), loss of control, financial worries and many other factors all affect the family's ability to cope. The suffering of other children and families often amplifies anxiety but it may also in a way be able to comfort some families. Helping parents to cope with their child's critical illness and the ICU environment is a central part of intensive care. Parents display many behaviors that help them cope, including excessive clinginess, intellectualizing the process, blaming others (including their spouses), minimizing, and seeking opinions everywhere (the internet, the unit social worker, etc.). To provide optimal care, these mechanisms must be understood. Helping the parents to be parents and educating them about their child's illness are essential. Parental support, support groups, psychological support, child and family therapy, and social workers are all part of the critical care team.

A more difficult question, for some clinicians, will be how to address the issue of parental presence during invasive procedures and cardiopulmonary resuscitation (CPR) efforts. In a recent review of 15 studies addressing the issue of parental presence during procedures or CPR, only two were conducted in the PICU environment [4]. Of the remainder, 10 studies were conducted in the emergency department and there may have been episodes where parents were asked to assist in comforting or restraining their child during placement of peripheral intravenous (IV) lines.

Currently, in some hospitals parents are given the option of staying in the room with their child during complex procedures and even CPR. This is helpful for parents coping with the trauma of a critically ill child. In response to questionnaires, a majority of parents indicated they would stay again in a similar circumstance. These ideas have become more common, leading the American Academy of Pediatrics to issue a policy statement supporting parental presence in the emergency department. There is limited evidence supporting similar policies in the PICU. As each PICU considers its own policy, there are several issues to consider. The concerns of the clinicians will need to be addressed. The limited literature does not indicate that parents are obstructive or interfere with procedures. Additionally, teaching trainees has not been compromised. Nevertheless, this decision cannot be forced on everyone and a means for declining on the part of the clinician as well as the parent must be available. Further, a mechanism to provide an attendant for family members during these events is necessary. This is similar to parental presence during induction of anesthesia. Arrangements need to be made in advance to inform and accompany the family so that clinical care is not interrupted. It has not been an issue for our unit during CPR as the unit social worker or member of the clergy is available to explain to the family what is occurring. Parental presence during procedures may pose a different type of challenge as these events occur more frequently compared to CPR. Yet it would seem logical that in the best interest of the patient and family, someone other than the person performing the procedure should be looking after the family. Given the changes that are occurring in this area, by the next edition of this book it will probably seem that there was never a time when we did not offer parents in the ICU the choice of whether or not to remain during these events.

Disclosure of medical errors

We believe disclosure of medical errors to families is ethically correct. Nevertheless, many continue to resist this due to concerns regarding litigation. Of the 1018 respondents in a recent survey of Illinois residents, 27% indicated they would sue, but 38% stated they would recommend the hospital if appropriate disclosure and remediation occurred. The conclusion drawn by Helmchen et al was: "Patients who are confident in their providers' commitment to disclose medical errors are not more litigious and far more forgiving than patients who have no faith in their providers' commitment to disclose" [5]. In our institution, explanations about medical errors come from the senior member of the team to the family. This is likely the current attending physician, but can be the medical director of the PICU, depending on the complexity of the incident and its outcome. The discussion includes a frank explanation of what happened and why, what the repercussions are, what change of care is planned for their child, and what will be done to prevent a similar error in the future. The ICU social worker is present or immediately available to help validate concerns and provide support. We remain present until all questions are answered or additional time is scheduled if necessary. Errors and outcome are tracked through our quality assurance program and when necessary, a "root cause analysis" is performed. Medical errors can be viewed as an opportunity to improve practice quality and prevent injury to any future patient. We believe families should be informed of errors, and that future research will further support the view that disclosure does not increase the risk of medical liability.

Of course, coping with death and dying is also a necessary function of the critical care environment [6]. Often when nothing medically can be done for the child, the provision of palliative care becomes even more important. Death is not necessarily a failure but should be a well-managed process ensuring minimal pain and suffering for the child and family. Of course, in every society there are multiple ethical issues that arise in providing care for critically ill children. Intensive caregivers must understand the basic principles of ethical care and when to allow families choice and support them over what may be their own beliefs and practices – as long as the goal remains to prevent further pain and suffering [7]. The concept of futility has received much attention in the last few years and is overshadowed by financial, societal, ethical, personal and religious opinions and feelings. It is a difficult concept to define but when the pain and suffering of continuing life are more severe than the inevitability of death, care may become futile. One caution – the term "futile care" should never be ascribed to pain relief, caring support for the child and family, and understanding.

Continuous quality improvement – how do we measure quality?

How good is an ICU? Does it provide the best quality of care? When there is one ICU in a given institution, to what does it compare itself? Are there objective standards of ICU care and outcomes practices? This is a challenging field, in large part because ICU practices vary widely. For units that have high mortality, high resource utilization and high emotional impact, how can the quality of care be determined? After all, death and poor outcomes can be expected in the face of devastating diseases.

Which ICU is better? One with 1% mortality or one with 5% mortality? Obviously, the answer to this question depends on a number of factors. If the expectation of the first unit is that all children should survive because it cares for children with a low-level severity of illness, then it is underperforming. If the second unit has a very high severity of illness, such that perhaps a 10% mortality might be expected, it is doing very well [8]. There are ways to compare units objectively due to multiple methods of determining severity of illness. Since the pioneering work of Dr Murray Pollock and development of the Pediatric Risk of Mortality Score (PRISM) system of determining severity of illness from physiological and other measures, it has been possible to compare populations of critically ill children for outcomes including mortality and length of stay [9]. Currently, systems including PRISM, the Pediatric Index of Mortality (PIM) and the Pediatric Logistic Organ Dysfunction (PELOD) allow objective ways of determining severity of illness [10,11]. In addition, it is possible to determine the ratio of actual outcomes to expected outcomes and thus have a standardized outcome score. For example, if comparing the two ICUs with 1% and 5% mortalities, we know that the predicted mortality for the first is 0.5% and the predicted mortality for the latter is 15% from their severity of illness scores, so the risk-adjusted mortality (or standardized mortality ratio (SMR)) is 2 for the first unit and 0.3 for the second – a greater than sixfold difference in this performance measure. The higher mortality-rate unit actually does a much better job. This example demonstrates the importance of comparing critical care among ICUs and of using severity of illness-adjusted comparisons.

Aggregating populations of care and comparing them among units permits a continuous degree of comparative effectiveness research among units and populations. Performance of a unit for a given disease, a given population, age group or demographic can be compared and the cause of these differences discovered. The existence of a system to prospectively collect information on all critically ill children admitted to an ICU and adjust the outcomes for severity of illness permits a national infrastructure for continuous quality improvement. Such a system exists in VPS, LLC (https://portal.myvps.org), a national organization of over 100 hospital ICUs with nearly 400,000 patient records. This allows the reporting of comparative quality reports for each member ICU and contributes to improving pediatric critical care nationally and continuously. Membership of such organizations for the purpose of research and quality improvement is a national, US Agency for Healthcare Research and Quality (AHRQ) recognized standard of excellence for critical care. In addition, it allows trending and improving of other quality measures such as failed extubations, unplanned extubations [12], average length of stay, ventilator-associated pneumonias, central line infections, and short-term readmissions. All of these are considered quality measures for pediatric critical care and as for all quality efforts, the first step in improving quality is having a measurable outcome.

This short overview of how PICUs work is far from exhaustive. Familiarity with the processes that run under the surface of an ICU and determine the quality of the care it delivers may help in sharing the care of critically ill children among medical specialists.

The remainder of this chapter will deal with specific disease processes that cause critical illness in children.

Organ system function and failure

Circulation
Assessment of cardiovascular function
Routine continuous monitoring of physiological variables occurs in the ICU, including heart rate, electrocardiogram, temperature, and end-tidal carbon dioxide ($ETCO_2$). Cardiac output should always be assessed by physical examination in addition to monitoring data, and using the invasive and non-invasive methods described below. Poor cardiac output is often heralded by tachycardia, poor heart tones, diminished pulses, cool extremities and, if cardiogenic in nature, presence of third or fourth heart sounds, and evidence of hepatic and pulmonary congestion.

Cardiac output can be measured by multiple methods such as Fick thermodilution or dye dilution, echocardiography, ultrasonic cardiac output monitor (USCOM), and magnetic resonanace imaging (MRI). The first three methods use a change in measured blood concentration of a substance to calculate cardiac output. The principle is that the change in concentration is proportional to the volume of blood that it is being diluted in.

Of the dilutional methods, thermodilution is the most frequently used in PICUs. A special thermistor-tipped catheter is inserted in a central vein and advanced to the pulmonary artery (PA). Cold saline of a known temperature and volume is injected via a proximal port on the catheter into the right atrium. The saline mixes with the blood as it passes into the ventricle and PA. In this process the blood is cooled a small amount. The thermistor-tipped catheter in the PA measures the temperature of blood as it passes. A computer acquires the temperature profile, integrates the area, and calculates the flow of blood. A very accurate and rapid assessment of cardiac output is obtained, but this technique can be expensive and placement of a pulmonary artery catheter is not without risks. In addition, interpretation of the results can be very difficult in patients with congenital heart disease who have intracardiac shunts. There are risks associated with the insertion, maintenance and removal of the catheter [13] and the risks may be greater in children [14]. The use of pulmonary artery catheters has decreased over time in pediatric critical care.

The Fick method of measuring cardiac output relies on precisely measuring oxygen consumption. The formula is:

$$CO = VO_2 / (C_a - C_v)$$

Where CO is cardiac output, VO_2 is oxygen consumption, C_a is arterial oxygen content, and C_v is mixed venous oxygen content. Measurement of oxygen consumption is technical, difficult, and requires a steady physiological state. In addition, the best site to measure venous oxygen content is in the pulmonary artery as measurements from a central venous catheter result in incomplete mixing of blood. The dye technique is not used in pediatrics as it requires injection of indocyanine green dye as the marker to measure change in concentration. See Chapter 17 for a further discussion of monitoring and vascular access.

Echocardiography provides a significant amount of information about cardiac function. M-mode echocardiography provides what looks like an ice pick view through the heart. There is a single line of information at a very high frame rate that can be used to measure fractional shortening of ventricular tissue. Normal left ventricle fractional shortening is 28–44%. However, M-mode echocardiography does not assess regional wall motion abnormalities. Two-dimensional echocardiography provides detailed analysis of the heart structure. The information available is good enough that few children born with congenital heart disease require cardiac catheterization to define the lesion prior to surgical intervention. Tracing the outline of the left ventricle in systole and diastole allows an estimate of ejection fraction to be made. Normal ejection fraction of blood from the left ventricle is 55–65%. Doppler echocardiography allows the velocity of blood moving in the heart to be measured. Using a simplification of the Bernoulli equation, the difference in pressure between two chambers of the heart can be estimated. The formula is $P_1 - P_2 = 4V^2$ where V is the measured velocity (cm/sec) between two chambers. As an

example, right ventricular pressure is estimated by measuring the velocity of a tricuspid regurgitation jet (squared and multiplied by 4) and then subtracting the measured right atrial pressure from a central venous line. In the same manner, pulmonary artery pressure can be measured. Cardiac output (CO) can be measured by echocardiography by taking the area of a valve (A) multiplied by the flow velocity (V) through the valve multiplied by the heart rate (HR) ($CO = A \times V \times HR$). Flow velocity is the integration of the area under the Doppler curve across the valve. Typically, the aortic valve is used.

Echocardiography is limited by available equipment and expertise. Typically, a cardiologist or echocardiography technologist is required to make these measurements. In addition, it is an intermittent event and if the patient has poor echocardiographic windows from a transthoracic approach, transesophageal echocardiography is required. Heavy sedation or anesthesia may be required for transesophageal echocardiography. See Chapter 25 for additional discussion of echocardiography.

An alternative ultrasonic device used to measure cardiac output is the ultrasonic cardiac output monitor (USCOM, Sydney, Australia, www.uscom.com.au), approved for use in the US in 2005. The USCOM is a portable continuous-wave Doppler device, which uses an ultrasonic transducer to measure the velocity of blood flow. The transducer is placed in the suprasternal notch and the Doppler signal directed at the pulmonary or aortic valves. Formulas are used to estimate valve area and the velocity is multiplied by the heart rate to provide cardiac output. The system also indirectly calculates stroke volume. The USCOM allows beat-to-beat quantitative evaluation of cardiac hemodynamics and repeated measures can help evaluate the effectiveness of medical therapies. The USCOM has been used in the management of children with septic shock, hypovolemia, and myocardial dysfunction. Studies validating the USCOM are mixed, with some reporting poor association between USCOM and thermodilution [15,16] and others demonstrating agreement with conventional echocardiography [17,18]. The device is much less expensive compared to echocardiography, the required training is limited, and it can be performed as needed in the PICU. Further studies will be needed to determine if this will become a clinically useful tool.

Magnetic resonance imaging provides very detailed pictures of the heart structure. In addition, cardiac output as well as flow velocities can be measured. However, the procedure takes more than an hour, requires sedation or anesthesia, and expert clinicians are needed to interpret the data. This is very rarely used as a technique to gather information on intensive care patients.

Pharmacology of the cardiovascular system

During periods of physiological stress, the body releases hormones from the adrenal gland, resulting in a rapid increase in the tissue level of cyclic AMP (cAMP). The same support can be provided via exogenous catecholamines. The most common vasoactive medications used in the PICU are those stimulating the β receptor (dopamine, dobutamine, epinephrine, isoproterenol) or inhibiting the breakdown of cAMP by phosphodiesterase (PDE) (milrinone). In rare circumstances medications producing pure vasoconstriction are needed (vasopressin, phenylephrine – an α agonist).

When the β1 receptor is stimulated, a series of G-protein mediated changes occur leading to activation of adenylate cyclase. This results in the formation of the adrenergic second messenger cAMP. Cyclic AMP via protein kinase A causes phosphorylation of calcium channel protein. This results in an increased probability of the calcium channel being open with a greater influx of calcium. In the cardiac muscle this influx of calcium results in an increase in the velocity and force of myocardial contraction (positive inotropy). There is also an increased reuptake of calcium into the sarcoplasmic reticulum resulting in increased myocardial relaxation (positive lusitropy). The effect of increased calcium on the sinus node is an increase in rate (chronotropy) [19] and rate of conduction (positive dromotropy). However, a rapid bolus of calcium can cause bradycardia. The reason for this is not definitively known. Some believe it occurs due to a vagal effect [20], others feel it is secondary to the Gibbs–Donnan effect where charged particles near a semi-permeable membrane sometimes fail to distribute evenly across the two sides. The imbalance of calcium causes a transient decrease in automaticity directly on the cardiac cells. See Table 37.1.

Dopamine

Dopamine is the metabolic precursor of both norepinephrine (NE) and epinephrine. In the heart it releases NE from stores in nerve endings. In the periphery, the activity of the prejunctional dopaminergic DA_2 receptors inhibits NE release, promoting vasodilation. Dopamine activates many receptors at various doses causing β1, β2 or α receptor stimulation. At doses of 5–10 μg/kg/min positive chronotropic and inotropic effects are seen through β receptor activation. These doses typically result in an increase in systolic blood pressure with minimal effect on diastolic blood pressure. At doses of 10–20 μg/kg/min there is α receptor stimulation with peripheral vasoconstriction. As the peripheral resistance increases, renal blood flow may fall. At low infusion rates of dopamine, increases in renal blood flow have been demonstrated in healthy volunteers. These low-dose dopamine effects have not been demonstrated in critically ill patients. There are age-dependent responses to dopamine that differ from preterm infant to infant to child [21]. Potentially, in sick preterm infants there can be decreased dopamine clearance and a blood pressure response at a lower value. Titration in preterm and term infants occurs on a case-by-case basis and dose response is more consistent in older children. Dopamine is only given intravenously, as a continuous infusion as it is rapidly metabolized. Dopamine should be given via a central venous line as extravasation into the tissues can cause damage. Emergency circumstances arise where dopamine is given via peripheral IV while a central venous line is being placed. The extremity should be observed closely and the infusion moved to the new central line as soon as possible.

Table 37.1 Continuous infusion mediciations for the heart

Drug	Dosing	α	β1	β2	Effect
Dopamine	5–10 μg/kg/min	0	++	++	More β effect at low dose
	10–20 μg/kg/min	+++	++	0	More vasoconstrictor effect at higher dose
Dobutamine	5–20 μg/kg/min	+	+++	++	More β effect, less vasopressor activity compared to dopamine
Epinephrine	0.05–0.1 μg/kg/min	++	++	++	Has some β2 effect at lower doses
	0.1–0.2 μg/kg/min	++++	++++	0	More vasoconstriction and inotropic effects at higher doses
Norepinephrine	0.1–0.5 μg/kg/min	++++	++	0	Increases systemic vascular resistance
Isoproterenol	0.05–0.5 μg/kg/min	0	++++	++++	Increases HR and contractility, smooth muscle relaxant
Phenylephrine	0.1–0.5 μg/kg/min	++++	0	0	Produces both venous and arterial vasoconstriction
Milrinone	0.5–1 μg/kg/min				Selective phosphodiesterase III inhibitor
Nesiritide	0.005–0.01 μg/kg/min				Recombinant B-type natriuretic peptide used to increase urine output
Levosimendan	0.1–0.2 μg/kg/min				Calcium-sensitizing agent; increases ejection fraction, reduces catecholamine dose, minimal effect on heart rate and blood pressure

Dobutamine

Dobutamine is structurally similar to dopamine and works at β and α receptors. Its pattern of activity is β1 > β2 > α. Dobutamine functions primarily as an inotropic agent but it has less vasopressor activity compared to dopamine. Further, for bradycardic patients it is less likely to increase heart rate compared to dopamine. It is used as a continuous infusion of 5–20 μg/kg/min. It can only be given intravenously and is rapidly metabolized. In some studies dobutamine increases myocardial oxygen demand and may be more likely to provoke arrhythmias compared to dopamine.

Epinephrine

Epinephrine has mixed β1 and β2 receptor activity as well as α receptor effects at higher doses. Due to vasodilator effects, it is possible to have a decrease in blood pressure at low doses (<0.01 μg/kg/min) but at higher doses blood pressure will increase due to inotropic and vasoconstrictor effects. Epinephrine is useful for the treatment of shock when there is myocardial dysfunction as well as hypotension. It is typically given at a dose of 0.05–0.2 μg/kg/min. Doses up to 1–2 μg/kg/min are used but are associated with significant vasoconstriction with decreased perfusion to abdominal organs as blood is shunted to the heart, brain and skeletal muscle; these very high doses should only be used for short periods, i.e. during ECMO cannulation.

Epinephrine is the principal drug used after cardiac arrest; it supports blood pressure during shock. It also has uses in the treatment of bronchospasm and anaphylaxis or hypersensitivity reactions. It is given as a continuous infusion via a central line for its cardiovascular effects and it is rapidly metabolized. It can be given as a subcutaneous medication but vasoconstriction may slow absorption. It can be delivered as an inhaled medication to treat respiratory conditions but the development of tachycardia is possible. Use of epinephrine may cause tachycardia or provoke arrhythmias.

Norepinephrine

Norepinephrine has strong activity at the α1 and β1 receptors with little activity at the β2 receptor. It will increase systemic vascular resistance (SVR) and therefore will increase blood pressure. However, there can be vasoconstriction of mesenteric blood vessels with decreased abdominal and liver perfusion. Blood pressure may be increased without improving perfusion in low cardiac output states. Norepinephrine may be the ideal drug for the treatment of vasodilatory or warm septic shock as well as spinal shock. The use of norepinephrine in pediatric ICUs is limited compared to adult ICUs. It is not entirely clear if this is the result of physiological differences between the age groups or because of personal practitioner choice.

Isoproterenol

Isoproterenol is a synthetic, potent, non-selective β receptor agonist that has very low affinity for the α-adrenergic receptors. Isoproterenol increases heart rate and contractility, and lowers systemic vascular resistance by peripheral vasodilation. It can be tried as a pharmacological means of increasing heart rate in cases of complete heart block but in practice the heart rate increases in this scenario are modest and not sufficient to prevent further intervention. Isoproterenol is often used in the immediate postoperative period after cardiac transplantation to maintain acceptable heart rates in the denervated donor heart. Isoproterenol relaxes smooth muscle and is used as a bronchodilator. With its β2-adrenergic receptor activity, it is also used as a potent pulmonary vasodilator. Isoproterenol can be given intravenously or inhaled.

Vasopressin

Vasopressin is a pituitary peptide hormone. In the renal tubules vasopressin controls water reabsorption. It also acts on the vasculature, causing vasoconstriction by stimulation of smooth muscle V1 receptors. This results in increased SVR and increased arterial blood pressure. Clinically this drug is used to treat diabetes insipidus, gastric hemorrhage and as a second- or third-line drug to treat hypotension. Vasopressin has been used in adult cardiac arrest with ventricular fibrillation. Pediatric advanced life support (PALS) guidelines do not support the use of vasopressin in pediatric resuscitation. In 2009, Duncan et al [22] published a review of the American Heart Asssociation's National Registry of CPR. Vasopressin was used infrequently in children in only 5% of cases of pulseless cardiac arrest. Children receiving vasopressin had prolonged resuscitation and decreased likelihood of return of spontaneous circulation.

Vasopressin continues to be used with other vasoactive medications in order to support blood pressure during episodes of vasodilatory shock. There is limited pediatric literature [23–25] regarding the use of vasopressin for this indication. The most recent randomized double-blind controlled trial by Choong et al showed no benefit of low-dose vasopressin in conjunction with other inotropic support in the treatment of pediatric septic shock [25]. It is also used to increase SVR after cardiac surgery early in the postoperative period during periods of vasomotor instability.

Phenylephrine

Phenylephrine is considered a pure α agonist that increases both venous and arterial constriction in a dose-related manner. It is used extensively in adult anesthesia to increase blood pressure. Its predominant use in pediatrics is to increase pulmonary blood flow in patients with tetralogy of Fallot during hypoxemic spells [26–29]. All other episodes of hypotension in children are likely best treated by volume expansion, other inotropic agents or decreasing anesthetic depth.

Milrinone

Milrinone selectively inhibit phosphodiesterase (PDE) III at the cell membrane and decreases the breakdown of cAMP. As cAMP levels increase, protein kinase is activated to promote phosphorylation. This results in increased inotropy as well as vasodilation. PDE inhibitors are remarkable in producing these effects without acting on α or β receptors. Milrinone is a derivative of the PDE inhibitor amrinone. Amrinone causes thrombocytopenia which limited its use in pediatrics. Milrinone is given as a continuous infusion, usually at a starting dose of $0.5\,\mu g/kg/min$ and titrated to clinical effect. A loading dose of $50\,\mu g/kg$ is advocated by some but may result in episodes of hypotension. Milrinone has a much more common usage following pediatric heart surgery but has been used in the treatment of vasoconstricted septic shock. In the future there may be a role for milrinone in the treatment of pulmonary hypertension [30–32].

Calcium

Calcium is essential for myocardial contraction and is commonly used as a functional inotropic agent, especially following surgery for congenital heart disease. It has short-term benefits on blood pressure, but this may be outweighed by long-term detrimental effects [33]. Hypocalcemia may be under-recognized in the ICU. In an adult study, 88% of critically ill patients had reduced serum ionized calcium levels [34]. When appropriate, hypocalcemia should be corrected.

Nesiritide

Nesiritide is a recombinant form of the human B-type natriuretic peptide. This is the same hormone that is liberated from the ventricles in response to volume overload and increased wall tension. B-type natriuretic peptide acts on guanylate cyclase, resulting in venous and arterial vasodilation. Further effects include myocardial relaxation (positive lusitropy) and increased natriuresis. The recombinant form has been used exogenously in adult critical care for patients with acute decompensated heart failure. The goal for use of nesiritide in adults is decreased right atrial pressure, decreased pulmonary capillary wedge pressure, decreased systemic vascular resistance and then improved cardiac output. Use of nesiritide in pediatrics is limited but the overall goal is an increased urine output and decreased mean central venous pressure. Ryan et al [35] published preliminary experience with nesiritide in children less than 12 months of age and

saw a significant increase in urine output even with decreased fluid intake. Usual dosage recommendations for children and adults are an initial $2\,\mu g/kg$ bolus followed by a continuous infusion of 0.005–$0.01\,\mu g/kg/min$. This can be increased to a maximum infusion rate of $0.03\,\mu g/kg/min$.

Levosimendan

Levosimendan is a novel agent that acts as an inotrope by binding to cardiac myocyte troponin C and increasing the sensitivity of the contractile apparatus to calcium. In the setting of cardiac failure or postcardiac surgery in children, this agent is effective at increasing ejection fraction in many patients, while allowing a reduced catecholamine dose and having minimal effect on blood pressure and heart rate. Central venous pressure is usually unchanged but serum lactate decreases, and central venous oxygen saturation and cerebral oxygen saturation increase. Adverse effects were not found in three recent small pediatric series. A loading dose of $612\,\mu g/kg$ followed by an infusion of 0.1–$0.2\,\mu g/kg/min$ is recommended.

As of this writing, levosimendan is not US Food and Drug Administration approved, but it is available in many other parts of the world and appears to be a promising agent in pediatrics; more study is warranted [36–38].

Disorders of cardiac rhythm

Sinus rhythm originates from the sinus node and has a sinus P-wave morphology. On a 12-lead ECG, the P-waves are upright in leads I, II, AVF, and inverted (negative deflection) in AVR. Sinus tachycardia is not an arrhythmia but patients with this rhythm may be among the most ill in the ICU. Causes include fever, anxiety, pain, hypovolemia, thyrotoxicosis, congestive heart failure and myocardial disease. The goal is to treat the etiology, not the tachycardia. Sinus heart rates up to 180 beats per minute are well tolerated in children without heart disease. The young child's cardiac output is more heart rate than stroke volume dependent. Artificially slowing a compensatory sinus tachycardia can provoke cardiac catastrophe.

Sinus arrhythmia is a phasic irregularity of heart rate seen with respiration. It is a sign of good cardiac reserve and demonstrates greater vagal than sympathetic tone in children. Sinus bradycardia is rarely clinically significant in children; the exception is the neonate, whose cardiac output is more heart rate dependent than the older child because they cannot increase the inotropic state of the heart as readily. Sinus bradycardia may occur in patients who are trained athletes. It is also associated with increased intracranial pressure, hypothermia, hyperkalemia, hypothyroidism, and profound hypoxia. Drugs that may cause it include digoxin or β-blockers. "Sick sinus syndrome" can occur in children following repair of congenital heart disease and may require placement of a pacemaker. When the sinus rate is significantly slowed, escape beats or escape rhythms can occur from the atrium, atrioventricular (AV) node or ventricle. Ventricular escape beats will have a wide complex QRS morphology.

Supraventricular tachycardia (SVT) describes an abnormally elevated heart rate from a variety of causes. This is distinguished from sinus tachycardia. Re-entrant tachycardias include orthodromic reciprocating tachycardia (ORT) and AV node re-entrant tachycardia (AVNRT), both usually thought of as SVT. These tachycardias occur because the electrical conduction is repeated through an apparent accessory pathway (Wolff–Parkinson–White (WPW)) or a concealed pathway (non-WPW ORT) or through AV nodal tissue (AVNRT). Other causes of SVT occur due to abnormal automaticity of cardiac muscle, including ectopic atrial tachycardia, atrial flutter, and atrial fibrillation. In WPW rapid conduction through the accessory pathway during atrial fibrillation can result in ventricular fibrillation and sudden death. This is a rare but fatal complication of WPW.

Unstable re-entrant SVT is heralded by hypotension, poor peripheral perfusion, and altered mental status, and treated with synchronized direct current (DC) cardioversion. If the patient is stable, i.e. blood pressure minimally affected, re-entrant SVT can be acutely treated with vagal maneuvers such as ice applied to the face or a Valsalva maneuver, which slows conduction through the AV node. Adenosine can be used to terminate re-entrant SVT as it blocks the sinus node for a period of time. Adenosine is a short-acting agent, metabolized by red blood cells. The initial dose is 25–50 μg/kg given rapidly through the most central venous access possible. Equipment should be immediately available to perform cardioversion if necessary. If the first dose is ineffective, 100 μg/kg may be given. If re-entrant SVT recurs other drugs may be necessary. Verapamil blocks the AV node for a longer period of time but the patient must be older than 2–5 years of age to reduce the risk of verapamil inducing other arrhythmias. The dose of verapamil is 0.1 mg/kg over 5 min. Procainamide will block the accessory pathway and it may speed or slow conduction through the AV node. The initial dose is 5–15 mg/kg over 15–45 min. If an infusion is necessary, start the procainamide at 20 μg/kg/min. Doses up to 60 μg/kg/min may be needed. Amiodarone blocks the accessory pathway and the AV node. The initial dose is 1 mg/kg over 10 min, repeated as needed up to 5 mg/kg. This can be followed with an infusion at 5 μg/kg/min. Cardiology consultation should be obtained for SVT evaluation and possible long-term management.

Junctional ectopic tachycardia (JET) is a rapid heart rate for age caused by a focus of abnormal automaticity within or around the atrioventricular junction. The QRS rate is by definition faster than the P-wave discharge rate in JET. This is a very uncommon arrhythmia in the absence of cardiac surgery. It appears occasionally following repair of congenital heart disease, most notably for tetralogy of Fallot. Treatment consists of cooling the patient, reducing exogenous catecholamine infusions as much as possible, and an antiarrhythmic agent, such as procainamide or amiodarone.

Ectopic atrial tachycardia (EAT) is consecutive fast atrial beats without sinus morphology. In multifocal or chaotic atrial tachycardia, different atrial origins may be seen. EAT is usually asymptomatic in the short term, but in the long term can lead to cardiomyopathy. Atrial flutter occurs due to re-entrant circuits around the tricuspid valve. It is very regular with many more atrial than ventricular beats. Atrial flutter is treated with DC cardioversion or pacing. Atrial fibrillation is usually caused by disorganized circuits from near the pulmonary veins. There are irregular difficult-to-see P-waves. Atrial flutter is treated with DC cardioversion.

Premature atrial contractions (PAC) are caused by automaticity of atrial tissue. Even if frequent, PACs are usually benign. Premature ventricular contractions (PVC) are an early occurring, wide complex beat associated with a compensatory pause if the sinus node is not reset. At times, the underlying stimulus for PVCs is the presence of a central venous catheter in the heart. If this catheter can be pulled back from the heart, doing so may reduce PVCs. Unifocal PVCs are usually benign but they can be reduced in frequency by correcting electrolytes including potassium, magnesium, and calcium. In addition, exogenous catecholamines should be decreased if possible. Treating pain or anxiety may reduce endogenous catecholamines, lessening the frequency of PVCs.

All wide complex tachycardias should be treated as ventricular tachycardia until proven otherwise. SVT with aberrant conduction of the QRS can be in the differential diagnosis, but initially the patient should be treated as ventricular tachycardia. If the patient is pulseless, begin CPR and defibrillate followed by medications from Pediatric Advanced Life Support (PALS). If the patient is stable with a pulse, DC cardioversion should be performed or the use of adenosine, amiodarone or procainamide can be considered. Ventricular fibrillation is always treated with CPR and defibrillation, followed by medications following the PALS guidelines. Magnesium should especially be considered if there is any possibility that the arrhythmia is torsade de pointes. See Chapter 12 for further discussion of cardiac arrest and resuscitation.

First-degree heart block is a prolongation of the PR interval. This can be seen in normal children and is almost always asymptomatic. Second-degree heart block has two forms: Mobitz type I and Mobitz type II. Mobitz type I or Wenckebach phenomenon is a gradual prolongation of the PR interval until there is a dropped QRS. This is because of delay in the AV node and can be benign. Mobitz type II is an all-or-nothing phenomenon, the PR interval remains constant but there are intermittent dropped beats. Every second or third beat is conducted, evidenced by a QRS complex. This is a sign of His–Purkinje disease and is much more common in adults. This can progress to complete heart block (CHB). Third-degree AV block or CHB is complete dissociation of atrial and ventricular beats. To be diagnosed as CHB, the atrial beats have to be faster than the ventricular beats. This can occur as congenital CHB in infants born to mothers with autoimmune disorders such as lupus. CHB can also be seen after surgery for congenital heart disease. The heart rate may be increased in response to intravenous isoproterenol, but more often requires transthoracic or transvenous pacing.

Shock

Shock is often described as an inability to provide adequate perfusion of blood and in turn oxygen to tissues that require it. The concept of shock is often explained as a problem of oxygen supply and demand. During periods of normal health, the body supplies excess oxygen to tissues. The amount of oxygen the blood carries to the body is dependent on the amount of oxygen bound to hemoglobin and the amount of oxygen dissolved in blood. The normal oxygen content of the blood is explained by the formula:

$$CaO_2 \text{ (mL/dL)} = (1.34\,\text{g/dL})(SaO_2)(Hb) + (PaO_2)(0.003)$$

where CaO_2 is the oxygen content, SaO_2 the measured oxygen saturation, Hb the hemoglobin, PaO_2 the arterial oxygen tension, and 0.003 is a factor used to calculate the dissolved oxygen content, in mL per mmHg PaO_2.

The normal carrying capacity is approximately 20 mL/dL. The delivery of oxygen (DO_2) to the tissues is dependent on this carrying capacity and cardiac output (CO): $DO_2 \text{ (mL/min)} = CaO_2 \times CO \times 0.01$. The demand portion of the equation is oxygen consumption. O_2 consumption ($\dot{V}O_2$) is independent of O_2 delivery above a critical point and over a wide range. Below a critical point, $\dot{V}O_2$ is $\dot{D}O_2$ dependent. For infants and young children, $\dot{V}O_2$ is estimated at 175 mL/min/m^2. Oxygen consumption is equal to oxygen delivery multiplied by oxygen extraction: $\dot{V}O_2 = \dot{D}O_2 \times O_2EX$, where O_2EX is oxygen extraction and is equal to $(CaO_2 - CvO_2)/CaO_2$. CaO_2 is the oxygen content of arterial blood and CvO_2 the oxygen content of venous blood. The difference between the two is predictably 4–6 mL/100 mL blood.

Initially, as oxygen delivery decreases, the oxygen consumption remains constant via increased extraction. Below a critical point in oxygen delivery, oxygen consumption becomes delivery dependent. When oxygen to meet the metabolic needs of the body cannot be delivered, non-essential metabolism is eliminated. Examples are metabolism to maintain growth, thermoregulation, and neurotransmitter synthesis. This allows the remaining oxygen to continue to provide substrate for mitochondria. Certain organs in the body (kidney, skin, skeletal muscle, and intestines) receive a high blood supply relative to their metabolic needs. These organs also have a high proportion of sympathetic nerve innervations, allowing for redistribution of blood flow to organs that do not have adequate O_2 reserves, such as brain and heart.

Classification of shock

Shock can be classified by several schemas. Within different classification schemas, disease states can fall into more than one category and in clinical scenarios several may be working together. One classification includes hypovolemic, cardiogenic, distributive or vasogenic, and extracardiac obstructive shock.

Hypovolemic shock may be due to hemorrhage in cases like trauma or gastrointestinal (GI) losses. Non-hemorrhagic hypovolemic shock includes external losses of fluid from vomiting, diarrhea, polyuria, and poor fluid intake. There can also be a fluid redistribution shock state in cases of burns, trauma, and anaphylaxis.

Cardiogenic shock may be myopathic where the heart muscle itself does not function appropriately. In adults this may be following myocardial infarction. In children myocarditis or cardiomyopathy are more common. As indicated in the extracardiac life support (ECLS) section, in many cases in the PICU this can occur from myocardial stunning (effects of prolonged ischemia during aortic cross-clamping) following bypass for repair of congenital heart lesions. Further subdivisions of cardiogenic shock include mechanical failure such as valvular regurgitation or obstruction. Significant arrhythmias may result in a type of cardiogenic shock as contractions may not be synchronized to the point where there is effective output.

Extracardiac obstructive shock results from a physical impairment preventing adequate forward circulatory flow. This can occur due to inadequate preload secondary to mediastinal masses, increased intrathoracic pressure from tension pneumothorax, constrictive pericarditis, and cardiac tamponade from pericardial effusions. There can also be obstruction to systolic contraction from pulmonary hypertension, pulmonary embolus, and aortic dissection.

Distributive shock is associated with poor peripheral vascular tone and a maldistribution of blood flow to organs within the body. In distributive shock, cardiac output can be increased but blood pressure may remain low due to a very low systemic vascular resistance. Septic causes of distributive shock can be related to bacterial, fungal, viral or rickettsial infections or toxins produced from these infections. Toxic shock syndrome would be an example of this latter cause. Aspects of anaphylactic or anaphylactoid reactions are a type of distributive shock. Systemic inflammatory response syndrome (SIRS) may present with a picture of distributive shock. Distributive shock can also occur on a neurogenic basis in the case of spinal shock. Adrenal insufficiency with low circulating cortisol results in distributive shock as the vascular bed has difficulty maintaining vascular tone.

Diagnosis of shock

A high index of suspicion is necessary to rapidly identify shock in pediatric patients. The history will provide clues to volume loss or poor oral intake. Fever and malaise may point to infection. However, the history accompanying cardiogenic shock may be vague, with reports of decreased activity and level of alertness. In addition, physical findings may be limited if the patient is currently compensating. A child with shock may present with just tachycardia, cold extremities, and poor capillary refill. In distributive shock, the child may remain warm and have isolated tachycardia. A brief pertinent physical examination should be performed evaluating level of alertness, peripheral perfusion, mucous membranes, pulse rate and quality, respiratory effort, urine output and blood pressure. In children, blood pressure may be maintained until the last possible moment. Hypotension is a sign of late and decompensated shock in children. Initially laboratory values may not show significant metabolic acidosis, depending on how far the illness has progressed.

Compensatory mechanisms

With onset of shock, the body applies compensatory mechanisms to maintain adequate tissue perfusion for as long as possible. Fluid is redistributed from the intracellular and interstitial spaces to the intravascular compartment. There is a decrease in glomerular filtration to decrease renal fluid losses. Aldosterone and vasopressin are released which also decrease renal fluid losses. Increased sympathetic activity and release of epinephrine decrease venous capacitance and attempt to support blood pressure. Heart rate is elevated in an effort to maintain cardiac output. Cardiac contractility is increased through circulating catecholamines and adrenal stimulation. As noted above, sympathetic tone shunts blood away from non-vital organs. At the tissue level, oxygen unloading is optimized by increased red blood cell 2,3-diphosphoglycerate (2,3-DPG), fever, and tissue acidosis.

Therapy and outcomes of shock

Outcomes associated with aggressive therapy to treat septic shock in pediatric patients have been studied. Septic shock is a good example for discussing therapy for shock in general. The overall goal of treatment of any type of shock is to treat the underlying cause, return the body to a state of adequate oxygen delivery to all the tissues, and remove the metabolic products that developed during anaerobic metabolism. It appears that the faster the body returns to a state of adequate perfusion, the better the overall outcome.

In 1991 Carcillo et al [39] described a population of 34 children who presented to an emergency department with septic shock. Sepsis was defined as positive blood or tissue culture and shock was diagnosed based on hypotension for age, with decreased perfusion, poor peripheral pulses, cool extremities and tachycardia. Within a period of 6 h of presentation, all the patients had a functioning pulmonary artery catheter in place. Overall mortality was 47%. However, in the group of patients who received more than 40 mL/kg of fluids in the first hour, there was only one death out of nine patients (11%). The authors go further to point out that this patient did not die during the initial therapy but with a second episode of sepsis 2 weeks later. In this study, rapid fluid administration was not associated with increased cardiogenic pulmonary edema or adult respiratory distress syndrome (ARDS).

In 2001 Rivers et al [40] published a study demonstrating that early, aggressive, goal-directed therapy in the first 6 h of care for adults with septic shock improved mortality; 263 adults were enrolled and of these, 133 received standard therapy based on clinician discretion in the emergency department. Those patients randomized to early goal-directed therapy followed protocols to address issues of hypovolemia and support blood pressure with vasoactive agents if necessary. If the patient remained hypotensive, inotropic support was initiated to maintain a mean arterial pressure (MAP) greater than 65 mmHg. If patients were hypertensive, they were given vasodilators and if central venous oxygen saturation was less than 70%, the patients were transfused to a hematocrit of at least 30%. If central venous saturations remained low, dobutamine was started. When necessary, patients for whom hemodynamics could not be optimized were intubated, ventilated, and sedated. There were no significant differences between the groups with regard to baseline characteristics. The in-hospital mortality was 30.5% in the group assigned to early goal-directed therapy compared to 46.5% receiving standard therapy (p < 0.01). Although it was carried out in adults, this work extends and supports the efforts of Carcillo et al from 1991.

The Rivers' publication [40] prompted the formation of a task force from members of the Society of Critical Care

Medicine to address shock in children. The result of their work was published in 2002 as "Clinical practice parameters for hemodynamic support of pediatric and neonatal patients in septic shock" [41]. The physiological differences between adults and children make adoption of adult guidelines challenging. The task force reviewed the literature and made recommendations for the diagnosis and treatment of pediatric shock. These guidelines, published by the American College of Critical Care Medicine (ACCM), are incorporated into the American Heart Association's (AHA) Pediatric Advanced Life Support (PALS) Provider Manual. From their work, septic shock can be defined as cold or warm shock. Decreased perfusion is present with decreased level of alertness. The capillary refill will be prolonged in cold shock (>2 sec) and pulses are diminished with cold mottled extremities. In episodes of warm shock, capillary refill is very brisk and pulses may be bounding. See Box 37.1.

The goals of therapy include rapid recognition of shock and early administration of intravenous crystalloid. Fluid should be given as a bolus of 20 mL/kg and repeated up to 60 mL/kg in the first 40 min with a goal of reducing heart rate and improving perfusion. When the heart rate does not improve with this volume of fluid, central venous access should be obtained and dopamine infusion initiated. Arrangements should be made to admit the child to a PICU. If shock persists despite fluid and dopamine up to 10 μg/kg/min, then epinephrine (cold shock) or norepinephrine (warm shock) is recommended (Fig. 37.1). The areas of the recommendation that have undergone further discussion and debate include the use of pulmonary artery catheters and use of hydrocortisone for concerns of adrenal insufficiency. There has been decreased use of PA catheters in children over time. In the

absence of PA catheters, many clinicians are using the central venous pressure, information from echocardiography, and other non-invasive measures of cardiac output such as central venous oxygen saturation (ScvO$_2$) or the USCOM to guide decisions. Clinicians currently in training are less likely to place PA catheters and, due to decreased familiarity, may be less able to use all the information provided. Whether PA catheters are of significant benefit seems to depend on the experience and needs of the practitioner.

With regard to adrenal insufficiency during septic shock, there certainly are instances where limited function of the adrenal axis is anticipated. Patients who have recently received glucocorticosteroids, ketoconazole or etomidate may be at increased risk. Disease states such as purpura fulminans or those affecting the hypothalamus, pituitary or adrenal glands will put patients at increased risk. These patients need supplemental corticosteroids to replace what their adrenal glands may not be able to produce. For the remaining children with septic shock, it is not clear whether the risk of relative insufficiency or treatment with systemic steroids alter outcome. Zimmerman presents an excellent review of the history of steroid use as well as the adult and limited pediatric literature for therapeutic use in sepsis [42]. As he indicates, adult studies have shown that high-dose short courses of steroids are associated with *decreased survival*. In addition, recent data from the CORTICUS trial [43] have shown that low-dose steroids as a physiological replacement during periods of vasopressor-resistant shock resolve shock more quickly but there is no change in mortality. Pediatric studies of low-dose steroids have not been done, but the information generated to date would indicate that steroids in sepsis do more harm than good. There remains institutional and individual bias to throw everything possible at patients to prevent mortality but there is not experimental evidence to indicate that steroids are effective.

The outcome in pediatric shock with adherence to the American Heart Association's guidelines was studied in 2003. Han et al [44] published a retrospective cohort study of children admitted to community hospitals with septic shock who were then transferred to a tertiary children's hospital. The overall mortality for the study was 29%. The study defined reversal of shock as return of normal systolic blood pressure and capillary refill time. For those patients in whom shock reversal was achieved by the time the transport team arrived (median time 75 min), survival was 96%. For each hour that shock persisted, there was a 2.29 times increased odds of mortality. This study indicates that the quicker shock is reversed, the better the outcome.

Further work has been done to evaluate whether the addition of central venous saturations as a goal-directed

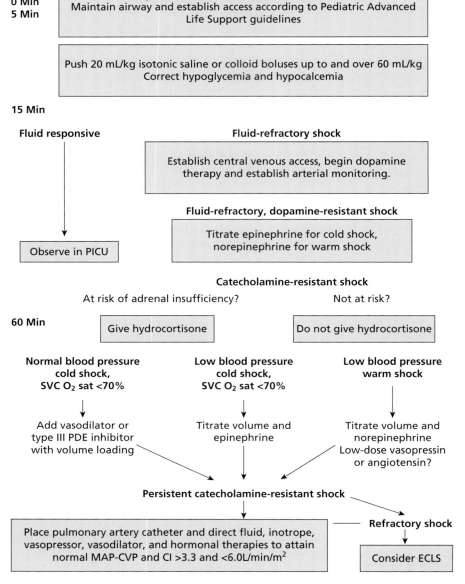

0 Min
5 Min

Recognize decreased mental status and perfusion
Maintain airway and establish access according to Pediatric Advanced
Life Support guidelines

Push 20 mL/kg isotonic saline or colloid boluses up to and over 60 mL/kg
Correct hypoglycemia and hypocalcemia

15 Min

Fluid responsive

Fluid-refractory shock

Establish central venous access, begin dopamine
therapy and establish arterial monitoring.

Fluid-refractory, dopamine-resistant shock

Titrate epinephrine for cold shock,
norepinephrine for warm shock

Observe in PICU

Catecholamine-resistant shock

At risk of adrenal insufficiency?   Not at risk?

60 Min

Give hydrocortisone   Do not give hydrocortisone

**Normal blood pressure
cold shock,
SVC O₂ sat <70%**

**Low blood pressure
cold shock,
SVC O₂ sat <70%**

**Low blood pressure
warm shock**

Add vasodilator or
type III PDE inhibitor
with volume loading

Titrate volume and
epinephrine

Titrate volume and
norepinephrine
Low-dose vasopressin
or angiotensin?

Persistent catecholamine-resistant shock

Refractory shock

Place pulmonary artery catheter and direct fluid, inotrope,
vasopressor, vasodilator, and hormonal therapies to attain
normal MAP-CVP and CI >3.3 and <6.0L/min/m²

Consider ECLS

Figure 37.1 Recommendations for stepwise management of hemodynamic support in infants and children with goals of normal perfusion and perfusion pressure (mean arterial pressure – central venous pressure [MAP – CVP]). Proceed to next step if shock persists. PALS, pediatric advanced life support; SVC O_2, superior vena cava oxygen saturation; PDE, phosphodiesterase; CI, cardiac index; ECLS, extracorporeal life support. Adapted from Carcillo and Fields [41] with permission from Lippincott Williams and Wilkins.

endpoint has an impact on mortality in pediatric septic shock. De Oliveira [45] in 2008 published a randomized trial using the ACCM/PALS guidelines for early correction of pediatric septic shock. One group had monitoring of central venous saturations (ScvO₂) with increased fluid resuscitation, transfusion of packed red blood cells (PRBCs) or inotropic support if ScvO₂ was less than 70%. The group with ScvO₂ goal-directed therapy had a mortality of 12% compared to 39% in the group treated by ACCM/PALS guidelines without this additional ScvO₂ goal. The ScvO₂ group received more crystalloid, transfusions, and inotropic support in the first 6h. The majority of patients with this level of acuity will require a central

venous catheter for inotropic support and stable vascular access. This study shows that more information can be gained from central lines than just venous pressure and guiding therapy to improve the balance of oxygen delivery and consumption will save lives. See Box 37.2 for etiologies of circulatory failure.

Systemic inflammatory response syndrome and multiple organ dysfunction syndrome
Systemic inflammatory response syndrome

Sepsis is one possible cause of the systemic inflammatory response syndrome (SIRS). SIRS is a non-specific inflammatory process occurring after trauma, burns,

Box 37.2 Etiology of circulatory failure in children

Hypovolemia: inadequate circulating blood volume

- Volume loss
  - Blood loss (trauma, surgical)
  - Plasma loss (burns, capillary leak, third-spacing of fluid)
  - Water loss (vomiting, diarrhea, decreased oral intake)
- Vasodilation
  - Anaphylaxis, drug intoxication
  - Sepsis
  - Neurogenic: sympathetic blockade, dysautonomia

Diminished cardiac function

- Myocardial dysfunction
  - Myocarditis, cardiomyopathy
  - Hypoxia, acidosis, electrolyte disturbance, toxins
  - Postoperative from heart surgery
- Anatomical obstruction to ventricular inflow or outflow
- Physiological obstruction to ventricular outflow
  - Increased systemic or pulmonary vascular resistance
- Shunt lesions (e.g. large arteriovenous malformations)
- Dysrhythmias
  - Bradycardia, ectopy, extreme tachycardia

Box 37.3 Systemic inflammatory response syndrome definition

1. Abnormality in core temperature
   Can be fever >38.5°C
   Can be hypothermia <36°C
2. Abnormality of heart rate
   Tachycardia with HR >2 SD for age
   Children <1 year can be bradycardic with HR <10th% for age
3. Abnormality of respiratory rate
   Respiratory rate >2 SD for age
4. Abnormality of white blood count
   Elevated or depressed for age

At least two of the four criteria must be present, of which one must be abnormal temperature or white blood count.

---

esses. Typically infection results in a raised temperature and production of the cytokine tumor necrosis factor (TNF). These events help to fight infections. SIRS may be an excess proinflammatory response by the body or an imbalance of proinflammatory to anti-inflammatory response. Clinically very few children respond to a specific insult with a SIRS response. Most manage their inflammatory insults without significant problem. Early work is demonstrating that there may be a genetic predilection determining which patients develop SIRS. Agbeko et al [47] in a prospective study demonstrated that "polymorphisms in the complement activation cascade modify the risk for early SIRS/sepsis in general pediatric critical care." In the future we might be able to identify which patients are at greater risk.

Development of multiple organ dysfunction syndrome and outcomes

Organ dysfunction represents a continuum of physiological abnormalities. It is not a simple issue of a normal organ versus a failed organ. Diagnostic criteria have been set forth to define organ failure for the purpose of description and research [48]. In turn, multiple organ failure is two or more organ systems meeting these criteria. Research supports the association between number of organs failing and increasing mortality [48,49].

The pediatric logistic organ dysfunction (PELOD) score was first described by Leteurtre et al in 1999 [50] and validated in 2003 [51]. The PELOD includes assessment of neurological, cardiovascular, renal, respiratory, hematological, and hepatic function (Box 37.4). Other organ dysfunction scoring systems exist incorporating different indicators, but PELOD is the most widely used. An excellent review by Proulx et al [52] in 2009 addressed the issue of multiple organ dysfunction syndrome (MODS) as well as the inflammatory spectrum covering sepsis, SIRS, MODS, and ARDS. A study by Typpo et al [53] using the virtual pediatric intensive care performance system

pancreatitis, cardiac bypass, surgery, infection, and other less frequent causes. In 2005 the International Pediatric Sepsis Consensus Conference [46] published their pediatric definitions for SIRS, sepsis and organ dysfunction. SIRS is defined by the presence of two of four criteria, of which one must be abnormal temperature or white blood count. The criteria are:

1. *abnormality in core temperature*: the patient can be febrile (>38.5°C) or hypothermic (<36°C)
2. *abnormality of heart rate*: the patient can be tachycardic with a HR >2 standard deviations (SD) for age or in children <1 year of age the patient can be bradycardic <10th percentile for age. The abnormal HR is in the absence of external stimulus such as pain or medications
3. *elevated respiratory rate* >2 SD for age
4. *abnormal white blood count* which is elevated or depressed for age.

See Box 37.3. The consensus definition of sepsis is SIRS in the presence of or as a result of suspected or proven infection. Septic shock is defined as sepsis and cardiovascular organ dysfunction.

Systemic inflammatory response syndrome currently is defined by clinical criteria, but in the future may include laboratory values. In SIRS a specific insult to the body results in an unbalanced inflammatory response that affects coagulation, white blood cell release, cytokine release, chemotaxis, and downstream biochemical proc-

Box 37.4 PELOD (pediatric logistic organ dysfunction) elements

- **Cardiovascular**
  - Heart rate (beats/min)
  - Systolic blood pressure (mmHg)
- **Neurological**
  - Pupillary reaction (both)
  - Glasgow Coma Scale
- **Hepatic**
  - Aspartate transaminase (IU/L)
  - International normalized ratio (INR)
- **Respiratory**
  - PaO_2/FIO_2 mmHg
  - $PaCO_2$ mmHg
  - Mechanical ventilation
- **Hematological**
  - White blood cell count ($\times 10^9$/L)
  - Platelet count
- **Renal**
  - Creatinine μmol/L

database analyzed 44,693 PICU admissions with complete data meeting their criteria. Of these, 18.6% (8303 patients) met criteria for MODS on day 1 of hospitalization. Mortality in the group with MODS was 10% compared to 1.2% in the patients not meeting MODS criteria. There was also a longer PICU length of stay and worse functional outcomes. Leteurtre et al [54] recently published results showing increased mortality with an elevated PELOD score on day 1, and a mortality of 50% if a high PELOD day 1 score rose further on day 2. MODS represents another area where consensus definitions and ongoing research studies have provided further information on outcome. Work will proceed using these tools to evaluate the impact of therapy on MODS.

Respiration

Assessment of monitoring of respiratory function

The cornerstones of ventilatory assessment remain clinical examination and the chest radiograph. In the non-intubated patient, respiratory rate, subcostal and sternal retractions, nasal flaring, grunting, use of accessory muscles, cyanosis, and SaO_2 >10% below baseline are signs of significant respiratory distress. Diminished breath sounds, rales, rhonchi, and wheezing on auscultation accompany respiratory compromise. Decreased level of consciousness due to hypoxemia or hypercarbia, and respiratory pauses are often harbingers of respiratory arrest. A variety of chest radiograph findings, including lobar or lung consolidation, pleural fluid, pneumothorax or severe hyperinflation due to bronchospasm, are seen in patients with compromised respiratory function. Similar findings may be seen in patients receiving either non-invasive ventilation or full mechanical ventilation, and these findings should be continually re-evaluated, even in the modern era of advanced respiratory monitoring.

The gold standard for measuring oxygenation is an arterial blood gas. Partial pressure of oxygen in arterial blood (PaO_2) is measured directly from blood. The percent oxyhemoglobin saturation (SaO_2) is calculated using pH, $PaCO_2$, PaO_2, and temperature but preferably is measured directly by blood oximetry, available on many modern blood gas machines. Capillary and venous blood gases do not measure or predict PaO_2. Pulse oximetry provides an accurate continuous measure of arterial oxygen saturations (SpO_2). Pulse oximeters are less accurate for saturations <60%, if there is poor perfusion where the probe is located or if there are other forms of hemoglobin present (methemoglobin, carboxyhemoglobin) interfering with the pulse oximeter. Methemoglobin and carboxyhemoglobin absorb light at the same wavelengths as oxyhemoglobin and deoxyhemoglobin, respectively.

The gold standard for measuring ventilation is the $PaCO_2$ from an arterial blood gas. As opposed to PaO_2, a free-flowing capillary blood gas adequately estimates $PaCO_2$. In addition, capnography and transcutaneous CO_2 (TCOM) devices are good non-invasive alternatives to monitor ventilation. Capnographs consist of an exhalation chamber, infrared light source, and detector connecting to the adapter end of the endotracheal tube. They produce waveforms of exhaled CO_2 that can either be time based or volumetric. Time-based CO_2 is the most commonly used method and what is normally seen on an anesthesia machine. Information available from capnography includes end-tidal CO_2 ($ETCO_2$), respiratory rate and pattern, confirmation of endotracheal tube (ETT) position, dead space calculations, cardiac output and presence of obstructive airways disease. Many PICUs now use continuous capnography as a standard of care in intubated patients in order to rapidly detect changes in ventilation or circuit disconnections.

When viewing the plateau of time-based capnography the level of CO_2 detected approaches $PaCO_2$ but will never equal it. As such, any elevation in $ETCO_2$ should be taken seriously and deserves further evaluation. For individuals without pulmonary disease, there is a 2–5 mmHg gradient between $ETCO_2$ and $PaCO_2$. This difference can be even greater in disease states where there is increased dead space, pulmonary vascular abnormalities, decreasing cardiac output, right-to-left intracardiac shunting or pulmonary overdistension. The ratio of relative dead space to tidal volume (V_D/V_T) can be calculated using capnography and arterial blood gas. $V_D/V_T = [PaCO_2 - \overline{E}CO_2]/PaCO_2$ where $\overline{E}CO_2$ = mean expired CO_2. Graphically $\overline{E}CO_2$ is the area under the curve of time-based capnography. Time-based capnography also demonstrates obstructive airways disease as an upslope to the plateau phase of the CO_2 curve. The accuracy of capnography improves if there is minimal leak around the ETT and with slower respiratory rates. It is also possible to use capnography to monitor the non-intubated patient, via a divided nasal cannula as is used during monitored anesthesia care.

Volumetric capnography is appearing as an additional feature on modern ventilators. This tracks the CO_2 concentration against exhaled volume. The technique allows a ready determination of dead space calculations and helps to determine optimal positive end expiratory pressure (PEEP) on the ventilator and response to bronchodilator therapy. The PEEP can be titrated to balance optimal oxygenation and lowest dead space fraction.

Transcutaneous CO_2 monitoring (TCOM) heats the skin in a small area underlying the sensor. The warmed capillary bed dilates and there is an increased CO_2 diffusion across the skin. The CO_2 is measured electrochemically. TCOMs require initial calibration compared to a blood gas but this can be a capillary sample. They are useful with high-frequency ventilation or non-intubated patients where capnography cannot be used.

Esophageal pressure monitoring is being incorporated into some ventilators and exists on free-standing devices. A balloon-tipped catheter is placed through the nose and advanced into the distal third of the esophagus. Due to transmitted forces, changes in esophageal pressure reflect changes in pleural or transpulmonary pressure. These changes can be followed while adjusting ventilator settings, providing an assessment of the patient's work of breathing.

Respiratory spirometry includes displaying flow–volume and pressure–volume loops, as well as flow–time, pressure–time, and volume–time graphs. Flow–volume loops measured by the ventilator or by free-standing devices can help diagnose the type of respiratory disease present based on characteristics of curve shapes. For spontaneously breathing patients, the classic presentations of flow–volume loops are inspiration negative and exhalation positive. However, the display on most mechanical ventilators places inspiration positive and exhalation negative (Fig. 37.2). Obstructive airways disease has a classic pattern of a scooped-out appearance on the exhalation portion of the curve (Fig. 37.3). Pressure–volume loops for mechanically ventilated patients help to identify recruitment of the lungs above an area of atelectasis (Fig. 37.4). Graphically, this is seen as a lower inflection point on the inspiratory curve from a flat area to an area of maximal compliance (greatest change in

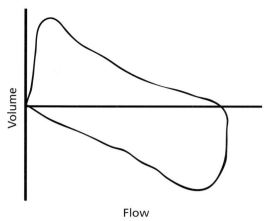

Figure 37.2 Flow volume loop during mechanical ventilation. Note that exhalation is negative.

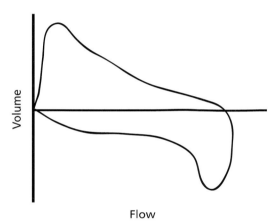

Figure 37.3 Flow volume loop with airway obstruction. Note the scooped-out appearance of exhalation.

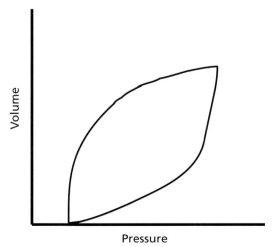

Figure 37.4 Pressure volume loop during mechanical ventilation.

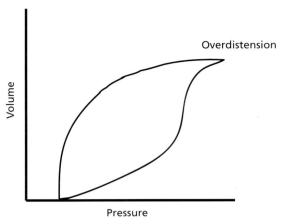

Figure 37.5 Pressure volume loop with overdistension of the lung. The area of the curve that looks like a bird's beak demonstrates an increase in pressure and significant change in volume. The lung is already at maximum inflation.

Table 37.2 Oxygen delivery by non-invasive means

Device	FIO₂	Flow (L/min)
Nasal cannula	Up to 40%	<5 L/min
Simple facemask	Up to 60%	6–10 L/min
High-flow humidified nasal cannula	Close to 100%	1–30 L/min
Non-rebreather mask with reservoir	Close to 100%	6–15 L/min
CPAP or BiPAP therapy	100%	As needed to deliver pressure

volume for change in pressure). Pressure–volume loops also contain an upper inflection point or an area above maximal compliance where the lung is overdistended by the current ventilator settings. This area of overdistension looks like a bird's beak and should prompt reductions in set ventilator peak pressure (Fig. 37.5). See Chapter 17 for additional discussion of respiratory monitoring.

Respiratory care

Nasal cannula oxygen can improve a patient's oxygenation by increasing their fraction of inspired oxygen (FIO₂). The formula for calculating the anticipated PaO₂ with completely normal lungs is the alveolar gas equation:

$$PAO_2 = (\text{barometric pressure mmHg} - \\ \text{water vapor pressure mmHg}) \times FIO_2 - \\ (PaCO_2 / \text{respiratory quotient}).$$

For example, with FIO₂ 0.40 at sea level, a PaCO₂ 40 mmHg, and respiratory quotient (CO₂ production/O₂ consumption, usually estimated to be 0.8), expected PaO₂ would be:

$$[(760 \text{ mmHg} - 47 \text{ mmHg}) \times 0.40] - (40 \text{ mmHg} / 0.8) \\ = 235 \text{ mmHg}$$

Nasal cannula can increase the FIO₂ up to approximately 40% when it is flowing at 5 L/min. Above this, the nasal cannula is uncomfortable after a short period of time, due to the non-humidified gas flow drying and irritating mucus membranes. FIO₂ cannot be increased further as room air is entrained during inspiration. However, of note, the smaller the patient, the lower their inspiratory

tidal volume and potentially the greater impact on FIO₂ is made by nasal cannula oxygen.

Using a properly fitted facemask can increase inspired oxygen further. Oxygen delivery with a simple facemask may not be as great as the open holes allow for entrainment of room air. Use of a non-rebreather facemask with an oxygen reservoir and one-way valve for exhalation allows for near 100% oxygen to be delivered. Many children may not tolerate a facemask for a prolonged period of time. Practically, many patients reach this level of support while on a pediatric ward and either show improvement with therapy or progress to requiring PICU admission and intubation. Few patients remain on a non-rebreather mask for long. These systems can be humidified, but do not provide positive pressure. See Table 37.2.

High-flow humidified nasal cannula (HFHNC) oxygen has been used over the past 5–8 years as a means of providing higher FIO₂. As the oxygen is heated to body temperature and humidified to 100% water vapor, higher flow of gas is much better tolerated than with just nasal cannula. As the flow of oxygen can be delivered at 10 L/min or more, close to 100% oxygen can be achieved. There is belief that HFHNC may produce some amount of positive airway pressure, especially in small infants, but this is inadequately studied. The means by which different systems saturate oxygen with water vapor vary and some are proprietary. Many hospitals limit HFHNC use to the ICU. The device provides a significant support of oxygenation while not looking much different from nasal cannula. Some clinicians have significantly underestimated the severity of respiratory failure in patients on HFHNC until they deteriorate further.

Positive airway pressure can be delivered non-invasively. A well-fitting nasal or full-face mask maintains a seal and allows the system to apply positive pressure. Modern ventilators can be set to deliver constant positive airway pressure (CPAP) or bilevel support. More often specific bilevel positive airway pressure (BiPAP) machines are used. Use of non-invasive ventilation requires a patient with ability to protect their airway and a central drive to breathe. With bilevel support a back-up rate can be set. However, if a patient is too dependent on this support, a more definitive airway should be considered. CPAP provides distending pressure and helps to overcome atelectasis, thereby decreasing dead space, improving ventilation/perfusion, and potentially reducing work of breathing. Initial starting pressures of 4–6 cmH$_2$O may be used and increased to the level tolerated and clinical improvement. More commonly, BiPAP therapy is used. The expiratory pressure again starts at 4–6 cmH$_2$O and can be increased to expand the lungs. The inspiratory pressure is set initially at 5–6 cmH$_2$O above expiratory pressure. Both settings as well as inspiratory and expiratory times can be adjusted. An FIO$_2$ of 1.0 can be delivered. Patients are at risk for aspiration and this is greatly increased with any episode of emesis. BiPAP therapy has been successfully used to treat asthmatics in an emergency department setting and improve aerosolized medication delivery. BiPAP is a common non-invasive therapy for patients with chronic respiratory failure, allowing them to be cared for at home. Pulmonologists often care for patients on night-time BiPAP for chronic respiratory failure or for central hypoventilation syndrome. If these patients are admitted for issues other than worsening respiratory distress, they may be cared for on a pulmonary ward, avoiding an ICU admission.

Short-term use of continuous BiPAP should be the expectation. In the best of circumstances, it is supportive while waiting for therapy to be effective. If used as a bridge to more definitive respiratory care, it should be short. The constant pressure of the mask will lead to tissue breakdown on the face. This is accelerated when the patient's global perfusion or skin integrity is poor. Patients remain nil per os (NPO) while on continuous BiPAP. Tracheal intubation and further respiratory support may allow initiation of enteral feeds. There are benefits to BiPAP therapy as it can be tried without requiring intubation and patients may tolerate BiPAP with little or no sedation.

There are many modes of mechanical ventilation. The preferred mode often depends on the clinical scenario and the intensivist's experience. For *volume-controlled* ventilation, a set tidal volume is chosen. As the ventilator delivers the set volume, changes in respiratory compliance or resistance alter the peak airway pressure to deliver the volume. If the changes to compliance or resistance are significant, as with partial obstruction of airways or endotracheal tube, then very high pressures can be deliv-

ered. However, ventilators are set with maximal pressure limits, and with obstruction or deteriorating respiratory compliance the ventilator will alarm and the volume delivered will be limited by peak pressure. For *pressure-controlled* ventilation, a set pressure is defined. As the ventilator delivers the set pressure, the tidal volume achieved will change depending on respiratory compliance and resistance. If the changes to compliance and resistance are significant, as in airway obstruction or worsening respiratory failure, decreasing tidal volumes may be delivered, resulting in underventilation of the patient. However, practically speaking, the ventilator will alarm for low minute ventilation. For differences between adult and pediatric normal respiratory parameters, see Table 37.3.

One advantage of pressure-controlled ventilation is that most ventilators have a decelerating inspiratory flow

Table 37.3 Respiratory mechanics

	Infant	Adult
Respiratory frequency (breaths/min)	30–40	12–16
Inspiratory time (sec)	0.4–0.5	1.2–1.4
I/E ratio	1/1.5–1/2	1/2–1/3
Inspiratory flow (L/min)	2–3	24
Tidal volume		
mL	18–24	500
mL/kg	6–8	6–8
Functional residual capacity (FRC)		
mL	100	2200
mL/kg	30	34
Vital capacity		
mL	120	3500
mL/kg	33–40	52
Total lung capacity		
mL	200	6000
mL/kg	63	86
Total respiratory compliance		
mL/cmH$_2$O	2.6–4.9	100
mL/cmH$_2$O/mL FRC	0.04–0.06	0.04–0.07
Lung compliance		
mL/cmH$_2$O	4.8–6.2	170–200
mL/cmH$_2$O/mL FRC	0.04–0.07	0.04–0.07
Specific airway conductance		
mL/sec/cmH$_2$O/mL FRC	0.24	0.28
Respiratory insensible water loss		
mL/24 h	45–55	300

pattern for gas delivery. Inspiratory flow is maximal early in inspiration and then gradually decreases to no flow when peak pressure is reached. For most patients, pressure control results in delivery of a tidal volume for a lower peak pressure relative to the pressure reached to deliver the same tidal volume in volume mode.

Modern ventilators have additional modes including a volume-guaranteed setting where the ventilator adjusts to the lowest pressure needed to deliver a set volume. Commonly, the mode is referred to as pressure regulated volume control (PRVC). After several consistent breaths, the ventilator will reduce the peak pressure over several breaths as long as the set volume is delivered. When it falls below the targeted volume, the pressure is increased until the volume is met. This may be an effective means of reducing pulmonary trauma from high peak pressures in patients with severe restrictive lung disease. However, this mode is most effective when patients are well sedated with or without muscle relaxants. Coughing or competing with the ventilator greatly affects the delivered volume.

The previously mentioned ventilator modes all address the means by which mandatory breaths are delivered. Typically the mandatory delivered breaths are synchronized to the patient's effort to initiate a breath. These triggers to initiate a breath occur by a change in flow or change in pressure in the ventilator circuit. A third triggering strategy has recently been developed by Maquet using the Servo-i® ventilator with NAVA® (Neurally Adjusted Ventilatory Assist). A small esophageal probe is placed in the patient, which senses the electrical activity of the diaphragm. The diaphragm activity is used as the trigger to start the ventilator. A possible benefit of NAVA is that patients may be ventilated more comfortably and will require less sedation. Improved synchrony has been shown in an animal study [55]. There is limited work in human infants [56] and further work evaluating the technique is ongoing.

In addition to set ventilator breaths triggered by the patient, further respiratory effort can be supported. When detecting a change in flow or pressure, the ventilator can deliver volume support or pressure support based on the patient's needs. During periods of worsening respiratory illness, the patient can receive additional respiratory support above the set ventilator rate. During periods of improvement some clinicians will use this as a mechanism of weaning from mechanical ventilation. As the patient improves, the set ventilator rate is serially weaned to the point where the patient is mostly or completely breathing with pressure support and PEEP. Pressure support is then gradually decreased to the point where the patient is tolerating just CPAP and then the trachea can be extubated.

High-frequency ventilation describes multiple modes of ventilation where the ventilator's respiratory cycle is far in excess of a normal physiological rate. The earliest published works referring to these systems appeared in the late 1960s with Sanders describing high flow jet ventilation (HFJV) in 1967 [57] and high-frequency positive pressure ventilation (HFPPV) by Oberg and Sjostrand in 1969 [58]. High-frequency oscillatory ventilation (HFOV) was described by Lunkenheimer in 1972 [59] and is the form of high-frequency ventilation most commonly used in pediatric ICUs today. HFOV allows a mean airway pressure to be set. The entire airway and ventilator circuit is pressurized to that value all the way back to a piston on the ventilator. The piston of the ventilator provides small positive and negative ventilatory cycles up to 840 times per minute. The set mean airway pressure maintains airway patency, preventing the cycle of alveolar collapse and overexpansion. A frequency of oscillation is usually chosen between 6 and 14 hertz (1 hertz = 60 cycles/sec) and adjustment of this frequency is a component of altering carbon dioxide removal. An amplitude or distance of piston movement is chosen which effectively wiggles the chest. This chest wiggle also contributes to carbon dioxide removal. FIO_2 is adjusted just as in a typical ventilator. The exact mechanism of gas transport with HFOV is not completely understood. Several proposed mechanisms exist, but due to difficulty of study none has been proven.

High-frequency oscillatory ventilation can be used as a rescue therapy for hypoxemia refractory to conventional mechanical ventilation. It is also used as a means of reducing the shear forces which the lung is exposed to with conventional ventilation. This causes HFOV to be used with air leak syndromes from ongoing pneumothorax or bronchopleural fistula. HFOV should not be used if there is obstruction to expiratory flow, as with bronchospasm. In moderate-to-severe obstructive lung disease, HFOV will frequently result in overdistension of the lung and likely pneumothorax. Randomized controlled trials of early use of HFOV in ARDS have been proposed and discussed, but are difficult to enact due to a lack of equipoise.

Weaning from mechanical ventilation

The pediatric literature is very limited with regard to providing guidance on weaning and extubating from mechanical ventilation. A recent review by Newth et al published in 2009 addresses what is known [60]. Attempts have been made to predict which children can be successfully weaned from mechanical ventilation. Most of the indices are used as research tools. One of the easiest to conceptualize is the Rapid Shallow Breathing Index (RSBI) devised by Yang and Tobin [61]. The RSBI = respiratory rate/tidal volume. When patients are breathing comfortably they have a decreased respiratory rate and are moving larger tidal volumes. Therefore the RSBI decreases.

There are many different techniques for weaning from ventilation. Possibilities include decreasing the set ventilator rate over time, a daily spontaneous breathing trial with pressure- or volume-supported breaths, or increasing cycles of reduced ventilator support until the patient tolerates the decreased support. No clear information exists supporting one means over another. Likely the best current answer is to ask the question on a daily basis whether the patient is able to be extubated. Evidence does show that a significant percentage of patients evaluated for weaning are actually ready for extubation [62,63].

There is an anticipated extubation failure rate; if the intensivist waits until absolutely certain that a patient will not fail, then many patients will be ventilated too long. A review of 16 ICUs for length of ventilation and extubation failure revealed a failure rate of 6.2% (range 1.5–8.8%) for patients intubated longer than 48h [64]. Spontaneous breathing trials are defined periods of decreased support where clinical signs are followed to evaluate respiratory distress. Depending on the institution, this may be pressure support, volume support, CPAP or T-piece ventilation. Some will challenge the patient for 2h and others as little as 15min. There should be no significant increase in respiratory rate, decrease in saturations, diaphoresis or clinical evidence of increased work of breathing or hemodynamic compromise. Blood gas values should not change significantly during these trials; if they do, it is assumed that the patient is not yet ready for extubation.

A common misconception is that patients with smaller endotracheal tubes are "breathing through a straw" when placed on CPAP or T-piece. This view has been refuted through the work of Manczur et al [65], Willis et al [66] and Hammer et al [67]. The ETT is smaller in diameter compared to an adult, but it is also shorter and the flow rate in infants is low compared to an adult. Flow rates are approximately 0.5 L/kg/min [68]. A 3 kg infant has a flow velocity of 1.5 L/min compared to 30 L/min for a 60 kg adult.

In general, criteria for extubation include intact airway reflexes, hemodynamic stability, manageable secretions, and an appropriate level of alertness. Negative inspiratory force (NIF) may be measured. However, many do not measure it appropriately with a calibrated manometer and inspiration from residual volume. However, a NIF of −30 cmH$_2$O or greater is associated with improved success. A leak around the ETT may give additional support that the extubation will be successful. Absence of a leak should not delay extubation if all other conditions are favorable. See Box 37.5 for criteria for extubation. Extubation failure is defined as reintubation within 24 h of a scheduled extu-

---

Box 37.5 Criteria for extubation

- Acceptable ABG or saturations on FIO$_2$ of 0.40 or less with CPAP of 5 cmH$_2$O or less and pressure support of 5 cm H$_2$O or less
- In the absence of cyanotic heart disease, acceptable PaO$_2$ >60 mmHg or saturations >95%
- PaCO$_2$ not elevated more than 20% of the child's baseline
- Comfortable breathing pattern, without tachypnea, retractions or excessive work of breathing
- Able to maintain and protect airway
- Appropriate level of alertness
- Able to cough, breathe deeply, and clear secretions
- Hemodynamic stability
- No major instability of other organ systems
- Able to generate an inspiratory force of −20 to −30 cm H$_2$O (if measurable)

---

bation attempt. Upper airway obstruction has been the stated cause in up to 37% of failed extubations [64]. For this reason, many intensivists pretreat the patient who is ready for extubation with a course of dexamethasone starting 6–12 h in advance. Further research is needed to define measures which may decrease subglottic edema.

Specific diseases of the respiratory system
Asthma
Estimates from the US Centers for Disease Control indicate the prevalence of childhood asthma is increasing. In 1980 it was estimated at 3.6%, in 2003 it was 5.8% and in 2008 it is estimated the percent of children who currently have asthma is 9.4%. It is fortunate that the majority of children with asthma attacks will never be ill enough to require intensive care. However, for the small percentage of children that do, the morbidity and mortality are much greater. In fact, prior ICU admission and history of intubation for asthma are strong indicators of severe or uncontrolled asthma.

Asthma is a disease of inflammation. The submucosal area of the airways is infiltrated with mast cells, eosinophils, and CD4 lymphocytes. When mast cells are degranulated, leukotrienes and histamine are released, resulting in edema, increased mucus production, and attraction of white blood cells. Asthma attacks and triggering of mast cells can be caused by allergens, infections (viral > bacterial), weather changes, and strong emotions. The inflammatory environment increases airway irritability and hyper-responsiveness. Severe spasm of the bronchial muscles adds to the edema and mucus to reduce the airway lumen. Resistance to laminar airflow is inversely proportional to the fourth power of the radius but with turbulent flow it is to the fifth power. Children experience much greater increases in airway resistance during asthma attacks than adults, due to the smaller caliber of their airways. There is greater resistance to exhalation and the clinical presentation is one of expiratory wheezing. Mucus plugging or complete obstruction of small airways can occur from edema and bronchospasm. The primary initial component is hypoxemia as a result of V/Q mismatch. Air trapping can lead to increased dead space. To compensate, respiratory rate is increased. Typically, the initial $PaCO_2$ is low. A normal or elevated $PaCO_2$ may indicate fatigue and impending respiratory failure.

It is important to recognize early that not all wheezing episodes are asthma, and that asthma can occur without wheezing. Wheezing is the sound of obstruction to airflow. In addition to asthma, wheezing can be caused by pneumonia, upper airway obstruction, aspiration of a foreign body, and congestive heart failure. All these conditions merit different therapies. Sudden onset of wheezing in a toddler with no prior history of asthma or atopy should prompt evaluation for foreign body aspiration.

Intermittently, we are surprised when a chest radiograph obtained for wheezing shows cardiomegaly rather than peribronchial cuffing. A chest radiograph is warranted for any first-time wheezing patient and any child admitted to the ICU with wheezing. Airflow is required to detect wheezing by auscultation. Children can present with such significant airflow restrictions that they are unable to wheeze. Such patients presenting with a quiet chest are concerning and require immediate action.

The typical presentation of a child with asthma may be one of a few days of upper respiratory infections (URI) symptoms followed by increased work of breathing. The patient has a decreased SpO_2 in room air and is frequently sitting up. There is accessory muscle use, a prolonged expiratory phase, and possibly pursed-lip breathing (also known as autopositive end expiratory pressure). If a child is able to speak it may only be in one- or two-word bursts. There should be no delay in starting therapy. Supplemental oxygen is given to address hypoxemia. If the child is alert and speaking, with a moderate expiratory wheeze, nasal cannula oxygen may be sufficient. If respiratory distress is more severe, oxygen should be delivered by either simple facemask or non-rebreather facemask. Inhaled β agonists are given to relax bronchial smooth muscles. Typically this is albuterol, but occasionally intravenous terbutaline is needed, as are subcutaneous terbutaline or epinephrine. Steroids should be given early in treatment as they will take time to become effective. If there is not significant improvement with initial therapy, arrangements for ICU admission should be considered. Arterial blood gases are often obtained but usually the clinical picture provides more information to direct care.

Therapy of asthma

Supplemental oxygen

Oxygen can be delivered by a standard nasal cannula, but concentration is limited. High-flow humidified nasal cannula may provide greater FIO_2 and delivery of β agonists with this device is becoming common. Simple facemasks or non-rebreather facemasks are frequently used.

Inhaled β agonists

Inhaled β agonists relax bronchial smooth muscles. Albuterol is most commonly used and is a racemic mixture of the R- and S-enantiomers. The active R-enantiomer is available (levalbuterol) and may be associated with less tachycardia, but is more expensive. Albuterol is β2 selective, available as metered dose inhaler and solution for nebulization. Initially in the ICU setting, continuous albuterol is preferred and the usual dose is 0.15–0.5 mg/kg/h or 10–20 mg/h. When there is improvement, intermittent doses can be given every 1–2 h. Inhaled terbutaline is less β2 selective compared to albuterol and therefore is used less commonly. Albuterol use is associated with tachycardia. Less often there can be dysrhythmias such as increased premature ventricular contractions. At higher doses diastolic hypotension has been observed. Central nervous system (CNS) stimulation occurs typically with agitation and tremors. β Agonists drive potassium into cells so hypokalemia can be seen on electrolyte panels. Ipratropium bromide is an inhaled anticholinergic that is sometimes paired with intermittent albuterol doses. Ipratropium bromide promotes bronchodilation without decreasing mucociliary clearance.

Corticosteroids

In an ICU setting intravenous steroids are preferred to oral due to concerns of decreased absorption. Inhaled steroids are of no benefit in the initial ICU setting. Methylprednisolone is commonly used because of its limited mineralocorticoid effects. The first dose is 2 mg/kg and then 0.5–1 mg/kg every 6 h. Some ICUs will prefer dexamethasone or hydrocortisone. Steroids are usually given for the duration of the acute asthma attack. If given for 5 days or less, they typically are not tapered. Hyperglycemia, hypertension and occasionally agitation are seen with systemic steroid use.

Intravenous fluids

Children admitted with status asthmaticus will likely be dehydrated from poor oral intake during their illness and higher insensible losses from increased respiratory effort. Patients should be rehydrated to a sufficient circulating volume. Excessive fluids should be avoided so as to not contribute to pulmonary edema, which could worsen both oxygenation and airway resistance. For children who require mechanical ventilation, additional fluid may be needed around the time of intubation to prevent hypotension.

Intravenous and subcutaneous β agonists

Severely reduced air exchange may prompt the use of IV β agonists. If there is limited ventilation albuterol distribution and absorption may be limited. Of the available drugs, terbutaline is often first choice. Terbutaline is relatively β2 selective compared to isoproterenol and epinephrine. For children without IV access it can be given subcutaneously with a dose of 0.01 mg/kg/dose up to a maximum of 0.3 mg. Intravenous terbutaline is given with a loading dose of 10 μg/kg over 10–20 min. The continuous infusion is given with a range of 0.1–10 μg/kg/min titrated to effect. Intermittently subcutaneous epinephrine is given for severe asthma exacerbation with a dose of 0.01 mg/kg of the 1:1000 solution with a maximum dose of 0.5 mg. Poor perfusion to extremities may limit absorption. Intravenous epinephrine may be an ideal drug for mechanically ventilated patients with hypotension. Isoproterenol is rarely used in status asthmaticus.

Methylxanthines

The decision as to whether the methylxanthine aminophylline or the β agonist terbutaline is a second-line drug appears to be regional. With the increased use of leukotriene inhibitors for maintenance asthma therapy, fewer children are receiving oral theophylline. Methylxanthines promote relaxation of the bronchial smooth muscle, but the exact mechanism of action is not completely known. IV aminophylline is loaded with a dose of 5–7 mg/kg over 30 min followed by a continuous infusion of 0.5–0.9 mg/kg/h. If the patient has received oral theophylline in the prior 24 h the loading dose is reduced by 50% or dosing is adjusted based on serum theophylline level. Generally, a loading dose of 1 mg/kg will raise the serum theophylline level by 2 μg/mL. The goal for theophylline is 10–20 μg/mL. Theophylline has a very narrow therapeutic window and levels above 20 μg/mL are often associated with nausea, tachycardia, restlessness or irritability. Higher levels have been associated with seizure activity.

Magnesium

Magnesium sulfate can be given intravenously to relax bronchial muscles. It causes smooth muscle relaxation due to its effect as a calcium channel blocker. Controversy exists as to whether magnesium has a significant clinical benefit and in turn its use is clinician dependent. A magnesium level should be measured with the initial set of electrolytes and hypomagnesemia should be treated. The dose for status asthmaticus or hypomagnesemia is 25–40 mg/kg given over 30 min. Toxicity of magnesium can include muscle weakness, decreased reflexes, cardiac arrhythmias, and respiratory depression.

Helium

Helium oxygen mixtures (heliox) are used to improve laminar flow of gas due to the decreased density of helium compared to nitrogen. Helium is about one-seventh as dense as air. Heliox may be potentially beneficial in the treatment of asthma by improving flow in very small airways. However, benefit from helium occurs when it is administered in a high ratio compared to oxygen. The most effective ratios would be 80:20 or 70:30 helium:oxygen. In clinical practice hypoxemia and the need for supplemental oxygen typically limit heliox use.

Ketamine

Ketamine is a dissociative anesthetic that produces bronchodilation. In usual doses it does not blunt the respiratory drive or cause significant myocardial depression. It does, however, increase oral and airway secretions. Ketamine is a good sedative in conjunction with a benzodiazepine for patients who are intubated and mechanically ventilated. It is still not clear whether ketamine used to treat anxiety is beneficial in preventing intubation in patients during an asthma attack. Ketamine is given as a bolus dose at 1 mg/kg, allowing time for effect before repeating. Ketamine as a continuous infusion is usually given as 5–30 μg/kg/min titrated to effect. As ketamine is a dissociative anesthetic causing dysphoria it is usually given with a benzodiazepine.

Non-invasive ventilation

There is very limited evidence that non-invasive ventilation (NIV) is effective in children with asthma [69]. Clinically, patients with effective air exchange who fight the mask and positive pressure do not benefit from NIV. Nevertheless, some children with very limited air exchange and fatigue take to NIV easily and appear more comfortable. Non-invasive ventilation may allow time for therapies to become effective (steroids) and may prevent intubation. This should not be used when the level of alertness or ability to protect the airway is diminished.

Tracheal intubation and mechanical ventilation

Asthmatic patients who require intubation are hypoxemic, acidotic, and greatly fatigued. They have limited reserve and decreased mental status, often from CO_2 narcosis that occurs with acutely elevated $PaCO_2$ above 80 mmHg. In this scenario, it is preferable to have the most experienced practitioner to intubate the patient. Good venous access is necessary and fluid boluses should be ready. Ketamine and a benzodiazepine titrated to effect are a good choice for many practitioners. In our unit a short-acting muscle relaxant such as rocuronium is preferred to allow the patient to breathe spontaneously as soon as possible. A cuffed endotracheal tube should be used as high peak pressures on the ventilator may be necessary. Slow hand ventilation after intubation will prevent alveolar overdistension and the risk of pneumothorax. Acute decompensation following intubation requires prompt evaluation. Causes include displacement or obstruction of the endotracheal tube, pneumothorax or decreased venous return from excessive positive pressure resulting in reduced stroke volume and cardiac output.

Mechanical ventilation

Controversy remains regarding the best means to mechanically ventilate patients with asthma. During pressure-controlled ventilation, changes in airway resistance occurring with asthma result in variable tidal volumes. However, volume-controlled ventilation may be suboptimal in that the same tidal volume can be delivered with a lower peak pressure in a pressure-controlled mode. The goal for intubated children with asthma is to achieve spontaneous ventilation as soon as possible. The patient then sets his or her own respiratory rates and inspired tidal volumes, and spontaneous breathing allows active exhalation as early as possible during weaning from mechanical assistance. Pressure support ventilation may be helpful in this scenario [70]. In the short term an increase in $PaCO_2$ is well tolerated as long as the patient is well oxygenated.

Classically PEEP was limited during treatment of obstructive airways disease such as asthma in view of the perceived risk of hyperinflation [71] and barotrauma. However, since 1988 there have been four studies in adults [72–75] and one [76] in children which suggested that adding extrinsic PEEP during mechanical ventilation is effective. The studies showed that extrinsic PEEP (PEEP added by the ventilator), up to a level matching intrinsic PEEP (residual pressure at the end of the ventilator cycle due to expiratory obstruction), improves effective triggering sensitivity of the ventilator. This in turn diminishes ventilatory work, and reduces mechanical work of breathing (WOB) during assisted and spontaneous breathing. This decrease in WOB reduces stress and improves comfort by reducing need for sedation. Matching PEEP may improve delivery of aerosol therapy via the endotracheal tube, and possibly allow earlier liberation from mechanical ventilation. However, it also carries the negative implication that application of increased levels of PEEP will overdistend the patient's lungs and increase the hazards of hyperinflation such as air leak syndrome [71,77]. According to our studies [66,76], during spontaneous breathing both application of PEEP and breathing with pressure-supported breaths lower WOB. However, the level of extrinsically applied PEEP at which hyperinflation will occur is unknown for any given patient. Theoretically, if the patient is breathing spontaneously, application of extrinsic PEEP to counteract intrinsic PEEP should not cause any increase in end-expiratory lung volume (EELV) until the former supersedes the latter [78]. Further, EELV may even decrease which would decrease dead space and increase compliance. In our current practice intrinsic PEEP is measured by allowing the patient to exhale completely with a ventilator pause and measuring final pressure before the next breath. Extrinsic PEEP is gradually added to the ventilator as respiratory rate and clinical work of breathing are observed. Extrinsic PEEP always kept at a level below intrinsic PEEP. These values are reassessed as the patient responds to therapy. Further research studies are necessary to determine the best means of applying mechanical ventilation to these patients.

Inhalational anesthetics

Inhaled anesthetics have been used as bronchodilators in critically ill intubated children with asthma. The largest reported case series is six patients [79]. Isoflurane has been used effectively in our ICU with the reduction of bronchospasm and the ability to decrease intravenous sedation, but there are difficulties associated with its use. Most ventilators are not designed to accept a vaporizer. ICU ventilators do not have a circle system so there is a tremendous use of anesthetic vapor. Scavenging is a significant concern to reduce contamination of the patient room. Details of its use and other therapies in the ICU are included in several recent reviews [80–82]. A good choice where available would be to use a modern anesthesia machine with a ventilator capable of performance matching standard ICU ventilators, while having a built-in vaporizer and anesthetic gas scavenging ability.

Extracorporeal life support

Extracorporeal life support (ECLS) has been used as a rescue therapy in near fatal asthma with some positive success. Given the nature of this therapy, the reports are very small in number. As there is usually no other associated disease state, the use of ECLS for asthma may be considered as there are no co-morbidities that would preclude its use. See Box 37.6.

Acute lung injury and acute respiratory distress syndrome
Consensus definitions

Consensus definitions of disease states from leaders in their fields improve research and clinical care through uniformity. Enrollment criteria and assessments can be standard across hospitals and providers. The American European Consensus Conference on ARDS defined acute

Box 37.6 Escalating asthma therapy

Supplemental oxygen

- Nasal cannula can deliver FIO_2 up to 40%
- May require facemask oxygen or high-flow humidified oxygen
- Mask BiPAP therapy may decrease work of breathing in co-operative patients

Inhaled β agonists

- Albuterol is most common, racemic β2-selective agonist
- Continuous albuterol dosing 0.15–0.5 mg/kg/h or 10–20 mg/h
- Xoponex is R-enantiomer of albuterol, expensive but less tachycardia

Corticosteroids

- Methylprednisolone used commonly due to limited mineralocorticoid effects
- First dose 2 mg/kg and then 0.5–1 mg/kg every 6 h
- Regional practice may use dexamethasone or hydrocortisone
- If given for less than 5 days, steroid taper usually not indicated

Intravenous fluids

- Patients should be rehydrated to a sufficient circulating volume
- Avoid excessive fluids

Intravenous or subcutaneous β agonist

- Terbutaline can be given subcutaneously if there is no IV access
- Subcutaneous terbutaline 0.01 mg/kg/dose up to max of 0.3 mg
- IV terbutaline load of 10 µg/kg over 10–20 min
- IV terbutaline drip 0.1–10 µg/kg/min titrated to effect

Methylxanthines

- Promote relaxation of bronchial smooth muscle
- IV aminophylline load of 5–7 mg/kg over 30 min
- IV aminophylline drip 0.5–0.9 mg/kg/h
- If the patient has been taking oral theophylline, load reduced by 50%
- Target theophylline level is 10–20 µg/mL

Magnesium

- IV bronchial smooth muscle relaxant
- IV dose for asthma or hypomagnesium is 25–40 mg/kg over 30 min
- Toxicity includes muscle weakness, decreased reflexes, arrhythmias, respiratory depression

Helium

- Reduces work of breathing due to improved laminar flow
- Helium is 1/7th as dense as nitrogen
- Typically 70% helium required for benefit so hypoxemia usually limits use

Ketamine

- Dissociative anesthetic that produces bronchodilation
- Usual doses do not blunt respiratory drive but do increase secretions
- Bolus dose 1 mg/kg, drip 5–30 µg/kg/min titrated to effect
- May cause dysphoria, usually given with a benzodiazepine

Non-invasive ventilation

- Mask BiPAP therapy may decrease work of breathing in co-operative patients

Intubation and mechanical ventilation

- Patients have limited reserve at this point; the most experienced person should intubate
- Ketamine and a benzodiazepine may be good induction agents
- Fluid boluses likely will be required
- Reversing muscle relaxants as early as possible may allow the patient to breath with PS/PEEP

Inhalational anesthetics

- Isoflurane is a potent bronchodilator
- Technical aspects limit delivery of inhaled anesthetics with modern ventilators

Extracorporeal life support (ECLS)

- Has been used as a rescue therapy in near fatal asthma
- Very few reported cases

---

lung injury (ALI) and acute respiratory distress syndrome (ARDS) in 1994 [83]. This acknowledges that respiratory distress can occur in all ages, as the disease had been known at times as adult respiratory distress syndrome [84]. ALI and ARDS are the acute onset of bilateral infiltrates on chest radiograph without evidence of left ventricular dysfunction and a diminished PaO_2/FIO_2 (PF) ratio. The PF ratio for ALI is ≤300 and the PF ratio for ARDS is ≤200. The concern for ventricular function follows from a higher incidence of myocardial infarction in adults leading to decreased cardiac contractility, resulting in pulmonary edema and a lower PF ratio. This would be a separate disease process. Cardiac dysfunction can occur in children, but is less common. Bilateral infiltrates on chest radiograph identify diffuse pulmonary inflammation. See Box 37.7.

Box 37.7 Acute lung injury (ALI) and acute respiratory distress syndrome (ARDS) definitions

- Acute onset of disease
- Bilateral infiltrates on chest radiograph
- No clinical evidence of left atrial hypertension or left ventricular dysfunction
- For ALI $PaO_2/FIO_2 \leq 300$
- For ARDS $PaO_2/FIO_2 \leq 200$
- In the absence of an arterial line:
  - ALI: pulse oximeter saturation $(SaO_2)/FIO_2 \leq 260$ has been used
  - ARDS: $SaO_2/FIO_2 \leq 200$ has been used

Morbidity and mortality

Acute lung injury and ARDS are associated with significant morbidity and mortality. Historical estimates had placed mortality at 50% or more. The length of time spent on a ventilator can be weeks or longer. Ventilator free days (VFD) is a term used to compare outcomes with therapy in lung injury. The ventilator free days are the number of days out of 28 that the patient is not mechanically ventilated. Estimates of mortality and decisions about management changed when the ARDS network published a landmark paper in the New England Journal of Medicine in 2000 [85]. For adult patients with ALI and ARDS, ventilation with a lower tidal volume of 6 mL/kg predicted bodyweight resulted in decreased mortality (31%) compared to a tidal volume of 12 mL/kg (39%). The clinical trial was stopped early due to these findings. Additionally, there was also a significant increase in ventilator free days using the lower tidal volume. Concerns were raised following this study that the larger tidal volume control arm did not reflect current care provided in most adult ICUs. Over a period of years clinicians had moved closer to 8–10 mL/kg and if a low tidal volume strategy was used, it was with 5–7 mL/kg. The ARDS network trial demonstrated a lower mortality for this disease process (31%), but some portion of this may have been improved overall care. In adult studies the degree of hypoxia at presentation is not associated with increased mortality. The changes to clinical practice following these reports have been significant. The take-home message was: lower peak pressures, smaller tidal volumes and oxygenation supported with increased PEEP. Many intensivists and ICUs have changed their practice.

Flori et al [86] reported a mortality rate for ALI and ARDS in children of 22%. This was significantly lower than adult mortality at the time. These children were enrolled in a time period from 1996 to 2000 at two major pediatric hospitals. In addition, it was demonstrated in children that the initial degree of hypoxemia was associated with mortality. This decreased mortality likely represents the first modern-era publication of pediatric ALI/ARDS. Albuali et al [87] published outcomes for ALI from a single center in two groups (1988–1992 and 2000–2004). The earlier group was ventilated with significantly higher tidal volumes (10 mL/kg), lower PEEP (6 cmH$_2$O), and higher inspiratory pressures (31.5 cmH$_2$O) and had a mortality of 35%. The later group used a tidal volume of 8 mL/kg, PEEP of 7 cmH$_2$O, and inspiratory pressures of 28. The mortality in this group was 21% and there was a significantly increased number of ventilator free days. A higher tidal volume was independently associated with increased mortality. This study also described significant increases in patients receiving adjuvant therapy to treat hypoxemia. There was increased use of inhaled nitric oxide, high-frequency oscillatory ventilation, prone positioning, surfactant administration and extracorporeal life support. Over the long run not all adjuvant therapies have proven efficacious; however, this does demonstrate that other interventions are available.

The similarities between children and adults include the primary causes of ALI/ARDS, which are pneumonia, aspiration and sepsis, and increased mortality for patients with more than one organ system disease. These studies also highlight the differences between adults and children. For pediatric lung injury, the initial degree of hypoxemia relates to mortality, which is not the case for adults. In turn, low tidal volume strategies may be helpful when using PEEP to recruit lungs in pediatric patients. Further, many pediatric studies take into account the amount of ventilator support needed to arrive at a degree of oxygenation. One measure is the oxygenation index (OI): $OI = (FIO_2 \times \text{mean airway pressure})/PaO_2$. The mode of ventilation used in respiratory failure also differs between intensivists caring for adults versus children. There are institutional and regional preferences but in general the majority of adults are ventilated with a volume mode and children are ventilated with a pressure mode. Data from our institution [88] assessing outcomes for patients with ALI or ARDS revealed that greater than 90% were ventilated with a pressure control mode.

Pediatric research

Pediatric research for acute lung injury (ALI) is limited by low incidence of disease and relatively low mortality. Recent population studies in Australia, New Zealand, and The Netherlands place the incidence of ALI between 2.2 and 2.9/100,000 for age <16 years [89,90]. Ventilator free days can be used as a surrogate outcome but quality of life indicators as an outcome measure are not common in children. Research groups have been formed to collaborate on research trials in the hope of providing more accurate or rapid answers to these questions. The Pediatric Acute Lung Injury and Sepsis Investigators (PALISI) held their first meeting in 2002 and currently have 78 PICUs participating. Recent studies have evaluated blood transfusion [91] and surfactant therapies with ALI [92]. One potential limitation to study enrollment is the need for an arterial PaO_2 to identify hypoxemia. The routine use of pulse oximetry has meant that many more patients are being managed without an arterial catheter. It has been shown in adults [93] and children [94] that a SpO_2/FIO_2 (SF) ratio provides a useful alternative to PF ratio for enrollment in trials and clinical care. Values to define lung injury using SF ratios are <260 for ALI and <200 for ARDS.

Therapy

There are a number of therapies providing temporary improvements in oxygenation, but no effect on mortality or ventilator free days. Such therapies include prone positioning and inhaled nitric oxide. Numa et al [95] demonstrated that prone positioning of children did not improve functional residual capacity (FRC) and only improved oxygenation in those with obstructive lung disease. However, prone positioning continued to be used to improve oxygenation in children with ALI or ARDS [96,97]. In 2005 PALISI [97] demonstrated no improvement in ventilator free days for children with ALI treated with prone positioning. Similarly, inhaled nitric oxide use may temporarily improve oxygenation but a review and meta-analysis [98] with mostly adult data showed no reduction in mortality.

Potential rescue therapies for hypoxemia unresponsive to conventional ventilation are high-frequency oscillatory ventilation (HFOV) and extracorporeal life support (ECLS). HFOV maintains a near constant mean airway pressure and oscillation of a piston provides movement of very low tidal volumes. A large randomized cross-over trial showed no improvement in ventilator free days or mortality with HFOV [99]. However, with little else to offer, HFOV remains common in many pediatric centers [100]. A similar effect is seen with ECLS for ARDS. Results of the CESAR trial (described in the ECLS section) for adults with ARDS showed that for patients treated with ECLS, 63% survived to 6 months without disability. This is compared to 47% treated with conventional ventilation. Given the significant resources used by ECLS and its associated risks, decisions regarding its use should take into account other disease states the patient has and their prognosis.

Surfactant use to treat ALI and ARDS has not been promising in adults [101]. A large randomized pediatric trial showed an improvement in mortality and ventilator free days with use of exogenous surfactant [102]. In a small subset of patients from this study who were immunocompromised, surfactant therapy showed potentially an even greater benefit [92]. Patients who develop ALI or ARDS following hematopoietic stem cell transplantation have significant mortality reported as 71% [103]. Clearly any reasonable therapy that could show promise deserves further study.

Transfusion of red blood cells increases oxygen-carrying capacity. Unfortunately, no pediatric data indicate that supranormal values for hemoglobin confer any benefit. In addition, work published by Lacroix et al [91] showed a hemoglobin target of 7.5 g/dL to be as safe as 10 g/dL in stable patients in pediatric ICUs. There are risks to transfusion including fluid overload and transfusion-related acute lung injury. See section on Hematology/oncology later in this chapter.

There is potential promise from adult studies using glucocorticosteroids in patients with ARDS improving mortality and ventilator free days [104]. However, there are no studies of corticosteroid use in pediatric patients for the treatment of ALI or ARDS.

Management recommendations

The underlying trigger for ARDS should be identified and eliminated if possible. Sources such as infection, pancreatitis, and tissue necrosis can cause lung injury through inflammation. Antibiotics should be given early for any suspected infection. The overall goal of ventilator management is not to achieve normal blood gases. A degree of hypercarbia and respiratory acidosis may be tolerated in an effort to reduce the lung injury that can occur with overzealous ventilator management. The goal range for pH can be 7.30–7.45. Lower than normal saturations (≥89%) are tolerated, but there are no long-term outcome data on this intervention. To avoid barotrauma and volutrauma, tidal volumes greater than 10 mL/kg and plateau pressures greater than 30 cmH₂O should be avoided if at all possible. In a pressure control mode of ventilation, adjust the peak pressure to achieve tidal volumes of 6–10 mL/kg. After possible fluid resuscitation for shock, overall fluid balance should be restricted if possible.

Extracorporeal life support

Background

Cardiopulmonary support in the PICU with extracorporeal life support (ECLS) grew from experience in the operating room. ECLS is also known as extracorporeal membrane oxygenation (ECMO); the latter term is perhaps more descriptive. Work started initially in the neonatal population to support infants with profound hypoxemia due to meconium aspiration, pneumonia, sepsis or persistent fetal circulation with pulmonary hypertension. Over the years, advances in respiratory support such as HFOV, surfactant use and inhaled nitric oxide have decreased ECLS in this population. There remains the need for support of respiratory failure in refractory hypoxemia as well as congenital diaphragmatic hernia and there has been a dramatic increase in ECLS for cardiac support following surgical repair of congenital heart defects.

Similar to cardiopulmonary bypass in the operating room, blood is drained from the body passively by gravity from the largest vein safely accessed in the child. The blood passes through a membrane oxygenator where carbon dioxide is removed and oxygen is added. Blood is warmed and pumped back into the body. Blood returns via the same double-lumen venous cannula in veno-venous (VV) ECLS or via an arterial cannula in veno-arterial (VA) ECLS. For respiratory support the decision to initially pursue VV or VA ECLS is usually based on the experience of the center. There are associated risks and benefits of each but VV ECLS relies on native cardiac output, whereas VA ECLS can completely support both pulmonary and cardiac function.

Cervical cannulation is preferred in infants and small children. In VV ECLS, a double-lumen catheter is placed in the right internal jugular (IJ) vein. The proximal portion of the catheter drains blood from the right atrium and blood is perfused back via the distal lumen towards the tricuspid valve. VV ECLS relies on the heart to function as the pump returning oxygenated blood to the lungs and body. In VA ECLS a drainage venous catheter is placed via the right IJ into the right atrium and blood is returned via a second arterial catheter placed in the right carotid artery. The return of blood is directed toward the descending portion of the aortic arch and away from the aortic valve. Some institutions will use a second drainage catheter placed retrograde in the internal jugular vein at the level of the jugular venous bulb to improve cerebral venous drainage and monitor jugular venous oxygen saturations.

In adolescents and adults it is possible to provide access for VA and VV ECLS via femoral blood vessels. Following repair of congenital heart defects, if there is respiratory or cardiac failure requiring support, cannulation can occur through the mediastinum. The venous catheter is typically placed via the right atrial appendage and the arterial catheter is placed in the aorta. If there are limitations to outflow via the aortic valve or severe left ventricular dysfunction, a left atrial drain may be placed into the left ventricle to prevent ventricular dilation.

Basic components of the ECLS circuit include a venous reservoir collecting blood draining from the patient, a pump to drive blood flow, and an oxygenator that provides for gas exchange. In the past, the majority of ECLS circuits use a rollerhead pump that produces non-pulsatile blood flow. Centrifugal pumps were used much less commonly and had a higher incidence of hemolysis. Modern pumps, such as the Rotaflow Centrifugal Pump (Maquet Inc., www.maquet.com), use modern designs to minimize blood heating and hemolysis, and are the preferred device in many centers. The other significant difference between

these types of pumps is that if there is a downstream obstruction, with a roller pump there is the risk of tubing or circuit rupture. This does not occur with centrifugal pumps, but the flow of blood still decreases. Membrane oxygenators consist of a silicone membrane envelope wound around a central spool. Blood is kept separate from gas and diffusion occurs across the membrane. Hollow fiber oxygenators were used less commonly in the past, but as technology improves they offer some advantages. The Quadrox D and Quadrox iD Pediatric (Maquet Inc., www.maquet.com) offer high gas transfer rates and a low pressure drop across the oxygenator that minimize blood trauma and have become the preferred devices in many centers.

Patients requiring ECLS and those caring for them receive great benefit from the Extracorporeal Life Support Organization (ELSO) and its registry. Since 1989 it has been maintaining a registry on the care and outcomes of patients receiving ECLS at active ELSO centers. There are details on greater than 40,000 national and international patients. The majority of the ECLS literature comes from the ELSO registry and large single-center studies.

Infant outcomes

Over time a significant improvement in outcomes for ECLS for meconium aspiration has occurred, with survival approximately 95% [105]. This is the best outcome for all ECLS indications and all age groups. With improvement in respiratory support and care, there has been a steady decrease in neonatal ECLS for respiratory failure. At the same time, use of ECLS for cardiac support has increased. In review of the ELSO data from 1996 to 2000 for cardiac ECLS in neonates, there was a 34.2% survival to discharge or transfer [106]. The diagnoses of transposition of the great arteries (TGA) and persistent pulmonary hypertension of the neonate (PPHN), and initiating ECLS at less than 3 days of age were associated with a greater likelihood of survival. Survival was also improved in patients with shorter ECLS runs. Evaluating the entire registry for neonates, survival to discharge was 75% for respiratory failure, 39% for cardiac failure, and 38% if placed on ECLS during cardiopulmonary resuscitation [105]. Due to the need for heparin therapy while on ECLS and its associated risk of intracranial hemorrhage, prematurity is a contraindication to ECLS.

Pediatric outcomes

Pediatric ECLS has been used in many fewer cases compared to neonates and the indications are very different. In children, the causes of respiratory failure are more varied and therefore compared to neonates the outcome in the total registry is worse. For ECLS for respiratory failure, neonatal survival is 75% and for older children

56% [105]. For children, the causes of cardiovascular failure include postoperative, cardiomyopathy or myocarditis. In a population of 1–16 year olds requiring ECLS for cardiac support, the indication was cardiomyopathy in 15.35% of the patients [107]. The overall ELSO registry of survival for pediatric cardiac ECLS is 47% and 39% if initiated during CPR [103]. Results are similar in a large single-center study of cannulation for ECLS during active resuscitation where there was a 33% survival to discharge [108].

Adult outcomes

The first randomized trial of ECLS in adult ARDS was published in 1979 [109]. Nine ECLS centers participated and the survival was 9.5% with ECLS and 8.3% with conventional therapy. There were significant concerns that inexperience with this new technique contributed to the mortality. In 1994, Morris et al [110] published the results of a randomized trial from one center where extracorporeal carbon dioxide removal was performed with mechanical ventilation versus conventional ventilation for adult ARDS. The 30-day survival was not significantly different between the two groups at 33% versus 42%. However, this was a significant improvement compared to the overall mortality for ARDS. There have been significantly more studies performed over the last several years and many more adults placed on ECLS. The CESAR trial (Conventional Ventilatory Support Versus Extracorporeal Membrane Oxygenation for Sever Adult Respiratory Failure) has recently been published. Of the patients allocated to consideration for ECLS treatment, 63% survived to 6 months without disability compared to 47% allocated to conventional therapy [111]. Potentially due to poor initial outcomes, the overall survival to discharge in adult patients placed on ECLS for respiratory failure is 52% from the ELSO registry [105]. Compared to pediatric patients, many of the adults placed on ECLS for cardiac causes have had cardiogenic shock following myocardial infarction. There is also a population of patients who fail to wean off bypass following cardiac surgery. In turn, the survival for adult cardiac ECLS is 34% and 27% when started during CPR [105].

Pediatric indications

Criteria defining both the use and exclusion of ECLS for children with cardiac, respiratory, or multiorgan failure are less structured compared to those for neonates. In addition, as ECLS programs grow in experience and technology changes, ECLS is initiated in patients who previously would have been excluded for secondary disease. It is clear that hypoxia not responding to conventional ventilation with lung recruitment strategies or to high-frequency ventilation is an indication for ECLS. However, at some point in the disease process the ventilator trauma

that has occurred before ECLS may preclude a successful outcome. In a retrospective review by Nance et al [112] of ELSO data for 2550 pediatric patients, survival decreased significantly as ventilator days prior to ECLS increased. For each additional day of pre-ECLS ventilation, the average decrease in survival was 2.9%. Their study also found a decrease in survival with increasing age, on average 2.5% per additional year of age.

Extracorporeal life support has been used as a rescue therapy for additional disease processes. In a single-institution study of ECLS used in septic shock, 21/45 patients survived to discharge [113]. ECLS has also been used sporadically to support patients with meticillin-resistant *Staphylococcus aureus* sepsis [114] and case reports occur for cardiovascular failure supported with ECLS for specific causes such as ibuprofen overdose [115] or anterior mediastinal mass [116].

Significant complications can occur with ECLS use. Patients will receive blood transfusions as their circulatory volume is now expanded and hemolysis occurs. To prevent thrombosis, the circuit is heparinized which increases the risk of bleeding or heparin-induced thrombocytopenia [117]. Bleeding is the most common complication of ECLS and of greater risk if the patient is status post cardiac surgery. In neonates there remains a risk of intracranial hemorrhage from anticoagulant use, but this is reduced in older populations. There can be significant neurological injury that occurs with ECLS [118] and this risk is greater if ECLS is initiated during CPR [119]. Patients are at risk for the development of systemic infections [120,121], liver and kidney dysfunction. There is an infrequent risk for mechanical components failure of ECLS equipment [122]. As with conventional mechanical ventilation or HFOV, ongoing medications are needed for sedation while on ECLS.

Cardiac ventricular assist devices as a bridge to recovery or transplant

The decision to use mechanical support for a failing myocardium can be a difficult one, depending on the underlying cause. Myocardial dysfunction can follow cardiopulmonary bypass (CPB) and is separated into those unable to separate from CPB in the operating room and those able to separate from CPB initially. There is a greater chance of a good outcome if there is a period of separation before needing cardiac support. In both cases, however, ECLS may be a reasonable means of support as recovery of myocardial function may occur in a period of several days. When the underlying myocardial dysfunction is secondary to chronic dysrhythmias, dilated cardiomyopathy, viral myocarditis or failed prior surgical palliation for complex congenital heart disease, the need for support may extend beyond a few weeks. Mechanical support may not be a bridge to recovery, but a bridge to transplantation. The possibility of whether the patient can be a candidate for transplantation must be included in the discussion. The need for daily immunosuppressant, medical follow-up, financial and social support for the patient as well as the limitation of donor organs all affect the decision to provide long-term support for a failing heart.

The devices available at each institution are primarily chosen by the cardiothoracic surgical service. Centrifugal ventricular assist devices are commonly chosen for short-term support. Children more often than adults have right heart failure and may need biventricular support. Equipment may be limited for infants due to their size. Implantable devices are used more commonly in adults but are appearing in pediatrics. Currently the HeartAssist 5™ is the only FDA-approved device for pediatric use. The Berlin Heart EXCOR VAD has been used extensively on a compassionate use basis by petitioning the FDA, and a multicenter trial of this device is under way.

Central nervous system

Baseline neurological examination

During admission to the pediatric ICU each child receives a neurological examination. Based upon the reason for admission, this may be a limited examination but key elements should always be present. When neurological deterioration is the cause for admission, the level of detail required will be much greater. A detailed exam includes evaluation of level of consciousness (Glasgow Coma Scale) and alertness in context of recent medications for sedation. Additional elements include evaluation of cranial nerve function, respiratory effort and synchrony, motor and sensory function, skin findings, reflexes and tone. Practically speaking, evaluation of alertness recurs each time a clinician is at the bedside. One should note upon entering the room if the patient is awake, alert and appears comfortable or uncomfortable. Can they be easily aroused with gentle stimulation? When they are awoken, are they appropriate? If more stimulation is required, are the responses purposeful? If the child is relatively sedated they should still withdraw from painful stimulation in an extremity. A stereotypical response to painful stimulation such as decorticate or decerebrate posturing indicates significant CNS malfunction and requires further investigation. Decorticate posturing of the upper extremities is flexion at the elbows with the hands clenched. Decerebrate posturing is extension at the elbows with the arms and hands pronated. If the patient does not respond to increasing stimulation, the ability to protect the airway should be assessed. This includes evaluating the presence of a cough adequate to clear the airway of secretions, gag, and handling of oral secretions. The bedside nurse likely will be able to provide a recent perspective for comparison.

The pupils should be examined for size, equality, and response to light. The pupillary reflex is well preserved and therefore unreactive pupils are an ominous sign. Small reactive pupils may indicate the presence of opioids or barbiturates, but may also be caused by damage to the pons. Large reactive pupils may be caused by atropine, tricyclic antidepressants or pharmacological withdrawal. A fundoscopic examination may show distortion of the optic cup, evidence of increased intracranial pressure. It may also point to signs of non-accidental injury if retinal hemorrhages are present. Due to significant medico-legal implications of diagnosing retinal hemorrhage, an ophthalmologist should confirm this. Additional physical findings can be elicited with further investigation. However, if there is a depressed neurological examination or a significant change, radiological imaging is warranted. A brain computed tomography (CT) scan is often the fastest to obtain but if it does not show any abnormalities and concern persists, it may be necessary to obtain a brain MRI.

Glasgow Coma Scale

The Glasgow Coma Scale (GCS) or Pediatric Glasgow Coma Scale can provide a numeric assessment of activity and function. This can allow care providers to easily discuss the patient's ongoing neurological function. This scale is helpful in studying neurological injury and outcomes. Due to the association between decreased GCS and ability to protect the airway, many clinicians will intubate the trachea electively if the GCS is 8 or less. The pediatric version of this scale has been modified for age-appropriate behaviors in a non-verbal child (Table 37.4).

Intracranial pressure

Once the cranial sutures have closed, the intracranial pressure (ICP) is determined by the relationship of the volume of the skull and its contents. The typical contents of the cranial vault are brain tissue, cerebral spinal fluid (CSF), and blood. The abnormal contents can include tumor, hemorrhage, and foreign body such as a projectile. Vasogenic or cytotoxic edema can expand brain tissue. The CSF and blood volume can expand if there is obstruction to drainage. The typical curve demonstrating intracranial pressure plotted against change in intracranial volume describes elastance of brain (Fig. 37.6). Elastance is a change in pressure divided by change in volume. As the intracranial volume increases, compensatory mechanisms occur that protect against an initial rise in ICP. Spinal fluid surrounding the brain can be redistributed to the area around the spinal cord or there can be increased absorption through the arachnoid granulations. In

Table 37.4 Glasgow Coma Scale

Activity	Adult/child response	Infant response	Score
Eye opening (E)	Spontaneous	Spontaneous	4
	To verbal stimuli	To verbal stimuli	3
	To pain	To pain	2
	None	None	1
Best verbal response (V)	Oriented, appropriate	Coos and babbles	5
	Confused conversation	Irritable cries	4
	Inappropriate words	Cries to pain	3
	Incomprehensible sounds	Moans to pain	2
	No response	None	1
Best motor response (M)	Obeys verbal command	Normal spontaneous movement	6
	Localizes stimulus	Withdraws to touch	5
	Withdraws from noxious stimulus	Withdraws to pain	4
	Decorticate flexion	Decorticate flexion	3
	Decerebrate extension	Decerebrate extension	2
	No response (flaccid)	No response (flaccid)	1

Total score is sum of E + V + M.
Minimum score is 1E + 1V + 1M = 3.
Maximum score is 4E + 5V + 6M = 15.

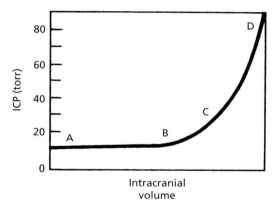

Figure 37.6 Intracranial pressure–volume relationship. Under normal circumstances, small increases in the volume of the intracranial contents (points A and B) cause only minimal increases in ICP. In pathological conditions that increase the volume of intracranial contents, a small further increase in volume (points C and D) causes a marked increase in ICP.

addition, the cerebral blood volume and CSF can be displaced extracranially. Blood and CSF together normally make up approximately 10% of the volume. When these mechanisms are exhausted, ICP increases. When this rise occurs slowly, the patient's level of alertness will be preserved longer than if it occurs suddenly. Initial presenting symptoms for a slow increase in ICP include nausea, vomiting, headache, decreased appetite, and malaise.

As pressure increases there may be focal neurological symptoms and a decreased level of alertness. Late findings include hypertension (attempt to maintain cerebral perfusion pressure) and then reflex bradycardia caused by the hypertension. If the expansion of brain tissue is asymmetrical there can be stereotypical neurological findings of impending brain herniation as different portions of the brain are compressed against ossified structures.

In the ICU measures can be used to lower ICP, but only to a certain extent. Basic management includes maintaining the head in a midline position and elevated to at least 30° to improve drainage of blood. The patient should be kept well sedated to decrease agitation and spikes in ICP. Some ICUs will premedicate the patient with bolus doses of sedatives or intravenous lidocaine prior to endotracheal suctioning as this may prevent spikes in ICP. This degree of ICP management typically implies that the patient is intubated and has their airway protected. In turn, some have used ventilation strategies to manipulate the ICP. Hyperventilation will effectively decrease cerebral blood flow through vasoconstriction. However, these effects are temporary, and cerebral blood flow regulation will reset to this lower value of $PaCO_2$ in a matter of hours. Current recommendations advocate adjusting ventilation to keep $PaCO_2$ at the lower range of normal, i.e. 34–36 mmHg. Hypoxia should be prevented as well as hypotension.

The cerebral perfusion pressure (CPP) is the mean arterial pressure minus the ICP or the central venous pressure (CVP), whichever is greater. An elevated CVP may be an issue with infants who have undergone palliative surgery for congenital heart disease. A value for minimum or ideal CPP can be described for adult patients, but this is a more difficult issue for pediatrics where the population can span preterm infants to teenagers and weights from less than 1 to over 100 kilograms. When necessary, the mean arterial pressure can be increased with inotropic support or judicious intravascular volume expansion.

The core body temperature should be monitored and fever treated aggressively. For each 1°C increase in temperature, the cerebral metabolism increases approximately 6%. However, data are not as clear regarding the benefits of active cooling. Some studies have demonstrated worse long-term outcome using cooling as a therapy following cardiac arrest. Further studies in pediatric patients are ongoing.

Intravenous fluids are typically decreased to two-thirds maintenance levels, but additional fluid boluses may be necessary. IV fluids should be isotonic and the patient's serum sodium should be followed and maintained at the high end of normal. Hypertonic or 3% normal saline can be used to raise serum sodium if necessary. Hypertonic saline is also used as a means to address elevations in ICP. Hyperglycemia should be avoided as this may result in further neuronal cell death. Diuretics may be used, both osmotic and loop, in an effort to reduce brain water and improve blood rheology.

Additional medications that may be helpful include muscle relaxants when necessary to prevent the patient from coughing or straining against the ventilator. Barbiturates may be necessary to induce EEG burst suppression and coma.

Invasive pressure monitoring of intracranial pressure

Many patients leaving the operating room following craniotomy will have an extraventricular drain in place. This allows ICU monitoring of ICP and CSF drainage as needed to lower ICP. When the lateral ventricles are very small in size, further drainage of CSF is ineffective. When necessary, ventriculostomy can be performed as a bedside procedure by a neurosurgeon in the ICU providing the same benefits. Following placement of a burrhole in the skull, a catheter is advanced into a lateral ventricle with return of CSF. Another type of pressure monitoring device consists of a fiber-optic catheter placed through the burrhole, but outside the dura under the skull. Changes in pressure are transmitted along this catheter to a measurement device. ICP is measured, but CSF cannot be drained. The ventricular catheter has a higher risk of infection, but allows drainage whereas the fiber-optic catheter has a lower risk of infection but the pressure measured can be subject to drift over several days. Some fiber-optic models cannot be recalibrated to 0mmHg once inserted.

Non-invasive measures

Non-invasive measures of brain perfusion are available. Transcranial Doppler (TCD) ultrasonography measures the blood flow velocity in the basal cerebral arteries, most typically the middle cerebral artery. TCD can help diagnose emboli, stenosis or vasospasm with subarachnoid hemorrhage. Placement of the device and interpretation of TCD readings require specialized training. Near infrared cerebral oximetry is a readily available alternative. These devices consist of a light source of known intensity and wavelength and a detector to measure the light exiting the tissues. The light or laser emitting diode and the detector are built into a sensor, which is placed on the forehead below the hairline. The device has an integrated computer converting changes in light intensity to clinical information such as regional tissue oxygen saturation. These are useful to follow as a trend monitor and provide information in addition to the clinical picture. These sensors are also being used to measure regional blood flow in somatic areas by placing them over the flank to assess renal perfusion. Studies correlating use of these devices and outcomes are ongoing.

Postoperative management

The management of children following neurosurgery depends on the type of procedure performed. Common surgeries in children involve shunting of CSF, craniofacial remodeling, repair of Chiari malformations, and treatment of CNS tumors. For every postoperative neurosurgery patient, ventilation should be monitored closely. Impaired ventilation will raise $PaCO_2$, increasing cerebral blood flow, which will impair ventilation further. Because of concern for respiratory depression, adequate pain control may be difficult to achieve. Many neurosurgeons forego continuous infusions of opioid medications and limit PRN doses significantly. Frequent neurological checks and titration of medications to effect may allow for improved pain relief.

Hydrocephalus is enlargement of brain ventricles not secondary to volume loss of brain tissue. Obstructive hydrocephalus results from obstructed drainage of CSF, and communicating hydrocephalus is the result of decreased reabsorption of CSF. In addition, there can be arachnoid cysts or collections of CSF which may cause mass effect. Hydrocephalus presents in infants with an enlarging head, full fontanelle, loss of appetite, vomiting and irritability. In children, the presentation is headaches, irritability, loss of appetite, and vomiting. Obstruction can be alleviated with either shunting or fenestration. In the immediate postoperative period these patients need to be followed closely with frequent neurological checks and vital signs as it is possible for acute obstruction to occur secondary to hemorrhage. If there is an acute change in condition neurosurgery consultation and an emergency head CT should be considered.

Postoperative ICU management of craniofacial remodeling is generally concerned with blood loss and hypovolemia. In shorter cases for just calvarial remodeling, there may not have been enough time to adequately resuscitate the patient intraoperatively. Frequent hematocrit measurements should be obtained and the patient transfused as necessary. Swelling will occur, but this rarely causes airway compromise. More complex surgeries involve correction of abnormalities of the calvarium, skull base or facial bones. These longer surgeries typically have greater blood loss and many patients will require further transfusion in the ICU. In addition, swelling is usually more severe and patients may remain intubated at the completion of the case to prevent airway compromise. It may be necessary for the patient to remain intubated for several days for swelling of the face to resolve prior to extubation. Because of difficulties with suctioning through a preformed curved endotracheal tube, many ICUs will have policies regarding the smallest preformed tube allowed. Acute obstruction of the ETT and the inability to suction will cause life-threatening consequences. In addition, these patients require ongoing sedation and pain relief during this time period. If it is anticipated that the patient will remain intubated for more than a day, it may be advisable to place a percutaneous central venous line.

Chiari malformations are disorders in which the posterior fossa structures are restricted in their space and are herniating caudally through the foramen magnum and rostrally through the incisura. Following surgery to correct these defects, ICU management involves maintaining airway patency and adequate ventilation. Following arterial blood gases may identify hypoventilation before it is detected clinically. The swallowing reflex and vocal cord control may be diminished from the disease process and surgery. These patients will need good pulmonary toilet. Vital signs are closely observed as a hematoma in the posterior fossa may result in airway compromise or apnea before a change in level of alertness becomes obvious.

Approximately 70% of the tumors in children present in the posterior fossa and the most common tumor type is astrocytoma. The ICU management after tumor resection, as noted above for other surgeries, focuses on frequent neurological assessment, vital signs, and attention to adequate ventilation. A change in condition is an indication for an immediate brain CT scan. Hemorrhage into the posterior fossa may cause respiratory compromise. If there is an extraventricular drain in place, ICP can be followed directly. Additional complications that occur include seizures, the syndrome of inappropriate antidiuretic hormone secretion (SIADH), cerebral salt wasting, and diabetes insipidus. Seizures should be treated promptly but taking care that boluses of drugs that may depress blood pressure or respiration, i.e. benzodiazepines, are not given too rapidly. If necessary, the airway may need to be secured. SIADH may occur 24–48 h following surgery. The retention of free water will result in a decreased serum osmolality, which may worsen cerebral edema. Electrolytes should be monitored as well as hematocrit in patients after craniotomy for this reason. Fluid restriction may be sufficient until this resolves but some may require therapy with 3% hypertonic saline.

Cerebral salt wasting occurs in some patients following neurological injury or insult. The urine output is greater than seen with SIADH but remains concentrated. There are significant urinary losses of sodium and 3% hypertonic saline may be required. Frequent monitoring of electrolytes and intake/output is required. Diabetes insipidus may follow removal of suprasellar tumors. This may occur 12–24 h after surgery when antidiuretic hormone stores are exhausted. The clinical picture is a sudden increase in urine output with a low urine specific gravity (<1.005). Initial therapy is volume replacement with isotonic fluids. A vasopressin infusion may be required with frequent monitoring of electrolytes, hourly intake and output, and urine specific gravity. If diabetes insipidus persists, endocrinology consultation is important to assist with anticipated long-term management. See Chapter 23 for a further discussion of neurosurgical procedures.

Status epilepticus

Status epilepticus (SE) is defined as seizures lasting longer than 30 min or recurring so frequently that there is no return of consciousness between episodes. However, the 30-min cut-off is relatively arbitrary and is not supported by clinical data. More importantly, seizure activity increases CNS energy demand and with loss of control of the airway there may be hypoxia limiting energy production. Data in children have shown that new-onset seizures cluster by duration. The majority of seizures last less than 5 min. In one study by Shinnar et al [123], 76% were less than 5 min. Seizures lasting longer than 5 min should be treated more aggressively as they can become status epilepticus or refractory status epilepticus. In addition, delay in treatment may make resolution of seizure activity more difficult.

Initial supportive care includes monitoring vital signs including saturations, providing oxygen and supporting the airway as necessary. Many patients arrive in the ICU after paramedic transport having received rectal diazepam as first-line therapy. When IV access is established lorazepam 0.1 mg/kg is usually regarded as the first step. Electrolyte levels including glucose, calcium and magnesium should be measured. Hypoglycemia is treated with IV glucose 0.5 g/kg followed by maintenance glucose-containing fluids. Hypocalcemia is treated with either calcium chloride 10–20 mg/kg or calcium gluconate 30–60 mg/kg. Calcium gluconate is the safer of the two as $CaCl_2$ may cause sclerosis of veins and tissue necrosis if the intravenous line is infiltrated. Calcium gluconate requires conversion by the liver into the active form. As medications to stop the seizure activity are given, it is common that the airway and ventilation will need to be supported. If the patient is to be intubated, either a short-acting muscle relaxant should be used or if possible none at all. Seizure activity may continue after intubation and in the presence of neuromuscular blockade the clinical exam is limited.

If seizure activity persists the patient can be given additional lorazepam 0.1 mg/kg and then loaded with either fosphenytoin or phenobarbital. Fosphenytoin is a water-soluble phenytoin prodrug and is used in preference to phenytoin, which can cause hypotension, arrhythmias, injection pain, and thrombophlebitis if given too quickly. Fosphenytoin is dosed in phenytoin sodium equivalent units (PE) and the loading dose is 10–20 mg PE/kg. If phenobarbital is used, the loading dose is 10–20 mg/kg. The majority of seizures likely will stop with the use of a benzodiazepine and phenobarbital or fosphenytoin.

Additional treatment of status epilepticus that is refractory to this therapy may include high-dose barbiturates, high-dose benzodiazepines, propofol, valproic acid, and inhalational agents and is beyond the scope of this chapter. These efforts should be performed in consultation with a pediatric neurologist.

Central nervous system infections

Infants and young children who develop acute central nervous systems infections present with acute onset of fever and altered level of consciousness. They may have headache, stiff neck, bulging fontanelle, photophobia, vomiting, decreased oral intake, and seizures. Patients may also present with signs of shock. The younger the child, the less reliable the secondary symptoms and a high index of suspicion is warranted.

The typical causes of bacterial meningitis in a neonatal population include group B streptococci, gram-negative bacilli, and *Listeria monocytogenes*. In infants greater than one-month old, this changes to *Streptococcus pneumoniae*, *Neisseria meningitides*, and *Haemophilus influenzae*. Since the introduction of the *Haemophilus influenzae* B vaccine the incidence of meningitis caused by this organism has dramatically decreased. Results from a lumbar puncture make the definitive diagnosis but at times the patient is too unstable to perform this or there is concern about a focal CNS mass lesion that would elevate the ICP. Antibiotics should not be delayed when the lumbar puncture cannot be performed rapidly. Antibiotics may alter some of the CSF findings but should not completely obscure the final diagnosis.

Over time penicillin-resistant strains of *Strep. pneumoniae* have emerged in some geographic regions. Empirical antibiotic coverage has changed to reflect this resistance.

Vancomycin and a cephalosporin dosed for meningitis is an appropriate initial therapy until bacterial identification and antibiotic sensitivities are known. Routine administration of dexamethasone to reduce inflammation in bacterial meningitis remains controversial. Current recommendations support the use of dexamethasone for bacterial meningitis with *H. influenzae* type B.

Nephrology

The kidney, in a resting state, receives 20–25% of the cardiac output. Autoregulation by the kidney maintains near constant renal blood flow and glomerular filtration rate. Creatinine is an end-product of skeletal muscle catabolism and is excreted solely by the kidneys. Blood urea nitrogen (BUN) is a by-product of protein metabolism. Values for BUN can increase independent of renal function as a result of dehydration, high protein intake, and degradation of blood from the GI tract.

Maintaining an appropriate fluid balance is very important in critical care. Even in patients who have normal renal function, diuretics are often used to limit lung water and help with cardiorespiratory dysfunction. After medications for sedation, the ascending loop diuretic furosemide is likely one of the most widely used drugs in pediatric intensive care. Furosemide is secreted into the tubular lumen by the proximal tubular cells and reaches the ascending loop of Henle by way of the tubular fluid. A prescribed starting dose of furosemide is typically 1 mg/kg up to approximately 10 mg total dose for patients who are naïve to diuretic therapy. The lowest dose necessary to increase urine output should be used. As renal dysfunction develops, potentially larger doses are needed to maintain the same diuretic effect. Furosemide can be used as a continuous infusion and some practitioners believe there are fewer electrolyte disturbances with this method of delivery.

As with all other patients in the ICU, strict intake and output measurements are necessary. In addition, frequent electrolytes need to be followed as diuretic therapy will cause hypokalemia and hypochloremia as well as other electrolyte wasting. In low albumin states, the delivery of furosemide to renal secretory sites is decreased. Diuresis may be improved by administering 25% albumin just before or with the diuretic. The typical dose is 0.5–1 g albumin/kg. When the patient fails to respond to furosemide or the urine output cannot keep up with the intake, larger doses of this loop diuretic can be given. Additional diuretics acting at other locations such as hydrochlorothiazide (distal tubule) can be added. The drug spironolactone, which blocks the hormone aldosterone, is a weak diuretic but may prevent potassium losses. Failure of increasing doses of diuretics to be effective likely represents worsening renal perfusion and/or renal failure.

Acute renal failure (ARF) is the abrupt onset of renal dysfunction where there is insufficient removal of nitrogenous wastes and problems with fluid and electrolyte balance. Toxins, drugs, inflammation, and autoimmune disorders can cause ARF. Commonly in the ICU, however, it is the result of insufficient renal blood flow or systemic hypoperfusion. This can result in peritubular edema mediated by prostaglandins or the renin-angiotensin system. Poor urine output can also result in intraluminal debris that takes time to clear after return of renal perfusion. The structural and functional changes to the kidney that occur with ARF are usually reversible but this may take days to weeks.

Acute renal failure is described by the area of obstruction and whether urine is still being made. The obstruction can be prerenal, in the kidney parenchyma, or postrenal. Decreased renal blood flow and perfusion result in prerenal azotemia. Azotemia is the term for the accumulation of nitrogenous by-products of protein metabolism. Intravascular fluids in the case of dehydration or fluids and inotropic support may be needed to reverse prerenal failure. True parenchymal renal disease may be due to toxicity caused by the renal excretion of drugs, toxins, or autoimmune processes. It may also be the result of hypoperfusion to the kidney over a long-standing duration. Postrenal obstruction is an obstruction to urine flow distal to the kidney. Posterior urethral valves or an obstructed Foley catheter can cause this. The urine collecting system is typically dilated on ultrasound examination. In non-oliguric renal failure, urine continues to be produced but is typically of poor quality, i.e. solutes are not being cleared well. Oliguric or anuric ARF is associated with no urine output and may be more concerning. Evaluation of urine sodium, specific gravity, and osmolality can help determine whether the cause of renal failure is prerenal or renal (Table 37.5).

In the circumstance of rising BUN, creatinine and decreased urine output, it is reasonable to try to support the patient to prevent impending renal failure. If possible, the circulating blood volume and renal perfusion should be improved. In many circumstances in the ICU, there may be a total body fluid overload and a decreased intravascular volume secondary to hypoproteinemia and capillary leak syndrome. Some practitioners will give moderate- to high-dose diuretics with some additional fluid in an effort to prevent oliguric renal failure. Whether this is effective is not well proven.

Hyperkalemia

As the patient develops renal failure, management needs to be directed at maintaining optimal fluid and electrolyte balance. Decreased renal function will cause decreased

Table 37.5 Laboratory differentiation of oliguria

Test	Prerenal oliguria	Intrinsic renal failure
Urine		
Sodium	Low (<20 mEq/L)	High (>40 mEq/L)
Specific gravity	High (>1.020)	Low (<1.010)
Osmolality	High (>500 mOsm/L)	Low (<350 mOsm/L)
Urine/plasma ratios		
Osmolality	>1.3:1	<1.3:1
Urea nitrogen	>20:1	<10:1
Creatinine	>40:1	<20:1
Urine sediment	Normal	Proteinuria; hematuria; casts
Fractional excretion of sodium (FE-NA)	<1%	>2%

excretion of potassium. Hyperkalemia may provoke cardiac arrhythmias leading to death and therefore requires immediate treatment. The potassium should be removed from any IV fluids immediately. Clinically there is a peak in the T wave at moderately elevated potassium levels; as the potassium level increases there may be ST segment depression and widening of the QRS complex. As the potassium rises further, there may be conduction abnormalities, bradycardia, ventricular fibrillation or asystole. Calcium in the form of calcium chloride 10–20 mg/kg or calcium gluconate 30–60 mg/kg should be given IV to stabilize the cardiac cell membrane. Sodium bicarbonate 1–2 mEq/kg IV will make the blood pH more basic, driving potassium into cells. Glucose and insulin also drive potassium into cells. Glucose is given as 1–2 g/kg IV with insulin 1 unit per 4 g of glucose IV. If the patient is intubated, increasing minute ventilation increases blood pH, driving potassium into the cells. None of these treatments actually reduces total body potassium. The ion exchange resin Kayexalate is sodium polystyrene sulfate which can bind potassium. It is given orally or rectally in suspension but does require excretion from the body. The dose is 1 g/kg orally and it can be given every 6 h; rectally, it can be given every 2–6 h. The enema route is less effective than oral administration. If severe hyperkalemia persists after all the above maneuvers, emergency dialysis (see below) is required.

Abnormalities of sodium

Severe hyponatremia and hypernatremia is another electrolyte disturbance that can be seen in the ICU.

Hyponatremia may present with seizure activity when the level is less than 120 mEq/L. Initial treatment would be to raise the serum sodium above 124 mEq/L with 3% hypertonic saline. However, in the absence of seizures, if a patient reached this low value slowly, it can be corrected slowly. The same condition applies to hypernatremia. Rapid correction of elevated serum sodium is likely more harmful than the value itself.

Oliguric renal failure

When oliguric renal failure is present the fluid intake should be reduced. At times, just meeting insensible fluid losses is appropriate. However, in many circumstances the ongoing need for blood products or fluid boluses to support blood pressure causes much more fluid than insensible losses to be given. In addition, achieving adequate nutrition may be difficult. In the face of ongoing fluid shifts and significant electrolyte disturbance, renal replacement therapy may be necessary. See Box 37.8 for indications for dialysis. The modality will depend on the experience and resources of the institution. If the decision has been made to begin renal replacement therapy, its initiation should not be delayed. There is evidence supporting improved outcomes when there is a shorter time from an ischemic insult to starting dialysis.

Peritoneal dialysis

Peritoneal dialysis (PD) has the benefits of being relatively low cost, causing less hemodynamic compromise compared with venovenous filtration, requires no central venous line and is technically simpler. Essentially the peritoneum is used as the dialysis filter. If long-term therapy is anticipated, a tunneled catheter may be placed by the pediatric or urology surgeons. For temporary therapy, pediatric surgeons may place a PD catheter at the bedside or nephrologists may place a percutaneous catheter. PD works well in infants and smaller children. The volume of fluid removal is a result of the volume of dia-

lysate infused, dialysate glucose percentage, the length of time it remains in the abdomen and frequency of exchange. As this therapy is relatively inefficient it is not the ideal choice for severe life-threatening pulmonary edema and hyperkalemia. Strict intake and outputs and frequent electrolytes will guide therapy.

Hemodialysis and continuous renal replacement therapy

Hemodialysis (HD) may be the therapy of choice for patients who are already on chronic dialysis and have vascular access. Portable dialysis machines are available in many hospitals. In other ICU settings, patients on chronic HD will be placed on continuous venovenous hemofiltration rather than transporting them to the dialysis center in the hospital. There appears to be better hemodynamic stability with continuous fluid removal rather than intermittent HD. The patient's overall condition and ability to be transported will best dictate the location of care.

Improvement in technology has allowed the use of continuous renal replacement therapy in smaller infants. Continuous venovenous hemofiltration (CVVHF) is likely the most common type of continuous renal replacement therapy (CRRT). This provides isotonic fluid removal but minimal solute clearance. These circuits can be easily converted to perform dialysis (CVVHD) providing more solute clearance. Arteriovenous filtration (CAVH) is possible but occurs less commonly. Accurate flow rates are important in circumstances where more than 15% of the patient's circulating blood volume can be sequestered in the CVVH tubing. The further limitation in small infants requiring dialysis is venous access. Modern CRRT devices machines can operate with two separate 5 Fr single-lumen catheters, but typically a dual-lumen 7 Fr catheter at a minimum is required. This size catheter can be difficult to place in an edematous infant, and thrombosis is a significant risk. Anticoagulation for CVVH can be provided either with heparin or with regional citrate administration. Citrate can be administered just proximal to the CRRT machine, which creates a regional area of hypocalcemia in the circuit, preventing activation of the coagulation cascade. Intravenous calcium is administered to the patient via a central line. Protocols are available which dictate the amount of citrate and calcium to be infused based on ionized calcium levels for the circuit and the patient. The use of regional anticoagulation with citrate avoids the concerns of systemic anticoagulation, which can be an issue in multiple organ failure.

In an effort to advance the field of pediatric CRRT, a prospective registry was developed in 2001 (ppCRRT) [124]. The registry was closed in 2005 with complete data on 344 patients [125]. Data from the ppCRRT cohort demonstrated a 58% survival. Current work is being directed

---

Box 37.8 Indications for dialysis

- Severe hyperkalemia
- Metabolic acidosis unresponsive to therapy
- Fluid overload with or without severe hypertension
- Fluid overload with or without congestive heart failure
- Uremia causing encephalopathy, pericarditis or bleeding
- Non-obstructive anuria
- Inborn errors of metabolism
- Certain drug overdoses
- Significantly elevated (>100) BUN may be a relative indication
- Some clinicians feel dialysis may reduce inflammation with sepsis or systemic inflammatory response syndrome

at introducing CRRT early in the patient's illness. It has been demonstrated that the degree of fluid overload at initiation of CRRT is associated with patient mortality [126]. This has been found to be independent of patient severity of illness scoring.

Hematology/oncology

Oncology in the pediatric intensive care unit

There has been significant improvement in survival rates for pediatric cancer over the past several decades. There has also been an expansion of number and types of diseases treated with bone marrow transplantation, and more centers now perform hematopoietic stem cell transplants. As a result, there has been a concomitant increase in the population of oncology patients in the pediatric ICU. Some of the critical care these patients receive will be on specialized oncology wards or bone marrow transplant units. The environmental isolation procedures employed in these specialized units are difficult to replicate in other areas. Depending on the institution, some oncology wards will allow the use of low doses of inotropic support, for example dopamine of up to $5\,\mu g/kg/min$. More ill patients require ICU admission for sepsis and shock not responding to fluid resuscitation and low-dose inotropic support, respiratory failure, and renal failure requiring CVVH. There is some evidence supporting improved outcomes for pediatric oncology patients requiring ICU care in recent years [127,128]. However, there remains an increased mortality in patients following hematopoietic stem cell transplantation.

During the course of their illness, there are times when patients with malignancy are left profoundly immunocompromised from disease and therapy. With a decreased ability to fight infection, they are at risk for sepsis. The first indication of sepsis may be fever while neutropenic and studies have looked at predicting which patients will go on to be bacteremic [129]. A recent study by Pound et al showed that ICU mortality for sepsis was not significantly different between oncology patients (15.9%) versus matched controls (11.6%) [130]. There was not a significant difference in survival between groups until 6 months post PICU discharge. This was similar to the overall ICU mortality in pediatric oncology patients published by Fiser et al in 2005 [131] for patients admitted to St Jude Children's Research Hospital. Information from this group also supports the clinically identified findings that patients after bone marrow transplantation fared worse (30% mortality) and patients requiring both mechanical ventilation and inotropic support had a high mortality (64%). Thankfully, it appears that the survival in oncology patients is improving over time. Again, data from St

Jude Children's Research Hospital published in 2008 by Tamburro et al [132] demonstrated improved survival for oncology patients requiring mechanical ventilation in later eras. In the time period 1996–1998 survival was 31%, in 1999–2001 46%, and in 2002–2004 61%. It is not possible to say how much of this improved survival is a result of improvements in technical and clinical care or a change in attitude resulting in patients being transferred to the PICU earlier. From a culture standpoint the shift to earlier admission to the ICU has occurred in many hospitals. From review of the literature, those patients admitted to the ICU after hematopoietic stem cell transplant have worse outcomes and the development of respiratory or multiple organ failure decreases survival. It is unlikely that this information would prevent resources being offered to an individual patient, but potentially it can guide discussions with the family and the primary service.

Transfusion therapy

Many patients in the PICU will require transfusions of blood components during their stay (Table 37.6). Anemia can be secondary to blood losses or bone marrow suppression. Thrombocytopenia may be secondary to platelet losses, poor production or sequestration in the spleen. Decreased coagulation factors may be secondary to underlying liver failure. All of these conditions result in the requirement for transfusion and its associated risks. Transfusion reactions can be classified into immune and non-immune mediated problems. The non-immune complications include viral or bacterial infections transmitted

Table 37.6 Blood component therapy

Product	Dose	Comments
Packed RBCs	10 mL/kg	Raises hemoglobin 2–3 g/dL; now tolerating hemoglobin 7–10 g/dL in absence of ongoing bleeding
Random donor platelets	1 unit/10 kg or 5–10 mL/kg	These are pooled units from multiple donors
Apheresis platelets	10 mL/kg	Donation from a single individual
Fresh frozen plasma	10–15 mL/kg	Will provide 20–30% of coagulation factors often resulting in normal clotting
Cryoprecipitate	1 unit/10 kg	Contains a significant amount of fibrinogen (60–80 mg/dL)

through blood components, volume overload, hypothermia, coagulopathy and electrolyte changes. Prolonged storage of packed red blood cells does result in erythrocyte hemolysis. This can lead to elevated potassium in the transfused unit. Rapid transfusion of red blood cells in trauma or acute blood loss during surgery can lead to hyperkalemia. If a unit of PRBCs is transfused over 2–4h, this is typically not a problem in the ICU as long as there is not renal failure. The immune-mediated reactions include those causing intravascular and extravascular hemolysis. These reactions are often regarded as the most severe and life threatening. These risks are reduced with blood cross-matching and careful patient and blood unit identification. Immune-mediated non-hemolytic reactions include febrile reactions, mild allergic, anaphylactic reactions, and transfusion-related acute lung injury (TRALI).

Transfusion-related acute lung injury

Transfusion-related acute lung injury is likely an underreported complication of transfusion. There are an increasing number of studies in the adult ICU literature regarding this complication but studies in pediatric ICU patients are limited [133–136]. The diagnosis relies on excluding other causes of pulmonary edema such as volume overload, sepsis, and cardiogenic pulmonary edema. There is a two-hit model of TRALI indicating that predisposing inflammation plays a role in the development of lung injury following transfusion. The first injury or hit is due to an inflammatory condition present in the lungs and the second hit is transfusion of a blood product. It is still unclear whether it is the presence of neutrophils, human lymphocyte antigen (HLA) antibodies or biologically active lipids present in older blood units that causes the damage. In a study published by Church et al [137], there was an association with increased mortality in pediatric patients with ALI who received transfusion of fresh frozen plasma. This effect was independent of the severity of hypoxemia, the presence of disseminated intravascular coagulation (DIC), or multiple organ dysfunction syndrome. Clearly, transfusion of any blood product has risk and the risk/benefit ratio should be carefully considered in each clinical situation. Lacroix et al [91] demonstrated reduced transfusion of PRBCs to patients in a PICU by adopting a restrictive transfusion strategy. They targeted a hemoglobin threshold of 7g/dL in one group versus 10g/dL in another and showed a 44% reduction in transfusion without an increase in adverse outcomes. These were patients with a blood pressure not less than 2 standard deviations below an age-appropriate mean and not on increasing doses of inotropic medication.

Coagulopathy

Sepsis, trauma, malignancy, pancreatitis, and liver failure are among conditions leading to coagulation problems for PICU patients (Table 37.7). The underlying inflammatory state resulting from infection can cause activation of coagulation and inhibit the natural anticoagulation mechanisms. Liver failure results in diminished production of clotting factors. In 2001 the International Society of Thrombosis and Hemostasis published a scoring system for DIC using platelet count, fibrin-related markers, prothrombin time, and fibrinogen [138]. Their definition separated the condition into non-overt DIC and overt DIC. In non-overt DIC the hemostatic system is stressed by inflammation or non-inflammatory disorders of the microvasculature but compensation is maintained. In overt DIC the hemostatic system is decompensated. A scoring system such as this allows research on DIC to be performed and provides the clinician a measure of response to therapy. In 132 PICU patients with sepsis or shock, Khemani et al [139] demonstrated an association with elevated DIC score and mortality. The DIC scale has a maximum of 8 total points. Points are given for lower platelet counts and fibrinogen, for prolongation of the prothrombin time, and for evidence of fibrin degradation. Patients with overt DIC (DIC score ≥5) had 50% mortality. Mortality was 20% for patients with a DIC score <5. The association for elevated DIC score and mortality remained

Table 37.7 Tests of clotting function

Test	Normal range	Interpretation
Platelet Count	100,000 to 400,00/µL	<50,000 may require transfusion to reduce surgical bleeding
Prothrombin time (PT)	10 to 12.5 seconds	Tests extrinsic and common pathways; prolonged in liver failure, vitamin K deficiency, DIC
Activated partial thromboplastin time (aPTT)	25 to 36 seconds	Tests intrinsic and common pathways; prolonged in liver failure, hemophilia A, Von Willebrand Disease, DIC
Fibrinogen	200 to 400mg/dL	Depleted in liver failure, DIC
Fibrin Split Product	Positive test: >40mcg/mL or titer 1:50	Elevated in DIC or other fibrinolytic process
D-dimer	Positive test: <1mg/mL	Indicates simultaneous activity of thrombin and plasmin; positive in DIC

Table 37.8 Components of the DIC score

	0	1	2	3	Max points possible
Platelet count (/mm³)	>100,000	51–100,000	≤50,000	–	2
Fibrinogen (mg/dL)	≥100	<100	–	–	1
FDP titer (mg/mL)	≤ 5	–	6–40	>40	3
Prolonged PT (sec)	<3	3–6	>6	–	2
Total score					8

All individual components are summed for a total of 8 possible points. If d-dimer is used instead of FDP titer, then cut-off values for the DIC score are (0: ≤2 mg/L, 2: 2.1–8 mg/L, 3: >8 mg/L)
Source: Khemani et al [139].

even after controlling for severity of illness or use of inotropic support (Table 37.8).

Treatment of DIC is aimed at resolving the underlying condition, which caused imbalance of the coagulation system. Given the findings of Church et al [137] with regard to increased mortality associated with fresh frozen plasma transfusion, it will be important to study outcomes with correction of DIC. The DIC score gives both the researcher and clinician a means of doing this.

Sickle cell disease

The most common of the hemoglobinopathies is hemoglobin S or sickle cell trait. Depending on the location of the PICU, a number of patients with various thalassemias may be admitted. Of the hemoglobinopathies, complications from sickle cell disease will cause the most frequent admission to the PICU. Hemoglobin S results from a point mutation in the β-chain at codon position 6 resulting in valine substitution instead of the normal glutamine. The abnormal β-chains produced from the mutation combine with normal α-chains to form abnormal hemoglobin S. When two copies of the gene are present, hemoglobin SS is produced. Deoxygenation of SS erythrocytes leads to intracellular hemoglobin polymerization, loss of deformability, and changes in cell morphology. In a deoxygenated state, the abnormal erythrocytes form the classic sickle cell. Patients with hemoglobin SS disease have chronic severe hemolytic anemia.

Sickle cell crisis

There are three types of crisis that occur in patients with sickle cell disease: hemolytic, aplastic, and vaso-occlusive. Hemolytic crises are characterized by increased hemolysis resulting in an acute decrease in hemoglobin. This is accompanied by a significant reticulocytosis in an effort to increase red cell production. Aplastic crises are characterized by acute decrease in hematocrit and hemoglobin, but are accompanied by a fall in reticulocytes. Bone marrow production of red cell precursors has slowed or stopped. Aplastic crises are most often associated with infections and greater than 90% are due to parvovirus B19. The vascular occlusive crisis is what is thought of as the classic sickle cell crisis. These crises may be precipitated by infection, acidosis, dehydration or hypoxia. Sickled RBCs block small vessels causing infarction, splenic sequestration, and priapism. Infarcts may occur in any organ but are most notable in bones, lungs, kidney, skin, spleen, eye and CNS.

Acute chest syndrome

Acute chest syndrome (ACS) is a vaso-occlusive crisis resulting from sickling of RBCs in the lungs. This is the second most common complication and leading cause of death in sickle cell disease. Acute chest syndrome is defined as a new pulmonary infiltrate on chest radiograph in combination with fever, chest pain, or respiratory symptoms. The clinical course for the patients can be quite variable. In a 30-center study performed by the National Acute Chest Syndrome Study Group, almost half of the patients who were later diagnosed with acute chest syndrome presented initially for another cause, mostly pain [140]. Pulmonary fat embolism to the lungs is reported frequently and is associated with a particularly severe course. It is believed the embolism most likely results from bone marrow necrosis with intravascular release of necrotic bone marrow fat. Infection is also a common etiology of ACS, with *Chlamydia pneumoniae* and *mycoplasma* being the most commonly identified pathogens.

Early recognition of ACS is imperative. Children may present with few symptoms, therefore a chest radiograph should be obtained in all febrile children with sickle cell disease. Therapy should start immediately after diagnosis. Antibiotic treatment should be cefuroxime or cefotaxime with a macrolide as well. Adequate hydration is necessary allowing for diuretic therapy if the patient becomes fluid overloaded. They should be supported with oxygen, incentive spirometry if able, and potentially bronchodilators. Pain needs to be adequately controlled. If the patient is anemic a simple red cell transfusion may be helpful but more likely an exchange transfusion will be needed. As hemoglobin rises, blood viscosity increases. Sickle cell blood has a much greater viscosity in the deoxygenated state. Red cell exchange can reduce overall viscosity of blood and improve oxygenation [141]. Improvements in microvascular perfusion may be more likely from reduced viscosity caused by exchange transfusion than from reduction of inflammatory mediators. Red cell exchange has been shown to reduce white blood count, platelet count, and soluble vascular cell adhesion molecule-1 in patients with sickle cell disease [142]. However, this effect was short-lived and there was no effect on interleukin-1α, interleukin-1β, interleukin-8, or tumor necrosis factor-α. Of the patients in the National Acute Chest Syndrome Study Group [140], 13% required mechanical ventilation and the mortality in the intubated group was 19%.

Neurological complications of sickle cell disease

Another area in which exchange transfusion is vital is in the treatment of neurological complications from sickle cell disease. The incidence of stroke in a population of patients with sickle cell disease under 20 years of age has been reported to be 0.44 per 100 patient-years [143]. Given the catastrophic nature of this type of brain injury, studies have been undertaken to identify patients at increased risk and to intervene before the development of stroke. The Stroke Prevention Trial in Sickle Cell Anemia (STOP) was undertaken to evaluate whether initial stroke could be prevented in children with sickle cell disease through chronic transfusion therapy. Patients were identified as at increased risk for stroke if they had an elevated velocity on transcranial Doppler. The study group was assigned to a transfusion regimen that maintained a hemoglobin S concentration of <30% [144]. Chronic transfusions reduced the risk for stroke development by more than 90% compared with the patients receiving standard of care. These results caused the trial to be stopped 16 months early. The long-term side-effects of this treatment include iron overload and alloimmunization [145].

While the management strategy for children with sickle cell in an outpatient setting may require further study, it appears clear that any child with an acute neurological change should receive exchange transfusion. In our institution this is often undertaken in the ICU.

From a practical standpoint, exchange transfusion is not without risk. Central venous access needs to be obtained in most cases. There is the risk of volume overload or hypovolemia, requiring great attention to volume withdrawn and replaced. There are all the associated risks of receiving blood products. There is the chance of hypothermia in small patients. Each center's method for handling these procedures will be based on the resources available with their hematology department and blood bank.

Endocrine disease in the pediatric intensive care unit

Hyperglycemia and diabetes mellitus

Hyperglycemia in the pediatric ICU has two major categories with distinct concerns and outcomes. The first is the population of patients with type 1 diabetes mellitus admitted to the ICU with their initial presentation of the disease, or those patients with known diabetes with recurrent problems of insulin balance, or non-compliance with insulin regimens. The second population with hyperglycemia is those children with critical illness who develop elevated glucose during treatment for their underlying disease process.

The management of type 1 diabetes has changed dramatically over the years with increased frequency of blood sugar monitoring, changes in insulin preparations, and the use of insulin infusion pumps. Fewer children who have previously been diagnosed are being admitted to the ICU with recurrent episodes of diabetic ketoacidosis (DKA). In addition, with the development of protocols to treat DKA, in some hospitals these patients may be cared for on the pediatric ward. At our institution, the criteria that prompt ICU admission include severe dehydration, significant hypo- or hypernatremia, blood pH <7.2, serum blood glucose >800, severe headache, altered level of consciousness, age <5 years, and uncertain treatment prior to arrival. These criteria help identify those patients at greatest risk for increased morbidity or mortality from diabetic ketoacidosis.

In insulin-deficient states, glucose will not enter cells, and fat or protein is metabolized for energy. Ketones and organic acids are the by-products of this metabolism and they accumulate in serum. Dehydration occurs from the osmotic diuretic effects of glucosuria and may be worsened by decreased oral intake and emesis. There are significant losses of water, sodium and potassium and this may result in decreased intravascular volume severe enough to result in poor tissue perfusion. Patients may often be 10–15% dehydrated. Metabolic acidosis is identified on admission by a low serum bicarbonate; compensation develops through the blood buffering system. The respiratory centers respond with hyperventilation in the face of low pH and this is seen as tachypnea or, when more severe, as Kussmaul respirations. As dehydration is a significant element of the disease, the initial history should include details of oral intake, and recent vomiting or diarrhea. New-onset DKA may be provoked by infection and this should be considered in the history and physical examination. Most importantly, due to the risk of cerebral edema, a neurological examination should be performed and the family should be questioned for any change from normal level of consciousness. Baseline labs include complete blood count, electrolytes, venous pH, glucose, BUN, and hemoglobin A1C level. If the patient has new-onset disease, a panel of insulin autoantibodies is often measured.

The goal of therapy is to provide insulin to allow glucose to enter the cells and intravenous fluids to correct the dehydration. It will take some time to resolve the metabolic acidosis and electrolyte disturbances. Therapy is tailored to prevent significant fluid or osmolar shifts. This relates to the most significant morbidity or cause of mortality in DKA, cerebral edema.

The cause of cerebral edema in DKA has not been completely elucidated. It occurs in approximately 1% of patients with DKA. The development of cerebral edema in this disease process is associated with significant mortality (reported as 21–25% in population-based studies) and residual neurological morbidity in survivors (reported as 15–35%) [146–148]. This complication remains difficult to study due to its low incidence, and most reports in the literature are case series or non-controlled studies. In addition, studying the *in vivo* metabolism of glucose and fluid shifts in the brain remains difficult. The use of MRI may be a good surrogate. Studies evaluating brain MRIs of patients undergoing treatment for DKA revealed narrowing of the lateral ventricles in 54%[149] and increases in whole-brain blood–brain barrier permeability in 77% [150]. In a large prospective case–control study, 43 cases of cerebral edema among 2940 episodes of DKA were identified over a 3-year period [151]. Cerebral edema was present in five of 43 cases at the time of admission and the median time to development in the remaining 38 patients was 7h after admission.

Predictors of the development of cerebral edema included degree of baseline acidosis as well as abnormalities of sodium, potassium, and BUN. In addition, early administration of insulin and large volumes of fluid resuscitation were associated with cerebral edema. The authors of this study point out that these types of studies cannot identify safe doses of fluid and insulin but only guiding principles. Consensus statements have been published [151–154] which address issues of monitoring, insulin delivery, and fluid/electrolyte replacement. Still, the majority of clinicians feel too rapid a correction of glucose may produce a rapid change in osmolarity, which could potentially initiate or aggravate cerebral edema. After a reasonable circulating intravascular volume is re-established, a majority of clinicians advocate a very slow correction of the patient's fluid deficit. Finally, fluid resuscitation should supply sufficient sodium so as not to cause a rapid change in osmolarity for the same reasons as above. The oversimplification of this therapeutic approach is: "Keep them dry, keep them sweet, and keep them salty."

With these goals stated, the DKA treatment protocol at our institution will limit patients to one bolus of 10mL/

kg of 0.9% normal saline over 30–60 min unless there is significant hypotension. Once urine output has been documented, maintenance fluids include potassium chloride at 40mEq/L with the possibility for potassium phosphate to help correct losses. Insulin is started as a continuous infusion at 0.1 units/kg/h but even smaller doses have been advocated in the literature [155]. Bicarbonate is rarely needed. Electrolytes are repeated every 4h and bedside blood glucose every hour. When the blood glucose approaches 250mg/dL, the maintenance fluids are changed to include 10% dextrose. Intravenous dextrose is added sooner if the blood glucose is falling too rapidly.

If there is any change in the neurological examination or a severe headache, a CT scan or MRI of the brain may be obtained.

It is very important to follow electrolytes closely. The potassium level may be normal initially but it will fall quickly once insulin is provided. If there is any evidence of infection from the history and physical examination and initial white blood count, cultures should be obtained and appropriate antibiotics for sepsis should be started.

Stress hyperglycemia

Hyperglycemia is common in critical illness. Stress hyperglycemia is often the cause of elevated blood glucose values in the ICU. The elevated glucose results from insulin resistance during illness, increased endogenous production of glucose or excessive administration with intravenous fluids. How best to manage hyperglycemia has been a significant issue over most of the past decade. The final answer with regard to whether tight glucose control is harmful or beneficial remains elusive. Significant changes in management in adult ICUs followed a landmark paper by van den Berghe et al [156]. In this study of 1548 patients, intensive insulin therapy (IIT) reduced mortality from 8% to 4.6% compared to conventional treatment. This article has been cited thousands of times in the literature and multiple studies have been undertaken to replicate this in other populations. In a large international adult medical population, the NICE-SUGAR trial [157], IIT to maintain serum glucose 81–108mg/dL (4.5–6.0mmol/L) was associated with increased mortality.

It is clear from most of these studies that attempts to regulate glucose very tightly result in an increased frequency of hypoglycemia. A review of the literature by Lipshutz and Gropper [158] summarizes the adult situation well: "We conclude that while avoidance of hyperglycemia is clearly beneficial, the appropriate glucose target and specific subpopulations who might benefit from IIT have yet to be identified." The situation remains as difficult in children. Studies have demonstrated that elevated serum glucose is associated with increased mortality in PICU patients [159–162]. Increased glucose variability results in higher mortality as well [161,162], potentially indicating loss of allostasis with disease progression. Whether control of glucose variability will improve outcome remains to be seen. In the United Kingdom a large randomized trial of glucose control is being undertaken: the Control of Hyperglycaemia in Paediatric Intensive Care (CHiP) study. Results of this study are likely several years away. In the meantime it seems prudent to avoid extremes of hyperglycemia and hypoglycemia; some PICUs are targeting serum glucose of 80–180 mg/dL as reasonable.

Adrenal dysfunction in the pediatric intensive care unit

The diagnosis of adrenal insufficiency in the PICU suffers from the lack of a consensus statement. Critical illness is associated with an increase in baseline serum cortisol level. In addition, there are ICU patients with normal serum cortisol levels who cannot increase their cortisol production in response to further stress or exogenous stimuli. Testing for adrenal dysfunction entails obtaining a baseline level and then providing adrenocorticotropin hormone (ACTH) and repeating the cortisol level at 30 min or 60 min or both. The standard dose of ACTH for this test is 250 μg, although an alternative test regimen of 1 μg has been proposed. Currently, there is no consensus on how much the cortisol level needs to rise to declare the function appropriate. Pizarro et al [163] published a study of 57 children with septic shock some of whom had adrenal insufficiency. Their study defined adrenal insufficiency as a change in serum cortisol <9 μg/dL following a 250 μg ACTH stimulation. Absolute adrenal insufficiency was defined as a baseline cortisol <20 μg/dL and relative adrenal insufficiency as >20 μg/dL. In their sample of 57 patients with septic shock, 18% had absolute adrenal insufficiency and 26% had relative adrenal insufficiency. They compared the incidence of adrenal insufficiency in their study to other criteria previously published and found it would vary between 9% and 44%.

To effectively study this disease process further, a consensus definition is needed. Until there is a single definition providing an understanding of the clinical picture, the criteria set by Pizarro et al seem like a reasonable starting point for the clinician. When the diagnosis of adrenal insufficiency is made, hydrocortisone should be given. The initial dose is 50 mg for small children and 100–150 mg for larger children and adults. Following the initial dose, hydrocortisone is added to the intravenous fluids at 100 mg/m²/day. Endocrinology consultation is advised for assistance and follow-up.

Gastroenterology and nutrition issues in the pediatric intensive care unit

Enteral feeding and parenteral nutrition

Nutrition and feeding in the pediatric ICU often occur as an afterthought. Unfortunately, there are many obstacles to appropriate nutrition in critically ill patients; lack of consideration of this need should not be one. Feeding should be approached in a similar manner as weaning and extubation from mechanical ventilation, and should be addressed proactively on a daily basis. If it is possible that a patient will be able to be fed enterally, this should be attempted. There is evidence that an ICU-based adoption of a feeding protocol allows patients to reach goal enteral nutrition more rapidly [164]. However, for other issues with nutrition in the ICU there is less clear-cut evidence. It should be reasonable to assume that early initiation of nutrition and enteral feeds should be associated with improved outcome but in fact this is very difficult to prove. In a prospective adult ICU study, Barr et al [165] demonstrated that patients enrolled in a nutritional management protocol reached goal enteral feeds earlier. However, by day 4 of the study the caloric intake was not different between the groups. They did show a significant reduction in mortality in patients who received enteral nutrition, but the reduction occurred in both groups. Regression analysis was used to control for confounders to demonstrate a reduction in length of mechanical ventilation with early enteral nutrition.

In a study using historic controls in a PICU, Gurgueira et al [166] demonstrated an increase in enteral nutrition after implementation of a nutritional support team. During the 11-year period of the study, there was a significant reduction in mortality for infants who received early enteral nutrition. There was no change in mortality for postoperative surgical patients after implementation of a nutritional support team. This highlights the very important aspect that patients with limited reserves such as infants are at greater risk for "starvation in the ICU." Given the 11-year period this study reviewed, it would be impossible to identify the change in nutritional support (which occurred recently) as the cause of decreased mortality. Certainly during the same time overall reduction in infant mortality would be anticipated.

A Cochrane database review was published by Joffe et al [167] in 2009 to address the "impact of enteral and total parenteral nutrition (PN) on clinically important outcomes for critically ill children." The authors were only able to identify one randomized clinical trial in pediatrics. The study by Gottschlich et al [168] from 2002 enrolled children with >25% body surface burns who were randomized to early versus late enteral nutrition. There were no clinically significant differences between groups based on early initiation of enteral feeds. The conclusion of Joffe et al [167] was that "there is little evidence to support or refute the need to provide nutrition to critically ill children in a pediatric intensive care unit during the first week of their critical illness." Certainly further research will be needed to correlate nutrition with outcome. Until that time reasonable decisions must be relied upon.

In supplying the basics to our patients, we must first assure their fluid balance is appropriate. Fever, tachypnea, diarrhea, diuretics, and the presence of nasogastric suctioning all increase fluid losses. Only some of these may be accounted for in strict intake and output measurements. Daily weights and BUN/creatinine ratios may help identify patients who are volume depleted or overloaded. Further basic provisions would be enough food. This includes enough calories to meet resting energy expenditure, enough protein to prevent proteolysis, and enough trace elements and vitamins to prevent further disease. The last basic tenet is providing enteral intake whenever possible to decrease complications. Possible complications include the metabolic, mechanical and infectious issues that are associated with parenteral nutrition. Enteral nutrition also helps prevent atrophy of the intestinal lining and may reduce translocation of bacteria out of the intestines into the bloodstream. Also, enteral feeds with fiber help avoid constipation, which can be a big problem in the ICU.

Estimating resting energy expenditure (REE) can be very difficult in ICU patients. Published values for REE in pediatric ICU patients are between 37 and 62 kcal/kg/day [169–171]. Values for individual patients may be widely different. Intubated and sedated patients and those with multiorgan system failure may have a lower REE. Further, sepsis or systemic inflammatory response syndrome may produce a hypermetabolic state with activation of the sympathetic nervous system and the hypothalamic-pituitary-adrenal axis. A decreased uptake of glucose leads to hyperglycemia and there is decreased lipid uptake as well. There is increased breakdown of protein. Unfortunately, simply supplying glucose during the stress response does not prevent this protein breakdown and nitrogen loss. To treat each patient's metabolic needs individually, the goal would be to measure their own caloric expenditure. This is very difficult in critically ill children. Indirect calorimetry may be the gold standard but requires accurately measuring oxygen consumption and carbon dioxide production. Difficulties include the need for a metabolic cart or mass spectrometer as well as a steady clinical condition. It is possible to calculate energy expenditure by giving oral water that has been labeled with ^2H_2O and $H_2^{18}O$ and measuring isotope output. This doubly labeled water method is also difficult. Finally, even initiating enteral feeds does not mean they can continue. Feeding interruptions are frequently necessary in the ICU to perform procedures requiring sedation or anesthesia that mandate a period of nil per os to minimize aspiration risk.

Studies estimate that 25% of patients admitted to the PICU are malnourished [172]. Infants have limited reserves as well. These groups should be targeted to initiate enteral feeds early. If procedures interrupt feeding, efforts should be made to pass the feeding tube beyond the pylorus so the limitations for procedures will be for a shorter duration. Concerns about reflux are another reason to attempt to feed into the small intestine. Nutrition consultation and obtaining a daily weight that is readily visible to the care team are important principles in these patients. If this group does not tolerate enteral feeds, parenteral nutrition will need to be considered sooner. Peripheral parenteral nutrition may be a temporary solution but the higher the dextrose or amino acid concentration, the greater the risk for phlebitis or infiltration of a peripheral intravenous line. There are risks to placing a central venous line for parenteral nutrition such as vessel injury, bleeding, malposition, and infection. There are additional risks to PN such as hepatic stenosis, cholestasis, elevated triglycerides, and electrolyte disturbances. Weighing the balance of risk benefit for PN in malnourished patients likely falls on the side of PN. For well-nourished children who are likely to return to feeding in 4–5 days, the benefit from PN is not so great as to outweigh its risks.

Immunity and infection

Infection control
Empiric antibiotic coverage
Recommendations for empiric antibiotic coverage are difficult in the current practice of pediatric critical care. Use of very broad-spectrum antibiotics in an indiscriminate manner may result in further antibiotic resistance. In addition, bacterial susceptibilities vary significantly based upon region, hospital, and patient population. Due to the incidence of meticillin-resistant *Staphylococcus aureus*, the first choice for antibiotics for a patient presenting with sepsis in our hospital is vancomycin and a third-generation cephalosporin. As culture results begin to return, antibiotic choices can be more selective, with final changes often waiting for culture sensitivities. For newly admitted patients with serious or unusual infections, infectious disease consultation is important to guide decisions about empiric antibiotic coverage based upon current culture isolates and antibiotic resistance.

Prevention of nosocomial infection
Hand washing with antiseptic soap or alcohol-based gels before and after contact with any patient, or any other surface or equipment that may be contaminated, is an

important priority in the care of critically ill patients. Lab coats and stethoscopes are frequently contaminated and often overlooked as potential sources of infection. Nosocomial or hospital-acquired infections are estimated to occur in 5–10% of all hospitalized patients. These infections are a significant cause of morbidity and mortality that can be avoided by adherence to guidelines for hand hygiene (HH). In studies physicians are less likely to adhere to HH compared to nurses. Interventions targeting improvement also have not shown sustained results. However, the impact of any individual on hand hygiene and preventing infection should not be underestimated.

In a unique study by Schneider et al [173], junior trainees (critical care fellows and nurse orientees) were paired with senior supervisors who were unaware they were being observed for HH adherence. With the clinicians unaware of their observation, HH adherence was 22% among trainees and 20% among senior supervisors. Still unaware of observation, the trainees were paired with senior clinicians who had been notified of the study. At this point the senior supervisors had 94% adherence to hand hygiene and the trainee percentage adherence rose to 54% (Table 37.9). This supports findings of other studies that HH compliance is greater when people know they are observed. Importantly, it is novel in demonstrating that role modeling positive behavior can have an impact on hand hygiene. Parents in our unit are instructed and reminded to ask clinicians to wash their hands if they have not seen them do this. We should not be afraid to remind our peers to wash their hands to protect our patients.

Ventilator-associated pneumonia

Patients benefit from ventilator support during episodes of respiratory failure. However, loss of airway protective mechanisms by the placement of an endotracheal tube through the vocal cords increases the risk of development of pneumonia. Patients previously uninfected are at risk for nosocomial infection and patients intubated for pneumonia are at risk for secondary infection. There is associated increased length of mechanical ventilation, mortality, and cost. In a study by Srinivasan et al [174], patients with

Table 37.9 Good role models influence hand hygiene. Percentage hand washing during period of observation

	Supervisor	Trainee
Control period	20%	22%
Study period	94%	54%

Source: Schneider et al [173].

ventilator-associated pneumonia (VAP) had longer ventilation, longer ICU stay, and an increase in absolute hospital mortality. Mortality was 10.5% in the group who developed VAP and 2.4% in the group who did not. The median difference in hospital cost incurred by the extended stay was greater than $50,000. This is consistent with the additional cost of $40,000 associated with adult VAP [175].

Ventilator-associated pneumonia is defined as a new onset of lower respiratory tract infection in patients ventilated for ≥48 h. Diagnostic criteria include fever or temperature instability, low or elevated white blood count, new infiltrate on chest x-ray, and positive respiratory culture. The incidence of VAP in intubated PICU patients was reported in 2002 as 5.1% [176] or 11.6/1000 ventilator days. The date is of note as potentially the incidence of VAP will decline in the coming years. The Institute for Healthcare Improvement (IHI) initiated a campaign to save 100,000 lives over the period of 2 years by starting evidence-based interventions in six specific clinical areas. Three of these areas deal with the prevention of infection: VAP, central line infection, and surgical site infection. It has been demonstrated that the use of bundles of interventions or information can reduce infections in these areas. These bundles have been tailored for use in pediatric patients [177] and the reduction in VAP has been significant. Bigham et al [178] observed a reduction in VAP rate from 5.6 to 0.3 infections per 1000 ventilator days following the introduction of a ventilator bundle. There was also a significant reduction in length of stay, mechanical ventilator days, and mortality rates. One of the interesting findings after institution of bundles is that the cumulative impact of the combined interventions is greater than the sum of individual parts.

The elements of a pediatric VAP bundle include those things which reduce bacterial colonization of the mouth, sinuses, and stomach as well as those preventing aspiration of contaminated secretions. Mouth care is performed every 2–4 h with chlorhexidine rinse. The oropharynx is suctioned prior to endotracheal tube suctioning or deflating its cuff. The condensation is drained out of the ventilator tubing every 2–4 h without disconnecting the circuit. The ventilator tubing is drained prior to repositioning or moving the patient. In-line suction catheters are used to reduce the number of airway circuit disconnections. The head of the bed is elevated to between 30° and 45° unless there is a specific contraindication. Our experience with bundles is they are relatively easy to perform and have a significant impact on the development of VAP.

Central line infections

Reliable venous access is necessary in critically ill patients and even more so when dependent on vasoactive infusion or other drugs which cause peripheral vein injury. The adage remains true, however, that if you do not place a central line you cannot get a central line infection. Catheter-associated bloodstream infections (CA-BSI) like VAP result in increased hospital stays, costs, morbidity, and mortality. Pediatric cardiac intensive care units may provide the best information regarding the impact of CA-BSI on mortality. The overall risk of sepsis and a bloodstream infection (BSI) in general is likely lower in a cardiac ICU compared to a medical ICU. In a prospective study, Abou et al [179] demonstrated an 11% mortality rate in patients with a BSI compared to 2% in non-BSI patients. It has been demonstrated that additional care during insertion and with daily catheter care will reduce the risk of CA-BSI. In a quality improvement study [180] initiated in 29 PICUs across the country, CA-BSI rates were reduced by 43% with the use of central line insertion and maintenance bundles. Bundle items were adapted using expert opinion from adult standards, in addition to information from the US Centers for Disease Control. Insertion bundles focused on use of chlorhexidine prep for patients ≥2 months and maintaining complete sterile barriers. This means mask, gown, glove, and full sterile drape of the patient bed. Maintenance bundles include daily assessment of a need for a central venous line as well as strict catheter site, hub, and tubing care guidelines. Dressing changes are performed with a 30-sec chlorhexidine scrub followed by 30-sec air dry. Our institution participated in this study and at one point had no CA-BSI for up to 500 days. As noted in the VAP section, it is strict attention to all the details that reduces the overall risk. The same care procedures are also used whenever a central venous catheter is accessed throughout our hospital in an effort to reduce nosocomial infections overall.

Urinary tract infection

The greatest risk factor for the development of a urinary tract infection (UTI) while in the ICU is the present of a bladder catheter. Removing these when not necessary reduces the chance of developing a UTI. Because of sedation, age, or developmental delay, many patients cannot indicate the symptoms of a developing UTI. Evaluation of fever or change in white blood cell count should include examination of the urine for microscopic analysis and culture. If removal of the catheter is not possible a bladder care bundle is necessary. In our unit periurethral cleaning with a chlorhexidine cloth occurs at least once a shift. The urine collection bag is always below the level of the bladder and is drained completely before moving the patient. Prior to this bundle it was possible to see urine reflux from the collecting tubing back into the patient's bladder as they were moved from transport gurney to ICU bed. This no longer occurs and catheter-associated UTIs have been significantly reduced.

Transport of the critically ill pediatric patient

There are two types of transport that concern the pediatric ICU physician. The first is the intrahospital transport of critically ill patients to other areas including the operating room or for radiological procedures. The second is interhospital transport of patients from referring hospitals. For transports within the hospital, the first issue to address is the risk/benefit of moving a critically ill patient. Is there enough information to be gained from a CT scan or MRI, which will help determine a course of therapy, which makes the transport necessary? The more the patient is dependent on technology, the more difficult or hazardous it will be to move them. Simply, intubated patients with central venous and arterial lines requiring inotropic infusions are at greater risk. The team providing care may include the bedside nurse, respiratory therapist, and ICU physician. All necessary medicines and equipment to resuscitate the patient should be brought on transport. One cannot rely on equipment being available and working in other areas of the hospital. Transport monitors have the ability to monitor heart rate, saturations, and non-invasive blood pressure. Some can measure arterial blood pressure, intracranial pressure, or end-tidal carbon dioxide. End-tidal CO_2 should be monitored if available to prevent hypocarbia from overaggressive hand ventilation.

The systems in place to address the needs of interhospital transport will depend on the goals and resources of the tertiary hospital receiving the patient. Information supports the use of ground transports as well as rotor or fixed wing flight. The location of the receiving and referring hospitals will affect the means of transport more than any study indicating that one is better than the other. By the same token, it is more important that the transport team is well organized and trained in pediatric care than whether it is nurse or physician led. There can be further discussion on both sides as to whether the tertiary hospital should send a team of experts or whether resources in the community are sufficient for a one-way transport. Distance from a tertiary center and the clinical scenario must be taken into account. Experience and culture of the particular unit likely will play a role in determining transport method. Details regarding the equipment necessary and development of a transport team are beyond the scope of this chapter and excellent textbooks have been written on this topic such as *Guidelines for Air and Ground Transport of Neonatal and Pediatric Patients* [181], most recently updated in 2006 and available through the American Academy of Pediatrics

The majority of care provided by emergency medical services is for adult patients. Children make up approximately 10% of paramedic calls. The number of times that each individual team member provides bag-valve mask ventilation to a child is limited. Their experience may be even more limited for intubation or other advance practice procedures. In addition, small community hospitals may have limited equipment or expertise to care for critically ill children. Arrangements should be made as soon as possible to transport these children to a pediatric facility. However, the concept of the "golden hour" was not to support the notion of scooping up the patient and running back to the tertiary care facility. Regardless of the resources, the referring hospital should resuscitate the child to the best of their ability prior to transport. It is likely that a call for transport will be made shortly after arrival of a child *in extremis*. Transport teams have been known to arrive while CPR is still ongoing. By common sense as well as policy, transport teams do not retrieve children from other hospitals while performing CPR. The ambulance or helicopter is a hostile environment. Intubation or placement of venous access should best occur before leaving the referring hospital. Medications can be given, inotropic support can be started, the ventilator can be changed while *en route* but it is best if this does not have to occur.

The control physician receiving the referring call should obtain information on the history and current physical examination of the child with complete vital signs. Ongoing efforts to resuscitate the patient should be noted. A decision is made regarding make-up of the transport team based on the information received. Telemedicine may provide a different picture of the patient's clinical status but we are more often relying on the impression of the physician caring for the child. Given their experience of caring for children, some have been known to overestimate the severity of illness. After accepting the patient, there should be contact with the referring hospital until the transport team arrives. Appropriate guidance should be given and clinical updates obtained.

Transport by helicopter requires a consideration of altitude physiology. The alveolar gas equation provides the relationship between barometric pressure, FIO_2, pressure of water vapor, $PaCO_2$, and respiratory quotient. $PAO_2 = (P_B - P_{H2O})(FIO_2) - (PaCO_2/R)$. At sea level P_B is 760 mmHg, but at an altitude of 8000 feet it is 565 mmHg. To maintain reasonable saturations, supplemental oxygen may be needed and with significant lung disease hypoxemia may remain despite an FIO_2 of 1.0. Further, at these altitudes there can be expansion of gas already contained in the body. This may mean the potential increase of a pneumothorax or, more commonly, endotracheal tube cuff pressure.

As a final word on transport, many tertiary pediatric hospitals view it as their responsibility to the community to help train and educate emergency medical practitioners. While working in the operating room, pediatric anesthesiologists are often asked to allow a paramedic or transport nurse to work with them to learn to manage the pediatric airway. As the true experts in this field, pediatric anesthesiologists can teach the skills that improve the care these first-line providers give to children.

CASE STUDY

The patient was a 3-year-old 20 kg girl who presented to the emergency department with a 3-day history of fever and rash. The patient was seen by her regular pediatrician one day after developing a fever to 38.5°C and she was noted to have a slight maculopapular rash. A blood culture, throat culture, and complete blood count were obtained and the patient was started on oral azithromycin. Two days later, as the symptoms persisted and the patient now complained of abdominal pain, the family returned to the pediatrician who referred them to the emergency department.

Initial vital signs in the emergency department were a temperature of 38°C, heart rate 150 beats/min, respiratory rate 24/min, and blood pressure 81/63 mmHg. She was described as being somnolent but appropriate when stimulated. Her skin exam was remarkable for a diffuse blanching maculopapular rash throughout her body and a newly developed petechial rash covering her wrists and ankles. In addition to the fever and rash, the patient complained of abdominal pain. Peripheral venous access was obtained and a bolus of 40 mL/kg of normal saline was given. There was a slight improvement in her systolic blood pressure with the initial fluid bolus but no improvement in her heart rate. Initial blood work obtained was significant for a white blood count of 2000 per μL, with an absolute neutrophils count of 1260/μL. Her hemoglobin was 10.6 g/dL, hematocrit 32.2%, and platelet count of 69,000 per μL. Her coagulation studies were mildly abnormal with a prothrombin time of 15.8 sec and partial thromboplastin time of 31 sec. Fibrinogen level was normal at 364 mg/dL but the D-dimer was elevated at greater than 8 μg/mL. With her laboratory values, a blood culture was obtained and intravenous cefotaxime and vancomycin were administered. The infectious disease consultation was obtained, and they agreed with the possibility of meningococcemia versus streptococcus or staphylococcus infection.

Shortly after receiving antibiotics, the patient's blood pressure decreased and she was given three 20 mL/kg normal saline fluid boluses. She temporarily required nasal cannula oxygen for an episode of desaturation. Arrangements were made to admit the patient to the intensive care unit. Upon arrival in the ICU, her vital signs were temperature of 40°C, heart rate 165 beats/min, respiratory rate 32/min, blood pressure 91/48 mmHg, and SpO$_2$ 99%. She was described as crying, uncomfortable, edematous, and with a diffuse rash over her body. Her neck exam had full range of motion without signs of meningismus. Cardiac examination was unremarkable other than tachycardia. She had 2+ distal pulses with a capillary refill less than 3 sec. Her hands and feet were cold. Her abdominal examination was without organomegaly or masses. She was diffusely tender to palpation but there was no guarding or rebound.

The patient continued to be tachycardic with cold extremities and at this point she had received 100 mL/kg of normal saline. Dopamine was started at 5 µg/kg/min through a peripheral vein while arrangements were made to obtain central venous access. Cefotaxime and vancomycin were continued at meningitic doses. Given the thrombocytopenia, lumbar puncture to rule out meningitis was delayed. After several hours in the ICU, her blood pressure improved and she was able to be weaned off dopamine.

The patient remained off inotropic support through the night but required further additional fluid boluses. In the morning her heart rate had returned to normal and she was awake and alert. From a respiratory standpoint, she was requiring 1 L/min of nasal cannula oxygen to maintain saturations. On her lung examination there were crackles at the lung bases. Radiological studies showed small bilateral pleural effusions at both lung bases. Morning laboratory examination revealed persistent thrombocytopenia, anemia, leukopenia, and neutropenia. There was a predominance of eosinophils on her peripheral blood smear. The C-reactive protein was elevated at 13. There were no positive cultures either from her regular pediatrician's office or from those obtained in the emergency department.

Viral studies including Epstein–Barr virus and cytomegalovirus were pending at this time.

The patient continued to convalesce in the ICU over the next few days. There was a gradual improvement in her fever curve and rash. Her neurological examination remained at an appropriate baseline. She had been 2.3 L fluid positive over the few days in the ICU and her urine output was increased. Her pleural effusions remained present on chest radiograph but she did not require increased FIO$_2$. The summary from the services involved described her as having systemic inflammatory response syndrome (SIRS) with some degree of bone marrow suppression. The etiology of her SIRS could have been from culture-negative sepsis. Bacterial cultures were all negative to date but the patient had received a few days of oral antibiotics prior to admission. There were no positive viral studies. Lumbar puncture was performed after her platelet counts began to increase and this showed a white blood count of 39/µL and red blood count of 7/µL. The Infectious Diseases Service recommended an empirical 10-day course of antibiotics at meningitic doses given the antibiotic pretreatment prior to cultures. A peripherally inserted central catheter was placed by interventional radiology for ongoing venous access. She was transferred to the pediatric ward service and was discharged home after completion of intravenous antibiotics.

This case demonstrates the presentation of an acute-onset systemic inflammatory response syndrome of infectious etiology, and rapid response to diagnostic studies, without delaying necessary hemodynamic management and monitoring with intravascular fluid resuscitation and intropic support. Importantly, broad-spectrum antibiotic therapy against the likely infecting organisms was administered without delay. Fortunately for this patient, she did not have full-blown multiorgan failure resulting in ARDS, renal, liver, and cardiac failure, as is often seen in this syndrome; she thus did not require mechanical ventilation, high-dose inotropic support (or even ECLS for sepsis), or renal replacement therapy.

Annotated references

A full reference list for this chapter is available at:
http://www.wiley.com/go/gregory/andropoulos/pediatricanesthesia

41. Carcillo JA, Fields AI. Clinical practice parameters for hemodynamic support of pediatric and neonatal patients in septic shock. Crit Care Med 2002; 30: 1365–78. Best practice guidelines to treat pediatric and neonatal patients in septic shock.

42. Zimmerman JJ. A history of adjunctive glucocorticoid treatment for pediatric sepsis: moving beyond steroid pulp fiction toward evidence-based medicine. Pediatr Crit Care Med 2007; 8: 530–9. Review of the use of glucocorticoid steroid treatment in pediatric sepsis.

60. Newth CJ, Venkataraman S, Willson DF et al. Weaning and extubation readiness in pediatric patients. Pediatr Crit Care Med 2009; 10: 1–11. A systematic review of the literature on weaning and extubation in pediatric patients.

86. Flori HR, Glidden DV, Rutherford GW, Matthay MA. Pediatric acute lung injury: prospective evaluation of risk factors associated with mortality. Am J Respir Crit Care Med 2005; 171: 995–1001. A significant work demonstrating lower mortality in pediatric acute respiratory distress syndrome compared to adult patients.

91. Lacroix J, Hebert PC, Hutchison JS et al. Transfusion strategies for patients in pediatric intensive care units. N Engl J Med 2007; 356: 1609–19. Demonstrates that a target hemoglobin of 7 is as safe as 10 in stable PICU patients.

97. Curley MA, Hibberd PL, Fineman LD et al. Effect of prone positioning on clinical outcomes in children with acute lung injury: a randomized controlled trial. JAMA 2005; 294: 229–37. An excellent example of a prospective randomized clinical trial of a therapeutic intervention where great care and detail were needed to demonstrate no improvement with prone positioning in acute lung injury.

102. Willson DF, Thomas NJ, Markovitz BP et al. Effect of exogenous surfactant (calfactant) in pediatric acute lung injury: a randomized controlled trial. JAMA 2005; 293: 470–6. A prospective randomized trial addressing the use of exogenous surfactant in acute lung injury. An immunocompromised subset of this population may show greater benefit with this therapy.

159. Srinivasan V, Spinella PC, Drott HR et al. Association of timing, duration, and intensity of hyperglycemia with intensive care unit mortality in critically ill children. Pediatr Crit Care Med 2004; 5: 329–36. Retrospective study addressing the increase in mortality associated with hyperglycemia of longer duration.

163. Pizarro CF, Troster EJ, Damiani D, Carcillo JA. Absolute and relative adrenal insufficiency in children with septic shock. Crit Care Med 2005; 33: 855–9. Addresses issue of prognosis with a test for a disease and may be the basis for a consensus definition of adrenal insufficiency.

177. Curley MA, Schwalenstocker E, Deshpande JK et al. Tailoring the Institute for Health Care Improvement 100,000 Lives Campaign to pediatric settings: the example of ventilator-associated pneumonia. Pediatr Clin North Am 2006; 53: 1231–51. An important review demonstating an approach to prevention of important ICU complications in the pediatric population.

CHAPTER 38

Anesthesia for the Patient with a Genetic Syndrome

David Mann, Priscilla J. Garcia & Dean B. Andropoulos

Department of Anesthesiology and Pediatrics, Baylor College of Medicine, and Texas Children's Hospital, Houston, TX, USA

General approach to the patient with a genetic syndrome

A syndrome is the occurrence of more than one recognizable phenotypical trait that occurs together in a specific association, with a cause that is thought to be a specific genetic defect. A geneticist or dysmorphologist is usually able to determine a diagnosis from the phenotype of the patient, but as the science of molecular genetics advances, more of these syndromes have a known genetic cause and inheritance. It is presumed that many of those without a known cause will have their genetic bases determined in the near future. Definitive diagnosis of the more common genetic disorders is most often made from conventional karyotyping, chromosomal microarray (CMA) or fluorescence *in situ* hybridization (FISH), from peripheral blood lymphocytes. An association is a constellation of several recognizable phenotypical traits, either without a known genetic cause or with a variety of genetic causes. The distinction between a syndrome and an association is often not clear, and this chapter will use these terms interchangeably. The term "sequence" is also often used, as in "Pierre Robin sequence," but in modern terminology this term is also normally replaced with "syndrome."

Because many of these children will require anesthesia or sedation for diagnostic or therapeutic procedures, the pediatric anesthesiologist will encounter patients with syndromes frequently, often almost on a daily basis. This chapter will first review the general approach to the patient with a genetic syndrome, and then review in more detail a few of the most common syndromes associated with challenges in anesthetic care. Finally, a listing of 103 syndromes associated with anesthetic management issues will be presented alphabetically.

Airway considerations

Management of the airway is always a central consideration for the pediatric anesthesiologist, and many patients with genetic syndromes have abnormal airways. Among the most common are syndromes with mandibular hypoplasia, including Pierre Robin sequence, Treacher Collins syndrome, and Goldenhar syndrome (hemifacial microsomia). Other conditions include cleft lip and palate, high arched palate with small mouth opening, cervical vertebral fusion limiting neck movement, and soft tissue obstruction from macroglossia or other causes. It is important to obtain a thorough preoperative history of airway problems, including snoring, airway obstruction during sleep, and acute life-threatening events. History of previous anesthetics and tracheal intubations is crucial and whenever possible, examination of previous anesthetic records or speaking to the patient's previous

---

anesthesiologist, otolaryngologist or craniofacial surgeon is very important. Examination of the airway for mouth opening, and visualization of the pharynx and soft palate, as well as neck range of motion, should be done carefully. Finally, any imaging studies such as chest, neck, and facial radiographs, computed tomography (CT) or magnetic resonance imaging (MRI) scans should be reviewed.

A management plan for the difficult airway should be developed. Details of difficult airway management are presented in Chapter 14. Details of anesthetic management for craniofacial surgery are presented in Chapter 32. Table 38.1 includes airway considerations for each of the 103 syndromes listed.

Cardiac manifestations

A number of genetic syndromes have a cardiac component, and the importance of a thorough cardiac history and physical examination cannot be overemphasized. In the presence of an abnormal cardiac examination consisting most often of systolic and/or diastolic murmurs, the cardiac anatomy and pathophysiology must be understood, and any recent diagnostic studies such as echocardiography must be reviewed. In neonates without a cardiac diagnosis presenting for some types of surgery, i.e. a patient with VACTERL association (see below) presenting for tracheo-esophageal fistula (TEF) repair, cardiac consultation and echocardiography should be obtained if possible because of the high incidence , 30–40%, of cardiac abnormalities [1]. Other common syndromes with frequent cardiac involvement in patients presenting for noncardiac surgery include CHARGE and velocardiofacial syndromes (see below). A discussion with the patient's cardiologist is indicated for severely affected patients. Details of cardiac development are reviewed in Chapter 5 and anesthetic management and pathophysiology in cardiac disease are discussed in Chapter 25.

Neurodevelopmental abnormalities

Many patients with genetic syndromes have malformations of the central or peripheral nervous systems, and for many without obvious malformations, there is associated neurodevelopmental delay. This may manifest as general intelligence lag, gross or fine motor problems, speech and language delay, and behavioral problems. It is important to understand neurodevelopmental status in any patient with a genetic syndrome; the chronological age may be very different from the developmental age and the approach to preoperative preparation, communication, premedication, and parental presence may need to be altered accordingly. Many of these patients have undergone multiple medical encounters and interventions, and may be very anxious in the preanesthetic period.

Vascular access

Patients with genetic syndromes may have limb abnormalities that preclude conventional intravenous access, and alternative sites may need to be planned. This may include external or internal jugular vein access if the limbs are not available. In addition, patients with genetic syndromes often have had multiple hospitalizations and procedures, and peripheral venous access may be very difficult, and central veins may also be thrombosed from previous catheters. Absence of typical superficial veins and presence of cutaneous collateral vessels should increase suspicion for difficult access. If indicated, additional studies, i.e. ultrasound, MRI or CT scanning, may be necessary to plan for vascular access.

Orthopedic considerations

Scoliosis, hip dysplasia, and limb contractures are common in patients with genetic syndromes. Severe scoliosis should prompt an evaluation of the respiratory and cardiac status of the patient and may alter plans for postoperative ventilation and intensive care. Positioning of anesthetized patients with these problems must be done very carefully so as not to injure affected areas.

Other considerations

Particularly with rare disorders or disorders that the anesthesiologist is not familiar with, it is important to consult a reference source whenever possible to become familiar with the basic problems of the particular syndrome and devise a rational anesthetic plan. Table 38.1 lists 103 syndromes, ranging from the most common (fetal alcohol syndrome, Down syndrome, autism spectrum disorder) to the most rare. Another excellent general source is the US National Institutes of Health website: health.nih.gov/category/GeneticsBirthDefects [2]. The US NIH online Mendelian Inheritance in Man database (www.ncbi.nlm.nih.gov/omim), and US Institutes of Health Genetic and Rare Diseases Information Center (http://rarediseases.info.nih.gov/GARD) also have excellent information including the gene map locus, if known. Many other published and electronic resources are available, including general review articles [3] and textbooks [4]. It behooves the pediatric anesthesiologist to have these resources at hand because of the frequent presentation of these patients on the day of surgery, when the luxury of time for a thorough search for information is not available. In addition, the parents and other caregivers are usually extremely knowledgeable about the patient, and often the condition itself, and can offer valuable information about how the patient has responded to particular interventions in the past. It is important to listen to the parents' and patient's requests and concerns when approaching the patient with a genetic syndrome.

Management of common important syndromes

Down syndrome

Down syndrome (DS), or trisomy 21, is the most commonly identified genetic form of mental retardation, and the leading genetic cause of specific birth defects and medical conditions [5]. Approximately 95% of children with DS have an extra chromosome 21 due to abnormal segregation of chromosomes during gamete formation – about 4% due to chromosome 21 translocations and 1% due to chromosome 21 somatic mosaicism [5]. The estimated maternal age-adjusted prevalence of DS in the United States is 14 per 10,000 livebirths, or one in 732, suggesting that approximately 5400 infants are born annually with DS. Advanced maternal age is by far the most significant risk factor for DS.

Down syndrome patients experience a number of problems that result in them presenting to the anesthesiologist for diagnostic and therapeutic reasons, and have common features which present a challenge to the anesthesiologist. All DS patients by definition have the characteristic facial features of upslanting palpebral fissures, flat facial profile, and relatively large tongue; they also have mental retardation and hypotonia (Fig. 38.1). About 50% of DS patients have congenital heart disease (CHD), consisting of complete atrioventricular canal in the majority of patients, but ventricular septal defect, tetralogy of Fallot, and other lesions are also seen. Neonates with DS should be screened for congenital heart disease, and parents questioned about cardiac history before any anesthetic. Of particular note is that for reasons incompletely understood, DS patients develop pulmonary hypertension much earlier, and to a more severe degree, than patients without DS with the same cardiac lesion. Especially in unrepaired CHD in DS, an assessment of pulmonary artery pressures should be considered; echocardiography is often sufficient for this purpose. Chapter 25 discusses anesthetic management in CHD.

Airway obstruction is common in children with DS, caused by the relative midface flattening with constricted oropharyngeal space, small nasal passages, relatively large tongue, tonsils, and adenoids [6]. This may lead to obstructive sleep apnea, which may further exacerbate any pulmonary hypertension. DS children present frequently for tonsillectomy and adenoidectomy, and may require special diagnostic testing, and postoperative admission and monitoring. Despite this propensity for upper airway obstruction, the vast majority of DS patients have a straightforward mask airway and tracheal intubation.

Atlanto-occipital instability occurs in up to 15% of DS patients, defined by excessive movement on cervical flexion-extension radiographs [6]. However, the vast majority of these patients are asymptomatic, and many infants with DS who present for an anesthetic have incompletely ossified cervical spine vertebrae and radiographs are not reliable. Therefore, cervical spine radiographs are not indicated in the asymptomatic DS patient before anesthesia. A careful history of neck pain or neurological symptoms, and previous anesthetics or tracheal intubations is important for every DS patient. If such a history is positive, elective anesthetics should be postponed until a thorough evaluation, often involving cervical spine radiography, CT scan or MRI, is done. Very careful handling of the cervical spine during airway management and surgical positioning is indicated. This includes avoiding extremes of flexion, extension, and rotation, and holding the cervical spine in neutral position whenever possible. The majority of DS patients' tracheas can be intubated easily by direct laryngoscopy with these precautions.

Gastrointestinal problems occur in about 10% of patients with DS, with duodenal atresia and annular pancreas accounting for the majority of these findings [5]. Esophageal atresia/tracheo-esophageal fistula may also be present in patients with DS. These conditions often result in a neonate with DS presenting for urgent surgery for bowel obstruction; a careful search for associated conditions, especially CHD, is important in such patients.

Down syndrome patients frequently have abnormal thyroid function, with about 2% having congenital hypothyroidism and up to 25% of patients from birth to 10 years having compensated hypothyroidism, with

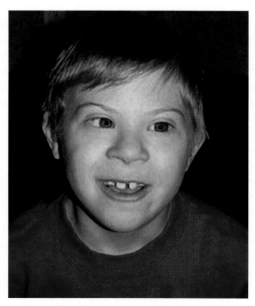

Figure 38.1 Typical facial features of Down syndrome. Note epicanthal folds, upslanting palpebral fissures, flat facial profile, and relatively large tongue. Reproduced from Davidson [35] with permission from Elsevier.

elevated thyroid-stimulating hormone (TSH) levels and low-normal T4 levels [7]. These patients often go undetected due to the other characteristics of DS, i.e. developmental delays, hypotonia, and obesity. Hypothyroidism is especially important in cardiac or other major surgery, where a subclinical state may be unmasked by the major stress in the perioperative period, which can affect myocardial function by desensitizing the heart to endogenous and exogenous catecholamines. Therefore, it is recommended that DS patients have screening thyroid function testing before major surgery.

Down syndrome children are at increased risk for acute leukemias, both myeloid (AML) and lymphocytic (ALL) [8]. DS children differ in their outcomes and response to treatments, as well as treatment toxicity and side-effects, compared to non-DS children. Survival and outcome are improved in DS patients with AML, but equivalent to non-DS patients in ALL. Side-effects, particularly mucositis and severe infections, are more frequent in DS patients undergoing intensive chemotherapy induction regimens. The anesthesiologist must evaluate the DS patient with leukemia for all of the other manifestations of DS noted above.

Finally, vascular access may be challenging in patients with DS, with peripheral venous access difficult because of increased adipose tissue, internal jugular access made difficult by a short webbed neck and increased adipose tissue, and radial arterial access difficult because of the small size of this artery [9].

In a recent study from a major US children's hospital, 9% of 479 anesthetics in children with complex special healthcare needs were for children with DS, representing 1.25% of all anesthetic cases [10]. This series indicates the frequency with which the pediatric anesthesiologist will encounter patients with DS, and a thorough understanding of the above noted disorders with DS is important in order to deliver appropriate anesthetic care to these patients.

VACTERL association

The VACTERL association was first proposed in 1972. The acronym comprises *V* for vertebral defects, *A* for anal or other intestinal atresia, *C* for cardiac defects, *TE* for tracheo-esophageal fistula, *R* for renal malformations, and *L* for limb defects. It was first proposed as the VATER association and this is occasionally still used; the frequent inclusion of cardiac and limb defects necessitated the change [11].

The genetics of this disorder are complex, but candidate genes in patients and animal models include defects or deletions in the sonic hedgehog gene on chromosome 7, *FOX* transcription gene cluster on chromosome 16, and *Gli2* gene on chromosome 2 [12,13]. Not all patients have all features of this association, but the TE fistula is often

accepted as essential for the diagnosis, along with at least one other major defect in one of the five additional categories. In the other categories, cardiac lesions are the most prevalent, seen in 30–50% of patients [13]. Ventricular septal defect and tetralogy of Fallot are common, and most CHD is acyanotic at presentation. In the case of the VACTERL association with complex CHD with patent ductus arteriosus-dependent systemic or pulmonary circulation, mortality after TEF repair exceeds 50% [14]. Vertebral anomalies are seen in about 25% of patients, including hemivertebrae, fused or butterfly vertebrae or extra vertebrae. Renal system anomalies are found in approximately 20% of patients and include horseshoe kidney, renal agenesis, vesicoureteral reflux, hypospadias, dysplastic kidney, and cryptorchidism. Atresias of the gastrointestinal tract are seen in approximately 15% of patients, with the significant majority of these being anal atresias. Limb anomalies are observed in about 10% of patients, with digital anomalies and absent radius the predominant defects.

The frequent and significant defects in the VACTERL association mean that these children are often presenting for repeated anesthetics for both diagnosis and treatment, necessitating a thorough preoperative evaluation encompassing an assessment of the lesions in all categories, and also of the developmental and emotional state of the child who has often endured multiple medical interventions. These children are most often developmentally normal.

CHARGE syndrome

The CHARGE syndrome was first described in 1979 and the acronym is *C* for coloboma, *H* for heart defect, *A* for atresia choanae, *R* for retarded growth and development, *G* for genital hypoplasia, and *E* for ear anomalies/deafness [15]. Further refinement of diagnostic criteria in 1998 designated major features seen in most all CHARGE patients, but rare in other patients, as the 4Cs: coloboma of iris or retina, microphthalmia (80% of patients); choanal atresia/stenosis either unilateral or bilateral or membranous or bony; cranial nerve anomalies – olfactory tract, facial paralysis, sensorineural deafness, and incoordination of swallowing; and characteristic ear anomalies – cup-shaped ear (80–100% of patients). The minor criteria, seen less frequently in CHARGE syndrome and less specific, include the cardiac malformations (75–80% of patients), most often conotruncal defects including tetralogy of Fallot, aortic arch anomalies, and also atrioventricular canal; genital hypoplasia including micropenis and cryptorchidism; cleft lip and palate; TE fisula; distinctive CHARGE facies and features – sloping forehead and flattened tip of nose; growth deficiency; and developmental delay [15].

The incidence of CHARGE syndrome is estimated to be approximately 1 per 10,000 livebirths [15]. A leading candidate gene, discovered recently, is the chromodomain helicase DNA binding protein 7 (*CHD7*) gene on the long arm of chromosome 8 which results in the expression of a protein that participates in chromatin remodeling during early development and allows a level of epigenetic control over target genes expressed in mesenchymal cells derived from the cephalic neural crest [16]. Mutations of this gene are found in 60–65% of individuals with CHARGE syndrome, and over 150 mutations have been discovered which encode for short, non-functional CHD7 protein.

A thorough evaluation of all organ systems is required before anesthetizing a patient with CHARGE syndrome. Neonatal choanal atresia or stenosis may be particularly challenging, requiring repeated anesthetics for imaging, the repair itself, and re-evaluation and follow-up procedures. The cardiac procedures are particularly common. With the advent and more widespread use of the cochlear implant, many CHARGE patients will also undergo this procedure. Although mental retardation and other developmental delays are common, these features are variable and some patients may have normal intelligence. Autism spectrum disorder behavioral syndromes are increasingly recognized in these patients [15].

Micrognathia syndromes: Pierre Robin sequence, Treacher Collins syndrome, Goldenhar syndrome

Among the most common causes for difficult airway management and tracheal intubation in pediatric patients is micrognathia, and an evaluation for this problem is done in every patient. There are a number of craniofacial syndromes leading to micrognathia, including the Pierre Robin sequence, Treacher Collins syndrome, and hemifacial microsomia (Goldenhar syndrome). Pierre Robin sequence (PRS) is defined as micro- or retrognathia, glossoptosis, and cleft soft palate. Isolated PRS does not have a known genetic cause and is not associated with other syndromes; the isolated form is seen in approximately half of the patients but the published series vary from 11% to 81%. Incidence is approximately 1 per 8500 livebirths, with mortality during childhood 2.2–26% [17]. PRS associated with genetic syndromes is most often seen with Stickler syndrome and velocardiofacial syndrome (see below and Table 38.1). Mildly affected patients may need minimal medical intervention, while severely affected patients manifest airway symptoms in the neonatal period. The constellation of upper airway anomalies frequently leads to obstructive apnea, and the intensity of medical intervention is proportional to the degree of upper airway obstruction. In significantly affected neonates, airway interventions such as prone positioning, nasal continuous positive airway pressure, endotracheal intubation or tracheostomy may be required. Feeding dif-

ficulties are common and feeding gastrostomy may be required. Airway surgery including cleft palate repair, veloplasty, and mandibular operations may be necessary. Details of difficult airway management are presented in Chapter 14.

Treacher Collins syndrome (TCS) is an autosomal dominant disorder of bilateral facial development, which affects approximately 1 in 50,000 livebirths; however, up to 60% of cases appear to be a *de novo* genetic mutation. TCS is a genetic developmental disorder of the first and second branchial arches, resulting in extensive neural crest cell abnormal development. The TCS phenotype includes hypoplasia of the maxilla, zygoma, and mandible, lateral downward sloping of the palpebral fissures, coloboma of the lower eyelids, defects of the external and middle ears, and sensorineural deafness (Fig. 38.2). The protein coded by this gene is called Treacle, and the hypothesis is that it assists in ribosomal DNA transcription during particular stages in embryonic development, particularly that of the structures of the head and face [18,19]. These patients may require extensive bony and soft tissue facial reconstruction over multiple procedures, including orbital and zygomatic reconstruction before age 10, external ear reconstruction, and mandibular advancement as teenagers when bony growth is complete. Difficulties in airway management for the anesthesiologist arise from the mandibular hypoplasia and high arched palate frequently encountered in TCS patients.

Goldenhar syndrome, also known as oculo-auriculo-vertebral syndrome or hemifacial microsomia, is a developmental disorder of the first and second branchial arches that affects approximately 1 in 5600 livebirths, is most frequently unilateral, and is characterized by malformations/hypoplasia of the external and middle ear often with sensorineural hearing loss, mandibular hypoplasia, eye abnormalities such as microphthalmos and epibulbar dermoids, and vertebral anomalies including cervical spine malformations and scoliosis (Fig. 38.3). Most cases of Goldenhar syndrome are sporadic, and heterogenous manifestations of the phenotype are common, ranging from very mild hemifacial asymmetry, preauricular ear tags or pits, to severe deformity and mandibular hypoplasia. Congenital heart disease is present in approximately one-third of patients, most commonly septal and conotruncal defects [20]. Developmental delay and autism spectrum disorder are seen in some patients [21]. Difficulties with airway management and tracheal intubation are common in this syndrome due to the mandibular hypoplasia and lack of space for direct laryngoscopy. These patients frequently present for anesthesia and sedation for diagnostic and therapeutic procedures for ear, facial, and cardiac anomalies. Techniques such as fiberoptic or video-assisted laryngoscopy are frequently required for airway management [22,23].

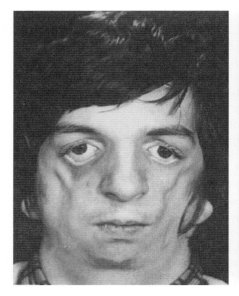
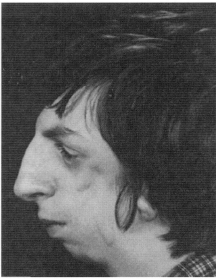

Figure 38.2 Treacher Collins syndrome in an adolescent. Note the hypoplasia of the maxilla, zygoma, and mandible, lateral downward sloping of the palpebral fissures, coloboma of the lower eyelids, and defects of the external and middle ears. Reproduced from Marszalek et al [18] with permission from Springer.

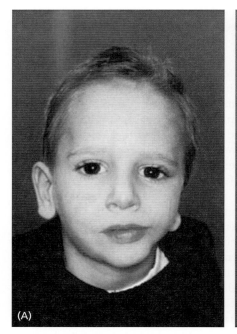
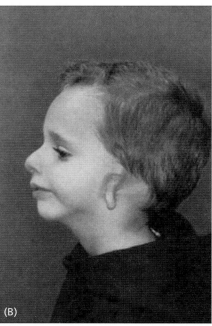
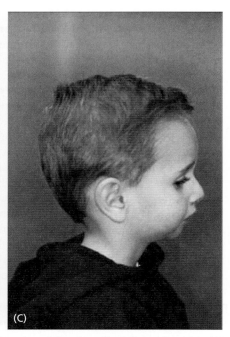

(A) (B) (C)

Figure 38.3 Goldenhar syndrome in a 7-year-old boy. Note facial asymmetry with hypoplastic mandible and ear deformity on the left side. Reproduced from Vendramini-Pittoli and Kokitsu-Nakata [36] with permission from Lippincott Williams and Wilkins.

Cardiac syndromes: Williams syndrome, Noonan syndrome, velocardiofacial syndrome (22.Q11.2 deletion)

Williams syndrome (WS) is a genetic syndrome whose phenotype involves supravalvular aortic stenosis and characteristic facial features including periorbital puffiness, flat nasal bridge, long philtrum, full cheeks, and full lower lip (Fig. 38.4). Other features include developmental delay, friendly or outgoing personality, hypercalcemia, hypotonia, joint laxity, and hypertension. WS affects approximately 1 in 10,000 livebirths and has been localized to a 1.5 Mb base pair deletion on one copy of chromosome 7, involving 26–28 genes, including the elastin gene, at 7q11.23 [24]. This deletion can arise from a spontaneous mutation or can be inherited as an autosomal dominant familial form. Fifty to 75% of WS patients have cardiac disease, most frequently supravalvar aortic stenosis, and peripheral pulmonary artery stenosis. These changes are

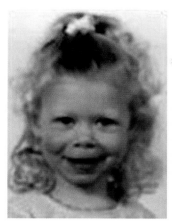

Figure 38.4 Williams syndrome facies in a young child. Note the periorbital puffiness, flat nasal bridge, long philtrum, wide smile, full cheeks and full lower lip. Reproduced from Waxler et al [24] with permission from Slack Incorporated.

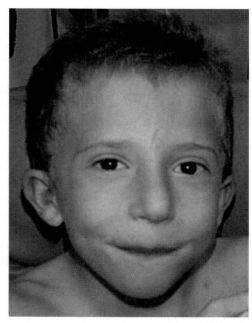

Figure 38.5 Facial features of velocardiofacial syndrome. Note small low-set posteriorly rotated ears and slight retrognathia; the patient also has a high arched palate with submucous cleft. Reproduced from Shprintzen [28] with permission from Wiley-Blackwell.

characterized as an elastin arteriopathy, and the usual large quantity of elastin present in the medial layer of large arteries is absent, resulting in limited distensibility and stenosis of the artery. In addition, adhesion of the aortic valve leaflet edges to the narrowed sinotubular junction can result in obstruction of the coronary artery ostia, leading to impaired coronary blood flow [25]. It is this feature which leads to sudden death in WS patients, both spontaneously and during diagnostic and therapeutic procedures requiring anesthesia and sedation [26]. Careful anesthetic management to balance myocardial oxygen supply and demand, including avoidance of excessive tachycardia, hypotension, and hypovolemia, is an important principle. The peripheral pulmonic stenosis is often present during infancy but improves over time. Details of anesthetic management for left heart obstructive lesions are presented in Chapter 25.

Noonan syndrome is characterized by cardiac disease and distinctive facial features including hypertelorism with downslanting palpebral fissures, ptosis, and low-set, posteriorly rotated ears. The cardiovascular manifestations are most commonly valvar pulmonary stenosis in about 60%, hypertrophic cardiomyopathy in 20%, atrial septal defects and ventricular septal defects in approximately 10% and 5%, respectively, and patent ductus arteriosus in 3% [27]. Other defects include webbed neck, shield chest, and abnormal lymphatic drainage resulting in lymphedema. The syndrome occurs in approximately 1 in 1000–2500 livebirths and may occur sporadically, or with an autosomal dominant inheritance, predominantly by maternal transmission. Approximately 50% of cases have a missense mutation in the *PTPN11* gene on chromosome 12, which encodes for a protein, tyrosine phosphatase SHP-2. This enzyme is involved in a variety of signal cascades for receptors for hormones, cytokines, and growth factors and in a number of developmental processes [27]. Intervention requiring anesthesia is most commonly balloon valvuloplasty or surgery for pulmonary valve stenosis.

Velocardiofacial syndrome (VCFS) is also known as DiGeorge syndrome or sequence, 22Q11 deletion syndrome, CATCH 22, and conotruncal anomalies face syndrome. This disorder has a wide spectrum of phenotypical findings with more than 180 clinical features. It is one of the most common multiple anomaly syndromes, with incidence estimates of approximately 1:2000 livebirths. VCFS is inherited as an autosomal dominant disorder and is caused by a microdeletion at chromosome 22q11.2 [28]. The phenotype is extremely variable and there is no single clinical feature present in 100% of cases, and so the diagnosis is defined by the chromosome defect itself. Congenital heart disease is present in 70% of cases, and constitutes a high percentage of all conotruncal cardiac anomalies, including more than 50% of cases of interrupted aortic arch, over 15% of patients with tetralogy of Fallot, about 50% of truncus arteriosus cases, and about one-third of posteriorly malaligned ventricular septal defects. Hemizygosity of the gene *TBX1* is responsible for the cardiac defects. Other defects commonly encountered are cleft palate, most commonly submucous clefts, facial anomalies, including high arched palate, low-set ears, and occasionally varying degrees of micrognathia (Fig. 38.5). Other important features present in a variable percentage of patients are partial hypoparathyroidism resulting in neonatal hypocalcemia and relative immunodeficiency from abnormal lymphocyte function. Developmental delay is common in VCFS, although in some patients intelligence may be normal.

Patients with the cardiac diseases noted above should be tested for the 22q11.2 deletion using FISH, and the other defects, especially hypocalcemia and immune dysfunction leading to increased infection risk, should be sought as well, as these may affect anesthetic management. In patients with simpler forms of CHD and VCFS, i.e. tetralogy of Fallot, VSD, and simple truncus arteriosus, surgical outcomes are not worse than in patients without a chromosome defect. However, in interrupted aortic arch, surgical outcomes are worse with the 22q11.2 deletion. Finally, the later neurodevelopmental outcomes at 1 year or more after cardiac surgery are definitely worse overall with 22q11.2 deletion [29]. In spite of the known mild craniofacial anomalies in this syndrome, airway management and tracheal intubation are most often straightforward.

Autism spectrum disorder

Autism spectrum disorder (ASD) is an increasingly recognized neurodevelopmental disorder of empathy that encompasses autism, Asperger syndrome, atypical autism, and pervasive developmental disorder not otherwise specified. ASD is characterized by impairments in social communication and social interaction of varying degrees, and also includes restricted and repetitive behaviors and impairments of imaginary thought [30]. The prevalence is now thought to be approximately 1:150 children, with boys affected four times more frequently than girls [31]. There is increasing evidence that ASD has a genetic basis, including data indicating that the relative risk to siblings is 25 times higher than the general population, and twin studies showing higher rates in concordant twins. Genome association studies have identified several candidate genes on different chromosome regions, including 2q, 7q, 15q, 15p14.1 and X. In addition, syndromes such as fragile X, Down syndrome, velocardiofacial syndrome, and others account for 1–2% of ASD patients [30].

Anesthetic management of patients with ASD, especially preoperative preparation, premedication, and induction of anesthesia, presents problems unique to this population [32]. When possible, parents of patients with ASD should be contacted in advance of the anesthetic to gain some understanding of the degree of the patient's ASD, their particular behaviors, and interventions to avoid. Outpatient surgery whenever possible, and returning the patient to their home environment and routines as soon as possible, are important for the ASD patient. Parental presence and/or premedication with oral mida-

zolam or ketamine, or in some cases intramuscular ketamine, are reported to be effective in this population.

The most common procedures in the ASD population include dental restorations, otorhinolaryngological procedures, and brain MRI scans [32]. Scheduling these patients first in the day, admitting them a short time before induction of anesthesia, admitting them to a quiet secluded recovery area, removing intravenous catheters whenever possible, parental presence in the recovery room, and discharging home as soon as possible all are reported to help in minimizing behavioral disruptions in the ASD population.

Epidermolysis bullosa

Epidermolysis bullosa (EB) is a group of hereditary bullous skin disorders distinguished by blister formation as a result of mechanical trauma. Although there are over 20 subtypes of EB, it can be divided into three major types: EB simplex (mutations in keratin 5 and 14 genes), where the epidermis only is affected; junctional EB (mutations in laminin 5 or type XVII collagen genes), where the basement membrane is involved; and dystrophic EB (mutations in type VII collagen genes) in which the dermis is primarily involved. Mutations in 10 additional genes encoding protein components of the basement membrane have also been implicated in various subtypes of EB [33].

Clinical manifestations vary from mild to severe, with dystrophic EB (DEB) the most severe and the form most frequently requiring surgical and anesthetic intervention (Fig. 38.6). The majority of patients with DEB have blisters and wounds that are present at birth or shortly after,

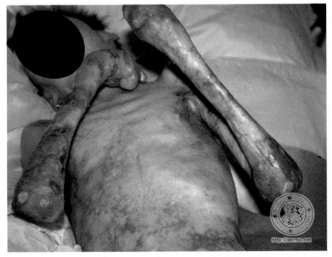

Figure 38.6 Dystrophic epidermolysis bullosa. Note severe blistering with hypertrophic scarring and contractures in axillae and antecubital foaase. Note also pseudosyndactyly from severe chronic contractures. Reproduced from DERMIS Dermatology Information System [37] with permission.

with a variety of blister sizes that heal with atrophic scars and development of contractions [34]. These occur commonly on the dorsum of the hands, feet, elbows, and knees. Friction caused by scratching or other mechanical forces is very damaging in EB. Oral, pharyngeal, and esophageal blistering is common in EB, leading to contractures of the mouth and tongue. The pain associated with these blisters leads to decreased oral intake and poor nutrition. Esophageal strictures, dental caries, and gum disease are also common in DEB. Contractures on the extremities can cause severe scarring to the point that a pseudosyndactyly is created. Corneal scarring can also occur.

General management of EB involves teaching the family to avoid friction and shearing forces, special clothing and feeding techniques, draining of blisters and treatment with silver sulfadiazine for large infected blisters, special dressings with hydrofiber foam with silicone coating, and topical corticosteroids. Feeding open gastrostomy, dental treatment, and analgesia as well as a multidisciplinary approach are crucial to optimize outcomes for this complicated patient population.

All of these problems lead to the need for anesthesia and sedation for diagnostic and therapeutic procedures, which can be very challenging and are best carried out in a specialized center that cares for large numbers of these patients. However, these patients may present in a number of settings, and may require emergency interventions and so the pediatric anesthesiologist must be familiar with their care. Common surgical procedures in EB include dressing changes, casting, repair of contractures and pseudosyndactyly, dental restoration, esophagoscopy and esophageal dilation, open gastrostomy, long-term indwelling central venous access, skin biopsy, and eye surgery [34].

The most important principle of anesthetic care of children with EB is that friction and shearing forces, and not direct pressure, are responsible for new bullae formation. Airway management problems are frequent, secondary to neck contractures and pharyngeal bullae. After thorough evaluation of preoperative condition, an oral premedication can be given if needed. Veins are often easily visualized and cannulated in these patients and are often an option for premedication and anesthetic induction. The number of transfers of the patients should be minimized, as sliding causing shearing forces between stretcher and operating room bed, for example, may contribute to bullae formation. For the attachment of monitors, IV cannulae or airway devices, adhesives should be assiduously avoided.

It is often preferable to secure a peripheral IV cannula with a single suture. A clip-on pulse oximetry probe is used and ECG electrodes can be used by cutting away the adhesive portion and laying only the gel part on the skin, or covering the skin with paraffin gauze or a gelpad. Non-invasive blood pressure monitoring is used, but the skin is first padded with Webril® soft gauze. Nasopharyngeal and rectal temperature probes are avoided.

Inhalation induction can be used, but the facemask must be thoroughly lubricated with petrolatum jelly or protected with paraffin gauze, and great care should be taken to avoid shearing forces on the skin of the face and neck. In general, tracheal intubation has been the preferred airway management method, with a tube half size smaller than normal; with gentle laryngoscopy the incidence of new laryngeal or pharyngeal bullae is low [34]. Anticipated difficult airway management because of contractures or severe intraoral bullae must be accompanied by a careful plan, including the availability of videolaryngoscopy, fiber-optic bronchoscopy, and laryngeal mask airways (LMA). The LMA can also be used for airway maintenance successfully with little risk of new severe intraoral bullae, but maintenance of the airway with a facemask for long periods of time should be avoided. Non-depolarizing muscle relaxants can be used, but succinylcholine should be avoided. Standard intravenous induction agents, maintenance agents, and opioid and regional anesthesia may be used safely in these patients. Emergence from anesthesia and tracheal extubation must be done carefully, again avoiding shearing forces on the face; intraoral suctioning must be done gently. Avoidance of use of conventional facemasks for oxygen administration in postanesthesia recovery is important; increasing oxygen concentration by blowing humidified oxygen over the face from a 22 mm corrugated oxygen tubing is an effective method. Evaluation for new bullae and communication with the patient's dermatologist about any changes in treatment plan after an anesthetic are very important.

Listing of 103 syndromes encountered by the pediatric anesthesiologist

Table 38.1 lists, in alphabetical order, 103 syndromes encountered by the pediatric anesthesiologist, with considerations for anesthesia noted by organ system, emphasizing airway, cardiac, pulmonary, and neurological disease associations.

CASE STUDY

A 6-month-old girl presented for an MRI of the brain, spine, and heart. She was born at 39 weeks' gestation weighing 3.4 kg with polyhydramnios and multiple congenital anomalies. Because an orogastric tube could not be passed, yet there was abdominal gas present on radiograph, a diagnosis of type C esophageal atresia with distal tracheoesophageal fistula (TEF) was made. She did not have respiratory distress, and room air oxygen saturation was 92%. Other findings included a systolic II/VI cardiac murmur, and echocardiogram revealed a double outlet right ventricle, with large subaortic ventricular septal defect and large patent ductus arteriosus, as well as a hypoplastic aortic arch. Additional findings on renal ultrasound were bilateral hydronephrosis with a multicystic and dysplastic right kidney and an enlarged and abnormally positioned left kidney. She also had imperforate anus and ambiguous genitalia. On chest and abdominal radiograph it was evident that she had vertebral anomalies, including partial fusion of C5 and C6 vertabrae, complete fusion of L3–L4 vetrbrae, and sacral agenesis beginning at the S4 level. Finally, she exhibited rocker bottom feet.

A diagnosis of VACTERL association was made. PGE1 infusion was begun in the neonatal period, and repair of the TEF was done as the first priority on the first day of life, via a right thoracotomy. No ventilation difficulties were encountered and a small TEF was ligated and divided, and the esophageal atresia was repaired primarily without problems. Then, a colostomy and a feeding gastrostomy were performed, again without incident. The patient's trachea was left intubated, and 5 days later she was taken to the cardiac operating room for an aortic arch repair, and pulmonary artery banding via median sternotomy on cardiopulmonary bypass, and again did well with postoperative oxygen saturations of 80–85% on room air, and an appropriate mean echocardiographic gradient of 3.5 m/sec across the pulmonary artery band. Ten days postoperatively from the cardiac repair, she underwent placement of a percutaneous left nephrostomy tube because of progressive hydronephrosis, to preserve renal function until more definitive surgery could be done. After a 4-week hospitalization she was discharged home.

On the day of the MRI the patient's only medication was trimethoprim/sulfamethoxazole for urinary tract infection prophylaxis. She had undergone three additional anesthetics to replace the nephrostomy tube, all without incident. The MRI was scheduled to image her spine defects in detail and rule out any brain anomalies. She was alert, afebrile and responsive, room air saturation was 76%, heart rate 135, respiratory rate 24. Weight was 6.5 kg (10th percentile). Examination of the airway revealed no abnormalities; mandible was normal size. Neck appeared slightly short but

had full range of motion. Lungs were clear to auscultation bilaterally, and she had no signs of respiratory distress. There was a long harsh IV/VI systolic murmur at the right sternal border. There were well-healed right thoracotomy and median sternotomy scars, as well as a colostomy and gastrostomy button, and a percutaneous nephrostomy tube. She had significant kyphoscoliosis. Echocardiogram done at cardiology clinic visit the week before revealed good biventricular function, large subaortic VSD measuring 12 mm, and a 4.8 m/sec pulmonary artery band gradient. Plans had been made for a complete biventricular repair versus bidirectional cavopulmonary connection when she was 8–9 months of age. Laboratory studies at that time included a hemoglobin concentration of 17 g/dL, normal electrolyes, BUN of 11 mg/dL and creatinine 0.3 mg/dL. Cardiac MRI was requested to further define the size of the left ventricle, and the anatomical relationship of the VSD to the great vessels, to assist in determining whether a full biventricular repair was possible.

Because of the approximately 3 h planned scan time, the patient's age and cardiac lesion with requested apnea for the cardiac imaging, general endotracheal anesthesia was chosen. Emergency drugs were available, including epinephrine, phenylephrine, and atropine, as well as isotonic crystalloid solutions and 5% albumin for intravascular volume expansion. After application of standard monitors, inhalation induction was initiated with sevoflurane in the MRI suite outside the scanner room. The pediatric anesthesia fellow managed the airway while the faculty anesthesiologist attempted peripheral intravenous access.

Inhalation induction proceeded slowly with FIO_2 1.0 and increasing inspired sevoflurane concentrations up to 5%. After three attempts a 22 G peripheral IV was started in the left foot. During induction systolic blood pressures were 60–80 mmHg, heart rate 120–150 with sinus rhythm. SpO_2 began at 65% with crying, but quickly improved to 80–85%. Rocuronium 1 mg/kg was administered and the trachea intubated with a 3.5 mm cuffed endotracheal tube. After a period of 5 min observation and ongoing stability, she was moved into the MRI scanner with MRI-compatible monitoring. The brain and spine scans were completed first, with 90 min scan time. Brain MRI was normal, and the vertebral anomalies were confirmed and tethered spinal cord noted. Anesthesia was maintained with 1.5–2% endtidal sevoflurane and FIO_2 at 0.5. Two periods of mild hypotension and arterial desaturation to SpO_2 70–75% were treated by decreasing the inspired anesthetic, and intravenous boluses of 10 mL/kg lactated Ringer's solution. Intravenous contrast was not used during this phase because of the concern over her renal function. During the cardiac MRI the patient was stable with SpO_2 80–85%. Two 30-sec periods of apnea were requested, and were accomplished with preoxygenation with FIO_2 1.0 and manual hyperventilation. A reduced dose of gadolinium MRI contrast was administered, and excellent cardiac images were obtained with the patient stable throughout. After a 3 h, 10 min anesthetic, the patient's trachea was extubated with the patient awake after reversal of neuromuscular blockade with neostigmine 70 µg/kg and glycopyrrolate 14 µg/kg. The patient spent 3 h in the recovery area, returned to baseline room air saturations of 75–80%, and was alert, responsive, in no distress, and had resumed gastrostomy and nipple feeds.

After the cardiac surgery, additional procedures planned were colostomy take-down and repair of imperforate anus, and repair of hydroureter. No interventions for the spine or feet were planned at this time.

This patient, with all the manifestations of VACTERL association, illustrates the complex multisystem nature of the disorders of some patients with syndromes, along with the need for multiple anesthetics for therapeutic and diagnostic procedures. A thorough evaluation of all systems, including access to all previous medical records, is important in planning care of these patients.

Annotated references

A full reference list for this chapter is available at:
http://www.wiley.com/go/gregory/andropoulos/pediatricanesthesia

2. United States National Institutes of Health Genetics/Birth Defects website: health.nih.gov/category/GeneticsBirthDefects. United States National Institutes of Health Mendelian Inheritance in Man database: www.ncbi.nlm.nih.gov/omim. United States Institutes of Health Genetic and Rare Diseases Information Center: http://rarediseases.info.nih.gov/GARD. National Institutes of Health websites that contain a wealth of clinical, genetic, and molecular genetic information, updated continually as new information is available.

3. Butler MG, Hayes BG, Hathaway MM et al. Specific genetic diseases at risk for sedation/anesthesia complications. Anesth Analg 2000; 91: 837–55. An outstanding, comprehensive review of multiple syndromes and anesthetic implications.

4. Baum VC, O'Flaherty JE (eds) Anesthesia for Genetic, Metabolic, and Dysmorphic Syndromes of Childhood, 2nd edn. Philadelphia: Lippincott, Williams and Wilkins. The standard textbook listing hundreds of syndromes in an easily readable, standard, alphabetically organized format.

10. Graham RJ, Wachendorf MT, Burns JP et al. Successful and safe delivery of anesthesia and perioperative care for children with complex special health care needs. J Clin Anesth 2009; 21: 165–72. An excellent case series and comprehensive review and listing of patients with complex needs, almost all of whom have genetic syndromes.

11. Keckler SJ, St Peter SD, Valusek PA et al. VACTERL anomalies in patients with esophageal atresia: an updated delineation of the spectrum and review of the literature. Pediatr Surg Int 2007; 23: 309–13. Review of a large series of patients with VACTERL association as well as a review of recent literature.

25. Burch TM, McGowan FX Jr, Kussman BD et al. Congenital supravalvular aortic stenosis and sudden death associated with anesthesia: what's the mystery? Anesth Analg 2008; 107: 1848–54. A superb review of the etiology, genetics, pathophysiology, and anesthetic management of patients with Williams syndrome and related disorders. Emphasizes anesthetic hemodynamic management to avoid coronary ischemia and death under anesthesia.

32. Van der Walt JH, Moran C. An audit of perioperative management of autistic children. Ped Anesth 2001; 11: 401–8. A review of anesthetic care in a large series of autistic children, and a review of the literature, and nicely done summary of the problems encountered in autism.

34. Herod J, Denyer J, Goldman A, Howard R. Epidermolysis bullosa in children: pathophysiology, anaesthesia, and pain management. Ped Anesth 2002; 12: 388–97. A comprehensive review of the problems encountered in epidermolysis bullosa, a description of the subtypes and genetic etiologies, a review of general care, and a very specific detailed review of the anesthetic considerations.

62. Papay FA, McCarthy VP, Eliachar I et al. Laryngotracheal anomalies in children with craniofacial syndromes. J Craniofac Surg 2002; 13: 351–64. An excellent review of airway anomalies in children with the major craniofacial syndromes.

Table 38.1 Genetic syndromes encountered by the pediatric anesthesiologist

No.	Syndrome: name, eponyms, inheritance, incidence, gene locus, gene product	Airway	Central nervous system	Cardiovascular
1	**Achondroplasia** (autosomal dominant, mutation chromosome 4p16.3, 1:25,000, fibroblast growth factor receptor 3 (FGFR3))	Upper airway stenosis, retruded chin, increased mandibular plane angle	Possible spinal cord compression from small foramen magnum/ intervertebral foramina	NA
2	**Adrenoleukodystrophy** (Siemerling-Creutzfeldt disease, Schilder disease, X-linked recessive, 1:42,000 males, mutation chromosome Xq218, ABCD1 transporter protein)	NA	Two types: (adult) non-inflammatory adrenomyeloneuropathy & (children) inflammatory cerebral myelinopathy Seizure disorder Hypotonia Altered somatosensory evoked potentials: central pathways in women/ peripheral & central pathways in men	Adrenocortical insufficiency
3	**Alagille syndrome** (autosomal dominant, 1:100,000, chromosome 20p12 microdeletion, JAG 1 signaling pore)	NA	Intracranial hemorrhage/ stroke; developmental delay	90% with cardiovascular anomalies; most commonly branch pulmonary artery stenosis Other cardiac lesions: tetralogy of Fallot, tricuspid atesia, patent ductus arteriosus, ventricular septal defect

Pulmonary	Other	Additional anesthetic considerations	References
Smaller than predicted lungs/ airways, reduced vital capacity but normal function; respiratory abnormalities from small thoracic cage, airway obstruction, or cervicomedullary compression	Obesity; joint laxity with bow-legs; transient thoracolumbar kyphosis usually resolves with independent gait	Few reports of difficult mask ventilation/ laryngoscopy/intubation; assess cervical spine for foramen magnum stenosis/ upper cervical canal narrowing; post-op respiratory complications reported: atelectasis, respiratory distress, pulmonary edema; reports of successful neuraxial analgesia/anesthesia; evaluate with rapid-ACTH test and/or stress dose steroid administration; altered response to non-depolarizing neuromuscular blocking drugs with upper motor neuron disease; possible hyperkalemia with hypotonia – avoid succinylcholine; altered drug metabolism with anti-seizure therapy	38–48
NA	NA	NA	
NA	Spontaneous bleeding of unknown etiology	Airway assessment: unusual facies, possible cervical spine abnormalities with no reports of difficult intubation	49
	Biliary excretion abnormalities more than synthetic/ metabolic hepatic abnormalities	Abdominal distension may predispose to gastroesophageal reflux	50
	Butterfly vertebrae; possible shortened interpedicular distance	Neurological assessment: avoid succinylcholine with myopathies	51
	Exocrine pancreatic insufficiency	Cardiac work-up	52
	Renal disease	Assess coagulation profile – caution with neuraxial analgesia/anesthesia	
	Vitamin K malabsorption – coagulopathies	Caution with positioning – rickets/hepatic osteodystrophy	

(Continued)

Table 38.1 (*Continued*)

No.	Syndrome: name, eponyms, inheritance, incidence, gene locus, gene product	Airway	Central nervous system	Cardiovascular
	Alagille syndrome (*continued*)			
4	**Angelman syndrome** (maternally inherited chromosome 15 deletion, chromosome 15q11-13 deletion, 1:10–20,000, UBE3A ubiquitin pathway)	Progressive microcephaly; brachycephaly after age 2 years	Developmental delay; happy disposition with bursts of laughter	Vagal hypertonia
		Macrostomia & mandibular prognathism worsening with age	Puppet-like movement: ataxia, hypotonia, hyper-reflexia	
		Protruding tongue improving with age	Seizure disorder	
			γ-Aminobutyric acid system disordered function; varies from hyper- to hypofunction	
5	**Antley-Bixler syndrome** (trapezoidocephaly-synostosis syndrome, autosomal recessive, very rare disorder, chromosome 10q26, fibroblast growth factor receptor 2 (FGFR2))	Midface hypoplasia +/− choanal stenosis/atresia	Craniosynostosis	Reports of cardiac defects; atrial septal defect
			Brachycephaly; trapezoidal when viewed from above	
			Large anterior fontanelle	
			Ocular proptosis	
6	**Apert syndrome** (acrocephalosyndactyly, 1:160–200,000, sporadic autosomal dominant, chromosome 10q26, fibroblast growth factor receptor 2 (FGFR2))	Flat elongated forehead; obtuse nasofrontal angle; maxillary retrusion/mandibular prominence	Achrocephalia due to synostosis of coronal suture	NA

Pulmonary	Other	Additional anesthetic considerations	References
	Vitamin D malabsorption – rickets/pathological fractures		
	Vitamin E malabsorption – peripheral myopathy/ neuropathy		
NA	NA	Caution using benzodiazapines/ halogenated anesthetic agents	53
		Altered drug metabolism with anti-seizure therapy	54
		Hypervagal tone predisposes to bradycardia	55
		Muscular atrophy – titrate neuromuscular blocking drugs to effect with monitoring	56
45–50% mortality from respiratory complications: choanal stenosis/atresia, or midface hypoplasia	Femoral bowing, radiohumeral synostosis	Definitive airway (tracheostomy) may be required for choanal atresia	57
	Urogenital abnormalities: ureteral obstruction/ hydronephrosis, hypoplastic/fused labia	Mask ventilation/endotracheal tube placement may be challenging with midface hypoplasia – no reported difficult airway cases	58
		Meticulous eye protection for proptosis	59
		Vascular/arterial access may be challanging with limb deformities	
		Normal intellegence with cranial vault remodeling	
Cleft soft palate; reports of closure causing frank airway obstruction	Symmetrical syndactyly involving 4 extremities	Possible increased intracranial pressure	60

(Continued)

Table 38.1 (*Continued*)

No.	Syndrome: name, eponyms, inheritance, incidence, gene locus, gene product	Airway	Central nervous system	Cardiovascular
	Apert syndrome (*continued*)	Upper/lower airway compromise, obstructive sleep apnea: lack of tracheal distensibility	Non-progressive ventriculomegaly, corpus callosum agenesis, others	
		Laryngotracheal anomalies: laryngomalacia, cartilaginous tracheal sleeve, bronchomalacia	>60% Cervical spine fusion; C5-6 most commonly	
		Tracheal intubation is more difficult following midface distraction surgery	Early craniosynostosis surgery correlates with improved mental function	
		Airway compromise may worsen with growth		
7	**Arnold-Chiari malformation** (1:1–5000, association with connective tissue disorders)	Vocal cord paralysis	Herniation of cerebellum portions through foramen magnum, medulla oblongata kinking – hydrocephalus	Heart rate dysregulation
		Laryngeal obstruction: vocal cord paralysis, paradoxical vocal cord motion, laryngomalacia	Chiari Type II associated with meningomyelocele	Arterial pressure dysregulation
			Brainstem dysfunction – velopharyngeal incompetence, gastroesophageal reflux, vagal hypertonia	
			Obstructive & central apnea	

Pulmonary	Other	Additional anesthetic considerations	References
Obstructive sleep apnea is common		Obstructive sleep apnea may complicate mask ventilation	61
Increased incidence of perioperative wheezing		Airway: possible direct laryngoscopy but caution with cervical spine instability	62
		Bronchoscopy may be necessary to diagnose cause of upper/lower airway compromise	63
		Radiographic studies to rule out craniovertebral abnormalities/instability	64
		Recommended fiber-optic intubation following midface distraction surgery	65
		Laryngeal mask airway may rescue airway and facilitate endotracheal tube placement	66
			67
			68
			69
			70
			71
NA	NA	Brainstem dysfunction may require surgical airway	72
		Dysphagia and vocal cord paralysis predispose to aspiration	73
		Neck flexion/extension may exacerbate brainstem compression	74
		Posterior fossa surgery in prone position predisposes to venous air embolism	75

(Continued)

Table 38.1 (*Continued*)

No.	Syndrome: name, eponyms, inheritance, incidence, gene locus, gene product	Airway	Central nervous system	Cardiovascular
	Arnold-Chiari malformation (continued)		Hypoxic/hypercapneic arousal response deficits	
8	**Arthrogryposis multiplex congenita** (1:3000, multiple causes)	Laryngotracheal anomalies: vocal cord paralysis	Possible aqueductal stenosis with internal hydrocephalus	Congenital heart defects reported: patent ductus arteriosus, aortic stenosis or coarctation
		Cleft lip/palate, short neck, trismus	Possible myelomeningocele	
		Micrognathia	Vertebral anomalies: spina bifida, sacral agenesis, scoliosis, kyphosis	
		Mandibulofacial dysostosis, macrostomia, decreased supraglottic tone	Muscle atrophy	
9	**Autism spectrum disorder** (Asperger syndrome, atypical autism, pervasive developmental disorder, 1/150, candidate genes chromosome 2q, 7q, 15q, 15q14.1 and X)	NA	Autism: profound impairment in language, social-emotional functioning, restricted repetitive behaviors	NA
			Asperger: hyperfunctioning language & motor control problems	
10	**Becker muscular dystophy** (benign pseudohypertrophic muscular dystrophy, X-linked recessive, 1:20,000 males, mutation dystrophin gene, Xp21.2)	NA	May have neurocognitive dysfunction	ECG changes, hypertrophic cardiomyopathy, dilative cardiomyopathy +/− preserved systolic function

Pulmonary	Other	Additional anesthetic considerations	References
		Acute sinus arrhythmias reported during surgery in 4th ventricle	76
		Autonomic dysfunction should resolve following decompression	77
		Ventilatory support may be necessary postoperatively for apnea	78
Thoracic deformities: hypoventilation, hypoplastic lungs, restrictive lung disease	Distal joint contractures; medially overlapping fingers, ulnar deviation, camptodactyly, foot deformities	Possible difficult intubation – micrognathia and trismus; usually easy bag-mask ventilation	
	Esophageal dysfunction and gastroesophageal reflux	Consider/evaluate cervical spine involvement	79
	Genitourinary abnormalities: renal fusion/absence, hypospadias, inguinal hernia	Possible difficult IV access	80
		Reports of hypermetabolism/hyperthermia distinct from malignant hyperthermia	81
		Avoid succinylcholine – myopathies; sensitive to non-depolarizing neuromuscular blocking drugs	
		Caution with positioning – contractures	
		Possible post-op respiratory complications – restrictive lung disease, poor cough/gag	
NA	Criteria: impaired social interaction, impaired verbal/non-verbal communication, restricted interest range, resistance to change	Behavioral problems may be challenging during induction/emergence from anesthesia	82
		Consider family participation, oral midazolam/ketamine for preoperative sedation	83
Respiratory muscle weakness may predispose to pulmonary infections	Dystrophinopathy – altered size or abundance of dystrophin protein – characterized by muscle weakness	Dysphagia may predispose to aspiration	84
	Predisposed to rhabdomyolysis and hyperkalemic cardiac arrest with "triggering" agent	Cardiac work-up for cardiomyopathy	85

(Continued)

Table 38.1 (*Continued*)

No.	Syndrome: name, eponyms, inheritance, incidence, gene locus, gene product	Airway	Central nervous system	Cardiovascular
	Becker muscular dystophy (*continued*)			
11	**Beckwith-Wiedemann syndrome** (sporadic, 1:13,700, chromosome 11p15.5 mutations, multiple variants, insulin-like growth factor 2 (IGF2) likely involved)	Macroglossia Upper airway obstruction: macroglossia, prognathism, adenotonsilar hypertrophy	NA	Chronic airway obstruction may predispose to cor pulmonale
12	**Carpenter syndrome** (acrocephalopolysyndactyly type II, autosomal recessive, 1:1 million, chromosome 6p11, RAB 23 gene, RAB guanosine triphosphatase family of vesicle transport proteins)	Cleft lip/palate Hypoplastic mandible/maxilla Short, thick neck	Craniosynostosis: midline sutures fuse before coronal sutures Variable intelligence	Congenital heart: ventricular/atrial septal defects, patent ductus arteriosus, pulmonic stenosis, tetralogy of Fallot most common

Pulmonary	Other	Additional anesthetic considerations	References
		Concern for hyperkalemic cardiac arrest with triggering agents	86
		No apparent relation with malignant hyperthermia	87
			88
NA	Abdominal wall defect: omphalocele	Smaller than expected endotracheal tube size – cuffed may be preferred	89
	Visceromegaly: nephromegaly, hepatomegaly, splenomegaly, pancreatomegaly	Glossomegaly – predisposes to upper airway obstruction on induction/ emergence from anesthesia	90
	Increased incidence of intra-abdominal tumors	Glossomegaly – relatively improves with growth	91
	Hypoglycemia likely from hyperinsulinemia	Hypoglycemia from increased insulin secretion	92
		Videolaryngoscope and laryngeal mask airway described for difficult airway control	
NA	Syndactyly upper/lower limbs	Small mandible, short obese neck may cause challenging intubation	93
	Obesity: proximal limbs, face, neck and trunk	Evaluate for congenital heart disease	94
		Report of abnormal anatomical features leading to unexpected/severe blood loss	95
			96
			97

(Continued)

Table 38.1 (*Continued*)

No.	Syndrome: name, eponyms, inheritance, incidence, gene locus, gene product	Airway	Central nervous system	Cardiovascular
13	**Cat eye syndrome** (trisomy 22, Schmid-Fracarro syndrome, chromosome 22 partial tetrasomy, sporadic-spontaneous 3 or 4 copies of short arm and section of long arm, 1:50,000 and 1:150,000, cat eye syndrome critical region gene-7 (CECR7) protein)	Micrognathia, microcephaly	Ocular coloboma and motility defect	Congenital heart defects: ventricular/atrial septal defect, total anomalous pulmonary venous return, tetralogy of Fallot, patent ductus arteriosus
		Cleft palate or absent uvula	Muscular tonus dysregulation, visual and hearing impairments	
14	**Catel-Manzke syndrome** (Pierre Robin syndrome with hyperphalangy and clinodactyly, X-linked recessive, 26 cases reported, gene defect not known)	Pierre Robin anomaly: micrognathia, glossoptosis, cleft palate	NA	Severe congenital heart disease: septal defects, aortic defects, dextrocardia
15	**Central core disease** (central core myopathy, autosomal dominant, chromosome 19q13.1, mutations in the ryanodine receptor-1 gene)	NA	NA	Structural abnormalities are rare
16	**Cerebrocostomandibular syndrome** (rib gap defects with micrognathia, sporadic inheritance, 65 cases reported, gene defect not known)	Pierre Robin: small mandible (micrognathia), cleft palate, glossoptosis	Mental retardation – likely from upper airway obstruction leading to neonatal hypoxia	Ventricular septal defect has been reported

Pulmonary	Other	Additional anesthetic considerations	References
Scoliosis or chest deformity	Preauricular skin tags/pits	Micrognathia may predispose to difficult intubation – reports of awake nasal fiber-optic and through laryngeal mask airway	98
Rib or sternal anomaly	Anal atresia with rectal fistulas	Cardiac work-up for congenital heart defects	99
	Urogenital malformations: external genitalia malformation, renal agenesis, hydronephrosis, VUR	Abnormal renal/hepatic function may alter anesthetic drug pharmacokinetics	100
	Limb deformity	Limb abnormalities may result in challenging arterial access	
	Vertebral anomaly		
	Intra/extrahepatic biliary atresia		
Pectus carinatum/excavatum	Bilateral hyperphalangy and clinodactyly of the index finger	Pierre Robin: difficult or impossible endotracheal intubation	101
	Vertebral/rib anomalies	Cardiac work-up for congenital heart defects	102
			103
Respiratory involvement is exceptional but severe	Myopathy: proximal (hip girdle) muscle weakness, but also axial muscles	RYR1 gene mutation – high malignant hyperthermia risk	104
	Ortho complications: hip dislocation, scoliosis, foot deformities, ligamentous laxity, rarely contractures	Closely linked to malignant hyperthermia susceptibility	105
	Elevated serum creatine kinase, selective muscle involvement pattern on MRI	Avoid triggering anesthetic agents/drugs	106
Scoliosis	Kidney abnormalities: cysts, persistent urinary tract infection, reflux and ectopia	Pierre Robin: difficult or impossible endotracheal intubation	107

(Continued)

Table 38.1 (*Continued*)

No.	Syndrome: name, eponyms, inheritance, incidence, gene locus, gene product	Airway	Central nervous system	Cardiovascular
	Cerebrocostomandibular syndrome (*continued*)	Possible tracheal ring anomalies	Absent olfactory bulb	
17	**Charcot-Marie-Tooth syndrome** (hereditary sensorimotor neuropathy, peroneal muscular atrophy, multiple modes of inheritance, 1:3000, duplication chromosome 17p12 (75%), PMP22, 38 other gene mutations in neuronal proteins: myelins or axons)	NA	Peripheral motor and sensory neuropathy – demyelinating	NA
			Primarily peroneal muscle atrophy with foot drop	
			Progressive muscle weakness beginning in legs	
			Autonomic dysfunction possible with postganglionic sympathetic involvement	
18	**CHARGE association** (parental gonadal mosaicism in some cases, spontaneous mutation, 1:10,000, mutation chromosome 7q21.11, chromodomain helicse DNA binding protein 7 (CHD7) gene–neural crest epigenetic chromatin remodeling)	Swallowing/sucking difficulties	Colobomata: typical iris coloboma to anophthalmos	Right-sided congenital heart disease: tetralogy of Fallot, pulmonic stenosis, double outlet right ventricle
		Cleft palate associated with congenital heart disease, mostly tetralogy of Fallot	Cranial nerve dysfunction: CNI – anosmia, CNVII – facial palsy, CNVIII – hearing loss, CNIX/CNX – velopharyngeal inco-ordination	Atrioventricular septal congenital heart disease: ventricular/atrial septal defect associated with tetralogy of Fallot

Pulmonary	Other	Additional anesthetic considerations	References
Thoracic insufficiency syndrome from "implosion" of the thorax from congenital posterior rib pseudoarthrosis		Thoracic insufficiency syndrome from rib pseudoarthrosis may necessitate mechanical ventilation	108
			109
			110
Respiratory insufficiency possible with severe disease	NA	Questionable response to neuromuscular blocking drugs – reports of successful use of non-depolarizing drugs	111
		Hyperkalemic arrest possible with succinylcholine – successful use reported	112
		Temperature dysregulation from impaired sweating with autonomic dysfunction	113
		Nitrous oxide does not worsen neuropathy	114
		Total intravenous anesthesia without muscle relaxants/triggering agents reported	115
Atresia choanae	Hypogenitalism	Possible difficult/impossible endotracheal intubation with micrognathia	116
Tracheoesophageal fistula associated with congenital heart disease, mostly tetralogy of Fallot	Renal anomalies (malrotation, hydronephrosis, reflux) associated with congenital heart disease, mostly atrioventricular septal defect	May require continuous positive airway pressure to maintain airway patency with laryngomalacia/velopalatal insufficiency	117

(Continued)

Table 38.1 (*Continued*)

No.	Syndrome: name, eponyms, inheritance, incidence, gene locus, gene product	Airway	Central nervous system	Cardiovascular
	CHARGE association (*continued*)	Hypoplastic mandible (micrognathia) associated with congenital heart disease, mostly tetralogy of Fallot Three major issues: micrognathia, laryngomalacia, subglottic stenosis	Delayed motor development, may involve truncal hypotonia	Aberrant subclavian artery and/or right aortic arch
19	**Cockayne syndrome** (Weber-Cockayne syndrome, Neill-Dingwall syndrome, autosomal recessive, 1:250,000, mutation chromosome 5q12, 10q11, ERCC6 or ERCC8 gene: proteins repairing damaged DNA transcription-coupled repair mechanism)	Microcephaly, micrognathia, dental overcrowding	Progressive neurological degeneration with spastic quadriparesis	Individual reports of aortic dilation and dilated cardiomyopathy
		Postcricoid narrowing (subglottic stenosis)	Developmental regression	Progressive arteriosclerosis with hypertension
		Bird-like face, beak-like nose, inappropriately large teeth	Photosensitivity	Hypertension with renal disease
				Reports of myocardial ischemia from hypertension
20	**Cornelia de Lange syndrome** (sporadic mutation, 1:30,000, mutation chromosome 5p13.1, NIPBL gene affecting cohesin complex)	Micrognathia, macroglossia, microbrachycephaly	Motor/mental retardation	Congenital heart disease: ventricular septal defect most common

Pulmonary	Other	Additional anesthetic considerations	References
	Vertebral anomalies (hemivertebrae, scoliosis) associated with congenital heart disease	May require smaller than expected endotracheal tube for subglottic stenosis	118
		Aspiration risk with swallowing dysfunction	119
		Cardiac work-up for congenital heart defects	120
		Thyroid/parathyroid functional studies for similarities between CHARGE and DiGeorge syndromes	121
		High incidence of post-operative airway events	
		Successful airway management with laryngeal mask airway has been reported	
NA	NA	Difficult intubation reports with successful use of laryngeal mask airway	122
		Aspiration risk, but mental retardation makes awake fiber-optic intubation challenging	123
		Reported cerebral ischemia with nifedipine	124
		Difficult intravenous access with contractures	125
			126
			127
Frequent pulmonary aspiration from severe gastroesophageal reflux	Micromelia +/– oligodactyly	Possible difficult intubation with aspiration risk	128

(Continued)

Table 38.1 (*Continued*)

No.	Syndrome: name, eponyms, inheritance, incidence, gene locus, gene product	Airway	Central nervous system	Cardiovascular
	Cornelia de Lange syndrome (*continued*)	Frequently narrow, arched palate or complete cleft	Strabismus	
		Short neck and cylindrical trunk	Neonatal hypertonia	
			Self-injurious behavior	
21	**Costello syndrome** (faciocutaneoskeletal syndrome, spontaneous mutation, 300 reported cases, mutation chromosome 11p15.5, mutation HRAS gene: proteins controlling cell growth and division)	Mucopolysaccharidosis-like: macrocephaly, bulbous nose, big mouth, large tongue	Possible seizure disorder	Cardiavascular malformation – pulmonic stenosis
		Possible choanal stenosis or congenital laryngeal web		Hypertrophic cardiomyopathy
		50% with perioral/ perinasal papillomas manifesting in childhood		Rhythm disturbances – supraventricular tachycardia
		Short neck		
		Abundant tracheobronchial secretions		
		Hypertrophied adenoids/ base of tongue		
22	**Cri du chat syndrome** (chromosome 5p deletion syndrome, 5p minus syndrome, Lejeune syndrome, sporadic deletion, 1:20–50,000, deletion chromosome 5p15.2)	Microcephaly, micrognathia	Hypotonia replaced by hypertonia with age	20–30% with congenital heart disease: ventricular septal defect, patent ductus arteriosus, tetralogy of Fallot
		Typical cry: small, narrow, diamond-shaped larynx; small hypotonic epiglottis	Psychomotor and mental retardation	

Pulmonary	Other	Additional anesthetic considerations	References
	Dystrophic dwarfism	Unco-operative patient making induction challenging	129
	Forearm and hand deformities	Reduced anesthetic requirements	130
			131
			132
			133
Connective tissue disorder-like: limb disorders with possible kyphosis and/or scoliosis	Hypoglycemia possible from growth hormone/ cortisol deficiency &/or hyperinsulinemia	Airway management with macroglossia, short neck, hypertrophied supraglottic tissue	134
		Possible change in drug metabolism from anti-seizure therapy	135
		Cardiac work-up for structure, function, & rhythm	136
		Reports of pulmonary hypertension, elevated catechols, hypertrophic cardiomyopathy, obstructive sleep apnea, pulmonary infiltrates, severe scoliosis	137
		Possible central temperature regulation defect	138
			139
Laryngotracheal anomalies: vocal cord paralysis	Metabolic anomalies: purine synthesis defect	Consider pre-op CT evaluation of airway	141
	Progressive scoliosis	Possible difficult intubation – successful laryngeal mask airway use reported	142

(Continued)

Table 38.1 (*Continued*)

No.	Syndrome: name, eponyms, inheritance, incidence, gene locus, gene product	Airway	Central nervous system	Cardiovascular
	Cri du chat syndrome (*continued*)	Laryngeal abnormalities: hypoplastic larynx, narrow laryngomalacia, diamond-shaped larynx Epiglottal abnormalities: long, curved, floppy, hypoplastic & hypotonic epiglottis		
23	**Crouzon syndrome** (craniofacial dysostosis, autosomal dominant, 1:60,000, mutation chromosome 10q26, fibroblast growth factor receptor 2 (FGFR2))	Maxillary hypoplasia, midface complex underdevelopment Severe airway obstruction: midface hypoplasia, adenotonsillar hypertrophy, laryngotracheomalacia Cervical "butterfly" vertebrae & some cervical fusion	Craniosynostosis, ocular proptosis and shallow orbits	NA
24	**Cystic fibrosis** (mucoviscidosis, autosomal recessive, 1:4000, chromosome 7q31.2 mutation, cystic fibrosis transmembrane conductance regulator (CFTR): chloride transporter channel protein)	NA	NA	Possible right ventricular enlargement from bronchiectatic lung disease via hypoxic pulmonary vasoconstriction and pulmonary vascular remodeling

Pulmonary	Other	Additional anesthetic considerations	References
		Pharyngeal muscle hypotonia may cause soft tissue airway obstruction	143
		Cardiac work-up for congenital heart disease	144
			145
			146
Laryngotracheal anomalies: cartilaginous tracheal sleeve	NA	Possible difficult intubation: abnormal facies & possible fused cervical vertebrae	147
		Possible increased intracranial pressure with craniosynostosis	148
		Possible obstructive airway with craniosynostosis	149
			150
Exocrine gland mucosal obstruction – small airway plug, poor ciliary clearance, chronic colonization/infection	Exocrine gland mucosal obstruction – pancreatic insufficiency, biliary obstruction, male infertility	Pulmonary bacterial colonization, apical blebs, and prone to pneumothoraces	151
Obstructive airway disease on PFTs: decreased FEV1, decreased peak exp flow, increased residual vol	Protein/fat malabsorption – fat-soluble vitamin deficiency with vitamin K-deficient coagulopathy	Assess pulmonary function/reactivity – airway patency may depend on muscle tone in older patients	152
Nasal polyps, chronic sinusitis	Diabetes mellitus and insulin resistance	Cardiac work-up to assess right ventricular function	153
	Neonatal meconium ileus from abnormally thick meconium	Glucose control	

(Continued)

Table 38.1 (*Continued*)

No.	Syndrome: name, eponyms, inheritance, incidence, gene locus, gene product	Airway	Central nervous system	Cardiovascular
	Cystic fibrosis (*continued*)			
25	**Diastrophic dysplasia** (autosomal recessive, 1:100,000, chromosome 5q32-q33.1, SLC26A2 gene: protein for normal cartilage formation)	50% with cleft palate	Normal intelligence	NA
		Dysmorphic facial features: retrognathic mandible	Cervicothoracic spina bifida occulta	
		Cervical kyphosis with substantial C1-C2 instability	Possible spinal cord compression from kyphoscoliosis	
		Laryngomalacia, laryngotracheal stenosis		
26	**DiGeorge (22q11-) syndrome** (velocardiofacial syndrome, CATCH-22, conotruncal anomalies face syndrome, sporadic or autosomal dominant, 1:2000, microdeletion chromosome 22q11.1, TXB1 deletion causes most cardiac defects)	Craniofacial anomalies: cleft palate, micrognathia, small mouth	Learning difficulties, other pyschiatric disorders	Cardiac defects: tetralogy of Fallot, interrupted aortic arch, ventricular septal defect, pulmonic stenosis, tricuspid atresia
		Small thyroid cartiledge with increased anterior angle		
		Short trachea with reduced number of cartilage rings		
		Laryngobronchomalacia		
		Tracheal bronchi		

Pulmonary	Other	Additional anesthetic considerations	References
	Distal intestinal obstruction syndrome with abdominal distension, nausea/vomiting	Coagulopathy/altered drug metabolism with hepatobiliary involvement	
	Fatty liver with 10% complicated by cirrhosis & portal HTN	Decreased bone density – positioning (fracture risk), kyphoscoliosis	
	Low bone mineral density	Consider alternatives to narcotic analgesia to avoid respiratory suppression	
Thoracolumbar kyphoscoliosis – may interfere with pulmonary function	Reduced height, hand/feet deformities, joint contractures	Smaller than expected blood pressure cuff	154
	One-third with scoliosis	CT evaluation of cervical spine	155
		Possible difficult intubation with micrognathia and cervical spine kyphosis	156
			157
			158
NA	Hypo- or aplasia of parathyroid gland resulting in hypocalcemia	Reports of vasomotor instability	159
	Hypo- or aplasia of thymus gland resulting in immune deficiencies	Cardiac work-up for congenital heart disease	160
	Renal & skeletal anomalies	Possible difficult airway with dysmorphic facies	161
	DiGeorge anomaly is likely a feature of velocardiofacial syndrome	Possible difficult extubation with velopharyngeal insufficiency	162
		Recurrent infection risk with thymic dysfunction	163
		Persistant hypocalcemia with parathyroid dysfunction leading to seizures	164
		Report of tachycardia from epinephrine injected with local anesthetics	165

(Continued)

Table 38.1 (*Continued*)

No.	Syndrome: name, eponyms, inheritance, incidence, gene locus, gene product	Airway	Central nervous system	Cardiovascular
27	**Down syndrome** (trisomy 21, meotic non-dysjunction event, maternal origin, 1/732)	High arched narrow palate, macroglossia, subglottic stenosis	Mental retardation	Congenital heart disease: endocardial cushion defects, ventricular septal defect, patent ductus arteriosus, tetralogy of Fallot
		Atlantoaxial subluxation	Possible altered response to opioids	Predisposed to pulmonary hypertension
		Smaller tracheal lumen diameter		Predisposed to bradycardia with inhaled induction; halothane, sevoflurane
				Possible difficult arterial/venous access
28	**Duchenne muscular dystrophy** (pseudohypertrophic progressive muscular dystrophy, recessive X-linked, 1:3500, mutation chromosome Xp21, absent dystrophin)	33% with macroglossia	Intellectual impairment	Cardiomegaly leading to dilated cardiomyopathy
				ECG changes: short PR interval, right ventricular hypertrophy, Q waves in leads II, III, aVF, V5, V6

Pulmonary	Other	Additional anesthetic considerations	References
Upper airway obstruction/sleep apnea	Dental abnormalities	Radiologic cervical spine abnormalities do not correlate to neurological symptoms	166
	Duodenal atresia, Hirschsprung disease with gastroesophageal reflux	Atlantoaxial instability may increase with loss of muscle tone under anesthesia	167
	Immunosuppression and hypothyroidism	Smaller enotracheal tube (0.5–1 mm) to avert tracheal trauma	168
	Hypotonia, hyperextensibility, dysplastic pelvis	Possible difficult vascular access	169
		Possible bradycardic response to high concentration volatile anesthetic agents	
Restrictive defect from diaphragm, intercostal, & accessory respiratory muscle weakness	Abnormal gait to difficulty climbing stairs to Gower sequence to wheelchair bound with muscle atrophy	Cardiac work-up for cardiomyopathy	170
Glottic dysfunction with inadequate intrathoracic pressure needed for adequate cough	Elevated serum creatine kinase from extensive skeletal muscle wasting	Avoid succinylcholine – hyperkalemic cardiac arrest	171
	Progressive scoliosis	Avoid volatiles – rhabdomyolysis & cardiac arrest	172
	Progressive dysphagia	No apparent relation with malignant hyperthermia	173
		Pulmonary insufficiency may complicate extubation	174
		Gastric dysmotility may predispose to aspiration	
		Non-depolarizing neurmuscular blocking drugs may have longer duration of action	
		Corticosteroids improve muscle function, cause obesity, hypertension, glucose intolerance, osteoporosis	

(Continued)

Table 38.1 (*Continued*)

No.	Syndrome: name, eponyms, inheritance, incidence, gene locus, gene product	Airway	Central nervous system	Cardiovascular
29	**Dutch-Kentucky syndrome** (Hecht-Beals syndrome, congenital contractural arachnodactyly, distal arthrogryposis type 9, sporadic inheritance, very rare syndrome, mutation chromosome 5q23-q31, fibrilin-2 gene: connective tissue protein)	Limited mouth opening Reports of mandibular prognathism & micrognathia	NA	NA
30	**Ehlers-Danlos syndrome (EDS)**	Dysphonia – hemi-laryngeal weakness	Mild/mod weakness, myalgia, and easy fatiguability in majority of patients	Bleeding symptoms for all EDS types
	EDS – classic type (autosomal dominant disorder type V collagen; 1:20–50,000)			Mitral valve prolapse, aortic root/sinus of Valsalva dilation, septal defects
	EDS – hypermobility type (autosomal dominant or recessive mutation in tanascin X gene)		Decreased/absent analgesic effect from lidocaine given subcutaneously, or local anesthetic cream	Mitral valve prolapse, aortic root/sinus of Valsalva dilation, septal defects
	EDS – vascular type (autosmal dominant mutation in type III collagen gene: 1:100–250,000)			Medium and large-size vessel fragility leading to rupture
	EDS – kyphoscoliosis type (autosomal recessive mutation in gene for lysyl hydroxylase: fewer than 60 cases)	Atlantoaxial subluxation may occur in type IV		
	EDS – arthrochalasia type (mutation in type I collagen gene; fewer than 30 cases)			

Pulmonary	Other	Additional anesthetic considerations	References
NA	Hand and feet deformities	Difficult intubation – trismus is unrelieved by general anesthesia, muscle relaxants, physical force	175
		Reports of retrograde guidewire-assisted FO intubation	176
		Reports of nasal (blind & FO) intubations	177
			178
			179
NA	NA	Bleeding symptoms are responsive to desmopressin	180
			181
	Classic: I and II – skin hyperextensibility, widened atrophic scars, joint hypermobility	Report of scoliosis correction using spinal fusion complicated by bleeding & wound dehiscence	182
			183
	Hypermobility: III – hyperextensibility +/– smooth, velvety skin, generalized joint hypermobility		184
			185
	Vascular: IV – translucent skin, arterial/intestinal/ uterine fragility, extensive bruising, characteristic facies:	Premature death from organ rupture (arterial, bowel, uterus)	186
		Report of success using recombinant factor VIIa	187
	Kyphoscoliosis: VI – joint laxity, muscle hypotonia, progressive scoliosis, scleral fragility	Report of scoliosis correction using spinal fusion complicated by arterial avulsion/ rupture	188
			189
	Arthrochalasia: VIIA/B – joint laxity with recurrent subluxations, congenital B/L hip dislocation		190

(Continued)

Table 38.1 (*Continued*)

No.	Syndrome: name, eponyms, inheritance, incidence, gene locus, gene product	Airway	Central nervous system	Cardiovascular
	Ehlers-Danlos syndrome (EDS) (*continued*) EDS – dermatosparaxis type (10 cases reported)			
31	**Epidermolysis bullosa (EB)** EB simplex (mutations keratin 5 and 14 genes) EB junctional (mutations laminin 5 or collagen XVII genes) EB dystrophic (mutation type VII collagen, 1:50,000 overall incidence)	Oral: cyclic blistering leads to milia, ankyloglossia, microstomia Larynx: trauma leads to supraglottic bullae/cysts, glottic VC cysts/webs, subglottic stenosis Pharyngoesophageal: blisters lead to odynophagia, esophageal scar/web/stenosis to dysphagia	EB simplex with plectin deficiency is associated with slowly progressive muscular dystrophy	Dilated cardiomyopathy associated with low plasma carnitine

Pulmonary	Other	Additional anesthetic considerations	References
			191
	Dermatosparaxis: VIIC – severe skin fragility, sagging, redundant skin	Gentle intubation with minimal inspiratory pressures to avoid airway hematomas	192
		Consider possible cervical instability	
		Cardiac work-up to assess valves and great vessels	
		Avoid central vascular access or place under U/S visualization	
		Prepare for significant blood loss	
		Caution with neuraxial anesthesia/ analgesia	
Respiratory tract lesions from mouth to bronchi with plectin deficiency	Poor nutrition and gastroesophageal reflux are common	Anemia likely but blood draws may be done post induction	193
	Cutaneous scarring causes joint contractions of fingers/toes	Gastroesophageal reflux may necesitate oral antacids	194
	Conjunctival bullae in cornea may compromise vision	"No touch" principle to minimize friction	195
	Anemia, glomerulonephritis, nephrotic syndrome are common	Avoid "sticky" items, lubricate eyes, diligent pressure point padding	196
	Epitheliomas (squamous cellular carcinomas) in 3rd/4th decade	Consider pulse-ox to monitor oxygen saturation and heart rate without ECG or use needle ECG probes	197
	Acute/chronic pain from wounds	Pad beneath blood pressure cuff; avoid intra-arterial monitoring to prevent wrist scarring	198
	Unrelated to porphyria – thiopental is no longer contraindicated	Microstomia may lead to difficult intubation	199
		Avoid oropharyngeal/laryngotracheal trauma from intubation – use uncuffed ETT, lubricate everything	
		Cardiac work-up for DCM may be indicated	
		Utilise regional analgesia whenever possible	

(Continued)

Table 38.1 (*Continued*)

No.	Syndrome: name, eponyms, inheritance, incidence, gene locus, gene product	Airway	Central nervous system	Cardiovascular
32	**Fabry disease** (Anderson-Fabry disease, angiokeratoma corporis diffusum, alpha-galactosidase A deficiency, X-linked recessive, 1:55,000 males, mutation chromosome Xq22, alpha-galactosidase A)	Possible angiokeratomas (raised, red, non-blanching telangiectases) in oral mucosa	Cerebrovascular complications: stroke, hemiplegia, hemianesthesia, transient ischemic attacks	Progressive hypertrophic infiltrative cardiomyopathy
			Acroparesthesia (as well as gastrointestinal and joint pain) responsive to enzyme replacement therapy	Valvular abnormalities
			Corneal verticillata (whorls) leading to "haze," retina vascular abnormalities	Arrhythmias and conduction abnormalities
				Atherosclerotic lesions and hypertension
				RV commonly involved – progress to severe diastolic/systolic RV dysfunction
33	**Familial dysautonomia (Riley-Day syndrome)** (hereditary sensory and autonomic neuropathy, type III, autosomal recessive, 1:3700 Ashkenazi Jewish ancestry, mutation chromosome 9q31-33, IKBKAP (inhibitor of kappa light polypeptide gene enhancer in B-cells); regulates transcription)	NA	Emotional lability – anxiety, depression	Baroreflex abnormal: efferent sensitivity to resistance vessels, efferent to heart
			Alacrima – absence of overflow tearing	Orthostatic hypotension without compensatory tachycardia
			Peripheral sensory deficits: abnormal pain/temperature, decreased deep tendon reflexes	Decreased heart rate variability
			Central sensory deficits: decreased cranial nerve V pain perception, diminished corneal reflexes	Supine hypertension

Pulmonary	Other	Additional anesthetic considerations	References
Dyspnea, cough/wheezing, hemoptysis, obstructive airway disease responsive to enzyme replacement therapy	Hypohydriasis	Caution anticholinergics with hypohydriasis	200
	Gastrointestinal disturbances: diarrhea, pain, nausea/vomiting	Avoid trauma to oral mucosa with angiokeratomas	201
	Nephropathy is dominant feature: from chronic to endstage renal disease	Cardiac work-up for ischemia, valvular dysfunction, arrhythmias	202
		Renal work-up for insufficiency, failure, end-stage renal disease	203
		Caution with positioning due to peripheral neuropathy	204
		Caution using neuraxial anesthesia/ analgesia due to peripheral neuropathy	205
			206
Insensitivity to hypoxia & hypercarbia	Oropharyngeal inco-ordination leading to dysphasia & aspiration	Aspiration risk with intubation	207
Cardiorespiratory dysregulation both awake/asleep likely representing alveolar hypoventilation	Incompetent lower esophageal sphincter leading to gastroesophageal reflux	Reports of general anesthesia with significant hemodynamic instability	208
Bronchial/interstitial inflammation consistent with chronic gastric aspiration	Esophageal dilation with fluid overload leading to aspiration	Reports of regional anesthesia minimizing hemodynamic instability	209
	Gastroesophageal reflux is independent of sensory dysfunction severity	Assess intravascular volume status	210

(Continued)

Table 38.1 (*Continued*)

No.	Syndrome: name, eponyms, inheritance, incidence, gene locus, gene product	Airway	Central nervous system	Cardiovascular
	Familial dysautonomia (*continued*)			"Sympathetic storm" – hypertension, tachycardia, diaphoresis, functional ileus
				Higher normalized QT variance – risk for ventricular arrhythmias
34	**Familial periodic paralysis (FPP)** (autosomal dominant myopathy; variable penetrance)	NA	NA	Dyskalemias leading to arrhythmias
	FPP: hypokalemic (mutation chromosome 1q32, HOKPP gene)		Flaccid weakness associated with decreased serum potassium	
	FPP: hyperkalemic (mutation sodium channel gene SCN4A on chromosome 17)		Flaccid weakness associated with increased serum potassium	
	FPP: Anderson syndrome (Anderson-Twail syndrome)	Dysmorphic features: micrognathia, cleft palate, macrocephaly	Periodic paralysis may be hyper-, normo- or hypokalemic	Long QT syndrome is primary cardiac manifestation, independent of periodic paralysis
				Ventricular ectopy: premature ventricular contractions, ventricular tachycardia from "triggered activity" by delayed afterdepolarizations
	Long QT syndrome 7			Reports of bicuspic aortic valve, coarctation, pulmonic stenosis
	Anderson cardiodysrhythmic periodic paralysis (mutation chromosome 17q23.1-q24.2)			

Pulmonary	Other	Additional anesthetic considerations	References
	Chronic kidney disease with significant orthostatic hypotension	High risk for postoperative pulmonary complications, including abnl response to hypoxia/hypercapnia	211
	Spine deformities: scoliosis/kyphosis	High risk for postoperative nausea/ vomiting with no reports of response to potent 5-HT3 antagonists	212
	Poor bone quality: osteopenia/osteoporosis		213
			214
Respiratory insufficiency during an attack	Progressive myopathy affecting pelvic girdle and proximal/distal lower extremity with fatty replacement		215
			216
		Theoretical risk of malignant hyperthermia without case reports	217
		Avoid exogenous insulin/glucose, alkalosis	218
		Reports of successful use of atracurium	219
		Reports of successful spinal anesthesia	220
		Avoid epidural mepivicaine as it lowers serum potassium	221
			222
		Avoid exogenous potassium, acidosis, succinylcholine	223
		Reports of successful use of propofol & propofol/remifentanil	224
	Proximal muscle atrophy without mytonic disorders	Possible difficult intubation with micrognathia	
	Bone deformities: wormian bones, scoliosis	Mandatory cardiac evaluation	
	Reports of unilateral renal dysplasia		

(Continued)

Table 38.1 (*Continued*)

No.	Syndrome: name, eponyms, inheritance, incidence, gene locus, gene product	Airway	Central nervous system	Cardiovascular
35	**Fibrodysplasia (myositis) ossificans progressiva syndrome** (autosomal dominant, 1:1.5 million, mutation chromosome 2q23-q24, ACVR1 gene)	Progressive muscle ossification: neck/paraspinal rigidity to shoulder/spine to hips/knees to jaw Variable cervical spine vertebral fusion +/− adjacent muscular ossification	NA	Cardiac muscle is spared from ossification ECG changes: right bundle branch block, T wave inversion, ST change
36	**Fetal alcohol syndrome** (teratogenic syndrome, 1/100)	Facial anomalies: short palpebral fissures, thin upper lip, smooth philtrum Possible flat midface	Microcephaly and structural brain anomalies Cognitive deficits: attention deficit hyperactivity disorder Delayed motor development and impaired fine/gross motor skills Maladaptive behaviors: poor judgment, distractibility, poor social cue perception	Cardiac defects: atrial/ventricular septal defect common

Pulmonary	Other	Additional anesthetic considerations	References
Severely restrictive chest wall disease suggesting diaphragmatic breathing dependence	Short laterally deviated great toes from birth	Trauma (surgery, biopsy, tourniquet) may initiate ossification	225
Diaphragm is spared from ossification	Heterotopic ossification: neck/spine/shoulder girdle proceeding axial to appendicular, cranial to caudal, proximal to distal	Chest wall restriction leads to respiratory failure, atelectasis, inadequate cough	226
		Awake FO intubation – DL avoided to prevent TMJ ankylosis	227
		Avoid tracheostomy – ossification at incision site may cause airway obstruction	228
		Avoid IM injection – ossification at injection site	229
		Avoid neuraxial techniques	230
		Successful U/S-guided peripheral nerve block has been reported	231
			232
			233
			234
			235
	Clinodactyly of 5th finger, camptodactyly, "hockey stick" palmar crease	Induction may be challenging with cognitive deficits	236
		No known association with upper airway abnormalities	237
		Single case report of difficult intubation	238
		Cardiac work-up as indicated	239
			240

(Continued)

Table 38.1 (*Continued*)

No.	Syndrome: name, eponyms, inheritance, incidence, gene locus, gene product	Airway	Central nervous system	Cardiovascular
37	**Fragile X syndrome** (X-linked dominant, 1:3600 males, 1:4–6000 females, mutation chromosome Xq27.3, FMR1 gene, involved in translation)	Increased risk for obstructive sleep apnea: adenotonsillar hypertrophy, narrow oropharyngeal cavity, hypoplastic midface	Most common form of inherited mental retardation	Mitral valve prolapse and/or aortic root dilation may occur in adolescence
		High arched palate	Behavior traits: tactile defensiveness, hand flapping/biting, perseverative speech	Fragile X tremor/ataxia syndrome: autonomic dysfunction
			Fragile X tremor/ataxia syndrome: normal intellect, progressive cerebellar ataxia, parkinsonism, dementia	
38	**Fraser syndrome** (autosomal recessive, 1:230,000, FRAS1 or FREM 2 genes, mutation chromosome 13q13.3 or 4q21)	Laryngotracheal anomalies: laryngeal atresia/stenosis	Ocular abnormalities: cryptophthalmos +/– microphthalmos, anophthalmos, corneal opacification	Reported: left ventricular hypertrophy, Ebstein anomaly, coarctation, atrial/ ventricular septal defect, tricuspid atresia, dextrocardia, transposition
		Glottic web or subglottic stenosis	Reports of hydrocephalus & structural abnormalities	
		Cleft lip/palate	Reports of developmental delay and hypotonia	
39	**Friedreich ataxia** (autosomal recessive, 1:50,000, mutation chromosome 9q13-q21, frataxin gene: protein involved in mitochondrial iron metabolism)	NA	Progressive ataxia, dysarthria, loss of joint position/ vibration, absent tendon reflexes, hypotonia	Possible cardiomyopathy
				Transition from hypertrophic to hypokinetic dilated cardiomyopathy occurs
40	**Glycogen storage diseases (GSD)**			

Pulmonary	Other	Additional anesthetic considerations	References
Possible pectus excavatum deformity	Male macro-orchidism	Cognitive deficits make induction challenging	241
	Hyperextensible metacarpophalangeal joints, plamar/hallucal crease, pale blue irises	Cardiac work-up as indicated: MVP, autonomic dysfunction	242
			243
			244
			245
Choanal stenosis or atresia	Syndactyly	Difficult/impossible intubation – consider microlaryngoscopic evaluation preoperatively	246
Pulmonary hyperplasia likely from fetal lung fluid retention with tracheal stenosis	Genitourinary malformations: imperforate anus, renal agenesis	Consider increased ICP	247
		Cardiac work-up and renal function	248
			249
NA	Possible scoliosis	Cardiac work-up	250
		Avoid neuromuscular blockade whenever possible	251
		Reports of successful use with monitoring	252
		Central neuraxial blockade is relatively contraindicated	253
		Reports of successful spinal anesthesia	254
	GSD-0: glycogen synthase deficiency, 2 subtypes – muscle, liver		255

(Continued)

Table 38.1 (*Continued*)

No.	Syndrome: name, eponyms, inheritance, incidence, gene locus, gene product	Airway	Central nervous system	Cardiovascular
	Glycogen storage diseases (*continued*)			
	GSD Type 0: glycogen synthase deficiency		Subject to hypoglycemic seizures with GYS2 (liver) GSD Cognitively and developmentally normal	Report of sudden cardiac death- mitochondrial compensatory phenomenon
	GSD Type I: von Gierke disease (glucose-6-phosphate deficiency, 1:50–100,000)		Subject to hypoglycemic seizures	Possible cardiomyopathy
	GSD Type II: Pompe disease (acid maltase deficiency, 1:60–140,000)	Infantile onset: macroglossia	Infantile onset: rapidly progressive muscle weakness – axial hypotonia, areflexia	Infantile onset: cardiomegaly/cardiomyopathy leading to cardiac failure

Pulmonary	Other	Additional anesthetic considerations	References
	GSD-I: Glucose-6-Phosphatase System Deficiency, 4 subtypes		
	GSD-II: defective lysosomal alpha-glucosidase, 4 onset forms		
	GSD-III: Amylo-1,6-Glucosidase Deficiency, 6 forms		
	GSD-IV: glycogen branching enzyme deficiency, numerous forms		
	GSD-V: Muscle Phosphorylase Deficiency, 2 forms		
	GSD-VI: liver phosphorylase deficiency		
	GSD-VII: phosphofructokinase deficiency, 2 forms		
	GSD-VIII (VIIa, IX, X): tissue-specific phosphorylase kinase deficiency		
	No apparent relation with MH		
	Wide fluctuation in glucose ,hypo- to hyperglycemia, in GSY2 (liver) GSD	Test exists to differentiate between GYS1 (muscle) and true mitochondrial disease	256
	Fasting ketotic hypoglycemia without muscle symptoms or hepatomegaly	Monitor blood glucose and limit NPO preoperatively	257
			258
	Hypoglycemia without dietary carbohydrate intake	Monitor blood glucose & limit NPO preoperatively	259
	Hepatomegaly, anemia, osteopenia, hyperuricemia, proteinuria	Maintain euglycemia and normal pH intraoperatively	260
	Gout, renal stones, nephropathy leading to proteinuria, hypertension, and renal dysfunction	Bispectral index score may not reflect anesthetic depth with hypoglycemia	261
	Acquired (reversible) platelet dysfunction (prolonged BT; abn aggregation, less adhesiveness) with hypoglycemia	Propofol infusion may exacerbate hyperuricemia	262
		Reports of propofol-induced pancreatitis	263
		Caution with regional anesthesia with possible platelet dysfunction	264
		Caution with positioning – osteopenia	265
Infantile onset: respiratory insufficiency with frequent infections	Infantile onset: hepatomegly , elevated creatine kinase	Respiratory insufficiency & hypertrophic cardiomyopathy pose significant anesthetic risk	266
		Maintain intravascular volume and diastolic blood pressure for coronary perfusion	267

(Continued)

Table 38.1 (*Continued*)

No.	Syndrome: name, eponyms, inheritance, incidence, gene locus, gene product	Airway	Central nervous system	Cardiovascular
	Glycogen storage diseases (continued)			
		Late onset: macroglossia is infrequent	Late onset: progressive proximal muscle weakness – lower>upper extremity, Gower sign, decreased deep tendon reflexes	Late onset: cardiomegaly/cardiomyopathy is uncommon
	GSD Type III: Debrancher deficiency (Cori or Forbes disease) (glycogen debrancher deficiency, 1:100,000)	Frequent midface hypoplasia		
		Possible macroglossia		
			Distal myopathy: mild sensory deficits and fasciculations	Distal myopathy: absence of severe cardiomyopathy
				Up to 50% with cardiomyopathy resembling idiopathic hypertrophic cardiomyopathy

Pulmonary	Other	Additional anesthetic considerations	References
		Reports of arrhythmias due to decreased coronary perfusion with propofol	268
		Reports of successful regional anesthetic techniques	269
Late onset: respiratory insufficiency/failure with infections, dyspnea on exertion, obstructive sleep apnea, orthopnea	Late onset: moderate hepatomegaly, scoliosis/kyphosis/lordosis	Respiratory insufficiency poses anesthetic risk	
		Hypotonia/wheelchair bound – avoid neuromuscular blocking drugs and succinylcholine for prolonged weakness and hyperkalemia	
		Reports of prolonged respiratory depression with volatile agents	
		Midface hypoplasia/macroglossia may contribute to difficult airway	270
			271
	Distal myopathy: adult onset, slowly progressive, involves calves/peroneal muscles with rare hepatic involvement	Assess sensory deficiets preoperatively	272
Respiratory muscle myopathy: myogenic respiratory failure	Respiratory muscle myopathy: adult onset, selective respiratory muscle involvement without limb muscle involvement	Report of respiratory myopathy reversal with high protein diet	273
		Assess respiratory function	274
	Severe generalized myopathy (juvenile onset): complete recovery at puberty		275
Severe generalized myopathy (adult onset): respiratory failure	Severe generalized myopathy (adult onset): progressive to wheelchair bound, hepatic involvement, neuropathy	Assess respiratory function	
		Assess hepatic function & monitor glucose intraoperatively	
		Avoid NMBD (hypotonia) & succinylcholine (hyperkalemia)	
		Assess neuropathy preoperatively, positioning consideration	
	Minimal variant myopathy: predominantly hepatic involvement, cardiomyopathy	Assess hepatic function & monitor glucose intraoperatively	

(Continued)

Table 38.1 (*Continued*)

No.	Syndrome: name, eponyms, inheritance, incidence, gene locus, gene product	Airway	Central nervous system	Cardiovascular
	Glycogen storage diseases (*continued*)			GSD cardiomyopathy has relative normal exercise stress/ECG results
	GSD Type IV: brancher deficiency (Andersen disease) (glycogen branching enzyme deficiency, very rare)			Possible cardiomyopathy
	GSD Type V: McArdle syndrome (muscle glycogen phosphorylase deficiency, 1:100,000)			
	GSD Type VI: Hers disease (liver glycogen phosphorylase deficiency, 1:65–85,000)			
	GSD Type VII: phosphofructokinase deficiency (Tarui disease) (muscle phosphofructokinase deficiency, very rare)		Progressive partial complex seizure, diplopia, decreased deep tendon reflexes, facial palsy, bradydiadochokinesia, distal UE weakness Increased calcium permeability in red blood cells possibly explaining diminished deformability leading to hemolysis	Progressive: low voltage ECG to supraventricular tachycardia, thick mitral valve to mitral valve insufficiency, left atrial enlargement/left ventricular hypertrophy to diastolic dysfunction

Pulmonary	Other	Additional anesthetic considerations	References
		Cardiomyopathy resembles idiopathic hypertrophy but with normal stress/exercise tolerance	
	Classic Anderson: hepatosplenomegaly, progressive liver cirrhosis (with portal hypertension) leading to death	Cardiac work-up for cardiomyopathy	276
	Phenotypic variant: with peripheral myopathy +/– cardiomyopathy, neuropathy, or cirrhosis	Coagulation profile as assessment for degree of liver failure	277
	Cardioskeletal variant with normal glycogen brancher enzyme activity leading to death from cardiac failure		
	Cardiomyopathy with deficienct glycogen brancher enzyme activity leading to death from cardiac failure		
	Exercise-induced muscle cramps, injury, and myoglobiniuria relieved by extramuscular glucose delivery	Caffeine halothane contracture test positive report; but no case reports of malignant hyperthermia – minimal risk	278
	Exercise induced creatine kinase elevation, hyperkalemia, and acute renal failure	Preoperative creatine kinase, lactate dehydrogenase, creatinine; avoid tourniquet/shivering	279
		Avoid malignant hyperthermia-triggers: succinylcholine, volatile agents	280
		Avoid sympathetic stim, increased temp, neuroleptics	
	Hepatosplenomegaly, hypotonia at young age; but minimal hypoglycemia	Limit NPO/monitor glucose	281
	Muscle cramps, exercise intolerance, rhabdomyolysis/myoglobinuria +/– hemolytic anemia/hyperuricemia	Cardiac work-up	282
		Reports of rhabdomyolysis leading to acute renal failure	283
		Glucose infusion is ineffective	284
			285
			286
			(Continued)

Table 38.1 (*Continued*)

No.	Syndrome: name, eponyms, inheritance, incidence, gene locus, gene product	Airway	Central nervous system	Cardiovascular
	Glycogen storage diseases (*continued*) GSD Type VIII (IX) (phosphorylase kinase deficiency, very rare)		Delayed motor development	Hypercholesterolemia/hypertriglyceridaemia
41	**Goldenhar syndrome** (hemifacial microsomia, oculo-auriculo-vertebral syndrome, sporadic mutation, 1:5600, genetics imcompletely analyzed, possible TCOF1 gene at 5q32)	Unilateral facial hypoplasia: prominent forehead, zygomatic hypoplasia, maxillar/mandibular hypoplasia	Epibulbar dermoid/lipodermoid, eye anomalies; microphthalmia, anophthalmia, etc.	30–60% CHD: 40% conotruncal, 30% septal, 15% targeted growth, 7% situs/looping, 4% left-sided obstruction
		Unilateral macrostomia – lateral facial cleft	Preauricular skin tag/blind fistulas, microtia or other external ear malformations	
		Vertebral anomalies: atlas occipitalization, synostosis	Vertebral anomalies; bifid spine	
		Laryngotracheal anomalies: cartilaginous tracheal sleeve	Often with occipital encephalocele	
		Significant incidence of C1-C2 instability	Oftern with complex retardation of development	
		Often with cleft lip/palate/tongue, unilateral tongue hypoplasia, parotid gland aplasia		
		Often with tracheoesophageal fistula/esophageal atresia		
42	**Hajdu-Cheney syndrome** (arthrodento-osteodysplasia, autosomal dominant, 50 cases reported, genetics not fully analyzed)	Micrognathia, progressive midface flattening to apparent prognathia	Wormian bones, open sutures, basilar invagination, bathrocephaly, platybasia, hydrocephalus	Possible congenital heart disease; patent ductus arteriosus, ventricular septal defect, valvular disorder
		High arched palate or cleft palate	Platybasia may cause: stretched cranial nerves, increased intracranial pressure, foramen magnum compression; syringomyelia may develop	Hypertension with renal cystic disease

Pulmonary	Other	Additional anesthetic considerations	References
	Hepatomegaly	Limit NPO/monitor glucose	287
	Fasting hyperketosis/hypoglycaemia		
NA	Vertebral anomalies: hemivertebrae, fused vertebrae, scoliosis	Difficult airway – reports of failed intubation	288
	Often with rib/extremity anomalies	Reports of successful intubation with multiple techniques	
	Genitourinary anomalies: ectopic kidney, renal agenesis, vesicoureteral reflux, ureteropelvic junction obstruction	Evaluate cervical spine for instability	289
		Cardiac work-up	291
			290
			291
NA	Acro-osteolysis, vertebral compression, scoliosis/kyphosis	Assess renal function and neurological deficits	292
	10% renal abnormalities: cystic disease, hypoplasia, vesicoureteral reflux, glomerulonephritis, hypertension, chronic renal failure	Possible difficult airway – micrognathia, C-spine instability, dental abnormalities	293

(Continued)

Table 38.1 (*Continued*)

No.	Syndrome: name, eponyms, inheritance, incidence, gene locus, gene product	Airway	Central nervous system	Cardiovascular
	Hajdu-Cheney syndrome (*continued*)	Abnormal dentition	Progressive paresthesia with acroosteolysis	
		Short neck	Occasionally associated with facial spasm & rarely trigeminal neuralgia	
43	**Hallermann-Streiff syndrome** (Francois dyscephalic syndrome, autosomal recessive, 200 reported cases, mutation chromosome 6q21-q23.2 in some patients, GJA1 gene)	Small face, brachycephaly with frontal/parietal bossing	Possible developmental delay, seizure disorder	5% congenital heart disease: pulmonic stenosis, atrial/ventricular septal defect, patent ductus arteriosus, tetralogy of Fallot
		Hypoplastic mandible, anteriorly displaced TMJ, high/narrow palate, dental anomalies	Ocular findings: microphthalmia, cataracts, nystagmus, strabismus	Reported biventricular failure from tracheomalacia causing respiratory insufficiency
		Laryngotracheal anomalies: tracheomalacia		
		Upper airway obstruction from micrognathia with glossoptosis may cause cor pulmonale		
44	**Hemophilia**	NA	Intracranial haemorrhage is significant cause of mortality	NA

Pulmonary	Other	Additional anesthetic considerations	References
		Reports of cervical instability	294
		Possible airway obstruction postoperatively	295
		Reports of upper airway obstruction	296
		Reports of vocal cord paralysis	297
		Prone to fractures (long bones and spine) – care with positioning	298
Narrow upper airway predisposing to infections & OSA	Possible skeletal deformities, hematopoietic (immunodeficient) defects	Difficult airway: mandibular hypoplasia/ microstomia, displaced TMJ, abnormal teeth	299
		Tracheostomy may be required but difficult with cricoid cartilage at/near suprasternal notch	
		Reports of successful intubation with multiple techniques	300
		Cardiac work-up	301
			302
			303
NA	Classification: both VIIIc or Ixc	Assess factor concentrations – treat as indicated	304
	Severe if <1% of normal activity – spontaneous joint/muscle bleeding, bleeding after injury	Arrange for specific factor therapy as indicated	305
	Moderate if 1–5% of normal activity – minor injury-induced joint/muscle bleeding, excessive bleeding post surgery/dental procedure	Oral intubation preferred to avoid nasal bleeding	306
	Mild if 5–40% of normal activity – no spontaneous bleeding, bleeding post surgery/dental procedures	Reports of successful use of multiple anesthetic techniques	

(Continued)

Table 38.1 (Continued)

No.	Syndrome: name, eponyms, inheritance, incidence, gene locus, gene product	Airway	Central nervous system	Cardiovascular
	Hemophilia (continued)			
	Hemophilia A (X-linked recessive, 1:5000 males, mutation chromosome Xq28, factor VIII gene)			
	Hemophilia B (Christmas disease, X-linked recessive, 1:50,000 males, mutation chromosome Xq27.1-q27.2, factor IX gene)			
45	**Hereditary angio-edema (C1 esterase inhibitor deficiency)** (hereditary angioneurotic edema, autosomal dominant, 1:10–50,000, mutation chromosome 11q11-q13.1, deficiency C1 esterase inhibitor gene)	Poor dentition	NA	NA
		Acute laryngeal edema is significant cause of mortality		

Pulmonary	Other	Additional anesthetic considerations	References
	X-linked trait: affects males but female carriers have 1/2 normal concentrations – may predispose to excessive bleeding	Neuraxial techniques relatively contraindicated; no "safe" factor level defined	
	Risk of human immunodeficiency virus/hepatitis infection from blood product replacement therapy prior to recombinant factor development		
	DDAVP raises VIIIc concentration effectively in mild hemophilia A	Report of non-operative splenic laceration therapy with recombinant factor VIII in Jehovah's Witness	307
	Recombinant factor VIIIc therapy for mod/sev hemophilia A	Reports of hyponatremia & seizures in young patients given DDAVP	308
	Inhibitors (antibodies to RF-VIIIc) develop in 30–50% hemophilia A patients	Report of recombinant factor VII use to achieve hemostasis with factor VIII inhibitor	309
		Report of successful peripheral nerve block in hemophilia A patient	310
	Recombinant factor Ixc therapy for hemophilia B	Significant risk of anaphylaxis in hemophilia B patients with inhibitors	311
	Inhibitors (antibodies to recombinant F-Ixc) develop in 1–3% hemophilia B patients	Report of acute hepatitis in hemophilia B patient after isoflurane anesthesia	312
NA	C1 esterase inhibitor inhibits many mediator cascades which result in plasma leakage	Prepare for upper airway obstruction due to oropharyngeal/laryngeal edema	313
	Postcapillary plasma leakage into dermis resulting in non-pitting edema of hands/feet, genitalia, face/tongue, larynx, bowel	Elective surgery: reports of successful monitored/regional/general anesthesia	314
	Bowel wall swelling leads to spasmodic abdominal pain with vomiting	Avoid airway manipulation, prophylaxis when airway manipulation is indicated	315
	Prophylaxis treatments: Danazol, epsilon aminocaproic acid		

(Continued)

Table 38.1 (*Continued*)

No.	Syndrome: name, eponyms, inheritance, incidence, gene locus, gene product	Airway	Central nervous system	Cardiovascular
	Hereditary angio-edema (*continued*)			
46	**Holt-Oram syndrome** (heart-hand syndrome, atriodigital dysplasia, autosomal dominant, 1:100,000, mutation chromosome 12q24.1, TBX5 gene mutation: promotes cardiomyocyte differentiation)	NA	NA	Congenital heart disease: septal defects
				Frequent cardiac conduction disease: bradycardia, atrioventricular block, atrial fibrillation
				Atrial sepal defect most common, but reports of endocardiac cushion defect with left ventricular hypoplasia
				Vascular abnormalities: persistant left superior vena cava, renal arterial malformations, absent radial artery
47	**Homocystinuria** (cystathionine beta-synthase deficiency, autosomal recessive, 1:344,000, mutation chromosome 21q22.3)	High arched palate, dental crowding with incisor protrusion	Eye: ectopia lentis leading to myopia, retinal detachment & glaucoma	Arterial/venous thrombosis, cutaneous flushing
			Frequent mental retardation, not seen in Marfan	Medium sized artery (coronary, renal subclavian, iliac, carotid) medial changes: dilation & thrombosis
48	**Hunter syndrome** (mucopolysaccharidosis type II, X-linked recessive, 1:110–320,000 males, mutation chromosome Zq28, deficient enzyme, iduronate-2-sulfatase)	Dural hyperplasia/ thickening ligamentum flavum lead to cervical myelopathy with UMN signs	Normal intelligence with progressive neurodegeneration leading to vegetative state as teenagers	Cardiac disease: cardiomyopathy, asymmetrical ventricle septal thickening, mitral/aortic valve thickening

Pulmonary	Other	Additional anesthetic considerations	References
	Acute treatments: C1 INH concentrate, fresh frozen plasma, epinephrine, diphenhydramine		
NA	Skeletal deformities: thenar/carpal bones, occasionally hypoplastic clavicles/shortened radii	Cardiac work-up: structure/function, internal cardiac defibrillator assessment	316
		Vascular access may be difficult	317
		Upper limb peripheral nerve blocks may be challenging	318
		Report of successful neuraxial anesthesia/analgesia	
Thorax: pectus excavatum, scoliosis	Marfanoid habitus – dolichostenomelia, "long, thin extremities"	Caution: arterial/venous puncture may initiate thrombosis	319
Rarely spontaneous pneumothorax	Generalized osteoporosis (not seen in Marfan) leading to codfish vertebrae and vertebral collapse	Avoid prolonged nitrous oxide – inhibits methionine synthase conversion homocysteine to methionine	320
		Measure to decrease thrombosis/embolization – hydration, hemodynamic stability	321
		Minimize time without anticoagulation therapy	
		Consider neuraxial analgesia/anesthesia if coagulation status is appropriate	
NA	Gastrointestinal dysfunction: idiopathic diarrhea, spontaneous gastric perforation, bowel pseduo-obstruction	Difficult airway: short neck, high larynx, large tongue, cervical instability	322

(Continued)

Table 38.1 (*Continued*)

No.	Syndrome: name, eponyms, inheritance, incidence, gene locus, gene product	Airway	Central nervous system	Cardiovascular
	Hunter syndrome (*continued*)	Coarse facies:	Narrowing of the bony neural canal predisposing to cervical cord compression	Sudden death – likely arrhythmia from coronary insufficiency
		Temperomandibular joint stiffness and short stiff neck	Compressive myelopathy from meningeal thickening causing communicating hydrocephalus	
		Adenotonsillar hypertrophy contributing to obstructive sleep apnea, progressive upper airway obstruction, infections		
		Glycosaminoglycan deposition in pharynx/ larynx wall – laryngeal inlet prolapse/stridor/ airway compromise		
		Progressive tracheal deformation; cricoid to lower bronchi		
		Trauma (airway instrumentation) may induce mucopolysaccharide deposition		
		C1 & C2 subluxation with odontoid dysplasia		
49	**Hurler syndrome** (mucopolysaccharidosis type I, autosomal recessive, 1:100,000, mutation chromosome 4p16.3, iduronidase deficiency)	Facial dysmorphism, obstructive sleep apnea is nearly universal	Normal intelligence	Cardiac disease: cardiomyopathy, asymmetrical ventricle septal thickening, mitral/aortic valve thickening
		Coarse facies:/gum hypertrophy, macroglossia	Possible hydrocephalus	Sudden death – likely arrhythmia from coronary insufficiency
		TMJ stiffness & short stiff neck	Ocular findings: corneal clouding, glaucoma	Mitral/aortic valve dysplasia, left ventricular hypertrophy, normal function – same or better following bone marrow transplant

Pulmonary	Other	Additional anesthetic considerations	References
		Reports of postobstructive pulmonary edema at induction/extubation	323
		Reports of successful intubation using multiple techniques: blind nasal, fiber-optic, LMA	324
		Reports of intubation failure using laryngeal mask airway	325
		Report of delayed awakening following single dose of opioid	326
			327
			328
			329
NA	Progressive joint stiffnes with decreased mobility, severe back pain, lumbar spondylolisthesis with cord compression	Difficult airway: short neck, high larynx, large tongue, cervical instability	330
	Poor hand function likely from carpal tunnel syndrome	Epiglottis tip behind soft palate – oral airway exacerbates rather than relieves obstruction	
	Hepatosplenomegaly – likely leading to high incidence of umbilical hernia	Reports of postobstructive pulmonary edema at induction/extubation	

(Continued)

Table 38.1 (*Continued*)

No.	Syndrome: name, eponyms, inheritance, incidence, gene locus, gene product	Airway	Central nervous system	Cardiovascular
	Hurler syndrome (*continued*)	Adenotonsillar hypertrophy contributing to obstructive sleep apnea, progressive upper airway obstruction, infections Glycosaminoglycan deposition in pharynx/larynx wall – laryngeal inlet prolapse/stridor/airway compromise		
50	**Jeune syndrome** (asphyxiating thoracic dystrophy, thoracic-pelvic-phalangeal dystrophy, autosomal recessive, very rare, mutation chromosome 15q13, gene product not yet known)	NA	Ocular abnormalities: retinitis pigmentosa	Absent
51	**Kearns-Sayre syndrome** (mitochondrial disease, ophthalmoplegia-plus, oculocraniosomatic disease, oculocraniosomatic neuromuscular disease with raggel red fibers, spontaneous inheritance, 1:125,000, various mitochondrial DNA deletions transmitted from mother)	Possible weak pharyngeal muscles: increased risk for aspiration	Progressive external ophthalmoplegia Pigmented retinal degeneration: visual loss Sensorineural hearing loss	Atrioventricular conduction defects: Heart block (second- or third-degree atrioventricular block): may need pacemaker Congestive cardiomyopathy

Pulmonary	Other	Additional anesthetic considerations	References
		Reports of successful intubation using multiple techniques	
		Report of failed epidural anesthesia – likely from mucopolysaccharide deposits on meninges	
			331
Respiratory distress: bell-shaped/long narrow small thorax with handlebar clavicles	Renal tubular-concentrating defect and proteinuria and diffuse interstitial fibrosis/glomerular sclerosis	Severe respiratory insufficiency – desaturate with agitation from asynchronous rib/abdominal motion	332
	Hepatic disease to portal hypertension to transplantation	Minimize airway pressures to avoid barotrauma	333
	Cystic pancreatic disease	Assess renal function to guide fluid management	334
	Short long bones, postaxial polydactyly, trident acetabulum	Assess hepatic function – abnormal drug metabolism	335
Decreased respiratory drive	Mitochondrial myopathy		336
Pes cavus		Lactic acidosis, worse with fasting: avoid excessive preoperative fasting and lactated Ringer's, include glucose with intravenous fluids	337
		Possibly more sensitive to rocuronium, atracurium, succinylcholine, and mivacurium	338

(Continued)

Table 38.1 (*Continued*)

No.	Syndrome: name, eponyms, inheritance, incidence, gene locus, gene product	Airway	Central nervous system	Cardiovascular
	Kearns-Sayre syndrome (continued)		Ataxia	
			Cranial nerve dysfunction	
			Bulbar and limb girdle muscle weakness	
			Myopathy with proximal limb weakness	
			Seizures	
			Dementia	
52	**King-Denborough syndrome** (malignant hyperthermia susceptibility-1, King syndrome, autosomal dominant, 1:5–15,000 children, mutation chromosome 19q13.1, RYR1: ryanadine receptor mutation)	Micrognathia, webbed neck, & dental crowding/malocclusion	Normal intelligence with delayed motor development	NA
			Myopathy: elevated resting creatine kinase, muscle weakness, decreased deep tendon reflexes	
53	**Klippel-Feil syndrome** (autosomal dominant and recessive forms, 1:1500–5000, mutation chromosome 8q22.1 (dominant) or 5q11.2 (recessive), GDF6 gene (dominant) or unknown gene (recessive)	Laryngotracheal anomalies: laryngeal stenosis, vocal cord stenosis	Vertebral fusion, spina bifida, some myeloencephalocele, syringohydromyelia, Chiari malformation	Congenital heart disease (14%): ventricular septal defect

Pulmonary	Other	Additional anesthetic considerations	References
		Consider avoiding succinylcholine in myopathic patient due to risk of exaggerated hyperkalemia	
		Possible impaired respiratory control: consider titration of narcotics and other respiratory depressants	
		Unclear, but unlikely, association between mitochondrial disorders and malignant hyperthemia. Only one reported case in literature links malignant hyperthermia and mitochondrial disorders	
		At risk for developing metabolic acidosis and myocardial failure after propofol infusion	
	Orthopedic abnormalities: Short stature Kyphoscoliosis Hirsutism Fatal hyperosmolar coma and hyperglycemia after steroid therapy Exercise intolerance		
Pectus carinatum/excavatum, scoliosis or kyphoscoliosis, lumbar hyperlordosis	Closely linked to malignant hyperthermia susceptibility	Multiple reports of KDS diagnosis following malignant hyperthermia event – use non-triggering anesthetic	339
		Succinylcholine is contraindicated due to hyperkalemic response in myopathies	106
		Report of successful epidural anesthesia	340
Scoliosis	Genitourinary anomalies (30%): renal agenesis, renal/pelvic/ureteral duplication	Difficult airway: cervical spine instability/ fusion, microtia, short/webbed neck, micrognathia	62

(Continued)

Table 38.1 (*Continued*)

No.	Syndrome: name, eponyms, inheritance, incidence, gene locus, gene product	Airway	Central nervous system	Cardiovascular
	Klippel-Feil syndrome (*continued*)	Malformation of laryngeal cartilages with voice impairment	Extraocular muscle palsies, lower extremity paresthesias, respiratory apnea, mental retardation, spasticity	
		Micrognathia, cleft palate, microtia, bifid uvula, facial asymmetry		
		cervical spine (C2-C3) vertebral fusion, short webbed neck, torticollis, cervical ribs		
54	**Klippel-Trenaunay-Weber syndrome** (angio-osteohypertrophy syndrome, sporadic inheritance, *de novo* translocation t(8:14) (q22.3;q13), rare, several hundred cases reported, AGGF1: angiogenic factor 1 gene may be involved)	NA	Glaucoma	Capillary malformations: port-wine stains
			Spinal cord arteriovenous malformations	Venous malformations: varicose veins +/− persistent lateral embryological veins
				Frequently: venous incompetence & lymphatic malformations
				Hemangiomas with thrombotic events, high output cardiac failure, and bleeding
55	**LEOPARD syndrome** (multiple lentigenes syndrome, autosomal dominant, very rare, approx. 100 reported cases, mutation chromosome 12q24, protein-tyrosine phosphatase, non-receptor type II (PTPNII): regulates intercellular signaling)	Prognathism	Sensorineural deafness	Electrocardiographic conduction abnormalities: consider preoperative ECG

Pulmonary	Other	Additional anesthetic considerations	References
Central respiratory apnea	Restricted extremity movement	Cervical spine evaluation	341
		Cardiac work-up	342
		Risk for postoperative apnea/obstruction: central respiratory apnea, micrognathia/cleft palate	343
		Reports multiple airway management techniques: fiber-optic, laryngeal mask airway, videolaryngoscopy	
NA	Unilateral soft tissue or bony hypertrophy	Avoid hypertension to prevent spontaneous bleed – blunt sympathetic response to direct laryngoscopy and endotracheal tube	344
	Occasional hip dysplasia or syndactyly	Avoid hypovolemia to prevent expanding hemangiomas with thrombocytopenia/DIC	345
	Scoliosis	Avoid hypervolemia to prevent increased perfusion to non-autoregulated vessels	346
	Chronic disseminated intravascular coagulation	Avoid scopolamine (interferes with aqueous humor drainage) with glaucoma	347
		Cardiac work-up for high-output failure as needed	
		Regional analgesia/anesthesia may be relatively contraindicated	
		Multiple successful neuraxial anesthetics reported with spinal imaging & coagulation status verified	
Pectus excavatum or carinatum	Multiple lentigenes (large freckles) on the skin	NA	348

(Continued)

Table 38.1 (*Continued*)

No.	Syndrome: name, eponyms, inheritance, incidence, gene locus, gene product	Airway	Central nervous system	Cardiovascular
	LEOPARD syndrome (*continued*)	Micrognathia	Possible mental retardation	Hypertrophic obstructive cardiomyopathy: consider preoperative screening echocardiography
		Flat nasal bridge	Learning difficulties	Pulmonic stenosis
		Cleft palate		Subaortic stenosis, mitral valve disease
		Dental abnormalities		Left atrial myxoma
56	**Long QT** (prolonged QT syndrome including Jervell-Lange-Nielson, Romano-Ward, and Andersen syndromes, autosomal dominant or recessive, approx. 1:10,000, at least 12 different mutations mostly of sodium and potassium channel protein genes)	Possible difficult intubation with Andersen syndrome: micrognathia, cleft palate, low-set ears, hypertelorism	Syncope during exertion, seizures	Prolonged QTc:
			Jervell-Lange-Nielson syndrome:	Sudden death due to ventricular tachyarrhythmia, classically torsade de pointes
			Congenital nerve deafness	
			Andersen syndrome:	
			Potassium-sensitive periodic paralysis: avoid succinylcholine due to risk of hyperkalemia	
				Andersen syndrome patients have congenital cardiac defects and a high incidence of sudden death

Pulmonary	Other	Additional anesthetic considerations	References
Restrictive lung disease with possible pulmonary hypertension	Characteristic facies:		349
	Ocular hypertelorism, low-set ears		350
	Flat nasal bridge		
	Orthopedic abnormalities:		
	Retardation of growth (growth deficiency)		
	Winged scapulae		
	Possible kyphoscoliosis		
	Genitourinary abnormalities:		
	Abnormal genitalia, cryptorchidism, hypospadias		
	Renal agenesis or hypoplasia		
NA	Andersen syndrome		351
	Orthopedic abnormalities: syndactyly, short stature, scoliosis, clinodactyly	Avoid drugs that increase QT interval: droperidol, ondansetron	352
		Avoid hypocalcemia, hypomagnesemia, hypokalemia	353
		Avoid adrenergic stimulation including loud environment	354
		Avoid hypothermia	
		Avoid light (or insufficient) anesthesia, hypertension, brady- or tachycardia, hypoxemia, hypo- or hypercapnia	
		Avoid reversal of neuromuscular blockade with anticholinergic and anticholinesterase medications	

(Continued)

Table 38.1 (*Continued*)

No.	Syndrome: name, eponyms, inheritance, incidence, gene locus, gene product	Airway	Central nervous system	Cardiovascular
57	**Marfan syndrome** (variable inheritance, often autosomal dominant, 1:3–10,000, mutation chromosome 15q21.1, mutation fibrilin-1 gene)	High arched palate	Widened lumbosacral canal may lead to increased cerebrospinal fluid volume: may need larger than normal doses of spinal or epidural anesthetics	Aortic dissection: avoid hypertension
		Crowded teeth	Spinal arachnoid cysts	Mitral valve prolapse
				Aortic or pulmonary artery dilation: consider preoperative echocardiography to confirm absence
				Aortic insufficiency
				Possible progressive narrowing of coronary arteries
58	**Maroteaux-Lamy syndrome** (mucopolysaccharidosis VI, arylsulfatase B deficiency, autosomal recessive, 1:238–433,000, mutation chromosome 5q11-q13, deficient arylsulfatase B)	Possible difficult to impossible direct laryngoscopy and intubation	Normal intelligence	Heart failure is most common cause of death
	Mucopolysaccharidosis VI	Frontal bossing	Spinal compression from dural thickening, usually cervical: avoid neck extension	Aortic valve calcifications
		Depressed nasal bridge	Communicating hydrocephalus from lumbar stenosis	Possible mitral valve involvement
		Enlarged tongue, gingival hypertrophy	Hearing loss: conductive and sensorineural	Hypertension
		Thick mucous secretions	Atlantoaxial instability from odontoid dysplasia	

Pulmonary	Other	Additional anesthetic considerations	References
Pectus excavatum	Characteristic facies:	Widened lumbosacral canal may lead to increased cerebrospinal fluid volume: may need larger than normal doses of spinal or epidural anesthetics	355
Pulmonary blebs with spontaneous pneumothoraces	Dolichocephaly, long and narrow facies:	Avoid hypertension	356
Obstructive sleep apnea	Lens dislocation, elongated globe, myopia		357
Possible tracheomalacia	Increased risk of glaucoma, retinal detachment		358
Possible emphysema and bronchogenic cysts	Orthopedic abnormalities:		
	Tall with arm span greater than height		
	Winged scapula		
	Joint laxity leading to recurrent dislocations		
	Ulnar deviation, arachnodactyly		
	Scoliosis, kyphosis		
	Congenital contractures, flat feet		
	Gastrointestinal/genitourinary abnormalities:		
	Inguinal, umbilical, and femoral hernias		
At risk for airway obstruction: possible postoperative respiratory distress, postobstructive pulmonary edema	Characteristic facies:	NA	359
Pectus carinatum	Coarse face, "tight" skin		360
Recurrent upper respiratory infections	Hirsutism		361
Sleep apnea	Corneal clouding		362
Restrictive lung disease	Orthopedic abnormalities:		

(Continued)

Table 38.1 (*Continued*)

No.	Syndrome: name, eponyms, inheritance, incidence, gene locus, gene product	Airway	Central nervous system	Cardiovascular
	Maroteaux-Lamy syndrome (*continued*)	Short, stiff neck		
		Possible atlantoaxial instability		
		Intubation difficulty worsens with age		
		At risk for airway obstruction due to mucopolysaccharide deposits in the lips, tongue, epiglottis, tonsils, adenoids, lower airway		
59	**MELAS syndrome** (mitochondrial myopathy–encephalopathy–lactic acidosis–stroke syndrome, spontaneous inheritance, rare, various mitochondrial DNA deletions transmitted from mother)	NA	Encephalopathy	Cardiomyopathy
			Stroke-like episodes with sudden onset of hemiparesis, hemianopsia, cortical blindness	Possible Wolff-Parkinson-White syndrome: consider preoperative ECG
			Encephalomalacia and degeneration with focal infarcts, cortical or cerebellar atrophy, or basal ganglia calcifications	
			Seizures	
			Recurrent headaches	

Pulmonary	Other	Additional anesthetic considerations	References
	Normal growth for first few years, then stops		
	Hypoplasia of hip acetabulae with small, flared iliac wings		
	Hypoplasia of L1–2 vertebrae with lumbar kyphosis		
	Proximal femoral dysplasia		
	Contractures of joints due to deposits of polysaccharide in ligaments		
	Restricted mobility of hips, knees, elbows		
	Carpal tunnel syndrome, claw hand		
	Hepatosplenomegaly with hypersplenism: results in anemia, thrombocytopenia, genitourinary abnormalities: umbilical and inguinal hernias		
Respiratory failure	Mitochondrial myopathy	Lactic acidosis, worse with fasting: avoid excessive preoperative fasting and lactated Ringer's, include glucose with intravenous fluids	363
	Exercise intolerance	Possibly more sensitive to rocuronium, atracurium, succinylcholine, and mivacurium	364
	Onset: childhood	Consider avoiding succinylcholine in myopathic patient due to risk of exaggerated hyperkalemia	365
	Orthopedic abnormality: short stature	Possible impaired respiratory control: consider titration of narcotics and other respiratory depressants	366
	Gastrointestinal abnormality: recurrent vomiting	Unclear, but unlikely, association between mitochondrial disorders and malignant hyperthemia. Only one reported case in literature links malignant hyperthermia and mitochondrial disorders	

(Continued)

Table 38.1 (*Continued*)

No.	Syndrome: name, eponyms, inheritance, incidence, gene locus, gene product	Airway	Central nervous system	Cardiovascular
	MELAS syndrome (*continued*)		Dementia	
			Myoclonus, peripheral neuropathy	
			Myopathy, muscle weakness	
			Reduced muscle mass	
			Blindness, cataracts, ophthalmoplegia	
			Progressive sensorineural hearing loss	
60	**Menkes kinky hair syndrome** (steely hair disease, copper transport disease, X-linked recessive, 1:254–357,000, mutation chromosome Xq12-q13, mutation in the gene encoding CU(2+)-transporting ATPase, alpha polypeptide)	Microcephaly or brachycephaly	Progressive cerebral and cerebellar deterioration	Vascular elongation and tortuosity
		Pudgy cheeks	Hypotonia at birth, then hypertonia	Capillary fragility due to lysyl oxidase deficiency: possible increased risk with regional techniques and increased risk of intraoperative bleeding
			Seizures	
			Possible occipital horns	
			Developmental regression around 5–6 months	

Pulmonary	Other	Additional anesthetic considerations	References
	Genitourinary abnormality: nephropathy	At risk for developing metabolic acidosis and myocardial failure after propofol infusion	
	Thin habitus: at risk for perioperative hypothermia		
	Hirsutism		
	Purpura		
Possible pectus excavatum or carinatum	Characteristic facies:	NA	367
	Hypopigmentation of skin and hair		368
	Abnormal kinky hair		369
	Sparse hair		370
	Pudgy cheeks		371
	Orthopedic abnormalities:		
	Growth retardation		
	Skeletal demineralization		
	Possible fractures		
	Hyperextensible joints, loose skin		
	Gastrointestinal abnormalities:		
	Gastroesophageal reflux with recurrent aspiration		
	Failure to thrive		
	Gastric polyps, gastrointestinal bleeding		
	Genitourinary abnormalities:		

(Continued)

Table 38.1 (*Continued*)

No.	Syndrome: name, eponyms, inheritance, incidence, gene locus, gene product	Airway	Central nervous system	Cardiovascular
	Menkes kinky hair syndrome (*continued*)			
61	**MERRF syndrome** (myoclonic epilepsy with ragged red fibers, spontaneous inheritance, 1:400,000, various mitochondrial DNA deletions transmitted from mother)	NA	Myoclonus	Cardiomyopathy
			Myopathy, muscle weakness	Wolff-Parkinson-White syndrome
			Spasticity	
			Degenerative changes in the cerebrum, cerebellum, spinal cord	
			Ataxia	
			Intention tremor	
			Epilepsy	
			Sensorineural hearing loss	
			Optic atrophy	
			Dementia	
62	**Miller syndrome** (postaxial acrofacial dysostosis syndrome, Genee-Wiedemann syndrome, sporadic inheritance, extremely rare, mutation chromosome 16q22, mutations in dihydro-orotate dehydrogenase gene: DHODH))	Possible difficult direct laryngoscopy and intubation	Possible hearing loss	Congenital cardiac defects:
		Malar hypoplasia: possible poor mask fit	Normal intelligence	Atrial and ventricular septal defects

Pulmonary	Other	Additional anesthetic considerations	References
	Small testes		
	Bladder diverticula		
	Prone to develop intraoperative hypothermia		
NA	Mitochondrial myopathy	Lactic acidosis, worse with fasting: avoid excessive preoperative fasting and lactated Ringer's, include glucose with intravenous fluids	372
		Possibly more sensitive to rocuronium, atracurium, succinylcholine, and mivacurium	
		Consider avoiding succinylcholine in myopathic patient due to risk of exaggerated hyperkalemia	373
		Possible impaired respiratory control: consider titration of narcotics and other respiratory depressants	
		Unclear, but unlikely, association between mitochondrial disorders and malignant hyperthemia. Only one reported case in literature links malignant hyperthermia and mitochondrial disorders	
	Orthopedic abnormality: short stature		
	Exercise intolerance		
Possible pectus excavatum	Characteristic facies:	NA	374
Rib anomalies	Malar hypoplasia		375

(Continued)

Table 38.1 (*Continued*)

No.	Syndrome: name, eponyms, inheritance, incidence, gene locus, gene product	Airway	Central nervous system	Cardiovascular
	Miller syndrome (*continued*)	Micrognathia		Patent ductus arteriosus
		Cleft lip or palate		
		Possible choanal atresia: cannot place nasal airway, perform nasal intubation, or place nasogastric tube		
63	**Moebius syndrome** (variable inheritance, 1:50,000, mutation chromosome 13q12.2-q13, gene product unknown) variable inhereitance	Possible difficult direct laryngoscopy and intubation	Congenital cranial nerve VI, VII palsies: protect eyes against corneal abrasions due to incomplete eye closure	Congenital cardiac defects
		Micrognathia	Peripheral neuropathy	
		Microstomia	Central hypoventilation	
		Tethered tongue	Hypotonia	
		Cleft lip or palate	Seizures	
		Flattened nasal bridge	Possible hearing loss	
		Poor swallow: may have copious secretions	Speech difficulties	

Pulmonary	Other	Additional anesthetic considerations	References
Absent hemidiaphragm	Absent superior orbital ridges		376
	Down-slanting palpebral fissures, eyelid coloboma		377
	Hypoplastic, low-set, cup-shaped ears		
	Orthopedic abnormalities:		
	Postaxial upper and lower limb defects including absent fifth digit in hands and feet		
	Forearm shortening due to radial and ulnar hypoplasia		
	Syndactyly, congenital hip dislocations		
	Gastrointestinal abnormalities:		
	Pyloric stenosis, malrotation, volvulus		
	Cryptorchidism, renal anomaly		
	Accessory nipples		
	Difficult venous access		
Weak cough and swallow: at risk for aspiration	Characteristic facies:	NA	378
Central hypoventilation: monitor postoperatively	Mask-like due to facial nerve palsy with incomplete closure of eyelids while asleep, drooling		379
Recurrent apnea: monitor postoperatively	Strabismus, ptosis		380
	Prominent ears		381
	Orthopedic abnormalities:		
	Clubfoot deformity, syndactyly		
	Digital contractures, limb reduction defects		
	Arthrogryposis		
	Gastrointestinal abnormalities: poor swallowing		
	Endocrine abnormalities: hypogonadotrophic hypogonadism		

(Continued)

Table 38.1 (*Continued*)

No.	Syndrome: name, eponyms, inheritance, incidence, gene locus, gene product	Airway	Central nervous system	Cardiovascular
64	**Morquio syndrome**	Possible difficult mask ventilation, direct laryngoscopy, and intubation	Cervical spine instability, odontoid hypoplasia with atlantoaxial subluxation: evaluate cervical spine preoperatively	Mitral and aortic valve disease, especially aortic insufficiency late in the disease
	Mucopolysaccharidosis IV	Short neck with limited movement	Sensorineural or mixed hearing loss	Possible pulmonary hypertension, cor pulmonale due to lung disease
	Mucopolysaccharidosis IVA (galactosamine-6-sulfatase deficiency, autosomal recessive, 1:216–640,000 (A and B), mutation chromosome 16q24.3)	Neck flexion may occlude the airway	Normal intelligence	
		Cervical spine instability		
		Possible limited mouth openining		
		Prominent mandible or maxilla		
		Redundant pharyngeal mucosa		
		Macroglossia		
		Tonsillar and adenoid hypertrophy		
	Mucopolysaccharidosis IVB (autosomal recessive, 1:216–640,000 (A and B), mutation chromosome 3p21.33, deficiency in beta-galactosidase)	Widely spaced maxillary anterior teeth		
		May require smaller than predicted endotracheal tube		
		Enamel hypoplasia with pitting (type A)		
		Possible copious tracheobronchial secretions: consider antisialagogue		

Pulmonary	Other	Additional anesthetic considerations	References
Restrictive lung disease from kyphoscoliosis	Type A: severe form	NA	382
Pectus carinatum, rib flaring	Type B: milder form		383
Obstructive or central sleep apnea	Characteristic facies:		384
Recurrent lower airway infections	Dense calvarium		
Susceptible to pulmonary hemorrhage after bone marrow transplant	Coarse facial features		
	Short, anteverted nose		
	Short neck with limited movement		
	Broad mouth with redundant pharyngeal mucosa		
	Macroglossia		
	Widely spaced maxillary anterior teeth		
	Corneal clouding, glaucoma		
	Orthopedic abnormalities:		
	Short stature due to shortened trunk and neck		
	Shortened long bones, short hands		
	Odontoid hypoplasia with atlantoaxial subluxation		

(Continued)

Table 38.1 (*Continued*)

No.	Syndrome: name, eponyms, inheritance, incidence, gene locus, gene product	Airway	Central nervous system	Cardiovascular
	Morquio syndrome (*continued*)			
65	**Myotonic dystrophy, type I** (Steinert disease, congenital myotonic dystrophy, autosomal dominant, variable penetrance, all forms 1:8000, congenital variety is a small proportion, mutation chromosome 19q13.2-q13.3, DMPK gene: myotonic dystrophy protein kinase)	NA	Facial, neck, distal musculature myotonia, with preservation of limb girdle strength until later in the disease	Greater than 90% of patients have conduction abnormalities, especially first-degree heart block and intraventricular conduction delays: recommend preoperative ECG
			Myotonia worsens after exercise	Sudden death with third-degree heart block and ventricular tachyarrhythmia
			Muscle wasting	Cardiac enlargement, interstitial fatty infiltration and fibrosis
			Generalized myotonia: can be induced by anesthetic or surgical manipulation, cold or shivering – keep normothermic	Left axis deviation and ST-T wave changes on ECG
			Myotonia is not prevented or reversed with muscle relaxants or regional anesthesia	Impaired ventricular function late in the disease
			Can infiltrate muscle with local anesthetic to attenuate contraction	Mitral valve prolapse
			Succinylcholine can induce sustained contraction of chest wall muscles, making positive pressure ventilation difficult even in intubated patients: avoid succinylcholine for this reason and for the risk of exaggerated hyperkalemia	

Pulmonary	Other	Additional anesthetic considerations	References
	Flattened vertebral bodies (platyspondyly)		
	Kyphoscoliosis, lumbar lordosis		
	Joint laxity and instability: needs careful intraoperative positioning		
	Genu valgum		
	Gastrointestinal abnormality: hepatosplenomegaly		
Recurrent aspiration pneumonia due to bulbar weakness	Most common myotonic syndrome	More likely to have apnea after intravenous anesthetics including propofol, benzodiazepines, opioids, barbiturates: needs postoperative monitoring for possible respiratory depression	385
Poor cough and alveolar hypoventilation due to weak diaphragm and intercostal muscles	Not associated with malignant hyperthermia		386
Central or obstructive sleep apnea	Characteristic facies:		387
	Premature frontal baldness		388
	Muscle wasting with hollowed cheeks and temporal fossa		
	Facial weakness, "expressionless" face		
	Extraocular muscle involvement, cataracts		

(Continued)

Table 38.1 (*Continued*)

No.	Syndrome: name, eponyms, inheritance, incidence, gene locus, gene product	Airway	Central nervous system	Cardiovascular
	Myotonic dystrophy, type I (*continued*)		Variable sensitivity to non-depolarizing muscle relaxants Avoid anticholinesterase drugs for reversal of non-depolarizing muscle relaxants as they can precipitate myotonia: use shorter acting muscle relaxants that do not need reversal Mild mental retardation	
66	**Nager syndrome** (mandibulofacial dysostosis with proximal limb anomalies, autosomal dominant and recessive, very rare disorder, approx. 100 reported cases, mutation chromosome 9q32 reported, ZFP37 candidate gene: protein for cartilage development)	Possible difficult direct laryngoscopy and intubation	Conductive hearing loss: atretic external auditory canals	Associated with congenital heart defects
		Absent zygomatic arches	Possible hydrocephalus	
		Malar hypoplasia	Possible agenesis of corpus callosum	
		Small mouth		
		Severe micrognathia with mandibular hypoplasia		
		Laryngeal or epiglottic hypoplasia		

Pulmonary	Other	Additional anesthetic considerations	References
	Neonates with congential myotonic dystrophy can have facial weakness with tent-shaped mouth		
	Orthopedic abnormality: clubfoot deformity		
	Gastrointestinal abnormalities:		
	Dysphagia, reduced peristalsis: at risk for perioperative aspiration		
	Intestinal pseudo-obstruction, pneumoperitoneum		
	Genitourinary abnormality: gonadal atrophy or ovarian failure		
	Endocrine abnormalities:		
	Possible insulin resistance		
	Possible increased incidence of colloid goiters		
	Obstetric abnormalities:		
	Associated with premature labor, uterine atony, and postpartum hemorrhage		
NA	Orthopedic abnormalities:	NA	389
	Radial limb hypoplasia: peripheral access and radial arterial catheter placement may be difficult		390
	Hypoplastic or aplastic thumbs		391
	Shortened humeral bones		
	Clubfoot deformity		
	Dysplastic hips		

(Continued)

Table 38.1 (*Continued*)

No.	Syndrome: name, eponyms, inheritance, incidence, gene locus, gene product	Airway	Central nervous system	Cardiovascular
	Nager syndrome (*continued*)	Choanal atresia: cannot place nasal airway, perform nasal intubation, or place nasogastric tube		
		Cleft palate, soft palate agenesis, velopharyngeal insufficiency		
67	**Neurofibromatosis**	Possible difficult mask ventilation and intubation		Renovascular hypertension from arterial vasculopathy of the abdominal aorta
		Cervical spine stiffness	Peripheral nerve involvement may preclude regional anesthesia	Hypertension secondary to pheochromocytoma
	Neurofibromatosis type 1 (von Recklinghausen disease, autosomal dominant; 50% arise as new mutations, 1:3500, mutation chromosome 17q11.2, neurofibromin gene 1: GTPase activating enzyme)	Macroglossia	NF1: peripheral and central nervous system neurofibromas	Aneurysm rupture
		Tumors of tongue or larynx	NF2 "central neurofibromatosis": bilateral schwannomas of CNVIII, brain meningiomas, schwannomas of dorsal roots of spinal cord	Pregnancy can worsen hypertension
		Dysplasia of sphenoid wing	Pregnancy can initiate or exacerbate growth of neurofibromas	Arterial vasculopathy
		Mediastinal extratracheal tumors	Spinal cord neurofibromas may erode spine and compress cord	
		Macrocephaly	Possible pituitary or hypothalamic dysfunction	

Pulmonary	Other	Additional anesthetic considerations	References
	Possible cervical vertebral anomalies		
	Possible scoliosis		
	Low-set ears		
	Down-slanting palpebral fissures		
	Absent eyelashes in medial third of lower lids		
Restrictive lung disease from kyphoscoliosis	NF1: 85% of patients – cutaneous café au lait spots, osseous abnormalities, possible pheochromocytomas, higher incidence of malignant disease	High incidence of spinal cord involvement – verify no cord lesions with imaging prior to spinal or epidural techniques	
Pulmonary fibrosis with pulmonary hypertension in adulthood	NF2: no cutaneous manifestations		392
Pectus excavatum	Other tumors: neurofibrosarcoma, parathyroid adenoma, rhabdomyosarcoma, duodenal carcinoid, somatostatinoma, pheochromocytoma		393
	Possible endocrinopathies: central precocious puberty, growth hormone deficiency		394
	Newer reports show normal response to succinylcholine and non-depolarizing muscle relaxants, not increased sensitivity		395
			396
			397

(Continued)

Table 38.1 (*Continued*)

No.	Syndrome: name, eponyms, inheritance, incidence, gene locus, gene product	Airway	Central nervous system	Cardiovascular
	Neurofibromatosis (*continued*)		Possible mental retardation, developmental delay, learning disabilities	
			Possible seizures	
	Neurofibromatosis type II (autosomal dominant; 50% arise as new mutations, 1:50–120,000, mutation chromosome 22q12.2, neurofibromin 2 gene – merlin: cytoskeletal protein)			
68	**Noonan syndrome** (autosomal dominant, 1:1000–2500, mutation chromosome 12q24.1 in 50%, PTPNII gene: protein tyrosine phosphatase SHP-2: modulates intercellular signaling including epidermal growth factor)	Possible difficult intubation	Arnold-Chiari malformation	Pulmonic stenosis
		Webbed, short neck	Cerebral arteriovenous malformation	Hypertrophic obstructive cardiomyopathy
		Micrognathia		Bleeding diathesis – coagulation factor deficiency, platelet dysfunction, thrombocytopenia
		Dental malocclusion	Possible hearing loss	Left ventricle hypertrophy
		Flat midface with depressed nasal bridge	Mild mental retardation	Patent ductus arteriosus
		High arched palate		Aortic stenosis
		Possible cervical cystic hygroma		Coarctation of the aorta

Pulmonary	Other	Additional anesthetic considerations	References
			398
			399
			400
			401
			402
			403
			404
Pectus excavatum	Characteristic facies:	May be difficult to place epidural due to relatively narrow spinal canal with normal sized spinal cord	405
Kyphoscoliosis, thoracic lordosis	Triangular face	Possible difficult peripheral intravenous access due to subcutaneous edema	406
Restrictive lung disease	High arched eyebrows		407
	Downward-slanting palpebral fissures		408
	Epicanthal folds		409
	Ptosis		410
	Myopia		411
	Strabismus		412
	Nystagmus		413
	Low-set ears with thickened helix		414
	Orthopedic abnormality: short stature		415
	Gastrointestinal abnormalities:		416

(Continued)

Table 38.1 (*Continued*)

No.	Syndrome: name, eponyms, inheritance, incidence, gene locus, gene product	Airway	Central nervous system	Cardiovascular
	Noonan syndrome (*continued*)			
69	**Oral-facial-digital syndrome**	Possible difficult intubation due to facial and oral abnormalities	Intracerebral cysts	NA
	OFDS type I (Papillon-Leage syndrome, Psaume syndrome, X-linked recessive, very rare, mutation chromosome Xp22.3-p22.2, CXORF5 gene: unknown gene product)	Oral abnormalities:	Corpus callosum agenesis: may have delayed awakening	
		Cleft palate	Cerebellar agenesis	
		Midline cleft tongue	Mental retardation	
		Hamartomas/papilliform protuberances of tongue	Seizures	
		Hyperplastic frenulum with possible multiple oral frenula	Hydrocephalus	
		Abnormal dentition with missing lateral incisors, dental caries, enamel hypoplasia, supernumerary teeth		
		Facial abnormalities:		
		Mandibular hypoplasia		
	OFDS type 2 (Mohr syndrome, sporadic inheritance, very rare, chromosome defect not identified)	Hypoplastic alae nasi		
		Midline cleft lip		
		Cleft alveolar ridge		
		Choanal atresia: cannot place nasal airway, perform nasal intubation, or place nasogastric tube		

Pulmonary	Other	Additional anesthetic considerations	References
	Hepatosplenomegaly		
	Poor feeding in infancy		
	Genitourinary abnormalities:		
	Renal dysfunction, cryptorchidism		
	Lymphatic dysplasia		
NA	Orthopedic abnormalities:		417
	Asymmetrical digit shortening		418
	Syndactyly, clinodactyly, or brachydactyly of hands		419
	Unilateral postaxial polydactyly of feet		420
	Irregular mineralization of bones of hand and feet		421
	Possible polycystic kidney disease (type I)		
	Most patients are female		

(Continued)

Table 38.1 (*Continued*)

No.	Syndrome: name, eponyms, inheritance, incidence, gene locus, gene product	Airway	Central nervous system	Cardiovascular
70	**Osler-Weber-Rendu syndrome** (hereditary hemorrhagic telangiectasia (HHT), autosomal dominant, 1:5–8000)	Telangiectasias of face, lips, tongue, nasopharynx, conjunctiva – avoid trauma during laryngoscopy	Paradoxical emboli or abscess formation due to pulmonary arteriovenous fistula	
		Recurrent epistaxis – avoid nasal intubation, nasogastric tubes, nasal trumpets	Neurovascular malformations in brain (fistula or aneurysms) and spinal cord	High output congestive heart failure due to hepatic or pulmonary arteriovenous fistula
			Bleeding from intracerebral telangiectasias	
	HHT 1 (mutation chromosome 9q34.1, ENG gene: endoglin, a receptor of TGF-beta 1)			
	HHT2 (mutation chromosome 12q11–14, ACVRL1 gene: codes for Alk-1, a TGF-beta 1 receptor)			
71	**Osteogenesis imperfecta** (brittle bone disease, autosomal dominant, 1:20,000, mutation chromosome 17q21.31-q22, 7p22.1, COL1A1 or 1A2 gene: abnormal amount collagen I)	Care during intubation – hyperextension of neck can result in fracture, laryngoscopy can fracture mandible, increased risk of tooth loss with dentinogenesis imperfecta – consider LMA	Atlantoaxial subluxation	Type I: possible aortic root dilation, aortic insufficiency, mitral valve prolapse, rare cor pulmonale from kyphoscoliosis
		Larynx may be difficult to visualize due to kyphoscoliosis or decreased neck mobility	Hydrocephalus	Type I: thin skin, easy bruising, functional platelet abnormality – desmopressin (DDAVP) has been used successfully in one case report

Pulmonary	Other	Additional anesthetic considerations	References
Pulmonary telangiectasias	Visceral arteriovenous malformations can lead to GI bleeding	Paradoxical emboli due to pulmonary arteriovenous fistula – avoid bubbles in IV fluids	422
Possible pulmonary bleeding	Hepatic arteriovenous fistulas can lead to portal hypertension and high-output heart failure		423
Pulmonary arteriovenous fistula can cause intrapulmonary right-to-left shunting leading to arterial desaturation	Hepatic cirrhosis		424
Pulmonary hypertension	Finger and fingertip telangiectasias		425
			426
			427
			428
			429
			430
Severe kyphoscoliosis leads to restrictive lung disease	Increased risk of fractures: careful positioning, insufflation of blood pressure cuff can result in fractures, succinylcholine-induced fasciculations may cause fractures	NA	431
	Type I: most common, mild		432

(Continued)

Table 38.1 (*Continued*)

No.	Syndrome: name, eponyms, inheritance, incidence, gene locus, gene product	Airway	Central nervous system	Cardiovascular
	Osteogenesis imperfecta (*continued*)	Macroglossia, short neck	Basilar impression or invagination syndrome	Possible bleeding diathesis thought due to abnormal collagen on platelet-endothelial cell interactions and capillary strength – consider platelet function tests and coagulation tests prior to neuraxial techniques
			Conductive hearing loss	
			Type II: hypotonia	
72	**Pallister-Hall syndrome** (hypothalamic hamartoblastoma, hypopituitarism, imperforate anus, postaxial polydactyly, autosomal dominant, very rare, mutation chromosome 7p13, GLI3 gene: protein controlling gene expression)	Possible difficult direct laryngoscopy and intubation:	Hypothalamic hamartoma	Congenital cardiac defects:
		Micrognathia	Pituitary dysplasia or aplasia results in panhypopituitarism	Patent ductus arteriosus, ventricular septal defect, endocardial cushion defects, mitral and aortic valve defects, coarctation of the aorta

Pulmonary	Other	Additional anesthetic considerations	References
	Head, ears, eyes, nose, throat: blue sclerae, dentinogenesis imperfecta, progressive conductive hearing loss, vertigo		433
	Orthopedic abnormalities: osteopenia, rapidly healing fractures but with deformities of the limbs, hyperextensible joints, progressive kyphoscoliosis		434
	Endocrine: possible hyperthyroidism		435
	Type II: most die *in utero* or in perinatal period		436
	Head, ears, eyes, nose, throat: blue sclerae, soft skull from poor mineralization, hypotelorism, low nasal bridge with small, beaked nose		437
	Orthopedic abnormalities: short long bones, multiple fractures, flat vertebra		438
	Type III: most severe, non-lethal form		439
	Head, ears, eyes, nose, throat: blue sclerae, soft skull, macrocephaly with triangular facies:		440
	Orthopedic abnormalities: short stature, osteopenia, multiple fractures with progressive deformities		441
	Type IV: moderate severity		442
	HEENT: normal sclera, normal hearing		443
	Orthopedic abnormalities: possible short stature, multiple fractures and bone deformities		
	Several reports of perioperative hypermetabolic state with fever thought not related to malignant hyperthermia, but possibly related to inhalational agents – some reports consider TIVA rather than inhalation agents to avoid this state		
	One report of lactic acidosis with propofol		
Hypoplastic or absent lung	Characteristic facies:	NA	444
Possible abnormal lung lobation	Flattened midface		445

(Continued)

Table 38.1 (*Continued*)

No.	Syndrome: name, eponyms, inheritance, incidence, gene locus, gene product	Airway	Central nervous system	Cardiovascular
	Pallister-Hall syndrome (*continued*)	Dysplastic tracheal cartilage (possible posterior subglottic web, laryngotracheal cleft) – may need smaller than expected endotracheal tube	Possible holoprosencephaly, polymicrogyria, occipital encephalocele, Dandy-Walker malformation	
		Bifid, hypoplastic, or absent epiglottis in greater than 50%	Possible seizures	
		Flattened midface	Vertebral anomalies	
		Microglossia, multiple oral frenula		
		Cleft lip, palate, or uvula		
		Choanal atresia: cannot place nasal airway, perform nasal intubation, or place nasogastric tube		

Pulmonary	Other	Additional anesthetic considerations	References
Possible rib anomalies	Downward-slanting palpebral fissures, ptosis, microphthalmia		446
	Flat nasal bridge, short nose, anteverted nares		447
	Orthopedic abnormalities:		448
	Postaxial polydactyly		
	Syndactyly, brachydactyly, oligodactyly, camptodactyly		
	Nail dysplasia		
	Short limbs		
	Congenital hip dislocation		
	Vertebral anomalies		
	Gastrointestinal abnormalities:		
	Anal defects including imperforate anus, rectal atresia		
	Hirschsprung disease		
	Endocrine abnormalities:		
	Hypoplasia of adrenal glands, pancreas, thyroid gland		
	Hypoparathyroidism		
	Precocious puberty		
	Panhypopituitarism from pituitary dysplasia or aplasia		
	Genitourinary/renal abnormalities:		
	Renal agenesis or dysplasia		
	Micropenis		
	Hypospadias		

(Continued)

Table 38.1 (*Continued*)

No.	Syndrome: name, eponyms, inheritance, incidence, gene locus, gene product	Airway	Central nervous system	Cardiovascular
73	**Pentalogy of Cantrell** (thoracoabdominal syndrome; Cantrell pentalogy, sporadic, very rare, mutation chromosome Xq25-q26.1 in some patients)	Cleft lip or palate	Hydrocephaly or anencephaly	Ectopia cordis (heart protrudes through open sternum)
		Cystic hygroma		Congenital heart defects:
				Ventricular septal defect, atrial septal defect, tetralogy of Fallot, left ventricular diverticulum
				Absent pericardium
74	**Pfeiffer syndrome** (acrocephalosyndactyly type V, autosomal dominant, 1:100,000, mutation chromosome 8p11.2-p11.1 in some patients, FGFR1 gene: fibroblast growth factor receptor 1, mutation chromosome 10q26 in some patients, FGFR2 gene)	Possible difficult intubation	Craniosynostosis	Congenital heart defects
		Craniosynostosis with maxillary hypoplasia	Conductive hearing loss due to atresia of external auditory canal	
		Fused vertebrae (usually upper cervical spine) limits mobility	Possible seizures, hydrocephalus, Arnold-Chiari malformation	
		Possible laryngomalacia, tracheomalacia, calcified trachea, tracheal stenosis		
		Rare choanal atresia: cannot place nasal airway, perform nasal intubation, or place nasogastric tube		

Pulmonary	Other	Additional anesthetic considerations	References
Failure of sternal fusion	Defects in midline fusion	NA	449
Diaphragmatic hernia	Gastrointestinal abnormalities: midline supraumbilical abdominal wall defect		450
Hypoplastic lungs	Omphalocele		451
Possible pulmonary hypertension	Diaphragmatic hernia		452
	Genitourinary/renal abnormalities:		453
	Renal agenesis		454
	Hypospadias		455
Obstructive sleep apnea related to midface hypoplasia and nasal obstruction – needs postoperative observation	Orthopedic abnormalities:	NA	456
	Craniosynostosis		457
	Mild syndactyly, polysyndactyly, radiohumeral synostosis of elbow		458
	Broad thumbs and great toes		
	Characteristic facies:		
	Kleeblattschaedel anomaly (cloverleaf skull)		
	Hypertelorism, shallow orbits, proptosis		

(Continued)

Table 38.1 (*Continued*)

No.	Syndrome: name, eponyms, inheritance, incidence, gene locus, gene product	Airway	Central nervous system	Cardiovascular
	Pfeiffer syndrome (*continued*)			
75	**PHACE association** (posterior fossa malformations–hemangiomas–arterial anomalies–cardiac defects–eye abnormalities–sternal cleft and supraumbilical raphe syndrome, very rare, gene defect not known)	Facial hemangiomas, including subglottic – may bleed with airway instrumentation	Posterior fossa brain malformations including Dandy-Walker malformation	Arterial anomalies – atresia, aneursyms, stenosis, aberrant arterial origins
		Possible micrognathia	Internal carotid artery aneurysm and anomalous branches	Cardiac anomalies including coarctation of the aorta
			Ischemic strokes	
			Agenesis of corpus callosum, cerebrum	
			Developmental delay	
			Seizures	
			Contralateral hemiparesis	
			Absent pitutitary or partially empty sella turcica	
			Spinal dysraphism	
76	**Pierre-Robin syndrome** (Robin sequence, sporadic if non-syndromic, familial if syndromic, 1:8500, mutation chromosome 17q24.3-q25.1 in some patients, candidate genes: SOX9, KCNJ2, KCNJ16, MAP2K6)	Possible difficult mask ventilation and intubation	Possible brainstem dysfunction with central apnea	Cor pulmonale from severe chronic airway obstruction
		Micrognathia		Possible vagal hyperactivity
		Glossoptosis		
		Cleft soft palate		

Pulmonary	Other	Additional anesthetic considerations	References
	Small nose with flat nasal bridge		
	Gastrointestinal abnormalities:		
	Prune belly syndrome, malrotation, duplication		
Possible sternal clefting, possible complete or partial agenesis of sternum	Hemangiomas of face	NA	459
	Eye abnormalities:		460
	Congenital cataracts, glaucoma		461
	Choroidal hemangiomas		462
	Cryptophthalmos, exophthalmos, microphthalmos		
	Colobomas		
	Esotropia		
	Optic atrophy, optic nerve hypoplasia		
	Possible supraumbilical raphe		
	Endocrine abnormalities:		
	Congenital hypothyroidism		
	Possible pituitary insufficiency		
	Marked female predominance		
Obstructive apnea leading to hypoxia	Characteristic facies:	NA	463
	Severe micrognathia		
	Glossoptosis		464
	Gastrointestinal abnormalities:		465

(Continued)

Table 38.1 (*Continued*)

No.	Syndrome: name, eponyms, inheritance, incidence, gene locus, gene product	Airway	Central nervous system	Cardiovascular
	Pierre-Robin syndrome (*continued*)	Obstructive apnea (airway obstruction usually improves with age) Neonates may require prone positioning, nasal airway, surgical fixation of tongue to lip or mandible		
77	**Prader-Willi syndrome** (sporadic, 1:10–25,000, absence of paternal genes from the 15q11-q13 segment, SNRPN, P, UBE3A and necdin gene involvement)	Possible difficult direct laryngoscopy and intubation	Abnormal hypothalamic function:	Pulmonary hypertension due to chronic hypoventilation
		Morbid obesity	Hyperphagia	Hypertension
		Viscous saliva	Temperature instability – hyper- or hypothermia	Possible arrhythmias, especially premature ventricular contractions
		High risk of gastric aspiration	Hypogonadotropic hypogonadism	NA
		Dental enamel hypoplasia	Short stature	
			Neurosecretory growth hormone deficiency	
			Labile temperament with outbursts of rage	
			Hypotonia, especially in neonatal period, but improves with age	
			Psychomotor retardation	
			Relatively insensitive to pain	

Pulmonary	Other	Additional anesthetic considerations	References
	Feeding difficulties due to anatomical abnormalities		
	Possible swallowing difficulties due to brainstem dysfunction		
Hypotonia leads to poor cough and restrictive lung disease	Orthopedic abnormalities:	NA	466
Possible Pickwickian (chronic pulmonary hypoventilation due to obesity) sleep apnea	Short stature		467
	Small hands and feet with tapered fingers		468
Reduced ventilatory response to hypoxia and hypercapnia	Hypermobile joints	NA	469
Blunted hypercapnic ventilatory response thought due to abnormal peripheral chemoreceptor function	Scoliosis, kyphosis		
	Gastrointestinal abnormalities:		
	Morbid obesity		
	Increased rumination		
	Insatiable hunger		
	Hypoglycemia in younger patients, non-insulin dependent diabetes mellitus in older patients		
	Genitourinary abnormalities:		
	Cryptorchidism, hypoplastic penis and scrotum		
	Hypoplastic labia		
	Hypogonadotropic hypogonadism		
	Precocious puberty		
	Myopia, strabismus		

(Continued)

Table 38.1 (*Continued*)

No.	Syndrome: name, eponyms, inheritance, incidence, gene locus, gene product	Airway	Central nervous system	Cardiovascular
78	**Progeria** (Hutchinson-Gilford syndrome, sporadic, 1:8 million, mutation chromosome 1q21.2, lamin A gene: component of nuclear envelope)	Possible difficult direct laryngoscopy and intubation	Childhood cerebrovascular disease	Early and progressive coronary artery disease leading to death in mid-teens from ischemic heart disease
		Micrognathia	Normal intelligence	Hypertension
		Decreased temporomandibular joint mobility	Possible conductive hearing loss	
		Limited mouth opening		
		May require smaller than expected endotracheal tube		
		Abnormal teeth – more susceptible to loss		
		Maxillar and mandibular hypoplasia with beak-like nose		
		Decreased subcutaneous fat: mask ventilation may be difficult		
79	**Proteus syndrome** (sporadic, very rare, about 200 reported case, mutation chromosome 10q23.31, PTEN gene: antagonizes PI3K and MAPK signaling)	Possible difficult direct laryngoscopy and intubation	Vertebral anomalies can cause spinal stenosis	Hypertrophic cardiomyopathy
		Macrocephaly, cranial hyperostosis	Seizures	Cardiac conduction defects
		Cervical spine abnormalities	Retinal or optic nerve abnormalities	Capillary, venous vascular malformations
		Thickened epiglottis	Meningiomas	Venous thrombosis
		Fixed torticollis		Lymphatic malformations
		Anomalous teeth		

Pulmonary	Other	Additional anesthetic considerations	References
Thin ribs	Accelerated aging	NA	470
Small thoracic cage	Progressive alopecia		471
	Decreased subcutaneous fat: monitor for hypothermia		472
	Fragile skin with sclerodermatous changes		473
	Orthopedic abnormalities:		
	Short stature		
	Arthritic, stiff joints		
	Skeletal degeneration		
	Osteoporosis and pathological fractures: must carefully position patients		
	High-pitched voice		
	Orthopedic abnormalities:	Cystic lung disease: avoid nitrous oxide, monitor peak airway pressures	474
Pectus excavatum	Partial gigantism, hemihypertrophy		475
Increased incidence of pulmonary embolism from venous thrombosis	Hyperostoses, often near epiphyses causes impaired mobility		476
	Macrodactyly, syndactyly		477
	Soft tissue hypertrophy of hands and feet		478
	Neck elongation from vertebal enlargement		
	Hemivertebrae, dysplastic vertebrae, dystrophic disks, spondylomegaly		

(Continued)

Table 38.1 (*Continued*)

No.	Syndrome: name, eponyms, inheritance, incidence, gene locus, gene product	Airway	Central nervous system	Cardiovascular
	Proteus syndrome (*continued*)			
80	**Prune belly syndrome** (Eagle-Barrett syndrome, triad syndrome, sporadic, 1:40,000, some cases associated with trisomy 18 or 21)	Micrognathia In utero compression from oligohydramnios can lead to Potter facies: (hypertelorism, epicanthal folds, low-set ears, flattened beaked nose)	NA	Congenital heart defects including patent ductus arteriosus, atrial septal defect, ventricular septal defect, and tetralogy of Fallot

Pulmonary	Other	Additional anesthetic considerations	References
	Scoliosis, kyphosis		
	Subcutaneous hamartomas		
	Thickened skin on palms and soles		
	Lipomas, lymphangiomas		
	Possible hypogammaglobulinemia		
	Possible renal abnormalities		
	Ovarian cystadenoma, testicular tumors		
Pulmonary hypoplasia due to distal urinary tract obstruction and oligohydramnios	Gastrointestinal abnormalities:	NA	479
Weak cough due to deficient abdominal musculature: at risk for postop atelectasis, respiratory failure	Absent abdominal wall musculature		480
Chronic bronchitis	Redundant folds of skin		481
Flat diaphragm, accessory muscles more important	Chronic constipation		482
Possible pectus excavatum	Possible imperforate anus		
	Possible malrotation of the gut		
	Genitourinary abnormalities:		
	Severe bladder and ureteral dilation		
	Cryptorchidism		
	Hydronephrosis with small dysplastic kidneys		
	Recurrent UTIs		
	Possible renal failure		
	Urethral atresia in females		
	Orthopedic abnormalities:		
	Congenital dislocation of the hips		
	Clubfoot deformity		
	Possible polydactyly, syndactyly		
	Scoliosis, torticollis		
	Possible lower limb defects due to compression of iliac vessels by the dilated urinary tract		

(Continued)

Table 38.1 (*Continued*)

No.	Syndrome: name, eponyms, inheritance, incidence, gene locus, gene product	Airway	Central nervous system	Cardiovascular
	Prune belly syndrome (continued)			
81	**Rett syndrome** (X-linked dominant, 1:15–20,000 females: surviving males have Klinefelter (XXY), mutation chromosome Xq28, MECP2 gene: lower epinephrine levels)	Progressive microcephaly (normal head circumference at birth) Upper airway obstruction	Developmentally normal until age 6 to 18 months, then regression to dementia and autism Behavior problems Choreo-athetosis, dystonia, ataxia, myoclonic jerks, stereotypical automatism Hand wringing Seizures	Prolonged QT interval: avoid drugs that prolong QT Possible increased risk of sudden death Tachybradyarrhythmias Vasomotor changes in lower extremities
82	**Rubinstein-Taybi syndrome** (broad thumb-hallux syndrome, broad thumbs and great toes, characteristic facies:, mental retardation, autosomal dominant, 1:10,000, mutation chromosome 16p13.3, CREB binding protein: a nuclear protein participating as a co-activator in cAMP-regulated gene expression)	Possible difficult direct laryngoscopy and intubation Microcephaly Hypoplastic maxilla Prominent forehead Broad nasal bridge with beaked nose and deviated nasal septum	Mental retardation Motor retardation Hypotonia with stiff and unsteady gait Seizures Hyper-reflexia	Congenital heart defects in one-third

Pulmonary	Other	Additional anesthetic considerations	References
	Male predominance 20:1		
While awake, abnormal respiration with intermittent hyperventilation and occasional apnea; this improves while asleep. Possible postoperative respiratory complications	Orthopedic abnormalities:	Very sensitive to sedative drugs and volatile anesthetics – patients have a faster onset and a prolonged emergence	483
Kyphoscoliosis can lead to restrictive lung disease	Short stature	High pain threshold: titrate analgesics	484
	Kyphoscoliosis	Hypotonia and limb spasticity: susceptible to perioperative aspiration with advanced disease	485
	Hip dislocation		486
	Osteopenia, pathological fractures		
	Small hands and feet		
	Thin body habitus: avoid hypothermia, needs careful positioning		
Obstructive sleep apnea	Characteristic facies:	NA	487
Sternal abnormalities, including pectus excavatum	Prominent forehead with large anterior fontanelle		488
Possible postoperative respiratory failure	Hypertelorism		489
Aspiration risk	Thick, arched eyebrows		
	Nasolacrimal duct stenosis		

(Continued)

Table 38.1 (*Continued*)

No.	Syndrome: name, eponyms, inheritance, incidence, gene locus, gene product	Airway	Central nervous system	Cardiovascular
	Rubinstein-Taybi syndrome (*continued*)	Possible choanal atresia: cannot place nasal airway, perform nasal intubation, or place nasogastric tube	Agenesis of corpus callosum	
		Short upper lip with pouting lower lip	Large foramen magnum	
		Microstomia	Possible spina bifida occulta	
		High-arched palate		
		Micrognathia with overcrowding of teeth		
		Easily collapsible larynx		
		Aspiration risk		
83	**Russell-Silver syndrome** (Russell-Silver dwarf, Silver-Russell dwarfism, sporadic or uniparental disomy (10%), 1:30–100,000, mutation chromosome 11p15.5, parental disomy 7p11.2, gene: methylation defects)	Possible difficult intubation and mask fit	Normal intelligence	NA
		Micrognathia	Weakness during infancy	
		Triangular facies: with large head in relation to the face (pseudohydrocephalus because head circumference is actually normal)		
		Facial asymmetry		

Pulmonary	Other	Additional anesthetic considerations	References
	Downward-slanting palpebral fissures, ptosis, glaucoma, strabismus, iris coloboma		
	Orthopedic abnormalities:		
	Short stature		
	Broad thumbs and first toes		
	Clinodactyly of fifth finger		
	Slipped capital femoral epiphyses		
	Flat feet		
	Scoliosis, cervical kyphosis		
	Genitourinary abnormalities:		
	Cryptorchidism, shawl scrotum, hypospadias		
	Occasional renal anomaly		
	Gastroesophageal reflux		
NA	Orthopedic abnormalities:	Possible fasting hypoglycemia from 10 months to 2 to 3 years old: avoid extended perioperative fasting, monitor glucose, use glucose-containing fluids	490
	Short stature, small for gestational age	Consider use of non-triggering anesthetics as malignant hyperthermia has been reported in these patients, although unknown if true malignant hyperthermia or abnormal thermoregulation	491
	Possible scoliosis		
	Skeletal asymmetry, limb length discrepancy		

(Continued)

Table 38.1 (*Continued*)

No.	Syndrome: name, eponyms, inheritance, incidence, gene locus, gene product	Airway	Central nervous system	Cardiovascular
	Russell-Silver syndrome (continued)	Use smaller than predicted endotracheal tube secondary to patient's small size		
		Inverted V-shaped mouth		
84	**Schwartz-Jampel syndrome** (chondrodystrophica myotonia, myotonic myopathy, dwarfism, chondrodystrophy, ocular and facial anomalies, autosomal recessive, very rare, mutation chromosome 1p34-p36, HSPG2 gene which codes for perlecan, a heparin sulfate proteoglycan)	Possible difficult direct laryngoscopy and intubation	NA	
	Chondrodystrophica myotonia	Micrognathia		
		Small mouth with pursed lips		

Pulmonary	Other	Additional anesthetic considerations	References
	Hemihypertrophy		
	camptodactyly, clinodactyly of fifth finger		
	Possible congenital hip dysplasia		
	Gastrointestinal abnormalities:		
	Feeding problems		
	Gastroesophageal reflux: at risk for aspiration		
	Esophagitis		
	Genitourinary abnormalities:		
	Cryptorchidism		
	Hypospadias, posterior urethral valves		
	Renal anomalies		
	Possible inguinal hernia		
	Associated with testicular seminoma, hepatocellular carcinoma, Wilms tumor, craniopharyngioma		
	Café au lait spots		
	Possible growth hormone deficiency		
	Excess sweating during infancy		
	Possible bluish sclearae during infancy		
	Prone to hypothermia		
Pectus carinatum			492
Kyphoscoliosis can lead to restrictive lung disease	Characteristic facies:	Generalized myotonia: can be induced by anesthetic or surgical manipulation, cold or shivering – keep normothermic	493
Possible aspiration pneumonia	Fixed, mask-like facies	Myotonia is not prevented or reversed with muscle relaxants or regional anesthesia	494

(Continued)

Table 38.1 (*Continued*)

No.	Syndrome: name, eponyms, inheritance, incidence, gene locus, gene product	Airway	Central nervous system	Cardiovascular
	Schwartz-Jampel syndrome (continued)	Short neck with decreased range of motion		
		Small larynx, high-pitched voice		
		Jaw muscle rigidity		
			Muscle hypertrophy or atrophy	
			Mental retardation	
85	**Sickle cell disease** (autosomal recessive, 1:5000 overall, 1:500 African Americans, mutation chromosome 11p15.5, beta globin)	Prominent maxilla from increased marrow space	Transient ischemic attacks	Congestive heart failure
			Strokes	Myocardial fibrosis
			Peripheral neuropathy	Hemolytic anemia
			Chronic pain syndrome	Increased risk of pre-eclampsia during pregnancy

Pulmonary	Other	Additional anesthetic considerations	References
Possible respiratory distress, postoperative complications	Narrow palpebral fissures, blepharophimosis, myopia	Can infiltrate muscle with local anesthetic to attenuate contraction	495
	Orthopedic abnormalities:	Avoid succinylcholine due to risk of hyperkalemia	496
	Short stature	Avoid anticholinesterase drugs for reversal of non-depolarizing muscle relaxants as they can precipitate myotonia: use shorter acting muscle relaxants that do not need reversal	
	Progressive joint contractures with joint limitation: need careful positioning	Possible resistance to rocuronium has been reported	
	Carpal tunnel syndrome		
	Bowing of long bones, ankle valgus, pes planus		
	Kyphoscoliosis, lumbar lordosis		
	"Marionette-like" gait		
	Gastrointestinal/genitourinary abnormalities:		
	Umbilical and inguinal hernias		
	Small testes		
Acute chest syndrome leads to pulmonary infarctions	Orthopedic abnormalities:	Perioperative recommendations:	497
Intrapulmonary right-to-left shunting from bronchopulmonary anastomoses	Aseptic necrosis of hip	Avoid cold, stasis, exertion, infection, dehydration, acidosis, and hypoxemia	498
Airway hyperreactivity	Skeletal deformities from marrow hyperplasia and pain crisis, including dactylitis	Treat hypotension with fluids rather than vasopressors	499
Pulmonary hypertension	Bone infarcts with arthropathies	Possible tolerance to narcotics from treatment of pain from vaso-occlusive crises, may require larger doses	500
Restrictive lung disease	Thoracic kyphosis, lumbar lordosis	Perioperative Transfusion in Sickle Cell Disease Study Group compared aggressive transfusion to hemoglobin S <30% to conservative regimen of preoperative transfusion to hemoglobin 10 g/dL with no specific hemoglobin S level. Conservative regimen was as effective in preventing perioperative complications as the aggressive regimen and was associated with fewer transfusion-related adverse events	501

(Continued)

Table 38.1 (*Continued*)

No.	Syndrome: name, eponyms, inheritance, incidence, gene locus, gene product	Airway	Central nervous system	Cardiovascular
	Sickle cell disease (*continued*)			
86	**Smith-Lemli-Opitz syndrome** (Rutledge lethal multiple congenital anomaly syndrome, polydactyly, sex reversal, renal hypoplasia, unilobar lung, lethal acrodysgenital syndrome, autosomal recessive, 1:20–40,000, mutation chromosome 11q12-q13, DHCR7 gene: reduces or eliminates the activity of 7-dehydrocholesterol reductase, preventing cells from producing enough cholesterol)	Possible difficult direct laryngoscopy and intubation	Hypotonia in young children, hypertonia in older children	Congenital heart disease, especially tetralogy of Fallot and ventricular septal defect
		Microcephaly	Demyelination of brain and peripheral nerves	
		Micrognathia	Hypoplasia and abnormal morphogenesis of brain structures	
		Cleft palate, small and hard tongue	Seizures	
		Short nose with anteverted nostrils	Mental retardation	

Pulmonary	Other	Additional anesthetic considerations	References
Obstructive sleep apnea due to adenotonsillar hypertrophy	Growth failure	Minor or low-risk surgeries may not require preoperative transfusion	502
	Gastrointestinal abnormalities:		503
	Splenic sequestration of red cells and platelets		
	Autoinfarction of spleen leading to immune incompetence against encapulated bacteria, including pneumococci and *Haemophilus*		
	Gallstones		
	Intrahepatic sickling can be painful		
	Genitourinary abnormalities:		
	Polyuria, proteinuria, inabilitiy to concentrate urine (avoid hypovolemia)		
	Chronic renal insufficiency		
	Pyelonephritis, glomerulonephritis		
	Renal papillary necrosis		
	Painful priapism		
	Increased risk of pre-eclampsia, placental abruption, placental previa, and intrauterine growth retardation during pregnancy		
Pulmonary hypoplasia, single-lobed lungs	Caused by an inborn error in cholesterol biosynthesis	NA	504
Recurrent aspiration leading to pneumonia	Charcteristic facies:		505
	Microcephaly		506
	High, square forehead		507
	Ptosis, epicanthal folds, strabismus, cataracts		

(Continued)

Table 38.1 (*Continued*)

No.	Syndrome: name, eponyms, inheritance, incidence, gene locus, gene product	Airway	Central nervous system	Cardiovascular
	Smith-Lemli-Opitz syndrome (*continued*)	Short neck Prominent incisors	Behavior problems	
87	**Spinal muscular atrophy (SMA) types I and II (Werdnig-Hoffmann disease)** (autosomal recessive, all types: 1:10,000 total incidence)	Type I: Difficulty handling secretions due to swallowing problems Tongue atrophy and fasciculations	Type I: Hypotonia, weakness, no deep tendon reflexes Normal intelligence	NA
	SMA I – acute Werdnig-Hoffmann disease, acute infantile SMA (autosomal recessive, 1:25,000, mutation chromosome 5q12.2-q13.3, SMN1 gene: regulates telomeres)	Type II:	Type II:	

Pulmonary	Other	Additional anesthetic considerations	References
	Low-set ears		
	Short nose with anteverted nostrils		
	Orthopedic abnormalities:		
	Syndactyly of second and third toes		
	Postaxial polysyndactyly		
	Simian crease, flexed fingers		
	Dislocated hips		
	Gastrointestinal abnormalities:		
	Feeding problems, failure to thrive		
	Gastroesophageal reflux, vomiting		
	Hepatic dysfunction		
	Hirschsprung disease, rectal atresia, pyloric stenosis		
	Genitourinary abnormalities:		
	Hypospadias, cryptorchidism		
	Ambiguity of external male genitalia with micropenis		
	bifid or hypoplastic scrotum		
	Male pseudohermaphroditism		
	Renal hypoplasia, renal duplication		
	Ureteropelvic junction obstruction		
	Hydronephrosis, renal cysts		
	Possible adrenal insufficiency		
Type I:	Type I:		508
Respiratory distress	Usually diagnosed age <6 mo		509
Shallow respirations	Death from respiratory failure by age 2 yr without mechanical ventilation		
Paradoxical respiratory pattern with diaphragmatic breathing	Type II:		

(Continued)

Table 38.1 (*Continued*)

No.	Syndrome: name, eponyms, inheritance, incidence, gene locus, gene product	Airway	Central nervous system	Cardiovascular
	Spinal muscular atrophy (SMA) types I and II *(continued)*	Tongue atrophy and fasciculations in half of patients	Fine tremor of hands	
			Decreased to absent deep tendon reflexes	
			Normal intelligence	
	SMA II – chronic Werdnig-Hoffmann disease, intermediate SMA (mutation chromosome 5q12.2-q13.3, SMN1 gene: regulates telomeres)			
88	**Spinal muscular atrophy type III (Kugelberg-Welander disease)** (juvenile spinal muscular atrophy, mild SMA, autosomal recessive, mutation chromosome 5q12.2-q13.3, SMN1 gene: regulates telomeres)	NA	Muscle atrophy and weakness initially affects the proximal limb muscles then progresses distally	NA
			Possible calf pseudohypertrophy	
89	**Stickler syndrome** (arthro-ophthalmopathy, hereditary progressive, autosomal dominant, 1:7500–9000, mutation chromosome 12q13.11-q13.2, genes: COL2A1 , COL11A1, COL11A2, COL9A1, abnormal collagen type II and XI)	Possible difficult direct laryngoscopy and intubation	Sensorineural or conductive hearing loss	Mitral valve prolapse
		Micrognathia		

Pulmonary	Other	Additional anesthetic considerations	References
Usually require respiratory support	Intermediate severity		
Type II:	Diagnosed from age 7 to 18 months		
Severe scoliosis leads to restrictive lung disease	Cannot walk independently but can sit unaided		
	Orthopedic abnormalities:	May require postoperative ventilation	
	Type II – kyphoscoliosis, possible calf hypertrophy	Avoid succinylcholine due to risk of exaggerated hyperkalemia	
		Variable sensitivity of non-depolarizing muscle relaxants: recommend avoidance or monitoring	
Decreased pulmonary function leads to recurrent pulmonary infections	Usually diagnosed in early toddler years to as late as adolescence	Avoid succinylcholine due to risk of exaggerated hyperkalemia	508
Disordered breathing while asleep	Normal life expectancy	Variable sensitivity of non-depolarizing muscle relaxants: recommend avoidance or monitoring	509
May require postoperative ventilation	Males more severely affected		510
	Orthopedic abnormalities:		
	Kyphoscoliosis and contractures		
Pectus excavatum	Connective tissue disorder	NA	511
	Characteristic facies:		512

(Continued)

Table 38.1 (*Continued*)

No.	Syndrome: name, eponyms, inheritance, incidence, gene locus, gene product	Airway	Central nervous system	Cardiovascular	
	Stickler syndrome (*continued*)	Midface hypoplasia with flat nasal bridge, anteverted nares			
		Cleft palate, tooth abnormalities			
		May have associated Pierre Robin syndrome			
90	**Sturge-Weber syndrome** (encephalotrigeminal angiomatosis, sporadic, unclear inheritance, 1:50,000, no chromosome abnormality identified)	Possible difficult mask ventilation and intubation	Capillary or cavernous hemangiomas (port wine stains, nevus flammeus) in the cutaneous distribution of the first or second division of the trigeminal nerve	High output heart failure due to shunting	
		Angiomas of tongue or larynx can interfere and rupture	Leptomeningeal angiomatosis usually ipsilateral to the facial cutaneous vascular malformation	Possible congenital heart defects	
		Angiomas of the mucous membranes	Spinal cord hemangiomas: verify absence prior to neuraxial anesthesia		
		Possible hypertrophy of bones and soft tissues in regions adjacent to areas of facial angioma	Seizures		
			Mental retardation		
			Linear intracranial calcifications		
			Hemiatrophy of brain		

Pulmonary	Other	Additional anesthetic considerations	References
	Flat facies: with flat nasal bridge, anteverted nares		513
	Epicanthal folds		
	Orthopedic abnormalities:		
	Hyperextensible joints, joint pains		
	Marfanoid habitus, arachnodactyly		
	Short stature, narrow long bones		
	Scoliosis, kyphosis, lumbar lordosis		
	Herniation of thoracic disks, flat vertebrae		
	Hip subluxation, clubfoot deformity		
	Early-onset osteo-arthritis		
	Ocular abnormalities:		
	Myopia, dislocated lens, glaucoma, chorioretinal degeneration		
	Retinal detachment, cataracts		
	Vision loss		
Vascular abnormalities in the lung	Characteristic facies:	NA	514
	Facial port-wine stain, or angioma, in distribution of trigeminal nerve		515
	Eye abnormalities:		516
	Glaucoma, retinal vessel varicosities		517
	Choroid hemangioma, retinal detachment		
	Optic atrophy		
	Gastrointestinal abnormalities:		

(Continued)

Table 38.1 (*Continued*)

No.	Syndrome: name, eponyms, inheritance, incidence, gene locus, gene product	Airway	Central nervous system	Cardiovascular	
	Sturge-Weber syndrome (*continued*)		Hemiplegia: avoid succinylcholine Behavior problems Headaches		
91	**Thrombocytopenia-absent radii (TAR) syndrome** (inheritance unclear, 1:250,000, chromosome deletion at 1q21.1, 11 candidate genes)	Possible micrognathia Avoid nasal intubation or nasal gastric tubes due to risk of epistaxis	Possible intracranial hemorrhage	Congenital heart defects: Tetralogy of Fallot Coarctation of the aorta Atrial septal defect	
92	**Treacher Collins syndrome** (mandibulofacial dysostosis; Franceschetti-Klein syndrome, autosomal dominant, 50% *de novo* mutations, 1:50,000, mutation chromosome 5q32-q33.1, TCOF1 gene (treacle: ribosomal DNA transcription)	Possible difficult to impossible direct laryngoscopy and intubation	Normal intelligence	Congenital heart defects possible	

Pulmonary	Other	Additional anesthetic considerations	References
	Colonic ischemia		
	Hematemesis from gastric bleeding		
	May be associated with Klippel-Trenaunay-Weber syndrome		
NA		Thrombocytopenia (congenital or develops in infancy); episodes decrease with age: need preoperative platelet count, hematocrit	518
	Characteristic facies:		519
	Port-wine stain on forehead		
	Ptosis, strabismus		
	Small, upturned nose		
	Orthopedic abnormalities:		
	Bilateral absence of radii with the presence of both thumbs		
	Hypoplastic or absent (unilateral or bilateral) ulnae		
	Abnormal humerus or shoulder		
	Dislocated hips, knee subluxation, coxa valga		
	Dislocated patella, femoral and tibial torsion		
	Small feet, abnormal toe placement, foot edema		
	Small stature		
	Arthritis of ankle and knees		
	Gastrointestinal abnormalities:		
	Pancreatic cysts, Meckel diverticulum, hepatosplenomegaly		
	Cow's milk intolerance		
	Various renal anomalies		
Sleep apnea	Characteristic facies:	NA	520

(Continued)

Table 38.1 (*Continued*)

No.	Syndrome: name, eponyms, inheritance, incidence, gene locus, gene product	Airway	Central nervous system	Cardiovascular	
	Treacher Collins syndrome (*continued*)	Malar hypoplasia with possible cleft zygoma			
		Mandibular and pharyngeal hypoplasia: leads to narrow airway			
		Small mouth			
		High arched palate, cleft palate or cleft lip			
		Teeth malocclusion			
		Patient may need to be placed in prone position to assist in spontaneous ventilation as tongue may fall back into pharynx			
93	**Trisomy 13** (Patau syndrome, sporadic, meotic non-dysjunction, 1:10,000, chromosome 13 trisomy)	Possible difficult direct laryngoscopy and intubation	Hypotonia	Congenital heart defects:	
		Microcephaly: may require smaller than predicted endotracheal tube size	Myelomeningocele	Ventricular septal defect, tetralogy of Fallot	
		Wide sagittal suture and fontanelles		Double-outlet right ventricle	
		May require smaller than predicted endotracheal tube size	Developmental delay		
		Cleft lip or cleft palate	Febrile seizures		
		Short neck	Holoprosencephaly with agenesis of corpus callosum		
		Micrognathia	Cerebellar hypoplasia		

Pulmonary	Other	Additional anesthetic considerations	References
	Malar hypoplasia		521
	Down-slanting palpebral fissures		522
	Colobomas of lower eyelid, partial to total absence of lower eyelashes		523
	Visual loss, microphthalmia		524
	Low-set ears with external canal atresia: conductive deafness		
	Absent parotid gland		
	Genitourinary abnormality:		
	Possible cryptorchidism		
Possible apnea: monitor postoperatively	Characteristic facies:	Spinal dysraphism: confirm absence prior to neuraxial technique	525
Pectus carinatum	Microcephaly with occipital scalp defect		526
Kyphoscoliosis	Low-set ears, abnormal helices		
	Broad, flat nose		
	Microphthalmia, anophthalmia, cataracts		
	Optic nerve hypoplasia, limited vision		
	Short neck		
	Capillary hemangioma on forehead		
	Gastrointestinal abnormalities:		

(Continued)

Table 38.1 (Continued)

No.	Syndrome: name, eponyms, inheritance, incidence, gene locus, gene product	Airway	Central nervous system	Cardiovascular
	Trisomy 13 (continued)			
94	**Trisomy 18** (Edwards syndrome, sporadic, meotic non-dysjunction, 1:6–8000, chromosome 18 trisomy)	Possible difficult direct laryngoscopy and intubation	Sensorineural hearing loss	Greater than 95% incidence of cardiac defects:
		Microcephaly, prominent occiput, narrow bifrontal diameter	Severe mental retardation	Ventricular septal defect, atrial septal defect, patent ductus arteriosus, bicuspid aortic valve
		Micrognathia	Hypotonia in neonatal period	Pulmonic stenosis, coarctation of the aorta
		Cleft lip or cleft palate	Hypertonia after neonatal period	Aberrant subclavian artery: confirm absence prior to placement of subclavian central venous line
			Possible holoprosencephaly	

Pulmonary	Other	Additional anesthetic considerations	References
	Microscopic pancreatic dysplasia		
	Malrotation, omphalocele, Meckel diverticulum		
	Genitourinary abnormalities:		
	Unilateral renal agenesis, renal and urogenital duplication		
	Hydronephrosis, polycystic kidneys		
	Renal insufficiency		
	Cryptorchidism, hypospadias		
	Hypoplastic ovaries, abnormal insertion of fallopian tubes		
	Orthopedic abnormalities:		
	Polydactyly of hands, possibly feet		
	Flexion deformities of hands, simian crease		
	Radial aplasia		
	Prominent heel, rockerbottom feet, clubfoot deformity		
	Joint subluxation		
Short sternum	Characteristic facies:	NA	527
Possible diaphragmatic muscle hypoplasia	Microcephaly, prominent occiput		528
Absent or malformed right lung	Short palpebral fissures		
Recurrent apnea in neonatal period	Epicanthal folds, ptosis, corneal opacity		
	Low-set, malformed ears		
	Gastrointestinal abnormalities:		
	Omphalocele, Meckel diverticulum, malrotation		
	Anal anomalies, ectopic pancreatic or splenic tissue		
	Failure to thrive		
	Genitourinary abnormalities:		
	Cryptorchidism		
	Ectopic kidneys, horseshoe kidney, polycystic kidney		
	Hydronephrosis, duplication of collecting system		

(Continued)

Table 38.1 (*Continued*)

No.	Syndrome: name, eponyms, inheritance, incidence, gene locus, gene product	Airway	Central nervous system	Cardiovascular
	Trisomy 18 (*continued*)			
95	**Tuberous sclerosis** (autosomal dominant, 1:12–14,000, mutation chromosome 9q34 (TSC1) or 16p12 (TSC2), genes: TSC1 hamartin, TSC2 tuberin – tumor-suppressing proteins)	Possible oropharyngeal or laryngeal tumors	Cognitive disability	Cardiac rhabdomyomas may obstruct blood flow, cause arrhythmias or heart block: need baseline assessment to verify absence
		Pitting of tooth enamel	Seizures	Possible Wolff-Parkinson-White
			Autism or behavior problems	Aneurysms of major arteries
			Giant cell astrocytomas amd subependymal periventricular nodules can calcify or cause hydrocephalus	
			Sacrococcygeal chordomas	

Pulmonary	Other	Additional anesthetic considerations	References
	Renal insufficiency		
	Orthopedic abnormalities:		
	Clenched hands at birth, index finger overlaps third finger, fifth finger overlaps the fourth		
	Short, hypoplastic, or absent thumb		
	Small, narrow pelvis with limited hip abduction		
	Clubfoot deformity, rockerbottom feet		
	Syndactyly of second and third toes		
	Short stature		
Pulmonary lymphangiomyomatosis	Characteristic facies:	NA	529
	Adenoma sebaceum (facial angiofibromas) usually on the malar areas of face		530
	Multiple retinal astrocytomas, choroid hamartomas		531
	Orthopedic abnormalities:		
	Periungual fibromas around the fingertips		
	Separation of periosteum from underlying bone in phalanges and long bones		
	Gastrointestinal abnormalities:		
	Tumors in mouth, esophagus, stomach, intestines, pancreas, or liver		
	Genitourinary abnormalities:		
	Adrenal angiolipomas		
	Renal angiomyolipomas which can spontaneously rupture		
	Renal cysts		
	Renal carcinomas		
	Papillary adenoma of the thyroid		
	Cutaneous manifestations:		
	Shagreen patches on lower trunk		

(Continued)

Table 38.1 (*Continued*)

No.	Syndrome: name, eponyms, inheritance, incidence, gene locus, gene product	Airway	Central nervous system	Cardiovascular
	Tuberous sclerosis *(continued)*			
96	**Turner syndrome** (XO syndrome, gonadal dysgenesis, meotic non-dysjunction, mosaicism, 1:2500 females, monosomy chromosome X)	Possible difficult intubation	Sensorineural hearing loss	Congenital heart anomalies:
		Short, webbed neck: possible endobronchial intubation		Coarctation of the aorta
		High arched palate		Bicuspid aortic valve
		Micrognathia		Aortic dissection
				Partial anomalous venous return
				Possible prolonged QT
				Hypertension
				Hypercholesterolism

Pulmonary	Other	Additional anesthetic considerations	References
	Hypopigmented elliptical shaped macule, "ash leaf spots"		
	Café au lait spots		
Broad, "shield-like" chest	Occurs in females	NA	532
Mild pectus excavatum	Characteristic facies:		533
	Webbed neck		534
	Ptosis, inner canthal folds		
	Protruding external ear		
	Strabismus, amblyopia		
	Orthopedic abnormalities:		
	Short stature		
	Increased carrying angle of elbows		
	Short fourth metacarpal and metatarsal		
	Narrow, deeply set nails		
	Dislocated hips, puffy hands and feet		
	Scoliosis, kyphosis		
	Dislocation of patella		
	Gastrointestinal abnormalities:		
	Crohn disease, ulcerative colitis		
	Genitourinary abnormalities:		
	Gonadal dysgenesis or agenesis with streak ovaries		
	Fertility is rare		
	Horseshoe kidney		
	Possible duplicated collecting system		
	Endocrine abnormalities:		
	Absent thelarche and menarche: may be on hormone therapy		
	Sometimes receive growth hormone replacement therapy		
	Insulin resistance with type II diabetes		

(Continued)

Table 38.1 (*Continued*)

No.	Syndrome: name, eponyms, inheritance, incidence, gene locus, gene product	Airway	Central nervous system	Cardiovascular
	Turner syndrome (*continued*)			
97	**VACTERL/VATER** (sporadic inheritance, 1:17,000, possible defects at chromosome 2, 7,16 (animal models), candidate genes: SHH, FOX gli)	Laryngeal stenosis Tracheal atresia Possible choanal atresia: cannot place nasal airway, perform nasal intubation, or place nasogastric tube	Vertebral anomalies: hemivertebrae, dysplastic vertebrae, vertebral fusion, tethered cord	Cardiac malformations
98	**Von Hippel-Lindau syndrome** (autosomal dominant, 1:36–45,000, mutation chromosome 3p26-p25, tumor suppressor gene)	NA	Cerebellar, medullary, spinal cord hemangioblastomas Spinal cord lesions are usually cervicothoracic, but have been reported lumbosacral and in cauda equina: verify absence prior to lumbar neuraxial technique Cerebellar tumors may lead to increased intracranial pressure	Episodic hypertension due to cerebellar tumors Type I: not associated with pheochromocytomas Type II: associated with pheochromocytomas

Pulmonary	Other	Additional anesthetic considerations	References
	Hypothyroidism		
	Obesity		
Tracheoesophageal fistula	Gastrointestinal abnormalities:	NA	535
Ectopic bronchus	Anal atresia		536
	Tracheo-esophageal fistula		
	Esophageal atresia		
	Duodenal atresia		
	Orthopedic abnormalities:		
	Radial dysplasia		
	Vertebral anomalies: hemivertebrae, dysplastic vertebrae, vertebral fusion		
	Dysplastic thumb		
	Preaxial polydactyly, syndactyly		
	Hip dysplasia		
	Genitourinary abnormalities:		
	Renal dysplasia		
	Defects of external genitalia		
Pulmonary cysts	Ocular abnormalities:	NA	537
Oat cell carcinoma	Retinal vascular hamartomas		538
	Capillary hemangiomas, exudative retinopathy		539

(Continued)

Table 38.1 (*Continued*)

No.	Syndrome: name, eponyms, inheritance, incidence, gene locus, gene product	Airway	Central nervous system	Cardiovascular
	Von Hippel-Lindau syndrome (*continued*)		Tumors of the endolymphatic sac of the ear: possible hearing loss, tinnitus, vertigo, cranial nerve VII dysfunction	
99	**Weaver syndrome** (Weaver-Smith syndrome, sporadic inheritance, very rare, mutation chromosome 5q35 in some patients, NSD1 gene in some patients)	Possible difficult direct laryngoscopy and intubation	Developmental delay	Possible atrial septal defect, ventricular septal defect
		Macrocephaly, flat occiput, broad forehead	Behavior problems	
		Short, broad neck with excess fat	Hypertonia	
		Depressed nasal bridge, long philtrum	Seizures	
		Large, thick tongue		
		Retrognathia		
		Prominent chin		
		Low-pitched, hoarse voice		
		Cleft palate		

Pulmonary	Other	Additional anesthetic considerations	References
	Retinal detachment		
	Gastrointestinal abnormalities:		
	Hepatic adenomas, hepatocellular carcinoma		
	Pancreatic cysts, islet cell tumors		
	Genitourinary abnormalities:		
	Hypernephromas, renal cell carcinomas		
	Adrenal adenomas		
	Cystadenomas of the epididymis		
NA	Characteristic facies:	NA	540
	Macrocephaly, flat occiput		541
	Short, broad neck with excess fat		542
	Depressed nasal bridge, long philtrum		
	Prominent chin		
	Low-set, large ears		
	Epicanthal folds, strabismus, down-slanting palpebral fissures		
	Sparse hair		
	Loose skin		
	Orthopedic abnormalities:		
	Accelerated growth		
	Advanced bone age		
	Camptodactyly, broad thumbs, prominent finger pads, deep set nails		
	Hyperextensible fingers, limited extension of elbows and knees		

(Continued)

Table 38.1 (*Continued*)

No.	Syndrome: name, eponyms, inheritance, incidence, gene locus, gene product	Airway	Central nervous system	Cardiovascular
	Weaver syndrome (*continued*)			
100	**Whistling face syndrome** (Freeman-Sheldon syndrome, craniocarpotarsal dysplasia, whistling face-windmill vane hand syndrome, craniocarpotarsal dystrophy, distal arthrogryposis type 2A, sporadic or autosomal dominant, very rare, mutation chromosome 17p13.1, gene: myosin heavy chain 3)	Possible difficult to impossible direct laryngoscopy	Myopathy: has been associated with muscle rigidity with exposure to halothane and hyperpyrexia with exposure to other volatile agents	Cor pulmonale due to chronic airway obstruction
		Fixed microstomia not relieved by muscle relaxants from increased tone and fibrosis of facial muscles	Hypertonia	
		Microcephaly	Mental retardation	
		Micrognathia, short neck	Hearing loss	
		Cephalad larynx due to muscle contractures	Possible spinal bifida occulta: verify absence prior to neuraxial technique	
		Pharyngeal muscle myopathy can lead to chronic airway obstruction	Possible seizures	
		High-arched palate with small tongue and limited palate movement		
		Broad nasal bridge		

Pulmonary	Other	Additional anesthetic considerations	References
	Kyphosis, scoliosis		
	Genitourinary abnormalities:		
	Inguinal or umbilical hernias		
	Cryptorchidism		
Intercostal myopathy: may result in postoperative pulmonary complications	Characteristic facies:	Myopathy: has been associated with muscle rigidity with exposure to halothane and hyperpyrexia with exposure to other volatile agents	543
Dysphagia with recurrent vomiting can lead to aspiration	Full forehead, prominent supraorbital ridges		544
Pectus excavatum	Microcephaly		545
Kyphosis can lead to restrictive lung disease	Immobile, mask-like facial expression		546
Sleep-disordered breathing	Epicanthal folds, ptosis, blepharophimosis		547
	Strabismus		
	Small nose, hypoplastic alae		
	Microstomia, pursed lips, long phitrum		
	H-shaped dimpling of chin		
	Orthopedic abnormalities:		
	Kyphoscoliosis		
	Joint contractures		

(Continued)

Table 38.1 (*Continued*)

No.	Syndrome: name, eponyms, inheritance, incidence, gene locus, gene product	Airway	Central nervous system	Cardiovascular
	Whistling face syndrome (*continued*)			
101	**Williams syndrome** (Williams-Beuren syndrome, autosomal dominant or spontaneous inheritance, 1:10,000, deletion chromosome 7q11.23, gene: elastin)	Possible difficult intubation	Cerebral artery stenosis	Congenital heart defects:
		Flat midface, wide mouth	Infantile hypotonia with hypertonia later	Aortic stenosis, usually supravalvular, can lead to sudden death
		Dental malocclusion, poor dentition	Visuospatial deficits	Bicuspid aortic valve, mitral valve prolapse, mitral insufficiency
			Attention deficit disorder	Left coronary artery stenosis, myocardial ischemia
			Hyperacusis	Peripheral pulmonary artery stenosis
			Seizures	Abdominal aortic coarctation
				Tetralogy of Fallot, ventricular septal defect
				Possible narrowing of celiac, mesenteric, or renal arteries
				Hypertension

Pulmonary	Other	Additional anesthetic considerations	References
	Camptodactyly, ulnar deviation, flexion contractures of fingers		
	Clubfoot, toe contractures		
	Hip dislocation		
	Gastrointestinal abnormalities:		
	Dysphagia with recurrent vomiting can lead to aspiration		
	GU abnormalities:		
	Inguinal hernia		
	Cryptorchidism		
NA	Characteristic facies:	High incidence of coronary artery abnormalities and obstruction even if supravalvular aortic stenosis is not severe. Avoid hypotension and hypovolemia, tachycardia. Avoid prolonged fasting and anesthetic drugs that excessively veno- and vasodilate. Have volume infusion and bolus vasoconstrictor agents available (phenylephrine)	548
	"Elfin" facies		549
	Puffy eyes, lacy iris pattern		550
	Hyperacusis		551
	Depressed nasal bridge with anteverted nares		
	Enamel hypoplasia with small teeth		
	Harsh voice		
	Orthopedic abnormalities:		
	Short stature		
	Hypoplastic nails		
	Hallux valgus, progressive joint limitation		
	Gastrointestinal abnormalities:		
	Chronic constipation, diverticulosis		
	Genitourinary abnormalities:		
	Renal structural anomalies		
	Nephrocalcinosis, recurrent UTIs		

(Continued)

Table 38.1 (*Continued*)

No.	Syndrome: name, eponyms, inheritance, incidence, gene locus, gene product	Airway	Central nervous system	Cardiovascular
	Williams syndrome (*continued*)			
102	**Wiskott-Aldrich syndrome** (eczema-thrombocytopenia-immunodeficiency syndrome, immunodeficiency 2, X-linked recessive, 1:250,000 males, mutation chromosome Xp11.23-p11.22, gene: Wiskott-Aldrich syndrome protein)	Epistaxis	Intracranial hemorrhage from thrombocytopenia	Autoimmune vasculitis can affect coronary arteries
		Recurrent oral infections	Autoimmune vasculitis can affect cerebral arteries	
		Reccurent sinusitis, otitis media		

Pulmonary	Other	Additional anesthetic considerations	References
	Renal artery stenosis		
	Endocrine abnormalities:		
	Neonatal hypercalcemia		
	Early menarche		
	Possible hypothyroidism		
	Musical ability		
	Friendly, "cocktail party" personalities		
Recurrent pulmonary infections	X-linked recessive disorder	Need aseptic technique	552
	Immune deficiency with recurrent infections	Transfused blood products need to be irradiated to prevent graft-versus-host disease	553
		Thrombocytopenia with small platelets:	554
		Need to evaluate preoperative platelet count, hematocrit	
		May need platelet transfusion	
		Verify platelet count prior to neuraxial technique	
		May require splenectomy to control thrombocytopenia	
	Increased incidence of autoimmune disorders: hemolytic anemia, vasculitis, idiopathic thrombocytopenic purpura		
	Increased incidence of malignancies: non-Hodgkin lymphoma, brain cancer		
	Eczema		
	Gastrointestinal abnormality: bloody diarrhea		
	Genitorurinary abnormality: renal insufficiency		

(Continued)

No.	Syndrome: name, eponyms, inheritance, incidence, gene locus, gene product	Airway	Central nervous system	Cardiovascular
103	**Zellweger syndrome** (cerebrohepatorenal syndrome, autosomal recessive, very rare, mutations chromosome 1p36.2, 1q22, 6p, 6q, 7q21, 8q, 12, genes: multiple peroxisome genes, PEX1 most common)	Long face with midface hypoplasia		Congenital heart defects:
		High arched palate, cleft palate	Failure of myelination and white matter development	Patent ductus arteriosus
		Micrognathia	Microgyria	Septal defects
			Poor suck	Aortic abnormalities
			Seizures	
			Neurocognitive delay	

References for gene mapping, gene product, incidence, and inheritance: United States National Institutes of Health Mendelian Inheritance in Man database: www.ncbi.nlm.nih.gov/omim.
United States Institutes of Health Genetic and Rare Diseases Information Center; http://rarediseases.info.nih.gov/GARD.

Pulmonary	Other	Additional anesthetic considerations	References
Respiratory insufficiency due to hypotonia: may result in postoperative pulmonary complications	Peroxisomal dysfunction and/or absence	Hypotonia: may need to avoid preoperative sedation	555
Apnea	Characteristic facies:		556
	Prominent forehead, wide anterior fontanelle		557
	Long, flat, shallow face with flat supraorbital ridges		558
	Epicanthal folds, puffy lids, corneal opacities		
	Gliosis of optic nerve		
	Extra neck skinfolds		
	Orthopedic abnormalities:		
	Simian crease, camptodactyly		
	Contractures, especially knees and fingers: needs careful intraoperative positioning		
	Gastrointestinal abnormalities:		
	Hepatomegaly, chronic liver disease, jaundice, cirrhosis, albuminuria: confirm absence of coagulopathy prior to neuraxial technique		
	Genitourinary abnormalities:		
	Impaired adrenal cortical function or atrophy: may need stress dose steroids		
	Renal cortical cysts		
	Cryptorchidism		
	Less severe forms include neonatal adrenoleukodystrophy and infantile Refsum disease		

CHAPTER 39
Pediatric Anesthesia in Developing Countries

Adrian T. Bosenberg
Department of Anesthesia, Seattle Children's Hospital, Seattle, WA, USA

Organization

Children constitute more than half the population in many developing countries [1–3]. Many of these children are victims of circumstance, orphaned by HIV [3,4], natural disasters, war, social unrest, economic crises, and famine (Figs 39.1, 39.2). Providing anesthesia for children in the developing world can be very challenging [5–9] because for the most part anesthetic practice has not kept pace with the advances made in the developed countries [7]. Our understanding of anesthesia in the developing world is based on personal experience or anecdotal reports provided by local healthcare workers or visitors on medical missions. This reflects the low incentive to publish in the face of a heavy clinical workload and staff shortages.

Many developing countries have a colonial history and were exploited for their raw materials. The infrastructure was developed for the benefit of the colonial power and not the country or region [2,3]. As a result, many of these countries are today characterized by poverty, poor housing and educational standards, limited health resources and social services [1,5,7–13]. Of the world's poorest countries, 70% are in sub-Saharan Africa [11–13], an area ravaged by HIV, malaria, and tuberculosis [4].

Access to safe anesthesia and pain relief following surgery is considered a basic human right in the 21st century. International standards for the safe practice of anesthesia, adopted by the World Federation of Societies of Anaesthesiologists (WFSA) in 1992, are seldom met in developing countries [5]. Provision of safe anesthesia requires trained anesthetists, essential equipment, consumables, and drugs [14–19]. All these essentials are seldom found in the operating rooms of the developing world [17–19]. The anesthetic issues published in previous decades persist and, in many instances, are remarkably similar to those seen today [2,13,20–23]. Improving the safety of surgery and anesthesia worldwide, but particularly in the developing world, has finally become the focus of the World Health Organization (WHO) and WFSA [17–21].

Different countries have different problems demanding different solutions. Conditions may even vary significantly within the same country [2,5]. The essential differences include the medical personnel and their level of training, the spectrum and nature of disease, the facilities, including access to electricity and running water, the equipment available, and access to cheap, generic and perhaps outmoded drugs [8,22–24] (Fig. 39.3). The ratio of anesthetists to population varies greatly (Table 39.1, Fig. 39.4). It is not surprising that perioperative mortality and morbidity are high by developed world standards and, not surprisingly, inversely related to the anesthetic manpower [25]. The expectations of the local population are often commensurate with the facilities and quality of the available care.

Anesthesia does not enjoy a high profile and lacks the voice to demand access to resources in developing countries. Anesthesia is not perceived to be an attractive career for many undergraduates [26–28] who receive little, if any, exposure to the specialty [29–31]. Indeed, very few developing countries can afford specialist anesthesiolo-gists, except perhaps in the principal hospitals. The "pediatric anesthesiologist" is invariably someone who may have a special interest or affinity for children or has simply been allocated to pediatric anesthesia for the day because there is no one else. Pediatric anesthesiologists *per se* are a luxury.

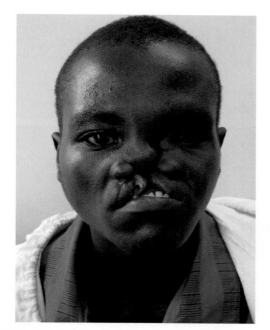

Figure 39.1 Victims of war. Mutilating injuries acquired almost two decades ago during the Rwandan genocide received basic treatment only. Child survivors face an intense struggle for survival as a consequence of displacement, separation from or loss of parents, poverty, hunger and disease in countries that are subject to total collapse of economic, health, social and educational infrastructures.

Table 39.1 Anesthetic mortality per 100,000 and the year reported

Year	Country	Anesthetic death rate	Hospital setting	Reference
1987	Zambia	1:1925	University/ teaching	21
2000	Malawi	1:504	Central	21
1994–2001	Zimbabwe	1:482	District	21
2006	Nigeria	1:387	Teaching	21
2005	Togo	1:133	Teaching	21
2007	Pakistan	1: 5556	University	21
2002	Ghana	1:1250		96
2007	Benin	1:103	University	106
1996–2004	Brazil	1:1020	Tertiary / teaching	107
1992–2006	Pakistan	1:2888	University/ teaching	108
1987	United Kingdom	1:185,000		21

Data from Walker and Wilson [21] and others [106–110].

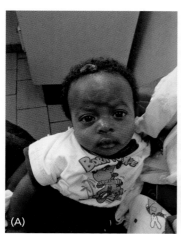
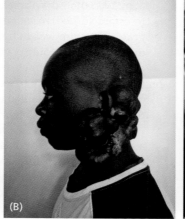
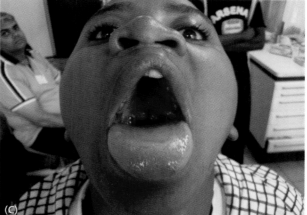

Figure 39.2 Traditional healers and tribal customs. Traditional healers play a significant role in healthcare. (A) A potion had been placed over this baby's fontanelle to close it. (B) Keloid. Extensive keloid formation after injury or tribal scarification is a common complication in Africa. Tribal ear piercing as a child led to this disfiguring keloid formation. Access to specialist treatment is limited. (C) Uvulectomy. This child had a uvulectomy performed to ward off "evil spirits" and treat a sore throat.

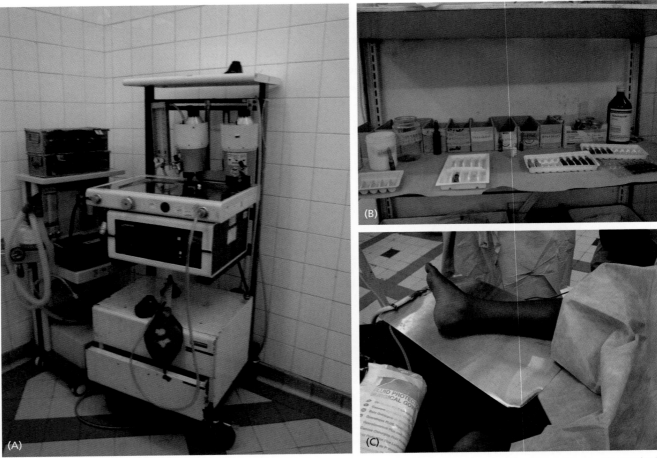

Figure 39.3 Anesthesia equipment. (A) Boyles machine. Considered obsolete in many developed countries, this machine was used to provide anesthesia for a newborn. The 2 L bag on the T piece was patched with zinc oxide tape and was used by the author to successfully resuscitate a newborn delivered by emergency caesarean section. (B) Drug cupboard. Anesthetic supplies are basic, similar colored glass ampoules are poorly labeled and almost illegible. The risks of administering the wrong drug, as a result, are high. (C) Diathermy. A steel plate with poor connections places the child at risk of an electrical burn.

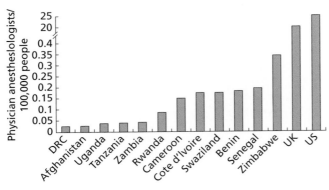

Figure 39.4 Anesthesia providers per 100,000 people. DRC, Democratic Republic of the Congo; UK, United Kingdom; US, United States. Data from Dubowitz et al [25] and Bridenbaugh [109].

In 1996 the Education Committee of the WFSA set out to establish pediatric anesthesia fellowship training programs. The aim was to train individuals from a medically disadvantaged country in a more medically advanced country, ideally in their own language [17]. Whether this training should take place on site within a given country or off site in an established program has been a topic of debate recently [31–39].

Through a WFSA-driven sponsorship program, a cohort of pediatric anesthesiologists is being trained in Chile [36], Tunisia, South Africa, and soon Kenya [17,32,35]. The advantage of this training is that the trainees are exposed to similar problems to those they would encounter in their own country. On completion of their training, they must return to their country of origin and champion the development of pediatric anesthesia as a speciality [2,17,32]. In those countries where a training program has been developed, the value of a pediatric anesthesiologist is enormous [17,35].

The vast majority of anesthetics are delivered by non-physicians [2,5,13,40], a reality that has remained constant over many decades. Supervision of "non-physician anesthetists" or "anesthetic officers" is invariably inadequate [31,32,41,42] and access to textbooks, journals or other medical literature is limited [2,5,13]. Internet access and communication, considered the norm in the developed world, are limited given that functional computers are scarce and electrical supplies and telecommunication networks are unreliable.

Some countries, such as Nigeria, Kenya and India, have trained significant numbers of physician anesthetists, but these physicians tend to practice in large hospitals in urban areas [2,6]. The majority of anesthetics in rural communities are still provided by nurses or unqualified personnel, with little medical background, who are "trained on the job" [2,5,13,40]. In many African [43] and Asian countries [44], the doctor/patient ratio is so low that the ideal of employing a physician specifically to provide routine anesthesia is out of the question [2,25,27]. Salaries are insufficient to attract suitably trained and qualified practitioners for more than short periods. Emigration of scarce trained personnel to developed countries in search of better salaries and an improved lifestyle exacerbates these shortages [2,26,27,45].

Equipment procurement and maintenance

Essential equipment to provide safe anesthesia for children, particularly neonates, is often lacking [2,12–14,16,40,46] (Fig. 39.3). Neonatal or pediatric ventilators are virtually non-existent outside the main centers [12]. Syringe pumps and other control devices are impractical in environments that have an erratic electricity supply. Laryngoscopes, both metal and plastic, are usually available but generally not well maintained. Even batteries may be in short supply and light bulbs unreliable. Endotracheal tubes in the full pediatric range are rarely found; disposable endotracheal tubes are consequently recycled [14] as there is little or no alternative. Laryngeal mask airways (LMA) in pediatric sizes are considered a luxury. Intravenous fluids are very expensive if not manufactured locally, and many developing countries do not have any local production facilities [6]. The choice of intravenous fluid is therefore limited and in relative short supply.

Unreliable electrical supplies add to the challenges in the developing world. In many hospitals, particularly in rural areas, neither mains electricity nor reliable and functional back-up generators are available [2,5,47]. General

facilities for infection control, such as running water, disinfectants or gloves (sterile or non-sterile), are not constantly available even though the reuse of disposable equipment is "normal" practice in many countries [5,13,14,48].

Anesthetic machines fall into two categories: modern sophisticated machines or simple low-maintenance equipment [47]. Modern electronic machines, provided by well-meaning international donors, have a poor track record in austere environments [1,2,12–14]. Sophisticated equipment needs to be understood but operating manuals provided in a foreign language are of no benefit. Sophisticated machines require maintenance and technicians trained to repair them. Service contracts are not considered viable. Unfortunately, these machines are consequently discarded when the first fault occurs. Guarantees are unlikely to be honored and faults are considered too expensive to repair. Poorly maintained equipment becomes hazardous and even life threatening in untrained hands [47].

Simplicity and safety have long been the key to anesthetic equipment in developing countries [6,13,14,49–51]. Ideally the anesthetic machine should be inexpensive, versatile, robust and able to withstand extreme climatic conditions (temperature (hot or cold), humidity, dust and altitude), able to function even if the supply of cylinders or electricity is interrupted, easy to understand and operate by those with limited training, economical to use, and easily maintained by locally available skills [51–53]. The cheapest, most practical, and most widely used anesthetic is inhalational anesthesia administered through an EMO (Epstein Macintosh Oxford) or OMV (Oxford miniature vaporizer) draw-over vaporizer [14]. Oxygen concentrators supplement oxygen delivery and eliminate the need for expensive oxygen cylinders whose reducing valves are often faulty or destroyed in austere environments. The most appropriate ventilator is the Manley multivent ventilator, which essentially functions like a mechanical version of the OIB (Oxford inflating bellows) and can be used with a draw-over system [53].

A general scheme for inhalation anesthesia in developing countries is shown in Figure 39.5 [54], first proposed by Ezi Ashi et al [55]. Four different modes can used and can be modified according to the available supplies and services. The basic mode A is for use when there is no electricity and no supply of compressed gases. The apparatus consists of a low-resistance vaporizer, linked by valves to the patient to act as a draw-over system with room air as the carrier gas. The self-inflating bag or hand bellows makes it possible to provide artificial ventilation while the vaporizer remains as a draw-over. The addition of low-flow oxygen to the inspired gas (mode B) is dependent on the availability of an oxygen cylinder. The addition of a length of reservoir tubing to the circuit

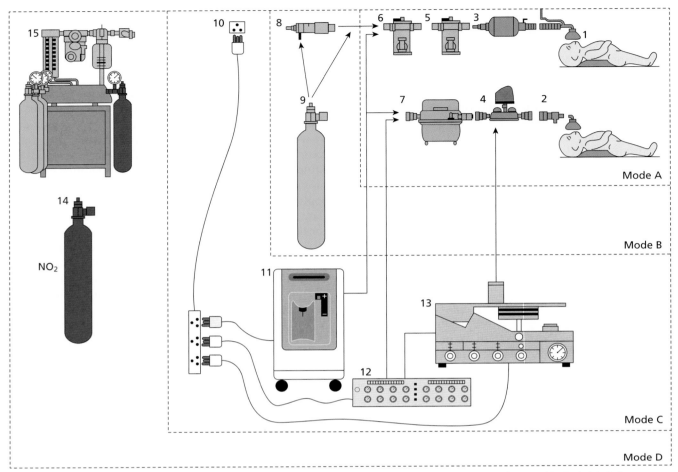

Figure 39.5 A schematic diagram of anesthetic systems that could be used depending on available resources. Mode A provides basic inhalation anesthesia with air, spontaneous ventilation or self-inflating bags. Draw-over vaporizers are required. Mode B provides oxygen enrichment but requires the availability of oxygen cylinders. Plenum vaporizers can be used. Mode C requires electricity to power the oxygen concentrator, air compressor, and/or ventilator. A mechanical ventilator, e.g. Manley, does not require electrical power. Mode D requires a Boyles machine and nitrous oxide cylinders. 1. T piece with reservoir tube and facemask; 2. Ambu Paedi valve; 3. self-inflating bag (Ambu); 4. Oxford inflating bellows (OIB); 5. Oxford miniature vaporizer (OMV) with halothane; 6. OMV with trichloroethylene; 7. EMO vaporizer with ether. These circuits and manual ventilators are interchangeable and ether, halothane, and trichloroethylene can be used on their own or in series. 8. Farman's entrainer with an oxygen cylinder (9) can be used to supplement oxygen or an electrical power source (10) is available with an oxygen concentrator (11), air compressor (12) or Manley ventilator (13). Nitrous oxide (14) and Boyles apparatus (15) allow anesthesia practice equivalent to that of developed countries.

enables oxygen to be stored on expiration, to be used on the next inspiration, making it substantially more economical [56].

When electricity is available (mode C) the operation of the anesthetic apparatus can be extended by permitting (a) the use of an air compressor to provide continuous gas flow (which in turn will allow the use of a Boyles apparatus and plenum vaporizer); (b) oxygen concentrator; and (c) ventilators. When nitrous oxide is available (mode D) all types of inhalation anesthesia currently available in developed countries can be practiced. In situations where services and supplies are interrupted even acutely, it is possible to change from one mode to another without requiring other anesthetic apparatus.

Draw-over anesthesia enables inhalation anesthesia to be administered using atmospheric air as the carrier gas [14]. The essential features of this system consist of a calibrated vaporizer with sufficiently low resistance (EMO and OMV) to allow the negative pressure created by the patient's inspiratory effort to draw room air through the vaporizer during spontaneous ventilation. Positive pressure ventilation can be provided by means of a self-inflating bag or bellows (OIB), with a valve to prevent the gas mixture re-entering the vaporizer, as well as a unidirectional valve at the patient's airway to direct expired gases to the atmosphere, preventing rebreathing (mode A, Fig. 39.5). In this way an anesthetic can be administered in the absence of compressed gases. The vaporizer has an inlet for supplementary oxygen that can be attached to the oxygen output tube of an oxygen concentrator, or oxygen cylinder if available (modes B and C, Fig. 39.5).

The EMO (Penlon Ltd) and the OMV (Penlon Ltd) are the more commonly used low-resistance vaporizers [14]. The EMO is only calibrated for ether but its performance is linear for other agents. The OMV is calibrated for a variety of agents [51,53]; despite the lack of temperature compensation, its performance is stable under most conditions. Both these vaporizers have been used successfully in pediatric anesthetic practice [23] but it is recommended that they be converted to form a T-piece for greater safety.

The OMV has been evaluated as a simple draw-over system for pediatric anesthesia. Wilson et al [46] showed that when a self-inflation bag is used in a draw-over mode, more efficient vaporization occurs despite vaporizer cooling. However, the respiratory efforts of neonates or weak infants are insufficient to operate the valve mechanisms of the self-inflating bag, e.g. Ambu bag, necessitating continuous assisted ventilation even in the presence of ether, which stimulates ventilation.

Oxygen concentrators can improve oxygen availability, independent of compressed gas and electrical power supply, by linking oxygen concentrators to a draw-over anesthetic apparatus as first described by Fenton [14,57]. Maintenance requirements are low and servicing is recommended only after approximately 10,000 hours of usage. The benefits are enormous but a reliable electricity supply is critical.

The concentrator functions by using a compressor to pump ambient air alternately through one of two canisters containing a molecular sieve of zeolite granules that reversibly absorbs nitrogen from compressed air [53,58]. The controls are simple and comprise an on/off switch for the compressor and a flow-control knob to deliver 0–5 L/min. Flow of oxygen continues uninterrupted as the canisters are alternated automatically so that oxygen from one canister is available while the other regenerates. A warning light on a built-in oxygen analyzer illuminates if the oxygen concentration is <85% and the concentrator switches off automatically when the oxygen concentration is <70%. This is heralded by visual and audible alarms. Air is then delivered as the effluent gas. Modern machines are relatively silent.

The oxygen output of the concentrator depends on the size of the unit, the inflow of oxygen, the minute volume, and pattern of ventilation. The addition of dead space (or oxygen economizer tube) at the outlet improves the performance, and predictable concentrations >90% oxygen can be obtained with flows between 1 and 5 L/min independent of the pattern of ventilation. Much lower concentrations and less predictability were noted when the dead space tubing was omitted [56].

The possible hazards of oxygen concentrators are few, provided they are positioned in the operating room so that the in-draw area is free from pollutants. Failure of power supply or failure of the zeolite canisters will result in the delivery of ambient air. A bacterial filter at the outlet combined with the use of dust-free zeolite should prevent contamination of the delivered gas. Dirty internal air filters may produce lower oxygen concentrations and must be checked. An oxygen storage tank and booster pumps afford protection against the vagaries in electrical supply.

Intravenous fluid administration must also be given careful consideration [2]. Small intravenous cannulas are a precious commodity and butterfly needles are still used (and in some cases reused!) [59]. Syringe pumps and other control devices are impractical in environments that have an erratic electricity supply [2]. Unmonitored IVs can have disastrous consequences including volume overload, sepsis, tissue loss, compartment syndrome or even loss of limb [2]. The choice of intravenous fluid is often limited and in short supply [2,53,60].

Evaluation of patients

The burden of disease in the poorest countries is formidable. Children of the developing world are victims of circumstance, natural disasters, war, social unrest, and economic crises [8,12,61–65]. An estimated 10 million children die annually before their 5th birthday [5,64,66]; that is one of every six children born in Africa, and one of every 12 children born in South Asia [5]. Approximately 50% of these deaths occur in the neonatal period [5] and birth asphyxia, prematurity, sepsis, and tetanus are the major causes. In the older child diarrhea, pneumonia, malaria, HIV/AIDS, measles, and trauma are major causes [5,64,67].

For many in rural areas, timely access to medical care is a remote possibility (Figs 39.1, 39.6) [59,60]. Fear, poor understanding, and lack of education often result in delayed presentation to medical facilities [13,68–70]. Illiterate people in rural areas may simply not be aware that surgical treatment is possible [14]. Superstition may also play a role in compounding the anesthetic risk. Frequently, well-meaning traditional healers have had prior involvement, exposing the child to additional risk (see Fig. 39.2) [2,15,71] caused by potions that may be hepatic-renal toxins or enemas that may perforate the bowel [72–74]. Further delays are engendered when patients have to undertake long journeys to hospital. As a result, dehydration, infection, sepsis, and complications compound the surgical problem and the anesthetic risk. Tertiary referral is often only made when complications arise [8,12,13,40,47,73–75].

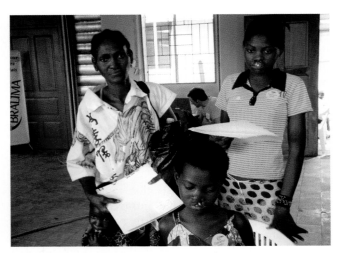

Figure 39.6 Cleft lip and palate. In many developing countries worldwide the failure to provide surgical services may lead to lifelong disability, social exclusion or even premature death. This family all had an isolated cleft lip that had remained unrepaired until they were successfully treated during a volunteer mission with Operation Smile.

Perinatal mortality in some parts of the developing world is 10 times greater than that in developed countries [5,66]. The common denominators include early child-bearing, poor maternal health and, above all, the lack of appropriate and quality medical services. One-third of pregnant women still have no access to medical services during pregnancy, and almost 50% do not have access to medical services for childbirth [12,61,65]. The majority of parturients deliver at home or in rural health centres [61] where basic neonatal resuscitation equipment is often deficient or non-existent [12]. Those who require surgery may need to be transferred, but specialized transport teams rarely exist.

The safe administration of anesthesia should take into account the pre-existing condition of the child. Preoperative investigations are generally limited, perhaps stretching to hemoglobin and screening for malarial parasites. There are few functional laboratories in the rural areas and trained technicians are virtually non-existent. Similarly, radiographic studies are often rudimentary and of poor quality [2,9,14]. Even an experienced anesthesiologist with minimal access to laboratory or radiographic investigations and limited in the choice of resuscitation fluid would be challenged to manage these children.

Co-morbidities need to be excluded or treated prior to elective surgery. Tuberculosis (TB) remains an important cause of morbidity and mortality [40,76]. The epidemiology of pediatric tuberculosis is shaped by risk factors such as age, race, immigration, poverty, overcrowding, and HIV/AIDS [48,76–79]. The emergence of drug-resistant tuberculosis adds to the burden and is a constant danger to healthcare workers in general and anesthesiologists in particular.

Primary TB infection usually does not produce clinical illness in well-nourished immunized children, whereas reactivated pulmonary tuberculosis is a chronic or subacute disease, which may present a variety of challenges for the anesthesiologist. These range from a need to prevent transmission by contamination of the anesthetic circuits to the risks associated with pleural effusions, pulmonary cavitation, and bronchiectasis. Mediastinal and hilar lymphadenopathy may severely compromise the airway.

Primary TB and its complications are more common in children than in adults. Once infected, young children are at risk of progression to extrapulmonary disease [76,77]. *Mycobacterium tuberculosis* can cause symptomatic disease in any organ, and is usually a reactivation of a latent site of infection. The most common sites of reactivation are lymph nodes, bones, joints, and the genitourinary tract. Less frequently, the disease may involve the gastrointestinal tract, peritoneum, pericardium or skin. TB meningitis and miliary TB, both more common in children, carry a high mortality [76]. In view of the high prevalence of HIV infection in tuberculous children, HIV testing should be performed on all children with TB; conversely TB should be sought in all HIV-positive children [78].

Rheumatic heart disease is more common than congenital heart disease in many developing countries, reflecting the socio-economic problems of poverty, overcrowding, malnutrition, and lack of antibiotics. Children often present late with life-threatening symptoms secondary to repeated infections and superimposed endocarditis. The acute deterioration precipitated by endocarditis may be the factor that prompts the search for medical attention. Valve replacement can be life saving but long-term follow-up of anticoagulant therapy is not feasible without laboratory facilities nearby.

Malaria is caused by one of four species of malaria parasites: *Plasmodium falciparum, P. vivax, P. ovale,* and *P. malariae.* Effective and safe prophylaxis against malaria has become increasingly difficult because the species that causes the most severe illness, *P. falciparum,* has become widely resistant to chloroquine and in some areas to other antimalarial drugs as well [80]. Severe malaria even when optimally treated carries a mortality of 10–25% [80]. Prompt diagnosis and early treatment are important determinants of outcome.

Uncomplicated malaria usually presents with flu-like symptoms (fever, headache, dizziness and arthralgia). Gastrointestinal symptoms may predominate and include anorexia, nausea, vomiting and abdominal discomfort or pain that may mimic appendicitis. Malaria in children can present with an acute life-threatening disease or run a chronic course with acute exacerbations. The acute manifestations include three overlapping syndromes: respiratory distress secondary to a severe underlying metabolic acidosis (pH <7.3), usually a lactic acidemia, severe anemia (Hb <5) that can develop hypovolemia very rapidly even within hours [81], and neurological impairment as a manifestation of cerebral malaria. Seizures are an important presenting feature in 60–80% of cases. Prolonged seizures that are refractory to treatment and those that occur on antimalarial treatment are ominous signs and are usually associated with neurological sequelae or death [81].

Children with chronic malaria adjust physiologically to low hemoglobin levels but may decompensate rapidly when challenged with a febrile illness or surgery. The characteristic physical findings in children with severe anemia are respiratory distress and a hyperdynamic circulation. Blood transfusion may be administered rapidly in these children with metabolic acidosis since most have a depleted intravascular volume. Although controversial, exchange transfusion has been advocated for severe malaria. Unfortunately, many malaria endemic areas also have a high prevalence of HIV, adding significantly to the risk of blood transfusions.

Chronic recurrent malarial infections may manifest with splenic enlargement. This may cause delayed gastric emptying and pose an aspiration risk on induction of anesthesia. The spleen may also enlarge acutely or rupture spontaneously during coughing, vomiting or defecation. Rupture during external cardiac massage has also been described. Malaria may cause bloody diarrhea with massive loss of fluid resembling dysentery in children. Development of renal failure with severe malaria is not uncommon. Malaria may present preoperatively or may complicate the postoperative course. Children in endemic areas who develop postoperative fever must be investigated for malaria. This is especially true if they have had a blood transfusion.

Types of surgery

It is estimated that 85% of children in developing countries will require surgery of some sort before their 15th birthday [4]. Congenital anomalies, trauma (road traffic accidents, assaults, falls, burns, bites, fractures), and infections (abscess, osteomyelitis) make up the bulk of the surgical workload [11–13,68,71]. Burns, particularly in young children, affect resources in many developing countries [60] but especially in sub-Saharan Africa [59].

While the burden of disease is dominated by infections and malnutrition [48], pediatric trauma has low advocacy and as such is given scant attention [5,12,40,68]. Socioeconomic advances in some countries have introduced a new danger in the form of faster, more powerful vehicles without the necessary maintenance culture or road discipline. Trauma prevention strategies are given low priority despite the acknowledged impact it has on the economy of any country. Road traffic accidents are thus inevitable.

Additionally, many developing countries are at war and this has led to massive trauma and injuries to children who are both participants in the fighting and innocent bystanders. Effective systems to handle the polytrauma victims that result are hard to find [40]. Even simple bone fractures may have disastrous outcomes. Inappropriate management by traditional bonesetters can result in compartment syndromes or even gangrene [71].

Many pathological conditions, seldom seen in industrialized countries, are more prevalent in developing countries because of poor health education, malnutrition, the close proximity of livestock to humans, earth-floored homes, poor sanitation, and contaminated water supplies.

In some hospitals, neonates are not considered candidates for surgery because "they always die" [56] whereas in others, they undergo surgery without anesthesia [82] because "it's safer" and some still believe that neonates do not feel pain. When surgery is performed on neonates, there are additional challenges, particularly in emergency situations [61]. Not only is there a lack of appropriately sized equipment [40] but it may be extremely difficult to maintain normothermia even in relatively warm climates, let alone provide ventilatory support.

Regrettably, even neonates who have skilful anesthesia and surgery may die because of inadequate postoperative care [13,83]. Overwhelming infection, sepsis, respiratory insufficiency, and surgical complications are the main causes of morbidity and mortality [12,61]. The development of highly specialized neonatal anesthetic and surgical services [51,82,83], essential for a good outcome after neonatal surgery [12,40,61], is a low priority.

Anesthesia monitoring and drugs

In a recent survey, only 13% of anesthesiologists were able to provide safe anesthesia for children [2]. In this survey the minimal requirements for anesthesia were an oxygen supply, suction apparatus, a pulse oximeter, a tilting table, a pediatric breathing circuit, a laryngoscope, facemasks, endotracheal tubes, oropharyngeal airways, and intravenous cannulas suitable for use in children [2]. Implausible as these findings may seem to those who have not experienced the austere conditions in some parts of the developing world, many anecdotal reports, both recent and in the past, bear witness to this stark reality.

Monitoring is therefore very basic – a precordial stethoscope or a finger on the pulse [6]. Electrocardiogram (ECG) monitoring is used when available but is also dependent on a constant supply of electricity, ECG pads, and proper maintenance. Appropriately sized blood pressure cuffs are scarce, non-invasive blood pressure monitors even more so. Even though pulse oximetry has been shown to be the most useful monitor, and should be available in all centers where pediatric surgery is performed [6,12], this ideal is far from reality. Recently global pulse oximetry has become the aim of a recent WHO initiative (Millennium Goal 4) [5,20]. The current standard of monitoring expected in the developed world is unrealistic.

The supply of anesthetic gases and drugs, particularly to rural medical facilities, is erratic and unreliable [5,14]. Furthermore, the cost of many drugs, particularly the modern agents, has risen beyond the reach of most health budgets. Anesthesiologists in developing countries therefore have to resign themselves to using cheaper agents or generics.

Ether and halothane remain the mainstay of anesthesia in many countries [2,9,13,23,58]. Unfortunately, ether, and more recently halothane, has virtually disappeared from operating rooms in the developed world. As a result, the demand for these cheaper agents has fallen and lack of profitability claimed by some manufacturers has threatened the withdrawal of halothane [1,14]. While this may make commercial business sense, these agents sustain the anesthesia services for millions of patients in the developing world and their loss would have a huge impact [1,14].

In many remote rural areas anesthesia for children remains largely ketamine based [5,13,14,82,84], even when halothane or ether is available. Lack of airway equipment such as tracheal tubes, facemasks or breathing circuits and the perception that intravenous access is not necessary are further reasons for its popularity in this setting [5,69,85]. Ketamine is simple to use, relatively inexpensive, provides anesthesia, analgesia, and cardiovascular stability and some preservation of the airway reflexes [2,6,69]. Ideally ketamine should be used with midazolam to reduce the hallucinatory side-effects. Benzodiazepines, however, are not commonly available.

For developing countries, the cost of nitrous oxide is prohibitive in terms of storage, erratic delivery, and budgetary constraints [55,57]. Closed or semi-closed anesthetic systems are considered dangerous in an environment where the oxygen supply is erratic [45] and agent monitors are not available [14,47]. The erratic supply of soda lime and compressed gas cylinders further limits it use. Consequently, the potential benefits and cost savings of low-flow anesthesia are lost [55]. Scavenging is almost non-existent.

The choice of muscle relaxants is also limited [13]. Suxamethonium, gallamine, curare, alcuronium, or pancuronium are the usual options, and the choice is dictated by their availability or the availability of reversal agents. For this reason, muscle relaxants are not commonly used. Other drugs considered basic to anesthesia are seldom available in the developing world [2,5,13,23]. These include induction agents (propofol), analgesics (morphine, pethidine), reversal agents (naloxone), and long-acting local anesthetics (bupivacaine, ropivacaine).

Opioid analgesia may not be permitted in some cultures. The ability to deal with complications, such as malignant hyperthermia, is virtually non-existent. Dantrolene is simply too expensive and the shelf-life too short to be cost-effective.

Regional anesthesia has many benefits, in terms of safety, cost savings, and immediate postoperative analgesia [6,12,40,41,61,83,86–89]. Generally, children in developing countries are very accepting of this form of analgesia. However, there seems to be a general reluctance to perform regional anesthesia in children [13,40,90] even in some institutions in the developed world. Possible reasons include lack of training or expertise, fear of failure, and the unavailability of drugs, disposables, and other ancillary equipment (nerve stimulators, portable ultrasound) [41]. Improvisation may be the key. Access to the epidural space can be obtained if the appropriate equipment is not available by using a technique first described before the introduction of pediatric epidural needles into clinical practice. A catheter can be threaded well into the epidural space through an intravenous cannula inserted into the caudal space via the sacral hiatus in neonates and small infants [91]. Furthermore, cheap non-insulated needles can be used, with a nerve stimulator, for peripheral nerve blocks when more expensive insulated needles are not available [92].

Postoperative pain relief

Pain management in children is another factor that divides the developed world from the developing world. Providing pain relief in the face of limited resources, a limited spectrum of analgesics, if available, and inadequately trained staff is a challenge [2,13,14]. Attempting to apply similar standards to those used in sophisticated units is fraught with difficulty. Illiteracy, malnutrition, poor cognitive development, differing coping strategies, pharmacogenetic, cultural, and language differences all add to the complexity of the problem [93,94].

Children of the developing world learn to cope with vastly different problems. Their attitude towards pain, and tolerance thereof, is different. Children from an impoverished background seem more stoical and indifferent to even severe pain. Following cardiac surgery, for example, some appear to need very little pain relief and are easily soothed by lollipops or play therapy [62].

Pain assessment of children from an impoverished background is difficult and may be inaccurate [93,94,95]. Many children in acute pain do not show facial expression. Is this stoicism or simply a reflection of malnutrition, lack of social stimulation, severity of illness or even cultural attitude? Language difficulties, cultural barriers, willingness to share information, emotional expressiveness, and outdated attitudes of the caregiver may sanction this quandary [93,94]. Some societies convey pain readily, while others teach that expression of pain is inappropriate. In many parts of Africa boys are not supposed to express pain. Reporting the pain of testicular torsion, for example, may be delayed and would be considered taboo if the boy lives with his mother only.

Although there are many pain assessment instruments available, few have been validated in children from the developing world [93,94]. There is an urgent need not only to make analgesics universally available but also to develop strategies that can be safely applied to the children of the developing world. Local conditions will dictate their use and applicability. Simple pain management strategies may produce the most benefit with the least risk whereas more complex techniques, that offer the most benefit, require a minimum standard of monitoring and regular reassessment to allow individualized titration of analgesia. These are seldom available. The final choice of analgesia, unfortunately, is dictated by economic pressures or by the facilities available rather than what would be considered in the best interest of the child. Nonetheless, it is morally, ethically and physiologically beneficial to provide children with effective analgesia despite the immense inequalities that exist in our world [93].

Follow-up care

Perioperative morbidity and mortality are understandably high by developed world standards [5,13,47,49,84]. Facilities considered mandatory for the surgical care of children, such as the provision of adequate analgesia, a recovery area for immediate postoperative observation, ventilatory support or high care following surgery [9,12–14], are inadequate or non-existent in many parts of the developing world. In some countries pediatric surgery is even considered too expensive to justify these additional needs [12,13].

There is precious little information on the anesthesia morbidity or mortality in developing countries [13,49,50,95]. Fisher et al reported on the incidence of anesthesia-related problems seen by volunteer services working over 18 months [49], which reflects the quality assurance data of trained anesthesia providers working in the developing countries. This is vastly different to the reality where the risks associated with surgery and anesthesia vary widely [22,25] (see Table 39.1). For example, in Ghana a 0.08% mortality for elective surgery was recently reported [96] while there was a 20% mortality for intestinal obstruction of the newborn in a Nigerian teaching hospital [97].

We have little idea of the incidence of problems associated with anesthesia provided by non-physicians,

nurses or unqualified personnel "trained on the job" [13,22,98,99]. In some areas, even today, neonatal surgery may be performed without anesthesia [83] or simply under local infiltration only [84,97,100,101] in an attempt to improve outcome. Understandably, late presentation, respiratory failure, infection or anesthetic complications [83,100,101] are still the major contributors to a poor outcome.

Follow-up care is generally poor. The follow-up visit is generally not considered worth the added financial burden. Long distances, lack of transport, and poor telecommunications prevent patients from returning. Even patients who live nearby are lost to follow-up and seldom return unless there are complications.

Conclusion

The practice of anesthesia in a developing country will always be challenging, particularly for those who provide anesthesia for children. The challenges vary and it is wise to expect the unexpected and have the flexibility to improvise in the face of an ever-changing world racked by famine, war, violence, natural disasters, and political unrest. The nuances of practice in different communities will inevitably vary and may even challenge some fondly held beliefs in pediatric anesthesia.

Different standards may emerge from different parts of the world. Such standards need not necessarily be considered inferior but may well open the way for the assimilation of new ideas [103]. A safe anesthetic is not necessary the most expensive one. After all, it is generally not the agents that we use but the skill with which we use them that determines outcome. It should never be necessary to depart from the dictum *primum non nocere*. Simplicity may be the key, but there is no place for double standards. Guidelines evolved over time in the UK, USA, and Australia [103,104] may be untenable in many parts of the world, but every attempt should be made to exercise the same standard of care as expected in the developed countries. Our children deserve no less!

What can be done to improve the lot of children who undergo anesthesia in the developing world? Audits of morbidity and mortality are the first steps towards improvement provided action is taken to address the problems uncovered. Publications reflecting outcomes in developing countries have increased over the past decade [105–108] (see Table 39.1). Sending money is another suggestion [105] but unfortunately, with all the goodwill in the world, there is no guarantee that money will ever reach the right people and be put to the best use. Purchasing equipment without subsequent maintenance is wasteful. Disposables are short-lived even if they are recycled. Human resources are needed!

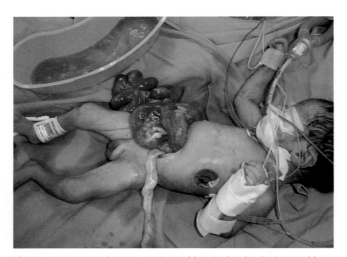

Figure 39.7 Gastroschisis is a major problem in the developing world. The outcome is poor because of a paucity of facilities for neonates. This baby with significant intrauterine growth retardation was not diagnosed antenatally and presented late for closure. The risk of sepsis is high. The bowel content (kidney dish) was emptied as far as possible to facilitate closure. Postoperative ventilatory support was not available.

Attracting trained anesthesiologists to work in the developing world is the challenge [1,108–110]. Temporary sojourns with volunteer medical groups are for the most part stimulating but few, if any, of these volunteers are likely to return for longer periods, let alone permanently. Is it the environment? Is it the lack of home comforts? Is it the family that finds it difficult? How much influence does political uncertainty have? Unfortunately, until these questions and many others can be addressed, anesthesia in the developing world, particularly for children, is unlikely to advance [1].

The WHO has also recognized that surgery is a public health issue and has launched the 'Safe Surgery Saves Lives' program. The WHO has also emphasized that safe surgery does not exist without safe anesthesia [2,19–21]. Training anesthesiologists in the skills required for pediatric anesthesia is a slow process. It is hoped that the WFSA program [105] will soon snowball so that children undergoing surgery in developing countries will reap the benefit.

CASE STUDY

A 1.8 kg newborn male with gastroschisis presented to the emergency room of the regional hospital. The baby had been delivered in a remote hut in a village some 5 h away. His mother, an 18-year-old primigravida, had not attended antenatal clinic because she lived at least a 1 h walk away from the nearest clinic. Her HIV status was unknown. The baby, whose gestational age was unknown, was delivered by a "traditional midwife" who after resuscitation had wrapped the baby in towels and sent the mother to the nearest clinic for further management. On arrival at the clinic after an hour's walk, the baby was clearly hypothermic, had a weak cry and the bowel, that had extruded further, was covered with a green film suggesting meconium staining.

At this point the baby's lower body was placed in a plastic bag and the local ambulance driver was notified that the baby needed to be transported to the regional hospital. The ambulance was undergoing repairs but would only be ready in an hour. There were no IV fluids or antibiotics available at the clinic. There were no laboratory facilities to check the blood glucose, hematocrit, electrolytes or acid–base status; the bottle of "Dextrostix" had expired. The initial examination had been conducted in semi-darkness because of another temporary power outage.

The ambulance finally arrived 2 h later and needed to refuel *en route*. On arrival at the regional hospital, the baby's temperature was 34.1°C. The blood glucose measured 25 mg/dL, the urea was elevated and the hematocrit was 54%. No incubator was available, but the child was warmed with an overhead radiant heater. The gastroschisis

was wrapped in cling film, and the child was prepared for surgery. The surgeon was not immediately available because he was busy with an ectopic pregnancy.

A peripheral IV line was started and a bolus of 10 mL/kg Ringer's lactate was given for resuscitation. Glucose was added after the initial resuscitation. Antibiotics in the form of ampicillin and gentamicin were given intravenously. The general surgeon, who had been working all night, became available after completion of the ectopic pregnancy. The baby was taken to the operating room, anesthesia was induced with halothane, and the trachea was intubated after suxamethonium administration. No other muscle relaxants were available. The lungs were hand-ventilated with a modified Ayre's T piece by the anesthetist who had recently completed his 6 months of "training on the job." There was no scavenging system or suitable ventilator for postoperative ventilatory support. The surgeon aimed to achieve primary closure to improve the chances of survival. A caudal block using 2.5 mL/kg 0.25% bupivacaine with epinephrine 1:400,000 was placed by the visiting anesthesiologist using a 22 G scalp vein needle. The surgeon, in an attempt to reduce the bowel volume, managed to "milk" approximately 30 mL of meconium from the bowel using normal saline irrigation through a Jacques red rubber catheter (Fig. 39.7). The bladder was also emptied (3 mL) using Crede's method since there were no urinary catheters available. If primary closure was not possible the surgeon aimed to fashion a "silastic" bag from an intravenous bag. Fortunately this was not needed.

Primary closure was achieved with difficulty. The abdomen was tense but the dorsalis pedis pulse was palpable and there was good capillary refill of both feet. The baby was able to breathe spontaneously but there was no way to measure the increase in airway pressure, blood gases or capnography to evaluate respiratory function. The residual effects of the caudal provided analgesia and some degree of motor block without respiratory depression. Ideally, a caudal catheter could provide continuous or intermittent blockade, but neither a caudal catheter nor a functional infusion pump was available.

The closure was completed within 9 h of delivery. Although closure was achieved as soon as possible, the delay was expected to have a negative influence on the outcome because of the high risk of sepsis [83,102]. The mother's positive HIV status became apparent and both mother and child were started on antiretroviral therapy. The HIV status was not expected to affect the baby's outcome [79].

Early initiation of total parenteral nutrition (TPN) would have been ideal but was not possible because of the budgetary limitations in the regional hospital. Furthermore, neither central venous access nor peripherally inserted central catheters (PICC) were available nor could they be performed at this hospital. Ten percent glucose in quarter normal saline was the only IV fluid available to provide some calories, but its use placed the infant at significant risk of hyponatremia-induced convulsions.

The postoperative course was stormy, punctuated by episodes of sepsis related to infiltrated peripheral IVs, wound sepsis, and minor dehiscence. Enteral nutrition was tolerated by 28 days of age and the baby was discharged after 40 days in hospital and referred for follow-up at the surgery and the HIV clinics.

Annotated references

A full reference list for this chapter is available at:
http://www.wiley.com/go/gregory/andropoulos/pediatricanesthesia

2. Hodges SC, Mijumbi C, Okello M, McCormick REM, Walker IA, Wilson IH. Anesthesia services in developing countries: defining the problems. Anaesthesia 2007; 62: 4–11. The shocking reality of the anesthetic services in the Ugandan health system is conveyed in the results of this survey. Twenty-three percent of anesthesia providers, representative of hospitals with an average annual surgical caseload of around 7500, could provide safe anesthesia for adults, 13% for children and only 6% for caesarean section. Lack of facilities, i.e. no electrical supply in 41% hospitals, unreliable oxygen source in 20% and running water in only 56%, affects the whole healthcare system.

4. Andrews G, Skinner D, Zuma K. Epidemiology of health and vulnerability among children orphaned and made vulnerable by HIV/AIDS in sub-Saharan Africa. AIDS Care 2006; 18: 269–76. The many aspects of the HIV/AIDS epidemic in poor countries are outlined. The social, economic, and health issues affect children in the poorest countries that cannot afford to their treat HIV-infected citizens. Difficult decisions need to be made based on the limited available resources.

5. Walker IA Morton NS. Pediatric healthcare – the role of anesthesia and critical care services in the developing world. Paediatr Anaesth 2009; 19: 1–4. Anesthesia is closely linked to intensive care. Limited resources (trained doctors and nurses, equipment) combine to challenge the delivery of critical care in countries where patients present with advanced disease. See also reference 13.

12. Mhando S, Lyamuya S, Lakhoo K. Challenges in developing paediatric surgery in sub-Saharan Africa. Pediatr Surg Int 2006; 22: 425–7. This paper gives the surgical perspective of the pathology and difficult challenges a pediatric surgeon in sub-Saharan Africa faces when managing a neonate or child with no trained anesthetists or facilities for the postoperative care management of their patients.

14. McCormick BA, Eltringham RJ. Anaesthesia equipment for resource poor environments. Anaesthesia 2007; 62(Suppl 1): 54–60. The choice of equipment is vital in developing countries. Simple, functional, reliable, and easily maintained equipment is vital to providing safe anesthesia in austere environments. This recent publication supports Ezi Ashi et al's suggestions (reference 55) made in 1983.

25. Dubowitz G, Detlefs S, McQueen KA. Global anesthesia workforce crisis: a preliminary survey revealing shortages contributing to undesirable outcomes and unsafe practices. World J Surg 2010; 34(3): 438–44. The authors provide up-to-date information on the level of training and anesthetic manpower in developing countries. The countries with the lowest anesthetists per capita working with limited resources not surprisingly have the greatest perioperative morbidity and mortality.

27. Eastwood JB, Conroy RE, Naicker S et al. Loss of health professionals from sub-Saharan Africa: the pivotal role of the UK. Lancet 2005; 365: 1893–900. Healthcare professionals who have the qualifications seek employment in developed countries for many reasons. Inadequate remuneration, huge student loans, inadequate resources, and heavy workload are some of the frustrations of medical practice in their home countries. They are welcomed in developed countries because they have broad clinical experience and are hardworking.

60. Forjuoh SN. Burns in low- and middle-income countries: a review of available literature on descriptive epidemiology, risk factors, treatment and prevention. Burns 2006; 32: 529–37. Burns are the scourge of healthcare systems in developing countries. The results of a Medline search are presented in this publication which gives insight into the causes, initial management, and prevention of burns in the developing world. The authors suggest that anesthetists should be involved in the resuscitation and pain management of these children. Unfortunately healthcare systems place little emphasis on prevention.

79. Karpelowsky JS, Leva E, Kelley B, Numanoglu A, Rode H, Millar AJ. Outcomes of human immunodeficiency virus-infected and -exposed children undergoing surgery – a prospective study. J Pediatr Surg 2009; 44(4): 681–7. HIV-infected patients have not been offered optimum care in developing countries because it is believed that the outcome after surgery is poor. This prospective study shows that there is no difference compared to those patients who are not HIV infected.

110. Dubowitz G. Global health and global anesthesia. Int Anesth Clin 2010; 48(2): 39–46. Current information with regard to global health and surgical outcome is provided together with strategies to improve the situation worldwide. Perhaps most importantly the adage that "safe surgery saves lives" has been recognized by those who have the resources to bring about a change.

CHAPTER 40
Clinical Complications in Pediatric Anesthesia

Randall Flick

Department of Anesthesiology, Mayo Clinic, Rochester, MN, USA

Introduction

Complications in the perioperative care of children range from very minor to devastating. This chapter describes some of the most common and severe complications that may be encountered in the day-to-day care of children in the perioperative environment. Limited space prohibits an exhaustive review of all the existing data pertaining to the topic, and for many complications, data, especially pediatric-specific data, are either lacking or insufficient to provide the reader with thoughtful guidance. Nonetheless, for many commonly encountered situations and most serious problems, data are available for clinicians to develop strategies and to stratify risk in a way that allows them to provide the best care possible to the children under their care. Covered in this chapter are cardiac arrest, malignant hyperthermia, toxicity to local anesthetics, propofol infusion syndrome, positioning injuries, latex allergy, and anaphylaxis.

Cardiac arrest in the pediatric perioperative period

It is widely recognized and a credit to the field that the risk of major morbidity or mortality experienced by both adults and children undergoing a procedure requiring anesthesia has declined dramatically over a generation. Mortality, the most robust measure of outcome in pediatric anesthesia, has declined along with a similar decline in adult perioperative mortality. Figure 40.1 shows the decline in mortality observed among children over the past 50 years [1–14]. Pediatric mortality rates have in the past been assumed to be greater than those for adults; however, recent data suggest that except for infants, rates for children and younger adults are similar. The mortality rates among children undergoing non-cardiac surgery range from 0.4 to 1.6 per 10,000 anesthetics [13,15]. However, among infants and especially those undergoing cardiac surgery, mortality rates are much higher [13,16].

Gregory's Pediatric Anesthesia, Fifth Edition. Edited by George A. Gregory, Dean B. Andropoulos.
© 2012 Blackwell Publishing Ltd. Published 2012 by Blackwell Publishing Ltd.

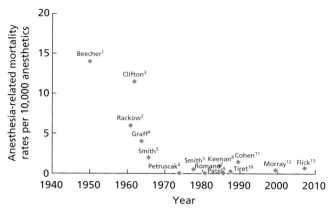

Figure 40.1 Anesthesia-related mortality rates in children from studies published between 1950 and 2000; the year of publication is indicated by the author's last name. Adapted from Morray [14] with permission from Elsevier.

Great care must be used when comparing rates of cardiac arrest (CA) or mortality because patient type, setting, procedure, and age distribution have a profound impact on the frequency and outcome of CA among pediatric patients. Also important are factors such as the span of time over which cases are ascertained and whether the cases are gathered from one or many institutions because practice varies over time and from one institution to another. Finally, of obvious importance is the accuracy of denominators because incidence can be determined only if total case volume is available. Recent studies have defined the incidence of CA in the pediatric population. Flick et al [13] at the Mayo Clinic reported the incidence of CA among more than 92,000 children undergoing anesthesia between 1988 and 2005. They found an overall rate of CA of 8.6 per 10,000 anesthetics, with those undergoing cardiac surgery having a dramatically higher incidence than that observed among those undergoing non-cardiac procedures (127 per 10,000 versus 2.9 per 10,000). These findings were similar to those of Odegard et al at Boston Children's [16], Tay et al in Singapore [17], and Braz et al in Brazil [18]. Each of these studies was derived from a single institution and therefore provides accurate estimates of incidence but they are less well suited to providing insight into cause and consequence of the events.

The most important contribution to the existing knowledge related to pediatric CA in the operative setting comes from the Pediatric Perioperative Cardiac Arrest (POCA) Registry. The POCA Registry was created at the University of Washington in 1994 as an extension of the American Society of Anesthesiologists (ASA) Closed Claims Project and was supported by the American Academy of Pediatrics Section on Anesthesiology and Pain Medicine. In 1985, the

ASA Committee on Professional Liability, with the co-operation of 28 insurance providers, began collecting data obtained from closed malpractice cases in the United States. In 1993, Morray and colleagues [19] reported a comparison of pediatric and adult closed claims and found that claims in children disproportionately involved infants, healthy children (ASA Physical Status (PS) I), death or permanent injury, and deficiencies in anesthesia care. Claims paid for malpractice involving pediatric care tended to be higher than those paid for adults.

To further study complications arising during the anesthetic care of children, the POCA Registry has subsequently provided valuable insights into the risk factors and outcomes associated with pediatric perioperative CA [12]. The registry, now closed, collected data from pediatric anesthesia practices throughout the United States and Canada and then reported their findings. The initial report was made in 2000 and provided data gathered from 63 institutions that had submitted a total of 289 cases of CA in children [12]. A subsequent report was published in 2007 [20].

The POCA Registry compiled CA data from as many as 79 primarily academic institutions and in its most recent report provided information on 397 cases covering a 7-year period. Reports from the POCA Registry grouped events as either related or unrelated to anesthesia and focused the analysis primarily on those judged to be anesthesia related. When comparing data from the first report (289 cases, 1994–1997) to the second report (397 cases, 1998–2004; 193 anesthesia related), the distribution of cases judged to be anesthesia related was similar at 52% and 49%, respectively. These rates are higher than those observed by Flick et al [13] (18%) when the POCA definition of anesthesia related was applied to the Mayo data. Likewise, in a series of 41 arrests among children undergoing cardiac procedures, Odegard et al [16] found that 26.8% were anesthesia related, and Braz et al [18] found that 20% were anesthesia related [21]. The designation of anesthesia related is obviously subjective but allows for the elimination of cases from review that might obscure important patterns, risk factors, or causes.

The children at greatest risk have been identified by Morray et al [12] and others [13,17,20] and include higher ASA PS rating, young age (neonates and infants), presence of congenital heart disease, and the need for emergency procedures. In the initial report from the POCA Registry, 32% of anesthesia-related CA occurred in children who were ASA PS classes 1 and 2, whereas in the subsequent report, the frequency of CA in PS 1 and 2 children had fallen to 25%. Over a similar time period, Braz et al [18] found in all CA that only four of 35 arrests (11%) occurred among the healthiest children. Flick et al [13] found that, among those undergoing non-cardiac surgery, half the 26 CAs occurred in children who were

ASA PS 3 or less. Clearly, the higher the ASA PS is, the greater the risk of complications of all types, including CA [10]. It would appear that fewer healthy children are experiencing CA than in the past. This has been attributed by some to the shift from the use of halothane to sevoflurane as the primary inhalational anesthetic used in children [14,22].

Co-existing disease, as reflected by the ASA PS, is without question the strongest predictor of risk for CA and death as an outcome, particularly for those children with congenital heart disease undergoing both cardiac and non-cardiac procedures. In a cohort of more than 92,000 patients at the Mayo Clinic, Flick and colleagues [13] described 26 CAs among patients undergoing non-cardiac procedures and 54 events during cardiac procedures. However, a total of 61 patients (87.5%) were known to have congenital heart disease, suggesting that for all procedures, the presence of congenital heart disease is a strong predictor of CA. Interestingly, the frequency of CA among children undergoing cardiac surgical procedures declined in the cohort over the study period of more than 15 years. This was attributed to the more aggressive use of extracorporeal membrane oxygenation (ECMO) for failure to wean from cardiopulmonary bypass (CPB) [23]. Patients who previously would have experienced CA during a cardiac procedure are now placed on ECMO and are no longer captured in analysis of perioperative CA. Morray et al [12] in the POCA Registry and Odegard et al [16] in a study of CA among patients undergoing cardiac surgical procedures at Children's Hospital Boston excluded most or all of those patients from their analysis. At the Children's Hospital Boston [16], the overall rate of CA during cardiac surgery was found to be 79 per 10,000 anesthetics, whereas at the Mayo Clinic, the rate was 127 per 10,000, probably reflecting the inclusion of those patients failing to wean from CPB in the Mayo series [13]. Regardless of the analysis, the presence of cardiac disease is a powerful predictor of not only CA but also mortality.

Unquestionably, neonates and infants are at greater risk. In the study by Olsson and Hallen [24], the risk of CA among infants was found to be 17 per 10,000 anesthetics, more than three times the risk for older children and almost six times that of adults less than 60 years old. More recent studies have found somewhat lower rates, ranging from 9 to 15 per 10,000 anesthetics [13,18]. Among neonates, CA rates are dramatically magnified to as high as 200 per 10,000 anesthetics [18]. Beyond 12 months, rates appear to decline rapidly to levels similar to those found in young adults.

Emergency procedures have been found by some to be associated with greater risk of CA and other major complications [13,17,24]. Additionally, Morray et al [12]

found in the initial report of the POCA Registry that the odds of mortality from CA increased almost fourfold among those experiencing CA during an emergency procedure. Similarly, time of day appears in some studies to affect risk such that those children undergoing procedures during off hours (typically after 5 p.m.) and on weekends are at increased risk for CA [25]. The cause of this elevated risk is unclear; however, one can speculate that the acuity of illness and the lack of availability of resources such as experienced personnel and equipment may affect procedures taking place during those times [13].

Of great interest to the pediatric anesthesia community is the question of provider and risk for CA. The benefit of specialty-trained pediatric anesthesiologists has been examined as has the presence of trainees. The data are not sufficient, however, to draw clear conclusions. Sprung et al [26] found in a study of adults and children that the provider at the time of the arrest was not predictive of ultimate survival after intraoperative CA. Alternatively, Olsson and Hallen [24] suggested that the incidence of CA was inversely proportional to the availability of specialist anesthetists. In a pediatric study, Keenan et al [27] examined the effect of subspecialty pediatric anesthesia care on the occurrence of CA among infants cared for at a major academic center. They found that of the four CAs observed in the cohort, all occurred in the non-pediatric anesthesiologist group (incidence 19.7 per 10,000 anesthetics; p = 0.048). A follow-up study [28] found a similar relationship when the frequency of bradycardia was compared between pediatric and non-pediatric anesthesiologists, and a large study by Mamie et al [29] demonstrated a reduction in critical events among children cared for by specialist pediatric anesthesiologists, especially during ear, nose, and throat surgery.

Analysis of correctable causes of CA may lead to improvements in anesthetic care. In the 1950s, deaths related to administration of curare were reported and led to changes in practice [1]. Later in the 1960s and 1970s, airway obstruction and aspiration were common antecedents to CA [3,4]. Over subsequent decades, improvements in care resulted in a reduction in the incidence of CA and also a predominance of inadequate ventilation and anesthetic overdose as frequent causes [8,24]. Data from the Closed Claims Project in the 1990s [19] suggested a decline in respiratory causes of CA; this decline was confirmed by subsequent analysis of POCA and other data [12,14,15,20]. The change may be attributable to the introduction of pulse oximetry and, later, capnography. Medication-related CA declined after the late 1990s and was reflected in the second report of the POCA Registry [14], suggesting that the conversion from halothane to sevoflurane may have been responsible.

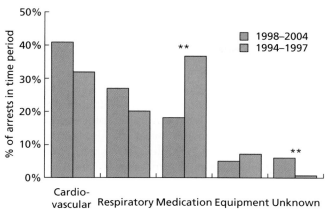

Figure 40.2 Causes of perioperative cardiac arrest from the Pediatric Perioperative Cardiac Arrest Registry, 1994–97 and 1998–2004. **p<0.01, 1998–2004 vs 1994–1997 by Z test. Reproduced from Bhananker et al [20] with permission from Lippincott Williams and Wilkins.

Table 40.1 Causes of cardiac arrest, 1998–2004

Cause	n = 193 No. (% of 193)
Cardiovascular	79 (41)
Hypovolemia associated with blood loss	23 (12)
Electrolyte imbalance	10 (5)
Hypovolemia (nonhemorrhage)	5 (3)
Air embolism	4 (2)
Other CV	11 (6)
Presumed CV unclear mechanism	26 (13)
Respiratory	53 (27)
Airway obstruction – laryngospasm	11 (6)
Airway obstruction – other	5 (3)
Inadequate ventilation or oxygenation	9 (5)
Inadvertent or premature extubation	7 (4)
Difficult intubation	4 (1)
Esophageal or endobronchial intubation	3 (2)
Bronchospansm	4 (2)
Pneumothorax	2 (1)
Aspiration	2 (1)
Other	1 (1)
Presumed respiratory, unclear mechanism	5 (3)
Medication	35 (18)
Halothane-induced CV depression	9 (5)
Sevoflurane-induced CV depression)	6 (3)
Other single medication[a]	9 (5)
Medication combination	7 (3)
Allergic reaction	2 (1)
Intravascular injection of local	2 (1)
Equipment	9 (5)
Central catheter	5 (3)
Kinked or plugged ET tube	2 (1)
Peripheral IV catheter	1 (1)
Breathing circuit	1 (1)
Multiple events	3 (2)
Miscellaneous	2 (1)
Unknown	12 (6)

CV, cardiovascular; ET, endotracheal; IV, Intravenous.

[a] Non-thalation agents.

Reproduced from Bhananker et al [20] with permission from Lippincott Williams and Wilkins.

The decline in respiratory- and medication-related CA was accompanied by a concomitant rise in the proportion of events related to cardiovascular causes in the data reported by Bhananker et al [20] from the POCA Registry. These were primarily related to blood loss and its replacement (hyperkalemia secondary to massive transfusion). Similar findings were observed in the Mayo Clinic series [13]. The findings reinforced the need for adequate hemodynamic and electrolyte monitoring as well as avoidance of the use of whole, irradiated, or old blood whenever possible (Fig. 40.2, Table 40.1).

Respiratory events, although proportionately less common, continue to be an important source of CA in children. Laryngospasm was the most frequent antecedent event identified in the POCA data. This is supported by other large series that examine adverse events such as those by Mamie et al [29], Tay et al [17], and Murat et al [15]. These arrests may be attributed to the failure to rapidly recognize and effectively treat laryngospasm before the onset of bradycardia that may be accentuated by the use of intramuscular or intravenous succinylcholine.

Outcomes of CAs among children in the perioperative setting are, not surprisingly, dependent on the cause. Overall survival ranges from 21% according to Flick et al [13] to 28% [20], 37% [18], 57% [17], and 92% [16]. The higher survival reported by Odegard et al [16] was among cardiac surgical cases and did not include those who failed to wean from CPB or were placed directly onto ECMO support. In general, the outcome of in-hospital CA among children is better than that of adults, and CA occurring in the operative setting has better outcome than CA occurring elsewhere in the hospital [30]. Cardiac arrest in children outside the hospital has a poor outcome, with only a 12% survival to discharge; this survival rate is based on a meta-analysis by Donoghue et al in 2005 [31].

As more robust methods of capturing clinical events become more widely available and organizations such as the Society for Pediatric Anesthesia and others develop and support methods of capturing these data across multiple institutions, the ability to quantify and study these rare events will improve and so will the care of children. See Chapter 43 for further discussion of databases and outcomes research. For treatment of cardiac arrest, see Chapter 12.

Control of temperature

Physiology of temperature control

The management of temperature is critical in the care of pediatric patients. Much more so than adults, children are susceptible to changes in environmental temperature and the effects of anesthetics on thermoregulatory responses. As mammals, humans are homeothermic and therefore maintain their body temperature within a narrow range. Core temperatures in humans are in general maintained at within 0.2°C around the thermal set point of 37°C. To achieve this precise temperature control, a complex array of thermoregulatory processes that are not completely understood are required.

From the earliest experiences in the use of general anesthetics, it has been recognized that these agents impair normal thermoregulatory mechanisms and without intervention will inevitably result in hypothermia in patients of all ages and sizes. Pickering [32], in a 1958 lecture to the Royal College of Physicians, discussed (among other things) the potential benefits of hypothermia and stated, "The practical difficulty in cooling men is to break through the defences of the body; the most effective means is to give an anaesthetic, which (as we have seen) has been shown to interrupt at some point or points the reflex arcs which protect against cooling, particularly shivering." Although perioperative hypothermia may have a benefit in selected patients and clinical settings, the effects of cold may have profound negative effects, including increased bleeding, infection, renal dysfunction, and alterations in the pharmacology of anesthetic agents and other medications [33–36]. Although relatively rare, severe hyperthermia is much less well tolerated than hypothermia and will, in settings such as malignant hyperthermia (MH), result in death unless effectively treated. In this section, the physiology of thermoregulation is discussed along with temperature measurement and disturbances encountered in the perioperative setting as well as strategies to prevent or manage these alterations.

Temperature regulation in homeotherms is highly complex and not completely understood. Clearly, temperature regulation is among the most closely guarded of all physiological processes and involves interplay among peripheral and central receptors and controllers distributed widely throughout virtually the entire organism. Temperature control is not symmetrical; that is, much greater control is exerted over increases in central temperature as opposed to central hypothermia. Temperatures higher than 44°C constitute the upper limit of survival in humans, whereas temperatures as low as 30°C are experienced in the operative setting without profound effect [37]. This asymmetry is, in all likelihood, related to the effect of high temperatures on the tertiary structure of proteins (Fig. 40.3).

The dominant control of temperature can be localized in the preoptic anterior hypothalamus (POAH) although the dorsomedial nucleus, periaquaductal gray matter of the midbrain, and the nucleus raphe pallidus in the medulla also play an important role [38]. In the most commonly described model, the POAH is at the center of a negative feedback loop that involves afferent input from superficial and deep temperature receptors and efferent output to effectors in the sweat glands, blood vessels (dilation-constriction), muscles (shivering), brown fat deposits (non-shivering thermogenesis), and respiratory centers (hyperpnea). The thalamus functions much like a thermostat to closely maintain core temperature by reducing heat loss and activating heat production in response to cold afferent input and dissipating heat and decreasing thermogenesis in response to warm afferent input [39]. The interthreshold range, i.e. the range over which the thalamus senses temperature as normal, is between 36.8°C and 37.2°C although there are diurnal variations and differences between men and women associated with menstruation. Temperatures within the thalamus outside the normal range will initiate an effector response to return the central temperature to the normal set point.

The POAH contains warm-sensitive, cold-sensitive, and temperature-insensitive receptors. However, warm sensors vastly outnumber cold and insensitive receptors, emphasizing the survival importance associated with guarding against hyperthermia. Warm sensors exert primary control over temperature by integrating thermal inputs from the periphery and by directly sensing thalamic temperature [40]. The dendrites of these warm sensor neurons lie adjacent to the third ventricle and therefore directly sense cerebrospinal fluid temperatures [41]. As temperature rises, these sensors increase firing rates and initiate autonomic responses to reduce core temperature as well as providing tonic inhibition of cold sensors. Likewise, reduced input to warm sensors is the primary mechanism of initiating sympathetic responses to thermogenesis and thermal preservation. Cold-sensitive neurons are relatively few in number and are much less important in temperature control within the POAH. Temperature-insensitive sensors function to provide inhibition to warm sensors in response to afferent input from the periphery as well as to activate cold sensor neurons. The integration of input to warm sensors, cold sensors, and insensitive neurons within the POAH establishes separate but highly integrated mechanisms for the response to cold and warm core temperatures. The response to cold relies predominantly on afferent input mostly from skin to inhibit warm sensor activity rather than a reduction in firing of central cold sensors. At temperatures 0.5°C lower than normal, warm sensor neurons essentially cease firing [42]. In contrast, a response to increasing core temperature relies primarily on the

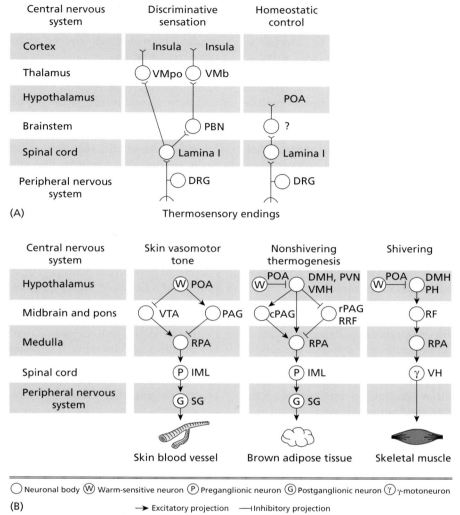

Figure 40.3 (A) Afferent neuronal pathways for discriminative sensation/localization of a thermal stimulus and for homeostatic control of body temperature. DRG, dorsal root ganglion; PBN, parabrachial nucleus; POA, preoptic anterior hypothalamus; VMb, basal part of the ventromedial nucleus of the thalamus (formerly known as the parvicellular part of the ventroposterior medial nucleus); VMpo, posterior part of the ventromedial nucleus of the thalamus; ?, unknown location(s) within the medulla, pons, and midbrain. (B) Efferent neuronal pathways for control of skin vasomotor tone, non-shivering thermogenesis in brown adipose tissue, and shivering in the rat. DMH, dorsomedial hypothalamus; IML, intermediolateral column; PAG, periaqueductal gray matter; cPAG, caudal PAG; rPAG, rostral PAG; PH, posterior hypothalamus; PVN, paraventricular nucleus; RF, reticular formation; RPA, raphe/peripyramidal area; RRF, retrorubral field; SG, sympathetic ganglia; VH, ventral horn; VMH, ventromedial hypothalamus; VTA, ventral tegmental area. Reproduced from Romanovsky [37] with permission from the American Physiological Society.

increased firing of warm sensor neurons and does not depend on peripheral input.

Afferent input into the central thermoregulatory controllers is derived from receptors distributed throughout the body, primarily in the skin and oral and urogenital mucosa. In contrast to the central sensors, peripheral receptors are predominantly cold sensors (a ratio of about 10:1) [42]. Traditionally, these sensors have been thought to provide input only to central sensors where these inputs are integrated and result in an effector response. More recently, however, this theory of negative feedback has been challenged to the extent that an alternative

model has been proposed suggesting that skin receptors may directly activate effectors in a feedforward rather than feedback loop [43]. Direct activation allows for pre-emptive control of temperature, primarily enabling defense against cold. This model of control suggests that the sensation of cold is a byproduct of control rather than an effector. Activation of cold sensors produces the sensation of cold and an effector response as a parallel process rather than a sequential one.

Regardless of the mechanism, input from peripheral sensors (primarily cold) located in the skin are sent to the brain via thin myelinated A δ fibers through the spinoreticulothalamic tract to the thalamus and other brain regions involved in thermal control. These sensors' peak firing rate occurs at temperatures between 25°C and 30°C. Peripheral sensors in the skin are exquisitely sensitive and respond to temperature changes as small as 0.0003°C. They are most sensitive to rapid rather than gradual change in temperature and are the major source of peripheral thermal input [44].

Sensors (predominantly warm) are found in deep tissues of the core and send afferent signals via unmyelinated C fibers with peak firing rates at temperatures between 40°C and 50°C [45]. These sensors also respond primarily to change in temperature rather than to absolute temperature. Firing rates increase with increasing or decreasing temperature and subsequently accommodate to a new stable temperature [37]. This phenomenon explains both adaptation to temperature change and also the observation that responses to temperature change are most vigorous when change occurs rapidly.

Efferent output to temperature effectors occurs via autonomic and behavioral mechanisms. In humans, behavioral mechanisms predominate either directly or, in the case of a young child, indirectly through the actions of a caregiver. Behavioral control of temperatures allows humans to survive temperatures lower than −100°C and higher than 2000°C (temperature on the surface of the moon and surrounding the shuttle during re-entry) [37]. Behavioral control allows for the use of deep hypothermic circulatory arrest and survival from MH. In day-to-day care of children in the perioperative setting, the pediatric anesthesiologist must provide indirect control of body temperature to avoid the negative consequences associated with both hypothermia and hyperthermia.

Autonomic control of temperature is achieved through thermoeffectors, including piloerection, sweating, cutaneous vasoconstriction or vasodilation, shivering, brown fat metabolism (non-shivering thermogenesis), and, to at least a minimal extent, hyperpnea. These effectors function to either conserve or dissipate heat, depending on the specific need. Outputs to the effectors are integrated within the POAH as well as at the level of the spinal cord and potentially through even more direct mechanisms. Clearly, the most effective non-behavioral means of both heat conservation and dissipation is vasodilation or vasoconstriction of cutaneous blood vessels. In adult humans, skin blood flow can be increased in response to hyperthermia to as high as 6–8 L/min and, when combined with sweating, is the most effective means of heat dissipation [39].

Given the large surface area-to-weight ratio of infants, heat loss and gain are much more rapid. The normal newborn has a surface area-to-volume ratio of approximately 1, whereas in the adult, the ratio is closer to 0.4. In the adult in a thermally neutral environment, cutaneous blood flow is approximately 250 mL/min, dissipating approximately 90 kcal/h. When core temperature rises, a gradient is created between the central and skin temperatures, resulting in a reduction in peripheral cold sensor activity and subsequent cutaneous vasodilation with a severalfold increase in blood flow. Heat is then effectively transferred from the core to the periphery, and the thermal set point is re-established. In cold environments, blood flow is shunted away from cutaneous vessels by closing arteriovenous shunts that are maximally open in a thermally neutral environment. Reducing blood flow up to tenfold may result in as much as a 50% reduction in heat loss [46].

Shivering increases heat production in adults by a factor of five for brief periods or by a smaller factor for sustained periods. It is involuntary muscular activity that is central in origin and can be reliably reproduced by cooling of the hypothalamus (POAH). In neonates and young infants, shivering is often believed not to occur although it is difficult to find a reference to that effect or to define the age at which shivering can be expected to occur. Darnall [47] has suggested that neonates can indeed shiver although shivering is a secondary mechanism of heat production much less efficient than non-shivering thermogenesis and therefore rarely observed. When β-blocking agents that inhibit non-shivering thermogenesis are given to guinea pigs, they demonstrate shivering at temperatures higher than normally observed [48]. Regardless, shivering, if it occurs in infancy, plays a relatively minor role in heat generation. Instead, neonates and infants are, to a large extent, dependent on non-shivering thermogenesis.

Non-shivering thermogenesis, resulting primarily from the metabolism of brown fat, is the most important means of thermal response to cold in hibernating animals as well as in neonates and infants. Once thought to occur only in infants, brown fat has been identified in adults and may be important in future research on weight management [49]. Brown fat is adipose tissue that is rich in mitochondria that have a unique capacity to uncouple oxidative phosphorylation, thereby generating large amounts of heat rather than adenosine triphosphate (ATP). The uncoupling of oxidative phosphorylation is dependent on uncoupling protein (UCP1), a 33 kD protein found on the inner membrane of the mitochondria in brown fat [50]. This tissue comprises approximately 2–6% of bodyweight in a newborn and is found in the mediastinum, between the scapulae, around the adrenals, and in the axillae. Non-shivering thermogenesis is mediated by sympathetic stimulation in response to cold stress and, as previously stated, can be inhibited by β-blocking agents. In addition to norepinephrine and epinephrine, thyroxin and glucocorticoids may also stimulate lipolysis of brown fat. Lipolysis of brown fat, compared with that of white adipose tissue, results in oxidation of approximately three times the amount of fatty acid (30% versus 10%) within the lipocyte [51]. A considerable proportion of free fatty acids is released into the bloodstream to be oxidized elsewhere in the body. Ultimately, the metabolic result of maximum oxidation of brown fat is a near doubling of heat production, with an increase in oxygen consumption from 5.4 mL/kg/min to 9.3 mL/kg/min [52]. The capacity for substantial heat production through non-shivering thermogenesis is present at birth and persists through the second year of life.

In animals, hyperpnea makes a major contribution to thermoregulation, especially of the brain. In humans, the role of panting is less pronounced but it is nonetheless important. There are two phases of the panting response. The first phase, thermal tachypnea, is characterized by increased respiratory frequency with reduced tidal volume, resulting in heat loss but no change in carbon dioxide tension [53]. This pattern produces preferential ventilation of anatomical dead space, including the nasopharynx, selectively cooling the brain. The second phase, thermal hyperpnea, produces a reduced respiratory rate coupled with an increased tidal volume, resulting in alveolar hyperventilation hypocapnia and alkalosis. In humans, thermal hyperpnea predominates and can at times account for 46% of cephalic heat loss [54]. Given the relative size of the infant cranium, it could be assumed that this figure may be larger, although no data support this assumption.

An interesting theory is related to the role of yawning in thermoregulation, especially with regard to selective brain cooling [55]. In a study group of college students, contagious yawning was eliminated by selective cooling of the forehead [56]. In preterm and near-term infants, yawning begins at approximately 20 weeks and decreases in frequency between 31 and 40 weeks, coincident with development of homeostatic control [57]. Also interesting is the role of opioids in yawning behavior. Opioids are known, through κ receptor activity, to produce hypothermia in animals and also to inhibit yawning. Additionally, the administration of naloxone increases yawning in opiate-dependent humans [58]. Ultimately, the importance of yawning is uncertain in humans and especially in neonates and infants.

Mechanisms of heat loss

Unintentional hypothermia is the major concern that motivates inclusion of a discussion of thermoregulation in this and every text of pediatric anesthesia. Although heat is lost and gained from the body in similar ways, heat gain is a relatively rare concern, whereas avoiding heat loss is part of the anesthetic management of every child. A basic understanding of the mechanisms of heat loss is central to the prevention of unintentional hypo-thermia. Hypothermia has beneficial effects in a few select clinical situations such as hypoxic ischemic brain injury, head trauma, CPB, and deep hypothermic circulatory arrest, but it has clear negative effects in most day-to-day perioperative situations. Hypothermia inhibits immune responses and is a source of renal dysfunction and coagulation abnormalities. It affects the action of various medications, including muscle relaxants, that are components of many anesthetics provided to adults and children.

Heat loss in the operating room environment occurs through radiation, convection, evaporation, and conduction, in order of importance. Radiant heat loss is the heat loss that occurs between two objects in the environment. All objects in the operating room, whether animate or inanimate, gain or transfer heat to one another in a process that would, in the absence of intervention, lead to equilibrium. The heat of the sun and the heat generated by an infrared warming light are typical examples of radiant heat sources. Radiant heat loss is somewhat less easy to imagine but much more important in the operating environment. Radiant heat is transferred as electromagnetic waves in the infrared spectrum and is unaffected by air currents, air temperature, or distance between the radiating surfaces. Radiant heat loss becomes an increasingly important source of heat loss as the temperature of surrounding objects and surfaces decreases. In a neutral thermal environment, radiant heat loss accounts for about 39% of total heat loss, whereas at 22°C, radiant losses increase to nearly 80% of the total [59].

Radiant heat loss can be calculated using a simplified formula that accounts for radiant properties of the two surfaces, surface area, and temperature difference between the objects. The radiant heat loss can be estimated for a typical young child on the basis of the following assumptions: if human skin has an emissivity coefficient of close to 1.0, a body surface area of 0.5 m² at a temperature of 22°C and skin temperature of 36°C would continuously radiate approximately 40 W. This energy loss can be greatly reduced by use of simple coverings such as clothing, sheets, or blankets. Even light clothing can dramatically reduce radiant heat losses. It may at times not be possible to cover the child. In this circumstance, the most effective means of maintaining temperature is increasing the temperature of objects within the environment (heating the operating room) or, alternatively, providing a source of radiant heat energy such as an infrared heat lamp or other radiant heater. In this example, increasing the ambient temperature to 30°C would reduce radiant heat loss by almost 50%, keeping in mind that in order to achieve this, the environment must be at equilibrium. Simply raising the air temperature briefly has little effect until all objects in the environment have had sufficient time to equilibrate.

Convective heat loss is second to radiation as a source of energy loss in the operating room environment. It accounts for approximately 34% of heat loss in a neutral thermal environment. Convection is the loss in heat that occurs as a result of mass motion of a fluid, typically either air or water. The amount of heat loss depends on the velocity of air (water) movement and the difference between the temperature of the object (person) and the surrounding fluid. For those living in northern latitudes, the concept of wind chill is a familiar example of the effects of convection on cooling or heat loss from one object to the surrounding air (termed *forced convection*). Although air currents in the indoor environment are minimal, it is important to keep in mind that a warm object heats the surrounding air (termed *natural convection*). The warmer air is less dense and rises away from the warm object, thus creating an air current that promotes convective heat loss. The addition of even light covering inhibits this air current and reduces convective heat loss. The rate of convective heat transfer ($\dot{Q}$) is determined by the following formula: $\dot{Q} = hA(T_s - T_b)$, where h is the constant heat transfer coefficient of the fluid, in this case air, A is the surface area in meters squared, T_s is the surface temperature, and T_b is the temperature of the fluid (air). The transfer coefficient is situationally dependent and must be determined for each setting, making use of this formula problematic in the clinical setting.

Heat loss through conduction occurs whenever the body comes in direct contact with a cooler object that is not in motion (air or water are objects in motion) such as the operating table or other solid. Similar to convection, the transfer of heat is dependent on the temperature difference between the two objects, the densities of the objects, and the area of contact. The greater the area of contact and the greater the density of the cooler object, the more heat is transferred. A soft mattress transfers less heat than a solid surface such as an x-ray table. The mathematical expression of this relationship is identical to that for convection: $\dot{Q} = hA(T_s - T_b)$. However, in this case, heat transfer is related to h, the conductivity or thermal properties of the solid, A, the area in contact, and the temperature difference between the body (T_s) and object (T_b) in contact. Heat loss via conduction is typically small and accounts for about 3% of heat loss in a neutral thermal environment.

Evaporative heat losses are encountered whenever a fluid evaporates from the surface of an object such as a patient whose abdomen has been prepared with a solution such as povidone-iodine. Evaporation is an important means of cooling the body when the body temperature exceeds 37°C. Heat loss through sweating, evaporation of another liquid from the skin (skin preparation solutions), or insensible losses from an open abdominal wound or via the respiratory tract depend on the vapor pressure

gradient between the skin and surrounding air and the velocity of air movement. The formula is familiar from the previous discussion; however, in the case of evaporation, the difference is not in temperature but rather vapor pressure between skin and surrounding air: $\dot{Q} = hA(P_s - P_a)$, where $\dot{Q}$ is heat transfer in watts, h is the coefficient of evaporation and accounts for the latent heat of vaporization of the liquid as well as the air flow velocity, A is the area covered by the liquid in meters squared, and P_s and P_a are the vapor pressures of the liquid at the skin surface and the surrounding air.

Evaporative heat loss accounts for approximately 25% of total heat loss, of which roughly half can be attributed to respiratory losses. In the infant, respiratory losses can be assumed to be greater given the increased minute ventilation per kilogram of bodyweight. The use of warm, humidified inspired gases eliminates this source of heat and free water loss. Table 40.2 summarizes the mechanisms of heat loss, and prevention and treatment in anesthetized children.

Anesthetics and thermoregulation

Anesthetic agents produce consistent effects on thermoregulation in infants, children, and adults. All agents act to increase the interthreshold range by both increasing the upper threshold and decreasing the lower threshold such that the range of temperatures within which thermoregulatory mechanisms are not initiated becomes much wider. Under normal circumstances, the poikilothermic range is limited to 0.2°C. Under anesthesia, that range increases to between 2°C and 4°C, depending on the agent. The interthreshold range is determined on the lower end by measuring the temperatures at which vasoconstriction and shivering are initiated and on the higher end by the initiation of sweating. Vasoconstriction and shivering track consistently at approximately 1°C difference, regardless of the effects of anesthesia, such that vasoconstriction is initiated at a 1°C higher temperature than shivering.

The effects of anesthetics on the interthreshold range are not symmetrical. The upper boundary of the range is increased only by 1–1.5°C, whereas the lower threshold is decreased by approximately 2.5°C. The effect is that hypothermia is much more likely to occur than hyperthermia, especially given the typical ambient temperature of most operating rooms. At this point, it is also important to recognize that the most effective responses to both hyperthermia and hypothermia are behavioral, and these responses are obviously absent under general anesthesia. Although the range over which no response to temperature change occurs increases under anesthesia, the intensity of response does not. Cutaneous vasoconstriction under isoflurane anesthesia in healthy volunteers occurred at 34.6°C and was similar in intensity to that

Table 40.2 Mechanisms of heat loss in anesthetized infants and children

Mechanism	Relative % of heat loss	Causes	Prevention/treatments
Radiation	39% in NTE (80% at 22°C)	Cold room temperature	Warm room as high as 26°C; heating lamp; cover with clothing, sheets, blankets, caps, wrap extremities – plastic, cotton wadding
Convection	34% in NTE	Motion of air/fluid	Cover with clothing, sheets, blankets, caps, wrap extremities – plastic, cotton wadding; forced-air warming; warmed IV fluids
Evaporation	25% in NTE	Respiratory losses; drying of skin, preparation fluids and other fluids on skin	Condenser humidifier or active warming/ humidification of gases; warm skin prep solutions
Conduction	3% in NTE	Direct contact with cooler object not in motion, e.g. OR table	Circulating water blankets; forced-air warming

NTE, neutral thermal environment. See text for detailed explanation.

achieved in awake volunteers. Shivering can also be observed in anesthetized patients, although it is much less common because it occurs at a temperature 1°C lower than vasoconstriction. Like vasoconstriction, the intensity of shivering observed is unchanged.

Non-shivering thermogenesis is the predominant means of heat generation in neonates and infants. It too is inhibited in the setting of general anesthesia. Halothane 1.5% inhibits non-shivering thermogenesis by 70% in rodents [60]. Human infants under propofol and fentanyl anesthesia fail to increase metabolic rate despite core temperatures 2°C below the vasoconstrictive threshold, suggesting that non-shivering thermogenesis is absent in this setting [61], although Ohlson et al [62] failed to demonstrate an inhibitory effect on non-shivering thermogenesis by propofol in hamsters.

Inhalational anesthetics affect the thermoregulatory threshold of infants and children in a manner similar to that observed in adults. Bissonnette and Sessler [63] showed that halothane and nitrous oxide reduce the thermoregulatory threshold in children to 35.7°C, whereas in a previous study [64], they found that under isoflurane, the threshold was further reduced to levels similar to those observed in adults (34.4–35.3°C). In both studies children were stratified by weight, and in neither study did threshold response vary significantly with weight. Sevoflurane and desflurane have been found to produce similar changes in thermoregulatory responses although desflurane is unique in that it reduces the magnitude or gain of the vasoconstrictive response to hypothermia [65–67]. Xenon has been shown to have a greater inhibitory effect on thermoregulation than isoflurane, whereas nitrous oxide is less inhibitory [68]. In general,

the thermoregulatory response to inhalational anesthetic agents appears to be similar in adults and children and is not determined by weight or age. Inhalational anesthetics, with the exception of nitrous oxide, appear to inhibit non-shivering thermogenesis [62].

The effects of intravenous anesthetics on thermoregulation vary. Propofol produces a linear decrease in the threshold temperature for vasoconstriction and shivering, while only slightly increasing the threshold for sweating in humans, as demonstrated by Matsukawa, Kurz, and colleagues [69,70]. Unlike volatile anesthetics, propofol does not appear to inhibit non-shivering thermogenesis. Ohlson et al [62] compared the effects of various anesthetic agents on brown fat metabolism and found that propofol and ketamine did not inhibit non-shivering thermogenesis in hamsters. Midazolam appears to impair thermoregulatory control only minimally compared to the effects of propofol and narcotics [71].

The individual thermoregulatory effects of opioids have not been widely studied. Spencer et al [72] showed that, in rats, different opioid agonists had differing effects on thermoregulation depending on the type of receptor stimulated (μ, κ, δ) with the μ agonist increasing the set point and κ and δ agonists reducing it. Kurz et al [73] examined the thermoregulatory effects of alfentanil in human volunteers and found a minimal increase in set point for sweating and a linear, serum concentration-dependent decrease in set point for vasoconstriction and shivering similar to those observed for other general anesthetics. Meperidine similarly reduces set point and also appears to diminish the threshold for non-shivering thermogenesis by its effects on the α2-adrenergic receptor [74–76]. Clonidine and dexmedetomidine also act as α2-agonists and reduce the threshold for vasoconstriction and shivering but have little or no effect on sweating [77].

Postoperative shivering is a problem that primarily affects older children and adults and occurs in two patterns termed *thermoregulatory* and *non-thermoregulatory*. Thermoregulatory shivering is related to hypothermia and appears similar to shivering that occurs in other settings. Non-thermoregulatory shivering seems to have an etiology separate from thermoregulation because it occurs in normothermic patients in the postoperative period and is also seen in patients such as laboring women who have not been exposed to an anesthetic and are not hypothermic. The exact mechanism of this type of shivering is not entirely clear; however, its appearance is distinct in that it is predominantly clonic, resembling the clonus seen in spinal cord-injured patients [78]. Postanesthetic shivering occurs in approximately 50% of patients allowed to become hypothermic and in 27% of non-hypothermic patients, 15% of whom display a primarily clonic pattern of shivering [79]. Pain appears to be a factor also; patients with lower pain scores are less likely to shiver postoperatively [80].

Shivering in children is not well studied; however, a few studies have been published that describe the problem. Akin et al [81] prospectively followed more than 1500 children in the postanesthetic care unit and found the incidence of shivering to be 3.5%. Older children, those undergoing long procedures, and those in whom anesthesia was induced with an intravenous agent appeared to be at greater risk, whereas those whose anesthetic was supplemented with a caudal block appeared to be a lower risk. Lyons et al [82] found a rate of almost 15% in a smaller study and found that anticholinergic use was also a risk factor.

The consequences of shivering are primarily confined to patients who do not have the cardiovascular reserve to tolerate as much as a 380% increase in oxygen consumption that may be associated with shivering [83]. Shivering may also increase intraocular and intracranial pressure and should certainly be treated in those settings. The majority of episodes in children, however, are brief and do not necessarily require treatment other than external warming. When pharmacological treatment is desired for comfort or safety, meperidine appears to be the most efficacious agent. Its usefulness may be the result of its activity as an α2-adrenergic receptor agonist based on its opioid activity. In keeping with this, other α2-agonists have been used successfully to treat shivering. Dexmedetomidine and clonidine have been successfully, although clonidine appears to be most useful in preventing rather than treating this problem. Other narcotics have been used but with mixed results and none with the efficacy of meperidine.

Thermoregulation and regional anesthesia

In children, regional anesthesia is nearly always combined with a general anesthetic, which is not usual in adults. The thermoregulatory effects of regional anesthesia are confined primarily to neuraxial techniques as the effects of extremity and other blocks tend not to involve a large enough area to greatly affect core temperature. The effects of neuraxial anesthesia on thermoregulation have been extensively studied by Sessler and others, mostly in adults [84–94]. Bissonnette and Sessler, in two studies [63,64], examined the effect of general anesthesia with regional block in children, a situation that has clear relevance to clinical pediatric practice. In the first study [64], in which isoflurane was used in combination with caudal blockade, the authors found that thermal responses in children were similar to those in adults and were independent of bodyweight and age. The use of combined neuraxial and general anesthesia was thought not to be an important factor in determining responses. In the second study [63], halothane was used in combination with either penile or caudal block. Thermal responses were not different between the two groups and were similar to those in adults and children under general anesthesia without regional anesthesia. It appears from these studies that the combination of regional anesthesia with general anesthesia has little impact on thermoregulation in children.

Temperature monitoring

The ASA requires that temperature monitoring be available for all patients under anesthesia. Accurate measurement of temperature in the operative period is primarily directed at the detection of hypothermia. Less common but no less important are instances of notable fever, especially those related to MH. Temperature is measured using various technologies at multiple sites with accuracy that varies widely. The appropriate unit of measure is degrees Celsius as the Fahrenheit scale is cumbersome and outmoded, and, like most aspects of the US customary system ("English units"), should be abandoned in clinical practice.

The measurement of temperature has a rich and fascinating history that cannot be covered in this text. One of the first thermometers, invented by Rhomer at the turn of the 18th century, used red wine as an indicator. Fahrenheit invented the mercury thermometer in 1714 and later the Fahrenheit scale, which unfortunately remains in use in the United States and a few other countries. The Celsius scale originally designated 0° as the boiling point and 100° as the freezing point of water. Linnaeus inverted the scale to its present format in the middle of the 18th century, and the scale became widely popular as the centigrade scale, later designated the Celsius scale in 1948. The official metric unit of temperature is the Kelvin named after its inventor Lord Kelvin in 1848. The Kelvin scale is based on absolute zero and uses the triple point of water (273.16°K) as a reference. The triple point of a substance is the temperature at which all three phases co-exist in equilibrium.

Monitoring temperature requires that an accurate instrument be used at an appropriate site that reflects the temperature of interest. Modern thermometers use thermistors, thermocouples, infrared, and liquid crystal technologies. All are sufficiently accurate for most applications although thermistors are probably the most accurate and liquid crystal thermometers the least accurate.

Typically in the operative setting the temperature of interest is an estimation of core temperature, although the ability to measure core temperature is often limited by the availability of appropriate sites and instruments. Core temperature is undefined but represents the major input into thermoregulation and therefore is of the greatest importance in terms of measurement. Sites such as the tympanic membrane, bladder, esophagus, nasopharynx, and rectum are typically considered to represent core temperature; each has limitations, however. It has been suggested that the core temperature is the temperature of the thalamus; however, the core temperature can more appropriately be described as the temperature at which the thalamus responds rather than its own intrinsic temperature. Since the thalamus receives input from throughout the body, core and thalamic temperatures may differ.

Peripheral temperature varies widely over time and by location and therefore is much more limited as a measure of thermoregulatory input or status. Skin temperature, including axillary measurement, is often the simplest and most accessible site for monitoring. When the sensor has been placed properly, axillary temperature correlates well with measures of core temperature in infants, making it useful for brief procedures during which marked temperature change is not anticipated [95]. Placement of skin temperature probes elsewhere on the skin surface is much less likely to reflect core temperature and should be used with that caveat in mind. Figure 40.4 shows the correlation of various temperature measurement sites as measured in children weighing between 5 and 30 kg. Esophageal, rectal, and axillary temperatures are similar, but forearm and fingertip temperatures are much lower and clearly do not reflect core temperature [95].

Hypothermia, hyperthermia, and internal heat transfer

Heat loss or gain in the operative setting results in the transfer of heat either to or from the core. Redistribution hypothermia results from the transfer of heat from the core to the periphery caused by vasodilation usually induced by anesthetic agents. This heat transfer is responsible for the initial drop in temperature of 1–1.5°C

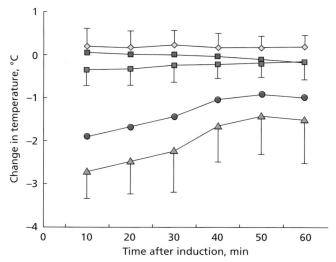

Figure 40.4 The average difference between temperatures at five different measurement sites and tympanic membrane temperature in 20 children weighing between 5 and 30 kg. The central sites (esophagus ◇, rectum ■, and axilla ▪) did not differ significantly, whereas the temperatures of the peripheral skin surface (forearm ▲ and fingertip ●) were significantly lower than the central temperatures. Vertical bars illustrate the standard deviation. Standard deviations of the rectal temperatures (omitted for clarity) were similar to those of the esophageal and axillary temperatures. Standard deviations of fingertip temperatures were similar to those of the forearm temperatures. Adapted from Bissonnette et al [95] with permission from Lippincott Williams and Wilkins.

typically observed in the first hour under anesthesia. Once initiated, the process is difficult to reverse; it can be prevented, however, through the use of prewarming and active warming immediately after the induction of anesthesia [96]. Active warming through the use of heated gases, heated forced air, heat lamps, heating pads, or heated intravenous fluids can be effective to slow or eliminate heat loss during the intraoperative period, but the most effective means of limiting heat loss is increasing the ambient temperature of the operating room.

Warming intravenous fluids is a relatively ineffective means of treating or preventing hypothermia except in situations such as rapid blood loss or CPB in which large volumes of blood are transferred to the patient in a very short time. The ineffectiveness of warming fluids is otherwise true for several reasons. Intravenous fluids can be warmed safely to temperatures only slightly above core temperature to prevent hemolysis, typical procedures require relatively small amounts of fluids, and finally, fluids warmed in an intravenous bag are often significantly cooler by the time they reach the patient. This is particularly true in small children, infants, and neonates with low intravenous flow rates and when warmed fluids are likely to cool prior to reaching the child. Whereas warm fluids are not an effective means of restoring normothermia, cold fluids are a much more effective means of cooling, primarily because cold or cool fluids have a much larger temperature gradient (15°C below core temperature for room temperature fluids) than warmed fluids (1–2°C above core temperature). Therefore, it is important to warm fluids when severe hypothermia can be anticipated, but warmed fluids are not an effective means of treating even mild hypothermia.

The use of a heated and humidified breathing circuit is also only modestly effective in either preventing or treating intraoperative hypothermia because heat loss through the respiratory tract accounts for only about 10% of total heat loss. Of that 10%, roughly two-thirds is accounted for in the process of humidifying inspired gases, suggesting that the use of a passive heat and moisture exchanger (artificial nose) is probably sufficient for most situations. In children, especially infants, the role of respiratory heat loss may be greater, given that minute ventilation is much higher than in adults. In a study in infants that compared active heating and humidification with either no intervention or passive humidification, Bissonnette and Sessler [97] found a marked difference in rectal temperature 2 h after induction. This difference suggests that, at least in infants and neonates, active heating and humidification may be useful, at least for longer or more extensive procedures. For shorter procedures that do not involve major body cavities, the use of an artificial nose (condenser humidifier) maintains sufficient airway humidity above the 50% needed for mucociliary function.

Surface warming using warm fluid-filled mattresses effectively reduces conductive heat losses, but these losses are a minor contributor to overall heat loss. As with heated airway gases and intravenous fluids, a major limitation of surface warming is the small increment between the temperature of the warming device and that of the patient. The use of high temperatures to warm externally creates an unacceptable risk of thermal injury. Therefore, the use of traditional hot water blankets has limited value in the management of hypothermia in the pediatric operative suite. Newer circulating-water devices have been developed that are more effective than either older systems or current forced-air systems [98]. This is due to the increased capacity of fluids to transfer heat and the increased surface area in contact with the skin.

The most widely used and effective means of external warming is forced-air (convective) warming devices. They have been in use for more than a decade and have an excellent safety record, despite reports of burns in children [99]. When a sufficient area of the body surface is covered, these systems can eliminate heat losses from the skin.

Despite the development of new technologies, the most effective means of preventing intraoperative hypothermia remains the maintenance of high ambient tempera-

tures and the use of simple insulators such as plastic sheeting or cloth coverings. Few data suggest that one type of covering is superior, but all are highly effective means of reducing surface heat loss and are of minimal cost. Ultimately, however, to maintain normothermia in infants, an ambient temperature of 26°C is required, which is uncomfortable, especially for the surgical team [100]. For longer or more invasive procedures in which major body cavities are exposed, active warming may be necessary and can be most comfortably and effectively achieved with the use of forced-air convective systems.

Hyperthermia in the operative setting is relatively rare compared with hypothermia. Temperatures exceeding 38°C may result from intrinsic processes such as infection, drug fever, transfusion reaction, or MH or may be the result of excessive warming. Children – especially infants and neonates – are most susceptible to hyperthermia induced by overly aggressive warming. It is important to investigate and eliminate the cause of the hyperthermia rather than to simply treat with antipyretics. Clearly, the most concerning cause of hyperthermia in the operative setting is MH.

Malignant hyperthermia

History of malignant hyperthermia
Malignant hyperthermia is a pharmacogenetic syndrome characterized by a hypermetabolic state of skeletal muscle, typically induced by exposure to specific anesthetic agents, including all the halogenated volatile agents as well as succinylcholine. The syndrome typically presents with fever, profound acidosis, rhabdomyolysis, and, if untreated, death in the majority of cases.

Malignant hyperthermia was first described in 1960 in a letter to the editor of *The Lancet* [101] and subsequently in an article in the *British Journal of Anaesthesia* entitled "Anaesthetic Deaths in a Family," reported by Denborough et al [102]. In that paper, the authors described the MH symptoms in a young man and several of his family members who had previously experienced unexplained anesthetic deaths. The young man survived a halothane anesthetic but displayed what are now known to be classic signs and symptoms of what later became known as MH. The term malignant hyperthermia was first used in a 1966 paper by Wilson et al [103] describing phosphorylation defects as a possible mechanism for MH. A subsequent 1972 report identified a characteristic phenotype for some affected individuals [104]. This entity was termed King–Denborough syndrome, and Britt et al [105] confirmed the heritability of the syndrome in a 1969 paper. Key to the understanding of MH was the early recognition of the pale soft exudative pork or porcine stress syndrome as an animal model for the human disorder.

Genetics and pathophysiology

Both contraction and relaxation of skeletal muscle are energy-requiring processes that depend on the coupling of excitation to contraction through acetylcholine-mediated depolarization of the muscle membrane and sarcoplasmic reticulum. Depolarization results in the release of calcium stored within the sarcoplasmic reticulum. The released calcium binds to actin thin filament proteins, allowing activation of myosin thick filaments and ultimately initiating muscle contraction. The sequestration of Ca^{2+} is active and required for relaxation of the motor unit. In MH, high levels of intracellular calcium persist, resulting in sustained contraction and continued consumption of ATP in a cellular attempt to restore Ca^{2+} homeostasis. This consumption of ATP leads to the production of heat and ultimately muscle breakdown that is characteristic of MH. Therapy with dantrolene is directed at reducing intracellular calcium, thereby allowing for muscle relaxation and elimination of uncontrolled ATP metabolism.

Over the generation since its original description, MH has been determined to be a pharmacogenetic syndrome related to abnormalities in the gene coding for the skeletal muscle ryanodine receptor (RyR1) and in a few cases in the *CACNA1S* gene. Both gene products control intracellular calcium metabolism. The *CACNA1S* gene codes for a voltage-gated skeletal muscle Ca^{2+} channel and accounts for less than 1% of cases [106]. The RyR1 receptor functions in skeletal muscle as a Ca^{2+} channel that regulates intracellular calcium in a bidirectional manner. The mechanism by which abnormal RyR1 channels fail is unclear but may be related to abnormalities in receptor sensitivity to normal or abnormal ligands. The channel may become hypersensitive to activators such as Ca^{2+}, is less sensitive to inhibitors including both Ca^{2+} and Mg^{2+}, or responds to a pharmacological agent (dantrolene, halothane) to alter calcium efflux or influx (Fig. 40.5).

The pattern of inheritance in MH is autosomal dominant although a considerable proportion of affected individuals appear to follow a recessive pattern or no identifiable inheritance pattern. This is likely the result of variable expression or reduced penetrance within or among affected families. Genetic diagnosis is increasingly available but cannot identify a large portion of susceptible individuals [106–108]. Therefore, accurate diagnosis continues to rely on the use of the caffeine-halothane contracture test (CHCT) first developed more than 30 years ago [109,110]. The test is called the *in vitro* contraction test in Europe and requires a muscle biopsy to obtain fresh muscle that can be exposed under controlled conditions to halothane and caffeine. Strict criteria are used to define positive, negative, or equivocal tests [111–114]. Regardless, the false-positive rate is approximately 6% using European guidelines and 9% using those from North America [114,115]. Testing is increasingly restricted to a few centers and can only be accurately performed using fresh muscle from adults and children older than about age 6 years [116]. Genetic testing may be performed on relatives of a known case (with positive or equivocal CHCT result) with a positive genetic test [117]. Although a negative genetic test among relatives does not preclude the remote possibility of another MH mutation not included in the test battery within the same family, it nonetheless provides a high degree of reassurance [113].

Epidemiology

Malignant hyperthermia is a rare disorder affecting fewer than 1:50,000 adults and as many as 1:3000 children [118], representing approximately 13 cases per million hospital discharges in the United States [119] or 1 per 100,000 in New York State in 2005 [120]. Although large epidemiological studies have not been performed recently, it appears that the frequency of MH has declined with increased awareness and a greater degree of certainty as to the agents that are and are not associated with the syndrome. MH may occur at any age although it is most common in children and young adults. It has been reported rarely in infants and among the elderly [121,122]. Concentrations of cases can be found among large extended families or among members of closed or relatively closed communities. In a recent review of data compiled by the Malignant Hyperthermia Association of the United States, Larach and colleagues [123] found that of 286 cases reported between 1987 and 2006, 75% were male, most were young (median age 22 years), a disproportionately large number were muscular (29%), and most were white (70%).

Acute presentation

In the past, agents known to trigger MH included ether, halothane, and enflurane. Currently, sevoflurane, isoflurane, desflurane, and succinylcholine are known to trigger an episode of MH. Desflurane and sevoflurane are weak triggers for MH and therefore may be associated with episodes that are less fulminant than those seen in association with older agents and succinylcholine [124–127]. The rate of triggering may also be slowed or even eliminated by other factors, including the use of non-depolarizing muscle relaxants, barbiturates, and hypothermia [128]. Nevertheless, specific pharmacological triggering agents are not necessary to initiate a reaction among susceptible individuals. Carr et al [129], in a series of more than 2000 biopsy-proven MH patients, observed a rate of triggering of 0.46% despite the use of a non-triggering anesthetic.

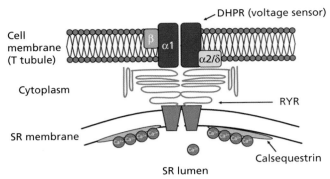

Figure 40.5 A schematic representation of the key structures involved in excitation-contraction coupling, including the ryanodine receptor (RYR) located on the sarcoplasmic reticulum (SR) membrane. DHPR indicates dyhydropyridine receptor. Adapted from Hopkins [205] with permission from Oxford University Press.

The clinical presentation of MH is highly variable and may at times be confused with other conditions such as rhabdomyolysis. The classic features of the disorder are non-specific and can be found in association with many other conditions. The combination of a highly variable presentation with non-specific signs and symptoms in a rare disorder explains the continued association of MH with poor outcomes, including death. This also explains the frequency with which MH is confused with other conditions. To assist in the clinical diagnosis of MH, Larach and colleagues [130] developed a clinical grading scale.

The presentation of MH relates to the underlying hypermetabolic state after exposure to a triggering agent such as a volatile anesthetic or succinylcholine. Hypermetabolism of skeletal muscle produces tachycardia, tachypnea, fever, muscle rigidity, acidosis (both respiratory and metabolic), hyperkalemia secondary to rhabdomyolysis with associated dysrhythmia, and ultimately cardiovascular collapse and death. Each of the symptoms can be traced to the calcium-induced hypermetabolic state within the skeletal muscle. Rigidity, occurring in approximately 40% of patients in the series described by Larach et al [123], is a function of sustained contraction that may lead to muscle breakdown and release of large amounts of potassium. The release of potassium in the setting of profound acidosis is often the proximate cause of ventricular dysrhythmia, CA, and ultimately death unless resuscitation efforts are successful. It must be kept in mind that acute hyperkalemia, fever, acidosis, and other manifestations of MH are associated with other conditions and may be confused with MH, although regardless of the etiology, treatment may be the same. Table 40.3 lists the order of appearance of clinical signs of MH in a series of 255 patients reported by Larach et al [123].

Laboratory evidence of MH reflects the underlying pathology. Thus, along with the aforementioned hyperkalemia and metabolic and respiratory acidosis, a rapid rise in creatine kinase (CK) and myoglobinuria reflect muscle destruction. Coagulopathy is common as are pulmonary edema and cardiac and hepatic dysfunction. Survivors of the acute phase will have evolving evidence of acute renal failure, with increasing serum creatinine and oliguria or anuria [123].

The onset of symptoms of MH is variable and may occur within minutes or may at times be delayed for hours [131–133]. Many patients with MH have had uneventful anesthetics in the past, with 30% having had as many as three previous exposures without triggering. Tachycardia and, in the spontaneously breathing patient, tachypnea are usually the first signs and are virtually always present, and the absence of tachycardia should cast doubt on the diagnosis of MH. In general, the more rapid the onset, the more severe the presentation; however, fulminant cases of MH have been described in patients whose first symptoms did not appear until after admission to the postanesthesia care unit or even many hours later [132,133]. Clearly, accurate and timely recognition requires a high degree of clinical suspicion and vigilance. As many as 20% of patients experience a recrudescence of symptoms an average of 13 h after the initial reaction. Those at greatest risk for recrudescence are those with delayed onset and muscular build [134].

Patients at risk

Recognition of MH must begin with an appreciation of the patient populations at greatest risk. Susceptibility to MH has been a subject of controversy since its original description. In a 1985 paper, Britt [135] described a series of features that suggest the potential for MH: "While some are perfectly healthy, others complain of: ptosis and strabismus in childhood; kyphoscoliosis or lumbar lordosis; club foot, various kinds of hernias . . . joint hypermobility . . . undescended testicle; calcium stones . . . poor dental enamel . . ." [135]. The author's extensive list reflected the lack of knowledge regarding the disorder available at that time. Currently, it is believed that MH is associated with only a few conditions, including central core disease, Evans myopathy, and King–Denborough syndrome [136–138]. The presence of strabismus, scoliosis, or other non-specific findings cannot be considered helpful in identification of those at risk.

Clearly succinylcholine-induced masseter spasm and susceptibility to MH are associated. The combination of halothane and succinylcholine produces masseter spasm in approximately 1% of children anesthetized for otolaryngological procedures [139]. Among those exhibiting masseter spasm, the association with MH depends to a large extent on the presentation. Those with mild jaw stiffness

Table 40.3 Order of appearance of clinical signs[a] during 255[b] malignant hyperthermia events

Clinical sign	Medial (first, third quartile) appearance number[c]	Range of appearance number[c]	No. (%) of patients with sign
Masseter spasm	1.00 (1.00, 1.00)	1.00–4.00	68 (26.7)
Hypercarbia	2.00 (1.00, 2.00)	1.00–8.00	235 (92.2)
Sinus tachycardia	2.00 (1.00, 2.00)	1.00–7.00	186 (72.9)
Generalized muscular rigidity	2.00 (1.00, 3.50)	1.00–6.00	104 (40.8)
Tachypnea	2.00 (1.00, 3.00)	1.00–6.00	69 (27.1)
Other	2.00 (1.00, 4.00)	1.00–7.00	43 (16.9)
Cyanosis	2.00 (2.00, 4.00)	1.00–7.00	24 (9.4)
Skin mottling	2.00 (1.00, 3.50)	1.00–7.00	16 (6.3)
Rapidly increasing temperature	3.00 (3.00, 4.00)	1.00–7.00	165 (64.7)
Elevated temperature[d]	3.00 (2.00, 4.00)	1.00–8.00	133 (52.2)
Sweating	4.00 (3.00, 5.00)	1.00–8.00	45 (17.6)
Ventricular tachycardia[d]	4.00 (2.00, 5.00)	1.00–7.00	9 (3.5)
Cola-colored urine	5.00 (3.00, 5.00)	2.00–9.00	35 (13.7)
Ventricular fibrillation[d]	5.50 (4.00, 8.00)	1.00–8.00	6 (2.4)
Excessive bleeding	6.00 (5.00, 6.00)	4.00–8.00	7 (2.7)

[a] Table lists the abnormal clinical sign and appearance order (judged to be inappropriate by the attending anesthesiologist or other physician) during malignant hyperthermia (MH) events. Clinical signs are listed in order of occurrence with the earliest signs listed first and the latest signs listed last. (No points on the clinical grading score are accumulated for the presence of the following adverse signs: cyanosis, skin mottling, sweating, excessive bleeding, and other.)

[b] For 31 cases, clinical sign appearance order was not known. (Appearance order is not required to calculate clinical grading scale score, and no additional points accrue for early appearance.)

[c] Appearance number is the numerical order in which a clinical sign appeared, e.g. the first clinical sign that appeared during an MH event would be assigned the appearance number of 1, the second clinical sign that appeared during an MH event would be assigned the appearance number of 2, and so on.

[d] An early version of the AMRA (adverse *m*etabolic/*m*usculoskeletal *r*eaction to *a*nesthesia) report form did not request these signs in one fatal case in which the maximum temperature was 41°C, but these findings were noted elsewhere in the AMRA report and have been counted in this table.

Adapted from Larach et al [123] with permission from Lippincott Williams and Wilkins.

appear to have only a slight increase in susceptibility to MH, whereas those exhibiting what has been termed "jaws of steel" are thought to have as high as an 80% concordance with MH. Patients with masseter spasm and an associated elevation of CK to more than 20,000 units/L have been demonstrated to have a 100% concordance with MH susceptibility [140]. As the use of succinylcholine has declined, especially in children, so has the frequency of masseter spasm. Larach et al [123] noted that, among subjects with probable or certain MH in their database, 20% had masseter spasm as a finding during their MH event.

For the clinician, a decision must be made about whether to continue with a procedure after a patient experiences masseter spasm. Some advocate canceling the planned procedure [140] and others recommend conversion to a non-triggering anesthetic and proceeding, provided no further evidence of MH is seen [140,141]. Although clear guidance cannot be given, the decision should probably be based on the severity of the masseter spasm, the urgency of the procedure, the environment (children's hospital versus free-standing surgical center),

and the resources available to provide care should the event progress to fulminant MH despite a change to a non-triggering anesthetic. A child experiencing masseter spasm should almost certainly be admitted for observation and a serum CK level determined, preferably before any surgical incision to assist in determining risk for MH in the future. Weglinski and colleagues [142] demonstrated that among children with idiopathic elevations of CK and no history of masseter spasm, 49% were found to be susceptible after biopsy and CHCT. As noted previously, the combination of masseter spasm and CK higher than 20,000 units/L is virtually diagnostic. Follow-up of the child who has experienced masseter spasm should probably include counseling with regard to the risk of MH, need for biopsy now or in the future, avoidance of triggering agents in the future for the child and first-degree relatives, and referral to pediatric neurology to evaluate for other potential causes of masseter spasm (e.g. congenital myotonia).

The association between various myopathies and MH remains an area of controversy. Specifically, are children with undiagnosed myopathies at increased risk? And are those patients with Duchenne-type muscular dystrophy also at increased risk? As previously stated, only three myopathic conditions can be clearly associated with MH: central core disease, Evans myopathy, and King–Denborough syndrome. Other myopathies have been associated with MH in the past but have not been clearly demonstrated to be linked and are no longer considered to require MH precautions. Osteogenesis imperfecta, Schwartz–Jampel syndrome, myotonia, and other myopathies have been at one time or another associated with MH, and previous editions of this and other texts have recommended the use of non-triggering anesthetics for children with a myopathy.

The relationship between MH and dystrophies, including Duchenne and Becker, however, remains uncertain. Reports in the past have described sudden CA and death in children known to have a muscular dystrophy and attributed those events to fulminant MH. It has become clear, though, that these events are more likely to be the result of rhabdomyolysis and subsequent hyperkalemic CA rather than true MH. The question remains as to whether volatile anesthetics are the cause of the rhabdomyolysis and consequently should be avoided in these patients. Clearly, succinylcholine is associated with this phenomenon and should never be used in a patient with a known or suspected dystrophy (or myopathy). In the young boy with Duchenne-type muscular dystrophy, the decision to avoid both succinylcholine and a volatile agent is relatively straightforward, as there are obvious alternatives. However, it is less clear how to approach the child with an undiagnosed myopathy, because the alternative, typically propofol, may be contraindicated in children with mitochondrial disorders [137,138].

Acute management

Successful management of an acute MH episode depends on early recognition and swift application of a treatment protocol that has been well thought out in advance of the need. Figure 40.6 is a poster from the Malignant Hyperthermia Association of the United States that describes the management of fulminant MH.

Specific management includes discontinuation of triggering agents and institution of therapy with dantrolene. Non-specific therapy is aimed at the effects of acidosis, fever, rhabdomyolysis, and consequent hyperkalemia, including correction of acidosis with hyperventilation and sodium bicarbonate; active cooling using cooling blankets, iced saline lavage, cooled fluids, etc.; maintenance of urine output with mannitol and furosemide; and management of hyperkalemia with bicarbonate, glucose, and insulin. Additional therapies directed against dysrhythmia such as procainamide and amiodarone may be useful; however, rhythm disturbance is almost certainly secondary to hyperkalemia, and therapy should be primarily directed at reducing serum potassium.

First available in the late 1960s as an oral muscle relaxant for use in patients with spasticity, dantrolene was recognized as an effective therapy for MH in pigs by Harrison in 1975 [143] and 2 years later in humans by Austin and Denborough [144]. The drug was of limited value for acute management, given the need to deliver it orally. It was extremely useful, however, for prophylaxis, and when solubility problems were resolved, it became available for intravenous use in 1979.

Dantrolene acts to inhibit excitation contraction coupling in skeletal muscle by inhibiting calcium release at the level of the sarcoplasmic reticulum. It depresses twitch height by more than 70% in humans when given intravenously in a dose of 2.5 mg/kg. Bio-availability of the oral form, once an issue of concern, is very similar to that of the intravenous form [145]. Elimination is by hepatic conversion to an active 5-hydroxy metabolite that is excreted in the urine, with a half-life of approximately 9 h for the parent and 15 h for the metabolite [146].

Dantrolene is used for either prophylaxis or acute management and is indicated as prophylaxis in adults and children with biopsy-proven MH. The drug is highly effective and, when used in sufficient doses early in the course of acute MH, is virtually 100% effective in preventing mortality. The trend in mortality associated with acute MH up to 1993 was described by Strazis and Fox [147]. Mortality declined dramatically in the years immediately after the introduction of dantrolene, from more than 60% to less than 10%. Currently, mortality has further declined to less than 5%.

Preparation and care of the susceptible patient

Identification of the patient at risk and the provision of a safe, non-triggering anesthetic environment are the primary goals for those providing care to those at risk for MH. Patients at risk have been discussed previously and include those with a previous history of MH or masseter spasm and a CK higher than 20,000 units/L within 24 h; those with one of the previously mentioned myopathies (central core, Evans, King–Denborough); those with an idiopathic elevation of CK; and first-degree relatives of a person with known or suspected MH. These patients should be managed as if they are known to have MH, regardless of whether they have been tested.

Testing consists of either the CHCT (in Europe, *in vitro* muscle contracture testing), considered to be the gold standard, or newer genetic testing to identify individuals who carry one of more than 29 different *RYR1* mutations. The CHCT is essentially 100% sensitive and approximately 80% specific but requires a surgical procedure, can only be done in a few centers around the world, is

MH Hotline
1-800-644-9737
Outside the US:
1-315-464-7079

EMERGENCY THERAPY FOR

MALIGNANT HYPERTHERMIA

Effective May 2008

DIAGNOSIS vs. ASSOCIATED PROBLEMS

Signs of MH:
- Increasing $ETCO_2$
- Trunk or total body rigidity
- Masseter spasm or trismus
- Tachycardia/tachypnea
- Mixed Respiratory and Metabolic Acidosis
- Increased temperature (may be late sign)
- Myoglobinuria

Sudden/Unexpected Cardiac Arrest in Young Patients:
- Presume hyperkalemia and initiate treatment (see #6)
- Measure CK, myoglobin, ABGs, until normalized
- Consider dantrolene
- Usually secondary to occult myopathy (e.g., muscular dystrophy)
- Resuscitation may be difficult and prolonged

Trismus or Masseter Spasm with Succinylcholine
- Early sign of MH in many patients
- If limb muscle rigidity, begin treatment with dantrolene
- For emergent procedures, continue with non-triggering agents, evaluate and monitor the patient, and consider dantrolene treatment
- Follow CK and urine myoglobin for 36 hours.
- Check CK immediately and at 6 hour intervals until returning to normal. Observe for dark or cola colored urine. If present, liberalize fluid intake and test for myoglobin
- Observe in PACU or ICU for at least 12 hours

ACUTE PHASE TREATMENT

1 GET HELP. GET DANTROLENE – Notify Surgeon
- Discontinue volatile agents and succinylcholine.
- Hyperventilate with 100% oxygen at flows of 10 L/min. or more.
- Halt the procedure as soon as possible; if emergent, continue with non-triggering anesthetic technique.
- Don't waste time changing the circle system and CO_2 absorbant.

2 Dantrolene 2.5 mg/kg rapidly IV through large-bore IV, if possible

To convert kg to lbs for amount of dantrolene, give patients 1 mg/lb (2.5 mg/kg approximates 1 mg/lb).

- Dissolve the 20 mg in each vial with at least 60 ml sterile, preservative-free water for injection. Prewarming (not to exceed 39° C.) the sterile water may expidite solublization of dantrolene. However, to date, there is no evidence that such warming improves clinical outcome.
- Repeat until signs of MH are reversed.
- Sometimes more than 10 mg/kg (up to 30 mg/kg) is necessary.

- Each 20 mg bottle has 3 gm mannitol for isotonicity. The pH of the solution is 9.

3 Bicarbonate for metabolic acidosis
- 1-2 mEq/kg if blood gas values are not yet available.

4 Cool the patient with core temperature >39°C. Lavage open body cavities, stomach, bladder, or rectum. Apply ice to surface. Infuse cold saline intravenously. Stop cooling if temp. <38°C and falling to prevent drift < 36°C.

5 Dysrhythmias usually respond to treatment of acidosis and hyperkalemia.
- Use standard drug therapy **except calcium channel blockers, which may cause hyperkalemia or cardiac arrest in the presence of dantrolene.**

6 Hyperkalemia – Treat with hyperventilation, bicarbonate, glucose/insulin, calcium.
- Bicarbonate 1-2 mEq/kg IV.
- For **pediatric,** 0.1 units insulin/kg and 1 ml/kg 50% glucose or for **adult,** 10 units regular insulin IV and 50 ml 50% glucose.
- Calcium chloride 10 mg/kg or calcium gluconate 10-50 mg/kg for life-threatening hyperkalemia.
- Check glucose levels hourly.

7 Follow $ETCO_2$, electrolytes, blood gases, CK, core temperature, urine output and color, coagulation studies. If CK and/or K+ rise more than transiently or urine output falls to less than 0.5 ml/kg/hr, induce diuresis to >1 ml/kg/hr and give bicarbonate to alkalanize urine to prevent myoglobinuria-induced renal failure. (See D below)
- Venous blood gas (e.g., femoral vein) values may document hypermetabolism better than arterial values.
- Central venous or PA monitoring as needed and record minute ventilation.
- Place Foley catheter and monitor urine output.

POST ACUTE PHASE

A Observe the patient in an ICU for at least 24 hours, due to the risk of recrudescence.
B Dantrolene 1 mg/kg q 4-6 hours or 0.25 mg/kg/hr by infusion for at least 24 hours. Further doses may be indicated.
C Follow vitals and labs as above (see #7)
- Frequent ABG as per clinical signs
- CK every 8-12 hours; less often as the values trend downward

D Follow urine myoglobin and institute therapy to prevent myoglobin precipitation in renal tubules and the subsequent development of Acute Renal Failure. CK levels above 10,000 IU/L is a presumptive sign of rhabdomyolysis and myoglobinuria. Follow standard intensive care therapy for acute rhabdomyolysis and myoglobinuria (urine output >2 ml/kg/hr by hydration and diuretics along with alkalinization of urine with Na-bicarbonate infusion with careful attention to both urine and serum pH values).
E Counsel the patient and family regarding MH and further precautions; refer them to MHAUS. Fill out and send in the Adverse Metabolic Reaction to Anesthesia (AMRA) form (www.mhreg.org) and send a letter to the patient and her/his physician. Refer patient to the nearest Biopsy Center for follow-up.

Non-Emergency Information
MHAUS
PO Box 1069 (11 East State Street)
Sherburne, NY 13460-1069
Phone
1-800-986-4287
(607-674-7901)
Fax
607-674-7910
Email
info@mhaus.org
Website
www.mhaus.org

Since 1981

MALIGNANT HYPERTHERMIA ASSOCIATION OF THE UNITED STATES

Dedicated to Patient Safety

CAUTION: This protocol may not apply to all patients; alter for specific needs.

ORPO 5/08/5K   Produced by the Malignant Hyperthermia Association of the United States (MHAUS). MHAUS is a non-profit organization under IRS-Code 501(c)3. It operates solely on contributed funds. All contributions are tax deductible. For more information, go to www.mhaus.org.

Figure 40.6 Poster prepared by the Malignant Hyperthermia Association of the United States (MHAUS) to provide the clinician with essential information for the care of the malignant hyperthermia patient. Reproduced with permission from reference [206] with permission from the Malignant Hyperthermia Association of the United States.

expensive, and cannot be done accurately on children under the age of 6 years (age criteria vary for each testing site). Genetic testing will not identify all those who are susceptible and therefore must be used in combination with muscle biopsy testing in those with a negative genetic test result. The test is especially useful to evaluate family members of a patient known to have MH; however, a negative test result does not rule out MH because not all the genetic mutations responsible for MH have been identified. Genetic testing is, however, much less expensive and does not require travel or a surgical procedure.

For the patient determined to be at risk, a non-triggering anesthetic should be provided, avoiding the use of volatile anesthetic agents and succinylcholine. The use of regional anesthesia is an excellent option because amide-type local anesthetics have not been found to carry risk either in animal models or in clinical practice. The anesthesia machine should be flushed of residual anesthetic, absorbant changed, agent and vaporizers either removed or otherwise rendered inoperable. Various protocols have been recommended for specific anesthesia machines. The Draeger Fabius machine (Draeger Medical Systems Inc, Telford, Pennsylvania) requires more than six times as long to adequately flush as the older Draeger Narkomed [148]. This is similar to the time required to flush the Draeger Primus compared to the Ohmeda Excel (GE Healthcare, Piscataway, New Jersey) [149]. Both new machines required more than 1 h to reduce the anesthetic agent concentration to less than 5 parts per million. This protracted preparation time may require that a clean machine be kept available or that MH-susceptible cases be cared for as the first case on the surgery schedule to avoid delays.

Summary

In summary, MH is a rare pharmacogenetic disorder that is likely to become increasingly rare, given its increased recognition, more frequent use of weak triggering agents, and less frequent use of succinylcholine. Prompt recognition and early treatment with dantrolene should make severe morbidity or mortality extremely rare. As genetic diagnosis becomes increasingly available and sensitive, this disorder will be more easily identified and managed in the future.

Propofol infusion syndrome

Propofol is an intravenous anesthetic agent used for the induction of general anesthesia in children and adults. Because of its rapid onset and offset of action, it is an ideal agent for sedation of mechanically ventilated patients. Developed in 1980, it had been used for a number of years in both adults and children without report of severe adverse events.

In 1992, Parke et al [150] reported on the deaths of five children in whom metabolic acidosis and myocardial failure developed after propofol infusion. All these children had upper respiratory tract infections, ranged in age from 4 weeks to 6 years, and were sedated with propofol at a rate ranging between 66 and 178 μg/kg/min (4–10.7 mg/kg/h) for between 66 and 115 h. The constellation of metabolic acidosis, bradyarrhythmia, and heart failure was typical for these patients. The dose range was within that recommended by the British Medical Association at that time, 150–2500 μg/kg/min (9–150 mg/kg/h). Parke was the first to suggest that propofol infusion, although safe in adults, perhaps should not be used for sedation for children.

In 1998, Bray [151] further characterized this constellation of symptoms as propofol infusion syndrome (PRIS) by review of information collected from the literature on 18 children who received propofol and had similar adverse effects. The majority of affected patients had respiratory tract infections, although other associations have been reported subsequently by other providers [5]. These other situations were found to occur in young, healthy patients who had sustained head trauma and had received intravenous steroids, as well as vasopressors. In Bray's series, the terminal event was myocardial failure, ventricular dysrhythmia, or, in some instances, a resistant and progressive bradycardia, which has further been identified as the Brugada syndrome [152].

Postmortem examination commonly reveals a fatty liver and myocardial fiber necrosis, metabolic acidosis is common, and plasma is lipemic. According to Bray [151], there appeared to be a definite association between PRIS and propofol infusions higher than a mean dose of 67 μg/kg/min (4 mg/kg.h) and lasting 48 h or longer.

Although the dose limits suggested by Bray [151] provide guidance, the rapid development of tolerance requires an increased rate of propofol infusion to maintain adequate sedation, and the relatively low dose suggested by Bray is often quickly exceeded. The catecholamine surge, present in acute neurological conditions or produced in various other stress models, may result in sympathetic overactivity with secondary endogenous catecholamine toxicity that may be responsible for decreasing the anesthetic effect of propofol as well as contributing to the direct myocytolytic effects of catecholamines [153].

The mechanism of the myocytotoxic effect of propofol given in prolonged doses has not yet been entirely elucidated. It is known that propofol uncouples oxidative phosphorylation and energy production in the mitochondria, impairs oxygen utilization, and inhibits electron flow along the mitochondrial electron transport chain.

These cellular effects result in a clinically apparent decrease in ventricular performance. Additionally, in this setting propofol may directly antagonize β-adrenoceptor binding and act directly on calcium channel proteins, resulting in diminished cardiac contractility [153].

Cardiac and peripheral muscle necrosis is often evident on postmortem examination. This may be the result of an imbalance of energy demand and supply [153]. Free fatty acids, derived from lipolysis of adipose tissues, are, under fasting conditions, the most important fuel for both the myocardium and skeletal muscle [153]. Oxidation within the mitochondria is the key process generating electrons, which are subsequently transferred to the respiratory chain. As propofol can impair the movement of electrons through this chain, the subsequent accumulation of free fatty acids can eventually lead to various grades of myocytolysis. Furthermore, the accumulation of unused free fatty acids has proarrhythmogenic properties that contribute to the overall clinical picture of dysrhythmia and myocardial failure observed in PRIS (Fig. 40.7) [153].

Although PRIS is most commonly observed after a prolonged propofol infusion, there have been some reports of development of this syndrome after just a few hours of continued propofol infusion in pediatric patients. Koch et al, in 2004 [154], reported the first case of suspected PRIS after short-term infusion of propofol in a child. The patient was a 5-year-old girl admitted to the hospital after endovascular coil embolization of a high-output arteriovenous malformation. Propofol infusion was started at 250 μg/kg/min (15 mg/kg/h). A progressive elevation in serum lactate developed within 6 h of admission, and a diagnosis of PRIS was considered. The lactic acidosis rapidly resolved after propofol infusion was tapered and discontinued, and the child subsequently recovered (Table 40.4).

There is some thought that, in patients receiving propofol infusion, frequent monitoring of acid–base status and lactate level may alert the clinician to early development of PRIS [155]. Veldhoen and colleagues [155] described a 17-year-old boy who sustained multiple skull fractures in a motor vehicle accident. A propofol infusion was initiated to allow continued endotracheal intubation, and over the ensuing hours, escalating doses were required to maintain adequate depth of sedation. A maximum of 8 mg/kg/h was administered for 14 h early in the hospital course. On the fourth day, propofol was discontinued as a progressive lactic acidosis was noted. Despite serial measurement of acid–base status and lactate and eventual discontinuation of propofol after lactate was noted to increase, albeit modestly, the child subsequently had CA and eventually died as a result of profound myocardial failure. This was the first report of mortality due to PRIS despite careful monitoring of metabolic parameters and prompt discontinuation of propofol

with increased lactate. It should be noted, however, that the child received a continuous infusion of propofol at a dose exceeding that recommended (67 μg/kg/min or 4 mg/kg/h for a limited duration of no longer than 48 h) [155]. Figure 40.8 details this patient's hospital course.

Some predictors have been identified for mortality in patients with suspected PRIS [156]. Patients with suspected PRIS who died were more likely to be younger than 18 years old, be male, have received propofol for more than 48 h, and have been concomitantly treated with catecholamine therapy. The presence of cardiac symptoms, hypotension, rhabdomyolysis, renal involvement, metabolic acidosis, or dyslipidemia also heralded increased mortality in these patients.

Because of the association with propofol and derangement of the flow of electrons through the respiratory chain in the mitochondria, it is also thought there may be a genetic susceptibility to PRIS manifested as a mitochondrial fatty acid oxidation abnormality.

Current recommendations for propofol administration are as follows: pediatric patients should not receive infusions of propofol that exceed 67 μg/kg/min (4 mg/kg/h) for more than 48 h. For those individuals with mitochondrial myopathies or known mitochondrial defects, it is probably prudent to avoid propofol infusions altogether unless there is no viable alternative or to use adjunctive medications to facilitate sedation and allow a lower dose of propofol as infusion. Regardless, it would certainly be recommended to monitor acid–base status as well as lactate level on a regular basis (every 6 h) to minimize the chance for development of PRIS. The development of a metabolic acidosis or rise in lactate without further cause would warrant discontinuation of propofol infusion and administration of an alternative sedating medication.

Local anesthetic toxicity and intralipid administration

Thousands of doses of local anesthetic medications are administered to pediatric patients every day in hospitals and outpatient surgical centers throughout the world. Local anesthetic medications may act not only as the sole agent for analgesia; more often, they serve as an important component of an anesthetic technique that uses a combination of both regional and general anesthesia.

Cocaine was the first local anesthetic, isolated from coca leaves in the 1860s by Albert Niemann, a German chemist. Cocaine was initially used by Sigmund Freud in 1884 to assist a patient in weaning from morphine. The first clinical use of cocaine for nerve block occurred in 1884 by Dr William Stewart Halsted to create surgical anesthesia. The first modern local anesthetic developed was lidocaine in the 1940s [157].

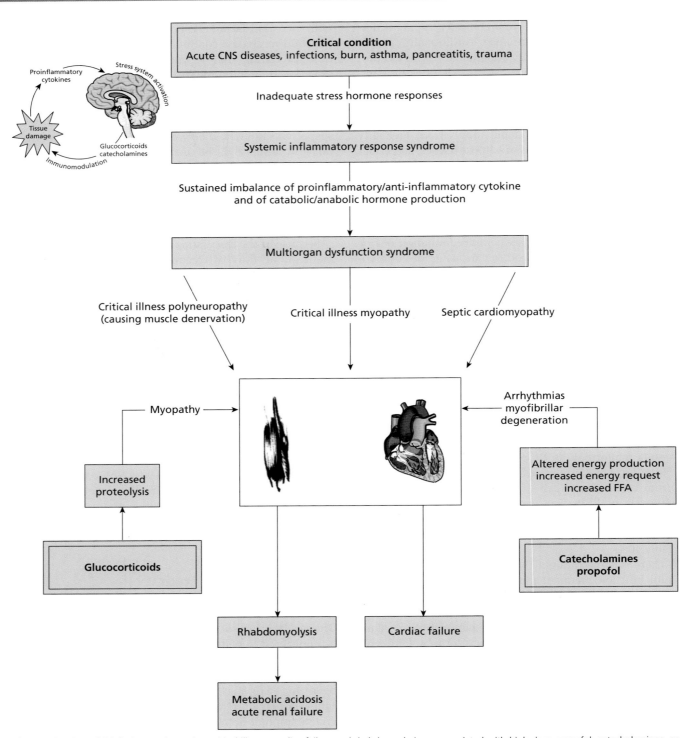

Figure 40.7 Propofol infusion syndrome is a critical illness; cardiac failure and rhabdomyolysis are associated with high-dose propofol, catecholamines, or steroids. CNS, central nervous system; FFA, free fatty acid. Adapted from Vasile et al [153] with permission from Springer.

Table 40.4 Evolution of propofol dose and acid–base status (hours after admission)

Dose and status	Admission	Time after admission, h						
		2	4	6	8	10	18	24
Propofol, mg/kg per h	15	15	15	15	6	6	0	0
pH	7.45	7.38	7.31	7.34	7.33	7.36	7.39	7.37
Paco₂, mmHg	33	36	42	36	41	41	40	39
Bicarbonate, mmol/L	22.8	20.9	20.7	19.1	21	23.1	23.7	22.1
Lactate, mmol/L	1.8	3.4	4.6	5.3	3.9	1.9	1.4	1.3
Base excess, mmol/L	−0.7	−3.4	−4.5	−5.6	−4	−1.6	−0.6	−2.4

Adapted from Koch [154] with permission from Springer.

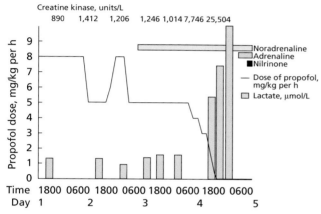

Figure 40.8 Time overview of propofol dose and laboratory results. See text for detailed explanation. Adapted from Veldhoen et al [155] with permission from Lippincott Williams and Wilkins.

Local anesthetics prevent neural transmission through inhibition of fast sodium channels as well as via inhibition of γ-aminobutyric acid in pathways located in the cerebral cortex [158]. Local anesthetics are of either the amide or the ester type and are metabolized via differing mechanisms. Local ester anesthetics are metabolized via plasma pseudocholinesterase; local amide anesthetics are metabolized via the liver. It is important to understand that the toxicities of local anesthetics are additive. Therefore, when two local anesthetics are combined, the maximum dose of the local anesthetics must be carefully determined, keeping in mind the overall ratio of each of these medications.

Ever since the first use of cocaine for medical purposes, there have been reports of its adverse reactions on the nervous, respiratory, and cardiac systems. In 1885, four publications dealt with serious adverse events, including death. A report by Mayer [159] in 1924 raised medical awareness of the toxic reactions to these medications with a report of 40 fatalities related to local anesthesia.

In pediatric patients, local anesthetic toxicity is relatively rare. Among the largest series that have reviewed complications of regional anesthetics in the pediatric population, Giaufre et al [160] reported a complication rate of four per 10,000 systemic toxic reactions after the performance of epidural injection of local anesthetic. In this series, no systemic toxicity was associated with peripheral nerve blocks.

When neurotoxicity occurs, it typically precedes the more severe cardiotoxicity. In awake patients, tinnitus, a metallic taste in the mouth, and circumoral tingling are frequent initial symptoms. As the blood level of local anesthetics increases, there is progression to motor twitching followed in some by grand mal seizures. In those who progress to cardiotoxicity, the manifestations include cardiac arrhythmia and hypotension, with eventual cardiovascular collapse [161]. McClenahan [162] reported the first pediatric death in 1955 after local anesthetic toxicity after the child consumed a dibucaine troche. He described a wide-complex bradycardia unresponsive to conventional treatment with sodium bicarbonate and other medications.

In 2006, Rosenblatt et al [163] reported the first successful use of a 20% lipid emulsion in a human patient during resuscitation after a presumed bupivacaine-related CA. The rationale for use of lipid emulsion had been introduced by Weinberg et al in 1998 [164] with initial studies in rats and subsequently dogs, demonstrating that lipid infusions both raise the threshold for cardiotoxicity and increase the likehood of survival in rodents receiving a large single intravenous dose of bupivacaine [164]. Ludot et al [165] presented the first case report of successful resuscitation after presumed local anesthetic toxicity in a child. A 13-year-old child received a lumbar plexus block under general anesthetic and subsequently experienced ventricular tachycardia 15 min after injection of lidocaine and ropivacaine with epinephrine. Plasma levels of local anesthetics were obtained during early resuscitation and indicated local anesthetic toxicity.

Within 2 min of intralipid administration, normal sinus rhythm was achieved [165].

Experience in animals and humans suggests that intravenous lipid emulsion increases the lethal threshold and decreases mortality after systemic overdose of local anesthetics and animals [166]. This finding represents an important advance in the care of both adults and children, given that cardiopulmonary bypass has traditionally been the therapy of last resort in adults and children with CA secondary to local anesthetic overdose [167].

Mechanism of action of lipid emulsion

The "lipid sink" theory described by Weinberg suggests that local anesthetic is sequestered in the plasma lipid fraction, thereby isolating tissue from the toxic effect [167]. Lipid may also have a direct inotropic effect on the heart and that effect may contribute positively to its ability to reverse bupivacaine-induced cardiac depression (Fig. 40.9) [167].

Clearly, evidence supports the early use of lipid emulsion in the treatment of local anesthetic toxicity. Rather than waiting for progression to a non-productive or unstable rhythm, treatment with lipid emulsion should be initiated as soon as possible. Weinberg [167] suggested that lipid emulsion should be used at the earliest signs of local anesthetic toxicity, for example, when the neurological signs and symptoms appear and before the onset of more serious cardiac manifestations. Subsequently, Shah et al [168] reported the successful use of a lipid emulsion

in a 40-day-old infant with presumed local anesthetic toxicity after caudal injection.

According to Weinberg's recommendations [167], the dose of 1 mL/kg of lipid emulsion 20% over 1 min could be repeated every 3–5 min for a maximum dose of 3 mL/kg. At the point of conversion to sinus rhythm, infusion of lipid emulsion 20%, at a rate of 0.25 mL/kg/min should be continued until hemodynamic recovery. Initiation of intralipid infusion is often needed because the sequelae of local anesthetic systemic toxicity can potentially persist or recur even hours after the initial exposure. Given this potential, monitoring of patients should continue for at least 12 h, particularly if there has been evidence of severe cardiovascular compromise. A number of lipid emulsions are available and have been used during resuscitation of local anesthetic systemic toxicity, including Intralipid (Baxter Healthcare Corporation, Deerfield Illinois), Liposyn (Hospira Inc, Lake Forest, Illinois), and Medialipid (Braun Medical, Boulogne, France) [169]. None has been demonstrated to be superior, and all are based on proprietary intravenous lipid formulations used for total parenteral nutrition. Medialipid was the formulation used by Ludot et al [165] in their 2008 report.

The role of more conventional medications used during resuscitation from local anesthetic overdose has been investigated. There is evidence for impairment of lipid-based resuscitation with a single dose of epinephrine of 10 μg/kg or greater. Dose–response trials suggest that small epinephrine doses (1–2.5 μg/kg) may be advantageous in terms of rapid recovery; however, higher doses of epinephrine appear to adversely affect both metabolic and hemodynamic recovery profiles. Although experimental animals treated with high-dose epinephrine had earlier return of circulation than the saline-treated or lipid-treated controls, this earlier return of circulation did not translate to sustained hemodynamic stability and, in fact, contributed to their mortality [170]. Likewise, studies in swine that included the use of vasopressin and epinephrine along with lipid administration demonstrated that survival was not improved with this practice [171]. Despite the fact that propofol is formulated in a 10% lipid emulsion, it should not be used as a substitute for lipid administration, because a fatal dose of propofol would have to be administered to achieve a therapeutic level of lipid. Propofol also may cause dose-related bradycardia and hypotension and can potentially further impair myocardial contractility in the setting of local anesthetic toxicity [158].

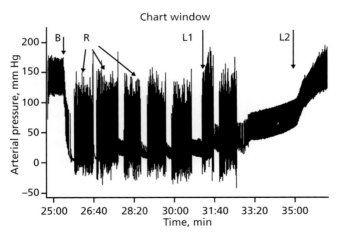

Figure 40.9 Hemodynamic response to lipid infusion. The arterial pressure trace of a rat is shown over approximately 12 min. The arrow at B indicates intravenous injection of bupivacaine, 20 mg/kg, over 20 sec. The arrows at R indicate resuscitation by closed chest compression. The L1 arrow indicates infusion of 30% soybean oil emulsion, 5 mL/kg, over 10 sec. Recovery of hemodynamic profile occurs after the second lipid bolus, L2 (*arrow*). Adapted from Weinberg [167] with permission from Lippincott Williams and Wilkins.

Summary

Local anesthetic systemic toxicity, although a rare event, can have devastating consequences. It has been suggested that every facility that administers local anesthetics to patients should assure the rapid availability of lipid emulsion for the treatment of toxicity [163]. Lipid emulsion should be used early in treatment, even before the devastating effects of cardiotoxicity have occurred. As previously described, the initial dose of lipid emulsion 20% is 1 mL/kg over 1 min. This dose could be repeated every 3–5 min for a maximum dose of 3 mL/kg. At the point of return of hemodynamic stability, consideration should be given to initiation of an infusion at the rate of 0.25 mL/kg/min. Because local anesthetic toxicity may recur even after hemodynamic stability, patients should be monitored for at least 12 h if there has been evidence of cardiovascular compromise. In addition, during resuscitative efforts, attention must be paid to the ABCs of standard cardiopulmonary resuscitation. The use of epinephrine in doses higher than 10 μg/kg, administered along with lipid emulsion therapy, may not translate to improved survival and may even contribute to higher mortality. Smaller doses of epinephrine limited to 1–2.5 μg/kg may be tolerated well during resuscitation. Similarly, the addition of vasopressin to this regimen may not be beneficial, although additional research may be necessary to fully elucidate the effects of more traditional therapy when combined with lipid emulsion therapy.

Nerve and positioning injuries

The anesthesiologist is primarily responsible for safe and comfortable positioning of the surgical patient during the operative period. Despite great care and attention, nerve injuries do occur and can lead to temporary or, rarely, permanent disability. Not surprisingly, few data directly address positioning injuries in children. Clinical practice is therefore primarily dependent on data extrapolated from adult studies to the pediatric population.

The incidence of peripheral nerve injuries in pediatric patients appears to be much lower than that among adults although data are limited to a handful of case reports. Morray et al [19], using the ASA Closed Claims database, found that the rate of peripheral nerve injuries in children was only 1% of claims, whereas in adults, the figure was 16%. Given that pediatrics represents about 10% of all anesthetics performed, these data tend to confirm the sense that positioning injury is recognized less frequently in children than in adults.

In an adult population, Welch et al [172] evaluated a total of 380,680 anesthetics administered over a 10-year period; only 112 were associated with a nerve injury (0.03%). In that study, nerve injury was defined as a new sensory and/or motor deficit. Nerve injuries from the surgical procedure itself were excluded. This series represents the largest number of consecutive patients ever reviewed for all types of perioperative peripheral nerve injuries. In the Welch et al study [172], as in others, it was difficult to define nerve injury related to positioning

because existing deficits, injuries occurring in the postoperative period, and predisposing conditions make case finding challenging. In that study, by far the most common of the positioning-related injuries was that affecting the ulnar nerve [172]. Box 40.1 is a simplified guide to the recognition of various nerve injuries [173].

The practice advisory for the prevention of perioperative peripheral neuropathies published by the ASA in 2002 provides guidance that, although directed primarily at adult patients, can be useful for children as well [174]. Even when the ASA guidelines are followed, however, injury cannot be prevented in all patients, most likely secondary to predisposing conditions. Welch et al [172] demonstrated that certain populations may be more likely to have perioperative positioning injuries due to co-morbid conditions. This study reported associations with the following surgical specialties: neurosurgery, cardiac surgery, general surgery, and orthopedic surgery. Medical co-morbid conditions such as hypertension, tobacco use, and diabetes mellitus were also associated with peripheral nerve injuries in the perioperative setting. It is interesting to note that the Welch et al study did not demonstrate an increased frequency in peripheral nerve injuries in patients maintained in a prolonged lithotomy position, although it has been shown in previous studies [175] that the lithotomy position for more than 2 h has been a major risk factor for injury. Upper extremity nerve injuries were more common than lower extremity injuries. During this study, three different databases were examined. Sensory deficits were slightly more frequent in one database, whereas motor deficits were more frequent in another, and, not surprisingly, patients with a motor component to their injury are more likely to pursue legal measures.

Ischemia and infarct are mechanisms of localized injury to the peripheral nerves of an anesthetized patient. Winfree and Kline [176] indicated that disruption of blood supply to the nerves is integral to the mechanism of injury. Thus, it is reasonable to consider that patients with disease states that affect changes in blood flow might have a higher frequency of positioning injuries. Pediatric patients, who are less likely to have some of the above co-morbid conditions, may have a lower frequency of peripheral nerve injuries due to positioning.

In addition to peripheral neuropathy and subsequent neurological deficits, the occurrence of postoperative vision loss (POVL) is of particular concern during the performance of particular procedures. The causes of POVL are threefold: ischemic optic neuropathy (including anterior and posterior types), central retinal occlusion, and cortical blindness [177]. A number of factors, which may be under the control of the anesthesiologist, have been identified as being associated with POVL, including patient positioning, intraoperative hypotension, and blood loss. Patients who had ischemic optic

Box 40.1 Simplified clinical identification of major peripheral nerve injuries

Arm

• Median nerve	Numbness over the index finger; weakness of abduction of the thumb
• Ulnar nerve	Numbness over the little finger; weakness of abduction and/or adduction of the fingers; weakness of flexion at the distal interphalangeal joints of the little and ring fingers if the lesion is at the elbow
• Radial nerve	Weakness of extension at the distal interplanalgeal joint of the thumb and of the wrist and finger extensors
• Musculocutaneous nerve	Weakness of flexion of the elbow
• Circumflex nerve	Weakness of abduction of the shoulder
• Brachial plexus	Various combinations of lesions within the median, ulnar, radial, musculocutaneous, and circumflex nerve territories

Leg

• Femoral nerve	Weakness of flexion of the hip; numbness over the thigh
• Obturator nerve	Weakness of adduction of the hip
• Sciatic nerve	Weakness of ankle dorsiflexion and plantarflexion; weakness of knee flexion, if the lesion is proximal; numbness below the knee
• Common peroneal nerve	Weakness of dorsiflexion of the ankle and toes
• Tibial nerve	Weakness of plantarflexion of the ankle and toes

Adapted from Sawyer et al [173] with permission from Elsevier.

neuropathy had longer periods in the prone position with a larger estimated blood loss compared with those patients with central retinal artery occlusion. The majority of patients with ischemic optic neuropathy had both eyes affected, whereas recovery was very unlikely in the group of patients who had central retinal artery occlusion. Recovery of vision is more likely in ischemic optic neuropathy, with 44% of patients recovering their vision compared with 0% recovery in the central retinal artery occlusion group [178].

Etiology of ischemic optic neuropathy is unknown and possibly multifactorial; it is more commonly associated with large blood loss, hypotension, anemia, the prone position, and/or vaso-occlusive disease, although specific etiologies for anterior and posterior ischemic optic neuropathy may differ [179,180]. Conversely, the etiology of central retinal artery occlusion is thought to be caused by direct pressure on the globe from facemasks or cushions when the patient is in the prone position, by emboli or by low perfusion pressure in the retina [179].

Postoperative vision loss is often thought of as being associated with spinal surgery; however, other surgical procedures may be complicated by problems similar to those encountered during prolonged spinal procedures and might also be associated with this complication. Indeed, Lee et al [181] reported on the first case of POVL caused by anterior ischemic optic neuropathy in a pediatric patient who underwent cranial vault reconstruction.

Because cranial vault reconstruction is often associated with the possibility of a large volume of blood loss, prolonged surgery, often in the prone position, and occasionally the need for controlled hypotension, these conditions do increase the chance for ischemic optic neuropathy. The child described by Lee et al [181] had an uneventful anesthetic and immediate postsurgical recovery but was readmitted on postoperative day 6 with bilateral blindness.

Although rare, the potential for nerve injury in children should not be ignored. Careful positioning, special attention to those at greatest risk, and awareness of nerve injury as a cause of postoperative pain, limited mobility or visual loss, even in the non-verbal or preverbal child, should be maintained.

Anaphylaxis and its treatment

Anaphylaxis is a progressive, potentially fatal, IgE-mediated reaction associated with histamine release into the systemic circulation. Upon histamine release, hypotension, edema, and hypoxia, even circulatory arrest and death may occur. To improve survival and outcome, rapid diagnosis and treatment are important. Multiple factors may lead to anaphylaxis (e.g. food allergies, insect stings, and drugs). Interestingly, 20% of patients treated for anaphylaxis had no identifiable cause [182]. This section focuses on drug-induced anaphylaxis in the perioperative period.

Definition

In 2006, the Second Symposium on the Definition and Management of Anaphylaxis recommended the following definition: "Anaphylaxis is a serious allergic reaction that is rapid in onset and may cause death" [183]. Due to the powerful sequelae of histamine release into the systemic circulation, immediate diagnosis and treatment are of utmost importance. Anaphylaxis is due to an IgE-mediated immediate hypersensitivity reaction, resulting in immediate release of potent chemical mediators from mast cells and basophils. Histamine is the predominant mediator being released, followed by prostaglandin D2, leukotrienes, platelet-activating factor, tryptase, and eosinophil and neutrophil chemotactic factors. In contrast, anaphylactoid reactions are not IgE mediated but cannot be distinguished clinically from anaphylaxis. The most important organ systems affected by anaphylactic reactions are cutaneous, respiratory, cardiovascular, and gastrointestinal [184].

Epidemiology

The incidence of anaphylactic reactions in the perioperative period ranges from 1 in 10,000 cases to 1 in 20,000 cases [185]. Unfortunately, incidence data are often underestimated because of under-reporting. Interestingly, 90% of anaphylactic reactions appear at anesthesia induction. Mortality rates are reported to be between 3% and 9%. Most of the deaths related to anaphylaxis are drug induced, followed by food- and insect sting-related causes. Data regarding pediatric anaphylaxis in the United States vary because of insufficient reporting in the pediatric population and discrepancies in the definition of anaphylaxis. Data from 2004 estimated the incidence of anaphylaxis among children and adolescents to be 10.5 episodes per 100,000 person-years [186], lower than the incidence in the general population.

The population of the United States seems to have a higher incidence of anaphylaxis compared with that in other countries. Factors such as expansion of diet and increasing use of peanut products in foods have been attributed to this finding. Children and adolescents with atopy, asthma, eczema, and a history of allergies are at an increased risk of anaphylaxis. Although male sex may be a predisposing factor for development of anaphylaxis, genetic factors and racial differences do not seem to play a role. However, any patient who has had an anaphylactic reaction is at increased risk of recurrence. The severity of the previous anaphylactic reaction does not predict the severity of the recurring reaction [184].

In regard to anaphylactic reactions within the perioperative period, non-depolarizing neuromuscular blocking agents (NMBAs), latex, and antibiotics are at the top of the list of offending agents.

Death from anaphylaxis is rare. However, lack of reporting and difficulty diagnosing anaphylaxis posthumously with any specific test contribute to inaccurate numbers related to morbidity and mortality.

Etiology

Although this section is focused on drug-induced anaphylaxis in the perioperative period, there is some relationship between food allergies and drug-induced anaphylaxis. Food is actually the most common cause of anaphylaxis in children, followed by medications, insect stings, blood products, latex, vaccines, and contrast dye [186,187]. While children can outgrow many food allergies, e.g. milk, eggs, and soybeans, certain food allergies persist. Foods causing persistent sensitivity include peanuts, tree nuts, and shellfish. These foods are responsible for more severe and near-fatal and fatal anaphylactic reactions [188].

Among drug-induced anaphylactic reactions, allergy to penicillin is the most common [186]. Among individuals with penicillin allergy, 4–10% have cross-reactivity to other penicillin-related drugs [187]. Some medications contain food-related substances to which food-allergic individuals may react. Propofol, marketed as Diprivan (AstraZeneca, Wilmington, Delaware), is used for sedation and general anesthesia in children. It contains egg and soybean products that increase the risk of anaphylaxis in individuals with these specific food allergies.

Pathophysiology

The IgE-mediated hypersensitivity reaction has been classically used to describe anaphylaxis. The body is introduced to different allergens via different routes including ingestion, skin contact, or intravenous injections or infusions. Interestingly, a small amount of allergen is sufficient for cells to react. On initial exposure to an allergen, IgE isotype antibodies are produced and bind to high-affinity FcεRI receptors located in the plasma membrane of tissue mast cells and blood basophils. Lymphocytes, eosinophils, and platelets bind IgE antibodies via low-affinity FcεRII receptors. This initial antigen sensitization is clinically silent. On re-exposure, epithelial and endothelial barriers break down. This allows the antigen to come into contact with its specific IgE antibodies. The multimeric allergen cross-links two specific IgE receptors, thereby creating a bridge between two IgEs. The two IgE receptors aggregate and induce a signal transduction cascade, releasing systemically preformed biochemical mediators. Histamine is being released predominantly from intracellular granules in cells within tissues and blood, followed by neutral proteases (tryptase, chymase), and proteoglycans (heparin). Proinflammatory phospholipid-derived mediators, including prostaglandin D2, leukotrienes, thromboxane A2, and platelet-activating factor, are released soon after. Thereafter, mast cells release numerous chemokines and cytokines that initiate recruitment and activation of additional inflammatory cells.

The release of these mediators mediates the symptoms of anaphylaxis, i.e. increased vascular permeability with erythema, edema, and pruritus, vasodilation, bronchospasm, and increased smooth muscle tone.

Mast cell and basophil activation with subsequent chemical mediator release can also be triggered via activation of the complement system and direct actions on mast cells and basophils. However, the symptoms are indistinguishable from those triggered via IgE.

Timing of reactions

While most anaphylactic reactions occur within minutes of exposure to the offending agent, an additional delayed response is also possible. Delayed reactions may occur up to 72h after the initial reaction. In addition, inadequate treatment of the initial reaction may predispose individuals to delayed reactions [189]. Route, quantity, and type of antigen do not seem to play a role in delayed reactions. Severity of the initial reaction does not predict the occurrence of a delayed reaction. Corticosteroid treatment specifically in delayed anaphylactic reactions has not been effective [190].

Causes of anaphylaxis in the perioperative period

The most common cause of anaphylaxis in the perioperative period is neuromuscular blocking agents (NMBAs), with an incidence ranging from 50% to 70% [182–191], followed by latex and antibiotics [192]. Usually, anaphylactic reactions occur shortly after induction, which is especially true for NMBAs and antibiotics, but may occur at any time with all potentially allergenic agents [192]. Latex allergy, which contributes to a high number of anaphylactic reactions in the perioperative period, is discussed separately in this chapter.

In NMBAs, the quarternary ammonium groups (NH_4^+) on the NMBAs are responsible for the anaphylactic reactions. Quarternary ammonium groups also exist in foods, cosmetics, and drugs. Prior contact with quarternary ammonium groups contained in foods, cosmetics, and drugs may lead to anaphylaxis on subsequent exposure to NMBAs. In addition, NMBAs may trigger mast cell degranulation through activation of nicotinic acetylcholine receptors on cell surfaces [182]. Cross-reactivity between NMBAs occurs in approximately 60–70% of those tested [192].

Antibiotics are also known to cause anaphylaxis, especially in the perioperative period. Specifically β-lactam antibiotics (e.g. penicillins and cephalosporins) and vancomycin seem to trigger anaphylaxis [193]. In regard to vancomycin, direct mast cell activation seems to be the cause. The specificity of skin testing with β-lactams is between 97% and 99%, whereas the sensitivity is about 50% [185].

Anaphylaxis in response to thiopental or propofol is reported infrequently, whereas anaphylaxis to etomidate and ketamine is extremely rare [191,192]. Anaphylaxis to opioids is very rare as well [191,192].

Anaphylaxis to local anesthetics is uncommon and has decreased in frequency as a result of the reduced use of the ester group of local anesthetics. Most allergic reactions are attributable to the common metabolic product of the ester local anesthetic, para-amino benzoic acid [191,192], which also leads to cross-reactivity among all local anesthetics belonging to the ester group. Allergic reactions to amide local anesthetics remain anecdotal. Ingredients included in local anesthetic solutions such as antioxidants or preservatives, including metabisulfite or parabens, may also elicit allergic or adverse reactions [193]. Cross-reactivity among esters is common, whereas it is rarely seen in the amide group and is absent between esters and amides.

Diagnosis

Because anaphylaxis may progress within minutes to a life-threatening condition, its immediate diagnosis is essential. The first line of evidence for the diagnosis of anaphylaxis includes the features and severity of clinical signs as well as the timing between the introduction of a suspected allergen and the onset of symptoms. The amount of resuscitative agents required to treat the occurrence gives insight into the severity of the reaction [192].

Dewachter et al [194] adapted a clinical severity scale from Ring and Messmer [195] to describe perioperative immediate hypersensitivity reactions. Although this scale does not take into account the pathophysiological mechanisms, it is appropriate for grading the clinical severity and guiding the clinical care of immediate reactions [192]. Grades I and II describe cutaneous and cutaneous-mucous signs. Although cutaneous symptoms such as flushing, pruritus, or urticaria may be the first indication of an anaphylactic reaction, these are often missed in the operating room where patients are covered with drapes and blankets. In addition, anesthetized patients cannot verbalize complaints regarding pruritus or nausea. Bronchospasm has been reported to be the first sign of anaphylaxis in the operating room followed by hypotension, hypoxemia, and angio-edema, which relates to a grade III reaction [182], followed by CA, which is grade IV. Grades I and II are usually not life-threatening conditions, whereas grades III and IV are emergency situations necessitating prompt resuscitation.

In cases of suspected anaphylaxis, the time of occurrence is important. Appearance of symptoms within minutes of anesthetic induction implicates an intravenous agent. Reactions 15 min or more after induction suggest skin or mucous membrane contact of the offending compounds. Biphasic reactions, with an initial event followed by a second delayed reaction, have been described to occur in 6–23% of patients with anaphylaxis [184]. Delayed reactions can occur up to 72h after the initial reaction. Insufficient treatment with epinephrine during the initial reaction increases the risk of a delayed reaction.

Box 40.2 shows the clinical criteria for diagnosing anaphylaxis. This was developed by the participants of the Second Symposium on the Definition and Management of Anaphylaxis, which was thought to capture at least 95% of the cases of anaphylaxis [183]. It is important to notice that the criteria listed refer to patients not undergoing anesthesia at the same time as there is suspicion for an anaphylactic reaction.

Laboratory tests

During acute management of anaphylaxis, no test is needed to confirm the diagnosis. However, if the diagnosis is uncertain, elevated levels of histamine, serum tryptase, or both may be helpful [184]. Histamine and tryptase are the major components being released during mast cell degranulation. While histamine is the major compound being released during anaphylaxis, its detection is difficult because of its short plasma half-life of 15–20 min. After a grade I or II reaction, blood samples for histamine measurement should be drawn within 30 min. After severe reactions (grades III and IV), histamine may still be increased 2 h after the reaction. Saturation of the enzymatic metabolism of histamine is the suggested mechanism that allows detection of increased histamine levels for this prolonged period after the reaction [196].

Tryptase is a mast cell neutral serine protease and a preformed enzyme. Two major forms – α-tryptase and β-tryptase – have been identified [191]. While α-tryptase is increased in mastocytosis, pro-β-tryptase serves as a measure of mast cell mass. Mature β-tryptase is preferentially stored in mast cell granules and, when systemically released, reflects mast cell activation with mediator release. Serum tryptase concentrations reach a peak between 15 and 60 min, with a half-life of approximately 2 h [191,192]. In grade I or II reactions, blood samples may be drawn within 15 and 60 min and within 30 min and 2 h in grade III or IV reactions [192]. An increase of total tryptase concentrations (i.e. the sum of α-tryptase and β-tryptase) is highly suggestive of mast cell activation as seen in anaphylaxis, but its absence does not preclude the diagnosis. Some studies have demonstrated low sensitivity of tryptase levels in the diagnosis of anaphylaxis [191].

As a result of an immediate non-allergic reaction (e.g. histamine release), histamine may be increased, whereas tryptase remains normal. Because histamine and tryptase concentrations correlate with the severity of the allergic reaction, combined histamine and tryptase measurements have been recommended for the diagnosis of immediate reactions, whereas others recommend only tryptase [191,192].

More specific testing should be done in patients who have more than just cutaneous symptoms. Specific IgE testing can be done 2–3 weeks after an anaphylactic reaction. Skin testing is more sensitive than measuring IgE-specific antibodies and remains the gold standard for the

---

Box 40.2 Clinical criteria for diagnosing anaphylaxis

Anaphylaxis is highly likely when any *one* of the following three criteria is fulfilled:
1. Acute onset of an illness (minutes to several hours) with involvement of the skin, mucosal tissue, or both (e.g. generalized hives, pruritus or flushing, swollen lips-tongue-uvula)
   AND AT LEAST ONE OF THE FOLLOWING:
   (a) Respiratory compromise (e.g. dyspnea, wheeze-bronchospasm, stridor, reduced PEF, hypoxemia)
   (b) Reduced BP or associated symptoms of end-organ dysfunction (e.g. hypotonia (collapse), syncope, incontinence)
2. Two or more of the following that occur rapidly after exposure *to a likely allergen for that patient* (minutes to several hours):
   (a) Involvement of the skin-mucosal tissue (e.g. generalized hives, itch-flush, swollen lips-tongue-uvula)
   (b) Respiratory compromise (e.g. dyspnea, wheeze-bronchospasm, stridor, reduced PEF, hypoxemia)
   (c) Reduced BP or associated symptoms (e.g. hypotonia (collapse), syncope, incontinence)
   (d) Persistent gastrointestinal tract symptoms (e.g. crampy abdominal pain, vomiting)
3. Reduced BP after exposure to *known allergen for that patient* (minutes to several hours):
   (a) Infants and children: low systolic BP (age specific) or greater than 30% decrease in systolic BP[a]
   (b) Adults: systolic BP of less than 90 mmHg or greater than 30% decrease from that person's baseline.

BP, blood pressure; PEF, peak expiratory flow.
[a] Low systolic BP for children is defined as less than 70 mmHg from 1 month to 1 year, less than (70 mmHg + [2 × age]) from 1 to 10 years, and less than 90 mmHg from 11 to 17 years.
Adapted from Sampson et al [183] with permission from Elsevier.

detection of IgE-mediated reactions by exposing the mast cells of the skin to the suspected allergen in patients who have had anaphylaxis [185].

Premedication with H1 or H2 receptor antagonists, with corticosteroids, or with a combination of these agents has not been proven to prevent anaphylaxis [192]. Therefore, skin tests allow identification of the offending agent and demonstrate the pathophysiological mechanism of the reaction (allergic versus non-allergic). A 4–6-week delay after the reaction is required to avoid a false-negative test result because of mast cell depletion [192]. After the final test results, patients should be given a detailed report to provide to caregivers prior to future anesthetic exposures.

Management and treatment

Management of patients in whom anaphylaxis develops in the perioperative period is challenging. Most of them will have received multiple medications and present with more advanced symptoms, and their condition progresses faster than in other settings. Anaphylaxis during anesthesia is especially challenging since most of the time the initial symptoms of urticaria or erythema are not observed because the patients are covered by drapes. It is important for all people involved in the care of these patients to help identify the cause so that future exposures can be avoided [182].

Due to its severity, the diagnosis and treatment of anaphylaxis must occur simultaneously. Treatment is directed toward managing the most severe symptoms, including cardiovascular collapse, bronchospasm, and airway edema. Initiation of intravenous epinephrine and other therapies and expeditious interruption of suspected causative agents must go hand in hand. In addition to ventilation with 100% oxygen, volume support and definitive airway managment are required [182]. Patients should be placed supine in the Trendelenburg position, and the surgical procedure abbreviated if possible when anaphylaxis occurs intraoperatively.

Administration of intravenous epinephrine and expansion of intravascular volume are essential to the perioperative management of anaphylaxis [191,192]. Epinephrine's α-agonistic effects reverse vasodilation, while its β-agonist effects treat bronchospasm and release of inflammatory mediators. Because epinephrine has a short half-life, repeated doses or a continuous infusion may be necessary. There is no absolute contraindication during anaphylaxis for the use of epinephrine, and early administration should be the rule [191,192].

Due to the increased vascular permeability, fluid therapy with crystalloid or colloid solutions should be initiated immediately. Bronchospasm is treated with an inhaled β2 agonist (salbutamol or albuterol) [191,192]. Given that cardiovascular collapse and bronchospasm

occur together, epinephrine remains the first-line therapy as it corrects both cardiovascular disturbances as well as bronchoconstriction through its β2-adrenergic effects. Intravenous corticosteroids early in the course of therapy are recommended because of their anti-inflammatory effects although the beneficial effects are delayed at least 4–6h [192]. Corticosteroids, H1 receptor antagonists, or both are often recommended, with varying success, in the management of anaphylaxis [191,192].

Affected patients are sometimes unresponsive to catecholamines, possibly because of desensitization of adrenergic receptors. The use of arginine vasopressin may be an alternative as its vasoconstrictive effects are mediated by non-adrenergic vascular arginine vasopressin V1 receptors [197].

Summary

Perioperative anaphylaxis is a severe and rapid clinical condition that can lead to mortality even in previously healthy patients. Because of its infrequent presentation and variable clinical presentation, perioperative anaphylaxis may not be diagnosed immediately. The severity of symptoms as well as the rapidity of symptom progression demand prompt and aggressive treatment. The combination of clinical, biochemical, and skin test evidence will identify the responsible agent and allow the patient to avoid it in the future.

Latex allergy

Natural rubber latex (NRL) is derived from the rubber tree, *Hevea brasiliensis*, one of over 200 lactifer-type plants belonging to the family Euphorbiaceae [198]. Among numerous compounds released by NRL, the heat-stable proteins retained in NRL are responsible for the adverse events. Although the risks of hypersensitivity as well as anaphylactic reactions to latex are well recognized, the frequency of events is increasing [199]. In addition to healthcare workers, children with atopy and spina bifida and those undergoing frequent procedures requiring surgical instrumentation are at increased risk. Among all the products containing NRL in the healthcare environment, surgical gloves made from NRL have the highest prevalence for latex sensitization. Overall, the continued use of latex and the resulting sequelae of allergic reactions impose a high cost in terms of patient risk as well as provider risk and a financial burden to the healthcare system [199].

History

Use of latex items can be tracked back to 1600 BCE in ancient Mesoamerica. However, surgical gloves came into common use in the early 20th century. Descriptions of allergic reactions to NRL appeared in the medical literature by 1927, but the description of an immediate allergic reaction to NRL was not published until 1979. Since 1980, the allergic potential of NRL has been more widely recognized, and different approaches have been taken to study latex sensitivity [200].

Epidemiology

Due to differences in populations studied and methods used to verify sensitization, the reported prevalence of latex allergy in the general population varies widely, ranging from less than 1% to 6.7% [199]. A French survey obtained between 1989 and 2001 reported that latex was the second highest cause of perioperative accidents, at a rate of 27%. The healthcare environment has the highest incidence of latex sensitivity, ranging form 3% to 17% [201]. Anesthesiologists themselves have a high prevalence of latex sensitization [202]. As mentioned above, gloves made from NRL have been associated with the greatest prevalence of sensitization in the hospital setting.

Mechanism of sensitization

Frequent exposure remains the main cause of sensitization. This finding resulted in the recommendation that children undergoing frequent surgical procedures, for example, children with spina bifida, should be handled latex free from the very beginning of their management. As a result of this initiative, these children are automatically listed as being latex sensitive. In addition, children with atopy are at increased risk, especially children with food allergies to tropical fruits such as avocado, kiwi, and banana who have been shown to be at increased risk. Some evidence suggests that genetic profiles may potentiate latex reactions to hevein (HLA-DR phenotypes) [199]. The route of exposure may also play a role. In the case of NRL, skin exposure and inhalation exposure are more common. Skin exposure is of particular importance because it may result in airway hyper-reactivity leading to allergen-induced asthma [203]. Independent of the exposure, patients with latex sensitivity develop increased levels of IgE-specific latex protein. Increased IgE levels are responsible for the symptoms, and IgE levels may increase with increased exposure frequency.

Identification of patients at risk

Identification of patients at risk relies primarily on the history but may be aided by the use of questionnaires developed specifically to identify these patients.

Although some patients initially present with only cutaneous symptoms, cardiovascular symptoms as well as bronchospasm are common clinical features. Cutaneous manifestations are often inapparent as patients in the operating room are typically covered by drapes. As a consequence, the initial manifestation may be increased airway resistance manifested by high airway pressures and wheezing, rapidly followed by cardiovascular collapse. Typically, these events occur within 30–60 min after induction [191].

Although some high-risk groups of patients are widely recognized to be at increased risk (e.g. those with myelomeningocele), others have been identified such as those with spina bifida, multiple surgical procedures during childhood, cerebral palsy, mental retardation, quadriplegia, and atopy, including allergies to avocado, banana, chestnut, kiwi, papaya, peach, and nectarine.

Diagnostic methods

Obtaining a thorough patient history may suggest the diagnosis of latex allergy; specific laboratory tests are needed to confirm the diagnosis. Currently two tests are available: skin prick test and detection of IgE specific to latex protein (radio-allergosorbent test). Skin prick tests are inexpensive, sensitive, and specific. However, they must be performed in the physician's office with appropriate precautions because of the real risk of anaphylaxis.

The sensitivity of the measurement of latex-specific IgE is lower than that for the skin prick test, being positive in only 60–90% of sensitized patients [199]. With first exposure, patients produce latex-specific IgE, and the levels increase with each subsequent exposure. Sensitivity of the measurement of latex-specific IgE depends on the number of prior exposures.

Prevention in patients at risk

The first line of prevention is identification of children at risk. Creation of a latex-free or latex-sensitive environment within the perioperative area is desirable and encouraged. Complete avoidance of latex products prevents severe anaphylactic reactions. Indeed, De Queiroz et al [199] reported that since creation of a latex-free environment in all operating rooms and perioperative areas in 2002, no latex anaphylactic reactions have occurred after more than 25,000 procedures over a period of 5 years.

A latex-free protocol should include a checklist on how to manage children with latex allergy in every department involved in the care of children. Arrangements for a latex-free environment need to be made not only for the operating room but also for the recovery room and postoperative period. Communication between the different care teams (anesthesiologist, surgeon, nurses) is crucial. In the operating room, there should be a cart with latex-free equipment readily available to be used in these patients. Box 40.3 summarizes the recommendations for prevention of latex allergy [199].

Aerosolized latex allergen from previous cases requires at least 90 min to clear. The recommendation is to schedule elective procedures as first cases since levels of aerosolized latex allergens are at their lowest. Otherwise, a

Box 40.3 Recommendations for primary prevention of latex allergy (reducing exposure to latex protein to prevent sensitization for latex)

- Bring a latex-free cart into the room
- Use a latex-free reservoir bag, airways, and endotracheal tubes, and laryngeal mask airways
- Use a non-latex breathing circuit with plastic mask and bag
- Ventilator must have non-latex bellows
- Use IV tubing without latex ports; utilize stopcocks if available
- Cover all rubber injection ports on intravenous bags with tape and label in the following way:
  - Do not inject or withdraw fluid through the latex port. Note: pulmonary artery catheters (especially the balloon), central venous catheters, and arterial lines may all contain latex components
- Use non-latex gloves
- Use non-latex tourniquets, electrodes, and examination gloves
- Draw medication directly from opened multidose vials (remove stoppers) if medications are not available in ampoules
- Utilize latex-free syringes, bladder catheter, and nasogastric tubes
- Use stopcocks to inject drugs rather than latex ports
- Minimize mixing/agitating lyophilized drugs in multidose vials with rubber stoppers

time gap of 90 min should be allowed to lower latex allergen levels between patients [199].

Pre-emptive use of medication to reduce allergic reactions is controversial. Although there have been recommendations to use medications such as diphenhydramine, cimetidine, and prednisone prophylactically, the current opinion is not to do so. In addition, premedication is not necessarily successful in preventing latex anaphylaxis and might even mask the initial immune response [199].

In children in whom latex exposure cannot be completely avoided, desensitization may be an option. Sublingual, subcutaneous, or percutaneous desensitization may improve cutaneous reactions as well as rhinitis and asthma.

Prevention: complete avoidance

Complete avoidance of latex in the perioperative care areas is the most effective way to prevent sensitization to latex. The American College of Allergy, Asthma, and Immunology released recommendations to avoid latex material in healthcare institutions [204]. Indeed, since children at risk are better identified, the incidence of latex allergy has markedly decreased. There are numerous reports of reduction of latex sensitization with the implementation of a latex-free perioperative environment. In addition, avoidance of latex can reduce latex-specific IgE in these patients and progression of symptoms.

Although latex is ubiquitous in medical equipment and devices, manufacturing of single-use latex-free items has improved tremendously. In addition, there is more emphasis by manufacturers on labeling items to identify potential latex content. To maintain a latex-free perioperative environment requires continuous meticulous effort by all healthcare workers involved as well as continuous education among healthcare staff. After all, anaphylactic reactions to latex are most commonly encountered in the perioperative period.

Annotated references

A full reference list for this chapter is available at:
http://www.wiley.com/go/gregory/andropoulos/pediatricanesthesia

13. Flick RP, Sprung J, Harrison TE et al. Perioperative cardiac arrests in children between 1988 and 2005 at a tertiary referral center: a study of 92,881 patients. Anesthesiology 2007; 106: 226–37. A major study of cardiac arrest at a single institution with a comprehensive anesthesia database and record-keeping system.
20. Bhananker SM, Ramamoorthy C, Geiduschek JM et al. Anesthesia-related cardiac arrest in children: update from the Pediatric Perioperative Cardiac Arrest Registry. Anesth Analg 2007; 105: 344–50. An important contemporary update on the causes and outcomes of perioperative cardiac arrest in children.
37. Romanovsky AA. Thermoregulation: some concepts have changed. Functional architecture of the thermoregulatory system. Am J Physiol Regul Integr Comp Physiol 2007; 292: R37–R46. An outstanding contemporary review of new concepts about thermal regulation in humans.
44. Sessler DI. Temperature monitoring and perioperative thermoregulation. Anesthesiology 2008; 109: 318–38. An important review article with a clinical emphasis on temperature monitoring, thermoregulation, adverse effects of hypothermia, and prevention and treatment of hypothermia.
119. Rosero EB, Adesanya AO, Timaran CH et al. Trends and outcomes of malignant hyperthermia in the United States, 2000 to 2005. Anesthesiology 2009; 110: 89–94. A modern review of malignant hyperthermia, its status, treatment, and outcomes.
130. Larach MG, Localio AR, Allen GC et al. A clinical grading scale to predict malignant hyperthermia susceptibility. Anesthesiology 1994; 80: 771–9. An important scale to assess likelihood of malignant hyperthermia based on observable clinical phenomena.
156. Fong JJ, Sylvia L, Ruthazer R et al. Predictors of mortality in patients with suspected propofol infusion syndrome. Crit Care Med 2008; 36: 2281–7. An important review of propofol infusion syndrome, and the multiple factors predicting poor outcome in this disease.
167. Weinberg GL. Lipid infusion therapy: translation to clinical practice. Anesth Analg 2008; 106: 1340–2. A short review of the translational research that made clinical use of lipid emulsion treatment for local anesthetic overdose a first-line therapy.
194. Dewachter P, Mouton-Faivre C, Emala CW. Anaphylaxis and anesthesia: controversies and new insights. Anesthesiology 2009; 111: 1141–50. A contemporary review of anaphylaxis and anesthesia, etiologies, mechanisms, diagnosis, and treatment and prevention.
199. De Queiroz M, Combet S, Berard J et al. Latex allergy in children: modalities and prevention. Paediatr Anaesth 2009; 19: 313–19. A modern review of the problem of latex allergy in pediatrics, prevention, and treatment.

CHAPTER 41

Impact of Pediatric Surgery and Anesthesia on Brain Development

Andreas W. Loepke[1] & Sulpicio G. Soriano[2]

[1]Departments of Anesthesia and Pediatrics, Cincinnati Children's Hospital Medical Center, and University of Cincinnati College of Medicine, Cincinnati, OH, USA
[2]Department of Anesthesiology, Perioperative and Pain Medicine, Children's Hospital Boston, Boston, MA, USA

Introduction

The ability to pharmacologically render patients insensible to noxious stimulation using general anesthetics and sedatives represents one of the greatest discoveries in medicine. Undoubtedly, life-threatening conditions have been mitigated by surgical interventions that could only be performed with advanced physiological monitoring and meticulous administration of anesthetic drugs. While the exact molecular mechanisms by which these medications provide immobility, analgesia, and amnesia remain under investigation, most are thought to provide their physiological effects either by potentiating neuronal activity involving γ-aminobutyrate (GABA) receptors, by inhibiting N-methyl-D-aspartate (NMDA) glutamate receptors, or by a combination of the two.

Worldwide, every year millions of children are exposed to $GABA_A$-agonists or NMDA-antagonists to ablate the stress response to noxious stimulation and to mitigate potential, stress-related morbidity during painful procedures and imaging studies. However, recent findings in laboratory animals have demonstrated a widespread increase in apoptotic brain cell death, an inborn cell suicide program, immediately following exposure to these drugs early in life. Moreover, several animal studies have also observed subsequent neurocognitive impairment. These findings in newborn animals have led to significant concerns among pediatric anesthesiologists.

Given the potentially serious consequences of long-term neurological sequelae following uneventful pediatric anesthesia, this chapter presents the pediatric anesthesia provider with an overview of this rapidly emerging field of research by summarizing the currently available data from animal models and human clinical studies. These findings will be moderated by a review of the neuroprotective effects of anesthetic drugs. Moreover, the impact of other perioperative events, such as pain, stress, inflammation, hypoxia-ischemia, co-morbidities, and genetic predisposition, on long-term neurological function will be discussed. Finally, the reader will be introduced to the phenomenon's putative mechanisms and to the currently proposed ameliorating strategies.

Historical perspective

General anesthetics have been widely used for more than 160 years and are administered to millions of children every year [1]. Prior to the 1980s, general anesthetics were routinely withheld from hemodynamically unstable premature and term neonates. The rationale for this practice was to avoid further hemodynamic deterioration in surgical neonates who were perceived to be unable to tolerate the myocardial depressant effects of anesthetic drugs. However, the denial of adequate doses of anesthetics or analgesics in these patients ignored the fact that the neonatal central nervous system is capable of sensing pain and mounting a stress response following a surgical stimulus, even in premature infants [2]. Subsequent studies by Robinson and Anand demonstrated that the administration of opioids blunted physiological responses to surgical stress without compromising hemodynamic stability and minimized postoperative morbidity in critically ill neonates [3–5]. These developments, along with more technological advances in hemodynamic monitoring and mechanical ventilation, have resulted in the current humane practice of administering anesthetics and analgesics even to the most critically ill neonates during and after surgery.

Nociception and stress in the neonate

Neonatal animal models testing the effects of stressful conditions and exposure to recurrent painful stimulation have demonstrated widespread neuronal cell death and adverse neurological outcome as a result from these deleterious conditions [6]. Both somatic as well as visceral noxious stimulation in the neonate appear to alter processing of nociceptive inputs in adulthood. Thus, neonatal injury can subsequently be associated with either hyperalgesia or hypoalgesia, depending upon the type and severity of injury and the sensory modality tested [7]. In addition to altered pain processing, repetitive or persistent pain in the neonatal period may lead to changes in brain development, widespread alterations in animal behavior, cognitive function, and increased vulnerability to stress and anxiety disorders or chronic pain syndromes [6,8,9]. Specifically, inflammatory pain associated with repeated injection of complete Freund's adjuvant (CFA) in rat pups resulted in hyperalgesia and lasting changes in nociceptive circuitry of the adult dorsal horn [10]. Rat pups receiving repeated formalin injections into the paw developed subsequent generalized thermal hypoalgesia [7]. Moreover, early adverse emotional experiences can induce long-lasting age-, brain region-, and neuronal subgroup-specific imbalances of the inhibitory nervous system [11], disturb development of the nociceptive system and cause long-term behavioral changes [12], as well as leading to persistent learning impairment [13]. Repetitive painful stimulation in neonatal animals has been shown to lead to decreased pain thresholds and increased anxiety later in life [8,14,15]. In addition to alterations of the central nervous system, repetitive

painful skin lacerations have also been found to lead to long-term, local sensory hyperinnervation [16]. Therefore, fetuses and neonates subjected to pain and stresses associated with painful procedures may be at risk for long-term adverse outcomes.

The pre-emptive administration of analgesics and sedatives, such as morphine or ketamine, in this context, has been found to ameliorate the deleterious effects of neonatal pain [6,13,15]. Importantly, painful stimulation in turn obviated adult behavioral impairment due to neonatally administered morphine [13].

Similar to these animal studies, clinical reports have demonstrated that neonates and infants can mount a metabolic and endocrine response to perioperative stress and painful stimulation [17,18] which includes increases in catecholamines, cortisol, β-endorphins, insulin, glucagon, and growth hormone [17,19,20]. Some of these markers, such as cortisol, can remain elevated for more than a year, potentially due to cumulative stress related to multiple painful procedures early in life [21]. Administration of potent anesthetics, opioid analgesics, and regional anesthesia has been shown to inhibit intraoperative stress and improve postoperative outcome [4,19,22], reduce the incidence of sepsis and disseminated intravascular coagulation, as well as decreasing mortality [5]. Even less invasive procedures, such as circumcisions, when performed without analgesia, can exaggerate pain responses later in life [23]. In contrast, topical or regional anesthesia for circumcision will blunt the immediate humoral stress response [24] and obviate long-term hyperalgesia [23].

In premature neonates, an association has been observed between painful stimulations early in life and subsequent diminished cognition and motor function [25]. At more than 1 year of age, children who were born at less than 32 weeks' gestational age without significant neonatal brain injury or major sensorineural impairment were compared with full-term controls regarding cognitive and motor development. Results demonstrated that the number of skin-breaking procedures from birth to term (including heel sticks, intramuscular injections, chest tube placements, and central line insertions) predicted lower subsequent cognitive and motor development as assessed using the Bayley Scales of Infant Development-II. Importantly, after controlling for severity of illness and days on intravenous morphine or dexamethasone, gestational age at birth was not significantly associated with cognitive or motor outcome. These findings suggest that repetitive pain-related stressful experiences and not prematurity *per se* were responsible for poor neurodevelopmental outcome [25].

While this study did not examine the effects of anesthetic or analgesic administration during painful stimulation on subsequent outcome, a small, retrospective study suggested improved outcome following anesthetic exposure during painful stimulation. In that study, painful stimulation during reduction of herniated bowel without anesthesia in infants suffering from gastroschisis tended to more frequently lead to serious adverse events, such as bowel ischemia, need for total parenteral nutrition, and unplanned reoperation than in infants undergoing the same procedure with general anesthesia [26]. However, despite the fact that large numbers of painful and stressful procedures are being performed in vulnerable neonates, recent data indicate that the majority of these are still not accompanied by analgesia [27].

Taken together, the data from animal and human studies suggest that pain-related stress experienced early in life is deleterious to the developing nervous system, that sedatives and analgesics may alleviate many of the degenerative effects, and that pain in children still remains undertreated.

Developmental anesthetic-induced neurotoxicity

Concerns regarding potentially deleterious effects of general anesthetics on neurological function were first raised after more than a century of their routine clinical use. Personality changes observed in young children following administration of vinyl ether, cyclopropane, or ethylchloride for otolaryngological surgery were interpreted as long-term neurological sequelae caused by the anesthetic agents [28]. While these findings were not immediately acted upon, approximately two decades later the focus of research into potentially deleterious effects of anesthetics shifted to occupational exposure of the unborn fetus during pregnancy [29–32]. Chronic exposure of pregnant rats to subanesthetic doses of halothane during their entire pregnancy led to delayed synaptogenesis and behavioral abnormalities in their offspring. However, it took almost another two decades until initial studies were carried out examining anesthetic exposure early in postnatal life, more closely representing pediatric anesthesia practice. In these ground-breaking studies, widespread neuronal degeneration was observed following prolonged ketamine exposure in neonatal rat pups [33]. The researchers likened this phenomenon to abnormalities observed in children suffering from fetal alcohol syndrome caused by the combined $GABA_A$-agonist/ NMDA-antagonist ethanol [34–36]. Accordingly, these findings were followed up by using a combination of the $GABA_A$-agonist midazolam, the combined $GABA_A$-agonist and NMDA-antagonist isoflurane, and the NMDA-antagonist nitrous oxide, demonstrating immediate brain structural abnormalities as well as long-term decreases in neuronal density and impaired neurocognitive function following a 6h exposure to the anesthetic

combination [37,38]. Acute neuronal degeneration immediately following exposure to all routinely used anesthetics and sedatives has now been confirmed by numerous laboratories in several immature animal models [39,40]. However, the link between neurodegeneration and long-term neurocognitive impairment remains controversial, because several studies have demonstrated extensive initial neurodegeneration without long-term functional impairment [41–44].

Given the serious implications of potential long-term cognitive impairment following exposure to sedatives or anesthetic early in life, the direct clinical applicability of these laboratory findings continues to be intensely debated [45,46]. These concerns led to a risk assessment by the United States Food and Drug Administration's Life-Support Advisory Committee in March of 2007, stating that the "existing and well-understood risks of anesthesia (hemodynamic and respiratory) continue to be the overwhelming considerations in designing an anesthetic, and the understood risks of delaying surgery are the primary reasons to determine the timing" (transcript available at www.fda.gov/ohrms/dockets/ac/07/transcripts/2007-4285t1.pdf.)

Experimental evidence for anesthetic neurotoxicity

To date, more than 100 articles and numerous abstracts have described brain structural abnormalities and/or functional impairment following exposure to the vast majority of clinically utilized sedatives and anesthetics in immature animal models, including chicks, mice, rats, guinea pigs, swine, sheep, and rhesus monkeys. While the exact molecular mechanisms by which anesthetics provide their therapeutic effects remain uncertain, two main putative targets are the NMDA and GABA receptors.

N-methyl-D-aspartate-antagonists

Glutamate represents the most ubiquitous excitatory neurotransmitter in the mammalian central nervous system. Drugs routinely used in clinical anesthesia and sedation practice that provide their hypnotic effects predominantly by inhibition of the NMDA-type glutamate receptor include ketamine and nitrous oxide [47], as well as the less frequently, clinically utilized noble gas xenon [48]. Pioneering animal studies carried out in the 1990s demonstrated widespread degeneration of brain cells in newborn rat pups following the repeated administration of ketamine [33]. These findings have subsequently been replicated and expanded upon by several other laboratories [39,49]. Most of these studies demonstrated deleterious effects on the developing brain structure following the administration of multiple doses of up to 75mg/kg of ketamine (Table 41.1). Conversely, a single dose of up

Table 41.1 Preclinical studies into structural and neurocognitive effects of anesthetic exposure in neonatal animals

Anesthetic agent	Dose and duration	Species, age	Pathology	Reference
Buprenorphine	1.5 mg/kg/d to dam	Rat, E7–21	Decrease in striatal nerve growth factor	Wu et al [91]
Chloral hydrate	50–300 mg/kg × 1	Mouse, P5	Increased neuroapoptosis, ameliorated by lithium	Cattano et al [92]
Clonazepam	0.5–4 mg/kg × 1	Rat, P7	Increased neurodegeneration	Bittigau et al [93]
Clonazepam	0.5–4 mg/kg × 1	Rat, P7	Increased neurodegeneration	Ikonomidou et al [35]
Desflurane	7% for 30–120 min	Rat, P16	No increase in neurodegeneration or gross changes in dendritic arborization, increase in number of dendritic spines	Briner et al [74]
Desflurane	7.4% for 6 h	Mouse, P7–8	Increased neuroapoptosis compared with no anesthesia, but similar to equi-anesthetic doses of isoflurane or sevoflurane	Istaphanous et al [75]
Dexmedetomidine	1–75 μg/kg × 3	Rat, P7	No increase in neuroapoptosis	Sanders et al [64]
Diazepam	10–30 mg/kg × 1	Rat, P7	Increased neurodegeneration	Ikonomidou et al [35]
Diazepam	5–30 mg/kg × 1	Rat, P7	Increased neurodegeneration above 10 mg/kg	Bittigau et al [93]
Diazepam	5 mg/kg × 1	Mouse, P10	No increased neurodegeneration in cortex, but increased in thalamus, no subsequent behavioral or learning deficits	Fredriksson et al [59]
Diazepam	20 mg/kg on P6 and on P8	Rat, P6 and P8	Inhibition of neurogenesis	Stefovska et al [94]
Enflurane	2–4% for 0.5 h	Mouse, prenatal E6–17	Learning impairment in adulthood	Chalon et al [95]
Fentanyl	50 μg/kg/h for 72 h	Rat, P14	Diminished morphine antinociceptive sensitivity in juvenile and adult animals	Thornton et al [85]
Halothane	10 ppm for 40 h/week	Rat, conception to P60	Learning deficits and decrease in synaptic density	Quimby et al [29]
Halothane	10 ppm for 40 h/week	Rat, conception to P60	Defects in visual and spatial learning tasks	Quimby et al [30]
Halothane	50–200 ppm continuously	Rat, conception to P28	Dose-dependent decrease in cerebral synapse density	Uemura et al [31]
Halothane	25–100 ppm continuously	Rat, conception to P60	Decrease in apical and basal dendritic length and numbers	Uemura et al [96]
Halothane	25–100 ppm continuously	Rat, conception to P60	Decrease in synaptic density, no learning impairment	Uemura et al [32]
Halothane	1–2% for 0.5 h	Mouse, prenatal E6–17	Learning impairment in adulthood	Chalon et al [95]
Heroin	10 mg/kg/d to dam	Mouse, E8–18	Hyperactivity and spatial learning deficits in adulthood	Yanai et al [97]
Heroin	10 mg/kg/d to dam	Mouse, E9–18	Increased neuronal apoptosis and impaired spatial learning and memory in juvenile animals	Wang et al [98]
Heroin	500 μg/mL	Rat, E16–17 cortical neuronal cultures	Decrease in neuronal viability, increase in apoptosis and DNA fragmentation	Cunha-Oliveira et al [99]

Table 41.1 (*Continued*)

Anesthetic agent	Dose and duration	Species, age	Pathology	Reference
Isoflurane	0.2–0.3 mM	Mouse, P14 and P60 hippocampal slices	Block of synaptic transmission more pronounced in P14 slices, compared with older animals	Simon et al [100]
Isoflurane+ nitrous oxide +midazolam	0.75% + 75% + 9 mg/kg for 6 h	Rat, P7	Increased neuroapoptosis and neurodegeneration, adult learning impairment	Jevtovic-Todorovic et al [37]
Isoflurane	0.75–1.5% for 6 h	Rat, P7	Increased neurodegeneration	Jevtovic-Todorovic et al [37]
Isoflurane+ midazolam+ thiopental	1.5% for 4 h + 1 mg/kg + 7 mg/kg to ewe	Sheep, prenatal E120	No increase in neuroapoptosis, as assessed 6 d postanesthesia	McClaine et al [101]
Isoflurane+ nitrous oxide +midazolam	0.75% + 75% + 9 mg/kg for 2–6 h	Rat, P1–14	Increased neuroapoptosis following exposure on P7, not P1–3 or P10–14	Yon et al [66]
Isoflurane+ nitrous oxide +midazolam	0.55% + 75% + 1 mg/kg for 4 h	Swine, P5	Increased neurodegeneration in neocortex	Rizzi et al [102]
Isoflurane	1.5% for 1–5 h	Rat, organotypic slice culture	Increased neurodegeneration only after 5 h of exposure	Wise-Faberowski et al [103]
Isoflurane	2.4% for 24 h	Rat, primary cortical neuron culture	Increased apoptosis	Wei et al [104]
Isoflurane+ nitrous oxide +midazolam	0.75% + 75% + 9 mg/kg for 2–6 h	Rat, P7	Increased neuroapoptosis	Lu et al [67]
Isoflurane+ nitrous oxide +midazolam	0.75% + 75% + 9 mg/kg for 6 h	Rat, P7	Increased neuroapoptosis, ameliorated by melatonin	Yon et al [68]
Isoflurane	0.75% for 4 h	Mouse, P5	Increased neuroapoptosis, ameliorated by pilocarpine	Olney et al [105]
Isoflurane	0.75% for 6 h	Rat, P7 and mouse organotypic hippocampal slices	Increased neuroapoptosis, exacerbated by nitrous oxide and ameliorated by xenon	Ma et al [62]
Isoflurane	0.75% for 6 h	Rat, P7 and mouse, P8 organotypic hippocampal slices	Increased neuroapoptosis, ameliorated by dexmedetomidine, not reversed by gabazine	[106]
Isoflurane	2.4% for 24 h	Rat, primary cortical neuron culture	Increased cellular degeneration, blocked by isoflurane or halothane preconditioning	Wei et al [107]
Isoflurane	1.3% for 6 h	Rat, prenatal E21	Decrease in neuroapoptosis, no impaired learning, improved memory retention in juvenile animals	Li et al [108]
Isoflurane+ nitrous oxide +midazolam	0.75% + 75% + 9 mg/kg for 6 h	Rat, P7	Decreased neuronal density in multiple brain areas in adulthood	Nikizad et al [38]

(*Continued*)

Table 41.1 (*Continued*)

Anesthetic agent	Dose and duration	Species, age	Pathology	Reference
Isoflurane+ nitrous oxide +midazolam	0.55% + 75% + 1mg/kg for 4h	Guinea pig, prenatal E20–50	Increased neuroapoptosis between E35–40 and decreased adult neuronal density, not after E50 or in fentanyl control group	Rizzi et al [109]
Isoflurane	0.75% for 4h, 1.5% for 2h, or 2% for 1h	Mouse, P5–7	Increased neuroapoptosis	Johnson et al [110]
Isoflurane+ nitrous oxide	0.75% + 75% for 6h	Rat, P7	Increased neuroapoptosis in spinal cord	Sanders et al [111]
Isoflurane		Mouse, P4	Increased neuroapoptosis, ameliorated by hypothermia	Olney et al [112]
Isoflurane	1.4%	Rat, cortical and hippocampal neuron culture, harvest P1, DIC 5	Increased neuroapoptosis, reduction in dendritic spines and number of synapses, ameliorated by administration of tPA or inhibition of p75^{NTR}	Head et al [113]
Isoflurane+ nitrous oxide	0.55% + 75% or individually for 2–8h	Rat, P7	Increased neuroapoptosis and neurodegeneration after exposure of 6 hours or longer, ameliorated by L-carnitine, no increase by either agent administered individually	Zou et al [114]
Isoflurane	1–2% for 10min	Mouse, P0	Neonatal and adolescent impairment in tests of body co-ordination and adult learning; decreased hippocampal cellularity and volume, more pronounced in males	Rothstein et al [115]
Isoflurane	1.2% for 12h	Rat, primary cortical neuron culture	Increased cytotoxicity, ameliorated by xestospongin C	Wang et al [116]
Isoflurane	0.75% for 6h	Rat, P7	Increased neuroapoptosis, ameliorated by dexmedetomidine	Sanders et al [64]
Isoflurane	1.5% for 6h	Mouse, P7	Increased neurodegeneration early after exposure, no adult learning impairment, no decreased adult neuronal density	Loepke et al [41]
Isoflurane	1 MAC for 1–4h	Rat, P7	Widespread brain cell death following exposure for >2h, not 1h; adult neurocognitive deficits only after 4h exposure	Stratmann et al [117]
Isoflurane	1 MAC for 4h	Rat, P7	Decreased progenitor proliferation, deficits in fear conditioning and memory impairment in adulthood	Stratmann et al [43]
Isoflurane	3.4% for 4h	Rat, neuronal progenitor culture, harvest P2, 2–12 weeks in culture	No neurodegeneration or activation of caspases 3 or 7, decrease in caspase 9, inhibition of proliferation, preferential differentiation to neurons	Sall et al [118]
Isoflurane+ nitrous oxide +midazolam	0.75% + 75% + 9mg/kg for 6h	Rat, P7	Decreased synaptic density in subiculum 2 weeks after treatment	Lunardi et al [119]
Isoflurane	1.6% for 5h	Rhesus monkey, P5	Increase in neocortical apoptotic cell death	Brambrink et al [70]

Table 41.1 (*Continued*)

Anesthetic agent	Dose and duration	Species, age	Pathology	Reference
Isoflurane	1.6% for 5 h	Rhesus monkey, P5	Increase in apoptotic cell death of neurons in neocortex and immature oligodendrocytes in white matter	Olney et al [120]
Isoflurane	1.3% or 3% for 1 h to dam	Rat, E21	No increase in neuroapoptosis or S100β blood levels following lower dose, but both increased following higher dose	Wang et al [121]
Isoflurane	1.7% for 35 min × 4 d	Rat, P14 Mouse, P14	No increased immediate hippocampal neuronal cell death, no difference in adult learning of easy task, impairment in adult learning of difficult learning and recognition tasks	Zhu et al [122]
Isoflurane	1.5% for 30–120 min	Rat, P16	No increase in neurodegeneration or gross changes in dendritic arborization, increase in number of dendritic spines	Briner et al [74]
Isoflurane	0.75% for 6 h	Mouse, P7	Increased neuroapoptosis and serum levels of S100β immediately following exposure, no long-term impairment in learning and memory tests	Liang et al [44]
Isoflurane	2% for 2 h and/or caffeine 80 mg/kg	Mice, P4	Increased neuroapoptosis following caffeine, worse than following isoflurane exposure, demonstrating potentiation following combination exposure	Yuede et al [123]
Isoflurane	1.5% for 6 h	Mouse, P7–8	Increased neuroapoptosis compared with no anesthesia, but similar to equianesthetic doses of desflurane or sevoflurane	Istaphanous et al [75]
Ketamine	20 mg/kg × 7	Rat, P7	Increased neurodegeneration	Ikonomidou et al [33]
Ketamine	25–75 mg/kg × 1–7	Rat, P7	Increased neurodegeneration only after 7 repeated doses of 25 mg/kg	Hayashi et al [50]
Ketamine	50 mg/kg × 1	Mouse, P10	Cortical neurodegeneration; hypo- and hyperactivity, abnormal habituation in adulthood	Fredriksson et al [124]
Ketamine	50 mg/kg × 1	Mouse, P10	Neurodegeneration, worsened by co-administration of diazepam	Fredriksson et al [59]
Ketamine	50 mg/kg × 1	Mouse, P10	Neurodegeneration and impairment in memory tasks in adulthood	Fredriksson et al [57]
Ketamine	10–25 mg/kg × 1–7	Rat, P7	Neurodegeneration observed after 7 repeated doses of 25 mg/kg, plasma levels 7 times higher than during human anesthesia	Scallet et al [125]
Ketamine	1.25–40 mg/kg × 1	Mouse, P7	Neurodegeneration after doses of 5 mg/kg or higher, no gross neurobehavioral abnormalities 7 days after treatment	Rudin et al [60]
Ketamine	0.1–10 μM for 6–48 h	Rat forebrain neuron culture	Increased DNA fragmentation after higher doses for longer periods of time	Wang et al [53]
Ketamine	10–40 mg/kg × 1	Mouse, P7	Increased neurodegeneration following doses of 20 mg/kg or higher, worsened by midazolam co-administration	Young et al [58]

(*Continued*)

Table 41.1 (*Continued*)

Anesthetic agent	Dose and duration	Species, age	Pathology	Reference
Ketamine	1–20 µM for 2–24 h	Rhesus monkey forebrain neuron culture	Increased DNA fragmentation and decreased mitochondrial function after higher doses for longer periods of time	Wang et al [55]
Ketamine	0.01–40 µg/mL for 1–48 h	Rat GABAergic neuron culture	Neuronal cell loss and decrease in dendritic length and branching with higher concentrations for longer exposure times	Vutskits et al [54]
Ketamine	100 µM for 48 h	Rat, cortical neuron culture	Increased apoptosis, ameliorated by NMDA, IGF-1, alsteropaullone, or iodoindirubin	Takadera et al [126]
Ketamine	0.1–30 µM for 24 h	Rat, cortical neuron culture	Decreased cell viability and increased DNA fragmentation, ameliorated by erythropoietin	Shang et al [127]
Ketamine	20–50 mg/kg/h × 24 h	Rhesus monkey, E122, P5 or P35	Increased neurodegeneration in two younger age groups, ketamine plasma levels higher than in humans	Slikker et al [51]
Ketamine	1–100 µg/mL for 1–24 h	Rat GABAergic neuron culture	Neuronal cell loss with higher concentrations or longer exposure times	Vutskits et al [56]
Ketamine	2.5 mg/kg × 2 for 4 d	Rat, P1–4	Minimal neurodegeneration, but ameliorated pain-induced neurodegeneration and subsequent learning abnormalities	Anand et al [6]
Ketamine or S-ketamine	1–8 mM or 0.6–4 mM for 24 h	Neuroblastoma cells	Increased apoptosis, but up to 80% less cell death following S-ketamine	Braun et al [128]
Ketamine	25 mg/kg × 1	Mouse, P10	No increase in neurodegeneration, but subsequent learning impairment, worsened by co-administration of thiopental or propofol	Fredriksson et al [61]
Ketamine	1–20 µM for 24 h	Rat forebrain neuron culture	Increased DNA fragmentation after higher doses, blocked by nitroindazole	Wang et al [129]
Ketamine	5–25 mg/kg × 1	Mouse, P10	Dose-dependent alterations in levels of developmentally expressed proteins and adult behavioral abnormalities	Viberg et al [130]
Ketamine	2.5 mg/kg × 2 for 4 d	Rat, P1–4	No increase in neuronal cell death, no change in adult learning and exploratory behavior and ameliorated pain-induced neurodegeneration and behavioral abnormalities	Rovnaghi et al [131]
Ketamine	20 mg/kg × 6	Rat, P7	Decreased body weight 1–3 days after exposure, no abnormal spontaneous behavior observed during first 4 days	Boctor et al [132]
Ketamine	30 mg/kg + 15 mg/kg every 90 min × 2	Mouse, P15–90	No increase in neurodegeneration, impairment in dendritic spine development following exposure on P20 or younger	Vutskits et al [133]
Ketamine	40 mg/kg	Mouse, P5	Increased neuroapoptosis, ameliorated by lithium co-administration	Straiko et al [72]
Ketamine	5–20 mg/kg × 1–6	Rat, P7	Increased apoptosis and neurodegeneration only observed following 6 repeated doses of 20 mg/kg	Zou et al [134]

Table 41.1 (*Continued*)

Anesthetic agent	Dose and duration	Species, age	Pathology	Reference
Ketamine	20 mg/kg × 7	Rat, P7	Increased apoptosis and neurodegeneration, decreased weight gain, increase in BDNF and TrkB cDNA	Ibla et al [135]
Ketamine	20–50 mg/kg/h for 3–25 h	Rhesus monkey, P5 or 6	Neuronal degeneration only in neocortex following 9 h exposure or longer, no degeneration in deeper brain areas	Zou et al [52]
Ketamine	30 mg/kg + 15 mg/kg every 90 min × 2	Mouse, P15	Increase in dendritic spine density and decrease in spine head diameter in the somatosensory cortex and hippocampus	De Roo et al [73]
Ketamine	5–20 mg/kg × 5	Rat, P7	Increased neuroapoptosis in neocortex and thalamus, increase in cell cycle proteins	Soriano et al [136]
Ketamine	0.1–1000 μM × 6–48 h	Rat, cortical neuron culture	Increase in expression of caspase 3 and cell cycle proteins	Soriano et al [136]
Methadone	10 mg/kg/d to dam	Rat, E5–21	Decreased brain monoamines in juveniles and hyper-responsive in adulthood	Rech et al [137]
Methadone	10–15 mg/kg/d to dam	Rat, E8–21	Increased excitability tested in juvenile animals using the acoustic startle reflex	Hutchings et al [138]
Methadone	9 mg/kg/d to dam	Rat, E7–21	Increased noradrenergic activity in hippocampus of male juveniles	Robinson et al [83]
Methadone	9 mg/kg/d to dam	Rat, P1–10	Reduced activity of dopaminergic neurons in frontal cortex of juvenile males	Robinson et al [83]
Methadone	9 mg/kg/d to dam	Rat, E7–21	Reduction in nerve growth factor, disruption of cholinergic neuronal activity	Robinson et al [84]
Midazolam	9 mg/kg × 1	Rat, P7	No increase in neurodegeneration	Jevtovic-Todorovic et al [37]
Midazolam	9 mg/kg × 1	Mouse, P7	Increased neuroapoptosis	Young et al [58]
Midazolam	9 mg/kg × 1	Mouse, P5	Increased neuroapoptosis	Olney et al [105]
Midazolam	3–9 mg/kg × 1	Rat, P1–14	No increase in neuroapoptosis	Yon et al [66]
Midazolam	0.25–25 μg/mL	Rat GABAergic neuron culture	No effect on neuronal survival	Vutskits et al [139]
Midazolam	25 mg/kg + 15 mg/kg every 90 min × 2	Mouse, P15–90	No increase in neurodegeneration, impairment in dendritic spine development following exposure on P20 or younger	Vutskits et al [133]
Midazolam	25 mg/kg + 15 mg/kg every 90 min × 2	Mouse, P15	Increase in dendritic spine density and decrease in spine head diameter in the somatosensory cortex and hippocampus	De Roo et al [73]
Midazolam	50 mg/kg	Mouse, P10	No impairment of learning and memory in adulthood	Xu et al [42]
Morphine	10 mg/kg/d to dam	Rat, E12–21	Gender- and region-specific changes in μ receptor density in neonatal rats	Hammer et al [81]
Morphine	5 mg/kg/d	Rat, P1–4	Decreased μ-opioid receptor density in striatum following exposure	Tempel el al. [80]

(*Continued*)

Table 41.1 (*Continued*)

Anesthetic agent	Dose and duration	Species, age	Pathology	Reference
Morphine	20 mg/kg/d to dam, except for E11; 10 mg/kg/d	Rat, E11–18	Decreased μ-opioid receptor density in adulthood	Rimanoczy et al [82]
Morphine	1 μM for 1–2 d	Mouse, P5–6 cerebellar neuronal precursor culture	Marked decrease in DNA synthesis, without effect on cell survival	Hauser et al [140]
Morphine	5 mg/kg × 3 doses, then 10 mg/kg twice a day to dam	Rat, E11–18	Impairment in spatial learning in adulthood	Slamberova et al [86]
Morphine	1–100 μM for 5 d	Human, GW16–22 fetal microglial, astrocyte, and neuronal cultures	Progressive increase in apoptosis in neurons after 2-d exposure, or microglia after 3 d but not in astrocytes	Hu et al [141]
Morphine	2 mg/kg/d to dam, progressively increased by 2 mg/kg/d	Rat, E0–P21	Impairment in spatial learning in young adulthood	Yang et al [87]
Morphine	20 mg/kg/d	Chick, E12–16	Impairment in long-term memory formation	Che et al [142]
Morphine	2 mg/kg/d	Rat, P3–7	Impairment in adult cognitive function	McPherson et al [88]
Morphine	15 μM for 7 d	Mouse, E16 hippocampal neuronal culture	Increased apoptosis, decreased neuronal density	Svensson et al [143]
Morphine	4 mg/kg/d	Mouse, P5–9	Impairment in reward-mediated learning in adulthood	Boasen et al [13]
Morphine	5 mg/kg × 3 doses, then 10 mg/kg twice a day to dam	Rat, E11–18	Decreased synaptic plasticity and impaired learning in juveniles	Niu et al [90]
Morphine	2 mg/kg/d to dam, progressively increased by 2 mg/kg/d, max. 14 mg/kg/d	Rat, E0–P21	Decreased performance in learning tasks in adulthood	Lin et al [89]
Nitrous oxide	50–150% for 2–6 h	Rat, P7	No increase in neurodegeneration	Jevtovic-Todorovic et al [37]
Nitrous oxide	50–150% for 2–6 h	Rat, P1–14	No increase in neuroapoptosis	Yon et al [66]
Nitrous oxide	75% for 6 h	Rat, P7 and mouse organotypic hippocampal slices	No increase in neuroapoptosis in rats, increased neuroapoptosis in mice	Ma et al [62]
Pentobarbital	5–10 mg/kg × 1	Rat, P7	Increased neurodegeneration	Bittigau et al [93]
Phenobarbital	40–100 mg/kg	Rat, P7	Increased neuroapoptosis, ameliorated by β-estradiol	Bittigau et al [93]
Phenobarbital	50 mg/kg	Rat, P7	Increased neuroapoptosis, ameliorated by β-estradiol	Asimiadou et al [144]

Table 41.1 (*Continued*)

Anesthetic agent	Dose and duration	Species, age	Pathology	Reference
Phenobarbital	30 mg/kg × 2	Mice, P6	Long-term alterations in brain protein expression	Kaindl et al [145]
Phenobarbital	75 mg/kg	Rats, P7–8	Increased neuroapoptosis, enhanced by lamotrigine administration	Katz et al [146]
Phenobarbital	25 mg/kg	Mice, P0	Neonatal and adolescent impairment in tests of body co-ordination and adult learning; decreased hippocampal cellularity and volume, more pronounced in males	Rothstein et al [115]
Phenobarbital	50 mg/kg (P6), 40 mg/kg (P8)	Rat, P6 and P8	Inhibition of neurogenesis	Stefovska et al [94]
Propofol	0.5–10 µg/mL for 8 h	Rat GABAergic neuron culture	Dose-dependent decrease in GABAergic enzyme GAD after higher doses	Honegger et al [147]
Propofol	10–100 µg/mL for 2 h–10 d	Rat dissociated neuronal culture P1 or P7	Increased cell death in P1 neurons following higher doses, no evidence for neurotoxic effects in organotypic hippocampal culture on P7	Spahr-Schopfer et al [148]
Propofol	1–50 µg/mL	Rat GABAergic neuron culture	Increased neuronal cell death following highest dose, altered dendritic development following lowest dose	Vutskits et al [139]
Propofol	5–500 µM for 2–24 h	Chick neuron explant culture	Dose-dependent neurite growth cone collapse	Al-Jahdari et al [149]
Propofol	10–60 mg/kg × 1	Mouse, P10	Increased neurodegeneration following highest dose	Fredriksson et al [61]
Propofol	25–300 mg/kg × 1	Mouse, P5–7	Increased neuroapoptosis following doses higher than 50 mg/kg	Cattano et al [71]
Propofol	6 mg/kg/h for 24 h	Swine, P0	No increased neurodegeneration	Gressens et al [150]
Propofol	5 µM for 5 h	Rat hippocampal neuron culture	Increased neuroapoptosis	Kahraman et al [151]
Propofol	50 mg/kg + 25 mg/kg every 90 min × 2	Mouse, P15–90	No increase in neurodegeneration, impairment in dendritic spine development following exposure on P20 or younger	Vutskits et al [133]
Propofol	25 mg/kg	Rat, P7	Increased neuroapoptosis, decrease in nerve growth factor,	Pesic et al [152]
Propofol	50–100 mg/kg	Mouse, P5	Increased neuroapoptosis, ameliorated by lithium co-administration	Straiko et al [72]
Propofol	0.01–1 mg/mL for 3–48 h	Rat, primary cortical neuron culture, harvested E18	Highest concentration improved cell viability after up to 6 h of exposure, but reduced cell viability after more than 12 h	Berns et al [153]
Propofol	30 mg/kg every 90 min × 3	Rat, P6	No increase in neurodegeneration in most brain areas, except for defined areas, subtle neurological impairment in adult animals	Bercker et al [154]
Propofol	50 mg/kg + 25 mg/kg every 90 min × 2	Mouse, P15	Increase in dendritic spine density and decrease in spine head diameter in the somatosensory cortex and hippocampus	De Roo et al [73]

(*Continued*)

Table 41.1 (*Continued*)

Anesthetic agent	Dose and duration	Species, age	Pathology	Reference
Sevoflurane	4% for 24 h	Rat, primary cortical neuron culture	No increase in apoptosis	Wei et al [104]
Sevoflurane	2% for 12 h	Rat, primary cortical neuron culture	No increase in cytotoxicity	Wang et al [116]
Sevoflurane	1.7% for 2 h	Mouse, P7	Increased neuroapoptosis	Zhang et al [155]
Sevoflurane	3% for 6 h	Mouse, P6	Increased neuroapoptosis, impairments in fear conditioning and social interaction in adulthood	Satomoto et al [69]
Sevoflurane	4% or 8% for 12 or 6 h, respectively	Rat, primary cortical neuron culture, E18	No difference in cell viability compared with untreated controls	Berns et al [156]
Sevoflurane	3–5% for 6 h	Rat, P6	No increase in neurodegeneration immediately after exposure, no long-term neurological impairment	Bercker et al [154]
Sevoflurane	2.1% for 0.5–6 h	Rat, P4–8	Seizure activity during exosure and neuroapoptosis partially blocked by administration of bumetanide	Edwards et al [157]
Sevoflurane	2.5% for 30–120 min	Rat, P16	No increase in neurodegeneration or gross changes in dendritic arborization, increase in number of dendritic spines	Briner et al [74]
Sevoflurane	1.1% for 6 h	Mouse, P7	Increased neuroapoptosis immediately following exposure, no long-term impairment in learning and memory tests	Liang et al [44]
Sevoflurane	2.1% or 3% for 2 h or 6 h	Mice, P6	Increased neuroapoptosis following the longer, but not the shorter exposure time. Transgenic Alzheimer disease mice more susceptible.	Lu et al [158]
Sevoflurane	2.9% for 6 h	Mouse, P7–8	Increased neuroapoptosis compared with no anesthesia, but similar to equi-anesthetic doses of desflurane or isoflurane	Istaphanous et al [75]
Thiopental	5–25 mg/kg × 1	Mouse, P10	No increase in neurodegeneration	Fredriksson et al [61]
Xenon	75% for 6 h	Rat, P7 and mouse organotypic hippocampal slices	No increase in neuroapoptosis	Ma et al [62]
Xenon	70% for 4 h	Mouse, P7	Increase in neuroapoptosis, decreased isoflurane-induced neuroapoptosis	Cattano et al [63]

DIC, days in culture; P, postnatal day; E, embryological day.

to 75 mg/kg of ketamine did not seem to lead to widespread cytotoxic effects [50]. Whole brain slices from neonatal rats receiving ketamine for at least 6 h demonstrate increased cleaved caspase-3 expression, which leads to apoptotic cell death (Fig. 41.1) Moreover, a dose-dependent increase in ketamine-induced neuronal cell death has recently also been observed in non-human primates [51,52]. In these studies, a 24-h infusion of ketamine (20–50 mg/kg/h) significantly increased neuronal cell death in prenatal (gestational age 122 days) or neonatal (5-day-old) rhesus monkeys. However, a ketamine infusion for 3 h did not lead to any increased neurodegeneration in these monkeys and even a 24-h infusion failed to cause neuronal degeneration in older, 35-day-old animals. Ketamine neurotoxicity has also been studied using *in vitro* preparations from neonatal rats and rhesus monkeys [53–55]. Primary cortical cells cultured in ketamine for 6h or longer led to an increase in neurodegeneration in both species, whereas shorter exposure times did not. However, lower concentrations of ketamine have been shown to decrease dendritic arborization in differentiated neurons in culture [56]. Microscopic images of primary neurons exposed to ketamine demonstrate a reduction in neurite length and the number of branching points (Fig. 41.2).

It currently remains unknown whether the seemingly large doses of injectable anesthetics used in animal neurotoxicity studies can be directly compared with the relatively smaller doses used in clinical practice (further discussed below). However, it should be noted that in

neonatal mice, lower concentrations than those found deleterious in rats and also single doses of ketamine and propofol have been found to induce neuroapoptosis, which may indicate differential susceptibilities among species [57,58].

Long-term neurological function following neonatal ketamine exposure has so far only been examined in a few studies. A single ketamine exposure of 50 mg/kg in newborn mice led to subsequent abnormal behavior as well as impaired learning and memory acquisition in adolescent animals [59]; however, in another study, albeit without formal tests of learning, no gross neurobehavioral abnormalities were observed 7 days after neonatal administration of up to 40 mg/kg [60]. Moreover, adult rats that were injected as neonates with four daily, relatively small doses of ketamine (5 mg/kg) performed as well as their unexposed peers in subsequent learning and

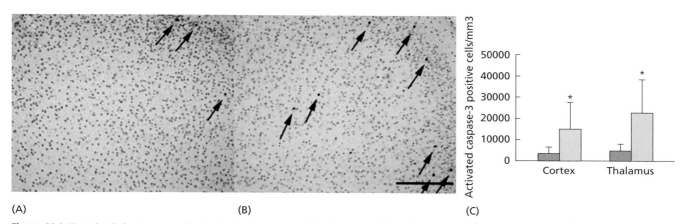

(A)   (B)   (C)

Figure 41.1 Ketamine induces caspase-3 activation *in vivo*. Immunohistochemistry with antibody to cleaved caspase-3 on cortical sections from P7 rat pups receiving either saline (A) or ketamine 20 mg/kg every 90 min for 6 h (B) (scale bar = 200 μm). (C) Quantitation of activated caspase-3-immunoreactive cells in P7 cortex and thalamus. Data are presented as mean ± standard deviation, * p < 0.05 compared to saline. Courtesy of Soriano Laboratory.

Figure 41.2 Ketamine stunted neurite arborization and branching points in primary neurons (scale bar = 100 μM). Courtesy of Soriano Laboratory.

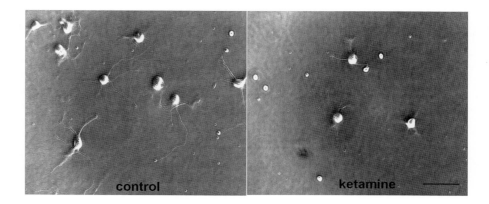

memory tasks [6]. Concomitant administration of GABA-mimetic drugs, such as midazolam, thiopental or propofol, a common practice during clinical anesthesia and sedation, significantly exacerbated the deleterious effects of ketamine [58,61].

Less information is available regarding the effects of the NMDA-antagonists nitrous oxide or xenon on brain development. Whereas nitrous oxide by itself, even under hyperbaric conditions, did not seem to increase neuronal cell death [37,62], xenon showed differential effects, being deleterious in one study [63] and not in another [62]. The two compounds, however, differed in their effects when co-administered with isoflurane; nitrous oxide exacerbated isoflurane-induced neurotoxicity [37,38,62,64] whereas xenon alleviated some of isoflurane's cytotoxic effects [62,63].

γ-Aminobutyrate$_A$-agonists

γ-Aminobutyrate represents the main inhibitory neurotransmitter in the adult central nervous system, while it has excitatory properties in the developing brain [65]. To date, the impact of this developmental switch on anesthesia-induced neurotoxicity remains unresolved. Regardless of these uncertainties, numerous GABA$_A$-agonists are commonly used as anesthetics or sedatives in young children and animal studies have demonstrated the harmful impact of exposure to these compounds during early development on brain cell structure and later neurological function. Several animal studies have been carried out in immature animal species examining the effects of isoflurane, sevoflurane, halothane, enflurane, thiopental, pentobarbital, clonazepam, diazepam, midazolam, chloral hydrate, or propofol (see Table 41.1).

Many of these studies have been carried out by the Jevtovic-Todorovic laboratory, which examines the combined administration of the GABA$_A$-agonist midazolam, the mixed GABA$_A$-agonist and NMDA-antagonist isoflurane, and the NMDA-antagonist nitrous oxide. This combination caused a widespread, dramatic increase in the rate of brain cell degeneration in newborn animals shortly after cessation of a 6h exposure [37,66–68]. In addition to the immediate deleterious effects on brain structure, long-term abnormalities in spatial learning tasks and decreased neuronal cell density were observed in adult rats exposed to the anesthetic combination as neonates [37,38]. Sevoflurane has been also shown to induce neuroapoptosis in neonatal mice and lead to learning deficits and abnormal social behaviors [69] while a recent report suggested that it may cause less immediate neuroapoptosis compared with isoflurane [44]. Neurostructural abnormalities have also been reported in neonatal rhesus monkeys following exposure to clinically relevant doses (0.75–1.5%) isoflurane for 5 h [70]. Subanesthetic doses of

the GABA$_A$-agonist propofol have also been shown to induce neuroapoptosis in postnatal day 5 mice [71,72].

Collectively, these reports demonstrate that the neuroapoptotic effect of anesthetic drugs peaks during the neonatal period in rodents. Older rats seem to be much less susceptible to the neuroapoptotic process, while still subject to anesthesia-induced disruption in dendritic spine architecture, as demonstrated in 15-day-old mice [73,74]. These findings suggest that juvenile rodents may experience anesthetic-induced alterations in synaptogenesis and neuronal cross-talk.

However, long-term correlates of neonatal brain cell death and dendritic alterations on subsequent neurological function remain unresolved. Our group has previously demonstrated that isoflurane as a single agent, while causing widespread neuronal degeneration in neonatal mice immediately following the exposure (Fig. 41.3), did not lead to long-term impairment in spatial learning and memory tasks or to alterations in neuronal density in adult animals [41]. Similar results have recently been observed following the single administration of midazolam [42], isoflurane [44] or sevoflurane [44], suggesting that under certain circumstances, the developing brain may either be able to recover from the neonatal neuronal degeneration or that neonatal brain cell loss may not be causatively linked to adult learning impairment. Studies by Stratmann and co-workers have indicated that hypercarbia during anesthetic exposure might contribute to the immediate neurodegenerative effects, while not necessarily being causatively linked to long-term neurocognitive impairment [43]. Recent work performed by the Loepke laboratory has demonstrated that neurodegeneration, observed immediately following a prolonged anesthetic exposure to desflurane, isoflurane or sevoflurane, is comparable among the three anesthetics (Figs 41.4, 41.5), suggesting that there might not be benefit of using one inhaled agent over another [75].

Other anesthetics and sedatives

Recently, the α2-agonist dexmedetomidine has gained more prominence in pediatric sedation practice. Only one animal study has examined its effects on the developing brain and found dexmedetomidine to be devoid of neurotoxic effects [64]. Moreover, the authors noted that dexmedetomidine might be useful in ameliorating isoflurane's deleterious consequences on neonatal brain structure and adult learning [64]. Further studies are needed to investigate whether dexmedetomidine causes neurodegeneration in other models and whether its protective effects extend to other anesthetics.

Opioid analgesics

Opioid analgesics are another class of potent medications commonly administered to young children before, during,

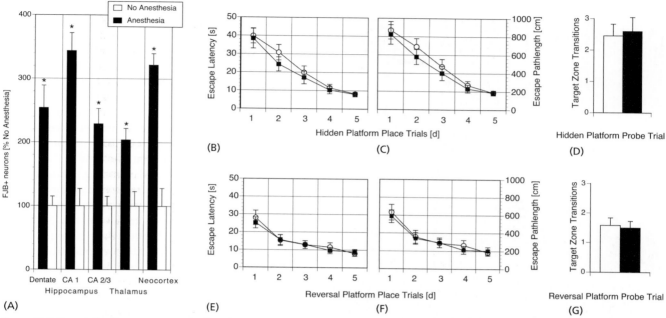

Figure 41.3 Neonatal isoflurane exposure significantly increases the number of dead or dying neurons in the neonatal mouse brain (A). Columns represent mean number of brain cells staining positive for the cell death marker Fluoro-Jade B (FJB+) for each brain region 2 h following 6-h exposure to 0.6 MAC of isoflurane (anesthesia, *black bars*) compared with littermates fasted for 6 h (no anesthesia, *white bars*). However, neuronal cell death in neonatal mice immediately following isoflurane exposure does not lead to impairment in spatial learning and memory in adulthood (B–G). Morris water maze place and probe trials in adult mice previously exposed as neonates to 6 h of fasting (no anesthesia, *open circles*) or to 0.6 MAC isoflurane (anesthesia, *black boxes*) using a hidden platform (B–D) or a more difficult reversal platform paradigm (E–G). Both groups significantly improved over the 5-d trial period and performed equally well in the memory retention tasks. Data are shown as mean ± SEM; n = 8–26 for each group; *$p < 0.05$. Reproduced from Loepke et al [41] with permission from Lippincott Williams and Wilkins.

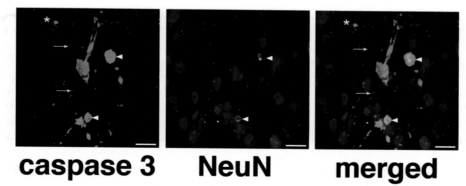

caspase 3   NeuN   merged

Figure 41.4 Representative, high-power magnification photomicrograph, obtained with laser confocal microscopy, demonstrating co-localization of the apoptotic cell death marker activated-caspase 3 (*green*) and the postmitotic neuronal marker NeuN (*red*) in neocortex. Brain section was obtained from a 7-d-old mouse pup following a 6 h to 0.6 MAC of isoflurane, depicting 9 μm image stack stained for activated-caspase 3 (*left*) and NeuN-stained single optical sections through each cell body, for clarity (*middle*). Apoptotic neurons, indicated by co-localization of caspase 3 and NeuN in merged images on right, demonstrate degenerative changes, such as dendritic atrophy (*arrows*), dendritic beading (*), and pyknotic neurons (*arrowheads*), and are surrounded by unaffected neurons; scale bar = 10 μm. Reproduced from Istaphanous et al [75] with permission from Lippincott Williams and Wilkins.

and after surgery, often in conjunction with anesthetics and sedatives [76,77]. Since opioids can reduce dose requirements for anesthetics and sedatives, their co-administration could lead to lower anesthetic requirements and thereby potentially assist in mitigating anesthesia-induced cytotoxicity. However, several animal studies have suggested that opioid exposure may also

have harmful effects in the developing brain (see Table 41.1) Moreover, opioid co-administration can enhance cell death of immature brain cells triggered by other apoptosis-inducing drugs [78]. Specifically, chronic perinatal exposure to morphine, fentanyl or methadone has been shown to induce acute neuronal degeneration in the neonatal animal brain [79], to alter brain opioid receptor density

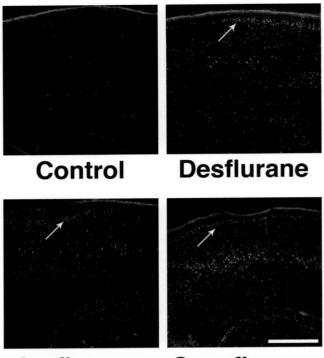

Control   Desflurane

Isoflurane   Sevoflurane

Figure 41.5 Six-hour exposure to desflurane, isoflurane, or sevoflurane similarly increases apoptotic cell death in neonatal mice, compared with fasted, unanesthetized littermates (control). Representative, low-magnification photomicrographs of coronal brain sections, obtained with laser confocal microscopy, demonstrate the pattern of apoptotic neuronal cell death. Brain sections from 7–8-d-old mouse pups were stained for the apoptotic cell death marker activated-caspase 3 (*bright green*) following a 6-h exposure to room air (control) or 0.6 MAC desflurane, isoflurane, or sevoflurane, respectively; arrows mark clusters of dying neurons in neocortical layers II/III; scale bar = 500 μm. Reproduced from Istaphanous et al [75] with permission from Lippincott Williams and Wilkins.

[80–82] and to disrupt nerve growth factor expression as well as dopaminergic, noradrenergic, serotonergic, and cholinergic activity [83,84]. Moreover, perinatal opioid administration can cause long-lasting desensitization to opioid analgesia in adult animals [85] and has also been shown to induce long-term behavioral changes, cognitive deficits, and learning impairment extending into adulthood [13,86–90]. However, as discussed previously, analgesics can diminish the deleterious effects of painful stimulation early in life.

Putative mechanisms of drug-induced neurotoxicity

The exact mechanisms of neurotoxicity induced by anesthetics, sedatives, and analgesics in the developing brain remain unresolved. Elucidating these mechanisms will be essential in assessing the relevance of toxicity for pediat-

ric anesthesia and neonatal critical care medicine and for devising mitigating therapies, if necessary. The currently prevailing hypothesis suggests that exposure to GABA$_A$-receptor agonists and/or NMDA-receptor antagonists during a vulnerable period in brain development may cause abnormal neuronal inhibition, triggering cell death in susceptible neurons, which in turn leads to adult learning impairment and decreased neuronal density [37,38,159]. However, several observations cast serious doubt on this hypothesis. While GABA$_A$-receptor stimulation results in decreased neuronal activity in the mature brain, it causes excitation in developing neurons [65], thereby contradicting the hypothesis that abnormal neuronal inhibition is the cell death trigger in developing neurons. Accordingly, recent studies in newborn rats have linked the neurotoxic effects of sevoflurane to brain excitatory properties and episodes of epileptic seizures [157]. Isoflurane has also been shown to cause excessive Ca^{2+} release from the endoplasmic reticulum via overactivation of inositol 1,4,5-triphosphate receptors (InsP3Rs) in neonatal rats *in vivo* and *in vitro* [160]. A similar mechanism may be linked to the production of Alzheimer-associated increases in β-amyloid protein levels [161]. Moreover, while xenon and hypothermia cause neuronal inhibition, they do not appear to exacerbate isoflurane-induced neuronal cell death, as expected by cumulative neuronal inhibition, but rather significantly reduce it [62,63,112].

Importantly, preliminary studies have failed to link the anesthetic and cell death mechanisms. Specifically, while racemic ketamine and S-ketamine both elicit their anesthetic effects via NMDA receptor blockade, S-ketamine induced up to 80% less cell death *in vitro* when compared with equipotent doses of racemic ketamine [128]. Moreover, concomitant administration of gabazine, a GABA$_A$-receptor antagonist, does not attenuate isoflurane-induced neuroapoptosis [64]. Decreases in neuronal activity induced by anesthetics may be less important than the disruption of the neuronal balance of excitation and inhibition, as demonstrated in triggering dendritic morphological changes in postnatal day 15 mice [73,74]. Accordingly, while simultaneous blockade of excitatory and inhibitory activity with tetrodotoxin did not lead to structural changes during synaptogenesis, as expected for a causative relationship between neuronal inhibition and structural damage, administration of GABA$_A$-agonistic or NMDA-antagonistic compounds did alter synaptogenesis [73].

Many of the animal studies using GABA-ergic compounds have clearly shown that anesthesia-induced neurodegeneration is not caused by cellular energy failure and necrosis, such as occurring during ischemic stroke, but rather predominantly involves a cellular suicide program, termed apoptosis [66]. Apoptosis, or programmed cell death, represents an inherent, energy-consuming process, which is highly conserved among species and culminates in self-destruction and elimination of cells that are functionally redundant or potentially detrimental to the organism, utilizing a cascade of enzymes called caspases [162]. As such, apoptotic cell death is an integral part of normal development, as demonstrated by the embryonal cell death of interdigital mesenchymal tissue separating the digits of the hands and feet, as well as during ablation of tail tissue as part of tadpole metamorphosis in amphibians. In the central nervous system, cells are also produced in excess and up to 50–70% of developing neurons are eliminated during normal brain development, be it in rodents, primates or humans [163,164]. This physiological apoptotic cell death establishes proper central nervous system structure and function, and any disruption of this process will lead to massive brain malformation and intrauterine demise [165]. However, apoptotic cell death can also be triggered by pathological insults, such as hypoxia and ischemia [166]. It currently remains unknown whether anesthesia-induced cell death hastens physiological neuroapoptosis or whether it eliminates cells not destined to die, i.e. pathological apoptosis. Normal adult neuronal density as observed following isoflurane exposure in neonatal mice may suggest accelerated physiological apoptosis [41] whereas decreased neuronal density demonstrated following a combination of isoflurane, nitrous oxide, and midazolam in neonatal rats supports the concept of anesthesia-induced, pathological apoptosis [38].

Anesthetic exposure has been shown to trigger both the intrinsic and extrinsic pathways of the apoptotic cascade [66] and to be associated with a decrease in brain-derived neurotrophic factor (BDNF) [67], a protein integral to neuronal survival, growth, and differentiation. Recently, exciting work on the cellular mechanism of anesthesia-induced neuronal cell death has highlighted reductions in synaptic tissue plasminogen activation (tPA) release and increases in proBDNF/p75[NTR]-mediated apoptosis following isoflurane exposure in newborn mice [113]. However, it is not entirely clear at this point whether cytotoxicity is a direct effect of the anesthetic exposure or whether it is triggered by anesthetic byproducts or by metabolic and respiratory derangements, such as hypercarbia and acidosis, which have been observed during anesthetic exposure in small rodents [41,43,167]. Importantly, recently published data have demonstrated that hypercarbia can trigger widespread neuronal cell death in unanesthetized neonatal rats, which was in several brain areas quantitatively indistinguishable from neurodegeneration observed in isoflurane-treated littermates, which were also hypercarbic. However, adult neurocognitive impairment was only observed in the isoflurane-exposed animals [43]. Studies by the Jevtovic-

Todorovic and Vutskits laboratories demonstrated prolonged cellular effects of anesthetic exposure beyond neuronal death, albeit with somewhat conflicting results [73,119]. While both studies demonstrated alterations in synaptic plasticity in neonatal animals following anesthetic exposure, Jevtovic-Todorovic et al found a decrease in synaptic density following anesthetic exposure in postnatal day 7 rats [119]. In slightly older, postnatal day 15 mice, however, anesthetic exposure increased density of dendritic spines [73,74]. These contradicting observations may indicate an age-dependent difference in the effects of anesthetics on dendritic morphology.

Regarding the neurodegenerative mechanisms for NMDA-antagonists in the immature brain, three potential causative pathways have been suggested. The first involves upregulation of the NMDA-receptor, whereby prolonged antagonism of the NMDA-receptor by ketamine results in accelerated neurodegeneration and upregulation of the NR1 receptor subunit as demonstrated in rodent and monkey primary neuronal cell cultures [53,55]. This line of investigation stipulates that a 6-h wash-out period after the prolonged exposure to ketamine results in an increased number of NR1 receptors. This upregulation of the NR1 receptor facilitates pathological calcium entry into the neuron, leading to excitotoxicity [51]. These data support an excitotoxic mechanism for ketamine-induced neurodegeneration, demonstrating a dose-dependent increase in nuclear translocation of NF-κB. Treatment of the neurons with SN-50, a peptide inhibitor of NF-κB translocation, attenuated neuronal cell death. Ketamine also affects other signaling kinases that influence neuronal viability. A second presumptive mechanism involves intracellular signaling by protein kinases. Straiko and colleagues reported that ketamine and propofol individually suppressed phosphorylation of extracellular signal-regulated protein kinase (ERK) and serine/threonine-specific protein kinase 473 (pAkt[473]) in neonatal mice [72]. They also demonstrated that lithium mitigated the decrease in pERK and neuroapoptotic response.

Lastly, experimental models of neurodegeneration have implicated re-entry of postmitotic neurons into the cell cycle, leading to cell death. These authors have demonstrated that ketamine induces aberrant cell cycle re-entry, leading to apoptotic cell death in the developing rat brain [136]. Certainly there are still many other mechanisms that induce neurodegeneration that have not been interrogated in the setting of anesthetic-induced neuroapoptosis [168].

Interspecies comparison

While abundant experimental evidence is available in developing animals implicating anesthetics and sedatives in triggering neurotoxicity, such as immediate brain structural damage and long-term neurocognitive impairment, the implications of these findings for clinical practice remain entirely unclear. Unlike animal studies, administration of anesthetics and analgesics in clinical pediatric medicine almost always coincides with significant noxious stimulation, such as during painful procedures and surgical operations. In this setting, some animal models have actually demonstrated therapeutic effects of analgesics or sedatives, without evidence for neurodegeneration [6,13]. Moreover, several studies have demonstrated significant discrepancies between the metabolic and respiratory effects of anesthetic exposure in small rodent species and those in humans, such as extensive hypercarbia, metabolic acidosis, and hypoglycemia in some animals [41,43,167]. Importantly, unlike during pediatric anesthesia, exposure to clinical doses of anesthetics for only 2–4h can be lethal in more than 20% of small rodents [41,43].

These findings seriously limit the immediate applicability of results obtained in small rodents to clinical pediatric anesthesia practice. Moreover, doses needed for injectable anesthetics to cause neuronal degeneration in animals are significantly higher than those used in clinical practice. Animal studies have shown that toxic doses for ketamine are 10 times higher and doses for propofol are up to 20–30 times higher than clinically used doses, using a weight-based comparison. Some of these discrepancies might be related to differences in body size and whole-body metabolic rates among species, resulting in higher dose requirements for smaller animals on a mg/kg basis, compared with larger animals [169]. However, even when allometric scaling is performed to account for differences

in body size [170], toxic doses in animal studies still remain higher than clinically used doses for many of these compounds (Table 41.2).

The significant differences of comparative doses used in animal studies and clinical practice are further emphasized by the fact that plasma concentrations of neurotoxic doses for ketamine, as measured in small rodents and monkeys, were approximately 3–10 times higher than those observed during clinical human practice [51,125].

Another important finding from animal studies is the narrow age window during which anesthetics trigger neurotoxicity. According to animal studies, exposure to ketamine or ethanol only inflicts significant damage in the developing brains of rodents aged 5–7 days or in monkeys aged 6 days or younger, but not in older animals [33,35,51]. Similarly, in the study of the cytotoxic effects of isoflurane, neurotoxicity did not seem to occur in 1-day-old animals, peaked in 7-day-olds, and dramatically subsided after 10 days of age [66]. Anesthetic exposure outside this period does not seem to trigger neuronal cell death. On the contrary, in prenatal rats, exposure to clinical doses of isoflurane may actually decrease physiological apoptosis and improve subsequent memory retention [108] whereas only isoflurane doses higher than during clinical anesthesia increase neuroapoptosis in this setting [121].

Given these findings of a narrow window of anesthetic neurotoxicity in animals, it is imperative to identify the corresponding developmental state of the human brain, in order to predict the age range for possible susceptibility in humans (Fig. 41.6). Previously, simple estimations of brain cell numbers and degree of myelination defined this period as spanning from the last trimester of preg-

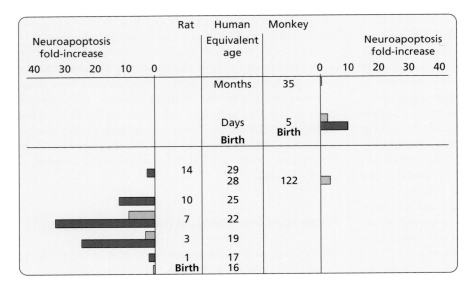

Figure 41.6 Quantification and developmental timing of anesthesia-induced neuroapoptosis. Brown bars signify relative increase in neuroapoptosis compared with physiological apoptosis (fold-increase) following an isoflurane-based anesthetic, yellow bars signify ketamine exposure. Ages indicate postnatal days for rats (left), embryological and postnatal days for rhesus monkeys (right) and estimated, equivalent gestational weeks in humans. Data derived from references [33,51,67,70]. Human developmental equivalency estimated using reference [173]. Reproduced from Istaphanous et al [49] with permission from Elsevier.

Table 41.2 Interspecies comparison of toxic and non-deleterious doses for injectable anesthetics

	Mouse	Rat	Monkey	Human
Toxic ketamine dose	20–40 or 50 mg/kg [58,59]	14–17 mg/kg/h for 11 h [33,50,125]	20–50 mg/kg/h for 24 h in 5 day old [51,52]	–
Estimated equivalent human dose	1.6–3.3 or 4.1 mg/kg	2.3–2.7 mg/kg/h for 11 h	6.5–16 mg/kg/h for 24 h	–
Safe ketamine dose	10 mg/kg [58]	75 mg/kg or 17 mg/kg/h for 6 h [50]	20–50 mg/kg/h for 24 h in 35 day old [51]	–
Estimated equivalent human dose	0.8 mg/kg	12.2 mg/kg or 2.7 mg/kg/h for 6 h	6.5–16 mg/kg/h for 24 h	–
				0.5–2 mg/kg or 0.1–1.2 mg/kg/h
Toxic propofol dose	60 mg/kg [61]	25 mg/kg [152]	–	–
Estimated equivalent human dose	4.9 mg/kg	4 mg/kg	–	–
Safe propofol dose	10 mg/kg [61]	n.d.	–	–
Estimated equivalent human dose	0.8 mg/kg	–	–	–
				2–3 mg/kg
Toxic diazepam dose	n.d.	10–30 mg/kg [35,93]	–	–
Estimated equivalent human dose	–	1.6–4.9 mg/kg	–	–
Safe diazepam dose	5 mg/kg [59]	5 mg/kg [93]	–	–
Estimated equivalent human dose	0.4 mg/kg	0.8 mg/kg	–	–
				0.1 mg/kg
Toxic midazolam dose	9 mg/kg [58]	n.d.	–	–
Estimated equivalent human dose	0.7 mg/kg	–	–	–
Safe midazolam dose	n.d.	9 mg/kg [37]	–	–
Estimated equivalent human dose	–	1.5 mg/kg	–	–
				0.1 mg/kg

n.d., no data.

nancy all the way to the third year of life [159,171,172]. However, using a more up-to-date neuroinformatics approach, the period of maximum neurotoxic susceptibility has been approximated as being closer to the 20th week of gestation until early postnatally (calculator available at www.translatingtime.net) [173]. If these calcula-tions prove correct, susceptibility to anesthesia-induced, neuroapoptotic cell death, if it occurred in humans, may seem more plausible in premature neonates, during fetal surgery, or in neonatal intensive care, and less likely during pediatric anesthesia in term infants and children [174].

Clinical evidence for anesthetic neurotoxicity

While neurotoxic properties of anesthetics are well documented in developing animals, sound clinical evidence for definitive neurological abnormalities in children following anesthetic exposure is much harder to obtain. Obvious ethical concerns preclude randomization of young children to undergo painful procedures with or without anesthesia and analgesia. Moreover, prolonged anesthetic exposures cannot be justified without any surgical or diagnostic indication. Hence, possible clinical evidence for the neurological effects of anesthetics and sedatives in young children has to be gathered from case reports of inadvertent overdoses, postoperative behavioral studies, epidemiological analyses, or from studies into long-term neurological outcome in children suffering from disorders requiring the administration of anesthetics and sedatives during life-saving surgery and intensive care at a very young age [39,40,49].

Postoperative behavioral abnormalities

While many studies investigating behavioral changes immediately postoperatively list the specific anesthetic drugs used and usually involve healthy patient cohorts, their neurological assessment frequently only consists of short-term, parent-reported behavioral questionnaires or observations (Table 41.3). It has long been known that surgery and anesthesia in young children can lead to prolonged behavioral abnormalities [28,175–184]. Reported behavioral abnormalities, such as attention seeking, crying, temper tantrums, sleep disturbance, and anxiety, occur in up to 50% of children early after anesthesia and decrease significantly during the first postoperative month. These symptoms have repeatedly been associated with younger patient age, severity of postoperative pain, and lack of sedation prior to induction of anesthesia [28,177,179,182,184]. While the phenomenon's exact mechanism remains unknown, psychological factors, rather than structural brain abnormalities, are generally believed to be the underlying etiology [175,176,185]. Importantly, the administration of a benzodiazepine prior to general anesthesia did not exacerbate postoperative behavioral abnormalities, as expected for a cytotoxic etiology, but rather significantly reduced abnormal behavioral symptoms [186]. However, since most postoperative behavioral studies rely on parental assessment of the child, no continuing professional observations and long-term neurocognitive assessments were incorporated in any of the behavioral studies. Therefore, the permanence of these neurological abnormalities remains uncertain.

Anesthesia in critically ill neonates

A patient population more closely followed with standardized neurodevelopmental tests are previously critically ill neonates, who may have undergone surgical procedures involving general anesthesia, such as ligation of patent ductus arteriosus, repair of esophageal atresia, inguinal hernia repair, neurosurgical operations, laparotomies, or tracheotomies [187–196]. However, none of these studies were designed to study the long-term effects of anesthetic exposure and accordingly, they consistently fail to specify the exact anesthetic agents used and oftentimes involve several potent confounders, such as severe prematurity, prolonged ventilator support, considerable pain and distress, significant co-morbidities, latent episodes of hypoxia or hypoxia-ischemia, and frequently include major surgical procedures with potentially significant postoperative inflammatory response (Table 41.4). In this context, long-term neurodevelopmental impairment, such as a reduction in IQ, increased incidence of cerebral palsy, deafness, or blindness, have frequently been observed [190–194,196]. Greater severity of illness and co-existing, congenital abnormalities were associated with worsening neurological outcome [188,193].

In an attempt to at least partially control for severity of illness, several case-control studies compared neurodevelopmental outcome in survivors of surgical therapy for necrotizing enterocolitis and patent ductus arteriosus with those receiving medical management alone. When compared with age-matched controls or medically treated patients in the same cohort, several investigators noticed an impairment in neurocognitive function in surgically treated survivors of laparotomy or thoracotomy [190–192,194,196] while others were unable to find these differences [187,189,195]. However, it remains difficult to separate the effects of neonatal stress and surgery from the effects of the anesthetics. Moreover, study designs did not include randomized controlled trials, but were rather designed as cohort studies or case–control studies. It therefore seems conceivable that, due to selection bias, some of the extremely premature neonates that needed surgery had more concomitant illnesses and were therefore sicker than their matched controls. This notion is underscored by the fact that some of the studies identified longer periods of hypotension, more common use of inotropic support, and longer periods of total parenteral nutrition in the postsurgical patients [190,192]. Accordingly, a prospective randomized trial of 117 preterm infants with necrotizing enterocolitis who were assigned to either laparotomy or to peritoneal drainage without surgery did not find any difference in patient survival and early outcomes [197].

Another patient population that has been followed for evaluation of long-term neurocognitive development fol-

Table 41.3 Behavioral assessment following anesthetic exposure in early childhood

Anesthetic agent	Dose or duration	Study design	Number of subjects	Age during exposure	Neurological sequelae on exam	Duration of symptoms and outcome	Reference
Midazolam (plus fentanyl)	0.07–0.94 mg/kg/h for up to 38 d	Case–control	45	0.03–19.2 years	After discontinuation of sedation, poor social interaction, decreased visual attentiveness, dystonic postures, and choreoathetosis in 11%	No sequelae 4 weeks after discontinuation	Bergman et al [232]
Midazolam (plus pentobarbital)	1–17 d	Retrospective cohort study	40	0.5–14 years	After discontinuation of sedation, agitation, anxiety, muscle twitching, sweating, tremor in 35%. Midazolam dose of >60 mg/kg strongly associated with symptoms	Symptoms abolished by pentobarbital treatment	Fonsmark et al [233]
Midazolam (plus opioid)	1.5–4 mg/kg for 10 d	Case series	6	1–6 years	Multifocal myoclonus, dystonia, chorea, facial grimacing, tongue thrusting without seizure activity on EEG. Chemotherapy for CNS malignancies, MRI abnormalities	3–7 days	Khan et al [234]
Midazolam (plus morphine)	0.025–0.72 mg/kg/h for 1–18 d	Cohort study	53	6 days to 11 years	After discontinuation, prolonged sedation for up to 1 week in 8%. Disorientation, hallucinations, and behavioral abnormalities in up to 11%	0.13–7 days	Hughes et al [235]
Midazolam (plus opioid)	0–0.014 mg/kg/min for 4–18 d	Cohort study	15	6 weeks to 2.3 years	After discontinuation, sleeplessness, tremors, agitation, movement disorder in up to 50%. Symptoms occured as late as 6 d after start of taper	3 days	Franck et al [236]
Lorazepam (plus opioid)	0.1–0.4 mg/kg/h for 11–30 d	Prospective, open-label study	29	0.2–3 years	During taper, 24% experienced agitation, irritability, abnormal movements, or hallucinations	Not specified	Dominguez et al [237]
Pentobarbital (plus midazolam)	1–17 d	Retrospective cohort study	40	0.5–14 years	After discontinuation of sedation, agitation, anxiety, muscle twitching, sweating, tremor in 35%. Pentobarbital >25 mg/kg associated with symptoms	Symptoms abolished by pentobarbital treatment	Fonsmark et al [231]
Pentobarbital (plus benzodiazepines and opioids)	1–5 mg/kg/h for 0.6–49 d	Case series	8	0.4–7 years	During sedation, one patient (12.5%) experienced choreiform movements with athetoid features, ataxia, facial twitching. Also received mathadone and phenobarbital	1 week	Yanay et al [238]
Pentobarbital	1–4 mg/kg/h for 4–28 d	Case series	6	0.17–1.4 years	None reported	Not applicable	Tobias et al [239]

(Continued)

Table 41.3 (Continued)

Anesthetic agent	Dose or duration	Study design	Number of subjects	Age during exposure	Neurological sequelae on exam	Duration of symptoms and outcome	Reference
Phenobarbital (plus phenytoin)	20–1800 mg/d in mother	Case–control	172	Fetal exposure	Greater need for special education, learnign difficulties, lower intelligence (WAIS), decreased attention on D-2, but not CPT test in adults after fetal exposure vs. controls. No difference in memory tasks (DS, ALT)	Not applicable	Dessens et al [240]
Phenobarbital	2.5–50 mg for 1–540 d	Cross-sectional, case–control	28	Neonate	No difference in Kaufman-ABC intelligence and D-2 tests between 8–14 year old children following neonatal treatment with phenobarbital and best-friend controls	Not applicable	Gerstner et al [241]
Ketamine	13–56 mg/kg	Case series	18	0.07–7 years	After inadvertent overdose, prolonged sedation and respiratory depression	Sedation for 3–24 h, no neurological sequelae on follow-up, where available	Green et al [242]
Propofol	200 mg/h for 48 h *in utero*	Case report	1	Premature neonate 33 wk GA	Prolonged sedation, no other neurological sequelae reported	12 h	Bacon et al [243]
Propofol	10.9 mg/kg/h for 11 d	Case report	1	23 months	Restlessness, muscle twitching limbs, functional blindness	Motor function impaired for 2 weeks, blindness for 33 days	Lanigan et al [244]
Propofol	Median infusion 2.7 mg/kg/h for >24 h	Case series	20	Median age 3.3 years	No neurological sequelae	Not applicable	Macrae and James[245]
Propofol	6–18 mg/kg/h for 2–4 d	Case report	2	2.5 and 4 years	Muscle weakness, twitching	9–18 days, full recovery	Trotter et al [246]
Propofol	10 mg/kg/h for 54 min	Case report	1	6 years	Seizure, ataxia, hallucinations starting 44h after discontinuation of propofol	5 d, recovered without overt long-term sequelae	Bendiksen et al [247]

Isoflurane	13–497 MAC-hours	Cohort study	10	0.06–19 years	Agitation, non-purposeful movement in 50% of patients; all received >70 MAC-hours isoflurane, plus benzodiazepines and opioids	Symptoms responded to treatment advocated for opioid withdrawal	Arnold et al [248]
Isoflurane	0.25–1.5% for 1–76h	Case series, case–control	12	0.5–10 years	Transient ataxia, agitation, hallucinations, and confusion after isoflurane administration >24h; no symptoms after benzodiazepines or isoflurane <15h	Normal follow-up exam 4–6 weeks after discharge	Kelsall et al [249]
Isoflurane	81 MAC-hours	Case report	1	2.5 years	Self-limiting, fine tremor in patient with myasthenia	46h	McBeth et al [250]
Isoflurane	0.4–0.9% for 6–8 d	Case series	3	4–11 years	Temporary involuntary movements, myoclonia, brief seizures, and ataxia	Resolution of symptoms within 4–5 d	Sackey et al [251]
Isoflurane (plus midazolam and morphine)	0.5–1% for 4 d	Case report	1	7 years	Disorientation, hallucinations, agitation, seizure	5 d; reportedly normal behavior	Hughes et al [252]
Sevoflurane	8% during induction	Prospective study	20	1.1–8.4 years	Seizure-like movement and epileptiform EEG in 10%, no neuro exam	Not applicable	Conreux et al [253]
Sevoflurane	8% during induction	Prospective study	31	2–12 years	Epileptiform discharge in 88% with controlled ventilation and 20% with spontaneous breathing. No neuro exam	Not applicable	Vakkuri et al [254]
Sevoflurane	7% during induction	Prospective, randomized trial	45	2–12 years	No seizure activity on induction. Neurological exam not performed	Not applicable	Constant et al [255]
Sevoflurane	2% after intravenous thiopental	Prospective study	30	3–8 years	No epileptiform EEG activity. Neurological exam not performed	Not applicable	Nieminen et al [256]
Sevoflurane	Dose not specified	Meta-analysis of prospective studies in one center	791	3.3±2.1 to 6.9±2.4 years	Increased "maladaptive" behavior in children who were younger and whose parents were more anxious on induction	Assessment up to 14 d postoperatively	Kain et al [182]
Sevoflurane or halothane	2–4% for 22 ± 17 min, 1–2% for 22 ± 15 min	Prospective, randomized trial	120	3.3 ± 2.6 to 4 ± 2.9 years	Negative behavioral changes, such as temper tantrums, loss of appetite or sleep disturbance in 38% for up to 30 d; no difference between sevoflurane or halothane	Assessment up to 30 d postoperatively	Keaney et al [181]

(Continued)

Table 41.3 (*Continued*)

Anesthetic agent	Dose or duration	Study design	Number of subjects	Age during exposure	Neurological sequelae on exam	Duration of symptoms and outcome	Reference
Sevoflurane or halothane	Doses not specified; outpatient surgery	Double-blinded, randomized, controlled trial	102	3–10 years	PHBQ: no difference between both anesthetics in regard to postoperative anxiety, sleep or appetite disturbance, strength, and energy	Up to 1 week postoperatively	Kain et al [183]
Pentobarbital, scopolamine, ether, nitrous oxide, and/or cyclopropane	Doses not specified; otolaryngological surgery	Survey study	612	2 to over 12 years	Parental assessment: negative behavioral changes, such as night terrors, temper tantrums, fears, bed-wetting most prevalent in under 3 year group (57%) compared with older group (8%)	Questionnaires mailed to parents 2 months postoperatively	Eckenhoff [28]
Pentobarbital, scopolamine, morphine, and ether or nitrous oxide	Doses not specified; otolaryngological, dental, or ophthalmological surgery	Survey, case–control	290	1–15 years	No differences in psychological upset after anesthesia, surgery, and hospitalization compared with siblings or healthy controls	Interview administered to patient's mother 2 weeks postoperatively	Davenport and Werry [257]
Halothane or ketamine	Dose not specified; scheduled and emergency surgery	Prospective randomized study, survey	103	1–12 years	Parental assessment: fear of strangers, sleep disturbance, nightmares, or bed wetting in 38% under 4 years vs 16% in 4 year olds and over	Parental assessment 1 month postoperatively	Modvig et al [176]
Thiopental, halothane, or methohexital induction and halothane, nitrous oxide maintenance	Methohexital 15 mg/kg PR, otherwise not specified; routine day-case ENT surgery	Survey study	86	2–10 years	PHBQ: problematic behavioral changes in 51% at 1 d and 34% at 1 month postoperatively. Temper tantrums tended to be more common following stormy induction vs calm induction of anesthesia	Questionnaires given to parents to report behavior 1 d, 1 week, and 1 month postoperatively	Kotiemi et al [178]
Thiopental or propofol, isoflurane, or halothane or enflurane. Midazolam or diazepam premed	Doses not specified; ENT or ophthalmological procedures with mean anesthesia time of 32.8 ± 17.9 min	Multicenter survey	551	0.3–13.4 years	PHBQ: behavioral problems in 47% on day of surgery, 9% after 4 weeks, including attention seeking, crying, temper tantrums, sleep problems, anxiety	Questionnaires given to parents to report behavior up to 4 weeks postoperatively	Kotiemi et al [179,180]

Drug	Details	Study type	N	Age	Findings	Outcome measure	Reference
Halothane/nitrous oxide	Dose not specified; elective minor head and neck surgery	Survey study	122	1–8 years	Parental assessment: behavioral abnormalities in up to 88% of children awake during induction and 58% of children asleep during induction	Questionnaires mailed to parents within first postoperative month	Meyers and Muravchick [177]
Predominantly halothane, nitrous oxide, ketamine, and/or thiopental	Doses not specified, stratified by number of exposures for mostly ENT and general surgery	Retrospective, epidemiological study	5357	0–4 years	Review of medical and educational records demonstrate a doubling of the risk of learning disabilities following 2 or more surgical procedures with anesthesia for more than a combined 2 h, compared with no or one exposure	Review of educational records several years after anesthetic exposure	Wilder et al [229]
Predominantly sodium thiopental, nitrous oxide, and halothane	Doses not specified, general or regional anesthesia for cesarean delivery vs spontaneous vaginal birth	Retrospective review of records	5320	Day of birth	The incidence of learning disabilities was similar among children delivered vaginally without anesthesia and via cesarean section with general anesthesia, but lower following cesarean section with regional anesthesia	Review of school records	Sprung et al [228]
No data	No data	Epidemiological case–control study	5050	0–3 years	Doubling of presence of diagnostic codes for developmental problems in children also carrying a billing code for inguinal hernia repair prior to 3 years of age, compared with those that did not carry this billing code	Presence of a diagnostic code for developmental or behavioral disorder, mental retardation, autism, and language or speech problems	DiMaggio et al [225]
No data	No data	Review of data from monozygotic twin pairs from Young Netherlands Twin Register	1143	0–3 years	Educational scores lower in concordant twin pairs exposed to anesthesia compared with unexposed pairs. However, no difference in educational achievement comparing both twins in discordantly exposed pairs	Educational achievement (Cito test administered at age 12) and Connor Teacher Rating Scale	Bartels et al [258]

ALT, associated learning task; CPT, continuous performance task for sustained attention; D-2, selective attention test; DS, digit span memory test; EEG, electroencephalogram; GA, gestational age; PNBQ, Vernon Post Hospitalization Behavioral Questionnaire; WAIS, Wechsler Adult Intelligence Scale.

Table 41.4 Neurocognitive performance following surgery and anesthesia in neonates and infants

Study design	Study group	Control group	Number of subjects	Age during exposure	Age during neurological assessment	Neurological assessment tool	Neurological sequelae in study group	Reference
Case–control study	PDA ligation, inguinal hernia repair, GI surgery, neurosurgery, tracheotomy	No surgical intervention	221	First hospitalization for <27 weeks PCA, ELBW	5 years	Neurological examination, WPPSI-R	Increased incidence of cerebral palsy, blindness, deafness, WPPSI-R >3 SD below mean	Victorian Infant Collaborative Study Group [191]
Case series	Repair esophageal atresia	None, comparison with general population	36	Neonatal	10.2 years	WISC-RN, ADQC, CBCL, TRF	10% reduction in IQ, SE five times as frequent; subgroup without major associated congenital anomalies had normal IQ	Bouman et al [193]
Case series	Repair esophageal atresia	None, comparison with general population	34	Neonatal	12.7 years	WISC, HFT, Rorschach Test	No statistical difference in IQ compared with age- and gender-matched general population	Lindahl et al [187]
Cohort study, case–control study	PDA ligation	Indometacin treatment	340	84% neonatal (25–29 weeks PCA), ELBW	18 months	Neurological examination, BSID2	Increase in cerebral palsy, cognitive delay, hearing loss, bilateral blindness	Kabra et al [196]
Cohort study, case–control study	Laparotomy	Peritoneal drain placement	245	Neonatal, ELBW	18–22 months	Neurological examination, BSID2	Blinded assessor: higher frequency of CP and lower BSID 2; no difference between medically treated patients with or without NEC	Hintz et al [194]
Case–control study	Laparotomy	Peritoneal drain placement	78	29 weeks PCA, ELBW	18–22 months post term	Neurological examination, BSID2	Less neurodevelopmental impairment and lower mortality	Blakely et al [195]
Case–control study	NEC	No NEC	802	30 weeks PCA, VLBW	20 months post term	SBIS, BSID	No blinded assessor: no significant difference in BSID scores; impairment more prevalent in survivors of most severe form of NEC, however, not stratified by surgical or medical management	Walsh et al [188]
Case–control study	NEC requiring laparotomy	No NEC or NEC managed medically	115	26–27 weeks PCA, VLBW	12 months, 3 years, and 5 years PCA	GMDS, SBIS	No blinded assessor: higher incidence of neurodevelopmental impairment; use of inotropes and TPN dependence more prevalent after laparotomy	Tobiansky et al [190]

Study type	Patient group	Controls	N	Population	Timing	Tests	Results	Reference
Case–control study	NEC requiring laparotomy	Gestational age-, birthweight-matched controls	30	26 weeks PCA, ELBW	5 and 7 years	GMDS, SBIS, CBCL, Peabody tests	No blinded assessor: NDI in 70% of survivors of NEC vs 25% in age-matched controls. NDI after laparotomy for NEC 66.6% vs 9.1% after NEC managed medically. Hypotension requiring inotropes more prevalent after laparotomy	Chacko et al [192]
Case–control study	NEC requiring laparotomy	NEC managed medically	18	Neonatal, VLBW	8, 15 months post term, 24 months	BSID, INFANIB, DDST	Assessor not blinded: higher prevalence of motor delays early after surgery; no differences detected at 2 years of age	Simon et al [189]
Prospective, randomized trial	ASO with DHCA	ASO with LF-CPB or general population	155	Neonatal	1, 2.5, 4, 8 years	WISC 3, WIAT, TRF, CBCL, WCST, TOVA, Mayo Test for Apraxia of Speech, Goldman-Fristoe Test of Articulation	Lower Full-Scale IQ, Perceptual Organization, and Freedom from Distractability scores, WIAT Reading and Mathematics Composites, Memory Screening Index, WCST, TOVA scores. Most differences were <1 SD	Bellinger et al [200,202,206]
Cohort study	Open heart surgery	None	59	Neonatal	≥2 years	SBIS or BSID	Cerebral palsy in 22%, mean IQ 90, but highly dependent on type of congenital heart disease	Miller et al [198,199]
Case series	ASO	None, comparison with general population	60	Neonatal	3–14 years	Kiphard and Schilling Body Co-ordination Test, Kaufman Assessment Battery for Children, Oral and Speech Motor Control Test, Mayo Test of Speech and Oral Apraxia	Assessor not blinded: increased prevalence of neurological impairment (27%), speech impairment (40%), motor dysfunction, language impairment; no difference in intelligence	Hövels-Gürich et al [208,214]

(Continued)

Table 41.4 (Continued)

Study design	Study group	Control group	Number of subjects	Age during exposure	Age during neurological assessment	Neurological assessment tool	Neurological sequelae in study group	Reference
Case-control study	ASO with limited DHCA	"Best friend" control group or general population	148	0–118 (median 9) d	9.1 ± 2.9 years	WPPSI-R or WISC 3, CBCL, Movement ABC	Lower IQ than control, but still above general population mean; higher prevalence of behavioral, language expression and comprehension problems	Karl et al [207]
Case series	Open heart surgery	None, comparison with general population	98	Infancy	1–3 years	PDMS, GMDS	Blinded assessor: abnormal neurological exam in 41%, motor delay in 42%, and global developmental delay in 23%	Limperopoulos et al [215]
Case series	HLHS	None, comparison with general population	28	Several procedures as neonates and early childhood	8.6 ± 2.1 years	WISC 3, WJPB, VMI, CELF-R, CBCL	Assessor not blinded: prevalence of mental retardation 18% and borderline IQ in 36%. Learning disability in over 14% of survivors. Performance IQ scores lower than verbal IQ	Mahle et al [204]
Cohort study, case-control study	Intrauterine exposure to nitrous oxide	No intrauterine exposure	159	Prenatal: third trimester	5 days postnatally	Prechtl's neurological and Brazelton's behavioral assessments	Weaker habituation to sound, stronger muscular tension and resistance to cuddle, fewer smiles	Eishima [213]
Case-control study	General or local anesthetics	No anesthetic exposure	39	Prenatal: first to third trimester	0.8–6 days postnatally	Measurement of visual-pattern preference	Prolongation of visual-pattern preference	Blair et al [211]
Case-control study	General or local anesthetics	No anesthetic exposure	14	Prenatal: 1st to third trimester	4 ± 0.08 years	PPVT, vocabulary parts of WPPS and SBIS	Lower PPVT IQ scores, no differences in WPPS or SBIS	Hollenbeck et al [212]
Prospective, case-control study	Thiopental, nitrous oxide for general anesthesia	Lidocaine 1.5% for epidural analgesia	30	Perinatal for cesarean section	1–7 days	Neurological assessment as per Prechtl and Beintema	Blinded assessor: abnormal neurological activity for up to 7 d in 47%, regardless of group assignment	Hollmen et al [210]
Cohort study	Elective procedures that required anesthesia		340	2–13 years	Up to 2 weeks after exposure	PHBQ, CBCL	Behavioral abnormalities in 34%, especially if age <5 years, postoperative pain or nausea, anxiety during induction, post-tonsillectomy, previous hospitalizations	Karling et al [216,217]

Study type	Surgery/anesthesia	Controls	n	Age at exposure	Follow-up	Tests	Outcome	Reference
Survey study	General anesthesia for general surgery, ENT, gastroenterology, plastics surgery, orthopedics	None, some sibling controls	1027	3–12 years	3 and 30 days postanesthesia	PHBQ	Behavioral changes in 24% on day 3 after surgery, 16% on day 30, including anxiety and regression, apathy or withdrawal, and separation anxiety	Stargatt et al [184]
Prospective poulation-based study	Prolonged sedation and/or analgesia for intensive care	No exposure to sedation or analgesia	1345	Neonatal: premature infants born 22–32 weeks PCA	Up to 5 years	MPC of Kaufman Assessment Battery for Children	No difference in disability after adjustment for severity of illness	Rozé et al [218]
Retrospective cohort study	General anesthesia for urological procedures	None, comparison with general population	243	0–6 years	Several years after surgery	CBCL/4–18	Incidence of behavioral disturbances higher in children operated on <2 years of age, compared with >2 y	Kalkman et al [219]
Prospective, longitudinal study	General anesthesia, intensive care for correction of congenital anomalies	None, comparison with general population	101	Neonatal period	Up to 2 years	BSID, MDI	Normal mental development, but impaired growth and delayed psychomotor development	Gischler et al [220]
Prospective, longitudinal case-control study	General anesthesia, intensive care, ventilator support following major emergency abdominal surgeries	Healthy controls and neonates requiring intensive medical care	19	Neonatal period	Up to 11 years	GMDS, Reynell Developmental Language Scales, British Picture Vocabulary Scales, Wallin B pegboard, compulsory national curriculum examinations	Continued impaired performance in previously critically ill patients requiring prolonged care, with significant improvements in medical group, but not surgical patients, especially following multiple procedures	Ludman et al [221–224]

ADQC, Abbreviated Depression Questionnaire for Children Self Assessment; ASO, Arterial Switch Operation; BSID, Bayley Scales of Infant Development; CBCL, Achenbach Child Behavior Checklist Parental Assessment; CELF-R, Clinical Evaluation of Language Fundamentals-Revised; DDST, Denver Developmental Screening Test; DHCA, deep hypothermic circulatory arrest; ELBW, extremely low birthweight (<1000 g); GMDS, Griffiths Mental Development Scales; INFANIB, Infant Neurological International Battery; LF-CPB, low flow-cardiopulmonary bypass; MDI, Bayley Mental Development Index; Movement ABC, Movement Assessment Battery for Children; MPC Mental Composite Score of the Kaufman Assessment Battery for Children; NDI, neurodevelopmental impairment; PDI, Bayley Psychomotor Developmental Index; PDMS, Peabody Developmental Motor Scales; PHBQ, Vernon Post Hospitalization Behavior Questionnaire; PPVT, Peabody Picture Vocabulary Test; SBIS Stanford-Binet Intelligence Scales; TOVA, Test of Variables of Attention; TRF, teacher's report form; VMI, Developmental Test of Visual Motor Integration; WCST, Wisconsin Card Sorting Test of problem solving; WJPB, Woodcock-Johnson Psychoeducational Battery; VLBW, very low birthweight (≤1500 g); WIAT, Wechsler Individual Achievement Test; WISC 3, Wechsler Intelligence Scale for Children, Third Edition; WISC-RN, Wechsler Intelligence Scale for Children; WPPS-R, Revised Wechsler Preschool and Primary Scales for Intelligence.

lowing surgical procedures early in life are neonates and infants undergoing congenital heart surgery, such as for hypoplastic left heart syndrome, transposition of the great arteries, or tetralogy of Fallot [198–208]. Neurocognitive impairment has been documented in many of these studies, compared with the general population [198–206,208] or with "best friend" control subjects [207]. However, the anesthetic regimen was not specified for any of these studies and in many of the patients confounding factors included preoperative neurological lesions, pre-existing or perioperative hypoxia and hypotension, as well as chronic postoperative hypoxemia. Interestingly, in the largest trial, the Boston Circulatory Arrest Trial with patient follow-up for 8 years after arterial switch operation, many outcome measures in a battery of neurodevelopmental tests were within normal population limits, despite major corrective cardiac surgery with anesthesia in the neonatal period [206]. In an important report in this population, Guerra et al studied 95 survivors of neonatal open heart surgery with normal chromosomes. They calculated the cumulative dose, dose per day, and number of days each patient received opioids, benzodiazepines, ketamine, and chloral hydrate in the intensive care unit and OR. They also calculated exposure to anesthetic gas in MAC-hours from end-tidal concentrations, and inspired concentrations in the sweep gas of the cardiopulmonary bypass circuit. At 18–24 months, none of the sedation or anesthetic variables was associated with poor performance on Bayley Scales of Infant Development, or other tests of adaptive behavior and vocabulary [209].

Several case–control studies try to address the neurocognitive implications of prenatal anesthetic exposure *in utero* [210–212]. Abnormal neurological activity observed in neonates early after delivery included increased motor tone and decreased interaction [212], visual test abnormalities [211] and motor weakness [210]. Interestingly, the incidence of early neurological abnormalities following cesarean section did not differ between neonates exposed to general anesthesia, including thiopental and nitrous oxide, or to maternal epidural analgesia using lidocaine [210]. In a small, 4-year follow-up after prenatal exposure to anesthetics for dental procedures [211], children demonstrated decreased intelligence scores compared with unexposed controls, but demonstrated similar performance on tests of their vocabulary [212]. However, anesthetic exposure was not quantified, spanned from the first to the third trimester of pregnancy, and consisted of such diverse agents as methohexital, sodium thiopental, lidocaine, or carbocaine.

In summary, while several cohort studies in premature and term neonates undergoing major surgical operations involving general anesthesia demonstrate neurodevelopmental impairment later in life, none of these studies specified the anesthetic technique utilized. Moreover, due to design limitations in these studies, the effects of concomitant disease and the impact of the surgical procedure cannot be separated from the effects of anesthesia.

Epidemiological studies

More recently, several research groups have utilized retrospective reviews of large-scale epidemiological data sets to investigate neurodevelopmental outcome following surgery and anesthesia.

One of these studies used billing codes to identify a birth cohort of children in the New York State Medicaid database who underwent inguinal hernia repair during the first 3 years of life and compared these patients with a sample of more than 5000 age-matched children without the same billing code [225]. After controlling for gender and birth-related complications, such as low birthweight, children who carried an ICD-9 procedure code for inguinal hernia repair were more than twice as likely as their age-matched peers without this procedural code to also possess diagnostic codes for developmental or behavioral disorder. Interestingly, highlighting the importance of co-morbidities in retrospective data sets, surgical patients were more likely to carry secondary diagnoses, including congenital anomalies of the central nervous system (10% of patients), birthweight less than 2500 g (32%), or perinatal hypoxia (17%) and were also more likely to be male and African-American. Accordingly, as the authors correctly pointed out, health and medical care utilization as well as the frequency of mental illness differ in this vulnerable Medicaid study group from the general population [226,227], significantly complicating the generalization of these findings to all patients undergoing surgery with anesthesia.

Two other epidemiological studies in more heterogeneous patient populations investigated the effects of anesthetic exposure either during cesarean delivery or for pediatric surgery prior to age 4 years of age on subsequent learning abilities [228,229]. After adjusting for gestational age, sex, birthweight, and American Society of Anesthesiologists physical status, children who underwent multiple surgical procedures with general anesthesia prior to age 4 were found to be at increased risk for learning disabilities (35% of children), while children who only underwent one operation with anesthesia did not differ from unexposed children (21% learning disabilities) [229]. While listing the anesthetic regimen as predominantly halothane, nitrous oxide, and ketamine, the study was not powered to specifically analyze learning disabilities according to anesthetic drug. The important confounding influence of co-morbidities in this patient cohort was highlighted by the fact that almost half the previously anesthetized patients diagnosed with developmental disability had suffered from serous otitis media prior to age 4, a controversial predictor of neurocognitive disabilities, whereas only one-third of children without learning disabilities had experienced chronic ear infections [230,231]. However, a more definitive analysis including the unanesthetized children will be needed to assess this potential association.

In a second retrospective review, the same research group collected school and health data from almost 5000 children born via vaginal delivery and compared them to almost 200 neonates delivered via cesarean section with either general anesthesia, consisting predominantly of sodium thiopental, halothane, and nitrous oxide, or with about 300 children undergoing cesarean delivery with regional anesthesia [228]. The overall rate of potential learning disability was found to be 26% in this study population and did not differ between those children delivered with or without anesthesia. This finding could not have been easily predicted, because neonates in the general anesthesia group experienced lower birthweights, lower gestational age, and lower Apgar scores. In addition, their delivery was more commonly complicated by hemorrhage and eclampsia/pre-eclampsia, and was more frequently performed due to an emergency indication. Importantly, other risk factors independent from anesthetic exposure, such as male gender and mother's educational status, were strongly correlated with subsequent learning impairment. Children born to mothers with only some high school education were three times more likely to acquire learning disabilities than children from mothers with college education, suggesting powerful genetic and/or socio-economic confounders. Interestingly, babies born with regional anesthesia were less likely to be diagnosed with a later learning disability than those born vaginally without anesthesia, most likely because their parents also tended to be better educated.

In a pilot study, Kalkman et al tried to control for the fact that there might be a causal relationship between the requirement for surgery and subsequent behavioral and learning impairment independent of anesthetic exposure [219]. They examined behavioral outcome following similar urological procedures, performed either before or after 2 years of age. In this small retrospective study involving fewer than 300 patients, parental evaluations of their children's competencies and behavioral/emotional issues were based on a combination of the child's activities, social relationships, and performance in school. There was a non-significant trend towards a relationship between timing of surgery and the risk for developing behavioral problems, even after adjusting for confounders such as parental education, number of total anesthetic exposures, gestational age, and birthweight. However, the authors correctly point out in their discussion that the indication for the surgery or the timing of the procedure may not be entirely independent of factors that could have also influenced neurobehavioral development, such as co-morbidities. In other words, the decision to operate on a child prior to age 2 years could depend on the sever-

ity of symptoms resulting from the anatomical anomaly, which in turn may influence neurobehavioral development independent of anesthetic exposure.

Arguably the most vulnerable group of patients potentially susceptible to the effects of prolonged exposure to anesthetics and sedatives during an immature state of brain developmental is not otherwise healthy pediatric patients undergoing brief, elective surgical procedures, but rather premature infants requiring neonatal intensive care [174]. In this exceptionally vulnerable patient population, Rozé and co-workers employed a prospective population-based study approach to evaluate the effects of prolonged sedation and analgesia on long-term neurological outcome, as measured by a validated, neurocognitive assessment tool [218]. A birth cohort of preterm infants born prior to 33 weeks gestational age who were subjected to mechanical ventilation and/or surgery were examined at 5 years of age using the Kaufman Assessment Battery for Children. While 74% of those treated with sedatives and/or analgesics for less than 7 days or not at all showed no disabilities, only 58% of those treated for more than 7 days were deemed without disability. However, after adjustment for significant confounders, such as birthweight, malformations, complications of pregnancy, characteristics of the delivering hospital, neonatal complications, need for surgery, and postnatal administration of corticosteroids, this association no longer remained statistically significant. While the study did not have the power to detect differences in disability of less than 10%, the long exposure times suggest that effect sizes during comparably briefer surgical anesthesia would be expected to be even smaller.

Confounders and anesthetic protection

The presence of powerful, confounding perioperative factors in infants and children undergoing surgery and anesthesia and the lack thereof in animal studies represent a serious limitation of directly applying findings of preclinical studies to humans. Given the overwhelming evidence for pharmacological interference with normal development of the central nervous system and the lack of anesthetics devoid of cytotoxic effects, one could be tempted to limit the use of suspect medications during medical interventions early in life. However, preclinical and human studies, as outlined above, have clearly demonstrated the increased morbidity and developmental abnormalities in animals and children exposed to unmitigated pain and stress. In this deleterious context, anesthetics have demonstrated protective abilities. Similarly, anesthetics may help alleviate the harmful effects from other perioperative stressors, such as inflammation and hypoxia-ischemia.

Inflammatory response

Following physical trauma or surgery, in addition to painful stimulation, neurological impairment of infants may also be related to long-term effects of the inflammatory response to the trauma or due to subsequent bacterial infections. Inflammation plays a major role in the evolution of cerebral injury after cerebral ischemia and traumatic brain injury (TBI). Within hours, transcription factors are activated locally in brain tissue and upregulate proinflammatory genes, including the cytokines, tumor necrosis factor (TNF)-α, interleukin (IL)-1β and chemokines such as IL-8, interferon inducible protein-10, monocyte chemoattractant protein-1, and fractalkine [259]. The production of these inflammatory cytokines promotes the transmigration of the inflammatory cells in the brain parenchyma. Experimental studies in animal models of focal ischemic stroke have suggested that leukocytes play an important role in the development of secondary injury after acute CNS injury [260].

In animal studies, local neonatal inflammation has led to excessive hyperalgesia in adulthood [261]. Chronic persistent inflammation experienced early during development is capable of altering behavior and sensitivity to pain later in life, especially in response to recurrent inflammatory events [262]. Systemic infection, as demonstrated in a mouse model of neonatal injection of live bacteria, leads to sustained increases in microglial activation in the brain [263]. In these animals, cytokine levels are exaggerated following an immune challenge in adulthood, which can lead to impairment in memory function [263]. Injection of lipopolysaccharides during a critical postnatal period can affect adult sensation and pain responses [264] and may also cause long-lasting increases in seizure susceptibility [265].

Several injectable and inhaled anesthetics have been found to modulate immune function. Inhaled anesthetics, such as isoflurane and sevoflurane, were shown to interfere with the leukocyte-mediated immune response, which may lead to immunosuppression following surgical procedures [266]. Ketamine and propofol have also been shown to play a role in modulating inflammatory or immune system function [267,268]. However, postoperative immune function may be influenced by dose and timing of the anesthetic drugs, pain, psychological state, perioperative blood loss, or hypothermia [269]. Similarly opioid analgesics, such as morphine, have been found to suppress natural killer cell activity, inflammatory cytokine production, and mitogen-induced lymphocyte proliferation [270–272]. However, this response is modulated by the presence or absence of noxious stimulation and the type of opioid used.

Importantly, in an adult mouse endotoxemia model, isoflurane anesthesia immediately following the injection of a lethal dose of *Escherichia coli* lipopolysaccharide dramatically improved survival by 300% compared with unanesthetized animals [273]. In these animals, the administration of isoflurane, pentobarbital, or ketamine/xylazine attenuated serum levels of the inflammatory markers TNF-α, IL-10, and IL-6. These findings suggest that anesthetic administration during endotoxemia may not only improve survival, but also lead to attenuation of the inflammatory process.

In children, abdominal surgery can lead to significant increases in blood levels of the cytokines C-reactive protein and IL-6 [274,275] which have been linked to increased complication rates in adult patients [276]. Moreover, invasive surgery in children has also been shown to depress the patients' immune system [274,277]. Neuromotor abnormalities 6 months following open heart surgery have been correlated with plasma levels of IL-6 that were measured immediately postoperatively [278]. These findings justify further investigations into the long-term effects of anesthetics on cytokine levels and their potential for improved outcome.

Hypoxia and hypoxia-ischemia

Due to the brain's limited ischemia tolerance, even relatively brief episodes of inadequate supply of oxygen or nutrients can lead to long-term neurological impairment in critically ill children, irrespective of anesthetic exposure. Several patient populations at increased risk for neurological sequelae, such as infants with congenital heart disease and premature neonates undergoing surgical procedures, have been studied regarding their long-term neurodevelopmental outcome. Many of these studies demonstrate neurobehavioral abnormalities, motor deficiencies, and decreased intelligence in many of these patients [191,205,279–281]. However, none of these studies describes the anesthetic and sedative regimens utilized or discusses their impact on subsequent neurological outcome. Conversely, neonatal animal models have repeatedly confirmed the protective properties of anesthetics when administered during episodes of brain hypoxia-ischemia [282–288]. These findings in immature animals suggest that critically ill human neonates might also benefit from these protective properties during clinical scenarios of neurological injury.

Co-morbidities and environmental factors

Even patients who do not suffer from life-threatening illnesses may have co-morbidities or be exposed to environmental factors outside the perioperative period that may act as confounders for neurodevelopmental outcome.

Chronic otitis media

Relatively subtle medical problems, such as chronic otitis media, have been implicated in causing neurological impairment. While this effect is controversial and the exact mechanism unresolved, some studies suggest impairment in language development, literacy, and school performance following chronic otitis media with persistent middle ear effusions before the age of 3 years, while others were unable to find this association [230,231,289–292]. A recent epidemiological review of anesthetic exposure in young children suggested a trend towards an association between serous otitis media prior to the age of 4 years and subsequent learning disabilities [229].

Chronic airway obstruction

In contrast to the contentious effects of chronic otitis media, the deleterious consequences of sleep-disordered breathing on neurocognition are well documented. Children with obstructive sleep apnea may face behavioral abnormalities, lower intelligence, and diminished academic performance, when compared to children with normal breathing patterns [293–295]. In these patients, surgical correction of the obstruction through adenotonsillectomy, which involves exposure to anesthetics, results in improved quality of life, behavior, and cognitive function [296]. Interestingly, even children with a pre-existing neurological condition, such as those with attention deficit hyperactivity disorder, demonstrated improved attention and decreased hyperactivity following surgical correction of mild sleep-disordered breathing, despite the obligatory exposure to surgery and anesthesia [297].

Environmental factors

Environmental factors and exposures outside the operating room can significantly interfere with normal brain development in humans. *In utero*, environmental compounds that may negatively influence subsequent neurocognition include such diverse substances as pesticides [298], methyl mercury, manganese, lead, and polychlorinated biphenyls [299]. Fetal exposure to prescription medications has also been found to lead to subsequent neurological sequelae, such as drugs for the treatment of acne [300], antihypertensives [301] and anticoagulants [302]. Prenatal exposure to alcohol and cocaine can impair children's speech, language, hearing, and cognitive development [303]. Intrauterine exposure to antiepileptic drugs, which share many pharmacodynamic properties with anesthetics, have been linked to brain structural abnormalities in young adults [304].

Other "environmental" factors known to affect learning and behavior in children are not as easily measured by subjective standards. Socio-economic aspects related to family dynamics, neighborhoods, and school environments all contribute to development and learning in children. In this context, factors negatively influencing neurodevelopment include economic deprivation, minority and/or immigrant status, exposure to violence, and chronic poverty [305]. Even when providing a strong community and positive family support, differences in school quality and negative encounters with teachers and/or peers can dramatically affect development and learning outcomes [305]. Moreover, negative influences on neurocognition have also been suggested by recreational activities, such as prolonged television viewing or video game play [306–308]. Due to this plethora of confounders, studies into the potential detrimental effects of anesthetic exposures need to take these socio-economic and environmental influences into account.

Genetic predisposition

Genetic composition can also affect neurodevelopment, even to a greater degree than environmental confounders. Close relationships have been demonstrated between genetic factors and cognitive abilities, including reading and mathematics skills, and intelligence [309]. Moreover, genetic predisposition can influence the effects of environmental stressors and vice versa [310].

Investigating the effects of anesthetic exposure on learning abilities in young children with an emphasis on genetic predisposition, a recent twin study found no causal relationship between anesthetic exposure and cognitive impairment [258]. A review of data from more than 1000 monozygotic twin pairs in The Netherlands Twin Registry demonstrated that, while children exposed to an anesthetic prior to age 3 years scored significantly lower on educational achievement tests and experienced more cognitive problems than children not exposed to anesthesia, cognitive performance of the unexposed co-twin did not differ from that of the exposed twin. These findings seem to suggest that the need for surgery with anesthesia may just represent a marker for subsequent learning abnormalities and not a causative factor leading to the impairment.

Potential alleviating strategies

While human applicability is not yet confirmed, as discussed above, numerous animal studies have suggested that all currently utilized general anesthetics as well as many analgesics may elicit a neurotoxic response in the immature brain, suggesting the judicious use of these compounds in young children. Conversely, though, inadequate alleviation of pain and distress may equally trigger neurodegenerative effects. Decreasing anesthetic doses by combinations of several deleterious anesthetics or concomitant administration of opioid analgesics may not obviate neurotoxicity, but rather exacerbate it, at least according to animal studies. Accordingly, a few animal studies have tested potentially alleviating strategies, ranging from concomitant administration of other anesthetics or sedatives, other drugs, to naturally occurring hormones. Moreover, whole-body hypothermia has also been proposed in the pursuit of reducing anesthesia-induced neurodegeneration.

Limited studies have found that the NMDA-antagonist xenon [62,63] and the α2-agonist dexmedetomidine [311] can reduce isoflurane-induced neuroapoptosis when administered concurrently. When administrated as a single drug, dexmedetomidine did not exhibit any neurotoxic effects in one study [311] whereas xenon demonstrated some neurotoxic properties in one study [63] but not in another [62]. One *in vitro* study has even suggested that pretreatment with isoflurane can protect from subsequent exposure to higher doses of the same drug [107]. Lithium has been found to alleviate neurodegeneration caused by propofol or ketamine in neonatal mice [72] whereas preliminary data may suggest that pilocarpine reduces neuroapoptosis triggered by the GABA-agonists midazolam or isoflurane [105] while it augments brain damage caused by the NMDA-antagonist phencyclidine [312]. Naturally occurring hormones, such as estradiol [67] and melatonin [68], have been successfully tested in newborn rats to reduce neuronal injury caused by the prolonged, combined administration of midazolam, isoflurane, and nitrous oxide. Head and co-workers have demonstrated that administration of tissue plasminogen activator, plasmin, or pharmacological inhibition of the neurotrophic receptor p75^{NTR} reduced neurotoxic effects of isoflurane in neonatal mice [113]. Most recently, it has been proposed that whole-body hypothermia to 24°C may reduce isoflurane-induced neuroapoptosis in neonatal mice [112,313].

While implementation of these proposed strategies during pediatric anesthesia appears premature, given the fact that human applicability of this phenomenon remains highly controversial, the safety of some of the proposed therapies has not been tested in young children. Estradiol may not be a feasible adjuvant prior to puberty or in boys, pilocarpine has demonstrated proconvulsant activity in some animals [314,315], lithium has been labeled as harmful for the human fetus [316] and may cause neurocognitive impairment in young children [317,318], and hypothermia of 24°C may only be feasible in procedures involving hypothermic cardiopulmonary bypass, but not during routine pediatric anesthesia or intensive care. While xenon's scarcity makes it a very expensive treatment, dexmedetomidine may be a valid option for light sedation or as an adjuvant for general anesthetics.

Ongoing and future research

Whereas animal studies seem to unequivocally demonstrate deleterious brain structural changes immediately following anesthetic exposure, long-term neurological abnormalities are not universally demonstrated. Moreover, human epidemiological studies examining developmental outcomes have returned ambiguous results. However, the potentially immense impact of neurotoxicity induced by anesthetics and sedatives on child health necessitates significant research efforts into this phenomenon. These efforts must include both preclinical studies investigating the exact structural changes, underlying molecular mechanisms, and the affected target cells, as well as carefully designed clinical studies delineating human susceptibility, while taking into full account the above-mentioned perioperative confounding variables. Given the public health impact of the potential neurotoxic effect of anesthetic drugs in pediatric patients, the United States Food and Drug Administration and the International Anesthesia Research Society created a public-private partnership called SmartTots (Strategies to Mitigate Anesthetic Related NeuroToxicity in Tots) to support clinical investigators in this area. (www.smarttots.org). This collaboration has provided funding for ongoing research studies (GAS and PANDA studies).

GAS study

This is an international, multi-site, randomized controlled trial, which compares the effects of regional and general anesthesia on neurodevelopmental outcome and apnea in infants in a projected cohort of 660 patients (Dr Andrew Davidson, personal communication, September 2009). The study, under the direction of Dr Andrew Davidson, includes pediatric hospitals in Australia, Canada, France, Italy, New Zealand, the United Kingdom, and the United States and proposes to assess patients' intelligence quotient 2 years following a neonatal inguinal hernia repair performed either with general anesthesia or with caudal or spinal anesthesia [319]. Dr Mary Ellen McCann directs the United States arm of the study and receives funding from the National Institutes of Health and the SAFEKIDS initiative. Advantages of the GAS study, which also enrolls premature neonates born as early as 26 weeks of gestation, include the prospective randomized approach, the use of contemporary anesthesia techniques, and the true separation of the effects of surgery and general anesthesia. The relatively brief exposure period, however, does not allow for the assessment of dose–response relationships. Moreover, neurobehavioral assessment cannot begin until at least 2 years into the study and definitive results may take even longer to collect [319].

PANDA study

A different approach of retrospective identification and prospective study of subjects has been taken in the Pediatric Anesthesia and NeuroDevelopmental Assessment (PANDA) study [1]. The PANDA study's aim is to assess the effects of anesthetic exposure for inguinal hernia repair within the first 3 years of life in a retrospectively identified cohort, excluding premature neonates, on prospectively measured neurodevelopmental outcome later in life. Neurodevelopment will be assessed with the NEPSY II (acronym for NEuroPSYchological Assessment, Pearson Education Inc., www.pearsonassessments.com) and the Wechsler Abbreviated Scale of Intelligence instruments and compared with an unexposed sibling control. The study, which is led by Dr Lena Sun at Columbia University, plans to enroll a total of 500 patients and 500 controls and includes several other major pediatric centers throughout the United States, such as in Boston, Chicago, Cincinnati, Iowa, Philadelphia, Pittsburgh, and Nashville. With the PANDA study's approach, neurobehavioral testing starts immediately after enrollment, socio-economic and genetic confounders are addressed using a sibling control, and anesthetic techniques are still within 10 years of current practice. However, due to the relatively brief surgical time, findings are limited to between 1 and 2 h of anesthetic exposure, which might still represent the length of the typical pediatric surgical procedure. However, the measured outcome is a function of both surgery and anesthesia.

Danish Registry

In an epidemiological approach, Hansen and co-workers are using a database of all 45,000 children who underwent surgical operations in Denmark from 1977 to 1990 before 1 year of age, comparing the academic achievement of exposed children with that of the general Danish population. The researchers are planning to achieve this goal by linking a nationwide demographic database with a national hospital discharge registry and compulsory school completion test scores. While this study is limited by the retrospective nature of an epidemiological approach and the relatively outdated anesthetic methods, the size of the cohort will help to control for many of the confounders discussed in this review [320].

Conclusion

In conclusion, neonatal exposure to numerous anesthetics causes widespread neurodegeneration in a dose- and duration-dependent fashion and can lead to long-term neurological impairment following administration of anesthetic combinations in newborn animals. However, the relevance of these findings to pediatric anesthesia is unknown. The phenomenon's exact underlying mechanism has not yet been determined, but does not seem to be entirely explained by anesthetic-induced neuronal inhibition. While animal studies reveal susceptibility to be limited to a very brief stage during brain development, the corresponding human maturational state has not been clearly defined; several lines of evidence point towards the prenatal or early postnatal period. Whereas anesthetic administration in animals differs significantly from pediatric anesthesia practice and numerous confounders exist in humans that do not occur in animal populations, emerging human epidemiological studies do not exclude anesthetics as a factor for impaired learning and neurodevelopment observed following surgical procedures. However, unlike the consistent neurodegeneration and neurological impairment demonstrated in anesthetized animals, neurological sequelae observed in retrospective epidemiological studies seem sporadic and do not affect all exposed individuals to the same degree, suggesting a potential genetic or other influence on this association. Since existing epidemiological studies are unable to establish causality and cannot distinguish between the differential effects of surgery and anesthesia on neurological outcome, further well-designed preclinical and clinical studies are needed to examine the phenomenon's mechanisms and its clinical relevance. Given the serious consequences of unopposed pain for the developing brain, current anesthetic practices should only be changed once results from these future studies become available.

- All currently used anesthetics have been found to be neurotoxic in neonatal animal studies.
- The phenomenon's clinical relevance is unknown.
- Animal and preliminary human studies suggest the maximum potential for susceptibility in humans to occur early in life, potentially prenatally.
- Pain and stress in unanesthetized, immature animals and humans have similarly been found to cause neuronal cell death and neurocognitive impairment.
- More studies into this phenomenon are needed before changes to current anesthetic and sedation practices can be recommended.

Annotated references

A full reference list for this chapter is available at:
http://www.wiley.com/go/gregory/andropoulos/pediatricanesthesia

2. Anand KJ, Hickey PR. Pain and its effects in the human neonate and fetus. N Engl J Med 1987; 317: 1321–9. The classic review article establishing the foundations of modern pain treatment in the neonate.

6. Anand KJ, Garg S, Rovnaghi CR et al. Ketamine reduces the cell death following inflammatory pain in newborn rat brain. Pediatr Res 2007; 62: 283–90. An important animal model study demonstrating that adequate treatment of pain with ketamine protects the developing brain.

33. Ikonomidou C, Bosch F, Miksa M et al. Blockade of NMDA receptors and apoptotic neurodegeneration in the developing brain. Science 1999; 283: 70–4. The first paper to demonstrate neuroapoptosis in the developing brain with ketamine.

39. Loepke AW, Soriano SG. An assessment of the effects of general anesthetics on developing brain structure and neurocognitive function. Anesth Analg 2008; 106: 1681–707. A thorough review of the problem of anesthetic neurotoxicity.

51. Slikker W Jr, Zou X, Hotchkiss CE et al. Ketamine-induced neuronal cell death in the perinatal rhesus monkey. Toxicol Sci 2007; 98: 145–58. An important demonstration of apoptosis in the subhuman primate; however, requiring very high and prolonged doses to produce this effect.

173. Clancy B, Finlay BL, Darlington RB et al. Extrapolating brain development from experimental species to humans. Neurotoxicology 2007; 28: 931–7. A novel neuroinformatics approach addressing the difference in animal species in brain development, and correlating chronological to developmental brain stages across species.

225. DiMaggio CJ, Sun LS, Kakavouli A et al. A retrospective cohort study of the association of anesthesia and hernia repair surgery with behavioral and developmental disorders in young children. J Neurosurg Anesthesiol 2009; 21: 286–91. A modern example of an epidemiological cohort study, retrospective in design, as one important approach to addressing the question.

229. Wilder RT, Flick RP, Sprung J et al. Early Exposure to anesthesia and learning disabilities in a population-based birth cohort. Anesthesiology 2009; 110: 796–804. An important retrospective cohort study establishing that multiple exposures to anesthesia may affect long-term school performance.

282. Loepke AW, Priestley MA, Schultz SE et al. Desflurane improves neurologic outcome after low-flow cardiopulmonary bypass in newborn pigs. Anesthesiology 2002; 97: 1521–7. One of the earliest papers to describe anesthetic neuroprotection against hypoxic-ischemic brain injury.

319. Davidson AJ, McCann ME, Morton NS et al. Anesthesia and outcome after neonatal surgery: the role for randomized trials. Anesthesiology 2008; 109: 941–4. An exposition of the crucial importance of actual human prospective randomized trials to answer the question of anesthetic neurotoxicity.

CHAPTER 42

Patient Simulation and Its Use in Pediatric Anesthesia

Anita Honkanen & Michael Chen

Department of Anesthesia, Stanford Hospital and Clinics, and Stanford University, Stanford, CA, USA

Introduction

Simulation has taken the medical world by storm but why has this type of approach to teaching, evaluation, and research become so popular in medicine? What does it have to offer us in improving the delivery of pediatric anesthesia care to our patients?

There are many types of simulation, requiring a wide range of facilities and equipment to perform, but all types can be neatly described as creation of an artificial environment that replicates a real-world situation to achieve a particular objective. In re-creating a critical event after the fact, the objective may be the ability to better understand factors that lead to the undesirable outcome. In developing a crisis scenario for an imaginary patient, it may be the training of a new resident in the management of the medical events portrayed. The set of possible goals is as infinite as the human imagination.

In today's world of shrinking budgets, limited hours for trainees, and dispersal of patients from the inpatient to the outpatient setting, the degree of exposure to a wide variety of patients and critical situations for our trainees in medicine has decreased steadily. The challenge, to ensure that our residents and students have the basic tools required to react appropriately to crisis situations or to diagnose rare illnesses, has increased. Private payers, the government, and the public are scrutinizing our medical system, demanding improved patient safety and a decrease in medical errors, and measuring the training and performance of our medical practitioners.

Using simulation, we can focus training hours for our residents and students to elicit the maximum exposure to the types of patients and events deemed critical for complete well-rounded training in any particular field. Skills required by the US Accreditation Council for Graduate Medical Education (ACGME) in communication, professionalism, patient care, and medical knowledge can be practiced and tested. Teams can be drilled on critical actions, helping to ensure that they will act together in appropriate ways when a real situation presents. And we can tease out problems in our care environments, changing processes, protocols, and equipment, prior to exposing our patients to imperfect systems.

Gregory's Pediatric Anesthesia, Fifth Edition. Edited by George A. Gregory, Dean B. Andropoulos.
© 2012 Blackwell Publishing Ltd. Published 2012 by Blackwell Publishing Ltd.

For all these reasons, it seems clear that simulation in medicine is here to stay. Putting it to good use will ultimately not only benefit our patients, but improve our own mastery of our field as well. This chapter will explore what simulation is, how and why it has grown in medicine, the many ways in which it is applied and finally, the applications and current state of simulation use in pediatric anesthesia.

History of simulation: development in aviation and beginnings in medicine and anesthesia

In order to remain competitive, increase safety, improve outcomes and become cost effective, the medical system has begun to borrow methods and techniques from successful business models. When dollars are at stake, approaches such as Toyota's "lean" manufacturing principles are used [1]. However, when looking to teach and train for-high risk, high-stakes activities, medicine has borrowed from fields with known extraordinary risks such as nuclear power, aviation, space exploration, and the military. These industries represent high-reliability organizations (HRO), institutions where positive results are consistently delivered with minimal error, despite the need for multiple individuals working together as a team in high-risk situations. Simulation exercises have been used in these areas both to train new practitioners and to expose experienced individuals to critical and rare events.

Development in aviation
Aviation in particular is often used as a metaphor for the practice of anesthesia. Both require a high degree of vigilance, attention to detail, and periods of relative inactivity interspersed with critical moments when the need to react quickly and effectively is mandatory to avoid poor outcomes. In both fields, lives are at risk if mistakes happen or if practitioners are unable to respond appropriately. Thus, it is helpful to understand the evolution of simulation in that field and to understand how those methods have been adapted to the anesthesia environment.

In aviation, simulation, in the form of mocked-up aircraft controls, was used as early as the manufacturing of the first aircraft, between 1920 and 1927. A more sophisticated, pneumatically driven flight simulator was invented by Edwin Link in 1929 [2]. Improvements have been made over time, and the modern, computer-assisted simulators include high-fidelity computer graphics to create the illusion of the real world outside the cockpit [3]. These simulators are routinely used for both training of new pilots and review of crisis situations for experienced pilots. In fact, it is clear that simulation is an expected part of aviation training in the public mind,

when it becomes the norm in cinematic representations. Futuristic flight simulation team training is dramatically depicted in the movie *Star Trek* (2009) [4], when trainee James Tiberius Kirk is subjected to the "Kobayashi Maru" test, a simulation exercise created by "professor" Spock, with the objectives of evaluating a cadet's performance and teaching how to deal with a failure in space.

Not all aviation simulation requires high-tech tools, however. In the military, dunker training, a simulated crash of an aircraft into water, is routinely used as a method both to train recruits in the appropriate reactions to survive such a crash and to weed out individuals that don't have what it takes to respond appropriately in such a situation. The movie *An Officer and a Gentleman* [5] includes a memorable scene with this training for Navy flight cadets, where one of the main characters fails the test. Army flight surgeon training includes a day of simulated water exercises, with long bouts in a pool in full flight gear, jumps from high boards into water, and escape from a simulated "downed helicopter" which flips underwater (personal experience, 1988, Army Aviation Medicine Course, Ft. Rucker, Alabama).

Team training in aviation began in earnest after a series of crashes in the 1970s that were clearly not related to technical or equipment failures. One of the most famous was the Tenerife Airport disaster that occurred in 1977, involving two jet airliners that crashed on the runway at take-off, killing 583 people in all. Review of the crashes clearly demonstrated multiple failures, including problems with communication and team work [6]. Crew resource management (CRM) training, teaching crews to work together through a crisis in a simulated environment, was developed as a method to reduce the system and communication errors inherent in these complex environments [7].

Beginnings in medicine and anesthesia
Just as in aviation, simulation in medicine started with simple task trainers and moved to complex high-fidelity simulation environments. Patient simulation was first explored in medicine by Asmund S. Laerdal, with Peter Safar and Bjorn Lind, who created a mannequin, Resusci Anne, for the training of mouth-to-mouth resuscitation [8]. She was introduced as the first patient simulator in 1960; her face was based on the death mask of a young girl pulled from the River Seine at the turn of the century [9]. These first simulation systems were simple and generally task oriented, looking to teach individuals medical skills. High-fidelity patient simulation with the replication of a real-world environment, using interactive mannequins, was introduced to anesthesia in the 1960s and 1970s with the Sim One Anesthesiological Simulator by Abrahamson and Denson [10]. David Gaba created the Virtual Anesthesiology Training Simulation System at the

Veterans Affairs Hospital in Palo Alto, California, in 1986 as the first center-based high-fidelity anesthesia simulator environment, allowing a full range of individual and team training, and research into the uses of simulation and the assessment of human performance [11].

In aviation, it took a series of disasters to stimulate the use of simulation and the birth of crew resource management training. In medicine, the widespread use of simulation was stimulated after a pivotal report from the Institutes of Medicine was released in 2000 that shocked the medical world. It publically exposed the high degree of medical error that routinely occurs, stating that between 44,000 and 98,000 patients die in US hospitals due to avoidable medical error each year. The report went on to recommend team training based on both aviation's crew resource management programs and simulation-based education and training in medicine, as a means to create a safer healthcare environment [12]. The widespread acceptance of these techniques and perceived utility in developing and maintaining critical skills are exemplified by the approach taken by Harvard's malpractice insurance carrier: in order to maintain a favorable insurance rate for the anesthesia department, all faculty participate in a simulation event on an annual basis [13]. This approach has since been taken by other malpractice carriers.

Uses of simulation

As the need for simulation in medicine has grown, its use has moved from specialized simulation centers into actual patient care areas, such as hospitals and clinics. It has also progressed from a focus on single medical specialties to involving all levels of healthcare professionals and disciplines, often working together. In the following section, the application of simulation to education, research, team training, professional evaluation, continuing medical education (CME), and systems evaluation will be reviewed.

Education

Medical schools are now using simulation as a regular part of their curricula, responding in part to the ethical dilemma of allowing novice students to learn techniques for the first time on real patients. From part-task trainers, which allow students to place intravenous catheter or sutures, to standardized patient actors who teach students how to approach a patient, communicate, and perform a physical exam, simulation has become an integral part of medical student education. Five factors have been cited by Issenberg and Gaba as contributing to the increased use of simulation in medical school curricula: "a. problems with clinical teaching, b. new technologies

for diagnosis and management, c. assessing professional competence, d. medical errors, patient safety and team training, and e. the role of deliberate practice"[14].

This trend toward simulation-based training has not been restricted to medical students. The continued shrinking of residency training hours is a worldwide trend [15]. In the US, it is limited by the ACGME to 80 hours per week, with strict rules about rest time between shifts [16,17]. While this may appear to be enough time to expose residents to the many cases required, the restrictions have been felt across all medical disciplines and reflected in residency programs looking for ways in which to accelerate learning apart from the usual "apprenticeship" model currently practiced [18–23]. More and more, simulation is being used to fill the gap.

In anesthesia training, these tools have been used for many years. The operating room represents a unique environment in medicine, full of complicated technology requiring facility in use for rapid responses when changes in patient status occur. Most medical students have very minimal exposure to this environment prior to residency training. Thus, there is a strong impetus for simulation's use in anesthesia education for development of trainees' skills, both in basic understanding of the equipment and in responding to critical events [23,24].

At Stanford, like many other programs, training for anesthesia residents includes regular simulation training with an increase in the difficulty of scenarios presented at each level of training. Trainees may spend a day in the simulation center, running through a series of simulation crisis scenarios and debriefing sessions, examining their own performance and that of their peers in a formative review [25]. *In situ* training, with short focused simulation events, is also becoming more common (Fig. 42.1).

Attempting to understand human performance factors, which are critical to achieving positive outcomes in crisis

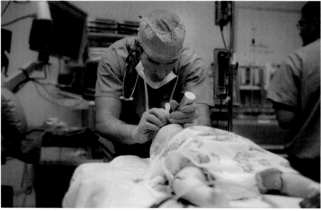

Figure 42.1 Anesthesia trainee intubating a Sim Baby mannequin during an *in situ* simulation scenario in the operating suite.

situations, has been a widely appreciated practice since it became a focus in evaluating a series of severe accidents in the aviation industry in the 1970s. These human performance factors have been heavily studied and described [26]. Recognizing their importance to a wide variety of situations in medicine, many of the factors are also listed as required competencies for all medical residents by the ACGME [27]. Gaba et al have also described a set of skills that correlate with successful performance during a simulated anesthesia crisis (anesthesia crisis resource management – ACRM) [28]. Many of these human performance skills, described as non-technical skills by Flin et al in *Safety at the Sharp End: A Guide to Non-Technical Skills*, are also noted as essential in team work during crisis for multiple industries [6]. The concurrency in the description of these skills is evident in listing of some of the factors from these three systems – ACGME, ACRM, non-technical team skills – in Table 42.1. They all have as key components aspects of human behavior and communication which are important in working together well in complex situations.

Simulation courses, such as the ACRM course based on aviation's CRM principles, are geared to help teach these critical human performance factors (see below) [14,29,30]. Simulation, with debriefing focused on these non-technical skills, can help improve overall competency while raising the awareness of the importance of team-work skills [31].

Most anesthesia residents may spend very little time in pediatric anesthesia training: often just 2–4 months during their 3 years of residency. The approach to patients and families, the method of preoperative sedation and preparation, the induction techniques, and the types of crisis that occur in pediatrics are very different from those in adult anesthesia. This limited clinical time, with an extensive behavioral knowledge set required, creates an ideal situation for the application of simulation training to enhance the rapid acquisition of this specialized skill set.

The reasons why simulation works as an effective means of education have been studied, with some inconsistent results. Issenberg et al searched the literature to extract the key factors of simulation noted to be associated with effective learning [14], listed in Table 42.2. The most common element seen in 47% of the journal articles they reviewed was "providing feedback." During high-fidelity patient simulation (HFPS), this is usually done during a debriefing session that follows the simulated scenario. Effective debriefing allows for a carefully guided introspective review of the scenario, how the event unfolded, and the outcomes, with input from all participants. Other common factors include "repetitive practice," cited in 39% of journal articles, and "curriculum integration" in 25%. These two factors require a standard design to scenario development, which allows for repetition and inclusion in standard curriculum, for standard

objectives and goals. Templates have been designed to facilitate standardization of scenario development and consistency in repeated use of single scenarios [32] (see below).

Performance of these types of dynamic interactive and interpersonal human performance skills is difficult to observe and evaluate in the normal testing situation. Simulation provides a venue to demonstrate or practice these skills, allowing feedback on effectiveness of leadership, communication, or decision-making abilities [33,34]. Use of simulation for evaluation of trainee performance has long been an area of considerable interest [35]. While it has been difficult to convincingly link performance measurements in simulation environments to real clinical situations, tools are beginning to be developed that demonstrate improved reliability and validity [36,37].

Finally, another factor driving the increased use of simulation in medical education is the perceived effectiveness of the learning method itself. By using high-fidelity patient simulation, the learner becomes immersed in the educational domain, participating actively in the learning environment rather than passively absorbing information. This type of performance learning has been shown to be more effective for adult learners, and information is retained at a higher rate than information imparted in passive learning sessions [38–41]. The evocation of emotional responses improves the learning process and increases retention as well [41]. Simulation provides just such a learning environment.

Research

Simulation's applicability to research is beginning to be fully realized. From answering basic questions in human performance to teasing out ways to improve protocols, procedures, and equipment, simulation can be used to answer multiple questions in practice sessions prior to the real event.

Research in human factors and performance is facilitated with the use of simulation. This has been a particularly fruitful area of investigation, because of the ability to recreate relatively uniform circumstances for testing with more than one practitioner group [42]. Theoretically, questions regarding practice performance can be answered, which otherwise might demand an approach using retroactive reviews of multiple charts, thereby including many uncontrolled assumptions. Investigations have been conducted into human interactions with the environment, fatigue, and response to the stressors inherent in caring for patients during a crisis [43–45]. Looking at the effectiveness of crew co-ordination and the ability to perform to task would be difficult or impossible without the use of a high-fidelity simulated environment in which to create a crisis scenario and elicit a team response [46].

Table 42.1 Comparison of non-technical and team skill characteristics from three systems: non-technical team skills as described by Flin et al [6], ACRM performance goals, and ACGME trainees' performance criteria (*includes only the subset of ACRM and ACGME areas for which there was some correlation with the other system behaviors noted)

Non-technical skills	Behaviors	ACRM key points	Behaviors	ACGME competency areas*	Interpretation: demonstrated behaviors for anesthesia residents at Stanford University
Situation awareness	• Gathering information • Interpreting information • Anticipating future states	Maintain situational awareness	• Anticipate and plan • Maintain vigilance • Know the environment • Assign team member to monitor patient if involved in task	Systems-based practice Patient care	• Acts to deliver anesthesia services efficiently • Able to call on system resources/providers to improve care • Gathers adequate preoperative information and recommends appropriate diagnostic steps/consults if preparation is inadequate
Communi-cation	• Sending information clearly and concisely • Including context and intent during information exchange • Receiving information, especially by listening • Identifying and addressing barriers to communication	Communicate effectively	• Clearly state requests and commands • Avoid statements into "thin air" • Close communication loop • Foster open exchange between team members • Deal with conflict: what is right for patient, not who is right	Interpersonal & communication skills	• Listens effectively, allows patients/families to ask questions • Leader in the healthcare team • Explains procedures and anesthesia plans appropriately for consent • Creates sound relationship with patient
Teamwork Leadership	• Supporting others • Solving conflicts • Exchanging information • Co-ordinating activities • Using authority • Maintaining standards • Planning and prioritizing • Managing workload and resources	Take an appropriate leadership role	• Ensure the team knows who is in charge • Prioritize and assign tasks • Make decisions • Elicit participation • Be assertive while respectful	Professionalism	• Takes responsibility and is appropriately self-confident • Respectful, courteous and compassionate • Adheres to professional ethics and respects patient privacy
Decision making	• Defining problem • Considering options • Selecting and implementing option • Outcome review	Utilize all available resources	• All team members • Equipment • Cognitive aids • External resources: call for help	Patient care	• Carries out safe and rational anesthetic after proper selection of drugs/ techniques and responds appropriately to changes in anesthetic course
Managing stress Coping with fatigue	• Identifying symptoms of stress • Recognizing effects of stress • Implementing coping strategies • Identifying symptoms of fatigue • Recognizing effects of fatigue • Implementing coping strategies	Distribute the workload	• Assign tasks appropriately to skill of individual • Delegate manual tasks unless particular skills required • Scan for overload or fatigue of team members	Patient care	• Possesses appropriate technical skills in airway management (mask, ETT, LMA, FOB) and vascular access (IV, CVP/PA, arterial line)

ACRM, anesthesia crisis resource management; ACGME, Accreditation Council for Graduate Medical Education; CVP, central venous pressure; ETT, endotracheal tube; FOB, fiber-optic bronchoscope; IV, intravenous line; LMA, laryngeal mask airway; PA, pulmonary artery catheter.

Table 42.2 Factors noted by Issenberg et al [14] to be associated with effective learning

Factor	No. of citations	% of journals	Description
Providing feedback	51	47%	Educational feedback
Repetitive practice	43	39%	Repeated practice of behavior
Curriculum integration	27	25%	Integration of simulation-based exercises into the standard medical school or postgraduate educational curriculum
Range of difficulty	15	14%	Range of task difficulty level
Multiple learning strategies	11	10%	Adaptability of high-fidelity simulations to multiple learning strategies
Capture clinical variation	11	10%	Capture a wide variety of clinical conditions
Controlled environment	10	9%	Controlled environment where learners can make, detect, and correct errors without adverse consequences
Individual learning	10	9%	Reproducible, standardized, educational experiences where learners are active participants, not passive bystanders
Defined outcomes	7	6%	Clearly stated goals with tangible outcome measures, appropriate to level of training
Simulator validity	4	3%	Degree of realism

Finally, not only has HFPS facilitated obtaining answers to many primary research questions, it has also been used by researchers to improve the effectiveness of their clinical trials. Problems in protocol design, procedures, and data collection tools can be exposed prior to the beginning of the trial, saving time and decreasing costs. Also using simulation to train evaluators and co-ordinators can help to decrease errors at the start of the trial, ensuring better compliance with trial rules [47,48].

Team training: review of Anesthesia Crisis Resource Management principles

Anesthesia crisis resource management (ACRM) refers to a system of appropriate team and individual responses to a crisis in a patient under anesthesia. This system is based on principles and techniques derived from aviation: crew resource management. Training in these techniques teaches crews to work together through a crisis in a simulated environment, and was developed as a method to reduce the system and communication errors inherent in the complex aviation environment [7,49–51]. The primary goal of crisis management is to detect problems early in their evolution, then mobilize an appropriate response in order to prevent an adverse outcome.

Many of the keys to ACRM revolve around maintenance of situation awareness and effective dynamic decision making. Leadership ability and communication among team members are essential, as is the effective use of all available resources. Figure 42.2, an example of a

Crisis Resource Management Key Points

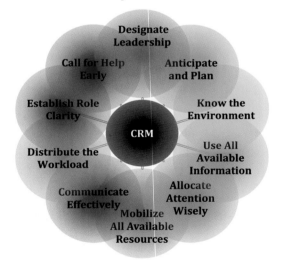

Figure 42.2 Cognitive aid developed to assist in recall of performance goals using the ACRM framework, by David Gaba, Steven Howard, and Sara Goldhaber-Fiebert (Stanford University School of Medicine and VA Palo Alto Health Care System).

cognitive aid, includes the behaviors that are associated with an improved team response to crisis as taught in ACRM [28].

One of the mechanisms that helps create an effective team is the concept of the "shared mental model"; that is, the mutually agreed upon set of knowledge and processes used to explain or predict events to achieve certain goals safely and effectively [52,53]. While team training began in the military in the 1950s, training based on the "shared mental model" concept was first instituted in the 1990s [29]. Crew resource management, used in aviation for many years, works with shared mental models, using a variety of training methods, including simulation, to teach appropriate team skills. These teamwork functions are fleshed out from work focused on the macrocognitive skill sets required to achieve effective team management of complex tasks [54]. Included are leadership and communication skills such as those outlined in Table 42.1, and others such as adaptability, back-up behavior, mutual trust, and team orientation. Simulation is an effective tool to create a situation in which these skills can be teased out and practiced [50].

Professional evaluation

The ability to grade performance in medicine has long been fraught with difficulty. Testing paradigms which focus on the ability to regurgitate medical knowledge in board examinations ignore the multiple skill sets known to affect performance in real patient care situations, including communication and professional skills, and ability to work in an acute crisis situation within a team structure. Across healthcare disciplines, simulation has been adopted for training and assessment, because of its ability to demonstrate these critical skill sets [55]. Both standardized patients and mannequin-based simulation have been used for summative assessment, and in some cases, are required to obtain certification and licensure [56,57].

Various simulation modalities, from part task trainers and mannequins to computer-based case management scenarios, have been adopted for professional assessment in anesthesiology. Using simulation, particular situations can be recreated for testing for competence. For limited situations, experts come together to develop checklists, which can be tested for reliability and validity, permitting "credentialing" for that particular situation [36,58–60]. Broadening evaluation in order to comment on a practitioner's ability to practice is fraught with difficulty because of the lack of a widely accepted assessment tool [61]. Despite the challenges, this model is already in place in some countries, and is being used to allow professional accreditation, such as passing of board exams [62]. Testing systems are being investigated and developed for residency training in several fields, including anesthesia [63].

While not being used for evaluation, the American Board of Anesthesia (ABA) has recently added simulation exposure as part of the core CME requirements in the Maintenance of Certification in Anesthesiology (MOCA) system for recertification of anesthesia boards in the US [64]. Understanding the value of exposure to teamwork skills and crisis management is a prime driver for including simulation in CME for anesthesiologists [57].

Continuing medical education

Exceptional performance and expertise have been shown to be linked both to practice and to repeated exposure to activities with strong teachers who give formative real-time feedback [65,66]. The American Society of Anesthesiologists (ASA) has taken a proactive approach to CME, encouraging both the retention of skills and the acquisition of new expertise in practicing anesthesiologists by the introduction of simulation training in CME requirements for recertification [64]. Simulation offers the opportunity to practice the responses required to any given situation again and again, enabling practice performance assessment and improvement by participants [57,67].

Systems evaluation

Simulation methods have been used to evaluate the effectiveness of hospital systems, allowing targeting of system fixes if needed. Team responses to disasters in which multiple patients arrive in the emergency department [68] have been evaluated, as has the ability to respond in a timely and appropriate way to hospital emergency codes [69]. The ability to respond to crisis in the use of extracorporeal membrane oxygenation (ECMO) for neonates has been practiced [70]. Simulation has also been used to review new spaces prior to them being used for patient care, ensuring adequate equipment, space, and familiarization of staff with the environment [71]. Prior to opening the new operating rooms at Lucile Packard Children's Hospital at Stanford University, simulations of the complex information technology systems created to assist with scheduling of surgical cases and recording of surgical care in nursing and anesthesia documentation, and of the ability to perform the anticipated surgical cases, were completed prior to using the new OR suite. All surgical services were used in a simulation session in which a test case was scheduled, all team members required were present, and all equipment and supplies were reviewed and obtained to ensure that no significant gaps remained prior to receiving the first patient. Issues revealed included critical equipment that was discovered to be missing, process and policy problems that interfered with effective communications, and poor patient flow. Identified problems were then addressed proactively, eliminating their possible impact on actual patients (Fig. 42.3).

Types of simulation

Part task trainers

Performance of procedures requires technical skills that rely on mechanical facility. An understanding of the basic mechanical steps can be acquired with the use of part task trainers, pieces of the whole picture that represent some part of a patient or physical reality. For instance, a mock arm, with tubing representing vessels, can be used to practice the steps required for starting an IV. A manne-

quin head, with tongue, pharynx, glottis, larynx, and trachea, can be used to practice mask ventilation and intubation. These trainers can be as simple as a block of gelatin encompassing a target for practice using ultrasound-guided regional blocks to sophisticated computer-driven, sensor-laden systems for practice of laparoscopic surgical manipulations [72,73]. Complex haptic devices are being developed that meld computer-based virtual simulation and hands-on control [74,75].

Just as adult simulation high-tech mannequins have "evolved" to smaller pediatric models, part task trainers are now being created to simulate pediatric patients. Limbs for vascular access, intubate-able neonatal heads, and ultrasound-guided central vascular access trainers are just some of the items that are available. Figure 42.4 represents some of the current pediatric task trainers being marketed. As interest in these systems has grown, the variety and scale of available models have increased greatly.

Computer-based simulation systems

Sophisticated computer programs have been written to enable practice of various anesthesia tasks and medical crisis scenarios in a virtual format. These types of systems have the advantage of being available at any time to allow learners the chance to practice whenever they have the time [76–78]. Using the input of large amounts of data, from systems such as magnetic resonance images (MRI),

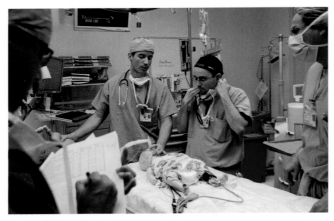

Figure 42.3 *In situ* simulation in the Lucile Packard operating room, team training for improved response time to critical events.

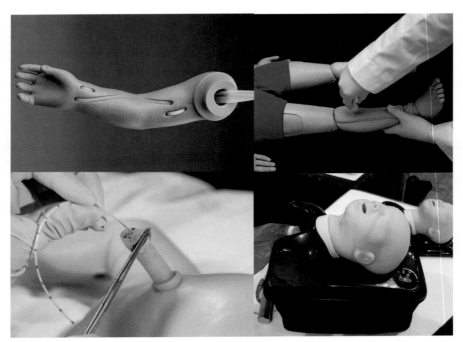

Figure 42.4 Part task/technical trainers. Clockwise from upper left corner: arm for IV starts (Gaumard Scientific), intraosseous needle placement (Gaumard Scientific), infant head for intubation and mask ventilation, umbilical catheter placement (Laerdal Medical).

models of human anatomy, based on various patients' idiosyncrasies, can finally be realized and used to present learners with the type of variety that they will see in practice [79,80]. Some internet-based systems, based on avatars, facilitate multiple users coming together in a virtual world to act as team members in various clinical scenarios. This keeps facility and material costs down, but relies on scheduling participants appropriately, having multiple access ports available, and a teacher/facilitator to guide the action [81].

Other systems allow for a melding of simulated transparency of functions in real time, enabling a deeper understanding of both mechanical anesthesia systems and simulated patient physiology [82]. Taking virtual systems and task trainers and combining them with a full-scale simulator allows for another twist on increasing the perceived reality of the scenario depicted [83,84].

As pediatric-based systems have yet to be developed and are likely to be difficult to pull together as basic vital signs and responses are so varied in pediatrics based on age and physical status, this area will not be discussed further in this chapter.

High-fidelity patient simulation

High-fidelity patient simulation (HFPS) refers to simulation scenarios that closely replicate real patients, making it easier for participants to believe in the reality of the situation depicted and thus to apply realistic responses. In any high-fidelity simulation, a learning or evaluative goal is selected, and a scenario is developed to create the opportunity for the goal to be achieved. Using a simulated environment and tools such as high-tech mannequins that both simulate a patient's responses to interventions and allow varying degrees of interaction with the participants, the scenario is played out. Expert facilitators in various roles encourage the participants to react to the cues supplied for the scenario and supply real-time feedback supporting the scenario as it unfolds.

High-tech mannequins

High-tech mannequins have been developed by several companies for use in simulation. These mannequins are made to represent patients of varying ages, from neonates to adults, and come equipped with mechanical and electrical parts to produce various effects from coughing and wheezing to hypotension and cyanosis. Heart tones, chest wall motion, palpable pulses, and closure of the airway can all be mimicked. Interventions are possible including bag-mask ventilation, tracheal intubation, IV placement, defibrillation, and in some cases chest tube insertion or cricothyrotomy. A vital signs monitor shows the patient's current status and can be manipulated by a technician in response to interventions by the simulation participants (Fig. 42.5).

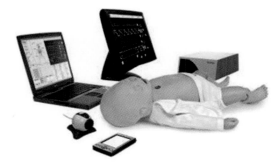

Figure 42.5 Elements of infant simulation mannequin by Laerdal Medical: mannequin with electrical and mechanical elements, control computer, monitor, remote control device, video camera, and relay box.

Some simulation systems include software which provides automatic realistic responses to interventions, including chest compressions, ventilation, and administered drugs. Table 42.3 provides a review of the features currently available in the more popular pediatric mannequins. Many of the mannequins have common features, which allow for basic interactions to control the airway and respirations. Some mannequins provide the ability to perform a variety of invasive interventions. The "consumable" parts, skin and bone, often need to be replaced after a certain number of uses. Setting some rules of engagement with the mannequins before beginning the simulation can allow for near realistic performance while saving the limited and costly resources of the mannequin parts.

Standardized patient actors

When communication skills were made one of the core competencies for ACGME, the central importance of clear and effective communication in medicine was emphasized. Team communication is very important and can be practiced during simulated scenarios involving mannequins, but effective communication with a patient or family member cannot be simulated well with these tools. Thus, standardized patient actors are frequently used in many simulated situations in both medical schools and other educational venues [85].

Using patient actors allows learners to interact with a "patient" or "family member" capable of evoking convincing emotions by improvising and adjusting their response based on the learner's input. This type of high-fidelity simulation can also create complex and subtle interactions, with the ability to practice the most basic features of medicine: effective history taking or developing a caring and empathetic approach. Videotaping of the interactions for review during debriefing also helps the learner to see how they come across and the non-verbal communication cues they may be using unknowingly (Fig. 42.6). This type of simulation has now been

Table 42.3 Comparison of some of the features offered in mannequins created to mimic various pediatric patients, from premature infants to 6 year olds

Product name	Laerdal SimBaby	Laerdal SimNewB	METI PediaSIM	METI BabySIM	Gaumard Pedi HAL	Gaumard Newborn HAL	Gaumard Premie HAL
Age	1-2 y	Neonate	6–7 y	3–6 mo	1 & 5 yr	Neonate	Premie
Model or instructor driven	Inst	Inst	Model	Model	Both	Both	Both
Airway & breathing							
Variable lung compliance	✓	✓	✓	✓	–	–	–
Tongue edema	✓	–	✓	✓	✓	–	–
Laryngospasm	✓	–	✓	✓	–	–	–
Needle cricothyrotomy	–	–	✓	–	–	–	–
See-saw respirations	✓	–	–	✓	–	–	–
Cyanosis	✓	✓	–	–	✓	✓	✓
Real CO_2 gas exhalation	✓	✓	✓	✓	–	–	–
Chest tube placement	✓	Thoracocentesis	✓	✓	–	–	–
Circulation							
Variable pulse with BP	✓	✓	✓	✓	✓	✓	✓
Palpable umbilical pulse	–	✓	–	–	–	✓	✓
Defibrillation/cardioversion	✓	–	✓	✓	✓	–	–
Pacing	✓	–	✓	✓	✓	–	–
Vascular access							
Umbilical vessel cannulation	–	✓	–	–	–	✓	✓
Intraosseous, tibial	✓	✓	✓	–	✓	✓	–
Intramuscular	–	–	–	–	✓	–	–
Sounds							
Coughing	✓	✓	–	✓	–	–	–
Stridor	✓	–	–	✓	✓	✓	✓
Speech library	✓	✓	✓	✓	✓	–	–
Bowel	–	–	✓	✓	✓	✓	–
General							
Palpable fontanelle	✓	–	–	✓	–	✓	✓
Eye, mouth, nasal secretions	–	Meconium	✓	✓	–	–	–
Reactive pupil or eyelids	–	–	✓	–	✓	–	–
Tetherless	–	–	–	–	✓	✓	✓
Wireless control	Limited	Limited	✓	–	Full	Full	Full
Limbs movement/seizure	–	✓	–	–	✓	✓	–

This table does not represent all the features that these simulators offer. Some features which were common to all the simulators were not included. All these high-fidelity models allow the users to place airway management devices, attach standard ASA monitors, and perform advanced life support interventions. In addition, all models have a vitals signs monitor that can produce a complete gamut of physiological states and a user input device that triggers the simulator to generate various heart sounds, breath sounds, and vocalizations. Some METI and Laerdal models offer a wider variety of advanced airway emergencies such as laryngospasm and airway edema, whereas the Gaumard models have the distinct advantage of being completely tetherless (i.e. not needing to be attached to compressed air source).

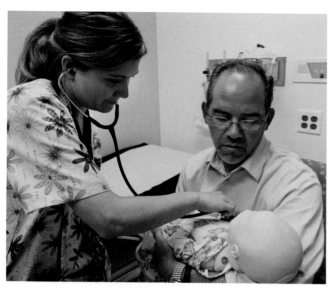

Figure 42.6 Depiction of actor as parent coupled with simulation mannequin in training exercise.

incorporated into Step 2 of the US Medical Licensing Examinations for medical students. Students must effectively interact with trained patient actors to obtain a history and physical, thereby demonstrating not only the technical medical knowledge but also the effective communication and interactive skills critical to becoming a physician [85,86].

Hybrid simulation

Hybrid simulations refer to the combination of any two types of simulation, whether the use of a part task trainer combined with a mannequin, or a patient actor and a simulated body part that can be manipulated by the participant to treat the simulated situation. For instance, a part task trainer arm can be attached to a patient actor's arm and used to start an IV, or a delivery task trainer can be combined with a patient actor for simulated infant delivery. The patient actor can then provide active and realistic responses to the participant as they attempt to provide the indicated care. This combination of task training and communication with the "patient," such as suturing of a wound or injection of a local anesthetic, creates a much more instructive and meaningful situation for the learner and allows a substantially greater understanding by an evaluator of the participant's skill set and patient management style. The tasks that are performed on patients never happen in a vacuum. Learning to deal with the patient's reactions to the procedures we perform is critical for effective patient care. This hybrid model allows the integration of these components for a much more realistic and effective training scenario.

Organization and running of high-fidelity simulation sessions

Elements of high-fidelity patient simulation
The introduction

Prior to starting a simulation scenario, the participants should be familiarized with the simulation environment, the tools to be used, and the roles they will play, elements critical in enabling a positive learning experience. Just as important is ensuring that all learners understand the goals of the exercise and how their performance will be assessed. Some essential points to cover include goals of the session, who will be participating, who will be facilitating, and how to engage and behave in the environment.

When the simulation scenario is focused on formative rather than summative assessment, removing any sense of threat from the session will help ensure a positive learning frame of mind. Many simulation centers ask the participants to sign a consent that emphasizes the importance of keeping the elements of the session, both the scenario and the performance of individuals, confidential. This can help decrease the concern that an "inadequate" performance will be talked about after the event. In these types of learning sessions, participants are told that there is no penalty for "failing" in a crisis simulation, allowing them to take risks in their interactions and actions during the scenario that will enable their learning.

The scenario

A scenario is created, somewhat like a storyboard for a movie, which sets the framework for the simulation session. It is based on both the goals and the anticipated participants. Content experts are critical in designing a realistic scenario, as an understanding of patient responses in various clinical situations is key to playing out any scenario. No matter what framework is set for the situation, the particular participants during the session will bring their own experience and knowledge base to the interpretation of the scenario, and will often react in unexpected ways. Thus, content experts are key during the running of the scenario as well, allowing credible manipulation of patient vital signs and reactions to any actions by the participants.

Debriefing

Arguably, the greatest learning from a simulation session occurs during the final section, called the debriefing. Debriefing has its roots in the military and aviation, where a group leader brings the unit together after an

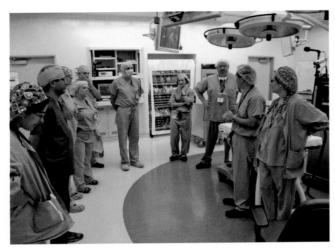

Figure 42.7 *In situ* team debrief after simulation in the Lucile Packard Children's Hospital operating room, aimed at improving response time and management effectiveness for patient crisis at induction.

Box 42.1 Factors that can facilitate or detract from the effectiveness of the debriefing portion of a simulation session

Thing to do	Things to avoid
Set expectations for crew participation	Don't lecture
Engage the team to facilitate achieving those expectations	Don't provide your own analysis before it is "discovered" by team's analysis
Cover all critical topics	Don't give impression that your observations are the most important
Balance the discussion: draw in quiet participants	Limit interruptions of team discussion
Cover teaching points to be made – integrate into discussion at appropriate times	Don't create the sense of an interrogation
Discuss positive actions and how they affected outcome	Avoid a rigid agenda
Consider using visual cues to track major discussion points	Don't cut sessions short when outcomes are positive

event or mission to review outcomes, both positive and negative, and to develop some lessons learned to apply to the next mission. Similarly, in medical simulations, this part of the session allows the team to discuss what occurred during the scenario and develop an understanding of how the crisis or situation unfolded (Fig. 42.7).

The goals of a debriefing session may vary but in ACRM, the technique is used to allow members of the team a chance to review their own performance, to evaluate the team's performance, to understand the drivers in the crisis, and to learn some general principles of crisis management that they may then use more effectively during future critical events [34,41].

Facilitated debriefing is the key to reaching learning goals from a simulation scenario. During a critical event, attention is intensely focused on managing the crisis and completing necessary tasks. It is only in the later analysis that an understanding of all the factors affecting the outcome can be gained. This then leads to learning from the event, its management, and any failures that occurred. A facilitator is important in guiding the debriefing and framing the learning points [41].

Ideally, the facilitator encourages reflective analysis, leading the participants in the crisis through the event, eliciting their own reactions and thus assisting them in developing their own analyses. Material covered in a group discussion is much more likely to be retained than that passively obtained in a lecture type presentation. In addition, when participants provide their own insights and observations, they feel that their input has been heard and then have more of a stake in the discussion and a sense that their ideas become part of the conclusion. These conclusions then become more acceptable and believable to the participants.

Facilitating a debriefing well takes time and practice. Box 42.1 includes actions that help create a positive learning session and several that can hinder the ability of the group to develop their own conclusions.

Debriefing sessions are most effective when the team members are able to guide their own discussion based on observations of their own, using the facilitator to initiate the discussion by setting the objectives and assist in leading the discussion minimally. Teams that have not previously participated in this type of analysis or group discussion will require much more guidance from the facilitator.

Starting the debriefing session with an introduction that outlines the expectations for the session and the ways in which the team members will participate allows creation of the proper framework for the learning session. Setting a format will then help the team develop an agenda for the session. The facilitator should be sure that all critical items are included in the agenda. Using the basic principles of ACRM to frame the analysis and evaluation can help deflect difficult feelings related to any perceptions of individual inadequate performance among participants. Finally, the lessons learned from the session should be explicitly reviewed and generalized if possible.

Some techniques that encourage active team member participation and in-depth analysis of events include the following.

- Ask questions: what, why, and how?
- Engage all team members in the discussion.
- Reword questions instead of answering – allow the team to answer the questions.
- Allow pauses and silence to encourage thoughtful analysis and time for answers.

In summary, debriefing creates the opportunity for members of a team involved in a crisis situation to reflect on their performance, review the elements that were active during the crisis, analyze how these factors affected the outcome, and develop some lessons to be carried away and used in future situations. In addition, basic concepts useful in approaching any crisis can be emphasized during the debriefing, allowing a review of important skills that can then enhance participants' performance in a wider set of circumstances.

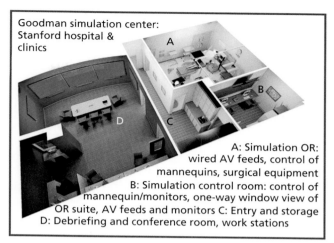

Goodman simulation center: Stanford hospital & clinics

A: Simulation OR: wired AV feeds, control of mannequins, surgical equipment
B: Simulation control room: control of mannequin/monitors, one-way window view of OR suite, AV feeds and monitors C: Entry and storage
D: Debriefing and conference room, work stations

Figure 42.8 Three-dimensional rendering of the simulation center at Stanford Hospital and Clinics.

Creating scenarios

The first step in creating a scenario is defining the participants who will be taking part in the scenario and the learning goals to be set. The resources available to run the simulation must also be considered, from location of the simulation to equipment, staffing, and facilitators. The particular clinical situation can then be set. A simple storyline for the scenario, identifying roles to be played by both participants and facilitators/confederates, an outline of the basic clinical situation, the crisis to be dealt with, and the key patient characteristics that will orient the participants to the situation at hand are all key elements to include. It is helpful to try and anticipate the types of reactions from the participants and map out the likely patient responses, vital signs changes, and other changes to those actions. A map is thus created that helps the technician running the mannequin and attached monitor to set the proper circumstances as the scenario plays out (Table 42.4).

Development of the scenario relies on experts, in the clinical situation being portrayed, to ensure realistic patient responses and a reasonable premise. In addition, running of the scenario must include confederate facilitators who are expert as well, allowing the team to modify scenario responses realistically based on the actions of the participants. Thus one of the challenges in creating scenarios that are generally applicable to a wide range of practitioners, particularly for evaluative purposes, is the ability to translate the expertise of one group to the expectations in another. Consensus must be developed around scenarios and performance goals.

Creating the environment: where simulations are run

Medical simulation training has traditionally occurred in simulation centers, which were designed to recreate specific patient environments such as operating rooms. They were often built with viewing rooms and debriefing conference rooms, allowing post-event review of the video and breakdown of the trainees' performance [11]. Many large academic centers now include a separate simulation center for education, incorporating multidisciplinary approaches and allowing for training of medical personnel at all levels of practice. From Stanford University, where simulation use in anesthesia training was first developed, to Duke University in North Carolina and the University of Florida in Jacksonville, these centers are now an integral part of the fabric of medical education [87–89]. Use of some of these centers is not limited to physician education but includes nursing education as well, partially in response to increased limits of access to patients for their training. Private free-standing centers are also beginning to be seen, a response to the growing demand by hospitals and physicians for reproducible and reliable training and testing (Fig. 42.8).

Taking simulations to the various areas in which actual patient care is provided is called *in situ* simulation and allows a unique ability not only to test the areas for process and equipment deficiencies, but also to see how the teams work in their usual environment. This helps create a highly realistic milieu for training and eliminates many confounders that otherwise inhibit the normal responses of participants. However, the ability to recreate the positive features available in full-blown simulation centers, including audio-video capture and playback of scenarios, could be a technical challenge. By using a mobile audiovisual cart, simulation can be used in any work environment without giving up video-facilitated debriefing that is used in analyzing center-based simulation scenarios. After experimenting with several prototypes, a system was developed and first demonstrated at

Table 42.4 Template of Vital Signs Changes for Lost Airway Scenario

Patient state: trigger	Physiologic parameter: di-dir glenn	Physiologic parameter: down's with repaired av canal, phn	Time	Step required	Team actions	Ideal steps and notes
Anesthetized: immediately after induction	HR 120 BP 80/45 RR 26 SpO2 86	HR 120 BP 80/45 RR 26 SpO2 98	t = 0	chaotic because primary anesthesiologist in extremis	circulating nurse escorts anesthesiologist from room	–
Drapes going up: prepped	HR 120 BP 82/48 RR 26 SpO2 85	HR 120 BP 80/45 RR SpO2 99	t = 2	review of work space, materials etc.	scrub arid surgeon place drapes, patient prepped just as scenario started	Patient ventilated on FiO2 30%
Antibiotic given	HR 122 BP 80/45 RR 26 SpO2 85	HR 122 BP 80/45 RR 26 SpO2 98	t = 3	Already drawn up and labeled on anesthesia machine	surgeon asks if antibiotic given; team proceeds with time out only if anesthesiologist asks for this step	–
Surgeon makes incision	HR 158 BP 100/56 RR SpO2 85	HR 158 BP 100/56 RR SpO2 99	t = 4	patient coughs/moves, requires more anesthetic	Surgeon states, patient is moving, can you give him more anesthesia?	Vitals return to baseline if candidate responds to deepen anesthesia
Desaturation	HR 164 BP RR SpO2 75	HR 164 BP RR SpO2 85	t = 5	Note changes, run through differential, adjust vent	Team continues with surgery unless anesthesiologist states need to stop	no/minimal increase in SpO2 if candidate goes to 100% fiO2
Hypotension	HR 180 BP 50/35 RR SpO2 70	HR 180 BP 50/35 RR SpO2 80	t = 5	Treat wheezing with appropriate meds, Epi vs Albuterol?	Surgeon talks with nurse about fact that has meeting with Dean in one hour, so need to proceed quickly	–
Wheezing and PIPs increase	HR 180 BP RR SpO2 65	HR 180 BP RR SpO2 75	t = 7	Differential, adjust anesthetics, communicate with surgeon	Team continues with surgery unless anesthesiologist states need to stop	–
Hives on torso	HR BP RR SpO2	HR BP RR SpO2	t = 12	narrow differential, work on premise of anahylaxis	Surgeon states notes hives in field	–
? Dysrhythmia and/or ischemia	HR BP RR SpO2	HR BP RR SpO2	t = 14	Support cardiac function, call code	Nurse brings in code cart, other participants respond when called	ST segment changes then pulseless VT
Management steps: meds, ventilator management, etc.	HR BP RR SpO2	HR BP RR SpO2	t = 15–20	Management of patient state, attempt to stabilize	Team works with direction of anesthesia leader	–
End of scenario: alive but surgery cancelled and prep for ICU	HR BP RR SpO2	HR BP RR SpO2	t = 15–20	Patient still with moderate hypotension, poor saturations, holding on but not stable enough to continue surgery	When calling ICU nurse notes antiobiotic allergy on page in chart, different information than on anesthesia preop record	–

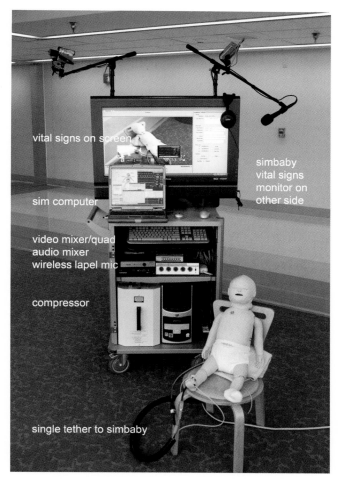

Figure 42.9 *In situ* simulation cart developed at Stanford, Lucile Packard Children's Hospital. Includes mechanical elements for a Sim Baby® (Laerdal Medical) with control computer, monitor, and large screen for display of multiple video and monitor channels to the simulation technical operator during simulations and after for debriefing. Audio elements are also integrated into the unit.

the 2006 Society for Pediatric Anesthesia Annual Winter Meeting by the Stanford Pediatric Anesthesia group [90] (Fig. 42.9). Commercial mobile audiovisual systems are now also available and have been used with positive results at other centers [91].

Facilitation: running a scenario

Prior to starting, participants must be briefed on the basic setting for the scenario, helping them to set the proper mental framework in which to play it out. Specific roles are assigned to each participant, allowing them to take part in the scenario as part of the care team. For instance, when the goal is improving medical management of a rare medical crisis in the OR, the learners may be assigned the role of the anesthesiologist, a member of a code team,

or a second anesthesiologist responder. However, if the goal is to develop an understanding of team dynamics in the operating rooms, participants may be asked to assume other roles within the team, such as the scrub-tech, which would allow them a different perspective on events as they unfold during the crisis.

Teaching facilitators will take other roles in the clinical team, such as the surgeon or circulating nurse, playing the parts as the scenario unfolds to help present the appropriate cues for the learner. The confederates feed information to the learners at appropriate times, guiding the understanding of the situation for participants or constraining their actions if needed.

A technician is required to run the computer that controls the mannequin throughout the scenario, allowing realistic "patient" responses to the actions of all participants. Communication between the confederates within the scenario and the technician controlling the mannequin is important to ensure the mannequin responses are made in an appropriate and timely manner.

An expert facilitator manages the flow of the scenario throughout, answering queries from the participants when environmental cues are unclear and giving absolute "truths" about the situation, which align with the rules set by the clinical situation being depicted.

Pediatric anesthesia simulation

Applications of pediatric anesthesia simulation

Simulation scenarios focused on pediatric anesthesia care can be created to serve many purposes: basic training of medical students or anesthesia residents, advanced training for pediatric anesthesia fellows, and refresher training for non-pediatric attending anesthesiologist or non-anesthesia specialists who might be called to sedate or resuscitate a pediatric patient.

With the continuing trend to centralize the surgical care of pediatric patients to large pediatric centers, anesthesiologists in community hospitals are exposed to fewer and fewer pediatric patients [92–94]. This could increase the demand for simulations related to pediatric care in order to maintain a sense of confidence in caring for these patients. Common crisis scenarios that depict relatively common and potentially critical events could help in this setting.

Pediatric anesthesia simulation centers and activities

Centers offering simulation experiences in pediatric anesthesia have multiplied over the last decade. Academic centers across the country have developed pediatric-focused groups, allowing training of fellows and residents, OR teams, and support personnel. Fellow training in pediatric anesthesia includes simulation to varying degrees. With the gradual decline in numbers of cases of neonatal emergency surgery in the past decade, some centers are beginning to develop scenarios targeted at exposing fellows in pediatric anesthesia to these rare cases critical to the complete training of consultants in pediatric anesthesia.

Factors in creating pediatric-specific anesthesia simulations

There are six major factors that affect the types of anesthesia simulations created for pediatrics versus adults: anatomy, psychology, physiology, procedural locations, types of surgery required, and parental involvement. The first relates simply to the size of the patients: children come in a large variety of sizes as a normal function of growth and development. This requires a whole different range of equipment, including mannequins specialized for the appearance of infants and small children. The second factor is that children present psychological challenges in IV access, co-operation, and the desire to avoid trauma. Therefore, they are frequently anesthetized using an inhalational mask induction, without IV access in place. The third factor relates to the propensity for children to exhibit rapid reactions and decompensation based on their physiology, such as rapid hypoxia following laryngospasm because of low functional residual capacity and high metabolic rate. These reactions present challenges in management, unique to pediatrics. The fourth factor is the relatively wide variety of locations in which anesthetics are administered to children routinely, because of their inability to co-operate with procedures or remain still, such as for diagnostic imaging. The limited equipment and support systems available in these diverse locations create opportunities for interesting scenarios. The fifth factor pertains to the types of surgery required by infants, which are often rare but require a high skill and focused knowledge set to manage well. Finally, the sixth factor acknowledges the parents' relation to and role in their children's lives: they have legal authority for their children and extremely strong emotional bonds. This relationship creates some unique situations ideal for simulation learning. See Box 42.2 for examples of scenarios created at Cincinnati Children's Medical Center.

The early patient simulation mannequins were developed with the adult model in mind. This not only targeted the vast majority of medical care delivered, but the larger mannequin provided more space for the mechanical and electrical components needed to create the various desired physical effects. With advances in computer technology and the miniaturization of components, smaller high-tech mannequins have become possible. Several companies now offer pediatric, newborn, and even premie- sized mannequins with a wide range of realistic

---

Box 42.2 Topics for some of the scenarios run at the Cincinnati Children's Medical Center, Cincinnati, Ohio (courtesy of Paul Samuels MD)

- Smoke inhalation
- Hemorrhage shock
- Supraventricular tachycardia
- Near drowning
- Head injury requiring RSI
- Status asthmaticus
- Seizures
- Opiate ingestion
- Meningococcal disease
- Anaphylaxis
- Spontaneous pneumothorax
- TCA overdose
- Cardiogenic shock
- Fentanyl reaction
- Ketamine reaction
- FBOA arrest
- Head injury requiring RSI - complication
- Malignant hyperthermia (PACU specific)
- Laryngospasm-induced pulmonary edema
- Pulseless electrical activity (no CPR initially)
- Child burn victim
- Child diabetic ketoacidosis

- Infant heat illness
- Pneumothorax (ECMO)
- Hypovolemia – basic (ECMO)
- Infant supraventricular tachycardia
- Airway trach crisis
- Child gunshot wound
- Infant near drowning
- Pediatric blunt trauma
- Infant blunt trauma
- Infant multiple trauma
- Respiratory failure
- VFIB arrest
- Arterial venous malformation
- Calcium channel blocker overdose
- Septic shock
- Hypertensive encephalopathy
- Ventricular tachycardia arrest

CPR, cardiopulmonary resuscitation; ECMO, extracorporeal membrane oxygenation; FBOA, foreign body obstructing the airway; PACU, postanesthesia care unit; RSI, rapid sequence intubation; TCA, tricyclic antidepressant; VFIB, ventricular fibrillation.

dynamic physical effects and interactive capabilities. For instance, the newborn simulator by Gaumard® (Gaumard Scientific, Miami, FL) not only delivers heart tones, breath sounds, peripheral pulses, and patient phonation, but will exhibit chest wall motion with either spontaneous or positive pressure ventilation, increased peak inspiratory pressures with various pathological conditions being simulated, and random rapid motion of the extremities to simulate a seizure. Advances in wireless signaling allow this mannequin to be picked up and moved without any tethers, allowing for an increased degree of realism and flexibility in creating scenarios, during which an infant might normally be moved from one location to another in a caregiver's arms.

Scenarios based on infants can only be realistically created using these appropriately sized mannequins. Everything in the environment is then appropriately sized as well, allowing the participant learner to more easily "suspend disbelief" and react to the crisis. Indeed, sizing of equipment and materials such as laryngoscopes and endotracheal tubes is one of the key elements in effectively working in any pediatric milieu. For applications in either learning or checking for proficiency, it was essential to overcome this size barrier before pediatric scenarios were possible.

Anatomy, psychology, and physiology affect another fundamental aspect of pediatric anesthesia, which is the induction technique. Pediatric patients have small veins, often masked by copious subcutaneous adipose tissue, making IV access difficult. They do not have the ability to understand the circumstances bringing them to our care, nor to co-operate and follow direction. These characteristics create a situation in which the child can become agitated and combative when attempting an IV start while awake. In addition, their physiology, including a high metabolic rate, heart rate, and respiratory rate, ensures rapid uptake of inhaled anesthetic agents, allowing for rapid induction using a mask technique. For these reasons, inhalation induction is commonly the method of choice when anesthetizing small children. Because there is no IV access for drug delivery yet available, this also creates some unique circumstances in which life-threatening reactions that are difficult to treat can occur during induction. Pediatric scenarios dealing with laryngospasm, bronchospasm, desaturation, bradycardia and hypotension during induction are both realistic and rich in teasing out both technical and non-technical skills for debriefing and learning. A practiced pediatric anesthesiologist becomes facile at the critical steps involved in these types of situations, and working through these reactions and steps in simulation scenarios with anesthesiologists who do not care for children every day or trainees is extremely useful.

The basic physiology in children is fundamentally different from that of adults in many ways, as noted above. In neonates, particularly if born prematurely, the airway reflexes are immaturely innervated, creating the propensity for apnea, laryngospasm, and bronchospasm, at times with no clear stimulation. Desaturation occurs very rapidly due to the limited functional residual capacity and rapid metabolic rate. Bradycardia is a common sequela of desaturation and, as opposed to adults, is commonly accompanied by significant hypotension due to the fixed ejection fraction of the still developing heart. These combined circumstances allow for a varied set of crises to deal with in simulated scenarios, often simply manipulating the patient's vital signs to create very realistic sequences. Also, the crisis can be attributed to minor triggers in healthy patients without major pathology, enabling a quick, rich scenario with full recovery of the patient and a sense of positive engagement and reinforcement for the learners.

When designing pediatric anesthetic scenarios, the full range of hospital locations can be utilized. Unlike the adult population, children often require anesthesia for painless imaging studies or minimally invasive procedures. As a result, it is common to anesthetize pediatric patients in various venues, such as MRI suites, radiation therapy rooms, endoscopic suites, and dental offices. Scenarios based on some of these remote locations can take advantage of the variable constellation of equipment available, unfamiliar personnel on hand, and unique environmental concerns. For example, one common scenario involves anesthetizing patients in the MRI suite, which requires special precautions around the magnetic field. Resuscitation cannot occur within the magnet, so the simulated patient must be removed to an adjacent locale for treatment.

In these remote locations, the availability of back-up support or help in the event of a crisis is likely to be markedly different as well. A focus on the system requirements in these locations during debriefing of these scenarios can open the participants' minds to the safeguards that have been put in place in their usual work environment and what might in fact be missing.

Pediatrics includes many types of surgery and procedures that are not seen in adults. Some of these operations are becoming rarer so it can be more difficult to acquire the skills needed to successfully navigate the appropriate anesthetic and to develop an understanding of the physiological aberrations that are commonly seen. Emergency operations in neonates, such as tracheo-esophageal fistula (TEF) repair, congenital diaphragmatic hernia repair, omphalocele and gastroschisis repair, are becoming less and less frequent. This, coupled with the increasing use of thoracoscopic and laparoscopic surgical approaches, which adds challenges for the anesthetic management, creates an ideal circumstance for the use of simulation training. For example, physiological aberrations, such as end-tidal CO_2 levels greater than 100 mmHg during thoracoscopic repair of TEF in a neonate, must often be tolerated. Simulation scenarios created to mimic normal circumstances in these rare operations can be used both for fellow trainees and for maintenance of skill in senior faculty.

Using high-fidelity simulation for this type of scenario can be extremely useful to practice the interdisciplinary communication and co-ordination that are key to successful management during these cases, whether sharing the airway with the otolaryngologist during a direct laryngoscopy and bronchoscopy or intermittently ventilating both lungs during a TEF repair, forcing a pause in the surgery for stabilization of the patient.

Finally, as children are minors and unable to consent to their medical care without an adult, working with the parents or guardians is a normal part of every pediatric anesthetic plan. Parents must be counseled for consent to proceed, co-opted to assist with the preparation of the patient, and at times assist the anesthesiologist with the patient through induction. Their own anxieties in facing the procedure or surgery for their child are often extreme.

Scenarios that incorporate a parental presence not only add a great deal of realism to pediatric simulations but can be used to create the crisis or circumstance that is the learning objective. Whether practicing effective communication before, during or after an event or successfully disengaging a parent as a crisis begins to unfold, much realism can be gained by adding this element. Scenarios are often derived from the real-world experiences of faculty members. One such case involved a parent-present induction in which the parent became panicked as the child went into laryngospasm on induction and fled with the baby from the operating room. In our adapted scenario, the patient developed a dysrhythmia and hypotension, forcing our participant-learner to effectively communicate with the parent, engage the team members for assistance in managing the crisis, and direct a team member to assist the parent out of the room, all while beginning effective management of the patient.

Pediatric-specific simulation equipment

An essential element of high-fidelity patient simulation is the creation of a realistic environment with appropriate equipment and props. Pediatric anesthesia simulations had to await the production of mannequins sized to approximate pediatric age ranges. Challenges in developing components small enough to fit into an infant mannequin delayed introduction of an infant mannequin for many years. In 1999, METI (Medical Education Technologies Inc., Sarasota, FL) was the first to introduce a pediatric mannequin known as the PediaSIM, approxi-

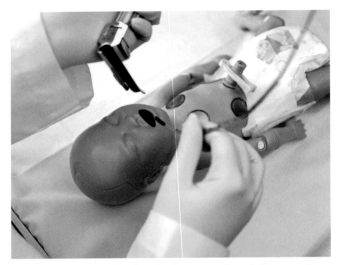

Figure 42.10 Gaumard wireless simulator created to mimic a premature infant.

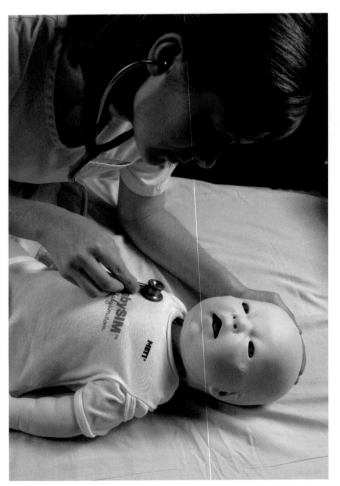

Figure 42.11 METI® infant simulator, created to mimic an infant 1–2 years of age.

Case title (<u>not</u> to be read to participants)	**Management of anaphylaxis in patient with congenital cardiac disease for hernia repair: inaccurate paperwork causes confusion about allergies, and wrong med given** *Note: scenario is preliminary for follow up scenario in which the "hot seat" anesthesiologist must disclose the events to the patient's mother*
Patient information MRN (will be changed)	Name: Baby Sim Packard Age: 13m Gender: Male Weight: 14Kg Height: 90cm Race: Caucasian
Case presentation (to be read to participants)	13 month-old-boy, scheduled for hernia repair one week after difficult reduction of incarcerated hernia
Past medical/surgical/family history	Original surgery planned for day of hernia reduction but patient with Down Syndrome, h/o AV Canal repair with small PFO, mild PHN, therefore surgery delayed for cardiac consult, now one week later, consult states patient is stable with no active cardiac symptoms and OK for surgery, "avoid hypotension and hypoxia"; URI and OM 2 weeks prior, no other medical history, family history negative for problems with anesthetics
Diagnostic tools	ASA monitors
Narrative case description (describe how the case unfolds, including major patient trends and consequences of interventions)	Patient in the OR and anesthesia already induced when "hot seat" participant comes in to take over care – original anesthesiologist acutely severely ill (chest pain, presyncopal); patient is stable at the time of handoff, immediately after intubation; surgeon is impatient to begin, draping completed and surgeon asks for antibiotics, which are already drawn up (Cefazolin), antibiotics given by hot-seat participant, surgeon states that patient moves with incision and anesthetic deepened, shortly thereafter desaturation and hypotension occur. Congenital cardiac disease, causes confusion about immediate diagnosis in OR, "red herring"/complicating factor. Wheezing, increased PIP's, and hives appear within next few minutes. Anaphylaxis treatment ensues, with patient not responding completely, requiring pressors/remain intubated, transfer to ICU for observation and treatment; the primary circulating nurse is not in the room at "time-out" to relay new allergy information to team, she presents this information when clear that allergic reaction is occurring and asks what antibiotic was given, this information does not correlate with information on anesthesia preop assessment form. Surgery cancelled with incision already made, transfer to ICU. Surgeon states will go speak with mother while team takes patient to ICU.
Clinical diagnosis and "correct" treatment	1. Recognize signs and symptoms of anaphylaxis 2. Understand likely manifestations of congenital heart condition 3. Manage ventilation, hypotension 4. Initiate post-op care plan
Educational objectives (with references to core competencies when applicable)	1. Understand the importance of timeout procedures 2. Increase understanding of congenital cardiac condition 3. Review of anaphylaxis manifestations and treatments 4. Understand critical behaviors for effective team performance in ACRM, leadership and communication in a crisis situation (communication & system based practice)
3–5 teaching/debriefing points (include references)	1. Proper steps for timeout (WHO checklist?) 2. Paperwork/system problems with mixed information 3. Team roles in crisis management – anaphylaxis 4. Sorting out differential diagnosis in patient with congenital heart disease
Staffing (roles – participants needed to reenact case)	1. Simulation facilitator (run computer) 2. Circulating nurse 3. Surgeon 4. Hand-off anesthesiologist (becomes computer facilitator)
Learners (med students, residents, etc.)	Participants: SPA attendees 1. Hot seat 2. First responder 3. Scrub technician 4. 2nd circulating nurse
Props needed	Simbaby, anesthesia machine, IV poles/sets, IV materials/supplies, syringes and needles for sim meds, airway equipment, suction, defibrillator (?), stethoscopes, drapes/surgical instruments
Timing	Scenario: 20 minutes Debriefing: 20 minutes

Figure 42.12 An example of a template used to capture and organize the critical elements in a scenario, from a short description of the basic clinical situation being depicted, to the staffing and equipment needs and the learning goals and objectives. Adapted from the Duke University Simulation Scenario Development Template available at http://simcenter.duke.edu/support.html and the Scenario-Preparation and Script by P. Dieckmann and M. Rall, TuPASS Germany, published in the IMSH 2008 Instructor Training Course manual [88].

mately the size of a 5–7-year-old child. In 2005, both Laerdal (Laerdal Medical, Stavanger, Norway) and METI brought infant mannequins to the market [92]. Their many features and the availability of connected vital sign monitors allowed for creation of complex and realistic scenarios. Now other companies, such as Gaumard, have also created infant and neonatal models (Figs 42.10, 42.11). Again, refer to Table 42.3 for a list of high-fidelity simulator mannequins, age ranges simulated, and features available.

Creating pediatric anesthesia scenarios

Various templates have been used to organize the diverse elements required to create and re-create a given scenario for high-fidelity patient simulation. All templates include the basic premise for the scenario to be acted out with a description of the patient's condition, the procedure or circumstance in which the patient is found, and the sequence of events that is planned to occur. This plan is created to specifically test the skills and teamwork of the participants, targeting particular learning goals. The roles for facilitators and participants must be carefully delineated. The supporting equipment required, either to create a realistic environment or for use in responding appropriately to the scenario, must be listed. Expected reactions to the script and the typical physiological responses are planned as well, so that any actions taken by participants will give realistic consequences. Figure 42.12 depicts a typical short template for a scenario, listing all critical elements required. The longer format adds detail to each element or includes references to support reactions depicted in various steps of the scenario. A "map" for the technician, to help guide them through the expected physiological reactions to different steps in the scenario, can also be included (see Fig. 42.8). Learning objectives are spelled out to ensure their inclusion during the debriefing section of the simulation.

Conclusion

Medical simulation has become a standard in education in medical schools and resident training, used for research, systems evaluations, and human performance evaluation. With the development of pediatric sized equipment, the use of simulation has been introduced to the area of pediatric anesthesia, with multiple and varied applications. It seems clear that these tools will continue to be developed and expand within medicine to improve education and ultimately patient care.

Annotated references

A full reference list for this chapter is available at:
http://www.wiley.com/go/gregory/andropoulos/pediatricanesthesia

11. Gaba D, DeAnda A. A comprehensive anesthesia simulation environment: re-creating the operating room for research and training. Anesthesiology 1988; 69: 387–94. The original description by the founder of the anesthesia simulation movement, a classic paper laying the foundation for modern anesthesia simulation paradigms.

12. Kohn LT, Corrigan JM, Donaldson MS. To Err is Human: Building a Safer Health System. Washington, DC: Institutes of Medicine, National Academy Press, 2000, p. 287. The seminal influential report by the Insitutes of Medicine that is the foundation for the modern patient safety movement. This report recommends team training based on aviation principles to improve patient safety.

22. Weinstock PH, Kappus LJ, Kleinman ME et al. Toward a new paradigm in hospital-based pediatric education: the development of an onsite simulator program. Pediatr Crit Care Med 2005; 6: 635–41. A description of an on-site simulation program inside a pediatric intensive care unit that was one of the early publications advocating the approach of taking the simulation session to the team as a way to facilitate scenarios that closely mimic actual situations.

24. Park CS, Rochlen LR, Yaghmour E et al. Acquisition of critical intraoperative event management skills in novice anesthesiology residents by using high-fidelity simulation-based training. Anesthesiology 2010; 112: 202–11. A very interesting, prospective, controlled crossover study demonstrating superior performance in specific scenarios of hypotension and hypoxemia when simulation-based training is used for new anesthesiology residents.

28. Gaba D, Fish K, Howard S. Crisis Management in Anesthesiology. New York: Churchill Livingstone, 1994. The seminal book describing team crisis management as it applies to the specialty of anesthesiology.

35. Gaba DM, Howard SK, Flanagan B et al. Assessment of clinical performance during simulated crises using both technical and behavioral ratings. Anesthesiology 1998; 89: 8–18. An early description of the non-technical factors that can be taught using anesthesia simulation scenarios. Paved the way for much of the later work in this area.

41. Fanning R, Gaba D. The role of debriefing in simulation-based learning. Simul Healthcare 2007; 2: 115–25. An excellent description of the importance of the debriefing process in simulation in healthcare.

52. Mathieu JE, Heffner TS, Goodwin GF et al. The influence of shared mental models on team process and performance. J Appl Psychol 2000; 85: 273–83. An important review of the concept of shared mental models in the functioning of teams, laying the foundation for the application of this model to healthcare teams.

85. Cantrell MJ, Deloney LA. Integration of standardized patients into simulation. Anesthesiol Clin 2007; 25: 377–83. An interesting and informative paper laying out the rationale for incorporating standardized patients into high-fidelity simulation scenarios, to more completely represent real-life situations.

91. Weinstock PH, Kappus LJ, Garden A, Burns JP. Simulation at the point of care: reduced-cost, in situ training via a mobile cart. Pediatr Crit Care Med 2009; 10: 176–81. An excellent description of a program and the benefits of mobile, *in situ* simulation delivered in the actual patient care units.

CHAPTER 43

Databases and Outcome Research in Pediatric Anesthesia

Donald C. Tyler, Laura Schleelein & Harshad Gurnaney

Department of Anesthesiology and Critical Care Medicine, The University of Pennsylvania School of Medicine, and The Children's Hospital of Philadelphia, Philadelphia, PA, USA

Introduction

Databases are playing an increasingly important role in research about care of patients, and this chapter will provide a background to what databases are and how they are used. We will then review some important anesthesia-related databases, and finally we will examine the growing importance of outcomes research and look at the approaches used in outcomes research. An important role for databases is in the evaluation of care and the quality and cost of care, and we will begin with an examination of this topic.

Introduction to medical databases

In the past the assessment of the quality of care provided by institutions and by individual physicians was based on word of mouth information, on subjective appraisals of physician–patient interactions and on the reputation of institutions and physicians. This method of evaluation is in the process of change, and society is moving toward attempts at objective measures of the quality of health systems and of physicians. As a result, physicians and healthcare systems are being challenged to provide objective measures of quality and safety. We are just in the infancy of using data to measure the quality of results produced by the healthcare system and also the performance of physician groups and individual physicians. Given that it is difficult for physicians to define quality in healthcare, the task of developing objective measures of a largely subjective concept is proving challenging.

There are several reasons for the drive toward objective measures of quality and performance. Beside the desire to select healthcare professionals based on the quality of the care that they provide, the ability to control costs, the elimination of unnecessary care and perhaps other motivations are involved. We are a long way from measurement systems that are equivalent to those available for the purchase of consumer goods such as automobiles, but the process is well under way. In this climate it is important that physicians are involved in the design of measurement tools so that the measurements will be meaningful and not based on inaccurate or biased data.

In evaluating the quality of care, one can use process measures or outcome measures. Process measures are activities that are carried out during the care of a patient. They might include whether we use a mask or intravenous induction, whether antibiotics are given, whether a surgical safety checklist is followed, or other similar items. Outcome measures, on the other hand, look at what happens to the patient; in the above examples, was the induction smooth and non-traumatic for the child or did the patient experience a surgical site infection? Because the outcomes of patients that anesthesiologists care for in the operating room depend to a great extent on both surgical care and anesthesia care, it is difficult to develop good outcome measures for anesthesia alone. The result is that process measures are often used as a measure of the quality of anesthesia care.

As an example of what is happening and of the difficulties involved, the 2006 Tax Relief and Health Care Act established a physician quality reporting initiative (PQRI) for physicians caring for patients in the Medicare program [1]. Since it is difficult to find objective measures that relate specifically to outcomes of anesthesia care, the measures developed so far are process measures and are inadequate measures of the quality of anesthesia. The current measures are timely administration of antibiotics, maintenance of patient temperature, and use of standard protocols during insertion of central venous catheters, all of which are important but do not by themselves define the quality of anesthesia care.

Since the number of measures for anesthesiology is so small and limited, it is likely that other more sophisticated tools will be used to measure the influence of anesthesia on patient outcomes. This process of evaluation will likely involve the use of data in databases and sophisticated statistical techniques to measure the influence of anesthesia on patient outcomes. In order to ensure that the measurements are meaningful and appropriately measure the quality of care, it is important to know from where the data that will be used in the measurements came and how the data are manipulated. Since most data used for these purposes are stored in databases, a basic understanding of databases is important for practicing physicians.

Database terminology

A number of terms are used in relation to management and storage of data. A *database* is defined as a large collection of data organized especially for rapid search and retrieval. Data in a database are obtained not by planned scientific experiment but come from data maintained for clinical care or other purposes. Medical databases are a logically coherent collection (which is often computerized) of observations and related information about a group of patients. Databases are designed to manage and archive large amounts of information that can be accessed or retrieved, and they help with collecting information in a standard format, which decreases redundancy of the data and reduces repeated data entry. Databases also improve data security and provide a means for retrieval of the data using query languages. The term *data warehouse* is often used. A data warehouse is a collection of a large amount of data. Data get into a data warehouse from one or more sources after the data are cleaned (cross-checked and corrected), transformed and catalogued.

*Database management system*s are a collection of software programs that allow users to define, construct and manipulate databases for various applications. Data can be extracted from data warehouses using so-called data mining techniques or other analytical processing techniques using database management systems. The structure of the stored data is maintained in a *data dictionary*, which provides information about data such as meaning, relationships to other data, origin, usage, and format. The data dictionary typically includes the names and description of various tables and fields in each database, plus additional details, such as the type and length of each data element.

Classification of databases

There are several ways in which databases can be classified. One way is classification based on the function they perform.

* *Analytical* databases are primarily used to keep track of statistics. They are used in online analytical processing, which provides improved speed compared to a relational database. Analytical databases differ from relational databases in their ability to look within the database at specific elements in which the end-user is interested.
* *Operational* databases are databases that let the user modify the data. These databases can store and update data such as employee personal information, employee training status, and previous work history and this information is updatable and retrievable across the company. An example of an operational database is a database used by a store to take orders, track completion of the order, and keep track of the inventory. Thus the user would change the database when an order is sent to a customer

Another way of classifying databases is by their data model. A data model describes how the data are stored in and retrieved from a database.

- *Flat-file database model.* In this system the data are stored in numerous files that are not linked. This type of database can perform basic record keeping of a limited number of data elements; for example, an Excel spreadsheet is a flat-file database model.
- *Hierarchical database model.* This system consists of a series of databases that are grouped together to resemble a family tree. The top database in the hierarchical model is called the parent database. The databases under it are called child databases. The child databases are all connected to the parent database via links creating a one-to-many ratio.
- *Network database model.* This model is designed to allow for links between the child databases but these kinds of databases are harder to use and maintain. A network database model is similar to the hierarchical database but the network model allows for multiple parent databases. Hierarchical and network databases have largely been replaced by relational databases which offer a higher degree of flexibility.
- *Relational database model.* In this model data are stored in any number of separate databases that are connected by a "key" field. The same key field is present in each dataset and allows for the tables to be related to each other. Use of a relational database makes it easy to extract data. Many of the commonly used databases such as Access, Oracle and MySQL are relational databases.
- *Object-oriented database model.* Object-oriented database models let databases store and manipulate text, sounds, images, and all sorts of media clips. Examples are Java and C++.
- *Client/server databases.* Client/server databases are the databases that are used for the Internet and for the World Wide Web

Administrative data versus clinical data

In the medical field, administrative data are usually collected from billing information that hospitals submit to payers, whereas clinical data are extracted from information used to care for a patient [2,3]. Administrative data have major problems when used for purposes for which they were not intended. They may lack clinically important information, such as significant pre-existing illnesses and other problems that might make one patient a higher risk than another. The primary and secondary diagnosis codes are based on the interpretation of the person entering the codes for billing purposes, and billers may not interpret medical issues correctly. Since higher severity of illness often results in higher payments, there could be a bias toward including insignificant or trivial diagnoses, but since there are penalties for "upcoding" there may be a bias to downcode some of the data elements in an administrative database. In addition, administrative data may not distinguish between conditions that were present on admission and those that occurred during the hospitalization.

Some other concerns that have been raised include such issues as data collection and sampling procedures, missing data, and erroneous data. In addition, more technical issues related to data distribution, data independence, data quality management, data integration, data access and data privacy may also be involved [4]. Analytical problems when using large administrative datasets include issues related to multiple testing on a particular dataset which increases the likelihood of observing a statistically significant result due to chance, making comparisons using datasets from different sources with data that may be represented differently. Finally, there is the problem of differentiating the statistically significant from the scientifically significant.

The accuracy and validity of the data used to calculate a measure's value are primarily determined by the match between the purpose for which the data were entered and the meaning ascribed to that data element when generating a report [5,6]. Using administrative data from billing systems to deduce clinical context can produce misleading results [6]. As an example of the problems associated with the use of administrative data, consider the measurement of the data element "complications of anesthesia." If a surgeon is doing a case with local anesthesia and administers an overdose of local anesthetic, that error would be labeled as a "complication of anesthesia" and could be attributed to the anesthesia department, when in fact no anesthesia provider was involved in the case.

Another problem with administrative data is the issue of risk adjustment [7]. If one group of patients is healthier than another before comparable operations, we would expect the healthier patients to have better outcomes. The differences in expected outcome because of differing prior health can be minimized by risk adjustment; that is, by using scoring systems to adjust expected outcome for the risk of the patient. For example, the risk of complications during an anesthetic for hernia repair is presumably greater in a 1500 g premature infant compared to a healthy 8-year-old child. If the quality of care were to be compared in this case, risk adjustment would use statistical techniques to take into account the difference in risk and expected outcomes of the two patients. The validity of risk adjustment systems that use only administrative data has been challenged and there is a need for additional data to increase the accuracy of predicting a patient's risk. The previously mentioned problems with coding of co-existing illness and other factors tends to make risk adjustment with administrative data difficult, but in some cases risk adjustment may appear to produce the expected results. The advantage of administrative data is the fact that they are readily available in electronic form, whereas clinical data may be scattered in many places, collected in different ways and may even use different definitions for the same concept. When good clinical data are available, though, it would seem preferable to use them. There are some robust clinical databases available such as those which collect data from cardiac surgery patients.

The value of good clinical data compared to administrative data has been shown by Welke et al [8] who compared mortality rates using administrative data with those of the Congenital Heart Surgeons Society and the Society for Thoracic Surgeons databases. They found that mortality rates based on data from administrative sources were higher than from those based on good clinical data. But sometimes administrative data may produce the expected result. Aylin et al [9] were concerned that administrative datasets might not have sufficient information for appropriate risk adjustment. They compared risk adjustment for mortality in coronary artery bypass grafting, repair of aortic aneurysm and colorectal procedures using administrative data and compared the results to those obtained when using clinical data and found that risk adjustment was equivalent. Since there is no validated comparison, though, their findings could mean that neither system did a good job with risk adjustment.

Limitations of databases

Database systems are complex, difficult, and time-consuming to design and involve substantial hardware and software start-up costs. They also involve initial training for users and continued manpower to maintain the database and facilitate data entry, check data accuracy and provide means for data extraction. There may be problems or limitations with the quality of the data that go into the database and the research based on databases is only as good as the data in the database. In addition, to some extent the interpretation of the results of database research depends on the assumptions used in generating the information. In evaluating research based on databases, it is important to understand how the data were obtained, how they were extracted, and how they were interpreted.

Privacy laws and data sharing

Research using databases depends on using scientific data over a period of time to support scientific observations. The use of these data has to comply with a host of regulatory directives at different levels (federal, state, local) [10]. The Privacy Rule in the US Health Insurance Portability and Accountability Act of 1996 (HIPAA) both created new procedural requirements for the use of protected health information (PHI) and defined PHI more broadly. The HIPAA rule requires that certain personal identifiers be stripped from a dataset prior to sharing. These include explicit identifiers (e.g. names), quasi-identifiers (e.g. dates and geocodes), and traceable elements (e.g. medical record numbers). An alternative to the use of data with these identifiers is to use a limited dataset, which allows sharing of some detailed data but requires the data recipient to enter into a contract that prohibits them from reidentification of a patient [11].

Uses of databases

In addition to attempts to measure quality of care, databases have been used in a number of ways. As we will discuss in more detail below, databases have been used for quality improvement, as in the National Surgical Quality Improvement Program. The have also been used in research on diseases and treatments, one notable example being cystic fibrosis. Other uses have been evaluation of risks of various treatments and techniques, especially with the anesthesia Closed Claims Project and the Pediatric Perioperative Cardiac Arrest Registry (POCA). Finally outcomes research, which we will discuss below, is another use of databases. The next section will review several initiatives involving databases in order to provide examples of how databases have been used.

Anesthesia databases

Two databases, the Closed Claims Project and the Pediatric Perioperative Cardiac Arrest Registry, have contributed to the safety of anesthesia, and it is important to discuss these before covering current and future anesthesia databases.

American Society of Anesthesiologists Closed Claims Project

The Closed Claims Project was an effort begun by Richard J. Ward MD and Ellison Pierce Jr MD, working with the American Society of Anesthesiologists Committee on Professional Liability. Under the direction of Frederick W. Cheney MD, the initiative was begun in 1984. In this initiative the researchers received clinical information from insurance companies on anesthesia malpractice claims that had been settled or adjudicated. Expert anesthesiologists reviewed the claims to analyze the cases and to look for errors in care, and the results of their reviews were entered into a database. It was then possible to use the database to analyze relatively rare but serious events [12,13]. The results of these analyses were published in a series of papers.

One of the first reports was by Caplan et al in 1988 [14]. From a review of the closed claims data, they found 14 cases of unexpected cardiac arrest during spinal anesthesia in ASA 1 or 2 patients undergoing relatively minor surgical procedures. These arrests appeared to occur in spite of what was judged to be adequate anesthesia care, and did not appear to be related to inappropriate care. In approximately half of the cases the reviewers found that the arrest was associated with sedation sufficiently deep to result in verbal unresponsiveness, and they felt that unrecognized respiratory insufficiency might have been the cause of the arrest. In the other half of the patients, it was assumed that an unexpectedly high sympathetic block was involved, and that the vasodilation might have interfered with resuscitation. The authors pointed out that recognition of this condition was important and they recommended that epinephrine be administered in cases of sudden bradycardia or cardiac arrest in this setting.

In 1990 the group reported on adverse outcomes related to respiratory events [15]. At the time of the review there were 1541 claims in the database, and of these 522 or 34% were classified as being respiratory in origin. The most common causes of respiratory problems were inadequate ventilation, esophageal intubation, and difficult tracheal intubation. Reviewers concluded that better monitoring could have prevented 72% of the events. Most of these events occurred before the widespread use of pulse oximetry and capnography and the results presented in this paper were important in demonstrating even to the most skeptical the value of routine pulse oximetry and capnography. One other important observation was the apparent presence of breath sounds in a significant number of cases of esophageal intubation.

Further reports followed, examining less common respiratory events (airway trauma, pneumothorax, airway obstruction, aspiration and bronchospasm) [16]. In the cases of airway trauma, 58% were not associated with difficult intubation. Some of the injuries noted were injury to pharynx or esophagus leading to mediastinitis. There were a number of injuries to the larynx in patients in whom intubation was thought to be routine. Pneumothorax was associated with blocks (mostly supraclavicular or intercostal) in 40% of cases, and also with airway management or barotrauma.

Another report from Caplan [17] focused on adverse outcomes related to malfunction or misuse of gas delivery equipment. This group comprised only 2% of events included in the closed claims database, and the majority were due to misuse of the equipment, not failure. Approximately 10% of the events were due to switches of oxygen lines. Most of the events were judged to be preventable with better monitoring, such as high airway pressure alarms.

Morray et al [18] compared pediatric closed claims with adult claims. Respiratory events, particularly those associated with inadequate ventilation, were more common in the pediatric cases than in adult cases, and mortality rate was higher. They found more claims in the group of

patients under 6 months of age than in any of the other age groups. More of those claims were thought to be preventable than in adult claims. Jimenez [19] provided an update on pediatric closed claims, looking at trends over time. She found that although there was a decrease in proportion of claims due to death or events with respiratory causes, nevertheless cardiovascular and respiratory causes were still major contributors to claims in the later period. There was an increase in the proportion of claims in younger children, and inadequate ventilation decreased from 26% of claims to 3% of claims, presumably as a result of the introduction of pulse oximetry and capnography. Cardiovascular events increased to 26% of claims in this later report, and the most common of these events involved blood loss and fluid resuscitation.

While closed claims analysis led to a significant number of findings and reports which initiated changes in anesthetic practice, there are limitations to this sort of research. These limitations include the lack of a denominator which prevents any determination of incidence of these adverse events. Another limitation was that the reviewers knew the outcomes and this fact led to bias in assessment of responsibility [20]. A further problem was that the only cases available to reviewers were those that came to litigation, and these represented only a limited sample of adverse events. Finally data collection was retrospective and some important data may have been missing or subject to misinterpretation.

Pediatric Perioperative Cardiac Arrest Registry

The Pediatric Perioperative Cardiac Arrest Registry (POCA) is a pediatric database that followed the Closed Claims Project. POCA was formed in 1994 in an attempt to determine the clinical factors and outcomes associated with cardiac arrest in anesthetized children [21]. Some institutions that provide anesthesia for children voluntarily enrolled in the POCA registry, and the investigators created a database of information about cardiac arrests that occurred in children. To create the database, a representative from each participating institution anonymously submitted a standardized data form for each cardiac arrest. Cardiac arrest for this registry was defined as the need for chest compressions or as death in anesthetized children 18 years or younger. The investigators used the database to try to determine the causes of the cardiac arrests, and published a series of reports. In the first 4 years of the POCA registry, 63 institutions enrolled and submitted 289 cases of cardiac arrest.

The Pediatric Perioperative Cardiac Arrest Registry provides an interesting example of changes in causes of cardiac arrest in children over time, presumably related to changes in anesthestic practice. The initial report in 2000 by Morray et al [21] divided the arrests into groups:

medication related, cardiovasular causes, respiratory events, and equipment related. Of the medication-related arrests, halothane-induced cardiovascular depression was the most common cause of arrest and significantly, a large number of these arrests occurred in patients who were ASA 1 or 2 status. The incidence of cardiac arrest was found to be 1.4 ± 0.45 per 10,000 anesthetics, calculated using the reported cardiac arrests as numerator and total number of anesthestics at participating institutions as denominator. A later report by Bhananker et al [22] showed a decrease in arrests due to halothane, presumably due to the replacement of halothane by sevoflurane as the most common induction agent. In the report by Bhananker, cardiovascular causes became more common, particularly hypovolemia from blood loss and hyperkalemia associated with transfusion of blood.

A final report detailed the higher risk surrounding cardiac arrest in children with heart disease. Ramamoorthy et al [23] compared findings associated with cardiac arrest in patients with heart disease with those who did not have heart disease. Ninety-two percent of the patients with heart disease were ASA 3 or higher, and 63% of the patients were less than 2 years of age; 54% of the arrests occurred in cases in which the operative procedure was non-cardiac. In looking at causes, the reviewers felt that cardiovascular depression was a contributing factor in some cases and that myocardial ischemia was a contributing factor in some cases.

The POCA registry has made some significant observations but as with the Closed Claims Project, it has some methodological weaknesses. POCA depended on voluntary reporting and for a variety of reasons, underreporting is likely. Selection bias is also possible, in that unexpected cardiac arrests or highly sensitive cases might not get reported. Furthermore, since the participants were for the most part large academic institutions, they may not be representative of all institutions that provide anesthesia care for children. This preponderance of large institutions could result in skewed statistics that are not representative of the actual population [21].

Other pediatric anesthesia databases

As with any good study, many questions arose after POCA, including questions about the incidence of cardiac arrest, and several institutions used local databases to provide more information about pediatric cardiac arrests. The use of databases for research often begins with a local database maintained by individual departments, and as the reports below indicate, it is possible for departments to maintain an effective database and to extract meaningful information from it. Several institutions have maintained databases relating to anesthesia, and reports from these databases are appearing in the scientific literature. Different types of data are maintained, and different structures often make comparing information from one database to another difficult. On the other hand, an advantage of local databases is the ability to maintain more control over the data, and to enter more extensive and specific data. Several of these databases are discussed below to point out some of the attractive features of local databases and to enumerate some of their limitations. This is not meant to be an exhaustive discussion of local anesthesia-related databases.

The cardiac anesthesia service at Boston Children's Hospital has maintained a database relating to anesthesia care of cardiac patients since January 2000. Extensive data including diagnosis, demographics, procedure, anesthetic technique and details of cardiopulmonary bypass were maintained on every case. Data on cardiac arrests were reported in 2007 by Odegard et al [24] who assessed procedures with and without cardiopulmonary bypass and also whether the arrests were anesthesia related or not. The incidence of cardiac arrest in this group was 79 per 10,000; 26.8% were possibly related to anesthesia. The anesthesia-related causes include airway management, monitoring issues, medication-related issues, and myocardial ischemia.

The Mayo clinic has maintained a quality assurance database since November 1988, and in a recent report the data were used to determine the incidence of cardiac arrest in children undergoing anesthesia [25]. They analyzed a total of 92,881 anesthetics, for both cardiac and non-cardiac procedures. In the non-cardiac cases the incidence of cardiac arrest was 2.9 per 10,000 anesthetics, while for cardiac cases the rate was 127 per 10,000. Most of the arrests were due to factors not related to anesthesia.

Baum [26] used the University Hospital Consortium (UHC) database to examine the influence of congenital heart disease on mortality after non-cardiac surgery in children. UHC is a group of more than 60 university hospitals in the US that share data in a database. They found increased mortality in those patients with congenital heart disease, especially in the youngest patients, and in those patients with more severe cardiac disease.

Current and future database research in anesthesia

The findings of the Closed Claims Project and POCA provided useful data about problems in the administration of anesthesia but they raised a number of questions that cannot be answered with the data available from these sorts of databases. For this reason and for the reasons discussed above relating to quality and outcomes measurement, a number of databases have been and are being developed that will be important in the future of anesthesia research.

The Congenital Cardiac Anesthesia Society is working with the Society for Thoracic Surgeons (STS) to include anesthesia-specific data in the STS Congenital Database. This database will be an important step forward as it will include both surgical and anesthesia information in a common database [27,28] (Table 43.1). Pediatric cardiac cases represent a specific subset of pediatric cases and a specialized database is important for understanding outcomes with this group of patients. The group is developing common definitions of events and complications, and also methods to track patients if one patient receives care from multiple institutions. As data are collected the common definitions and quality control of data should provide a valuable resource for understanding the contribution of anesthesia to outcomes in pediatric cardiac surgery patients.

Pediatric Sedation Research Consortium

Several other initiatives in pediatric anesthesia are collecting data for the purpose of conducting research. The Pediatric Sedation Research Consortium (PSRC) was created in 2003 in an effort to improve pediatric sedation process and outcomes [29]. It initially was a collaboration of 35 institutions that wanted a more comprehensive approach to the study of the safety and reliability of pediatric sedation. Only 26 institutions actually submitted data to the database before the first publication of the data in 2006. The consortium wanted the participating institutions to share their prospective observational outcome data on procedural encounters. As of October 2010, there were more than 200,000 encounters in the database [30]. There are no selection criteria for participation and, as a result, the PSRC consists of data from sedation administered by a mix of anesthesiologists, pediatric medical subspecialists, emergency physicians, pediatric intensivists, nurses, physician assistants, and healthcare research personnel. The data are collected through a self-report system. The National Patient Safety Foundation supports the development and management of the database [31]. The future analysis of the database will focus on evaluating the association of adverse outcomes with various provider types, monitoring standards, and medications used [32].

The Sedation Consortium reported on the use of propofol for sedation or anesthesia in 49,836 procedures outside the operating room (OR). There were no deaths and cardiopulmonary resuscitation (CPR) was required twice. Apnea or airway obstruction occurred in 575 per 10,000 cases. The group concluded that propofol sedation is unlikely to yield serious adverse outcomes in the settings in which it was used in the study, that is, in highly motivated institutions with established protocols and

with training for the providers of sedation. These factors of motivation and training limit the degree to which the findings in this study are generalizable to other situations. Furthermore, there is no assurance that all adverse outcomes are reported. Leaders of the consortium have tried to address this issue by using blinded data submission [32].

Pediatric Regional Anesthesia Network

The Pediatric Regional Anesthesia Network (PRAN) was organized in 2006 in an effort to facilitate multi-institutional studies of regional anesthesia in children. The goal of this group is to create an online data collection network that can facilitate the conduct of large-scale multi-institutional studies involving regional anesthesia in infants and children. The network began with six pilot sites, after which one withdrew from the project and five continued. All regional anesthetics performed at each institution by an anesthesiologist are entered into the database on a self-report system. Blocks performed by surgeons are excluded from the database. In addition to the details of the block, any intraoperative and postoperative complications are recorded as well as age, gender, and ASA physical status [33]. Completeness and accuracy of data submission are verified by the investigator at each institution through a monthly random audit of 10% of charts that are checked against the submitted data [34]. As of October 2010, there were more than 17,000 regional anesthetics in the database. Data from the PRAN are now being utilized to strengthen recommendations for regional anesthesia in children, for example the safety of epidural catheter placement under general anesthesia [35].

Wake Up Safe

Wake Up Safe is a quality improvement initiative sponsored by the Society for Pediatric Anesthesia (SPA) and founded in 2006. The database is a registry of serious adverse events, an analysis of why the event occurred, and in addition, demographic data on all anesthetics at participating institutions. Initially 10 institutions participated in the start-up phase, and as of December 2010, 14 institutions participate with approximately 250,000 anesthetics per year.

Almost immediately after data collection began, five cases of wrong side procedure were reported, three surgical cases and two anesthesia blocks. In the analysis it was determined that no "time out" occurred prior to the blocks. For the surgical procedures, there were protocols in place to protect against wrong side/site procedures, but the protocols were not followed. For example, one case occurred when the site was marked but the marking was not visible when the patient was prepped and draped for the procedure. Information about the wrong side procedures was transmitted to the members of the Society

Table 43.1 Anesthesia fields for the Congenital Cardiac Anesthesia Society-Society of Thoracic Surgeons joint congenital heart surgery database

Patient Information	
Location of procedure	
Primary Anesthesiology attending	Name
Secondary Anesthesiology attending	Name
Fellow or Resident present	Yes/No
CRNA/SRNA present	Yes/No
Patient body surface area	Calculated
Preoperative medications	
Preoperative medications	Drop down list of common medications patient is on for 24 hours prior to OR
Preoperative sedation	Yes/No; medication used
Time of transport from ICU/Floor	Hours:Minutes (HH:MM)
Time of induction	Hours:Minutes (HH:MM)
Monitoring	
Preoperative baseline oxygen saturation	%
Arterial line	Percutaneous/Cutdown/None
Central pressure monitoring	Percutaneous/Cutdown/Transthoracic/None
Neurologic monitoring	None/BIS/NIRS/TCD/SSEP/EEG
Lowest recorded core intraoperative temperature	Degrees Celsius
Transesophageal echocardiography	Yes/No
Anesthetic technique	
Induction	Inhalation/Intravenous/Intramuscular
Primary induction agent	List of medications
Primary maintenance agent	List of medications
Regional anesthetic	Yes/No: type (caudal/epidural/spinal); single/continuous
Airway	
Airway type	None/Nasal cannula/Endotracheal tube (ETT)/Double lumen endobronchial tube (EBT)/Laryngeal mask airway (LMA)/Other
Airway size	
Cuffed	
Airway site	None/Oral/Nasal/Tracheostomy
Transfusion	No/Yes (if Yes than continue below)
Packed red blood cells (PRBC)	Volume or units
Platelets	Volume or units
Fresh frozen plasma (FFP)	Volume or units
Cryoprecipitate	Volume or units
Whole blood	Volume or units
Activated Factor VII	Yes/No

Table 43.1 *(Continued)*

Intraoperative pharmacology	
Drop down list of medications	All common intraoperative/intraprocedural medications
Pharmacology at transfer to ICU/PACU	
Drop down list of medications	All common intraoperative/intraprocedural medications
ICU/PACU care	
Time of ICU/PACU arrival	Hours:Minutes (HH:MM)
Initial FiO2	
ECMO	Yes/No
Initial pH	
Initial SpO2	%
Temperature on arrival	Degrees Celsius
Need for pacemaker	Yes/No
Morbidity/Mortality	
None	No/Yes (if Yes than continue below)
Anesthesia-related morbidity	(only events occurring during time of anesthetic care or related directly to anesthetic care)
Airway – pulmonary	Dental injury
	Respiratory arrest either pre-operatively, intra- or post-operatively requiring unanticipated airway support
	Unanticipated difficult intubation/reintubation
	Post-extubation stridor or sub-glottic stenosis requiring therapy
	Unintended extubation in Operating Room or during patient transfer
	Endotracheal tube migration requiring repositioning
	Airway/pulmonary injury related to ventilation
Vascular	Arrhythmia during central venous line placement requiring therapy
	Difficult vascular access (> one hour of attempted access)
	Hematoma requiring cancellation or additional surgical exploration
	Inadvertent arterial puncture with hematoma or hemodynamic consequence
	Myocardial perforation or injury with central venous line placement
	Vascular compromise secondary to line placement (such as blue leg or venous obstruction)
	Pneumothorax during central venous line placement
Regional anesthetic	Bleeding at site or with aspiration
	Inadvertent intrathecal puncture
	Local anesthetic toxicity
	Neurologic injury
Pharmacology	Anaphylaxis/anaphylactoid reaction
	Non-allergic drug reaction
	Inadvertent drug administration (wrong drug)

(Continued)

Table 43.1 (Continued)

	Inadvertent drug dosing (right drug, wrong dose)
	Intraoperative recall
	Malignant hyperthermia
	Protamine reaction requiring pharmacologic intervention
Cardiac*	Cardiac arrest after admit to operating room and prior to incision
	Unexpected cardiac arrest not related to surgical manipulation
	*Cardiac arrest defined as the sudden abrupt loss of heart function
Transesophageal echocardiography	Esophageal bleeding or rupture during transesophageal echocardiographic probe placement or manipulation
	Esophageal chemical burn
	Airway or vascular compromise during transesophageal echocardiographic probe placement/manipulation requiring removal of transesophageal echocardiographic probe
	Accidental extubation during transesophageal echocardiographic probe manipulation
Positioning	Patient falling out of either transport bed or Operating Room table to floor
	Neurologic injury resulting from patient positioning during anesthetic care

Reproduced from Vener et al [28] with permission from Cambridge University Press. See text for full explanation.

for Pediatric Anesthesia with recommendations for ways to avoid wrong side/site procedures [36]. Another early finding from Wake Up Safe was a warning concerning syringe swaps; that is, using one syringe mistaking it for another with a different drug, particularly with non-color coded pharmacy-produced syringes [37].

Wake Up Safe plans to increase the number of institutions participating, and to use the reports of adverse events to develop quality improvement initiatives to decrease the frequency of occurrence of serious adverse events.

Other anesthesia databases

Other anesthesia subspecialty societies are also starting databases to examine outcomes.

The Society for Ambulatory Anesthesia (SAMBA) was founded in 1985 in an effort to advance the field of ambulatory anesthesia. In 2009, the society announced the launching of the SAMBA Clinical Outcomes Registry or SCOR. The goal is to develop a registry that will serve to build a national database of patient outcomes in both ambulatory surgical centers and office-based surgical suites. The society hopes to use the database to establish benchmarks for accepted standards of care, for example, best practices to deal with postoperative nausea and vomiting, delayed awakening, and perioperative glucose

management [38,39]. It is collecting a large number of data elements including information about the type of ambulatory center, the anesthesia provider model, demographic information on patients, co-morbidities, and type of anesthesia. It will also collect current "pay for performance" elements and operational data such as operative times. For outcomes, it will track emesis, use of pain medications, urinary retention and significant adverse events such as death, cardiac arrest and sentinel events. It will also collect information about readmission or emergency room visits, pain and patient satisfaction.

The Society for Obstetric Anesthesia and Perinatology (SOAP) started the Serious Complication Repository Project (SCORE) in 2005 to track adverse complications in obstetric anesthesiology. The society recognized that characteristics associated with rare complications can best be identified using a large population base rather than from prospective clinical studies that typically enroll few patients. Furthermore, the goal was to avoid assessing the incidence of complications at any individual institution because this may be more indicative of practice patterns unique to that institution and may occur more or less frequently than in the general population. The ultimate goals of the repository are to reliably estimate the incidences of serious complications and to improve patient safety by identifying factors associated with each complication. The data are collected by a self-report mechanism and institutional confidentiality is maintained by pooling all the data [40].

The American Society for Regional Anesthesia/Pain Medicine (ASRA) is also in the process of starting a database. It will collect basic demographic information on all patients, information about surgeon and anesthesiologist, type of anesthesia, and discharge information. With regard to regional anesthesia, it will collect information about the modalities used, the effectiveness of pain therapy and side-effects, follow-up information such as pain at home and major complications and will also ask the important question of whether the patient would want the same technique for a subsequent procedure [41].

The Malignant Hyperthermia Association of the United States (MHAUS) was founded in 1981 to educate the medical and lay communities about malignant hyperthermia (MH) and serve as a resource for families affected. In an effort to start a database, MHAUS merged with the North American MH Registry in 1995. The Registry, originally established in 1987, collected and recorded information about clinical episodes and the results of laboratory tests concerning MH in order to learn about the manifestations of the disorder [42]. As a result of these two organizations, a wealth of information has been obtained and recorded from clinical experiences. The data are obtained by self-report and the database is unique in that data are mostly collected while the crisis is occurring. When there is a case of malignant hyperthermia, a caller rings the MH hotline, where an expert will help the caller manage the situation that is occurring. All calls are logged at the time of the initial contact. There is attempted follow-up for each call, but this is difficult to obtain for every case. As a result, in most cases entered into the database, the final diagnosis is never known.

The Anesthesia Patient Safety Foundation (APSF), developed in 1985, has also been an advocate for outcomes research specifically in the field of anesthesia and has recognized the need for aggregate databases. A major initiative by this foundation started in 2001 when the APSF endorsed the use of anesthesia information management systems (AIMS) as a means of collecting data in order to easily review patient records for the purpose of research and practice analysis. It soon encountered a barrier to meeting the goal when it discovered that there is a lack of standardization for terms in different AIMS systems, and this problem inhibits the sharing of data across institutions. This was the same barrier that the National Center for Clinical Outcomes Research (NCCOR) encountered in the late 1990s when that organization embarked on the same mission of developing a data warehouse to which participants would send their perioperative records. In 2002, the APSF announced the launch of the Data Dictionary Task Force (DDTF) to define and address the problem of consistency and communication in surgical anesthesia. The long-term goal is to develop an active data dictionary that will direct database systems to obtain outcome data and to link to computer-based anesthesia record keepers nationwide [43].

The most recent investment by the specialty of anesthesiology in making a national clinical database has been made by the American Society of Anesthesiologists (ASA). This organization announced the launch of the Anesthesia Quality Institute (AQI) in October 2008. The mission of the AQI is to develop and maintain an ongoing registry of case data that helps anesthesiologists assess and improve patient care. The eventual goal is to provide a resource for anesthesiologists to obtain patient safety and quality management data and to meet regulatory requirements designed to improve patient care. The data will be useful for activities ranging from education to outcomes measurement to emerging federal efforts to ensure performance improvement [44].

The impetus for the formation of this quality database came from several quarters. Not only was there a desire to form a national database to permit research about clinical quality, but the ASA wanted to respond to the growing need for objective measures of anesthesia performance. As the public desire for transparency grows, the drive for reporting performance data increases. The AQI has accepted the responsibility to determine that the metrics by which the public and government judge anesthesiologists are legitimate and meaningful. The belief is that individual anesthesiologists or groups of anesthesiologists will need to document their performance metrics and outcomes against benchmark data. Therefore, a strong and validated anesthesia process and outcome database will become a necessity for future practice [45].

The AQI national database is called the National Anesthesia Clinical Outcomes Registry (NACOR). The NACOR goal is to eventually capture data on all of the anesthetics and pain clinic procedures performed each year by anesthesiologists in the United States. These data will be evaluated and analyzed by the AQI, and then the information will be reported back to the providers in an effort to guide approaches to anesthesia. After the data are assimilated, the information will be disseminated to the wider anesthesia community for education purposes.

Electronic anesthesia information system and databases

The electronic anesthesia information management system (AIMS), although utilized currently in less than

50% of anesthesia departments, is expected to gain more widespread use fairly quickly in the next several years [46] (see Chapter 44 for a complete discussion of AIMS). The collection of electronic anesthesia records, pre- and postoperative anesthesia documentation into larger databases with computerized search capabilities has made both clinical and outcomes research possible, as demonstrated by recent publications.

Kraemer et al [47] assessed the incidence of bradycardia and hypotension during sevoflurane induction in children with Down syndrome, with a case–control retrospective analysis. Using an electronic anesthesia record-keeping system (Compurecord, Phillips Healthcare, Bothell, WA), they searched for patients meeting study criteria with Down syndrome and sevoflurane induction. They selected a control group of patients without Down syndrome. They then used the database's computerized searching capabilities to assess the incidence of bradycardia, using predefined criteria, in the first 360 sec of administration of sevoflurane, in the electronic data which were stored every 15 sec. They then used the search capabilities to extract additional data, including sevoflurane end-tidal concentrations, other drugs administered, demographic data, co-existing conditions, and ASA physical status. They determined that bradycardia and hypotension were significantly more frequent with Down syndrome (57% versus 12%), and that Down syndrome conferred a relative risk ratio of 54 (95% confidence interval 14–206, p < 0.001), after multivariable analysis.

Large-scale anesthesia and perioperative outcomes research has now become possible with pooled AIMS databases from multiple institutions [48]. One such effort is the Multicenter Perioperative Outcomes Group (MPOG), formed in 2008 by the University of Michigan Department of Anesthesiology and several other large departments with well-developed AIMS [49]. Requirements for membership include deployment of an AIMS system capable of collecting a minimum electronic data set, contribution of at least 10,000 anesthetic cases to the consortium, obtaining local institutional review board approval for collection and transmission of data, developing and configuring electronic data interfaces to transfer data, and completing data transfer agreements with MPOG. Over 40 institutions are now participating, including several large children's hospital departments of anesthesia. Research projects can be initiated by individuals or institutions with permission of the MPOG leadership. This approach has the potential to pool tens or even hundreds of thousands of anesthetics, with complete electronic data for objective assessment, for high-quality outcomes research in anesthesia in response to specific research questions.

Perioperative databases

National Surgical Quality Improvement Program (NSQIP)

The National Surgical Quality Improvement Program (NSQIP) is an important database run by the American College of Surgeons (ACS). This program grew out of a congressionally mandated requirement that the Veterans Administration (VA) compare its surgical outcomes with national norms [50]. As a result, in the early 1990s VA nurses collected numerous preoperative, intraoperative and postoperative data points on surgical patients. After risk adjustment of presurgery status, the data were used to compare actual outcome with expected outcome developed from performance of the group as a whole. These data allowed risk-adjusted analysis of surgical outcomes. Those hospitals with poor outcomes were able to take steps to improve their outcomes [51].

The success of the VA program led to interest in the private sector, and a pilot group of 14 hospitals began to collect data. With these data the hospitals attempted to improve in areas where their actual outcomes were not as good as the expected outcomes. A study of the hospitals who adopted the program demonstrated reductions in morbidity, surgical site infections, and renal complications [51]. Seeing the successful results of the study in 14 hospitals, in the mid/late 1990s the ACS developed the NSQIP. Currently NSQIP collects 136 variables in a rigidly defined sample of both inpatient and outpatient surgical patients in participating hospitals. The data include demographic data, preoperative risk factors, laboratory values, operative information, and outcome data. What makes this database important is that the data are clinical data, and that they are collected carefully, and rigid data quality monitoring is carried out. Data gatherers are extensively trained, and periodic audits of data gathering are conducted on site [51]. Tests of inter-rater reliability are carried out periodically. Another benefit is that the data include 30-day outcomes, not just outcomes while the patient is in the hospital.

From the data, using statistical methods, the program determines expected risk-adjusted outcomes and determines the observed/expected ratio. This information provides risk-adjusted outcomes and allows comparison of a hospital's outcomes with external benchmarks. These data can then be used in programs to improve the quality of care. The value of NSQIP has been reported by Hall et al [52]. They looked at whether the observed/expected ratios reduced over time. In 118 hospitals 66% of hospitals had improvement of O/E ratios over 3 years.

Once the database had been established with reliable clinical data, many useful clinical studies were completed. One of the values of this database is that it represents everyday clinical practice and not the somewhat unusual circumstances often seen with patients involved in clinical trials. For example, Kiran et al [53] compared surgical site infection rates after colorectal surgery using open surgical approaches and laparoscopic approaches. They studied 3414 laparoscopic cases and 7565 open cases submitted in 2006–07 to the ACS NSQIP. The overall infection rate was 9.5% for laparoscopic cases and 16.1% for open cases. An interesting finding that is available because of the extensive data in the database is that the risk based on co-morbidities was higher in those patients with open procedures, presumably because sicker patients were offered open surgery more often.

Page et al [54] used the database to examine whether the laparoscopic approach to appendectomy has benefits over the open approach. In this situation, the benefits of laparoscopy are not as clear, as the complication rate with open procedures is relatively small and a large number of cases is required to demonstrate the superior technique. Page et al studied data from 17,199 patients who underwent appendectomy, 3025 open and 14,174 laparoscopic. Laparoscopic patients had shorter length of stay, lower incidence of wound disruptions, and lower perioperative mortality.

Another use of a database such as NSQIP is to prioritize quality improvement efforts. One group carried out such an effort in orthopedic surgery [55]. They reasoned that it is important to direct quality improvement efforts to those areas where the need is greatest, as defined as those procedures that generate the greatest number of adverse events. They examined the database first to find orthopedic procedures and then to find those procedures that contributed most to the occurrence of adverse events and to excess length of stay in hospital. They found that 10 procedures (hip fractures, total hips and knees, and others) accounted for 70% of adverse events and 65% of excess hospital days. They recommend that orthopedic surgeons and hospitals use these data to focus quality improvement efforts toward those areas that will benefit the most.

Merkow et al [56] examined variability in reoperation rates as a target for quality improvement efforts. Using NSQIP data, they examined reoperation rates in patients who had colorectal procedures. Reoperations occurred more often than expected in 16 hospitals and less often than expected in seven. The following factors were associated with a higher risk of reoperation: higher ASA class, male gender, contaminated wounds, surgical extent, surgical indication, and smoking.

Pediatric National Surgical Quality Improvement Program

The patients whose data have been submitted to NSQIP have largely been adults, but recently several pediatric hospitals have joined NSQIP in a pediatric model. As of October 2010, 27 institutions are submitting pediatric data, using a sampling model that is similar to adult NSQIP. The program is currently in a β-test mode. The pediatric model samples patients under 18 years of age and it is different from the adult NSQIP in that it includes more subspecialty cases. Thus, it includes cases from general surgery, thoracic surgery, orthopedic, ENT, urology, plastic surgery, and neurosurgery. It does not include trauma. Data from the α-test were published in 2010 [57]. The purpose of the report was to provide a summary of phase I results, identify variables associated with postoperative occurrences, and outline potential areas of focus as the ACS NSQIP Pediatric moves toward the use of data for surgical quality improvement.

A total of 7287 patients were evaluated during the initial phase. There were 22 deaths captured (0.3%). A total of 287 patients (3.9%) had one or more postoperative complications. These complications were four times more likely in patients undergoing inpatient procedures versus outpatient procedures. Factors associated with a higher likelihood of postoperative occurrences included a nutritional or immune history such as preoperative weight loss or chronic steroid use and a history of physiological compromise, such as sepsis or inotrope use before surgery. Operative factors associated with occurrences included multiple procedures under the same anesthetic and ASA classification category 4 or 5 versus 1. Variability in outcomes was demonstrated across participating sites as well as across surgical specialties. This finding supported the potential of the project to identify improvement targets in the future, although risk-adjusted performance evaluation of the small number of pilot sites was not attempted.

Several specific challenges to developing a quality improvement program for children's surgery were identified in this preliminary report. First, mortality and morbidity event rates after surgery are low in the pediatric patient population. A second challenge to measuring surgical quality in children is that the procedures for which morbidity and mortality are high are uncommon. The last challenge to measuring surgical quality in children involves the data burden associated with data collection, the number of variables needed for risk adjustment, and the duration of follow-up [57].

While the adult NSQIP data are being effectively used for evaluation of surgical care, and there is promise with pediatric data, less is being done with anesthesia care. As noted above, the AQI is still in the start-up phase, and anesthesia comparative effectiveness research has had to rely on other, administrative databases.

Outcomes and effectiveness research using databases

Outcomes research was established in 1988 when the Health Care Financing Administration (HCFA) of the US Department of Health and Human Services proposed an "Effectiveness Initiative." In this case, the initiative was in response to work on geographic variations in medical practice, appropriateness of care, the poor quality of medical evidence, congressional reluctance to fund health services research, and Medicare costs [58]. The initiative was the first attempt at finding a solution to these interrelated problems.

To start the initiative, the HCFA requested that the Institute of Medicine, National Academy of Sciences recommend those clinical conditions that should receive initial priority attention. The first five high-priority medical conditions that the outcomes research initiative focused on were acute myocardial infarction, angina (stable and unstable), breast cancer, congestive heart failure, and hip fracture. The goal of the initiative was to assess the success of different interventions in treating the identified clinical conditions in an effort to guide clinicians in the management of patients and to aid policy makers in allocating Medicare resources. In return, the HCFA would make the information gathered in its database available to the medical community for analysis of effectiveness. Any new information gathered from clinical demonstrations or trials would be available for review. As a result, the first outcomes research national database was established.

One goal of a national program is to collect information in a common database in order to conduct comparative effectiveness research. The definition of outcomes and effectiveness research has been described in numerous ways. One group reviewed all seminal and contemporary descriptions of outcomes and effectiveness research in order to arrive at an encompassing definition of the topic. The definition they arrived at was as follows.

Outcomes and effectiveness research evaluates the impact of healthcare (including discrete interventions such as particular drugs, medical devices, and procedures as well as broader programmatic or system interventions) on the health outcomes of patients and populations. It may include evaluation of economic impacts linked to health outcomes, such as cost effectiveness and cost utility. Outcomes and effectiveness research emphasizes health problem- (or disease-) oriented evaluations of care delivered in general, "real-world" settings; multidisciplinary teams; and a wide range of outcomes, including mortality, morbidity, functional status, mental well-being, and other aspects of health-related quality of life. Outcomes and effec-

tiveness research may entail any in a range of primary data collection methods and secondary (or "synthetic") methods that combine data from primary studies [59].

The importance of this definition is that it encompasses all aspects of a patient's care. The definition includes evaluating whether a traditional biomedical measure, such as the result of a laboratory test, determines if a health intervention is necessary or successful, but it goes beyond that. This research also measures how people function and the patient's experiences with care. These outcomes are sometimes what matter most to patients. This is the key to understanding how to improve the quality of care.

In 1989, the initiative took legislative form in a law called the Omnibus Budget Reconciliation Act (OBRA). This law created the Agency for Health Care Policy and Research (AHCPR) which accepted the primary responsibility for carrying the initiative forward. The mandate was that the AHCPR would focus heavily on researching the outcomes and effectiveness of medical care and on the development and dissemination of practice guidelines. This represented an important hypothesis: guidance for optimal medical practice could be gleaned from analysis of data routinely gathered in the process of delivering and paying for patient care. This was the start of the trend in thinking that evidence instead of opinion should guide clinical decision making [58].

Essentially, a decade later, in 1999, the AHCPR was renamed the Agency for Healthcare Research and Quality (AHRQ). "Policy" was explicitly removed from the name because the agency did not want to be viewed as a regulatory body. Today, the AHRQ still makes advances towards its mission to improve the quality, safety, efficiency, and effectiveness of the nation's healthcare system. One of its successes has been through the Healthcare Cost and Utilization Project (HCUP) which has created a family of healthcare databases that focus on the data collection efforts of state data organizations, hospital associations, private data organizations, and the federal government to create a national information resource on patient care [60]. The HCUP includes the largest collection of longitudinal hospital care data in the United States, dating as far back as 1988. It contains six databases, three at the national level and three at the state level.

The Nationwide Inpatient Sample (NIS) collects inpatient data from over 1000 hospitals. It is the largest all-payer inpatient database in the US, dating back to 1988, and contains more than 100 clinical and non-clinical elements per hospital stay. These include, but are not limited to, primary and secondary diagnoses, primary and secondary procedures, admission and discharge status, patient demographics (e.g. gender, age, race, median income for ZIP code), expected payment source, total charges, length of stay, hospital characteristics (e.g. ownership, size, teaching status). The data are administrative data. The NIS is based on the data collection efforts of data organizations in participating states that maintain state-wide data systems and that have partnered with AHRQ.

The data are most commonly used to examine trends in healthcare costs, access, practice variation, and quality of care. Lee and Morell noted the limitations in using such a database to evaluate quality of care. For example, they reviewed two papers recently published using the NIS database about the rare complication of postoperative visual loss (POVL). While the strengths of the national database are the volume of entries and the breadth of sampling, limitations for this study of the database include incomplete data entry, lack of any intraoperative data from the anesthesia record, inability to verify POVL diagnosis, and inability to determine whether a condition was pre-existing. The process of how the data are collected and entered into the database merits scrutiny if used for something like evaluating quality of care. For example, commonly there are hospital employees who review hospital records to look for codes that may upgrade a patient's acuity status for reimbursement purposes. Hypothetically, this could result in the diagnoses of hypotension and POVL being entered in the patient's medical record, which could lead to potential conclusions that are arbitrary. It may be implied that intraoperative hypotension caused the POVL, without considering the baseline blood pressure or associated factors during the surgery. The search for associated factors in the medical record is much more intense when a complication arises [61].

The Kids' Inpatient Database (KID) [62] is the only all-payer inpatient care database for children in the United States. The KID contained data from 2–3 million hospital discharges for children. There has been greater success with data collection as the years have passed. The 1997 KID contained data drawn from 22 state inpatient databases on children 18 years of age and younger. By 2006, KID contained data drawn from 38 state inpatient databases on children 20 years of age and younger. The disadvantage for medical research purposes is that the KID database consists of administrative data. The data are collected in the same way as the NIS database and record the same 100 non-clinical and clinical elements.

The last national database developed through this project is the Nationwide Emergency Department Sample (NEDS). The NEDS is the largest all-payer emergency (ED) database in the United States. It was constructed using records from both the HCUP state emergency department databases (SEDD) and the state inpatient databases (SID). The SEDD captures information on ED visits that do not result in an admission (i.e. treat-and-release visits and

transfers to another hospital). The SID contains information on patients initially seen in the emergency room and then admitted to the same hospital [63]. This is an administrative database that records elements like primary and secondary ICD-9-CM diagnoses, primary and secondary ICD-9-CM and CPT-4 procedures, discharge status from the ED, patient demographics (e.g. gender, age, median income for ZIP code), expected payment source, total ED charges (for ED visits) and total hospital charges (for inpatient stays for those visits that result in admission), hospital characteristics (e.g. region, trauma center indicator, urban-rural location, teaching status).

The three state-level databases are the SID, SEDD, and the state ambulatory surgery database (SASD). The SID and SEDD database information contribute to make up the NEDS database.

The SID contains inpatient discharge abstracts in participating states, translated into a uniform format to facilitate multi-state comparisons and analyses. It is well suited for research that requires complete enumeration of hospitals and discharges within market areas or states. Researchers and policy makers use the SID to investigate questions unique to one state; to compare data from two or more states; to conduct market area research or small area variation analyses; and to identify state-specific trends in inpatient care utilization, access, charges, and outcomes. For example, one article that used the SID as a resource was published by Coben et al [64]. They compared motorcycle-related hospitalizations across states with differing helmet laws, looking at hospital discharge data from 33 states. Results revealed that motorcyclists hospitalized from states without universal helmet laws are more likely to die during the hospitalization, sustain severe traumatic brain injury, be discharged to long-term care facilities, and lack private health insurance. However, a major limitation to this study was the lack of specific helmet use information on individual cases.

The SEDD is an administrative database that captures discharge information on all emergency department visits that do not result in an admission. It has not been used as frequently as the SID for publishing thus far. Potential areas of research include injury surveillance, access to healthcare in a changing healthcare marketplace, trends and correlations between emergency department use and environmental events, emerging infections, occurrence of non-fatal, preventable illness, and community assessment and planning.

The state ambulatory surgery databases (SASD) are a powerful set of databases, from data organizations in participating States, that capture surgeries performed on the same day in which patients are admitted and released. It is an administrative database that has not been used as much as the SID for publishing thus far. However, it has potential to aid in areas needed to identify state-specific trends in ambulatory surgery utilization, access, charges, and outcomes [61].

Another national administrative database is managed by the National Association of Children's Hospitals and Related Institutions (NACHRI). This organization is made up of children's hospitals with members from the United States, Canada, Australia, the United Kingdom, Italy, China, and Mexico. In addition to hospitals, this organization also has representation from large pediatric units of medical centers and related health systems, including those that specialize in rehabilitative care of children with serious chronic or congenital illnesses. The purpose of the association is to provide a voice for health systems to ensure children's access to healthcare and the continuing ability of children's hospitals to provide services needed by children. To accomplish this, the NACHRI developed the Case Mix Comparative Data Program, a pediatric inpatient discharge database for children's hospitals in the United States [65].

Historically, the only indicator to monitor quality of care and utilization of services in the hospital setting was diagnosis-related groups (DRGs). However, DRGs have been criticized because they do not take into account the acuity of patients. For example, a child who is admitted with pneumonia and also had cystic fibrosis would be simply listed as having a diagnosis of pneumonia despite the significant co-morbidity. The NACHRI has developed all-patient refined DRGs (APR-DRGs) which take into account severity of illness and risk of mortality. In doing so, the NACHRI APR-DRG case mix comparative database now has the ability to separate out acuity levels within a diagnosis. The result is a sensitive tool to determine variances in care [66]. Using the only pediatric acuity measures available, the database helps target quality improvement activities, enhance hospital utilization, develop pricing strategies and evaluate the likely effects of alternative prospective payment systems.

An example of how the NACHRI database has been used in a real setting was demonstrated at the University of Michigan Mott Children's Hospital (UMMCH). Sedman et al [66] reported using the NACHRI APR-DRG case mix comparative database to research non-complicated asthma cases (level 1 severity). The data showed that the UMMCH average length of hospital stay was longer than the NACHRI data for the same population (2.16 days versus 2.14 days). Also, the UMMCH cost per case was higher ($2824 versus $2738). Furthermore, their cases of moderate, major, and extreme severity were lower than the national aggregate. This showed that the APR-DRG system is sensitive enough to distinguish variances of care within a diagnosis according to severity level. The UMMCH went on to redesign its clinical processes to improve quality in the level 1 severity group.

Another database for practice improvement has come from the Virtual Pediatric Intensive Care Unit (VPICU) that started in 1997. The VPICU was started with the vision of creating a common information space for the international community of caregivers providing critical care for children. After the VPICU was initiated, it collaborated with the NACHRI to develop a database to define, understand, and improve pediatric critical care. Today, there are over 250,000 patient admissions to the database. The database is unique in that it utilizes severity of illness adjustment tools in an effort to insure that patients with similar severity of illnesses are compared. The core purpose of the prospective data collection is quality improvement. This effort includes comparative data reporting and the availability of comprehensive quality reports and tracking for individual institutions [67].

A recent trend in perioperative safety research is to look at not just issues traditionally associated with anesthesia but the entire encounter. As anesthesia becomes safer, it is important to look at potential contributions of anesthesia to the healing and recovery process. This sort of research is an important part of comparative effectiveness research, and extends the concept to looking at what happens in everyday practice as opposed to what happens in controlled clinical trials, where as many factors as possible are controlled [48]. Memtsoudis et al [68] examined perioperative outcomes after unilateral and bilateral total knee arthroplasty. The question is if a patient needs bilateral total knees, is it best to do them together, staged during the same hospitalization, or totally separately? Memtsoudis et al used the national inpatient sample to examine this question and found that there were worse outcomes with simultaneous procedures or procedures done during the same hospitalization. Kheterpal uses this as an example of the kinds of research that anesthesiologists should start getting involved in [48].

The important question is, does anesthesia have effects on recovery and later outcomes that we are not currently tracking? For pediatrics, one important current question is: is there an impact of anesthetic exposure by neonates on longer term neural and cognitive development? The use of databases has the potential to shed some light on these issues. See Chapter 41 for a complete discussion of anesthesia neurotoxicity.

Study design issues for outcomes research: comparison of non-inferiority (equivalence) statistics to traditional superiority statistics

Compared to a superiority trial whose aim is to determine if one intervention is superior to another (control) intervention, non-inferiority trials aim to determine if one intervention is similar to another [69]. In superiority trials, the null hypothesis is that the treatments are equally effective and the alternative hypothesis is that they differ. In a non-inferiority or equivalence trial, the null hypothesis is that the treatments differ and the alternative hypothesis is that they are equally effective [70] (Fig. 43.1). An important point is that a superiority trial should not conclude that the groups are equivalent if the null hypothesis is true. If the primary objective of a study is to prove equivalence then the study design, conduct, and data analysis should be based on the null hypothesis that the treatments differ.

Non-inferiority designs are useful when the new treatment is more favorable than standard therapy in other ways than the one being tested (economic benefit, ease of use, etc.). In this case, even showing that the two treatments are equivalent would justify the use of the new treatment. For example, an equivalence trial comparing hydroxyethyl starch (HES) and hetastarch showed that the two treatments are equally effective as plasma volume substitutes but HES has less of an effect on coagulation [71].

It is important when reviewing outcomes and effectiveness research to understand who is influencing the drive behind the research and who is interpreting the results. Organizations may serve as producers, consumers, or sponsors of research. The nature and intensity of this involvement vary dramatically as a function of the type, size, commitment, and history of the organization. This overlap of interest becomes apparent, for instance, when a managed care plan funds its own research for use in internal policy decisions. The interest of each group drives production in what areas will be researched. It is for this reason that the topics of research in the public and private sectors do not significantly overlap. The research is used in a focused way to promote business goals and other organizational objectives.

Departmental and institutional requirements for database participation

As noted throughout this chapter, information collected in the course of routine clinical anesthetic care is often not in a form that is organized and accessible for databases, and thus not useful for clinical or outcomes research. Databases, whether organized from data entered by clinicians or researchers or collected automatically from AIMS, require significant institutional and departmental commitments in the form of infrastructure (hardware and software), information technology expertise, a clear strategy and standards for entering and auditing data, and personnel to maintain the systems. Most of these elements are not provided for in routine clinical care, and the additional financial and personnel resources require a long-term commitment. The benefit to patient care, quality and outcomes, and contribution to research in these areas need to be demonstrated to department and hospital leadership. Box 43.1 lists the components needed for departmental participation in anesthesia and perioperative databases.

Conclusion

Databases for pediatric anesthesiology are in their infancy. New initiatives within the subspecialty and participation in larger anesthesiology and perioperative databases are increasing, and hold promise to hasten the pace of data-driven improvement in care and outcomes, with properly performed studies with valid data in adequate numbers of patients to draw valid conclusions. As a subspecialty, pediatric anesthesiology will need to commit to acquiring expertise in databases to maximally affect the improvements available in this rapidly advancing field.

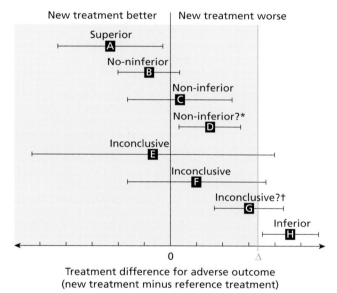

Figure 43.1 Possible scenarios of observed treatment differences for adverse outcomes (harms) in non-inferiority trials. Error bars indicate two-sided 85% confidence intervals (CIs). Tinted area indicates zone of inferiority. (A) If the CI lies wholly to the left of zero, the new treatment is superior. (B,C) If the CI lies to the left of Δ and includes zero, the new treatment is non-inferior but not shown to be superior. (D) If the CI lies wholly to the left of Δ and wholly to the right of zero, the new treatment is non-inferior in the sense already defined, but it is also inferior in the sense that a null treatment difference is excluded. This puzzling case is rare, since it requires a very large sample size. It can also result from having too wide a non-inferiority margin. (E,F) If the CI includes Δ and zero, the difference is non-significant but the result regarding non-inferiority is inconclusive. (G) If the CI includes Δ and is wholly to the right of zero, the difference is statistically significant but the result is inconclusive regarding possible inferiority of magnitude Δ or worse. (H) If the CI is wholly above Δ, the new treatment is inferior. Reproduced from Piaggio et al [70] with permission from the American Medical Association.

Box 43.1 Necessary components for departmental and institutional participation in anesthesia databases

- Leadership
  - Departmental vision and strategy for databases; anesthesiologist expertise in database design, management, maintenance
  - Strategies and processes for integration with institutional databases and hospital electronic medical records
- Information technology expertise
  - Database designers working with clinical and research staff to maximize efficiency and accuracy of data entry according to purpose of database; collect data over and above standard clinical and administrative databases
- Anesthesia information management systems
  - Interface for collection of clinical data into research database; search capabilities of clinical database for research and outcomes projects
- Computer hardware and software
  - Proper software to collect and organize data locally and allow connection to local networks and databases as well as transmission to national data warehouses
  - Hardware, including adequate computing power and speed, and high-capacity redundant data storage capacity
- HIPAA , legal, and IRB compliance
  - Patient permission for data collection for research, appropriate de-identified data, IRB approval for research
  - Compliance with hospital, institutional, local, state, and federal requirements for data collection and sharing
- Participation in national databases
  - Institutional legal agreements for participation, financial costs of participation, permission for research projects, benchmarking of institutional data versus de-identified data from outside institutions
- Local database personnel to enter data
  - Clinicians (attendings, fellows, residents, OR nurses, research nurses and other personnel)
- Audit procedures
  - Well-defined criteria for auditing or correcting data before analysis or transmission to national data consortia
- Financial resources
  - Realistic budget and business plan; calculated return on investment in databases: quality and outcomes, research, financial

Annotated references

A full reference list for this chapter is available at:
http://www.wiley.com/go/gregory/andropoulos/pediatricanesthesia

8. Welke KF, Diggs BS, Karamlou T, Ungerleider RM. Comparison of pediatric cardiac surgical mortality rates from national administrative data to contemporary clinical standards. Ann Thorac Surg 2009; 87: 216–23. An important discussion of the differences between large administrative databases and detailed clinical databases for mortality research.

11. Malin B, Karp D, Scheuermann RH. Technical and policy approaches to balancing patient privacy and data sharing in clinical and translational research. J Invest Med 2010; 58: 11–18. A recent discussion of problems with data sharing and patient privacy in clinical databases used for research.

13. Cheney FW. The American Society of Anesthesiologists Closed Claims Project. Anesthesiology 2010; 113: 957–60. A description of the design and accomplishments of the landmark database in anesthesiology.

22. Bhananker SM, Ramamoorthy C, Geiduschek JM et al. Anesthesia-related cardiac arrest in children: update from the Pediatric Perioperative Cardiac Arrest Registry. Anesth Analg 2007; 105: 344–50. An important update from the longest standing pediatric anesthesia registry.

25. Flick RP, Sprung J, Harrison TE et al. Perioperative cardiac arrests in children between 1988 and 2005 at a tertiary referral center: a study of 92,881 patients. Anesthesiology 2007; 106: 226–37. An important example of a large, single institutional database used to study infrequent events in pediatric anesthesia.

26. Baum VC, Barton DM, Gutgesell HP. Influence of congenital heart disease on mortality after noncardiac surgery hospitalized children. Pediatrics 2000; 105: 332–35. Example of a large national administrative database used to study mortality in pediatric perioperative care.

28. Vener DF, Jacobs JP, Schindler E, Maruszewski B, Andropoulos D. Databases for assessing the outcomes of the treatment of patients with congenital and paediatric cardiac disease – the perspective of anaesthesia. Cardiol Young 2008; 18 (Suppl. 2): 124–9. A description of the design and rationale of the combined Congenital Cardiac Anesthesia Society/Society of Thoracic Surgeons database.

32. Cravero JP, Beach ML, Blike GT et al. The incidence and nature of adverse events during pediatric sedation/anesthesia with propofol for procedures outside the operating room: a report from the Pediatric Sedation Research Consortium. Anesth Analg 2009; 108: 795–804. An important outcome research study from a large consortium of sedation providers voluntarily submitting quality data.

47. Kraemer FW, Stricker PA, Gurnaney HG et al. Bradycardia during induction of anesthesia with sevoflurane in children with Down syndrome. Anesth Analg 2010; 111: 1259–63. An important recent example of clinical research with electronic anesthesia record data.

57. Raval MV, Dillion PW, Bruny JL et al. American College of Surgeons National Surgical Quality Improvement Program Pediatric: a Phase 1 report. J Am Coll Surg 2011; 212: 1–11. A new report on the perioperative quality database initiative in pediatric patients.

CHAPTER 44

Electronic Anesthesia and Medical Records

James Edward Caldwell & David Robinowitz

Department of Anesthesia and Perioperative Care, University of California San Francisco, San Francisco, CA, USA

Medical electronic databases: usefulness, drawbacks

Documentation in medicine is moving inexorably from the paper to the electronic realm. An electronic medical record (EMR) is the legal record created by a hospital or health care institution. The EMR is the data source for the electronic health record (EHR) and is a different concept [1]. The EHR represents the vehicle by which medical information can be shared between stakeholders and will allow a patient's information to follow them through the various areas of their care. Stakeholders include patients, providers, employers, and third party payers.

Anesthesia documentation is also moving in the direction of electronic records, but perhaps more slowly than in other areas of medicine, despite being advocated for over 20 years ago [2]. To reflect the fact that these systems have potential that goes beyond simply documentation, the term commonly used is anesthesia information management system (AIMS). The relatively slow progress in converting anesthesia to an electronic system is because there are some very specific aspects of anesthesia documentation that make conversion from the paper to the electronic medium particularly challenging. This chapter discusses the overall movement of health documentation to the electronic realm, with special focus on anesthesia records.

Computers are the tools used to implement electronic systems and have actually been used in medicine for several decades. In the era of mainframe computers in the 1960s, a decision support system was developed at the University of Leeds to aid in the diagnosis of acute abdominal pain. In the 1970s, the minicomputer arrived, and significant computing power was available at the level of clinical departments. The personal computing era arrived in the 1980s and individual physicians have had access to computers of ever increasing power and at decreasing cost.

With this computational ability, many individuals and departments developed and used home-grown electronic record systems in their practice. However, the healthcare industry as a whole has been relatively slow to adopt enterprise-wide electronic systems for managing health information. Even now, less than 5% of healthcare institutions have enterprise-wide electronic medical documentation, and only 17% have computerized physician order entry (CPOE) for medications [3]. The penetration for electronic records has increased over the past few years and the pace of change will likely accelerate [4]. Powerful external forces are driving the adoption of electronic systems in healthcare.

There is a strong, though not yet well-substantiated belief that use of electronic systems such as CPOE systems will improve quality of care and patient safety. As a result, there is encouragement (in some cases a mandate) at both the federal and state level for healthcare institutions to adopt electronic information systems.

In 2004, then President George W. Bush ordered the Department of Health and Human Services to develop a national health information network [5]. The task was to be complete within 10 years and was allocated to a newly created entity, the Office of the National Coordinator for Health Information Technology. In 2009 President Barack Obama called for a national system of electronic health records by 2014. The Health Information Technology for Economic and Clinical Health Act (HITECH) of 2009 was a part of the American Recovery and Reinvestment Act (ARRA). This "stimulus" bill authorized incentive payments to hospitals that used EHRs in a "meaningful" way [6].

It is unlikely that a national system will be in place by 2014. In the meantime, regional networks of electronic health information are being created [7]. These regional networks will then feed into state networks which will in turn feed into the proposed national database. This patchwork approach raises the question of "interoperability," i.e. how well these various systems interact. This question is receiving a lot of national attention, but the problems are far from solved [5,7].

In addition to these outside forces, our own professional bodies, such as the Anesthesia Patient Safety Foundation (APSF), endorse the use of electronic records: "The APSF endorses and advocates the use of automated record keeping in the perioperative period and the subsequent retrieval and analysis of the data to improve patient safety." Finally, major purchasers of healthcare, such as the Leapfrog Group (an alliance of large corporations), have strongly advocated the use of CPOE systems. In the not too distant future, payments for services will be linked to use of electronic information systems.

Why convert from paper to electronic records?

By and large, clinicians are comfortable with the systems that they use every day. Where the systems don't work well, people have developed workarounds. Most clini-

Table 44.1 Paper versus electronic records: comparison of cardinal properties

	Paper	Electronic
Legibility	Variable, often poor	Excellent
Accessibility	One location only	Multiple access points
Reliability	May be lost	Backed up
Clinician comfort	High – familiarity	Wariness for change
Training required	Minimal	May be extensive
Data entry	Very unstructured	Structured
Viewing options	Limited	Extensive
Searching records	Labor intensive	Easy after initial set-up

cians use and are familiar and comfortable with paper records; less than 25% have used electronic documentation [3]. Consequently, clinicians may have a hard time giving up paper. To help make the case for electronic records, it is worth comparing the strengths of paper and electronic records.

Paper and electronic records compared

First, let's consider paper records (Table 44.1). They are familiar, probably the property that makes change most difficult. Data can be entered quickly and simply, the process of data entry is very flexible plus the whole record can be viewed easily. No special training is required. Finally, paper records do not break, i.e. they do not go "down" like electronic systems can.

On the downside, paper records are available in only one location, and this may not be where they are needed. Paper records can also be lost irretrievably, as was the personal experience of the current Surgeon General Regina Benjamin from Alabama after a destructive hurricane [8]. Legibility may be poor, space to enter information is restricted, there is no systematic standardized format of data entry, and ability to collect, monitor, and analyze information is poor [3]. The unused record looks pristine (Fig. 44.1A), but that property is lost as soon as documentation is started (Fig. 44.1B). This is an example of a real (de-identified) patient paper record at the University of California San Francisco. All the problems listed above are clearly demonstrated.

While a paper record is the traditional method of record keeping, it cannot be considered a "gold standard." The accuracy and completeness of data entry on a paper record are often inadequate [9], and the deficiencies are independent of the experience of the clinician [10]. In addition, adverse events are commonly under-reported on paper records [11]. Many of these deficiencies can be alleviated with electronic record keeping (Box 44.1). While an electronic record does not cram as much information on a single page as a paper record, the ability to

UCSF Medical Cer

☐ UCSF Medical Center San Francisco, CA (Check hospital location) ☐ UCSF / Medical San Fra

DATE | AGE | WT. (Kg) | HCT | NPO | ASA | OR RM

I/We verify attendance at all critical portions of the procedure.
Anesthesiologists:
(1)
(2)
(3)
START : END :
Resident/CRNA (1)
Resident/CRNA (2)
Attending Surgeon:
MEDICAL EVALUATION:
PREMED EFFECT ALLERGIES
(A)
DIAGNOSIS:
PERFORMED OPs:

UNIT NUMBER
PT. NAME
BIRTHDATE
LOCATION DATE

☐ FiO₂ ☐ ECG ☐ Disc Alarm ☐ PNS ☐ A-line
☐ PET CO₂ ☐ BP Auto: (arm/leg: R / L) ☐ TEE ☐ CVP
☐ SpO₂ ☐ Temp ☐ Steth:ES/PCS ☐ EEG-EP ☐ PA
☐ Anes Agent ☐ HME ☐ Forced Air Wm ☐ Level 1 ☐ Fluid Warm
Anes Equipment, Drug, Gas Supply Checked by ________ (initial)

TIME TOTAL
AGENTS
N₂O / O₂ / Air

Pre-Induction
BP
P
Sp O₂
Induction
☐ Pre Oxygenation
☐ Intravenous
☐ Inhaled
☐ LTA: Lidocaine
☐ Cricoid Pressure
Airway Mgmt.
☐ Oral airway
☐ Nasal airway
☐ Mask
☐ LMA ______
Tracheal Intubation
☐ Oral ☐ Nasal
☐ Easy ☐ Difficult
☐ Atraumatic
Comments:
☐ Fiberoptic
Blade(s)
Cuff
Tube Size
☐ BS ☐ CO₂
☐ Eyes taped
☐ Pressure Points Padded

200
B.P. CUFF
150
ART LINE
100
M.A.P. ×
PULSE ●
SPONT. RESP. ⊙ 50
VT
f
PIP
FiO₂
Sp O₂
ET CO₂
ET %
ECG
TEMP.
URINE
EBL
Reference:
Positions: ☐ Supine ☐ Prone ☐ Sitting ☐ Lateral ☐ Jack-Knife ☐ Lithotomy

PACU
ICU
(circle unit)
BP:
P:
R:
SpO₂:
CONDITION
Stable
Unstable
TRANSPORT
O₂
ECG
SpO₂
A-line
ETT

ANES CARE
: TO :
ANES OR
START LEAVE END
: : :
COMMENTS
REMARKS:

Size-LOC Placed by Anesth.
IV ______ L R
IV ______ L R
IV ______ L R
Size-LOC Placed by Anesth.
ART ______ L R
CVP ______ L R
PA ______ L R
TEE: Inserted by ______ initial
☐ Adult ☐ Pediatric
Epidural / Block used for Post-op pain relief. ______ Initial

Reg. Block | Prep | Needle | Epidural Space ___ cm | Cath dpth @ skin ______ cm
Position | Interspace | Parasthesia | CSF/Blood

ANESTHESIA RECORD

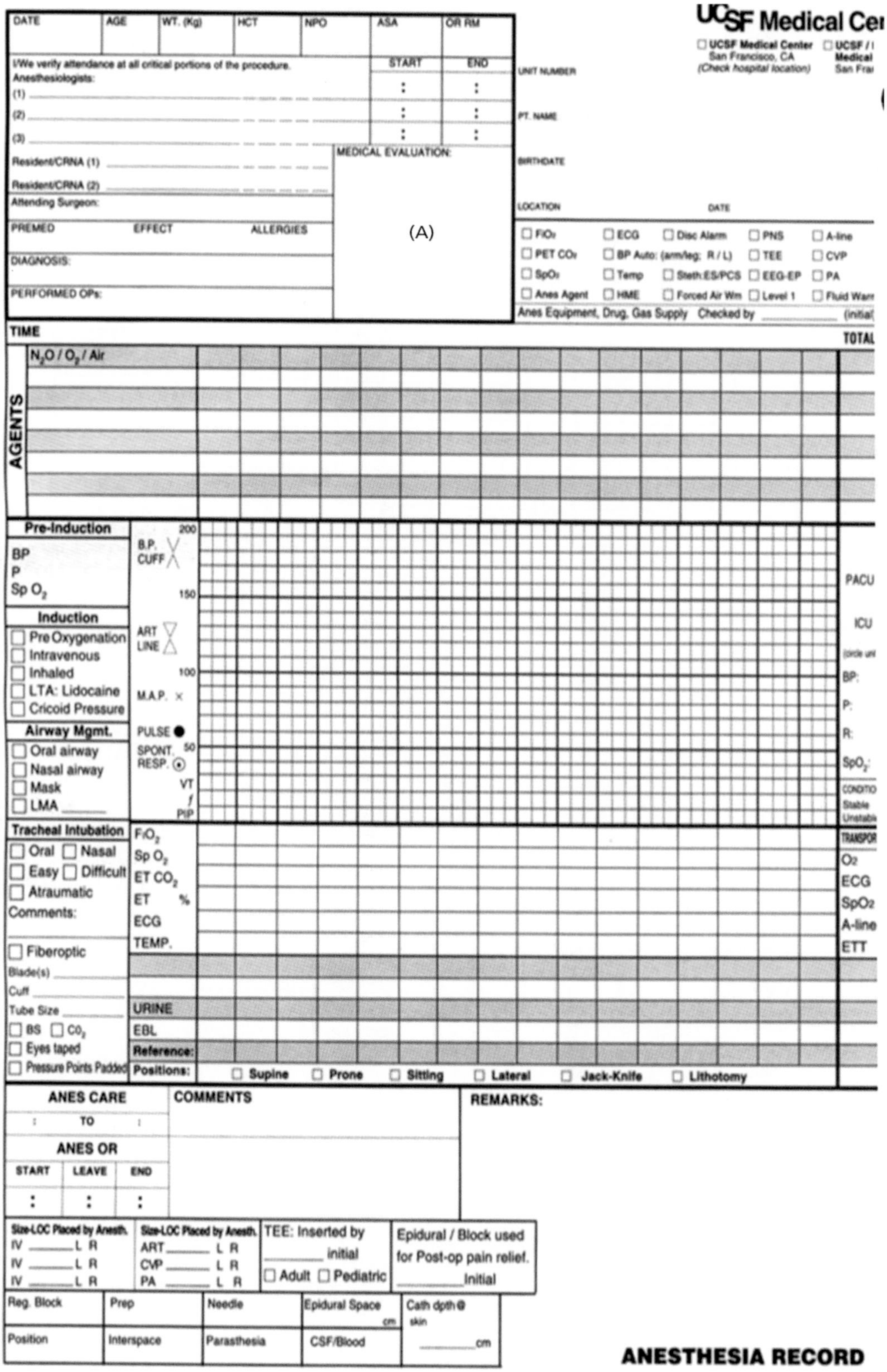

Figure 44.1 (A) Paper record before any entries are made. It appears well structured and clear. (B) The apparent structure of the empty record has disappeared. Many entries are barely legible. There is little space for entries, such as laboratory results. Someone looking at the record for the first time would not know where to find items such as antibiotics or a consistent description of procedures, events, etc. Many critical elements, such as pulse oximetry values, are entered only every 15 min.

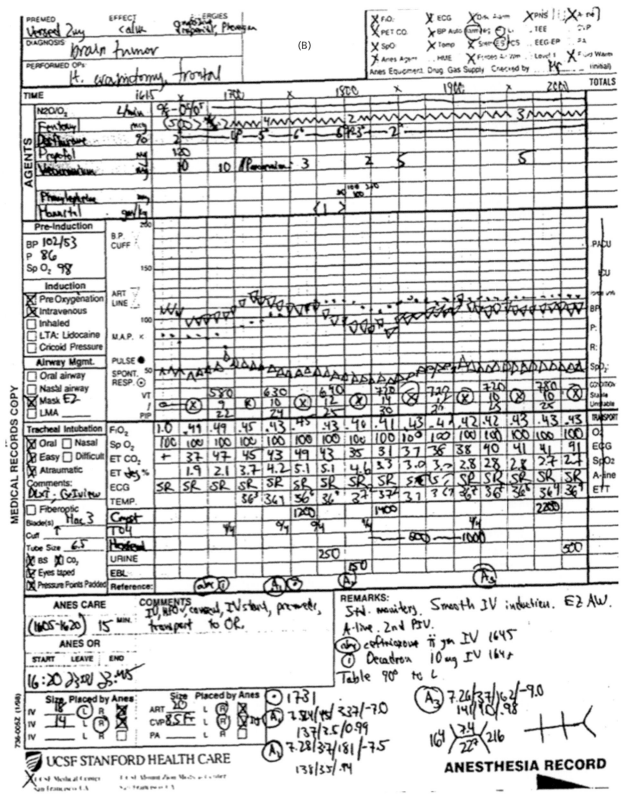

Figure 44.1 (Continued)

Box 44.1 The specific data elements that constitute protected health information (PHI)

- Names
- All geographic subdivisions smaller than a state
- All elements of dates and the age of patients over 89
- Telephone numbers
- Fax numbers
- Email addresses
- Social Security numbers
- Medical record numbers
- Health plan beneficiary numbers
- Account numbers
- Certificate/license numbers
- Vehicle identifiers and serial numbers
- Device identifiers and serial numbers
- Web Uniform Resource Locators (URLs)
- Internet protocol (IP) address numbers
- Biometric identifiers, including finger and voice prints
- Full-face or comparable photographic images
- Any other identifying number, characteristic (e.g. a tattoo), or code

view multiple screens allows for better legibility and data presentation (Fig. 44.2).

Electronic records are accessible from many locations, allow structured and standardized data input, allow multiple views and trending of the data, are legible, can link to other hospital systems, and allow for ongoing monitoring and systematic analysis of data [11–16]. Electronic records can be backed up in multiple locations so that they are never lost. Disadvantages of these records are that they are unfamiliar to many clinicians, require training, need ongoing support, and can go "down" for a variety of technical reasons. However, the eventual adoption of electronic records is inevitable and it is important that clinicians have influence in the process of choosing and implementing an electronic record-keeping system that they, the clinicians, must use.

Reasons to adopt an electronic anesthesia system
Enhance quality of patient care
This should always be the number 1 criterion driving change. It is easy to justify electronic medical record keeping on this one issue alone. Safety is enhanced by the easy accessibility and legibility of previous records, and by the ability to track outcomes and improve record keeping for quality improvement initiatives [17–19]. Electronic record keeping is a necessary first step in the move towards evidence-based practice and decision support. A good example of enhanced safety comes from the Children's Hospital of Philadelphia. Their electronic tracking of adverse events, specifically bronchos-

pasm, led the clinicians to stop using rapacuronium 8 months before it was withdrawn from the market by the company [20].

Increased provider satisfaction
With few exceptions, anesthesia providers embrace technology and believe that electronic records are an indication that they are working in a modern facility. Medical records are more readily available, data can be entered directly from other hospital systems, and the amount of time devoted to record keeping is decreased [21]. This leads to a perception that the overall quality of work is improved [16].

The financial case
Electronic information systems are very expensive to install and maintain, and it is difficult to demonstrate financial gains to offset these costs [22]. As described above, patient safety is enhanced and this has real but hard-to-quantify financial benefit [22]. Within anesthesia, the areas where financial benefits may be quantifiable are revenue and costs.

Increased revenue
Automated electronic error detection systems enhance anesthesia professional fee billing [23]. The identification of additional diagnoses and co-morbidities from an electronic anesthesia preoperative evaluation system allowed the use of additional ICD-9 codes in 12% of cases that increased hospital revenue 1.5% [24]. Additional areas of increased revenue are enhanced charge capture for specific high-cost drugs and for technical fees for anesthesia services.

Decreased costs
There is clear evidence that giving providers feedback on their drug costs, compared to those of their colleagues or other institutions, can bring down the average cost per case by 20% [12,13]. The problem is that the effect is transient and reverts to previous costs after 3 months without reinforcement. There is no way, using paper records, that the effort of gathering and disseminating drug use information to individuals can be sustained. In contrast, generating recurring drug and supply use reports is simple with electronic information systems [14]. Finally, there is accumulating evidence that electronic records decrease medico-legal liability and costs [25].

Potential problems with an electronic anesthesia system
The disadvantages of an electronic system relate mostly to costs, effort, and resources needed for implementation, maintenance, and upgrading. In addition, if data entry imposes significant additional workload on the clinician

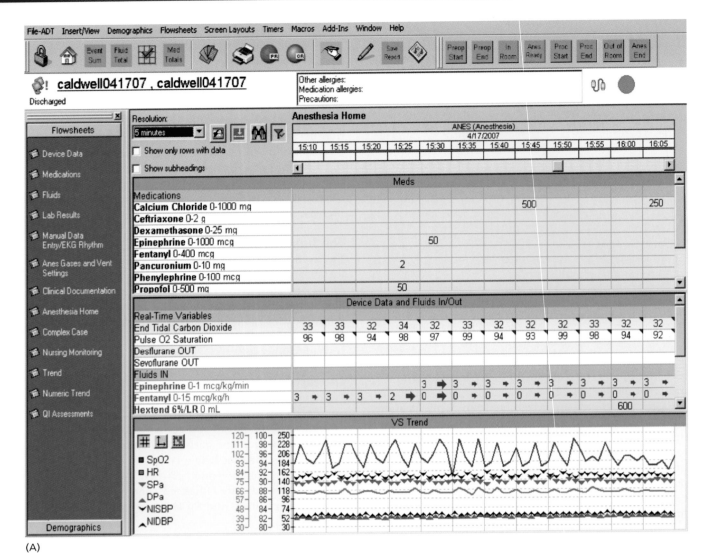

(A)

Figure 44.2 These illustrations are taken from the AIMS used at the University of California San Francisco. Their use in this figure does not imply an endorsement of the product. (A) This is an example of the default home screen in an electronic anesthesia system. All entries are legible and vital signs data are displayed at a 5-min resolution. The data display can be compressed by increasing the interval to 30 min, allowing for a summary view of a long case. Alternatively, the resolution can be increased to every 10 sec to allow very close inspection of rapidly changing events. Data are actually saved to the database at 1-min intervals. (B) Computer screens do not display the totality of information as a paper record does. Rather different pages are used to view different data summaries. This is a medication summary review. All the medications administered can be viewed by individual doses and totals. (C) This screen is a summary view of all fluids administered during the procedure. Individual totals and current fluid balance are automatically calculated by the application. (D) This shows a summary of procedures, e.g. airway management, performed by the anesthesia provider. In this example, all the entries are in structured data fields and so can be searched after the fact for purposes of analysis and reporting.

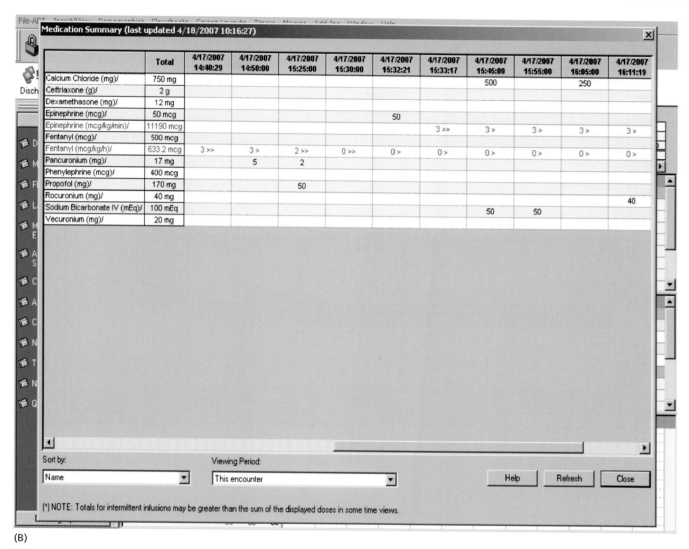

	Total	4/17/2007 14:40:29	4/17/2007 14:50:00	4/17/2007 15:25:00	4/17/2007 15:30:00	4/17/2007 15:32:21	4/17/2007 15:33:17	4/17/2007 15:45:00	4/17/2007 15:55:00	4/17/2007 16:05:00	4/17/2007 16:11:19
Calcium Chloride (mg)/	750 mg							500		250	
Ceftriaxone (g)/	2 g										
Dexamethasone (mg)/	12 mg										
Epinephrine (mcg)/	50 mcg					50					
Epinephrine (mcg/kg/min)/	11190 mcg						3 >>	3 >	3 >	3 >	3 >
Fentanyl (mcg)/	500 mcg										
Fentanyl (mcg/kg/h)/	633.2 mcg	3 >>	3 >	2 >>	0 >>	0 >	0 >	0 >	0 >	0 >	0 >
Pancuronium (mg)/	17 mg		5	2							
Phenylephrine (mcg)/	400 mcg										
Propofol (mg)/	170 mg			50							
Rocuronium (mg)/	40 mg										40
Sodium Bicarbonate IV (mEq)/	100 mEq							50	50		
Vecuronium (mg)/	20 mg										

Sort by:

Name

Viewing Period:

This encounter

Help   Refresh   Close

[*] NOTE: Totals for intermittent infusions may be greater than the sum of the displayed doses in some time views.

(B)

Figure 44.2 (Continued)

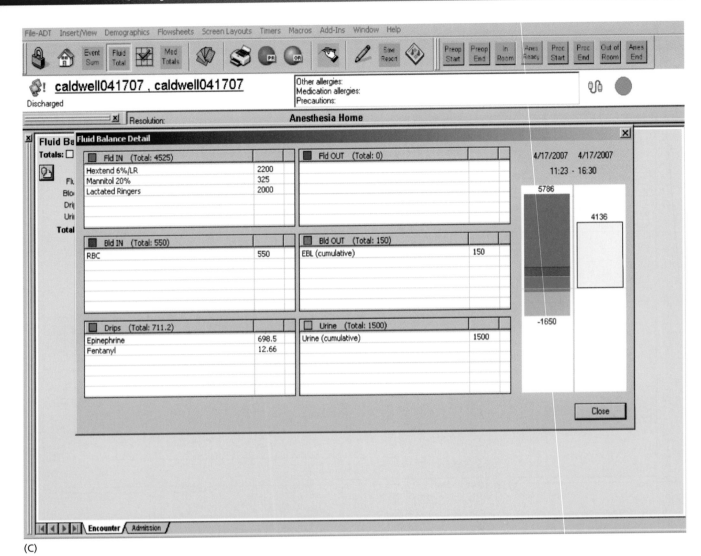

(C)

Figure 44.2 (*Continued*)

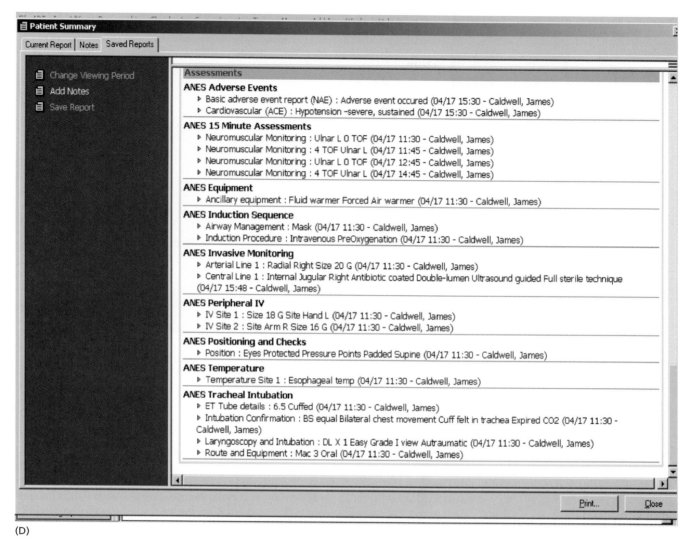

Figure 44.2 (*Continued*)

Computers in medicine

or the electronic infrastructure is unstable and the system goes down frequently, clinicians will soon become dissatisfied. Computers, screens, and keyboards may take up very valuable space within the clinical workspace (Fig. 44.3). Finally, it is possible to generate more paper after implementation of an electronic system due to printouts, and a specific printout may be required for your own institution [26].

Computers in medicine

Computers are the vehicles used to enable electronic documentation. Perhaps the most compelling reason to incorporate computer-based electronic information systems in anesthesia and medicine is that it is the only way to manage and effectively utilize the already large and rapidly increasing amount of information available. A

simple example is the proliferation of medications and the information on their interactions. An individual physician cannot keep details of drugs and their interactions in their head the way an earlier generation once did. There are more tests and services available and more tests performed on patients than ever before. Turnover of patients in hospitals has increased, and resident work hours require multiple transfers of care in a single day. The only way to manage the array of data and to pass it on safely between the members of the care team is by electronic means.

Standards

The use of computers to manage and share information has many consequences. The first of these is that common standards of information transfer need to be developed.

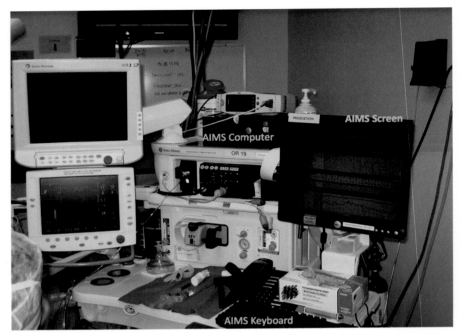

Figure 44.3 An electronic information system takes up a significant amount of real estate in the usually tight confines of the anesthesia workspace. In addition, the devices need network connection to the central database. This is a tough environment with risks to the equipment of damage from impact, fluids, and electrical interference. A good inventory of readily available spare parts, mouse, keyboards, cables, etc. is essential to keep the system up and running.

A simple definition of what constitutes a standard is that it is "what most people do." Standards familiar to most clinicians are the ICD-9 (International Classification of Diseases, version 9) and the CPT-4 (Current Procedural Terminology version 4) standards for describing diseases and medical procedures, respectively. Standards may be developed in several ways. The first and simplest way is that the dominant vendor in an area sets the standard. An example of this is the iPhone operating system. Second, a government agency, such as the Centers for Medicare and Medicaid Services (CMS) or National Institute for Standards and Technology (NIST), may mandate the use of an existing system. Finally, groups of interested parties can meet and develop standards independently. If the process has been sufficiently open and rigorous, these recommendations are adopted as standards, for example the Health Level 7 (HL7) standard for clinical data interchange.

There are many areas where standards have been developed and adopted in medicine, but there are several crucial areas, including AIMS, where there are no standards [26]. The most complex problem is perhaps that of medical terminology. Take, for example, the terms "heart attack," "cardiac infarction," "myocardial infarction." To a clinician they all mean the same thing but to a computer they are three different entities. Structured systems such

as the Unified Medical Language System (UMLS) and Systemized Nomenclature of Human and Veterinary Medicine (SNOMED) exist, but none has gained universal acceptance. Within the SNOMED systems, a subgroup of anesthesia-related terms is under development [27]. Developing standardized terminology is compounded by the problem that systems of nomenclature are required for all areas of healthcare, e.g. nursing, and in all applicable languages. Terminology must not just be standardized within a system; it must also be standardized across systems in different areas of healthcare.

Devices: why electronic anesthesia systems are different

There are two characteristics of anesthesia documentation that separate it from other areas in medicine. The first is that data are directly recorded in real time from devices, for example vital signs monitors and mechanical ventilators [28]. The second is that these devices and the associated computer workstation are connected to and can be linked with only one patient at a time. Consequently, if the system develops a problem, one cannot delay data entry or go to another workstation to enter the data. These characteristics impose unique demands for high data transfer capabilities, the reliability of the system, and the need for 24/7 immediate technical support.

Medical records

What is the medical record in the electronic world? The legal definition of the health record is "the composite documentation of healthcare services provided to an individual during any aspect of healthcare delivery in any type of healthcare organization." When all documentation was on paper and x-ray images were all on film, identifying the legal health record was easy. The contents of the paper chart (including the paper anesthesia record) plus x-rays formed the healthcare provider's legal business (medical) record. The advent of the EHR has complicated matters considerably.

Now the legal health record comprises a wide variety of individually identifiable data stored on any medium, electronic, paper or a hybrid. The purpose of the legal record remains the same: to support decisions made in the patient's care, to provide justification for revenue claims to payers, and to support legal testimony pertinent to both of these. The legal health record is not the totality of the patient's EHR; rather, it is a subset of records, which serves as the legal business record for the organization.

Medico-legal issues in electronic records

Concerns over electronic record systems and medical liability were raised back in 1997 at a time when very few institutions had electronic medical records. At the time, the question did not generate much urgency [29]. However, with the rapid expansion of the use of EHRs, the question is now receiving a lot of attention [30]. From a medico-legal perspective, EHRs confer both benefit and risk.

Discoverability and electronic records

Since the legal health record is now a subset of a potentially much larger dataset comprising the full EHR, the legal issue arises of how much of the EHR is discoverable. The courts are in the process of defining limits to discoverability, but many issues remain unsettled. Some areas have been identified that generally are not discoverable in litigation. Examples include fragmented information on hard drives, items that are temporary, such as cookies, and other transient information that would require extraordinary efforts to preserve. Exceptions can be made when justified, but the courts will likely discourage "fishing expeditions" through the EHR by attorneys.

Another question relates to the format in which the 'discoverable" data will be produced. In the days of paper records this was simple; the patient's chart or a photocopy of the original record could be produced. It is a very different situation with an electronic record. With paper, what constitutes the anesthesia record is obvious. With an AIMS, there are tens of thousands of individual electronic data elements stored in every patient's record. In what format should that be produced for litigation? In practical terms, most AIMS include some form of clinical summary of the record that can be read much as a paper record would be. While it will depend on an individual institution's policies and procedures, and on some degree of negotiation between parties to the litigation, it is most likely that this is the form of the record that would be produced for discovery [31].

Medico-legal benefit of electronic records

As described earlier, electronic records are more legible than paper records, documentation is standardized and likely to be more complete, and other information, such as pertinent laboratory results, is likely to be included. A survey by the Medical Records Institute of practitioners using EHRs found that 50% felt they were better protected against malpractice claims, and 20% reported a reduction in their malpractice premiums. Of the anesthesia departments that were using an AIMS and were also involved in a malpractice lawsuit, the majority viewed the electronic record as helpful [25].

Areas of possible medico-legal risk with electronic records

An inevitable area of risk with electronic records is the privacy and security of the patient's protected health information (PHI). These risks will be covered more fully in the following section on privacy. Specifically in the realm of anesthesia, it is common to print summaries of the preoperative evaluation or anesthesia record for easier reading, or as an *aide-memoire*. Since these printouts no longer go into the patient chart, it is easy to discard them in an unsecure way, e.g. left lying around in a lounge. This is a clear violation of the Health Insurance Portability and Accountability Act (HIPAA), and one of which anesthesia providers should be very aware.

Anesthesia information management systems incorporate audit trails so all entries into the record bear a stamp of the time of the entry and the electronic identity of the person logged into the system. Providers should be very careful to annotate any significant alterations to the record with an explanation for the change. Likewise, any information entered after the fact may require explanation.

Errors in, or omission of, required documentation is very obvious in an electronic anesthesia record. Asynchronous timelines of events, e.g. anesthetic induction recorded as occurring before the patient entered the operating room, will create medico-legal problems down the road. Clinicians are heavily reliant on the AIMS for automatically documenting vital signs. If, for example, any vital signs values are not recorded and this is not noticed, then the record appears deficient and non-compliant with standard of care [32].

In conclusion, the medico-legal issues around EMRs and AIMS are in a phase of development and definition.

The overall consensus is that an AIMS will decrease medico-legal liability, but as with anything in anesthesia, attention to detail, vigilance, and proper training are keys to success [33].

Implementing an AIMS at your hospital

The majority of hospitals do not have an AIMS and, as mentioned earlier, there is a great deal of pressure to adopt electronic records in medicine. Consequently, it is likely that many anesthesiologists will be involved in or even lead the implementation of an AIMS at their institution some time in the next few years. It is vital to the ultimate success of electronic documentation that the clinicians who will be the end users are involved in the choice and design of the system [34]. Useful guidelines to help in the implementation of AIMS are already available as original articles or online reports [35,36]. It is vital that clinicians drive the process, since there are significant differences in the priorities for the medical documentation process between hospitals and medical professionals [37].

Should you find yourself leading or otherwise being involved in a project to implement an electronic anesthesia record system, you are in an enviable position because you will be leading your colleagues on a major step into the future of anesthesia practice. It is also a difficult position because of the number of headaches that are in your own future. Before considering the challenge, you should ask yourself a couple of questions.

First, are you passionate about the need for electronic record-keeping systems? You will be leading a significant cultural change and you need to feel committed to it. Second, do you feel you can recruit the support of sufficient numbers of your colleagues to give the project enough momentum to overcome some inevitable clinician opposition? The answer to both questions should be yes.

Criteria for evaluating a system

There are several electronic anesthesia record systems on the market. The choice should take into account the needs of both the clinicians and the institution. The following is a brief overview of priorities in evaluation; the order of priority will not be the same for all institutions.

- *Enhance quality of patient care.* This should always be the number 1 criterion. It is not difficult to justify electronic medical record keeping on this one issue alone. Safety is enhanced by the easy accessibility and legibility of old records and the ability to track outcomes and improve record keeping for quality improvement initiatives. In addition, electronic systems are a necessary first step in the move towards evidence-based practice and decision support.

- *Vendor history.* These systems must be robust and reliable. The best guarantee of this is a vendor with a long track record in the field, a commitment to the future of their products, and the successful implementation of the system in many centers similar to your own.

- *Interoperability.* The system should integrate with other hospital systems. One of the principal advantages of an electronic anesthesia system (easy access to all the patient's medical data) is lost in "stand-alone" systems that do not have outside connectivity. In particular, the system should link with the operating room scheduling and management system, with the hospital admission, discharge and transfer (ADT) system, and with the clinical laboratory (Fig. 44.4). The Centers for Medicare & Medicaid Services (CMS) and the Joint Commission (TJC) are particularly concerned by the phenomenon of the "fractured" medical record. This is where a hospital has put in multiple different systems that do not communicate, and clinicians are limited in their ability to access the totality of a patient's record.

- *Accessibility (information retrieval).* The system should be easily accessible from many locations, including outside the operating room. Many systems now have web-based front ends to allow such accessibility, but the need to protect patients' medical information is paramount. Although enhanced accessibility of patient medical information was an important core goal in the original intention of the HIPAA legislation, it has sadly been largely ignored in the pursuit of privacy and security.

- *Scalability.* The system should be capable of adapting easily to operating suites of different sizes. A system that requires a large up-front investment for infrastructure and technology may be financially unjustifiable for a small institution. The initial cost and maintenance costs should be in rough proportion to the size of installation.

- *Improve compliance.* Because electronic systems encourage standardization of data entry and record keeping, there is significant potential to enhance compliance for billing and regulatory agencies.

- *Analytical tools.* Part of the power of electronic systems is their ability to analyze data to improve billing and compliance, to monitor outcomes, and to improve efficiency. Such analysis tools may or may not be provided with the system. At the very least, the system must be capable of interfacing with the reporting and analysis tools used by the hospital.

Forming the project group

It is unlikely that clinicians have sufficient expertise in information technology, budgeting, project management, etc. to put together an AIMS proposal by themselves. Your principal role is to provide clinical insights and to

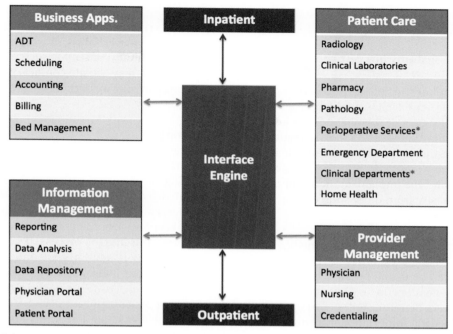

Business Apps.		Inpatient	Patient Care	
ADT			Radiology	
Scheduling			Clinical Laboratories	
Accounting			Pharmacy	
Billing			Pathology	
Bed Management			Perioperative Services*	

Interface Engine

			Emergency Department	
			Clinical Departments*	
Information Management			Home Health	
Reporting				
Data Analysis			Provider Management	
Data Repository			Physician	
Physician Portal			Nursing	
Patient Portal		Outpatient	Credentialing	

Figure 44.4 Anesthesia information systems do not exist in isolation. Hospitals have many electronic systems, both clinical and administrative. An AIMS would exist as a subsystem in the section of "Patient Care" under "Perioperative Services*" and/or "Clinical Departments*." It is easy to see why there is always competition for IT resources, and why issues that are priorities for clinical departments such as anesthesia may not get the attention we think they deserve.

set clinical needs and priorities. Clinicians should insist that the hospital put together a project group that will oversee the project. The following are key members of this group.

- *Clinician colleague.* There should be at least one other clinician on the group to ensure representation of more than just your views. This colleague should be someone who has the respect of you and your colleagues.
- *Information technology.* The committee should have a representative from the hospital information technology department who can address issues such as the state of the existing or planned IT infrastructure, available human resources, etc.
- *Hospital administration.* A high-level representative of hospital administration is required to give the support needed to champion the project through to completion. One of the principal reasons why initiatives fail is because the project lacks support in the high levels of the administration.
- *Project manager.* In an ideal world the hospital has a department dedicated to project management. An individual from this group should be appointed to organize the resources and shepherd the project from inception to completion. If such an individual is not available, someone from information technology or the hospital administration will often act in this capacity.

- *Business/finance.* Since much of the financial justification of the project will be improved billing, enhanced compliance, and increased efficiency, a representative of the business side of the administration is very useful to the project.
- *Others.* The above comprises the core members of the group. If the project is to involve integration with other systems, such as the OR management/scheduling system, then someone from those projects should be closely involved from the beginning.

Setting the scope

The first crucial goal for the project group is to define the scope of the project. Will the system be used only in the main operating room suite? Will it be used in remote areas, e.g. interventional radiology, labor and delivery? Will it be an operating room system only or will it have a preoperative evaluation and a postanesthesia care unit (PACU) component? Will the new system require the upgrading of all the existing monitoring systems? What are the essential interfaces that will be required: the hospital ADT system, clinical labs, pharmacy, materials management, and billing? All are desirable, but all cost dollars and human resources. The scope should be settled pretty firmly before the project moves forward. It is really important to involve your clinical colleagues in discussion about the scope and what they see as essential requirements for the system versus functions that would be merely "nice to have."

Determining what systems are out there
Personal contacts

There are several avenues to follow to determine what systems are available and which might best suit your needs. You, your colleagues or members of the information technology unit may know individuals in institutions with electronic anesthesia systems already installed. Personal contacts may provide information about a system, the vendor, and the implementation process that cannot be obtained easily from other sources.

Professional publications

There are several publications in the area of medical information technology. While they often have a significant industry bias, they can be useful because they have sections listing all the vendors in a particular area. The medical and anesthesia literature will occasionally have reviews related to medical information systems.

The internet

Simply typing "anesthesia information systems" into Google will bring up many sites for vendors of interest. Browsing these sites will often give background information (albeit slanted towards putting their system in a favorable light) about the system's capabilities.

Formal requests for information

You can make formal requests to vendors for information and proposal for a system or even a quotation for cost. Institutions usually have rules about soliciting such information. The IT department or a specific contracting group within the hospital may be the ones to make the contact. Before asking for this information, you should have specified your needs and the scope of the project.

Evaluating systems

Close attention must be paid to several areas when evaluating systems and vendors. These include the software itself, the quality of vendor support and responsiveness, and the level of resources needed to install and maintain the system. The IT representatives on your steering group will have had experience installing other hospital systems and should guide this process.

References

The prospective vendor should provide information about systems that have been installed in institutions comparable to yours. They should be able to provide names of individuals from the IT and clinical side of the system who are willing to talk with you and describe their experience.

Site visit

It is also very informative to visit sites that have the prospective systems installed. A very eager vendor might offer to pay the expenses for such a visit but this is not the norm and may violate conflict of interest and ethical guidelines at your institution.

Summary

Anesthesiologists will be involved one way or another with an AIMS implementation over the next few years. Installing a system and gathering the vast amount of data generated by these systems are just the first steps [38]. Whether you are a passionate advocate for electronic record keeping or not, it is important that, as a clinician, you have input into the process. If you are a leader in the project, you will have a great influence on the future practice of your colleagues, the majority of whom will much prefer an AIMS to paper [16]. You will also be embarking on a significant personal learning experience. It will probably take more effort and a greater commitment of time than you realize. Make sure to negotiate support from the hospital for the significant time commitment this will require of you.

Protecting electronic information

The use of computers for collecting, storing and exchanging patient information opens up the possibility of those data falling into the wrong hands. All clinicians have an obligation to ensure that the data are only available to those for whom it is appropriate to access patient information. An example of a breach of privacy would be prurient examination of the medical information of a "celebrity patient" by curious healthcare workers. A quote by Hippocrates is apposite.

> Whatever, in connection with my professional practice or not in connection with it, I see or hear, in the life of men, which ought not to be spoken of abroad, I will not divulge, as reckoning that all such should be kept secret. (Hippocrates 400 BCE, translated by Francis Adams)

In a somewhat chilling piece of legislation, the state of California has made healthcare providers individually liable up to $250,000 for breaches of patient privacy. The individual's employer or malpractice insurance carrier does not cover this liability! In addition, in April 2010 a former employee at the University of California Los Angeles became the first person in the country sentenced to federal prison for a violation of HIPAA.

Heath Insurance Portability and Accountability Act

In the United States 12 cents of every insurance premium dollar goes to support the insurance company; in Canada it is 1 cent. Healthcare providers in the US spend about 20% of total revenues on billing and administrative costs related to dealing with the very large number of insurance entities. In 1991, President Bush reached an agreement with the insurance industry that they would *voluntarily* convert to a system of standardized transactions. This did not happen!

In 1993 the Clinton administration introduced legislation to provide standardized transactions. Because such simplification would make patient-identifiable information more accessible, Congress argued for the inclusion of provisions for added privacy and security. The HIPAA was passed into law on 21 August 1996.

Amongst its many provisions are several relating to the use of electronic healthcare information. The requirements of the HIPAA apply to all "covered entities." A covered entity is one in which any patient information is transmitted electronically, no matter how small a proportion it represents of the overall data management by the entity. Thus, hospitals, physicians, other healthcare providers, health plans, plus their employees are covered entities. That means any clinician using any electronic means to use or access patient information is covered by the HIPAA and requires some basic knowledge of its provisions. The two areas of most relevance are privacy and security.

The HIPAA covers three areas: insurance portability, fraud, and administrative simplification. It is administrative simplification that is addressed in this chapter. Under administrative simplification the topics relevant to this discussion are privacy, security and standardized transactions.

Privacy

If a covered entity transmits any data electronically, then all protected health information (PHI), whether electronic or not, must be handled in accordance with the privacy rule. This means essentially that every healthcare establishment falls under the HIPAA regulations. PHI includes all information that can be matched to a patient, is created in the process of caring for the patient, and is kept or used in any manner, written, oral, or electronic. For a list of all information that is PHI, see Box 44.1. Research records of patient care are also PHI. If all the identifiers listed in Box 44.1 are removed then the material is no longer PHI.

All patients must be provided with an official notice of privacy rights and practices, and a good faith attempt must be made to obtain a written acknowledgment of receipt of these materials. It is usually not the responsibility of an anesthesia provider to give this notice and obtain

consent. Thereafter, routine use of PHI for treatment, payment or healthcare operations is permitted, without further consents being necessary.

Authorization is required for release of specific elements of PHI for specific purposes outside routine use or disclosure, e.g. application for insurance coverage, for an employment physical examination, for marketing or fundraising, or for clinical research. The authorization document must be signed by the patient and specify an expiration date or event. Authorization is required for any clinical research that involves access to or collection of PHI.

The clinician may both use (share data within the institution) and disclose (share data outside the institution) PHI. An example of the former is looking up results of tests in the clinical laboratory database. An example of the latter would be communicating with a patient's primary physician outside your institution. The Minimum Necessary Standard covers many exchanges of data, i.e. do not transmit more information than is absolutely necessary. However, this standard does not apply to treatment-related exchanges between healthcare providers. As an anesthesia provider, you have full access to any part of a patient's medical record (in any medium) that you consider necessary to provide care.

Business associate contract

An entity is not responsible for monitoring compliance of other entities with which it shares PHI. It must, however, have a contract with the other entity stating that the entity will comply with the Privacy Rule. As an anesthesia provider, you may be involved with industry representatives regarding devices, equipment, etc. The HIPAA applies to all interactions you have, and you should be aware of the requirement to ensure that the proper agreements are in place if those representatives will have any exposure to PHI.

Patients' rights under the HIPAA

Patients have an unlimited right to restrict or amend the use or disclosure of PHI. However, the clinician is under no obligation to treat that patient if the restrictions are considered to compromise the quality of care delivery. Patients have a right to access their records if they are part of a designated record set. A designated set is defined as any data that were used to make a decision about an individual. This applies to records held by the entity and by any business associate.

Security

Strong security is required to ensure that persons not authorized to have access to it cannot obtain PHI. A good security system emphasizes three areas: confidentiality, integrity, and availability. Confidentiality means that only appropriately authorized individuals have access to PHI.

Box 44.2 Questions to ask yourself about your own approach to data security

- Do you store any patient information in publicly accessible areas? Is it posted where the public can see it?
- Do you send any patient information over email or fax?
- Do you share any patient information with anyone over the phone?
- Do you store any patient information on paper? Is it in a secure area?
- Are patient data stored on your computer or on a server?
- Can anyone access patient information on your computer without your permission?
- Do you send patient information to anyone outside your institution?
- Can you track who accesses your databases and what they view?

Box 44.3 Good practices to safeguard the security of PHI

- Do not share passwords under any circumstances
- Always use a "strong" password (at least 6 characters with at least 3 of them being a capital letter, number or symbol), and change it at least every 90 days
- Log off computer stations when finished with use
- Destroy all papers containing PHI in shredder or locked disposal bins (never in a trash can)
- Do not leave PHI, in any form, lying around
- Do not send PHI over an unsecured email system (e.g. to outside physicians)
- Do not send PHI to an unsecured fax machine
- Do not leave PHI messages on voicemail
- Password protect all electronic devices with PHI

Integrity means that data can be altered only by those authorized to do so. Availability means that data are readily accessible by those who need them.

The basis of strong security lies in creating both a culture and an infrastructure that make security possible. The world of electronics has opened up many new opportunities for breaches of PHI security. Box 44.2 lists the questions you should ask yourself if you handle, store or transmit any PHI (paper or electronic). Your hospital or clinical department should have IT professionals who can advise you how to make your data as secure as possible. Some states, such as California, take security of PHI so seriously that they have laws making individuals (not their employer) personally liable for breaches of PHI security.

Security starts with an appropriate culture of human behavior (Box 44.3); this leads to an appropriate computer policy, which in turn determines the technical mechanisms (infrastructure) to be used. Inappropriate individual behavior will defeat even the best electronic security systems. An example of human behavior that will defeat the system might be a physician who carries unprotected PHI in a personal digital assistant that is then left in a public place. Another example is careless discussion about patients by providers in public areas (such as elevators). Unless the human/organizational culture changes first, technical solutions will fail to provide security.

Standardized transactions
Transactions
The intention of the HIPAA was that simplification brought about by having standards for transactions and codes, should decrease administrative overheads in healthcare. The standards apply to all health plans, clearing houses and any providers that transmit electronic data under the umbrella of the HIPAA. A standard is simply "what most people use." For example, Health Level 7 (HL7) is a current standard for clinical data inter-

change and the Institute of Electrical and Electronics Engineers (IEEE) publish standards for clinical instruments. These are the data transmission standards used when connecting vital signs monitors to an AIMS.

Code sets
Several code sets are mandated for use in electronic transactions. For diseases, the *International Classification of Diseases*, 9th edition, clinical modification (ICD-9-CM) will be used. For physician services, e.g. surgical procedures, the Current Procedural Terminology, 4th edition (CPT-4) is used. These code sets will also change over time. ICD-10-CM has recently been released in the United States, and the Department of Health and Human Services has mandated that it be used to replace the ICD-9-CM codes effective October 1, 2013.

Identifiers
An initial intention of the HIPAA was to introduce unique identifiers for individuals, providers, employers and health plans. Because of a strong negative response from the public, implementation of the individual identifier has been postponed indefinitely. This was a significant setback for any attempt to create a national data repository of patient healthcare information. The unique national provider identifier (NPI) is a 10-digit number issued to healthcare providers under the National Plan and Provider Enumeration System (NPPES) mandated under the HIPAA. For a healthcare organization, the identifier is their income tax code.

Patient care

One of the earliest questions asked about electronic systems was whether they enhance or detract from patient care [39]. The detractors will contend that poorly designed or unreliable systems take more time and are a distraction from patient care; this is indeed true [40]. They will argue also that manual entry of vital signs on a paper record requires the clinician to actually pay some attention to the monitors and recorded values; this also is a valid argument [41]. Proponents of electronic documentation take the position that more attention can be paid to direct observation of the patient by the clinician who is freed from the task of writing on a paper record and that this occurs without loss of vigilance [42]. They will contend that data recording is more timely and complete, and that electronic systems enhance evidence-based practice and decision support [27,43].

Compliance

One of the most onerous tasks facing anesthesia practitioners is keeping up with the increasing mandates for documentation needed to comply with the requirements of the various regulatory agencies and payers. Not only must these required elements be documented, but com-

pliance must also be tracked and reported. Many elements of performance must be documented in a very specific and complete manner. An example would be the requirements for insertion of a central venous catheter. There are elements of performance that constitute good clinical practice, and the clinician must not only adhere to the practice guidelines, but must document the individual elements performed. Using an AIMS can facilitate data entry, tracking, and reporting if the elements are built into the protocol for that procedure in the record (Fig. 44.5) [44,45].

Enhanced documentation

Electronic systems can provide automated reminders for necessary documentation or intervention. This enhances patient care by, for example, improved documentation of allergies or timing of antibiotic administration (Fig. 44.6) [46–48]. Real-time recording of data is important for accuracy and completeness, but timely documentation is

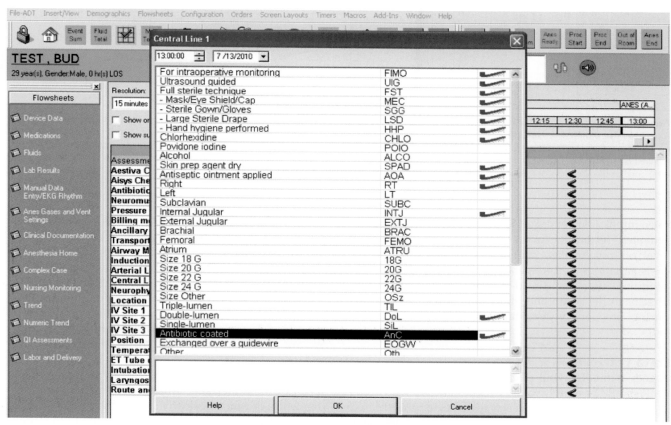

Figure 44.5 Electronic systems can greatly enhance the clinician's ability to fulfill regulatory requirements for following, tracking and reporting compliance with clinical guidelines. This shows a screen allowing checkbox documentation of the required elements for inserting a central venous catheter using good clinical practice. The checkboxes serve as an *aide mémoire* to good practice, and are in a highly structured data format that can be easily tracked and reported on, and modified as guidelines and regulations change. This illustration is taken from the AIMS used at the University of California San Francisco. Its use in this figure does not imply an endorsement of the product.

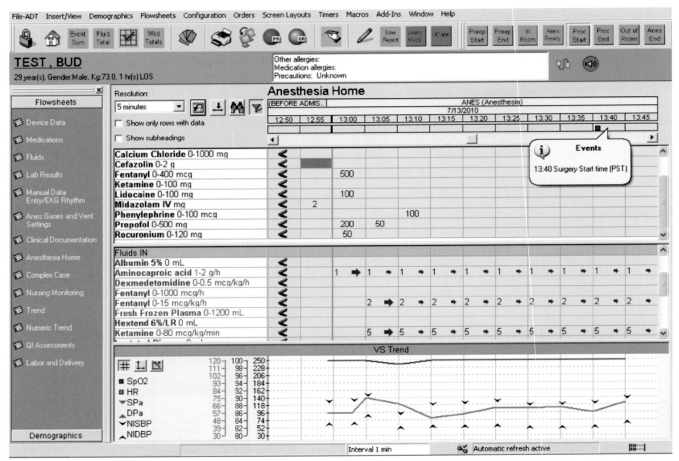

Figure 44.6 Electronic systems can also incorporate reminders to the clinician to perform certain tasks. In this illustration, the red box in the cefazolin row shows that prophylactic antibiotic has not been given. Once the antibiotic is charted, the red box disappears. If the procedure goes on sufficiently long, then a red box will reappear at the appropriate interval to prompt redosing of the antibiotic. In a similar manner, prompts can be given for required data entries, e.g. an attending signature, or to draw attention to events that are out of chronological order. This illustration is taken from the AIMS used at the University of California San Francisco. Its use in this figure does not imply an endorsement of the product.

often impossible, for example, in crisis situations. Speech-activated recording to an AIMS has now reached a level of functionality that makes its use practical for crisis situations in the operating room [49]. Outside the operating room, hand-held devices can be used to link directly to the AIMS and allow data entry by clinicians during preoperative evaluations or anesthesia rounds [50].

Data retrieval

It goes without saying that information in an AIMS or EMR should be easily available to the clinician who needs it. There are two main obstacles to achieving this desired state. First is the fact that only about 1% of hospitals have a truly integrated EHR so that all data in the record are available through a single source. Most hospitals have a multitude of different systems, all with different levels of security, usernames, passwords, and types of worksta-

tions on which they are available. This is a problem of real concern when the universal system, which is the paper record, is replaced by multiple and poorly interacting electronic systems. The ideal data retrieval system would tailor information to specific providers (e.g. residents on specialties) and provide it on media (e.g. PDA, tablet) most useful to the provider. In addition, it should be available wherever the provider happens to be working. We are a long way from achieving that vision in any widespread sense.

Data retrieval can also be affected by the stability and speed of the underlying system. Systems that go down frequently or function slowly significantly impair the clinician's ability to retrieve data. Lack of ability to retrieve data can actually lead to patient harm, and a particularly vulnerable time is when a new system is implemented and clinicians are not yet comfortable and competent with it [51].

Evidence-based medicine

Evidence-based medicine (EBM) has been defined as "the conscientious, explicit, and judicious use of current best evidence in making decisions about the care of individual patients. The practice of evidence based medicine means integrating individual clinical expertise with the best available external clinical evidence from systematic research" [52]. The optimal application of EBM requires two things. The first is clinical expertise in the acquiring of information from the patient via history, physical examination and performance of appropriate tests. The second is combining those results with the best available external knowledge (the medical literature) and applying this information to the patient's diagnosis and treatment. EBM gives less importance to intuition and more to a systematized approach to healthcare. This does not devalue individual clinical expertise, but rather supplements it.

Clinicians can perform their own *ad hoc* searches for clinical guidelines and evidence-based recommendations. The American College of Cardiology, American Heart Association, and Anesthesia Patient Safety Foundation all have websites that provide evidence-based guidelines for preoperative cardiac assessment and perioperative β-blockade management. However, the information on different sites may at times be conflicting and outdated. Evidence-based practice with an AIMS works best if the institution arrives at a consensus practice for the areas where there is strong and current evidence for best practice and embeds those into the EMR and even the AIMS.

Decision support

There are two general categories of information – patient-specific information and knowledge-based information. Patient-specific information is generated from the care of an individual patient. This comprises a careful, thorough history and physical examination plus the results of all tests and interventions. In the computerized world this information resides in the electronic medical record. The other category is knowledge-based information which consists of the scientific literature of healthcare. Computers provide the means for information retrieval and evidence-based medicine. When those two information systems are combined you have a decision support system. Decision support can also be defined as "the application of information from knowledge-based systems to an individual patient."

While clinicians may initially be wary of such systems, there are design characteristics that encourage acceptance [53]. The system should guide practice, not coerce it. The systems should not block nor lock out the physician. Systems should be perceived as being helpful in compensating for human failure. Computer-based clinical deci-

sion support systems can enhance drug dosing, reduce errors, enhance safety, and improve compliance with clinical guidelines [17,18,54]. To date, the preponderance of evidence suggests that computerized clinical decision support systems improve practitioner performance [55]. However, improved patient outcome from use of these systems is yet to be convincingly demonstrated [55].

Protocols for anesthesia technique can be built into the AIMS. For example, this might automatically load all the required drugs, fluids, and monitors that would be used in a given case. Included in this, for example, might be practice guidelines for prophylactic antibiotic administration. Such systems have been shown to improve timeliness in the administration of preoperative antibiotics [56]. The system can also be automated to include reminders to redose intraoperative antibiotics (see Fig. 44.6). Other protocols might include a set of advanced cardiac life support guidelines to facilitate resuscitation procedures.

There are significant consequences to implementing clinical guidelines and recommended best practices. They require constant maintenance to keep up with advancing knowledge and changing regulations. There must be acceptance that the clinician has the ultimate authority to determine the care for an individual patient. Inherent in this principle is the clear understanding that deciding to adopt a plan different from the guideline or protocol is not *per se* practicing below normal standard of care.

Using the system for perioperative management support

Installing a system and gathering the vast amounts of electronic data available are just the first steps. Greater advantage is obtained from the system if it is used to analyze the information and to guide perioperative management decisions.

Staffing plans

An example of this might be in optimizing human resource use. Operating rooms do not keep regular hours, and planning how many providers are required at different times of the day is a difficult problem. Programs exist that use case start and end times to analyze and project staffing needs at different times of the day [57]. Enhanced scheduling of staff may be a significant advantage of the installation of the electronic information system.

Quality improvement

Anesthesia-related adverse events are under-reported chronically [11,58]. Voluntary reporting can be facilitated by building it into normal workflow as an integral part of the EMR. Clinicians in general support such a system

[45,59]. Electronic information systems can increase the detection of some adverse events by automated scanning and extraction [60,61]. There is a strong association between adverse events and in-hospital mortality [58], so improved detection of and corrective measures for adverse events should lead to enhanced quality of care.

Potential pitfalls with electronic documentation

Documenting on wrong patient

It is very difficult with a paper record to enter information under the wrong patient name. Usually the record is blank and the correct name will be written or stamped on the paper by the clinician. Should a mistake be made, the record can be corrected by judicious scoring out of the erroneous data and appropriate correction made. The situation is not so simple with an electronic record. If the wrong patient is selected at the beginning of the record entry, then thousands of pieces of data will be entered into the wrong record. Retrieving and reassigning data inthis case are very difficult. The easiest fix is usually to delete the electronic record entirely and create a paper record instead, a far from elegant solution.

Data entry errors

Garbage in, garbage out is the operative phrase here. All AIMS require a significant amount of manually entered data, drug doses, descriptions of procedures, perhaps laboratory values, etc. Some systems use checkboxes to document events, and it is easy to check the wrong box. Such errors may go unnoticed since many data entry pages exist in the background, and once the entry is made they will not be looked at again.

Artifacts

It is the nature of clinical monitoring that many values are clearly incorrect. Such artifacts may be due to electrical interference with, for example, the ECG, movement artifact with the pulse oximeter reading, or incorrect arterial blood pressure readings when the line is flushed [62]. With a paper record, these values were simply not recorded, but with automatic electronic data collection they may be. It is possible to automatically filter some but not all of these artifacts [62]. Other options include deleting the value, altering the value, or annotating the record to explain the artifacts. The authors recommend the annotation approach rather than deletion or alteration. In an electronic system, all entries, modifications, and deletions are tracked and retained in the record. Deletions or alterations may be hard to defend (especially if not explained), while a simple annotation of the reason for the artifact will leave the issue quite clear.

Missing data

Data enter the electronic record in two ways. First, they are automatically transmitted from devices, vital signs monitors, and interfaces with other systems, e.g. ADT. While usually robust, the data flow may be interrupted and not noticed by the clinician for a period of time. This can lead to vital sign data being absent from the record and creates medico-legal liability [32]. Second, the clinician is required to enter many data elements manually. When this is not done records are often incomplete [63]. Designing manual data entry in logical sequences and providing prompts to enter the data where possible can mitigate, but probably not eliminate this problem.

Self-population of entries

One of the real advantages of an AIMS is that "boilerplate" type documentation can be entered automatically by the system. One of the consequences of living in a world obsessed with regulatory requirements is that every single element of care must be documented, or it is considered never to have happened. A simple example might be the meeting with the patient in the preoperative holding area. Providers will, for example, check the patient's identity, confirm the surgery, ask about NPO status, examine the airway, discuss the anesthesia plan, and obtain informed consent. Each of these interactions must be documented individually. With an electronic system, one press of a key or click on an icon and all the necessary statements are entered in the record. This is now complete and standardized, and fulfils compliance requirements. Of course, each of the items that are documented should in fact have been done. Overuse of automatic data entry can lead to problems if some of the documented interventions have not actually been performed.

Cloning

This is a term for the process whereby old data entries are replicated uncritically and automatically from one record to the next. Electronic records enable "copy forward" procedures and this is in many cases valid and useful. However, incorrect information may be promulgated, and items that should be updated are left unchanged. Unless this process is controlled by professional behavior or electronic means, there is a potential for what amounts to documentation fraud.

Research

Information retrieval

One advantage of hospitals with an EMR and AIMS is that computer workstations are usually easily accessible.

As a consequence, the clinician who wishes to search the literature has access to a vast array of online data. There are two major pitfalls. The first is searching in such a way that the actual information you seek will be found in a short period of time. The second is judging the quality of the information retrieved. When planning a search, the goal should be to optimize both the sensitivity of the search (i.e. the chance of finding what you want) and the specificity (i.e. avoid being inundated with non-relevant information).

The simplest way of finding information is to go to one of the many websites that offer clinically relevant information directly. Sites such as MDConsult (mdconsult.com), UpTodate (uptodate.com) and AccessMedicine (accessmedicine.com) are invaluable tools in finding answers to basic clinical care questions. In anesthesia there are many sites that specifically give expert practical information. Examples (out of many such sites) are directions on placing regional blocks (nysora.com) or performing a bronchoscopy (thoracic-anesthesia.com). Navigating these sites is simple, and the information is to a large degree vetted by experts and therefore reliable. The process gets a lot more complicated when you start to search the online medical literature.

Online literature search strategies

A good strategy for efficient searching is to start in a site that has a focus on the type of information that you seek. For the medical science literature, PubMed (www.ncbi.nlm.nih.gov/pubmed/) is still the definitive source. If your question involves specifically evidence-based medicine, then the Cochrane Library (www.cochrane.org), the Agency for Health Care Research and Quality (www.ahrq.gov) and the National Guidelines Clearing House (www.guidelines.gov) are excellent resources. Scirus (www.sciris.com) limits itself to searches of science-specific web pages. Alternatively, you can start your search at a site that deals with the specific disease entity or organ system in which you are interested, for example, the National Cancer Institute: CancerNet (www.cancer.gov). Finally you can start at specific sub-specialty websites. For example, the website for the American Society of Anesthesiologists (www.asahq.org) has up-to-date information on standards, guidelines, consensus statements, etc. related specifically to the practice of anesthesiology.

If you use general web search engines, Google for example, there is so much information available (much of it non-scientific) that it is quite possible to be inundated by both useful and non-useful data. It will save a lot of time if you plan your search before starting. For example, in Google, typing in the query *awareness under anesthesia* will generate over 4 million hits. Switching to the Google Scholar search engine decreases this number to a mere 102,000 hits. Putting quotation marks around the phrase limits the search to the exact phrase only and reduces the number of hits to about 370. Other modifiers such as preceding the search phrase in Google with "allintitle:" further limits the search to web pages with the exact title and results in only 18 hits.

The order in which the hits are presented may not exactly match the quality of the content. Judging the quality of the information recovered in searches is a necessary skill in this era when vast quantities of information are so easily available [64]. A comprehensive description of methods for analyzing and validating scientific papers is beyond the scope of this chapter, but an online guide to evaluating the literature (www.vetmed.wsu.edu/courses-jmgay/EvalGuide.htm) that was produced by the College of Veterinary Medicine at Washington State University is a good place to start.

A more in-depth discussion is provided in the excellent series of papers by Trisha Greenhalgh published in the *British Medical Journal* and gathered in a book entitled *How to Read a Paper: The Basics of Evidence Based Medicine* [65]. Since the publication of these articles in 1997 [66,67], much has changed in the world of medical literature. The internet, as we know it, and e-publishing did not exist when the articles were first published. The explosive growth of non-peer reviewed articles has made it more important than ever that the reader critically assess the validity of the work, and the principles espoused by Greenhalgh are as relevant as ever.

Data repositories

The proliferation of electronic data capture facilitates the creation of large data repositories that provide opportunities for new avenues of outcomes research. Multicenter outcomes research in anesthesia is not new; in fact, in 1954 Beecher and Todd published the first such study on deaths associated with anesthesia and surgery [68]. However, with manually collected and recorded data, the effort and resources involved in such multicenter studies limited the number and scope that could be performed. The advent of AIMS and EMRs has provided the opportunity to ask many more and wider-ranging outcome questions from data automatically uploaded into large data repositories from many sources.

There are several efforts under way to create anesthesia data repositories. Some individual institutions, such as the Cleveland Clinic, already have their own extensive clinical information data repositories. In other areas, national anesthesia data repositories are being created.

The Multicenter Perioperative Outcomes Group (MPOG) was formed by a group of academic anesthesia departments that use an AIMS. Its purpose is to "promote multi-institutional collaboration on outcomes research to advance knowledge and improve patient care in perioperative medicine." Leaders of the University of Michigan Department of Anesthesia initiated the project, and the MPOG data repository is hosted at the University of Michigan.

In 2008, the American Society of Anesthesiologists (ASA) created the Anesthesia Quality Institute (AQI). Under AQI, the National Anesthesia Clinical Outcomes Registry (NACOR) was created. The aim of the NACOR is to cast a very wide net, essentially to take all available electronic data elements from any anesthesia practitioner willing to upload it. The gathering of small amounts of data from wide-ranging sources by AQI complements the MPOG's gathering of rich datasets from a limited number of institutions.

Informatics

Managing the vast amount of data in these repositories involves the science of informatics. The term is a contraction of "information science" and is defined by the Merriam-Webster dictionary as "the collection, classification, storage, retrieval, and dissemination of recorded knowledge treated both as a pure and as an applied science." Medical or health informatics is the science of informatics as it relates to the fields within healthcare and biomedicine. Medical informatics is a relatively new science; the term was first coined in the late 1970s. There are several subcategories under the general umbrella of medical informatics, and one of the most recently created is "anesthesia informatics" [69].

The pure science of medical informatics relates to theoretical aspects of information and knowledge management, and is not within the scope of this chapter [70]. The applied component deals with how information is used in the service of patients and clinicians. It makes more sense when you realize that fundamentally, clinicians gather information and use their knowledge to make diagnoses and decide on interventions. The amounts of both information and knowledge are increasing beyond the capacity of individuals to manage them. Therefore, medical informatics is a vital tool for optimizing this process and for analyzing the vast amounts of data to create useful information for the clinician [71]. The judicious use of informatics in medicine promises, amongst other things, the possibility of decreasing medical errors [17].

Healthcare professionals with knowledge of informatics raise the quality of information processing, and the quality of information processing influences the quality of healthcare itself. This is particularly true in anesthesia where only anesthesia professionals who can speak the languages of both informatics and clinical care can optimize design of the information-gathering, data retrieval, and decision support systems to function in the real-time, immediate environment of anesthesia practice.

Annotated references

A full reference list for this chapter is available at:
http://www.wiley.com/go/gregory/andropoulos/pediatricanesthesia

14. McNitt JD, Bode ET, Nelson RE. Long-term pharmaceutical cost reduction using a data management system. Anesth Analg 1998; 87: 837–42. This paper showed that a financial case can be made for electronic anesthesia record keeping.

16. Quinzio L, Junger A, Gottwald B et al. User acceptance of an anaesthesia information management system. Eur J Anaesthesiol 2003; 20: 967–72. This paper showed that users of an electronic system felt that it improved the quality of their work and that they did not wish to return to paper.

19. Chaudhry B, Wang J, Wu S et al. Systematic review: impact of health information technology on quality, efficiency, and costs of medical care. Ann Intern Med 2006; 144: 742–52. A significant paper since it demonstrated that using electronic health information technology produced real, as opposed to theoretical, improvements in quality and efficiency of care.

23. Spring SF, Sandberg WS, Anupama S et al. Automated documentation error detection and notification improves anesthesia billing performance. Anesthesiology 2007; 106: 157–63. This paper is important since it provided hard evidence of financial benefit for an electronic anesthesia record system.

25. Feldman JM. Do anesthesia information systems increase malpractice exposure? Results of a survey. Anesth Analg 2004; 99: 840–3. A reassuring paper for those concerned about medico-legal risk with electronic anesthesia documentation.

36. Muravchick S, Caldwell JE, Epstein RH et al. Anesthesia information management system implementation: a practical guide. Anesth Analg 2008; 107: 1598–608. A good starting point for anyone involved in planning the implementation of an electronic anesthesia record system.

46. Sandberg WS, Sandberg EH, Seim AR et al. Real-time checking of electronic anesthesia records for documentation errors and automatically text messaging clinicians improves quality of documentation. Anesth Analg 2008; 106: 192–201. Demonstrates that real-time feedback with consequent enhancement of documentation compliance is possible with an electronic anesthesia system.

48. Wax DB, Beilin Y, Levin M et al. The effect of an interactive visual reminder in an anesthesia information management system on timeliness of prophylactic antibiotic administration. Anesth Analg 2007; 104: 1462–6. An illustration of how quality of care, using a very concrete measurement, can be improved using automated reminders in an electronic anesthesia system.

51. Han YY, Carcillo JA, Venkataraman ST et al. Unexpected increased mortality after implementation of a commercially sold computerized physician order entry system. Pediatrics 2005; 116: 1506–12. A cautionary paper identifying the risks to patients during the initial, learning stages of implementing a new electronic documentation system.

60. Grant C, Ludbrook G, Hampson EA et al. Adverse physiological events under anaesthesia and sedation: a pilot audit of electronic patient records. Anaesth Intensive Care 2008; 36: 222–9. This paper demonstrated that automated review of electronic anesthesia records could identify patterns of adverse outcome that were amenable to corrective action.

68. Beecher HK, Todd DP. A study of the deaths associated with anesthesia and surgery: based on a study of 599,548 anesthesias in ten institutions 1948–1952, inclusive. Ann Surg 1954; 140: 2–35. A seminal paper that was one of the first major multi-instititional outcome studies.

CHAPTER 45

Operating Room Safety, Communication, and Teamwork

Thomas L. Shaw & Stephen A. Stayer

Department of Anesthesiology and Pediatrics, Baylor College of Medicine, and Texas Children's Hospital, Houston, TX, USA

Introduction

"In solo or group practice, teamwork is a major part of the anesthesiologist's life. Whether a vital part of a surgical team, a member of an interdisciplinary group of diagnosticians at a pain clinic, or a partner on a research team or teaching faculty, an anesthesiologist works continuously with a variety of medical professionals" [1]. This quote from the American Society of Anesthesiologists career information webpage summarizes the importance of teamwork in the daily life of all anesthesiologists. Teamwork can be defined as "the ability of team members to work together, communicate effectively, anticipate and meet one another's demands, and inspire confidence resulting in a co-ordinated collective action" [2]. In 1999, the Institute of Medicine published a report entitled *To Err Is Human: Building a Safer Health System* [3]. This highlighted the fact that systemic failures in healthcare delivery account for more errors than poor performance by individuals. The Institute of Medicine recommended interdisciplinary team training to reduce the incidence of such medical errors. Effective teamwork can provide a safety net that can often prevent human errors from becoming a patient safety issue. This chapter will review the basic principles of operating room and anesthesia safety as they apply to pediatric patients, emphasizing the non-technical skills of communication and teamwork as crucial to patient outcomes.

Non-technical skills

In the 1970s, the investigation of several airplane crashes concluded that no mechanical failure of the aircraft or technical failure of the pilot had occurred. So why did these planes crash? The investigators blamed deficits in other human factors, characterized as non-technical skills [4]. Non-technical skills are defined as "the cognitive, social, and personal resource skills that complement technical skills, and contribute to safe and efficient task performance" [5]. These skills do not directly relate to medical knowledge, technical expertise, drugs, or equipment. For example, a surgeon could demonstrate excellent technical skills during the amputation of the wrong foot (lack of situational awareness). Non-technical skills have been increasingly recognized as crucial to maintaining patient safety. Non-technical skills can be classified as (i) cognitive and mental skills (such as decision making, planning, and situation awareness) and (ii) social and interpersonal skills (such as communication, teamwork, and leadership) [6]. Traditionally, medical training has not formally taught these skills and deficiencies in these skills have

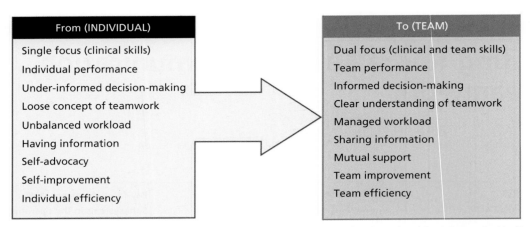

Figure 45.1 The mental shift needed to move from an individual perspective to a team perspective. Reproduced from Agency for Healthcare Research and Quality [13].

been reported amongst anesthesiologists [6,7]. Medical team training focuses on the cultivation of these non-technical skills.

Medical team training

Clinical training usually focuses on the individual execution of tasks. Safe and efficient patient care requires the co-ordination of activity amongst physicians, nurses, respiratory therapists, pharmacists, and other healthcare professionals. However, all of these team members are rarely trained together. Effective teamwork is not reliably learned without formal training and cultivation. Team training teaches a set of tools and strategies that requires a mental shift from an individual perspective to a team perspective, as shown in Figure 45.1.

Several different medical team training programs have been developed. Medical team training programs can be categorized into high-fidelity simulator-based programs and classroom-based programs. The high-fidelity simulator-based programs rely upon patient simulators and include courses such as anesthesia crisis resource management (ACRM) [7] and team-oriented medical simulation (TOMS) [8]. The classroom-based team training programs rely upon lectures, videos, demonstrations, and role play. Classroom-based programs include TeamSTEPPS® (Team Strategies and Tools to Enhance Performance and Patient Safety) [9], MedTeams® [10], medical team management, Lifewings™, and geriatric interdisciplinary team training.

There is considerable overlap between all of these training programs, and there is no evidence that one training program or method is superior to another. Advocates of high-fidelity simulator-based programs list several advantages [11]. Simulators provide hands-on training in a realistic environment. The environment mandates the

integration of decision skills, procedural skills, and teamwork skills in a scenario that actually challenges and stresses the clinician. Advocates of classroom-based programs highlight the lower cost, mobility, and ability to train large numbers of students simultaneously [12]. A detailed discussion of ACRM and TeamSTEPPS® follows.

Anesthesia Crisis Resource Management

In 1989, David Gaba and his colleagues at Stanford University and the Palo Alto Veterans Affairs Medical Center pioneered the adaptation of aviation crew resource management to the practice of anesthesiology, resulting in the curriculum for anesthesia crisis resource management (ACRM) [7]. The phrases "crew resource management," "crisis resource management," and "cockpit resource management" are used interchangeably throughout the literature. Crew resource management can be defined as a management system which makes optimum use of all available resources (equipment, procedures, and people) to promote safety and focuses on teaching nontechnical skills. The ACRM course begins with didactic presentations regarding anesthesia safety, decision making, specific anesthesiology crisis scenarios, and system-related failures that affect patient safety and human performance. Also, course participants critically analyze a video of an aviation accident. The bulk of the course consists of simulations followed by detailed debriefings. The simulator sessions feature a realistic patient simulator in an operating room environment in which each participant is the primary anesthesiologist managing critical event scenarios. Significant interaction between nursing and surgical personnel (role-played by instructors) is required during the scenarios. Emphasis is placed on working more effectively with different leadership, followership, and communication styles. The simulation sessions are video recorded and analyzed by the team during debriefing sessions with the help of an

Box 45.1 Anesthesia crisis resource management: key points in healthcare

1. Know the environment
2. Anticipate and plan
3. Call for help early
4. Exercise leadership and followership with assertiveness
5. Distribute the workload
6. Mobilize all available resources
7. Communicate effectively – speak up
8. Use all available information
9. Prevent and manage fixation errors
10. Cross-check and double-check
11. Use cognitive aids
12. Re-evaluate repeatedly
13. Use good teamwork – co-ordinate with and support others
14. Allocate attention wisely
15. Set priorities dynamically

Reproduced from Rall and Gaba [83].

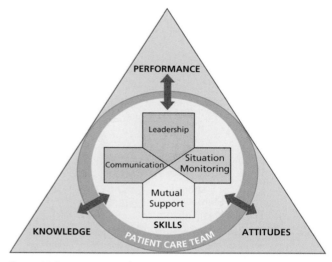

Figure 45.2 TeamSTEPPS® four core competencies. Source: Agency for Healthcare Research and Quality [13].

instructor. The key points emphasized in ACRM are listed in Box 45.1. See Chapter 42 for a more detailed discussion of simulation in pediatric anesthesiology.

TeamSTEPPS®

TeamSTEPPS® (Team Strategies and Tools to Enhance Performance and Patient Safety) is another resource for training healthcare professionals in better teamwork practices. The Patient Safety Program of the Department of Defense and the Agency for Healthcare Research and Quality collaborated for 20 years to explore the field of medical teamwork. TeamSTEPPS® is an evidence-based teamwork training system focusing on four complementary competency areas: leadership, situation monitoring, mutual support, and communication [9]. These are all teachable and learnable skills and should not be viewed as skills that a person "either has or does not have." TeamSTEPPS® offers a free public domain toolkit that can be tailored to any healthcare setting [13]. The free educational material on the TeamSTEPPS® website includes presentations, group exercises, and videos. The Agency for Healthcare Research and Quality also offers a free TeamSTEPPS® instructor course so that an institution can develop in-house expertise on team training. TeamSTEPPS® can be used by all healthcare organizations and all medical specialties. This open availability may allow the entire medical field to begin using a common language and approach to team training.

TeamSTEPPS® teaches specific tools and strategies to overcome barriers to team effectiveness. The tools and strategies are intimately linked to the four core competencies of the TeamSTEPPS® framework: team leadership, situation monitoring, mutual support, and communication, shown in Figure 45.2.

Leadership

"Leadership is the ability to direct and co-ordinate activities of team members, assess team performance, assign tasks, develop team knowledge and skills, motivate team members, plan and organize, and establish a positive team atmosphere" [14]. Effective team leaders organize the team, articulate clear goals, and make decisions through the collective input of members. They also delegate tasks, empower members to speak up and ask questions, actively promote and facilitate good teamwork, and are skillful at conflict resolution. Three strategies that leaders use to promote team information sharing are briefs, huddles, and debriefs.

A brief, also known as a team meeting, is held for planning purposes and lets everyone on the team know what is planned and why. It is a short planning session to discuss subjects such as a patient's current condition, diagnosis, the role of team members, team goals, potential complications, and back-up plans. Briefs open the lines of communication so that everyone can contribute their unique knowledge to the task. The team leader usually initiates the briefing, but any member of the team can do so. A huddle is an *ad hoc* discussion that focuses on problem solving. Huddles provide team members with an opportunity to update each other on changes in the status of the patient so that all team members can adapt. Huddles are used to re-establish situation awareness, reinforce plans already in place, and assess the need to adjust the plan. A debrief takes place after a procedure or event and focuses on process improvement. It is an informal information exchange session designed to improve team performance and effectiveness. Debriefs are most effective in an environment where

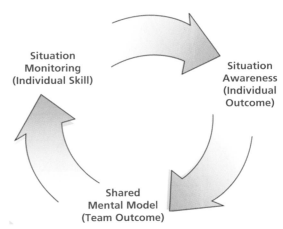

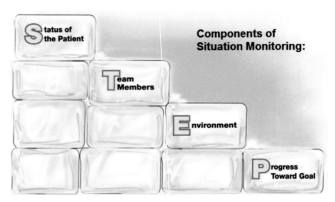

Figure 45.4 The STEP mnemonic for situation monitoring. Reproduced from Agency for Healthcare Research and Quality [13].

Figure 45.3 Continuum of situation monitoring, situation awareness, and a shared mental model. Reproduced from Agency for Healthcare Research and Quality [13].

honest mistakes are viewed as learning opportunities and the focus is not placed on individual blame.

Situation monitoring

Situation monitoring is the process of continually scanning and assessing what is going on around you to maintain situation awareness [14]. Situation awareness is "knowing what is going on around you." When everyone maintains their situation awareness and shares relevant facts to ensure that all team members are "on the same page," a shared mental model is formed. There is a continuum that begins with the individual skill of situation monitoring that leads to situation awareness and collectively results in a shared understanding of the situation (referred to as a shared mental model) (Fig. 45.3).

Situation awareness can be undermined by one team member's failure to share information, request information, and direct information to specific team members. Cross-monitoring involves monitoring the actions of other team members and provides a safety net within a team. It involves "watching each other's back." Cross-monitoring can help catch mistakes early before they compromise patient safety. The STEP mnemonic (Fig. 45.4) is a situation monitoring tool that is a mental reminder to constantly monitor the Status of the patient, Team members, Environment, and Progress towards goal.

Mutual support

Mutual support (or back-up behavior) is the ability to anticipate other team members' needs and to shift workload among members to achieve balance. Task assistance is a form of mutual support where team members protect each other from work overload situations. Some medical professionals are conditioned to avoid asking for help due to the fear of suggesting a lack of knowledge or con-

fidence. Effective teams place all offers and requests for assistance in the context of patient safety and team members foster a climate where it is expected that assistance will be actively sought and offered.

Feedback is another type of mutual support. Feedback provides information to improve team performance. Effective feedback is timely (the behavior is still fresh in the mind of the receiver), respectful (should not be personal and should focus on behavior and not personality), specific (should relate to a specific situation), and directed (goals are set for improvement). Feedback can also be used to reinforce positive behaviors. Personal feedback is more effective when it is given in private as it causes less defensiveness on the part of the recipient.

Advocacy and assertion tools and strategies should be used when a team member's viewpoint does not coincide with that of the decision maker. The team member thus has the opportunity to correct errors or the loss of situation awareness. Failure to advocate and assert is frequently identified as a primary contributor to malpractice cases, sentinel events, and aviation disasters. If the safety of the patient is at risk, even an unpopular viewpoint that questions authority should be advocated. The two-challenge rule was initially developed to help airline pilots prevent disasters caused by momentary lapses in judgment. The two-challenge rule states that if there is concern for potential harm to a patient, that concern should be asserted at least twice. If after two attempts the concern is still disregarded, a stronger course of action should be taken using the chain of command. This overcomes the natural tendency to believe that the team leader must always be right. It is the responsibility of the person challenged to acknowledge the safety concerns and resolve any safety issues. Leaders must foster an environment where all team members feel empowered to speak up when they notice a safety issue, knowing that their inputs are welcomed.

The healthcare environment is susceptible to frequent and sometimes disruptive conflict. This is not surprising given that it is an environment with a number of highly educated, experienced individuals with different training, backgrounds, and priorities. TeamSTEPPS® teaches two basic conflict resolution strategies. Two different scripts are taught that can aid communication during times of conflict. The CUS (Concerned, Uncomfortable, Safety) script uses signal words to catch an individual's attention. First, a *concern* is stated, next the speaker states why they are *uncomfortable*, and finally they state that they believe there is a *safety* issue. The DESC (Describe, Express, Suggest, Consequences) script can be used to communicate effectively during all types of conflict. The specific situation is *described*. Concerns about the action are *expressed*. Other alternatives are *suggested*. Finally, potential *consequences* are stated. A private discussion between the individuals who have conflict will lead to more focus on resolving the conflict instead of a focus on saving face. The focus should be on *what* is right, not *who* is right. When resolving conflict, the goal should be to achieve collaboration, which means working together to achieve a mutually satisfying solution yielding a win-win situation.

Communication

Communication includes the efficient exchange of information and consultation with other team members. Communication is defined as the "exchange of information between sender and a receiver . . . the process by which information is clearly and accurately exchanged between two or more team members in the prescribed manner and with proper terminology and the ability to clarify or acknowledge the receipt of information" [15]. Communication is the lifeline of an effective team and the glue that holds all the team skills together. Improving the quality of information exchange decreases communication-related errors. In order for communication to be effective, it must be complete, clear, concise, and timely. How does communication relate to the other team skills? Effective leaders must communicate clear information so that team members are aware of their roles and responsibilities. Team members monitor situations and communicate any changes to keep the team informed. Finally, communication facilitates a culture of mutual support.

The Joint Commission on Accreditation of Healthcare Organizations (now officially the Joint Commission) has set specific safety goals related to communication, including the need for standardized hand-offs with the opportunity to ask and respond to questions. Closed-loop communication is highly recommended and is defined as information exchange behavior whereby a sender initiates a message, a receiver acknowledges the message, and the message is verified by the initial sender, as depicted in Figure 45.5.

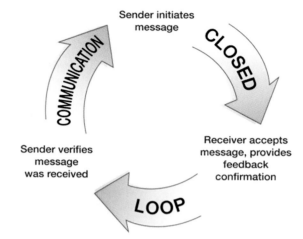

Figure 45.5 Closed-loop communication. Reproduced from Agency for Healthcare Research and Quality [13].

TeamSTEPPS® teaches four communication strategies and tools that have the potential to reduce errors associated with miscommunication. SBAR communication is described as one effective tool. SBAR is a mnemonic that stands for *situation, background, assessment, and recommendation*. SBAR was originally developed by the United States Navy and adapted for use in the medical setting [16]. Many leading healthcare institutions support the use of SBAR, including the Institute for Healthcare Improvement and the Joint Commission. SBAR is a standardized communication technique that allows the speaker to be clear and concise. Call-out is a communication strategy exemplified when a team member verbally states what they are doing, observing, or thinking in real time. A call-out is used to communicate important or critical information during a crisis so that all team members know what is occurring. Examples of call-outs include stating the ability to visualize the larynx during emergency laryngoscopy and intubation, or announcing "clear!" before defibrillation during cardiac arrest. A read-back (checkback) is a process of employing closed-loop communication to ensure that information conveyed by the sender is understood by the receiver as intended. Read-backs avoid orders being given without being acknowledged and ensure proper understanding of orders. Hand-offs are emphasized as important communication processes that can result in patient harm if performed ineffectively. Hand-offs are discussed in detail in the following section.

Many barriers to effective communication exist. These include language barriers, distractions, varying communication styles, workload, and conflict. The teamwork tools and strategies can be used to overcome these barriers to effective communication. Figure 45.6 summarizes the barriers to team effectiveness, the tools and strategies

Barriers to Team Effectiveness

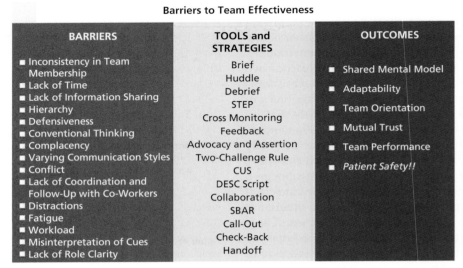

Figure 45.6 Barriers to team effectiveness. Tools and strategies to overcome these barriers, and the desired team outcomes. Reproduced from Agency for Healthcare Research and Quality [13].

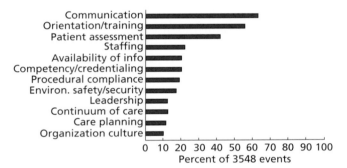

Figure 45.7 Frequency of communication problems as the root cause of sentinel events. Reproduced from Joint Commission on Accreditation of Healthcare Organizations [19].

to mitigate these barriers, and the desired outcomes of team training as taught by TeamSTEPPS®.

Hand-offs

A sentinel event is defined by the Joint Commission as "an unexpected occurrence involving death or serious physical or psychological injury" [17]. Examples of sentinel events include surgery on the wrong body part or the unintended retention of a foreign body such as a surgical instrument. The Joint Commission determined that between 1995 and 2006, nearly 70% of all sentinel events were caused by communication problems [18,19] (Fig. 45.7). More than half of the communication problems analyzed by the Joint Commission occurred during hand-offs. An analysis of one closed claim database showed that 40% of communication problems occurred during hand-offs [20].

A hand-off (also referred to as a handover, sign-out, transition, or sign-over) is defined as the transfer of accountability and responsibility of a patient from one healthcare provider to another. The Joint Commission states that the "primary objective of a hand-off is to provide accurate information about a patient's care, treatment, and services, current condition and any recent or anticipated changes. The information communicated during a hand-off must be accurate in order to meet patient safety goals" [18]. The daily workflow of anesthesiologists involves hand-offs to and from other anesthetists, surgeons, neonatologists, critical care physicians, emergency physicians, respiratory therapists, and perioperative nurses. Pediatric patients are particularly vulnerable to ineffective hand-offs due to their reduced capacity to advocate for themselves and provide information regarding their medical history [21]. Surprisingly, anesthesiologists are seldom formally taught how to perform this duty effectively.

Many specialties including anesthesiologists, surgeons, pediatricians, internists, and emergency medicine physicians have undertaken the qualitative evaluation of hand-offs, finding that they frequently lack a formalized structure [22–30]. They also note frequent omissions and distortions of important information. One study noted that pediatric interns overestimate the effectiveness of the hand-offs that they give [29]. The same study showed that almost 40% of the recipients felt that the most important information about the patient was not reported.

The Joint Commission has commented on the negative consequences of ineffective hand-offs based on the relationship with sentinel events. Analysis of closed claims databases has also demonstrated the contribution of ineffective hand-offs to wrong site surgery, wrong patient surgery, and unintended retention of foreign bodies [20,31]. Ineffective hand-offs have also been shown to result in medication errors, delays in diagnosis and treatment [32], completely missed diagnoses [33], and omission of handed over tasks [25]. Studies have also demonstrated the frequent inability of the incoming physician to find the missing information by means of the medical record [26].

There are many barriers to effective hand-offs. Most important is the lack of formal teaching of the hand-off process. Other barriers include interruptions, noise, distractions, and the time constraints on performing hand-offs in a busy practice [21,34,35]. Outgoing physician fatigue also can decrease the quality of a hand-off. Social hierarchy can also have a negative impact on the quality of a hand-off. It is commonly noted that when receiving a hand-off from a more senior person, the more junior person is reluctant to ask questions and ask for clarification [21,34,36]. This is because the junior person fears the perception that they are questioning a superior.

Controversy exists amongst anesthesiologists regarding whether hand-offs should be formally structured. One survey of anesthesiologists reflected the perspective that standardization is burdensome and not needed, arguing that extra paperwork is an impediment to clinical care [37]. Another group of surveyed anesthesiologists felt that standardization would be valuable [38,39].

Regardless of the desire for or perceived need for standardization of the hand-off process, it is clear that standardization and inclusion of a written and verbal component decreases omissions and distortions, and improves recipient satisfaction with hand off quality [22–25,27,28,34,40]. Another feature of high-quality hand-offs is the inclusion of a read-back (also referred to as a check-back) [21,35,41–44]. A read-back takes place when the incoming provider (recipient of the hand-off) repeats what they heard during the hand-off to the outgoing practitioner who confirms accuracy or clarifies errors. This two-way feedback technique double-checks information accuracy and verifies that the recipient was actually listening during the hand-off. Finally, face-to-face communication during a hand-off is ideal due to the nonverbal information that can be conveyed via facial expressions, body language, gestures, and eye contact. Box 45.2 summarizes the characteristics of effective hand-offs [30,35,44].

It may be useful for an institution to consistently use one mnemonic throughout the hospital so that when surgeons, nurses, anesthesiologists, neonatologists, critical care physicians, and emergency medicine physicians communicate, they utilize a similar communication struc-

---

Box 45.2 Characteristics of effective hand-offs

- Format is standardized
- Contains a verbal and written component
- Read-back used to verify understanding
- Allows the opportunity to ask questions
- Pending studies are emphasized
- Hierarchy is flattened
- Interactive
- Information is up to date
- Contingency plans discussed
- Free of interruptions
- Quiet environment
- Face to face

Box 45.3 Sample protocol for hand-off in SBAR format

Receiving/incoming provider is first given ample time to review the preoperative evaluation, intraoperative record, and surgical note before the hand-off begins

- Situation
  - Patient age, weight, diagnosis, and medical/surgical procedure stated
- Background
  - Allergies, medications, medical history, and surgical history stated
- Assessment
  - *Airway/breathing*: baseline respiratory status, airway management details
  - *Circulation*: hemodynamic stability, vasoactive infusions
  - *Central nervous system*: opioid doses, muscle relaxants, regional anesthesia techniques
  - *Fluids/electrolytes/nutrition*: aspiration risk, dextrose-containing fluids, electrolytes
  - *Hematology*: last hematocrit, estimated blood loss, blood availability
  - *Infectious disease*: antibiotic schedule, contact precautions
  - *Renal*: urine output
  - *Lines*: intravenous access, central lines, arterial lines
- Recommendations
  - Pending tasks and studies are emphasized
  - Recommendations for further management given
  - Read-back performed
  - Questions are solicited and encouraged from receiving/incoming provider

---

ture. At least 24 different mnemonics for hand-offs have been described in the medical literature [45]. SBAR is the most frequently cited mnemonic. SBAR is one format that can be used to standardize hand-offs. Box 45.3 displays a sample hand-off protocol in SBAR format.

Effective team members are expected to ensure that their colleagues are well informed when sharing the care of a patient. Providing an effective standardized hand-off prevents lapses in information that can lead to mistakes.

Checklists

In 1978, a study revealed that 14% of anesthetic mishaps could be attributed to failure of the anesthesia machine [46]. In 1987, the American Society of Anesthesiologists and the United States Food and Drug Administration collaborated to produce a generic anesthesia machine checklist to increase detection of malfunctions.

A checklist is a simple tool designed to reduce error and encourage compliance with best practice. Checklists are memory aids that list action items or criteria that have been determined to be essential to the success of a process or procedure. Indeed, "a short pencil is better than a long memory." Utilization of checklists is considered essential to safety in the industries of aviation, nuclear power, construction, and manufacturing [47]. Recent studies have also demonstrated positive applications in the medical field. Checklists are a proven component of interventions to reduce the incidence of central venous line-associated bloodstream infections, intensive care unit length of stay, and surgical morbidity and mortality.

Central venous line-associated bloodstream infections occur frequently, may result in death, and are considered mostly preventable [48]. In 2001, Pronovost and colleagues undertook a quality improvement project aimed at reducing the incidence of central line-associated infections [49]. The project included a checklist designed to ensure adherence to the infection control protocol. The checklist contained infection control guidelines that most practitioners recognize, but do not always follow. Use of the checklist resulted in a reduction in the mean rate of infections from 7.7 per 1000 catheter-days to 1.4 per 1000 catheter-days. Subsequent studies have reproduced these results, showing significant reductions in line-associated infection rates when a checklist is used [50–54]. Typical components of a central line insertion checklist are shown in Box 45.4.

Box 45.4 Central venous line insertion checklist

- Equipment assembled and supplies verified before procedure begins
- Nurse observes procedure and is empowered to intervene to ensure compliance
- Provider washes hands with antibacterial soap or waterless hand cleaner
- Provider wears hat, mask, sterile gown, and sterile gloves
- Insertion site scrubbed with 2% chlorhexidine (age >2 months) or povidone iodine (<2 months)
- Patient covered from head to toe with sterile drape
- Sterile dressing applied and dated immediately after procedure

---

The intensive care unit is an environment where multidisciplinary co-ordination and communication are vital to patient safety and throughput. The entire care team must clearly understand the goals of care, list of tasks, and communication plan. The intensive care unit daily goals form is a type of checklist designed to improve communication between team members [55–57]. The top two priorities of the daily goals form are the conditions necessary to discharge the patient from the intensive care unit and reducing the patient's greatest safety risk. Several studies have demonstrated that the use of this form results in significant improvements in team understanding of the daily goals for a patient and significant reductions in patient length of stay [55,57,58].

The World Health Organization (WHO) recognizes that surgical complications are common and often preventable. It has been estimated that over 230 million major surgeries take place per year [59]. Of these, 7 million major complications occur, including 1 million deaths. A team of experts created the WHO Surgical Safety Checklist, designed to improve teamwork and prevent common causes of perioperative morbidity and mortality (Fig. 45.8). The WHO Surgical Safety Checklist promotes and facilitates good teamwork by helping the team develop a shared mental model with the use of a brief before anesthesia induction and a time out before skin incision. Before the procedure begins, the entire team introduces themselves by name in order to flatten hierarchy. The checklist also empowers team members to speak up if they notice any safety concerns.

Several components of the WHO Surgical Safety Checklist are related to the practice of anesthesiologists. The Checklist specifically encourages vigilance related to the presence of a difficult airway, risk of aspiration, risk of significant blood loss, the presence of allergies, and timely administration of prophylactic antibiotics.

The effect of the Checklist was evaluated in eight hospitals across the world, including several in developing nations and others in highly developed academic teaching settings. Implementation of the Checklist resulted in a reduction of death from 1.5% to 0.8% and a reduction in inpatient complications from 11.0% to 7.0% [60]. Considering the high volume of worldwide surgeries and the high complication rates [59], global implementation of the WHO Surgical Safety Checklist could lead to substantial reductions in surgical mortality and morbidity. One criticism of this landmark safety study is that although there was improvement in all hospitals, more of the improvement in outcome could be attributed to the hospitals in developing nations.

A recent study of a comprehensive perioperative safety checklist was conducted in six intervention hospitals and five control hospitals in The Netherlands, all tertiary care and academic hospitals with previously demonstrated

Surgical Safety Checklist

World Health Organization | **Patient Safety**
A World Alliance for Safer Health Care

Before induction of anaesthesia	Before skin incision	Before patient leaves operating room
(with at least nurse and anaesthetist)	(with nurse, anaesthetist and surgeon)	(with nurse, anaesthetist and surgeon)

Before induction of anaesthesia

Has the patient confirmed his/her identity, site, procedure, and consent?
☐ Yes

Is the site marked?
☐ Yes
☐ Not applicable

Is the anaesthesia machine and medication check complete?
☐ Yes

Is the pulse oximeter on the patient and functioning?
☐ Yes

Does the patient have a:

Known allergy?
☐ No
☐ Yes

Difficult airway or aspiration risk?
☐ No
☐ Yes, and equipment/assistance available

Risk of >500ml blood loss (7ml/kg in children)?
☐ No
☐ Yes, and two IVs/central access and fluids planned

Before skin incision

☐ **Confirm all team members have introduced themselves by name and role.**

☐ **Confirm the patient's name, procedure, and where the incision will be made.**

Has antibiotic prophylaxis been given within the last 60 minutes?
☐ Yes
☐ Not applicable

Anticipated Critical Events

To Surgeon:
☐ What are the critical or non-routine steps?
☐ How long will the case take?
☐ What is the anticipated blood loss?

To Anaesthetist:
☐ Are there any patient-specific concerns?

To Nursing Team:
☐ Has sterility (including indicator results) been confirmed?
☐ Are there equipment issues or any concerns?

Is essential imaging displayed?
☐ Yes
☐ Not applicable

Before patient leaves operating room

Nurse Verbally Confirms:
☐ The name of the procedure
☐ Completion of instrument, sponge and needle counts
☐ Specimen labelling (read specimen labels aloud, including patient name)
☐ Whether there are any equipment problems to be addressed

To Surgeon, Anaesthetist and Nurse:
☐ What are the key concerns for recovery and management of this patient?

This checklist is not intended to be comprehensive. Additions and modifications to fit local practice are encouraged.   Revised 1 / 2009   © WHO, 2009

Figure 45.8 World Health Organization Surgical Safety Checklist. Reproduced from World Health Organization [82] with permission.

high standards and quality of care [61]. In 3760 patients studied before implementation of the checklist and 3820 patients after implementation, the total number of complications decreased from 27.3 to 16.5 per 100 patients (p < 0.001), and in-hospital mortality decreased from 1.5% to 0.8% (p < 0.001). These outcomes did not change in the control hospitals. Surgical safety checklists should be modified according to local institutional needs, including those of a children's hospital, where the surgical briefing may need to be done in the preoperative holding area with the parent present. One such modification is shown in Figure 45.9.

Checklists are important components of comprehensive patient safety interventions. It would be an oversimplification to state that checklists alone reduce central venous line-associated infections, ICU length of stay, and surgical morbidity [62]. Team education must first take place to build faith in the practices reinforced by the checklist. Barriers to the use of the checklist must be identified and eliminated or the checklist will often be left unused. Outcomes must be measured and feedback should be provided. Institutions should customize

checklists to fit the needs and culture of their own organization.

One survey revealed that some physicians remain skeptical about whether or not checklists truly improve patient safety. The fact that almost all of those same skeptics wanted the checklist used if they themselves were having surgery speaks for itself [47]. The use of checklists that have shown evidence in improvements in patient outcomes should be embraced.

Medication safety

The practice of anesthesia requires titration of multiple medications in order to safely produce the anesthetized state while maintaining hemodynamic and respiratory stability. Anesthesia providers also must have multiple medications immediately available to treat potential emergency situations that may develop during surgery. The environment is frequently chaotic and requires effective focus and skills in multitasking to avoid potentially life-threatening medication errors. In modern medical systems,

Texas Children's Hospital Surgical Safety Checklist- (VERSION 6.6)

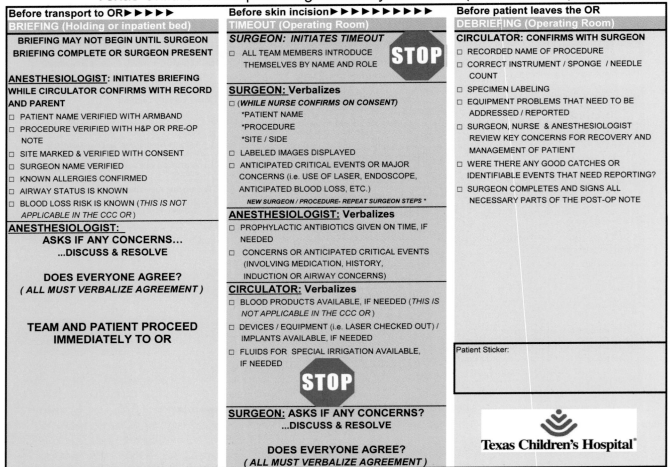

Before transport to OR►►►►►

BRIEFING (Holding or inpatient bed)

BRIEFING MAY NOT BEGIN UNTIL SURGEON
BRIEFING COMPLETE OR SURGEON PRESENT

**ANESTHESIOLOGIST: INITIATES BRIEFING
WHILE CIRCULATOR CONFIRMS WITH RECORD
AND PARENT**

☐ PATIENT NAME VERIFIED WITH ARMBAND
☐ PROCEDURE VERIFIED WITH H&P OR PRE-OP
  NOTE
☐ SITE MARKED & VERIFIED WITH CONSENT
☐ SURGEON NAME VERIFIED
☐ KNOWN ALLERGIES CONFIRMED
☐ AIRWAY STATUS IS KNOWN
☐ BLOOD LOSS RISK IS KNOWN (*THIS IS NOT
  APPLICABLE IN THE CCC OR*)

ANESTHESIOLOGIST:

**ASKS IF ANY CONCERNS...
...DISCUSS & RESOLVE**

DOES EVERYONE AGREE?
(*ALL MUST VERBALIZE AGREEMENT*)

**TEAM AND PATIENT PROCEED
IMMEDIATELY TO OR**

Before skin incision►►►►►►►►►►

TIMEOUT (Operating Room)

SURGEON: INITIATES TIMEOUT
☐ ALL TEAM MEMBERS INTRODUCE
  THEMSELVES BY NAME AND ROLE **STOP**

SURGEON: Verbalizes
☐ (*WHILE NURSE CONFIRMS ON CONSENT*)
  *PATIENT NAME
  *PROCEDURE
  *SITE / SIDE
☐ LABELED IMAGES DISPLAYED
☐ ANTICIPATED CRITICAL EVENTS OR MAJOR
  CONCERNS (i.e. USE OF LASER, ENDOSCOPE,
  ANTICIPATED BLOOD LOSS, ETC.)
  *NEW SURGEON / PROCEDURE- REPEAT SURGEON STEPS **

ANESTHESIOLOGIST: Verbalizes
☐ PROPHYLACTIC ANTIBIOTICS GIVEN ON TIME, IF
  NEEDED
☐ CONCERNS OR ANTICIPATED CRITICAL EVENTS
  (INVOLVING MEDICATION, HISTORY,
  INDUCTION OR AIRWAY CONCERNS)

CIRCULATOR: Verbalizes
☐ BLOOD PRODUCTS AVAILABLE, IF NEEDED (*THIS IS
  NOT APPLICABLE IN THE CCC OR*)
☐ DEVICES / EQUIPMENT (i.e. LASER CHECKED OUT) /
  IMPLANTS AVAILABLE, IF NEEDED
☐ FLUIDS FOR SPECIAL IRRIGATION AVAILABLE,
  IF NEEDED **STOP**

SURGEON: ASKS IF ANY CONCERNS?
  ...DISCUSS & RESOLVE

DOES EVERYONE AGREE?
(*ALL MUST VERBALIZE AGREEMENT*)

Before patient leaves the OR

DEBRIEFING (Operating Room)

CIRCULATOR: CONFIRMS WITH SURGEON
☐ RECORDED NAME OF PROCEDURE
☐ CORRECT INSTRUMENT / SPONGE / NEEDLE
  COUNT
☐ SPECIMEN LABELING
☐ EQUIPMENT PROBLEMS THAT NEED TO BE
  ADDRESSED / REPORTED
☐ SURGEON, NURSE & ANESTHESIOLOGIST
  REVIEW KEY CONCERNS FOR RECOVERY AND
  MANAGEMENT OF PATIENT
☐ WERE THERE ANY GOOD CATCHES OR
  IDENTIFIABLE EVENTS THAT NEED REPORTING?
☐ SURGEON COMPLETES AND SIGNS ALL
  NECESSARY PARTS OF THE POST-OP NOTE

Patient Sticker:

Texas Children's Hospital®

Figure 45.9 The Texas Children's Hospital Surgical Safety Checklist. The surgical briefing is done in the holding area or intensive care unit bedside, and initiated by the anesthesiologist with the parent present to verify information. The surgeon must be present for the briefing or have communicated to the anesthesiologist verbally or via written communication his/her plans and concerns for the case.

the anesthesiologist is in a unique situation with regard to medication administration: single-handedly responsible for ordering, preparing, and administering medications without a second person to cross-check. Pediatric patients are particularly vulnerable to medication dosing errors since most medications are administered on a dose per weight basis and incorrect measurement of weight, recording of weight, or calculation of dose can lead to significant overdosing or underdosing of medications.

Incidence

Medication errors are common in healthcare systems and are reported to be the seventh most common cause of death overall. In 1999 the Institute of Medicine (IOM) issued a report indicating that 44,000–98,000 patients die each year as a result of medical errors, and a large portion are medication related [3,63]. A survey of members of the Canadian Society of Anaesthesiologists reported that 85%

of respondents had experienced at least one drug error or near miss [64]. Similarly, 89% of respondents to a survey of anesthesiologists in New Zealand reported making a drug administration error at some stage of their career and 12.5% had actually harmed the patient [65]. Several prospective studies have found the incidence of drug errors during anesthesia to be between one per 133 anesthetics and one per 274 anesthetics, with major morbidities being rare [66–68].

Types of medication errors

Various groups have classified medication errors, and Table 45.1 is a classification scheme proposed by Webster et al [66].

A report from the ASA Closed Claims Project compared medication error claims between 1990 and 2001, finding that pediatric patients had a higher proportion of claims compared to adults and incorrect dosing was the most

Table 45.1 Classification scheme proposed by Webster et al [66]

Type of medication error	Definition
• Omission	Drug not given
• Repetition	Extra dose of an intended drug
• Substitution	Incorrect drug instead of the desired drug: a swap
• Insertion	A drug that was not intended to be given at a particular time or at any time
• Incorrect dose	Wrong dose of an intended drug
• Incorrect route	Wrong route of an intended drug
• Others	Usually a more complex event, not fitting the above categories

common type of error (44% of errors) [69]. A recent report from New Zealand also found the most common type of error to be incorrect dosing [66].

Risk factors

The large study from New Zealand evaluated many contributing factors to medication errors, finding a failure to check to be the most common (23%), followed by distraction (16%), inattention (13%), and haste or production pressure (10%) [66]. Interestingly, several studies have evaluated the risk of emergency surgery and this does not appear to be a contributing factor with medication errors.

Prevention

Webster and colleagues evaluated the baseline incidence of medication errors in two hospitals, both of which used a standard color-coding labeling system for medications used by anesthesiologists [66]. They evaluated the effect of implementing a new system designed to reduce such errors in one of the hospitals. This system included:

- labels with the class and generic name of each drug in large, clear lettering and incorporating a barcode
- alerts for known allergies and expired drugs
- custom software and a barcode scanner to allow a drug–identity cross-check before each administration, by redisplay of the drug name and its international color code on a computer screen and an auditory announcement of the drug name
- reorganization of the workspace using syringe trays and a color-coded drug tray, prefilled, standardized syringes for many commonly used medications
- a complete, automated anesthetic record
- operational rules designed to decrease human error and facilitate safe practice. The two principal operating rules were: to scan each drug before administration

and to retain used ampules and syringes in designated zones on the new trays as a physical "record" of what had been given
- additional labeling system for the accurate preparation of infusion drugs.

On 26 January 2010, the Anesthesia Patient Safety Foundation (APSF) convened a consensus conference of 100 stakeholders from many different backgrounds to develop new strategies for "predictable prompt improvement" of medication safety in the operating room. Their recommendations are summarized in Box 45.5 [70].

Pay-for-performance

Many evidence-based clinical processes that are known to improve patient outcomes are not consistently achieved or are implemented slowly [71]. In the United States, Medicare and many other healthcare plans have adopted pay-for-performance (P4P) methods to incentivize reporting of quality data and achieving quality goals. P4P initiatives create financial incentives for physicians to achieve quality goals by linking a portion of payments to performance on quality measures. The quality goals are based on evidence (or consensus in the absence of data) and strive for the efficient use of resources. For example, the Physician Quality Reporting Initiative was established by the Centers for Medicare and Medicaid Services. This was done to incentivize physicians to report data on various quality measures. By doing so, a group practice may qualify to earn an incentive payment equal to 2% of their total Medicare allowed charges. Currently, participation in Medicare P4P initiatives is voluntary and only requires the reporting of quality data to achieve financial incentives. The ASA has developed a set of five proposed "quality incentives" that can be the basis for performance measures [72]. These ASA measures parallel several Medicare measures [73] and are shown in Box 45.6.

Pay-for-performance initiatives are in the early phases of adoption. The actual effect that P4P has on quality improvement is currently unclear. Studies have generally shown that P4P initiatives have no effect or minimal effect on improving quality measures [74–77]. Even as many third party payers are moving forward with P4P initiatives, caution may be warranted due to the fact that the data regarding effectiveness are weak at best.

Safe systems in the operating room

Operating room (OR) safety can potentially be improved through the application of technology and knowledge. Recent advances in technology have moved the traditional surgical suite toward one that is more efficient

Box 45.5 Consensus recommendations for improving medication safety in the operating room.

Standardization

- High alert drugs (such as phenylephrine and epinephrine) should be available in standardized concentrations/diluents prepared by pharmacy in a ready-to-use (bolus or infusion) form that is appropriate for both adult and pediatric patients. Infusions should be delivered by an electronically-controlled smart device containing a drug library.
- Ready-to-use syringes and infusions should have standardized fully compliant machine-readable labels.
- *Additional ideas*
  - Interdisciplinary and uniform curriculum for medication administration safety to be available to all training programs and facilities.
  - No concentrated versions of any potentially lethal agents in the operating room.
  - Required read-back in an environment for extremely high alert drugs such as heparin.
  - Standardized placement of drugs within all anesthesia workstations in an institution.
  - Convenient required method to save all used syringes and drug containers until case concluded.
  - Standardized infusion libraries/protocols throughout an institution.
  - Standardized route-specific connectors for tubing (IV, arterial, epidural, enteral).

Technology

1. Every anesthetizing location should have a mechanism to identify medications before drawing up or administering them (bar code reader) and a mechanism to provide feedback, decision support, and documentation (automated information system).
2. *Additional ideas*
   a. Technology training and device education for all users, possibly requiring formal certification.
   b. Improved and standardized user interfaces on infusion pumps.

c. Mandatory safety checklists incorporated into all operating room systems.

Pharmacy/prefilled/premixed

1. Routine provider-prepared medications should be discontinued whenever possible.
2. Clinical pharmacists should be part of the perioperative/operating room team.
3. Standardized pre-prepared medication kits by case type should be used whenever possible.
4. *Additional ideas*
   a. Interdisciplinary and uniform curriculum for medication administration safety for all anesthesia professionals and pharmacists.
   b. Enhanced training of operating room pharmacists specifically as perioperative consultants.
   c. Deployment of ubiquitous automated dispensing machines in the operating room suite (with communication to central pharmacy and its information management system).

Culture

1. Establish a *"just culture"* for reporting errors (including near misses) and discussion of lessons learned.
2. Establish a culture of education, understanding, and accountability via a required curriculum and CME and dissemination of dramatic stories in the *APSF Newsletter* and educational videos.
3. Establish a culture of cooperation and recognition of the benefits of STPC within and between institutions, professional organizations, and accreditation agencies.

Reproduced from Eichhorn [70] with permission from the Anesthesia Patient Safety Foundation.

CME, continuing medical eduation; APSF, Anesthesia Patient Safety Foundation; STPC, Standardization, Technology, Pharmacy/Prefilled/Premixed, and Culture.

Box 45.6 Proposed anesthesiology pay-for-performance measures

American Society of Anesthesiologists recommended quality incentives	2010 Physician Quality Reporting Initiative List (Medicare)
1. Timely administration of antibiotic prophylaxis	1. Timely administration of antibiotic prophylaxis
2. Perioperative normothermia	2. Perioperative temperature management
3. Comprehensive planning for chronic pain management	3. Pain assessment prior to initiation of patient therapy
4. Prevention of ventilator-associated pneumonia	4. Venous thromboembolism prophylaxis
5. Prevention of catheter-related bloodstream infections	5. Prevention of catheter-related bloodstream infections

and safe. However, the practice in most operating rooms does not differ greatly from operating rooms 50 years ago. The Health Information Technology for Economic and Clinical Health (HITECH) Act as part of the American

Recovery and Reinvestment Act (ARRA) of 2009 pledges billions of dollars to improve access to data through technology and improve overall quality of care [78,79]. Yet, to date, electronic information systems do not have a common platform and do not effectively share data elements (pertinent patient information). Effective anesthesia information systems (AIMS) should enhance patient care by more than simply providing a legible record. In fact, although legible, most current information systems produce records that will automatically add data and descriptive text with the push of a button. Such a record may actually lead to inaccurate data entry, or produce a lengthy record that will fatigue users in the same way that sorting through a voluminous paper chart is inefficient. Also, the addition of complex technology to the operating room can increase hazards by distracting the anesthesiologist from the patient and surgical procedure. An effective anesthesia information system is easy to use and provides decision support to the user in order to enhance patient care (Box 45.7) [80]. See Chapter 44 for a more detailed presentation of the electronic anesthesia record.

Box 45.7 Examples of decision support from anesthesia information management systems

- Quality assurance
  - Maintenance of normothermia notifications
  - Presurgical antibiotic management notifications
- Medication support
  - Drug–drug interaction checking
  - Drug–dose calculations
  - Drug re-dosing reminders
  - Drug–allergy checking
- Regulatory and compliance support
  - Concurrency checking
  - Ensuring electronic records contain elements required for billing
  - Attending physician attestation statements
  - Case times (start of anesthesia care, end of anesthesia care)
  - Case type (general/monitored anesthesia care/regional)
  - Patient details (ASA physical status)
- Support around critical events
  - Algorithm display and guidance (malignant hyperthermia, advanced cardiac life support, ASA difficult airway algorithm)
  - Critical event detection
    1. Chaotic electrocardiogram + no pulse-ox wave form → consider ventricular fibrillation
    2. ↓Blood pressure + ↑heart rate + ↓end-tidal CO_2 → consider ↓cardiac output from hypovolemia

Other technologies that are being tested in the operating room to improve patient safety include the use of barcodes, radiofrequency identification (RFID), and smart imaging. As described above, barcodes can be used to perform as a second check on medication administration. Additionally, they can track instruments used in the surgical field.

Most commercial warehouses and supermarkets track their inventories more effectively than healthcare providers do in the perioperative environment. Modern retailers easily track the inventory of inexpensive items, while a charge nurse in a typical operating suite might have to search for a $20,000 ultrasound machine. RFID can be used to track, plan, and send shared equipment for operating room procedures, thereby improving efficiency. RFID can be inexpensively incorporated into the patient's armband so that when the patient enters the operating room, the most recent labs, images, planned surgical procedure, ordered antibiotics, and allergies are automatically displayed on a common screen. Adding RFID tags to surgical sponges and instruments could potentially eliminate retained foreign material in the surgical wound, and an RFID label on blood products could identify an incorrect unit as it is brought into the operating room. At the time of this writing, these technologies remain in the early phases of development.

Conclusion

The Institute of Medicine's seminal report *To Err is Human*, first published in 1999 [3], started the patient safety revolution in healthcare that continues to this day. That study used previously collected data from large population-based studies to determine that there were between 44,000 and 98,000 preventable hospital deaths, and up to 1 million patient injuries each year in the United States during the decade of the 1990s. In a recent report retrospectively reviewing adverse events from 2002 to 2007 in 10 randomly selected North Carolina general acute care hospitals, there was no reduction in patient harms on an annual basis over the 6 years of the study [81], averaging 25.1 harms per 100 admissions. The perioperative period was a significant source of patient harms.

These new data demonstrate that despite all the recent emphasis on patient safety and improving outcomes, medical error is still common and there is still a very significant amount of work to be done. The Institute of Medicine's stated goal of 50% reduction in medical error has clearly not been met. Although data specific to pediatric care are sparse, the same issues are identified in pediatric practice as in medical care in general. Pediatric anesthesiologists are in a unique position, interfacing with all members of the perioperative care team, to take a leadership role in teamwork, communication, and patient safety, to prevent adverse events and deaths in our vulnerable pediatric population.

Annotated references

A full reference list for this chapter is available at:
http://www.wiley.com/go/gregory/andropoulos/pediatricanesthesia

6. Fletcher GC, McGeorge P, Flin RH et al. The role of non-technical skills in anaesthesia: a review of current literature. Br J Anaesth 2002; 88: 418–29. The evidence base for the current emphasis on non-technical skills to improve team functioning in anesthesia care.

13. Agency for Healthcare Research and Quality. TeamSTEPPS Fundamentals Course. www.ahrq.gov/teamsteppstools/instructor/fundamentals/index.html. The publicly available team functioning training guide of the US Agency for Healthcare Research and Quality, with evidence-based principles to improve healthcare outcomes by enhancing team functioning.

21. Streitenberger K, Breen-Reid K, Harris C. Handoffs in care – can we make them safer? Pediatr Clin North Am 2006; 53: 1185–95. The pediatric perspective of hand-offs of care, emphasizing the pediatric patient's particular vulnerability to errors because of their inability to communicate and advocate for their own care.

47. Gawande A. The Checklist Manifesto: How to Get Things Right. New York: Metropolitan Books, 2009. An important book documenting the parallels between medicine and the industries of aviation, nuclear power, construction, and manufacturing.

49. Pronovost P, Needham D, Berenholtz S et al. An intervention to decrease catheter-related bloodstream infections in the ICU. N Engl J Med 2006; 355: 2725–32. The seminal article documenting a

dramatic decrease in central line infection with the introduction of a checklist for sterile insertion and maintenance of the catheters.

55. Pronovost P, Berenholtz S, Dorman T et al. Improving communication in the ICU using daily goals. J Crit Care 2003; 18: 71–5. An important study documenting an improvement in outcomes and resource utilization in ICUs when a daily goal system was formalized.

60. Haynes AB, Weiser TG, Berry WR et al. A surgical safety checklist to reduce morbidity and mortality in a global population. N Engl J Med 2009; 360: 491–9. A landmark article documenting significant reductions in morbidity and mortality in adult surgery, in eight major hospitals across the world.

61. De Vries EN, Prins HA, Crolla RM et al. Effect of a comprehensive surgical safety system on patient outcomes. N Engl J Med 2010; 363: 1928–37.An important contemporary follow-up documenting that a perioperative checklist reduces surgical morbidity and mortality even in very high-quality, sophisticated tertiary academic medical centers.

66. Webster CS, Larsson L, Frampton CM et al. Clinical assessment of a new anaesthetic drug administration system: a prospective, controlled, longitudinal incident monitoring study. Anaesthesia 2010; 65: 490–9. An important study of a new anesthesia drug administration paradigm, both classifying errors under a conventional system and improvement under a sytem using evidence-based principles.

75. Lindenauer PK, Remus D, Roman S et al. Public reporting and pay for performance in hospital quality improvement. N Engl J Med 2007; 356: 486–96. A clear explanation of the principles of pay for performance, using publicly available data.

APPENDIX A

Pediatric Anesthesia Drugs and Other Treatments in the Perioperative Period

Dean B. Andropoulos

Department of Anesthesiology and Pediatrics, Baylor College of Medicine, and Texas Children's Hospital, Houston, TX, USA

Drug doses and treatments are those commonly recommended; each patient's treatment must be individualized, drug doses double-checked for accuracy, and drug concentrations and modes of administration used according to local guidelines. Information is current at the time of publication; however, the practitioner must always be aware of new recommendations, and is responsible for determining the best course of treatment. Consult the textbook, hospital formulary, or authoritative internet resources for a complete listing of indications, contraindications, interval dosing schedules, and side-effects of these drugs and treatments. All drugs are intravenous unless otherwise noted. Drugs denoted with an asterisk (*) are not US FDA approved as of August 2011. Source for dosing information is the Texas Children's Hospital Drug Formulary, current as of August 2011, except where otherwise noted in the references.

Gregory's Pediatric Anesthesia, Fifth Edition. Edited by George A. Gregory, Dean B. Andropoulos.
© 2012 Blackwell Publishing Ltd. Published 2012 by Blackwell Publishing Ltd.

Category	Drug/treatment	Bolus/loading dose	Infusion/continuous dose
Anesthetic, sedative, and analgesic agents			
Opioids	Fentanyl	1–10 µg/kg; 50–200 µg/kg total dose	5–20 µg/kg/h
	Remifentanil	0.25–1 µg/kg	0.05–2 µg/kg/min
	Sufentanil	0.1–5 µg/kg	0.1–3 µg/kg/h
	Morphine	0.03–0.2 mg/kg	0.01–0.05 mg/kg/h
	Meperidine (shivering)	1–2 mg/kg	NA
	Methadone	0.1 mg/kg	NA
	Hydromorphone	0.02 mg/kg	0.006 mg/kg/h
Benzodiazepines	Midazolam IV	0.03–0.1 mg/kg	0.05–0.1 mg/kg/h
	Midazolam PO	0.5–1 mg/kg	NA
	Lorazepam	0.25–0.1 mg/kg	NA
	Diazepam IV	0.05–0.3 mg/kg, max 10 mg	NA
	Diazepam PO	0.04–0.3 mg/kg, max 10 mg	NA
Barbiturates	Thiopental	1–6 mg/kg	NA
	Pentobarbital	1–6 mg/kg	NA
	Methohexital	1–3 mg/kg	NA
Other sedative/analgesic agents	Ketamine IV	1–2 mg/kg	NA
	Ketamine IM	5–10 mg/kg	NA
	Etomidate	0.1–0.3 mg/kg	NA
	Propofol	1–3 mg/kg	50–200 µg/kg/min
	Scopolamine	10 µg/kg	NA
	Dexmedetomidine	0.3–1 µg/kg	0.3–0.7 µg/kg/h
Neuromuscular blocking drugs and reversals	Vecuronium	0.1–0.3 mg/kg	0.05–0.1 mg/kg/h
	Rocuronium IV	0.6–1.2 mg/kg	NA
	Rocuronium IM	2 mg/kg	NA
	Atracurium	0.4–0.5 mg/kg	NA
	Cisatracurium	0.15–0.2 mg/kg	NA
	Pancuronium	0.1–0.2 mg/kg	NA
	Succinylcholine IV	1–2 mg/kg	NA
	Succinylcholine IM	4 mg/kg	NA
	Neostigmine	40–80 µg/kg	NA
	Glycopyrrolate	8–16 µg/kg	NA
	Sugammadex*[1]	2–4 mg/kg	NA

Category	Drug/treatment	Bolus/loading dose	Infusion/continuous dose
Vasoactive drugs			
Inotropes/vasoconstrictors	Epinephrine	0.5–10 µg/kg	0.03–0.1 µg/kg/min
	Atropine IV	10–20 µg/kg	NA
	Atropine IM	20–40 µg/kg	NA
	Phenylephrine	0.5–3 µg/kg	0.05–0.5 µg/kg/min
	Ephedrine	0.05–0.2 mg/kg	NA
	Calcium chloride	10 mg/kg	5–10 mg/kg/h
	Calcium gluconate	30 mg/kg	NA
	Dopamine	NA	3–20 µg/kg/min
	Dobutamine	NA	3–20 µg/kg/min
	Milrinone	25–75 µg/kg	0.25–0.75 µg/kg/min
	Norepinephrine	NA	0.05–0.1 µg/kg/min
	Vasopressin	NA	0.02–0.05 units/kg/h
	Isoproterenol	NA	0.01–0.1 µg/kg/min
	Levosimendan [2-4]	6–12 µg/kg	0.1–0.2 µg/kg/min
	Tri-iodothyronine (T3)[5]	NA	0.05 µg/kg/h
Vasodilators/ antihypertensives	Sodium nitroprusside	NA	0.3–5 µg/kg/min
	Nitroglycerine	NA	0.3–5 µg/kg/min
	Prostaglandin E1	NA	0.0125–0.05 µg/kg/min
	Prostacyclin (Flolan, epoprostenol, PGI2)	NA	2–5 ng/kg/min
	Nesiritide	NA	0.01–0.03 µg/kg/min
	Fenoldopam	NA	0.025–0.3 µg/kg/min initially, titrate to max 1.6 µg/kg/min
	Nicardipine	NA	0.1–0.3 mg/kg/h, max 15 mg/h
	Hydralazine	0.1–0.2 mg/kg	NA
	Phentolamine	0.1–0.2 mg/kg on CPB	NA
	Phenoxybenzamine	0.25–1 mg/kg on CPB	
	Labetalol	0.25–0.5 mg/kg	NA
	Enalaprilat	5–10 µg/kg	NA
	Sildenafil [6,7]	0.35–0.44 mg/kg over 1–3 h	0.067 mg/kg/h

(Continued)

Category	Drug/treatment	Bolus/loading dose	Infusion/continuous dose
Antiarrhythmics/β-blockers	Lidocaine	1–2 mg/kg	20–50 µg/kg/min
	Procainamide	10–15 mg/kg	20–80 µg/kg/min
	Esmolol	250–500 µg/kg	50–300 µg/kg/min
	Propranolol	0.01–0.1 mg/kg	NA
	Amiodarone	5 mg/kg over 10–15 min, may repeat × 2 to max 15 mg/kg	NA
	Verapamil	0.1–0.3 mg/kg	NA
	Adenosine	25–50 µg/kg, double if ineffective	NA
	Magnesium sulfate	25–50 mg/kg over 30–60 min	NA
	Digoxin	8–10 µg/kg 1st loading dose	NA
Antibiotics	Cefazolin	25 mg/kg, max 1 g	NA
	Ampicillin	50 mg/kg, max 1 g	NA
	Vancomycin	15 mg/kg, max 1 g	NA
	Gentamicin	2.5 mg/kg, max 120 mg	NA
	Nafcillin	50 mg/kg, max 2 g	NA
	Clindamycin	10 mg/kg	NA
	Cefuroxime	25–30 mg/kg	NA
	Cefoxitin	30–40 mg/kg, max 2 g	NA
	Pipericillin/tazobactam	100 mg/kg piperacillin component, max 4 g	
Non-steroidal anti-inflammatory drugs/non-opioid analgesics	Ketorolac	0.5 mg/kg, max 30 mg	NA
	Acetaminophen PO	15 mg/kg, max 1000 mg	NA
	Acetaminophen PR	20–30 mg/kg (one time)	NA
	Acetaminophen IV	12.5–15 mg/kg, max 1000 mg	NA
	Ibuprofen IV	5–10 mg/kg, max 400 mg	NA
	Ibuprofen PO	5–10 mg/kg, max 400 mg	NA
Malignant hyperthermia treatment	Dantrolene	2.5 mg/kg; may repeat × 3 up to 10 mg/kg	NA
Local anesthetics	Lidocaine	Max 5 mg/kg	NA
	Bupivacaine	Max 2.5 mg/kg	NA
	Levobupivacaine	Max 2.5 mg/kg	NA
	Ropivacaine	Max 2 mg/kg	NA
	Tetracaine (spinal – infants <6 months)	0.4–0.8 mg/kg	NA
Local anesthetic toxicity	20% Intralipid [8]	1 ml/kg; repeat × 2 to max 3 mL/kg	0.25 mL/kg/min
Corticosteroids	Methylprednisolone	1–30 mg/kg depending on indication	5.4 mg/kg/h × 23 h for spinal cord injury
	Dexamethasone	0.25–1 mg/kg, max 20 mg	NA
	Hydrocortisone	1–2 mg/kg	NA

Category	Drug/treatment	Bolus/loading dose	Infusion/continuous dose
Anticoagulants	Heparin	CPB: 300–400 units/kg	NA
	Bivalirudin [9,10]	Interventional cardiac cath: 0.75 mg/kg CPB: 1 mg/kg, plus 1 mg/kg CPB prime	Cath: 1.75 mg/kg/h CPB: 2.5 mg/kg/h
	Argatroban	CPB: 35–100 µg/kg (ACT > 400 sec)	2–10 µg/kg/min
	Antithrombin III	50 units/kg; target levels 80–120% of normal	NA
Hemostasis agents	ε-Aminocaproic acid	75 mg/kg patient; 75 mg/kg CPB prime	75 mg/kg/h
	Tranexamic acid	10–100 mg/kg	1–10 mg/kg/h
	Recombinant factor VIIa	30–90 µg/kg; may repeat × 2	
Diuretics	Furosemide	0.5–1 mg/kg, max 40 mg	0.1–0.4 mg/kg/h
	Bumetanide	0.015–0.1 mg/kg, max 2.5 mg	NA
	Mannitol	0.25–1 g/kg	NA
Perioperative nausea and vomiting/ gastrointestinal prophylaxis	Ondansetron	0.1 mg/kg, max 4 mg	NA
	Granisetron	10–20 µg/kg	NA
	Metoclopramide	0.1–0.2 mg/kg, max 10 mg	NA
	Promethazine (over age 2 years only)	0.25–0.5 mg/kg, max 25 mg	
	Sodium citrate PO	30 mL	NA
Antihistamines	Diphenhydramine	1–2 mg/kg, max 50 mg	NA
	Ranitidine	1 mg/kg, max 50 mg	NA
	Famotidine	0.5 mg/kg, max 40 mg	NA
Alkalinizing agents	Sodium bicarbonate (dilute 1:1 sterile H_2O for neonates)	1–2 meq/kg	NA
	Tromethamine (THAM) 0.3 M solution	3–6 mL/kg	NA
Inhaled agents/ bronchodilators			Inspired dose
	Sevoflurane		1–8%
	Isoflurane		0.5–3%
	Desflurane		2–12%
	Nitrous oxide (N_2O)		50–75%
	Nitric oxide (NO)		5–20 ppm
	Levalbuterol	8–12 MDI puffs per ETT; 0.075–0.15 mg/kg nebulized in 3 mL normal saline	NA
	Racemic epinephrine	0.25–0.5 mL of 2.25% racemic epinephrine in 3 mL normal saline	NA
	Prostacyclin (Iloprost, PGI2) [11]	2.5–5 µg nebulized in 3 mL normal saline	NA

(Continued)

Category	Drug/treatment	Bolus/loading dose	Infusion/continuous dose
Electrolytes/dextrose	25% Dextrose in water (50% dextrose diluted 1:1)	0.25–0.5 mL/kg	NA
	Potassium chloride (KCl)	0.5–1 meq/kg	NA
	3% NaCl	3–5 mL/kg	NA
Insulin (regular)	Dose based on plasma glucose levels	0.02–0.1 units/kg	0.02–0.1 units/kg/h
Sedation/analgesia reversal	Naloxone	1–10 µg/kg	NA
	Flumazenil	1–5 µg/kg; repeat as needed, max dose 1 mg	NA
Immunosuppressants (transplant)	Basiliximab	<35 kg: 10 mg >35 kg: 20 mg	NA
	Mycophenolate	15 mg/kg, max 1.5 g	NA
Miscellaneous drugs	Caffeine citrate	10–20 mg/kg	NA
Transfusions	Packed red blood cells	10–15 mL/kg	NA
	Whole blood	10–15 mL/kg	NA
	Platelets	1 unit/5 kg will increase platelet count by 50,000; 1 pheresis unit = 6 random donor units	NA
	Cryoprecipitate	1 unit per 5 kg, max 4 units	NA
	Fresh frozen plasma	10–20 mL/kg	NA
Intravascular volume expansion	5% albumin	10–20 mL/kg	NA
	25% albumin	2–4 mL/kg; 0.5–1 g/kg	NA
	6% hetastarch	10–20 mL/kg, max 15 ml/kg/24 h	NA
Direct current cardioversion/ defibrillation	External synchronized cardioversion	0.5 J/kg; increase to max 1 J/kg; max 100 kg	NA
	External defibrillation	2–5 J/kg; increase if ineffective; max 200 J biphasic, 360 J monophasic	NA
	Internal defibrillation	5 J; increase to 10 if ineffective	NA
	Internal synchronized cardioversion	2 J; increase to 5 J if ineffective	NA

ACT, activated clotting time; CPB, cardiopulmonary bypass; ETT, endotracheal tube; IM, intramuscular; IV, intravenous; J, joules; µg, microgram; max, maximum; MDI, metered dose inhaler; meq, milliequivalents; mg, milligram; NA, not applicable; ng, nanogram; PO, oral (per os).

References

1. Paton F, Paulden M, Chambers D, et al. Sugammadex compared with neostigmine/glycopyrrolate for routine reversal of neuromuscular block: a systematic review and economic evaluation. Br J Anaesth 2010; 105: 558–67.
2. Osthaus WA, Boethig D, Winterhalter M et al. First experiences with intraoperative Levosimendan in pediatric cardiac surgery. Eur J Pediatr 2009; 168: 735–40.
3. Di Chiara L, Ricci Z, Garisto C et al. Initial experience with levosimendan infusion for preoperative management of hypoplastic left heart syndrome. Pediatr Cardiol 2010; 31: 166–7.
4. Namachivayam P, Crossland DS, Butt WW, Shekerdemian LS. Early experience with Levosimendan in children with ventricular dysfunction. Pediatr Crit Care Med 2006; 7: 445–8.
5. Mackie AS, Booth KL, Newburger JW et al. A randomized, double-blind, placebo-controlled pilot trial of triiodothyronine in neonatal heart surgery. J Thorac Cardiovasc Surg 2005; 130: 810–16.
6. Steinhorn RH, Kinsella JP, Pierce C et al. Intravenous sildenafil in the treatment of neonates with persistent pulmonary hypertension. J Pediatr 2009; 155: 841–7.

7. Stocker C, Penny DJ, Brizard CP et al. Intravenous sildenafil and inhaled nitric oxide: a randomised trial in infants after cardiac surgery. Intensive Care Med 2003; 29:1996–2003.

8. Weinberg GL. Lipid infusion therapy: translation to clinical practice. Anesth Analg 2008; 106: 1340–2.

9. Forbes TJ, Hijazi ZM, Young G et al. Pediatric catheterization laboratory anticoagulation with bivalirudin. Catheter Cardiovasc Interv 2011 Jan 4 (Epub ahead of print).

10. Anand SX, Viles-Gonzalez JF, Mahboobi SK, Heerdt PM. Bivalirudin utilization in cardiac surgery: shifting anticoagulation from indirect to direct thrombin inhibition. Can J Anaesth 2010; 58(3): 296–311.

11. Tissot C, Beghetti M. Review of inhaled iloprost for the control of pulmonary artery hypertension in children. Vasc Health Risk Manag 2009; 5: 325–31.

APPENDIX B
Pediatric Normal Laboratory Values

Dean B. Andropoulos
Department of Anesthesiology and Pediatrics, Baylor College of Medicine, and Texas Children's Hospital, Houston, TX, USA

For conversion of conventional (US) units to SI units, see: www.soc-bdr.org/rds/authors/unit_tables_conversions_and_genetic_dictionaries/e5196/index_en.html

Values are reference values from Texas Children's Hospital Clinical Laboratory, current as of August 2011. All practitioners are urged to consult the normal laboratory values for their local laboratory, as these may differ from those listed below. They are also advised to continually check for updated normal ranges.

Test	Reference range (United States/conventional units)	
Albumin (CSF)	10–30 mg/dL	
Albumin (S, P)		
Age	g/dL	
0–30 days	2.9–5.5	
1–3 months	2.8–5.0	
4–11 months	3.9–5.1	
≥1 yr	3.7–5.5	
Albumin (random urine)	<37 mg/L or <3.7 mg/dL	
Albumin/creatinine ratio (random urine)	<16 mg/g	
α1-Antitrypsin(S)		
Age	mg/dL	
0–1 yr	92–282	
1–4 yrs	94–156	
4–13 yrs	102–159	
>14 yrs	97–203	
α-Fetoprotein (AFP) (S)		
Adult	<10 ng/mL	
Birth	Up to 86,000 ng/mL	
1 month or less	May be >10,000 ng/mL	
2–3 months	Up to 1000 ng/mL	

Alanine aminotransferase (S, P)		
Age	M/F (U/L)	
0–11 months	6–50	
1–3 yrs	6–45	
4–6 yrs	10–25	
7–9 yrs	10–35	
	Male (U/L)	Female (U/L)
10–11 yrs	10–35	10–30
12–13 yrs	10–55	10–30
14–15 yrs	10–45	6–30
16–18 yrs	10–40	6–35
≥19 yrs	21–72	9–52

Alkaline phosphatase (S, P)		
Age	M/F (U/L)	
0–5 days	110–300	
6 days–11 months	110–320	
1–3 yrs	145–320	
4–6 yrs	150–380	
7–9 yrs	175–420	
	Male (U/L)	Female (U/L)
10–11 yrs	135–530	130–560
12–13 yrs	200–495	105–420
14–15 yrs	130–525	70–230
16–18 yrs	65–260	50–130
> 19 yrs	38–126	38–126

Ammonia (P)		
Age	μmol/L	
0–7 days	54–94	
8–30 days	47–80	
1–12 months	15–47	
1–15 yrs	22–48	
≥16 yrs	9–26	

(Continued)

Test	Reference range (United States/conventional units)	
Amylase (S, P)	30–115 U/L	
Amylase (U) – timed	4–37 U/2 h	
Amylase (U) – random	No reference range	
Anticardiolipin IgG (S)	<23.0 GPL	
Anticardiolipin IgM (S)	<11.0 MPL	
Anti-Dnase-B		
Age		
0–5 yrs	≤1:60	
6–18 yrs	≤1:170	
≥19 yrs	≤1:85	
Antistreptolysin-O (ASO)	<250 IU/mL	
Antithrombin (ATIII) (P)	85–130%	
Normal ranges for healthy full-term infants		
Day 1	63% (39–87%)	
Day 5	67% (41–93%)	
Day 30	78% (48–108%)	
Day 90	97% (73–121%)	
Day 180	104% (84–124%)	

Aspartate aminotransferase (S, P)		
Age	*M/F (U/L)*	
0–5 days	35–140	
6 days–3 yrs	20–60	
4–6 yrs	15–50	
7–9 yrs	15–40	
	Male (U/L)	*Female (U/L)*
10–11 yrs	10–60	10–40
12–15 yrs	15–40	10–30
16–18 yrs	10–45	5–30
≥19 yrs	17–59	14–36

Bilirubin (S, P)		
	Premature (mg/dL)	*Full-term (mg/dL)*
Age	*Total*	*Total*
Up to 23 h	1–8	2–6
24–48 h	6–12	6–10
3–5 days	10–14	4–8
≥1 month	*mg/dL*	
Bc conjugated	<0.35	
Bu unconjugated	<1.0	
Total	0.2–1.0	

B-hydroxybutyrate (S, P)	<0.30 mmol/L (12 h fast)	

Blood gases		
pH		
Capillary/arterial		
Age		
Newborn	7.33–7.49	
1 day	7.25–7.43	
2–30 days	7.32–7.43	
1 month	7.34–7.43	
2 months–1 yr	7.34–7.46	
≥2 yrs		

Test	Reference range (United States/conventional units)		
Male	7.35–7.45		
Female	7.36–7.44		
Venous			
All ages	7.32–7.42		
pCO$_2$			
Capillary/arterial			
Age	*mmHg*		
0–1 month	27–40		
2 months–1 yr	26–41		
≥2 yrs			
Male	36–46		
Female	33–43		
Venous			
All ages	40–50		
pO$_2$	*mmHg*	*mmHg*	*mmHg*
Age	*Capillary*	*Arterial*	*Venous*
0–1 yr	60–70	65–76	25–40
≥2 yrs	80–90	88–105	40–47
Oxygen saturation	85–100%		

B-type natriuretic peptide (BNP) (EDTA plasma)	0–100 pg/mL

BUN – see Urea nitrogen	

Complement (CH$_{50}$), total (S)	23–46 CH$_{50}$ U/mL

Complement C3,C4 (S)		
Age	*C3 (mg/dL)*	*C4 (mg/dL)*
0–30 days	54–128	8–28
1 month	60–153	8–32
2 months	66–134	10–31
3 months	63–179	9–43
4 months	66–171	8–41
5 months	75–176	10–48
6–8 months	77–170	12–42
9–11 months	86–179	14–45
1 yr	83–174	10–39
2 yrs	78–176	12–41
3–4 yrs	89–170	14–36
5–7 yrs	90–160	14–36
8–9 yrs	92–200	12–45
≥10 yrs	86–182	17–51

C-reactive protein (CRP)	<1.0 mg/mL

Ca^{2+}(ionized) (WB)	
Age	*mmol/L*
0–30 days	0.90–1.45
1–5 months	0.95–1.50
≥6 months	1.10–1.30

Carboxyhemoglobin (WB)	<1.5% of tHb

(Continued)

Test	Reference range (United States/conventional units)	
Calcium (S)		
Age	*mg/dL*	
0–11 months	8.0–10.7	
1–3 yrs	8.7–9.8	
4–11 yrs	8.8–10.1	
12–13 yrs	8.8–10.6	
14–15 yrs	9.2–10.7	
≥16 yrs	8.9–10.7	
Calcium (U) – timed	42–353 mg/24 h	
Calcium (U) – random	No reference range	
Ceruloplasmin (S)		
Age	*mg/dL*	
0–1 month	3–25	
1–11 months	14–44	
1 yr–9 yrs	23–51	
≥10 yrs	18–46	
Chloride (S, P)	95–105 mmol/L	
Chloride (SWT) sweat test	*≤6 months*	*>6 months*
	Normal = ≤29 mmol/L	Normal = ≤39 mmol/L
	Intermediate = 30–59 mmol/L	Intermediate = 40–59 mmol/L
	Positive = ≥60 mmol/L	Positive = ≥60 mmol/L
Chloride (CSF)	122–132 mmol/L	
Chloride (U) – timed		
Age	*mmol/24 h*	
0–11 months	2–10	
1–15 yrs	15–40	
≥16 yrs	110–250	
Chloride (U) – random	No reference range	
Cholesterol (S, P)		
Age	*mg/dL*	
0–11 months	50–120	
1 yr	70–190	
2–15 yrs	135–200	
≥16 yrs	130–200	
Cholesterol, HDL (S, P)		
Age	*Male (mg/dL)*	*Female (mg/dL)*
6–15 yrs	38–75	35–73
≥16 yrs	30–64	35–80
Cholesterol, LDL		
Age	*Male (mg/dL)*	*Female (mg/dL)*
6–16 yrs	64–130	60–140
17–18 yrs	63–135	59–141
19–21 yrs	65–145	60–155
≥22 yrs	65–161	62–162
CO$_2$ content (S, P)		
Age	*mmol/L*	
0–15 yrs	20–28	
≥16 yrs	25–35	
Cold agglutinins (S)	≤1:40	
Cortisol (S)		
Age	*μg/dL*	
1–7 days	2–11	
1–12 months	2.8–23	

Test	Reference range (United States/conventional units)	
1–16 yrs (8 am)	3–21	
≥16 yrs (8 am)	8–19	
(4 pm)	4–11	

Creatine kinase (CPK) (S, P)

	M/F (U/L)	
Age		
0–3 yrs	60–305	
4–6 yrs	75–230	
7–9 yrs	60–365	
	Male (U/L)	*Female (U/L)*
10–11 yrs	55–215	80–230
12–13 yrs	60–330	50–295
14–15 yrs	60–335	50–240
16–18 yrs	55–370	45–230
≥19 yrs	55–170	30–135

Creatine kinase MB band (S, P)   Normal: <5 ng/mL
Borderline: 5–10 ng/mL
Abnormal: >10 ng/mL

Creatinine (S, P)	0.12–1.06 mg/dL
Creatinine (U) – timed	0.8–2.8 g/24 h
Creatinine (U) – random	<500 mg/dL

Creatinine clearance (U)

Age	*mL/min*
0–30 days	25–55
1–5 months	50–90
6–11 months	75–125
≥1 yr	90–150

D-dimer (P)

Adult	≤0.40 µg/mL FEU
Neonatal reference range from cord blood	<3.40 µg/mL FEU

Diluted Russell viper venom test (DRVVT) (P)

DRVVT S/C ratio	<1.35
DRVVT result	Negative

Factor 2 (P)	50–150% normal activity
Factor 5 (P)	69–132% normal activity
Factor 7 (P)	58–150% normal activity
Factor 8 (P)	47–169% normal activity
Factor 9 (P)	67–141% normal activity
Factor 10 (P)	65–142% normal activity
Factor 11 (P)	48–139% normal activity
Factor 12 (P)	41–140% normal activity

Ferritin (S)

Age	*ng/mL*
1 day–6 months	36–391
7–12 months	36–100
1–5 yrs	36–84
>6 yrs	
Male	36–311
Female	36–92

Fibrinogen (P)

Adult	220–440 mg/dL
Neonatal reference range from cord blood	135–283 mg/dL

(Continued)

Test	Reference range (United States/conventional units)	
Follicle-stimulating hormone (FSH) (S)		
	Male (mIU/mL)	*Female (mIU/mL)*
Infants	<10	<50
Prepubertal	<7	<11
Adult	1.6–17.2	0.4–15.1
Follicular/luteal	–	3.5–16.9
Midcycle	–	11.9–32.7
Fibrin split product (FSP) (P)	1:2 Dilution = Negative (<5 µg/mL)	
γ-Glutamyl transferase (GGT) (S, P)		
Age	*M/F (U/L)*	
0–5 days	34–263	
6 days–2 months	10–160	
3–11 months	11–82	
1–3 yrs	10–19	
4–6 yrs	10–22	
7–9 yrs	13–25	
	Male (U/L)	*Female (U/L)*
10–11 yrs	17–30	17–28
12–13 yrs	17–44	14–25
14–15 yrs	12–33	14–26
16–18 yrs	11–34	11–28
≥19 yrs	10–78	10–78
Glucose (S, P)(WB): glucose conversion factor for mg/dL to mmol/L: divide mg/dL value by 18		
Age	*mg/dL*	
1–12 h	30–65	
12–23 h	30–80	
1 day	50–58	
2 days	58–60	
≥3 days	70–110	
Glucose (CSF)	50–70% of serum glucose	
Glucose (U) – timed	<500 mg/24 h	
Glucose (U) – random	<30 mg/dL	
Glycosylated hemoglobin (WB)	Without diabetes	4.0–6.8%
	With diabetes	6.0–22.0%
Haptoglobin (S)		
Age	*mg/dL*	
0–1 yr	34–175	
2–3 yrs	30–140	
4–5 yrs	30–191	
≥6 yrs	35–181	
Human chorionic gonadotropin (HCG) (S)	*Postconception normals (mIU/mL)*	
	1 Week = 5–50	
	2 Weeks = 40–1,000	
	3 Weeks = 100–5000	
	4 Weeks = 600–10,000	
	5–6 Weeks = 1500–100,000	
	7–8 Weeks = 16,000–200,000	
	Second trimester = 24,000–55,000	
	Third trimester = 6000–48,000	

Test	Reference range (United States/conventional units)		
Hematocrit (B)			
Age	*%*		
0–30 days	44–70		
1 month	32–42		
2–6 months	29–41		
7 months–2 yrs	33–39		
3–6 yrs	34–40		
7–12 yrs	35–45		
13–18 yrs/female	36–45		
13–18 yrs/male	37–49		
≥19 yrs/female	36–46		
≥19 yrs/male	41–53		
Hemoglobin (B)			
Age	*g/dL*		
0–30 days	15.0–22.0		
1 month	10.5–14.0		
2–6 months	9.5–13.5		
7 months–2 yrs	10.5–14.0		
3–6 yrs	11.5–14.5		
7–12 yrs	11.5–15.5		
13–18 yrs/female	12.0–16.0		
13–18 yrs/male	13.0–16.0		
≥19 yrs/female	12.0–16.0		
≥19 yrs/male	13.5–17.5		
Hemoglobin fractionation, HPLC (WB)	*A*	*A$_2$*	*F*
Age	*(%)*	*(%)*	*(%)*
0–30 days	10–35	–	65–90
1–3 months	30–50	–	50–70
4–5 months	>90	<4	<10
≥6 months	>90	<4	≤3
Heparin level, unfractionated (P)			
Treatment	0.35–0.7 U/mL		
Hexagonal phase phospholipid neutralization test			
Staclot Diff Tube 1–Tube 2	<8.0 sec		
Staclot result	Negative		
Homocysteine			
Age	*M/F (μmol/L)*		
2 months–10 yrs	3.3–8.3		
11–15 yrs	4.7–10.3		
16–18 yrs	4.7–11.3		
	Male		*Female*
≥19 yrs	5.9–16.0		3.4–20.4
Immunoglobulin E (IgE) (S)			
Age	*IU/mL*		
0–1 yrs	<15		
1–5 yrs	<60		
6–9 yrs	<90		
10–15 yrs	<200		
16 yrs	<100		
Immunoglobulin G (IGG) (CSF)	0.4–5.2 mg/dL (10% of total protein)		

(Continued)

Test	Reference range (United States/conventional units)			
IGG subclasses (S)	IgG1	IgG2	IgG3	IgG4
Age	(mg/dL)	(mg/dL)	(mg/dL)	(mg/dL)
0–1 month	240–1060	87–410	14–55	4–55
1–4 months	180–670	38–210	14–70	3–36
4–6 months	180–700	34–210	15–80	3–23
6–12 months	200–770	34–230	15–97	3–43
1–1.5 yrs	250–820	38–240	15–107	3–62
1.5–2 yrs	290–850	45–260	15–113	3–79
2–3 yrs	320–900	52–280	14–120	3–106
3–4 yrs	350–940	63–300	13–126	3–127
4–6 yrs	370–1000	72–340	13–133	3–158
6–9 yrs	400–1080	85–410	13–142	3–189
9–12 yrs	400–1150	98–480	15–149	3–210
12–18 yrs	370–1280	106–610	18–163	4–230
18 yrs	490–1140	150–640	20–110	8–140
International normalized ratio (INR) (P)				
Adult	0.8–1.2			
Neonatal reference range from cord blood	1.0–1.4			
Immunoglobins (S)	IgG	IgA	IgM	
Age	(mg/dL)	(mg/dL)	(mg/dL)	
0–30 days	252–909	0.83–50	18–80	
1 month	207–904	2–45	15–96	
2 months	177–583	5–43	22–82	
3 months	196–560	4–69	25–93	
4 months	173–817	7–80	30–99	
5 months	216–706	7–65	32–94	
6–8 months	218–907	10–85	31–116	
9–11 months	346–1217	13–100	40–159	
1 yr	425–1054	13–116	44–155	
2 yrs	442–1139	21–150	43–184	
3–4 yrs	464–1240	22–146	40–180	
5–7 yrs	635–1284	32–191	44–190	
8–9 yrs	610–1577	42–223	48–222	
≥10 yrs	641–1353	66–295	40–180	
Iron, total (S, P)	55–150 µg/dL			
Lactate (P, WB, CSF)	Mmol/L			
Plasma (venous)	0.2–2.0			
Plasma (arterial)	0.3–0.8			
CSF	0.6–2.2			
Whole blood	0.2–1.7			
Lactate dehydrogenase (LDH) (S, P)				
Age	M/F (U/L)			
0–5 days	934–2150			
6 days–3 yrs	500–920			
4–6 yrs	470–900			
7–9 yrs	420–750			
	Male (U/L)	Female (U/L)		
10–11 yrs	432–700	380–770		
12–13 yrs	470–750	380–640		
14–15 yrs	360–730	390–580		
16–18 yrs	340–670	340–670		
≥19 yrs	313–618	313–618		

Test	Reference range (United States/conventional units)	
LDH (CSF)		
Age		
0–30 days	2.3–8.4 U/L	
≥1 month	Approximately 10% of serum value	
Lovenox level (P)		
Prophylactic	0.20–0.40 U/mL	
Treatment:	0.50–1.00 U/mL	
Luteinizing hormone (S)		
	Male (mIU/mL)	*Female (mIU/mL)*
Infants	<3	<3
Prepubertal	<7	<7
Adult	0.9–10.6	–
Follicular	–	1.1–11.1
Midcycle	–	17.5–72.9
Luteal	–	0.4–15.1
Postmenopausal	–	6.8–46.6
Lipase (S, P)		
Age	*U/L*	
0–9 yrs	25–120	
10–13 yrs	15–110	
14–18 yrs	25–110	
≥19 yrs	23–300	
Magnesium (S, P)		
Age	*mg/dL*	
0–6 days	1.2–2.6	
7–30 days	1.6–2.4	
1 month–1 yr	1.6–2.6	
2–5 yrs	1.5–2.4	
6–9 yrs	1.6–2.3	
10–13 yrs	1.6–2.2	
≥14 yrs	1.5–2.3	
Magnesium (U) – timed	12.4–191.9 mg/24 h	
Magnesium (U) – random	No reference range	
Mean corpuscular hemoglobin (MCH)		
Age	*pg*	
0–30 days	33.0–39.0	
1 month	28.0–40.0	
2–6 months	25.0–35.0	
7 months–2 yrs	23.0–31.0	
3–6 yrs	25.0–30.0	
7–12 yrs	26.0–30.0	
13–18 yrs	26.0–32.0	
>19 yrs	27.0–31.0	
Mean corpuscular hemoglobin concentration (MCHC)		
Age	*g/dL*	
0–30 days	32.0–36.0	
1 month	33.0–38.0	
2–6 months	28.0–36.0	
7 months–2 yrs	30.0–34.0	
3–6 yrs	32.0–36.0	
7–12 yrs	32.0–36.0	

(Continued)

Test	Reference range (United States/conventional units)
13–18 yrs	32.0–36.0
>19 yrs	32.0–36.0
Mean corpuscular volume (MCV)	
Age	*fL*
0–30 days	86.0–115.0
1 month	72.0–88.0
2–6 months	72.0–82.0
7 months–2 yrs	76.0–90.0
3–6 yrs	76.0–90.0
7–12 yrs	76.0–90.0
13–18 yrs	78.0–95.0
>19 yrs	78.0–100.0
Methemoglobin (WB)	<2% of tHb
Microalbumin (random urine)	0–37 mg/L or 0–3.7 mg/dL
Microalbumin (U) – timed	<20 µg/min
	<30 mg/24 h
Osmolality (S, P)	275–295 mOsm/kg H_2O
Osmolality (U)	300–1000 mOsm/kg H_2O
Phosphorus, inorganic (S, P)	
Age	*mg/dL*
Premature	5.6–8.0
Term	5.0–7.8
0–3 months	4.8–8.1
4–11 months	3.8–6.7
1–4 yrs	3.5–6.8
5–7 yrs	3.1–6.3
8–11 yrs	3.0–6.0
12–16 yrs	2.5–5.0
≥17 yrs	2.3–4.8
Phosphorus, inorganic (U) – timed	0.9–1.3 g/24 h
Phosphorus, inorganic (U) – random	No reference range
Plasma hemoglobin (P)	≤4 mg/dL
Plasma hemoglobin (U)	None detected
Plasminogen activity	56–148%
Platelet count (B)	150,000–450,000/µL
Platelet function assay (WB)	
Collagen/epinephrine	84–183 sec
Collagen/ADP	69–126 sec
Potassium (S, P)	
Age	*mmol/L*
0–30 days	4.5–7.0 (venous or arterial)
	4.5–7.5 (heel stick)
1–2 months	4.0–6.2
3–11 months	3.7–5.6
≥1 yr	3.5–5.5
Potassium (U) – timed	40–80 mmol/24 h
Potassium (U) – random	No reference range
Potassium (WB)	
Age	*mmol/L*
Premature	4.5–7.0

Test	Reference range (United States/conventional units)
0–11 months	5.0–5.7
≥1 yr	3.5–5.5

Pre-albumin (S)

Age	*mg/dL*
0–6 days	4–20
7–41 days	8–25
≥42 days	18–44

Prolactin (S)

	ng/mL
Newborn	>10 x adult levels
Nursing female	<40
Follicular female	<23
Luteal female	5–40
Pregnancy	
1st trimester	<84
2nd trimester	18–306
3rd trimester	34–386

Protein, total (S, P)

Age	*g/dL*
0–30 days	4.4–7.6
1–3 months	4.2–7.4
4–11 months	5.6–7.2
≥1 yr	6.0–8.0

Protein (CSF)

Age	*mg/dL*
Premature	40–300
0–30 days	<100
≥1 month	15–45

Protein C (P)   80–175%

Normal ranges for healthy full-term infants:

Day 1	35% (17–53%)
Day 5	42% (20–64%)
Day 30	43% (21–65%)
Day 90	54% (28–80%)
Day 180	59% (37–81%)

(Am J Pediatr Hematol Oncol 1990;12:95–104)
Please note that these ranges were not established using the current reagent and analyzer at TCH Coagulation Lab

Protein S (P)   51–157%

Normal ranges for healthy full-term infants

Day 1	36% (12–60%)
Day 5	50% (22–78%)
Day 30	63% (33–93%)
Day 90	86% (54–118%)
Day 180	87% (55–119%)

(Am J Pediatr Hematol Oncol 1990;12:95–104)
Please note that these ranges were not established using the current reagent and analyzer at TCH Coagulation Lab

Protein, total (U) – timed	28–141 mg/24 h
Protein, total (U) – random	No reference range

Prothrombin time (PT) (P)

Adult	12.2–15.5 sec
Neonatal reference range from cord blood	12.9–16.9 sec

(*Continued*)

Test	Reference range (United States/conventional units)
Partial thromboplastin time (PTT) (P)	
Adult	26.5–35.5 sec
Neonatal reference range from cord blood	28.7–53.7 sec
Red blood cell count (RBC) (B)	
Age	*×10⁶/μL*
0–30 days	4.1–6.7
1 month	3.0–5.4
2–6 months	2.7–4.5
7 months–2 yrs	3.7–5.3
3–6 yrs	3.9–5.3
7–12 yrs	4.0–5.2
13–18 yrs /female	4.1–5.1
13–18 yrs /male	4.5–5.3
≥19 yrs/female	4.2–5.4
≥19 yrs/male	4.7–6.0
Red cell distribution width – coefficient of variation (RDWCV)	
Age	*%*
0–30 days	13.0–18.0
1 month	13.0–18.0
2–6 months	13.0–18.0
7 months–2 yrs	11.5–16.0
3–6 yrs	11.5–15.0
7–12 yrs	11.5–14.0
13–18 yrs	11.5–14.0
>19 yrs	11.5–14.0
Red cell distribution width – standard deviation (RDWSD)	
Age	*fL*
0–30 days	38.5–49.0
1 month	38.5–49.0
2–6 months	38.5–49.0
7 months–2 yrs	38.5–49.0
3–6 yrs	38.5–49.0
7–12 yrs	38.5–49.0
13–18 yrs	38.5–49.0
>19 yrs	38.5–49.0
Reticulocyte count % (B)	
Age	*%*
0–2 days	3.0–7.0
3–4 days	1.0–3.0
>4 days	0.5–1.5
Reticulocyte count absolute (B)	
Age	*×10⁶/μL*
0–2 days	0.140–0.220
3–4 days	0.040–0.110
>4 days	0.020–0.080
Reticulocyte hemoglobin content (B)	
Age	*pg*
<2 years	24.5–35.2
≥2 yrs	27.1–35.4
Sedimentation rate (B)	0–20 mm/h

Test	Reference range (United States/conventional units)
Sirolimus/rapamycin (P)	3–12 ng/mL
Sodium (S, P) (WB)	
Age	*mmol/L*
Premature	132–140
0–11 months	133–142
≥1 yr	136–145
Sodium (U) – timed	
Age	*mmol/24 h*
0–11 months	0.3–3.5
1–15 yrs	40–180
≥16 yrs	80–200
Sodium (U) – random	No normals
Free thyroxine (T4) (S)	1.0–2.5 ng/dL
T4 (S)	
Age	*µg/dL*
Cord blood	8.0–13
0–7 days	11.5–24
8 days–4 yrs	7.0–15
5 yrs–9 yrs	6.4–13.3
≥10 yrs	5.0–12
Free thyroxine index (T7) (S)	
Age	
0–7 days	9.1–26.6
8 days–4 yrs	5.5–16.6
5–9 yrs	5.1–14.7
≥10 yrs	4.0–13.3
Thromboelastogram (TEG) with kaolin	
Reaction time	4.4–11.0 min
Angle	49.1–74.7°
Max amplitude	53.6–70.3 mm
Fibrinolysis	0.0–7.5%
Clot strength	5.2–11.3
Thrombin time	15.0–19.0 sec
Thyroid stimulating hormone (TSH) (S)	
Age	*µIU/mL*
Cord blood	3–22
0–7 days	<40.00
8 –14 days	<25.00
≥15 days	0.32–5.00
Tri-iodothyronine (T3) uptake (S)	25–35%
Age	*ng/dL*
Cord blood	30–70
0–7 days	65–275
8 days–9 yrs	90–260
10–14 yrs	80–210
≥15 yrs	115–195
Transferrin (S)	169–300 mg/dL
Transferrin saturation (S)	
Age	*%*
0–11 yrs	15–39

(*Continued*)

Males 12–17 yrs	16–44
Females 12–17 yrs	11–44
Males >18 yrs	21–52
Females >18 yrs	11–44

Triglycerides (S, P)	20–150 mg/dL

Troponin I (S, P)	<0.15 ng/mL

Urea nitrogen (S, P)

Age	mg/dL
0–1 yr	8–28
2–15 yrs	5–25
≥16 yrs	5–20
Urea nitrogen (U) – timed	12–20 mg/24 h
Urea nitrogen (U) – random	No reference range

Uric acid (S, P)	2.0–6.2 mg/dL
Uric acid (U) – timed	250–750 mg/24 h
Uric acid (U) – random	No reference range

Urinalysis (U)

Specific gravity	1.001–1.035
pH	4–9
Protein	Neg
Glucose	Neg
Ketone	Neg
Bilirubin	Neg
Urobilinogen	<2.0
WBC	0–4/HPF
RBC	0–4/HPF
EPI (epithelial cells)	0–4/LPF

Von Willebrand ristocetin coactor activity (P)	48–142%
Von Willebrand factor antigen (P)	56–176%

White blood cell count (WBC) (B)

Age	×10³/μL
0–30 days	9.1–34.0
1 month	5.0–19.5
2–11 months	6.0–17.5
1–6 yrs	5.0–14.5
7–12 yrs	5.0–14.5
13–18 yrs	4.5–13.5
≥19 yrs	4.5–11.0

Age	Seg (%)	Band (%)	Lymphs (%)	Monos (%)	EOS (%)	BASO (%)	ANC
0–30 days	32–67	0–8	25–37	0–9	0–2	0–1	6.0–23.5
1 month	20–46	0–4.5	28–84	0–7	0–3	0–1	1.0–9.0
2–11 months	20–48	0–3.8	34–88	0–5	0–3	0–1	1.0–8.5
1–6 yrs	37–71	0–1.0	17–67	0–5	0–3	0–1	1.5–8.0
7–12 yrs	33–76	0–1.0	15–61	0–5	0–3	0–1	1.5–8.0
13–18 yrs	33–76	0–1.0	15–55	0–4	0–3	0–1	1.8–8.0
≥19 yrs	33–76	0–0.7	14–54	0–4	0–3	0–1	1.8–7.7

A, arterial; ADP, adenosine diphosphate; ANC, absolute neutrophil count; B, blood; band, banded neutrophils; BASO, basophils; C, capillary; CSF, cerebrospinal fluid; EOS, eosinophils; F, female; FEU, fibrinogen equivalent units; GPL, gG phospholipid units/mL; HPF, high power field; IU, international units; lymphs, lymphocytes; LPF, low power field; M, male; monos, monocytes; MPL, IgM phospholipid units/mL; P, plasma; S, serum; seg, segmented neutrophils; SWT, sweat; U, urine; WB, whole blood.

Index

Note: page numbers in *italics* refer to figures; those in **bold** to tables or boxes.

Gregory's Pediatric Anesthesia, Fifth Edition. Edited by George A. Gregory, Dean B. Andropoulos.
© 2012 Blackwell Publishing Ltd. Published 2012 by Blackwell Publishing Ltd.